KU-286-131
369 0160470

Textbook of Diabetes

COMPANION WEBSITE

Purchasing this book entitles you to access to the companion website:

textbookofdiabetes.com

The website includes:

- Interactive Multiple-Choice Questions for each chapter
- Reference lists with external links
- Figures from the book for downloading
- All chapters online

How to access the site:

- Scratch off the label below to see your unique PIN number
- Go to the website textbookofdiabetes.com and follow the registration instructions

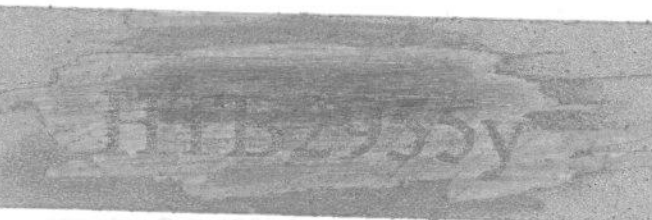

Please note that the book cannot be returned once the label is scratched off, and the unique (personal) PIN cannot be shared. The site is for individual use by purchasers only and cannot be networked.

We dedicate this book to all people living with diabetes and the healthcare professionals who look after them. We would also like to dedicate this book to our families without whose support and encouragement the book would never have been finished.

Textbook of Diabetes

EDITED BY

RICHARD I.G. HOLT MA, MB BChir, PhD, FRCP, FHEA
Professor in Diabetes & Endocrinology
Developmental Origins of Health and Disease Division
University of Southampton School of Medicine
Southampton, UK

CLIVE S. COCKRAM MB BS, BSc, MD (Lond), FRCP, FRACP, FHKAM (Med)
Emeritus Professor of Medicine
Chinese University of Hong Kong
Hong Kong SAR
People's Republic of China

ALLAN FLYVBJERG MD, DMSc
Professor of Clinical Endocrinology and
Chair, Department of Endocrinology and Internal Medicine
The Medical Research Laboratories
Aarhus University Hospital – Aarhus University
Aarhus, Denmark

BARRY J. GOLDSTEIN MD, PhD, FACP, FACE
Therapeutic Area Head, Diabetes and Obesity
Vice President, Clinical Research, Metabolism
Merck Research Laboratories
Rahway, NJ, USA

FOURTH EDITION

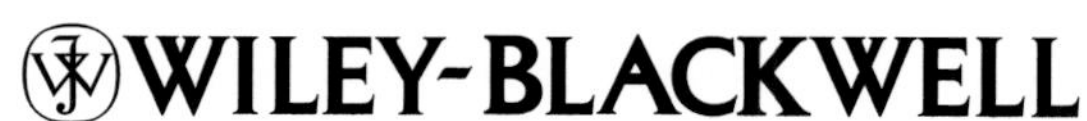

A John Wiley & Sons, Ltd., Publication

Blackwell Publishing was acquired by John Wiley & Sons in February 2007. Blackwell's publishing program has been merged with Wiley's global Scientific, Technical and Medical business to form Wiley-Blackwell.

Registered office: John Wiley & Sons Ltd, The Atrium, Southern Gate, Chichester, West Sussex, PO19 8SQ, UK

Editorial offices: 9600 Garsington Road, Oxford, OX4 2DQ, UK
111 River Street, Hoboken, NJ 07030-5774, USA
The Atrium, Southern Gate, Chichester, West Sussex, PO19 8SQ, UK

For details of our global editorial offices, for customer services and for information about how to apply for permission to reuse the copyright material in this book please see our website at www.wiley.com/wiley-blackwell.

ISBN: 9781405191814

A catalogue record for this book is available from the British Library.

Library of Congress Cataloging-in-Publication Data

Textbook of diabetes. – 4th ed. / edited by Richard I.G. Holt ... [et al.].
p. ; cm.
Includes bibliographical references and index.
ISBN 978-1-4051-9181-4 (hardback : alk. paper)
1. Diabetes. I. Holt, Richard I.G.
[DNLM: 1. Diabetes Mellitus. WK 810 T355 2010]
RC660.T467 2010
616.4'62–dc22

2010013907

Set in 9.25/12 pt Minion by Toppan Best-set Premedia Limited
Printed and bound in Singapore by Fabulous Printers Pte Ltd

1 2010

Contents

Part 5 Managing the Patient with Diabetes

Part 6 Treatment of Diabetes

Part 7 Microvascular Complications in Diabetes

Part 8 Macrovascular Complications in Diabetes

Part 9 Other Complications of Diabetes

A companion website for this book is available at: **textbookofdiabetes.com**

List of Contributors

Alan M. Adelman MS, MD
Professor of Family and Community Medicine, Vice Chair for Academic Affairs and Research, Penn State Milton S. Hershey Medical Center, Penn State College of Medicine, Hershey, PA, USA

Angela Alberga MSc
Faculty of Health Sciences, University of Ottawa and Ottawa Hospital Research Institute, Ottawa, Ontario, Canada

K. George M.M. Alberti DPhil, FRCP
Senior Research Fellow, Imperial College, London; Emeritus Professor of Medicine, University of Newcastle, Newcastle, UK

Mohammed K. Ali MBChB, MSc
Assistant Professor, Hubert Department of Global Health, Rollins School of Public Health, Global Diabetes Research Center, Emory University, Atlanta, GA, USA

Joseph A. Aloi MD
Associate Professor of Internal Medicine, The Strelitz Diabetes Center for Endocrine and Metabolic Disorders, Eastern Virginia Medical School , Norfolk, VA, USA

Mazen Alsahli MD
Professor of Medicine, University of Rochester School of Medicine, Rochester, NY, USA

Colum F. Amory MD, MPH
Mount Sinai School of Medicine, New York, NY, USA

John Ayuk MD
Centre for Endocrinology, Diabetes and Metabolism, University of Birmingham and Queen Elizabeth Hospital Birmingham, Birmingham, UK

Clifford J. Bailey PhD, FRCP(Edin), FRCPath
Professor in Clinical Science and Head of Diabetes Research, School of Life and Health Sciences, Aston University, Birmingham, UK

Anita Banerjee BSc, MBBS, MRCP
Obstetric Physician, Diabetes and Endocrinology, Princess Royal University Hospital, London, England UK

Andreea R. Barbu PhD
Department of Medical Cell Biology and Department of Medical Sciences, Uppsala University, Uppsala, Sweden

Adil E. Bharucha MD
Professor of Medicine, Division of Gastroenterology and Hepatology, Clinical Enteric Neuroscience Translational and Epidemiological Research Program, Mayo Clinic, Rochester, MN, USA

Andrew J.M. Boulton MD, DSc (Hon), FRCP
Professor of Medicine, University of Manchester and Manchester Royal Infirmary, Manchester, UK; Miller School of Medicine, University of Miami, Miami, FL, USA

George A. Bray MD, MACP
Boyd Professor, Pennington Biomedical Research Center, Louisiana State University, Baton Rouge, LA, USA

Michael Brownlee MD
Anita and Jack Saltz Professor of Diabetes Research, Albert Einstein College of Medicine, New York, NY, USA

Michael Camilleri MD
Atherton and Winifred W. Bean Professor, Professor of Medicine and Physiology, College of Medicine, Mayo Clinic and Clinical Enteric Neuroscience Translational and Epidemiological Research Program, Division of Gastroenterology and Hepatology, Mayo Clinic, Rochester, MN, USA

Riccardo Candido MD, PhD
Diabetic Centre, Trieste, Italy

Christine M. Chan MD
Barbara Davis Center for Childhood Diabetes, University of Colorado Denver, School of Medicine, Aurora, CO, USA

Juliana C.N. Chan MBChB MD FRCP
Professor of Medicine and Therapeutics, Director, Hong Kong Institute of Diabetes and Obesity, The Chinese University of Hong Kong, The Prince of Wales Hospital, Hong Kong SAR, China

Shuibing Chen PhD
Postdoctoral Fellow, Department of Stem Cell and Regenerative Biology, Harvard University, Cambridge, MA, USA

Bernard M.Y. Cheung MD, PhD
Chair of Clinical Pharmacology and Therapeutics, Department of Clinical Pharmacology, University of Birmingham, Birmingham, UK

Jae-Hyoung Cho MD
Assistant Professor, Department of Endocrinology, Seoul St. Mary's Hospital, College of Medicine, The Catholic University of Korea, Seoul, Korea

Mark E. Cooper MD, PhD
Director, Danielle Alberti JDRF Centre for Diabetes Complications, Head, Vascular Division – Baker IDI Heart Research Institute, Melbourne, Australia

Philip E. Cryer MD
Irene E. and Michael M. Karl Professor of Endocrinology and Metabolism in Medicine, Washington University School of Medicine, St. Louis, MO, USA

Nicola Dalbeth MD, FRACP
Department of Medicine, University of Auckland, Auckland, New Zealand

Ahmed J. Delli MD, MPH
Clinical Research Center (CRC), Lund University, Department of Clinical Sciences/Diabetes and Celiac Disease, University Hospital MAS, Malmö, Sweden

Anne Dornhorst BSc, DM, FRCP, FRCPath
Consultant Physician, Honorary Senior Lecturer, Department of Medicine, Imperial College Healthcare NHS Trust, Hammersmith Hospital, London, UK

Barbara Eichorst MS,RD,CDE
Healthy Interactions Global Conversation Map™ Facilitator, Chicago, IL, USA

Andrew J. Farmer DM, FRCGP
University Lecturer, Department of Primary Health Care, University of Oxford, Oxford, UK

Robin E. Ferner MSc, MD, FRCP
Professor, West Midlands Centre for Adverse Drug Reactions, City Hospital, Birmingham, UK

Brian M. Frier BSc(Hons), MD, FRCPE, FRCPG
Professor, Department of Diabetes, Royal Infirmary of Edinburgh, Edinburgh, UK

Philippe Froguel MD, PhD
Institut de Biologie de Lille, Institut Pasteur de Lille, Lille, France; Section of Genomic Medicine, Imperial College London, London, UK

Robert A. Gabbay MD, PhD
Director, Penn State Institute for Diabetes and Obesity; Professor of Medicine and Molecular Medicine, Penn State College of Medicine; Director, Diabetes Program, Penn State Milton S. Hershey Medical Center, Hershey, PA , USA

W. Timothy Garvey MD
Butterworth Professor and Chair, Department of Nutrition Sciences; Director, UAB Diabetes Research and Training Center, University of Alabama at Birmingham; Birmingham Veterans Affairs Medical Center, Birmingham, AL, USA

John E. Gerich MD
Professor of Medicine, University of Rochester School of Medicine, Rochester, NY, USA

Ferdinando Giacco PhD
Postdoctoral Fellow, Diabetes Research and Training Center, Departments of Medicine and Endocrinology, Albert Einstein College of Medicine, New York, NY, USA

Neil J.L. Gittoes MD
Senior Lecturer in Medicine, Centre for Endocrinology, Diabetes and Metabolism, University of Birmingham and Queen Elizabeth Hospital Birmingham, Birmingham, UK

Steve Gough
Professor of Diabetes, Oxford Centre for Diabetes Endocrinology and Metabolism, University of Oxford; Consultant Physician, Churchill Hospital, Oxford, UK

Andrew Grey MD
Department of Medicine, University of Auckland, Auckland, New Zealand

Maggie Sinclair Hammersley MB, FRCP
Consultant Physician and Senior Lecturer, Nuffield Department of Medicine, University of Oxford, Oxford, UK

Neil A. Hanley MBChB, PhD
Professor of Medicine, Endocrinology and Diabetes Group, University of Manchester, Manchester, UK

Troels Krarup Hansen MD, PhD
Associate Professor, Department of Endocrinology and Internal Medicine, Aarhus University Hospital, Aarhus, Denmark

Valma Harjutsalo PhD
Folkhälsan Institute of Genetics, Folkhälsan Research Center, Biomedicum Helsinki; Diabetes Prevention Unit, National Institute of Health and Welfare, Helsinki, Finland; Division of Nephrology, Department of Medicine, Helsinki University Central Hospital, Helsinki, Finland

Andrew T. Hattersley MD
Diabetes and Vascular Medicine, Peninsula Medical School, Exeter, UK

Hans Hauner MD
Director, Else Kröner-Fresenius-Center for Nutritional Medicine, Klinikum rechts der Isar, Technical University of Munich, Munich, Germany

Jens Juul Holst MD, DMSc
Professor of Medical Physiology, Department of Biomedical Sciences, The Panum Institute, University of Copenhagen, Denmark

Sten–A. Ivarsson MD, PhD
Clinical Research Center (CRC), Lund University and Department of Clinical Sciences/Paediatric Endocrinology, University Hospital MAS, Malmö, Sweden

June James MSc, BA (Hons) Dip Nursing, NP RGN
Consultant Nurse in Diabetes, University Hospitals of Leicester, Leicester, UK

Karin A.M. Jandeleit-Dahm MD, PhD, FRACP
Baker IDI Heart and Diabetes Institute, Co-head, Diabetes Division; Professor of Medicine (Adjunct), Monash University, Melbourne, Australia

Peter Jones PhD
Professor of Endocrine Biology, King's College London, London, UK

Angus Jones MBBS, MRCP
Diabetes and Vascular Medicine, Peninsula Medical School, Exeter, UK

Maria Kambourakis BSc(Hons)
Research Officer/Type 1 Diabetes Program Officer, Type 1 Diabetes Program, Diabetes Australia, Victoria, Australia

Glen P. Kenny MD
Ottawa Hospital Research Institute and Laboratory of Human Bioenergetics and Environmental Physiology, School of Human Kinetics, Faculty of Health Sciences, University of Ottawa, Ottawa, Ontario, Canada

Angela Koh MBBS (Singapore), MRCP (UK)
Assistant Professor, Department of Medicine (Endocrinology), Attending Physician, Clinical Islet Transplant Program, University of Alberta, Edmonton, Canada

Alice P.S. Kong MBChB, MRCP (UK), FRCP (Glasg)
Associate Professor, Department of Medicine and Therapeutics, The Chinese University of Hong Kong, Hong Kong SAR, China

Debbie Kralik PhD, RN
General Manager, Research and Strategy, Royal District Nursing Service, South Australia; Associate Professor, University of South Australia and University of Adelaide, Glenside, Australia

Andrew J. Krentz MD, FRCP
Formerly Southampton University Hospitals NHS Trust, Southampton, UK

Helena Elding Larsson MD, PhD
Clinical Research Center (CRC), Lund University; Department of Clinical Sciences/Paediatric Endocrinology, University Hospital MAS, Malmö, Sweden

Nelson Lee MD,FRCP(Edin)
Associate Professor, Head, Division of Infectious Diseases, Department of Medicine and Therapeutics, Faculty of Medicine, The Chinese University of Hong Kong, Hong Kong SAR, China

Åke Lernmark PhD
Professor of Experimental Diabetes, Lund University/CRC, Department of Clinical Sciences, University Hospital MAS, Malmö, Sweden

Naomi S. Levitt MBChB, MD, FCP(SA)
Professor and Head of Division of Diabetic Medicine and Endocrinology, Department of Medicine, University of Cape Town and Groote Schuur Hospital, Cape Town, South Africa

Ee Lin Lim MRCP
Diabetes Research Group, Institute of Cellular Medicine, University of Newcastle, Newcastle upon Tyne, UK

Ronald C.W. Ma MB BChir, MRCP
Associate Professor, Division of Endocrinology and Diabetes, Department of Medicine and Therapeutics, The Chinese University of Hong Kong, Prince Of Wales Hospital, Hong Kong SAR, China

Sten Madsbad MD, DMSc
Professor of Diabetology, Department of Endocrinology, Hvidovre Hospital, Hvidovre, Denmark

Sally M. Marshall MD
Professor of Diabetes, Diabetes Research Group, Institute of Cellular Medicine, Newcastle University, Newcastle upon Tyne, UK

Bob Mash MBChB, MRCGP, PhD
Professor, Division of Family Medicine and Primary Care, Stellenbosch University, Tygerberg, South Africa

Jean-Claude Mbanya MD, PhD, FRCP
Professor of Medicine and Endocrinology, Faculty of Medicine and Biomedical Sciences, University of Yaounde I, Yaounde, Cameroon

Anthony L. McCall MD, PhD
James M. Moss Professor of Diabetes in Internal Medicine, Diabetes and Hormone Center of Excellence, University of Virginia School of Medicine, Charlottesville, VA, USA

Margaret McGill RN, MSc(med)
Diabetes Centre, Royal Prince Alfred Hospital, Camperdown, Sydney, New South Wales, Australia

Douglas A. Melton
Thomas Dudley Cabot Professor in the Natural Sciences, Department of Stem Cell and Regenerative Biology; Harvard Stem Cell Institute; Investigator, Howard Hughes Medical Institute, Harvard University, Cambridge, MA, USA

Carolé R. Mensing RN, MA, CDE
Joslin Diabetes Center, Boston, MA, USA

Viswanathan Mohan MD, FRCP(UK), FRCP(Glasg), PhD, DSc, FNASc
Chairman and Chief Diabetologist, Dr. Mohan's Diabetes Specialities Centre, WHO Collaborating Centre for Non Communicable Diseases Prevention and Control, IDF Centre of Education; President and Chief of Diabetes Research, Madras Diabetes Research Foundation, ICMR Advanced Centre for Genomics of Diabetes, Gopalapuram, Chennai, India

Niels Møller MD, DMSc
Professor, Department of Endocrinology and Internal Medicine, The Medical Research Laboratories, Arhus University Hospital, Arhus, Denmark

Elena Moltchanova PhD
Diabetes Unit, Department of Health Promotion and Chronic Disease Prevention, National Institute for Health and Welfare, Helsinki, Finland

K. M. Venkat Narayan MD, MSc, MBA, FRCP
Ruth and O.C. Hubert Professor of Global Health, Professor of Epidemiology and Medicine, Rollins School of Public Health, Emory University, Atlanta, GA, USA

Parth Narendran
Institute of Biomedical Research, The Medical School, University of Birmingham, Birmingham, UK

Peter M. Nilsson MD
Professor of Clinical Cardiovascular Research, Department of Clinical Sciences, Lund University, University Hospital, Malmö, Sweden

Jane Overland MPH, PhD
Nurse Practitioner, Diabetes Centre, Royal Prince Alfred Hospital, Campderdown, New South Wales, Australia; Clinical Associate Professor, The Faculty of Nursing and Midwifery, The University of Sydney, Sydney, Australia

Shanta J. Persaud PhD
Professor of Diabetes and Endocrinology, King's College London, London, UK

Robert C. Peveler MA, DPhil, BM, BCh, FRCPsych
Clinical Neurosciences Division, School of Medicine, University of Southampton and Royal South Hants Hospital, Southampton, UK

David Price MD, FRCP
Department of Diabetes and Endocrinology, Morriston Hospital, Swansea, UK

Jayaraj Rajagopal
Center for Regenerative Medicine, Massachusetts General Hospital; Principal Investigator, Harvard Stem Cell Institute, Boston, MA, USA

Marian Rewers MD, PhD
Professor, Pediatrics and Preventive Medicine; Clinical Director, Barbara Davis Center for Childhood Diabetes, University of Colorado Denver, School of Medicine, Aurora, CO, USA

Robert A. Rizza MD
Professor of Medicine, Division of Endocrinology, Diabetes, Metabolism and Nutrition, Mayo Clinic, Rochester, MN, USA

Christopher M. Ryan PhD
Professor of Psychiatry, University of Pittsburgh School of Medicine, Pittsburgh, Pennsylvania, USA

Lars Rydén MD, FRCP, FESC, FACC, FAHA
Professor Emeritus, Cardiology Unit, Department of Medicine, Karolinska Institute, Stockholm, Sweden

Peter H. Scanlon MD, MRCOphth, DCH, FRCP
Consultant Ophthalmologist, Gloucestershire and Oxford Eye Units; Lecturer, Harris Manchester College, University of Oxford, Oxford, UK

Ole Schmitz MD, DMSc
Professor of Clinical Pharmacology, Department of Clinical Pharmacology, Aarhus University Hospital, Denmark

Peter A. Senior BMedSci, MBBS, PhD, MRCP(UK)
Clinical Islet Transplant Program, University of Alberta, Edmonton, Alberta, Canada

A.M. James Shapiro MD PhD DSc (Hon) FRCS(Eng) FRCSC MSM
Professor of Surgery, Director, Clinical Islet Transplant Program, AHFMR Scholar, University of Alberta, Edmonton, Canada

Graham R. Sharpe MBChB, BA, PhD, FRCP
Consultant Dermatologist, Department of Dermatology, Broadgreen Hospital, Liverpool, UK

Judy Shih MD, PhD
Joslin Diabetes Center, Boston, MA, USA

Ronald J. Sigal MD, MPH, FRCPC
Professor of Medicine, Cardiac Sciences, and Community Health Sciences, Faculties of Medicine and Kinesiology, The University of Calgary, Canada

Henrik H. Sillesen MD, DMSc
Head, Department of Vascular Surgery, Rigshospitalet, University of Copenhagen, Copenhagen, Denmark

Alan J. Sinclair MSc, MD, FRCP
Deputy Dean and Professor of Medicine, Bedfordshire and Hertfordshire Postgraduate Medical School; Geriatric and Diabetes Research Centre, University of Bedfordshire, Luton, UK

Wing-Yee So MBChB, MD, FRCP
Associate Consultant, Prince of Wales Hospital, Hong Kong SAR, China

Lars C. Stene PhD
Division of Epidemiology, Norwegian Institute of Public Health, Oslo, Norway; Oslo Diabetes Research Centre, Oslo University Hospital, Oslo, Norway

Mark W. J. Strachan MD, FRCP (Edin)
Consultant in Diabetes and Endocrinology, Metabolic Unit, Western General Hospital, Edinburgh, UK

Robert B. Tattersall MB, ChB, MD, FRCP
Emeritus Professor of Clinical Diabetes, University of Nottingham, Nottinghamshire, UK

Roy Taylor MD, FRCP
Professor of Medicine and Metabolism, and Director, Newcastle Magnetic Resonance Centre, Newcastle University, Newcastle upon Tyne, UK

Inga S. Thrainsdottir MD, PhD
Department of Cardiology, Landspitali University Hospital, Reykjavik, Iceland

Monika Toeller MD
German Diabetes Center, Heinrich Heine University Düsseldorf and Leibniz Center for Diabetes Research, Düsseldorf, Germany

Peter C.Y. Tong MBBS, PhD, BPharm, FRCP
Professor, Division of Endocrinology and Diabetes, Department of Medicine and Therapeutics, The Chinese University of Hong Kong and Prince Of Wales Hospital, Hong Kong SAR, China

Jaakko Tuomilehto MD, MA, PhD
Hjelt Institute, University of Helsinki and Diabetes Prevention Unit, Department of Health Promotion, National Institute for Health and Welfare, Helsinki, Finland, and South Ostrobothnia Central Hospital, Seinäjoki, Finland

Ranjit Unnikrishnan MD
Director and Consultant Diabetologist, Dr. Mohan's Diabetes Specialities Centre, WHO Collaborating Centre for Non Communicable Diseases Prevention and Control and IDF Centre of Education, Madras Diabetes Research Foundation, ICMR Advanced Centre for Genomics of Diabetes, Chennai, India

Nigel Unwin BA, MSc, DM, FRCP, FFPH
Professor of Public Health and Epidemiology, Faculty of Medicine, University of the West Indies, Barbados

Martine Vaxillaire PharmD, PhD
Research Director at Pasteur Institute, CNRS 8090 and Pasteur Institute, Lille, France

Adrian Vella MD, FRCP(Edin)
Associate Professor of Medicine, Division of Endocrinology, Diabetes, Metabolism and Nutrition, Mayo Clinic, Rochester, MN, USA

Adie Viljoen MBChB, MMed, FCPath (SA), FRCPath, MBA
Consultant Chemical Pathologist, Department of Chemical Pathology, Lister Hospital, Stevenage, UK

Mary Beth Weber MPH
Nutrition and Health Sciences Program, Graduate Division of Biological and Biomedical Sciences, Global Diabetes Research Center, Emory University, Atlanta, GA, USA

Jesse Weinberger MD
Department of Neurology, Mount Sinai School of Medicine, New York, NY, USA

Nils Welsh MD, PhD
Professor in Molecular Inflammation Research, Department of Medical Cell Biology, Uppsala University, Uppsala, Sweden

Anthony S. Wierzbicki DM, DPhil, FRCPath, FAHA
Consultant Metabolic Physician and Chemical Pathologist, Guy's and St Thomas Hospitals, London, UK

Howard Wolpert MD
Joslin Diabetes Center, Boston, MA, USA

Xuxia Wu MD, PhD
Department of Nutrition Sciences, University of Alabama at Birmingham, Birmingham, AL, USA

Jane E. Yardley MSc
Faculty of Health Sciences, University of Ottawa and Ottawa Hospital Research Institute, Ottawa, Ontario, Canada

Paul D. Yesudian MB, MD, MRCP
Consultant Dermatologist, Department of Dermatology, University of Liverpool and Broadgreen Hospital, Liverpool, UK

Hannele Yki-Järvinen MD, FRCP
Professor of Medicine, Department of Medicine, Division of Diabetes, University of Helsinki, Helsinki, Finland

Kun-Ho Yoon MD, PhD
Professor, Department of Endocrinology and Metabolism, Seoul St. Mary's Hospital, College of Medicine, The Catholic University of Korea, Seoul, Korea

Dennis K. Yue MBBS, FRACP, PhD
Diabetes Centre, Royal Prince Alfred Hospital; University of Sydney, Sydney, New South Wales, Australia

Qiao Zhou
Assistant Professor, Department of Stem Cell and Regenerative Biology, Principle Investigator, Harvard Stem Cell Institute, Havard University, Cambridge, MA, USA

Dan Ziegler MD, FRCPE
Professor of Internal Medicine, Institute for Clinical Diabetology, German Diabetes Center at the Heinrich Heine University, Leibniz Center for Diabetes Research; Department of Metabolic Diseases, University Hospital, Düsseldorf, Germany

Preface to the Fourth Edition

The management of diabetes is a major health challenge, and its prevalence is increasing at an alarming rate, especially in the developing world. According to the International Diabetes Federation, diabetes currently affects more than 285 million people worldwide, a figure that is expected to rise to 435 million by 2030. During the writing of this book over the last 18 months, approximately 15 million people will have developed diabetes. Although treatments continue to improve, many people die as a result of their diabetes. Between 6–16% of all deaths are attributable to diabetes and around 900 will have died in the 2 hours taken to write this preface. Diabetes accounts for about 6% of total global mortality, on a par with that seen in HIV/AIDS. Many of these deaths will result from cardiovascular disease which occurs at least twice as often in diabetes as in people without diabetes. Diabetes continues to cause suffering through its complications. It is the commonest cause of kidney failure in developed countries where it is also the leading cause of blindness in adults of working age. Diabetes is also a major cause of non-traumatic lower limb amputation. As well as the personal cost, diabetes places a huge burden on health economies. In 2010, it is estimated that worldwide, at least US$ 376 billion will be used to treat and prevent diabetes and its complications. Never have the challenges in providing diabetes healthcare been larger.

During the eight years since the publication of the previous edition of this textbook, there have been great strides in the management and understanding of diabetes. International collaborations using large and varied cohorts with increasingly sophisticated technologies have allowed a greater appreciation of the genetic factors that predispose to diabetes. Our molecular understanding of insulin resistance and the regulation of insulin secretion has increased as has our appreciation of the mechanisms underlying complications.

The diagnostic criteria look set to be changed again and may incorporate hemoglobin A1c (HbA_{1c}) while the units of the latter have also recently changed to reflect the development of more reliable and traceable assays. As HbA_{1c} remains the currency of everyday diabetes practice, these changes will provide major educational challenges for patients and professionals alike.

Alongside the developments in the pathophysiology of diabetes have come major advances in the treatment of diabetes. Some of these therapeutic innovations have been withdrawn, such as inhaled insulin, but many have been adopted in clinical practice. The development of new oral agents to treat type 2 diabetes has diversified choices for clinicians and people with diabetes. Drugs affecting glucagon-like peptide 1 (GLP-1) and the incretin axis that were mentioned briefly as future treatments in the last edition are now firmly established as effective treatments of type 2 diabetes. Many studies have highlighted the advantages and disadvantages of the newer agents making the choice of treatment more complicated than ever. Beyond the gluco-centric view of diabetes, major cardiovascular trials continue to show the benefits of statin therapy in people with diabetes.

The publication of this new edition is timely given the rapid advances in knowledge. This edition has a new editorial team drawn from the UK, Europe, USA and Asia to reflect the global nature of the diabetes epidemic. The new team has experienced a big learning curve and we are profoundly grateful that we could stand on the shoulders of John Pickup and Gareth Williams, the editors of the previous three editions. The new book has retained many of the excellent author team brought together by John and Gareth and the structure is similar to the previous editions. Nevertheless like any new teams we have tried to improve the book while keeping the sound ideas from the previous book. The book has been shortened into one volume to make it easier to use. We have emphasized the clinical aspects of diabetes to a greater extent than previous editions and reflecting the diverse locations of the editors, the chapter authors are also dispersed throughout the globe making this a truly international textbook which crosses continents and highlights both developed and developing health systems.

As editors we are only too aware of the work that many people have contributed to the book, without which our endeavors would have been much harder, if not impossible. The chapter authors are at the top of our list for our gratitude. Their willingness to devote their time and effort into compiling scholarly and relevant chapters, while tolerating nagging e-mails from us, has been humbling. In an age where book writing often comes fourth behind grant and paper writing and clinical work, we are grateful for the way that the authors met the deadlines set by us. We are also grateful for the immense help we have received from our publisher, Wiley-Blackwell. Our Commissioning Editor Oliver Walter, who took over from Alison Brown shortly into the book's development, has provided encouragement, support and guidance as has Jennifer Seward, the Development Editor. Often just at the time when things appeared to be insurmountable, Oliver or Jennifer took steps to get the project moving again. Our thanks also go to Rob Blundell (Production Editor) and Helen Harvey (Project Manager) in the production team.

We hope you enjoy reading the book and find it useful whether this is helping people with diabetes or teaching physicians and other health professionals how best to manage this disease and its complications.

Richard I.G. Holt
Clive S. Cockram
Allan Flyvbjerg
Barry J. Goldstein

Foreword

The face of diabetes is forever changing. Scientific knowledge increases exponentially and our understanding slowly improves although there are still massive gaps in many fundamental aspects of the diabetes story, such as the mechanisms underlying the development of type 2 diabetes. Trying to keep up with all the advances is an ever increasing burden, but with a large array of means to achieve this. Many people use the web, both specific websites and more general search engines, but there are still a large number of people who prefer the printed word and the collection together of an accessible compendium where you can expect to obtain answers to your questions. This volume provides exactly that; namely a series of up-to-date, well referenced, learned articles covering the manifold manifestations of diabetes together with the basic underlying science. It is truly comprehensive and I would challenge any reader to find missing aspects of the pathophysiology, treatment and care of people with diabetes.

The book begins with a fascinating historical essay which should be read by anybody who picks up the book. It reminds us that much valuable information is forgotten and many lessons can be learned by going back to pre-internet days! The possibility of using HbA_{1c} for the diagnosis of diabetes is discussed reflecting a potentially seismic shift in our diagnostic armamentarium that has relied on the measurement of glucose since that became available routinely a century ago. The world pandemic of diabetes is described with few populations spared and then each type of diabetes is described together with what is known of their pathophysiology. Particularly valuable are the essays on non-classical type 1 and type 2 diabetes.

The management and treatment of diabetes from education through lifestyle modification and the use of oral agents and insulin is dealt with exhaustively with useful chapters on the oft ignored psychological and social aspects of the disorder. Different models of care are also well discussed. Complications are dealt with comprehensively and again the book is of particular value in going beyond the classical complications and dealing with a range of less well defined problems found in people with diabetes. The book finishes with crystal ball gazing: a look at future drugs for both type 1 and type 2 diabetes, as well as the potential for stem cell therapy, islet cell transplantation and gene therapy, all of which are thought provoking and informative.

Overall I feel that this volume fulfils a major need for anyone with an interest in diabetes; it should be available in every setting where people with diabetes receive their care and will serve as an excellent vade mecum.

K. George M.M. Alberti
Imperial College London

List of Abbreviations

AA	arachidonic acid
AAA	abdominal aortic aneurysm
AACE	American Association of Clinical Endocrinologists
AADE	American Association of Diabetes Educators
ABI	ankle brachial index
ACA	acetyl co-enzyme A
ACC	acetyl-CoA carboxylase
ACCORD	Action to Control Cardiovascular Risk in Diabetes
ACE	American College of Endocrinology
ACE	angiotensin-converting enzyme
ACEi	angiotensin-converting enzyme inhibitor
ACR	albumin : creatinine ratio
ACS	acute coronary syndromes
ACTH	adrenocorticotropic hormone
ADA	American Diabetes Association
ADASP	autoimmune diabetes in adults with slowly progressive β-cell failure
ADI	acceptable daily intake
AGE	advanced glycation end-product
AGRP	agouti-related peptide
ALT	alanine aminotransferase
AMI	acute myocardial infarction
AMPK	adenosine 5′-monophosphate-activated protein kinase
APC	antigen-presenting cell
ARB	angiotensin receptor blocker
AST	aspartate aminotransferase
AT	angiotensin
ATG	antithymocyte globulin
BB	bio-breeding
BCG	bacille Calmette–Guérin
BIPSS	bilateral inferior petrosal sinus sampling
BMD	bone mineral density
BMI	body mass index
BNP	B-type natriuretic peptide
BP	blood pressure
BUN	blood urea nitrogen
CABG	coronary artery bypass grafting
CAD	coronary artery disease
CaMK	calcium/calmodulin-dependent kinase
cAMP	cyclic adenosine monophosphate
CA-MRSA	community-associated methicillin-resistant *Staphylococcus aureus*
CAP	Cbl associated protein
CAPD	continuous ambulatory peritoneal dialysis
CART	cocaine and amfetamine-related transcript
CBF	cerebral blood flow
CBT	cognitive–behavioral therapy
CCA	calcium-channel antagonist
CCK	cholecystokinin
CCM	Chronic Care Model
CD	celiac disease
CDC	Centers for Disease Control and Prevention
CDFC	comprehensive diabetic foot examination
CDK	cyclin-dependent kinase
CEL	carboxyl ester lipase
CETP	cholesterol ester transfer protein
CFTR	cystic fibrosis transmembrane conductance regulator
CGM	continuous glucose monitoring
cGMP	cyclic guanosine monophosphate
CGMS	continuous glucose monitoring systems
CGRP	calcitonin gene-related peptide
CHD	coronary heart disease
CHF	congestive heart failure
CHO	Chinese hamster ovary
CI	confidence interval
cIMT	carotid intima-media thickness
CKD	chronic kidney disease
CML	carboxymethyl lysine
CN	Charcot neuroarthropathy
CNV	copy number variant
CoA	coenzyme A
COX	cyclo-oxygenase

$cPLA_2$	cytosolic PLA_2
CPT	carnitine palmitoyltransferase
CRH	corticotropin releasing hormone
CRP	C-reactive protein
CRS	congenital rubella syndrome
CSII	continuous subcutaneous insulin infusion
CsA	cyclosporine A
CT	computed tomography
CTGF	connective tissue growth factor
CVD	cardiovascular disease
DAG	diacylglycerol
DASP	Diabetes Antibody Standardization Program
DAWN	Diabetes Attitudes, Wishes, and Needs study
DCCT	Diabetes Control and Complications Trial
DD	disc diameter
DEND	developmental delay, epilepsy and neonatal diabetes
DEXA	dual-energy X-ray absorptiometry
DHA	docosahexanoic acid
DHEA	dehydroepiandrosterone
DIDMOAD	diabetes insipidus, diabetes mellitus, optic atrophy and deafness
DIGAMI	Diabetes mellitus, Insulin Glucose infusion in Acute Myocardial Infarction
DISH	diffuse idiopathic skeletal hyperostosis
DKA	diabetic ketoacidosis
DM	diabetic maculopathy
DNSG EASD	Diabetes and Nutrition Study Group of the European Association for the Study of Diabetes
DPN	distal symmetrical sensory or sensorimotor polyneuropathy
DPP	Diabetes Prevention Program
DPP-4	dipeptidyl peptidase 4
DQOL	Diabetes Quality of Life
DR	diabetic retinopathy
DRS	Diabetic Retinopathy Study
DSA	digital subtraction angiography
DSME	diabetes self-management education
DVLA	Driver and Vehicle Licensing Agency
DVT	deep venous thrombosis
DZ	dizygotic
eAG	estimated average glucose measurement
EASD	European Association for the Study of Diabetes
ECG	electrocardiography/electrocardiogram
ED	erectile dysfunction
EDHF	endothelium-derived hyperpolarizing factor
EDIC	Epidemiology of Diabetes Interventions and Complications
EDNOS	eating disorder not otherwise specified
EEG	electroencephalography/electroencephalogram
eGFR	estimated glomerular filtration rate
ELISA	enzyme-linked immunosorbent assay
ELISPOT	enzyme-linked immunospot assay
EMEA	European Medicines Agency
eNOS	endothelial nitric oxide synthase
EPA	eicosapentaenoic acid
EPAC	exchange protein activated by cyclic AMP
EPC	endothelial progenitor cell
ER	endoplasmic reticulum
ERCP	endoscopic retrograde cholangiopancreatography
ERK	extracellular signal-regulated kinase
ERM	ezrin-radixin-moesin
ESCS	electrical spinal cord stimulation
ESRD	end-stage renal disease
ESRF	end-stage renal failure
ET	endothelin
ETDRS	Early Treatment Diabetic Retinopathy Study
EVAR	endovascular aneurysm repair
$FADH_2$	flavine adenine dinucleotide
FAS	fatty acid synthase
FCPD	fibrocalculous pancreatic diabetes
FDA	Food and Drug Administration
FDG	$[^{18}F]$-2-deoxy-2-fluoro-D-glucose
FDGF	fibroblast-derived growth factor
FDR	first-degree relative
FFA	free fatty acid
FHWA	Federal Highways Administration
FPD	fibrous proliferation at the disc
FPE	fibrous proliferation elsewhere
FPG	fasting plasma glucose
FPIR	first-phase insulin release
FSGS	focal segmental glomerular sclerosis
FSH	follicle stimulating hormone
GABA	γ-aminobutyric acid
GAD	glutamine acid decarboxylase
GAG	glycosaminoglycan
GAPDH	glyceraldehyde-3 phosphate dehydrogenase
GAS	group A streptococcus
GDM	gestational diabetes mellitus
GFA	glutamine : fructose-6-amidotransferase
GFR	glomerular filtration rate
GH	growth hormone
GHb	glycated hemoglobin
GHBP	growth hormone-binding protein
GHD	growth hormone deficiency
GHRH	growth hormone-releasing hormone
GI	glycemic index
GIP	glucose-dependent insulinotropic peptide
GK	glucokinase
GLP	glucagon-like peptide
GLUT	glucose transporter
GMP	good manufacturing practice
GNSO	S-nitrosoglutathione
GP	general practitioner
GRP	gastrin-releasing polypeptide
G_s	stimulatory G-protein
GSH	glutathione

GSK	glycogen synthesis kinase
GSSG	glutathione disulfide
GWA	genome-wide association
GWL	genome-wide familial linkage
HAAF	hypoglycemia-associated autonomic failure
HAART	highly active antiretroviral therapy
HBO	hyperbaric oxygen
HBV	hepatitis B virus
HCV	hepatitis C virus
HDL	high density lipoprotein
HETES	hydroxyeicosatetrenoic acids
HFCS	high-fructose corn syrup
HGF	hepatocyte growth factor
hGH	human recombinant growth hormone
HH	hyperosmolar non-ketotic hyperglycemia
HIC	high income country
HIF	hypoxia-inducible factor
HLA	human leukocyte antigen
HMa	small hemorrhage or microaneurysm
HMG	high mobility group
HNF	hepatic nuclear factor
HOMA	homeostasis model assessment
HONK	hyperosmolar non-ketotic coma
HPA	hypothalamic-pituitary-adrenal
HPETES	hydroperoxyeicosatetrenoic acids
HR	hazard ratio
hrIFN	human recombinant interferon
HRT	hormone replacement therapy
HSL	hormone sensitive lipase
HSS	hyperosmolar hyperglycemic syndrome
IA-2	insulinoma-associated antigen 2
IAA	insulin autoantibody
IAPP	islet amyloid polypeptide
IBGMS	Internet-based glucose monitoring system
IBMIR	immediate blood mediated inflammatory reaction
ICA	islet cell antibody
ICAM	intercellular adhesion molecule
ICC	interstitial cells of Cajal
ICCC	Innovative Care for Chronic Conditions
ICSA	islet surface antibody
IDDM	insulin-dependent diabetes mellitus
IDF	International Diabetes Federation
IDMPS	International Diabetes Management Practice Study
IENF	intra-epidermal nerve fiber
IFCC	International Federation of Clinical Chemistry
IFG	impaired fasting glucose
Ig	immunoglobulin
IGF	insulin-like growth factor
IGFBP	insulin-like growth factor binding protein
IGF1R	insulin-like growth factor 1 receptor
IGT	impaired glucose tolerance
IHD	ischemic heart disease
IKKβ	inhibitor κ-B kinase-β
IL	interleukin
INR	International Normalized Ratio
IOB	insulin-on-board
IP_3	inositol 1,4,5-trisphosphate
IPAN	intrinsic primary afferent neuron
IPF	insulin promoter factor
iPS	induced pluripotent cell
IR	insulin resistance
IRE	inositol-requiring kinase
IRE	insulin response element
IRMA	intraretinal microvascular abnormality
IRS	insulin receptor substrate
ISH	International Society of Hypertension
IUD	intrauterine contraceptive device
IVGTT	intravenous glucose tolerance test
JaK	Janus kinase
JDRF	Juvenile Diabetes Research Foundation
JNK	c-Jun N-terminal kinase
Km	Michaelis constant
KO	knockout
LADA	latent autoimmune diabetes of adults
LADC	latent autoimmune diabetes in children
LADY	latent autoimmune diabetes in the young
LAR	leukocyte antigen-related phosphatase
LD	linkage disequilibrium
LDL	low density lipoprotein
LEAD	Liraglutide Effect and Action in Diabetes
LGV	large goods vehicle
LH	lactic hydrogenase
LI	lability index
LMIC	low and middle income countries
LOX	lipoxygenase
LPL	lipoprotein lipase
LVH	left ventricular hypertrophy
MACE	major adverse cardiovascular event
MAPK	mitogen activated protein kinase
MBL	mannose-binding lectin
MCH	melanin-concentrating hormone
MCP	metacarpophalangeal
MCP	monocyte chemotactic protein
MDI	multiple daily injection
MELAS	mitochondrial encephalomyopathy, lactic acidosis and stroke-like episodes
MEN	multiple endocrine neoplasia
MHC	major histocompatibility complex
MI	myocardial infarction
MIBI	methyloxybutylisonitrile
MIDD	maternal inherited diabetes and deafness
MMP	matrix metalloproteinase
MnSOD	manganese superoxide dismutase
MODY	maturity-onset diabetes of the young
MR	modified release
MRA	magnetic resonance angiography

MRDM malnutrition-related diabetes mellitus
MRI magnetic resonance imaging
MRSA methacillin-resistant *Staphylococcus aureus*
MSH melanocyte stimulating hormone
MSU monosodium urate
mTOR mammalian target of rapamycin
MTP microsomal triglyceride transfer protein
MUFA monounsaturated fatty acid
MZ monozygotic
NAA N-acetyl aspartate
NAC N-acetylcysteine
NADPH nicotinic acid adenine dinucleotide phosphate
NAFLD non-alcoholic fatty liver disease
NAION non-arteritic anterior ischemic optic neuropathy
NASH non-alcoholic steatohepatitis
NCD non-communicable disease
NDDG National Diabetes Data Group
NEFA non-esterified fatty acid
NFG normal fasting glucose
NFκB nuclear factor κB
NGF nerve growth factor
NGT nasogastric tube
NGT normal glucose tolerance
NHANES National Health and Nutrition Examination Survey
NICE National Institute for Health and Clinical Excellence
NIDDM non-insulin-dependent diabetes mellitus
NIH National Institutes of Health
NIMGU non-insulin-mediated glucose uptake
NINDS National Institute of Neurologic Disorders
NK natural killer
NLD necrobiosis lipoidica diabeticorum
NNH number needed to harm
NNRTI non-nucleoside reverse-transcriptase inhibitor
NNT number needed to treat
NO nitric oxide
NOD non-obese diabetic
NOS nitric oxide synthase
NPDR non-proliferative diabetic retinopathy
NPH neutral protamine Hagedorn
NPWT negative pressure wound therapy
NPY neuropeptide Y
NRTI nucleoside reverse-transcriptase inhibitor
NSAID non-steroidal anti-inflammatory drug
NTD neural tube defect
NVD new vessels on and/or within 1 disc diameter of the disc
NVE new vessels elsewhere
NYHA New York Heart Association
OCP oral contraceptive pill
OCT optical coherence topography
OGT *O*-linked *N*-acetylglucosamine transferase
OGTT oral glucose tolerance test(ing)
OPG osteoprotegerin
OR odds ratio
ORP oxygen-regulated protein
PACAP pituitary adenylate cyclase-activating polypeptide
PAD peripheral arterial disease
PAI plasminogen activator inhibitor
PARP poly(ADP-ribose) polymerase
PCOS polycystic ovary syndrome
PCV passenger-carrying vehicle
PDE phosphodiesterase
PDGF platelet-derived growth factor
PDK 3-phosphoinositide-dependent protein kinase
PDR proliferative diabetic retinopathy
PDX pancreatic duodenal homeobox
PEG percutaneous endoscopic gastrostomy
PEPCK phosphoenolpyruvate carboxykinase
PET positron emission tomography
PFC perflurodecalin
PFC prefrontal cortex
PGE prostaglandin
PH pleckstrin homology
PHHI persistent hyperinsulinemic hypoglycemia of infancy
PI protease inhibitor
PI$_3$ phosphoinositide 3′
PID pelvic inflammatory disease
PIP proximal interphalangeal
PIP$_2$ phosphoinositol 4,5-bisphosphate
PIP3 phosphatidylinositol 3,4,5-trisphosphate
PK protein kinase
PLC phospholipase C
PLP periodate-lysine-paraformaldehyde
PNDM permanent neonatal diabetes mellitus
PNMT phenylethanolamine-*N*-methyltransferase
POMC pro-opiomelanocortin
POP progesterone-only pill
PP pancreatic polypeptide
PPAR peroxisome proliferator-activated receptor
PPG post-prandial plasma glucose
PPRE peroxisome proliferator response element
PRA panel reactive antibody
PRH preretinal hemorrhage
PTA percutaneous transluminal angioplasty
PTB phosphotyrosine binding
PTDM post-transplantation diabetes mellitus
PTEN phosphatase and tensin homolog
PTSD post-traumatic stress disorder
PTH parathyroid hormone
PTP protein tyrosine phosphatase
PVD peripheral vascular disease
PVN paraventricular nucleus
QALY quality-adjusted life year
QST quantitative sensory testing

RAGE	receptor for advanced glycation end-product
RAI	rapid acting analog
RANKL	receptor activator of nuclear factor κB ligand
RAS	renin angiotensin system
RBP	retinol-binding protein
RCAD	renal cysts and diabetes syndrome
RCW	removable cast walker
rhIGF	recombinant human insulin-like growth factor
RMR	resting metabolic rate
ROC	receiver operator characteristic
ROS	reactive oxygen species
RRT	renal replacement therapy
RT-CGM	real-time continuous glucose monitoring
SADS	seasonal affective depressive syndrome
SARS	severe acute respiratory syndrome
SCID	severe combined immunodeficiency
SD	standard deviation
SDF	stromal cell-derived factor
SDH	sorbitol dehydrogenase
SGLT	sodium-glucose co-transporter
SH2	Src homology 2
SHBG	sex hormone-binding globulin
SHIP	SH2-containing inositol phosphatase
SHORT	short atature, hyperextensibility of joints, ocular depression, Reiger anamoly, teething delay (syndrome)
SHP2	SH2-domain-containing tyrosine phosphatase 2
SMBG	self-monitoring of blood glucose
SMI	serious mental illness
SMR	standardized mortality ratio
SNARE	soluble N-ethylmaleimide-sensitive factor attachment protein receptor
SNP	single nucleotide polymorphism
SNRI	serotonin noradrenaline reuptake inhibitor
SOCS	suppressor of cytokine signaling
SoHo	sorbin homology
SPECT	single photon emission computed tomography
sRAGE	soluble receptor for advanced glycation end-product
SREBP	sterol regulatory element-binding protein
SSRI	selective serotonin reuptake inhibitor
SST	somatostatin
SSTR	somatostatin receptor
STAT	signal transducer and activator of transcription
SUR	sulfonylurea receptor
$t_{1/2}$	half-life
T1DM	type 1 diabetes mellitus
T2DM	type 2 diabetes mellitus
TCA	tricarboxylic acid
TCA	tricyclic antidepressant
TCC	total contact cast
TCC	transition case coordinator
TCF	transcription factor
TCR	T-cell receptor
TDI	tissue Doppler imaging
TENS	transcutaneous electrical nerve stimulation
TG	triglyceride
TGF	transforming growth factor
TIA	transient ischemic attack
TKA	tyrosine kinase activity
TLR	toll-like receptor
TNDM	transient neonatal diabetes mellitus
TNF	tumor necrosis factor
t-PA	tissue plasminogen activator
TRAIL	tumor necrosis factor related apoptosis inducing ligand
TSC	tuberous sclerosis complex
TSH	thyroid stimulating hormone
TZD	thiazolidinedione
UAE	urinary albumin excretion
UCP	uncoupling protein
UDP	uridine diphosphate
UKPDS	UK Prospective Diabetes Study
USDA	US Department of Agriculture
UT	urotensin
UTI	urinary tract infection
UW	University of Wisconsin solution
VADT	Veterans Affairs Diabetes Trial
VB	venous beading
VCAM	vascular cell adhesion molecule
VEGF	vascular endothelial growth factor
VH	vitreous hemorrhage
VIP	vasoactive intestinal polypeptide
VLCD	very low calorie diet
VLDL	very low density lipoprotein
VNTR	variable number tandem repeat
$\dot{V}O_{2max}$	maximal oxygen consumption
VPT	vibration perception threshold
VSMC	vascular smooth muscle cell
WHI	Women's Health Initiative
WHO	World Health Organization

1 Diabetes in its Historical and Social Context

1 The History of Diabetes Mellitus

Robert B. Tattersall

University of Nottingham, Nottingham, UK

Keypoints

- Polyuric diseases have been described for over 3500 years. The name "diabetes" comes from the Greek word for a syphon; the sweet taste of diabetic urine was recognized at the beginning of the first millennium, but the adjective "mellitus" (honeyed) was only added by Rollo in the late 18th century.
- The sugar in diabetic urine was identified as glucose by Chevreul in 1815. In the 1840s, Bernard showed that glucose was normally present in blood, and showed that it was stored in the liver (as glycogen) for secretion into the bloodstream during fasting.
- In 1889, Minkowski and von Mering reported that pancreatectomy caused severe diabetes in the dog. In 1893, Laguesse suggested that the pancreatic "islets" described by Langerhans in 1869 produced an internal secretion that regulated glucose metabolism.
- Insulin was discovered in 1921 by Banting, Best, Macleod and Collip in acid-ethanol extracts of pancreas. It was first used for treatment in January 1922.
- Diabetes was subdivided on clinical grounds into *diabète maigre* (lean subjects) and *diabète gras* (obese) by Lancereaux in 1880, and during the 1930s by Falta and Himsworth into insulin-sensitive and insulin-insensitive types. These classifications were the forerunners of the etiological classification into type 1 (insulin-dependent) and type 2 (non-insulin-dependent) diabetes.
- Insulin resistance and β-cell failure, the fundamental defects of type 2 diabetes, have been investigated by many researchers. The "insulin clamp" method devised by Andres and DeFronzo was the first accurate technique for measuring insulin action. Maturity-onset diabetes of the young was described as a distinct variant of type 2 diabetes by Tattersall in 1974.
- Lymphocytic infiltration of the islets (insulitis) was described as early as 1901 and highlighted in 1965 by Gepts who suggested that it might be a marker of autoimmunity. Islet cell antibodies were discovered by Doniach and Bottazzo in 1979.
- The primary sequence of insulin was reported in 1955 by Sanger and the three-dimensional structure by Hodgkin in 1969. Proinsulin was discovered by Steiner in 1967, and the sequence of the human insulin gene by Bell in 1980. Yalow and Berson invented the radioimmunoassay for insulin in 1956. The presence of insulin receptors was deduced in 1971 by Freychet, and the receptor protein was isolated in 1972 by Cuatrecasas.
- The various types of diabetic retinopathy were described in the second half of the 19th century as were the symptoms of neuropathy. Albuminuria was noted as a common abnormality in patients with diabetes in the 19th century and a unique type of kidney disease was described in 1936 by Kimmelstiel and Wilson. The concept of a specific diabetic angiopathy was developed by Lundbaek in the early 1950s.
- Milestones in insulin pharmacology have included the invention of delayed-action preparations in the 1930s and 1940s; synthetic human insulin in 1979; and in the 1990s novel insulin analogs by recombinant DNA technology.
- The first sulfonylurea carbutamide was introduced in 1955, followed by tolbutamide in 1957 and chlorpropamide in 1960. The biguanide phenformin became available in 1959 and metformin in 1960.
- That improved glucose control in both type 1 and type 2 diabetes was beneficial was proved by the Diabetes Control and Complications Trial (1993) and the UK Prospective Diabetes Study (1998).
- Landmarks in the treatment of complications include photocoagulation for retinopathy first described by Meyer-Schwickerath; the importance of blood pressure to slow the progression of nephropathy (demonstrated by Mogensen and Parving); the introduction of low-dose insulin in the treatment of diabetic ketoacidosis in the 1970s; and improvements in the care of pregnant women with diabetes pioneered by White and Pedersen.

Ancient times

Diseases with the cardinal features of diabetes mellitus were recognized in antiquity (Table 1.1). A polyuric state was described in an Egyptian papyrus dating from *c.* 1550 BC, discovered by Georg Ebers (Figure 1.1), and a clearly recognizable description of what would now be called type 1 diabetes was given by Aretaeus of Cappadocia in the 2nd century AD (Figure 1.2a). Aretaeus was the first to use the term "diabetes," from the Greek word for a syphon, "because the fluid does not remain in the body, but uses the man's body as a channel whereby to leave it." His graphic account of the disease highlighted the incessant flow of urine,

Textbook of Diabetes, 4th edition. Edited by R. Holt, C. Cockram, A. Flyvbjerg and B. Goldstein.

Table 1.1 Milestones in the clinical descriptions of diabetes and its complications.

Clinical features of diabetes	
Ebers papyrus (Egypt, 1500 BC)	Polyuric state
Sushrut and Charak (India, 5th century BC)	Sugary urine; thin and obese patients distinguished
Aretaeus (Cappadocia, 2nd century AD)	Polyuric state named "diabetes"
Chen Chuan (China, 7th century)	Sugary urine
Avicenna (Arabia, 10th century AD)	Sugary urine; gangrene and impotence as complications
Diabetic ketoacidosis	
William Prout (England, 1810–1820)	Diabetic coma
Adolf Kussmaul (Germany, 1874)	Acidotic breathing
Hyperlipidemia	
Albert Heyl (Philadelphia, 1880)	Lipemia retinalis
Retinopathy	
Eduard von Jaeger (Germany, 1855)	General features
Stephen Mackenzie and Edward Nettleship (England, 1879)	Microaneurysms
Edward Nettleship (England, 1888)	New vessels, beading of retinal veins
Julius Hirschberg (Germany, 1890)	Classification of lesions; specific to diabetes
Neuropathy and foot disease	
John Rollo (England, 1797)	Neuropathic symptoms
Marchal de Calvi (France, 1864)	Neuropathy is a complication of diabetes
William Ogle (England, 1866)	Ocular nerve palsies in diabetes
Frederick Pavy (England, 1885)	Peripheral neuropathy
Julius Althaus (Germany, 1890)	Mononeuropathy
Thomas Davies Pryce (England, 1887)	Perforating foot ulcers
Nephropathy	
Wilhelm Griesinger (Germany, 1859)	Renal disease in patients with diabetes
Paul Kimmelstiel and Clifford Wilson (USA, 1936)	Glomerulosclerosis associated with heavy proteinuria

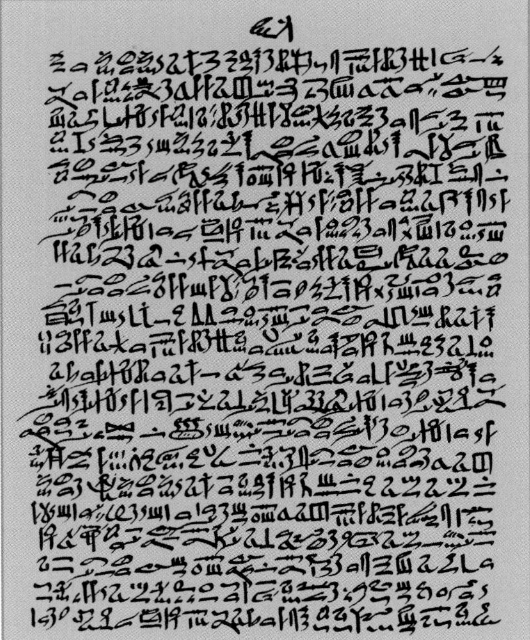

Figure 1.1 The Ebers papyrus. Courtesy of the Wellcome Library, London.

(a)

Diabetes is a dreadful affliction, not very frequent among men, being a melting down of the flesh and limbs into urine. The patients never stop making water and the flow is incessant, like the opening of aqueducts. Life is short, unpleasant and painful, thirst unquenchable, drinking excessive, and disproportionate to the large quantity of urine, for yet more urine is passed. One cannot stop them either from drinking or making water. If for a while they abstain from drinking, their mouths become parched and their bodies dry; the viscera seem scorched up, the patients are affected by nausea, restlessness and a burning thirst, and within a short time, they expire.

(b)

Figure 1.2 (a) Clinical description of diabetes by Aretaeus of Cappadocia (2nd century AD). Adapted from Papaspyros NS (1952) *The History of Diabetes Mellitus*. (b) Sushrut (Susrata), an Indian physician who wrote medical texts with Charak (Charuka) between 500 BC and 400 BC.

unquenchable thirst, the "melting down of the flesh and limbs into urine" and short survival.

The Hindu physicians, Charak and Sushrut, who wrote between 400 and 500 BC, were probably the first to recognize the sweetness of diabetic urine (Figure 1.2b). Indeed, the diagnosis was made by tasting the urine or noting that ants congregated round it. Charak and Sushrut noted that the disease was most prevalent in those who were indolent, overweight and gluttonous, and who indulged in sweet and fatty foods. Physical exercise and liberal quantities of vegetables were the mainstays of treatment in the obese, while lean people, in whom the disease was regarded as more serious, were given a nourishing diet. The crucial fact that diabetic urine tasted sweet was also emphasized by Arabic medical texts from the 9–11th centuries AD, notably in the medical encyclopedia written by Avicenna (980–1037).

The 17th and 18th centuries

In Europe, diabetes was neglected until Thomas Willis (1621–1675) wrote *Diabetes, or the Pissing Evil* [1]. According to him, "diabetes was a disease so rare among the ancients that many famous physicians made no mention of it … but in our age, given to good fellowship and guzzling down of unallayed wine, we meet with examples and instances enough, I may say daily, of this disease." He described the urine as being "wonderfully sweet like sugar or honey" but did not consider that this might be because it contained sugar.

The first description of hyperglycemia was in a paper published in 1776 by Matthew Dobson (1735–1784) of Liverpool (Figure 1.3) [2]. He found that the serum as well as the urine of his patient Peter Dickonson (who passed 28 pints of urine a day) tasted sweet. Moreover, he evaporated the urine to "a white cake [which] smelled sweet like brown sugar, neither could it by the taste be distinguished from sugar." Dobson concluded that the kidneys excreted sugar and that it was not "formed in the secretory organ but previously existed in the serum of the blood."

The Edinburgh-trained surgeon, John Rollo (*d.* 1809) was the first to apply the adjective "mellitus" (from the Latin word meaning "honey"). He also achieved fame with his "animal diet," which became the standard treatment for most of the 19th century. Rollo thought that sugar was formed in the stomach

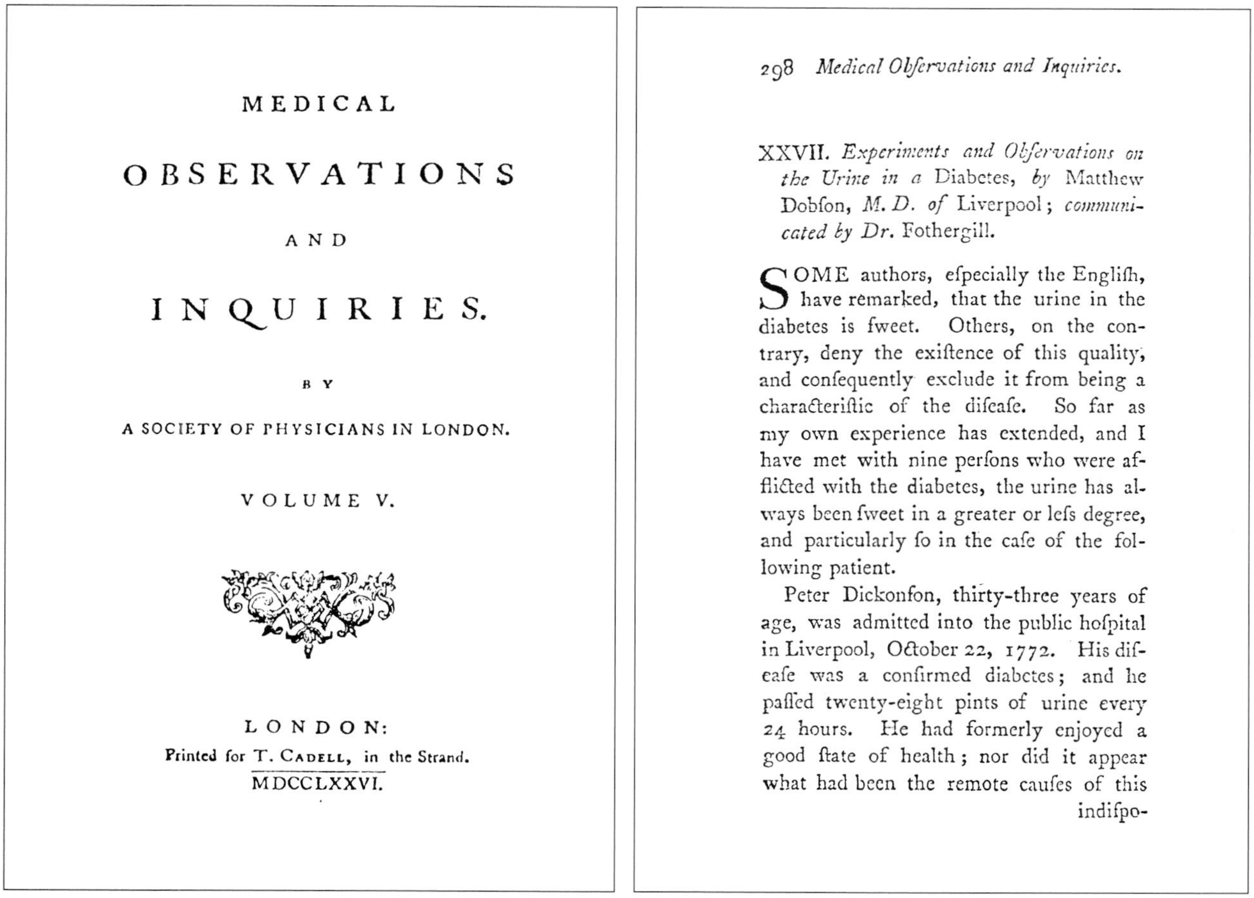

MEDICAL

OBSERVATIONS

AND

INQUIRIES.

BY

A SOCIETY OF PHYSICIANS IN LONDON.

VOLUME V.

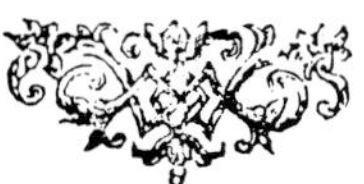

LONDON:

Printed for T. CADELL, in the Strand.

MDCCLXXVI.

298 *Medical Obſervations and Inquiries.*

XXVII. *Experiments and Obſervations on the Urine in a* Diabetes, *by* Matthew Dobſon, *M. D. of* Liverpool; *communicated by Dr.* Fothergill.

SOME authors, eſpecially the Engliſh, have remarked, that the urine in the diabetes is ſweet. Others, on the contrary, deny the exiſtence of this quality, and conſequently exclude it from being a characteriſtic of the diſeaſe. So far as my own experience has extended, and I have met with nine perſons who were afflicted with the diabetes, the urine has always been ſweet in a greater or leſs degree, and particularly ſo in the caſe of the following patient.

Peter Dickonſon, thirty-three years of age, was admitted into the public hoſpital in Liverpool, October 22, 1772. His diſeaſe was a confirmed diabetes; and he paſſed twenty-eight pints of urine every 24 hours. He had formerly enjoyed a good ſtate of health; nor did it appear what had been the remote cauſes of this indiſpo-

Figure 1.3 Frontispiece and opening page of the paper by Matthew Dobson (1776), in which he described the sweet taste of both urine and serum from a patient with diabetes [2].

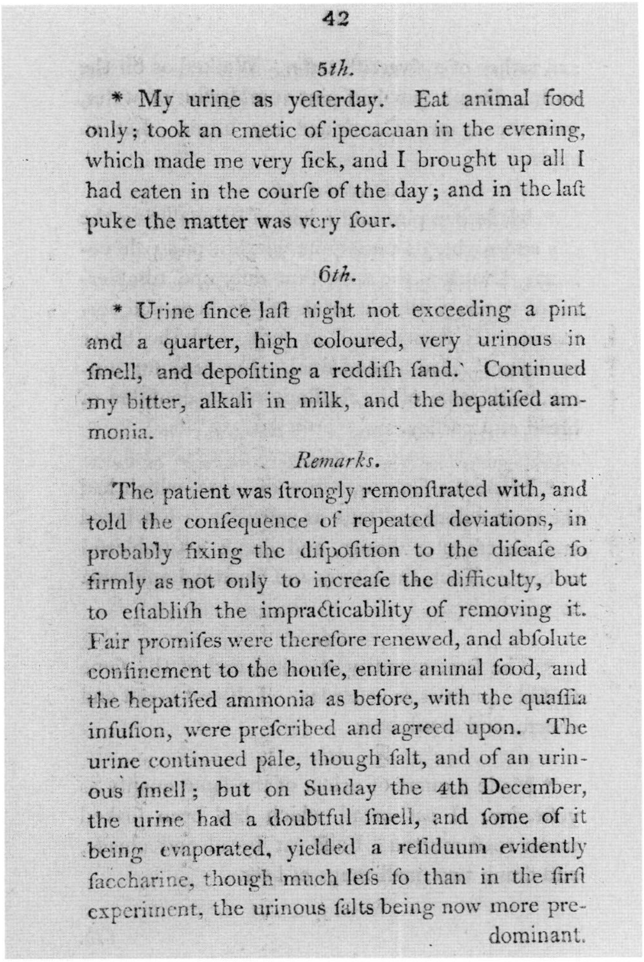

42

5th.

* My urine as yeſterday. Eat animal food only; took an emetic of ipecacuan in the evening, which made me very ſick, and I brought up all I had eaten in the courſe of the day; and in the laſt puke the matter was very ſour.

6th.

* Urine ſince laſt night not exceeding a pint and a quarter, high coloured, very urinous in ſmell, and depoſiting a reddiſh ſand. Continued my bitter, alkali in milk, and the hepatiſed ammonia.

Remarks.

The patient was ſtrongly remonſtrated with, and told the conſequence of repeated deviations, in probably fixing the diſpoſition to the diſeaſe ſo firmly as not only to increaſe the difficulty, but to eſtabliſh the impracticability of removing it. Fair promiſes were therefore renewed, and abſolute confinement to the houſe, entire animal food, and the hepatiſed ammonia as before, with the quaſſia infuſion, were preſcribed and agreed upon. The urine continued pale, though ſalt, and of an urinous ſmell; but on Sunday the 4th December, the urine had a doubtful ſmell, and ſome of it being evaporated, yielded a reſiduum evidently ſaccharine, though much leſs ſo than in the firſt experiment, the urinous ſalts being now more predominant.

Figure 1.4 Extract from John Rollo's account of two cases of diabetes (1797). Rollo was well aware of the problem of non-compliance. Note that "the patient was strongly remonstrated with, and told of the consequences of repeated deviations." Courtesy of the Wellcome Library, London.

from vegetables, and concluded that the obvious solution was a diet of animal food. Thus, the regimen described in his 1797 book, *An Account of Two Cases of the Diabetes Mellitus* [3], allowed his patient Captain Meredith to have for dinner "Game or old meats which have been long kept; and as far as the stomach may bear, fat and rancid old meats, as pork." Rollo was probably the first to note the difficulty that some patients find in adhering to treatment – a difficulty he blamed for the death of his second patient (Figure 1.4).

The 19th century

In 1815, the French chemist Michel Chevreul (1786–1889) proved that the sugar in diabetic urine was glucose [4]. In the middle of the century, tasting the urine to make the diagnosis was superseded by chemical tests for reducing agents such as glucose as introduced by Trommer in 1841, Moore in 1844 and – the best known – Fehling in 1848. Measurement of blood glucose could only be done by skilled chemists but needed so much blood that it was rarely used in either clinical care or research. It only became practicable with the introduction in 1913 of a micromethod by the Norwegian-born physician Ivar Christian Bang (1869–1918) and it was the ability to measure glucose repeatedly which led to development of the glucose tolerance test between 1913 and 1915.

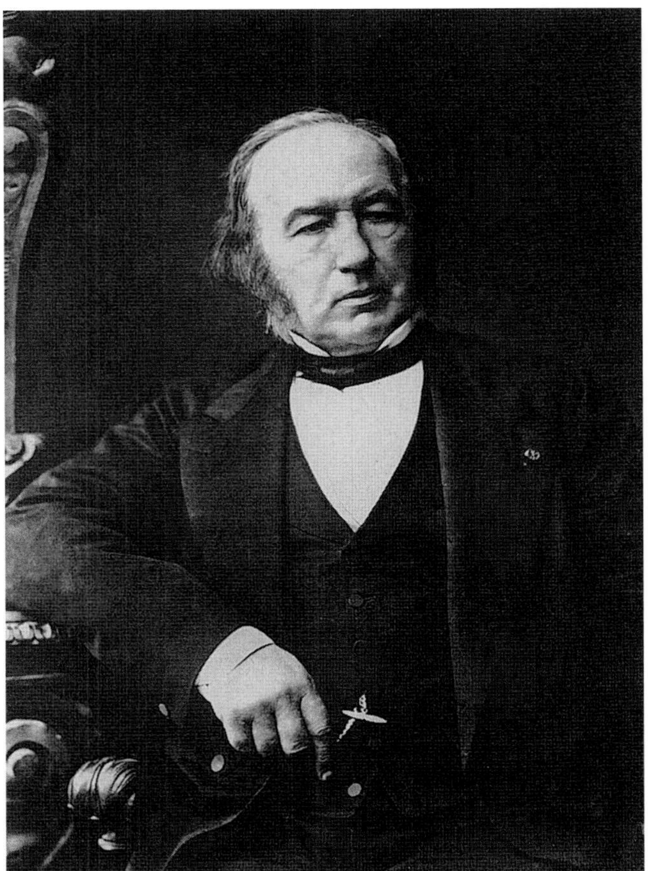

Figure 1.5 Claude Bernard (1813–1878). Courtesy of the Wellcome Institute Library, London.

Glucose metabolism was clarified by the work of Claude Bernard (1813–1878) [5], the Frenchman whose numerous discoveries have given him a special place in the history of physiology (Figure 1.5). When Bernard began work in 1843, the prevailing theory was that sugar could only be synthesized by plants, and that animal metabolism broke down substances originally made in plants. It was also thought that the blood only contained sugar after meals, or in pathologic states such as diabetes. Between 1846 and 1848, Bernard reported that glucose was present in the blood of normal animals, even when starved. He also found higher concentrations of glucose in the hepatic than in the portal vein, and "enormous quantities" of a starch-like substance in the liver which could be readily converted into sugar. He called this "gly-

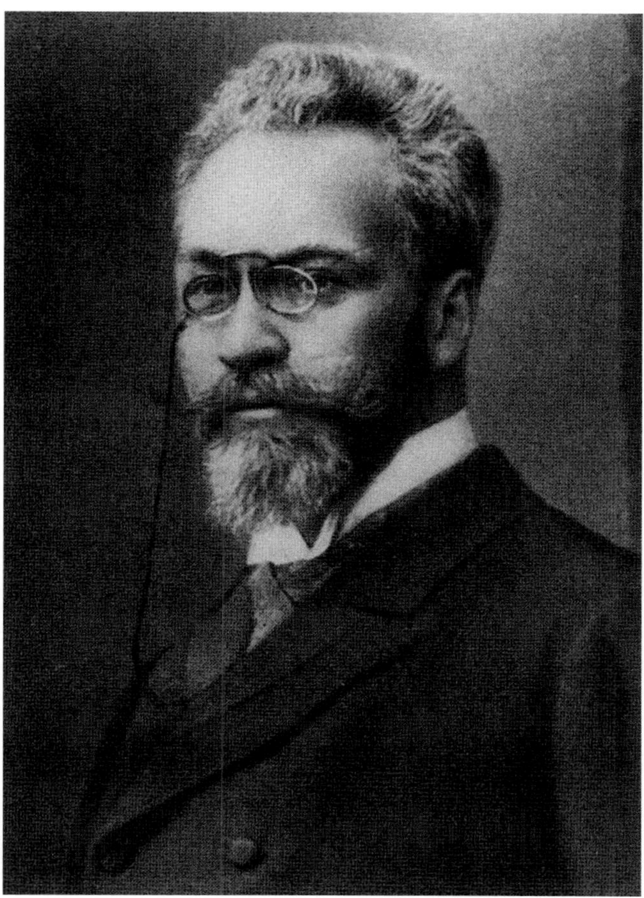

Figure 1.6 Oskar Minkowski (1858–1931).

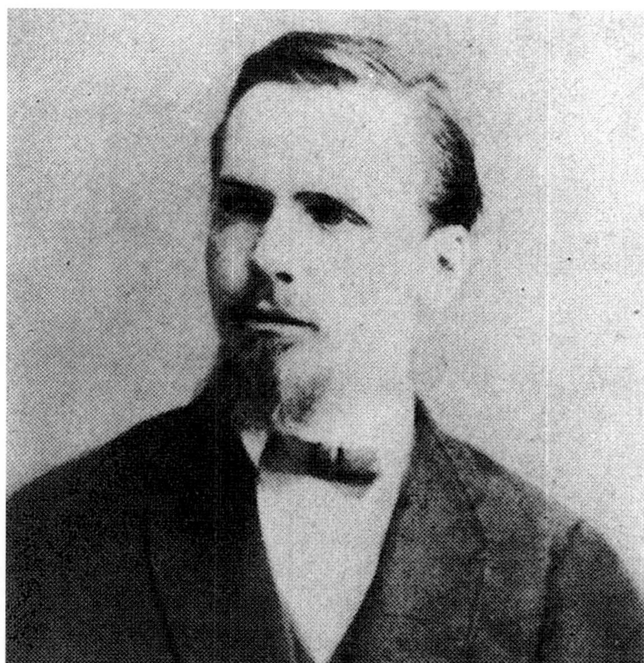

Figure 1.7 Paul Langerhans (1847–1888). Courtesy of the Wellcome Institute Library, London.

cogen" (i.e. sugar-forming) and regarded it as analogous to starch in plants. His hypothesis – the "glycogenic" theory – was that sugar absorbed from the intestine was converted in the liver into glycogen and then constantly released into the blood during fasting.

Another discovery by Bernard made a great impression in an era when the nervous control of bodily functions was a scientifically fashionable concept. He found that a lesion in the floor of the fourth ventricle produced temporary hyperglycemia (*piqûre* diabetes) [6]. This finding spawned a long period in which nervous influences were thought to be important causes of diabetes; indeed, one piece of "evidence" – cited by J.J.R. Macleod as late as 1914 – was that diabetes was more common among engine drivers than other railway workers because of the mental strain involved [7].

In the first part of the 19th century the cause of diabetes was a mystery, because autopsy usually did not show any specific lesions. A breakthrough came in 1889 when Oskar Minkowski (Figure 1.6) and Josef von Mering (1849–1908) reported that pancreatectomy in the dog caused severe diabetes [8]. This was serendipitous, because they were investigating fat metabolism; it is said that the laboratory technician mentioned to Minkowski that the dog, previously house-trained, was now incontinent of urine. Minkowski realized the significance of the polyuria, and tested the dog's urine.

Possible explanations for the role of the pancreas were that it removed a diabetogenic toxin, or produced an internal secretion that controlled carbohydrate metabolism. The concept of "internal secretions" had been publicized in June 1889, by the well-known physiologist Charles-Édouard Brown-Séquard (1817–1894), who claimed to have rejuvenated himself by injections of testicular extract [9]. It was given further credence in 1891, when Murray reported that myxoedema could be cured by sheep thyroid extract by injection or orally.

In 1893, Gustave Laguesse suggested that the putative internal secretion of the pancreas was produced by the "islands" of cells scattered through the gland's parenchyma [10], which had been discovered in 1869 by the 22-year-old Paul Langerhans (1847–1888) (Figure 1.7). Langerhans had described these clusters of cells, having teased them out from the general pancreatic tissue, but had not speculated about their possible function [11]; it was Laguesse who named them the "islets of Langerhans." At this time, the glucose-lowering internal secretion of the islets was still hypothetical, but in 1909 the Belgian Jean de Meyer named it *insuline* (from the Latin for "island") [12].

It would be wrong to give the impression that Minkowski's experiments immediately established the pancreatic origin of diabetes. In fact, during the next two decades, it was widely agreed that diabetes was a heterogeneous disorder with various subtypes, and that its pathogenesis involved at least three organs: the brain, pancreas and liver [13]. The discovery by Blum in 1901 that injec-

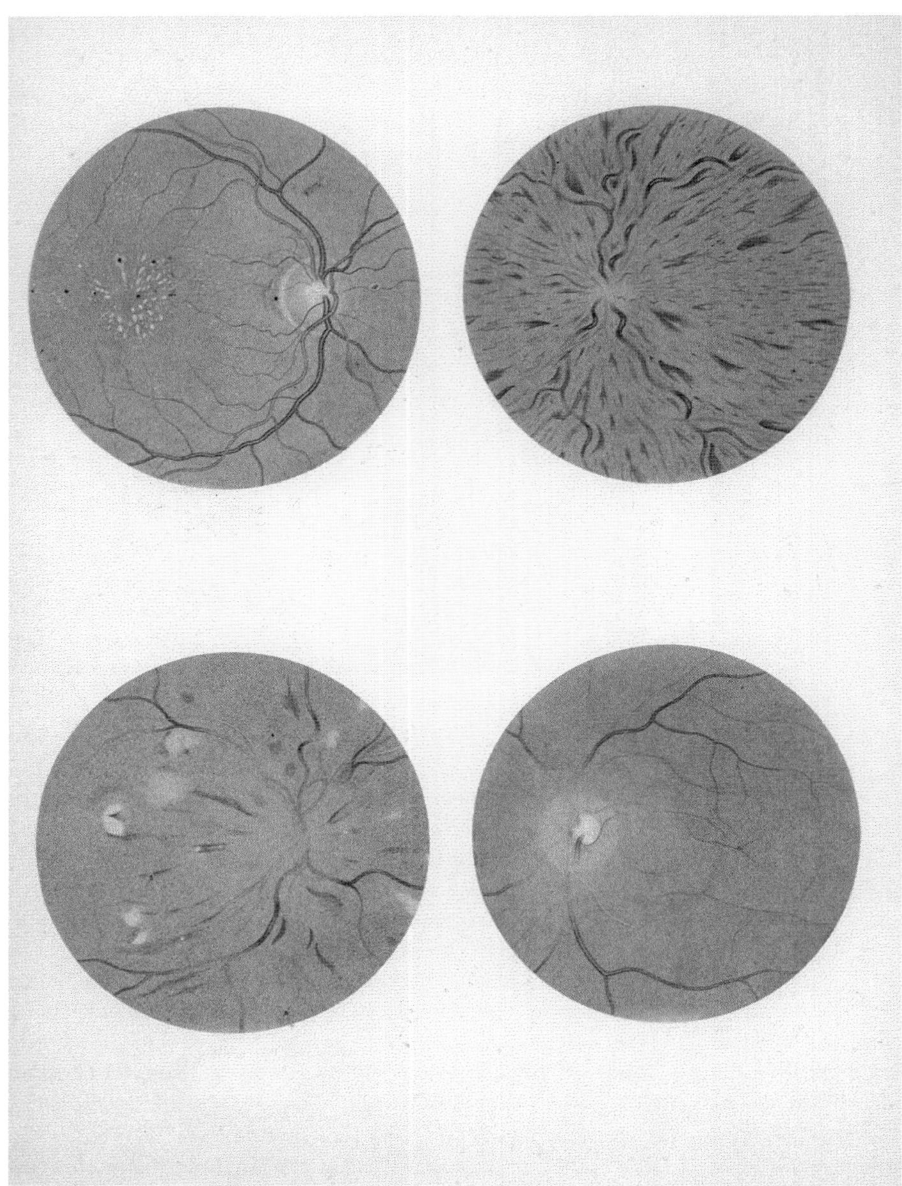

Figure 1.8 Pictures from *Jaeger's Atlas of the Optic Fundus,* 1869 [14]. Top left: Bright's disease. Top right: Jaeger's retinitis hemorrhagica is now recognized as central retinal vein occlusion. Bottom left: A 22-year-old man with suspected diabetes. Bottom right: Central retinal artery occlusion. Courtesy of W.B. Saunders.

tion of an adrenal extract caused glycosuria implicated other glands, and led to the "polyglandular theory" of Carl von Noorden (Vienna), who proposed that the thyroid, pancreas, adrenals and parathyroids controlled carbohydrate metabolism.

Clinical diabetes in the 19th century

Doctors in the 19th century were therapeutically impotent; their main role was as taxonomists who described symptom complexes and the natural history of disease. As a result, most of the major complications of diabetes were well described before 1900.

Eduard von Jaeger (1818–1884) is credited with the first description of diabetic retinopathy, in his beautiful *Atlas of Diseases of the Ocular Fundus*, published in 1869 [14]. In fact, the features illustrated (Figure 1.8), from a 22-year-old patient, look more like hypertensive retinopathy. In 1879, Stephen Mackenzie (1844–1909) and Sir Edward Nettleship (1845–1913) found microaneurysms in flat preparations of the retina and, in 1888, Nettleship described new vessels and the beaded appearance of retinal veins [15]. The full picture of diabetic retinopathy was described in 1890 by Julius Hirschberg (1843–1925) who was the first to claim that it was specific to diabetes [16].

Neuropathic symptoms in patients with diabetes had been mentioned by Rollo at the end of the 18th century, and in 1864 Charles Marchal de Calvi (1815–1873) concluded that nerve damage was a specific complication of diabetes. In 1885, the Guy's Hospital physician, Frederick Pavy (1829–1911), gave a description of neuropathic symptoms which would grace any modern textbook [17]:

"The usual account given by these patients of their condition is that they cannot feel properly in their legs, that their feet are numb, that their legs seem too heavy – as one patient expressed it, "as if he had 20 lb weights on his legs and a feeling as if his boots were great deal too large for his feet." Darting or "lightning" pains are often complained of. Or there may be hyperaesthesia, so that a mere pinching of the skin gives rise to great pain; or it may be the patient is unable to bear the contact of the seam of the dress against the skin on account of the suffering it causes. Not infrequently there is deep-seated pain located, as the patient describes it, in the marrow of the bones which are tender on being grasped, and I have noticed that these pains are generally worse at night."

Pavy also recorded unusual presentations, including a 67-year-old who complained of "lightning pains on the right side of the waist" and cases in which the third nerve was affected with "dropped lid and external squint" [18].

Kidney disease was known to be relatively common in diabetes. In 1859, Wilhelm Griesinger (1817–1868) reported 64 autopsies in adults, half of whom had renal changes which he attributed to hypertension and atherosclerosis [19]; however, the histologic features of diabetic kidney disease and the importance of renal complications were not reported until the 1930s.

In the latter part of the 19th century it was becoming apparent that there were at least two clinically distinct forms of diabetes. In 1880, the French physician Etienne Lancereaux (1829–1910) identified lean and obese patients as having *diabète maigre* and *diabète gras* [20], and this observation laid the foundations for subsequent etiologic classifications of the disease.

The 20th century

Murray's cure of myxoedema in 1891 led to a belief that pancreatic extract would soon result in a cure for diabetes, but, in the face of repeated failures over the next 30 years, even believers in an antidiabetic internal secretion were depressed about the likelihood of isolating it, and diverted their attention to diet as a treatment for the disease.

Best known was the starvation regimen of Frederick Madison Allen (1876–1964), which Joslin (Figure 1.9) described in 1915 as the greatest advance since Rollo's time [21]. This approach was

(a)

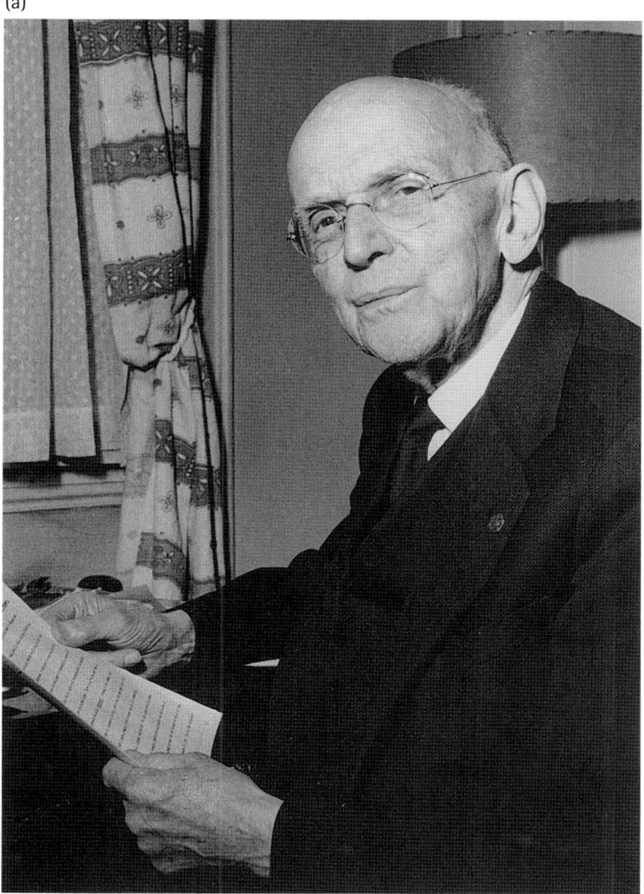

(b)

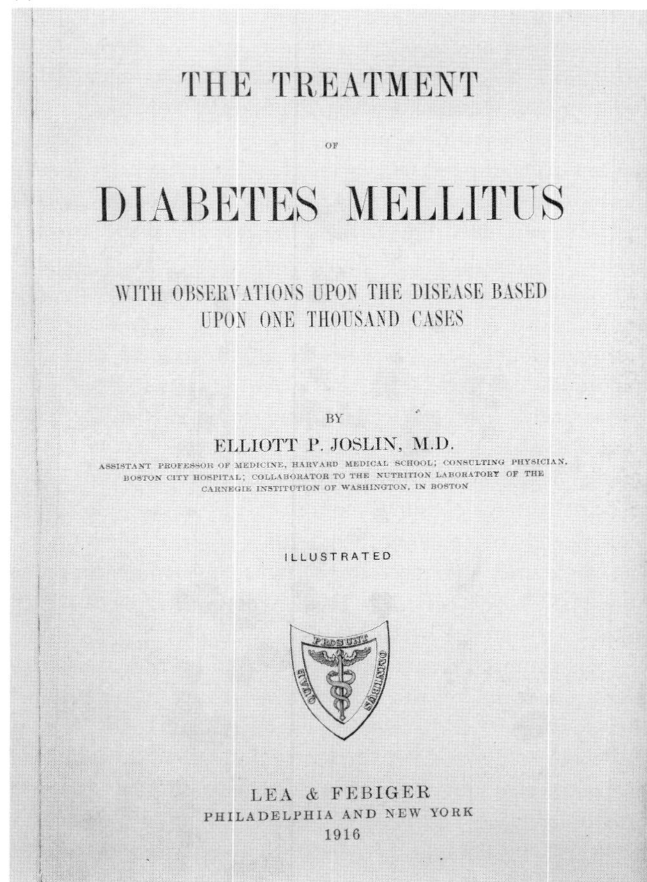

THE TREATMENT

OF

DIABETES MELLITUS

WITH OBSERVATIONS UPON THE DISEASE BASED UPON ONE THOUSAND CASES

BY

ELLIOTT P. JOSLIN, M.D.

ASSISTANT PROFESSOR OF MEDICINE, HARVARD MEDICAL SCHOOL; CONSULTING PHYSICIAN, BOSTON CITY HOSPITAL; COLLABORATOR TO THE NUTRITION LABORATORY OF THE CARNEGIE INSTITUTION OF WASHINGTON, IN BOSTON

ILLUSTRATED

LEA & FEBIGER
PHILADELPHIA AND NEW YORK
1916

Figure 1.9 Elliott P. Joslin (1869–1962), arguably the most famous diabetes specialist of the 20th century and the frontispiece to his 1916 textbook [22]. Courtesy of the Wellcome Library, London.

an extreme application of one that had been proposed as early as 1875 by Apollinaire Bouchardat (1806–1886), who advocated intensive exercise and "*manger le moins possible*." Starvation treatment did work in a limited sense, in that some patients could survive for many months or even years, instead of a few weeks or months with untreated type 1 diabetes. The quality of life, however, was very poor, and some patients died of malnutrition rather than diabetes. In 1921, Carl von Noorden (1858–1944) – proponent of the "oatmeal cure" – turned away in disapproval when he saw Joslin's prize patient, 17-year-old Ruth A, who at just over 1.52 m in height weighed only 24.5 kg (a body mass index of 10.6 kg/m^2).

Discovery of insulin

Many attempts were made between 1889 and 1921 to isolate the elusive internal secretion of the pancreas. These largely failed because the extracts were inactive or had unacceptable side effects; some preparations may have had limited biologic activity, but this was not recognized, either because hypoglycemia was misinterpreted as a toxic reaction or because blood glucose was not measured. Those who came closest were the Berlin physician, Georg Zuelzer (1840–1949) in 1907 [23], Ernest Scott (1877–1966) in Chicago in 1911 [24] and Nicolas Paulesco (1869–1931) in Romania in 1920–1921 [25] (Figure 1.10).

The story of how insulin was discovered in Toronto in 1921 is well known, at least superficially (Figure 1.11). A young orthopedic surgeon, Frederick Banting, inspired after reading an article by the pathologist Moses Barron (1884–1975), wondered whether the antidiabetic pancreatic principle was digested by trypsin during extraction, and decided to prevent this loss by ligating the pancreatic duct, thus causing the exocrine tissue to degenerate. He approached the Professor of Physiology in Toronto, J.J.R. Macleod, an authority on carbohydrate metabolism, who poured scorn on the idea and suggested that the only likely outcome would be "a negative result of great physiological importance."

Eventually, Macleod relented and installed Banting in a rundown laboratory, later leaving for Scotland and a fishing holiday. A student, Charles Best, was chosen by the toss of a coin to help Banting. Within 6 months of this unpromising start, Banting and Best (referred to in Toronto academic circles as B^2) had discovered the most important new therapy since the antisyphilitic agent Salvarsan. These events are described in detail in the excellent book by Michael Bliss [26].

Their approach began with the injection of extracts of atrophied pancreas (prepared according to Macleod's suggestions) into dogs rendered diabetic by pancreatectomy). Subsequently, they discovered that active extracts could be obtained from beef pancreas which Best obtained from the abbatoir. The extraction procedure (using ice-cold acid-ethanol) was greatly refined by James B. (Bert) Collip, a biochemist who was visiting Toronto on sabbatical leave.

The first clinical trial of insulin (using an extract made by Best) took place on January 11, 1922, on 14-year-old Leonard Thompson, who had been on the Allen starvation regimen since 1919 and weighed only 30 kg (Figure 1.12). After the first injection, his blood glucose level fell slightly, but his symptoms were unchanged and he developed a sterile abscess. On January 23, he was given another extract prepared by Collip, and this normalized his blood glucose by the next morning; further injections over the next 10 days led to marked clinical improvement and complete elimination of glycosuria and ketonuria. Initial clinical results in seven cases were published in the March 1922 issue of the *Canadian Medical Association Journal* [27], which concluded dramatically that:

1 Blood sugar can be markedly reduced, even to normal values;

2 Glycosuria can be abolished;

3 The acetone bodies can be made to disappear from the urine;

4 The respiratory quotient shows evidence of increased utilization of carbohydrates;

5 A definite improvement is observed in the general condition of these patients and, in addition, the patients themselves report a subjective sense of well-being and increased vigor for a period following the administration of these preparations.

The term "insulin" was coined by Macleod, who was unaware of de Meyer's earlier suggestion of *insuline*. News of its miraculous effects spread astonishingly rapidly [28]. In 1922, there were only 19 references in the world literature to "insulin" or equivalent terms such as "pancreatic extract"; by the end of 1923, there were 320 new reports, and a further 317 were published during the first 6 months of 1924.

By October 1923, insulin was available widely throughout North America and Europe. International recognition followed rapidly for its discoverers, and the 1923 Nobel Prize for Physiology or Medicine was awarded jointly to Banting and Macleod. Banting was angered by the decision, and announced publicly that he would share his prize with Best, whereupon Macleod decided to do the same with Collip.

The postinsulin era

It was confidently anticipated that insulin would do for diabetes in the young what thyroid extract had done for myxoedema, but it soon became obvious that insulin was a very different type of treatment. Thyroid was given once a day by mouth and at a fixed dosage. Insulin had to be injected in measured amounts which varied from day to day, and carried the ever-present danger of hypoglycemia. One often reads that insulin "revolutionized" the treatment of diabetes; it did so in the sense that it saved the lives of many who would otherwise have died, but its unforeseen effect was to transform an acute, rapidly fatal illness into a chronic disease with serious long-term complications. For example, only 2% of deaths among Joslin's young patients with diabetes before 1937 were caused by kidney disease, while over 50% dying between 1944 and 1950 had advanced renal failure. Strategies to avoid and prevent the chronic complications of diabetes remain important scientific and clinical priorities today.

(a)

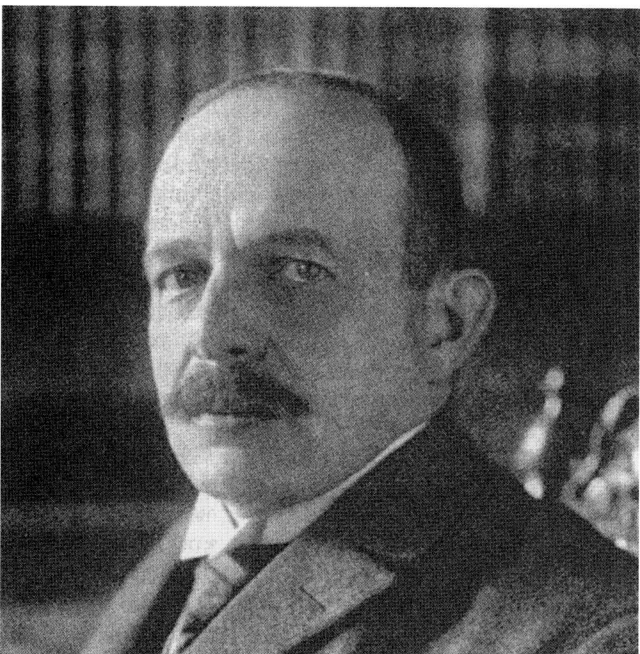

(b)

Experimentelle Untersuchungen über den Diabetes.[1])

Kurze Mitteilung.[2])

Von

G. Zuelzer.

F. Blum hat vor einigen Jahren gezeigt, dass subkutane oder intravenöse Injektion von Nebennierensaft bei den verschiedensten Tieren Glykosurie hervorruft, die 48 bis 74 Stunden anhalten kann. Ich, und kurze Zeit darauf Metzger wiesen nach, dass gleichzeitig eine Hyperglykämie besteht, dass es sich beim Nebennierendiabetes also nicht etwa um ein Analogon des Phloridzindiabetes, um einen sogenannten Nierendiabetes handeln könne. Während ich mich dahin aussprach, dass dieser Diabetes seiner ganzen Natur nach dem richtigen Diabetes ähnele, nur durch die Dauer seines Bestehens von ihm unterschieden sei und naturgemäss auch keine Tendenz zum Fortschreiten zeigen, i. e. niemals das Endstadium des gewöhnlichen schweren menschlichen Diabetes darbieten könne, wurde die in Frage stehende Glykosurie von den meisten anderen Autoren als eine ziemlich belanglose toxische Glykosurie aufgefasst.

Es schien mir nicht sehr wahrscheinlich, dass ein Körper, der anscheinend unverändert, wie er normalerweise produziert und dauernd[3]) dem Säftestrom des Organismus zugeführt wird, dass ein solcher, quasi physiologischer Körper eine vollkommen unphysiologische Wirkung sollte hervorbringen können. Ich habe also versucht, den Ort des Angriffs des Nebennierensaftes[4]), sowie die Ursachen seiner toxischen Wirkung näher zu erforschen. Ich folgte dabei, wie gesagt, stets dem Gedanken, in dem Nebennierendiabetes ein, wenn auch nur flüchtiges Bild gewisser menschlicher Diabetesformen zu finden.

So untersuchte ich zuerst, welchen Einfluss hat der Nebennierensaft auf die Leber als dasjenige Organ, welches, allgemein ansgedrückt, mit der Zuckerregulierung im Körper in erster

1) Die Untersuchungen wurden zum Teil mit Unterstützung der Gräfin Bose-Stiftung im physiologischen Institut der Berliner Universität, und zwar noch unter Mithilfe der verstorbenen Proff. I. Munk und Paul Schultz ausgeführt.

2) Diese kurze Mitteilung wurde der Redaktion bereits vor ca. 3 Jahren eingereicht. Die Drucklegung unterblieb auf Wunsch des Verf. in der bisher nicht erfüllten Erwartung, dass es gelingen würde, aus den theoretischen Untersuchungen praktisch-therapeutische Resultate zu erzielen.

3) Durch Versuche von Ehrmann, Archiv f. experim. Pathol. u. Pharmakol., Bd. 55, ist inzwischen der Nachweis erbracht worden, dass die Adrenalinsekretion konstant vor sich geht.

4) In meinen ersten Versuchen bediente ich mich des von mir selbst hergestellten Nebennierensaftes. In den zahlreichen späteren Versuchen habe ich inzwischen genau die gleichen Wirkungen mit den verschiedenartig hergestellten käuflichen Adrenalinpräparaten feststellen können.

(c)

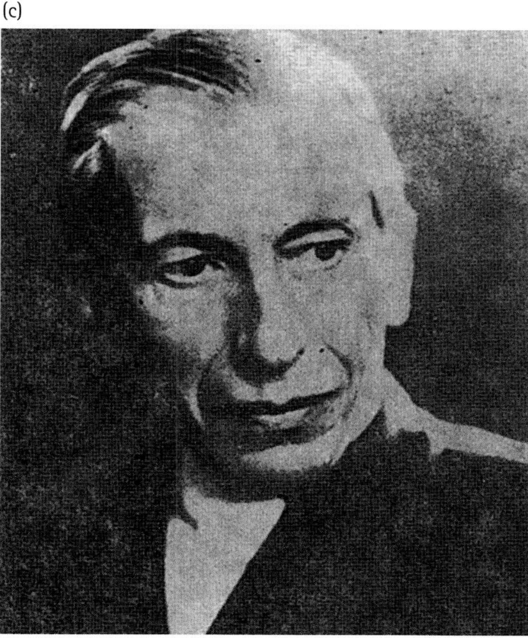

Figure 1.10 (a) Georg Zuelzer (1840–1949) and (b) the title page from his paper (1907) reporting that a pancreatic extract reduced glycosuria in pancreatectomized dogs [23] (top). (c) Nicolas Paulesco (1869–1931).

The rest of this chapter highlights some developments that can be regarded as landmarks in the understanding and management of the disease: to some extent, this is a personal choice, and it is obvious from the other chapters in this book that the "history" of diabetes is being rewritten all the time.

Causes and natural history of diabetes

The recognition that diabetes was not a single disease was important in initiating research that has helped to unravel the causes of hyperglycemia.

The broad etiologic subdivision into type 1 (juvenile-onset, or insulin-dependent) and type 2 diabetes (maturity-onset, or

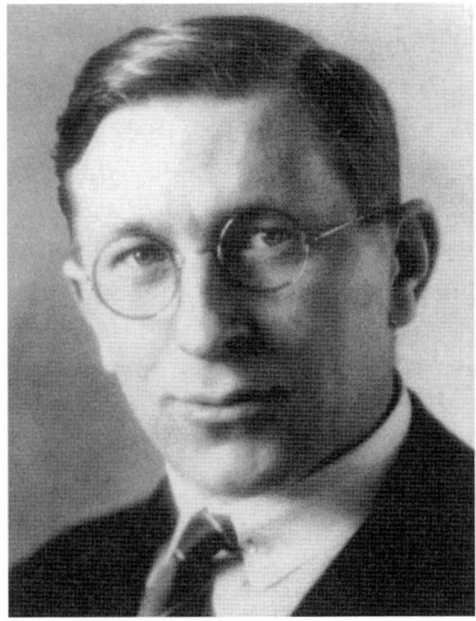

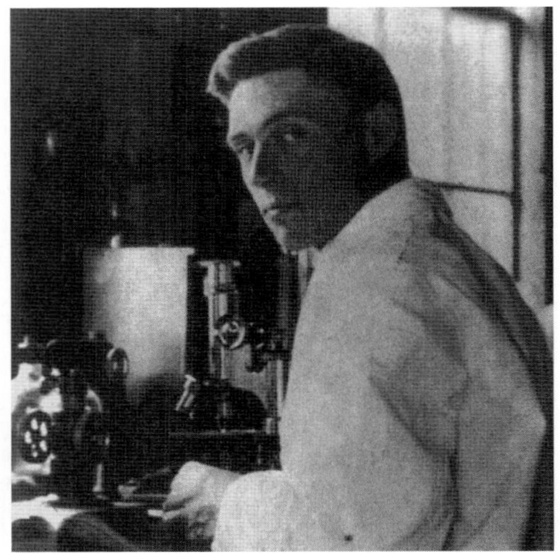

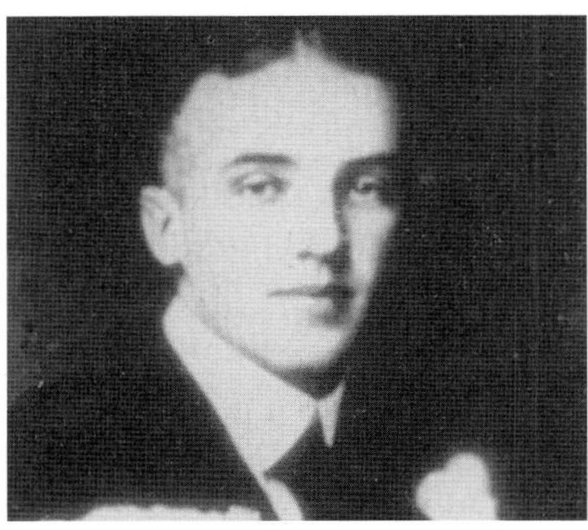

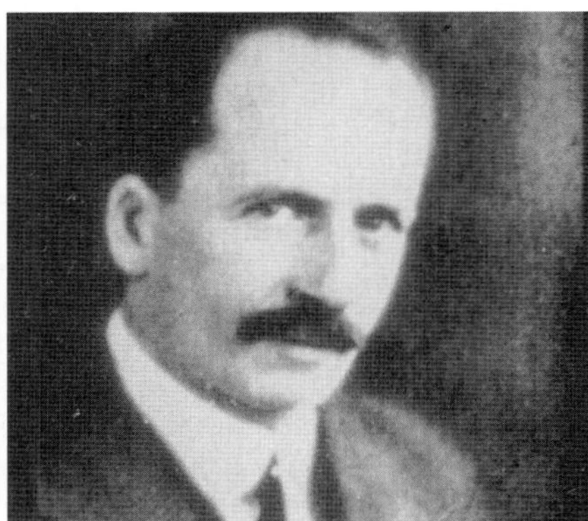

Figure 1.11 The discoverers of insulin. Clockwise from top left: Frederick G. Banting (1891–1941); James B. Collip (1892–1965); J.J.R. Macleod (1876–1935); and Charles H. Best (1899–1978). Courtesy of the Fisher Rare Book Library, University of Toronto.

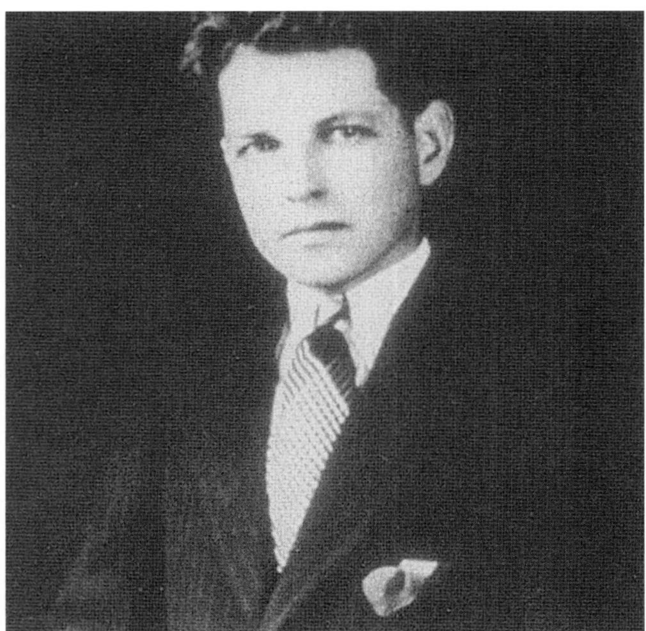

Figure 1.12 Leonard Thompson, the first patient to receive insulin, in January 1922. Courtesy of the Fisher Rare Book Library, University of Toronto.

non-insulin-dependent) stemmed ultimately from Lancereaux's *diabète maigre* and *diabète gras* distinction, as well as observations soon after the discovery of insulin that some patients did not react "normally" to insulin. In the 1930s, Wilhelm Falta (1875–1950) in Vienna [29] and Harold Himsworth (1905–93) in London [30] proposed that some individuals with diabetes were more sensitive to the glucose-lowering effects of insulin, whereas others were insulin-insensitive, or insulin-resistant. The former were usually thin and required insulin to prevent ketoacidosis, while the latter were older, obese and ketosis-resistant.

The "insulin clamp" technique developed in the 1970s by Ralph DeFronzo *et al.* [31] in the USA was the first to measure rigorously the hypoglycemic action of insulin, and has led to countless studies of insulin resistance and its relationship to type 2 diabetes and vascular disease. Various groups, including DeFronzo's, have helped to clarify the role of β-cell failure in type 2 diabetes, and how it relates to insulin resistance. Maturity-onset diabetes of the young (MODY) was recognized in 1974 by Robert Tattersall (*b.* 1943) as a distinct, dominantly inherited subset of type 2 diabetes [32]; since 1993, five different molecular defects have been identified in this condition.

The causes of the profound β-cell loss that led to the severe insulin deficiency of type 1 diabetes remained a mystery for a long time. "Insulitis", predominantly lymphocytic infiltration of the islets, was noted as early as 1901 by Eugene L. Opie (1873–1971) and colleagues [33], but because it was apparently very rare, found in only six of 189 cases studied by Anton Weichselbaum (1845–1920) in 1910, its importance was not appreciated. The possible role of insulitis in β-cell destruction was not suggested until 1965, by the Belgian Willy Gepts (1922–1991) [34]. The theory that type 1 diabetes results from autoimmune destruction of the β cells was first made in 1979 by Deborah Doniach (1912–2004) and GianFranco Bottazzo (*b.* 1946) [35]. Unlike other autoimmune endocrine diseases where the autoantibody persists, islet cell antibodies (ICA) turned out to be transient and disappeared within a year of the onset of diabetes. An unexpected finding from the Barts–Windsor prospective study of the epidemiology of diabetes in childhood started by Andrew Cudworth (1939–1982) was that ICA could be detected in siblings of young people with diabetes up to 10 years before they developed apparently acute-onset diabetes. This long lead-in period raised the possibilty of an intervention to prevent continuing β-cell destruction. Cyclosporine in people with newly diagnosed type 1 diabetes prolongs the honeymoon period but without permanent benefit once the drug is stopped [36]. Nicotinamide and small doses of insulin (together with many other interventions) prevent diabetes in the non-obese diabetic (NOD) mouse but were without effect in relatives of people with type 1 diabetes with high titers of ICA [37,38].

From 1967, when Paul Lacy (1924–2005) showed that it was possible to "cure" diabetes in inbred rats with an islet cell transplant, it always seemed that the problem of islet cell transplantation in humans was about to be solved. Hope was rekindled in 2000 by a team in Edmonton, Canada. After 5 years 80% of their transplanted patients were producing some endogenous insulin but only 10% could manage without any injected insulin [39].

Table 1.2 Milestones in the scientific understanding of diabetes and its complications.

Matthew Dobson (England, 1776)	Diabetic serum contains sugar
Michel Chevreul (France, 1815)	The sugar in diabetic urine is glucose
Claude Bernard (France, 1850s)	Glucose stored in liver glycogen and secreted during fasting
Wilhelm Petters (Germany, 1857)	Diabetic urine contains acetone
Paul Langerhans (Germany, 1869)	Pancreatic islets described
Adolf Kussmaul (Germany, 1874)	Describes ketoacidosis
Oskar Minkowski and Josef von Mering (Germany, 1889)	Pancreatectomy causes diabetes in the dog
Gustave Edouard Laguesse (France, 1893)	Glucose-lowering pancreatic secretion produced by islets
M.A. Lane (USA, 1907)	Distinguished A and B islet cells
Jean de Meyer (Belgium, 1909)	Hypothetical islet secretion named "*insuline*"
Frederick Banting, Charles Best, J.J.R. Macleod, James Collip (Canada, 1922)	Isolation of insulin
Richard Murlin (USA, 1923)	Discovered and named glucagon
Bernado Houssay (Argentina, 1924)	Hypophysectomy enhances insulin sensitivity
Frederick Sanger (England, 1955)	Determined primary sequence of insulin
W.W. Bromer (USA, 1956)	Determined primary sequence of glucagon
Rosalyn Yalow and Solomon Berson (USA, 1959)	Discovered radioimmunoassay for insulin
Donald Steiner (USA, 1967)	Discovered proinsulin
Dorothy Hodgkin (England, 1969)	Determined three-dimensional structure of insulin
Pierre Freychet (USA, 1971)	Characterized insulin receptors
Pedro Cuatrecasas (USA, 1972)	Isolated insulin receptor protein
Axel Ullrich (USA, 1977)	Reported sequence of rat insulin
Ralph DeFronzo and Reuben Andres (USA, 1979)	Invented insulin clamp technique
Graham Bell (USA, 1980)	Reported sequence of human insulin gene

Chronic diabetic complications

It had been assumed that arteriosclerosis caused chronic diabetic complications, but this notion was challenged by two papers published in the mid-1930s, which pointed to specific associations of diabetes with retinal and renal disease (Table 1.2). In 1934, Henry Wagener (1890–1961) and Russell Wilder (1885–1959) from the Mayo Clinic reported patients who had retinal hemorrhages but no other clinical evidence of vascular disease [40], and concluded that "The very existence of retinitis in cases in which patients have no other signs of vascular disease must mean that diabetes alone does something to injure the finer arterioles or venules of the retina, probably the latter."

In 1936, Paul Kimmelstiel (1900–1970) and Clifford Wilson (1906–1997) described the striking histologic finding of "intercapillary glomerulosclerosis" – large hyaline nodules in the glomeruli – in the kidneys of eight subjects at autopsy (Figure 1.13) [41]. Seven of the eight patients had a known history of diabetes, and Kimmelstiel and Wilson noted the common features of hypertension, heavy albuminuria with "oedema of the nephrotic type," and renal failure. In fact, this paper led to considerable confusion during the next 15 years: according to one writer, the "Kimmelstiel–Wilson syndrome" came to mean all things to all men [42]. Nonetheless, it was significant because it drew attention to a specific diabetic renal disease.

Acceptance of the concept that diabetic angiopathy was specific to the disease owed much to the work of Knud Lundbæk of Aarhus in Denmark (Figure 1.14), who published his findings in a book in 1953–1954 and a paper in the *Lancet* in 1954 [43,44]. His key arguments were that long-standing diabetic vascular disease differed fundamentally from atherosclerosis, in that both sexes were equally affected and that microaneurysms, ocular phlebopathy and Kimmelstiel–Wilson nodules were unique to diabetes and usually occurred together.

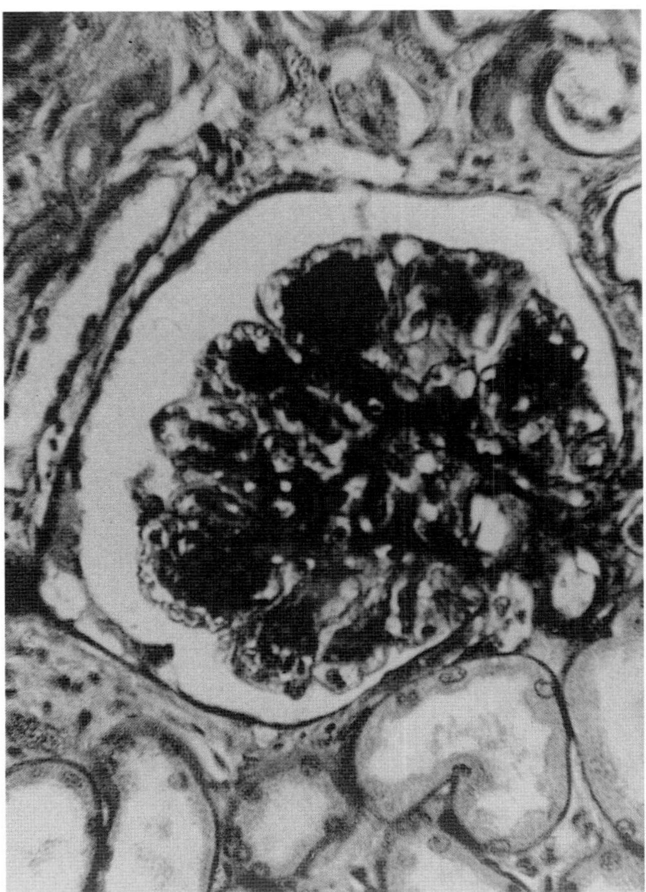

Figure 1.13 Nodular glomerulosclerosis. Figure from the paper by Kimmelstiel and Wilson, 1936 [41]. Courtesy of the British Medical Association Library.

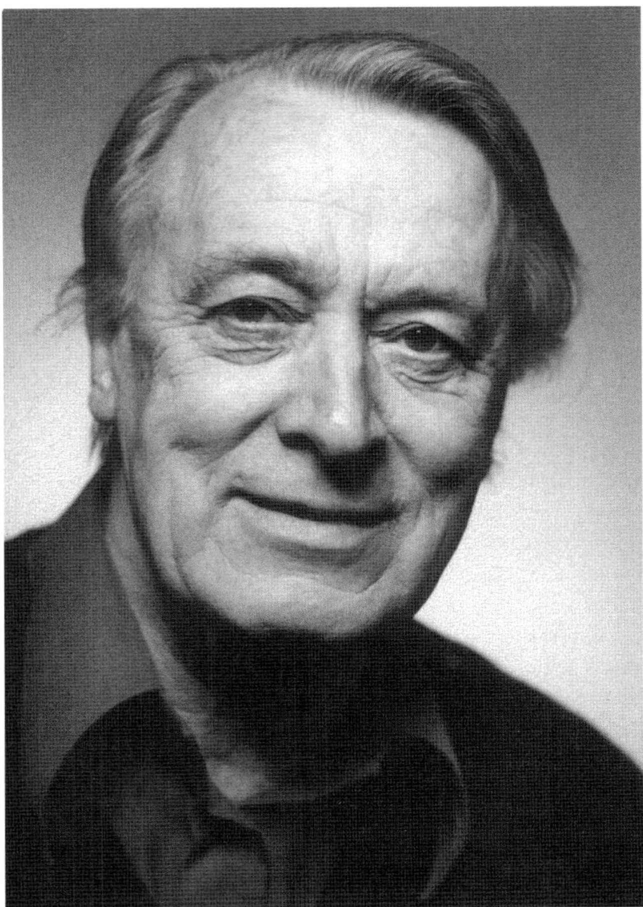

Figure 1.14 Knud Lundbæk (1912–1995). Courtesy of Dr Carl Erik Mogensen.

The molecular and cellular mechanisms underlying diabetic tissue damage remain controversial after decades of intensive research. One of the early landmarks in this field was the work of J.H. Kinoshita (*b.* 1922) during the early 1970s, which pointed to the involvement of the polyol pathway in the formation of diabetic cataracts [45].

Physiology

In 1907, M.A. Lane, a student of Robert Bensley (1867–1956), Professor of Antatomy in Chicago, used conventional histologic techniques to distinguish two different cell types in the islet of Langerhans, which he termed A and B [46]. The hormones secreted by these respective cell types were not identified until much later (Table 1.2). Frank Young (1908–1988) and colleagues reported in 1938 that injections of anterior pituitary extract could induce permanent diabetes in the dog, and that this was accompanied by selective degranulation and loss of the β-cells [47]; it was surmised that these cells produced insulin, and this was finally confirmed using immuno-histochemistry by Paul Lacy in 1959 [48]. Glucagon was similarly localized to the α-cells in 1962 by John Baum and colleagues [49].

Table 1.3 Milestones in the understanding of the causes of diabetes.

Thomas Willis (England, 17th century)	Overindulgence in food and drink
Thomas Cawley (England, 1788)	Pancreatic stones cause diabetes
Oskar Minkowski and Josef von Mering (Germany, 1889)	Pancreatectomy causes diabetes in the dog
Etienne Lancereaux (France, 1880)	Lean and obese diabetic subtypes distinguished
Eugene Opie (USA, 1900)	Hyaline degeneration (amyloidosis) of islets (type 2 diabetes)
Eugene Opie (USA, 1910)	Lymphocytic infiltration of islets ("insulitis"; type 1 diabetes)
Wilhelm Falta (Vienna) and Harold Himsworth (England; early 1930s)	Distinguished insulin-resistant and insulin-sensitive forms of diabetes
Willy Gepts (Belgium, 1965)	Suggested that insulitis caused β-cell destruction (type 1 diabetes)
Deborah Doniach and GianFranco Bottazzo (England, 1979)	Suggested that insulin-dependent diabetes is an autoimmune disease
Andrew Cudworth and John Woodrow (England, 1975)	Insulin-dependent diabetes associated with specific HLA antigens

(a)

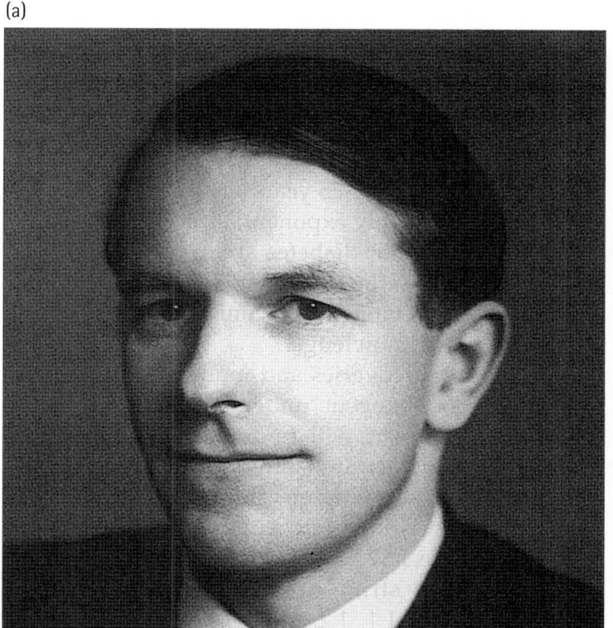

(b)

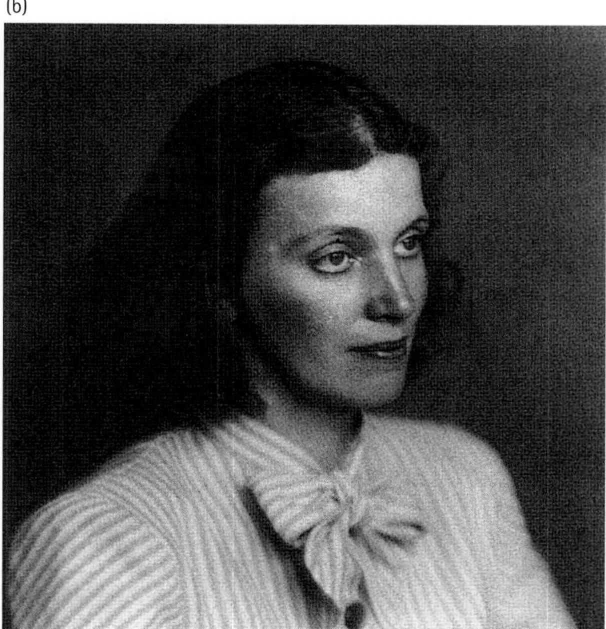

Figure 1.15 Frederick Sanger (*b.* 1918) and Dorothy Hodgkin, *née* Crowfoot (1910–1994). Courtesy of Godfrey Argent Studio, London.

The amino acid sequence of insulin was reported in 1955 by Frederick Sanger in Cambridge, UK [50], and the three-dimensional structure of the molecule in 1969 by Dorothy Hodgkin, in Oxford [51]; both discoveries were recognized by the award of Nobel Prizes (Figure 1.15). The complete insulin molecule was synthesized from amino acids by Wang Ying-lai (1908–2001) and colleagues in Shanghai in 1965 [52]. The insulin precursor, proinsulin, was described in 1967 by Donald Steiner (*b.* 1930) in Chicago [53]. The first bioassay for insulin, based on the hormone's ability to lower blood glucose in the alloxan-diabetic rat, was reported in 1950 by the Australian Joseph Bornstein (1918–1994), working in London with Robin D. Lawrence (see Fig. 1.20) [54]. This method was superseded in 1956 by Rosalyn Yalow and Solomon Berson in the USA, who discovered that insulin was antigenic; they exploited the binding of the hormone to anti-insulin antibodies to develop the first radio-immunoassay [55]. This assay method revolutionized endocrinology – and indeed, many areas of physiology and medicine – and was also rewarded with a Nobel Prize (Figure 1.16).

The sequence of rat insulin genes was described in 1977 by Axel Ullrich (*b.* 1945) and colleagues [56], and the human sequence by Graham Bell (*b.* 1948) and his group in 1980 [57]. The existence of insulin receptors was inferred from the insulin-binding characteristics of liver-cell membranes by Pierre Freychet (*b.* 1935) and colleagues in 1971 [58], and the receptor protein was isolated by Pedro Cuatrecasas (*b.* 1936) in the following year [59]. The gene encoding the insulin receptor was cloned and sequenced in 1985 by two groups [60,61]. In recent years, numerous advances have helped to clarify how insulin exerts its biologic actions. Among these was the discovery in 1985 of the first of the glucose transporter (GLUT) proteins by Mueckler and colleagues in the USA [62].

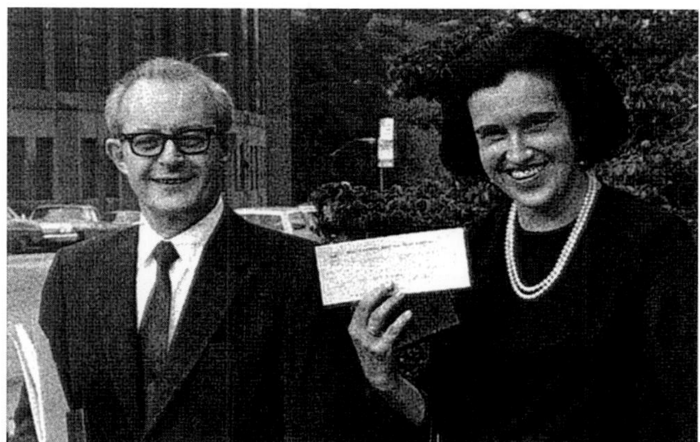

Figure 1.16 Solomon Berson and Rosalyn Yalow.

Management of diabetes

An objective observer surveying clinical diabetes during the half-century after the discovery of insulin and the "resurrection" (a word used by Joslin) of young people with diabetes would have been dismayed by what he saw (Table 1.4). In particular, young people were dying of complications that had previously been assumed to be the preserve of the elderly. Two particularly depressing papers were published in 1947 and 1950. First, Henry Dolger (1909–1997) in New York described 20 patients who fulfilled the then-accepted criteria for excellent diabetic control, but

Table 1.4 Selected milestones in the management of diabetes.

Lifestyle modification	
Li Hsuan (China, 7th century)	Avoid wine, sex and salty cereals
Thomas Willis (England, 17th century)	Food restriction
John Rollo (England, 1797)	Animal diet
Apollinaire Bouchardat (France, 1875)	Food restriction and increased exercise
Carl von Noorden (Germany, 1903)	"Oatmeal" cure
Frederick Allen (USA, 1913)	Starvation diet for early-onset diabetes
Karl Petrén (Sweden, 1915)	High-fat, low-carbohydrate diet
Insulin treatment	
Georg Zuelzer (Germany, 1907) and Nicolas Paulesco (Romania, 1921)	Isolated pancreatic extracts with hypoglycemic activity
Frederick Banting, Charles Best, J.J.R. Macleod, and James Collip (Canada, 1922–1923)	Isolation and first clinical use of insulin
Hans Christian Hagedorn (Denmark, 1936)	Protamine insulin, the first long-acting insulin
David Goeddel (USA, 1979)	Synthetic human-sequence insulin produced by recombinant DNA technology
John Pickup (London, 1978)	Described continuous subcutaneous insulin infusion
John Ireland (Scotland, 1981)	Invented pen injection device
Oral hypoglycemic agents	
Avicenna (Arabia, 10th century)	Recommended lupin, fenugreek and zedoary seeds
Willhelm Ebstein (Germany, 1876)	Recommended sodium salicylate
E. Frank (Germany, 1926)	Biguanide derivative (Synthalin) introduced, but withdrawn because of toxicity
Celestino Ruiz (Argentina, 1930)	Noted hypoglycemic action of some sulfonamides
Auguste Loubatières (France, 1942)	Discovered hypoglycemic action of prototype sulfonylurea
H. Franke and J. Fuchs (Germany, 1955)	Carbutamide introduced
G. Ungar (USA, 1957)	Phenformin introduced
Diabetic monitoring and treatment targets	
University Group Diabetes Program (USA, 1969)	First randomized trial in diabetes
Peter Sönksen and Robert Tattersall (1978)	Introduction of home blood glucose monitoring
R. Flückiger and K.H. Winterhalter (Germany, 1975)	Showed that HbA_{1c} was glycated hemoglobin
World Health Organization (1991)	St Vincent Declaration identified targets for diabetes care
Diabetes Control and Complications Trial (USA, 1993)	Proved that improved glycemic control prevents and slows progression of microvascular complication in type 1 diabetes
UK Prospective Diabetes Study (UK, 1998)	Proved that improved glycemic and blood-pressure control improve microvascular and macrovascular outcomes in type 2 diabetes
Management of complications	
Gerd Meyer-Schwickerath (Germany, 1964)	Use of xenon arc lamp to treat diabetic retinopathy
University of Minnesota Team (USA, 1966)	First combined kidney–pancreas transplants
Carl-Erik Mogensen and Hans-Henrik Parving (Denmark, 1980s)	Strict blood pressure controls slows progression of diabetic neuropathy

who all developed severe retinopathy after 6–22 years [63]; among these was the first patient ever to receive insulin at Mount Sinai Hospital, New York, who also had heavy albuminuria and hypertension by the age of 32. Second, Ruth Reuting reported a cohort of 50 young patients originally identified in 1929 [64]. By 1949, one-third had died (mostly from cardiovascular and renal disease) at an average age of 25 years, after only 18 years of diabetes, and the survivors showed "ominous signs of hypertension, azotemia and proteinuria in significant numbers." This had occurred despite the introduction of more versatile insulin preparations (see below); the situation was so hopeless that it inaugurated 20 years of treatment with "heroic" measures such as adrenalectomy and hypophysectomy.

These and other studies raised questions about whether lowering blood glucose levels to normal could prevent diabetic complications or reverse them once they had appeared. The hypothesis remained untestable for four more decades, until the means to achieve tight glycemic control and measure it had been devised.

Insulin

For the first decade after its discovery, insulin was available only in its soluble (regular) formulation, whose short-action profile required multiple daily injections. The first delayed-action preparation, protamine insulinate, was introduced in 1936 by Hans Christian Hagedorn in Denmark (Figure 1.17) [65]. This was followed by protamine zinc insulin later the same year, then

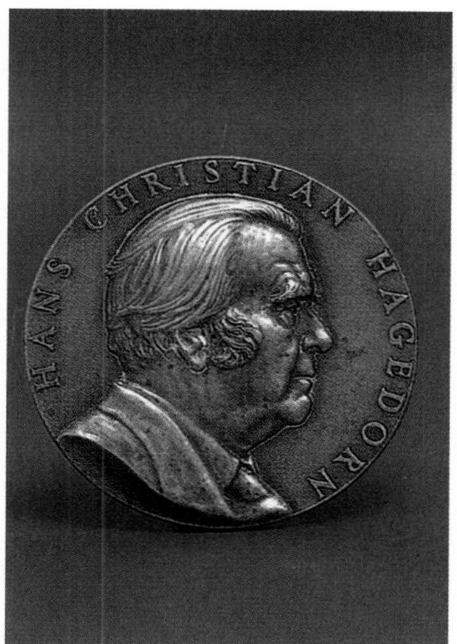

Figure 1.17 Hans Christian Hagedorn (1888–1971) from the Hagedorn Medal. Courtesy of C. Binder, Steno Institute, Hvidovre, Denmark.

globin insulin in 1939, NPH (neutral protamine Hagedorn, or isophane) in 1946, and the lente series in 1952. Long-acting insulins were welcomed by diabetes specialists and patients, but their use as a single daily injection probably produced worse glycemic control than three or four injections of soluble insulin. Indeed, delayed-action preparations were initially condemned by some diabetes specialists, such as Russell Wilder of the Mayo Clinic, because the patient could slip without apparent warning into hypoglycemia.

The number and variety of insulin preparations proliferated, but the main advances were in methods to produce highly purified preparations from porcine or bovine pancreas, which remained the source for therapeutic insulin until the early 1980s. Insulin was the first therapeutic protein to be produced by recombinant DNA technology, initially by David Goeddel (*b.* 1951), who expressed synthetic genes encoding the A- and B-chains separately in *Escherichia coli* and then combined these chemically to produce human-sequence insulin [66]. From there, genetic engineering has been used to produce "designer" insulins such as the fast-acting insulin analogs lispro and aspart and the "peakless" basal insulins such as glargine and detemir. How much these will improve glycemic control in the generality of people with diabetes is debatable; weekend golfers do not become champions when given expensive clubs!

Most people with diabetes still inject insulin subcutaneously. From the patient's viewpoint, major milestones were the replacement of glass and steel syringes by disposable plastic syringes with fine-gauge needles, and then by "pen" injection devices invented by John Ireland (1933–1988) in Glasgow, Scotland, in 1981 [67]. Portable insulin infusion pumps were developed by John Pickup (*b.* 1947) and colleagues in London during the late 1970s [68], and have become progressively smaller and more sophisticated. Patients and manufacturers hope that there will eventually be an insulin that can be given without injection. The first inhaled insulin was marketed in 2006 but withdrawn a year later because of lack of demand and concerns about safety [69].

Oral hypoglycemic agents

The first orally active glucose-lowering drug, synthalin, a guanidine derivative, was developed by Frank and colleagues in Breslau in 1926 [70], but had to be withdrawn because of toxicity (a recurrent problem for oral hypoglycemic drugs). The sulfonylureas originated from the work of Auguste Loubatières (1912–1977) in France during the early 1940s on the glucose-lowering action of a sulfonamide derivative, 2254RP. Loubatières made the crucial observations that proved that these drugs act as insulin secretagogues and that they were effective in intact, but not in pancreatectomized, animals [71]. In 1955 carbutamide was the first sulfonylurea to enter clinical practice and tolbutamide followed in 1957. Phenformin, the first biguanide, was introduced in 1959 following research into the metabolic effects of guanidine derivatives which had built on Frank's initial studies [72]. Metformin appeared on the European market in 1960 but was not marketed in the USA until 1994. Troglitazone, the first of a new class of antidiabetic drugs, the glitazones, was also marketed in 1994 but withdrawn because of liver damage. It was followed by rosiglitazone and pioglitazone. Another new class of drugs, acting on the incretin system, were introduced in 2005. These are either glucagon-like peptide 1 (GLP-1) agonists (such as exenatide) or inhibitors of the enzyme dipeptidylpeptidase-4 (DPP-4) which breaks down GLP-1 (gliptins).

Tolbutamide, phenformin and insulin were compared in the treatment of maturity-onset diabetes in the first randomized controlled trial, the University Group Diabetes Program [73–75]. This much-criticized study concluded that the death rate was higher for both oral agents than for placebo, and that insulin (whether given in a fixed or variable dose) was no better than placebo [75]. These findings were interpreted by some as suggesting that treatment of maturity-onset diabetes was a waste of time – a myth that was only laid finally to rest by the UK Prospective Diabetes Study.

Glucose control and treatment targets

During the 1920s, opinion leaders advocated normalizing blood glucose in young patients with diabetes, the rationale being to "rest" the pancreas, in the hope that it might regenerate. The only way of monitoring diabetic control was by testing the urine for glucose, and attempts to keep the urine free from sugar inevitably resulted in severe hypoglycemia and often psychologic damage. This led to the so-called "free diet" movement – linked particularly with Adolf Lichtenstein (Stockholm) and Edward Tolstoi (New York) – which encouraged patients to eat whatever they liked and not to worry about glycosuria, however heavy. Tolstoi's view [76] was that a life saved by insulin should be worth living, and that patients should be able to forget that they had diabetes after each morning's injection; it seems likely that many physicians followed this policy for the next 40 years.

Adult physicians were similarly ambivalent about the importance of good glycemic control. Only one-third of diabetes physicians questioned in England in 1953 thought that normoglycemia would prevent diabetic complications, and only one-half advised urine testing at home [77].

Practical monitoring of diabetic control became feasible in the late 1970s with the introduction into clinical practice of test strips for measuring blood glucose in a fingerprick sample and the demonstration that ordinary patients could use them at home [78,79]. The discovery of hemoglobin A_{1c} by Samuel Rahbar (*b.* 1929) paved the way for glycated hemoglobin (HbA_{1c}) assays which gave an objective measure of overall glucose control [80]. These methods in turn made possible the North American Diabetes Control and Complications Trial, which in 1993 finally established that good control prevents and delays the progression of microvascular complications in type 1 diabetes [81]. For type 2 diabetes, the importance of good glycemic control was definitively proved by another landmark study, the UK Prospective Diabetes Study (UKPDS), masterminded in Oxford, UK, by Robert Turner (Figure 1.18). The UKPDS reported in 1998, and not only showed a beneficial effect of improved glycemic control on microvascular complications [82], but also established the importance of treating hypertension [83]. By the late 1990s it was clear that reducing glucose levels, high blood pressure or cholesterol separately would reduce the frequency of heart disease and death and it was natural to wonder whether tackling them simultaneously (multiple risk factor intervention) would be even better. The Steno 2 study, which began in Denmark in 1992, enrolled patients with type 2 diabetes with microalbuminuria and after 13 years of follow-up showed that multiple risk factor intervention reduced the risk of death by 20% and the risk of developing nephropathy, retinopathy and neuropathy by 50% [84].

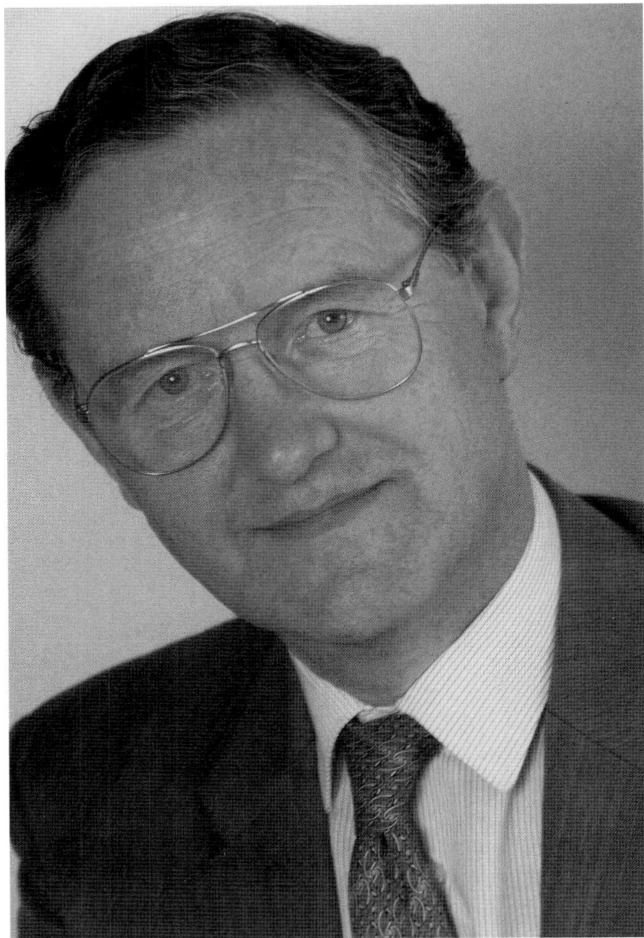

Figure 1.18 Robert Turner (1939–1999), instigator of the UKPDS, the first study to show that good control of blood glucose and blood pressure was beneficial in type 2 diabetes. Courtesy of the British Diabetic Association.

Diabetic complications

Apart from the general benefits of controlling blood glucose, some specific treatments have emerged for certain chronic complications. Well-conducted clinical trials during the late 1970s showed the effectiveness of laser photocoagulation in preventing visual loss from both maculopathy and proliferative retinopathy [85]. This technique was derived from the xenon arc lamp originally described in the late 1950s by Gerd Meyer-Schwickerath (1921–92) of Essen, Germany [86].

The importance of blood pressure control in preventing the progression of nephropathy is now fully recognized, and angiotensin-converting enzyme inhibitors may be particularly beneficial; that blood pressure control slowed the progression of nephropathy was shown in studies by Carl-Erik Mogensen (*b.* 1938) and Hans-Henrik Parving (*b.* 1943) published in the early 1980s [87]. The measurement of low albumin concentrations in urine (microalbuminuria), now used throughout the world to screen for and monitor the course of diabetic nephropathy, is derived from a radioimmunoassay developed in 1969 by Harry Keen and Costas Chlouverakis, at Guy's Hospital in London [88].

Diabetic ketoacidosis

The introduction of insulin was only one aspect of the management of this acute and previously fatal complication of diabetes. Of the first 33 cases treated by Joslin and his colleagues between January 1, 1923 and April 1, 1925, 31 survived – an excellent outcome, even by modern standards, which Joslin [89] attributed to: "Promptly applied medical care, rest in bed, special nursing attendance, warmth, evacuation of the bowels by enema, the introduction of liquids into the body, lavage of the stomach, cardiac stimulants, and above all the exclusion of alkalis."

Sadly, other centers did not pay so much attention to detail. In 1933, the death rate from ketoacidosis in Boston was only 5%, but elsewhere in North America and Europe it averaged 30% and could be as high as 75%. An important advance in management was the acceptance of relatively low-dose insulin replacement, following the example of Ruth Menzel and colleagues in Karlsburg, Germany [90]. This broke with the tradition of high-dose regimens such as that proposed by Howard Root in the USA, which had recommended an average of 1200 U insulin during the first 24 hours of treatment [91]. Another step forward was the recognition by Jacob Holler in 1946 of the danger of hypokalemia [92]. Holler's observation helped to establish the need for monitoring plasma potassium levels, which became feasible with the introduction of the flame photometer, and replacing potassium accordingly.

Diabetic pregnancy

As late as 1950, the outcome of pregnancy in women with diabetes was still very poor in most units, with perinatal fetal losses of 45–65%, some 10 times higher than in the general population. Exceptions to this depressing rule were the units run by Priscilla White at the Joslin Clinic in Boston, who had published excellent results as early as 1935 [93], and by Jørgen Pedersen in Copenhagen (Figure 1.19). Pedersen identified the common features underpinning success as good diabetic control and care provided by an experienced and dedicated team consisting of a physician, obstetrician and pediatrician [94]. Pedersen's target of a fetal mortality rate of 6% was not achieved in most European or US units until the 1980s.

Delivery of care for people with diabetes

From the earliest days of insulin injection and urine testing, it was apparent that people with diabetes needed knowledge and practical skills to manage their disease effectively. Lip-service was often paid to the importance of diabetes education, but most patients were badly informed. In 1952, Samuel Beaser (1910–2005) questioned 128 patients attending the Boston Diabetes Fair, and found that "all were distinctly deficient in knowledge of their disease" [95]; he felt that responsibility lay with both doctors and administrators. Further studies during the 1960s by Donnell Etzwiler (1927–2003) in Minneapolis showed that many doctors and nurses were also ignorant about managing diabetes. Since the

(a)

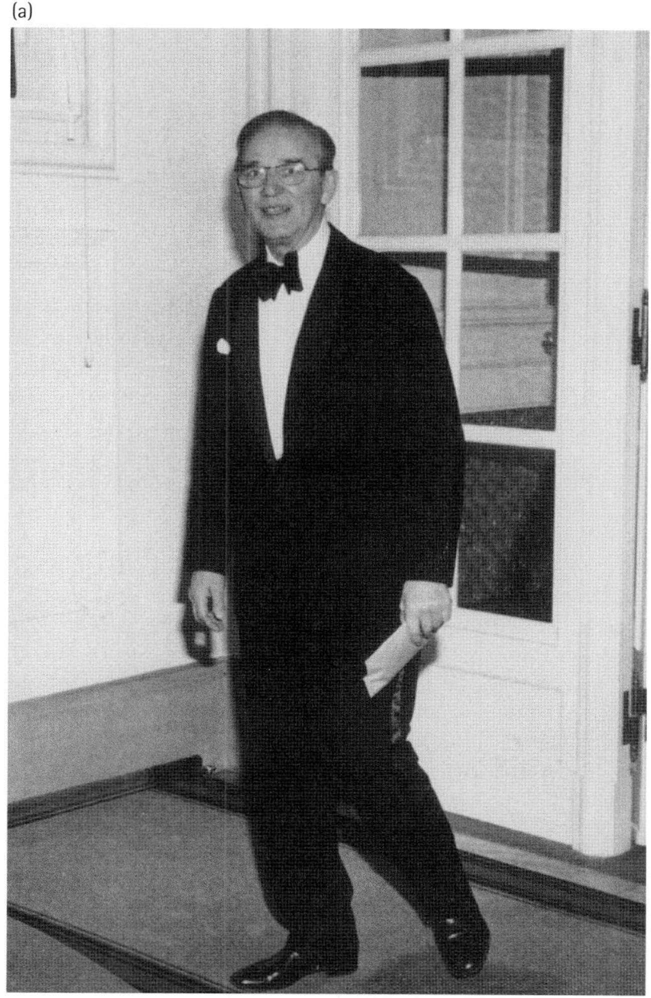

(b)

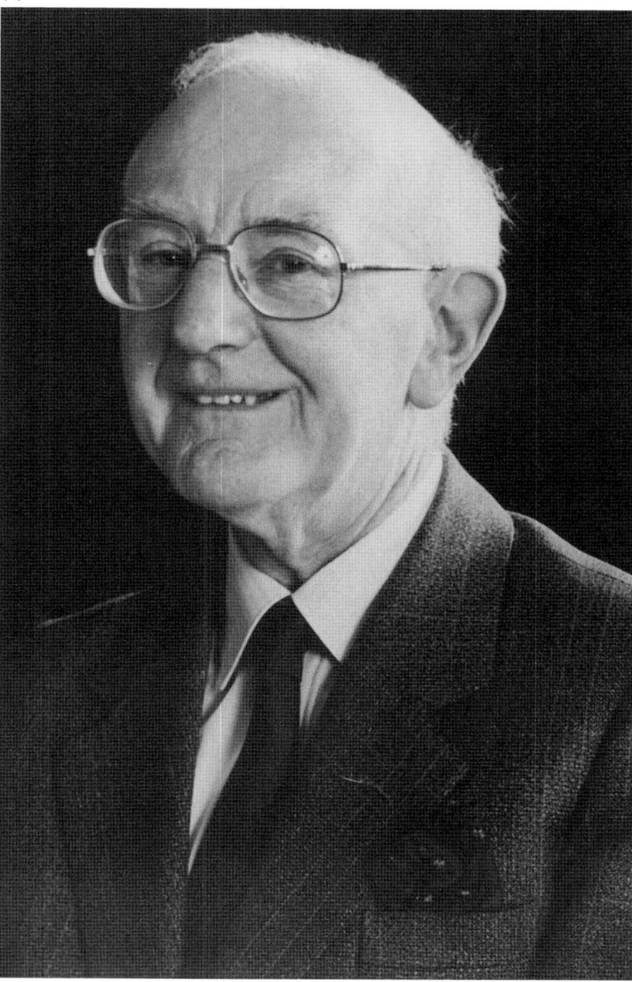

Figure 1.19 Jørgen Pedersen (1914–1978) and Ivo Drury (1905–1988), pioneers, with Priscilla White (1900–1989), in the management of pregnancy in women with type 1 diabetes. Courtesy of Dr. Carl Erik Mogensen and the Royal College of Physicians of Ireland.

(a)

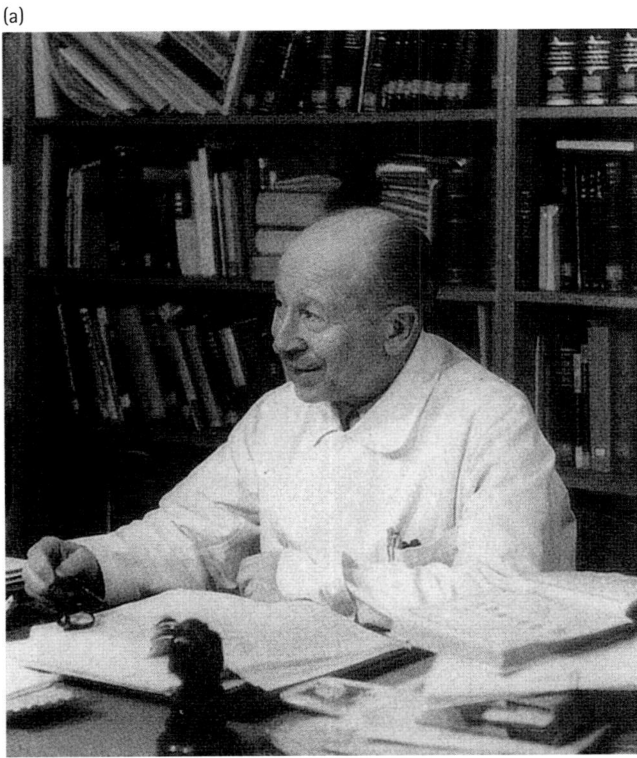

(b)

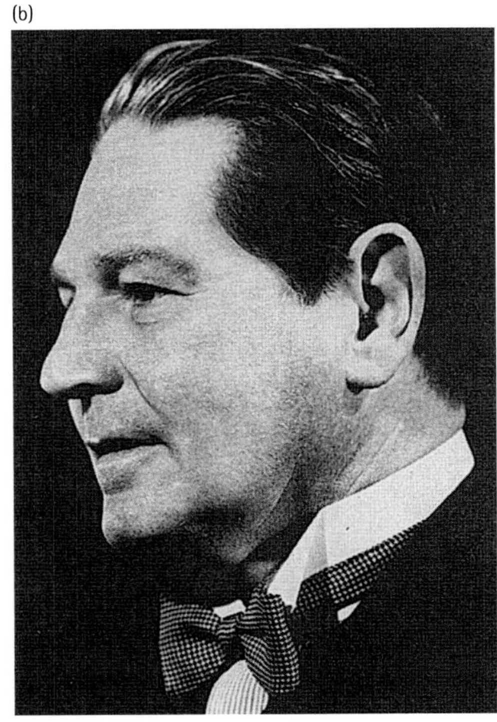

Figure 1.20 Ernesto Roma (1887–1978) and (right) Robin D. Lawrence (1892–1968). Photograph of Dr. Roma by courtesy of Manuel Machado Sá Marques and the Associação Protectura das Diabéticos de Portugal.

1980s, diabetes specialist nurses and nurse educators have been appointed in increasingly large numbers – thus fulfilling a suggestion originally made by Joslin in 1916.

National and international diabetes associations have also played an important part by supporting scientific and clinical research, providing practical and moral help for patients, and lobbying governments on patients' behalf. The first of these organizations was the Portuguese Association for the Protection of Poor Diabetics, founded in 1926 by Ernesto Roma of Lisbon after an inspiring visit to Joslin's clinic in Boston (Figure 1.20). The Association's aim was to provide free insulin and education for people with diabetes and their families. In the UK, the Diabetic Association (later the British Diabetic Association, and now Diabetes UK) was established in 1934 by Robin Lawrence of King's College Hospital, London, helped by the novelist H.G. Wells (Figure 1.20). Similar organizations were later founded in France (1938), the USA (1940) and Belgium (1942), and now exist in most countries.

On a wider scale, the International Diabetes Foundation was established in 1950 and the European Association for the Study of Diabetes (EASD) in 1964. These organizations are devoted to the practice of diabetes care as well as the basic and clinical science of the disease, and have been valuable in coordinating treatment targets and strategies at international level; an important example was the St. Vincent Declaration, issued jointly in 1990 by the EASD and the World Health Organization [96].

References

1 Willis T. *Pharmaceutice Rationalis; sive, Diatriba de Medicamentorum Operationibus in Humano Corpore* [2 parts in 1 vol]. Oxford: Sheldonian Theatre, 1674.

2 Dobson M. Experiments and observations on the urine in diabetes. *Med Obs Inq* 1776; **5**:298–316.

3 Rollo J. *An Account of Two Cases of the Diabetes Mellitus, With Remarks as They Arose During the Progress of the Cure.* London: C. Dilly, 1797. [A 2nd edition with more cases was published in 1798 and a 3rd edition in 1806.]

4 Chevreul ME. Note sur le sucre du diabète. *Ann Chim (Paris)* 1815; **95**:319–320.

5 Olmsted JMD. Claude Bernard, 1813–79. *Diabetes* 1953; **2**:162–164.

6 Bernard C. Chiens rendus diabétiques. *C R Seances Soc Biol (Paris)* 1850; **1**:60.

7 Macleod JJR. Recent work on the pathologic physiology of glycosuria. *JAMA* 1914; **113**:1226–1235.

8 Von Mering J, Minkowski O. Diabetes mellitus nach Pankreasextirpation. *Arch Exp Pathol Pharmacol Leipzig* 1890; **26**:371–387.

9 Tattersall RB. Charles-Édouard Brown-Séquard: double hyphenated neurologist and forgotten father of endocrinology. *Diabet Med* 1994; **11**:728–731.

10 Laguesse GE. Sur la formation des îlots de Langerhans dans le pancréas. *C R Séances Mem Soc Biol* 1893; **45**:819–820.

11 Langerhans P. *Beiträge zur mikroskopischen Anatomie der Bauchspeicheldrüse* [dissertation]. Berlin: Gustave Lange, 1869.

12 De Meyer J. Sur la signification physiologique de la sécrétion interne du pancréas. *Zentralbl Physiol* 1904; **18**:S826.

13 Saundby R. The Bradshaw Lecture on the morbid anatomy of diabetes mellitus. *Lancet* 1890; **ii**:381–386.

14 Jaeger E. *Jaeger's Atlas of Diseases of the Ocular Fundus: with New Descriptions, Revisions, and Additions*, tr. and ed. Albert DM. [Translation of *Ophthalmoskopischer Hand-Atlas*, rev. ed. Salzmann M., Leipzig, 1890; 1st edn. 1869.] Philadelphia: Saunders, 1972.

15 Nettleship E. Haemorrhagic retinitis in a patient with diabetes, varicose swellings on a retinal vein in the right eye. *Trans Opthalmol Soc UK* 1888; **8**:161.

16 Hirschberg J. Über diabetische Netzhautentzündung. *Dtsch Med Wochenschr* 1890; **16**:1181.

17 Pavy FW. Introductory address to the discussion on the clinical aspect of glycosuria. *Lancet* 1885; **ii**:1085–1087.

18 Pavy FW. On diabetic neuritis. *Lancet* 1904; **ii**:17–19.

19 Griesinger W. Studien über Diabetes. *Arch Physiol Heilkd* 1859; **3**:1–75.

20 Lanceraux E. Le diabète maigre: ses symptomes, son évolution, son pronostic et son traitement. *Union Méd Paris* 1880; **20**:205–211.

21 Joslin EP. Present-day treatment and prognosis in diabetes. *Am J Med Sci* 1915; **150**:485–496.

22 Joslin EP. *The Treatment of Diabetes Mellitus: with Observations Based upon One Thousand Cases*. Philadelphia: Lea & Febiger, 1916.

23 Zuelzer GL. Experimentelle Untersuchungen über den Diabetes. *Berlin Klin Wochenschr* 1907; **44**:474–475.

24 Richards DW. The effect of pancreas extract on depancreatized dogs: Ernest L. Scott's thesis of 1911. *Perspect Biol Med* 1966; **10**: 84–95.

25 Paulesco NC. Recherche sur le rôle du pancréas dans l'assimilation nutritive. *Arch Int Physiol* 1921; **17**:85–109.

26 Bliss M. *The Discovery of Insulin*. Chicago: University of Chicago Press, 1982.

27 Banting FG, Best CH, Collip JB, Campbell WR, Fletcher AA. Pancreatic extracts in the treatment of diabetes mellitus: preliminary report. *Can Med Assoc J* 1922; **12**:141–146.

28 Hetenyi G. The day after: how insulin was received by the medical profession. *Perspect Biol Med* 1995; **38**:396–405.

29 Falta W. *Die Zuckerkrankheit*. Berlin: Urban und Schwarzenberg, 1936.

30 Himsworth HP. Diabetes mellitus: its differentiation into insulinsensitive and insulin-insensitive types. *Lancet* 1936; **i**:127–30.

31 DeFronzo RA, Tobin JD, Andres R. Glucose clamp technique: a method for quantifying insulin secretion and resistance. *Am J Physiol* 1979; **237**:E214–E223.

32 Tattersall RB. Mild familial diabetes with dominant inheritance. *Q J Med* 1974; **43**:339–357.

33 Opie EL. On the relation of chronic interstitial pancreatitis to the islands of Langerhans and to diabetes mellitus. *J Exp Med* 1901; **5**:393–397.

34 Gepts W. Pathologic anatomy of the pancreas in juvenile diabetes. *Diabetes* 1965; **14**:619–633.

35 Bottazzo GF, Florin-Christensen A, Doniach D. Islet-cell antibodies in diabetes mellitus with autoimmune polyendocrine deficiencies. *Lancet* 1974; **ii**:1279–1283.

36 Feutren G, Papoz L, Assan R, Vialettes B, Karsenty G, Vexiau P, *et al.* Cyclosporin increases the rate and length of remissions in insulin-dependent diabetes of recent onset: results of a multicentre double-blind trial. *Lancet* 1986; **2**:119–124.

37 Gale EA, Bingley PJ, Emmett CL, Collier T, European Nicotinamide Diabetes Intervention Trial (ENDIT) Group. European Nicotinamide Diabetes Intervention Trial (ENDIT): a randomised controlled trial of intervention before the onset of type 1 diabetes. *Lancet* 2004; **363**:925–931.

38 Diabetes Prevention Trial – Type 1 Diabetes Study Group. Effects of insulin in relatives of patients with type 1 diabetes mellitus. *N Engl J Med* 2002; **346**:1685–1691.

39 Ryan EA, Paty BW, Senior PA, Bigam D, Alfadhli E, Kneteman NM, *et al.* Five-year follow-up after clinical islet transplantation. *Diabetes* 2005; **54**:2060–2069.

40 Wagener HF, Dry TJS, Wilder RM. Retinitis in diabetes. *N Engl J Med* 1934; **211**:1131–1137.

41 Kimmelstiel P, Wilson C. Intercapillary lesions in the glomeruli of the kidney. *Am J Pathol* 1936; **12**:83–97.

42 Bloodworth JMB. A re-evaluation of diabetic glomerulosclerosis 50 years after the discovery of insulin. *Hum Pathol* 1978; **9**:439–453.

43 Lundbæk K. *Long-Term Diabetes: the Clinical Picture in Diabetes Mellitus of 15–25 Years' Duration with a Follow Up of a Regional Series of Cases*. London: Lange, Maxwell and Springer, 1953.

44 Lundbæk K. Diabetic angiopathy: a specific vascular disease. *Lancet* 1954; **i**:377–379.

45 Kinoshita JH. Mechanisms initiating cataract formation. *Invest Ophthalmol* 1974; **13**:713–724.

46 Lane MA. The cytological characters of the areas of Langerhans. *Am J Anat* 1907; **7**:409–421.

47 Young FG. Permanent experimental diabetes produced by pituitary (anterior lobe) injections. *Lancet* 1937; **ii**:372–374.

48 Lacy PE. Electron microscopic and fluorescent antibody studies on islets of Langerhans. *Exp Cell Res* 1959; **7**:296–308.

49 Baum J, Simmons BE, Unger RH, Madison LL. Localization of glucagon in the A-cells in the pancreatic islet by immunofluorescence. *Diabetes* 1962; **11**:371–378.

50 Brown H, Sanger F, Kitai R. The structure of pig and sheep insulin. *Biochem J* 1955; **60**:556–565.

51 Adams MJ, Blundell TL, Dodson EJ, Hodgkin DC. Structure of 2 zinc insulin crystals. *Nature* 1969; **224**:491–495.

52 Kung K, Huang W, *et al.* Total synthesis of crystalline insulin. *Sci Sinica* 1966; **15**:544–561.

53 Steiner DF, Oyer PE. The biosynthesis of insulin and probable precursor of insulin by a human islet cell adenoma. *Proc Natl Acad Sci U S A* 1967; **57**:473–480.

54 Bornstein J, Lawrence RD. Two types of diabetes, with and without available plasma insulin. *Br Med J* 1951; **i**:732–735.

55 Yalow RS, Berson SA. Assay of plasma insulin in human subjects by immunological methods. *Nature* 1958; **184**:1648–1649.

56 Ullrich A, Shrine J, Chirgwin J, Pictet R, Tischer E, Rutter WJ, *et al.* Rat insulin genes: construction of plasmids containing the coding sequences. *Science* 1977; **196**:1313–1319.

57 Bell GI, Pictet RL, Rutter WJ, Cordell B, Tischer E, Goodman HM. Sequence of the human insulin gene. *Nature* 1980; **284**:26–32.

58 Freychet P, Roth J, Neville DM Jr. Insulin receptors in the liver: specific binding of [^{125}I] insulin of the plasma membrane and its relation to insulin bioactivity. *Proc Natl Acad Sci U S A* 1971; **68**:1833–1837.

59 Cuatrecasas P. Affinity chromatography and purification of the insulin receptor of liver cell membrane. *Proc Natl Acad Sci U S A* 1972; **62**:1277–1281.

60 Ullrich A, Bell JR, Chen EY, Herrera R, Petruzzelli LM, Dull TJ, *et al.* Human insulin receptor and its relationship to the tyrosine kinase family of oncogenes. *Nature* 1985; **313**:756–761.

61 Ebina Y, Ellis L, Jarnagin K, Edery M, Graf L, Clauser E, *et al.* The human insulin receptor cDNA: the structural basis for hormone-activated transmembrane signalling. *Cell* 1985; **40**:747–758.

62 Mueckler M, Caruso C, Baldwin SA, Panico M, Blench I, Morris HR, *et al.* Sequence and structure of a human glucose transporter. *Science* 1985; **229**:941–945.

63 Dolger H. Clinical evaluation of vascular damage in diabetes mellitus. *JAMA* 1947; **134**:1289–1291.

64 Reuting RE. Progress notes on fifty diabetic patients followed 25 or more years. *Arch Intern Med* 1950; **86**:891–897.

65 Deckert T. *H.C. Hagedorn and Danish Insulin.* Herning, Denmark: Kristensen, 2000.

66 Goeddel DV, Kleid DG, Bolivar F. Expression in *Escherichia coli* of chemically synthesized genes from human insulin. *Proc Natl Acad Sci U S A* 1979; **76**:106–110.

67 Paton JS, Wilson M, Ireland JT, Reith SBM. Convenient pocket insulin syringe. *Lancet* 1981; **i**:189–190.

68 Pickup JC, Keen H, Parsons JA, Alberti KGMM. Continuous subcutaneous insulin infusion: an approach to achieving normoglycaemia. *Br Med J* 1978; **i**:204–207.

69 Mathieu C, Gale EAM. Inhaled insulin: gone with the wind? *Diabetologia* 2008; **51**:1–5.

70 Frank E, Nothmann M, Wagner A. Über synthetisch dargestellte Körper mit insulinartiger Wirkung auf den normalen und den diabetischen Organismus. *Klin Wochenschr* 1926; 2100–2107.

71 Loubatières A. *Thèse Doctorat Sciences Naturelles*, no. 86. Montpellier, 1946. Montpellier: Causse, Graille et Castelnau, 1956.

72 Tyberghein JM, Williams RH. Metabolic effects of phenylethyldiguanide, a new hypoglycemic compound (23386). *Proc Soc Exp Med Biol* 1957; **96**:29–32.

73 Tattersall RB. The quest for normoglycaemia: a historical perspective. *Diabet Med* 1994; **11**:618–635.

74 Marks HM. *The Progress of Experiment: Science and Therapeutic Reform in the United States.* New York: Cambridge University Press, 1997: 197–228.

75 University Group Diabetes Program. A study of the effects of hypoglycemic agents on vascular complications in patients with adult onset diabetes. *Diabetes* 1970; **19**(Suppl.):789–830.

76 Tolstoi E. The objective of modern diabetic care. *Psychosom Med* 1948; **10**:291–294.

77 Walker GF. Reflections on diabetes mellitus: answers to a questionnaire. *Lancet* 1953; **ii**:1329–1332.

78 Sonksen P, Judd S, Lowy C. Home monitoring of blood glucose: method for improving diabetic control. *Lancet* 1978; **1**:729–732.

79 Walford S, Gale EAM, Allison SP, Tattersall RB. Self-monitoring of blood glucose: improvement of diabetic control. *Lancet* 1978; **1**:732–735.

80 Rahbar S. An abnormal hemoglobin in the red cells of diabetics. *Clin Chim Acta* 1968; **22**:296–298.

81 Diabetes Control and Complications Trial Research Group. The effect of intensive treatment of diabetes on the development and progression of long-term complications in insulin-dependent diabetes mellitus. *N Engl J Med* 1993; **329**:977–986.

82 UK Prospective Diabetes Study (UKPDS) Group. Intensive blood-glucose control with sulphonylureas or insulin compared with conventional treatment and risk of complications in patients with type 2 diabetes (UKPDS 33). *Lancet* 1998; **352**:837–853.

83 UK Prospective Diabetes Study (UKPDS) Group. Tight blood pressure control and risk of macrovascular and microvascular complications in type 2 diabetes: UKPDS 38. *Br Med J* 1998; **317**:703–713.

84 Gaede P, Vedel P, Larsen N, Jensen GV, Parving HH, Pedersen O. Multifactorial intervention and cardiovascular disease in type 2 diabetes. *N Engl J Med* 2003; **348**:383–393.

85 Diabetic Retinopathy Research Group. Photocoagulation treatment of proliferative diabetic retinopathy. The second report of Diabetic Retinopathy Study Findings. *Ophthalmology* 1978; **85**:82–106.

86 Meyer-Schwickerath G. *Light Coagulation* (Drance SM, trans). St Louis: Mosby, 1960.

87 Mogensen CE. Long-term antihypertensive treatment inhibiting progression of diabetic nephropathy. *Br Med J* 1982; **285**:685–688.

88 Keen H, Chlouverakis C. An immunoassay for urinary albumin at low concentrations. *Lancet* 1963; **ii**:913–916.

89 Joslin EP, Root HF, White P. Diabetic coma and its treatment. *Med Clin North Am* 1925; **8**:1873–1919.

90 Menzel R, Zander E, Jutzi E. Treatment of diabetic coma with low-dose injections of insulin. *Endokrinologie* 1976; **67**:230–239.

91 Root HF. The use of insulin and the abuse of glucose in treatment of diabetic coma. *JAMA* 1945; **127**:557–563.

92 Holler JW. Potassium deficiency occurring during the treatment of diabetic acidosis. *JAMA* 1946; **131**:1186–1188.

93 White P. Pregnancy complicating diabetes. *Surg Gynecol Obstet* 1935; **61**:324–332.

94 Pedersen J, Brandstrup E. Foetal mortality in pregnant diabetics: strict control of diabetes with conservative obstetric management. *Lancet* 1956; **i**:607–610.

95 Beaser SB. Teaching the diabetic patient. *Diabetes* 1956; **5**:146–149.

96 Anon. Diabetes care and research in Europe: the Saint Vincent Declaration. *Diabet Med* 1990; **7**:360.

Further reading

Bliss M. *The Discovery of Insulin.* Toronto: McClelland and Stewart, 1982; and Edinburgh: Paul Harris Publishing, 1983.

Deckert, T. *HC Hagedorn and Danish Insulin.* Copenhagen: Poul Kristensen, 2000.

Feudtner C. *Bitter Sweet, Diabetes, Insulin and the Transformation of Illness.* Chapel Hill and London: University of North Carolina Press, 2003.

Feudtner C, Gabbe S. Diabetes and pregnancy: four motifs of modern medical history. *Clin Obstet Gynecol* 2000; **43**:4–16.

Goldner MG. Historical review of oral substitutes for insulin. *Diabetes* 1957; **6**:259–262.

Ionescu-Tirgoviste C. *The Rediscovery of Insulin.* Bucharest: Geneze, 1996.

Loubatières A. The hypoglycaemic sulphonamides: history and development of the problem from 1942 to 1955. *Ann N Y Acad Sci* 1957; **71**:4–28.

Medvei VC. *A History of Endocrinology.* Lancaster: MTP Press, 1982.

Tattersall R. *Diabetes: the biography*, Oxford: Oxford University Press, 2009.

von Engelhardt, D. *Diabetes: its Medical and Cultural History.* Berlin: Springer, 1989.

Websites

General history of diabetes

http://pr15.mphy.lu.se/Diahistory1.html
http://www.diabetes/living.com/basics/histdev.htm

Discovery of insulin

Discovery of Insulin website: http://web.idirect.com/~discover
Banting Digital Library: http://www.Newtecumseth.library.on.ca.banting/main.html
Nobel Prize Website: http://www.nobel.se/medicine/laureates/1923

Archives

The notebooks and personal papers of the discoverers of insulin are preserved at the Thomas Fisher Rare Book Library, University of Toronto, Canada.

2 The Classification and Diagnosis of Diabetes Mellitus

K. George M.M. Alberti

Endocrinology and Metabolism, Imperial College St Mary's Campus, London, UK

Key points

- The classification of diabetes mellitus is based on four main categories: Type 1, Type 2, other specific types, and gestational diabetes mellitus
- Impaired glucose tolerance and impaired fasting glycemia are high-risk states collectively termed "intermediate hyperglycemia"
- Type 2 diabetes is a diagnosis by exclusion and as more specific causes are found these will move out of the type two category into other specific types
- Measurement of glucose continues to be the mainstay of diagnosis. In the symptomatic person a single abnormal value, either casual or fasting, is often enough to confirm the diagnosis. In asymptomatic individuals two abnormal values are required and an oral glucose tolerance test may be needed
- The diagnosis of diabetes can not be excluded by measuring fasting plasma glucose alone
- HbA_{1c} has major advantages over glucose testing in terms of convenience and lack of variability, although it is not adequately quality assured or standardized in many places, and is costly. Nonetheless, it is already recommended in some countries as an alternative diagnostic test. This is likely to become more widespread

Introduction

Diabetes mellitus is a disease of antiquity (see Chapter 1). A treatment was described in the Ebers papyrus and as long ago as 600 BC two main types were distinguished. Perhaps the most famous description was by Arateus the Cappadocian who talked of the melting down of flesh into urine and of the end being speedy. Over the ensuing centuries sporadic descriptions were noted, with Maimonides in Egypt pointing out its relative rarity. It was attributed to a salt-losing state although the sweetness of the urine had long been known. Undoubtedly, virtually all of these accounts referred to type 1 (T1DM) or late type 2 diabetes (T2DM).

Diabetes was better recognized in the 17th and 18th centuries, with the association with obesity noted in some cases. The obvious breakthrough came in the 17th century with the demonstration of excess glucose in the urine and later also in blood.

The presence of excess ketones was shown in the 19th century. A clear description of the two main types of diabetes appeared at the end of the 19th century, with the distinction being made between that occurring in young people with a short time course before ketoacidosis supervened, and that found in older people who were obese. Over the next decades these became known as juvenile-onset diabetes and maturity-onset diabetes, although it was generally stated that the latter was just a milder form of the disease. Diagnosis now depended on glucose measurement with some using glucose tolerance tests. There were no standard criteria for these initially, although glucose levels were clearly above normal. Diagnosis usually occurred after clinical development of the disease with the combination of symptoms with raised glucose in the blood or glycosuria being diagnostic, together with ketonuria in the juvenile-onset form.

A further breakthrough occurred with the work of Himsworth in 1936. Himsworth's work showed that people with diabetes could be divided into insulin-resistant and insulin-sensitive types, with the former much more common in those with the maturity-onset variety [1]. The next milestone was the development of the radioimmunoassay for insulin which allowed the unequivocal demonstration of insulin deficiency, or indeed absence, in those with juvenile-onset diabetes while levels were apparently normal or raised in those with maturity-onset diabetes.

At that time, diabetes was still considered to be a relatively uncommon disorder occurring predominantly in Europids. The World Health Organization (WHO) began to take note and held its first Expert Committee meeting in 1964 [2]. The real breakthrough, however, in terms of diagnosis and classification came in 1980 with the publication of the second Expert Committee report [3] shortly after the report from the National Diabetes Data Group (NDDG) in the USA in 1979 [4]. These events form the starting point for the diagnostic criteria and classification used today.

Textbook of Diabetes, 4th edition. Edited by R. Holt, C. Cockram, A. Flyvbjerg and B. Goldstein.

Definitions

Diabetes mellitus is a metabolic disorder of multiple etiologies. It is characterized by chronic hyperglycemia together with disturbances of carbohydrate, fat and protein metabolism resulting from defects of insulin secretion, insulin action or both [6]. The relative contribution of these varies between different types of diabetes. These are associated with the development of the specific microvascular complications of retinopathy, which can lead to blindness, nephropathy with potential renal failure, and neuropathy. The latter carries the risk of foot ulcers and amputation and also autonomic nerve dysfunction. Diabetes is also associated with an increased risk of macrovascular disease.

The characteristic clinical presentation is with thirst, polyuria, blurring of vision and weight loss. This can lead to ketoacidosis or hyperosmolar non-ketotic coma (see Chapter 19). Often, symptoms are mild or absent and mild hyperglycemia can persist for years with tissue damage developing, although the person may be totally asymptomatic.

Classification

There was awareness of different grades of severity of diabetes for many centuries; however, the possibility that there were two distinct types only emerged at the beginning of the 20th century. Even then there was no real clue to distinct etiologies. In the 1930s, Himsworth suggested that there were two phenotypes. The first real attempt to classify diabetes came with the first WHO Expert Committee on Diabetes Mellitus which felt that the only reliable classification was by age of onset and divided diabetes into juvenile-onset and maturity-onset disease [2]. There were many other phenotypes in vogue at that time including brittle, gestational, pancreatic, endocrine, insulin-resistant and iatrogenic diabetes, but for most cases there was no clear indication of etiology. Clarity began to emerge in the 1970s with the discovery of the human leukocyte antigen (HLA) genotypes common in juvenile-onset diabetes and the discovery of islet call antibodies. This gave a clear indication that younger patients with diabetes, all of whom required insulin therapy, had an autoimmune disorder.

The beginning of the modern era came with the second WHO Expert Committee [3] which reviewed and modified the revised classification published by the National Diabetes Data Group [4]. This proposed two main classes of diabetes: insulin-dependent diabetes mellitus (IDDM; type 1) and non-insulin-dependent diabetes (NIDDM; type 2) together with "other types" and gestational diabetes. There were also two risk classes: previous abnormality of glucose intolerance (PrevAGT) and potential abnormality of glucose tolerance (PotAGT) which replaced previous types known as pre-diabetes or potential diabetes.

The 1980 classification was revised further in 1985 [5] and reverted to clinical descriptions with retention of IDDM and NIDDM but omission of type 1 and type 2. Malnutrition-related diabetes mellitus was also introduced in recognition of a different phenotype found particularly in Asia and sub-Saharan Africa. Impaired glucose tolerance (IGT) was also introduced as a high risk class.

Table 2.1 Etiologic classification of disorders of glycemia. Adapted from World Health Organization [6].

Type 1 diabetes (β-cell destruction)
• Autoimmune
• Idiopathic
Type 2 diabetes (insulin resistance with insulin hyposecretion)
Other specific types (Table 2.2)
Gestational diabetes (includes former categories of gestational IGT and gestational diabetes)

IGT, impaired glucose tolerance.

Based on increasing knowledge, WHO revisited the classification in 1999 [6] as did the American Diabetes Association (ADA) [7]. It was recognized that the terms IDDM and NIDDM, although superficially appealing, were often confusing and unhelpful – as in patients with insulin-treated T2DM. The new classification attempted to encompass both etiology and clinical stages of the disease as well as being useful clinically. This was based on the suggestion of Kuzuya and Matsuda [8]. This acknowledges that diabetes may progress through several clinical stages (e.g. from normoglycemia to ketoacidosis) while having a single etiologic process such as autoimmune attack on the β-cells. Similarly, it is possible that someone with T2DM can move from insulin requirement to no pharmaceutical intervention through modification of lifestyle. The main classes are T1DM, T2DM, other specific types and gestational diabetes (Table 2.1). It should be noted that T2DM is largely categorization by exclusion. As new causes are discovered so they will be included under "other specific types" as has occurred for maturity-onset diabetes of the young (MODY).

The classification was revisited by WHO in 2006, but no further modification was introduced, and it will be examined again in 2010 when at most minor amendments will be made. IGT was removed from the formal classification of types of diabetes – logically, as it is not diabetes – but was retained as a risk state. Impaired fasting glycemia (IFG) was introduced as another risk state. This was particularly important in many countries where glucose tolerance tests are rarely performed in practice outside of pregnancy so that IGT was not diagnosed and IFG, although not strictly equivalent, has been used as an easily obtained risk marker.

Type 1 diabetes

T1DM is primarily caused by β-cell destruction although some insulin resistance is also present (see Chapter 9). After the initial stages, insulin is required for survival. In Europids >90% show evidence of autoimmunity with anti-glutamine acid decarboxylase (anti-GAD), anti-insulin and/or islet cell antibodies detectable. It shows strong association with specific alleles at the DQ-A and DQ-B loci of the HLA complex [9]. Not all subjects with the clinical characteristics of T1DM show these associations with autoimmunity although they are ketosis-prone, non-obese and generally under the age of 30 years. In non-Europid populations, up to 80% may show no measurable autoantibodies [10]; these are referred to as having idiopathic T1DM. As with autoimmune diabetes, however, there is clear loss of β-cell function as measured by low or absent C-peptide secretion. Diabetes occurring before the age of 6 months is most likely to be monogenic neonatal diabetes rather than autoimmune T1DM (see Chapter 15) [11].

In addition to the typically young people with acute-onset T1DM, there is an older group with slower onset disease. They may present in middle age with apparent T2DM but have evidence of autoimmunity as assessed by GAD antibody measurements and ultimately become insulin-dependent. This is referred to as latent autoimmune diabetes of adults (LADA) [12].

Type 2 diabetes

By far the majority of people with diabetes worldwide have T2DM. This is characterized by insulin resistance with relative insulin deficiency (i.e. patients secrete insulin, but not enough to overcome the insulin resistance) (see Chapters 10 and 11). Typically, they do not require insulin to survive but often will eventually need insulin to maintain reasonable glycemia control, often after many years.

The precise molecular mechanisms underlying T2DM are not known. Major efforts have been made to discover underlying genetic abnormalities but with only modest success (see Chapter 12). The most promising to be date has been TCF7L2 [13] which may have a role in insulin secretion but this does not explain diabetes susceptibility in the majority of subjects. What is clear is that T2DM is closely associated with obesity and physical inactivity, and the westernization of lifestyles. The dramatic increase in T2DM over the past two decades has been closely paralleled by the rise in obesity worldwide. Both obesity, particularly visceral adiposity, and physical inactivity cause insulin resistance which will result in diabetes in those with only a small capacity to increase insulin secretion. The incidence of T2DM also increases with age, which may be related to decrease in exercise and muscle mass; however, as the incidence increases so T2DM is being found at younger ages and it is now not uncommon in adolescence in many ethnic groups.

T2DM occurs in families so that those with a first-degree relative with diabetes have an almost 50% life-time risk. There is also marked variation between different ethnic groups. Thus, those of Polynesian, Micronesian, South Asian, sub-Saharan African, Arabian and Native American origin are much more prone to develop diabetes than Europids.

T2DM is a diagnosis by exclusion and the prevalence may fall as causes are identified, but this is likely to be a slow process.

Other specific types of diabetes

Diabetes occurs both as a result of specific genetic defects in insulin secretion and action and in a range of other conditions (Table 2.2).

Table 2.2 Other specific types of diabetes. Adapted from World Health Organization [6].

Genetic defects of β-cell function
Chromosome 20, HNF4α (MODY 1)
Chromosome 7, glucokinase (MODY 2)
Chromosome 12, HNF1α (MODY 3)
Chromosome 13, IPF-1 (MODY 4)
Mitochondrial DNA 3243 mutation
Others
Genetic defects in insulin action
Type A insulin resistance
Leprechaunism
Rabson–Mendenhall syndrome
Lipoatrophic diabetes
Others
Disease of the endocrine pancreas
Fibrocalculous pancreatopathy
Pancreatitis (particularly chronic)
Trauma/pancreatectomy
Neoplasia
Cystic fibrosis
Hemachromatosis
Others
Endocrinopathies
Cushing syndrome
Acromegaly
Pheochromocytoma
Glucagonoma
Somatostatinoma
Others
Drug- or chemical-induced
Nicotinic acid
Glucocorticoids
Thyroxine/triiodothyronine
α-Adrenergic agonists
Thiazides
Pentamidine
Vacor
Others
Infections
Congenital rubella
Cytomegalovirus
Mumps
Others
Uncommon forms of immune-mediated disease
Insulin autoimmune syndrome
Anti-insulin receptor antibodies
"Stiff man" syndrome
Others
Other genetic syndromes
(see Table 2.3)

The best known of the defects in insulin secretion are the MODY family, which are a group of autosomal-dominant inherited disorders where there is hyperglycemia at an early age, generally of a mild nature. The most common concerns a mutation in the HNF-1α gene on chromosome 12 (MODY 3) while another is caused by mutations in the glucokinase gene on chromosome 7p. These account for a small number of people with diabetes but are important in determining therapeutic approaches.

The association of diabetes with defects in insulin action has long been known, particularly in type A insulin resistance, leprechaunism and lipoatrophic diabetes. Not surprisingly, diseases of the exocrine pancreas often cause diabetes through destruction of the islets. Pancreatitis secondary to alcohol is probably the most common of these (see Chapter 18). Hemochromatosis and cystic fibrosis also commonly result in diabetes.

Fibrocalculous pancreatitis is also included in this category. Originally, this was part of malnutrition-related diabetes mellitus where there were two proposed variants: one associated with cassava consumption in malnourished people but without evidence of calculi, while the other was found after tropical pancreatitis and presented with fibrocalculous disease. The latter is akin to the diabetes found with other forms of chronic pancreatitis. In 1999 it was felt that this latter form would fit into the category of "other specific types" and that more evidence was needed before a specific malnutrition-related diabetes category could be included.

Several endocrinopathies are associated with diabetes: Cushing syndrome, acromegaly, pheochromocytoma, glucagonoma and hyperthyroidism (see Chapter 17). In general, the diabetes will disappear if the endocrinopathy is treated. Many drugs and chemicals cause diabetes (Table 2.2, Chapter 16). Some of these cause β-cell destruction but others will cause diabetes by increasing insulin resistance in susceptible individuals.

Infections are also associated with the development of diabetes; classically, mumps, congenital rubella, coxsackie B and cytomegalovirus are the main ones implicated. Many genetic syndromes are also associated with diabetes (Table 2.4).

There are other types of diabetes that do not fit conveniently into any of the current classes. These include "Flatbush" diabetes found in Afro-Americans [14] and so-called ketosis-prone T2DM found in Africans in sub-Saharan Africa [15]. These are both characterized by periods of ketosis with absolute insulin dependence and other times when the diabetes can be controlled by diet alone.

Gestational diabetes mellitus

Gestational diabetes mellitus (GDM) is hyperglycemia first detected during pregnancy (see Chapter 53). This is distinct from women with diabetes undergoing pregnancy, who have diabetes in pregnancy rather than gestational diabetes. Plasma glucose levels, both fasting and post-prandial, are lower than normal in early pregnancy so that raised levels at this stage are almost certainly caused by previously undetected T2DM. Screening for GDM is generally undertaken at around 28 weeks (see below for diagnostic criteria). There is significant morbidity associated with GDM including intrauterine fetal death, congenital malformations, neonatal hypoglycemia, jaundice, prematurity and macrosomia. Risk factors for GDM include certain ethnic groups, those with previous GDM or abnormalities of glucose tolerance, age, obesity and previous large babies.

Risk states

Prior to the 1979 and 1980 reports, the state of "borderline" diabetes had been recognized for cases where there was uncertainty about the diagnosis of diabetes but where plasma glucose was above accepted normal levels. This was formalized by the NDDG and WHO [3,4] as IGT, a higher than normal plasma

Table 2.3 Other genetic syndromes associated with diabetes. Adapted from World Health Organization [6].

Down syndrome
Friedreich ataxia
Huntington chorea
Klinefelter syndrome
Lawrence–Moon–Biedl syndrome
Myotonic dystrophy
Porphyria
Prader–Willi syndrome
Turner syndrome
Wolfram syndrome
Others

Table 2.4 World Health Organization (WHO) recommended criteria for the diagnosis of diabetes and intermediate hyperglycemia.

Diabetes
Fasting plasma glucose ≥7.0 mmol/L (126 mg/dL)
and/or
2-hour post-glucose load ≥11.1 mmol/L (200 mg/dL)
plasma glucose
Impaired glucose tolerance
Fasting plasma glucose <7.0 mmol/L (126 mg/dL)
and
2-hour post-glucose load
plasma glucose ≥7.8 and <11.1 mmol/L (140 and 200 mg/dL)
Impaired fasting glycemia
Fasting plasma glucose 6.1–6.9 mmol/L (110–125 mg/dL)
and (if measured)
2-hour post-glucose load <7.8 mmol/L (140 mg/dL)
plasma glucose

NB. All values refer to venous plasma glucose. Capillary plasma glucose values would be the same fasting but 1 mmol/L (18 mg/dL) higher than venous levels after the glucose load. The glucose load is 75 g anhydrous glucose.

glucose 2 hours after a glucose load but below the diagnostic cutoff for diabetes. Later, both the ADA and WHO introduced the concept of IFG as a fasting plasma glucose above normal but below the diabetes diagnostic level [6,7]. Both IFG and IGT are associated with a two- to threefold increased risk of developing diabetes, while IGT is also a cardiovascular risk marker. IFG was welcomed as it could indicate an at-risk individual without the need to perform a glucose tolerance test. Collectively, IFG and IGT became known as "pre-diabetes" – a misleading term as not everyone with pre-diabetes develops diabetes, and it diminishes the importance of other risk markers such as family history. The term "intermediate hyperglycemia" is preferred by WHO [16]. IGT and IFG are more likely in older people, those who are obese, people from particular high risk ethnic groups and those with cardiovascular disease or other features of the metabolic syndrome, such as dyslipidemia, hypertension or visceral adiposity.

Diagnostic criteria

The diagnosis of diabetes mellitus has lifelong implications for the individual. Thus, both the clinician, and person tested, must have full confidence in the diagnosis. In the symptomatic individual this is easier but in asymptomatic people once an abnormal test has been found it must be confirmed by a further test. This is increasingly important as screening programs spread and also because 30–50% of people with T2DM are asymptomatic and unaware that they have the disorder.

Clinical diagnosis of diabetes in symptomatic individuals

The search for diabetes in an individual is often driven by the presence of characteristic symptoms such as thirst, polyuria, weight loss, recurrent infections and, in more severe cases, precoma. In such individuals, a single elevated casual plasma glucose value is sufficient to confirm the diagnosis. A definite diagnosis can be assumed if the venous plasma glucose level is greater than 11.1 mmol/L (200 mg/dL) or 12.2 mmol/L (220 mg/dL) in capillary plasma [5]. WHO describes values of 5.0–11.0 mmol/L as uncertain. Further testing is then required as described below.

Diagnostic tests for diabetes

A raised blood glucose has been the hallmark of diabetes mellitus for over 100 years. The oral glucose tolerance test (OGTT) was developed in the early years of the 19th century but only came into common use as methods for measuring blood glucose became easier. When the first WHO Expert Committee on Diabetes reviewed diagnostic tests [2] they first of all stated that glycosuria was an unsatisfactory test and that neither the presence of glycosuria nor its absence could rule in or rule out diabetes. They also commented on the wide range of glucose tolerance tests available at the time and recommended strongly that only the 50-g or the 100-g OGTT should be used. They suggested that a fasting venous blood glucose level over 130 mg/dL (7.2 mmol/L) indicated the probability of diabetes. This was for whole blood so that in terms of plasma this would equate to about 150 mg/dL (8.3 mmol/L); however, at that time, most blood glucose chemical tests in use overestimated true glucose by at least 20 mg/dL (1.1 mmol/L). They placed most reliance on the OGTT. They examined both values at 1 and at 2 hours after the glucose load but decided that the 2-hour value on its own was adequate – and this was the key diagnostic test suggested. The value selected was 130 mg/dL (7.2 mmol/L) for venous whole blood and that was to be applied regardless of whether the 50-g or the 100-g glucose load was given. They also introduced the important concept of "borderline" diabetes – the forerunner of IGT – where values were to be above normal but less than those diagnostic for diabetes: 110 mg/dL (6.1 mmol/L) to 129 mg/dL (7.2 mmol/L) for venous whole blood 2 hours after the glucose load.

One further important comment is the need for people to be prepared for the OGTT with at least 250 g carbohydrate consumed for 3 days before the test. This still applies and is rarely adhered to, which may explain the large number of older people with normal fasting glucose but elevated 2-hour values. Many of these could well have "starvation" diabetes rather than genuine diabetes.

The modern era

The big change and rationalization came in 1979 and 1980 with the work of NDDG and WHO [3,4]. They reviewed all available data and concluded that a 75-g load would be appropriate and that this should be consumed in 300 mL water over 5 minutes. They based the diagnostic levels for fasting and 2-hour values largely on bimodality observations in high prevalence groups such as the Pima Indians and on some observations of risk for retinopathy. Fasting and 2-hour venous plasma levels of 140 mg/dL (7.8 mmol/L) and 200 mg/dL (11.1 mmol/L) were recommended by NDDG and these were – somewhat unfortunately – rounded up to 8 mmol/L and 11 mmol/L by the WHO Committee. IGT was defined as a fasting venous plasma value <8 mmol/L with a 2-hour value of 8–11 mmol/L. Confusion was rife and a further evaluation took place in 1985 [5] when the WHO group adjusted their values to match the NDDG values precisely.

The next big change occurred in 1997 and 1999 with the publication of the ADA and the new WHO report. This time a considerable amount of data were available to look at risk of retinopathy at different glucose levels. The data were cross-sectional but reasonable agreement was shown between studies of Egyptians, US citizens from NHANES III and Pima Indians (for review see Expert Committee on the Diagnosis and Classification of Diabetes Mellitus [7]). Although there was some tolerance on the precise values, the existing 2-hour cut point of 11.1 mmol/L (200 mg/dL) seemed reasonable but the fasting value was lowered to 7.0 mmol/L (126 mg/dL; Table 2.4). At the same time, the concept of IFG was introduced. This was equivalent to IGT but for the fasting state and was meant to indicate a risk state for diabetes. The values chosen were 6.1–6.9 mmol/L (110–125 mg/dL).

There was one major difference between the ADA and WHO proposals. ADA recommended that a fasting glucose alone could be used for diagnostic purposes and that an OGTT was unnecessary. Similarly, the implication was that fasting glucose could be used as a screening test to identify people at risk without requiring a glucose tolerance test. This was not agreed by the WHO group who continued to promote the use of the OGTT where necessary. Part of the reason is that a considerable number of people with diabetes by the 2-hour value have normal or IFG values when fasting.

The final changes came in 2003 when a new ADA group recommended lowering the threshold for IFG to 100 mg/dL (5.6 mmol/L) which was considered by WHO in 2006 but not supported [17].

Problems with glucose tests

Measurement of glucose has been the cornerstone and bedrock of diabetes diagnosis for the last 100 years; however, it does have problems. Initially, the assays measured reducing sugars and were not specific. Enzyme assays have largely negated this problem. Accuracy and precision are not problems in well-run laboratories with appropriate quality assurance in place but the advent of glucose meters has caused problems. They are efficient if carefully used, properly controlled and calibrated but the coefficient of variation can often be as high as 20% in field use, making them unsuitable for diagnostic purposes. There are other problems: unless blood is separated immediately after withdrawal from the subject there is a steady loss of glucose even when fluoride or other preservatives are present. This can range from 5 to 20%.

There are also potential problems with the subject tested. Fasting glucose is reasonably reproducible but can be influenced by drugs or coexisting conditions, or the patient may not have fasted appropriately. The OGTT is notoriously variable from day to day within the same individual and is unreliable when they are close to the threshold for diagnosis. It has long been deemed the gold standard but this is more by common usage and because there was no alternative. This has become more important as more screening programs take place and people with asymptomatic diabetes are sought.

Use of HbA_{1c} as a diagnostic test for diabetes

The introduction of HbA_{1c} as a means to test glycemic control has had an enormous impact on patient care. It has been proposed many times that it could prove a useful means of diagnosing diabetes as it requires neither fasting nor an OGTT. It also represents glycemic status over weeks and gives real certainty that a person is indeed hyperglycemic. It is also subject to fewer errors within an individual patient although it can obviously be affected by conditions such as anemias and hemoglobinopathies. The arguments against, which were reaffirmed by WHO in 2006 and ADA in 2003, were that the test was not sufficiently standardized, the quality of assays was variable, the test is expensive and it is not available at all in many parts of the world.

Recently, the situation has changed. There is now an international standard that is coming into widespread use and assays are reliable and show only small variation within and between assays in good laboratories. In the USA, the situation has been helped by the National Glycohemoglobin Standardization Program which has promoted standardized assays based on data from the Diabetes Control and Complications Trial. Several other countries also have standardized programs in place.

A groundswell of support has appeared suggesting that it would indeed be a useful addition to the diagnostic armamentarium for diabetes. Several authors have suggested its use in addition to fasting glucose [18]. In particular, an Expert Committee led by the ADA has endorsed the use of HbA_{1c} as a new means of diagnosing diabetes and identifying those at high risk of developing the disorder [19]. One problem concerns the appropriate diagnostic level at which to diagnose diabetes. Many suggestions have been made but that proposed by the Expert Committee [18] of 6.5% (47.5 mmol/mol) is gaining acceptance. This is based primarily on three cross-sectional studies that looked at fasting glucose, 2-hour glucose and HbA_{1c} in relation to retinopathy [7,20,21]. These were the same studies that were used to confirm the diagnostic glucose levels, fasting and after a glucose load. This has been supported by a recent analysis of 13 studies including the earlier three which showed that moderate retinopathy was virtually never found at levels below 6.5% (<47.5 mmol/mol) [22]. One problem is that the methods to detect retinopathy are much more sensitive now than previously and recent studies show background retinopathy occurs in 10% of normoglycemic individuals [23]. It is thus probably wise to use moderate retinopathy to determine cutoff diagnostic values. It has also been suggested that HbA_{1c} levels of 6.0–6.4% (42–47 mmol/mol) or 5.7–6.4% (39–47 mmol/mol) could be used to indicate those at high risk – similar to the use of IGT and IFG.

It seems likely that HbA_{1c} will be accepted for use as a diagnostic test. This should only be done in countries where stringent quality assurance and standardization against international standards are possible. It is also unsuitable in pregnancy. A new WHO Expert Committee has met to consider the use of HbA_{1c} but has not yet reported. Nevertheless, there are still various concerns about the use of HbA_{1c}. It is likely that some different individuals will be identified by HbA_{1c} and glucose. There is also the likelihood that prevalences of diabetes will be different. It is assumed by many that the glucose derived data are correct but the 2-hour glucose is a somewhat tarnished gold standard. It is indeed possible that HbA_{1c} will give more accurate diagnosis as it reflects a longer period of hyperglycemia rather than a single point in time and it is not subject to the same analytical and pre-analytical problems as glucose.

In most places glucose – casual, fasting and after a glucose load – will continue to be used routinely for the diagnosis of diabetes; in some countries (e.g. USA, Australia, Japan and Northern European countries), however, HbA_{1c} is likely to be the preferred test in the near future. This has indeed now been recommended by the ADA [24].

Gestational diabetes mellitus

Two different tests are widely used for the diagnosis of GDM. WHO recommends that the normal 75-g glucose load be given after an overnight fast and that those with either IGT or diabetes by non-pregnant criteria are deemed to have GDM [6].

In the USA, a two-step procedure is employed. First, a 50-g glucose load is given. If the 1-hour venous plasma glucose is ≥140 mg/dL (7.8 mmol/L) then the patient returns for a further test using either a 100 or 75 g glucose load. The cutoffs for venous plasma glucose are 95 mg/dL (5.3 mmol/L) fasting, 180 mg/dL (10 mmol/L) at 1 hour and 155 mg/dL (8.6 mmol/L) at 2 hours, regardless of which glucose load is used [17]. The WHO protocol is obviously simpler and has gained widespread acceptance; however, new recommendations are expected imminently in light of the results from the recent Hyperglycemia and Pregnancy Outcomes Study [25].

References

1 Himsworth HP. Diabetes mellitus: its differentiation into insulin-sensitive and insulin-insensitive types. *Lancet* 1936; **i**:117–119.

2 World Health Organization (WHO) Expert Committee on Diabetes Mellitus. *First Report: Technical Report Series 310.* Geneva: WHO, 1964.

3 World Health Organization (WHO) Expert Committee on Diabetes Mellitus. *Second Report: Technical Report Series 646.* Geneva: WHO, 1980.

4 National Diabetes Data Group. Classification and diagnosis of diabetes mellitus and other categories of glucose intolerance. *Diabetes* 1979; **28**:1039–1057.

5 World Health Organization (WHO). *Diabetes Mellitus: Report of a Study Group. Technical Report Series 727.* Geneva: WHO, 1985.

6 World Health Organization (WHO). *Report of a WHO Consultation. Definition, diagnosis and classification of diabetes mellitus and its complications. 1. Diagnosis and classification of diabetes mellitus.* WHO/NCD/NCS/99.2. Geneva: WHO, 1999.

7 Expert Committee on the Diagnosis and Classification of Diabetes Mellitus. Report of the expert committee on the diagnosis and classification of diabetes mellitus. *Diabetes Care* 1997; **20**:1183–1197.

8 Kuzuya T, Matsuda A. Classification of diabetes on the basis of etiologies versus degree of insulin deficiency. *Diabetes Care* 1997; **20**:219–220.

9 Concannon P, Rich SS, Nepom GT. Genetics of type 1A diabetes. *N Engl J Med* 2009; **360**:1646–1654.

10 McLarty DG, Athaide I, Bottazzo GF, Swai AM, Alberti KG. Islet cell antibodies are not specifically associated with insulin-dependent diabetes in Tanzanian Africans. *Diabetes Res Clin Pract* 1990; **9**:219–224.

11 Pearson ER, Starkey BJ, Powell RJ, Gribble FM, Clark PM, Hattersley AT. Genetic causes of hyperglycaemia and response to treatment in diabetes. *Lancet* 2003; **362**:1275–1281.

12 Tuomi T, Groop LC, Zimmet PZ, Rowley MJ, Knowles W, Mackay IR. Latent autoimmune diabetes mellitus in adults with a non-insulin-dependent onset of disease. *Diabetes* 1993; **42**:359–362.

13 Grant SF, Thorleifsson G, Reynisdottir I, Benediktsson R, Manolescu A, Sainz J, *et al.* Variant of transcription factor 7-like 2 (TCF7L2) gene confers risk of type 2 diabetes. *Nat Genet* 2006; **38**:320–323.

14 Banerji MA, Chaiken RI, Huey H, Tuomi T, Norin AJ, Mackay IR. GAD antibody negative NIDDM in adult black subject with diabetic ketoacidosis and increased frequency of human leukocyte antigen DR3 and DR4: Flatbush diabetes. *Diabetes* 1994; **43**:741–745.

15 Sobngwi E, Mauvais-Jarvis F, Vexiau P, Mbanya JC, Gautier JF. Diabetes in Africans. 2. Ketosis-prone atypical diabetes mellitus. *Diabetes Med* 2002; **28**:5–12.

16 World Health Organization (WHO) Consultation. *Definition and Diagnosis of Diabetes Mellitus and Intermediate Hyperglycemia.* Geneva: WHO, 2006.

17 Expert Committee on the Diagnosis and Classification of Diabetes Mellitus. Follow-up report on the diagnosis of diabetes mellitus. *Diabetes Care* 2003; **26**:3160–3167.

18 Barr RG, Nathan DM, Meigs JB, Singer DE. Tests of glycemia for the diagnosis of diabetes mellitus. *Ann Intern Med* 2002; **137**:263–272.

19 Expert Committee Report on the Diagnosis of Diabetes. The role of glycated haemoglobin (A1C) assay in the diagnosis of diabetes in non-pregnant persons. *Diabetes Care* 2009; **32**:1327–1334.

20 McCance DR, Hanson RL, Charles MA, Jacobsson LT, Pettitt DJ, Bennett PH, *et al.* Comparison of tests for glycated haemoglobin and fasting and two hour plasma glucose concentrations as diagnostic methods for diabetes. *Br Med J* 1997; **308**:1323–1328.

21 Engelau MM, Thompson TJ, Herman WH, Boyle JP, Aubert RE, Kenny SJ, *et al.* Comparison of fasting and 2-hour glucose and HbA_{1c} levels for diagnosing diabetes: diagnostic criteria and performance revisited. *Diabetes Care* 1997; **20**:785–791.

22 DETECT-2 Collaboration. Is there a glycemic threshold for diabetic retinopathy? *Diabetologia* 2010; in press.

23 Wong TY, Liew G, Tapp RJ, Schmidt MI, Wang JJ, Mitchell P, *et al.* Relation between fasting glucose and retinopathy for diagnosis of diabetes: three population-based cross-sectional studies. *Lancet* 2008; **371**:736–743.

24 American Diabetes Association. Diagnosis and classification of diabetes mellitus. *Diabetes Care* 2010; **33**(Suppl 1):S62–S69.

25 Metzger BE, Lowe DP, Dyer AR, Trimble ER, Chaovarindr U, Coustan DR, *et al.* Hyperglycemia and adverse pregnancy outcomes. *N Engl J Med* 2008; 3**58**:1991–2002.

3 Epidemiology of Type 1 Diabetes

Lars C. Stene,[1,2] Valma Harjutsalo,[3,4,5] Elena Moltchanova[3] & Jaakko Tuomilehto[3,6]

[1] Division of Epidemiology, Norwegian Institute of Public Health, Oslo, Norway
[2] Oslo Diabetes Research Center, Oslo University Hospital Ullevål and Aker, Oslo, Norway
[3] Diabetes Prevention Unit, Department of Health Promotion, National Institute of Health and Welfare, Helsinki, Finland
[4] Folkhälsan Institute of Genetics, Folkhälsan Research Center, Biomedicum Helsinki, Finland
[5] Division of Nephrology, Department of Medicine, Helsinki University Central Hospital, Helsinki, Finland
[6] Department of Public Health, University of Helsinki, Helsinki, Finland

Keypoints

- Type 1 diabetes mellitus (T1DM) develops in genetically susceptible individuals after a preclinical phase of variable length usually with immune-mediated destruction of pancreatic β-cells, and requires lifelong treatment with insulin.
- The disease can occur at any age, but the incidence peaks around puberty. Classification of T1DM vs type 2 diabetes (T2DM) becomes increasingly difficult with age.
- In childhood, the incidence is similar in females and males, but there is a 1.3- to 2.0-fold male excess in incidence after about 15 years of age in most populations.
- The incidence in childhood varies enormously between countries. Some Asian and South American populations have low incidences (approximately 0.1–8 per 100 000/year), while Finland (>40 per 100 000/year), Sardinia (approximately 38 per 100 000/year) and Sweden (approximately 30 per 100 000/year) have high incidences. North America (15–25 per 100 000/year) and Australia (approximately 15 per 100 000/year) have moderate to high incidences, while eastern countries in Europe have low to moderate incidences (4–10 per 100 000/year).
- About 10–20% of newly diagnosed childhood cases of T1DM have an affected first-degree relative. Those with an affected sibling or parent have a cumulative risk of 3–7% up to about 20 years of age, compared to cumulative risks of 0.2–0.8% in the respective general populations. The cumulative incidence among the monozygotic co-twins of persons with T1DM is less than 50%, even after >30 years' follow-up.
- Some of the geographic differences and familial aggregation may be explained by human leukocyte antigen haplotypes.
- The incidence of childhood-onset T1DM has increased 3–4% per calendar year, and there is a tendency towards younger average age at onset over time which cannot be explained by genetic factors. The causes of this increasing trend are not known.
- Virus infections and nutritional factors have been implicated, but no specific environmental factor has been established as a risk factor.
- Even though insulin replacement therapy and other advances in the management of T1DM have improved the prognosis of patients with T1DM, their mortality is still at least two times (approximately 2- to 10-fold) higher than in the background population. This is because of both acute and chronic complications of the disease, including cardiovascular disease after about 30 years of age.

Introduction

Type 1 diabetes mellitus (T1DM) requires lifelong treatment with insulin, and in the majority of cases results from a cell-mediated autoimmune destruction of the β-cells in susceptible individuals. This occurs after a long but variable preclinical period when islet autoantibodies to insulin, glutamine acid decarboxylase (GAD) and insulinoma-associated antigen 2 (IA-2) and other autoantigens can be detected [1]. Autoantibodies are not thought to cause the disease, but are markers of ongoing β-cell destruction. In general, the distinction between autoimmune T1DM (type 1 A according to the WHO [2]) and non-autoimmune T1DM (type 1 B) is not necessarily useful for clinicians or epidemiologists. Problems with measurement error of autoantibodies, the likely existence of additional autoantibodies (as indicated by the recent discovery of zinc transporter 8 autoantibodies [3]) and, perhaps equally important, the transient nature of autoantibodies, make accurate estimates of the proportion of autoimmune T1DM problematic. From longitudinal studies such as DAISY, it is known that some patients with newly diagnosed T1DM are negative for all autoantibodies at diagnosis while having previously been positive.

Genetic factors influence the susceptibility to T1DM, particularly human leukocyte antigen (HLA) genes [4,5]. It is particularly the combination of HLA DR3-DQ2 and DR4-DQ8 that confers very high risk of T1DM, while those who carry only one

Textbook of Diabetes, 4th edition. Edited by R. Holt, C. Cockram, A. Flyvbjerg and B. Goldstein.

of the two risk haplotypes have moderately increased risk. More details on the role of genetic factors and the pathologic process are covered in the first part of Chapter 9. Diagnosis of T1DM among children is considered relatively simple, typically with very high glucose levels and clear dependence upon insulin, but classification and early detection becomes increasingly difficult with increasing age.

Occurrence of T1DM by age, sex, place and time

The World Health Organization (WHO) DIAMOND Study (Multinational Project for Childhood Diabetes) [6] and the EURODIAB ACE Study [7,8] have collected standardized incidence data for T1DM among children aged under 15 years, based on notification by the diagnosing physician and date of diagnosis, defined as the date of first insulin injection. In both projects, the degree of undercounting of cases has been estimated using a second source of information [9].

Incidence rates are calculated as the number of new cases per 100 000 person-years, where person-years are estimated as the number of individuals in the population contributing the incident patients during the study period (mean population size in each calendar year, sex and age group) multiplied by the number of years covered by the age group in question. The proportion of the population expected to develop the disease by a certain age can be approximated by multiplying the average incidence rate in an age group by the number of years covered by the age group, the cumulative incidence rate. For instance, if the average incidence rate among 0- to 14-year-olds is 20 per 100 000 person-years, then ($[20/100\,000] \times 15 = 0.003 =$) 0.3% of children in that population will develop disease before they reach 15 years of age. The prevalence of disease among 0- to 14-year-olds is thus less than the cumulative incidence up to 15 years of age.

Most of the incidence data available today come from studies of children in European countries. Incidence data from Africa are still sparse, but increased information on the incidence of T1DM among Asian and South American populations has changed the understanding of the global patterns in variation in incidence.

Occurrence of T1DM by age

In principle, T1DM may occur at any age, but it is very rare in the first year of life and becomes increasingly difficult to distinguish from other types of diabetes after about 30 years of age. Essentially all populations display a steady increase in incidence rate with age up to around 10–15 years [6], but recent data from Finland indicate an incidence in 0- to 4-year-olds that is nearly as high as that in 10- to 14-year-olds [10]. The incidence rate increases from birth to peak at around puberty (Figure 3.1) and in most populations is lower among 15- to 29-year-olds than among 0- to 14-year-olds [11–15]. In some populations there seems to be a second rise in incidence after the age of about 25–30 years [16–18].

In the Swedish nationwide prospective incidence study of 15- to 34-year-olds, 78% of the newly diagnosed patients were classified as having T1DM and 15% as having type 2 diabetes mellitus (T2DM) at the time of the diagnosis [19]. The follow-up showed that 92% of patients diagnosed before 30 years of age were treated with insulin at a later date [20]. These findings are consistent with recent incidence data from Finland among 15- to 39-year-olds [21,22]. In these studies, the incidence of T2DM exceeded that of T1DM by the age of about 30 years. By contrast, in Turin, Italy, which has a much lower incidence of T1DM, the incidence of T2DM is about three times higher than that of T1DM at the age of 30 years [16]. Although beyond the scope of this chapter, it is important to consider the possible clinical heterogeneity and increasing difficulty of classification of diabetes with increasing

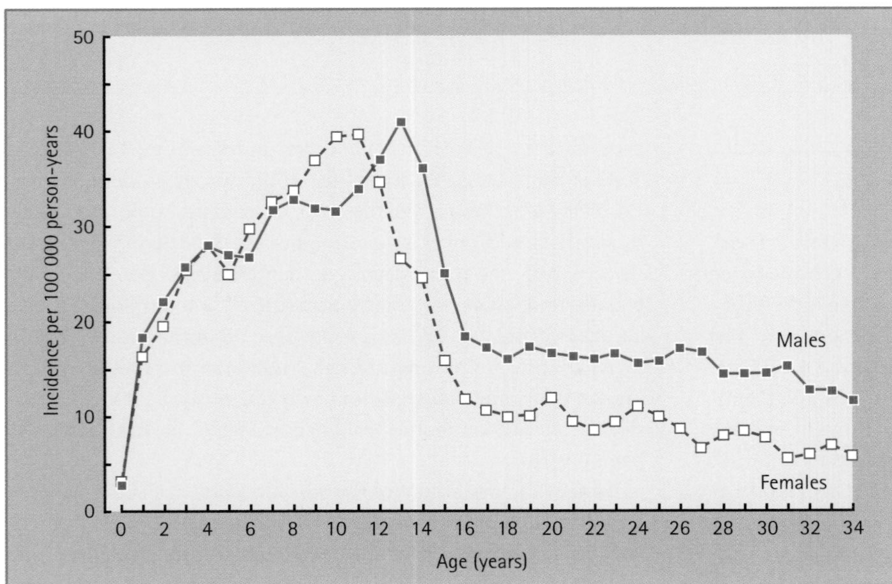

Figure 3.1 Incidence rate of type 1 diabetes per 100 000/year in Swedish males and females by age during 1983–1998. Reproduced from Pundziute-Lyckå *et al.* [14], with permission from Springer-Verlag.

age [23,24]. A proportion of the apparent heterogeneity may represent extremes within a continuum, although there is a need for more data in this field [24].

There is a lack of population-based incidence data for age groups above 35 years of age. The only published population-based incidence studies covering the incidence of T1DM over the whole age span is one from Rochester, Minnesota, 1945–1969 [25] and from Denmark, 1973–1977 [26]. The latter study indicated that the cumulative probability of developing T1DM before age 80 years is in the range of 1–1.5%.

Incidence by sex

The peak in incidence rate among children occurs slightly earlier in girls than boys (Figure 3.1), suggesting an influence of puberty. During the 1970s there was a male excess of T1DM in children in populations of European origin and a female excess in populations of African and Asian origin [27]; however, during the early 1990s, the sex-specific pattern in incidence among children changed towards more modest differences. Of 112 centers with data during 1990–1999, only six showed a significantly excess of females (Beijing, Hong Kong and Zunyi in China, New South Wales in Australia, Puerto Rico and the Afro-American ethnic group in the USA) and six centers showed a significant male excess (West Bulgaria, Finland, Attica in Greece, Switzerland, Oxford in the UK and the Dominican Republic), and all differences were generally of modest magnitude [6]. The general impression is still that it is the high incidence countries that tend to have a slight male excess, while the opposite is seen in low incidence countries. Many studies have shown a male excess in the incidence of T1DM among young adults [15,28]. While the male : female ratio among children in most populations is 0.9–1.1 [6], the male : female ratio among young adults ranges from about 1.3 up to 2.0 in many populations [15,28].

Incidence by country

The incidence rate of T1DM among childhood populations shows a vast geographic variation worldwide (Figure 3.2) [6–8,29]. Over the period 1990–1999, the age-adjusted incidence rate of T1DM ranged globally from 0.1 in Zunyi (China) and Caracas (Venezuela) to 37.8 in Sardinia and 40.9 per 100 000/year in Finland [6]. The most recent data from Finland indicate an incidence rate of nearly 60 per 100 000 in 2006 [10], the highest incidence ever recorded.

European countries are well represented with registries, and there is an approximately 10-fold difference between highest and lowest incidence countries in Europe [7], with the apparently lowest rate of 3.6 per 100 000/year in Macedonia during 1989–1994. Sweden has a high incidence rate (30 per 100 000/years). Centers from France and mainland Italy, for instance, report intermediate incidence rates around 10 per 100 000/year, while some other European countries have intermediate to high incidence rates [6]. In general, the incidence rates are low in eastern European countries, although the most recent EURODIAB data show that for several countries where the incidence rate previously was below 10 per 100 000/year, the incidence rate during 1999–2003 has increased to 10 per 100 000/year or more, for example in Lithuania, Bucharest in Romania and in Katowice in Poland [8].

Standardized data for the age group 15–29 years from European centers (in Belgium, Lithuania, Romania, Sardinia, Slovakia, Spain, Sweden and the UK) during 1996–1997 showed incidence rates between 5 and 12 per 100 000/year [15]. Incidence rates among 15- to 29-year-olds within this range have also been reported, albeit from earlier time periods, in other European centers, such as 5.5 per 100 000/year in Rzeszow, Poland, 1980–1992 [30], appproximately 7 per 100 000/year in Turin, mainland Italy 1984–1991 [16,31] and approximately 13 per 100 000/year in two regions of Denmark, 1970–1976 [11].

While Sweden and Sardinia have higher incidence rates among children, the incidence rate among young adults was not much higher in Sardinia and Sweden than the other centers in the multicenter study [15]. Older data from Norway (1978–1982) [13] indicated a higher incidence rate of 17 per 100 000/year and recent data from Finland (1992–2001) [21] indicated an incidence rate of 18 per 100 000/year among 15- to 29-year-olds. Differences between countries in the incidence among young adults should be interpreted with caution until more data are collected using comparable methodology.

The USA is represented with the data collected during the 1990s from Allegheny County in Pennsylvania, Chicago and Jefferson County in Alabama, with incidence rates in the range 11–18 per 100 000/year among children. Alberta and Calgary in Canada had slightly higher rates (about 23 per 100 000/year; Figure 3.2) [6], while the data from the Avalon Peninsula, Newfoundland, indicated a higher incidence rate of 35.9 per 100 000/year [32].

In South America, children in centers in Venezuela, Paraguay and Colombia had incidence rates of less than 1 per 100 000/year, Chile (Santiago) had around 4 per 100 000/year, while Argentina and Brazil had an average of around 8 per 100 000/year. Many centers in Central America and the West Indies (except Puerto Rico and St. Thomas) generally have low to intermediate incidence rates, with indications of decreasing time trends [6].

Data from New Zealand and parts of Australia show moderate to high incidence rates (15–25 per 100 000/year) among children [6]. Data from other Pacific Island countries are lacking, and would be difficult to interpret because the populations in most island countries are small. In Asia, the mean incidence rate among the 23 centers in China during the early 1990s was 0.8 per 100 000/years. Japan has a slightly higher average incidence rate of 1.7 per 100 000/year among three centers, while Kuwait stands out with a high incidence rate of 22 per 100 000/year.

There is limited information on the incidence rate of T1DM from sub-Saharan Africa [33]. The five DIAMOND centers are all in North Africa (Algeria, Libya, Sudan and Tunisia) or Mauritius, an island off the coast of Madagascar. Incidence rates reported from these centers range from low to intermediate, but these countries cannot be said to be representative of Africa.

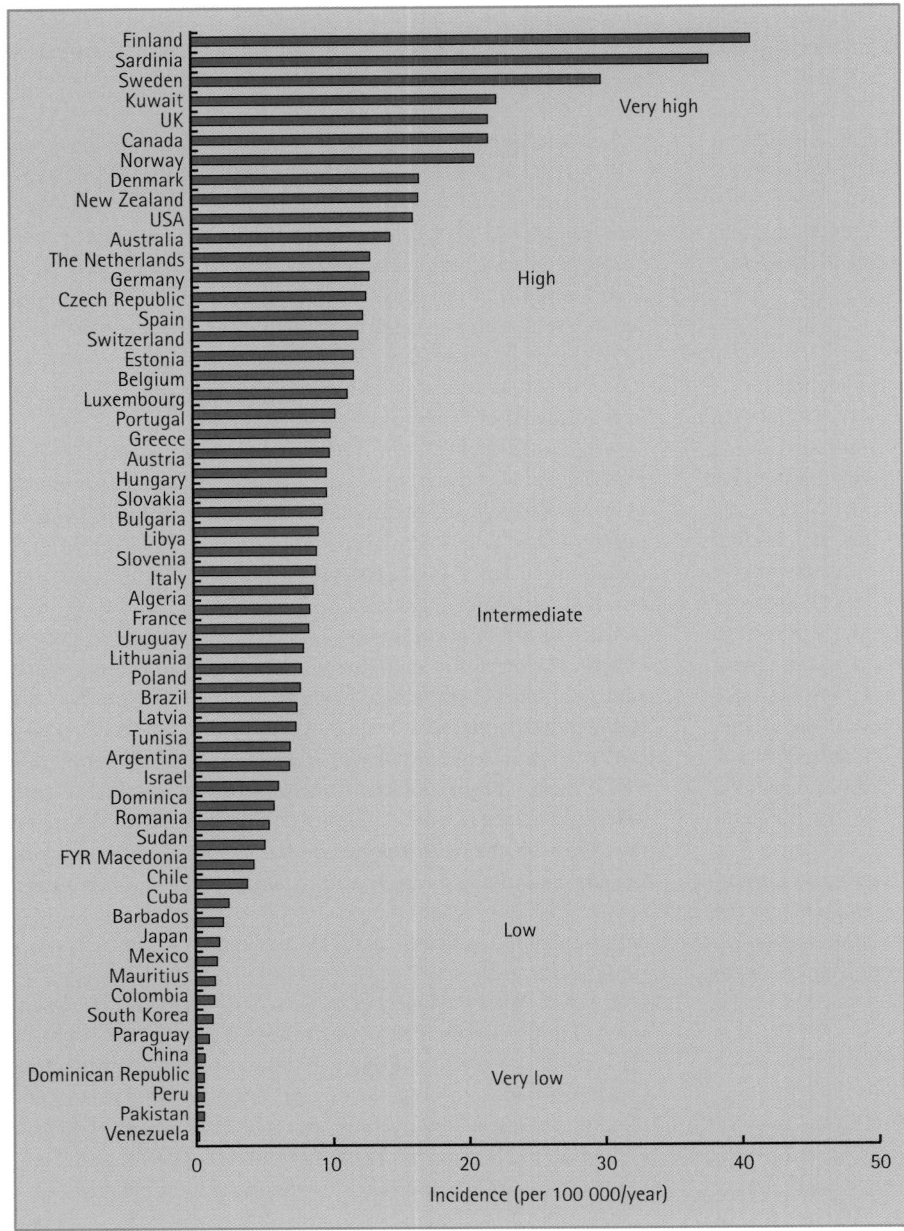

Figure 3.2 Geographic variation in childhood onset type 1 diabetes incidence rates, 1990–1999. Note that most registries were not nationwide and that several countries display within-country variation. Reproduced from the Diamond Project Group [6] with permission from John Wiley & Sons Ltd, Chichester.

Variation in incidence within countries, including by ethnic group

In several countries, marked within-country variations in the incidence rate of T1DM have been reported. For instance, up to 1.5-fold differences have been described within relatively homogenous populations, such as Finland, Sweden and Norway [34–36]. In Italy, the incidence rate among children in Sardinia 1990–1999 (38 per 100 000/year) was three to six times higher than the average in mainland Italy, where the incidence rates vary twofold from 6.3 in Campania to 12.2 per 100 000/year in Pavia in the same period [37]. In China, there was a 12-fold geographic variation (0.13–1.61 per 100 000), generally with higher incidence in the north and the east. In addition, there was a sixfold difference between the Mongol (1.82 per 100 000) and the Zhuang (0.32 per 100 000/year) ethnic groups [38].

The variation in incidence within some countries may in part be because of ethnic heterogeneity of populations. For instance, the 1.5-fold higher incidence among children in the South Island of New Zealand compared with that in the North Island was largely explained by the 4.5 times higher incidence among children of European origin compared to that among Maoris [39].

Several methodological problems arise when making inferences based on epidemiologic studies of different ethnic groups and immigrants. These include differential ascertainment and

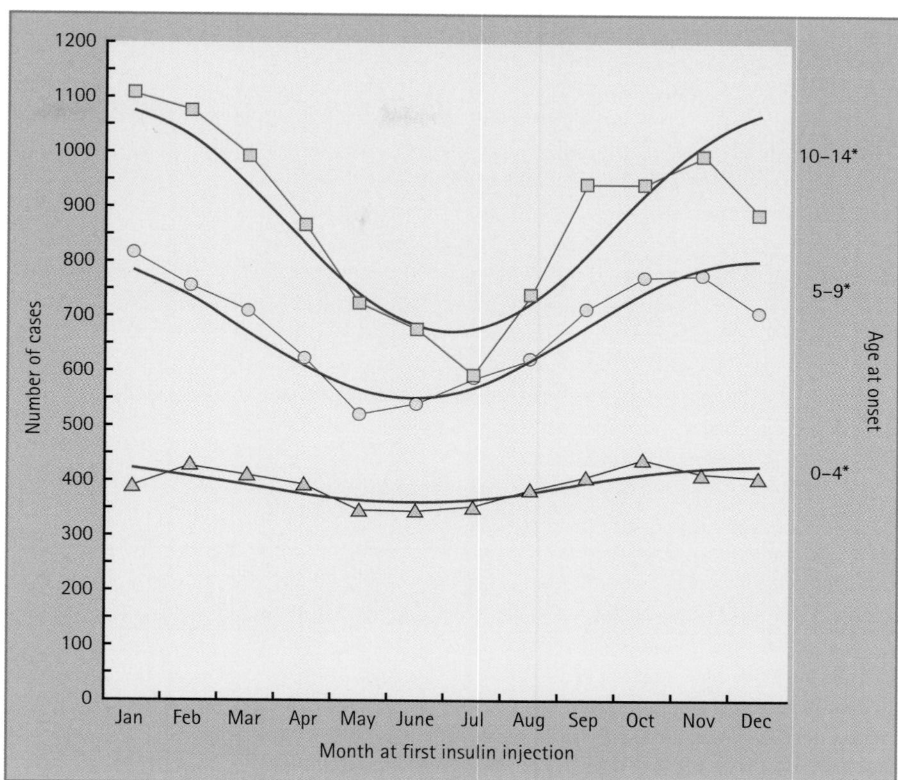

Figure 3.3 Seasonal variation in diagnosis of type 1 diabetes among >22 000 children diagnosed 1989–1998 in European centers, by age at onset. *Age (years) at first unsulin injection. Reproduced from Green & Patterson [7], with permission from Springer-Verlag.

definition of ethnic group, underestimation of the base population in some ethnic groups, genetic admixture and possible heterogeneity in clinical presentation [24,40,41]. Among childhood onset cases, however, it seems that the large majority, even in Japan [42], have classic autoimmune T1DM. Historically, the incidence of T1DM has been higher in populations of European origin, particularly those living in Europe, than that among populations of non-European origin [40,41]. Despite the previously reported lower incidence among African-American and Latino populations in the USA, the incidence among these groups in the USA seems currently not very different from children of European origin in the USA [6,41]. The incidence rates of T1DM in most South American studies with standardized registries seems to be much lower than that among Latino people in the USA and lower than that among Spaniards living in Spain [40].

The incidence of T1DM among children of immigrant parents to Germany, Sweden and mainland Italy has been shown to correlate with the incidence in the country or region of origin of their parents, whether the incidence in the country of origin is higher or lower [43–45]; however, the incidence among immigrants from Pakistan to the UK (or their children) is similar to that among the native Britons [46,47], despite the very much lower incidence recorded in Karachi, Pakistan [6].

In summary, although there are clear ethnic differences in incidence rate of T1DM and strong evidence for a role of genetic factors, some of the abovementioned studies also support a role for yet unidentified environmental factors.

Seasonal variation in diagnosis of T1DM

Several studies have reported a peak in the number of cases diagnosed in the autumn and winter, and a smaller proportion of the cases diagnosed in the spring or summer, consistent both in the northern and southern hemispheres [7,12]. Although reasonably consistent, there is some variation in exact peak and nadir between countries, age groups, sexes and periods. Generally, the degree of seasonal variation is stronger among those diagnosed at age 10–14 years than in younger children (Figure 3.3) [7]. Different methods have been used in the analysis of seasonal variations, and often with data covering relatively short periods of time and limited number of cases; the results are therefore not necessarily comparable. Interpretation of seasonal variation must be carried out in light of the long and variable preclinical period in T1DM, and it is speculated that viral or other periodic factors have a role in the timing of the precipitation or onset of the disease in susceptible individuals who would develop it sooner or later.

Trends in incidence over time

The methodology for population-based incidence registries was not standardized until the late 1980s, but a number of older data sources have been reviewed to assess possible time trends. There is a general impression that the incidence of T1DM increased strongly after the middle of the 20th century [48,49], although in Denmark, the incidence among 0- to 29-year-olds seemed stable from 1924 to the 1970s [11]. An analysis of incidence trends of

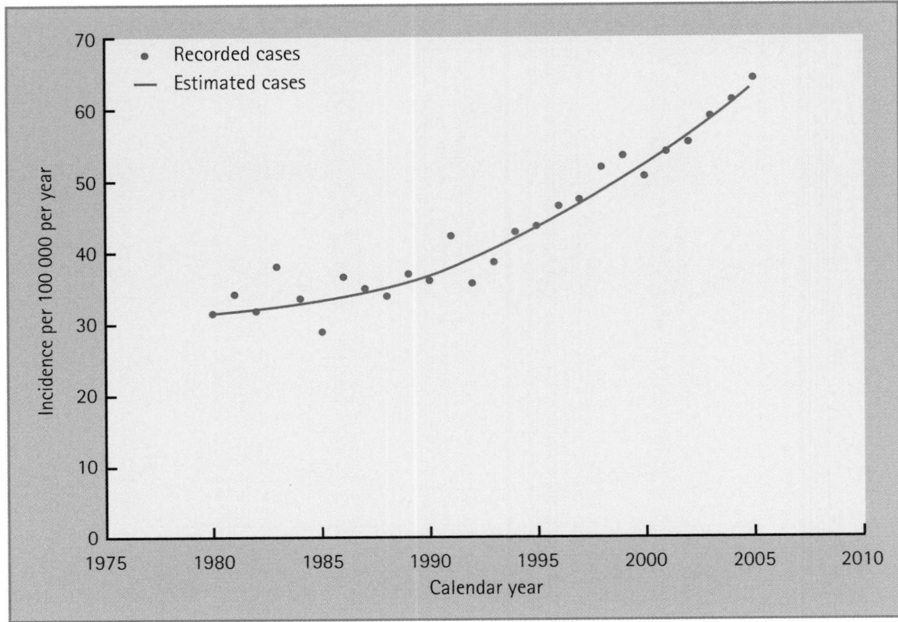

Figure 3.4 Time trend in incidence rate of type 1 diabetes diagnosed before 15 years of age in Finland. Reproduced from Harjutsalo *et al.* [10], with permission from Elsevier.

more standardized registry data from 1960 to 1996 in 37 populations worldwide showed a significant increase in incidence rate over time in the majority of populations, with a steeper relative increase in low-incidence than in high-incidence populations [50]. In Finland, the incidence rate has increased linearly from the mid 1960s to the mid 1990s [51] and thereafter even more steeply, reaching almost 60 per 100 000/year in 2006 (Figure 3.4) [10].

In the 103 centers participating in the WHO DIAMOND project for at least 3 years during 1990–1999, the overall relative increase in incidence rate was 2.8% per year [6]. By continent, overall increasing trends per year were estimated at 5.3% in North America, 3.2% in Europe and 4.0% in Asia [6]. The only region with an overall decreasing trend was Central America and the West Indies [6].

In general, the increasing trend appeared to be strongest in the centers with high and very high incidence rates during the 1990s. In the centers with low and very low incidence rates, there were no significant increases in incidence rates over time. However, the 15-year (1989–2003) time trends in Europe reported to EURODIAB indicated an overall mean increase in incidence rate of 3.9% per year, with a tendency towards stronger relative increases in the countries with lowest average incidence rates during the first 5 years (1989–1994) [8].

Overall, the relative increase over time during the 1990s among the DIAMOND centers was most pronounced in the younger age group: 4.0% among 0- to 4-year-olds, 3.0% in the 5- to 9-year-olds and 2.1% in the 10- to 14-year-olds, similar for boys and girls in most centers. The pattern of a steeper relative increase among the youngest was seen in Europe and Oceania, but not in Asia and North America [6]. A smaller relative increase in incidence rate over time among older individuals than among younger ones has also been seen in European studies covering wider age ranges [14,17,18,52,53]. This latter observation is in line with a model where a certain pool of genetically susceptible individuals contract the disease at younger ages [14,17,54]. The few available data, however, are not entirely consistent with this idea. An increasing incidence rate has been seen also among older age groups in some populations [18,22,31], but the lack of standardized incidence data covering the whole age range makes it difficult to draw firm conclusions. Note that despite the time trends indicated in Sweden with decreasing average age of onset, the peak incidence rate remained around the age of puberty [14].

Familial clustering and twin studies

Besides providing clues regarding the relative importance of genetic and non-genetic factors in the etiology of disease, data on risk of T1DM among people with affected relatives may also aid the clinician in counseling of family members of newly diagnosed patients. Around 80–90% of newly diagnosed T1DM patients do not have any affected siblings or parents, but first-degree relatives of a person with T1DM are at increased risk. By the age of 20 years, approximately 4–6% of siblings of T1DM probands have been reported to develop T1DM in European origin populations [55–57], compared with around 0.2–1.0% in the corresponding background populations. The offspring of affected fathers have

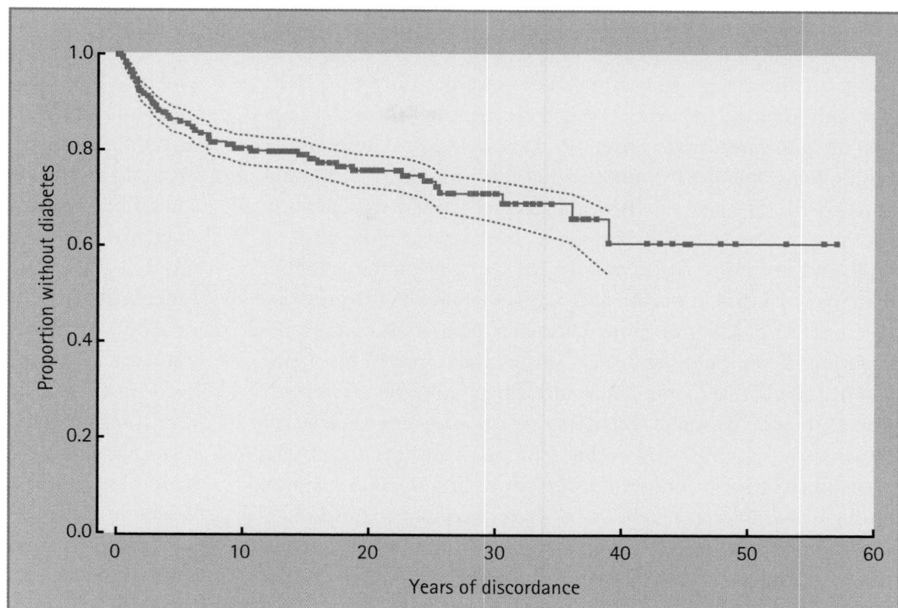

Figure 3.5 Diabetes-free survival in non-diabetic monozygotic twins whose co-twin had type 1 diabetes, after several years of follow-up. Dotted lines represent 95% confidence intervals. Reproduced from Redondo *et al.* [63], with permission from Springer-Verlag.

1.5–3 times increased risk of T1DM compared with the offspring of affected mothers [58,59]. By 20 years of age, 5–8% of the offspring of men with diabetes, but only 2–5% of the offspring of women with diabetes have been found to be affected. There is currently no accepted explanation for this phenomenon.

Given the well-established effect of genetic factors, there is no surprise that the concordance rate for T1DM in monozygotic (MZ) twins is much higher than that in dizygotic (DZ) twins [60,61]. In one study from North America, the estimated cumulative risk 10 years after onset in the proband (diagnosed before age 40 years) was about 25% in MZ twins and about 11% in DZ twins [62]. Corresponding 10-year cumulative risks from Finland were estimated to 32% for MZ twins and 3.2% for DZ twins [61]. Comparable estimates were also found in the Danish twin registry, although the exact age at onset was not known in this study [60]. In general, the risk for the co-twins was higher and the discordance time shorter the earlier the onset in the proband [61–63]. In a long-term follow-up of discordant MZ twins from the USA and the UK, more than 50% of MZ pairs remained discordant for T1DM (Figure 3.5) [63]. Because MZ twins share 100% of their genomic DNA, this suggests that genetic susceptibility is in most cases not sufficient for the development of disease.

Despite the relatively high proportion of MZ twins being discordant for clinical T1DM, many of the non-diabetic co-twins of patients with T1DM develop islet autoimmunity [64]. Together with the limited variation in prevalence of positivity for islet autoantibodies between countries [54] and animal studies suggesting a two-stage disease process [65], this supports the idea that environmental factors may have a more important role in the progression from islet autoimmunity to overt disease.

Environmental risk factors for T1DM: clues from epidemiologic studies

The time trends described above must be ascribed to some change in the environment, even in the event that the increase is brought about by a change in the age distribution. Some of the variation in incidence rate between European countries can be explained by differences in the frequency of HLA susceptibility genotypes [66], but clearly not all [67]. It has recently been suggested that the proportion of newly diagnosed patients with T1DM who carry the highest risk genotype (DR3-DQ2/DR4-DQ8) has decreased over time (reviewed in [68]). It may be speculated that increased exposure to some risk factor or decreased exposure to some protective factor have caused more individuals with moderate risk ("permissive") genotypes (e.g. either DR3-DQ2 or DR4-DQ8, but not both) to develop T1DM in recent years. Although there is overwhelming evidence for an essential role of genetic factors in the etiology of T1DM, available evidence strongly suggests that one or more non-genetic factors are also involved; however, the nature of these putative factors are not well known.

In general, environmental factors may be envisioned to have a role in the following:

1 Initiating of the autoimmune disease process;

2 Modulating the progression from islet autoimmunity to clinical T1DM; or

3 "Precipitating" disease in individuals with advanced preclinical disease.

Little is known about the initiation of autoimmunity in humans [69], but some form of immune-mediated mechanism leading to the breakdown of self-tolerance is likely to be involved. Limited geographic variation in the prevalence of islet autoimmunity despite the large differences in incidence of T1DM between countries suggests a major importance of environmental factors in the progression from islet autoimmunity to T1DM [54], although the hypothesis that there are environmental triggers of autoimmunity cannot be discarded [70]. Responsible factors may operate by modulating the immune system and metabolism. *In vitro* experiments have suggested that actively insulin-secreting β-cells hyperexpress islet autoantigens such as GAD, and are more susceptible to toxic effects of the cytokine interleukin 1β (71). It may be speculated that factors that increase the stress on β-cells may non-specifically contribute to the precipitation of clinical disease [71]. This includes insulin resistance or other mechanisms implied in infections, puberty and growth spurts. Insulin resistance is not easy to measure reliably in humans, but several studies have found measures of insulin resistance relative to first-phase insulin response to an intravenous glucose tolerance test to be predictive of progression to T1DM (reviewed in [72]). Below, some of the most frequently studied non-genetic factors with a potential role in the etiology of human T1DM are discussed.

Specific putative environmental factors

Viral infections

There is a large body of literature linking infections and T1DM, ranging from *in vitro* studies [73], experiments with various animal models [74], clinical and pathologic studies of patients with disease [73,75–77] and epidemiologic case–control and cohort studies [12,70,78]. Congenital rubella syndrome (CRS) has been associated with a several-fold increase in the incidence of T1DM [79]. Although not contributing to the incidence of T1DM in most countries today, this observation has been cited as a proof of principle that intrauterine factors and viral infections in general can influence the risk of T1DM in humans. It probably remains the best example of a non-genetic factor contributing to increased risk of T1DM in humans, but the consistency of the available evidence and the absolute risk associated with CRS may have been overstated [80,81].

Several early studies based on assays for antibodies to enteroviruses in cases with T1DM and controls initially seemed promising, but systematic review of the data showed too much heterogeneity in methodology and results to draw any conclusion [78]. Prospective study design and detection of enterovirus RNA represent important contributions to the methodology of such studies in recent years. Increased risk of childhood onset T1DM has been associated with evidence of maternal enterovirus infections during pregnancy in some studies, but not in all [82]. Using both serum enterovirus antibodies and RNA as indications of postnatal infection, independent prospective studies from Finland have found enterovirus to be associated with increased risk of islet autoimmunity and T1DM [70], while other similar studies have not found any significant association [83]. A recent immunohistochemical study of stored sections of pancreatic biopsies obtained postmortem in young individuals with recent onset T1DM found that the β-cells of multiple islets stained positive for enterovirus capsid protein VP1 in 44 of 72 cases. Very few of the controls in that study stained positive [77]. This study substantiated previous evidence based on one or a few patients [73,74] and indicated problems with the methods used in a previous study of a similar material where no such evidence was found [84]. Nevertheless, to confirm these findings in the future, *in situ* hybridization should be used to assess the presence of enterovirus RNA (rather than protein) in a larger number of islets from people with recent onset T1DM and the lack thereof in appropriate controls. Enterovirus infections are common and there is evidence that the frequency of infection has decreased with improved hygiene in the recent decades, opposite to the trend seen for T1DM. It has been postulated that the increasing incidence of T1DM in children may in part be explained by decreased protection from maternal enterovirus antibodies [85]. A more direct test of this hypothesis is still lacking.

The so-called "hygiene hypothesis" comes in different versions but essentially proposes that the decline in microbial exposure in many populations over the past few decades has caused the concomitant increase in incidence of immune-mediated diseases including T1DM [86]. Some infections and microbial agents reduce the incidence of autoimmune diabetes in experimental animals [74]. Epidemiologic studies have investigated non-specific infections and infectious symptoms, but the results have been inconsistent. Daycare attendance is usually associated with increased exposure to microbial agents, and a recent meta-analysis concluded that there is some evidence for a lower risk of T1DM among children who attended daycare centers early in life, but the results were not sufficiently homogenous to allow a strong conclusion [87].

There are many promising observations supporting a possible role of viral infections in the etiology of T1DM, but the current evidence that infections have an important and causal role in human T1DM is not conclusive. Although the problem of identifying the potential strain of enterovirus that might be diabetogenic would pose an additional problem, vaccine development towards such a strain might be envisioned in the future as a preventive measure, but it is currently unknown whether or when this could be feasible.

Toxins

The rodenticide Vacor has been associated with T1DM in humans after ingestion of large doses [88]. There are structural and mechanistic similarities between Vacor and streptozotocin and alloxan [88], which are specifically toxic to β-cells, and used to induce diabetes in experimental animals [88,89]. Some epidemiologic studies have assessed intake of nitrates and nitrites, which may be converted to related N-nitroso-compounds, but most studies have used ecologic study designs and assessed levels in community drinking water, which is probably a poor indicator of total exposure. A potential diabetogenic role of *in utero* exposure to bafilomycin, a toxin produced by bacteria growing on the skin of root vegetables such as potatoes, has been suggested based on experiments with rodents and *in vitro* studies [90]. In a prospective study there was no support for the idea that frequent potato consumption during pregnancy could increase the risk of islet autoimmunity in the offspring, but it is unknown whether frequency of potato intake really is a marker for bafilomycin exposure [91]. In conclusion, there is little direct evidence for a widespread role of toxins in human T1DM, but this may reflect the lack of well-conducted studies.

Nutritional factors

Several possible plausible mechanisms have been proposed to link dietary factors to T1DM, including "molecular mimicry" and a detrimental effect of bovine insulin in cow's milk (reviewed in [92]). A reduced risk conferred by prolonged breastfeeding and/or delayed introduction of cow's milk has been suggested in many case–control studies, but most of these studies were susceptible to recall bias and the issue is controversial [93]. In the largest prospective study to date involving multiple islet autoantibodies or T1DM as the endpoint, there was no significant association with duration of exclusive or total breastfeeding [94]. Duration of breastfeeding was also not associated with self-reported T1DM up to age 30 years in a recent prospective study including 61 cases [95]. It is hoped that an ongoing randomized controlled trial (TRIGR) will provide an answer to whether delayed introduction of cow's milk protein can reduce the risk of islet autoimmunity and T1DM [96]. Two prospective studies of islet autoimmunity have provided some evidence for a role of age at introduction of cereals or gluten [97,98], although the relation is complex and difficult to interpret.

The immunomodulatory effects of vitamin D and preventive effect of pharmacologic (hypercalcemic) doses of 1,25-dihydroxyvitamin D on diabetes development in experimental animals have been documented in several studies [99]. Systemic concentration of 1,25-dihydroxyvitamin D is tightly controlled by hydroxylation of 25-hydroxyvitamin D, and this must be taken into account when evaluating experimental results from animal models. Vitamin D is also produced in the skin upon exposure to ultraviolet light, and no prospective study has yet been published of serum 25-hydroxyvitamin D, which is an established marker of vitamin D status, and risk of T1DM. A multicenter case–control study found a significantly lower risk of T1DM associated with reported use of vitamin D supplement in early life [100], although recall and selection bias may have affected these findings; however, this was also supported by a prospective Finnish study [101]. Prospective studies of maternal intake of vitamin D via food during pregnancy and risk of islet autoimmunity in children have not produced convincing evidence for any relation [102].

A case–control study in Norway found an association between use of cod liver oil in the first year of life and lower risk of T1DM [103]. Cod liver oil, which is commonly used in Norway, is an important source of both vitamin D and long-chain n-3 fatty acids docosahexaenoic acid (DHA) and eicosapentaenoic acid (EPA) in this population. The lack of association with other vitamin D supplements in these studies supports a role of n-3 fatty acids rather than vitamin D. Although recall bias cannot entirely be ruled out from the latter study, support for the hypothesis that intake of dietary n-3 fatty acids may prevent islet autoimmunity and/or T1DM recently came from a prospective study including both dietary assessment and analysis of fatty acid composition of red cell membranes, which is a biomarker of n-3 fatty acid status [104]. Plans are underway to initiate a randomized intervention trial to prevent islet autoimmunity and/or T1DM using DHA supplements.

Despite previous indications from two prospective studies that serum alfa-tocopherol (vitamin E) could be associated with lower risk of T1DM, there was no association with advanced islet autoimmunity or T1DM in early life in the DIPP study [105]. In conclusion, the role of nutritional factors in T1DM remains uncertain.

Perinatal factors and postnatal growth

Offspring of non-diabetic mothers aged 35 years or more when giving birth have an approximately 20–30% increased risk compared with offspring of mothers who are 25 years or less [106–108]. Results for birth order and for paternal age have been less consistent [106,108]. Birth by cesarean section was recently associated with an approximately 20% increased risk of T1DM in children according to meta-analysis of 20 published studies [109]. Although there is some potential for selection bias in the case–control studies included, and the mechanism is unknown, it was speculated that delayed colonization of the infant's intestine associated with cesarean section may be involved.

Increased birth weight has been associated with a relatively weak but significant increase in risk of childhood onset T1DM in large cohort studies based on linkage of population registries, independent of maternal diabetes and other potential confounders [108,110–112]. There are also studies reporting no significant association, but these were generally smaller case–control studies. The association seems in most cases to be independent of gestational age. Indirect data suggest that the association with birth weight may in part be explained by HLA genes [113], but a study directly testing this idea found that this was not the case [114]. Birth weight is certainly only a marker of some other phenomenon and the mechanisms involved remain to be defined.

Associated factors such as postnatal growth or excess body weight might be of relevance. A number of studies have indicated that children developing T1DM are taller, heavier or gain more weight or height prior to diagnosis compared to their peers [95,115–121]. Because of the numerous size and growth variables included and the various methods of analysis used in these studies, a systematic review of the consistency of these associations is warranted.

In summary, environmental factors may influence individuals quite differently, depending on the genetic background, although direct evidence for specific gene–environment interactions from humans is scarce [80]. No specific single factor has been identified thus far. Taking into account the multifactorial nature of T1DM, specific environmental risk factors with sufficiently large impact to be of clinical importance and detectable in epidemiologic studies may not exist; however, identification of potential environmental risk factors and their role in the disease process is important in the potential prevention of T1DM in the future, and lack of consistent findings may reflect lack of properly conducted prospective studies. There are several randomized controlled trials ongoing with various interventions that are aiming at reducing the risk of islet autoimmunity or progression from islet autoimmunity to T1DM (see the first part of Chapter 9). Given the enormous amount of resources necessary for such efforts and the negative results of completed trials, it may be wise to initiate such trials based on consistent findings from properly conducted prospective observational studies. The large multicenter longitudinal TEDDY study may contribute towards this goal (http://www.niddk.nih.gov/patient/teddy/teddy.htm).

Mortality

Before the discovery of insulin in 1922, T1DM meant an almost certain death soon after its onset. After the initiation of insulin replacement therapy, a dramatic improvement in survival occurred [122]. Another major improvement in survival occurred in cases of diabetes diagnosed in the 1950s [123]; however, even today T1DM is associated with an approximately 2- to 10-fold excess risk of premature mortality [121,124–128]. A large variation in relative mortality has been reported from different countries. For instance, the standardized mortality ratio (SMR) for patients with T1DM in Finland was lower than that in Lithuania, Estonia and in Japan [129,130]. A higher mortality in African-American compared to white patients with T1DM in the USA has been reported, and this difference seems to be attributable to acute complications [131].

Recent data from Europe showed that the short-term mortality was two times higher in patients followed from diagnosis of T1DM in childhood than the respective general populations, with variation in the SMR from about 1.1 to 4.7 in different countries [128]. In a nationwide cohort of patients with T1DM in Norway followed from onset before 15 years of age and up to 30 years' duration (mean 24.2 years), the SMR was 4.0 [126]. In a UK cohort of more than 7000 prevalent cases of T1DM with mean age of 33 years at baseline, the SMR after up to 7 years of follow-up (mean 4.5 years) was 3.7 [125]. Many studies have reported that the SMR varies with age and with diabetes duration, or both, but results are not consistent among studies [122].

Ascertainment of cause of death is difficult, but around one-third of the early deaths in the recent European multicenter study were clearly attributable to diabetic ketoacidosis (DKA), while about half of the relatively few deaths among young people with T1DM seems to be unrelated to diabetes [127,128]. Hypoglycemia as a cause of death is currently rare compared to DKA, but potentially increasing because of the more vigorous glycemic control suggested for the prevention of long-term complications [132]. After about 10–15 years of diabetes duration, microvascular and macrovascular chronic diabetes complications start to make an impact, and after about 30 years of age cardiovascular causes become increasingly important. The relative mortality from cardiovascular causes is at least as high for women as for men. SMRs for cardiovascular causes of death of 8–40 have been reported in patients with T1DM, and it depends strongly on nephropathy (reviewed in [133]).

There is growing evidence that better glycemic control and improved risk factor control such as lowering of blood pressure and lipids is associated with reduced risk of late complications and improved survival (reviewed in [122,133]). The trend in mortality among patients with long-term T1DM seems to be improving [122], but there is a paucity of large cohorts with long-term follow-up of incident cases of T1DM covering long time periods to assess general trends after the late 1980s. Another challenge is the continued deaths of undiagnosed cases of T1DM and patients without access to care in the developing world.

Conclusions

T1DM is one of the most common chronic diseases diagnosed in childhood, but the disease can occur at any age. Its incidence varies drastically between populations and even within populations. T1DM has a strong genetic component and familial clustering, but the majority of cases have no affected siblings or parents. Only a minority of carriers of the susceptibility genes develop T1DM. The incidence of T1DM is increasing in most studied populations at an average rate of approximately 3–4% per year. The causes of this increase are not known. It is believed that some environmental factors may have contributed to it, but no definite causal environmental factor for autoimmune T1DM has yet been identified.

T1DM was a fatal disease before the insulin era. Although mortality in patients with diabetes has drastically decreased, both acute and late complications lead to increased morbidity and premature mortality in T1DM. Primary prevention of T1DM would be the only solution to these problems, but unfortunately no practical preventive measures are currently available.

Acknowledgment

We would like to apologize to the authors of the many original papers we were unable to cite because of space limitations.

References

1 Eisenbarth GS. Update in type 1 diabetes. *J Clin Endocrinol Metab* 2007; **92**:2403–2407.

2 World Health Organization (WHO). *Definition, diagnosis and classification of diabetes mellitus and its complications: report of a*

WHO consultation. Part 1: Diagnosis and classification of diabetes mellitus. Geneva: WHO, 1999.

3 Wenzlau JM, Juhl K, Yu L, Moua O, Sarkar SA, Gottlieb P, *et al.* The cation efflux transporter ZnT8 (Slc30A8) is a major autoantigen in human type 1 diabetes. *Proc Natl Acad Sci USA* 2007; **104**:17040–17045.

4 Undlien DE, Lie BA, Thorsby E. HLA complex genes in type 1 diabetes and other autoimmune diseases: which genes are involved? *Trends Genet* 2001; **17**:93–100.

5 Todd JA, Walker NM, Cooper JD, Smyth DJ, Downes K, Plagnol V, *et al.* Robust associations of four new chromosome regions from genome-wide analyses of type 1 diabetes. *Nat Genet* 2007; **39**:857–864.

6 DIAMOND Project Group. Incidence and trends of childhood type 1 diabetes worldwide 1990–1999. *Diabet Med* 2006; **23**:857–866.

7 Green A, Patterson CC. Trends in the incidence of childhood-onset diabetes in Europe 1989–1998. *Diabetologia* 2001; **44**(Suppl 3):B3–B8.

8 Patterson CC, Dahlquist G, Gyürüs E, Green A, Soltesz G; EURODIAB Study Group. Incidence trends for childhood type 1 diabetes in Europe during 1989–2003 and predicted new cases 2005–20: a multicentre prospective registration study. *Lancet* 2009; **373**:2027–2033.

9 LaPorte RE, McCarty D, Bruno G, Tajima N, Baba S. Counting diabetes in the next millennium: application of capture–recapture technology. *Diabetes Care* 1993; **16**:528–534.

10 Harjutsalo V, Sjöberg L, Tuomilehto J. Time trends in the incidence of type 1 diabetes in Finnish children: a cohort study. *Lancet* 2008; **371**:1777–1782.

11 Christau B, Kromann H, Christy M, Andersen OO, Nerup J. Incidence of insulin-dependent diabetes mellitus (0–29 years at onset) in Denmark. *Acta Med Scand Suppl* 1979; **624**:54–60.

12 Gamble DR. The epidemiology of insulin dependent diabetes, with particular reference to the relationship of virus infection to its etiology. *Epidemiol Rev* 1980; **2**:49–70.

13 Joner G, Søvik O. The incidence of type 1 (insulin-dependent) diabetes mellitus 15-29 years in Norway 1978–1982. *Diabetologia* 1991; **34**:271–274.

14 Pundziute-Lyckå A, Dahlquist G, Nyström L, Arnqvist H, Björk E, Blohmé G, *et al.* The incidence of type I diabetes has not increased but shifted to a younger age at diagnosis in the 0–34 years group in Sweden 1983 to 1998. *Diabetologia* 2002; **45**:783–791.

15 Kyvik KO, Nystrom L, Gorus F, Songini M, Oestman J, Castell C, *et al.* The epidemiology of type 1 diabetes mellitus is not the same in young adults as in children. *Diabetologia* 2004; **47**:377–384.

16 Bruno G, Runzo C, Cavallo-Perin P, Merletti F, Rivetti M, Pinach S, *et al.* Incidence of type 1 and type 2 diabetes in adults aged 30–49 years: the population-based registry in the province of Turin, Italy. *Diabetes Care* 2005; **28**:2613–2619.

17 Weets I, De Leeuw IH, Du Caju MV, Rooman R, Keymeulen B, Mathieu C, *et al.* The incidence of type 1 diabetes in the age group 0–39 years has not increased in Antwerp (Belgium) between 1989 and 2000: evidence for earlier disease manifestation. *Diabetes Care* 2002; **25**:840–846.

18 Pundziute-Lyckå A, Urbonaite B, Ostrauskas R, Zalinkevicius R, Dahlquist GG. Incidence of type 1 diabetes in Lithuanians aged 0–39 years varies by the urban–rural setting, and the time change differs for men and women during 1991–2000. *Diabetes Care* 2003; **26**:671–676.

19 Arnqvist HJ, Littorin B, Nyström L, Scherstén B, Ostman J, Blohmé G, *et al.* Difficulties in classifying diabetes at presentation in the young adult. *Diabet Med* 1993; **10**:606–613.

20 Littorin B, Sundkvist G, Hagopian W, Landin-Olsson M, Lernmark A, Ostman J, *et al.* Islet cell and glutamic acid decarboxylase antibodies present at diagnosis of diabetes predict the need for insulin treatment: a cohort study in young adults whose disease was initially labeled as type 2 or unclassifiable diabetes. *Diabetes Care* 1999; **22**:409–412.

21 Lammi N, Taskinen O, Moltchanova E, Notkola IL, Eriksson JG, Tuomilehto J, *et al.* A high incidence of type 1 diabetes and an alarming increase in the incidence of type 2 diabetes among young adults in Finland between 1992 and 1996. *Diabetologia* 2007; **50**:1393–1400.

22 Lammi N, Blomstedt PA, Moltchanova E, Eriksson JG, Tuomilehto J, Karvonen M. Marked temporal increase in the incidence of type 1 and type 2 diabetes among young adults in Finland. *Diabetologia* 2008; **51**:897–899.

23 Fourlanos S, Dotta F, Greenbaum CJ, Palmer JP, Rolandsson O, Colman PG, *et al.* Latent autoimmune diabetes in adults (LADA) should be less latent. *Diabetologia* 2005; **48**:2206–2212.

24 Leslie RD, Kolb H, Schloot NC, Buzzetti R, Mauricio D, De Leiva A, *et al.* Diabetes classification: grey zones, sound and smoke: Action LADA 1. *Diabetes Metab Res Rev* 2008; **24**:511–519.

25 Melton LJ, Palumbo P, Chu-Pin C. Incidence of diabetes mellitus by clinical type. *Diabetes Care* 1983; **6**:75–86.

26 Mølbak AG, Christau B, Marner B, Borch-Johnsen K, Nerup J. Incidence of insulin-dependent diabetes mellitus in age groups over 30 years in Denmark. *Diabet Med* 1994; **11**:650–655.

27 Karvonen M, Pitkaniemi M, Pitkaniemi J, Kohtamaki K, Tajima N, Tuomilehto J. Sex difference in the incidence of insulin-dependent diabetes mellitus: an analysis of the recent epidemiological data. World Health Organization DIAMOND Project Group. *Diabetes Metab Rev* 1997; **13**:275–291.

28 Gale EA, Gillespie KM. Diabetes and gender. *Diabetologia* 2001; **44**:3–15.

29 Karvonen M, Tuomilehto J, Libman I, LaPorte R. A review of the recent epidemiological data on the worldwide incidence of type 1 (insulin-dependent) diabetes mellitus. World Health Organization DIAMOND Project Group. *Diabetologia* 1993; **36**:883–892.

30 Grzywa MA, Sobel AK. Incidence of IDDM in the province of Rzeszow, Poland, 0- to 29-year-old age-group, 1980–1992. *Diabetes Care* 1995; **18**:542–544.

31 Bruno G, Merletti F, Biggeri A, Cerutti F, Grosso N, De Salvia A, *et al.* Increasing trend of type I diabetes in children and young adults in the provice of Turin (Italy): analysis of age, period and birth cohort effects from 1984 to 1996. *Diabetologia* 2001; **44**:22–25.

32 Newhook LA, Curtis J, Hagerty D, Grant M, Paterson AD, Crummel C, *et al.* High incidence of childhood type 1 diabetes in the Avalon Peninsula, Newfoundland, Canada. *Diabetes Care* 2004; **27**: 885–888.

33 Gill GV, Mbanya JC, Ramaiya KL, Tesfaye S. A sub-Saharan African perspective of diabetes. *Diabetologia* 2009; **52**:8–16.

34 Nyström L, Dahlquist G, Östman J, Wall S, Arnqvist H, Blohmé G, *et al.* Risk of developing insulin-dependent diabetes mellitus (IDDM) before 35 years of age: indications of climatological determinants for age at onset. *Int J Epidemiol* 1992; **21**:352–358.

35 Rytkönen M, Ranta J, Tuomilehto J, Karvonen M. Bayesian analysis of geographical variation in the incidence of type I

diabetes in Finland. *Diabetologia* 2001; **44**(Suppl 3):B37–B44.

36 Aamodt G, Stene LC, Njølstad PR, Søvik O, Joner G; the Norwegian Childhood Diabetes Study Group. Spatiotemporal trends and age-period-cohort modeling of the incidence of type 1 diabetes among children aged <15 years in Norway 1973–1982 and 1989–2003. *Diabetes Care* 2007; **30**:884–889.

37 Carle F, Gesuita R, Bruno G, Coppa GV, Falorni A, Lorini R, *et al.* Diabetes incidence in 0- to 14-year age-group in Italy: a 10-year prospective study. *Diabetes Care* 2004; **27**:2790–2796.

38 Yang Z, Wang K, Li T, Sun W, Li Y, Chang YF, *et al.* Childhood diabetes in China: enormous variation by place and ethnic group. *Diabetes Care* 1998; **21**:525–529.

39 Campbell-Stokes PL, Taylor BJ. Prospective incidence study of diabetes mellitus in New Zealand children aged 0 to 14 years. *Diabetologia* 2005; **48**:643–648.

40 Serrano-Rìos M, Goday A, Martinez Larrad T. Migrant populations and the incidence of type 1 diabetes mellitus: an overview of the literature with a focus on the Spanish-heritage countries in Latin America. *Diabetes Metab Res Rev* 1999; **15**:113–132.

41 Lipton RB. Epidemiology of childhood diabetes mellitus in non-caucasian populations. In: Ekoé J-M, Rewers M, Williams R, Zimmet P, eds. *The Epidemiology of Diabetes Mellitus*. Chichester: Wiley-Blackwell, 2008: 385–402.

42 Kawasaki E, Matsuura N, Eguchi K. Type 1 diabetes in Japan. *Diabetologia* 2006; **49**:828–836.

43 Muntoni S, Fonte MT, Stoduto S, Marietti G, Bizzarri C, Crinò A, *et al.* Incidence of insulin-dependent diabetes mellitus among Sardinian-heritage children born in Lazio region, Italy. *Lancet* 1997; **349**:160–162.

44 Neu A, Willasch A, Ehehalt S, Kehrer M, Hub R, Ranke MB. Diabetes incidence in children of different nationalities: an epidemiological approach to the pathogenesis of diabetes. *Diabetologia* 2001; **44**(Suppl 3):B21–B26.

45 Hjern A, Söderström U. Parental country of birth is a major determinant of childhood type 1 diabetes in Sweden. *Pediatr Diabetes* 2008; **9**:35–39.

46 Raymond NT, Jones JR, Swift PG, Davies MJ, Lawrence G, McNally PG, *et al.* Comparative incidence of type I diabetes in children aged under 15 years from South Asian and white or other ethnic backgrounds in Leicestershire, UK, 1989 to 1998. *Diabetologia* 2001; **44**(Suppl 3):B32–B36.

47 Feltbower RG, Bodansky HJ, McKinney PA, Houghton J, Stephenson CR, Haigh D. Trends in the incidence of childhood diabetes in south Asians and other children in Bradford, UK. *Diabet Med* 2002; **19**:162–166.

48 Krolewski AS, Warram JH, Rand LI, Kahn CR. Epidemiologic approach to the etiology of type 1 diabetes mellitus and its complications. *N Engl J Med* 1987; **317**:1390–1398.

49 Gale EA. The rise of childhood type 1 diabetes in the 20th century. *Diabetes* 2002; **51**:3353–3361.

50 Onkamo P, Väänänen S, Karvonen M, Tuomilehto J. Worldwide increase in incidence of type 1 diabetes: the analysis of the data on published incidence trends. *Diabetologia* 1999; **42**:1395–1403.

51 Tuomilehto J, Karvonen M, Pitkäniemi J, Virtala E, Kohtamäki K, Toivanen L, *et al.* Record high incidence of type 1 (insulin-dependent) diabetes mellitus in Finnish children. *Diabetologia* 1999; **42**:655–660.

52 Charkaluk ML, Czernichow P, Lévy-Marchal C. Incidence data of childhood-onset type I diabetes in France during 1988-1997: the case for a shift toward younger age at onset. *Pediatr Res* 2002; **52**: 859–862.

53 Feltbower RG, McKinney PA, Parslow RC, Stephenson CR, Bodansky HJ. Type 1 diabetes in Yorkshire, UK: time trends in 0–14 and 15–29-year-olds, age at onset and age-period-cohort modelling. *Diabet Med* 2003; **20**:437–441.

54 Gale EA. Spring harvest? Reflections on the rise of type 1 diabetes. *Diabetologia* 2005; **48**:2445–2450.

55 Lorenzen T, Pociot F, Hougaard P, Nerup J. Long-term risk of IDDM in first-degree relatives of patients with IDDM. *Diabetologia* 1994; **37**:321–327.

56 Gillespie KM, Gale EA, Bingley PJ. High familial risk and genetic susceptibility in early onset childhood diabetes. *Diabetes* 2002; **51**:210–214.

57 Harjutsalo V, Podar T, Tuomilehto J. Cumulative incidence of type 1 diabetes in 10,168 siblings of Finnish young-onset type 1 diabetic patients. *Diabetes* 2005; **54**:563–569.

58 Warram JH, Krolewski AS, Gottlieb MS, Kahn CR. Differences in risk of insulin-dependent diabetes in offspring of diabetic mothers and diabetic fathers. *N Engl J Med* 1984; **311**:149–152.

59 Harjutsalo V, Reunanen A, Tuomilehto J. Differential transmission of type 1 diabetes from diabetic fathers and mothers to their offspring. *Diabetes* 2006; **55**:1517–1524.

60 Kyvik KO, Green A, Beck-Nielsen H. Concordance rates of insulin dependent diabetes mellitus: a population based study of young Danish twins. *Br Med J* 1995; **311**:913–917.

61 Hyttinen V, Kaprio J, Kinnunen L, Koskenvuo M, Tuomilehto J. Genetic liability of type 1 diabetes and the onset age among 22,650 young Finnish twin pairs: a nationwide follow-up study. *Diabetes* 2003; **52**:1052–1055.

62 Kumar D, Gemayel NS, Deapen D, Kapadia D, Yamashita PH, Lee M, *et al.* North-American twins with IDDM: genetic, etiological, and clinical significance of disease concordance according to age, zygosity, and the interval after diagnosis in first twin. *Diabetes* 1993; **42**: 1351–1363.

63 Redondo MJ, Yu L, Hawa M, Mackenzie T, Pyke DA, Eisenbarth GS, *et al.* Heterogeneity of type I diabetes: analysis of monozygotic twins in Great Britain and the United States. *Diabetologia* 2001; **44**: 354–362.

64 Redondo MJ, Jeffrey J, Fain PR, Eisenbarth GS, Orban T. Concordance for islet autoimmunity among monozygotic twins (letter). *N Engl J Med* 2008; **359**:2849–2850.

65 Katz JD, Wang B, Haskins K, Benoist C, Mathis D. Following a diabetogenic T cell from genesis through pathogenesis. *Cell* 1993; **74**:1089–1100.

66 Rønningen KS, Keiding N, Green A. Correlations between the incidence of childhood-onset type I diabetes in Europe and HLA genotypes. *Diabetologia* 2001; **44**(Suppl 3):B51–B59.

67 Kondrashova A, Viskari H, Kulmala P, Romanov A, Ilonen J, Hyöty H, *et al.* Signs of beta-cell autoimmunity in nondiabetic schoolchildren: a comparison between Russian Karelia with a low incidence of type 1 diabetes and Finland with a high incidence rate. *Diabetes Care* 2007; **30**:95–100.

68 Rewers M, Zimmet P. The rising tide of childhood type 1 diabetes: what is the elusive environmental trigger? *Lancet* 2004; **364**:1645–1647.

69 Green EA, Flavell RA. The initiation of autoimmune diabetes. *Curr Opin Immunol* 1999; **11**:663–669.

70 Knip M, Veijola R, Virtanen SM, Hyöty H, Vaarala O, Åkerblom HK. Environmental triggers and determinants of type 1 diabetes. *Diabetes* 2005; **54**(Suppl 2):S125–S136.

71 Brown RJ, Rother KI. Effects of beta-cell rest on beta-cell function: a review of clinical and preclinical data. *Pediatr Diabetes* 2008; **9**: 14–22.

72 Pang TT, Narendran P. Addressing insulin resistance in type 1 diabetes. *Diabet Med* 2008; **25**:1015–1024.

73 Ylipaasto P, Klingel K, Lindberg AM, Otonkoski T, Kandolf R, Hovi T, *et al.* Enterovirus infection in human pancreatic islet cells, islet tropism *in vivo* and receptor involvement in cultured islet beta cells. *Diabetologia* 2004; **47**:225–239.

74 von Herrath M. Can we learn from viruses how to prevent type 1 diabetes?: the role of viral infections in the pathogenesis of type 1 diabetes and the development of novel combination therapies. *Diabetes* 2009; **58**:2–11.

75 Yoon JW, Austin M, Onodera T, Notkins AL. Isolation of a virus from the pancreas of a child with diabetic ketoacidosis. *N Engl J Med* 1979; **300**:1173–1179.

76 Dotta F, Censini S, van Halteren AG, Marselli L, Masini M, Dionisi S, *et al.* Coxsackie B4 virus infection of β cells and natural killer cell insulitis in recent-onset type 1 diabetic patients. *Proc Natl Acad Sci U S A* 2007; **104**:5115–5120.

77 Richardson SJ, Willcox A, Bone AJ, Foulis AK, Morgan NG. The prevalence of enteroviral capsid protein VP1 immunostaining in pancreatic islets in human type 1 diabetes. *Diabetologia* 2009; **52**: 1143–1151.

78 Green J, Casabonne D, Newton R. Coxsackie B virus serology and type 1 diabetes mellitus: a systematic review of published case–control studies. *Diabet Med* 2004; **21**:507–514.

79 Forrest JM, Turnbull FM, Sholler GF, Hawker RE, Martin FJ, Doran TT, *et al.* Gregg's congenital rubella patients 60 years later. *Med J Aust* 2002; **177**:664–667.

80 Stene LC, Tuomilehto J, Rewers M. Global epidemiology of type 1 diabetes. In: Ekoé J-M, Rewers M, Williams R, Zimmet P, eds. *The Epidemiology of Diabetes Mellitus.* Chichester: Wiley-Blackwell, 2008: 355–383.

81 Gale EA. Congenital rubella: citation virus or viral cause of type 1 diabetes? *Diabetologia* 2008; **51**:1559–1566.

82 Viskari HR, Roivainen M, Reunanen A, Pitkäniemi J, Sadeharju K, Koskela P, *et al.* Maternal first-trimester enterovirus infection and future risk of type 1 diabetes in the exposed fetus. *Diabetes* 2002; **51**:2568–2571.

83 Graves PM, Rotbart HA, Nix WA, Pallansch MA, Erlich HA, Norris JM, *et al.* Prospective study of enteroviral infections and development of beta-cell autoimmunity. Diabetes autoimmunity study in the young (DAISY). *Diabetes Res Clin Pract* 2003; **59**:51–61.

84 Foulis AK, McGill M, Farquharson MA, Hilton DA. A search for evidence of viral infection in pancreases of newly diagnosed patients with IDDM. *Diabetologia* 1997; **40**:53–61.

85 Viskari HR, Koskela P, Lönnrot M, Luonuansuu S, Reunanen A, Baer M, *et al.* Can enterovirus infections explain the increasing incidence of type 1 diabetes? [Letter] *Diabetes Care* 2000; **23**:414–416.

86 Bach JF. The effect of infections on susceptibility to autoimmune and allergic diseases. *N Engl J Med* 2002; **347**:911–920.

87 Kaila B, Taback SP. The effect of day care exposure on the risk of developing type 1 diabetes: a meta-analysis of case–control studies. *Diabetes Care* 2001; **24**:1353–1358.

88 Karam JH, Lewitt PA, Young CW, Nowlain RE, Frankel BJ, Fujiya H, *et al.* Insulinopenic diabetes after rodenticide (Vacor) ingestion: a unique model of acquired diabetes in man. *Diabetes* 1980; **29**:971–978.

89 Lenzen S. The mechanisms of alloxan- and streptozotocin-induced diabetes. *Diabetologia* 2008; **51**:216–226.

90 Myers MA, Mackay IR, Zimmet PZ. Toxic type 1 diabetes. *Rev Endocr Metab Disord* 2003; **4**:225–231.

91 Lamb MM, Myers MA, Barriga K, Zimmet PZ, Rewers M, Norris JM. Maternal diet during pregnancy and islet autoimmunity in offspring. *Pediatr Diabetes* 2008; **9**:135–141.

92 Virtanen SM, Knip M. Nutritional risk predictors of β cell autoimmunity and type 1 diabetes at a young age. *Am J Clin Nutr* 2003; **78**:1053–1067.

93 Harrison LC, Honeyman MC. Cow's milk and type 1 diabetes: the real debate is about mucosal immune function. *Diabetes* 1999; **48**:1501–1507.

94 Virtanen SM, Kenward MG, Erkkola M, Kautiainen S, Kronberg-Kippilä C, Hakulinen T, *et al.* Age at introduction of new foods and advanced beta cell autoimmunity in young children with HLA-conferred susceptibility to type 1 diabetes. *Diabetologia* 2006; **49**:1512–1521.

95 Viner RM, Hindmarsh PC, Taylor B, Cole TJ. Childhood body mass index (BMI), breastfeeding and risk of type 1 diabetes: findings from a longitudinal national birth cohort. *Diabet Med* 2008; **25**:1056–1061.

96 TRIGR Study Group. Study design of the Trial to Reduce IDDM in the Genetically at Risk (TRIGR). *Pediatr Diabetes* 2007; **8**: 117–137.

97 Norris JM, Barriga K, Klingensmith G, Hoffman M, Eisenbarth GS, Erlich HA, *et al.* Timing of initial cereal exposure in infancy and risk of islet autoimmunity. *JAMA* 2003; **290**:1713–1720.

98 Ziegler AG, Schmid S, Huber D, Hummel M, Bonifacio E. Early infant feeding and risk of developing type 1 diabetes-associated autoantibodies. *JAMA* 2003; **290**:1721–1728.

99 Mathieu C, Badenhoop K. Vitamin D and type 1 diabetes mellitus: state of the art. *Trends Endocrinol Metab* 2005; **16**:261–266.

100 EURODIAB Substudy 2 Study Group. Vitamin D supplement in early childhood and risk for type 1 (insulin-dependent) diabetes mellitus. *Diabetologia* 1999; **42**:51–54.

101 Hyppönen E, Läärä E, Reunanen A, Järvelin MR, Virtanen SM. Intake of vitamin D and risk of type 1 diabetes: a birth-cohort study. *Lancet* 2001; **358**:1500–1503.

102 Niinistö S, Virtanen SM, Kenward MG, *et al.* Maternal intake of vitamin D during pregnancy and risk of advanced beta-cell autoimmunity in the offpring. [Abstract] *Acta Diabetol* 2007; **44**(Suppl 1): S35–S36.

103 Stene LC, Joner G; the Norwegian Childhood Diabetes Study Group. Use of cod liver oil during the first year of life is associated with lower risk of childhood-onset type 1 diabetes: a large, population based, case–control study. *Am J Clin Nutr* 2003; **78**: 1128–1134.

104 Norris JM, Yin X, Lamb MM, Barriga K, Seifert J, Hoffman M, *et al.* Omega-3 polyunsaturated fatty acid intake and islet autoimmunity in children at increased risk for type 1 diabetes. *JAMA* 2007; **298**:1420–1428.

105 Uusitalo L, Nevalainen J, Niinistö S, Alfthan G, Sundvall J, Korhonen T, *et al.* Serum α- and γ-tocopherol concentrations and risk of advanced beta cell autoimmunity in children with HLA-conferred

susceptibility to type 1 diabetes mellitus. *Diabetologia* 2008; **51**:773–780.

106 Stene LC, Magnus P, Lie RT, Søvik O, Joner G; the Norwegian Childhood Diabetes Study Group. Maternal and paternal age at delivery, birth order, and risk of childhood onset type 1 diabetes: population based cohort study. *Br Med J* 2001; **323**:369–371.

107 EURODIAB Substudy 2 Study Group. Perinatal risk factors for childhood type 1 diabetes in Europe. *Diabetes Care* 1999; **22**:1698–1702.

108 Cardwell CR, Carson DJ, Patterson CC. Parental age at delivery, birth order, birth weight and gestational age are associated with the risk of childhood type 1 diabetes: a UK regional retrospective cohort study. *Diabet Med* 2005; **22**:200–206.

109 Cardwell CR, Stene LC, Joner G, Cinek O, Svensson J, Goldacre MJ, *et al.* Caesarean section is associated with an increased risk of childhood onset type 1 diabetes: a meta-analysis of observational studies. *Diabetologia* 2008; **51**:726–735.

110 Dahlquist G, Bennich SS, Källén B. Intrauterine growth pattern and risk of childhood onset insulin dependent (type 1) diabetes: population based case–control study. *Br Med J* 1996; **313**:1174–1177.

111 Stene LC, Magnus P, Lie RT, Søvik O, Joner G, the Norwegian Childhood Diabetes Study Group. Birth weight and childhood onset type 1 diabetes: population based cohort study. *Br Med J* 2001; **322**:889–892.

112 Dahlquist GG, Pundziute-Lyckå A, Nyström L. Birthweight and risk of type 1 diabetes in children and young adults: a population-based register study. *Diabetologia* 2005; **48**:1114–1117.

113 Larsson HE, Lynch K, Lernmark B, Nilsson A, Hansson G, Almgren P, *et al.* Diabetes-associated HLA genotypes affect birthweight in the general population. *Diabetologia* 2005; **48**:1484–1491.

114 Stene LC, Thorsby PM, Berg JP, Rønningen KS, Undlien DE, Joner G; Norwegian Childhood Diabetes Study Group. The relation between size at birth and risk of type 1 diabetes is not influenced by adjustment for the insulin gene (-23HphI) polymorphism or *HLA-DQ* genotype. *Diabetologia* 2006; **49**:2068–2073.

115 Baum JD, Ounsted M, Smith MA. Weight gain in infancy and subsequent development of diabetes mellitus in childhood. *Lancet* 1975; **2**:866.

116 Hyppönen E, Virtanen SM, Kenward MG, Knip M, Åkerblom HK; Childhood Diabetes in Finland Study Group. Obesity, increased linear growth, and risk of type 1 diabetes in children. *Diabetes Care* 2000; **23**:1755–1760.

117 EURODIAB Substudy 2 Study Group. Rapid early growth is associated with increased risk of childhood type 1 diabetes in various European populations. *Diabetes Care* 2002; **25**:1755–1760.

118 DiLiberti JH, Carver K, Parton E, Totka J, Mick G, McCormick K. Stature at time of diagnosis of type 1 diabetes mellitus. *Pediatrics* 2002; **109**:479–483.

119 Larsson HE, Hansson G, Carlsson A, Cederwall E, Jonsson B, Jönsson B, *et al.* Children developing type 1 diabetes before 6 years of age have increased linear growth independent of HLA genotypes. *Diabetologia* 2008; **51**:1623–1630.

120 Lammi N, Moltchanova E, Blomstedt PA, Tuomilehto J, Eriksson JG, Karvonen M. Childhood BMI trajectories and the risk of developing young adult-onset diabetes. *Diabetologia* 2009; **52**:408–414.

121 Couper JJ, Beresford S, Hirte C, Baghurst PA, Pollard A, Tait BD, *et al.* Weight gain in early life predicts risk of islet autoimmunity in children with a first-degree relative with type 1 diabetes. *Diabetes Care* 2009; **32**:94–99.

122 Barr EL, Zimmet PZ, Shaw JE. Mortality and life expectancy associated with diabetes. In: Ekoé J-M, Rewers M, Williams R, Zimmet P, eds. *The Epidemiology of Diabetes Mellitus.* Chichester: Wiley-Blackwell, 2008: 603–625.

123 Borch-Johnsen K, Kreiner S, Deckert T. Mortality of type 1 (insulin-dependent) diabetes mellitus in Denmark: a study of relative mortality in 2930 Danish type 1 diabetic patients diagnosed from 1933 to 1972. *Diabetologia* 1986; **29**:767–772.

124 Dahlquist G, Källén B. Mortality in childhood-onset type 1 diabetes: a population-based study. *Diabetes Care* 2005; **28**:2384–2387.

125 Soedamah-Muthu SS, Fuller JH, Mulnier HE, Raleigh VS, Lawrenson RA, Colhoun HM. All-cause mortality rates in patients with type 1 diabetes mellitus compared with a non-diabetic population from the UK general practice research database, 1992–1999. *Diabetologia* 2006; **49**:660–666.

126 Skrivarhaug T, Bangstad HJ, Stene LC, Sandvik L, Hanssen KF, Joner G. Long-term mortality in a nationwide cohort of childhood-onset type 1 diabetic patients in Norway. *Diabetologia* 2006; **49**:298–305.

127 Bruno G, Cerutti F, Merletti F, Novelli G, Panero F, Zucco C, *et al*; Piedmont Study Group for Diabetes Epidemiology. Short-term mortality risk in children and young adults with type 1 diabetes: the population-based Registry of the Province of Turin, Italy. *Nutr Metab Cardiovasc Dis* 2009; **19**:340–344.

128 Patterson CC, Dahlquist G, Harjutsalo V, Joner G, Feltbower RG, Svensson J, *et al.* Early mortality in EURODIAB population-based cohorts of type 1 diabetes diagnosed in childhood since 1989. *Diabetologia* 2007; **50**:2439–2442.

129 Podar T, Solntsev A, Reunanen A, Urbonaite B, Zalinkevicius R, Karvonen M, *et al.* Mortality in patients with childhood-onset type 1 diabetes in Finland, Estonia, and Lithuania. *Diabetes Care* 2000; **23**:290–294.

130 Asao K, Sarti C, Forsen T, Hyttinen V, Nishimura R, Matsushima M, *et al.* Long-term mortality in nationwide cohorts of childhood-onset type 1 diabetes in Japan and Finland. *Diabetes Care* 2003; **26**:2037–2042.

131 Bosnyak Z, Nishimura R, Hagan Hughes M, Tajima N, Becker D, Tuomilehto J, *et al.* Excess mortality in Black compared with White patients with type 1 diabetes: an examination of underlying causes. *Diabet Med* 2005; **22**:1636–1641.

132 Egger M, Davey Smith G, Stettler C, Diem P. Risk of adverse effects of intensified treatment in insulin-dependent diabetes mellitus: a meta-analysis. *Diabet Med* 1997; **14**:919–928.

133 Orchard TJ, Costacou T, Kretowski A, Nesto RW. Type 1 diabetes and coronary artery disease. *Diabetes Care* 2006; **29**:2528–2538.

4 Epidemiology of Type 2 Diabetes

Ronald C.W. Ma & Peter C.Y. Tong

Division of Endocrinology and Diabetes, Department of Medicine and Therapeutics, The Chinese University of Hong Kong, Prince of Wales Hospital, Shatin, Hong Kong

Keypoints

- The prevalence of type 2 diabetes is increasing worldwide.
- Approximately 285 million people worldwide have diabetes in 2010, making it one of the most common non-communicable diseases globally.
- The largest increase is observed in regions with rapidly developing economies and urbanization.
- The aging population, with an increase in the proportion of people aged over 65 years in most countries, has contributed significantly to this increase in prevalence.
- The age of onset of diabetes is also decreasing in many countries, giving rise to an increasing proportion of young people of working age being affected by the disease.
- Several risk factors are known to be associated with increased risk of type 2 diabetes. Many of these risk factors are associated with a westernized lifestyle and increase with urbanization.
- Areas with a high ratio of impaired glucose tolerance : diabetes are at an earlier stage of the diabetes epidemic, and thus may be a particular target for preventive strategies.
- The region with the highest diabetes prevalence rate at present is in the Eastern Mediterranean and Middle East Region.
- The largest increase in diabetes prevalence is predicted to occur in India and China.
- Diabetes is associated with approximately twofold increased mortality in most populations, with the excess risk decreasing with increasing age.
- The increase in diabetes prevalence, particularly among young adults, along with the increased morbidity and mortality associated with microvascular and macrovascular complications, is likely to lead to an escalation of health care costs and loss of economic growth.

Introduction

Type 2 diabetes mellitus (T2DM) is one of the most common forms of chronic disease globally and few societies or ethnic groups are spared. It accounts for about 85% of cases of diabetes in Caucasians and virtually all in certain non-Caucasian ethnic groups. In 2010, it was estimated that 285 million people worldwide have diabetes, of whom 80% live in less developed countries and areas [1]. Among those aged 20–79 years, about 6.6% have diabetes globally [1]. The highest number of people with diabetes is in the Western Pacific Region, with 76 million, and the region with the highest prevalence rate, at 11.7%, is North America and the Carribean [1].

The number of people with diabetes is expected to reach 438 million by 2030, an increase of 54% compared to predicted figures for 2010 [1]. The largest increases will be in countries with rapidly growing economies, such as India and China. With the increasing consumption of high-energy food, increasing adoption of sedentary lifestyles and urbanization, increasing numbers of individuals develop T2DM, and the age of diagnosis is decreasing. Individuals exposed to longer periods of hyperglycemia will undoubtedly have increased risks of developing vascular complications related to diabetes. The potential health care costs and burden of diabetes in these regions will have a significant impact on the economic growth of these regions, as discussed further in Chapter 5.

The epidemiology and prevalence of diabetes is partly determined by the diagnostic criteria used to diagnose diabetes, and these have been modified on a number of occasions. The diagnostic criteria for diabetes and impaired glucose tolerance (IGT) is based on epidemiologic evidence relating microvascular complications to specific degrees of hyperglycemia, and the fasting glucose cut-off has been modified as new data emerge. These changes have major implications on the interpretations of current and future epidemiologic studies on diabetes. In 1999, the diagnostic threshold of fasting glucose was lowered from 7.8 to 7.0 mmol/L. A fasting glucose between 6.0 and <7 mmol/L was previously considered to be pre-diabetic and the term "impaired fasting glucose" (IFG) was used. Subsequent lowering of the "normal" fasting glucose level to 5.6 mmol/L further increases the number of patients with "pre-diabetes." IGT, however, is a state of intermediate hyperglycemia that is only identified by oral

Textbook of Diabetes, 4th edition. Edited by R. Holt, C. Cockram, A. Flyvbjerg and B. Goldstein.

glucose tolerance testing (OGTT), with a post-load glucose level of 7.8–11.1 mmol/L. It is estimated that about 344 million or 7.9% in the 20–79 age group have IGT in 2010 [1]. Abnormal glucose tolerance is frequently associated with visceral obesity, hypertension and dyslipidemia, a collection of cardiovascular risk factors known as metabolic syndrome. While these subjects are at high risk of developing diabetes and coronary artery disease, interventions with increased physical activity, reduced fat and energy intake can substantially reduce these risks by 40–60%.

Risk factors for type 2 diabetes

Several risk factors are known to be associated with increased risk of T2DM. These include increasing age, obesity (especially central obesity), dietary excess, dietary factors such as increased intake of animal fats, carbonated drinks, sedentary lifestyle, a positive family history, history of gestational diabetes, polycystic ovary syndrome, severe mental illness, presence of hypertension, hyperlipidemia or cardiometabolic risk factors (Figure 4.1) (see Chapters 11, 12 and 14). The clustering of some of these risk factors – hypertension, elevated blood glucose, elevated triglyceride, low high-density lipoprotein (HDL) cholesterol, and abdominal obesity – is termed the metabolic syndrome. Many of these risk factors are associated with a westernized lifestyle and increase with urbanization and mechanization. The recognition of the role of these factors in the pathogenesis of T2DM has led to recommendations for selective screening for T2DM in subjects with these risk factors [2].

Obesity accounts for 80–85% of the overall risk of developing T2DM, and underlies the current global spread of the disease [3]. The risk of T2DM increases as body mass index (BMI) increases above 24 kg/m^2, although the risk appears to be present in association with lower BMI cut-offs in Asians [4,5]. While central obesity is a particularly strong factor, it can impart further risk regardless of the overall level of general obesity. This obesity-related risk is particularly marked in certain ethnic populations such as Native Americans, African-Americans, South Asians, Chinese (and other Asian populations) and Pacific Islanders [6–9], and may be related to increased visceral adiposity. Obesity, particularly central adiposity, is associated with insulin resistance, as well as β-cell dysfunction, partly through increased free fatty acids and lipotoxicity (see Chapter 14). Obesity is also associated with other metabolic abnormalities such as dyslipidemia and hypertension. Presence of the metabolic syndrome, according to the different definitions, is associated with two- to five-fold increased risk of developing diabetes in most populations [10]. Epidemiologic studies have suggested that early life events such as low birth weight and fetal malnutrition may also be associated with increased risk of diabetes and cardiovascular disease later in life [11].

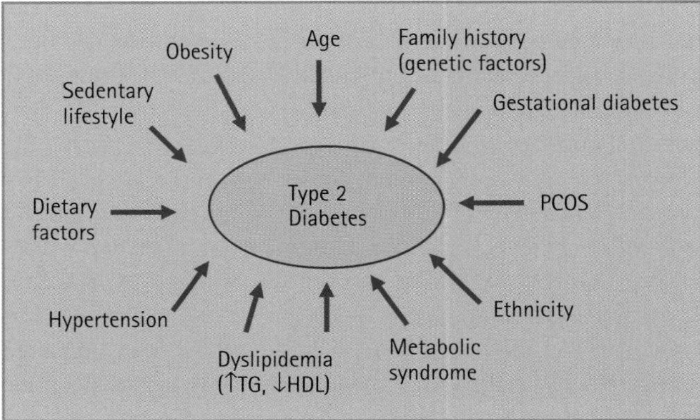

Figure 4.1 Risk factors in the development of type 2 diabetes. HDL, high density lipoprotein cholesterol; PCOS, polycystic ovarian syndrome; TG, triglycerides.

Recent emerging risk factors

Decreased sleep

In addition to changes in diet and level of physical activity, it is recently recognized that short sleep duration, another facet of our modern lifestyle, may also be an important contributing factor to the increasing prevalence of T2DM. Early seminal work has highlighted the detrimental effects of sleep deprivation on glucose tolerance and insulin sensitivity [12]. Subsequent cross-sectional studies have suggested an association between short sleep duration and diabetes [13] and obesity [14]. In a prospective study of more than 70 000 women in the Nurses Health Study, short sleep duration was associated with approximately 57% increase in the risk of diabetes diagnosis over the 10-year study period [15]. Similar data were obtained from the first National Health and Nutrition Examination Survey (NHANES I), which noted that subjects who have sleep durations of 5 hours or less had a 47% increase in the incidence of diabetes over a 10-year period [16]. The exact mechanism whereby sleep restriction increases diabetes risk is not clear, although it may be related to activation of the sympathetic nervous system, decrease in cerebral glucose utilization, changes in the hypothalamic-pituitary-adrenal axis as well as other neuroendocrine dysregulation [16].

Drug-induced metabolic changes

There is increasing recognition that some commonly used medications may be associated with adverse metabolic effects and increased risk of diabetes (see Chapter 16) [17]. High dose thiazide diuretics are known to worsen insulin resistance and beta-blockers can impair insulin secretion. More recently, the use of antipsychotic agents, particularly second generation (atypical) antipsychotics, have been linked with hyperglycemia and diabetes [18]. The increasing use of highly active antiretroviral therapy (HAART) has dramatically reduced the mortality of patients with HIV infection; however, protease inhibitors and, to a lesser extent, nucleoside reverse transcriptase inhibitors, have been found to be associated with insulin resistance, deranged glucose and lipid metabolism and an increased risk for T2DM. The increasing use of such agents will likely have a significant impact on the epidemiology of diabetes in areas where HIV/AIDS is endemic such as Africa (see Chapter 50) [19].

Environmental pollutants

While most studies on the increasing burden of diabetes with westernized lifestyle have focused on changes in dietary patterns and the increasingly sedentary lifestyles, recent studies suggest environmental pollutants may represent a previously unrecognized link between urbanization and diabetes [20,21]. For example, there is strong cross-sectional association between serum concentrations of chlorinated persistent organic pollutants with diabetes [22], as well as components of the metabolic syndrome [23]. More recently, brominated flame-retardants have emerged as another class of organic pollutants that are associated with diabetes [24]. It is believed that these environmental toxins may accumulate in adipose tissue and act as endocrine disruptors, leading to dysregulation of glucose and lipid metabolism.

Low birth weight and fetal malnutrition

There is now increasing evidence to support a relationship between intra-uterine environment, fetal malnutrition and the risk of diabetes and cardiovascular disease later in life [11,25]. Maternal undernutrition, low infant birth weight, along with rapid postnatal growth, has been found to be associated with increased risk of diabetes in the offspring. This "mismatch" of a metabolic phenotype programmed during intra-uterine development and the nutritionally rich postnatal environment may be most important in regions that are undergoing rapid economic development. In addition, offspring of obese women or women with diabetes have an increased risk of diabetes and cardiometabolic abnormalities [26,27]. With increasing numbers of women with young-onset diabetes, this is likely to exacerbate further the epidemic of diabetes by setting up a vicious cycle of "diabetes begetting diabetes" [1,11,28].

Despite the increasing recognition of these novel risk factors, the main risk factors associated with diabetes remain the traditional ones of increasing age, adiposity, physical inactivity, dietary factors, positive family history and presence of other cardiometabolic risk factors, as outlined in Figure 4.1.

Methodologic issues in the epidemiology of type 2 diabetes

In comparing epidemiologic data in T2DM, one must be aware of the importance of the study methodology. Survey methods must be robust, to allow comparison and standardization. A large, truly random sample of a community, with a good response rate, is best; workplace samples may demonstrate "healthy worker" effects, while selective samples (e.g. volunteers, or subjects with another disease) are the least useful because of inbuilt recruitment bias. The age distribution of sample populations is crucial in studying T2DM, whose prevalence rises with age; study populations must be age-stratified and any comparisons age-adjusted, either within the data set, or standardized against a reference population. Finally, ascertainment methods are important – for example, whether subjects undergo an OGTT, with or without preliminary blood glucose screening.

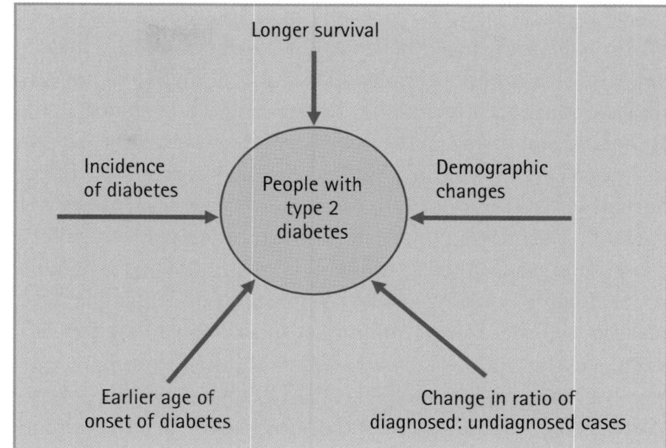

Figure 4.2 Diabetes epidemiologic model. Factors directly affecting the prevalence of diabetes included in the present analysis. Adapted from Colagiuri *et al.* [29] with permission from Springer Science and Business Media.

Studies conducted in different regions of the world have highlighted an increase in the prevalence of T2DM. While few would argue that this translates into increasing burden associated with diabetes, it is important to recognize the factors that have contributed to this increased prevalence. Several factors directly affect the prevalence of diabetes, and may partly account for the increasing prevalence (Figure 4.2):

1 Changes in the ratio of diagnosed : undiagnosed cases of diabetes;
2 Population demographic changes with an aging population;
3 Earlier age at onset of diabetes;
4 Longer survival in patients with diabetes than before;
5 Increasing incidence of diabetes [29].

The different factors may have different contributions depending on the population being studied, although most if not all are of some importance in most populations.

Effects of changes in the definition of diabetes

While it has long been established that diabetes is a condition associated with elevated levels of glucose in the bloodstream, there was no widespread accepted definition of the syndrome until the 1980s, when the World Health Organization (WHO) Expert Committee on diabetes mellitus defined the diabetic state as a state of chronic hyperglycemia that may result from many environmental and genetic factors, often acting together [30]. The precise degree of hyperglycemia that defines diabetes has evolved with time, and relies on epidemiologic studies regarding the distribution of glucose levels within various populations.

There are several consequences of the changes in the definition of diabetes with time on the epidemiology of the condition. First, with the American Diabetes Association (ADA) and WHO classification of 1999, the threshold of fasting glucose diagnostic of diabetes was lowered from 7.8 to 7.0 mmol/L, thereby increasing the number of individuals in any given population that fulfills a diagnosis of diabetes. Furthermore, it is important to appreciate that in any epidemiologic survey, whether the diagnosis was based on elevated fasting glucose or post-load values during an OGTT. While the lower fasting glucose values was chosen to resemble more closely the diagnostic significance of the 2-hour post-load concentration, numerous studies have demonstrated that the fasting glucose criteria and post-load criteria identify slightly different subjects in most populations [31–33], and the use of fasting glucose alone will reduce the overall prevalence of diabetes compared with that identified by 2-hour post-load glucose criteria [34]. Furthermore, there is an increasing number of epidemiologic studies that utilize measurement of HbA_{1c} as an indicator of dysglycemia [35]. Although HbA_{1c} is not at present considered a suitable diagnostic test for diabetes or intermediate hyperglycemia, this is under active discussion [36].

The WHO recommendations for the diagnostic criteria for diabetes and intermediate hyperglycemia is summarized in Table 4.1 (see Chapter 2). While the lower threshold for diagnosing IFG in the recommendation by the ADA will result in a larger number of subjects diagnosed to have intermediate hyperglycemia than the WHO recommendation, increased diagnostic activity (e.g. through use of the OGTT) will lead to an increasing ratio of diagnosed : undiagnosed diabetes, and may impact on the prevalence rate reported in epidemiology studies.

In a comprehensive report on the global prevalence of diabetes [37], it was noted that the most important demographic change

Table 4.1 Comparison of the 2006 WHO recommendations for the diagnostic criteria for diabetes and intermediate hyperglycemia.

	WHO (2006)	ADA (2003)
Diabetes		
Fasting plasma glucose	≥7.0 mmol/L (126 mg/dL)	≥7.0 mmol/L (126 mg/dL)
	or	
2-h plasma glucose* or random plasma glucose	≥11.1 mmol/L (200 mg/dL)	
Impaired glucose tolerance		
Fasting plasma glucose	<7.0 mmol/L (126 mg/dL)	
	and	
2-h plasma glucose*	≥7.8 and <11.1 mmol/L (140 mg/dL and 200 mg/dL)	
Impaired fasting glucose		
Fasting plasma glucose	6.1–6.9 mmol/L (110–125 mg/dL)	5.6–6.9 mmol/L (100–125 mg/dL)
	and (if measured)	
2-h plasma glucose*	<7.8 mmol/L (140 mg/dL)	

*Venous plasma glucose 2-h after ingestion of 75 g oral glucose load.

to diabetes prevalence across the world was the increase in proportion of people over 65 years of age. Another major factor that has impacted on the prevalence of diabetes is the increasing age-specific prevalence of diabetes, especially in the younger age groups [37]. This suggests an earlier age of onset of diabetes, which may be of particular importance in low and middle income countries. It is also worthwhile noting the tendency for the prevalence rates of IGT to decline as that of diabetes rises, perhaps suggesting that areas with a high ratio of IGT : diabetes are at an earlier stage of the diabetes epidemic and thus may be a particular target for preventative strategies. Changes and variations in the ratio of IGT : diabetes prevalence – the so-called "epidemicity index," may provide a useful marker for the scale of the epidemic in that particular region, as illustrated in Figure 4.3 [38].

Regional and ethnic patterns of type 2 diabetes worldwide

This section considers the geographic distribution and secular changes in the prevalence of T2DM and intermediate hyperglycemia in the major regions of the world. Whenever possible, the most comprehensive and up-to-date source of data is the *Diabetes Atlas* produced by the International Diabetes Federation [1]. In addition, a review by Wild *et al.* [37] utilized age- and sex-specific estimates for diabetes prevalence from available epidemiologic surveys to extrapolate prevalence in related countries using a combination of criteria including geographic proximity, ethnic and socioeconomic similarities.

Current estimates of the total number of people with diabetes in each region of the world and in those countries with the highest overall numbers are shown in Figure 4.4. A list of countries with the highest prevalence and projected prevalence is listed in Table 4.2, and a list of countries with the most number of people with diabetes in Table 4.3.

Africa

T2DM in the African continent provides contrasting pictures between regions that are more urbanized and the more rural areas. While poverty and malnutrition is still a major problem affecting sub-Saharan Africa, a region where diabetes is comparatively rare, urbanized areas such as North Africa are reporting increasing prevalence rates [39]. It has been estimated that, overall, 3.8% of the adult population in the African region in 2010 are currently affected by diabetes, which is projected to increase to 4.7% by 2030 [1]. Other important epidemiologic issues in the region include a low incidence of type 1 diabetes (T1DM), which is complicated by the occurrence of atypical "ketosis-prone" diabetes, an atypical presentation of diabetes characterized by an initial clinical presentation of apparent T1DM with severe hyperglycemia and ketosis, and subsequent long-term remission with a clinical course more compatible with T2DM [40]. In addition, there is also a form of early onset diabetes termed malnutrition-related diabetes mellitus (MRDM) that is associated with past or

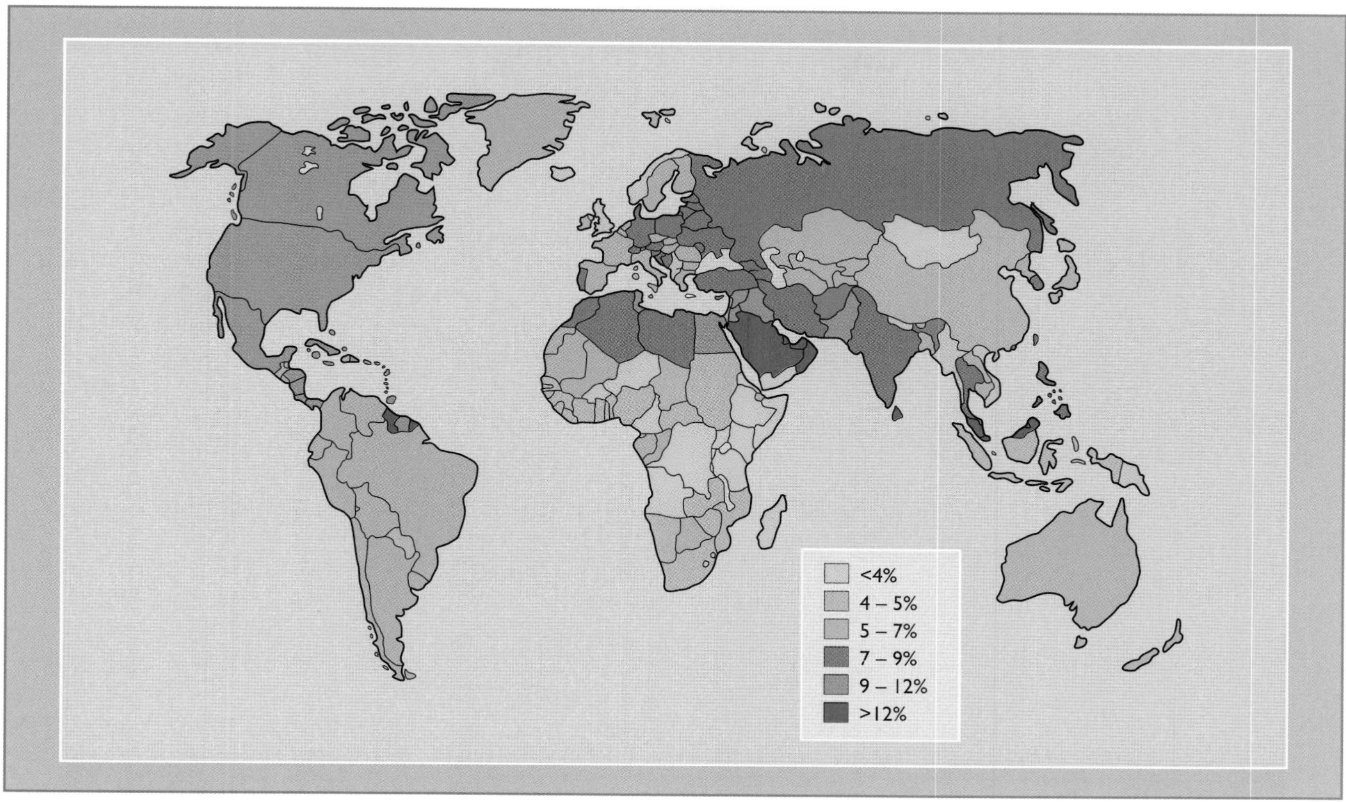

Figure 4.3 Global prevalence estimates of diabetes (20–79 years), 2010. Adapted from International Diabetes Federation [1].

present malnutrition and sometimes accompanied by pancreatic calcification [19]. Although infective diseases such as HIV infection and tuberculosis are currently the main causes of mortality in sub-Saharan Africa, the increasing prevalence of diabetes and other non-communicable diseases is likely eventually to overtake infections as major causes of mortality. In sub-Saharan Africa, only a small proportion of the population at present reaches ages at which T2DM becomes a major health problem. While greater access to HAART has lead to markedly reduced mortality, the improvement in life expectancy, coupled with the adverse metabolic effects of HAART, are likely to contribute to further increases in the prevalence of T2DM within the region [19,41].

North Africa

Prevalence rates are relatively high (4.2–9.3%) in Sudan and Tunisia as well as Egypt. The Egyptian study, of adults aged over 20 years, also showed an IGT prevalence rate of 10% [42]. Interesting urban–rural differences were also demonstrated; in Cairo city, diabetes was more common (prevalence 14–20%, depending upon socioeconomic status), while the IGT prevalence was lower (6–9%). The converse applied in a rural setting, with a diabetes prevalence of only 5% but a higher IGT prevalence of 13%. This may reflect the diabetes epidemic being at an earlier stage in rural populations (Figure 4.4). In the recent Tunisian National Nutrition Survey, prevalence of diabetes was 9.9%, giving age-adjusted prevalence of 8.5%, with marked urban–rural differences [43].

Sub-Saharan Africa

There is a paucity of prevalence data from sub-Saharan Africa, with most of the prevalence data derived from studies in Ghana, Cameron, Nigeria, Tanzania and South Africa [39]. In a recent systematic review of prevalence data from Ghanaians and Nigerians, diabetes was rare at 0.2% in urban Ghana in 1963 and 1.65% in urban Nigeria in 1985. The prevalence of diabetes had risen to 6.8% in Nigeria in 2000 (for adults aged ≥40 years) and 6.3% in Ghana in 1998 (for adults aged ≥25 years) [44,45]. In Cameroon (West Africa), adults aged 24–74 years had an overall diabetes prevalence of 1.1%, with an IGT rate of 2.7%. Prevalence rates in the capital of Cameroon (Yaounde) were 1.3% for diabetes and 1.8% for IGT, compared with rural prevalences of 0.8% for diabetes and 3.9% for IGT [46]. Undiagnosed cases accounted for the majority of cases in these studies, again reflecting a region at the early stages of a looming diabetes epidemic.

In South Africa, both diabetes and IGT are more common in both urban and rural communities. In Cape Town, age-adjusted prevalences were 8% for diabetes and 7% for IGT [47]. A recent study conducted in a rural South African community based on a 75-g OGTT and the 1998 WHO criteria reported an overall age-adjusted prevalence of diabetes of 3.9%, IGT 4.8% and IFG 1.5%.

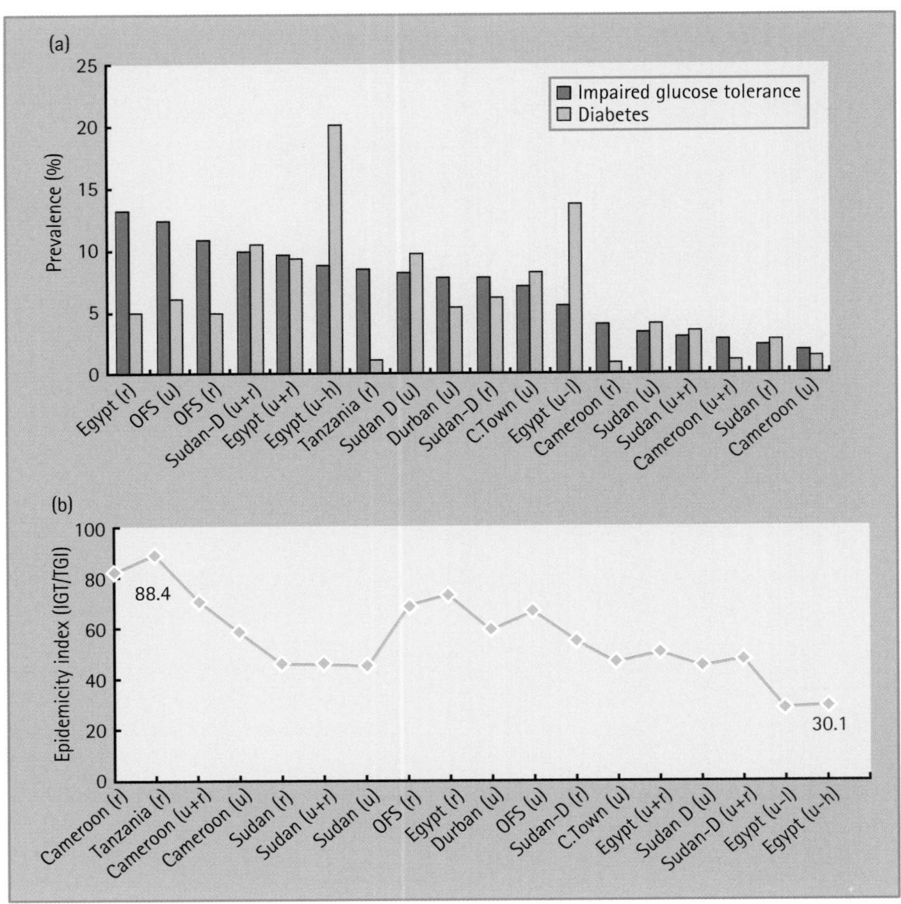

Figure 4.4 Relationship between impaired glucose tolerance (IGT) prevalence and diabetes prevalence and the relationship to the Epidemicity Index. h, high socioeconomic status; l, low socioeconomic status; r, rural; u, urban; Sudan-D, Dangla tribe; OFS, South Africa Free State. Adapted from Dowse *et al.* [38].

Table 4.2 Prevalence of diabetes (20–79 age group) in 2010 and 2030. Data from International Diabetes Federation, 2009 [1].

Rank	Country	2010 Prevalence (%)	2030 Prevalence (%)
1	Nauru	30.9	33.4
2	United Arab Emirates	18.7	21.4
3	Saudi Arabia	16.8	18.9
4	Mauritius	16.2	19.8
5	Bahrain	15.4	17.3
6	Reunion	15.3	18.1
7	Kuwait	14.6	16.9
8	Oman	13.4	14.9
9	Tonga	13.4	15.7
10	Malaysia	11.6	13.8

Notably, 85% of the cases with diabetes were uncovered by the survey [48].

In addition to exposure to urban environment, other factors that determine the risk of T2DM in African populations include positive family history, ethnic origin, central adiposity and physical inactivity [39]. Possible ethnic differences have been examined in several studies. In both Tanzania and South Africa, migrant Asians have higher diabetes prevalence rates than indigenous Africans [49] but this could reflect lifestyle differences. In Tanzania the difference was particularly marked (1.1% in Africans vs 9.1% in Asians), which again emphasizes the low prevalence in urban East Africans.

The emerging epidemic of T2DM is further compounded by the various problems hampering the delivery of effective diabetes care within this region. This has resulted in poor glycemic control among most patients, as well as a high frequency of chronic microvascular complications. Better access to health care and treatment, improvement in infrastructure to support services and health care information systems as well as primary prevention measures are urgently needed in order to reduce the burden of acute and chronic complications of diabetes in the region [19,39,41].

The Americas

North America (USA and Canada)

Diabetes and its complications are common and a significant cause of morbidity in North America. The NHANES study

Table 4.3 Estimated numbers of people with diabetes in 2010 and 2030 in the 20–79 year age group. Data from International Diabetes Federation, 2009 [1].

Rank	Country	Persons (millions) 2010	Rank	Country	Persons (millions) 2030
1	India	50.8	1	India	87.0
2	China	43.2	2	China	62.6
3	United States of America	26.8	3	United States of America	36.0
4	Russian Federation	9.6	4	Pakistan	13.8
5	Brazil	7.6	5	Brazil	12.7
6	Germany	7.5	6	Indonesia	12.0
7	Pakistan	7.1	7	Mexico	11.9
8	Japan	7.1	8	Bangladesh	10.4
9	Indonesia	7.0	9	Russian Federation	10.3
10	Mexico	6.8	10	Egypt	8.6

reported a crude prevalence of total diabetes in 1999–2002 as 9.3%, consisting of 6.5% diagnosed and 2.8% undiagnosed [50]. This was significantly increased compared with a crude prevalence of total diabetes in 1988–1994 of 5.1%, mainly because of an increase in diagnosed diabetes. There was marked variation in prevalence in different ethnic groups, with age- and sex-standardized prevalence of diagnosed diabetes approximately twice as high in non-Latino African-Americans (11%) and Mexican-Americans (10.4%) compared with White people of Northern European ancestry (5.2%). The prevalence of diabetes among the elderly of these minority groups was particularly high, exceeding 30% [50].

The high prevalence rates in US Latino people and African-Americans is well documented. In 1991, the age-adjusted prevalence of diabetes was 6% in White people, 9% in Cubans, 10% in African-Americans, 13% in Mexican-Americans and 13% in Puerto Ricans [51]. Rates have risen in all groups, but these differences appear to persist. Between 1987 and 1996, the 7- to 8-year incidence of T2DM approximately tripled in both Mexican-Americans and White people of Northern European ancestry, although the absolute rate was twice as high in the Mexican-Americans [52]. T2DM is also significantly more common among older Puerto Ricans (38%) and Dominicans (35%) than among White people of Northern European ancestry (23%) [53]. Economic disadvantage may explain much of the excess prevalence of T2DM among African-American women [54].

Other populations in the USA that are particularly at risk of T2DM are the Native American Indian communities, notably the Pima Indians, of whom 50% have diabetes [55]. Reports have highlighted the developing epidemic of T2DM in Native American Indian youth [56]. Among 15- to 19-year-olds, diabetes now affects 5.1% of Pima Indians (a sixfold increase in prevalence over the last 20 years) and 0.2% for Canadian Cree and Ojibway Indians. The overall prevalence among all US Native American Indians of this age is 0.5%. This epidemic of T2DM in young Native American Indians is supported by secular trends in the incidence rate of T2DM over the past 40 years in Pima Indians, which showed a more than fivefold increase in incidence rates among Pima Indians aged 5–14 years [57].

A similar situation was seen in Canada, where aboriginal peoples living in Canada had more than twofold increase in prevalence compared with the non-aboriginal population [58]. Other minority groups are also not spared. Among native Hawaiians (Polynesians), the crude (i.e. not age-adjusted) prevalence rates of T2DM and IGT were reported in 1998 to be 20% and 16%, respectively. The age-adjusted rate for T2DM was four times higher than among the US NHANES II study population [59]. In 1991, second-generation Japanese-Americans had prevalence rates of 16% (diabetes) and 40% (IGT) [60], and incidence rates remain high at 17.2 per 1000 person-years [61]. This is believed to be a result of the increase in visceral adiposity in a population predisposed to impaired β-cell function [62]. Other Asian populations living in the USA that are particularly prone to diabetes include Chinese-Americans, in whom linguistic barriers may be a particularly relevant barrier to diabetes education and effective care delivery [63].

It has been estimated that the number of Americans with diagnosed diabetes will rise from 11 million in 2000 (overall prevalence, 4.0%) to 29 million in 2050 (prevalence 7.2%). The fastest growth is expected to be among African-Americans. The projected increase of 18 million is accounted for by approximately similar contributions from changes in demographic composition, population growth and secular rises in prevalence rates [64]. In 2010, it is estimated that 26.8 million people in the USA have diabetes, of which 5.7 million is undiagnosed. The direct and indirect medical costs attributed to diabetes in the USA in 2007 was $174 million [65].

An increasing number of younger people will be affected. In the SEARCH for Diabetes in Youth Study, a multi-ethnic population-based study, the incidence of diabetes was 24.3 per 100 000 person-years. The incidence rates of T2DM was highest among Native American Indians and African-American adolescents, with incidence rates of 17–49.4 per 100 000 person-years,

Table 4.4 National estimates of diabetes and IGT prevalence in Europe in 2010. Data from International Diabetes Federation, 2009 [1].

Country	Prevalence (%)		Prevalence IGT (%)	
	National population*	Comparative population†	National population	Comparative population
Albania	4.8	4.5	2.6	2.4
Cyprus	10.4	9.1	6.7	5.9
Denmark	7.7	5.6	15.2	12.4
Finland	8.3	5.7	8.8	5.9
France	9.4	6.7	7.6	6.6
Germany	12.0	8.9	7.2	6.2
Greece	8.8	6.0	7.4	5.9
Iceland	2.1	1.6	7.3	5.9
Ireland	5.7	5.2	1.9	1.7
Israel	7.1	6.5	5.5	5.1
Italy	8.8	5.9	5.9	4.7
Malta	9.7	6.7	7.8	6.0
Netherlands	7.3	5.2	6.0	4.7
Norway	4.7	3.6	8.6	7.3
Poland	9.3	7.6	16.9	15.3
Spain	8.7	6.6	7.5	6.6
Sweden	7.3	5.2	9.0	7.3
Turkey	7.4	8.0	6.3	6.6
United Kingdom	4.9	3.6	5.1	4.7

* Prevalence based on current age/gender composition.
† Prevalence standardized to global age/gender composition.

compared with 5.6 per 100 000 person-years in White people of Northern European ancestry [66].

Central and South America

Data from these regions are scarce. In the Mapuche native people from rural Chile, the prevalence of T2DM estimated in 2001 was 3% in men and 5% in women [67]. This represents a substantial rise above the very low prevalence (<1%) reported in 1985 [68]. Diabetes is clearly much more common in urban communities, for example 14% in Mexico City in 1994 [69], compared with 5–10% prevalence nationwide [70]. Surveys in Brazil and Colombia in the early 1990s indicated age-adjusted prevalence rates of approximately 7% [71,72]. A high prevalence of abdominal obesity was noted in these populations, affecting more than 80% of women [70].

Caribbean

Studies from Jamaica exemplify the secular trend in the West Indies. Rates in the 1960s (underestimated because of the screening procedure used [73]) were low but rose in the 1970s to 4% in those aged 44 and 8–10% in those aged 45–64 years [74,75], and to an overall rate of 7.4% in 1996 [76]. The most recent report, which dates from 1999, indicates prevalence rates of 16% in women and 10% in men (13% overall). As elsewhere, this exceeds the rate of rise among European-origin populations and parallels the spread of obesity [77].

Europe

This region contains a diverse mix of countries that have marked differences in affluence, and includes some of the most developed countries in the world. Nevertheless, updated nationwide survey data are only available in some of the countries. In the recent *Diabetes Atlas*, less than half of the 54 European countries and territories in the European region had recently published data on national prevalence of diabetes, which ranged from 2.1% in Iceland to 12% in Germany (Table 4.4).

UK

T2DM imposes particular burdens in inner cities with multiethnic populations, as those originating from the Indian subcontinent have a high prevalence of the disease. In typical studies [78,79], the age-adjusted prevalence rates were 3% and 5% in Caucasian males and females, respectively, compared with 12% and 11% in their Asian counterparts in the UK. Asians also show a higher prevalence of IGT, a male preponderance, a younger age at diagnosis and a lower proportion of undiagnosed diabetes [79].

Poverty and social deprivation apparently contribute to the increasing prevalence of T2DM among inner-city residents. This was manifest in all ethnic groups in inner-city Manchester, including a surprisingly high age-standardized prevalence rate of 20% among White people) [80]. Social deprivation, obesity, physical inactivity and smoking tend to co-segregate, which may explain this phenomenon. The importance of dietary factors was highlighted by two recent studies, which demonstrated association between high dietary energy density or unhealthy dietary patterns characterized by high intake of soft drinks, sugar-sweetened beverages, burgers, sausages and snacks with incident T2DM [81,82]. In the Ely study, a population-based longitudinal study, the 10-year cumulative incidence of diabetes was 7.3 per 1000 person-years [83].

Scandinavia

In Scandinavia, the more homogenous population may indicate more accurately the true prevalence of T2DM among white Caucasians. A survey in Northern Sweden revealed a prevalence of diabetes of 8.1% [84]. Similar data were obtained in a recent study in Finland, with age-standardized prevalence of diabetes in 45- to 64-year-olds being 10.2% for men and 7.4% for women [85]. Lower prevalence data were noted for Iceland [86].

In the early 1990s, T2DM was rare in Northern Finland but the prevalence of IGT was 29% in men and 27% in women [87], comparable with that in a homogeneous white Caucasian female Swedish population aged 55–57 years (28%) [88]. In Denmark, around 15% of the population have IGT [89]. The high prevalence of IGT in Finland prompted the Finnish Diabetes Prevention Study [90], which examined whether lifestyle changes could prevent the development of T2DM. Strikingly, nutritional advice and increased physical activity were shown to reduce the risk of developing diabetes by 58% in subjects with IGT, and the effect was sustained over subsequent follow-up [90]. A more recent study in three regions in Finland noted prevalence of IGT of 10.5% in men and 9.2% in women, which was substantially lower then the previous reported figures from Northern Finland. It is unclear whether this difference is a result of regional differences or changes in the diabetes : IGT ratio [85].

Using a register of patients with diabetes, it was calculated that the incidence rate of diabetes in Denmark was 1.8 per 100 000 at age 40 years and 10 per 100 000 at age 70. The incidence rate increased 5% per year before 2004 but then stabilized. The lifetime risk of diabetes was estimated at 30% [91]. A recent study in Finland noted an alarming increase in the incidence of T2DM among young adults, with age-adjusted incidence of T2DM among 15- to 39-year-olds being 11.8 per 100 000/year. The incidence rate increased by 7.9% per year. Interestingly, despite having the highest incidence of childhood T1DM in the world, the incidence of T2DM among young adults in Finland is approaching that of T1DM among the 15–39 year age group (age-adjusted incidence of T1DM 15.9 per 100 000/year) [92].

Continental Europe

A population-based survey in Verona, Italy, revealed an overall prevalence of T2DM of 2.5% which increased significantly after the age of 35 years [93]. In northern Italy, the age-adjusted prevalence of T2DM was 9% in males and 8% in females over the age of 44 years [94]. In a study that compared the prevalence of diabetes in Casale Monferrato in northwest Italy in 1988 and 2000, it was noted that the age- and sex-adjusted prevalence of diabetes had increased from 2.13% in 1988 to 3.1% in 2000, with higher age-specific prevalence rates of diabetes in every age group in the later survey, including a twofold increase in the risk for those aged ≥80 years [95].

In France, the MONICA study estimated the adjusted prevalence of T2DM to be 7% in men and 5% in women aged 35–65 years, and the adjusted prevalence of IFG as 12% in men and 5% in women [96]. The prevalence of diabetes increases to 19% in males and 9% in females aged over 60 years [97].

In the Netherlands, T2DM affects 8% of elderly Caucasians [98]; 65% of those with IFG and post-load glucose levels went on to develop diabetes within 6 years [99]. In a prospective population-based study between 1998 and 2000, age- and sex-adjusted prevalence of diagnosed diabetes was 2.2% at baseline and 2.9% after 2 years of follow-up, with elderly patients aged 70 or over accounting for 50% of the T2DM population [100].

In Greece, the prevalence of diabetes increased from 2.4% in 1974 to 3.1% in 1990 [101], and aging and obesity were associated with both T2DM and IGT [102,103]. Prevalence of T2DM was 7.6% in men and 5.9% in women in a survey conducted in 2001–2002 [104]. In a follow-up study of those free of cardiovascular disease at baseline, the incidence rate of diabetes within a 5-year period was 5.5% [105]. In Turkey, the overall prevalence rates of T2DM and IGT were 6% and 9%, respectively. Low levels of occupational activity, family history and obesity were all associated risk factors [106,107]. Adherence to a Mediterranean diet may also have protective effects against diabetes [108].

Prevalence data from Eastern Europe are comparatively sparse. The age-adjusted prevalence of T2DM for men and women in Fergana, Uzbekistan, is estimated to be 8% in both urban men and women, with IGT affecting 5% of men and 6% of women. Lower prevalence rates for both T2DM and IGT are reported for semi-rural inhabitants [109]. A survey in the rural area in the Sirdaria province of Uzbekistan confirmed similar age-adjusted prevalence rates of diabetes for men (10%) and women (7.5%); however, prevalence rates of IGT in Sirdaria women (14%) and in men (11%) were higher than for semi-urban or urban inhabitants in Fergana [110]. In Russia, the estimated prevalences were 6% in males and 7% in females for diabetes, and 6% and 13%, respectively, for IGT; clustering of hyperlipidemia, obesity, hypertension and low 10-year survival were observed among subjects with diabetes [111]. A survey conducted in Moscow reported low incidence of reported diagnosis of diabetes (2%) [112], which was supported by another study based on self-reported doctor diagnosis [113]. In addition to underdiagnosis, undertreatment and infrequent insulin use are also likely to contribute to the burden of morbidity [113]. Much of the estimated prevalence data in other Eastern European countries have been extrapolated from data from Poland, where prevalence of T2DM increased from 3.7% to 10.8% between 1986 and 2000, with a similar increase in prevalence of IGT from 2.9% to 14.5% during this period [114].

Asia

India

India is the second most populous country in the world, but currently has the highest number of people with diabetes, with an estimated 40.9 million affected in 2007, a figure that is set to rise to 69.9 million by 2025 [115]. Sequential surveys from India indicate that the prevalence of diabetes has risen steadily since the 1970s [116–119], although methodologic differences hamper comparisons between these studies.

The National Urban Diabetes Survey, carried out in six cities in 2001, found age-standardized prevalence rates of 12% for diabetes (with a slight male preponderance) and 14% for IGT; subjects under 40 years of age had a prevalence of 5% (diabetes) and 13% (IGT) [119]. Diabetes was positively and independently associated with increasing age, BMI and waist : hip ratio, and also with a family history of diabetes, a higher monthly income and physical inactivity. IGT showed associations with age, BMI and family history of diabetes. Subsequent studies showed increasing prevalence, with prevalence rates of 14.3% reported in the Chennai Urban Rural Epidemiology Study (CURES-17) [120], and 18.6% in the city of Chennai in the most recent study [121]. In addition to the increasing prevalence of diabetes, there appears to be a decreasing prevalence of IGT (120). Another secular trend is the shift towards younger onset of diabetes, especially in urban areas, where up to 36% of those with diabetes are aged 44 years or less [120,121].

Urban–rural differences in the prevalence of diabetes have been consistently reported by different studies in India. A study from Chennai noted a progressive increase in prevalence rate with increasing urbanization; 2.4% in rural areas, 5.9% in semi-urban areas and up to 11.6% in urban areas [118,122]. Likewise, the most recent data revealed a prevalence of 18.6% in the city of Chennai compared with 16.4% in a town and 9.2% in peri-urban villages [121]. In a study carried out in 77 centers in India (40 urban and 37 rural), the standardized prevalence rate for diabetes in the total Indian, urban and rural, populations was 4.3, 5.9 and 2.7%, respectively. While the prevalence rates of diabetes and IGT are significantly higher in urban compared with rural areas, it appears that the rural–urban gradient is becoming increasingly attenuated [123].

The Chennai Population Study (CUPS) has recently revealed alarming rates of incident diabetes, which occurred at a rate of 20.2 cases per 1000 person-years [124]. Identification of high-risk subjects and increasing the awareness of the population is much needed. A risk score specific for Indian population, the Indian Diabetes Risk Score has been developed. It utilizes four clinical variables (age, family history, regular exercise and waist circumference) and a score of >21 is able to identify subjects with diabetes with a sensitivity and specificity of close to 60% [125]. This will help identify high-risk subjects for early intervention, because lifestyle modification has been shown to be effective in reducing progression from IGT to diabetes in the Indian population [126]. Recently, the pilot phase of a National Program on Diabetes, Cardiovascular Diseases and Stroke (NPCDS) has been launched in seven states in January 2008. It is hoped that this will help coordinate the multisectoral effort that is urgently needed in order to address the epidemic of obesity and diabetes in India [127].

Pakistan, Bangladesh and Sri Lanka

The situation in these countries largely mirrors that in India. Diabetes is particularly common (16% of men, 12% of women) in the rural Sindh Province in Northern Pakistan [128]. A more recent study from Pakistan indicates similar prevalence rates of 10–11% in urban and rural males and urban women, although lower rates were seen in rural females (5%); however, IGT rates in females were twice those in males [129]. Combining data from the four provinces of Pakistan, the prevalence of diabetes in the urban areas was 6.0% and 3.5% in women, with a total of 22% of the urban population estimated to have some degree of glucose intolerance [130]. Using data from the National Diabetes Survey, the WHO has estimated a marked increase in T2DM in Pakistan from 4.3 million in 1995 to 14.5 million in 2025 [37]. In rural Bangladesh, diabetes prevalence is 2.1% compared with an IGT prevalence of 13% despite the mean BMI being only 20.4 kg/m^2 [131].

In addition to urbanization, the main factor for the high prevalence of diabetes and metabolic abnormalities among Asians is the tendency to central obesity and insulin resistance [5,118,132–134]. Despite being born smaller, with lower birth weight, Indian babies have more body fat, which persists into adulthood, thus putting them at increased risk of cardiometabolic complications [135]. Interestingly, a recent study showed maternal nutrition, and in particular, low maternal vitamin B_{12} and high folate might be associated with increased adiposity and risk of T2DM in the offspring [136], suggesting that in addition to increased intake of fat and calorie-rich foodstuffs, other dietary factors may also have a contributory role.

Mauritius

The high prevalences of diabetes and cardiovascular disease on the island of Mauritius, in the India Ocean, have been intensively studied. Here, diabetes is common in an urbanized setting, across several ethnic groups (Asian Indian, Chinese and Creole); prevalence rates are 10–13% among the different ethnic groups, rising to 20–30% in those aged 45–74 years [137]. A repeat survey in 1998 revealed a rise in prevalence of T2DM to 17.9%. In both studies, the highest prevalence was seen in the Asian Indians [137,138].

The Middle East

Marked socioeconomic changes in many countries in the region, especially among the affluent oil-producing countries, has led to dramatic changes in lifestyle with changes in nutritional intake, decreased physical activity, increased obesity and smoking. This, coupled with increasing urbanization and improved life expectancy, has led to a marked increase in the prevalence of diabetes and IGT (Table 4.5). Compared with European patients, immigrants from the Middle East were noted to have an earlier onset of disease, more rapid decline in islet β-cell function, and have a stronger family history [139]. In terms of prevalence rate, the United Arab Emirates, Saudi Arabia, Bahrain, Kuwait, Oman and Egypt all feature among the top 10 countries with the highest prevalence rate of diabetes [115], highlighting this region as one that requires concerted public health action in order to reduce the potential impact of diabetes [140].

Western Pacific region

Australia

The Report of the AusDiab Study [141], published in 2000, provides up-to-date information about diabetes in a developed country. The overall prevalence of diabetes in Australians aged ≥25 years was 7.5% (8% for males and 7% for females), rising from 2.5% in those aged 25–44 years to 24% among subjects aged ≥75 years; the prevalence has more than doubled since 1981 [142,143]. Fifty percent of cases discovered in this survey were previously undiagnosed. The combined prevalence of IFG and IGT was 16% (males 17%, females 15%); thus, almost 25% of Australians aged 25 years or more have abnormal glucose metabolism. In Australia, T2DM accounts for over 85% of cases and T1DM for 10%. Using data from the AusDiab study, it has been estimated that the prevalence of diabetes is likely to rise from 7.6% in 2000 to 11.4% by 2025 [144].

T2DM is more common in Native Australian populations (e.g. 16–30% of adults in the Aborigine and Torres Strait Islander communities) [145]. In this population, diabetes was associated with higher rates of hypertension (69% vs 21%), obesity (44% vs 16%), elevated triglyceride and lower HDL cholesterol concentrations than subjects who have normal glucose tolerance.

Table 4.5 Prevalences of diabetes in selected countries from the Middle East.

Year	Country	Prevalence (%)	
		T2DM	IGT
1998	Lebanon [220]	13.2	6
2000	Oman [221]		
	Males	11.8	7.1 (IFG)
	Females	11.6	5.1 (IFG)
1995	Oman [222]		
	Males	9.7	8.1
	Females	9.8	12.9
2000	Saudi Arabia [223]		
	Males	26.2	14.4
	Females	21.5	13.9
1995	Saudi Arabia [224]		
	Males	11.8	10
	Females	12.8	9
1992	Iran [225]		
	Urban males	7.1	8.9
	Urban females	7.6	14.9
	Rural	7.3	7.2

IFG, impaired fasting glucose; IGT, impaired glucose tolerance; T2DM, type 2 diabetes mellitus.

New Zealand

In New Zealand, T2DM is consistently more common among Polynesians (Maoris and Pacific Islanders) than in Caucasians; it accounts for 89% of diabetes in Caucasians and 95% in Polynesians. Polynesians are also diagnosed, on average, 5–10 years younger than Caucasians and have a four- to eightfold higher prevalence of diabetic nephropathy. Strikingly high prevalence rates of 37–75% were reported for unemployed males, again emphasizing the role of socioeconomic status [146]. In the 2006–2007 New Zealand Health Survey, prevalence rates reported for adults aged >30 years were 4.3% for Europeans, 5.8% for Maoris, 6.5% for Asians and 10.0% for Pacific Islanders [147,148].

Pacific Island countries

The Melanesian, Micronesian and Polynesian populations of the Pacific Islands show great variations in diabetes prevalence, largely attributable to differences in economic development and lifestyle. Some of the highest prevalence rates worldwide come from this region, notably from Nauru and Papua New Guinea. The Micronesian population of Nauru, made wealthy by bauxite mining and with a longer history of westernization than other Pacific Island countries, currently have an age-standardized prevalence rate of 40%. High prevalence rates in Nauru have been maintained since the late 1970s, but now appear to have stabilized [149].

Fiji has a largely bi-ethnic population consisting of native Fijians of Melanesian ancestry together with migrants from India. Recent surveys from Fiji are lacking, but a survey conducted 20 years ago showed that diabetes prevalence rates were already higher among Indian migrants than in Melanesians. In adults above 20 years of age, crude prevalence rates were 13% among the Indian migrants (with no significant urban–rural gradient), but 7% and 1.7% among urban and rural Melanesians, respectively [150]. At the time, these results were thought to indicate a difference in ethnic (genetic) predisposition but this conclusion has since been tempered by the finding of high prevalence rates in urbanized Melanesians in Papua New Guinea.

The situation in Papua New Guinea provides an excellent example of the damage inflicted by rapid urbanization; diabetes is virtually non-existent in highland populations [151], a stark contrast to the age-standardized prevalence rate of over 40% among urbanized Koki people (Melanesians) in Port Moresby [152]. Intermediate rates are reported in Austronesians of coastal ancestry.

High prevalence rates have also been reported in Polynesian populations, conspicuously associated with obesity, both of which are particularly common in Polynesian women. In Western Samoa, diabetes prevalence was reported in 1991 to be 7–9% in two rural communities and 16% in Apia; the prevalence had doubled since 1978 [153]. In the Kingdom of Tonga, situated south of Samoa, the age-standardized prevalence of diabetes was 15.1% [154].

Evidence suggests that diabetes remains undiagnosed in most Pacific Island people with the disease – perhaps 80–100% in some communities – compared with less than 50% in developed countries [143]. This is likely to contribute to high rates of complications and frequent presentation with diabetes-related problems such as foot sepsis [155].

Japan

T2DM has become more common in Japan since the 1960s, and data from rural parts of Japan suggested a prevalence of 9.1% in men and 10.8% in women, with corresponding IGT prevalence of 12% and 16.5% for Japanese men and women, respectively [156]. A National Diabetes Survey conducted in 2002 estimated a prevalence of 9% [157]. The emerging problem of T2DM among Japanese children is now recognized as a critical problem. T2DM outnumber T1DM in children and adolescents by a ratio of 4:1 [158], and the incidence rate of T2DM for 1981–1990 was 4.1 per 100 000 person-years, approximately twice the incidence rate of T1DM [159]. Nutritional factors are believed to play an important part, with the prevalence of diabetes among Japanese-Americans approximately twice that of Japanese in Japan [160].

The causes of death in people with T2DM have also shifted, possibly because of westernization of diet and increased fat and total calorie intake; higher death rates from renal disease than in Caucasian populations are now being supplanted by rising deaths from coronary artery disease [161]. In order to reduce the burden of diabetes, the Japanese government has launched a large national strategic research project named J-DOIT to reduce diabetes, improve patient adherence to follow-up and to reduce complications of diabetes [162].

Korea

In the Korean National Health and Nutrition Survey conducted in 2001, age-adjusted prevalence of diabetes was reported to be 7.6%. The prevalence of IFG was an alarming 23.9% [163], thus predicting a future epidemic of diabetes in the Korean population, similar to other Asian countries [164].

China and Chinese populations

The rapid increase in prevalence of T2DM in China provides one of the most striking examples of the impact of urbanization on increasing diabetes prevalence. The People's Republic of China, with its population of 1.3 billion, is the world's most populous country. Diabetes used to be rare; prevalence rates reported between 1980 and 1990 were consistently 1.5% or less, even in urban areas such as Shanghai [165], and as low as 0.3% in rural Guangdong Province. Recently, however, the prevalence has risen rapidly, a trend first demonstrated by studies conducted in the Da Qing area of north-eastern China. There, the prevalence in 1986 was 1.0% but by 1994 this had increased over threefold to 3.5% [166,167]. The 1994 survey of 200 000 subjects aged 25–64 years in 19 provinces that included Da Qing found overall prevalence rates of 2.3% for diabetes and 2.1% for IGT. A community-based survey of 40 000 people aged 20–74 years in China between 1995 and 1997 confirms this rising trend and also demonstrates urban–rural gradients in prevalence rates. Age-standardized prevalence rates were 3.2% for diabetes and 4.8% for IGT, with the highest prevalence in provincial cities and the lowest in rural areas [168]. The International Collaborative Study of Cardiovascular Disease in Asia, conducted in 2000–2001, revealed a further increase in prevalence of diabetes (undiagnosed and diagnosed) to 5.5%, with another 7.3% affected by IGT (Figure 4.5) [169]. Furthermore, amongst the 20 million Chinese people estimated to have diabetes based on fasting blood glucose, only 30% were previously diagnosed [169]. The large proportion of subjects with IGT is particularly alarming. In the community-based Shanghai Diabetes Study, subjects with IGT and/or IFG had 11.7-fold increased risk of diabetes compared with those with normal glucose tolerance over a 3-year follow-up period [170].

Chinese populations in affluent societies such as Hong Kong, Singapore, Taiwan and Mauritius all show higher prevalence rates compared with the People's Republic of China. In Hong Kong, prevalence of diabetes has been reported to have increased from 8% to 10% between 1990 and 1995 [171,172]. Recent studies from Taiwan indicate prevalence rates of 9–11%, although methodological discrepancies make direct comparisons difficult [165]. The annual incidence rate in Taiwan has been reported to be 1.8% [173]. In a review summarizing the findings from prevalence studies conducted in Chinese populations, it was noted that Chinese in Hong Kong and Taiwan have a 1.5- to 2.0-fold increased risk of diabetes adjusted for age and diagnostic criteria when compared with their mainland counterparts [174].

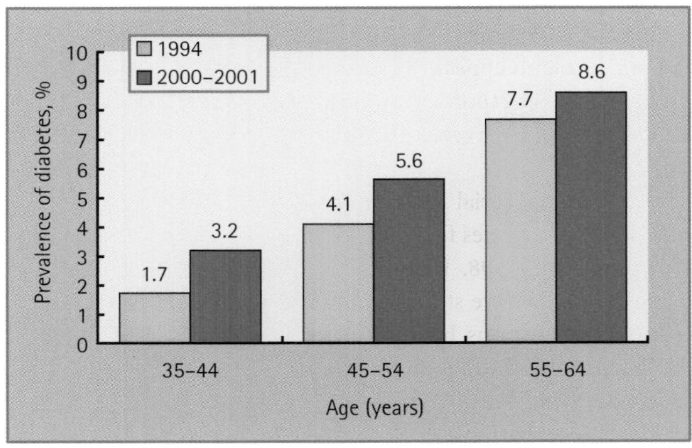

Figure 4.5 Changes in prevalence of diabetes among Chinese adults aged 35–64 years. Data from the 1994 Chinese National Survey and the 2000–2001 InterASIA study. Reproduced from Gu *et al.* [169], with permission from Springer Science and Business Media.

The rapid increase in diabetes prevalence in China is likely to be driven by the increase in obesity, particularly among children and adolescents [5,175]. Analysis of data from the 2002 National Nutrition and Health Survey noted prevalence of overweight among children aged 7–12 years of 4.1%, and 5.6% for those aged 12–18 years, with obesity prevalence of 2.5% and 1.6%, respectively, for the two age groups [176]. In Hong Kong, a community-based study involving more than 2000 adolescents aged 11–18 years found alarming rates of obesity, with 8–10% of those aged 12–13 years fulfilling criteria for obesity [177]. In a national screening program among schoolchildren in Taiwan, 1992–1999, the rate of newly identified diabetes was 9.0 per 100 000 for boys and 15.3 per 100 000 for girls. Obesity was found to be the major risk factor for the development of T2DM, whereby children with BMI in the 95th percentile or higher had an approximately 19-fold increased risk of T2DM compared with those with BMI <50th percentile [178].

Such alarming data from Chinese populations highlight the potential for future rises within China itself. Unless effective measures can be implemented, given the huge population in China, the consequences could be devastating. The International Diabetes Federation has forecasted that by 2030, there will be 67 million people affected by diabetes in China [1].

South-East Asian Peninsula

There is considerable economic diversity within this region, although the recent emerging data from this region showed that despite the relatively traditional lifestyle in many of the countries, diabetes is increasingly common within the region. A survey performed in two villages in Cambodia in 2004 revealed a diabetes prevalence rate of 5% in the rural community in Siemreap but up to 11% in a semi-urban community [179]. A study conducted in adults in Ho Chi Minh City in Southern Vietnam indicated that the prevalence of diabetes has increased substantially from 2.5% in 1993 to 6.9% in 2001 [180]. Similar increases has been reported in Indonesia [181] and the Philippines [182]. Prevalence rates in Thailand appear to be approaching those reported from Malaysia and Singapore, with prevalence of diabetes and IGT in a recent national survey reported to be 6.7% and 12.5%, respectively [183].

In Singapore, serial studies since 1975 have shown a rising prevalence of diabetes from 2% in 1975 to 4.7% in 1984, 8.6% in 1992 and 9% in 1998. Two most recent surveys indicate that the rate of rise may have stabilized. Ethnic Malays (especially Malay women) and Indians have the highest rates of diabetes (14.3–16.7%) and also the highest rates of obesity. A further 15% of the adult population have IGT. In a recent survey conducted in 2004 by the Ministry of Health, Singapore, the prevalence of diabetes among the adult population is estimated to be 8.2% [184]. Obesity and adoption of a westernized diet and lifestyle are again closely associated. T2DM in childhood is also highlighted as an emerging problem.

Impact of diabetes

The epidemic of diabetes is having major impacts on both individuals and societies. These impacts are discussed in Chapter 5. The major burden is from the treatment cost of its complications, such as stroke, blindness, coronary artery disease, renal failure, amputation and infection. In 2007, about 3.8 million people died of diabetes and its related diseases. Most patients die from cardiovascular disease (particularly coronary artery disease and stroke) and end-stage renal disease. There are geographic differences in both the magnitude of these problems and their relative contributions to overall morbidity and mortality. In Caucasian populations, macrovascular complications such as coronary artery disease and amputation are major causes of disability. In contrast, end-stage renal disease and stroke are prevalent among Chinese and Asian ethnic groups. Other issues include the apparent vulnerability of Pacific Island populations to neuropathy and metabolic problems, and South Asian to coronary artery disease.

It is well established that the occurrence of vascular complications of diabetes is related to the duration of hyperglycemia. With the earlier onset of T2DM, most patients will have increased risk of developing these devastating complications. Despite the high prevalence of complications of diabetes and hence the high costs of management, simple low-cost measures are effective in preventing the development of diabetes and its vascular complications. Rather than merely focusing on the control of hyperglycemia, global risk reduction with attention on cardiovascular risk factors has been proved to be the most effective way of reducing the burden of diabetes. The challenge is to provide a platform whereby effective care can be delivered at an affordable cost.

Mortality and morbidity

Diabetes is associated with approximately twofold increased mortality in most populations, with the excess risk decreasing with increasing age [185–187]. While initial data suggest the excess mortality associated with diabetes may be higher in Asian populations, this is probably related to differences in death certificates coding practices [188–190]. It was recently estimated that about 4 million deaths in the 20–79 age group may be attributed to diabetes in 2010, accounting for 6.8% of global all-cause mortality in this age group. Over two-thirds of these deaths attributable to diabetes are believed to have occurred in low and middle income countries [1].

Most patients with T2DM die from cardiovascular disease (particularly ischemic heart disease and stroke) and end-stage renal disease [191]. Geographic differences exist in both the magnitude of these problems and their relative contributions to overall morbidity and mortality.

The most systematic comparative data, using standardized methodology, originate from the WHO Multinational Study of Vascular Disease in Diabetes, which has drawn from 14 centers in 13 countries since the 1980s. A follow-up report from 10 of these centers [192] shows that coronary heart disease and limb amputation rates varied 10- to 20-fold among different centers; there was also marked variation in prevalence of clinical proteinuria and renal failure, but less variation in retinopathy and severe visual impairment. Striking features include the relative rarity of ischemic heart disease and lower extremity amputation in Hong Kong and Tokyo, contrasting with a high incidence of stroke, especially in Hong Kong. A high incidence of stroke was also found in Arizona and Oklahoma, the two Native American Indian centers. The highest rates of ischemic heart disease were seen in the European centers, notably among women from Warsaw. Myocardial infarction was also common in Native American Indians, especially among men, while renal failure and proteinuria rates were highest among Native American Indians and in Hong Kong.

Other issues include the apparent vulnerability of Pacific Island populations to diabetic foot problems associated with neuropathy and of South Asians to coronary heart disease. Importantly, the risk of coronary heart disease is already increased twofold at the stage of IGT [193].

Another cause of morbidity and mortality is the increased risk of cancer in patients with diabetes. Various epidemiologic studies from different populations have suggested a link between diabetes and increased risk of pancreatic, hepatocellular, endometrial, breast and colorectal carcinoma [194–196]. While some of this may be because of the presence of common risk factors such as obesity and dietary factors, it has been shown in a large prospective study that cancer risk increases with increasing fasting glucose at baseline [197].

Intensive multifactorial intervention to reduce cardiovascular risk factors has been shown to be effective in reducing cardiovascular mortality in diabetes [198,199]. While intensive blood glucose control has not been shown to lower cardiovascular mortality in the short term [200,201], it may have beneficial effects in reducing cardiovascular and total mortality in the longer term, as suggested by recent long-term follow-up data from the UK Prospective Diabetes Study [202]. It appears that the relative mortality of diabetes is decreasing in some countries [203,204], and this may be related to the increased utilization of drugs to control hyperlipidemia, hyperglycemia and hypertension [205].

Health care burden and economic costs

The increase in diabetes prevalence, particularly among young adults, along with the increased morbidity and mortality associated with microvascular and macrovasuclar complications, is likely to lead to escalation of health care costs and loss of economic growth. WHO predicts that between 2005 and 2015, net losses in national income from diabetes and cardiovascular disease will reach international dollars (ID) 557.7 billion in China, ID303.2 billion in the Russian Federation, ID336.6 billion in India, ID49.2 billion in Brazil and ID2.5 billion in the United Republic of Tanzania [115]. The annual global health expenditure for diabetes in 2007 is estimated to fall between $232.0 and $421.7 billion, of which half will be spent in the USA (around $119.4 billion) and one-quarter in Europe ($64 billion). In the USA, the estimated total costs (direct and indirect) of diabetes increased from $23 billion in 1969 to $132 billion in 2002 [206,207]. The cost of diabetes in the USA in 2007 was estimated by the ADA to be $174 billion, which includes $116 billion in excess medical expenditures and $58 billion in reduced national productivity (Figure 4.6). The largest components of medical expenditures attributed to diabetes are hospital inpatient care, accounting for 50% of total costs, and medications and supplies (12%) [208]; however, the actual burden is likely to be even

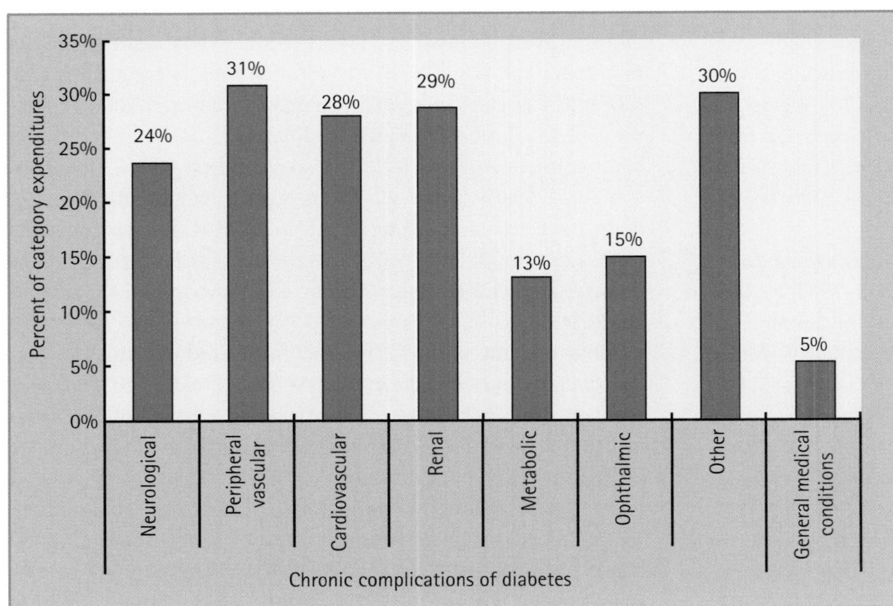

Figure 4.6 Economic costs of diabetes in the USA according to different cost of care for different diabetes-related complications [208]. Reproduced from American Diabetes Association (2008), with permission from American Diabetes Association.

Table 4.6 Estimated direct medical costs of diabetes by region, 2003. Adapted from Narayan *et al.* [226].

Region	Direct medical costs (millions)	
	Low estimate	High estimate
Developing countries	**$12 304**	**$23 127**
East Asia and the Pacific	$1368	$2656
Europe and Central Asia	$2884	$5336
Latin America and the Caribbean	$4592	$8676
Middle East and North Africa	$2347	$4340
South Asia	$840	$1589
Sub-Saharan Africa	$273	$530
Developed countries	**$116 365**	**$217 760**
World	**$128 669**	**$240 887**

greater, because other non-monetary effects such as changes in quality of life, disability and suffering, care provided by non-paid caregivers cannot be included in such analyses. The burden of diabetes affects all sectors of society; higher insurance premiums paid by employees and employers, reduced earnings through productivity loss and reduced overall quality of life for people with diabetes and their families and friends. The cost of medical care for diabetes varies greatly among the different regions (Table 4.6). While diabetes is a very costly disease, interventions used to prevent or control diabetes differ greatly in their cost-effectiveness [209]. The cost-effectiveness and feasibility of diabetes interventions in low and middle income countries, as assessed by the World Bank, is listed in Table 4.7. Cost-effective interventions that are technically and culturally feasible should be implemented with the highest priority [210].

Prevention of type 2 diabetes

"There are entirely too many diabetic patients in the country. Statistics for the last thirty years show so great an increase in the number that, unless this were in part explained by a better recognition of the disease, the outlook for the future would be startling. Therefore, it is proper at the present time to devote attention not alone to treatment, but still more, as in the campaign against the typhoid fever, to prevention. The results may not be quite so striking or as immediate, but they are sure to come and to be important". [Elliot Joslin, 1921]

T2DM is a very expensive disease. As illustrated above, a significant proportion of health care expenditure in developed countries is spent on the treatment of diabetes and its complications. It is therefore beneficial to prevent diabetes or delay its onset, thereby also reducing its associated complications. With improved understanding of the natural history of the development of T2DM and the role of various modifiable risk factors in its pathogenesis, a number of randomized clinical trials have been performed to examine the effect of lifestyle intervention on prevention of T2DM. A large body of evidence has accumulated from these studies on the effectiveness of lifestyle measures in the prevention of diabetes, summarized in Table 4.8. Most of these interventions include structured education and exercise programs, reducing fat intake and increasing fiber intake, moderate exercise for 30 minutes per day or more, and moderate weight reduction of 5% or more. Importantly, in addition to being highly cost-effective, the effect of structured lifestyle intervention on reduction of diabetes risk appears to be maintained over a long duration of follow-up [211,212]. In a follow-up of the Chinese Da Qing Diabetes Prevention Study, participants who received lifestyle intervention had a 51% lower incidence of diabetes during the 6-year active intervention period, and 43% lower incidence of diabetes over the 20-year period [212].

In addition to lifestyle intervention, several agents used in the treatment of T2DM and obesity have been evaluated in clinical trials and found to be effective in preventing diabetes. These include meformin, the thialozolidinedione class of compounds, acarbose and orlistat (Table 4.9). In addition, several clinical trials indicated that angiotensin-converting enzyme (ACE) inhibitors and angiotensin receptor blockers may reduce incident diabetes in high-risk patients with hypertension [213–217]. A large randomized clinical trial compared the ACE inhibitor ramipril with placebo in subjects with IGT or IFG. It did not show a significant reduction in incident diabetes after median follow-up of 3 years, although ramipril was associated with increased regression to normoglycemia [218]. A large number of pharmacologic agents are currently in development or undergoing clinical trials for the treatment of T2DM or obesity. This should provide a constant supply of promising agents for evaluation in their effectiveness for preventing T2DM. At present, however, lifestyle intervention remains more cost-effective as a strategy for diabetes prevention.

More detailed discussion on epidemiologic aspects of diabetes can be found elsewhere [219].

Conclusions

The interaction between genetic predisposition, popularization of fast food and sedentary lifestyle has a major role in the increase in the prevalence of impaired glucose tolerance and T2DM globally. Countries in the Asia Pacific regions with a growing economy will bear the major burden in the increase in number of subjects with diabetes. The significant increase in macrovascular and microvascular complications of diabetes induces a heavy burden on the health care resources. Recent studies confirmed the benefit of intensive multifactorial risk management in reducing all-cause mortality and cardiovascular adverse events. Measures such as dietary restriction and exercise have been shown to be effective in preventing the progression of IGT to

Table 4.7 Summary of cost-effectiveness of interventions for treatment and prevention of diabetes in developing countries. Reproduced from Narayan *et al.* [226].

Intervention	Cost/QALY (2001 US$)							
	East Asia and the Pacific	Europe and Central Asia	Latin America and the Caribbean	Middle East and North Africa	South Asia	Sub-Saharan Africa	Feasibility*	Implementing priority†
Level 1								
Glycemic control in people with HbA_{1c} higher than 9%	Cost saving	Cost saving	Cost saving	Cost saving	Cost saving	Cost saving	++++	1
Blood pressure control in people with pressure higher than 160/95 mmHg	Cost saving	Cost saving	Cost saving	Cost saving	Cost saving	Cost saving	++++	1
Foot care in people with a high risk of ulcers	Cost saving	Cost saving	Cost saving	Cost saving	Cost saving	Cost saving	++++	1
Level 2								
Preconception care for women of reproductive age	Cost saving	Cost saving	Cost saving	Cost saving	Cost saving	Cost saving	++	2
Lifestyle interventions for preventing T2DM	80	100	130	110	60	60	++	2
Influenza vaccinations among the elderly for T2DM	220	290	360	310	180	160	++++	2
Annual eye examination	420	560	700	590	350	320	++	2
Smoking cessation	870	1170	1450	1230	730	660	++	2
ACE inhibitor use for people with diabetes	620	830	1020	870	510	460	+++	2
Level 3								
Metformin intervention for preventing T2DM	2180	2930	3630	3080	1820	1640	++	3
Cholesterol control for people with total cholesterol higher than 200 mg/dL	4420	5940	7350	6240	3680	3330	+++	3
Intensive glycemic control for people with HbA_{1c} higher than 8%	2410	3230	4000	3400	2000	1810	++	3
Screening for undiagnosed diabetes	5140	6910	8550	7260	4280	3870	++	3
Annual screening for microalbuminuria	3310	4450	5510	4680	2760	2500	++	3

* Feasibility was assessed based on difficulty of reaching the intervention population (the capacity of the health care system to deliver an intervention to the targeted population), technical complexity (the level of medical technologies or expertise needed for implementing an intervention), capital intensity (the amount of capital required for an intervention), and cultural acceptability (appropriateness of an intervention in terms of social norms and/or religious beliefs). ++++ indicates feasible for all four aspects, +++ indicates feasible for three of the four, ++ indicates feasible for two of the four, and + indicates feasible for one of the four.

† Implementing priority was assessed by combining the cost-effectiveness of an intervention and its implementation feasibility; 1 represents the highest priority and 3 represents the lowest priority.

diabetes. Hence, despite being one of the most common chronic diseases, diabetes can be prevented or controlled effectively with interventions that are relatively cost-effective compared with the cost of treating vascular complications.

> *"Some 246 million people worldwide have diabetes in 2007. It is now one of the most common non-communicable diseases globally. Diabetes is the fourth or fifth leading cause of death in most developed countries and there is substantial evidence that it is epidemic in many developing and newly industrialized nations.*
>
> *Complications from diabetes, such as coronary artery and peripheral vascular disease, stroke, diabetic neuropathy, amputations, renal failure and blindness are resulting in increasing disability, reduced life expectancy and enormous health costs for virtually every society. Diabetes is certain to be one of the most challenging health problems in the 21st century".* [115]

Table 4.8 Summary of randomized clinical trials using lifestyle intervention in the prevention of T2DM.

Study	No. of participants	Study participants	Duration (years)	Incidence in control	RRR	Reference
Da Qing (1997)	577	IGT	6	15.7	38	Pan [227]
DPS (2001)	522	IGT, BMI >25 kg/m^2	3.2	6	58	Tuomilehto [90]
DPP (2002)	3234	IGT, BMI >24 kg/m^2 FG >5.3 mmol/L	3	10	58	Knowler [228]
IDPP-1 (2006)	531	IGT	3	18.3	29	Ramachandran [126]
Japanese (2005)	458	IGT (men) BMI >24 kg/m^2	4	9.3	67	Kosaka [229]

BMI, body mass index; DPP, Diabetes Prevention Program (USA); DPS, Diabetes Prevention Study (Finland); FG, fasting glucose; IDPP-1, Indian Diabetes Prevention Program; IGT, impaired glucose tolerance.

Table 4.9 Randomized controlled trials assessing the effect of pharmacologic interventions in the prevention of type 2 diabetes.

Study	No. of participants	Follow-up duration (years)	Drug	Total dose (mg/day)	RR (95% CI)	Reference
DPP (2002)	2155	2.8	Metformin	1700	0.69 (0.57–0.83)	Knowler [228]
CDPS (2001)	261	3		750	0.23	Wenying [230]
IDPP-1 (2006)	531	2.5		500	0.74 (0.65–0.81)	Ramachandran [126]
			TZD			
TRIPOD (2002)	236	2.5	Troglitazone	400	0.45 (0.25–0.83)	Buchanan [231]
DPP	585	0.9		400	0.25	
DREAM (2006)	5269	3.0	Rosiglitazone	8	0.40 (0.35–0.46)	DREAM [232]
STOP-NIDDM (2002)	1368	3.2	Acarbose	300	0.75 (0.63–0.9)	Chiasson [233]

CDPS, Chinese Diabetes Prevention Study; CI, 95% confidence interval; DPP, Diabetes Prevention Program (USA); DREAM, Diabetes REduction Assessment with ramipril and rosiglitazone Medications; IDPP-1, Indian Diabetes Prevention Program; RR, relative risk; TRIPOD, The Troglitazone in Prevention of Diabetes trial.

References

1 International Diabetes Federation. *Diabetes Atlas*, 4th edn. International Diabetes Federation, 2009.

2 American Diabetes Association. Screening for type 2 diabetes. *Diabetes Care* 2004; **27**(Suppl 1):S11–14.

3 Ma R, Chan J. *Metabolic complications of obesity*. In: Williams G, Fruhbeck G, eds. *Obesity: Science to Practice*. John Wiley & Sons Ltd, 2009: 235–270.

4. WHO Expert Consultation. Appropriate body mass index for Asian populations and its implications for policy and intervention strategies. *Lancet* 2004; **363**:157–163.

5 Ramachandran A, Ma RC, Snehalatha DC. Diabetes in Asia. *Lancet* 2009 Oct 27. [Epub ahead of print].

6 Fujimoto WY, Bergstrom RW, Boyko EJ, Leonetti DL, Newell-Morris LL, Wahl PW. Susceptibility to development of central adiposity among populations. *Obes Res* 1995; **3**(Suppl 2):179S–186S.

7 Fujimoto WY, Abbate SL, Kahn SE, Hokanson JE, Brunzell JD. The visceral adiposity syndrome in Japanese-American men. *Obes Res* 1994; **2**:364–371.

8 Raji A, Seely EW, Arky RA, Simonson DC. Body fat distribution and insulin resistance in healthy Asian Indians and Caucasians. *J Clin Endocrinol Metab* 2001; **86**:5366–5371.

9 Ko GT, Liu KH, So WY, Tong PC, Ma RC, Ozaki R, *et al.* Cutoff values for central obesity in Chinese based on mesenteric fat thickness. *Clin Nutr* 2009 Jun 25. [Epub ahead of print]

10 Kahn R, Buse J, Ferrannini E, Stern M, American Diabetes Association, European Association for the Study of Diabetes. The metabolic syndrome: time for a critical appraisal: joint statement from the American Diabetes Association and the European Association for the Study of Diabetes. *Diabetes Care* 2006; **28**:2289–2304.

11 Gluckman PD, Hanson MA, Cooper C, Thornburg KL. Effect of *in utero* and early-life conditions on adult health and disease. *N Engl J Med* 2008; **359**:61–73.

12 Spiegel K, Leproult R, Van Cauter E. Impact of sleep debt on metabolic and endocrine function. *Lancet* 1999; **354**:1435–1439.

13 Gottlieb DJ, Punjabi NM, Newman AB, Resnick HE, Redline S, Baldwin CM, *et al.* Association of sleep time with diabetes mellitus and impaired glucose tolerance. *Arch Intern Med* 2005; **165**:863–867.

14 Ko GT, Chan JC, Chan AW, Wong PT, Hui SS, Tong SD, *et al.* Association between sleeping hours, working hours and obesity in Hong Kong Chinese: the "better health for better Hong Kong" health promotion campaign. *Int J Obes (Lond)* 2007; **31**:254–260.

15 Ayas NT, White DP, Al-Delaimy WK, Manson JE, Stampfer MJ, Speizer FE, *et al.* A prospective study of self-reported sleep duration and incident diabetes in women. *Diabetes Care* 2003; **26**:380–384.

16 Gangwisch JE, Heymsfield SB, Boden-Albala B, Buijs RM, Kreier F, Pickering TG, *et al.* Sleep duration as a risk factor for diabetes incidence in a large US sample. *Sleep* 2007; **30**:1667–1673.

17 Ma RC, Kong AP, Chan N, Tong PC, Chan JC. Drug-induced endocrine and metabolic disorders. *Drug Saf* 2007; **30**:215–245.

18 Buchholz S, Morrow AF, Coleman PL. Atypical antipsychotic-induced diabetes mellitus: an update on epidemiology and postulated mechanisms. *Intern Med J* 2008; **38**:602–606.

19 Gill GV, Mbanya JC, Ramaiya KL, Tesfaye S. A sub-Saharan African perspective of diabetes. *Diabetologia* 2009; **52**:8–16.

20 Jones OA, Maguire ML, Griffin JL. Environmental pollution and diabetes: a neglected association. *Lancet* 2008; **371**:287–288.

21 Lee DH, Steffes MW, Jacobs DR Jr. Can persistent organic pollutants explain the association between serum gamma-glutamyltransferase and type 2 diabetes? *Diabetologia* 2008; **51**:402–407.

22 Lee DH, Lee IK, Song K, Steffes M, Toscano W, Baker BA, *et al.* A strong dose–response relation between serum concentrations of persistent organic pollutants and diabetes: results from the National Health and Examination Survey, 1999–2002. *Diabetes Care* 2006; **29**:1638–1644.

23 Lee DH, Lee IK, Porta M, Steffes M, Jacobs DR Jr. Relationship between serum concentrations of persistent organic pollutants and the prevalence of metabolic syndrome among non-diabetic adults: results from the National Health and Nutrition Examination Survey, 1999–2002. *Diabetologia* 2007; **50**:1841–1851.

24 Lim JS, Lee DH, Jacobs DR Jr. Association of brominated flame retardants with diabetes and metabolic syndrome in the US population, 2003–2004. *Diabetes Care* 2008; **31**:1802–1807.

25 Hales CN, Barker DJ, Clark PM, Cox LJ, Fall C, Osmond C, *et al.* Fetal and infant growth and impaired glucose tolerance at age 64. *Br Med J* 1991; **303**:1019–1022.

26 Silverman BL, Metzger BE, Cho NH, Loeb CA. Impaired glucose tolerance in adolescent offspring of diabetic mothers: relationship to fetal hyperinsulinism. *Diabetes Care* 1995; **18**:611–617.

27 Tam WH, Ma RC, Yang X, Ko GT, Tong PC, Cockram CS, *et al.* Glucose intolerance and cardiometabolic risk in children exposed to maternal gestational diabetes mellitus *in utero*. *Pediatrics* 2008; **122**:1229–1234.

28 Ma RC, Chan JC. Pregnancy and diabetes scenario around the world: China. *Int J Gynaecol Obstet* 2009; **104**:S42–S45.

29 Colagiuri S, Borch-Johnsen K, Glumer C, Vistisen D. There really is an epidemic of type 2 diabetes. *Diabetologia* 2005; **48**:1459–1463.

30 World Health Organization Expert Committee. *Diabetes Mellitus*, 1st report. Geneva: World Health Organization, 1965.

31 DECODE Study Group on behalf of the European Diabetes Epidemiology Study Group. Will new diagnostic criteria for diabetes mellitus change phenotype of patients with diabetes? Reanalysis of European epidemiological data. *Br Med J* 1998; **317**:371–375.

32 de Vegt F, Dekker JM, Stehouwer CD, Nijpels G, Bouter LM, Heine RJ. The 1997 American Diabetes Association criteria versus the 1985 World Health Organization criteria for the diagnosis of abnormal glucose tolerance: poor agreement in the Hoorn Study. *Diabetes Care* 1998; **21**:1686–1690.

33 Janus ED, Watt NMS, Lam KSL, Cockram CS, Siu STS, Liu LJ, *et al.* The prevalence of diabetes, association with cardiovascular risk factors and implications of diagnostic criteria (ADA 1997 and WHO 1998) in a 1996 community based population study in Hong Kong Chinese. *Diabet Med* 2000; **17**:741–745.

34 Qiao Q, Nakagami T, Tuomilehto J, Borch-Johnsen K, Balkau B, Iwamoto Y, *et al.* Comparison of the fasting and the 2-h glucose criteria for diabetes in different Asian cohorts. *Diabetologia* 2000; **43**:1470–1475.

35 Bennett CM, Guo M, Dharmage SC. HbA(1c) as a screening tool for detection of type 2 diabetes: a systematic review. *Diabet Med* 2007; **24**:333–343.

36 World Health Organization. *Definition and Diagnosis of Diabetes Mellitus and Intermediate Hyperglycaemia*. Geneva, Switzerland: World Health Organization International Diabetes Federation, 2006.

37 Wild S, Roglic G, Green A, Sicree R, King H. Global prevalence of diabetes: estimates for the year 2000 and projections for 2030. *Diabetes Care* 2004; **27**:1047–1053.

38 Dowse GK, Zimmet PZ, King H. Relationship between prevalence of impaired glucose tolerance and NIDDM in a population. *Diabetes Care* 1991; **14**:968–974.

39 Motala AA. Diabetes trends in Africa. *Diabetes Metab Res Rev* 2002; **18**(Suppl 3):S14–20.

40 Dodu SR. Diabetes in the tropics. *Br Med J* 1967; **2**:747–750.

41 Mbanya JC, Kengne AP, Assah F. Diabetes care in Africa. *Lancet* 2006; **368**:1628–1629.

42 Herman WH, Ali MA, Aubert RE, Engelgau MM, Kenny SJ, Gunter EW, *et al.* Diabetes mellitus in Egypt: risk factors and prevalence. *Diabet Med* 1995; **12**:1126–1131.

43 Bouguerra R, Alberti H, Salem LB, Rayana CB, Atti JE, Gaigi S, *et al.* The global diabetes pandemic: the Tunisian experience. *Eur J Clin Nutr* 2007; **61**:160–165.

44 Amoah AG, Owusu SK, Adjei S. Diabetes in Ghana: a community based prevalence study in Greater Accra. *Diabetes Res Clin Pract* 2002; **56**:197–205.

45 Abubakari AR, Bhopal RS. Systematic review on the prevalence of diabetes, overweight/obesity and physical inactivity in Ghanaians and Nigerians. *Public Health* 2008; **122**:173–182.

46 Mbanya JC, Ngogang J, Salah JN, Minkoulou E, Balkau B. Prevalence of NIDDM and impaired glucose tolerance in a rural and an urban population in Cameroon. *Diabetologia* 1997; **40**:824–829.

47 Levitt NS, Katzenellenbogen JM, Bradshaw D, Hoffman MN, Bonnici F. The prevalence and identification of risk factors for NIDDM in urban Africans in Cape Town, South Africa. *Diabetes Care* 1993; **16**:601–607.

48 Motala AA, Esterhuizen T, Gouws E, Pirie FJ, Omar MA. Diabetes and other disorders of glycemia in a rural South African community: prevalence and associated risk factors. *Diabetes Care* 2008; **31**:1783–1788.

49 Ramaiya KL, Swai AB, McLarty DG, Bhopal RS, Alberti KG. Prevalences of diabetes and cardiovascular disease risk factors in Hindu Indian subcommunities in Tanzania. *Br Med J* 1991; **303**:271–276.

50 Cowie CC, Rust KF, Byrd-Holt DD, Eberhardt MS, Flegal KM, Engelgau MM, *et al.* Prevalence of diabetes and impaired fasting glucose in adults in the US population: National Health And Nutrition Examination Survey 1999–2002. *Diabetes Care* 2006; **29**:1263–1268.

51 Harris MI. Epidemiological correlates of NIDDM in Hispanics, whites, and blacks in the US population. *Diabetes Care* 1991; **14**:639–648.

52 Burke JP, Williams K, Gaskill SP, Hazuda HP, Haffner SM, Stern MP. Rapid rise in the incidence of type 2 diabetes from 1987 to 1996:

results from the San Antonio Heart Study. *Arch Intern Med* 1999; **159**:1450–1456.

53 Tucker KL, Bermudez OI, Castaneda C. Type 2 diabetes is prevalent and poorly controlled among Hispanic elders of Caribbean origin. *Am J Public Health* 2000; **90**:1288–1293.

54 Robbins JM, Vaccarino V, Zhang H, Kasl SV. Excess type 2 diabetes in African-American women and men aged 40–74 and socioeconomic status: evidence from the Third National Health and Nutrition Examination Survey. *J Epidemiol Community Health* 2000; **54**:839–845.

55 Knowler WC, Bennett PH, Hamman RF, Miller M. Diabetes incidence and prevalence in Pima Indians: a 19-fold greater incidence than in Rochester, Minnesota. *Am J Epidemiol* 1978; **108**: 497–505.

56 Harwell TS, McDowall JM, Moore K, Fagot-Campagna A, Helgerson SD, Gohdes D. Establishing surveillance for diabetes in American Indian youth. *Diabetes Care* 2001; **24**:1029–1032.

57 Pavkov ME, Hanson RL, Knowler WC, Bennett PH, Krakoff J, Nelson RG. Changing patterns of type 2 diabetes incidence among Pima Indians. *Diabetes Care* 2007; **30**:1758–1763.

58 Horn OK, Jacobs-Whyte H, Ing A, Bruegl A, Paradis G, Macaulay AC. Incidence and prevalence of type 2 diabetes in the First Nation community of Kahnawake, Quebec, Canada, 1986–2003. *Can J Public Health* 2007; **98**:438–443.

59 Grandinetti A, Chang HK, Mau MK, Curb JD, Kinney EK, Sagum R, *et al.* Prevalence of glucose intolerance among Native Hawaiians in two rural communities. Native Hawaiian Health Research (NHHR) Project. *Diabetes Care* 1998; **21**:549–554.

60 Fujimoto WY, Leonetti DL, Bergstrom RW, Kinyoun JL, Stolov WC, Wahl PW. Glucose intolerance and diabetic complications among Japanese-American women. *Diabetes Res Clin Pract* 1991; **13**:119–129.

61 Hara H, Egusa G, Yamakido M. Incidence of non-insulin-dependent diabetes mellitus and its risk factors in Japanese-Americans living in Hawaii and Los Angeles. *Diabet Med* 1996; **13**(Suppl 6):S133–1342.

62 Fujimoto WY, Bergstrom RW, Boyko EJ, Chen K, Kahn SE, Leonetti DL, *et al.* Type 2 diabetes and the metabolic syndrome in Japanese Americans. *Diabetes Res Clin Pract* 2000; **50**(Suppl 2):S73–76.

63 Hsu WC, Cheung S, Ong E, Wong K, Lin S, Leon K, *et al.* Identification of linguistic barriers to diabetes knowledge and glycemic control in Chinese Americans with diabetes. *Diabetes Care* 2006; **29**:415–416.

64 Boyle JP, Honeycutt AA, Narayan KM, Hoerger TJ, Geiss LS, Chen H, *et al.* Projection of diabetes burden through 2050: impact of changing demography and disease prevalence in the US. *Diabetes Care* 2001; **24**:1936–1940.

65 Centers for Disease Control and Prevention. *National diabetes fact sheet: general information and national estimates on diabetes in the United States, 2007.* Atlanta, GA: US Department of Health and Human Services, Centers for Disease Control and Prevention, 2008.

66 Dabelea D, Bell RA, D'Agostino RB Jr, Imperatore G, Johansen JM, Linder B, *et al.* Incidence of diabetes in youth in the United States. *JAMA* 2007; **297**:2716–2724.

67 Perez-Bravo F, Carrasco E, Santos JL, Calvillan M, Larenas G, Albala C. Prevalence of type 2 diabetes and obesity in rural Mapuche population from Chile. *Nutrition* 2001; **17**:236–238.

68 Larenas G, Arias G, Espinoza O, Charles M, Landaeta O, Villanueva S, *et al.* [Prevalence of diabetes mellitus in a Mapuche community of Region IX, Chile.] *Rev Med Chil* 1985; **113**:1121–1125.

69 Llanos G, Libman I. Diabetes in the Americas. *Bull Pan Am Health Organ* 1994; **28**:285–301.

70 Sanchez-Castillo CP, Velasquez-Monroy O, Lara-Esqueda A, Berber A, Sepulveda J, Tapia-Conyer R, *et al.* Diabetes and hypertension increases in a society with abdominal obesity: results of the Mexican National Health Survey 2000. *Public Health Nutr* 2005; **8**:53–60.

71 Aschner P, King H, Triana de Torrado M, Rodriguez BM. Glucose intolerance in Colombia: a population-based survey in an urban community. *Diabetes Care* 1993; **16**:90–93.

72 Malerbi DA, Franco LJ. Multicenter study of the prevalence of diabetes mellitus and impaired glucose tolerance in the urban Brazilian population aged 30–69 yr. The Brazilian Cooperative Group on the Study of Diabetes Prevalence. *Diabetes Care* 1992; **15**:1509–1516.

73 Tulloch J. *Diabetes in the Tropics.* Churchill Livingstone, 1953.

74 Florey Cdu V, McDonald H, McDonald J, Miall WE. The prevalence of diabetes in a rural population of Jamaican adults. *Int J Epidemiol* 1972; **1**:157–166.

75 Florey CV. Blood sugar and serum insulin levels in Jamaica, West Indies. *Adv Metab Disord* 1978; **9**:65–91.

76 Cruickshank J, Riste L, Jackson M, Wilks R, Bennett F, Forrester T, *et al.* Standardized comparison of glucose tolerance and diabetes prevalence in 4 African/African-Carribean populations in Britain, Jamaica, and Cameroon. *Diabet Med* 1996; **13**:S18.

77 Wilks R, Rotimi C, Bennett F, McFarlane-Anderson N, Kaufman JS, Anderson SG, *et al.* Diabetes in the Caribbean: results of a population survey from Spanish Town, Jamaica. *Diabet Med* 1999; **16**:875–883.

78 Mather HM, Keen H. The Southall Diabetes Survey: prevalence of known diabetes in Asians and Europeans. *Br Med J (Clin Res Ed)* 1985; **291**:1081–1084.

79 Simmons D, Williams DR, Powell MJ. The Coventry Diabetes Study: prevalence of diabetes and impaired glucose tolerance in Europids and Asians. *Q J Med* 1991; **81**:1021–1030.

80 Riste L, Khan F, Cruickshank K. High prevalence of type 2 diabetes in all ethnic groups, including Europeans, in a British inner city: relative poverty, history, inactivity, or 21st century Europe? *Diabetes Care* 2001; **24**:1377–1383.

81 Wang J, Luben R, Khaw KT, Bingham S, Wareham NJ, Forouhi NG. Dietary energy density predicts the risk of incident type 2 diabetes: the European Prospective Investigation of Cancer (EPIC) Norfolk Study. *Diabetes Care* 2008; **31**:2120–2125.

82 McNaughton SA, Mishra GD, Brunner EJ. Dietary patterns, insulin resistance, and incidence of type 2 diabetes in the Whitehall II Study. *Diabetes Care* 2008; **31**:1343–1348.

83 Forouhi NG, Luan J, Hennings S, Wareham NJ. Incidence of type 2 diabetes in England and its association with baseline impaired fasting glucose: the Ely study 1990–2000. *Diabet Med* 2007; **24**:200–207.

84 Eliasson M, Lindahl B, Lundberg V, Stegmayr B. No increase in the prevalence of known diabetes between 1986 and 1999 in subjects 25–64 years of age in northern Sweden. *Diabet Med* 2002; **19**:874–880.

85 Yliharsila H, Lindstrom J, Eriksson JG, Jousilahti P, Valle TT, Sundvall J, *et al.* Prevalence of diabetes and impaired glucose regulation in 45- to 64-year-old individuals in three areas of Finland. *Diabet Med* 2005; **22**:88–91.

86 Vilbergsson S, Sigurdsson G, Sigvaldason H, Hreidarsson AB, Sigfusson N. Prevalence and incidence of NIDDM in Iceland: evidence for stable incidence among males and females 1967–1991: the Reykjavik Study. *Diabet Med* 1997; **14**:491–498.
87 Rajala U, Keinanen-Kiukaanniemi S, Uusimaki A, Reijula K, Kivela SL. Prevalence of diabetes mellitus and impaired glucose tolerance in a middle-aged Finnish population. *Scand J Prim Health Care* 1995; **13**:222–228.
88 Larsson H, Ahren B, Lindgarde F, Berglund G. Fasting blood glucose in determining the prevalence of diabetes in a large, homogeneous population of Caucasian middle-aged women. *J Intern Med* 1995; **237**:537–541.
89 Glumer C, Jorgensen T, Borch-Johnsen K. Prevalences of diabetes and impaired glucose regulation in a Danish population: the Inter99 study. *Diabetes Care* 2003; **26**:2335–2340.
90 Tuomilehto J, Lindstrom J, Eriksson JG, Valle TT, Hamalainen H, Ilanne-Parikka P, *et al.* Prevention of type 2 diabetes mellitus by changes in lifestyle among subjects with impaired glucose tolerance. *N Engl J Med* 2001; **344**:1343–1350.
91 Carstensen B, Kristensen JK, Ottosen P, Borch-Johnsen K. The Danish National Diabetes Register: trends in incidence, prevalence and mortality. *Diabetologia* 2008; **51**:2187–2196.
92 Lammi N, Taskinen O, Moltchanova E, Notkola IL, Eriksson JG, Tuomilehto J, *et al.* A high incidence of type 1 diabetes and an alarming increase in the incidence of type 2 diabetes among young adults in Finland between 1992 and 1996. *Diabetologia* 2007; **50**:1393–1400.
93 Muggeo M, Verlato G, Bonora E, Bressan F, Girotto S, Corbellini M, *et al.* The Verona diabetes study: a population-based survey on known diabetes mellitus prevalence and 5-year all-cause mortality. *Diabetologia* 1995; **38**:318–325.
94 Garancini MP, Calori G, Ruotolo G, Manara E, Izzo A, Ebbli E, *et al.* Prevalence of NIDDM and impaired glucose tolerance in Italy: an OGTT-based population study. *Diabetologia* 1995; **38**:306–313.
95 Bruno G, Merletti F, Bargero G, Melis D, Masi I, Ianni A, *et al.* Changes over time in the prevalence and quality of care of type 2 diabetes in Italy: the Casale Monferrato surveys, 1988 and 2000. *Nutr Metab Cardiovasc Dis* 2008; **18**:39–45.
96 Gourdy P, Ruidavets JB, Ferrieres J, Ducimetiere P, Amouyel P, Arveiler D, et *al.* Prevalence of type 2 diabetes and impaired fasting glucose in the middle-aged population of three French regions: the MONICA study 1995–97. *Diabetes Metab* 2001; **27**:347–358.
97 Defay R, Delcourt C, Ranvier M, Lacroux A, Papoz L. Relationships between physical activity, obesity and diabetes mellitus in a French elderly population: the POLA study. Pathologies Oculaires liees a l' Age. *Int J Obes Relat Metab Disord* 2001; **25**:512–518.
98 Mooy JM, Grootenhuis PA, de Vries H, Valkenburg HA, Bouter LM, Kostense PJ, *et al.* Prevalence and determinants of glucose intolerance in a Dutch Caucasian population: the Hoorn Study. *Diabetes Care* 1995; **18**:1270–1273.
99 de Vegt F, Dekker JM, Jager A, Hienkens E, Kostense PJ, Stehouwer CD, *et al.* Relation of impaired fasting and postload glucose with incident type 2 diabetes in a Dutch population: the Hoorn Study. *JAMA* 2001; **285**:2109–2113.
100 Ubink-Veltmaat LJ, Bilo HJ, Groenier KH, Houweling ST, Rischen RO, Meyboom-de Jong B. Prevalence, incidence and mortality of type 2 diabetes mellitus revisited: a prospective population-based study in the Netherlands (ZODIAC-1). *Eur J Epidemiol* 2003; **18**:793–800.
101 Katsilambros N, Aliferis K, Darviri C, Tsapogas P, Alexiou Z, Tritos N, *et al.* Evidence for an increase in the prevalence of known diabetes in a sample of an urban population in Greece. *Diabet Med* 1993; **10**:87–90.
102 Papazoglou N, Manes C, Chatzimitrofanous P, Papadeli E, Tzounas K, Scaragas G, *et al.* Epidemiology of diabetes mellitus in the elderly in northern Greece: a population study. *Diabet Med* 1995; **12**:397–400.
103 Lionis C, Bathianaki M, Antonakis N, Papavasiliou S, Philalithis A. A high prevalence of diabetes mellitus in a municipality of rural Crete, Greece. *Diabet Med* 2001; **18**:768–769.
104 Panagiotakos DB, Pitsavos C, Chrysohoou C, Stefanadis C. The epidemiology of type 2 diabetes mellitus in Greek adults: the ATTICA study. *Diabet Med* 2005; **22**:1581–1588.
105 Panagiotakos DB, Pitsavos C, Skoumas Y, Lentzas Y, Stefanadis C. Five-year incidence of type 2 diabetes mellitus among cardiovascular disease-free Greek adults: findings from the ATTICA study. *Vasc Health Risk Manag* 2008; **4**:691–698.
106 Erem C, Yildiz R, Kavgaci H, Karahan C, Deger O, Can G, *et al.* Prevalence of diabetes, obesity and hypertension in a Turkish population (Trabzon city). *Diabetes Res Clin Pract* 2001; **54**:203–208.
107 Kelestimur F, Cetin M, Pasaoglu H, Coksevim B, Cetinkaya F, Unluhizarci K, *et al.* The prevalence and identification of risk factors for type 2 diabetes mellitus and impaired glucose tolerance in Kayseri, central Anatolia, Turkey. *Acta Diabetol* 1999; **36**:85–91.
108 Panagiotakos DB, Tzima N, Pitsavos C, Chrysohoou C, Zampelas A, Toussoulis D, *et al.* The association between adherence to the Mediterranean diet and fasting indices of glucose homoeostasis: the ATTICA Study. *J Am Coll Nutr* 2007; **26**:32–38.
109 King H, Abdullaev B, Djumaeva S, Nikitin V, Ashworth L, Dobo MG. Glucose intolerance and associated factors in the Fergana Valley, Uzbekistan. *Diabet Med* 1998; **15**:1052–1062.
110 King H, Djumaeva S, Abdullaev B, Gacic Dobo M. Epidemiology of glucose intolerance and associated factors in Uzbekistan: a survey in Sirdaria province. *Diabetes Res Clin Pract* 2002; **55**:19–27.
111 Chazova LV, Kalinina AM, Markova EV, Pavlova LI. [Diabetes mellitus: its prevalence, relationship to the risk factors for IHD and prognostic importance (an epidemiological study).] *Ter Arkh* 1996; **68**:15–18.
112 State Science Research Centre of Preventive Medicine (Ministry of Health). *Moscow Behavioural Factor Survey 2000–2001*. Ministry of Health, 2002.
113 Perlman F, McKee M. Diabetes during the Russian transition. *Diabetes Res Clin Pract* 2008; **80**:305–313.
114 Szurkowska M, Szybinski Z, Nazim A, Szafraniec K, Jedrychowski W. [Prevalence of type II diabetes mellitus in population of Krakow.] *Pol Arch Med Wewn* 2001; **106**:771–779.
115 International Diabetes Federation. *Diabetes Atlas*, 3rd edn. International Diabetes Federation, 2006.
116 Ahuja M. Epidemiological studies on diabetes mellitus in India. In: Ahuja M, ed. *Epidemiology of Diabetes in Developing Countries*. New Delhi: Interprint, 1979: 29–38.
117 Verma NP, Mehta SP, Madhu S, Mather HM, Keen H. Prevalence of known diabetes in an urban Indian environment: the Darya Ganj diabetes survey. *Br Med J (Clin Res Ed)* 1986; **293**:423–424.
118 Ramachandran A, Snehalatha C, Dharmaraj D, Viswanathan M. Prevalence of glucose intolerance in Asian Indians: urban–rural difference and significance of upper body adiposity. *Diabetes Care* 1992; **15**:1348–1355.

119 Ramachandran A, Snehalatha C, Kapur A, Vijay V, Mohan V, Das AK, *et al.* High prevalence of diabetes and impaired glucose tolerance in India: National Urban Diabetes Survey. *Diabetologia* 2001; **44**:1094–1101.

120 Mohan V, Deepa M, Deepa R, Shanthirani CS, Farooq S, Ganesan A, *et al.* Secular trends in the prevalence of diabetes and impaired glucose tolerance in urban South India: the Chennai Urban Rural Epidemiology Study (CURES-17). *Diabetologia* 2006; **49**:1175–1178.

121 Ramachandran A, Mary S, Yamuna A, Murugesan N, Snehalatha C. High prevalence of diabetes and cardiovascular risk factors associated with urbanization in India. *Diabetes Care* 2008; **31**:893–898.

122 Ramachandran A, Snehalatha C, Latha E, Manoharan M, Vijay V. Impacts of urbanisation on the lifestyle and on the prevalence of diabetes in native Asian Indian population. *Diabetes Res Clin Pract* 1999; **44**:207–213.

123 Sadikot SM, Nigam A, Das S, Bajaj S, Zargar AH, Prasannakumar KM, *et al.* The burden of diabetes and impaired glucose tolerance in India using the WHO 1999 criteria: prevalence of diabetes in India study (PODIS). *Diabetes Res Clin Pract* 2004; **66**:301–307.

124. Mohan V, Deepa M, Anjana RM, Lanthorn H, Deepa R. Incidence of diabetes and pre-diabetes in a selected urban south Indian population (CUPS-19). *J Assoc Physicians India* 2008; **56**:152–157.

125 Ramachandran A, Snehalatha C, Vijay V, Wareham NJ, Colagiuri S. Derivation and validation of diabetes risk score for urban Asian Indians. *Diabetes Res Clin Pract* 2005; **70**:63–70.

126 Ramachandran A, Snehalatha C, Mary S, Mukesh B, Bhaskar AD, Vijay V. The Indian Diabetes Prevention Programme shows that lifestyle modification and metformin prevent type 2 diabetes in Asian Indian subjects with impaired glucose tolerance (IDPP-1). *Diabetologia* 2006; **49**:289–297.

127 Siegel K, Narayan KM, Kinra S. Finding a policy solution to India's diabetes epidemic. *Health Aff (Millwood)* 2008; **27**:1077–1090.

128 Shera AS, Rafique G, Khwaja IA, Ara J, Baqai S, King H. Pakistan National Diabetes Survey: prevalence of glucose intolerance and associated factors in Shikarpur, Sindh Province. *Diabet Med* 1995; **12**:1116–1121.

129 Shera AS, Rafique G, Khawaja IA, Baqai S, King H. Pakistan National Diabetes Survey: prevalence of glucose intolerance and associated factors in Baluchistan province. *Diabetes Res Clin Pract* 1999; **44**:49–58.

130 Shera AS, Jawad F, Maqsood A. Prevalence of diabetes in Pakistan. *Diabetes Res Clin Pract* 2007; **76**:219–222.

131 Sayeed MA, Khan AR, Banu A, Hussain MZ, Ali SM. Blood pressure and glycemic status in relation to body mass index in a rural population of Bangladesh. *Bangladesh Med Res Counc Bull* 1994; **20**:27–35.

132 Chandalia M, Abate N, Garg A, Stray-Gundersen J, Grundy SM. Relationship between generalized and upper body obesity to insulin resistance in Asian Indian men. *J Clin Endocrinol Metab* 1999; **84**:2329–2335.

133 Mohan V, Sandeep S, Deepa R, Shah B, Varghese C. Epidemiology of type 2 diabetes: Indian scenario. *Indian J Med Res* 2007; **125**:217–230.

134 Ramachandran A, Snehalatha C. Epidemiology of diabetes in South East Asia. In: Ekoe J-M, Rewers M, Williams R, Zimmet P, eds. *The Epidemiology of Diabetes Mellitus*, 2nd edn. Chichester: John Wiley & Sons Ltd, 2008: 207–224.

135 Yajnik CS. Early life origins of insulin resistance and type 2 diabetes in India and other Asian countries. *J Nutr* 2004; **134**:205–210.

136 Yajnik CS, Deshpande SS, Jackson AA, Refsum H, Rao S, Fisher DJ, *et al.* Vitamin B_{12} and folate concentrations during pregnancy and insulin resistance in the offspring: the Pune Maternal Nutrition Study. *Diabetologia* 2008; **51**:29–38.

137 Dowse GK, Gareeboo H, Zimmet PZ, Alberti KG, Tuomilehto J, Fareed D, *et al.* High prevalence of NIDDM and impaired glucose tolerance in Indian, Creole, and Chinese Mauritians. Mauritius Noncommunicable Disease Study Group. *Diabetes* 1990; **39**:390–396.

138 Soderberg S, Zimmet P, Tuomilehto J, de Courten M, Dowse GK, Chitson P, *et al.* Increasing prevalence of type 2 diabetes mellitus in all ethnic groups in Mauritius. *Diabet Med* 2005; **22**:61–68.

139 Glans F, Elgzyri T, Shaat N, Lindholm E, Apelqvist J, Groop L. Immigrants from the Middle East have a different form of type 2 diabetes compared with Swedish patients. *Diabet Med* 2008; **25**:303–307.

140 Alwan A, King H. Diabetes in the Eastern Mediterranean (Middle East) region: the World Health Organization responds to a major public health challenge. *Diabet Med* 1995; **12**:1057–1058.

141 International Diabetes Institute. The Australian Diabetes, obesity and lifestyle study (AusDiab). *Diabetes and Associated Disorders in Australia.* Melbourne, Australia: International Diabetes Institute, 2001.

142. Glatthaar C, Welborn TA, Stenhouse NS, Garcia-Webb P. Diabetes and impaired glucose tolerance: a prevalence estimate based on the Busselton 1981 survey. *Med J Aust* 1985; **143**:436–440.

143 Dunstan DW, Zimmet PZ, Welborn TA, De Courten MP, Cameron AJ, Sicree RA, *et al.* The rising prevalence of diabetes and impaired glucose tolerance: the Australian Diabetes, Obesity and Lifestyle Study. *Diabetes Care* 2002; **25**:829–834.

144 Magliano DJ, Shaw JE, Shortreed SM, Nusselder WJ, Liew D, Barr EL, *et al.* Lifetime risk and projected population prevalence of diabetes. *Diabetologia* 2008; **51**:2179–2186.

145 DeCourten M, Hodge AM, Dowse GK, King I, Vickery J, Zimmet P. *Review of the epidemiology, aetiology, pathogenesis and preventability of diabetes in Aboriginal and Torres Strait Islander populations.* Commonwealth of Australia: Office for Aboriginal and Torres Strait Islander Health Services, 1998.

146 Simmons D. The epidemiology of diabetes and its complications in New Zealand. *Diabet Med* 1996; **13**:371–375.

147 Ministry of Health NZ. *A Portrait of Health: Key Results of the 2006/07 New Zealand Health Survey.* 2008: 137–142.

148 Joshy G, Simmons D. Epidemiology of diabetes in New Zealand: revisit to a changing landscape. *N Z Med J* 2006; **119**:U1999.

149 Dowse GK, Zimmet PZ, Finch CF, Collins VR. Decline in incidence of epidemic glucose intolerance in Nauruans: implications for the "thrifty genotype". *Am J Epidemiol* 1991; **133**:1093–1104.

150 Zimmet P, Taylor R, Ram P, King H, Sloman G, Raper LR, *et al.* Prevalence of diabetes and impaired glucose tolerance in the biracial (Melanesian and Indian) population of Fiji: a rural–urban comparison. *Am J Epidemiol* 1983; **118**:673–688.

151 King H, Finch C, Collins A, Koki G, King LF, Heywood P, *et al.* Glucose tolerance in Papua New Guinea: ethnic differences, association with environmental and behavioural factors and the possible emergence of glucose intolerance in a highland community. *Med J Aust* 1989; **151**:204–210.

152 Dowse GK, Spark RA, Mavo B, Hodge AM, Erasmus RT, Gwalimu M, *et al.* Extraordinary prevalence of non-insulin-dependent

diabetes mellitus and bimodal plasma glucose distribution in the Wanigela people of Papua New Guinea. *Med J Aust* 1994; **160**: 767–774.

153 Collins VR, Dowse GK, Toelupe PM, Imo TT, Aloaina FL, Spark RA, *et al.* Increasing prevalence of NIDDM in the Pacific island population of Western Samoa over a 13-year period. *Diabetes Care* 1994; **17**:288–296.

154 Colagiuri S, Colagiuri R, Na'ati S, Muimuiheata S, Hussain Z, Palu T. The prevalence of diabetes in the kingdom of Tonga. *Diabetes Care* 2002; **25**:1378–1383.

155 Colagiuri S, Palu T, Viali S, Hussain Z, Colagiuri R. The epidemiology of diabetes in Pacific Island populations. In: Ekoe J-M, Rewers M, Williams R, Zimmet P, eds. *The Epidemiology of Diabetes Mellitus*, 2nd edn. Chichester: John Wiley & Sons Ltd, 2008: 225–240.

156 Sekikawa A, Eguchi H, Tominaga M, Igarashi K, Abe T, Manaka H, *et al.* Prevalence of type 2 diabetes mellitus and impaired glucose tolerance in a rural area of Japan: the Funagata diabetes study. *J Diabetes Complications* 2000; **14**:78–83.

157 Ministry of Health Law. *The Report of the National Diabetes Survey in 2002* [in Japanese]. 2002.

158 Owada M, Kitagawa T. Diabetes screening in school health system. *Chiryo* 1995; **77**:3047–3053.

159 Kitagawa T, Owada M, Urakami T, Yamauchi K. Increased incidence of non-insulin dependent diabetes mellitus among Japanese schoolchildren correlates with an increased intake of animal protein and fat. *Clin Pediatr (Phila)* 1998; **37**:111–115.

160 Hara H, Egusa G, Yamakido M, Kawate R. The high prevalence of diabetes mellitus and hyperinsulinemia among the Japanese-Americans living in Hawaii and Los Angeles. *Diabetes Res Clin Pract* 1994; **24**(Suppl):S37–42.

161 Tajima N. Japan. In: Ekoe J-M, Rewers M, Williams R, Zimmet P, eds. *The Epidemiology of Diabetes Mellitus*, 2nd edn. Chichester: John Wiley & Sons Ltd., 2008: 171–178.

162 Yazaki Y, Kadowaki T. Combating diabetes and obesity in Japan. *Nat Med* 2006; **12**:73–74.

163 Kim SM, Lee JS, Lee J, Na JK, Han JH, Yoon DK, *et al.* Prevalence of diabetes and impaired fasting glucose in Korea: Korean National Health and Nutrition Survey 2001. *Diabetes Care* 2006; **29**:226–231.

164 Yoon KH, Lee JH, Kim JW, Cho JH, Choi YH, Ko SH, *et al.* Epidemic obesity and type 2 diabetes in Asia. *Lancet* 2006; **368**:1681–1688.

165 Cockram CS. The epidemiology of diabetes mellitus in the Asia-Pacific region. *Hong Kong Med J* 2000; **6**:43–52.

166 Hu YH, Li GW, Pan XR. [Incidence of NIDDM in Daqing and forecasting of NIDDM in China in 21st century.] *Zhonghua Nei Ke Za Zhi* 1993; **32**:173–175.

167 Pan XR, Hu YH, Li GW, Liu PA, Bennett PH, Howard BV. Impaired glucose tolerance and its relationship to ECG-indicated coronary heart disease and risk factors among Chinese: Da Qing IGT and diabetes study. *Diabetes Care* 1993; **16**:150–156.

168 Wang K, Li T, Xiang H. [Study on the epidemiological characteristics of diabetes mellitus and IGT in China.] *Zhonghua Liu Xing Bing Xue Za Zhi* 1998; **19**:282–285.

169 Gu D, Reynolds K, Duan X, Xin X, Chen J, Wu X, *et al.* Prevalence of diabetes and impaired fasting glucose in the Chinese adult population: International Collaborative Study of Cardiovascular Disease in Asia (InterASIA). *Diabetologia* 2003; **46**:1190–1198.

170 Jia WP, Pang C, Chen L, Bao YQ, Lu JX, Lu HJ, *et al.* Epidemiological characteristics of diabetes mellitus and impaired glucose regulation in a Chinese adult population: the Shanghai Diabetes Studies, a cross-sectional 3-year follow-up study in Shanghai urban communities. *Diabetologia* 2007; **50**:286–292.

171 Janus ED, for the Hong Kong Cardiovascular Risk Factor Prevalence Study Group. Epidemiology of cardiovascular risk factors in Hong Kong. *Clin Exp Pharmacol Physiol* 1997; **24**:987–988.

172 Cockram CS, Woo J, Lau E, Chan JCN, Chan AYW, Lau J, *et al.* The prevalence of diabetes mellitus and impaired glucose tolerance among Hong Kong Chinese adults of working age. *Diabetes Res Clin Pract* 1993; **21**:67–73.

173 Chou P, Li CL, Kuo HS, Hsiao KJ, Tsai ST. Comparison of the prevalence in two diabetes surveys in Pu-Li, Taiwan, 1987–1988 and 1991–1992. *Diabetes Res Clin Pract* 1997; **38**:61–67.

174 Wong KC, Wang Z. Prevalence of type 2 diabetes mellitus of Chinese populations in Mainland China, Hong Kong, and Taiwan. *Diabetes Res Clin Pract* 2006; **73**:126–134.

175 Chan JC, Cockram CS. Epidemiology of diabetes mellitus in China. In: Ekoe J-M, Rewers M, Williams R, Zimmet P, eds. *The Epidemiology of Diabetes Mellitus*, 2nd edn. Chichester: John Wiley and Sons Ltd, 2008: 179–206.

176 Li Y, Yang X, Zhai F, Piao J, Zhao W, Zhang J, *et al.* Childhood obesity and its health consequence in China. *Obes Rev* 2008; **9**(Suppl 1):82–86.

177 Ko GT, Ozaki R, Wong GW, Kong AP, So WY, Tong PC, *et al.* The problem of obesity among adolescents in Hong Kong: a comparison using various diagnostic criteria. *BMC Pediatr* 2008; **8**:10.

178 Wei JN, Sung FC, Lin CC, Lin RS, Chiang CC, Chuang LM. National surveillance for type 2 diabetes mellitus in Taiwanese children. *JAMA* 2003; **290**:1345–1350.

179 King H, Keuky L, Seng S, Khun T, Roglic G, Pinget M. Diabetes and associated disorders in Cambodia: two epidemiological surveys. *Lancet* 2005; **366**:1633–1639.

180 Duc Son LN, Kusama K, Hung NT, Loan TT, Chuyen NV, Kunii D, *et al.* Prevalence and risk factors for diabetes in Ho Chi Minh City, Vietnam. *Diabet Med* 2004; **21**:371–376.

181 Sutanegara D, Budhiarta AA. The epidemiology and management of diabetes mellitus in Indonesia. *Diabetes Res Clin Pract* 2000; **50**(Suppl 2):S9–S16.

182 Baltazar JC, Ancheta CA, Aban IB, Fernando RE, Baquilod MM. Prevalence and correlates of diabetes mellitus and impaired glucose tolerance among adults in Luzon, Philippines. *Diabetes Res Clin Pract* 2004; **64**:107–115.

183 Aekplakorn W, Abbott-Klafter J, Premgamone A, Dhanamun B, Chaikittiporn C, Chongsuvivatwong V, *et al.* Prevalence and management of diabetes and associated risk factors by regions of Thailand: Third National Health Examination Survey 2004. *Diabetes Care* 2007; **30**:2007–2012.

184 National Health Survey 2004. September 2005.

185 Gu K, Cowie CC, Harris MI. Mortality in adults with and without diabetes in a national cohort of the US population, 1971–1993. *Diabetes Care* 1998; **21**:1138–1145.

186 DECODE Study Group (Diabetes Epidemiology: Collaborative analysis Of Diagnostic criteria in Europe)/European Diabetes Epidemiology Group. Glucose tolerance and mortality: comparison of WHO and American Diabetes Association diagnostic criteria. *Lancet* 1999; **354**:617–621.

187 Khaw KT, Wareham N, Luben R, Bingham S, Oakes S, Welch A, *et al.* Glycated haemoglobin, diabetes, and mortality in men in

Norfolk cohort of European Prospective Investigation of Cancer and Nutrition (EPIC-Norfolk). *Br Med J* 2001; **322**:15–18.

188 Nakagami T. Hyperglycaemia and mortality from all causes and from cardiovascular disease in five populations of Asian origin. *Diabetologia* 2004; **47**:385–394.

189 Tseng CH. Mortality and causes of death in a national sample of diabetic patients in Taiwan. *Diabetes Care* 2004; **27**:1605–1609.

190 McEwen LN, Kim C, Haan M, Ghosh D, Lantz PM, Mangione CM, *et al.* Diabetes reporting as a cause of death: results from the Translating Research Into Action for Diabetes (TRIAD) study. *Diabetes Care* 2006; **29**:247–253.

191 Morrish NJ, Wang S, Stevens LK, Fuller JH, Keen H. Mortality and causes of death in the WHO Multinational Survey of Vascular Diseases in Diabetes. *Diabetologia* 2001; **44**(Suppl 2):S14–21.

192 Keen H. The WHO Multinational Study of Vascular Disease in Diabetes. *Diabetologia* 2001; **44**(Suppl 2):S1–2.

193 Eschwege E, Richard JL, Thibult N, Ducimetiere P, Warnet JM, Claude JR, *et al.* Coronary heart disease mortality in relation with diabetes, blood glucose and plasma insulin levels: the Paris Prospective Study, ten years later. *Horm Metab Res Suppl* 1985; **15**:41–46.

194 Khandwala HM, McCutcheon IE, Flyvbjerg A, Friend KE. The effects of insulin-like growth factors on tumorigenesis and neoplastic growth. *Endocr Rev* 2000; **21**:215–244.

195 Hu FB, Manson JE, Liu S, Hunter D, Colditz GA, Michels KB, *et al.* Prospective study of adult onset diabetes mellitus (type 2) and risk of colorectal cancer in women. *J Natl Cancer Inst* 1999; **91**:542–547.

196 Yang X, So W, Ko GT, Ma RC, Kong AP, Chow CC, *et al.* Independent associations between low-density lipoprotein cholesterol and cancer among patients with type 2 diabetes mellitus. *CMAJ* 2008; **179**:427–437.

197 Jee SH, Ohrr H, Sull JW, Yun JE, Ji M, Samet JM. Fasting serum glucose level and cancer risk in Korean men and women. *JAMA* 2005; **293**:194–202.

198 Gaede P, Vedel P, Larsen N, Jensen GV, Parving HH, Pedersen O. Multifactorial intervention and cardiovascular disease in patients with type 2 diabetes. *N Engl J Med* 2003; **348**:383–393.

199 Gaede P, Lund-Andersen H, Parving HH, Pedersen O. Effect of a multifactorial intervention on mortality in type 2 diabetes. *N Engl J Med* 2008; **358**:580–591.

200 UK Prospective Diabetes Study (UKPDS) Group. Intensive blood-glucose control with sulphonylureas or insulin compared with conventional treatment and risk of complications in patients with type 2 diabetes (UKPDS 33). *Lancet* 1998; **352**:837–853.

201 Patel A, MacMahon S, Chalmers J, Neal B, Billot L, Woodward M, *et al.* Intensive blood glucose control and vascular outcomes in patients with type 2 diabetes. *N Engl J Med* 2008; **358**:2560–2572.

202 Holman RR, Paul SK, Bethel MA, Matthews DR, Neil HA. 10-year follow-up of intensive glucose control in type 2 diabetes. *N Engl J Med* 2008; **359**:1577–1589.

203 Gulliford MC, Charlton J. Is relative mortality of type 2 diabetes mellitus decreasing? *Am J Epidemiol* 2009; **169**:455–461.

204 Ringborg A, Lindgren P, Martinell M, Yin DD, Schon S, Stalhammar J. Prevalence and incidence of type 2 diabetes and its complications 1996–2003: estimates from a Swedish population-based study. *Diabet Med* 2008; **25**:1178–1186.

205 Charlton J, Latinovic R, Gulliford MC. Explaining the decline in early mortality in men and women with type 2 diabetes: a population-based cohort study. *Diabetes Care* 2008; **31**:1761–1766.

206 Hogan P, Dall T, Nikolov P. Economic costs of diabetes in the US in 2002. *Diabetes Care* 2003; **26**:917–932.

207 Ettaro L, Songer TJ, Zhang P, Engelgau MM. Cost-of-illness studies in diabetes mellitus. *Pharmacoeconomics* 2004; **22**:149–164.

208 Economic costs of diabetes in the US in 2007. *Diabetes Care* 2008; **31**:596–615.

209 Zhang P, Engelgau MM, Norris SL, Gregg EW, Narayan KM. Application of economic analysis to diabetes and diabetes care. *Ann Intern Med* 2004; **140**:972–977.

210 Narayan KM, Zhang P, Williams D, Engelgau M, Imperatore G, Kanaya A, *et al.* How should developing countries manage diabetes? *CMAJ* 2006; **175**:733.

211 Lindstrom J, Ilanne-Parikka P, Peltonen M, Aunola S, Eriksson JG, Hemio K, *et al.* Sustained reduction in the incidence of type 2 diabetes by lifestyle intervention: follow-up of the Finnish Diabetes Prevention Study. *Lancet* 2006; **368**:1673–1679.

212 Li G, Zhang P, Wang J, Gregg EW, Yang W, Gong Q, *et al.* The long-term effect of lifestyle interventions to prevent diabetes in the China Da Qing Diabetes Prevention Study: a 20-year follow-up study. *Lancet* 2008; **371**:1783–1789.

213 Barzilay JI, Davis BR, Cutler JA, Pressel SL, Whelton PK, Basile J, *et al.* Fasting glucose levels and incident diabetes mellitus in older nondiabetic adults randomized to receive 3 different classes of antihypertensive treatment: a report from the Antihypertensive and Lipid-Lowering Treatment to Prevent Heart Attack Trial (ALLHAT). *Arch Intern Med* 2006; **166**:2191–2201.

214 Heart Outcomes Prevention Evaluation Study Investigators. Effects of ramipril on cardiovascular and microvascular outcomes in people with diabetes mellitus: results of the HOPE study and MICRO-HOPE substudy. *Lancet* 2000; **355**:253–259.

215 Vermes E, Ducharme A, Bourassa MG, Lessard M, White M, Tardif JC. Enalapril reduces the incidence of diabetes in patients with chronic heart failure: insight from the Studies Of Left Ventricular Dysfunction (SOLVD). *Circulation* 2003; **107**:1291–1296.

216 Lindholm LH, Ibsen H, Dahlof B, Devereux RB, Beevers G, de Faire U, *et al.* Cardiovascular morbidity and mortality in patients with diabetes in the Losartan Intervention For Endpoint reduction in hypertension study (LIFE): a randomised trial against atenolol. *Lancet* 2002; **359**:1004–1010.

217 Preiss D, Zetterstrand S, McMurray JJ, Ostergren J, Michelson EL, Granger CB, *et al.* Predictors of development of diabetes in patients with chronic heart failure in the Candesartan in Heart Failure Assessment of Reduction in Mortality and Morbidity (CHARM) Program. *Diabetes Care* 2009; **32**:915–920.

218 Bosch J, Yusuf S, Gerstein HC, Pogue J, Sheridan P, Dagenais G, *et al.* Effect of ramipril on the incidence of diabetes. *N Engl J Med* 2006; **355**:1551–1562.

219 Ekoe JM, Rewers M, Willaims R, Zimmet P. *The Epidemiology of Diabetes Mellitus*, 2nd edn. Chichester, UK: John Wiley & Sons Ltd, 2008.

220 Salti S, Khogali M, Alam S, Abu Haidar N, Masri A. Epidemiology of diabetes mellitus in relation to other cardiovascular risk factors in Lebanon. *East Mediterr Health J* 1997; **3**:462–471.

221 Al-Lawati JA, Al Riyami AM, Mohammed AJ, Jousilahti P. Increasing prevalence of diabetes mellitus in Oman. *Diabet Med* 2002; **19**:954–957.

222 Asfour MG, Lambourne A, Soliman A, Al-Behlani S, Al-Asfoor D, Bold A, *et al.* High prevalence of diabetes mellitus and impaired glucose tolerance in the Sultanate of Oman: results of the 1991 national survey. *Diabet Med* 1995; **12**:1122–1125.

223 Al-Nozha MM, Al-Maatouq MA, Al-Mazrou YY, Al-Harthi SS, Arafah MR, Khalil MZ, *et al.* Diabetes mellitus in Saudi Arabia. *Saudi Med J* 2004; **25**:1603–1610.

224 Al-Nuaim AR. Prevalence of glucose intolerance in urban and rural communities in Saudi Arabia. *Diabet Med* 1997; **14**:595–602.

225 Musaiger AO. Diabetes mellitus in Bahrain: an overview. *Diabet Med* 1992; **9**:574–578.

226 Narayan KMV, Zhang P, Kanaya AM, Williams DE, Engelgau MM, Impperatore G, Ramachandran A. Diabetes: the pandemic and potential solutions. In: Jamison DT, Breman JG, Measham AR, Alleyne G, Claeson M, Evans DB, Jha P, Mills A, Musgrove P, eds. *Disease Control and Priorities*, 2nd edn. The International Bank of Reconstruction and Development/The World Bank, 2006.

227 Pan XR, Li GW, Hu YH, Yang WY, An ZX, Hu ZX, *et al.* Effects of diet and exercise in preventing NIDDM in people with impaired glucose tolerance. The Da Qing IGT and Diabetes Study. *Diabetes Care* 1997; **20**(4):537–44.

228 Knowler WC, Barrett-Connor E, Fowler SE, Hamman RF, Lachin JM, Walker EA, *et al.* Reduction in incidence of type 2 diabetes with lifestyle intervention or metformin. *N Engl J Med* 2002; **346**:393–403.

229 Kosaka K, Noda M, Kuzuya T. Prevention of type 2 diabetes by lifestyle intervention: A Japanese trial in IGT males. *Diabetes Res Clin Pract* 2005; **67**:152–162.

230 Wenying Y, Lixiang L, Jinwu Q, *et al.* The preventive effect of acarbose and metformin on the progression to diabetes mellitus in the IGT population: a 3-year multi-centre prospective study. *Chin J Endocrinol Metab* 2001; **17**:131–135.

231 Buchanan TA, Xiang AH, Peters RK, Kjos SL, Marroquin A, Goico J, *et al.* Prevention of pancreatic beta-cell function and prevention of type 2 diabetes by pharmacological treatment of insulin resistance in high-risk Hispanic women. *Diabetes* 2002; **51**:2796–2803.

232 DREAM (Diabetes Reduction Assessment with Ramipril and Rosiglitazone Medication) Investigators, Gerstein HC, Yusuf S, Bosch J, Pogue J, Sheridan P, *et al.* Effect of rosiglitazone on the frequency of diabetes in patients with impaired glucose tolerance or impaired fasting glucose: a randomized controlled trial. *Lancet* 2006; **368**:1096–1105.

233 Chiasson JL, Josse RG, Gomis R, Hanefeld M, Karasik A, Laakso M. Acarbose for prevention of type 2 diabetes mellitus: the STOP-NIDDM randomized trial. *Lancet* 2002; **359**:2072–2077.

5 The Global Burden of Diabetes

Mohammed K. Ali,[1,2] **Mary Beth Weber**[2] **& K.M. Venkat Narayan**[1,3]

[1] Hubert Department of Global Health, Rollins School of Public Health, Emory University, Atlanta, GA, USA
[2] Global Diabetes Research Center, Emory University, Atlanta, GA, USA
[3] Department of Epidemiology, Rollins School of Public Health, Emory University, Atlanta, GA, USA

Keypoints

- Diabetes results in a range of distressing symptoms, altered daily functioning (requiring attentive monitoring and treatments), changed family roles, higher costs, lost productivity and premature mortality, which are felt by households, communities, and national economies.
- Diabetes is the fifth leading cause of death in the world (4 million deaths annually), outnumbering global deaths from HIV/AIDS; 80% of this mortality occurs in low and middle income countries, disproportionately affecting the young and economically active populations.
- Cost appraisal methods require epidemiologic, clinical, and economic data, and utilize different approaches to calculate the direct medical costs (of treatment, diagnosis, monitoring), indirect costs (of lost outputs from disability and premature death) and intangible losses (psychosocial burdens) attributable to diabetes.
- Even though there are large variations in methods of cost appraisal, cost items incorporated and purchasing power, as well as accessibility to and patterns of clinical care resulting in widely varied between-country per capita expenditures, it is clear that the presence of diabetes results in excess consumption of resources worldwide.
- Progressive severity of disease complications, co-morbidities and complexity of therapy all increase the monetary, infrastructural and human resource costs of care.
- Individuals in vulnerable subpopulations are at an elevated risk of developing diabetes and progression toward significantly harmful outcomes, and devote a large proportion of resources toward their therapies and diabetes care; confronting the increased susceptibility and burdens will require addressing the underlying political, socioeconomic and behavioral factors that perpetuate disparities.

Introduction

Diabetes has emerged as a major health problem worldwide, with serious health-related and socioeconomic impacts on individuals and populations alike. Furthermore, the pandemic growth of diabetes is being spurred on by transitioning demographic (e.g. population aging), socioeconomic, migratory, nutritional and lifestyle patterns, and an affiliated proliferation in overweight and obese adults and children [1–2]. The International Diabetes Federation estimates there are 285 million people with diabetes worldwide in 2010 [3], and projects the absolute number will surpass 400 million in the coming twenty years. The overwhelming majority of this escalation will be attributable to growth of type 2 diabetes (T2DM). Rapid socioeconomic transformations seen with globalization, increasing urbanization, industrialization and marketization of developing regions will also result in a parallel growth of diabetes precursors (impaired fasting glucose [IFG] and impaired glucose tolerance [IGT]) and ensuing health consequences [4–6].

Textbook of Diabetes, 4th edition. Edited by R. Holt, C. Cockram, A. Flyvbjerg and B. Goldstein.

Current estimates suggest that two-thirds of those affected by diabetes live in low and middle income countries (LMIC). This challenges traditional paradigms that segregated chronic non-communicable diseases (NCDs) as problems of affluent countries alone. Eight out of the top 10 countries with the highest absolute numbers of people with diabetes are developing or transitioning economy countries [3]. While this burden of greater absolute numbers may be partially explained by larger population size, the rates at which NCDs are increasing in these countries amid transition are much steeper when compared with those in more developed affluent countries [7]; by 2025, the number of diabetes cases will increase by 170% in low and middle income countries, compared to a 41% increase in developed countries [8].

Thus far, the attention on health burdens in the developing world has focused justifiably on the persistence of infectious diseases and nutritional deficiencies; however, these same countries must also contend with 80% of global mortality associated with chronic diseases [9,10]. Projections suggest that this already overwhelming "double burden" will be exacerbated by the growth of NCDs. Altogether, projected increases in diabetes in all corners of the globe will result in corresponding escalation of burdens in the form of serious morbidity, disability, diminished life expectancy, reduced quality of life, loss of human and social capital, as well as individual and national income losses. This chapter describes these burdens in a global context, and systematically introduces data regarding regional patterns and associated themes.

Distribution and trends

Epidemiologic evidence quantifies the impacts and predictors of disease, identifies vulnerable populations and their needs, and facilitates formulation of appropriate disease prevention and control strategies; however, there are still limited representative epidemiologic data originating from a great many LMICs. Moreover, the utility of currently available estimates is hampered by methodological deficiencies (inconsistent diagnostic criteria, poor standardization of methods) and limited coverage (regional sampling with a predominance of urban studies whereas the vast majority of the populations in question are rural inhabitants). Despite this, notable patterns can be discerned and can be described by giving examples from regions where they are particularly noteworthy.

In Africa, there is:

- A general lack of awareness about chronic diseases and their risk factors.
- Limited data originating from a few localized centers in certain regions (western, eastern and southern) of the continent. The latest data (1998–2004) show prevalence rates of 1–3% in rural areas and 6–10% in urban environments [11].
- A growing double burden of communicable diseases and nutritional deficiencies, along with NCDs, especially where there is rapid economic development and globalization. Between-country differences in NCD prevalence likely reflect different stages of socioeconomic and epidemiologic transitions [12].
- A tendency for cultural (perceptions of excess weight and imported processed foods as symbols of status and luxury) and societal (stigmas regarding loss of weight as a sign of HIV infection) factors to influence health-seeking behavior [11,13].
- Variation in risk by ethnicity, with Black Africans showing a greater preponderance toward hypertension, while those of Egyptian and Asian Indian origin demonstrate higher prevalence of diabetes [14].

In Europe, the USA and Canada:

- Available data are derived from population studies, records of insulin and antidiabetic medication sales and/or reimbursement claims. Estimates still suggest 30–50% of people in these high income countries (HIC) have undiagnosed diabetes [4].
- Annual incidence of type 1 diabetes (T1DM) is increasing in Europe (+3.2% per year) and North America (+5.3% per year); the highest reported incidence rate is in Finland (40.9/100,000 per year) [15,16].
- Prevalence of T2DM is highest and growing fastest in vulnerable subgroups such as lower socioeconomic groups and the elderly [4].
- Life expectancy of people with diabetes, although reduced when compared with the general population, is markedly higher than in developing regions of the world. This is largely attributable to differences in access to self blood glucose monitoring and therapies to control glycemia.
- Uptake and costs related to newer and more expensive investigations and therapies are associated with inflated national health expenditures.

In Latin America:

- There is wide variation in prevalence rates (1.2–8%) of diabetes, reflecting the diversity of ethnicities and stage of development between countries.
- The pattern of T1DM incidence seems to correspond to the size of the population of Caucasoid origin.
- Diagnosis of diabetes frequently occurs late in the course of disease. Thus, complications may be present in 30–40% of cases at time of presentation for health care.
- Poor accessibility to health services results in only 30–40% of cases actually receiving therapy [17].

Asia is emerging as the epicenter of the cardiometabolic pandemic, because:

- Populous countries in this region are confronted with diabetes risk being manifest at younger ages and at lower body mass indices compared with populations in other regions.
- Patterns of genetic and/or ethnic propensity; South Asians and peninsular Arabs have markedly elevated metabolic risk [18]; Japanese are reported to have the highest prevalence of genetic polymorphisms [19]. Rural–urban differences in prevalence together suggest both gene–environment interactions and influences of the "thrifty" genotype.
- Estimates suggest a three- to fivefold increase in prevalence of T2DM over the last three decades, and an increasing prevalence of T2DM in children, with major implications for future burden in this region [20,21].
- India is estimated to have 50.8 million people living with diabetes [3], the highest absolute number in any country [22] and projections suggest that one-fifth of all people with T2DM will be living in the Indian subcontinent by 2030 [23].
- The "Asian Indian phenotype" is characterized by a preponderance to deposition of metabolically active visceral adiposity which may explain the greater vulnerability to diabetes in this population [24–26], while Western Pacific Islanders also demonstrate a markedly elevated risk.

Diabetes is renowned as a "silent epidemic" [22]. The slow progression and lack of symptoms in the early stages of disease preclude seeking medical attention and preventative care. As such, reported prevalence reflects an underestimate of the number of cases because it does not account for undiagnosed cases. Population studies estimate that 30–50% of diabetes cases are as yet unrecognized, even in the most advanced countries [4,17]. Also, almost half of all newly diagnosed cases will have already developed diabetes-related complications in the form of nerve, eye, kidney, and/or vascular diseases [23,27,28]. Target organ damage of this nature can be life-threatening and/or seriously disabling [29].

The traditional socioeconomic gradient associated with chronic diseases may itself be transitioning. As the world's urban population size begins to outnumber those living in rural areas, many developing economies face enormous challenges related to the growth of peri-urban slums and squatter settlements, the disparities in provision of basic amenities and lack of adequate sanitation and nourishment. Further challenges include subsequent exposure to contemporary dietary choices, tobacco use and mechanization of transport with consequent growth in the incidence of NCDs. Thus, the paradigm is shifting *globally* towards the inverse relationship found in established market economies where the greatest burdens of NCDs are felt by the least well-off segments of the population [30–35]. In India for example, Ramachandran *et al.* [36] demonstrated that although family history and prevalence of glycemic abnormalities in high-income groups were double those of low-income groups, the reverse was true for smoking, alcohol consumption, prevalence of co-morbid cardiovascular risks and occurrence of complications (macrovascular disease, cataracts, proteinuria and neuropathy). Recent prevalence and trend data show greater disease susceptibility in lower socioeconomic groups in India [37,38], mimicking patterns in wealthier nations [39–42]. As this chapter progresses, it will become evident that the countries with the greatest burdens of disease are also those least equipped to manage the growing epidemics.

Box 5.1 Evaluation of burden

Health-related burdens
- Health seeking and utilization (frequency and costs)
- Disease events and/or ill health
- Morbidity (physical and psychosocial)
- Mortality

Social implications of disease
- Disability
- Alteration of social roles or family structure
- Caregiver or "intangible" burdens

Economic costs of disease
- Direct medical expenditure
- Ancillary expenses of health seeking and care
- Indirect costs (losses in productivity)

Major burdens

The burden of any disease, including diabetes, can be described by its health-related impacts: the morbidity and mortality caused, and the social and economic costs to individuals, families, communities and national economies (Box 5.1). Evaluation of resources utilized or lost, be they human, social, monetary or infrastructural, and placing objective "values" on them may be inherently partial to the perspective taken. The term "value" may be used to describe the measured and/or perceived net worth of resources consumed or lost because of illness and/or infirmity which is the mode used in this chapter. Economists use this term to express the net benefit derived from an investment in health care in proportion to the amount of resources used [43].

Acute and chronic disease complications

The patterns of major health-related burdens of diabetes vary by the type of disease. T2DM accounts for 90–95% of all cases worldwide. Both T1DM and T2DM, the two most common forms, may be associated with acute and chronic metabolic consequences, but the frequency of events varies according to the underlying pathophysiology and level of glycemic control.

Acute fluctuations in serum glucose may rapidly spiral into emergency situations, with potentially fatal repercussions if untreated. Episodes of severe acute hyperglycemia (e.g. diabetic ketoacidosis [DKA] and hyperosmolar hyperglycemic syndrome) or, conversely, severe hypoglycemia, most often require immediate medical management. Longer term follow-up is then intended to promote better blood glucose regulation and avoidance of precipitants of diabetic emergencies (e.g. infection, non-compliance with treatments, missing meals, alcohol abuse). Apart from atypical variants such as ketosis-prone T2DM in African subjects [11], the vast majority of acute complications occur in patients with T1DM, while approximately 10–12% occur in subjects with T2DM. When treated properly, the mortality from acute hyperglycemic episodes such as DKA is extremely low (e.g. DKA mortality in Taiwan, USA and Denmark were estimated to occur in 0.67–4.0% of cases) [44,45]. In contrast, in some African countries, mortality from DKA can be as high as 25–33% [46], although the incidence of these complications from LMIC settings is limited [47]. Individual patient (e.g. age, additional co-morbidities) and resource (e.g. hospital facilities, experience of staff) characteristics may also modify the outcomes. In underresourced settings for example, complex, cumulative and interconnected barriers (poor accessibility, inadequate therapeutic instruments and medication, and insufficient numbers of trained staff) result in poor glycemic control and higher risk of mortality [48]. As such, early life mortality in patients with T1DM in low-resource settings is commonplace. The post-diagnosis life expectancy in some regions of Africa is just 1 year [49].

Apart from glucose dysregulation, both T1DM and T2DM are associated with damaging effects on tissues, with eventual progression to devastating complications. Diabetes increases the risk of macrovascular diseases (cardiovascular diseases [CVD], which comprise coronary heart disease and cerebrovascular disease or "stroke," and peripheral vascular disease [PVD]), microvascular diseases (retinopathy and nephropathy), neuropathies, and the consequences that stem from these (e.g. congestive heart failure, diabetic foot). These complications are associated with considerable morbidity, reduced quality of life, disability, premature mortality and high economic costs.

In addition, T2DM is associated with the "metabolic syndrome," a collection of cardiovascular risk factors (abdominal obesity, hyperinsulinemia, hypertension, dyslipidemia, proinflammatory and procoagulant states). It is believed that these biochemical and inflammatory derangements are intimately linked, possibly by a central mediating factor. In Latin America, it is estimated that 53–69% of people with diabetes have abnormal serum lipid subfractions, and 34–67% have hypertension [17]. As such, these factors increase the likelihood of developing additional risks, and with each added risk, predispose one to an exponentially increasing risk of atherosclerotic vascular disease events and mortality [50].

Moreover, T2DM has a distinctive association with coronary heart disease (CHD). Those with diabetes have a two- to fourfold higher risk of developing CHD than people without diabetes [51]. More significantly, however, the age- and sex-adjusted cardiovascular mortality risk in patients with diabetes is equivalent to that of individuals without diabetes who have had a previous myocardial infarction (MI) [50,52,53]. Precursors common to both T2DM and CVD (insulin resistance, visceral adiposity and excess inflammation) [54–58], and a complex mix of mechanistic processes such as oxidative stress, enhanced atherogenecity of cholesterol particles, abnormal vascular reactivity, augmented hemostatic activation and renal dysfunction, cumulatively confer this elevated risk of CHD [59]. As such, simply controlling glucose has not been found to reduce CVD events and mortality in large randomized controlled trials at least in the short term [60–62]. The implications therefore are that individualized comprehensive multifactorial risk management, involving the treatment of all co-morbidities, has been advocated for people with T2DM [63,64], adding to the burdens placed on patients, providers and health systems.

Diabetes also increases the risk of renal dysfunction. In Africa, it is estimated that within 5–10 years following diagnosis, 32–57% of people with diabetes will have developed microalbuminuria [48,65]. Also, diabetes is the primary cause in approximately 45% of patients with end-stage renal disease (ESRD) requiring dialysis or transplantation in the USA [66,67]. Meanwhile, approximately one in four persons with diabetes have some visual impairment, and 5% of all cases of blindness globally are caused by diabetes [68]. Particularly in the case of retinopathy and nephropathy, duration of disease, age, glycemic control and blood pressure control have all been found to be prominent modifying factors of disease onset, progression and outcomes.

Neuropathies are also common consequences of diabetes. One-third of Sri Lankan people with diabetes surveyed had lower extremity sensory loss putting them at risk of ulceration [69], while a similar proportion of people with diabetes in African countries were found to have either neuropathy or compromised peripheral vascular circulation [70,71]. The combination of neuropathy, increased susceptibility to infection, poor wound healing and poor distal circulation increases the risk of lower extremity amputation 15- to 40-fold [67,72].

The most significant repercussion of the asymptomatic early natural history of the diabetes and low community awareness is that subclinical disease results in progressive tissue injury. Microvascular and macrovascular complications cause morbidity, greater health-seeking and increased mortality risk in all regions of the world [23,27,73].

Health utilization patterns

Health seeking and health utilization behaviors are influenced by a number of individual, provider and system level factors. In the case of diabetes, ill health and morbidity as well as preventative care motives result in incrementally more health service utilization. In Costa Rica, for example, people with diabetes made 55% more medical visits than those without diabetes, and German patients with diabetes averaged 31 yearly consultations with general practitioners (GPs) and/or specialists [74,75]. In Sweden and Italy, approximately half of diabetes-related consultations were at hospital outpatient departments or dedicated diabetes centers, respectively, and the remainder were with GPs [76,77]. In Latin America, diabetes accounts for an estimated 35 million medical visits annually [74].

Various studies have shown that having diabetes doubles one's risk of hospitalization compared to not having diabetes, and this risk is amplified by the development of diabetes-related complications. The presence of poor peripheral circulation increases the risk of hospitalization by 70%, while CVD increases this risk by 310% [67]. The Cost of Diabetes in Europe Type II Study (CODE-2) reported 13% of people with T2DM were hospitalized (with an average stay of 23 days) over the 6-month study follow-up, while Germany's Cost of Diabetes Mellitus (CoDiM) study reported that 28.8% of people with diabetes had at least one hospital admission in 2001 [75]. Although studies from most regions of the world report late-stage macrovascular or microvascular complications as the leading cause of diabetes-related hospitalizations, lower income settings such as Ethiopia confront a greater proportion (almost two-thirds) of admissions in the form of acute episodes of dysglycemia.

Health care infrastructure and financing have strong impacts on health seeking and utilization. In India, estimates suggest that 85–95% of all health care costs are borne by individuals and their families from household income [78–81]. In Latin America, 40–60% of diabetes expenses are derived from out-of-pocket payments. A survey in Jamaica showed that 57% of the sample reported financial difficulties as a result of illness, and of these, half disclosed that they had avoided therapy because of economic constraints [74]. Financial limitations to accessing treatment are not confined to LMICs, as illustrated by 19% of elderly Americans revealing curtailed purchases of diabetes medications as a result of costs [82,83].

When one considers that the average number of medications used by people with diabetes in India is 3.5 [79], the cost implications are substantial. These drugs include antihypertensives, lipid-lowering, antidepressant medications and aspirin in addition to glucose-lowering drugs). The use of oral hypoglycemics increases health expenditure by 40% compared to the general population, while regular insulin use is a further twofold greater expense. As such, data from Germany show that use of insulin with or without oral agents increases total costs 3.1–3.4 times [75,84].

Increased health seeking and utilization in people with diabetes and associated complications result in greater medical costs incurred, compared to the general non-diabetic population.

Disability

Aside from the medical or biologic dysfunction caused by disease, there are implications of ill health for individual and interactive functioning in society. This concept of "disability" is distinctive from simple biomedical models of disease and signifies that psychosocial illness or physical deviations from generally accepted norms of anatomical structure or physiologic function may impair one's ability to perform domestic and occupational activities, and assume societal roles. As a result, diabetes may inhibit one's general utility and ability to integrate fully in society.

Diabetes can lead to disability through a variety of ways. Excluding the medical aspects of diabetes-related complications that directly restrict bodily function, diabetes may be considered a "hidden" disability, whereby the individual concerned is hampered from routine activities, but displays no physical manifestation of this illness. For example, children with diabetes may be unable to participate in all activities their contemporaries are engaged in and may suffer wrongful discrimination. Adults in the workplace may have lower work performance by virtue of any number of symptoms (impaired fine motor skills and concentration, grogginess, urinary frequency) [85] or even decline in cognitive functioning [86–88]. Those requiring insulin may be limited additionally by highly structured activities of daily living (the requirement of meticulous glucose monitoring, insulin administration, timed eating), recurrent hospitalizations, hyperglycemic and hypoglycemic episodes, and by regular preventative or therapeutic medical visits.

Indeed, the physical manifestations of diabetes become more significant with the development of complications. As such, visual impairment, restricted mobility (from shortness of breath, chest pain or even amputation) and general ill health (ranging from increased susceptibility to infection all the way to uremia related to irreversible renal dysfunction) are all considerable impediments to productive work and engagement in socially valuable activity. Cross-sectional studies in the USA have demonstrated that elevated glycated haemoglobin (HbA_{1c}) is associated with a higher likelihood of missing work, greater hours absent [89] and reduced at-work efficiency [85].

Depending on the health status of the individual and severity of disease, disability can be temporary or permanent. There is limited country-specific data on the permanent disability resulting from diabetes, although diabetes is the leading cause of adult-onset blindness, non-traumatic amputations and irreversible kidney failure worldwide [22]. Data from Chile showed that 8% of people with diabetes had some form of permanent disability [74].

Less tangible, but no less severe, are the psychosocial burdens that may accompany diabetes and affect functioning [90,91]. In a health maintenance organization cohort of 1642 people with diabetes, 12% were unemployed, 7% of those employed had missed more than 5 working days in the previous month and 4% of employed subjects reported difficulties with completing work tasks. Of those with any form of work disability inducing absence and/or poor productivity, over half had minor and/or major signs and symptoms of depression [92].

The complexity of disability as a limitation of individual and societal function is in quantifying this shortcoming. There are several methods that have been used which factor in age, education and occupation, but most have at least some imperfection because of the necessity of making judgments about the value of activities. This is especially difficult where there are cultural and ideological dissimilarities between the evaluator and the population being appraised.

Mortality

Ascertaining the global mortality attributable to diabetes is no easy task. Most mortality statistics rely on documented causes of death and do not acknowledge the roles of glucose dysregulation in underlying mortality associated with CVD and renal diseases. Danaei *et al.* [29] have therefore argued that evaluating actual diabetes-related mortality should take into account that diabetes contributes to 21% of CHD and 13% of stroke mortality worldwide. The World Health Organization (WHO) incorporated these sentiments into calculating that diabetes is the fifth leading cause of death worldwide in 2000 [93]. The International Diabetes Federation's most recent *Diabetes Atlas* approximates that diabetes is responsible for 6.8% of total global mortality (4 million deaths) annually [22,94]. In addition, the mortality attributable to diabetes would be even higher if deaths related to IGT were also included. This diabetes precursor independently increases the risk of mortality, and has a prevalence of 15–40% in adults [6].

Altogether, diabetes is associated with premature mortality, shortening life expectancy by approximately 7–15 years [95,96]. In developed countries, CVDs account for an overwhelming 65–75% of deaths in people with diabetes [97,98]. In low-resource settings, infections and acute metabolic emergencies are still the prevailing causes of death in people with diabetes [11,12,65,99]. ESRD also carries inexorably high mortality, mainly because of inaccessibility (physical and financial) of treatment (dialysis and/or transplantation) in most LMICs [11]. As a result, globally, CVD and nephropathy are the most prominent fatal endpoints, and occurrence is analogous to duration of disease in that early life survival and long-standing diabetes increase susceptibility to succumbing from these illnesses [27].

There is regional variation in the global distribution of diabetes-related mortality. Estimates for the percentages of deaths attributable to diabetes by region are shown in Table 5.1. Although the proportion of deaths in LMICs is lower than in more developed countries, the absolute numbers of deaths, by virtue of larger population size, outnumber those in economically developed countries. South Asia is currently reported to have the highest absolute number of diabetes-related deaths annually [100]. Also, there is a noticeably greater proportion of deaths in

Table 5.1 Estimated percentage of deaths attributed to diabetes by age and World Health Organization (WHO) region. All figures are presented as male/female percentages. Adapted from Roglic *et al.* [93].

Region	Age (0–34 years)		Age (35–64 years)		Age (≥65 years)		All ages	
	Male	Female	Male	Female	Male	Female	Male	Female
African Region	0.5	0.8	7.1	7.9	2.7	4.1	2.2	2.5
Region of the Americas	0.4	0.5	11.6	17.8	5.4	7.7	6.0	8.6
Eastern Mediterranean	0.5	0.8	14.8	22.3	6.6	10.0	6.1	8.8
European Region	1.0	0.9	9.5	11.3	5.8	4.4	6.5	5.1
Southeast Asia Region	0.8	0.9	12.7	18.2	5.1	8.2	5.4	6.9
Western Pacific Region	0.2	0.3	6.4	9.2	3.01	5.1	3.4	4.8

younger age groups in LMICs, resulting in higher loss of life years, and affecting the economically active subpopulations in these countries.

It must be mentioned that in Africa, the HIV/AIDS epidemic has already altered patterns of mortality and life expectancy and is projected to modify these further. Irrespective of the fact that sub-Saharan Africa accounts for 72% of HIV-related deaths worldwide [101], projections based on demographic trends alone suggest that the prevalence of diabetes will continue to grow in this region. Widespread use of antiretroviral therapy will also directly (in the form of pancreatic dysfunction associated with therapy) and indirectly (increasing longevity of life) affect diabetes prevalence. The scarcity of data emanating from this continent does not allow a greater comprehension of the relative impacts of these forces versus contemporary sociodemographic and epidemiologic transitions.

Economic and social implications

The prototypical chronic nature of diabetes requires empowered self- and clinician-guided management for the duration between diagnosis and death. Forestalling complications and premature mortality is the central theme underlying glucose control and preventative management. Together, the care and serious consequences of diabetes are burdensome and costly. Quantifying the costs of diabetes from the perspectives of diabetes patients as well as national resource use and losses are critical towards informing appropriate health care planning, resource allocation and response strategies.

Approaches used to estimate economic costs of disease vary, not only by the perspective taken, but also by methodology applied, data sources used, year of estimation, as well as purchasing power and clinical practice patterns in different settings (Table 5.2). Needless to say, between-country comparisons are even more problematic where issues emerge regarding uncertainty of incidence and prevalence estimates, and standardization of measures and criteria. General principles and concepts of estimating cost are described [1,67,102,103].

Table 5.2 Examples of different treatment patterns in high-income countries.

Country	Proportion of diabetes patients receiving treatment			
	Diet and/or exercise (%)	OHA (%)	Insulin (%)	Both OHA and insulin (%)
USA [124]	16	57	14	13
Germany [75]	28	44	16	11
France [84]	–*	80	14.7	5.3

OHA, oral hypoglycemic agents.
* Database query only recognizes medications prescribed for diabetes.

Types of costs

Direct costs (inputs)

These include costs of treatment and care of the disease, broadly encompassing all outpatient consultations, inpatient care, diagnostic investigations, therapeutic procedures, pharmacotherapy, paramedical care (e.g. home nursing, physiotherapy), patient time, transportation and rehabilitation.

Indirect costs (lost output)

These costs represent the present and future value of economic productivity lost by society on account of temporary or permanent disability, excess morbidity and premature mortality from disease; they are typically calculated by estimating foregone income by investigating the cumulative impacts of absenteeism, employment status and income, for both the individual and caregiver(s).

Intangible costs

Costs are associated with the psychosocial impacts (e.g. stress, depression, emotional problems) and altered quality of life from an illness; they may include diminished family role, informal care and foregone income by family members; these costs are typically difficult to estimate because of relative lack of standardized methods.

Cost appraisal methods

Cost-of-illness method

This is the most widely used approach to describe the direct and indirect costs of disease to society and is conducted by exploring costs in a group of selected persons either over a defined finite period (e.g. 1 year) or through the natural progression of the disease.

Human capital approach
This is a method of estimating indirect costs of disease, with an emphasis on foregone earnings and employment; it is criticized as a tool because of the tendency for overestimating future values, accepting wage disparities and disregarding socially valuable activities such as housekeeping and volunteer work.

Friction cost approach
This approach is a more conservative measure of indirect costs that considers lost productivity as finite where restoration of productivity (return to work or replacement of worker) occurs within a timeframe and therefore limits production losses; it does, however, require detailed data.

"Top-down" approach
This calculatates costs from national databases and/or estimates, partitioning costs of different illnesses according to diagnoses; it requires accurate data entry, especially when indirect costs are being investigated but avoids the risk of double counting.

"Bottom-up" approach
This follows the trail of illness-related costs of a defined subpopulation with the illness, over a finite period.

Studies that have examined costs of diabetes vary in their estimates of the excess costs generated through resource consumption. The major drivers of direct health care costs include health service utilization (outpatient or ambulatory care comprising health practitioner consultations as well as inpatient care); medication usage; diagnostic tests; self glucose monitoring and therapeutic medical devices; and therapeutic procedures. In more developed settings, auxiliary services such as paramedical care (dietitians, physiotherapists, occupational therapists and home nursing) and preventative checks (foot care, urine and eye testing) may contribute to costs. The relative contributions of these cost drivers in various regions of the world are shown in Table 5.3. Themes that surface from these studies affirm the high costs of complications and associated hospitalization in developed countries, but also point to higher relative costs of purchasing medications in LMICs. Indeed, the supplemental costs of drugs for co-morbid CVD risk management are also pronounced.

Demographic and clinical characteristics have profound influences on costs. In Germany, compared to the diabetes-free population of the same age, younger people with diabetes (under 40 years of age) had greater incremental costs (4.1 times) than the people in the elderly age group (only 1.5 times higher) [75]. The types of diabetes have different costs. T1DM accounts for 5.7% of people with diabetes in the USA; medical costs of US$10.5 billion (bn) and indirect losses amount to US$4.4 bn, totaling US$14.9 bn. This is comparatively much lower than the US$159.5 bn that cumulatively account for T2DM care and lost productivity, but the cost burden per case is greater for T1DM [104]. It has been postulated that more consultations and faster progression to retinopathy and nephropathy are the main drivers of cost and mortality risk in those with T1DM [27,76]. In T2DM, coexistence of hypertension and dyslipidemia have relatively more significant roles in mediating risk, outcomes and associated costs.

The presence of diabetes-related complications greatly increases both the magnitude and duration of resource consumption. In particular, CVD and nephropathy are associated with the highest health care costs in most regions of the world. In the USA, medical costs increase by a factor of 1.5 when early CVD manifestations develop, and escalate to 3.6 times with the occurrence of a serious CVD event. Similarly, early renal dysfunction is the basis for 65% more costs, and the onset of ESRD signifies a 771% increase in costs [105–107]. Brandle *et al.* estimated that 1-year direct costs of suffering and surviving a major vascular event in the USA totaled US$24 500 for a myocardial infarction, US$26 600 for a stroke and US$37 600 for an amputation [130]. The Diabetes Health Economics Study Group estimated that complications contribute up to 60% of all direct costs, and 80–90% of indirect losses from absenteeism and lost productivity [108]. A rudimentary, but possibly practical finding by Gilmer *et al.* [109] reports that for every 1% (11 mmol/mol) increase in HbA_{1c} over 7% (>53 mmol/mol), there is a corresponding 10% increase in costs.

National perspectives reveal large differences in the health care expenditure in developed and developing country settings. Although the metrics used are different, per capita expenditure on health in Tanzania (US$4) and South Africa (US$158), as well as annual direct costs of diabetes from Argentina (US$330), France (US$675) and Denmark (US$3535) demonstrate sizeable between-country disparities [110]. Industrialized countries are also advantaged in the organization of health care infrastructure, as well as the financing of the system. For example, nationalized insurance and social security schemes in France and Germany cover 83.4% and 86% of these populations, respectively, which ensures high accessibility to care for citizens [75,84].

The imbalance between resource expenditure and needs is further exemplified by estimates that only 20% of global expenditure occurs in the regions where 80% of people with diabetes live [111], demonstrating that Julian Tudor Hart's [112] "inverse care law" is very relevant to global diabetes burden. This states that "the availability of good medical care tends to vary inversely with the need for it in the population served". As a result of inadequate public spending on health in LMICs (e.g. in India, only 2% of the government's annual budget is devoted to health care), sizeable proportions of household income are spent on health care costs. In Africa, 40% of people are said to earn less than US$1 per day (~$300 per annum) [11,12], and in countries such as Sudan, almost two-thirds of family incomes are required to pay for the care of one child with diabetes [113]. In Mozambique, less than one-fifth of all health facilities have the wherewithal to offer blood glucose and urinary ketone measurement [49]. The other end of

Table 5.3 Regional and country estimates of costs of diabetes.

Country	Year	Method	Annual total cost per patient	Annual total costs for country/region	Main drivers of cost	Limitations
Europe						
8 countries (Belgium, France, Germany, Italy, Netherlands, Spain, Sweden, UK) – CODE-2 Study [125]	1999	Cost-of-illness, prevalence-based study, patient and practitioner surveys, n = 7000 T2DM	€2834 (range: €1305–3576)	€29 billion	Hospitalizations (55%); other drugs – mainly cardiovascular (21%); ambulatory care (18%); antidiabetic drug costs (7%)	6-month retrospective design subject to recall bias, extrapolation error that excludes seasonal variation
France [84]	1998–2000	Retrospective patient reimbursement data (national database)	€3680 (1998) – €3914 (2000)	€5.7 bn (2000); €2.4 bn directly on diabetes care	Inpatient care (42%), outpatient care (58%); ambulatory care (18%); antidiabetic drug costs (7%)	Excluded patients with diabetes controlled on lifestyle measures; excluded indirect and intangible costs
Sweden [77]	1994	Cost-of-illness, top-down, prevalence design	n/a	US$766.1 million (43% direct, 57% indirect)	Direct: hospital care (58%), drugs (18%), ambulatory care (13%), devices (11%) Indirect: early retirement (55%), absenteeism (24%), mortality (22%)	Excluded costs of other illnesses related to diabetes; excludes those treated by dietary modification alone
Italy [76]	1998	Cost-of-illness, bottom-up, multicenter, retrospective database query of OPD costs; n = 2260	2 month costs: €136.8 (T1DM) and €123.3 (T2DM)	n/a	T1DM patients (n = 592) had more consultations; T2DM patients (n = 1668) had more diagnostic tests and day-hospital procedures Drug costs: 32–36% (T1DM) and 13–24% (T2DM)	Study limited to 2 months; Excluded costs of hospital care (known to be 30–50%); excluded indirect costs
Germany – CoDiM Study [75]	2001	Cost-of-illness, prevalence-based, retrospective database query; n = 26 971	€10 281; €5262 (direct) and €5019 (indirect)	€30.6 bn (including €14.6 bn directly due to diabetes)	Excess costs related to: inpatient care, medications (insulin, drugs to treat co-morbidities, and complications); increasing age; use of medical devices	Indirect costs not included; data protection requirements preclude validating diagnoses; cross-sectional observation; illness severity varied
Africa						
Sudan [113]	2001	Cost-of-illness, bottom-up approach: parent interviews of 147 children with T1DM	US$283 per child	n/a	Direct costs: insulin (36%), glucose testing, physician visits Indirect costs: poor school performance, 65% of family expenses were used for care of one T1DM child	Subject to recall bias; sample may not be representative of wider population (private clinics); subjects had ≤5 years duration of diabetes

South Asia						
India (South India) [80]	Pre-1998	Cost-of-illness, bottom-up approach: interviews and billing data; private (n = 422) and government-funded (n = 174) clinics	Median Rs.4510 (surgery = Rs.13 880; inpatients = Rs.7505; OPD = Rs.3310)	Estimated Rs.90.2 bn (~US$ 2.2 bn)	Surgical or inpatient care; duration of diabetes	Quality and costs at government-funded institutions are unknown (no fee charged)
Other studies in India: North India [79]; CODI study; others [81,126,127]	Unknown	Cost-of-illness, bottom-up approach: questionnaires and disability assessments; n = 50 at OPD Community-based surveys of diabetes costs (national perspective)	Rs.14 508 (€264); direct (68%), indirect (29%) Rs.19 914; direct (36%), indirect (64%)	n/a	Direct: drug costs (62%), dietary changes (20%), travel costs, investigations Indirect: loss of income, loss of caregiver income (education and income correlates such that higher levels result in greater loss) Direct: hospitalization (35%), monitoring and doctor visits (34%), drug costs (31%)	Small sample size; short follow-up (6 months) with extrapolation; did not evaluate intangible and social burdens Wide variation in annual cost-per-patient estimates (e.g. Rayappa *et al.* [122] Rs.8595 = $191–208; Bjork *et al.* [129] Rs.7189)
Pakistan [129]	2006	Cost-of-illness: questionnaires; human capital approach; n = 345 (age = 20–60) at 6 OPD clinics	PKR 11 580 (= US$197)	Direct costs projection = PKR 71 bn (= US$1.21 bn) annually	Direct: medication (46%), laboratory investigations (32%); age, complications, and duration of disease were drivers of cost	Inclusion restricted to 20–60 year age group; did not include costs of self-monitoring; calculation of lost productivity limited to those employed
Americas						
USA [130]	2000–2001	Cost-of-illness study: surveys, chart reviews, and claims data; n = 1364 T2DM subjects from Michigan HMO	US$1684 (for diet-controlled, no CVD risks or complications) to US$10 500 (obese, insulin-treated, high BP, renal, and vascular disease)	n/a	Multipliers: ESRD with dialysis (×10.53), history or MI (×1.9), insulin treatment (×1.59), PVD (×1.31), CbvD (×1.3), treated BP (×1.24) † Redekop *et al.* showed age, insulin use, micro- and macrovascular complications, and dyslipidemia are cost drivers	Analysis limited to T2DM; not representative of general population of USA; costs excluded out-of-pocket expenses and indirect costs
USA [131	2007	Cost-of-illness, prevalence-based study: Cost of Diabetes Model utilizing national surveys and claims database (16.3 million people in 2006)	US$ 11 774 ($6649 directly for diabetes care)	US$174 bn; $116 bn (direct), $58 bn (indirect costs)	Direct medical costs: complications (50%), diabetes care (23%), general medical costs (27%) Indirect: premature mortality (46%), disability and lost productivity (54%)	Estimates do not include: intangible costs, caregiver opportunity costs and undiagnosed diabetes

Continued on p.78

Table 5.3 *Continued*

Country	Year	Method	Annual total cost per patient	Annual total costs for country/region	Main drivers of cost	Limitations
Latin America and Caribbean [74]	2000	Cost-of-illness, prevalence-based study: cost estimates for groups of countries and human capital approach	US$703 (range: $442–1219)	US$ 65.2 bn; $10.7 bn (direct), $54.5 bn (indirect)	Direct: drug costs (44%), consultations (24%), complications (23% – especially nephropathy) Indirect: disability and productive life years lost (93%), mortality (7%)	General lack of data forced use of estimates in heterogeneous countries Diabetes-related deaths undercounted on death certificates; high indirect cost may reflect poor access to medical care
Mexico [132]	2003–2005	Extracted data for a standard case and natural history; human capital approach; 50% of population are insured, 40% are low-income uninsured	Villareal-Rios *et al.* [134] report US$708–1488 per patient	US$317 m; $140 m (direct), $177 m (indirect) Phillips *et al.* [135]: US$100 m (direct); $330 m (indirect)	Direct: drug costs (39%), complications (32%, especially nephropathy), hospitalizations (12%), consultations (11%) Indirect: permanent disability (94%), mortality (4.5%), temporary disability (1.5%)	Restricted to T2DM and patients attending public institutions; excludes out-of-pocket expenses and the private sector
Canada [135]	1998	Cost-of-illness, prevalence-based, top-down, national database query	n/a	CAN$3.7 bn; 70% (direct), 30% (indirect); CAN$ 4.8–5.2 bn if undiagnosed cases included	Direct: hospital costs (50%), medications (31%), physician care (19%) – medical costs of complications 1.6 times more than diabetes alone Indirect: diabetes (45%), complications (55%)	Reliance on coding of cases subject to error; limited indirect cost evaluations; prevalence estimates and practice patterns vary across provinces; home, nursing care, and glucose testing not included in costs
Australia						
Australia [136]	2000	Cost-of-illness, prevalence-based, bottom-up study; n = 1294 T2DM	n/a	A$636 m	Age, co-morbidities	Changes in practice patterns between recruitment and cost appraisal may bias results; indirect costs or hospitalization for other illnesses not included
Australia – DiabCost Study	2003	Cost-of-illness, bottom-up: T2DM patients; self-reported surveys	A$9625 (if no complications); $15 580 (with complications)	A$3 bn	–	Data were self-reported; costs not associated with DM could not be separated out

A$, Australian dollar; BMI, body mass index; bn, billion; BP, blood pressure; CAN$, Canadian dollar; CbvD, cerebrovascular disease or stroke; DM, diabetes mellitus; €, European Union Euro; ESRD, end-stage renal disease; GP, general practitioner or primary care doctor; HMO, health maintenance organization; m, million; MI, myocardial infarction; OHA, oral hypoglycaemic agent; OPD, outpatient department; PKR, Pakistani rupee; PVD, peripheral vascular disease; QOL, quality of life; Rs., Indian rupee; SES, socioeconomic status; T1DM, type 1 diabetes mellitus; T2DM, type 2 diabetes mellitus; US$, US dollar.

the spectrum comprise developed countries such as Germany and the USA, which spend €31.3 billion and US$116 billion annually on direct costs of diabetes, respectively. Of the estimated US$2.2 trillion in health care expenditures in the USA in 2007, one out of every US$7 spent was for diabetes [114]. These expenses are partially related to differences in pricing and prescription, but are also linked to the high costs of new diagnostic and therapeutic options (e.g. while annual cost of treating a patient with maximal daily doses of metformin is US$46, the equivalent costs of using thiazolidinediones are US$710–980) [115].

Additional considerations with regard to national economic impact concern the distribution of diabetes burden *within* populations. In low and middle income countries, diabetes and its complications disproportionately affect the economically productive age range (15–69 years), while in mature market economies, the disease affects the older (≥65 years), disadvantaged and ethnic minority subpopulations. The implications emanating from these trends are that economic development in transitioning countries may be subdued because of loss of unrealized productivity, while direct health costs for the aging and uninsured populations in developed countries will continue to escalate [1].

In LMICs, the lowest income groups bear the greatest burdens, paying a larger proportion of their household incomes towards diabetes care (34% and 27% for the urban and rural poor, respectively, vs 4.8% and 5.0% for the high income urban and rural groups in India, respectively) [116]. Year-on-year increases in this proportion are greater in impoverished groups, and worsen with duration of diabetes, presence of complications, hospitalization, surgical therapy and glycemic control requiring insulin [81,116,117].

Furthermore, LMICs contain large and growing populations of people with pre-diabetes, as well as groups of people unaware that they have an asymptomatic metabolic disorder. Pre-diabetes is independently associated with the development of complications and increased specialist consultations, adding up to at least US$443 in supplementary expenses per person in the USA [118]. For individuals with undiagnosed diabetes, proxy measures of health service utilization suggest that annual costs are approximately US$2864, and may escalate depending on the severity of complications that have developed by the time of recognition and formal diagnosis [119].

Augmented expenditures associated with complications further perpetuate destitution and socioeconomic disadvantage (i.e. opportunity costs of health care expenses are often endured by foregoing children's education). Meanwhile, hardship amplifies vulnerability to disease. The Cost of Diabetes in India (CODI) [43] and Bangalore Urban District (BUD) [120,121] diabetes studies showed a later age at diagnosis of diabetes and occurrence of disabling complications were associated with lack of awareness, and being unemployed and less educated (e.g. a 7-year difference in age of diagnosis was demonstrated between illiterate people and those with college education). Similar observations substantiate a bidirectional link between poor health and poverty (Figure 5.1).

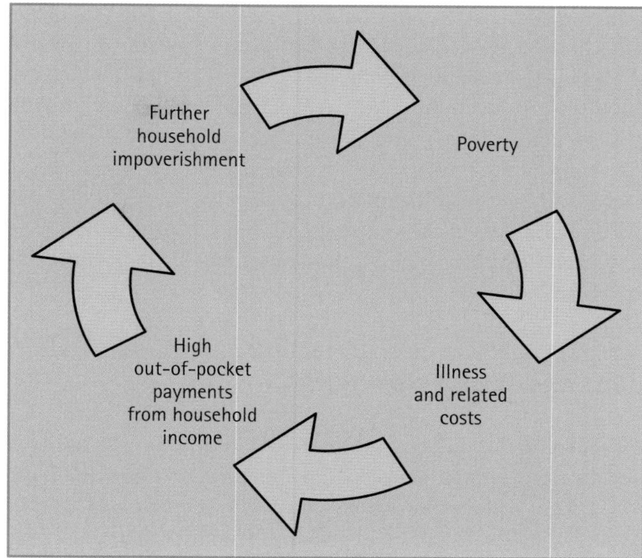

Figure 5.1 Cycle of poverty and ill health. Poverty predisposes one to illness, and costs of illness in a system of fee-for-service care have the potential to impoverish households, further perpetuating poverty.

Broadly speaking, diabetes results in roughly 1.5–5 times greater health care expenditure than the general population, depending on the context and the cost appraisal methodology employed [75,77,80,84,103,114]. In addition, it is important to note that the complex overlaps and interconnections between the underlying pathophysiology of T2DM and associated co-morbidities of the broader metabolic syndrome may alter the scope of costs. As such, depending on the viewpoint and chosen values, resource use attributable to diabetes alone may in fact underestimate the broader range of costs associated with diabetes-related illnesses as a group. Also, undiagnosed diabetes may not be described as a contributor to morbidity, mortality and resource use, suggesting that we may be underestimating the true burden of this disease. This is particularly relevant in regions of the world where there are few or no representative data regarding disease prevalence and causes of death. Finally, the value placed on the opportunity cost of diabetes-related infirmity has not been widely quantified or even qualitatively described.

Changing trends in costs

The global burdens associated with diabetes have been growing rapidly, and are projected to escalate even further in the future. The hypothesized explanations for this trend of increasing burden include, and are not limited to, the rising prevalence of diabetes and pre-diabetes worldwide; aging and longevity accompanied by costly co-morbidities; lowered diagnostic thresholds; more attentive detection of cases; availability of newer, more costly treatment methods on the basis of industry research and development; and changes in clinical management, especially growth in use of self glucose monitoring and medical devices, new therapeutic drugs and increasing demand for paramedical services. While it is evident that these latter reasons are more relevant in HICs, the continued epidemiologic transitions will no doubt affect LMICs too. It is unfortunate that scarcity of resources and inadequate access in these settings will result in greater disability and mortality, perpetuating the obstacles to socioeconomic development.

Gaps and future directions

Diabetes imposes serious health, social and economic burdens worldwide. Quantitative calculations suggest that direct and indirect costs of diabetes worldwide cumulatively total US$376 bn in 2010 [111]. Almost half of all global expenditure occurred in the USA, which is home to only 8% of those affected by diabetes worldwide. Given the disparities in burdens, access and expenditures described previously, more widespread and reliable data are a first step towards greater equity [122]. In addition, studies are needed that include both long-understood and emerging diabetes complications, such as cognitive function, in the models, to create better estimates of diabetes-attributable mortality, morbidity and cost. Assessing burdens using reliable consistent methods will aid our comprehension of the complex mix of programmed, predisposing and modifiable factors associated with diabetes, and lays a foundation for policy development and advocacy for greater global consciousness.

Despite varied estimates of expenditure, the pattern is consistent: people with diabetes experience greater symptoms, morbidity, co-morbidities and mortality than those without diabetes; they have diminished functional capacity and psychosocial illness; and incur greater costs for health care, self-care and losses in earning potential and societal role. While reductions in quality of life are less numerically evident, they are no less distressing. Needless to say, intervening before diabetes onset may hold great benefit in reducing global burdens; however, although there is evidence from large trials demonstrating that prevention can forestall conversion from pre-diabetes to diabetes, widespread translation of these findings is hampered by multiple levels of barriers (political, social, cultural, behavioral and economic factors).

In the future, preparation for the increasing diabetes burden requires progress in wider collection of reliable data (especially assuaging the scarcity from low and middle income countries regarding diabetes-related mortality, complications, disability and costs), and a greater emphasis on cost-effectiveness studies which may inform better resource allocation. On the shoulders of compelling evidence, greater investment and political will are required to overcome low accessibility and awareness, as well as to translate the evidence into practical real-life implementation of proven and effective prevention strategies [123].

References

1 Narayan KMV, Gregg EW, Fagot-Campagna A, Engelgau MM, Vinicor F. Diabetes: a common, growing, serious, costly, and potentially preventable public health problem. *Diabetes Res Clin Pract* 2000; **50**(Suppl 2):S77–S84.

2 Wild S, Roglic G, Green A, Sicree R, King H. Global prevalence of diabetes: estimates for the year 2000 and projections for 2030. *Diabetes Care* 2004; **27**:1047–1053.

3 International Diabetes Federation. *Diabetes Atlas*, 4th edn. International Diabetes Federation, 2009. Available from: http://www.diabetesatlas.org. Accessed on 4 March, 2009.

4 Cowie CC, Rust KF, Ford ES, Eberhardt MS, Byrd-Holt DD, Li C, *et al.* Full accounting of diabetes and pre-diabetes in the US population in 1988–1994 and 2005–2006. *Diabetes Care* 2009; **32**:287–294.

5 Gerstein HC, Santaguida P, Raina P, Morrison KM, Balion C, Hunt D, *et al.* Annual incidence and relative risk of diabetes in people with various categories of dysglycemia: a systematic overview and meta-analysis of prospective studies. *Diabetes Res Clin Pract* 2007; **78**:305–312.

6 Haffner SM. Abdominal obesity, insulin resistance, and cardiovascular risk in pre-diabetes and type 2 diabetes. *Eur Heart J Suppl* 2006; **8**:B20–25.

7 Popkin BM. An overview on the nutrition transition and its health implications: the Bellagio meeting. *Public Health Nutr* 2002; **5**:93–103.

8 King H, Aubert RE, Herman WH. Global burden of diabetes, 1995–2025: prevalence, numerical estimates, and projections. *Diabetes Care* 1998; **21**:1414–1431.

9 Abegunde DO, Mathers CD, Adam T, Ortegon M, Strong K. The burden and costs of chronic diseases in low-income and middle-income countries. *Lancet* 2007; **370**:1929–1938.

10 Strong K, Mathers C, Leeder S, Beaglehole R. Preventing chronic diseases: how many lives can we save? *Lancet* 2005; **366**:1578–1582.

11 Levitt NS. Diabetes in Africa: epidemiology, management and healthcare challenges. *Heart* 2008; **94**:1376–1382.

12 Beran D, Yudkin JS. Diabetes care in sub-Saharan Africa. *Lancet* 2006; **368**:1689–1695.

13 Kruger HS, Puoane T, Senekal M, van der Merwe MT. Obesity in South Africa: challenges for government and health professionals. *Public Health Nutr* 2005; **8**:491.

14 Motala AA. Diabetes trends in Africa. *Diabetes Metab Res Rev* 2002; **18**(Suppl 3):S14–S20.

15 Passa P. Diabetes trends in Europe. *Diabetes Metab Res Rev* 2002; **18**(Suppl 3):S3–S8.

16 Incidence and trends of childhood type 1 diabetes worldwide 1990–1999. *Diabet Med* 2006; **23**:857–866.

17 Aschner P. Diabetes trends in Latin America. *Diabetes Metab Res Rev* 2002; **18**(Suppl 3):S27–S31.

18 Pugh RN, Hossain MM, Malik M, El Mugamer IT, White MA. Arabian Peninsula men tend to insulin resistance and cardiovascular risk seen in South Asians. *Trop Med Int Health* 1998; **3**:89–94.

19 Kawamori R. Diabetes trends in Japan. *Diabetes Metab Res Rev* 2002; **18**(Suppl 3):S9–S13.

20 Yoon K-H, Lee J-H, Kim J-W, Cho JH, Choi Y-H, Ko S-H, *et al.* Epidemic obesity and type 2 diabetes in Asia. *Lancet* 2006; **368**:1681–1688.

21 Mohan V, Jaydip R, Deepa R. Type 2 diabetes in Asian Indian youth. *Pediatr Diabetes* 2007; **8**(Suppl 9):28–34.

22 Economic Intelligence Unit. *The Silent Epidemic: An economic study of diabetes in developed and developing countries.* New York, London, Hong Kong: The Economist, June 2007.

23 Chaturvedi N. The burden of diabetes and its complications: trends and implications for intervention. *Diabetes Res Clin Pract* 2007; **76**(Suppl 1):S3–12.

24 Ghaffar A, Reddy KS, Singhi M. Burden of non-communicable diseases in South Asia. *Br Med J* 2004; **328**:807–810.

25 Mohan V, Sandeep S, Deepa R, Shah B, Varghese C. Epidemiology of type 2 diabetes: Indian scenario. *Indian J Med Res* 2007; **125**:217–230.

26 Diaz VA, Mainous AG 3rd, Baker R, Carnemolla M, Majeed A. How does ethnicity affect the association between obesity and diabetes? *Diabet Med* 2007; **24**:1199–1204.

27 Zimmet P. Preventing diabetic complications: a primary care perspective. *Diabetes Res Clin Pract* 2009; **84**:107–116.

28 Raheja BS, Kapur A, Bhoraskar A, Sathe SR, Jorgensen LN, Moorthi SR, *et al.* DiabCare Asia: India Study: diabetes care in India – current status. *J Assoc Physicians India* 2001; **49**:717–722.

29 Danaei G, Lawes CM, Vander Hoorn S, Murray CJ, Ezzati M. Global and regional mortality from ischaemic heart disease and stroke attributable to higher-than-optimum blood glucose concentration: comparative risk assessment. *Lancet* 2006; **368**:1651–1659.

30 Albert MA, Glynn RJ, Buring J, Ridker PM. Impact of traditional and novel risk factors on the relationship between socioeconomic status and incident cardiovascular events. *Circulation* 2006; **114**: 2619–2626.

31 Avendano M, Kunst AE, Huisman M, Lenthe FV, Bopp M, Regidor E, *et al.* Socioeconomic status and ischaemic heart disease mortality in 10 western European populations during the 1990s. *Heart* 2006; **92**:461–467.

32 Cox AM, McKevitt C, Rudd AG, Wolfe CD. Socioeconomic status and stroke. *Lancet Neurol* 2006; **5**:181–188.

33 Ferrie JE, Martikainen P, Shipley MJ, Marmot MG. Self-reported economic difficulties and coronary events in men: evidence from the Whitehall II study. *Int J Epidemiol* 2005; **34**:640–648.

34 Kurian AK, Cardarelli KM. Racial and ethnic differences in cardiovascular disease risk factors: a systematic review. *Ethn Dis* 2007; **17**:143–152.

35 Singh GK, Siahpush M. Increasing inequalities in all-cause and cardiovascular mortality among US adults aged 25–64 years by area socioeconomic status, 1969–1998. *Int J Epidemiol* 2002; **31**:600–613.

36 Ramachandran A, Snehalatha C, Vijay V, King H. Impact of poverty on the prevalence of diabetes and its complications in urban southern India. *Diabet Med* 2002; **19**:130–135.

37 Misra A, Pandey RM, Devi JR, Sharma R, Vikram NK, Khanna N. High prevalence of diabetes, obesity and dyslipidaemia in urban slum population in northern India. *Int J Obes Relat Metab Disord* 2001; **25**:1722–1729.

38 Gupta R, Gupta VP, Sarna M, Prakash H, Rastogi S, Gupta KD. Serial epidemiological surveys in an urban Indian population demonstrate increasing coronary risk factors among the lower socioeconomic strata. *J Assoc Physicians India* 2003; **51**:470–477.

39 Gupta R, Gupta VP, Sarna M, Prakash H, Rastogi S, Gupta KD. Serial epidemiological surveys in an urban Indian population demonstrate increasing coronary risk factors among the lower socioeconomic strata. *J Assoc Physicians India* 2003; **51**:470–477.

40 INCLEN Multicentre Collaborative Group. Socio-economic status and risk factors for cardiovascular disease: a multicentre collaborative study in the International Clinical Epidemiology Network (INCLEN). *J Clin Epidemiol* 1994; **47**:1401–1409.

41 Steyn K, Bradshaw D, Norman R, Laubscher R. Determinants and treatment of hypertension in South Africans: the first Demographic and Health Survey. *S Afr Med J* 2008; **98**:376–380.

42 Yu Z, Nissinen A, Vartiainen E, Song G, Guo Z, Tian H. Changes in cardiovascular risk factors in different socioeconomic groups: seven year trends in a Chinese urban population. *J Epidemiol Community Health* 2000; **54**:692–696.

43 Gray JAM. *How To Get Better Value Healthcare.* Oxford: Oxford Press; 2007.

44 Lin SF, Lin JD, Huang YY. Diabetic ketoacidosis: comparisons of patient characteristics, clinical presentations and outcomes today and 20 years ago. *Chang Gung Med J* 2005; **28**:24–30.

45 Otto MH, Michael ERd, Julie BP, Ole Lander S. Diabetic ketoacidosis in Denmark: incidence and mortality estimated from public health registries. *Diabetes Res Clini Pract* 2007; **76**:51–56.

46 Rwiza HT, Swai AB, McLarty DG. Failure to diagnose diabetic ketoacidosis in Tanzania. *Diabet Med* 1986; **3**:181–183.

47 Osei K, Schuster DP, Amoah AG, Owusu SK. Diabetes in Africa: pathogenesis of type 1 and type 2 diabetes mellitus in sub-Saharan Africa – implications for transitional populations. *J Cardiovasc Risk* 2003; **10**:85–96.

48 Majaliwa ES, Munubhi E, Ramaiya K, Mpembeni R, Sanyiwa A, Mohn A, *et al.* Survey on acute and chronic complications in children and adolescents with type 1 diabetes at Muhimbili National Hospital in Dar es Salaam, Tanzania. *Diabetes Care* 2007; **30**:2187–2192.

49 Beran D, Yudkin JS, de Courten M. Access to care for patients with insulin-requiring diabetes in developing countries: case studies of Mozambique and Zambia. *Diabetes Care* 2005; **28**:2136–2140.

50 Stamler J, Vaccaro O, Neaton JD, Wentworth D. Diabetes, other risk factors, and 12-yr cardiovascular mortality for men screened in the Multiple Risk Factor Intervention Trial. *Diabetes Care* 1993; **16**:434–444.

51 Kannel WB, McGee DL. Diabetes and cardiovascular disease. The Framingham study. *JAMA* 1979; **241**:2035–2038.

52 Haffner SM, Lehto S, Ronnemaa T, Pyorala K, Laakso M. Mortality from coronary heart disease in subjects with type 2 diabetes and in nondiabetic subjects with and without prior myocardial infarction. *N Engl J Med* 1998; **339**:229–234.

53 Donahoe SM, Stewart GC, McCabe CH, Mohanavelu S, Murphy SA, Cannon CP, *et al.* Diabetes and mortality following acute coronary syndromes. *JAMA* 2007; **298**:765–775.

54 Plutzky J, Viberti G, Haffner S. Atherosclerosis in type 2 diabetes mellitus and insulin resistance: mechanistic links and therapeutic targets. *J Diabetes Complications* 2002; **16**:401–415.

55 Haffner SM. Abdominal adiposity and cardiometabolic risk: do we have all the answers? *Am J Med* 2007; **120**(Suppl 1):S10–16; discussion S16–17.

56 Barnett AH. The importance of treating cardiometabolic risk factors in patients with type 2 diabetes. *Diab Vasc Dis Res* 2008; **5**:9–14.

57 Laakso M, Kuusisto J. Epidemiological evidence for the association of hyperglycaemia and atherosclerotic vascular disease in

non-insulin-dependent diabetes mellitus. *Ann Med* 1996; **28**:415–418.

58 Haffner SM. Epidemiology of insulin resistance and its relation to coronary artery disease. *Am J Cardiol* 1999; 84:11J–14J.

59 Deedwania PC, Fonseca VA. Diabetes, prediabetes, and cardiovascular risk: shifting the paradigm. *Am J Med* 2005; **118**:939–947.

60 Duckworth W, Abraira C, Moritz T, Reda D, Emanuele N, Reaven PD, *et al.* Glucose control and vascular complications in veterans with type 2 diabetes. *N Engl J Med* 2009; **360**:129–139.

61 Gerstein HC, Miller ME, Byington RP, Goff DC Jr, Bigger JT, Buse JB, *et al.* Effects of intensive glucose lowering in type 2 diabetes. *N Engl J Med* 2008; **358**:2545–2559.

62 Patel A, MacMahon S, Chalmers J, Neal B, Billot L, Woodward M, *et al.* Intensive blood glucose control and vascular outcomes in patients with type 2 diabetes. *N Engl J Med* 2008; **358**:2560–2572.

63 Gaede P, Lund-Andersen H, Parving HH, Pedersen O. Effect of a multifactorial intervention on mortality in type 2 diabetes. *N Engl J Med* 2008; **358**:580–591.

64 Gaede P, Vedel P, Larsen N, Jensen GV, Parving HH, Pedersen O. Multifactorial intervention and cardiovascular disease in patients with type 2 diabetes. *N Engl J Med* 2003; **348**:383–393.

65 Mbanya JC, Kengne AP, Assah F. Diabetes care in Africa. *Lancet* 2006; **368**:1628–1629.

66 US Renal Data System. *USRDS 2008 Annual Data Report: Atlas of Chronic Kidney Disease and End-Stage Renal Disease in the United States.* Bethesda, MD: National Institute of Diabetes and Digestive and Kidney Diseases of National Institutes of Health, 2008.

67 Björk S. The cost of diabetes and diabetes care. *Diabetes Res Clin Pract* 2001; **54**(Suppl 1):13–18.

68 Kocur I, Resnikoff S. Visual impairment and blindness in Europe and their prevention. *Br J Ophthalmol* 2002; **86**:716–722.

69 Fernando DJ. The prevalence of neuropathic foot ulceration in Sri Lankan diabetic patients. *Ceylon Med J* 1996; **41**:96–98.

70 Boulton AJ, Vileikyte L, Ragnarson-Tennvall G, Apelqvist J. The global burden of diabetic foot disease. *Lancet* 2005; **366**: 1719–1724.

71 Boulton AJM. The diabetic foot: a global view. *Diabetes Metab Res Rev* 2000; **16**:S2–S5.

72 Oyibo SO, Jude EB, Tarawneh I, Nguyen HC, Armstrong DG, Harkless LB, *et al.* The effects of ulcer size and site, patient's age, sex and type and duration of diabetes on the outcome of diabetic foot ulcers. *Diabet Med* 2001; **18**:133–138.

73 Kengne AP, Amoah AG, Mbanya JC. Cardiovascular complications of diabetes mellitus in sub-Saharan Africa. *Circulation* 2005; **112**:3592–3601.

74 Barceló A, Aedo C, Rajpathak S, Robles S. The cost of diabetes in Latin America and the Caribbean. *Bull World Health Organ* 2003; **81**:19–27.

75 Koster I, vonFerber L, Ihle P, Schubert I, Hauner H. The cost burden of diabetes mellitus: the evidence from Germany: the CoDiM Study. *Diabetologia* 2006; **49**:1498–1504.

76 Garattini L, Tediosi F, Chiaffarino F, Roggeri D, Parazzini F, Coscelli C; Gruppo di Studio R. The outpatient cost of diabetes care in Italian diabetes centers. *Value Health* 2001; **4**:251–257.

77 Henriksson F, Jönsson B. Diabetes: the cost of illness in Sweden. *J Intern Med* 1998; **244**:461–468.

78 Chow J, Darley S, Laxminarayan R. *Cost-effectiveness of Disease Intervenions in India.* Washington DC: Resources for the Future, 2007.

79 Grover S, Avasthi A, Bhansali A, Chakrabarti S, Kulhara P. Cost of ambulatory care of diabetes mellitus: a study from north India. *Postgrad Med J* 2005; **81**:391–395.

80 Shobhana R, Rama Rao P, Lavanya A, Williams R, Vijay V, Ramachandran A. Expenditure on health care incurred by diabetic subjects in a developing country: a study from southern India. *Diabetes Res Clin Pract* 2000; **48**:37–42.

81 Kapur A. Economic analysis of diabetes care. *Indian J Med Res* 2007; **125**:473–482.

82 Piette JD, Heisler M, Wagner TH. Problems paying out-of-pocket medication costs among older adults with diabetes. *Diabetes Care* 2004; **27**:384–391.

83 Piette JD, Wagner TH, Potter MB, Schillinger D. Health insurance status, cost-related medication underuse, and outcomes among diabetes patients in three systems of care. *Med Care* 2004; **42**:102–109.

84 Ricordeau P, Weill A, Vallier N, Bourrel R, Schwartz D, Guilhot J, *et al.* The prevalence and cost of diabetes in metropolitan France: what trends between 1998 and 2000? *Diabetes Metab* 2003; **29**:497–504.

85 Lavigne JE, Phelps CE, Mushlin A, Lednar WM. Reductions in individual work productivity associated with type 2 diabetes mellitus. *PharmacoEconomics* 2003; **21**:1123–1134.

86 Arvanitakis Z, Wilson RS, Bienias JL, Evans DA, Bennett DA. Diabetes mellitus and risk of Alzheimer disease and decline in cognitive function. *Arch Neurol* 2004; **61**:661–666.

87 Gregg EW, Yaffe K, Cauley JA, Rolka DB, Blackwell TL, Narayan KMV, *et al*; for the Study of Osteoporotic Fractures Research G. Is diabetes associated with cognitive impairment and cognitive decline among older women? *Arch Intern Med* 2000; **160**:174–180.

88 Testa MA, Simonson DC. Health economic benefits and quality of life during improved glycemic control in patients with type 2 diabetes mellitus: a randomized, controlled, double-blind trial. *JAMA* 1998; **280**:1490–1496.

89 Tunceli K, Bradley CJ, Lafata JE, Pladevall M, Divine GW, Goodman AC, *et al.* Glycemic control and absenteeism among individuals with diabetes. *Diabetes Care* 2007; **30**:1283–1285.

90 McKellar JD, Humphreys K, Piette JD. Depression increases diabetes symptoms by complicating patients' self-care adherence. *Diabetes Educ* 2004; **30**:485–492.

91 Piette JD, Richardson C, Valenstein M. Addressing the needs of patients with multiple chronic illnesses: the case of diabetes and depression. *Am J Manag Care* 2004; **10**(Part 2):152–162.

92 Von Korff M, Katon W, Lin EHB, Simon G, Ciechanowski P, Ludman E, *et al.* Work disability among individuals with diabetes. *Diabetes Care* 2005; **28**:1326–1332.

93 Roglic G, Unwin N, Bennett PH, Mathers C, Tuomilehto J, Nag S, *et al.* The burden of mortality attributable to diabetes: realistic estimates for the year 2000. *Diabetes Care* 2005; **28**:2130–2135.

94 International Diabetes Federation. Global Burden: Mortality and Morbidity. In: *Diabetes Atlas*, 4th edn., International Diabetes Federation, 2009. Available from http://www.diabetesatlas.org/content/diabetes-mortality. Accessed December, 2009.

95 Morgan CL, Currie CJ, Peters JR. Relationship between diabetes and mortality: a population study using record linkage. *Diabetes Care* 2000; **23**:1103–1107.

96 Franco OH, Steyerberg EW, Hu FB, Mackenbach J, Nusselder W. Associations of diabetes mellitus with total life expectancy and life

expectancy with and without cardiovascular disease. *Arch Intern Med* 2007; **167**:1145–1151.

97 Moss SE, Klein R, Klein BE. Cause-specific mortality in a population-based study of diabetes. *Am J Public Health* 1991; **81**:1158–1162.

98 Geiss LS, Herman WM, Smith PJ. Mortality in non-insulin-dependent diabetes. In: National Diabetes Data Group, ed. *Diabetes in America*, 2nd edn. NIH & NIDDK; 1995:233–255.

99 Zargar AH, Wani AI, Masoodi SR, Laway BA, Bashir MI. Mortality in diabetes mellitus: data from a developing region of the world. *Diabetes Res Clin Pract* 1999; **43**:67–74.

100 International Diabetes Federation. *Diabetes Atlas*, 3rd edn. Brussels, 2006.

101 UNAIDS. Report on the global AIDS epidemic: sub-Saharan Africa [Website]. Available at: http://data.unaids.org/pub/EpiReport/2006/04-Sub_Saharan_Africa_2006_EpiUpdate_eng.pdf. Accessed March 27, 2009.

102 Valdmanis V, Smith DW, Page MR. Productivity and economic burden associated with diabetes. *Am J Public Health* 2001; **91**:129–130.

103 Zhang P, Engelgau MM, Norris SL, Gregg EW, Narayan KMV. Application of economic analysis to diabetes and diabetes care. *Ann Intern Med* 2004; **140**:972–977.

104 Dall T MS, Zhang U, Martin J, Chen Y. Distinguishing the economic costs associated with type 1 and type 2 diabetes. Paper presented at: Innovation in Health Care: The Economics of Diabetes; in Population Health Management (Mary Ann Liebert Inc., New Rochelle, New York). Commissioned by the National Changing Diabetes® Program, a program of Novo Nordisk, Inc.

105 Brown JB, Pedula KL, Bakst AW. The progressive cost of complications in type 2 diabetes mellitus. *Arch Intern Med* 1999; **159**:1873–1880.

106 Brown AF, Ettner SL, Piette J, Weinberger M, Gregg E, Shapiro MF, *et al.* Socioeconomic position and health among persons with diabetes mellitus: a conceptual framework and review of the literature. *Epidemiol Rev* 2004; **26**:63–77.

107 Selby JV, Ray GT, Zhang D, Colby CJ. Excess costs of medical care for patients with diabetes in a managed care population. *Diabetes Care* 1997; **20**:1396–1402.

108 Gruber W, Lander T, Leese B, Songer T, Williams R, eds. *The Economics of Diabetes and Diabetes Care: a report of Diabetes Health Economics Study Group*. IDF and WHO, 1997.

109 Gilmer TP, O'Connor PJ, Manning WG, Rush WA. The cost to health plans of poor glycemic control. *Diabetes Care* 1997; **20**:1847–1853.

110 Joshi SR. Cardio-metabolic burden of native asian Indian: India the global capital. *J Assoc Physicians India* 2004; **52**:359–361.

111 International Diabetes Federation. Global Burden: Economic Impacts of Diabetes. In: *Diabetes Atlas*, 4th edn., International Diabetes Federation, 2009. Available from http://www.diabetesatlas.org/content/economic-impacts-diabetes. Accessed December, 2009.

112 Hart JT. The inverse care law. *Lancet* 1971; **1**:405–412.

113 Elrayah H, Eltom M, Bedri A, Belal A, Rosling H, Östenson C-G. Economic burden on families of childhood type 1 diabetes in urban Sudan. *Diabetes Res Clin Pract* 2005; **70**:159–165.

114 Rubin RJ, Altman WM, Mendelson DN. Health care expenditures for people with diabetes mellitus, 1992. *J Clin Endocrinol Metab* 1994; **78**:809A–809F.

115 Gale EA. Dying of diabetes. *Lancet* 2006; **368**:1626–1628.

116 Ramachandran A, Ramachandran S, Snehalatha C, Augustine C, Murugesan N, Viswanathan V, *et al.* Increasing expenditure on health care incurred by diabetic subjects in a developing country: a study from India. *Diabetes Care* 2007; **30**:252–256.

117 Khowaja LA, Khuwaja AK, Cosgrove P. Cost of diabetes care in out-patient clinics of Karachi, Pakistan. *BMC Health Serv Res* 2007; **7**:189.

118 Zhang Y DT, Mann SE, Martin J, Chen Y. Medical cost associated with pre-diabetes. Paper presented at: Innovation in Health Care: The Economics of Diabetes; in Population Health Management (Mary Ann Liebert Inc., New Rochelle, New York). Commissioned by the National Changing Diabetes® Program, a program of Novo Nordisk, Inc.

119 Zhang Y DT, Mann SE, Martin J, Chen Y. The economic cost of undiagnosed diabetes. Paper presented at: Innovation in Health Care: The Economics of Diabetes; in Population Health Management (Mary Ann Liebert Inc., New Rochelle, New York). Commissioned by the National Changing Diabetes® Program, a program of Novo Nordisk, Inc.

120 Kapur A. Cost of diabetes in India: The CODI Study. Paper presented at: Proceedings of the Novo Nordisk Diabetes Update, Bangalore, 2000.

121 Rayappa PH, Raju KNM, Kapur A, Bjork S, Sylvest C, Kumar KD. Economic cost of diabetes care: the Bangalore urban district diabetes study. *Int J Diabetes Developing Countries* 1999; **19**:87–96.

122 Gostin LO, Powers M. What does social justice require for the public's health? Public health ethics and policy imperatives. *Health Affairs (Project Hope)* 2006; **25**:1053–1060.

123 Narayan KMV, Zhang P, Kanaya AM, Williams DE, Engelgau MM, Imperatore G, *et al.* Diabetes: the pandemic and potential solutions. In: Jamison DT, Breman JG, Measham AR, Alleyne G, Claeson M, Evans DB, *et al.* eds. *Disease Control Priorities in Developing Countries*, 2nd edn. New York: Oxford University Press, 2006: tables 30.33 and 30.34.

124 National Institute of Diabetes and Digestive and Kidney Diseases (National Institutes of Health). Graph: Treatment with insulin or oral medication among adults with diagnosed diabetes, United States, National Health Interview Survey, 2004 to 2006. Available at: http://diabetes.niddk.nih.gov/dm/pubs/statistics/index.htm#what.

125 Jonsson B. Revealing the cost of type II diabetes in Europe. *Diabetologia* 2002; **45**:S5–S12.

126 Kapur A, Bjork S, Nair J, Kelkar S, Ramachandran A. Socioeconomic determinants of the cost of diabetes in India. *Diabetes Voice* 2004; **49**:18–21.

127 Ramachandran A, Ramachandran S, Snehalatha C, Augustine C, Murugesan N, Viswanathan V, *et al.* Increasing expenditure on health care incurred by diabetic subjects in a developing country: a study from India. *Diabetes Care* 2007; **30**:252–256.

128 Björk S, Kapur A, King H, Nair J, Ramachandran A. Global policy: aspects of diabetes in India. *Health Policy* 2003; **66**:61.

129 Khowaja LA, Khuwaja AK, Cosgrove P. Cost of diabetes care in out-patient clinics of Karachi, Pakistan. *BMC Health Serv Res* 2007; **21**:189–196.

130 Brandle M, Zhou H, Smith BRK, Marriott D, Burke R, Tabaei BP, *et al.* The direct medical cost of type 2 diabetes. *Diabetes Care* 2003; **26**:2300–2304.

131 Dall T, Mann SE, Zhang Y, Martin J, Chen Y. Economic costs of diabetes in the US in 2007. *Diabetes Care* 2008; **31**:596–615.

132 Arredondo A, Zuniga A. Economic consequences of epidemiological changes in diabetes in middle-income countries: the Mexican case. *Diabetes Care* 2004; **27**:104–109.

133 Villarreal-Ríos E, Salinas-Martínez AM, Medina-Jáuregui A, Garza-Elizondo ME, Núñez-Rocha G, Chuy-Díaz ER. The cost of diabetes mellitus and its impact on health spending in Mexico. *Arch Med Res* 2000; **31**:511–514.

134 Phillips M, Salmeron J. Diabetes in Mexico: a serious and growing problem. *World Health Stat Q* 1992; **45**:338–346.

135 Keith GD, Daniel G, James FB, Kristijan HK. The economic cost of diabetes in Canada, 1998. *Diabetes Res Clin Pract* 2000; **50**:7.

136 Davis WA, Knuiman MW, Hendrie D, Davis TME. The obesity-driven rising costs of type 2 diabetes in Australia: projections from the Fremantle Diabetes Study. *Intern Med J* 2006; **36**:155–161.

2 Normal Physiology

6 Islet Function and Insulin Secretion

Peter M. Jones & Shanta J. Persaud

Diabetes Research Group, King's College London, UK

Keypoints

- Regulation of fuel homeostasis in mammals is dependent on numerous small endocrine organs known as islets of Langerhans, which are located in the pancreas.
- Islets contain β-cells which are the only source of the polypeptide hormone insulin.
- β-Cells are equipped to detect changes in circulating nutrients.
- β-Cells respond to elevated levels of nutrients by initiating an insulin secretory response which will induce the storage of circulating nutrients in liver, muscle and adipose tissue.
- β-Cells can also respond to a wide range of other signals including hormones, neurotransmitters and neuropeptides, which modify the insulin secretory response to circulating nutrients.
- Complex interactions between islet cells, the autonomic nervous system and gastrointestinal incretin hormones allow precise integration between metabolic fuel intake, usage and storage.

Introduction

The German anatomy student Paul Langerhans first described in 1869 the "islands of clear cells" distributed throughout the pancreas [1] but he did not realize the physiologic significance of these cell clusters, which are today known as islets of Langerhans. We now know that islets are the endocrine compartment of the pancreas, comprising around 2–3% of the total pancreatic volume. Islets are approximately spherical (Figure 6.1a), with an average diameter of 100–200 μm, and a healthy human pancreas may contain up to a million individual islets, each having its own complex anatomy, blood supply and innervation.

Islet structure and function

Islet anatomy

A typical mammalian islet comprises several thousand endocrine cells including the insulin-expressing β-cells (~60% of adult human islet cells), glucagon-expressing α-cells (20–30%), somatostatin-expressing δ-cells (~10%), pancreatic polypeptide-expressing cells (<5%), and ghrelin-expressing cells (~1%). The anatomic arrangement of islet cells varies between species. In rodents, the majority β-cell population forms a central core surrounded by a mantle of α-cells and δ-cells (Figure 6.1a), but human islets show less well-defined organization with α-cells and δ-cells also being located throughout the islet (Figure 6.1b) [2].

Islets are highly vascularized, and receive up to 15% of the pancreatic blood supply despite accounting for only 2–3% of the total pancreatic mass. Each islet is served by an arteriolar blood supply that penetrates the mantle to form a capillary bed in the islet core. Earlier studies using vascular casts of rodent islets suggested that the major route of blood flow through an islet was from the inner β-cells to the outer α and δ-cells [3], but more recent studies using optical imaging of fluorescent markers to follow islet blood flow *in vivo* [4] reveal more complex patterns of both inner-to-outer and top-to-bottom blood flow through the rodent islet.

Islets are well supplied by autonomic nerve fibers and terminals containing the classic neurotransmitters acetylcholine and norepinephrine, along with a variety of biologically active neuropeptides [5]. Vasoactive intestinal polypeptide (VIP) and pituitary adenylate cyclase-activating polypeptide (PACAP) are localized with acetylcholine to parasympathetic nerves, where they may be involved in mediating prandial insulin secretion and the α-cell response to hypoglycemia [6]. Other neuropeptides, such as galanin and neuropeptide Y (NPY), are found with norepinephrine in sympathetic nerves where they may have a role in the sympathetic inhibition of insulin secretion, although there are marked inter-species differences in the expression of these neuropeptides [5].

Intra-islet interactions

The anatomic organization of the islet has a profound influence on the ability of the β-cells to recognize and respond to physio-

Textbook of Diabetes, 4th edition. Edited by R. Holt, C. Cockram, A. Flyvbjerg and B. Goldstein.

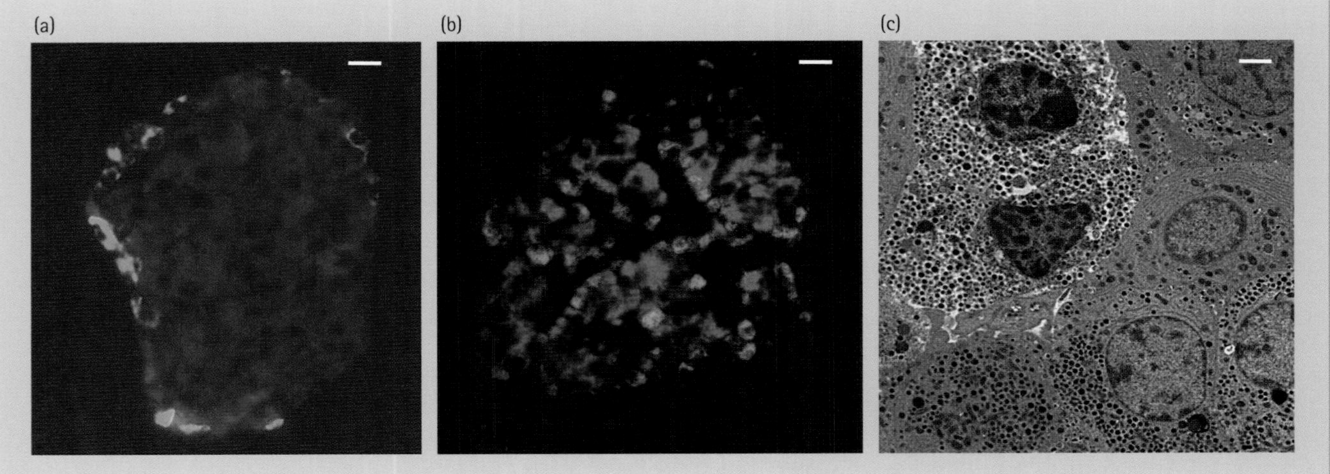

Figure 6.1 Anatomy of the islet of Langerhans. (a) Mouse islet. The figure shows a section through a mouse pancreas in which insulin and glucagon are identified by red and green immunofluorescence, respectively, demonstrating the typical β-cell core surrounded by a thin mantle of α-cells. In mouse islets β-cells comprise approximately 80% of the endocrine cell mass. Scale bar is 10 μm. Image courtesy of V. Foot, King's College London. (b) Human islet. The figure shows a section through a human pancreas in which insulin and glucagon are identified by red and green immunofluorescence respectively, demonstrating the less organized structure of the human islet when compared with mouse islets. In human islets β-cells comprise approximately 50–60% of the endocrine cell mass. Scale bar is 10 μm. Image courtesy of V. Foot, King's College London. (c) Transmission electron micrograph of human islet cells. The figure shows a transmission electron micrograph of several cells within a human islet. The two cells in the top left with the electron dense secretory granules surrounded by a clear halo are β-cells. The cells in the lower half of the micrograph are α-cells. Scale bar is 2 μm. Data from Jones & Persaud, unpublished.

logic signals [7–9]. There are a number of mechanisms through which islet cells can communicate, although the relative importance of the different mechanisms is still uncertain [10]. Islet cells are functionally coupled through a network of gap junctions, and gene deletion studies in mice have highlighted the importance of gap-junctional coupling via connexin 36 in the regulation of insulin secretory responses [11,12]. Cell–cell contact through cell surface adhesion molecules offers an alternative communication mechanism, and interactions mediated by E-cadherin [13,14] or ephrins [15] have been implicated in the regulation of β-cell function. A further level of control can be exerted via intra-islet paracrine and autocrine effects in which a biologically active substance released by one islet cell can influence the functional status of a neighboring cell (paracrine), or of itself (autocrine). Figure 6.2 shows some of the molecules that have been implicated in this type of intra-islet cell–cell communication. Thus, islet cells can interact with each other via the classic islet hormones – insulin, glucagon and somatostatin [16–19]; via other products secreted by the endocrine cells, such as neurotransmitters or adenine nucleotides and divalent cations that are co-released with insulin [20–23]; and via other less well-known mechanisms, including the generation of gaseous signals such as nitric oxide and carbon monoxide [24–27]. The wide range of intra-islet interactions presumably reflects the requirement for fine-tuning and coordinating secretory responses of many individual islet cells to generate the rate and pattern of hormone secretion appropriate to the prevailing physiologic conditions.

Insulin biosynthesis and storage

The ability to release insulin rapidly in response to metabolic demand, coupled with the relatively slow process of producing polypeptide hormones, means that β-cells are highly specialized for the production and storage of insulin, to the extent that insulin comprises approximately 10% (~10 pg/cell) of the total β-cell protein.

Biosynthesis of insulin

In humans, the gene encoding preproinsulin, the precursor of insulin, is located on the short arm of chromosome 11 [28]. It is 1355 base pairs in length and its coding region consists of three exons: the first encodes the signal peptide at the N-terminus of preproinsulin, the second the B chain and part of the C (connecting) peptide, and the third the rest of the C peptide and the A chain (Figure 6.3). Transcription and splicing to remove the sequences encoded by the introns yields a messenger RNA of 600 nucleotides, translation of which gives rise to preproinsulin, an 11.5-kDa polypeptide. The cellular processes and approximate timescales involved in insulin biosynthesis, processing and storage are summarized in Figure 6.4.

Preproinsulin is rapidly (<1 min) discharged into the cisternal space of the rough endoplasmic reticulum, where proteolytic enzymes immediately cleave the signal peptide, generating proinsulin. Proinsulin is a 9-kDa peptide, containing the A and B chains of insulin (21 and 30 amino acid residues, respectively) joined by the C peptide (30–35 amino acids). The structural

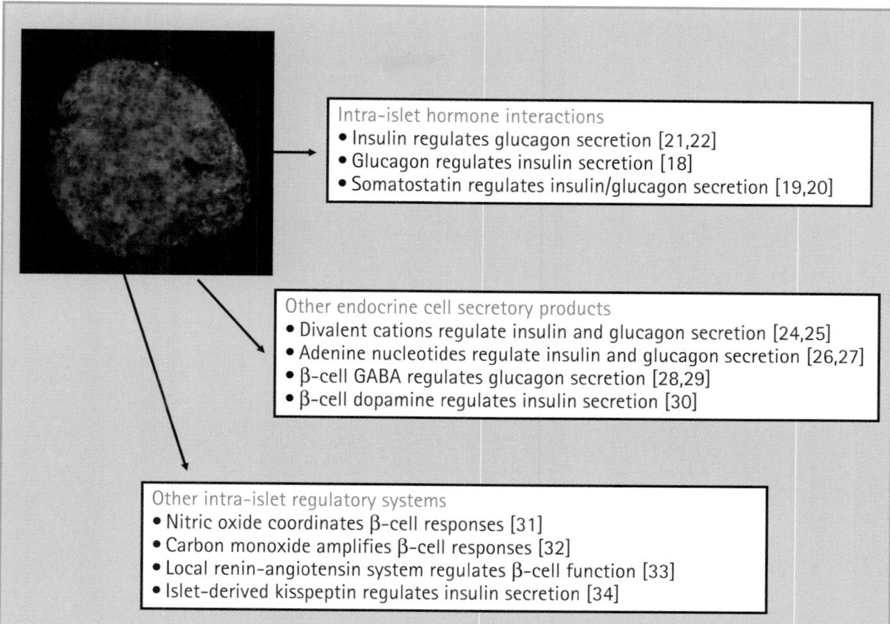

Figure 6.2 Intra-islet autocrine–paracrine interactions. The heterogeneous nature and complex anatomy of the islet enables numerous interactions between islet cells that are mediated by the release of biologically active molecules.

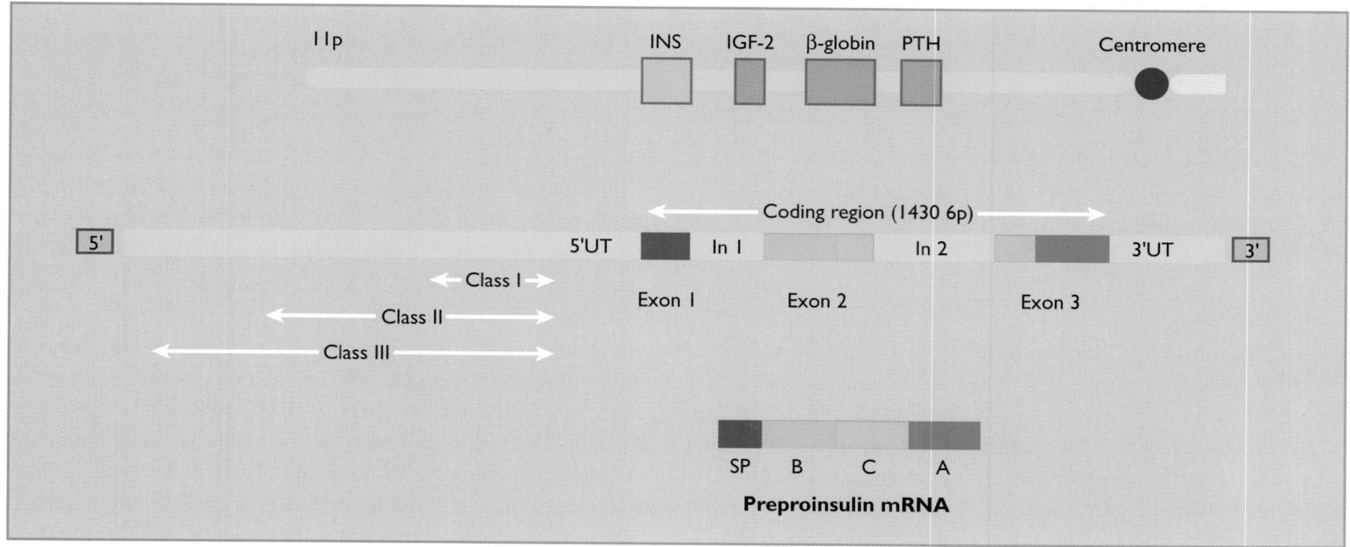

Figure 6.3 Structure of the human insulin gene. The coding region of the human insulin (INS) gene comprises three exons, which encode the signal peptide (SP), the B chain, C peptide and A chain. The exons are separated by two introns (In1 and In2). Beyond the 5′ untranslated region (5′UT), upstream of the coding sequence, lies a hypervariable region in which three alleles (classes I, II and III) can be distinguished by their size.

conformations of proinsulin and insulin are very similar, and a major function of the C peptide is to align the disulfide bridges that link the A and B chains so that the molecule is correctly folded for cleavage (Figure 6.5). Proinsulin is transported in microvesicles to the Golgi apparatus, where it is packaged into membrane-bound vesicles known as secretory granules. The conversion of proinsulin to insulin is initiated in the Golgi complex and continues within the maturing secretory granule through the sequential action of two endopeptidases (prohormone convertases 2 and 3) and carboxypeptidase H [29], which remove the C peptide chain, liberating two cleavage dipeptides and finally yielding insulin (Figure 6.5). Insulin and C peptide are stored together in the secretory granules and are ultimately released in equimolar amounts by a process of regulated exocytosis. Under normal conditions, >95% of the secreted product is insulin (and C peptide) and <5% is released as proinsulin. However, the secre-

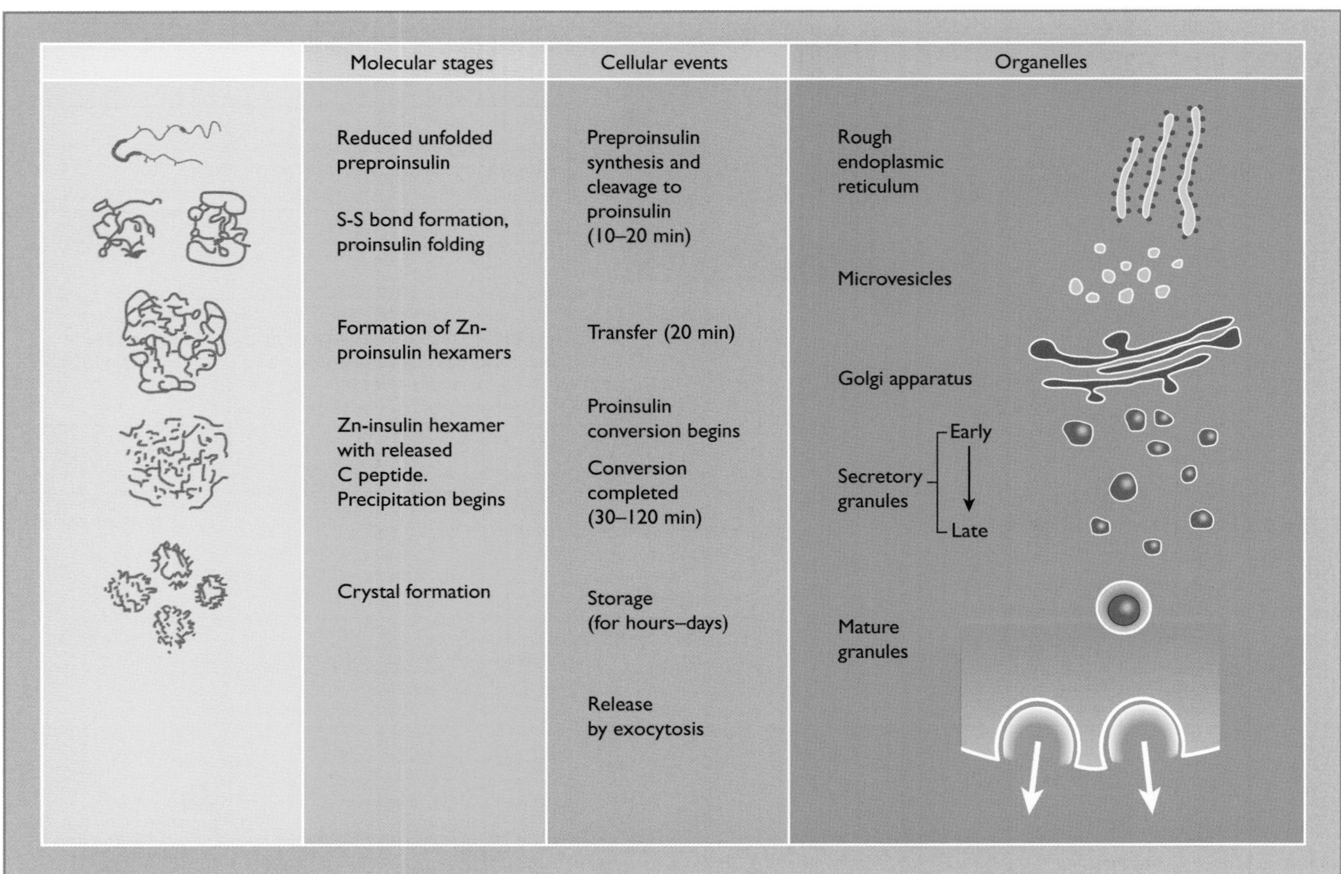

Figure 6.4 The intracellular pathways of (pro)insulin biosynthesis, processing and storage. The molecular folding of the proinsulin molecule, its conversion to insulin and the subsequent arrangement of the insulin hexamers into a regular pattern are shown at the left. The time course of the various processes, and the organelles involved are also shown.

tion of incompletely processed insulin precursors (proinsulin and its "split" products; Figure 6.5) is increased in some patients with type 2 diabetes.

The β-cell responds to increases in the circulating concentrations of nutrients by increasing insulin production in addition to increasing insulin secretion, thus maintaining insulin stores [30]. Acute (<2 hours) increases in the extracellular concentration of glucose and other nutrients result in a rapid and dramatic increase in the transcription of preproinsulin mRNA and in the rate of proinsulin synthesis [31]. There is a sigmoidal relationship between glucose concentrations and biosynthetic activity, with a threshold glucose level of 2–4 mmol/L. This is slightly lower than the threshold for the stimulation of insulin secretion (~5 mmol/L), which ensures an adequate reserve of insulin within the β-cell.

Storage and release of insulin

The insulin secretory granule has a typical appearance in electron micrographs, with a wide space between the crystalline electron-opaque core and its limiting membrane (Figure 6.1c). The major protein constituents of the granules are insulin and C peptide, which account for approximately 80% of granule protein [31], with numerous minor components including peptidases, peptide hormones and a variety of (potentially) biologically active peptides of uncertain function [32,33]. Insulin secretory granules also contain high concentrations of divalent cations, such as zinc (~20 mmol/L), which is important in the crystallization and stabilization of insulin within the granule [34,35]. The intra-granular function(s) of calcium (~120 mmol/L) and magnesium (~70 mmol/L) are uncertain, but as they are co-released with insulin on exocytosis of the secretory granule contents they may have extracellular signaling roles via the cell surface calcium-sensing receptor [20]. Similarly, the adenine nucleotides found in insulin secretory granules (~10 mmol/L) may have a signaling role when they are released into the extracellular space [21].

The generation of physiologically appropriate insulin secretory responses requires complex mechanisms for moving secretory granules from their storage sites within the cell to the specialized sites for exocytosis on the inner surface of the plasma membrane, and the role of cytoskeletal elements, notably microtubules and microfilaments, in the intracellular translocation of insulin

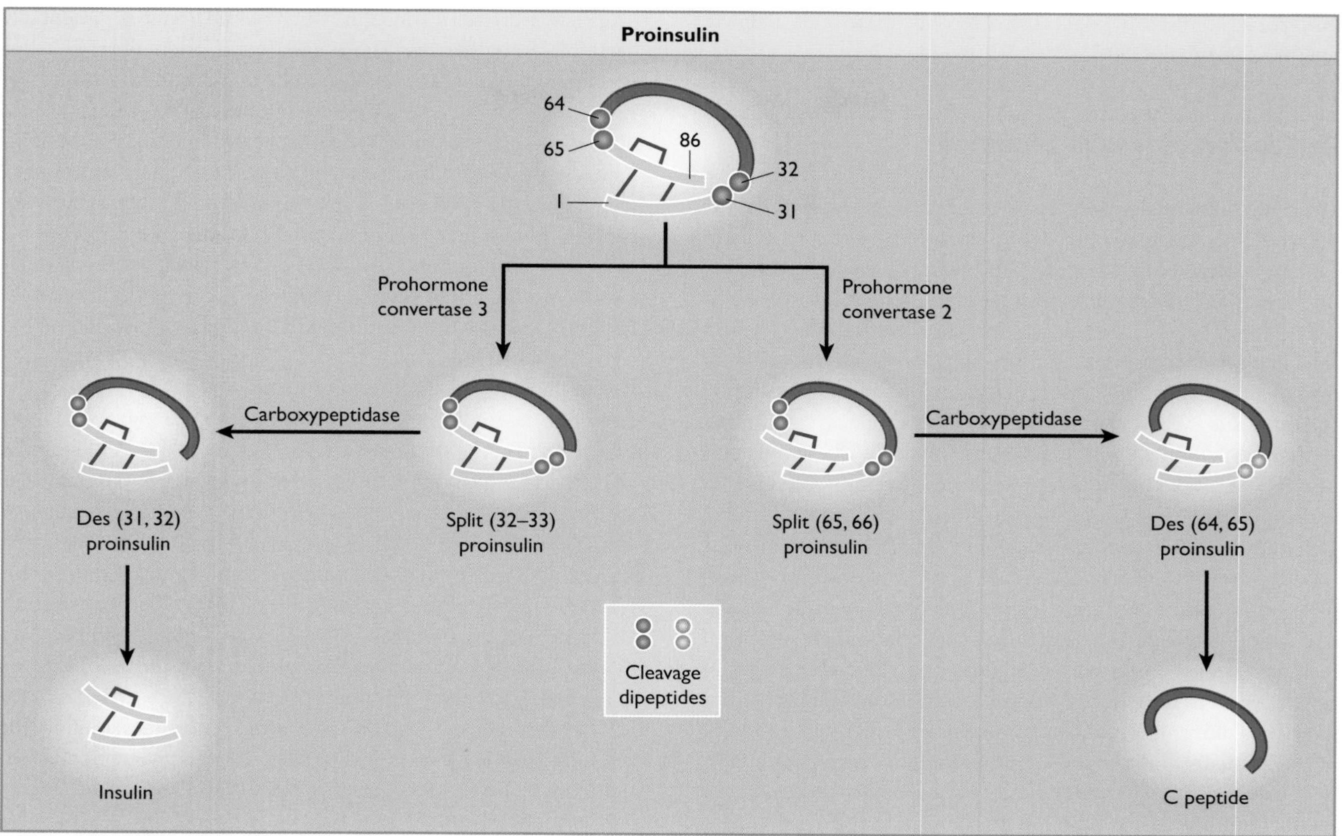

Figure 6.5 Insulin biosynthesis and processing. Proinsulin is cleaved on the C-terminal side of two dipeptides, namely Arg^{31}–Arg^{32} (by prohormone convertase 3) and Lys^{64}–Arg^{65} (prohormone convertase 2). The cleavage dipeptides are liberated, so yielding the "split" proinsulin products and ultimately insulin and C peptide.

storage granules has been studied extensively [36,37]. Microtubules are formed by the polymerization of tubulin subunits and normally form a network radiating outwards from the perinuclear region [38]. The microtubular network is in a process of continual remodeling and the dynamic turnover of tubulin, rather than the total number of microtubules, is important for the mechanism of secretion. The microtubule framework may provide the pathway for the secretory granules but microtubules do not provide the motive force [39] so other contractile proteins are likely to be involved. Actin is the constituent protein of microfilaments which exists in cells as a globular form of 43 kDa and as a filamentous form which associates to form microfilaments. Microfilament polymerization is regulated by agents that alter rates of insulin secretion [40], and the pharmacologic disruption of microfilament formation inhibits insulin secretion. Myosin light and heavy chains are expressed at high concentrations in β-cells, suggesting that actin and myosin may interact to propel granules along the microtubular network. It also seems likely that other molecular motors, including kinesin and dynein [41–43], are also involved in the movement of secretory granules, and perhaps other organelles, in β-cells.

Insulin is released from secretory granules by exocytosis, a process in which the granule membrane and plasma membrane fuse together, releasing the granule contents into the interstitial space. Much of our knowledge of the molecular mechanisms of exocytosis is derived from studies of neurotransmitter release from nerve cells, and similar mechanisms operate in β-cells. The docking of the granules at the inner surface of the plasma membrane is via the formation of a multimeric complex of proteins known as the SNARE (soluble N-ethylmaleimide-sensitive factor attachment protein receptor) complex, which consists of proteins associated with secretory granules and the plasma membrane, and soluble fusion proteins [44,45]. The docked granules will only fuse with the membrane and release their contents in the presence of elevated levels of intracellular calcium which is sensed by synaptotagmins, a class of calcium-binding granule proteins [44,46]. Secretory granules are distributed throughout the β-cell cytoplasm (Figure 6.1c), and it is likely that the transport of granules from distant sites to the plasma membrane is regulated independently from the final secretory process, with a reservoir of granules stored close to the inner surface of the plasma membrane. Fusion of this "readily-releasable" pool of granules may account for the rapid first-phase release of insulin in response to glucose stimulation [39,40]. Direct electrophysiologic measurements have demonstrated that the β-cell exocytotic response consists of a short-lived first phase, with a very rapid rate of granule exocytosis, followed by a sustained second phase with a slower rate of exocytosis [45,46].

Regulation of insulin secretion

To ensure that circulating levels of insulin are appropriate for the prevailing metabolic status β-cells are equipped with mechanisms to detect changes in circulating nutrients, in hormone levels, and in the activity of the autonomic nervous system. Moreover, β-cells have fail-safe mechanisms for coordinating this afferent information and responding with an appropriate secretion of insulin. The major physiologic determinant of insulin secretion in humans is the circulating concentration of glucose and other nutrients, including amino acids and fatty acids. These nutrients possess the ability to initiate an insulin secretory response, so when nutrients are being absorbed from the gastrointestinal system the β-cell detects the changes in circulating nutrients and releases insulin to enable the uptake and metabolism or storage of the nutrients by the target tissues. The consequent decrease in circulating nutrients is detected by the β-cells, which switch off insulin secretion to prevent hypoglycemia. The responses of β-cells to nutrient initiators of insulin secretion can be modified by a variety of hormones and neurotransmitters which act to amplify, or occasionally inhibit, the nutrient-induced responses (Table 6.1). Under normoglycemic conditions these agents have little or no effect on insulin secretion, a mechanism that prevents inappropriate secretion of insulin which would result in potentially harmful hypoglycemia. These agents are often referred to as potentiators of insulin secretion to distinguish them from nutrients which initiate the secretory response. The overall insulin output depends on the relative input from initiators and potentiators at the level of individual β-cells, on the synchronization of secretory activity between β-cells in individual islets, and on the coordination of secretion between the hundreds of thousands of islets in a human pancreas. This section considers the mechanisms employed by β-cells to recognize and respond to nutrient initiators and non-nutrient potentiators of insulin secretion.

Table 6.1 Non-nutrient regulators of insulin secretion.

Stimulators	Inhibitors
Islet products	
Glucagon	SST-14
Adenine nucleotides	Ghrelin
Divalent cations	
Neurotransmitters	
Acetylcholine	Norepinephrine
VIP	Dopamine
PACAP	NPY
GRP	Galanin
Gastrointestinal hormones	
CCK	SST-28
GIP	Ghrelin
GLP-1	
Adipokines	
Adiponectin	Leptin
	Resistin

CCK, cholecystokinin; GIP, glucose-dependent insulinotropic peptide; GLP-1, glucagon-like peptide-1; GRP, gastrin-releasing polypeptide; NPY, neuropeptide Y; PACAP, pituitary adenylate cyclase activating polypeptide; SST; somatostatin; VIP, vasoactive intestinal polypeptide.

Nutrient-induced insulin secretion

Nutrient metabolism

Pancreatic β-cells respond to small changes in extracellular glucose concentrations within a narrow physiologic range and the mechanisms through which β-cells couple changes in nutrient metabolism to regulated exocytosis of insulin are becoming increasingly well understood. Glucose is transported into β-cells via high capacity glucose transporters (GLUT; GLUT2 in rodents, GLUT1, 2 and 3 in humans [47,48]), enabling rapid equilibration of extracellular and intracellular glucose concentrations. Once inside the β-cell glucose is phosphorylated by glucokinase which acts as the "glucose sensor," coupling insulin secretion to the prevailing glucose level [49]. The dose–response curve of glucose-induced insulin secretion from isolated islets is sigmoidal (Figure 6.6) and is determined primarily by the activity of glucokinase. Concentrations of glucose below 5 mmol/L do not affect rates of insulin release, and the rate of secretion increases progressively at extracellular glucose levels between 5 and ~15 mmol/L, with half-maximal stimulation at ~8 mmol/L. The time-course of the insulin secretory response to elevated glucose is characterized by

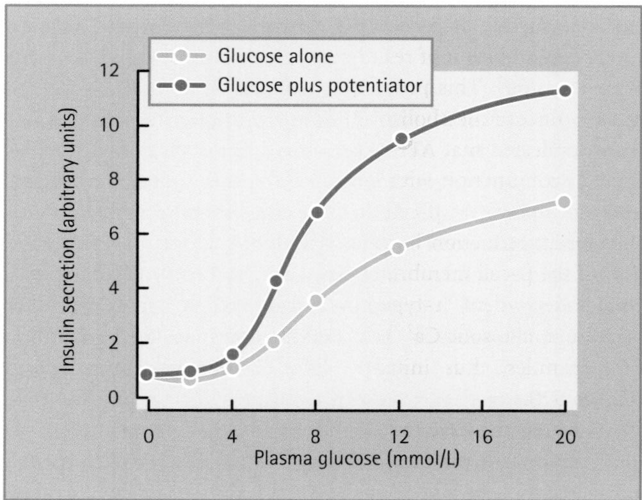

Figure 6.6 Glucose-induced insulin secretion from islets of Langerhans. No stimulation is seen below a threshold value of approximately 5 mmol/L glucose. Potentiators amplify insulin secretion at stimulatory concentrations of glucose, but are ineffective at subthreshold glucose levels.

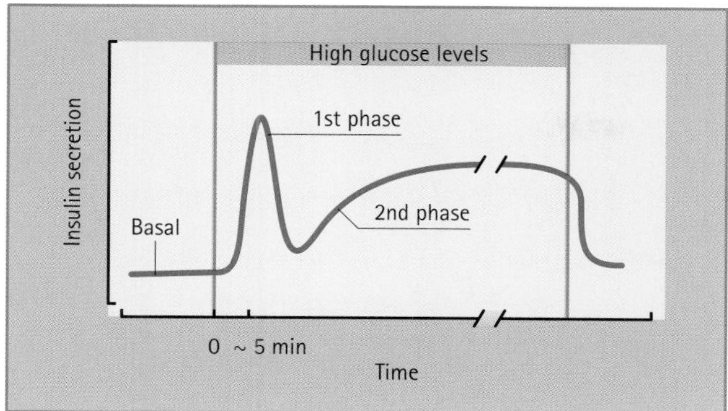

Figure 6.7 Glucose-induced insulin release *in vitro*. The figure shows the pattern of glucose-induced insulin secretion from perfused pancreas, in response to an increase in the glucose concentration. An acute first phase, lasting a few minutes, is followed by a sustained second phase of secretion which persists for the duration of the high-glucose stimulus.

a rapidly rising but transient first phase, followed by a maintained and prolonged second phase, as shown in Figure 6.7. This profile of insulin secretion is obtained whether insulin levels are measured following a glucose load *in vivo*, or whether the secretory output from the perfused pancreas or isolated islets is assessed, suggesting that the characteristic biphasic secretion pattern is an intrinsic property of the islets.

ATP-sensitive potassium channels and membrane depolarization

In the absence of extracellular glucose, the β-cell membrane potential is maintained close to the potassium equilibrium potential by the efflux of potassium ions through inwardly rectifying potassium channels. These channels were called ATP-sensitive potassium (K_{ATP}) channels because application of ATP to the cytosolic surface of β-cell membrane patches resulted in rapid, reversible inhibition of resting membrane permeability to potassium ions [50]. This property of the K_{ATP} channel is pivotal in linking glucose metabolism to insulin secretion. Thus, it is now well established that ATP generation following glucose metabolism, in conjunction with concomitant lowering of ADP levels, leads to closure of β-cell K_{ATP} channels. Channel closure and subsequent reduction in potassium efflux promotes depolarization of the β-cell membrane and influx of calcium ions through voltage-dependent L-type calcium channels. The resultant increase in cytosolic Ca^{2+} triggers the exocytosis of insulin secretory granules, thus initiating the insulin secretory response (Figure 6.8).

At around the time that the K_{ATP} channels were established as the link between the metabolic and electrophysiologic effects of glucose, they were also identified as the cellular target for sulfonylureas. The capacity of sulfonylureas to close K_{ATP} channels explains their effectiveness in type 2 diabetes where the β-cells no longer respond adequately to glucose, as the usual pathway for coupling glucose metabolism to insulin secretion is bypassed. The β-cell K_{ATP} channel is a hetero-octamer formed from four potassium channel subunits (termed Kir6.2) and four sulfonylurea receptor subunits (SUR1) [51]. The Kir6.2 subunits form the pore through which potassium ions flow and these are surrounded by the SUR1 subunits which have a regulatory role (Figure 6.8, inset). ATP and sulfonylureas induce channel closure by binding to Kir6.2 and SUR1 subunits, respectively, while ADP activates the channels by binding to a nucleotide-binding domain on the SUR1 subunit. Diazoxide, an inhibitor of insulin secretion, also binds to the SUR1 subunit to open the channels. The central role of K_{ATP} channels in β-cell glucose recognition makes them obvious candidates for β-cell dysfunction in type 2 diabetes. Earlier studies in patients with type 2 diabetes, maturity-onset diabetes of the young (MODY) or gestational diabetes, failed to detect any Kir6.2 gene mutations that compromised channel function [52,53]. Since then, larger scale studies of variants in genes encoding Kir6.2 and SUR1 have demonstrated polymorphisms associated with increased risk of type 2 diabetes [54]. Similarly, activating mutations in the Kir6.2 gene have recently been shown to be causal for cases of permanent neonatal diabetes (PNDM) [55], which has enabled insulin-dependent PNDM patients to achieve glycemic control with sulfonylurea treatment alone. In contrast, loss of β-cell functional K_{ATP} channel activity has been implicated in the pathogenesis of persistent hyperinsulinemic hypoglycemia of infancy (PHHI) [56], a condition characterized by hypersecretion of insulin despite profound hypoglycemia. Numerous mutations in both the Kir6.2 and SUR1 subunits have been identified in patients with PHHI and these are thought to be responsible for the severe impairment in glucose homeostasis in these individuals [57].

Calcium and other intracellular effectors

Intracellular calcium is a principal effector of the nutrient-induced insulin secretory response, linking depolarization with exocytosis of insulin secretory granules (Figure 6.8). A large electrochemical concentration gradient (~10 000-fold) of calcium is maintained across the β-cell plasma membrane by a combination of membrane-associated calcium extruding systems and active calcium sequestration within intracellular organelles. The major route through which calcium is elevated in β-cells is by influx of extracellular calcium through voltage-dependent L-type calcium channels that open in response to β-cell depolarization, and it has been estimated that each β-cell contains about 500 L-type channels [58].

Studies with permeabilized β-cells have demonstrated that elevations in intracellular calcium are alone sufficient to initiate insulin secretion [59], and conditions that elevate intracellular calcium usually stimulate insulin release. An increase in cytosolic calcium is essential for the initiation of insulin secretion by glucose and other nutrients: preventing calcium influx by removal of extracellular calcium or by pharmacologic blockade of voltage-dependent calcium channels abolishes nutrient-induced insulin secretion. Glucose and other nutrients also induce a calcium-dependent activation of β-cell phospholipase C (PLC) [60],

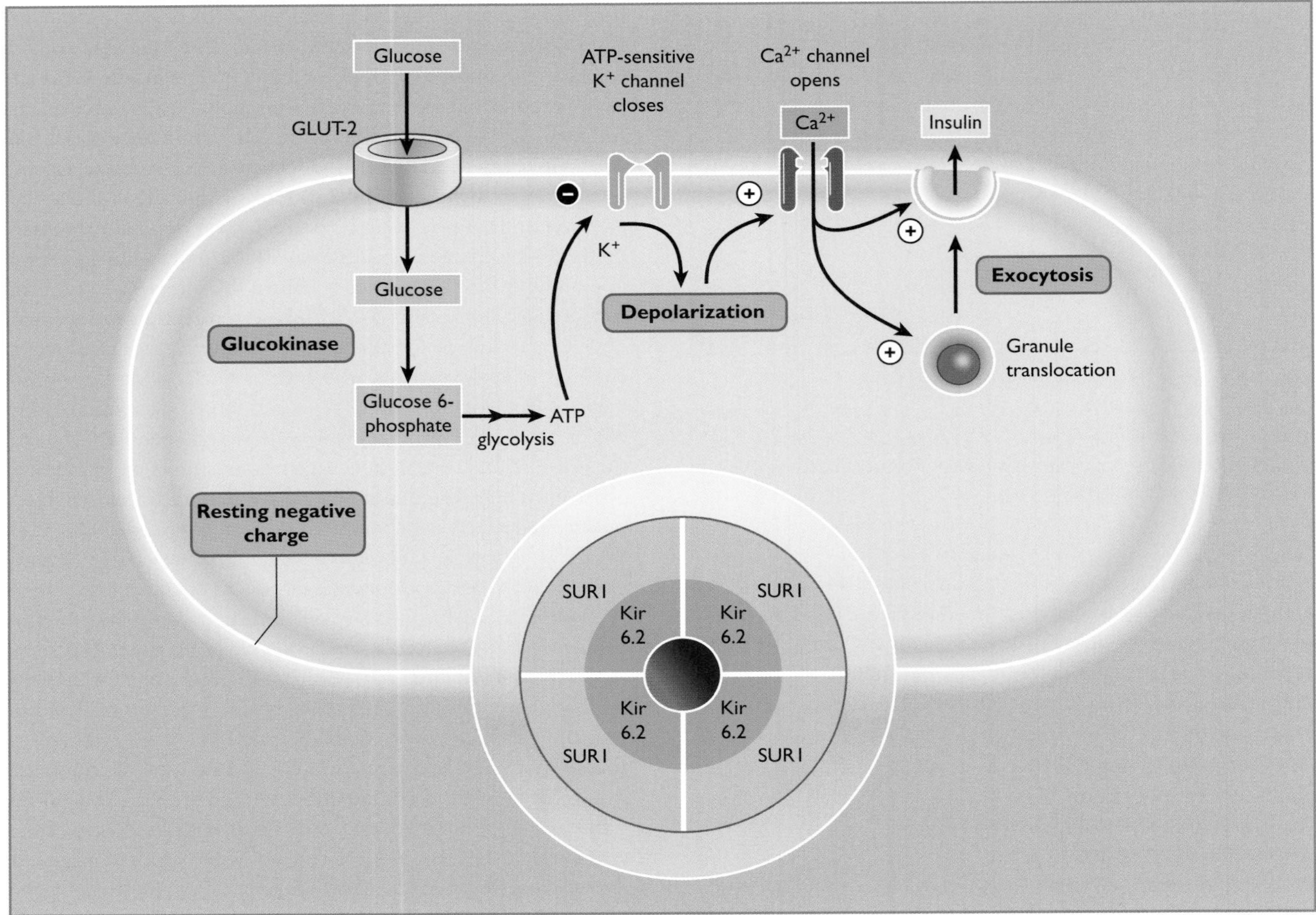

Figure 6.8 Intracellular mechanisms through which glucose stimulates insulin secretion. Glucose is metabolized within the β-cell to generate ATP, which closes ATP-sensitive potassium channels in the cell membrane. This prevents potassium ions from leaving the cell, causing membrane depolarization, which in turn opens voltage-gated calcium channels in the membrane and allows calcium ions to enter the cell. The increase in cytosolic calcium initiates granule exocytosis. Sulfonylureas act downstream of glucose metabolism, by binding to the SUR1 component of the K_{ATP} channel (inset). GLUT, glucose transporter.

leading to the generation of inositol 1,4,5-trisphosphate (IP_3) and diacylglycerol (DAG), both of which serve second-messenger functions in β-cells [61]. The generation of IP_3 leads to the rapid mobilization of intracellular calcium, but the significance of this in secretory responses to nutrients is uncertain, and it is likely to have little more than a modulatory role, amplifying the elevations in cytosolic calcium concentration induced by the influx of extracellular calcium.

The elevations in intracellular calcium are transduced into the regulated secretion of insulin by intracellular calcium sensing systems within β-cells. Important among these are the calcium-dependent protein kinases, which include myosin light chain kinases, the calcium/phospholipid-dependent kinases and the calcium/calmodulin-dependent kinases (CaMKs). CaMKs are protein kinases that are activated in the presence of calcium and the calcium-binding protein, calmodulin, and a number of studies have implicated CaMK II in insulin secretory responses [61]. It has been proposed that CaMK II activation is responsible for the initiation of insulin secretion in response to glucose and other nutrients, and for enhancing nutrient-induced secretion in response to receptor agonists that elevate intracellular calcium [61]. Cytosolic PLA_2 ($cPLA_2$) is another β-cell calcium-sensitive enzyme. It is activated by concentrations of calcium that are achieved in stimulated β-cells, and it generates arachidonic acid (AA) by the hydrolysis of membrane phosphatidylcholine. AA is capable of stimulating insulin secretion in a glucose and calcium-independent manner, and it is further metabolized in islets by the cyclo-oxygenase (COX) pathways to produce prostaglandins and thromboxanes, and by the lipoxygenase (LOX) pathways to generate hydroperoxyeicosatetrenoic acids (HPETES), hydroxyeicosatetrenoic acids (HETES) and leukotrienes.

The precise roles(s) of AA derivatives in islet function remains uncertain because experimental investigations have relied on COX and LOX inhibitors of poor specificity, but earlier reports that prostaglandins are largely inhibitory in rodent islets [62] have not been supported by more recent studies using human islets [63]. Calcium sensors are also important at the later stages of the secretory pathway, where the calcium-sensitive synaptotagmin proteins are involved in the formation of the exocytotic SNARE complex, as described above, to confer calcium sensitivity on the initiation and rate of exocytotic release of insulin secretory granules [44].

The elevations in intracellular calcium induced by nutrients activate other effector systems in β-cells, including PLC and $cPLA_2$, as discussed above, and calcium-sensitive adenylate cyclase isoforms, which generate cyclic AMP from ATP. Although these signaling systems are of undoubted importance in the regulation of β-cells by non-nutrients, their role in nutrient-induced insulin secretion is still uncertain. Thus, DAG generated by glucose-induced PLC activation has the potential to activate some protein kinase C (PKC) isoforms. PKC was first identified as a calcium and phospholipid sensitive, DAG-activated protein kinase, but it has become apparent that some isoforms of PKC require neither calcium nor DAG for activation. The isoforms are classified into three groups: calcium and DAG sensitive (conventional); calcium independent, DAG-sensitive (novel); and calcium and DAG independent (atypical), and β-cells contain conventional, atypical and novel PKC isoforms [64]. The early literature on the role of PKC in nutrient-induced insulin secretion is confusing but several studies have shown that glucose-induced insulin secretion is maintained under conditions where DAG-sensitive PKC isoforms are depleted, suggesting that conventional and novel PKC isoforms are not required for insulin secretion in response to glucose [61,65].

The role of cyclic AMP in the insulin secretory response to nutrients is similarly unclear. Cyclic AMP has the potential to influence insulin secretion by the activation of cyclic AMP-dependent protein kinase A (PKA), or via the cyclic AMP-regulated guanine nucleotide exchange factors known as exchange proteins activated by cyclic AMP (EPACs) [66]. However, elevations in β-cell cyclic AMP do not stimulate insulin secretion at substimulatory glucose concentrations, and the secretagogue effects of glucose can be maintained in the presence of competitive antagonists of cyclic AMP binding to PKA or EPACs [67]. These observations suggest that cyclic AMP does not act as a primary trigger of nutrient-stimulated β-cell secretory function, but more recent observations linking glucose-induced oscillations in β-cell cyclic AMP to oscillations in insulin secretion [68] suggest that a role for this messenger system in nutrient-induced insulin secretion cannot be ruled out.

K_{ATP} channel-independent pathways

Since the early reports linking K_{ATP} channel closure to the exocytotic release of insulin, it has become apparent that β-cells also possess a K_{ATP} channel-independent stimulus–secretion coupling pathway: this is termed the amplifying pathway to distinguish it from the triggering pathway that is activated by K_{ATP} channel closure [69]. Studies in which β-cell calcium is elevated by depolarization and K_{ATP} channels maintained in the open state by diazoxide have indicated that glucose, at concentrations as low as 1–6 mmol/L, is still capable of stimulating insulin secretion [70]. The mechanisms by which glucose stimulates insulin secretion in a K_{ATP} channel-independent manner have not been established [71]. However, it is clear that glucose must be metabolized and there is convincing evidence that changes in adenine nucleotides are involved [72], while it has been established that activation of PKA and PKC is not required. It has been suggested that the K_{ATP}-independent amplifying pathway is impaired in type 2 diabetes and that identification of novel therapeutic strategies targeted at this pathway may be beneficial in restoring β-cell function in patients with type 2 diabetes [69].

Amino acids

Several amino acids stimulate insulin secretion *in vivo* and *in vitro*. Most require glucose, but some, such as leucine, lysine and arginine, can stimulate insulin secretion in the absence of glucose, and therefore qualify as initiators of secretion. Leucine enters islets by a sodium-independent transport system and stimulates a biphasic increase in insulin release. The effects of leucine on β-cell membrane potential, ion fluxes and insulin secretion are similar to, but smaller than, those of glucose [73]. Thus, metabolism of leucine within β-cells decreases the potassium permeability, causing depolarization and activation of L-type calcium channels through which calcium enters the β-cells and initiates insulin secretion. Leucine is also able to activate the amplifying pathway of insulin secretion in a K_{ATP} channel-independent manner, as described above for glucose. The charged amino acids, lysine and arginine, cross the β-cell plasma membrane via a transport system specific for cationic amino acids. It is generally believed that the accumulation of these positively charged molecules directly depolarizes the β-cell membrane leading to calcium influx.

Regulation of insulin secretion by non-nutrients

The complex mechanisms that have evolved to enable changes in extracellular nutrients to initiate an exocytotic secretory response are confined to pancreatic β-cells, and perhaps to a subset of hypothalamic neurons [74]. However, the mechanisms that β-cells use to recognize and respond to non-nutrient potentiators of secretion are ubiquitous in mammalian cells, and so are covered only briefly in this section, followed by a review of the physiologically relevant non-nutrient regulators of β-cell function.

Most, if not all, non-nutrient modulators of insulin secretion influence the β-cell by binding to and activating specific receptors on the extracellular surface. Because of its central role in coordinating whole body fuel homeostasis the β-cell expresses receptors for a wide range of biologically active peptides, glycoproteins and neurotransmitters (Table 6.1). However, receptor occupancy generally results in the activation of a limited number of intracellular effector systems, which were introduced in the section on nutrient-induced insulin section (Figures 6.9 and 6.10).

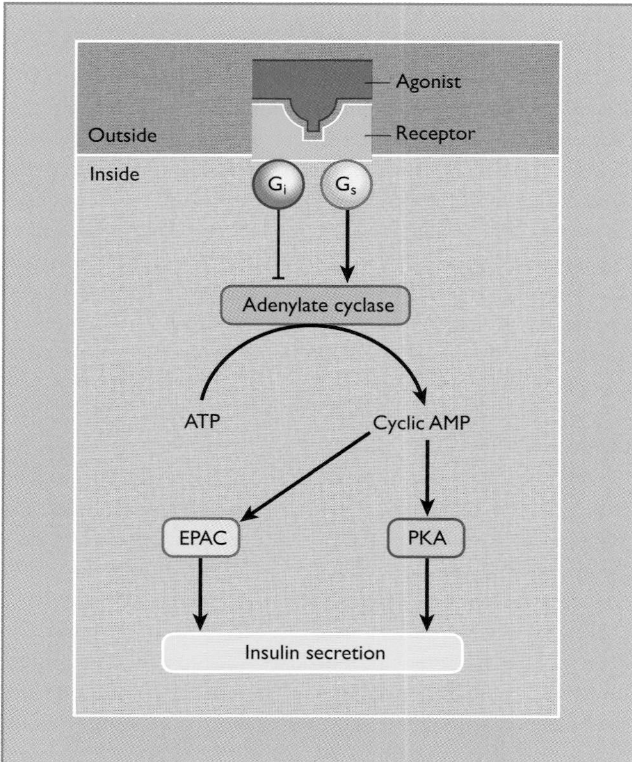

Figure 6.9 Adenylate cyclase and the regulation of insulin secretion. Some receptor agonists (e.g. glucagon, glucagon-like peptide 1, pituitary adenylate cyclase activating polypeptide) bind to cell-surface receptors that are coupled to adenylate cyclase (AC) via the heterotrimeric GTP-binding protein Gs. Adenylate cyclase hydrolyses ATP to generate adenosine 5′ cyclic monophosphate (cyclic AMP), which activates protein kinase A (PKA) and exchange proteins activated by cyclic AMP (EPACs). Both of these pathways potentiate glucose-stimulated insulin secretion. Glucose also activates adenylate cyclase, but increases in intracellular cyclic AMP levels in response to glucose are generally smaller than those obtained with receptor agonists. Some inhibitory agonists (e.g. norepinephrine, somatostatin) bind to receptors that are coupled to adenylate cyclase via the inhibitory GTP-binding protein G_i, resulting in reduced adenylate cyclase activity and a decrease in intracellular cyclic AMP.

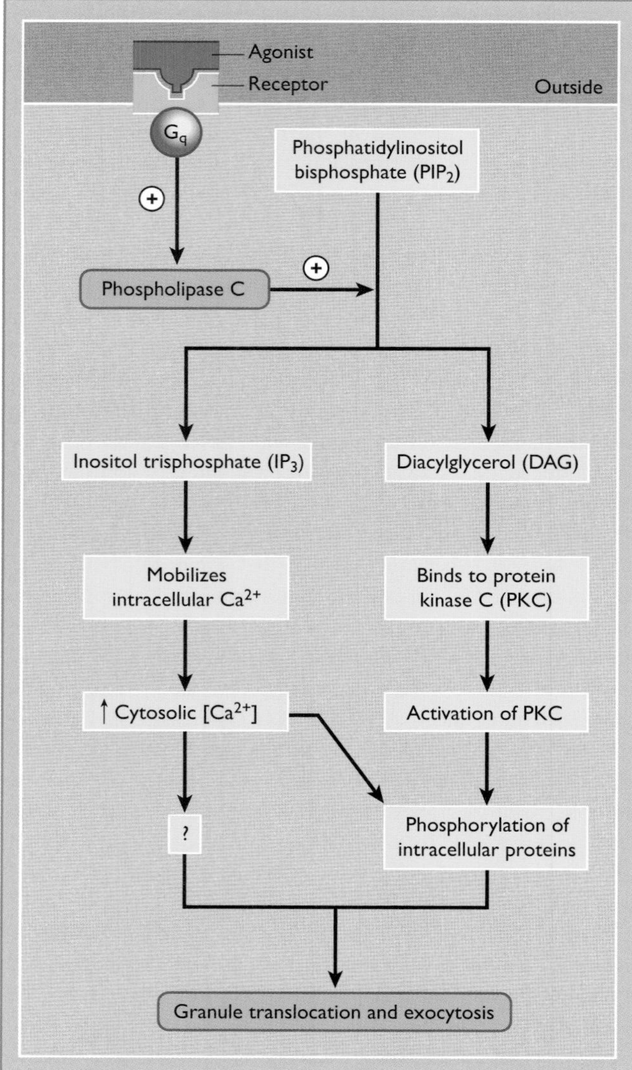

Figure 6.10 Phospholipase C and the regulation of insulin secretion. Some receptor agonists (e.g. acetylcholine, cholecystokinin) bind to cell-surface receptors that are coupled to phospholipase C (PLC) via the heterotrimeric GTP-binding protein G_q. Phospholipase C hydrolyzes phosphoinositol bisphosphate (PIP_2), an integral component of the membrane, to generate inositol 1,4,5-trisphosphate (IP_3) and diacylglycerol (DAG). IP_3 mobilizes calcium from the endoplasmic reticulum and DAG activates protein kinase C (PKC), both of which enhance insulin secretion. Nutrients also activate PLC in a calcium-dependent manner but the importance of IP_3 and DAG in nutrient-induced insulin secretion is uncertain.

Islet hormones

There is convincing evidence for complex intra-islet interactions via molecules released from islet endocrine cells (Figure 6.2). The physiologic relevance of some of these interactions is still uncertain, but some of the intra-islet factors that are thought to influence insulin secretion are discussed briefly in this section.

It is now clear that β-cells express insulin receptors and the associated intracellular signaling elements, suggesting the existence of autocrine and/or paracrine feedback regulation of β-cell function [19,75]. Earlier suggestions that secreted insulin regulates insulin secretion [76] have not been confirmed [19,77], and the main feedback function of insulin on β-cells is to regulate β-cell gene expression [75,78] and β-cell mass through effects on proliferation and apoptosis [19,79].

Glucagon is a 29 amino acid peptide secreted by islet α-cells. The precursor, proglucagon, undergoes differential post-translational processing in the gut to produce entirely different peptides with different receptors and biologic activities. These include glucagon-like peptide 1 (GLP-1) (7–36) amide, an "incretin" hormone that is discussed below, and GLP-2, which promotes growth of the intestinal mucosa. Glucagon secretion is regulated by nutrients, islet and gastrointestinal hormones and the autonomic nervous system, with hypoglycemia and sympathetic nervous input being important stimulators of glucagon secretion [80]. Glucagon enhances insulin secretion through the stimulatory G-protein (G_s) coupled activation of adenylate cyclase and the consequent increase in intracellular cyclic AMP (Figure 6.9).

Somatostatin (SST) is expressed by islet δ-cells and in numerous other sites, including the central nervous system and D cells of the gastrointestinal tract, where it acts predominantly as an inhibitor of endocrine and exocrine secretion [81]. The precursor, prosomatostatin, is processed by alternative pathways: in islets and the CNS SST-14 is generated, and SST-28, the major circulating form of SST in humans, is produced in the gastrointestinal tract [82]. SST secretion is regulated by a variety of nutrients, endocrine and neural factors [17,81,83]. Islets express five different somatostatin receptor (SSTR) subtypes, and SST-14 released from islet δ-cells has a tonic inhibitory effect on insulin and glucagon secretion [17], via activation of SSTR5 and SSTR2, respectively [84,85]. SST receptors are coupled via an inhibitory G-protein(s) to the inhibition of adenylate cyclase and decreased formation of cyclic AMP [86], and to ion channels that cause hyperpolarization of the β-cell membrane and reductions in intracellular calcium [87].

Pancreatic polypeptide (PP) is a 36 amino acid peptide produced by PP cells that are found in the mantle of islets, predominantly those located in the head of the pancreas. PP secretion is mainly regulated via cholinergic parasympathetic stimulation [81], but the physiologic function of PP as a circulating hormone, or as an intra-islet signal, remains uncertain [88].

Ghrelin is a 23 amino acid peptide first identified in the gastrointestinal system, but now known to also be expressed in islet ε-cells, which are localized to the islet mantle in rodents, and which appear to be developmentally distinct from the classic islet endocrine cells [89,90]. The physiologic function of ε-cell-derived ghrelin has not been established, but most experimental evidence suggests an inhibitory role in the regulation of insulin secretion [91], analogous to that of δ-cell SST [17].

Neural control of insulin secretion

The association of nerve fibers with islets was shown over 100 years ago by silver staining techniques [92], and since that time it has become well established that islets are innervated by cholinergic, adrenergic and peptidergic autonomic nerves. Parasympathetic (cholinergic) fibers originating in the dorsal motor nucleus of the vagus, and sympathetic (adrenergic) fibers from the greater and middle splanchnic nerves penetrate the pancreas and terminate close to the islet cells. The autonomic innervation of the islets is important in regulating insulin secretion, with enhanced insulin output following activation of parasympathetic nerves and decreased insulin secretion in response to increased sympathetic activity. The autonomic nervous regulation of islet hormone secretion is thought to be involved in the cephalic phase of insulin secretion during feeding, in synchronizing islets to generate oscillations of hormone secretion, and in regulating islet secretory responses to metabolic stress [5].

Neurotransmitters: acetylcholine and norepinephrine

The numerous parasympathetic nerve fibers that innervate islets are postganglionic and originate from the intra-pancreatic ganglia, which are controlled by preganglionic fibers originating in the dorsal vagal nucleus [5]. Acetylcholine is the major postganglionic parasympathetic neurotransmitter, and it stimulates the release of insulin and glucagon in a variety of mammalian species [5,93,94]. In β-cells, acetylcholine acts predominantly via M3 receptors [93,95] to activate PLC (Figure 6.10), generating IP_3 and DAG, which act to amplify the effects of glucose by elevating cytosolic calcium and activating PKC [61]. Activation of β-cell muscarinic receptors can also lead to the activation of PLA_2, with the subsequent generation of AA and lysophosphatidylcholine, which can further enhance nutrient-induced insulin secretion. Acetylcholine also depolarizes the plasma membrane by affecting Na^+ conductivity, and this additional depolarization induces sustained increases in cytosolic calcium [93].

Islets also receive an extensive sympathetic innervation from postganglionic nerves whose cell bodies are located in the celiac or paravertebral ganglia, while the preganglionic nerves originate from the hypothalamus [5]. The major sympathetic neurotransmitter, norepinephrine (noradrenaline), can exert positive and negative influences on hormone secretion. Thus, norepinephrine can exert direct stimulatory effects on the β-cell via β_2-adrenoreceptors [96], or inhibitory effects via α_2-adrenoreceptors [97], and the net effect of norepinephrine may depend on the relative levels of expression of these receptor subtypes. Differences between species in the expression levels of adrenoreceptor subtypes probably account for the differential effects of β-adrenergic agonists on human islets, where they are stimulatory, and rodent islets, where they are ineffective [98]. The stimulatory effects mediated by β_2-receptors occur by activation of adenylate cyclase and an increase in intracellular cyclic AMP (Figure 6.9) [99], while the inhibitory effect of α_2-receptor activation involve reductions in cyclic AMP and of cytosolic calcium [86,100], and an unidentified inhibitory action at a more distal point in the stimulus–secretion coupling mechanism [101]. In contrast, norepinephrine has direct stimulatory effects on glucagon secretion from α-cells mediated by both β_2 and α_2-receptor subtypes [5]. Circulating catecholamines secreted by the adrenal medulla (mainly epinephrine) also have the potential to influence islet hormone secretion through interactions with the adrenoreceptors expressed on the α and β-cells.

Neuropeptides

Parasympathetic nerve fibers in islets contain a number of biologically active neuropeptides, including VIP, PACAP and gastrin-releasing polypeptide (GRP), all of which are released by vagal activation and all of which stimulate the release of insulin and glucagon.

VIP (28 amino acids) and PACAP (27 or 38 amino acids) are abundantly expressed neuropeptides that are widely distributed in parasympathetic nerves that supply the islets and gastrointestinal tract [6,102]. VIP and PACAP have similar structures, and VIP1 and VIP2 receptors also have an affinity for PACAP. The stimulatory effects of VIP and PACAP on insulin secretion *in vitro* and *in vivo* are through β-cell VIP2 and PAC1 receptors, respectively, and are thought to involve increases in intracellular cyclic AMP (Figure 6.9) and cytosolic calcium [6,103,104]. GRP is a 27 amino acid peptide that also stimulates the secretion of insulin, glucagon, SST and PP [5,94]. These effects of GRP are mediated through specific receptors, and involve the activation of PLC and the generation of IP_3 and DAG (Figure 6.10) [102,105].

Sympathetic nerves contain different neuropeptides to parasympathetic nerves, and these include NPY and galanin, both of which have inhibitory actions within islets. NPY (36 amino acids) and galanin (29 amino acids) are expressed in fibers innervating both the endocrine and exocrine pancreas [5,106]. Both neuropeptides inhibit basal and glucose-stimulated insulin secretion [86,106,107], although differences between species have been reported. Both NPY and galanin act through specific G_i-coupled receptors to inhibit adenylate cyclase [108,109], and galanin may have additional inhibitory effects at an undefined late stage of exocytosis [86].

Incretin and adipokine regulation of insulin secretion

It has been known for over 40 years that insulin secretion from islets is greater following oral rather than intravenous administration of glucose [110], and it is now known that this enhanced insulin secretory output is a consequence of the release of gastrointestinal-derived "incretin" hormones [111]. The main incretins that have been implicated in an elevated insulin response to absorbed nutrients after food intake are glucagon-like peptide 1 (GLP-1), glucose-dependent insulinotropic peptide (GIP) and cholecystokinin (CCK), all of which are hormones secreted by specialized endocrine cells in the gastrointestinal tract in response to the absorption of nutrients [111,112]. These hormones are carried to the islets in the blood and they interact with specific receptors on the β-cell surface to stimulate insulin secretion.

Glucagon-like peptide 1

After food intake, intestinal L-cells secrete GLP-1 in response to elevated levels of nutrients derived from carbohydrates, lipids and protein in the intestinal lumen [112,113]. GLP-1 is generated by prohormone convertase 1–3 cleavage of proglucagon in the L-cells and it is highly conserved in mammals, with identical amino acid sequences in humans and mice [82,113]. GLP-1 is degraded by dipeptidyl protease 4 (DPP-4), which cleaves two amino acids from its N-terminus. Full length GLP-1 (1–37) does not show biologic activity, but the truncated peptides GLP-1 (7–36) amide and GLP-1 (7–37) are potent stimulators of insulin secretion *in vitro* and *in vivo* [114]. Observations that infusion of the peptide into individuals with type 2 diabetes before food intake improved insulin output and reduced the post-prandial increase in circulating glucose led to studies to determine whether GLP-1 or related peptides may be useful as therapies for type 2 diabetes. Reports of other beneficial effects of GLP-1, including its capacity to inhibit glucagon secretion, delay gastric emptying and decrease food intake indicated its positive effects on normalizing post-prandial glycemia, but its half-life of less than 2 minutes precludes its use as a diabetes therapy. Nonetheless, exenatide, a synthetic version of a GLP-1 analogue present in the saliva of the Gila monster lizard, has been developed for clinical use for type 2 diabetes [115]. It has approximately 50% amino acid homology with GLP-1 thus allowing it to exert the same effects on islets as native GLP-1, but its resistance to degradation by DPP-4 increases its half-life to around 2 hours *in vivo*, which ensures effective regulation of blood glucose levels. Another GLP-1 analogue, liraglutide, has a greatly extended half life (>12 hours) as a result of incorporation of the fatty acid palmitate into the GLP-1 sequence, allowing it to bind to plasma albumin and reducing its exposure to DPP-4. Selective DPP-4 inhibitors such as sitagliptin are used clinically to normalize blood glucose levels in type 2 diabetes by extending the half-life of endogenous GLP-1.

GLP-1, exenatide and liraglutide act at specific G-protein coupled receptors [111] that are linked, via G_s, to adenylate cyclase activation which ultimately increases insulin secretion (Figure 6.9) [114]. Although cyclic AMP has been implicated in the majority of effects of GLP-1 in islets, it may also close rat β-cell K_{ATP} channels in a cyclic AMP-independent manner [116].

Glucose-dependent insulinotropic peptide

Glucose-dependent insulinotropic peptide (GIP), a 42 amino acid peptide, is released from K-cells in the duodenum and jejunum in response to the absorption of glucose, other actively transported sugars, amino acids and long-chain fatty acids [112]. It was originally called "gastric inhibitory polypeptide" because of its inhibitory effects on acid secretion in the stomach, but its main physiologic effects are now known to be stimulation of insulin secretion in a glucose-dependent manner [102,111]. Like GLP-1, GIP binds to G_s-coupled receptors on the β-cell plasma membrane, with essentially the same downstream cascades leading to stimulation of insulin secretion (Figure 6.9) [102,111]. GIP is also reported to increase insulin release through generation of AA via phospholipase A_2 activation [117], and closure of K_{ATP} channels [111]. Although GLP-1 and GIP both enhance insulin output following their release in response to food intake, it seems unlikely that GIP-related peptides will be developed as therapies for type 2 diabetes because GIP stimulates glucagon secretion and inhibits GLP-1 release, and its infusion in individuals with type 2 diabetes is reported to worsen post-prandial hyperglycemia [118].

Cholecystokinin

CCK is another incretin hormone that is released from I-cells in the gastrointestinal tract in response to elevated fat and protein levels [112]. It was originally isolated from porcine intestine as a 33 amino acid peptide and the truncated CCK-8 form stimulates insulin secretion *in vitro* and *in vivo* [119]. CCK-8 acts at specific G_q-coupled receptors on β-cells to activate PLC (Figure 6.10) [102], and its potentiation of insulin secretion is completely dependent on PKC activation [120]. However, the physiologic role of CCK as an incretin has not been established because high concentrations are required for its effects on insulin secretion, and it is possible that its major function is in digestion in the duodenum.

Adipokines

Obesity is a risk factor for diabetes, and hormones (adipokines) released from fat depots have been implicated in insulin resistance associated with obesity and type 2 diabetes [121]. Some adipokines such as leptin, resistin and adiponectin are also reported to influence islet function. Thus, β-cells express Ob-Rb leptin receptors which, when activated by leptin, lead to inhibition of insulin secretion [122], and specific deletion of β-cell Ob-Rb receptors is associated with enhanced insulin secretion [123]. The inhibitory effects of leptin on glucose-stimulated insulin secretion have been attributed to activation of β-cell K_{ATP} channels [124] or of c-Jun N-terminal kinases (JNKs) [125]. Leptin may also further impair β-cell function through reductions in β-cell mass [123,125]. Resistin, another adipocyte polypeptide, also inhibits glucose-stimulated insulin release [126] and stimulates apoptosis of rat β-cells [127], suggesting that it has similar functions to leptin. However, resistin is not considered to be a true adipokine because although it is secreted at high levels from mouse adipocytes it is not produced by human adipocytes, and high plasma resistin levels do not correlate with reduced insulin sensitivity [128]. However, it is possible that resistin has paracrine effects on β-cell function in humans as it has been identified in human islets [129]. Unlike leptin and resistin, adiponectin has protective effects by improving insulin sensitivity, and decreased plasma adiponectin levels may contribute to the development of type 2 diabetes [130]. The functional effects of adiponectin in β-cells have not been fully established, but human and rat β-cells express adiponectin receptors [131,132], and adiponectin is reported to stimulate insulin secretion [131,132] and protect against β-cell apoptosis [133]. The signaling cascades that couple adiponectin receptors to downstream effects in β-cells are currently unknown.

Conclusions

Pancreatic islets of Langerhans are complex endocrine organs containing several different types of endocrine cells, with extensive vasculature and autonomic nerve supply. Interactions between the islet cells, the autonomic nervous system and hormones secreted by the gastrointestinal system and adipose tissue enable the appropriate release of islet hormones to regulate metabolic fuel usage and storage.

The insulin-secreting β-cells within islets respond to changes in circulating nutrients by linking changes in nutrient metabolism to β-cell depolarization and the calcium-dependent exocytotic release of stored insulin. β-Cells can also respond to a wide range of hormones and neurotransmitters through conventional cell surface receptors that are linked to a variety of intracellular effectors systems regulating the release of insulin. The ability to detect nutrient, hormonal and neural signals allows β-cells to integrate information about the prevailing metabolic status, and to secrete insulin as required for glucose homeostasis.

This detailed understanding of islet cell biology has informed the development of new treatments for type 2 diabetes, as exemplified by the recent introduction of GLP-1 agonists and DPP-4 inhibitors. Recent studies have suggested associations between type 2 diabetes and polymorphisms in genes associated with β-cell development or function, so current understanding of normal β-cell function may assist in identifying the β-cell pathologies in type 2 diabetes.

References

1 Langerhans P. Beitrage zur mikroskopischen Anatomie der Bauchspeicheldruse. Inaugural dissertation, Gustav Lange ed. 1869.

2 Cabrera O, Berman DM, Kenyon NS, Ricordi C, Berggren PO, Caicedo A. The unique cytoarchitecture of human pancreatic islets has implications for islet cell function. *Proc Natl Acad Sci U S A* 2006; **103**:2334–2339.

3 Bonner-Weir S. Anatomy of the islet of Langerhans. In: Samols E, ed. *The Endocrine Pancreas*. New York: Raven Press, 1991; 15–27.

4 Nyman LR, Wells KS, Head WS, McCaughey M, Ford E, Brissova M, *et al.* Real-time, multidimensional *in vivo* imaging used to investigate blood flow in mouse pancreatic islets. *J Clin Invest* 2008; **118**:3790–3797.

5 Ahren B. Autonomic regulation of islet hormone secretion: implications for health and disease. *Diabetologia* 2000; **43**:393–410.

6 Winzell MS, Ahren B. Role of VIP and PACAP in islet function. *Peptides* 2007; **28**:1805–1813.

7 Halban PA, Wollheim CB, Blondel B, Meda P, Niesor EN, Mintz DH. The possible importance of contact between pancreatic islet cells for the control of insulin release. *Endocrinology* 1982; **111**: 86–94.

8 Halban PA, Powers SL, George KL, Bonner-Weir S. Spontaneous reassociation of dispersed adult rat pancreatic islet cells into aggregates with three-dimensional architecture typical of native islets. *Diabetes* 1987; **36**:783–790.

9 Hopcroft DW, Mason DR, Scott RS. Insulin secretion from perifused rat pancreatic pseudoislets. *In Vitro Cell Dev Biol* 1985; **21**:421–427.

10 Carvell MJ, Persaud SJ, Jones PM. An islet is greater than the sum of its parts: the importance of intercellular communication in insulin secretion. *Cellscience Rev* 2006; **3**:100–128.

11 Ravier MA, Guldenagel M, Charollais A, Gjinovci A, Caille D, Sohl G, *et al.* Loss of connexin 36 channels alters beta-cell coupling, islet synchronization of glucose-induced Ca^{2+} and insulin oscillations, and basal insulin release. *Diabetes* 2005; **54**:1798–1807.

12 Serre-Beinier V, Bosco D, Zulianello L, Charollais A, Caille D, Charpantier E, *et al.* Cx36 makes channels coupling human pancreatic beta-cells, and correlates with insulin expression. *Hum Mol Genet* 2009; **18**:428–439.

13 Carvell MJ, Marsh PJ, Persaud SJ, Jones PM. E-cadherin interactions regulate beta-cell proliferation in islet-like structures. *Cell Physiol Biochem* 2007; **20**:617–626.

14 Jaques F, Jousset H, Tomas A, Prost AL, Wollheim CB, Irminger JC, *et al.* Dual effect of cell–cell contact disruption on cytosolic calcium and insulin secretion. *Endocrinology* 2008; **149**:2494–2505.

15 Konstantinova I, Nikolova G, Ohara-Imaizumi M, Meda P, Kucera T, Zarbalis K, *et al.* EphA-Ephrin-A-mediated beta cell communication regulates insulin secretion from pancreatic islets. *Cell* 2007; **129**:359–370.

16 Van Schravendijk CF, Foriers A, Hooghe-Peters EL, Rogiers V, De MP, Sodoyez JC, *et al.* Pancreatic hormone receptors on islet cells. *Endocrinology* 1985; **117**:841–848.

17 Hauge-Evans AC, King AJ, Carmignac D, Richardson CC, Robinson IC, Low MJ, *et al.* Somatostatin secreted by islet delta-cells fulfills multiple roles as a paracrine regulator of islet function. *Diabetes* 2009; **58**:403–411.

18 Ravier MA, Rutter GA. Glucose or insulin, but not zinc ions, inhibit glucagon secretion from mouse pancreatic alpha-cells. *Diabetes* 2005; **54**:1789–1797.

19 Persaud SJ, Muller D, Jones PM. Insulin signalling in islets. *Biochem Soc Trans* 2008; **36**:290–293.

20 Kitsou-Mylona I, Burns CJ, Squires PE, Persaud SJ, Jones PM. A role for the extracellular calcium-sensing receptor in cell–cell communication in pancreatic islets of Langerhans. *Cell Physiol Biochem* 2008; **22**:557–566.

21 Detimary P, Jonas JC, Henquin JC. Stable and diffusible pools of nucleotides in pancreatic islet cells. *Endocrinology* 1996; **137**:4671–4676.

22 Rorsman P, Berggren PO, Bokvist K, Ericson H, Mohler H, Ostenson CG, *et al.* Glucose-inhibition of glucagon secretion involves activation of GABAA-receptor chloride channels. *Nature* 1989; **341**:233–236.

23 Rubi B, Ljubicic S, Pournourmohammadi S, Carobbio S, Armanet M, Bartley C, *et al.* Dopamine D2-like receptors are expressed in pancreatic beta cells and mediate inhibition of insulin secretion. *J Biol Chem* 2005; **280**:36824–36832.

24 Hellman B, Grapengiesser E, Gylfe E. Nitric oxide: a putative synchronizer of pancreatic beta-cell activity. *Diabetes Res Clin Pract* 2000; **50**:S148.

25 Henningsson R, Alm P, Ekstrom P, Lundquist I. Heme oxygenase and carbon monoxide: regulatory roles in islet hormone release – a biochemical, immunohistochemical, and confocal microscopic study. *Diabetes* 1999; **48**:66–76.

26 Ramracheya RD, Muller DS, Wu Y, Whitehouse BJ, Huang GC, Amiel SA, *et al.* Direct regulation of insulin secretion by angiotensin II in human islets of Langerhans. *Diabetologia* 2006; **49**:321–331.

27 Hauge-Evans AC, Richardson CC, Milne HM, Christie MR, Persaud SJ, Jones PM. A role for kisspeptin in islet function. *Diabetologia* 2006; **49**:2131–2135.

28 Bell GI, Pictet RL, Rutter WJ, Cordell B, Tischer E, Goodman HM. Sequence of the human insulin gene. *Nature* 1980; **284**:26–32.

29 Hutton JC. Insulin secretory granule biogenesis and the proinsulin-processing endopeptidases. *Diabetologia* 1994; **37**(Suppl 2):S48–S56.

30 Andrali SS, Sampley ML, Vanderford NL, Ozcan S. Glucose regulation of insulin gene expression in pancreatic beta-cells. *Biochem J* 2008; **415**:1–10.

31 Ashcroft SJ, Bunce J, Lowry M, Hansen SE, Hedeskov CJ. The effect of sugars on (pro)insulin biosynthesis. *Biochem J* 1978; **174**:517–526.

32 Hutton JC. The insulin secretory granule. *Diabetologia* 1989; **32**:271–281.

33 Hickey AJ, Bradley JW, Skea GL, Middleditch MJ, Buchanan CM, Phillips AR, *et al.* Proteins associated with immunopurified granules from a model pancreatic islet beta-cell system: proteomic snapshot of an endocrine secretory granule. *J Proteome Res* 2009; **8**:178–186.

34 Howell SL, Young DA, Lacy PE. Isolation and properties of secretory granules from rat islets of Langerhans. 3. Studies of the stability of the isolated beta granules. *J Cell Biol* 1969; **41**:167–176.

35 Dunn MF. Zinc–ligand interactions modulate assembly and stability of the insulin hexamer: a review. *Biometals* 2005; **18**:295–303.

36 Li G, Rungger-Brandle E, Just I, Jonas JC, Aktories K, Wollheim CB. Effect of disruption of actin filaments by *Clostridium botulinum* C2 toxin on insulin secretion in HIT-T15 cells and pancreatic islets. *Mol Biol Cell* 1994; **5**:1199–1213.

37 Thurmond DC, Gonelle-Gispert C, Furukawa M, Halban PA, Pessin JE. Glucose-stimulated insulin secretion is coupled to the interaction of actin with the t-SNARE (target membrane soluble N-ethylmaleimide-sensitive factor attachment protein receptor protein) complex. *Mol Endocrinol* 2003; **17**:732–742.

38 Boyd AE III, Bolton WE, Brinkley BR. Microtubules and beta cell function: effect of colchicine on microtubules and insulin secretion *in vitro* by mouse beta cells. *J Cell Biol* 1982; **92**:425–434.

39 Howell SL, Tyhurst M. The cytoskeleton and insulin secretion. *Diabetes Metab Rev* 1986; **2**:107–123.

40 Howell SL. The mechanism of insulin secretion. *Diabetologia* 1984; **26**:319–327.

41 Meng YX, Wilson GW, Avery MC, Varden CH, Balczon R. Suppression of the expression of a pancreatic beta-cell form of the kinesin heavy chain by antisense oligonucleotides inhibits insulin secretion from primary cultures of mouse beta-cells. *Endocrinology* 1997; **138**:1979–1987.

42 Varadi A, Ainscow EK, Allan VJ, Rutter GA. Molecular mechanisms involved in secretory vesicle recruitment to the plasma membrane in beta-cells. *Biochem Soc Trans* 2002; **30**:328–332.

43 Bai JZ, Mon Y, Krissansen GW. Kinectin participates in microtubule-dependent hormone secretion in pancreatic islet beta-cells. *Cell Biol Int* 2006; **30**:885–894.

44 Gauthier BR, Wollheim CB. Synaptotagmins bind calcium to release insulin. *Am J Physiol Endocrinol Metab* 2008; **295**:E1279–E1286.

45 Eliasson L, Abdulkader F, Braun M, Galvanovskis J, Hoppa MB, Rorsman P. Novel aspects of the molecular mechanisms controlling insulin secretion. *J Physiol* 2008; **586**:3313–3324.

46 Gut A, Kiraly CE, Fukuda M, Mikoshiba K, Wollheim CB, Lang J. Expression and localisation of synaptotagmin isoforms in endocrine beta-cells: their function in insulin exocytosis. *J Cell Sci* 2001; **114**:1709–1716.

47 De VA, Heimberg H, Quartier E, Huypens P, Bouwens L, Pipeleers D, *et al.* Human and rat beta cells differ in glucose transporter but not in glucokinase gene expression. *J Clin Invest* 1995; **96**:2489–2495.

48 Richardson CC, Hussain K, Jones PM, Persaud S, Lobner K, Boehm A, *et al.* Low levels of glucose transporters and K^+ATP channels in

human pancreatic beta cells early in development. *Diabetologia* 2007; **50**:1000–1005.

49 Van SE. Short-term regulation of glucokinase. *Diabetologia* 1994; **37**(Suppl 2):S43–S47.

50 Cook DL, Hales CN. Intracellular ATP directly blocks K^+ channels in pancreatic B-cells. *Nature* 1984; **311**:271–273.

51 Miki T, Nagashima K, Seino S. The structure and function of the ATP-sensitive K^+ channel in insulin-secreting pancreatic beta-cells. *J Mol Endocrinol* 1999; **22**:113–123.

52 Zhang Y, Warren-Perry M, Sakura H, Adelman J, Stoffel M, Bell GI, *et al.* No evidence for mutations in a putative beta-cell ATP-sensitive K^+ channel subunit in MODY, NIDDM, or GDM. *Diabetes* 1995; **44**:597–600.

53 Sakura H, Wat N, Horton V, Millns H, Turner RC, Ashcroft FM. Sequence variations in the human Kir6.2 gene, a subunit of the beta-cell ATP-sensitive K-channel – no association with NIDDM in while Caucasian subjects or evidence of abnormal function when expressed *in vitro*. *Diabetologia* 1996; **39**:1233–1236.

54 Gloyn AL, Weedon MN, Owen KR, Turner MJ, Knight BA, Hitman G, *et al.* Large-scale association studies of variants in genes encoding the pancreatic beta-cell KATP channel subunits Kir6.2 (KCNJ11) and SUR1 (ABCC8) confirm that the KCNJ11 E23K variant is associated with type 2 diabetes. *Diabetes* 2003; **52**:568–572.

55 Sagen JV, Raeder H, Hathout E, Shehadeh N, Gudmundsson K, Baevre H, *et al.* Permanent neonatal diabetes due to mutations in KCNJ11 encoding Kir6.2: patient characteristics and initial response to sulfonylurea therapy. *Diabetes* 2004; **53**:2713–2718.

56 Thomas PM, Cote GJ, Wohllk N, Haddad B, Mathew PM, Rabl W, *et al.* Mutations in the sulfonylurea receptor gene in familial persistent hyperinsulinemic hypoglycemia of infancy. *Science* 1995; **268**:426–429.

57 Sharma N, Crane A, Gonzalez G, Bryan J, Guilar-Bryan L. Familial hyperinsulinism and pancreatic beta-cell ATP-sensitive potassium channels. *Kidney Int* 2000; **57**:803–808.

58 Barg S, Ma X, Eliasson L, Galvanovskis J, Gopel SO, Obermuller S, *et al.* Fast exocytosis with few Ca^{2+} channels in insulin-secreting mouse pancreatic B cells. *Biophys J* 2001; **81**:3308–3323.

59 Jones PM, Persaud SJ, Howell SL. Time-course of Ca^{2+}-induced insulin secretion from perifused, electrically permeabilised islets of Langerhans: effects of cAMP and a phorbol ester. *Biochem Biophys Res Commun* 1989; **162**:998–1003.

60 Thore S, Wuttke A, Tengholm A. Rapid turnover of phosphatidylinositol-4,5-bisphosphate in insulin-secreting cells mediated by Ca^{2+} and the ATP-to-ADP ratio. *Diabetes* 2007; **56**:818–826.

61 Jones PM, Persaud SJ. Protein kinases, protein phosphorylation, and the regulation of insulin secretion from pancreatic beta-cells. *Endocr Rev* 1998; **19**:429–461.

62 Robertson RP. Dominance of cyclooxygenase-2 in the regulation of pancreatic islet prostaglandin synthesis. *Diabetes* 1998; **47**:1379–1383.

63 Persaud SJ, Muller D, Belin VD, Papadimitriou A, Huang GC, Amiel SA, *et al.* Expression and function of cyclooxygenase and lipoxygenase enzymes in human islets of Langerhans. *Arch Physiol Biochem* 2007; **113**:104–109.

64 Tian YM, Urquidi V, Ashcroft SJ. Protein kinase C in beta-cells: expression of multiple isoforms and involvement in cholinergic stimulation of insulin secretion. *Mol Cell Endocrinol* 1996; **119**:185–193.

65 Biden TJ, Schmitz-Peiffer C, Burchfield JG, Gurisik E, Cantley J, Mitchell CJ, *et al.* The diverse roles of protein kinase C in pancreatic beta-cell function. *Biochem Soc Trans* 2008; **36**:916–919.

66 Szaszak M, Christian F, Rosenthal W, Klussmann E. Compartmentalized cAMP signalling in regulated exocytic processes in non-neuronal cells. *Cell Signal* 2008; **20**:590–601.

67 Persaud SJ, Jones PM, Howell SL. Glucose-stimulated insulin secretion is not dependent on activation of protein kinase A. *Biochem Biophys Res Commun* 1990; **173**:833–839.

68 Dyachok O, Idevall-Hagren O, Sagetorp J, Tian G, Wuttke A, Arrieumerlou C, *et al.* Glucose-induced cyclic AMP oscillations regulate pulsatile insulin secretion. *Cell Metab* 2008; **8**:26–37.

69 Henquin JC. Triggering and amplifying pathways of regulation of insulin secretion by glucose. *Diabetes* 2000; **49**:1751–1760.

70 Gembal M, Gilon P, Henquin JC. Evidence that glucose can control insulin release independently from its action on ATP-sensitive K^+ channels in mouse B cells. *J Clin Invest* 1992; **89**:1288–1295.

71 Ravier MA, Nenquin M, Miki T, Seino S, Henquin JC. Glucose controls cytosolic Ca^{2+} and insulin secretion in mouse islets lacking adenosine triphosphate-sensitive K^+ channels owing to a knockout of the pore-forming subunit Kir6.2. *Endocrinology* 2009; **150**:33–45.

72 Detimary P, Gilon P, Nenquin M, Henquin JC. Two sites of glucose control of insulin release with distinct dependence on the energy state in pancreatic B-cells. *Biochem J* 1994; **297** (Part 3):455–461.

73 Henquin JC, Meissner HP. Cyclic adenosine monophosphate differently affects the response of mouse pancreatic beta-cells to various amino acids. *J Physiol* 1986; **381**:77–93.

74 Minami K, Miki T, Kadowaki T, Seino S. Roles of ATP-sensitive K^+ channels as metabolic sensors: studies of Kir6.x null mice. *Diabetes* 2004; **53**(Suppl 3):S176–S180.

75 Muller D, Huang GC, Amiel S, Jones PM, Persaud SJ. Identification of insulin signaling elements in human beta-cells: autocrine regulation of insulin gene expression. *Diabetes* 2006; **55**:2835–2842.

76 Khan FA, Goforth PB, Zhang M, Satin LS. Insulin activates ATP-sensitive K^+ channels in pancreatic beta-cells through a phosphatidylinositol 3-kinase-dependent pathway. *Diabetes* 2001; **50**:2192–2198.

77 Zawalich WS, Zawalich KC. Effects of glucose, exogenous insulin, and carbachol on C-peptide and insulin secretion from isolated perifused rat islets. *J Biol Chem* 2002; **277**:26233–26237.

78 Leibiger B, Leibiger IB, Moede T, Kemper S, Kulkarni RN, Kahn CR, *et al.* Selective insulin signaling through A and B insulin receptors regulates transcription of insulin and glucokinase genes in pancreatic beta cells. *Mol Cell* 2001; **7**:559–570.

79 Muller D, Jones PM, Persaud SJ. Autocrine anti-apoptotic and proliferative effects of insulin in pancreatic beta-cells. *FEBS Lett* 2006; **580**:6977–6980.

80 Gromada J, Franklin I, Wollheim CB. Alpha-cells of the endocrine pancreas: 35 years of research but the enigma remains. *Endocr Rev* 2007; **28**:84–116.

81 Williams G, Bloom SR. Somatostatin and pancreatic polypeptide. In: Albert KGMM, DeFronzo RA, Keen H, Zimmett P, eds. *International Textbook of Diabetes Mellitus*. Chichester: Wiley, 1992; 341–355.

82 Holst JJ, Orskov C, Bersani M. Heterogeneity of islet hormones. In: Samols E, ed. *The Endocrine Pancreas*. New York: Raven Press, 1991; 125–152.

83 Vieira E, Salehi A, Gylfe E. Glucose inhibits glucagon secretion by a direct effect on mouse pancreatic alpha cells. *Diabetologia* 2007; **50**:370–379.

84 Kumar U, Sasi R, Suresh S, Patel A, Thangaraju M, Metrakos P, *et al.* Subtype-selective expression of the five somatostatin receptors (hSSTR1-5) in human pancreatic islet cells: a quantitative double-label immunohistochemical analysis. *Diabetes* 1999; **48**:77–85.

85 Strowski MZ, Parmar RM, Blake AD, Schaeffer JM. Somatostatin inhibits insulin and glucagon secretion via two receptors subtypes: an *in vitro* study of pancreatic islets from somatostatin receptor 2 knockout mice. *Endocrinology* 2000; **141**:111–117.

86 Sharp GW. Mechanisms of inhibition of insulin release. *Am J Physiol* 1996; **271**:C1781–C1799.

87 Nilsson T, Arkhammar P, Rorsman P, Berggren PO. Suppression of insulin release by galanin and somatostatin is mediated by a G-protein: an effect involving repolarization and reduction in cytoplasmic free Ca^{2+} concentration. *J Biol Chem* 1989; **264**:973–980.

88 Degano P, Peiro E, Miralles P, Silvestre RA, Marco J. Effects of rat pancreatic polypeptide on islet-cell secretion in the perfused rat pancreas. *Metabolism* 1992; **41**:306–309.

89 Wierup N, Svensson H, Mulder H, Sundler F. The ghrelin cell: a novel developmentally regulated islet cell in the human pancreas. *Regul Pept* 2002; **107**:63–69.

90 Andralojc KM, Mercalli A, Nowak KW, Albarello L, Calcagno R, Luzi L, *et al.* Ghrelin-producing epsilon cells in the developing and adult human pancreas. *Diabetologia* 2009; **52**:486–493.

91 Dezaki K, Sone H, Yada T. Ghrelin is a physiological regulator of insulin release in pancreatic islets and glucose homeostasis. *Pharmacol Ther* 2008; **118**:239–249.

92 Gentes M. Note sur les terminaisons nerveuses des islots de Langerhans du pancreas. *Soc Biol* 1902; **54**:202–203.

93 Gilon P, Henquin JC. Mechanisms and physiological significance of the cholinergic control of pancreatic beta-cell function. *Endocr Rev* 2001; **22**:565–604.

94 Porte D Jr, Seeley RJ, Woods SC, Baskin DG, Figlewicz DP, Schwartz MW. Obesity, diabetes and the central nervous system. *Diabetologia* 1998; **41**:863–881.

95 Iismaa TP, Kerr EA, Wilson JR, Carpenter L, Sims N, Biden TJ. Quantitative and functional characterization of muscarinic receptor subtypes in insulin-secreting cell lines and rat pancreatic islets. *Diabetes* 2000; **49**:392–398.

96 Ahren B, Lundquist I. Effects of selective and non-selective beta-adrenergic agents on insulin secretion *in vivo*. *Eur J Pharmacol* 1981; **71**:93–104.

97 Morgan NG, Chan SL, Lacey RJ, Brown CA. Pharmacology and molecular biology of islet cell adrenoceptors. In: Flatt PR, Lenzen S, eds. *Frontiers of Insulin Secretion and Pancreatic B-cell Research.* London: Smith-Gordon, 1994; 359–368.

98 Lacey RJ, Berrow NS, London NJ, Lake SP, James RF, Scarpello JH, *et al.* Differential effects of beta-adrenergic agonists on insulin secretion from pancreatic islets isolated from rat and man. *J Mol Endocrinol* 1990; **5**:49–54.

99 Kuo WN, Hodgins DS, Kuo JF. Adenylate cyclase in islets of Langerhans: isolation of islets and regulation of adenylate cyclase activity by various hormones and agents. *J Biol Chem* 1973; **248**:2705–2711.

100 Yamazaki S, Katada T, Ui M. Alpha 2-adrenergic inhibition of insulin secretion via interference with cyclic AMP generation in rat pancreatic islets. *Mol Pharmacol* 1982; **21**:648–653.

101 Jones PM, Fyles JM, Persaud SJ, Howell SL. Catecholamine inhibition of Ca^{2+}-induced insulin secretion from electrically permeabilised islets of Langerhans. *FEBS Lett* 1987; **219**:139–144.

102 Winzell MS, Ahren B. G-protein-coupled receptors and islet function-implications for treatment of type 2 diabetes. *Pharmacol Ther* 2007; **116**:437–448.

103 Wahl MA, Straub SG, Ammon HP. Vasoactive intestinal polypeptide-augmented insulin release: actions on ionic fluxes and electrical activity of mouse islets. *Diabetologia* 1993; **36**:920–925.

104 Straub SG, Sharp GW. Mechanisms of action of VIP and PACAP in the stimulation of insulin release. *Ann N Y Acad Sci* 1996; **805**:607–612.

105 Wahl MA, Plehn RJ, Landsbeck EA, Verspohl EJ, Ammon HP. Gastrin releasing peptide augments glucose mediated $45Ca^{2+}$ uptake, electrical activity, and insulin secretion of mouse pancreatic islets. *Endocrinology* 1991; **128**:3247–3252.

106 Dunning BE, Ahren B, Veith RC, Bottcher G, Sundler F, Taborsky GJ Jr. Galanin: a novel pancreatic neuropeptide. *Am J Physiol* 1986; **251**:E127–E133.

107 Moltz JH, McDonald JK. Neuropeptide Y: direct and indirect action on insulin secretion in the rat. *Peptides* 1985; **6**:1155–1159.

108 Morgan DG, Kulkarni RN, Hurley JD, Wang ZL, Wang RM, Ghatei MA, *et al.* Inhibition of glucose stimulated insulin secretion by neuropeptide Y is mediated via the Y1 receptor and inhibition of adenylyl cyclase in RIN 5AH rat insulinoma cells. *Diabetologia* 1998; **41**:1482–1491.

109 Cormont M, Le Marchand-Brustel Y, van OE, Spiegel AM, Sharp GW. Identification of G protein alpha-subunits in RINm5F cells and their selective interaction with galanin receptor. *Diabetes* 1991; **40**:1170–1176.

110 McIntyre N, Holdsworth CD, Turner DS. New interpretation of oral glucose tolerance. *Lancet* 1964; **2**:20–21.

111 Drucker DJ. The role of gut hormones in glucose homeostasis. *J Clin Invest* 2007; **117**:24–32.

112 Karhunen LJ, Juvonen KR, Huotari A, Purhonen AK, Herzig KH. Effect of protein, fat, carbohydrate and fibre on gastrointestinal peptide release in humans. *Regul Pept* 2008; **149**:70–78.

113 Kieffer TJ, Habener JF. The glucagon-like peptides. *Endocr Rev* 1999; **20**:876–913.

114 Drucker DJ, Nauck MA. The incretin system: glucagon-like peptide-1 receptor agonists and dipeptidyl peptidase-4 inhibitors in type 2 diabetes. *Lancet* 2006; **368**:1696–1705.

115 Kolterman OG, Kim DD, Shen L, Ruggles JA, Nielsen LL, Fineman MS, *et al.* Pharmacokinetics, pharmacodynamics, and safety of exenatide in patients with type 2 diabetes mellitus. *Am J Health Syst Pharm* 2005; **62**:173–181.

116 Suga S, Kanno T, Ogawa Y, Takeo T, Kamimura N, Wakui M. cAMP-independent decrease of ATP-sensitive K^+ channel activity by GLP-1 in rat pancreatic beta-cells. *Pflugers Arch* 2000; **440**:566–572.

117 Ehses JA, Lee SS, Pederson RA, McIntosh CH. A new pathway for glucose-dependent insulinotropic polypeptide (GIP) receptor signaling: evidence for the involvement of phospholipase A2 in GIP-stimulated insulin secretion. *J Biol Chem* 2001; **276**:23667–23673.

118 Chia CW, Carlson OD, Kim W, Shin YK, Charles CP, Kim HS, *et al.* Exogenous glucose-dependent insulinotropic polypeptide worsens post-prandial hyperglycemia in type 2 diabetes. *Diabetes* 2009; **58**:1342–1349.

119 Morgan LM. The entero-insular axis. *Biochem Soc Trans* 1980; **8**:17–19.

120 Persaud SJ, Jones PM, Howell SL. Stimulation of insulin secretion by cholecystokinin-8S: the role of protein kinase C. *Pharmacol Commun* 1993; **3**:39–47.

121 Catalan V, Gomez-Ambrosi J, Rodriguez A, Salvador J, Fruhbeck G. Adipokines in the treatment of diabetes mellitus and obesity. *Expert Opin Pharmacother* 2009; **10**:239–254.

122 Cases JA, Gabriely I, Ma XH, Yang XM, Michaeli T, Fleischer N, *et al.* Physiological increase in plasma leptin markedly inhibits insulin secretion *in vivo*. *Diabetes* 2001; **50**:348–352.

123 Morioka T, Asilmaz E, Hu J, Dishinger JF, Kurpad AJ, Elias CF, *et al.* Disruption of leptin receptor expression in the pancreas directly affects beta cell growth and function in mice. *J Clin Invest* 2007; **117**:2860–2868.

124 Kieffer TJ, Heller RS, Leech CA, Holz GG, Habener JF. Leptin suppression of insulin secretion by the activation of ATP-sensitive K^+ channels in pancreatic beta-cells. *Diabetes* 1997; **46**:1087–1093.

125 Maedler K, Schulthess FT, Bielman C, Berney T, Bonny C, Prentki M, *et al.* Glucose and leptin induce apoptosis in human beta-cells and impair glucose-stimulated insulin secretion through activation of c-Jun N-terminal kinases. *FASEB J* 2008; **22**:1905–1913.

126 Nakata M, Okada T, Ozawa K, Yada T. Resistin induces insulin resistance in pancreatic islets to impair glucose-induced insulin release. *Biochem Biophys Res Commun* 2007; **353**:1046–1051.

127 Gao CL, Zhao DY, Qiu J, Zhang CM, Ji CB, Chen XH, *et al.* Resistin induces rat insulinoma cell RINm5F apoptosis. *Mol Biol Rep* 2009; **36**:1703–1708.

128 Arner P. Resistin: yet another adipokine tells us that men are not mice. *Diabetologia* 2005; **48**:2203–2205.

129 Minn AH, Patterson NB, Pack S, Hoffmann SC, Gavrilova O, Vinson C, *et al.* Resistin is expressed in pancreatic islets. *Biochem Biophys Res Commun* 2003; **310**:641–645.

130 Hotta K, Funahashi T, Arita Y, Takahashi M, Matsuda M, Okamoto Y, *et al.* Plasma concentrations of a novel, adipose-specific protein, adiponectin, in type 2 diabetic patients. *Arterioscler Thromb Vasc Biol* 2000; **20**:1595–1599.

131 Gu W, Li X, Liu C, Yang J, Ye L, Tang J, *et al.* Globular adiponectin augments insulin secretion from pancreatic islet beta cells at high glucose concentrations. *Endocrine* 2006; **30**:217–221.

132 Okamoto M, Ohara-Imaizumi M, Kubota N, Hashimoto S, Eto K, Kanno T, *et al.* Adiponectin induces insulin secretion *in vitro* and *in vivo* at a low glucose concentration. *Diabetologia* 2008; **51**:827–835.

133 Rakatzi I, Mueller H, Ritzeler O, Tennagels N, Eckel J. Adiponectin counteracts cytokine- and fatty acid-induced apoptosis in the pancreatic beta-cell line INS-1. *Diabetologia* 2004; **47**:249–258.

7 Insulin Action

Xuxia Wu & W. Timothy Garvey

Department of Nutrition Sciences, University of Alabama at Birmingham and the Birmingham Veterans Affairs Medical Center, Birmingham, AL, USA

Keypoints

- Insulin signaling is accurately viewed as involving a matrix of interacting pathways, allowing for extensive modulation and divergence in signal transduction, rather than a linear cascade of sequential reactions.
- Diverse cell types commonly share the proximal steps in insulin signal transduction, including the insulin receptor, insulin receptor substrate molecules (IRS), phosphatidylinositide 3 kinase and Akt/protein kinase B.
- Insulin action is negatively modulated by multiple cellular mechanisms that impair tyrosine phosphorylation of insulin receptors and IRS; foremost among these are serine–threonine kinases and protein tyrosine phosphatases.
- The tissue-specific biologic effects of insulin are explained by effector systems which are uniquely expressed in differentiated target tissues such as the insulin-responsive glucose transport system in skeletal muscle, enzymatic systems mediating antilipolysis in adipose tissue and regulated gene expression leading to suppression of gluconeogenesis in liver.
- Insulin action is highly regulated by three pathways for nutrient sensing: the hexosamine biosynthetic signaling pathway; the mammalian target of rapamycin signaling pathway; and the AMP-activated protein kinase signaling pathway.
- Oxidative stress, inflammation and endoplasmic reticulum stress are associated with insulin resistance, obesity and metabolic syndrome, and impair insulin action via activation of serine–threonine protein kinases.

General aspects of insulin action

The peptide hormone insulin is exclusively synthesized in and secreted from pancreatic β-cells. Insulin exerts a broad spectrum of anabolic effects in multiple tissues. The regulation of whole body fuel homeostasis primarily involves insulin action in skeletal muscle, adipose tissue, and liver where insulin promotes uptake and storage of carbohydrate, fat, and amino acids, while at the same time antagonizing the catabolism of these fuel reserves. In skeletal muscle, insulin stimulates glucose transport and glucose storage as glycogen, as well as glycolysis and tricarboxylic acid cycle activity. Insulin lowers hepatic glucose output by inhibiting glycogenolysis and gluconeogenesis, and augments glycogen formation. In adipocytes, insulin promotes glucose uptake, glycerol synthesis, and triglyceride formation, while at the same time exerting an antilipolytic effect. During periods of fasting, a fall in circulating insulin combined with increased secretion of counter-regulatory hormones leads to breakdown of stored fuels and increased availability of metabolic substrates for cellular energy. In this way, alterations in insulin levels in the fed and fasting states have a key role in fuel metabolism and maintain blood glucose levels within a narrowly defined range. Insulin diminishes protein catabolism and increases translation, and also enhances cell growth, differentiation, and survival as a consequence of mitogenic and anti-apoptotic processes. Thus, the action of insulin at the level of cells and tissues affects substrate flux and coordinates the function of multiple organs as whole organisms adapt to the nutritional environment.

In mediating its pleiotropic actions, insulin binds to cell surface receptors, activates multiple signal transduction networks, and engages effector systems responsible for specific biologic functions. Over the last decade it has become clear that the classic perspective of insulin signaling as a linear cascade of sequentially interacting signal transduction molecules is short-sighted. Rather, the promulgation of insulin action is more accurately viewed as alterations in a network of interactions involving a matrix of signal cascades that engage in cross-talk. The final biologic action represents the net synergism of the combined facilitative, inhibitory and complementary signaling pathways that interact with more terminal functional systems in cell biology. While there is relative commonality in signal transduction networks, differentiated insulin target cells express a variety of unique effector systems, which are primarily responsible for mediating the cell-

Textbook of Diabetes, 4th edition. Edited by R. Holt, C. Cockram, A. Flyvbjerg and B. Goldstein.

specific and organ-specific biologic functions of insulin. Effector systems include rate-limiting enzymes, enzymatic pathways, membrane transport systems, gene expression, processes regulating the cellular trafficking of proteins and vesicles, and systems governing the translation, post-translational modification and degradation of proteins. Certain aspects of linear insulin signal transduction are evolutionarily conserved; however, complex patterns of interactions between signal and evolved effector systems are more pronounced in mammals and allow for greater plasticity in adaptive responses [1].

This chapter first discusses insulin signaling pathways and networks that are common to multiple target cell types. Recent advances in our understanding of cell processes and pathways that inhibit insulin signaling are delineated. Subsequently, unique aspects of insulin action are described, in particular key effector systems, which are properties of skeletal muscle, adipocytes, and liver, and explain the distinct effects on biologic functions in these tissues. Finally, nutrient sensing pathways and cell stress responses are discussed in terms of their interaction with insulin signaling and role in the pathogenesis of insulin resistance.

Insulin action: proximal signaling pathways

Proximal steps in insulin signaling, including the insulin receptor, insulin receptor substrate proteins (IRS), phosphatidylinositol 3 (PI_3) kinase, Akt/protein kinase B (Akt/PKB), and mitogen activated protein kinase (MAPK) are globally operative in multiple cell types. These proteins also serve as points of divergence or nodes in an expanding matrix of signal transduction pathways, and are highly regulated, both positively and negatively, via cross-talk with other signaling systems and modulatory pathways (Figure 7.1).

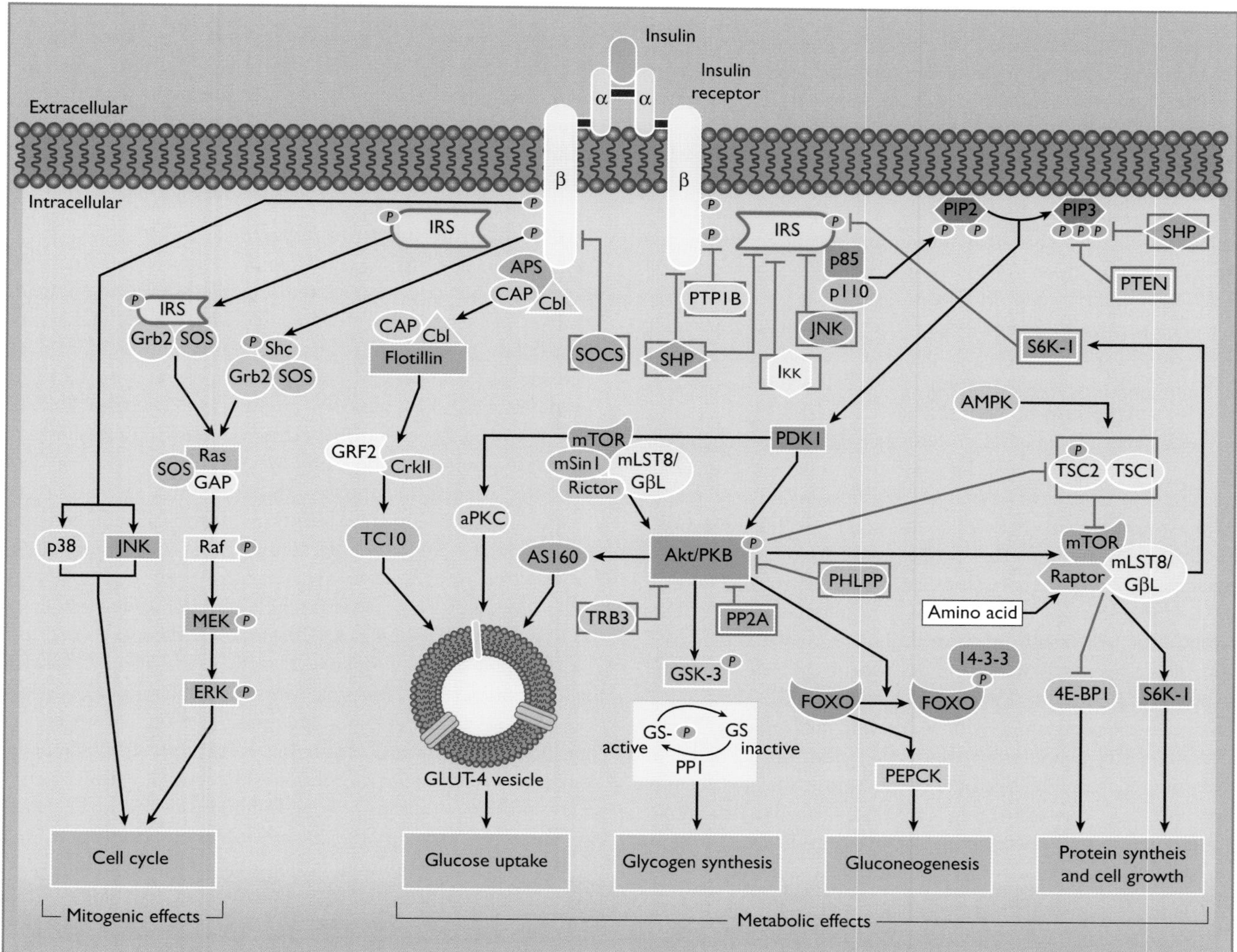

Figure 7.1 A schematic illustration of insulin signaling pathways involved in both metabolic and mitogenic effects. Arrows represent an activation process; blocked arrows represent an inhibition process.

Insulin receptor molecules

Insulin action is initiated by specific binding to high-affinity receptors on the plasma membrane of its target cells. The insulin receptor is a large transmembrane glycoprotein consisting of two α- and two β-subunits which form a heterotetramer. The insulin receptor is synthesized from a single gene that consists of 22 exons and 21 introns. Following translation of its mRNA, it is processed into two separate subunits (α and β) that assemble as a disulfide-linked holoenzyme of $(\alpha\beta)_2$ stoichiometry [2]. The 135 kDa α-subunits, derived from the amino-terminal portion of the proreceptor, reside entirely on the outside of the cell, tethered to the membrane via the 95 kDa β-subunits that span the membrane. Insulin binds to the extracellular α-subunits. This binding results in conformational changes that bring the α-subunits closer together, and enables ATP to bind to the intracellular domain of the β-subunit leading to autophosphorylation of distinct tyrosine residues on the β-subunit. Autophosphorylation augments the intrinsic activity of the β-subunit as a tyrosine kinase, directed against other tyrosines within the receptor as well as tyrosine phosphorylation of exogenous substrates. Ligand-dependent stimulation of the β-subunit tyrosine kinase activity is critical for promulgation of the insulin signal. At least six tyrosine residues in the β-subunit undergo phosphorylation and have been shown to serve different roles in insulin signaling. They lie within three functional groups. Phosphorylation of Tyr^{972} establishes a recognition motif and docking site that provides sufficient stability of the receptor–substrate complex for intracellular substrate phosphorylation. Tyrosine phosphorylation sites at positions Tyr^{1158}, Tyr^{1162} and Tyr^{1163} are essential for mediating an increase in subunit tyrosine kinase activity and signal transduction. Phosphorylation sites Tyr^{1328} and Tyr^{1334} affect the sensitivity of Ras/MAPK pathway activation, and are thus involved in the receptor's mitogenic responses [3].

The number of cell-surface insulin receptors is downregulated by chronic exposure to high insulin concentrations *in vitro*, and receptor loss is observed in target cells from hyperinsulinemic insulin-resistant humans. Receptor loss per se can impair maximal insulin responsiveness. This is illustrated in the extreme by genetic ablation of the insulin receptor in mice which results in lethality at 4–5 days after birth as a result of severe diabetic ketoacidosis [4]. Insulin-stimulated glucose uptake and activation of glycogen synthase in muscle are severely impaired in muscle-specific insulin receptor knockout mice [5]. These latter animals also have features of the metabolic syndrome including increases in fat mass, serum triglycerides and serum free fatty acids, but retain normal basal and contraction-stimulated glucose transport [6]. Transgenic mice expressing dominant-negative insulin receptors also develop obesity, hyperinsulinemia, glucose intolerance, and hypertriglyceridemia. These phenotypes are analogous to those seen in insulin-resistant humans. Patients with genetic mutations in the insulin receptor gene (type B insulin resistance) or circulating antibodies directed against the insulin receptor that block ligand binding (type A insulin resistance) develop severe insulin resistance, acanthosis nigricans and glucose intolerance. In addition to receptor downregulation, the intrinsic activity of the insulin receptor tyrosine kinase is impaired in insulin-resistant humans and patients with type 2 diabetes mellitus (T2DM) via a number of regulatory and pathophysiologic processes which are described in this chapter. Clearly, the number and functional activity of insulin receptors is critical for effective insulin action.

The insulin receptor is similar in structure to the insulin-like growth factor 1 receptor (IGF1R) and several other growth factor and cytokine receptors, which have in common an extracellular ligand-binding domain that activates an intracellular tyrosine kinase domain. The mammalian insulin-like signaling system includes three well-defined ligands: insulin, insulin-like growth factor 1 (IGF-1), and insulin-like growth factor 2 (IGF-2), and all three ligands can bind and activate cell-surface insulin receptors [7]. Alternative splicing involving exon 11 of the insulin receptor gene determines the insertion or deletion of 12 amino acids near the COOH-terminus of the α-subunit. Isoform A lacking the 12 amino acids has high affinity for IGF-2, predominates during fetal development, and promotes growth as a consequence of IGF-2 binding. Isoform B containing the 12 amino acids predominates postnatally and is activated mainly by insulin. Some evidence supports the contention that dysregulated expression towards the fetal pattern could occur in adult tissues and result in insulin resistance [8].

Insulin receptor substrate molecules

Following insulin binding and receptor autophosphorylation, the next committed step in signal transduction is tyrosine phosphorylation of intracellular proteins. At least 11 intracellular substrates have been identified that are rapidly phosphorylated on tyrosine residues by ligand-bound insulin receptors, including six insulin receptor substrate (IRS) proteins, Grb2-associated binder 1 (Gab1), Cas-Br-M (murine) ecotropic retroviral transforming sequence homolog (Cbl), and the various isoforms of Src-homology-2-containing protein (Shc) [9].

The IRSs are immediate substrates for the insulin receptor tyrosine kinase, and are of predominant importance for insulin action. IRS proteins have an N-terminal pleckstrin-homology (PH) domain, a phosphotyrosine-binding (PTB) domain and a COOH-terminal region of variable length that contains multiple tyrosine and serine phosphorylation sites [10]. The PH domain helps position IRS for coupling with the insulin receptor, possibly by binding to charged headgroups of certain phosphatidylinositides in adjacent membrane structures. PTB domains recognize the phosphotyrosine in the amino acid sequence asparagine-proline-any amino acid-phosphotyrosine (NPXpY), which encompasses Tyr^{972} in the juxtamembranous domain of the insulin receptor β-subunit, and facilitates the formation of the IRS–insulin receptor complex. The center and C-terminus of IRS proteins contain up to 20 potential tyrosine phosphorylation sites that, after phosphorylation by the insulin receptor, bind to other intracellular molecules that contain Src-homology-2 domains (SH2 domains). The SH2-containing proteins that bind to phosphorylated IRS proteins could be adaptor molecules, such as the regulatory subunit of PI_3 kinase and the adaptor molecule Grb2, or enzymes with kinase or phosphatase activities such as SH2-domain-containing tyrosine phosphatase 2 (SHP2) and the cytoplasmic tyrosine kinase Fyn. Non-covalent attachment of multiple SH2-containing signaling molecules allows IRS to function as a docking protein that physically apposes proteins involved in downstream transduction cascades. Thus, IRS propagates insulin signal transduction via the docking, apposition, interaction, and activation of downstream signal molecules, rather than as a consequence of any intrinsic enzymatic activity per se. Thus, IRSs provide a major point of divergence of insulin signal transduction pathways, for example, leading to activation of mitogenic (Ras/MAP kinase) and metabolic (PI_3 kinase) pathways [11].

Among the family of IRS proteins, IRS1 and IRS2 exhibit a wide range of tissue expression, including muscle, fat, liver, and pancreatic islets. IRS3 is expressed in adipose tissue, fibroblasts, and liver, while IRS4 is detected in brain, thymus, and embryonic kidney. IRS5 is ubiquitously expressed but most abundant in kidney and liver. IRS6 expression is highest in skeletal muscle. Deletion of IRS1 produces small insulin-resistant mice with nearly normal glucose homeostasis because of β-cell expansion and compensatory hyperinsulinemia. Mice lacking IRS2 display nearly normal growth but develop life-threatening diabetes at 8–15 weeks of age because of reduced β-cell mass and insufficient compensatory insulin secretion. IRS3 knockout mice do not have an obvious phenotype, and IRS4 null mice also appear normal with the exception of reduced fertility. Therefore, IRS1 and IRS2 are considered to be the IRS isoforms critically important in glucose homeostasis. IRS1 functions as the principal IRS in skeletal muscle, and IRS2 predominates in liver and β-cell, where insulin action is required for normal β-cell growth and development.

IRS proteins are a key locus for regulation of insulin action. One mechanism occurs at the level of IRS protein expression; for example, IRS1 and IRS2 proteins are decreased by hyperinsulinemia [12]. Cell loss of IRS could occur through accelerated protein degradation by induction of ubiquitin-mediated degradation of IRS1 and IRS2 by suppressor of cytokine signaling (SOCS) proteins [13], or by inhibition of IRS gene transcription. Regardless of the mechanism, decreased levels of IRS proteins in hyperinsulinemic states, coupled with downregulation of the insulin receptor itself, certainly contribute to the insulin resistance in diabetes [14]. The function of IRS proteins can also be negatively regulated by serine–threonine kinases and protein tyrosine phosphatases such as such as PTP1B and SHP2, as described below [15]. In addition, IRS1 can be post-translationally modified by either O-linked N-acetylglucosamine adducts (O-GlcNAc) on serine–threonine residues under hyperglycemic conditions [16], or S-nitrosylation as a consequence of nitric oxide generation [17]. These modifications induce the proteasomal downregulation of IRS1 and insulin resistance.

PI_3 kinase

Among several proteins that to bind to IRS1/2, PI_3 kinase is critical for signal transduction mediating the metabolic effects of insulin, including stimulation of glucose uptake into skeletal muscle and adipose tissues. PI_3 kinase activity represents a family of related enzymes that are capable of phosphorylating the hydroxyl groups in the inositol ring of membrane-associated phosphatidylinositol (PtdIns) [18]. The generation of $PI(3,4,5)P_3$ propagates the insulin signal, and therefore the class I subset of PI3K is responsible for the downstream action of receptor tyrosine kinases (including the insulin receptor) and Ras/MAPK [19]. Class I PI_3 kinases are heterodimeric molecules composed of one regulatory and one catalytic subunit. There are currently five known regulatory subunits, designated p85α, p55α, p50α, p85β or p55γ (known collectively as the p85 subunit), and one of these regulatory subunits is conjoined with one of four known p110 catalytic subunits, p110α, p110β, p110δ or p110γ [20]. Under normal conditions, p85 regulatory subunits are present in excess compared with the amount of the p85–p110 complex, and can serve as negative regulators of insulin action. One explanation pertains to the stoichiometry of free p85 and p85–p110 complexes because free p85 may be able to compete with the p85–p110 complex for recruitment to IRS phosphotyrosine docking sites (i.e. the "free p85" model) [21]. Accordingly, increased expression of p85 can worsen insulin sensitivity as demonstrated in patients with gestational diabetes or obesity who have increased levels of p85 in skeletal muscle. The p85 subunit can also exert negative modulatory effects via cross-talk with stress-kinase pathways. Recent studies have shown that p85 is required for the insulin-stimulated activation of c-Jun NH_2-terminal kinase (JNK) that occurs in states of insulin resistance, including high-fat diet-induced obesity and JNK overexpression [22]. Because the JNK pathway suppresses insulin action, the involvement of p85 in JNK activation provides a mechanism for cross-talk between the PI_3 kinase signaling pathway and JNK-mediated stress or inflammatory responses. Also, p85 is able to suppress insulin action via positive regulation of the phosphatase and tensin homolog (PTEN), a phosphoinositide phosphatase that degrades $PI(3,4,5)P_3$ and inhibits downstream insulin signaling [23].

3-Phosphoinositide-dependent protein kinase 1

Insulin-mediated activation of PI_3 kinase results in phosphorylation of the inositol ring at the 3′ position of phosphatidylinositol in membrane glycolipids, generating $PI(3,4,5)P_3$. This leads to recruitment of certain signaling proteins with PH domains to the plasma membrane. Binding to membrane-associated phosphoinositides both activates these proteins and positions them for downstream signal transduction. 3-Phosphoinositide-dependent protein kinase 1 (PDK1) can interact with $PI(3,4,5)P_3$, and is responsible for downstream activation of Akt/PKB and aPKCs. PDK1 phosphorylates the activation loops of Akt/PKB on Thr^{308}, and PKCζ on Thr^{410}, enhancing the activity of these kinases.

Akt/protein kinase B

Phosphorylation and activation of Akt/PKB mediates various insulin- and growth factor-induced cellular responses, such as the stimulation of GLUT-4 translocation to the plasma membrane, the inhibition of glycogen synthase kinase 3 (GSK-3), induction of triglyceride synthesis via increasing the expression of sterol regulatory element-binding proteins 1c (SREBP-1c), and the promotion of cell survival by inhibiting apoptosis. Akt/PKB is a serine–threonine kinase with multiple substrates including kinases, signaling proteins, and transcription factors, such as cyclin-dependent kinase inhibitor p21kip, GSK3β, Bcl-2 antagonist of cell death, AS160, endothelial NO synthase, forkhead box class O1 (Foxo 1) and others. There are three isoforms of Akt/PKB in mammals, each encoded by a different gene (Akt1, Akt2 and Akt3). Akt1 and Ak2 are widely distributed; however, Akt2 is predominant in insulin-sensitive tissues such as liver and fat. Akt3 is largely expressed in the nervous system and testis.

Several lines of evidence implicate a role for Akt/PKB activation in the stimulation of glucose transport and other insulin-induced biologic processes. Expression of constitutively active membrane-bound forms of Akt/PKB results in persistent translocation of GLUT-4 to the plasma membrane in muscle and fat cells [24]. Deletion of Akt1 results in growth retardation and reduced lifespan without metabolic abnormalities [25]. In contrast, Akt2-deficient mice display insulin resistance and develop diabetes as a result of the inability of insulin to stimulate glucose utilization and decrease hepatic glucose output [26]. Mechanistic studies have suggested that Akt2 is the key isoform transducing effects on GLUT-4 glucose uptake; however, Akt/PKB activity alone cannot fully explain the ability of insulin to promote GLUT-4 translocation and stimulate glucose transport [27].

Akt/PKB activation is involved in multiple other insulin responses. One of the first substrates indentified for Akt/PKB was GSK3β. Phosphorylation of GSK3β decreases its activity towards glycogen synthase, which leads to increased glycogen synthesis [28]. Akt/PKB seems to stimulate glucose transport concomitant with the phosphorylation of Akt substrate of 160 kDa (AS160), a Rab-GTPase-activating protein (GAP) [29]. Under basal conditions, a functional GAP domain within AS160 is necessary to maintain the intracellular localization of GLUT-4 [30]. Following insulin stimulation, phosphorylation of AS160 shuts off its GAP activity, shifting the equilibrium of its target Rab(s) to an active GTP-bound form, and this enables GLUT-4 translocation by releasing GLUT-4 from intracellular retention mechanisms [30]. As expected, this effect is blocked by pre-exposure to the PI_3 kinase inhibitor wortmannin, indicative of signaling through PI_3 kinase. This response involving AS160 is impaired in skeletal muscle collected from insulin-resistant patients.

Atypical protein kinase C

Protein kinase C isoforms are categorized as conventional (α,β,γ) (cPKC), novel (δ,θ,ε,η,μ) (nPKC), and atypical (ζ,λ) (aPKC) depending on their ability to be activated by calcium and diacylglycerol (DAG). cPKCs and nPKCs serve primarily as negative feedback inhibitors of the insulin receptor and IRS, and are discussed below. The aPKCs participate in signal transduction, and like Akt/PKB, are activated by the PI_3 kinase pathway and help mediate insulin's metabolic effects. The two aPKC isoenzymes ζ and λ vary in their tissue-specific expression and among various mammals; for example, PKCλ is the main aPKC in the skeletal muscle and adipose tissue of the mouse, whereas PKCζ is more prominent in rats, monkeys, and humans. Activation of PKCζ and PKCλ occurs proximal to Akt/PKB as a result of direct interaction with 3′ phosphoinositides and/or through phosphorylation and activation by PDK1. aPKCs have been shown to have a role in insulin-stimulated glucose uptake and GLUT-4 translocation in adipocytes and muscle [31]. Stimulation of glucose transport and translocation of GLUT-4 vesicles by aPKC may be brought about by effects on the actin cytoskeleton, because PKCλ/ζ can impinge on Rac and actin dynamics [32]. Overexpression of constitutively active forms of PKCζ and PKCλ increases, and expression of dominant negative forms of these aPKCs reduces, both glucose transport activity and GLUT-4 translocation in response to insulin (31). Decreased activation of aPKCs has been reported in the muscle of humans with T2DM and rodents with insulin resistance [33]. Compellingly, a mouse model with a muscle-selective PKCλ gene deletion displays whole-body insulin resistance, impaired insulin-stimulated glucose uptake into muscle and reduced GLUT-4 translocation. The mechanism by which aPKC participates in metabolic signaling remains to be fully elucidated.

CAP/Cbl/TC10 pathway

In parallel to the PI_3 kinase pathway, substantial evidence has confirmed the participation of the CAP/Cbl/TC10 pathway in glucose transport stimulation [34]. This pathway diverges at the level of the insulin receptor kinase, which mediates tyrosine phosphorylation of the Cbl proto-oncogene through a process that does not involve IRSs. This phosphorylation step requires recruitment of the adapter protein APS, which contains SH2 and PH domains, to the insulin receptor β-subunit and the subsequent binding of Cbl to APS [35]. APS interacts via its SH2 domain with phosphotyrosines in the activation loop of the insulin receptor. Upon binding to the receptor, APS is phosphorylated on a C-terminal tyrosine, which permits the recruitment of Cbl to APS via the SH2 domain of Cbl, and subsequent tyrosine phosphorylation of Cbl. The Cbl associated protein (CAP) is also recruited with Cbl to the insulin receptor–APS complex via tandem SH3 domains in the COOH-terminus of CAP that bind to a proline-rich domain in Cbl. CAP also contains a sorbin homology (SoHo) domain in the NH2-terminal region. After disengagement of CAP/Cbl from the insulin receptor, the CAP SoHo domain binds to flotillin in caveolin-containing lipid rafts in the plasma membrane. Lipid rafts are plasma membrane domains, enriched in cholesterol, glycolipids, and sphingolipids, that coordinate signaling events by accumulating specific protein constituents.

Once the CAP/Cbl complex is bound to flotillin, tyrosine phosphorylated Cbl presents a recognition site for recruitment of the CrkII–C3G complex to the lipid raft. CrkII binds to specific phosphorylation sites on Cbl via its SH2 domain and is constitutively associated with the nucleotide exchange factor C3G via its SH3 domain. C3G is a guanyl nucleotide exchange factor for TC10 and other small molecular weight GTP-binding proteins. TC10 is a member of the Rho family of GTPases, and can target to lipid raft domains as a result of its capacity to undergo post-translational modification by farnesylation and palmitoylation. The Rab proteins cycle between GTP- and GDP-bound states to affect vesicle budding from donor membranes and fusion with acceptor membranes. TC10 is known to regulate the actin cytoskeleton [36], and downstream effectors of TC10 have been identified which have been proposed to have a role in the translocation of GLUT-4 [37].

Ras-p38 MAPK pathway

Another component of signal divergence emanating from IRS docking proteins is the engagement of the Ras/MAPK signaling pathway, which has a critical role in cell growth and mitogenesis. Following insulin-mediated tyrosine phosphorylation of IRS, one of the SH2 domain-containing proteins that docks with IRS is Grb-2, a small cytosolic adapter protein. Grb-2 also contains an SH3 binding domain that binds proteins containing proline-rich sequences, and one of these proteins is SOS (mammalian homolog of the *Drosophila* son-of-sevenless protein), a GDP/GTP exchange factor. This interaction positions SOS for activation of the Ras/MAPK pathway. SOS facilitates GTP activation of membrane-bound Ras, the 21 kDa small molecular weight GTPase, and the GTP-bound form of Ras complexes with and activates Raf-1 kinase. Raf-1 kinase then initiates a cascade leading to sequential phosphorylation and activation of the dual-specificity kinase MEK (MAPK/ERK kinase), which in turn phosphorylates extracellular regulated kinases (ERK1 and ERK2) on threonine and tyrosine residues in their activation loops. Activated ERKs phosphorylate multiple targets that mediate the mitogenic actions of the Ras/MAPK pathway and the growth promoting effects of insulin [38]. Insulin receptors can also mediate activation of the Ras/MAPK pathway through another substrate docking molecule, SHC. Independent of IRS, SHC can also activate the Ras/Raf-1/MEK phosphorylation cascade by forming a complex with Grb-2/SOS in response to insulin. Whether activated through IRS or SHC, ERK1/2 translocates into the nucleus and phosphorylates transcription factors, such as ELK-1, thus modulating DNA binding properties and regulation of gene transcription. ERK also phosphorylates p90 ribosomal protein S6 kinase (p90 S6 kinase), which can phosphorylate and regulate the activity of transcription factors such as c-fos. In addition, the MAPK cascade is one of the pathways with the potential to stimulate glycogen synthase because p90 S6 kinase is able to activate the glycogen-associated protein phosphatase-1, which in turn dephosphorylates and activates glycogen synthase [39]. In this way, the MAPK pathway has the potential to interact with metabolic signaling pathways. However, the MAPK pathway is not necessary for stimulation of glucose transport, and is not viewed as being critically related to the metabolic effects of insulin [40].

Inhibition of insulin signal transduction

The promulgation of insulin signaling pathways does not proceed unabated; rather, there is an extensive array of mechanisms that dampen or inhibit signal transduction. These inhibitory mechanisms can represent normal dynamic functioning of insulin action as organisms adapt to changing physiologic conditions, or, when unbalanced, can lead to pathophysiologic consequences and the development of insulin resistant states. The elucidation of inhibitory processes has provided insight into the extensive network of regulated insulin action pathways, and has also identified potential therapeutic targets because blocking these inhibitory mechanisms could enhance insulin sensitivity.

Inhibition of the insulin receptor

As the first critical component in the insulin signaling network, there are also multiple mechanisms that can desensitize insulin action at the level of the insulin receptor. For example, it has long been known that persistent insulin stimulation can lead to loss of cell surface insulin receptors and this downregulation event impairs insulin sensitivity. In addition, multiple cellular proteins and processes can negatively regulate the intrinsic tyrosine kinase activity of the insulin receptor. Two mechanisms (serine–threonine phosphorylation and protein tyrosine phosphatases) act to impair both insulin receptors and IRS docking molecules.

Downregulation of insulin receptor number

Chronic exposure to high insulin concentrations leads to loss of insulin receptors, resulting in a rightward shift in insulin dose–response curves (i.e. impaired insulin sensitivity). This is caused by increased ligand-mediated internalization of insulin receptors followed by lysosomal degradation, as well as diminished gene expression. Insulin stimulation results in phosphorylation of Foxo1, which disrupts its interaction with the insulin receptor promoter, decreasing insulin receptor gene transcription, thus contributing to receptor loss and insulin resistance [41].

Plasma differentiation factor 1

Plasma differentiation factor 1 (PC-1), also referred to as ectonucleotide pyrophosphatase phosphodiesterase 1, is a membrane glycoprotein with pyrophosphatase activity that appears to act as an intrinsic inhibitor of the insulin receptor tyrosine kinase [42]. PC-1 binds to amino acids 485–599 of the insulin receptor connecting domain, a region required for the conformational change in receptor β-subunits that permit autophosphorylation upon insulin binding. This interaction with PC-1 interferes with the close opposition of the two β-subunits required for transphosphorylation. Muscle expression of PC-1 is elevated in patients with diabetes and in obesity, and it correlates with diminished insulin receptor tyrosine phosphorylation and muscle glucose uptake. Analysis of PC-1 gene polymorphisms in a variety of individuals and family cohorts suggests that alterations in this gene are associated with the risk for development of childhood and adult obesity as well as T2DM [43].

Grb proteins

The growth factor receptor-bound proteins (Grb proteins) constitute a family of structurally related multi-domain adapters with diverse cellular functions but lacking intrinsic enzymatic activity. Grb10 and Grb14 can bind to phosphotyrosine residues on the insulin receptor and alter receptor tyrosine kinase activity [44]. Overexpression of Grb10 and Grb14 in cells inhibits insulin-stimulated phosphorylation of IRS1, IRS2 and Shc [45]. However, the physiologic role of Grb proteins is not fully clear, and their actions may be tissue specific with capabilities as an inhibitory factor or a positive mediator in the insulin signaling pathway.

Inhibition of insulin receptor substrate proteins

Protein phosphotyrosine phosphatases

Endogenous protein phosphotyrosine phosphatases (PTPases) are able to dephosphorylate tyrosine residues on the insulin receptor β-subunit and insulin receptor substrate docking molecules, resulting in a dampening of insulin signal transduction. Two PTPases in particular, PTP-1B and leukocyte common antigen-related phosphatase (LAR), contribute to insulin receptor dephosphorylation in insulin target cells [46]. Membrane-associated PTPase activity is increased in skeletal muscle from patients with T2DM [47], principally because of increments in cytosolic PTPase-1B and membrane-associated LAR [48]. The ability of PTPases to modulate insulin signaling has been demonstrated in mice with genetic ablation of PTPase-1B, which exhibit enhanced insulin sensitivity, increased insulin-mediated tyrosine phosphorylation of the receptor and of IRS1, and a failure to develop insulin resistance when fed a high fat diet [46]. Muscle-specific overexpression of PTP-1B in mice induces tissue insulin resistance with decreased capacity for insulin receptor autophosphorylation [49]. Thus, available data consistently demonstrate that PTPase-1B is able to modulate insulin signaling negatively through dephosphorylation of tyrosine residues in the insulin receptor and IRSs. The role of the LAR in insulin receptor function remains less well defined.

Serine–threonine phosphorylation

Serine–threonine phosphorylation of insulin receptors and IRS docking proteins is a major mechanism for negative modulation of insulin signal transduction. Serine phosphorylation diminishes insulin receptor tyrosine kinase activity and decreases receptor–IRS coupling by inhibiting insulin-mediated tyrosine phosphorylation of IRS-1, binding and activation of PI_3 kinase, and stimulation of glucose transport. There are consensus sequences in IRS-1 that make it susceptible to a wide variety of serine–threonine kinases including PKC, PKA, Akt/PKB, MAPK, S6 kinase, GSK3, casein kinase II, Cdc2 kinase, JNK and IκB kinase (IKKβ). Several of these kinases have been shown to function as physiologic modulators causing desensitization of insulin signaling pathways under conditions of nutrient excess, inflammation and cell stress responses. For example, JNK and IKKβ are activated by inflammatory stimuli (e.g. TNFα) contributing to insulin resistance, and PKC is activated by DAG which accumulates with increased availability of free fatty acids.

Protein kinase C

PKCs are serine–threonine kinases with multiple substrates, including IRS docking proteins and the insulin receptor [50]. Serine–threonine phosphorylation of IRS impairs its ability to associate with the insulin receptor and with PI_3 kinase, resulting in desensitization of the PI_3 kinase pathway. Hyperinsulinemia, hyperglycemia and elevated circulating free fatty acids (e.g. nutrient excess) leads to increased intracellular DAG, which in turn activates conventional and novel PKC isoforms principally via recruitment to the plasma membrane. These conditions are associated with increased serine–threonine phosphorylation and diminished function of insulin receptors and IRS proteins. In addition, insulin activates atypical PKCs, such as PKCζ, via the PI_3 kinase pathway, which is also capable of phosphorylating and desensitizing IRS [51].

Tumor necrosis factor α

Tumor necrosis factor α (TNF-α) is a cytokine produced by immune cells and also by adipocytes and muscle tissue. While having little impact on systemic circulating concentrations, TNF-α expression is increased in adipose and muscle tissues as a function of insulin resistance [52]. In adipose tissue, TNF-α and other proinflammatory cytokines are produced by adipocytes and also by macrophages that infiltrate adipose tissue under conditions of obesity and insulin resistance. This raises the possibility that the cytokine could be inducing cellular insulin resistance via autocrine and/or paracrine effects. TNF-α induces serine phosphorylation of IRS1, thereby decreasing its ability to be phosphorylated by the insulin receptor tyrosine kinase and impairing downstream insulin signal transduction [53]. Several pathways activated by TNF-α are implicated in increased serine phosphorylation of IRS-1, including the stress-induced kinases, JNK and IKKβ.

JNK

Three JNK-encoding genes have been described in mammals; JNK1 and JNK2 are expressed ubiquitously, whereas JNK3 expression is restricted to neuronal tissues. The JNK isoforms belong to the extended family of MAPKs, and control many cellular functions through regulation of activator protein 1 (AP-1). In addition to TNF-α signaling, insulin also activates JNK1 and JNK2 [54], which then display increased serine kinase activity against multiple intracellular substrates including IRS1, IRS2 and Shc. The ability of insulin to activate JNK represents a negative feedback mechanism by which insulin inhibits its own signaling.

JNK activity is also augmented during cellular stress responses, such as endoplasmic reticulum stress, and is increased in insulin-resistant states. Illustrative data include the observation that high-fat diets increase Ser^{307} phosphorylation of IRS1 in wild-type mice but not in JNK1–/– mice, while the JNK1–/– mice are characterized by decreased adiposity, increased insulin receptor signaling and improved insulin sensitivity [55]. Thus, JNK has been implicated in the pathogenesis of insulin resistance in the metabolic syndrome and T2DM.

NF-κB

Activation of NF-κB-mediated pathways has been shown to inhibit insulin signaling through enhanced serine phosphorylation of IRS1 [56]. NF-κB is a transcription factor that functions as a proinflammatory "master switch" during inflammation, upregulating the transcription of a wide range of inflammatory mediators. NF-κB is normally retained in the cytoplasm by binding to members of the inhibitor of κB (IκB) protein family. During inflammatory or metabolic stress, NF-κB is activated by the IκB kinase (IKK) complex, which consists of two catalytic subunits, IKKα and IKKβ, and a regulatory subunit, IKKγ. The IKKβ subunit phosphorylates IκB, resulting in its ubiquitination and subsequent proteasomal degradation and in the release of NF-κB. The free NF-κB is then able to translocate into the nucleus and activate the transcription of at least 125 genes, most of which are proinflammatory [57]. There exists a substantial body of data implicating NF-κB in the pathogenesis of insulin resistance. Activation of NF-κB accompanies insulin resistance following high fat feeding and obesity, and in the metabolic syndrome. Proinflammatory cytokines such as TNF-α and interleukin 6 (IL-6) can also activate NF-κB. Circulating mononuclear cells in the obese display increased transcription of proinflammatory genes regulated by NF-κB with a decrease in IκB. Weight loss, caloric restriction and exercise training can lead to a reduction in transcription of the proinflammatory genes regulated by NF-κB [58]. Drugs with anti-inflammatory properties, such as thiazolidinediones, statins and salicylates, can inhibit proinflammatory cytokine secretion by interferring with the NF-κB pathway.

IκB kinase-β

IKKβ is a serine kinase that has the ability to desensitize insulin signaling through serine phosphorylation of IRS or the insulin receptor. The desensitizing effect of TNF-α, as a consequence of IRS serine phosphorylation, may in part be mediated through IKKβ. Consistent with this hypothesis, heterozygous ablation of the IKKβ gene in mice fed a high-fat diet, or in obese leptin-deficient *ob/ob* mice, prevents insulin resistance [59,60]. Mice that selectively express constitutively active IKKβ in hepatocytes (LIKK mice) exhibit a T2DM phenotype, characterized by hyperglycemia, profound hepatic insulin resistance, and moderate systemic insulin resistance including effects in muscle [56]. The hepatic production of proinflammatory cytokines, including IL-6, IL-1β and TNF-α, is increased in LIKK mice to a similar extent as induced by high-fat feeding in wild-type mice. However, no difference in obesity-induced insulin resistance is detectable in muscle-specific IKKβ knockout mice compared with wild type [61], which suggests that IKKβ may be more directly involved in the development of hepatic insulin resistance rather than in skeletal muscle.

An important biologic effect of salicylates is the inhibition of the IKKβ [62]. Predictably, salicylates would then enhance insulin sensitivity by causing a subsequent decrease in IKKβ-mediated serine phosphorylation of IRS. In fact, treatment with high doses of salicylates improves glucose tolerance and enhances insulin sensitivity in humans and rodents [59].

Accelerated catabolism of PI(3,4,5)P_3 by phosphoinositide phosphatases

Increased production of PI(3,4,5)P_3 as a result of activated PI_3 kinase is key to metabolic insulin signaling, and the downstream activation of PDK1. PTEN can dephosphorylate PI(3,4,5)P_3 on the 3 position, and SH2-containing inositol phosphatases (SHIPs) can dephosphorylate PI(3,4,5)P_3 on the 5 position of the inositol ring; in either instance, the ability of PI(3,4,5)P_3 to stimulate PDK1 is lost. Therefore, PTEN and SHIP can exert negative regulatory influences on insulin signaling, particularly with respect to its metabolic actions [63]. While multiple studies support the view that PTEN can participate as a negative regulator of insulin action in pathophysiologic states, its role in human insulin resistance is yet to be defined.

Inhibition of insulin signaling by protein–protein interactions

Suppressor of cytokine signaling 3

The SOCS family of proteins (CIS and SOCS 1–7) was originally described as a negative feedback loop for cytokine receptors involving Janus kinase (JaK). Following ligand activation of cytokine and growth factor receptors, JaK phosphorylates and activates signal transducer and activator of transcription (STAT), and these phosphorylated STAT family members then form homodimers or heterodimers that translocate to the cell nucleus where they act as transcription activators. In the nucleus, STAT augments SOCS gene expression. SOCS proteins then feedback to inhibit tyrosine-phosphorylated cytokine receptors, via either competitive binding through their SH2 domain preventing phosphorylation of cytokine receptor substrates, or by binding and inhibiting the action of JaK tyrosine kinases. Evidence suggests that a similar mechanism may be operative for the insulin receptor [46]. Studies have indicated that SOCS-1, SOCS-3 and SOCS-6 can bind to the COOH-terminus of the insulin receptor β-subunit, and block interaction between the insulin receptor and IRS [64]. Interestingly, several factors that induce cellular insulin resistance also induce SOCS-3 expression, including TNF-α, growth hormone, and leptin.

Tribbles

The Tribbles (TRB) gene family in mammals is comprised of three proteins that have a truncated kinase domain lacking an

ATP binding site. Accordingly, TRBs are "pseudokinases" that lack detectable kinase activity, but can bind to kinase substrates in phosphorylation cascades and inhibit their phosphorylation. TRB proteins, for example, can bind to Akt/PKB and inhibit its phosphorylation and activation in response to insulin [65], while downregulation of TRB3 improves insulin sensitivity [66].

Tissue-specific insulin action: the role of insulin effector systems

Insulin regulates whole-body fuel homeostasis via specific effects in multiple target tissues. The nature of these biologic actions varies dramatically from tissue to tissue, and these variations, for the most part, are not brought about by differences in insulin signal transmission (described above). Rather, tissue-specific insulin effects are principally explained by effector systems that are uniquely expressed in a variety of differentiated target cells. The biochemical basis of these effects is described in skeletal muscle, adipose tissue, and liver, three organs primarily responsible for fuel storage and oxidation as well as counter-regulatory metabolism.

Skeletal muscle

Insulin stimulation of glucose transport

Skeletal muscle accounts for the bulk of insulin-stimulated glucose uptake *in vivo*, and the hallmark of insulin action in this tissue is the ability to stimulate the glucose transport effector system (Figure 7.2). Glucose transport across the plasma membrane is facilitated by glucose transport proteins (GLUT); to date, 13 members of the GLUT/SLC2 family have been identified. All GLUT proteins are intimately embedded in membranes, and the most highly conserved regions are the putative membrane-spanning domains that serve a common function, the creation of a pore for facilitative diffusion of monosaccharides. Each glucose transporter isoform has a specific role in glucose metabolism determined by its pattern of tissue expression, substrate specificity and affinity, transport kinetics, and regulated expression in different physiologic conditions.

The major transporter isoforms that mediate glucose transport in cells with an insulin-responsive glucose transport system are GLUT-1 and GLUT-4. In unstimulated cells, GLUT-1 predominates at the cell surface and facilitates glucose diffusion across the plasma membrane into the cytosol where glucose is rapidly phosphorylated by hexokinase and metabolized. GLUT-4 contributes minimally to glucose transport in unstimulated target cells, because >90% of the cell content of GLUT-4 resides in intracellular membranes in the basal state. The mechanism by which insulin augments glucose transport activity is by recruiting intracellular GLUT-4 to the plasma membrane, a rate-limiting step for insulin-stimulated glucose uptake and metabolism in peripheral target tissues. Upon dissipation of the insulin signal, deactivation of glucose transport activity is the result of a net reverse translocation of GLUT-4 transporters back into the cell interior. Thus, GLUT-4 is the major transporter mediating insulin-stimulated glucose transport activity in tissues such as skeletal and cardiac muscle and adipose tissue.

In unstimulated muscle or adipose cells, a component of GLUT-4 resides in an inducible tubulo-vesicular storage compartment that includes the trans-Golgi network and endosomal vesicles located near the endofacial surface of the plasma membrane. However, another component of cellular GLUT-4 exists in an active endocytosis–endosomal recycling pathway that cycles GLUT-4 between endosomes and the plasma membrane. The recycling pathway results in the localization of approximately 4–10% of GLUT-4 in the basal plasma membrane, and this steady-state distribution is the balance of rapid endocytosis and slow recycling. Insulin shifts the distribution of GLUT-4 from intracellular pools towards the plasma membrane, both by elevating the exocytotic rate of GLUT-4 in the recycling pathway and by recruiting GLUT-4 from the inducible storage compartment to the cell surface. Deactivation of transport is accomplished via a slowing of the exocytotic rate and an acceleration of the endocytotic rate, as GLUT-4 is retrieved from the plasma membrane through clathrin-dependent and -independent mechanisms [67,68].

GLUT-4 vesicle trafficking involves the actin and microtubule cytoskeletons. Regarding actin, insulin stimulates cytoskeletal rearrangement with the appearance of cortical β-actin fiber projections that subtend the plasma membrane, and this actin remodeling is under the control of small G-proteins in the Rho, Rab and Rac families. Microtubules surround the inducible intracellular depot of GLUT-4 and microtubule proteins such as dynein and kinesin have been co-purified with GLUT-4. Inhibition of actin remodeling or disruption of microtubules using depolymerizing agents inhibits GLUT-4 translocation and glucose transport stimulation. Data suggest that exocytotic movement of GLUT-4 begins with its transfer to actin scaffolds that connect the microtubule cytoskeleton with the plasma membrane, which positions GLUT-4 vesicles for docking and membrane fusion.

The complete pathway linking insulin signal transduction to stimulation of the glucose transport system has not been fully elucidated. Activation of transport is critically dependent on insulin-mediated autophosphorylation of insulin receptors, tyrosine phosphorylation of IRS1 and activation of PI_3 kinase. The production of $PI(3,4,5)P_3$ by PI_3 kinase activates PDK1. At this point, PDK1 activates two separate kinase pathways that contribute to GLUT-4 translocation and stimulation of glucose transport activity, Akt2 and atypical PKCs (PKCζ and PKCλ). Akt2 then phosphorylates and inhibits AS160 (TBC1D4) and TBC1D1 [69], which are Rab-GTPase-activating proteins. The modulation of AS160 activates Rab small GTPases that in turn regulate aspects of GLUT-4 vesicle docking and cytoskeletal organization [70]. At the same time, the ligand-bound insulin receptor activates the CAP/Cbl/TC10 pathway upstream of IRS1 phosphorylation, and activates TC10, a Rho family member that regulates the actin cytoskeleton. Importantly, the factors

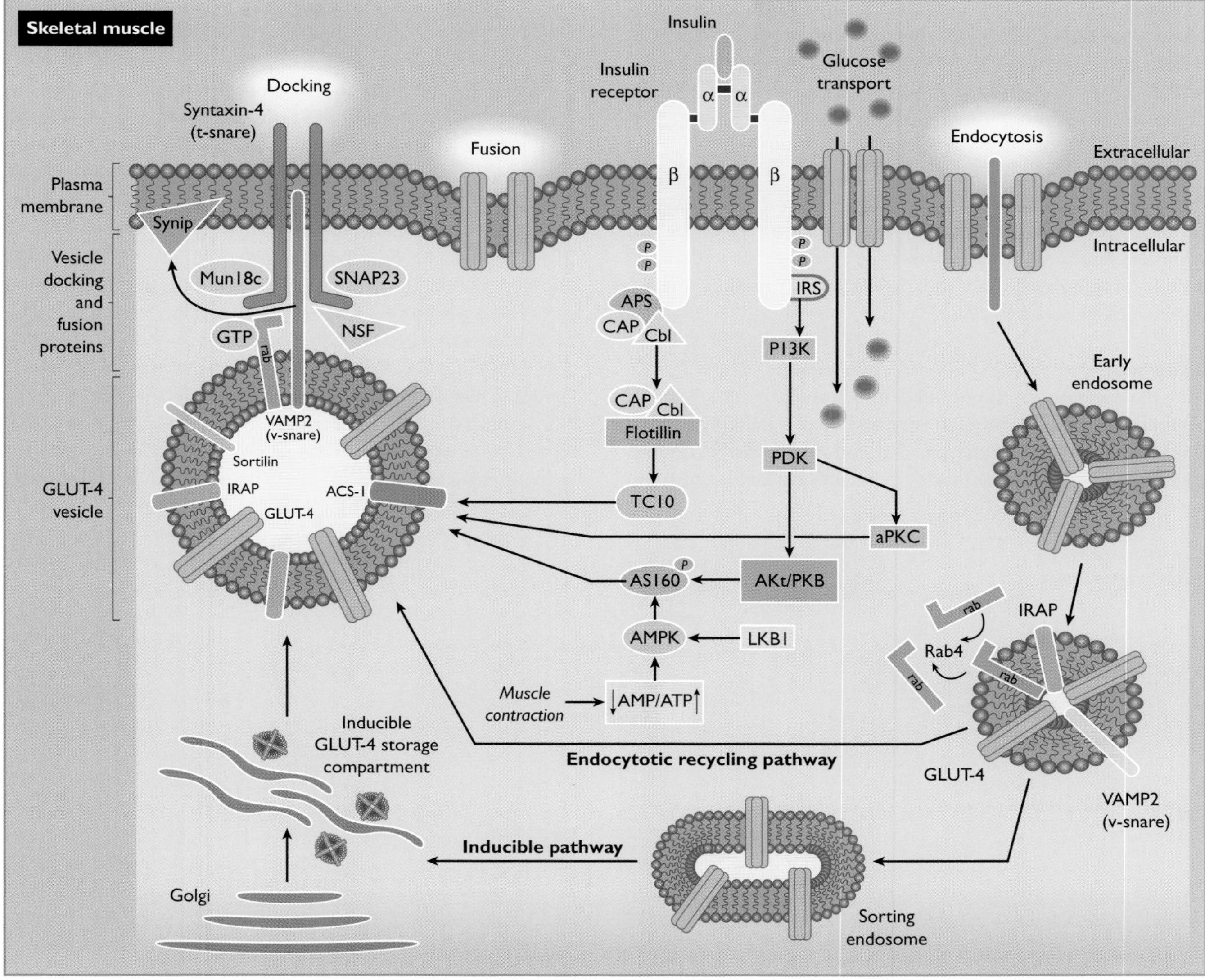

Figure 7.2 An overview of insulin signaling pathways in skeletal muscle. Arrows represent an activation process.

that link TC10, AS160, atypical PKCs, and other relevant factors with the glucose transport effector system, and which impel the complex changes in GLUT-4 vesicle trafficking associated with transporter translocation, are unknown.

Muscle contraction: stimulation of glucose transport independent of insulin signaling

Muscle contraction results in GLUT-4 translocation and stimulates muscle glucose transport activity [71]. This effect occurs without any change in serum insulin concentration and does not involve activation of insulin receptors, PI_3 kinase or Akt/PKB. The mobilization of GLUT-4 to the cell surface by acute exercise involves a different intracellular pool of GLUT-4 than that recruited by insulin, and the effects of acute exercise and insulin are partially additive. These observations indicate that signaling systems mediating glucose transport stimulation are different in response to acute exercise versus insulin [72]. This is underscored by the finding that, in muscle from insulin resistant humans and rodents, GLUT-4 translocation is impaired in response to insulin but normal in response to acute exercise.

While signal transduction mechanisms are not fully understood, this response appears to be at least partially dependent on increments in intracellular 5′AMP, and subsequent activation of adenosine 5′monophosphate-activated protein kinase (AMPK) [73]. AMPK is a serine–threonine kinase that responds to fluctuations in cellular energy levels and functions to maintain energy homeostasis. When ATP levels are low and 5′AMP is elevated, AMPK activates pathways for ATP regeneration and limits further ATP utilization by modifying activity of multiple metabolic enzymes, including acetyl-CoA carboxylase (ACC), hydroxymethylglutaryl-CoA reductase, creatine kinase, and hormone sensitive lipase. Exercise, ischemia, and hypoxia will activate AMPK via increments in AMP:ATP and creatine:phosphocreatine ratios. AMPK can also be activated, however, though allosteric modification and α-subunit phosphorylation by one or more upstream kinases, including LKB1.

Adipose tissue

Adipose tissue is the predominant site for fuel storage as triglyceride, and effector systems responsible for the anabolic effects of insulin on lipogenesis and antilipolysis are key aspects of adipocyte biology (Figure 7.3).

Lipogenesis

Fat accumulation in adipocytes is determined by the balance between triglyceride synthesis (fatty acid uptake and lipogenesis) and breakdown (lipolysis/fatty acid oxidation). Insulin is a critical stimulator of lipogenesis. Insulin augments availability of both glycerol and fatty acids for triglyceride synthesis by increasing the uptake of glucose in the adipose cell as well as by activating lipogenic and glycolytic enzymes. These enzymes constitute the effector system for the biologic effects of insulin on lipogenesis, and are modulated by insulin both through post-translational modifications and alteration of gene expression. Regarding post-translational effects, insulin activates Akt/PKB via phosphorylation, and its role in lipogenesis as illustrated by the observation that constitutively active Akt results in high levels of lipogenesis in 3T3-L1 adipocytes. Substrates for activated Akt/PKB include the phosphorylation and inhibition of GSK3, and this in turn abrogates GSK3 inhibition of ATP citrate lyase; the resulting increase in ATP citrase lyase activity enhances conversion of citrate to acetyl-CoA in the cytosol. Acetyl-CoA is then available as the "building block" for fatty acid synthesis.

Insulin also induces gene expression of two key lipogenic proteins: fatty acid synthase (FAS) and SREBP-1. FAS is the central enzyme participating in *de novo* lipogenesis and catalyzes the

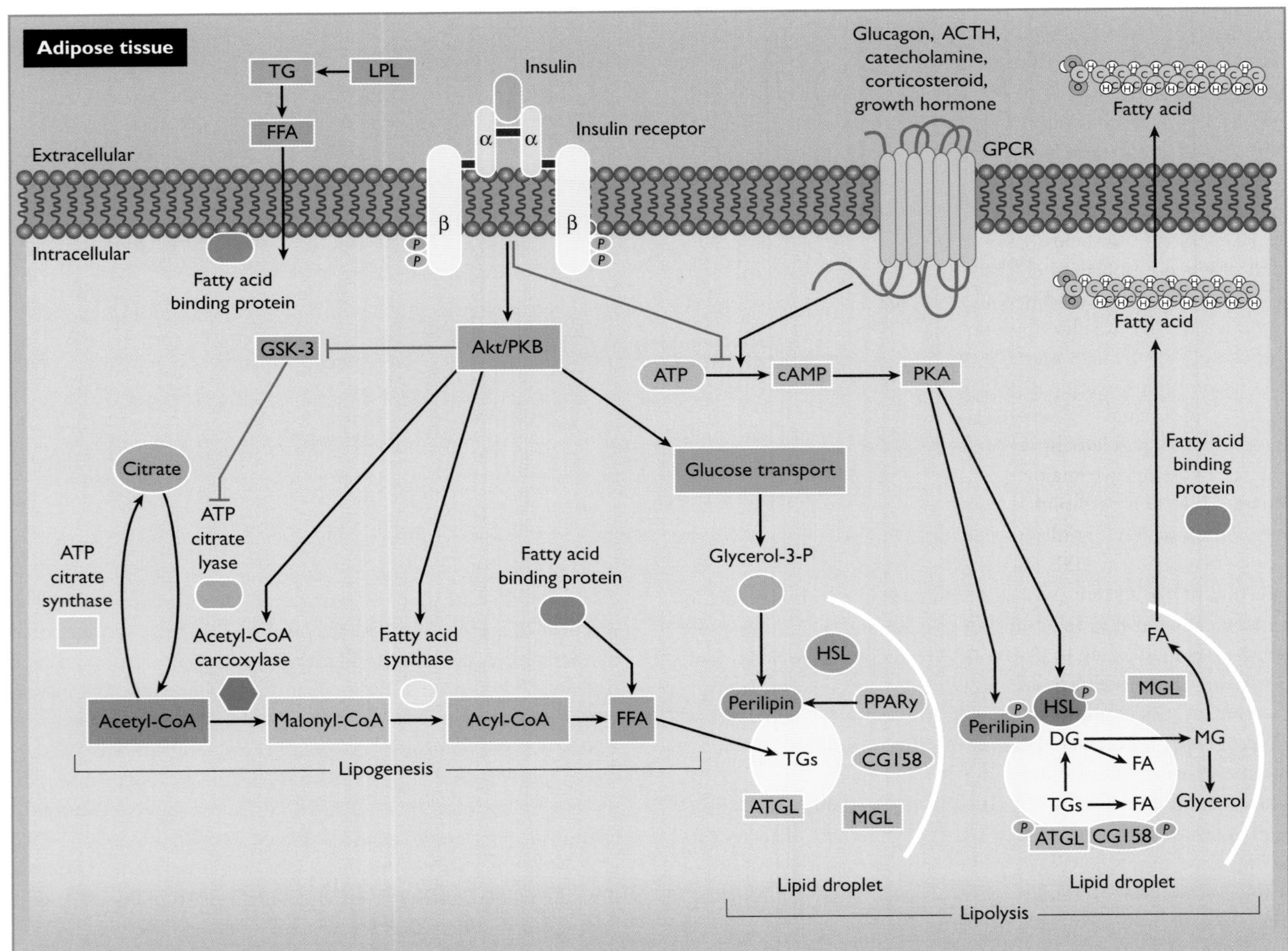

Figure 7.3 Summary of insulin function involved in lipogeneis and lipolysis in adipose tissue. Arrows represent an activation process; blocked arrows represent an inhibition process.

conversion of malonyl-CoA and acetyl-CoA to long-chain fatty acids. Regulation of FAS activity by insulin occurs mainly at the level of gene transcription. SREBP-1 belongs to the class C bHLH (helix-loop-helix) transcription factor family based on its ability to bind to the sterol regulatory element (SRE) of the low-density lipoprotein receptor gene promoter. It activates a battery of genes involved in the uptake and synthesis of fatty acids and triacylglycerides. SREBP-1c is under transcriptional control by insulin [74], and overexpression of SREBP-1c mimics the effect of insulin on the expression of FAS. SREBP-1 also regulates FAS expression as evidenced by the failure of FAS and other lipogenic enzyme genes to be induced by fasting/refeeding in SREBP-1c–/– mice [75].

Lipolysis and antilipolysis

Lipolysis in adipose tissue is tightly regulated to assure that partitioning of metabolic fuels, glucose and free fatty acids (FFA), is adapted to energy needs. During fasting, lipolysis is enhanced to make available FFAs that are the main oxidative fuel for the liver, the heart and skeletal muscle, and are metabolized by the liver to ketones that replace glucose as the principal fuel for nervous tissue. Upon feeding, lipolysis is abated and adipocytes convert to triglyceride storage. The rise (after a meal) and fall (with fasting) of insulin has a central role in this regulatory process as a result of its antilipolytic action in adipocytes. Lipolysis in normal subjects is exquisitely sensitive to inhibition by insulin, such that half-maximal suppression of lipolysis occurs at insulin concentrations well below those needed for significant stimulation of glucose uptake by skeletal muscle. Higher concentrations of insulin can reduce adipocyte release of FFA to nearly zero, although at high insulin concentrations there will still be some appearance of glycerol and FFA from the stimulatory effect of insulin on lipoprotein lipase which acts on triglycerides in circulating lipoproteins.

Hormones regulate lipolysis in adipocytes via coordinated action involving two major effector systems: hormone sensitive lipase (HSL) and perilipins localized to the surface of lipid droplets. Lipolytic and antilipolytic (i.e. insulin) hormones exert opposite effects on HSL and perilipins by determining cAMP availability and protein kinase A (PKA) activity. By way of illustration, catecholamines induce lipolysis and release FFAs from adipocytes by binding to β-adrenergic receptors coupled by heterotrimeric G-proteins to adenylate cyclase, which increases production of cAMP and activates PKA. The two main targets for PKA phosphorylation are HSL and the perilipins [76]. The ability of insulin to antagonize hormone-induced lipolysis is to a large extent accounted for by its ability to lower cAMP levels and thereby reduce PKA activity. The decrease in cAMP is mainly the result of an insulin-mediated phosphorylation and activation of phosphodiesterase 3B (PDE3B) via Akt/PKB. HSL is a key enzyme for the mobilization of triglycerides deposited in adipose tissue following its activation by cAMP/PKA-dependant phosphorylation [77]. HSL is an enzyme with three isoforms ranging from 84 to 130 kDa, yet all isoforms have three domains, a catalytic domain, a regulatory domain with several serine phosphorylation sites required for activation, and an N-terminal variable domain involved in protein–protein and protein–lipid interactions [78]. HSL in muscle can also be stimulated by adrenaline via β-adrenergic activation of PKA, or by muscle contraction via phosphorylation by PKC at least partly activated through the ERK pathway.

Perilipins are localized at the surface of the lipid droplet in adipocytes [79], and are essential in the regulation of triglyceride deposition and mobilization. In the absence of lipolytic stimulation, perilipin inhibits lipolysis by acting as a barrier against hydrolysis of the triacylglycerol by lipases. When PKA is activated, perilipin becomes phosphorylated and translocates away from the lipid droplet, which allows HSL to hydrolyze the lipid droplet triglyceride core [80]. Insulin blocks lipolysis by inhibiting PKA-mediated phosphorylation of HSL and perilipin, thus reducing both HSL activity and its access to triglycerides in the lipid droplet. In adipocytes there are two forms of perilipin, perilipin A and perilipin B, with perilipin A present at a higher concentration. Adipocyte perilipin content has an inverse correlation with lipolytic rates and a positive correlation with plasma glycerol in humans, and is reduced in obese women. Perilipin knockout mice are lean with increased basal lipolysis and are resistant to diet-induced obesity; however, these mice develop glucose intolerance and insulin resistance more readily, probably because of elevated levels of serum FFAs [81]. In addition, perilipin has a peroxisome proliferator-activated receptor γ (PPARγ) responsive element in its promoter region and is induced by thiazolidinedione agonists of PPARγ [82].

Liver

Insulin regulates hepatic metabolism through acute post-translational modifications of enzymes, such as phosphorylation, and through changes in gene expression. The stimulation of glycogen formation and regulation of gluconeogenesis by insulin are the critical determinants of hepatic glucose output. In addition, because regulation of gene transcription is critical for the biologic effects of insulin on hepatic metabolism, mechanisms pertinent to transcriptional regulation are discussed (Figure 7.4).

Glycogenesis/glycogenolysis

Insulin exerts dramatic effects on pathways of intracellular glucose metabolism. Under conditions of insulin stimulation, the major portion of glucose uptake is stored as glycogen in humans. Insulin promotes glycogen synthesis in muscle, adipocytes, and liver by activating glycogen synthase, which adds activated glucosyl groups to growing polysaccharide chains and thus catalyzes the final step in glycogen synthesis. The regulation of glycogen synthase is complex. It involves allosteric activators, translocation of glycogen synthase to the plasma membrane in the presence of glucose metabolites and insulin [83], inhibition by phosphorylation on serine residues by different kinases, and activation by dephosphorylation by serine–threonine phosphatases such as

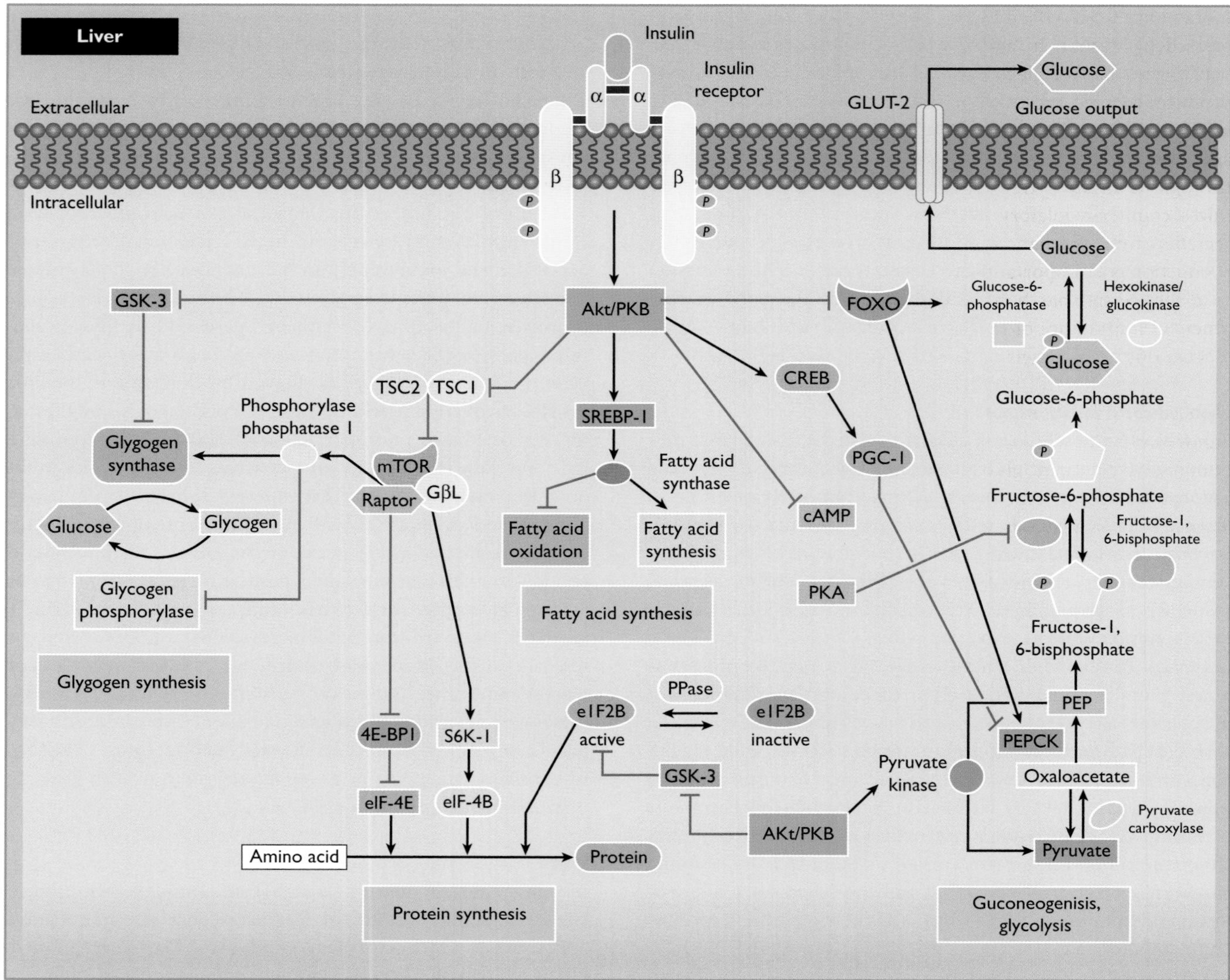

Figure 7.4 Summary of insulin signaling pathways in the liver that are involed in glycogen synthesis, gluconeogenesis and glycolysis, and protein synthesis, respectively. Arrows represent an activation process; blocked arrows represent an inhibition process.

protein phosphatase 1 (PP1). The ability of insulin to stimulate glycogen synthase requires proximal signaling through activation of PI_3 kinase and Akt/PKB. One downstream pathway that activates glycogen synthase involves Akt/PKB-mediated phosphorylation and inactivation of GSK3, which results in a reduction in net phosphorylation of glycogen synthase. The reduction in glycogen synthase phosphorylation augments its activity. GSK3β inhibition is not insulin's only mechanism for stimulating glycogen accumulation. In 3T3-L1 adipocytes, insulin is capable of stimulating glycogen synthase even under experimental conditions when GSK3β is either not detectable or present in very low amounts. Moreover, lithium, a GSK3β inhibitor, is additive with insulin in activating glycogen synthesis and glycogen synthase activity [84]. These studies indicate the existence of additional pathways for glycogen synthase activation.

Inhibition of gluconeogenesis and hepatic glucose output

Hepatic glucose production is stimulated under fasting conditions by the counter-regulatory hormones glucagon, catecholamines, and glucocorticoids, which augment glucose output by promoting glycogenolysis and gluconeogenesis. During feeding and in response to exogenous insulin injections, hepatic glucose output is potently suppressed by insulin as a result of inhibition of glycogenolysis and gluconeogenesis. Gluconeogenesis is predominantly regulated through changes in gene expression for two key enzymes: phosphoenolpyruvate carboxykinase (PEPCK) and glucose-6-phosphatase (G-6-Pase). PEPCK catalyzes one of the rate-limiting steps of gluconeogenesis, whereas G-6-Pase catalyzes the final step producing free glucose for transport out of liver via GLUT-2 glucose transporters. Gene transcription of PEPCK is tightly regulated by cAMP; counter-regulatory hormones increase cAMP and induce PEPCK, whereas both are suppressed by insulin. In addition to direct hormonal effects on hepatocytes, hepatic glucose output is modulated by the delivery of gluconeogenic substrates to the liver such as lactate, amino acids, and FFA. For example, a reduction in FFA availability contributes to suppression of hepatic glucose output by insulin through its antilipolytic action in adipocytes, and insulin minimizes counter-regulatory effects of glucagon by inhibiting its secretion from the pancreatic α cell. Increased hepatic glucose production is an important determinant of fasting hyperglycemia in diabetes, and has been given greater focus because of the potential importance of regulatory pathways controlling hepatic glucose output as targets of drug therapy.

General considerations pertaining to gene regulation by insulin

Suppression of hepatic glucose output by insulin relies heavily on induced changes in gene transcription. The ability of insulin to regulate gluconeogenesis via effects on gene transcription was first reported in 1963, with the observation that PEPCK expression is under negative regulation by insulin [85]. Over the ensuing five decades, it has become clear that insulin influences the expression of more than 800 genes in both positive and negative manners. Regulation of gene transcription can be brought about by effects on transcription factors that are directly modified via insulin signaling mechanisms, or that are indirect as the result of effects of substrate metabolism. The promoter elements (*cis*-acting sequences) that mediate changes in gene transcription are referred to as insulin response elements (IRE), of which multiple distinct consensus sequences have been defined. These include the serum response element, the activator protein 1 (AP-1) motif, the Ets motif, the E-box motif, and the thyroid transcription factor 2 (TTF-2) motif. All of these IREs mediate stimulatory effects of insulin on gene transcription. In contrast, an element with the consensus sequence T(G/A)TTT(T/G)(G/T), which can be referred to as the PEPCK-like motif, mediates the inhibitory effect of insulin on transcription of genes such as PEPCK, insulin-like growth factor binding protein 1 (IGFBP-1), tyrosine aminotransferase, and the G-6-Pase catalytic subunit. In addition, multiple insulin-responsive genes harbor an IRE containing GC-rich region, which binds the ubiquitous transcription factor Sp1, and this IRE is similarly considered to be an important mediator of insulin action [86].

Together with the *cis*-acting promoter sequences, it is also important to consider the identity of the transcription factors (*trans*-acting factors) activated by insulin that bind to the IREs and alter gene transcription rates. Inhibition of gluconeogenesis by insulin follows receptor-mediated tyrosine phosphorylation of IRS2, the IRS isoform that predominates in transducing the insulin signal in liver. Subsequent activation of PI_3 kinase and Akt/PKB are also required, and activation of Akt2 is critical because Akt2 knockout mice [26], but not Akt1 null mice [25], display hepatic insulin resistance, increased hepatic glucose output, and hyperglycemia. Activated Akt2 then phosphorylates and inhibits GSK-3, resulting in hepatic glycogen synthesis, and also suppresses PEPCK and G-6-Pase gene expression through a complex process involving multiple transcription factors including Foxo, SREBP-1c, liver X-activated receptor (LXR), Sp1, and others. The interplay of *cis*- and *trans*-acting factors in the regulation of hepatic metabolism is complex and remains to be fully elucidated.

Foxo transcription factors

The Foxo family in mammals is composed of three expressed genes: Foxo1, Foxo3 and Foxo4, although Foxo1 is the most highly expressed isoform in insulin-responsive tissues such as liver, adipose tissue, and pancreatic β-cells. Foxo proteins, contain a winged-helix motif, comprising the DNA binding domain. Under basal conditions, Foxo proteins reside within the nucleus and actively regulate gene transcription. Upon stimulation by insulin, Akt/PKB phosphorylates Foxo family members at three different conserved serine and threonine residues (Thr^{24}, Ser^{253} and Ser^{319} in Foxo1), which is followed by the dissociation of Foxo proteins from their DNA binding sites and exclusion from the nucleus [87]. Nuclear exclusion appears to involve the binding of protein 14-3-3 to the phosphorylated Akt/PKB sites of Foxo, thus masking the nuclear localization signal [88]. The relocation of Foxo out of the nucleus represents an effective mechanism by which insulin can suppress transcriptional activity. The dependence on Akt/PKB phosphorylation for this effect is highlighted by the observation that replacement of Thr^{24} or Ser^{253} by alanine results in loss of phosphorylation, lack of Foxo1 nuclear export, and failure of insulin-mediated promoter suppression [89].

The G-6-Pase and PEPCK promoters contain IREs which mediate transcriptional activation by Foxo1 and Foxo3 in the liver. Phosphorylation of Foxo by Akt/PKB impairs Foxo binding to this *cis* element, results in nuclear exclusion of Foxo, and suppression of G-6-Pase and PEPCK gene expression. Foxo is not involved in the regulation of all genes suppressed by insulin, however, and cannot account fully for suppression of G-6-Pase and PEPCK. Under physiologic conditions, there is strong evidence that SREBP-1, LXR, and peroxisome proliferator-activated receptor gamma coactivator 1 (PGC-1) all contribute to regulation of gluconeogenic genes by insulin [90].

The importance of Foxo transcription factors in cell differentiation related to whole body metabolic homeostasis is being increasingly recognized. Foxo1 is involved in pancreatic β-cell proliferation and regulation of pancreatic-duodenal homeobox 1 (Pdx1) expression by insulin [91]. Foxo1 appears to contribute to the complex coordination of transcriptional events involved in adipocyte differentiation. Constitutively active Foxo1 prevents the differentiation of pre-adipocytes, while dominant-negative Foxo1 restores adipocyte differentiation of fibroblasts from insulin receptor deficient mice [92]. The binding of Foxo to its co-activator, PGC-1α, is disrupted by the phosphorylation of Foxo, and the disruption of this complex can in itself suppress effects on gene transcription [93].

Sterol response element binding protein 1c

The SREBP family of transcription factors is classically viewed as being involved in the regulation of genes in response to cholesterol availability; however, SREBP-1c is regulated primarily by insulin [92]. This protein is also involved in adipocyte differentiation which explains its alternative designation as adipocyte determination and differentiation factor 1 (ADD1). SREBP-1c/ADD1 is most highly expressed in liver, white adipose tissue, muscle, adrenal gland, and brain.

Insulin stimulates the transcription, post-translational processing, and nuclear translocation of SREBP-1c in cell lines and in adipose, liver, and muscle tissues. In the nucleus, SREBP-1c contributes to a positive autofeedback loop where SREBP-1 augments its own transcription in response to insulin involving a coordinated interaction of multiple transcription factors including LXRα, Sp1, and SREBP-1c itself [94]. This insulin effect is mediated through PI_3 kinase and Akt/PKB, although downstream targets and transcription factors mediating induction of SREBP-1c gene transcription have not been fully clarified. In addition, insulin signal transduction via the Ras/MAPK pathway plays a contributory part by increasing SREBP-1c expression independent of changes in its mRNA levels [94].

While multiple mechanisms may contribute to stimulation of SREBP-1 activity, once in the nucleus, SREBP-1c has an important role in the regulation of specific genes in response to insulin. Insulin suppresses gluconeogenesis and PEPCK expression in part through SREBP-1c. In experiments involving overexpression of wild-type, constitutively active and dominant interfering mutants, SREBP-1c has also been shown to be involved in the induction of FAS and leptin in adipose cells, and glucokinase, pyruvate kinase, FAS, and acetyl CoA carboxylase in the liver [95]. While these insulin-regulated genes contain SREs in their promoter regions, multiple additional hormones, metabolic substrates and transcription factors participate in their transcriptional regulation. Thus, SREBP-1c mediates a positive transcriptional effect on genes promoting glycolysis and lipogenesis, while suppressing genes involved in gluconeogenesis, and seems to prepare the liver for carbohydrate availability following a meal. In fact, excessive and persistent SREBP-1c action has been implicated in intrahepatocellular lipid accumulation and hepatic steatosis.

Liver X receptors

Liver X receptors (LXRs) are ligand-activated nuclear receptors that regulate genes involved in lipid and carbohydrate metabolism. The endogenous agonists are oxidized cholesterol derivatives referred to as oxysterols, and, when activated, LXR receptors stimulate reverse cholesterol transport and excretion of cholesterol as bile acids to protect hepatocytes from cholesterol excess. LXR activators are also known to stimulate lipogenesis through the concerted action of activated LXR and SREBP-1c resulting in intrahepatocellular triglyceride synthesis and storage. Despite this lipogenic effect, LXR agonism or hyperexpression also increases hepatic insulin sensitivity and lowers glycemia in diabetic animals [96], largely through suppression of genes encoding the key gluconeogenic enzymes PEPCK and G-6-Pase [96]. Insulin augments expression of LXRα primarily through stabilization of LXRα transcripts, consistent with the conclusion that LXRα contributes in part to the reductions in gluconeogenesis and hepatic glucose output in response to insulin [96]. In addition to its modulatory effects in liver metabolism, activation of pancreatic β-cell LXRβ with a synthetic agonist increased glucose-induced insulin secretion and insulin content, whereas deletion of the nuclear receptor in LXRβ knockout mice severely blunted insulin secretion [97]. Downregulation of SREBP-1 expression with specific small interfering RNA blocked LXRβ-induced expression of pancreatic duodenal homeobox 1, insulin, and GLUT-2 genes. Thus, activation of LXRβ in pancreatic β-cells increases insulin secretion and insulin mRNA expression via a SREBP-1-regulated pathway. These data support the role of LXR and SREBP-1 pathways in both the regulation of gluconeogenesis in liver and insulin secretion in pancreatic β-cells.

PGC-1

PEPCK and G-6-Pase gene expression is regulated not only by transcription factors, but also by co-activator proteins, such as PGC-1 [98]. PGC-1 was first identified as a factor involved in brown fat adipogenesis [99]; however, it also has an important role in the expression of gluconeogenic enzymes at physiologic concentrations within hepatocytes [98]. PGC-1 is induced in the liver by glucagon and glucocorticoids in the context of fasting, insulin deficiency, and diabetes, and then participates in the induction of the gluconeogenic program. Glucagon increases expression of PGC-1 via a cAMP-dependent process, and PGC-1 participates as a co-activator with Foxo1 to increase the Foxo1-dependent transcriptional activity of G-6-Pase and PEPCK expression. In this role, both Foxo1 and PGC-1 cooperate to promote fully the induction of gluconeogenic genes in liver.

Sp1 transcription factors

Sp1 also participates in a complex interplay with other nuclear receptors and co-factors to mediate the effects of insulin on hepatic expression of several genes [86]. There are three different known mechanisms by which Sp1 mediates insulin action: Sp1 may act alone in mediating the effects of insulin; Sp1 binding sites may be closely juxtaposed to those of other insulin-responsive transcription factors, effecting a cooperative interaction required for insulin induction; and Sp1 binding to an insulin-responsive promoter may lead to basal activity, but dissociation of Sp1 from this site may permit other factors to modulate gene activity in response to insulin.

Nutrient sensing and insulin action

Fuel metabolism can interact with hormone signaling pathways to regulate a broad range of cell functions. With respect to insulin action, states of chronic nutrient excess, including glucose, amino acids, and fatty acids, impair signal transduction via transcriptional and post-transcriptional mechanisms. These processes link nutrient availability with the ability of insulin to regulate metabolism together with cell growth and differentiation. There are three predominant pathways for nutrient sensing that are highly relevant to the regulation of insulin action: the hexosamine biosynthetic signaling pathway; the mammalian target of rapamycin (mTOR) signaling pathway; and the AMPK signaling pathway.

Hexosamine biosynthetic signaling pathway

Defects in insulin signaling and impaired insulin secretion in T2DM have long been known to be at least partially reversible following a period (approximately 2–3 weeks) of therapeutic normalization of glycemia [100]. These observations, coupled with findings that elevated glucose concentrations can recapitulate these defects in cultured cell systems and rodent models, has given rise to the concept of "glucose toxicity" [101]. Marshall [102] and others have demonstrated that one important mechanism underlying glucose-induced insulin resistance involves glucose metabolism through a minor intracellular pathway, the hexosamine biosynthetic pathway. Glutamine: fructose-6-phosphate amidotransferase (GFA), the rate-limiting enzyme of this pathway transfers the amide group of glutamine to fructose 6-phosphate resulting in the production of glucosamine-6-phosphate. Glucosamine-6-phosphate is then metabolized to UDP-*N*-acetylglucosamine (UDP-GlcNAc). UDP-GlcNAc serves as the substrate for the enzyme *O*-linked *N*-acetylglucosamine transferease (OGT), which catalyzes the attachment of *O*-GlcNAc to proteins. The counterpart of OGT, *O*-GlcNAcase, catalyzes removal of the *O*-linked glycosyl adduct. Thus, increased glucose flux through the hexosamine biosynthetic pathway leads to increased post-translational modification of cytoplasmic and nuclear proteins by *O*-GlcNAc [103], which can modulate their enzyme activities, proteasomal degradation, and interaction with other proteins or DNA. UDP-GlcNAc levels can fluctuate with the availability of non-esterified fatty acids, uridine, glutamine and glucose, and in this way the hexosamine biosynthetic pathway acts as a nutrient sensor and regulator.

Increased glucose flux through the hexosamine biosynthetic pathway results in impaired ability of insulin to stimulate the glucose transport effector system in adipocytes and muscle cells, and represents a biochemical process by which hyperglycemia can induce insulin resistance [104]. In rodents, hyperglycemia induced by streptozotocin or by glucose infusions, and elevations in circulating FFAs induced by lipid infusion or high-fat feeding, lead to an increase in muscle UDP-GlcNAc levels and insulin resistance as demonstrated in hyperinsulinemic glucose clamp studies. In addition, overexpression of GFA in skeletal muscle and adipose tissue of transgenic mice enhanced glucose metabolism by the hexosamine biosynthetic pathway and induced insulin resistance. The mechanisms by which products of the hexosamine biosynthetic pathway induce insulin resistance, however, have not been fully elucidated. Increased metabolic flux through this pathway results in increased O-glycosylation of the insulin receptor, IRS1, Akt/PKB, GLUT-4 and GSK3β, and this can impair the functional capabilities of these proteins or accelerate their proteasomal degradation. For example, increased *O*-glycosylation of the insulin receptor is accompanied by a decrease in insulin-stimulated receptor autophosphorylation [105]. Glycosylation can also affect activities of nuclear transcription factors. O-GlcNAc adducts can decrease transcriptional activity of Sp1 but increase DNA binding and transcriptional regulation by Foxo1. *O*-glycosylation can impair phosphorylation and DNA binding of C/EBPβ, and decrease NK-κB binding with IκB freeing NF-κB for relocation to the nucleus thereby including transcription of proinflammatory genes. Finally, increased intracellular accumulation of glucosamine-6-P inhibits hexokinase and glycogen synthase activity rapidly via an allosteric interaction with these enzymes. Nevertheless, the extent to which these processes contribute to insulin resistance in patients with diabetes requires further study.

Mammalian target of rapamycin signaling pathway

The mTOR signaling pathway, also known as FK506 binding protein 12-rapamycin associated protein 1 (FRAP1), is an evolutionarily conserved serine–threonine protein kinase and a member of the PI_3 kinase-related kinase (PIKK) family [106]. It is a central signal integrator that receives signals arising from growth factors, nutrients and cellular energy metabolism, and then activates pathways that control cell growth, proliferation and survival. mTOR contains a COOH-terminal region with strong homology to the catalytic domain of PI_3 kinase, functions as a protein kinase [107], and exists in two functionally distinct complexes dubbed mTOR complex 1 (mTORC1) and mTORC2. mTORC1 is a heterotrimeric protein kinase that consists of the mTOR catalytic subunit and two associated proteins, regulatory associated protein of mTOR (raptor) and mammalian LST8/G-protein β-subunit like protein (mLST8/GβL). Nutrients modulate the activity of the mTORC1 complex by affecting the interaction and association of the mTOR catalytic subunit with raptor. mTORC1 determines the activity of eukaryotic initiation factor 4E binding protein (4E-BP1) and ribosomal S6 kinase (S6K). The mTORC2 complex is comprised of mTOR, mLST8/GβL, rapamycin-independent companion of mTOR (rictor) and MAPK-associated protein (mSin1). The rictor-mTOR complex directly phosphorylates Akt/PkB on Ser^{473} and facilitates Thr^{308} phosphorylation by PDK1 [108]. This phosphorylation of Akt occurs at Ser^{473} which is distinct from activation by PDK1 which phosphorylates Thr^{308}.

mTORC1 can impair insulin signaling via its ability to activate S6K, which then can phosphorylate serine residues of IRS1 resulting in desensitization of the PI_3 kinase/Akt pathway [109]. Indeed, IRS1 Ser^{302}, which is proximal to the IRS1 PTB domain, contains an S6K recognition motif and is able to be phosphorylated by S6K. In this way, an increase in mTOR activity can contribute to insulin resistance. A surfeit of glucose and amino acids, especially leucine, leads to an increase in mTOR activity, while depletion of these metabolic substrates or mitochondrial (e.g. oligomycin) and glycolytic (e.g. 2-deoxyglucose) inhibitors attenuate mTOR activity [110]. Thus, activation of S6K by mTOR activity serves as a mechanism by which nutrient excess can desensitize insulin action through serine phosphorylation of IRS1. Data in rodent models are consistent with this formulation. S6K1 activity is enhanced in insulin resistant mice fed a high-fat diet and in genetically obese mouse models, while S6K1–/– mice maintained on a high-fat diet remained insulin sensitive [111].

Insulin and amino acids can activate the mTOR pathway in a wortmannin-sensitive manner indicative of signaling through PI_3 kinase; however, the wortmannin target is not class I PI_3 kinases. Rather, the wortmannin target is the class III PI_3 kinase, hVps34. This is substantiated by the observation that knockdown of hVps34 blocks amino acid- and insulin-induced S6K1 activation but has no effect on Akt/PKB activation [112]. Rapamycin can inhibit mTOR through association with its intracellular receptor FKBP12. The FKBP12–rapamycin complex binds directly to a FKBP12–rapamycin binding (FRB) domain in mTOR, and this interaction inhibits mTOR activity. A recent study demonstrated that rapamycin enhances insulin-mediated glucose uptake by inhibiting mTOR-mediated S6K phosphorylation and reducing IRS serine phosphorylation [113]. The proximal signaling component immediately responsible for activating the mTOR pathway is the tuberous sclerosis complex (TSC). TSC can integrate information from the insulin signaling cascade and the AMPK signaling pathway. These multiple steps involved in nutrient sensing by the mTOR signaling pathway are attractive targets for treating insulin resistance in metabolic diseases cause by nutrient excess, such as T2DM and obesity.

AMPK signaling pathway

The AMPK signaling pathway is activated by elevation of the AMP:ATP ratio. The pathway is switched on by nutrient deprivation leading to accumulation of AMP, or by perturbations that interfere with ATP synthesis, such as glucose deprivation, hypoxia, metabolic inhibitors (2-deoxyglucose, arsenite), and disruption of oxidative phosphorylation. Hardie has described AMPK as a “fuel gauge” that regulates responses to extremes of nutrient availability at the levels of cells, tissues and the whole body [114]. Once activated, it switches on fuel metabolism pathways that generate ATP, while inhibiting anabolic processes that consume ATP. AMPK is a heterotrimeric enzyme complex comprised of α, β and γ-subunits, and each subunit has two or more isoforms that exhibit tissue-specific expression. The α-subunit is the catalytic component, and contains the Thr^{172} residue that is phosphorylated by activating upstream kinases. The β-subunit has glycogen-binding C-terminal domains that help cement the trimolecular complex, and can also interact with high glycogen stores to exert an inhibitory effect on AMPK activity. The γ-subunit of AMPK allosterically binds one molecule of AMP or ATP in a mutually exclusive manner allowing for regulation of AMPK activity by changing ratios of AMP to ATP.

The upstream cascade leading to phosphorylation of Thr^{172} in the AMPK α-subunit is initiated by the LKB1 complex. LKB1 is apparently not regulated by AMP and is constitutively active. The binding of AMP to the AMPK γ-subunit results in a net augmentation of phospho-Thr^{172} by making this site less susceptible to phosphatases, as well as by allosterically activating the phosphorylated form of the kinase. These two mechanisms create a “multiplier effect” for AMPK activity, allowing a small increase in AMP to produce a large effect on kinase activity. Both effects are antagonized by high ATP concentrations, so that the AMP:ATP ratio becomes a sensitive regulator of AMPK. AMPK is also activated in response to cytosolic Ca^{2+} levels via phosphorylation of Thr^{172} by calmodulin-dependent kinase kinase-β (CaMKKβ); however, this action of CaMKKβ is independent of the AMP level.

AMPK switches on catabolic processes that generate ATP such as glucose uptake, glycolysis, fatty acid oxidation, and mitochondrial biogenesis, while switching off anabolic processes that consume ATP such as fatty acid and cholesterol biosynthesis, gluconeogenesis and glycogenesis. To conserve ATP, AMPK activation suppresses protein synthesis by inhibiting the mTOR pathway and initiation of translation, and by inhibiting translational elongation of proteins via activation of elongation factor 2 kinase. To enhance the capacity for ATP generation, AMPK appears to promote mitochondrial biogenesis through concerted action with another metabolic sensor, the NAD^+-dependent deacetylase SIRT1. Evidence indicates that AMPK can enhance SIRT1 activity by increasing cellular NAD^+ levels. SIRT1 then deacetylates various AMPK substrates and modulates their activity including PGC-1α and Foxo1. In this way, AMPK, SIRT1 and PGC-1α can act in an orchestrated way to regulate energy metabolism. In skeletal muscle, AMPK stimulates lipid oxidation, increases insulin sensitivity and mediates contraction-induced increments in glucose uptake during exercise [115]. In liver, AMPK activation suppresses gluconeogenic enzyme expression and leads to decreased blood glucose values, while fatty acid oxidation is stimulated and cholesterol and triglyceride biosynthesis is blocked. These biologic actions are the result of phosphorylation and inactivation of both ACC and 3-hydroxy-3-methylglutaryl coenzyme A reductase (HMG-CoA reductase) by AMPK. The phosphorylation of ACC is central to the ability of AMPK to promote fatty acid oxidation, because this reduces its activity and results in decreased production of malonyl-CoA, an inhibitor of carnitine palmitoyltransferase I (CPT1). The reduction in malonyl-CoA relieves the inhibition of CPT1 and promotes CPT1-mediated transport of fatty acids into the mitochondria for oxidation. At the transcriptional level, AMPK blocks lipogenesis by limiting endogenous LXR ligand production, which inhibits LXR-dependent transcription of SREBP-1 [116]. AICAR is used experimentally to study the effects of AMPK activation on glucose and lipid metabolism and insulin signaling pathways. AICAR is an adenosine analog that is taken up by adenosine transporters and subsequently phosphorylated to ZMP (5-aminoimidazole-4-carboxamide-1-β-D-furanosyl

5′-monophosphate) within the cell, which mimics AMP and activates AMPK signaling through direct binding. In adipocytes, AICAR stimulates glucose uptake, increases adiponectin secretion, and inhibits production of cytokines such as TNF-α and IL-6. Two existing classes of antidiabetic drugs, biguanides (e.g. metformin) and the thiazolidinediones (e.g. rosiglitazone), both act (at least in part) by activation of AMPK. Furthermore, AMPK is activated by the insulin sensitizing hormones leptin and adiponectin. These actions are proof-of-principle that pharmacologic activators of AMPK could be used to treat patients with the metabolic syndrome and T2DM.

Cell stress and insulin action

Oxidative stress

Oxidative stress caused by increased reactive oxygen species (ROS) generation and/or compromised antioxidant systems represents an important factor in the development of insulin resistance and the related diseases of obesity, metabolic syndrome, and T2DM [117]. Nutrient excess, physical inactivity and hyperglycemia can lead to oxidative stress and low-grade inflammation. A considerable portion of total body oxidant stress and ROS production are generated by dysfunctional mitochondria in skeletal muscle. It is not clear, however, whether mitochondrial dysfunction is the consequence or the cause of increased ROS production. Production of excess ROS can occur in response to diverse stimuli including inflammation and proinflammatory cytokines (e.g. TNF-α). Oxidative stress can also be self-reinforcing, because ROS activates NF-κB and upregulates expression of proinflammatory genes such as TNF-α, IL-6, and C-reactive protein (CRP) [118]. Oxidants are believed to impair insulin signal transduction by inducing serine phosphorylation of IRS which impairs tyrosine phosphorylation and increases IRS protein degradation.

Inflammation

Human insulin resistance is frequently accompanied by low-grade systemic inflammation, evidenced by elevated circulating markers of inflammation in these disorders such as white blood cell count, sedimentation rate, CRP, adhesion molecules (e.g. e-selectin), cytokines such as IL-6 and IL-8, and serum amyloid A. In adipose tissue, obesity and insulin resistance are associated with an infiltration of activated macrophages and paracrine cross-talk between macrophages and adipocytes involving multiple secreted factors (e.g. cytokines, adipokines). This process can influence secretion patterns of circulating adipokines that can affect other organs and generate aspects of the metabolic syndrome trait cluster. This includes secretion of IL-1 and IL-6 which helps mediate inflammation in metabolic disorders. For example, IL-1α and IL-1β exert strong proinflammatory functions [119] and the latter is able to reduce IRS-1 expression. Interestingly, in humans with T2DM, treatment with recombinant human IL-1 receptor antagonist improves glycemic control [120]. Circulating IL-6 levels are highly correlated with insulin resistance, and related studies demonstrate how proinflammatory cytokines can compromise insulin action, by a mechanism involving recruitment and activation of Jak, STAT proteins, and SHP-2 which helps to activate the ERK/MAP kinase pathway. Subsequent steps include increased transcription of SOCS genes, whose protein products induce insulin resistance at a proximal step at the insulin receptor or IRS proteins.

Endoplasmic reticulum stress

Although endoplasmic reticulum (ER) stress has been recognized as an adaptive cellular response to an accumulation of unfolded or misfolded proteins in its lumen, the ER stress response can also be triggered by other factors, including chronic nutrient excess, high fatty acid concentrations, and oxidative stress, which are found in insulin resistant states. ER stress activates the JNK pathway with subsequent inhibitory serine phosphorylation of IRS-1, and the development of insulin resistance. The mechanism for JNK activation involves transmembrane ER proteins with luminal domains responsive to ER stress signals and cytoplasmic effector domains that influence intracellular pathways. One of these stress transducers, known as IRE1, links ER stress to JNK activation. Obesity and extended periods of high fat feeding can induce the ER stress response in adipose tissue and liver, as indicated by ER stress markers such as PERK, eIF2α phosphorylation, and JNK activation. Interestingly, small molecular weight "chemical chaperones" such as phenyl butyric acid which attenuate ER stress, can normalize fasting blood glucose, enhance insulin sensitivity and reduce ER stress in *ob/ob* mice [121]. In diabetes, ER stress has also been implicated in pancreatic β-cell failure [122]. Finally, oxidative stress, caused by excess availability of saturated fatty acids for mitochondrial oxidation, is linked to exacerbation of ER stress.

Acknowledgments

Dr. Garvey credits grant support from the National Institutes of Health (DK-038764, DK-083562, PO1 HL-055782) and the Merit Review program of the Department of Veterans Affairs. Dr. Wu credits grant support from the American Heart Association and the University of Alabama at Birmingham (UAB) Clinical Nutrition Research Center. The authors also acknowledge support from the Diabetes Research and Training Center (P60 DK079626) and the Clinical Nutrition Research Unit (P30-DK56336) at UAB. The authors are grateful to Kate Kosmac and Stephanie Rudolph, graduate students at UAB, for assistance with the figures, and to Dr. Barry Goldstein, our editor, for excellent editorial assistance.

References

1 Taniguchi CM, Emanuelli B, Kahn CR. Critical nodes in signaling pathways: insights into insulin action. *Nat Rev Mol Cell Biol* 2006; **7**:85–96.

2 Jacobs S, Cuatrecasas P. Insulin receptor: structure and function. *Endocr Rev* 1981; **2**:251–263.

3 Cheatham B, Kahn CR. Insulin action and the insulin signaling network. *Endocr Rev* 1995; **16**:117–142.

4 Okamoto H, Nakae J, Kitamura T, Park BC, Dragatsis I, Accili D. Transgenic rescue of insulin receptor-deficient mice. *J Clin Invest* 2004; **114**:214–223.

5 Bruning JC, Michael MD, Winnay JN, Hayashi T, Horsch D, Accili D, *et al.* A muscle-specific insulin receptor knockout exhibits features of the metabolic syndrome of NIDDM without altering glucose tolerance. *Mol Cell* 1998; **2**:559–569.

6 Wojtaszewski JF, Higaki Y, Hirshman MF, Michael MD, Dufresne SD, Kahn CR, *et al.* Exercise modulates postreceptor insulin signaling and glucose transport in muscle-specific insulin receptor knockout mice. *J Clin Invest* 1999; **104**:1257–1264.

7 Ullrich A, Bell JR, Chen EY, Herrera R, Petruzzelli LM, Dull TJ, *et al.* Human insulin receptor and its relationship to the tyrosine kinase family of oncogenes. *Nature* 1985; **313**:756–761.

8 Leibiger B, Leibiger IB, Moede T, Kemper S, Kulkarni RN, Kahn CR, *et al.* Selective insulin signaling through A and B insulin receptors regulates transcription of insulin and glucokinase genes in pancreatic beta cells. *Mol Cell* 2001; **7**:559–570.

9 Saltiel AR, Kahn CR. Insulin signalling and the regulation of glucose and lipid metabolism. *Nature* 2001; **414**:799–806.

10 Virkamaki A, Ueki K, Kahn CR. Protein–protein interaction in insulin signaling and the molecular mechanisms of insulin resistance. *J Clin Invest* 1999; **103**:931–943.

11 Khan AH, Pessin JE. Insulin regulation of glucose uptake: a complex interplay of intracellular signalling pathways. *Diabetologia* 2002; **45**:1475–1483.

12 Hirashima Y, Tsuruzoe K, Kodama S, Igata M, Toyonaga T, Ueki K, *et al.* Insulin down-regulates insulin receptor substrate-2 expression through the phosphatidylinositol 3-kinase/Akt pathway. *J Endocrinol* 2003; **179**:253–266.

13 Rui L, Yuan M, Frantz D, Shoelson S, White MF. SOCS-1 and SOCS-3 block insulin signaling by ubiquitin-mediated degradation of IRS1 and IRS2. *J Biol Chem* 2002; **277**:42394–42398.

14 Shimomura I, Matsuda M, Hammer RE, Bashmakov Y, Brown MS, Goldstein JL. Decreased IRS-2 and increased SREBP-1c lead to mixed insulin resistance and sensitivity in livers of lipodystrophic and ob/ob mice. *Mol Cell* 2000; **6**:77–86.

15 Stoker AW. Protein tyrosine phosphatases and signalling. *J Endocrinol* 2005; **185**:19–33.

16 Ball LE, Berkaw MN, Buse MG. Identification of the major site of O-linked beta-N-acetylglucosamine modification in the C terminus of insulin receptor substrate-1. *Mol Cell Proteomics* 2006; **5**:313–323.

17 Carvalho-Filho MA, Ueno M, Carvalheira JB, Velloso LA, Saad MJ. Targeted disruption of iNOS prevents LPS-induced S-nitrosation of IRbeta/IRS-1 and Akt and insulin resistance in muscle of mice. *Am J Physiol Endocrinol Metab* 2006; **291**:E476–482.

18 Rameh LE, Cantley LC. The role of phosphoinositide 3-kinase lipid products in cell function. *J Biol Chem* 1999; **274**:8347–8350.

19 Katso R, Okkenhaug K, Ahmadi K, White S, Timms J, Waterfield MD. Cellular function of phosphoinositide 3-kinases: implications for development, homeostasis, and cancer. *Annu Rev Cell Dev Biol* 2001; **17**:615–675.

20 Antonetti DA, Algenstaedt P, Kahn CR. Insulin receptor substrate 1 binds two novel splice variants of the regulatory subunit of phosphatidylinositol 3-kinase in muscle and brain. *Mol Cell Biol* 1996; **16**:2195–2203.

21 Luo J, Cantley LC. The negative regulation of phosphoinositide 3-kinase signaling by p85 and its implication in cancer. *Cell Cycle* 2005; **4**:1309–1312.

22 Taniguchi CM, Aleman JO, Ueki K, Luo J, Asano T, Kaneto H, *et al.* The p85alpha regulatory subunit of phosphoinositide 3-kinase potentiates c-Jun N-terminal kinase-mediated insulin resistance. *Mol Cell Biol* 2007; **27**:2830–2840.

23 Taniguchi CM, Tran TT, Kondo T, Luo J, Uek K, Cantley LC, *et al.* Phosphoinositide 3-kinase regulatory subunit p85alpha suppresses insulin action via positive regulation of PTEN. *Proc Natl Acad Sci U S A* 2006; **103**:12093–12097.

24 Kohn AD, Summers SA, Birnbaum MJ, Roth RA. Expression of a constitutively active Akt Ser/Thr kinase in 3T3-L1 adipocytes stimulates glucose uptake and glucose transporter 4 translocation. *J Biol Chem* 1996; **271**:31372–31378.

25 Cho H, Thorvaldsen JL, Chu Q, Feng F, Birnbaum MJ. Akt1/PKBalpha is required for normal growth but dispensable for maintenance of glucose homeostasis in mice. *J Biol Chem* 2001; **276**:38349–38352.

26 Cho H, Mu J, Kim JK, Thorvaldsen JL, Chu Q, Crenshaw EB 3rd, *et al.* Insulin resistance and a diabetes mellitus-like syndrome in mice lacking the protein kinase Akt2 (PKB beta). *Science* 2001; **292**:1728–1731.

27 Gonzalez E, McGraw TE. Insulin signaling diverges into Akt-dependent and -independent signals to regulate the recruitment/docking and the fusion of GLUT4 vesicles to the plasma membrane. *Mol Biol Cell* 2006; **17**:4484–4493.

28 Frame S, Zheleva D. Targeting glycogen synthase kinase-3 in insulin signalling. *Expert Opin Ther Targets* 2006; **10**:429–444.

29 Sano H, Kane S, Sano E, Mîinea CP, Asara JM, Lane WS, *et al.* Insulin-stimulated phosphorylation of a Rab GTPase-activating protein regulates GLUT4 translocation. *J Biol Chem* 2003; **278**:14599–14602.

30 Larance M, Ramm G, Stockli J, van Dam EM, Winata S, Wasinger V, *et al.* Characterization of the role of the Rab GTPase-activating protein AS160 in insulin-regulated GLUT4 trafficking. *J Biol Chem* 2005; **280**:37803–37813.

31 Farese RV. Function and dysfunction of aPKC isoforms for glucose transport in insulin-sensitive and insulin-resistant states. *Am J Physiol Endocrinol Metab* 2002; **283**:E1–11.

32 Liu LZ, Zhao HL, Zuo J, Ho SK, Chan JC, Meng Y, *et al.* Protein kinase Czeta mediates insulin-induced glucose transport through actin remodeling in L6 muscle cells. *Mol Biol Cell* 2006; **17**:2322–2330.

33 Farese RV, Sajan MP, Standaert ML. Atypical protein kinase C in insulin action and insulin resistance. *Biochem Soc Trans* 2005; **33**:350–353.

34 Watson RT, Pessin JE. Subcellular compartmentalization and trafficking of the insulin-responsive glucose transporter, GLUT4. *Exp Cell Res* 2001; **271**:75–83.

35 Baumann CA, Ribon V, Kanzaki M, Thurmond DC, *et al.* CAP defines a second signalling pathway required for insulin-stimulated glucose transport. *Nature* 2000; **407**:202–207.

36 Kanzaki M, Pessin JE. Caveolin-associated filamentous actin (Cav-actin) defines a novel F-actin structure in adipocytes. *J Biol Chem* 2002; **277**:25867–25869.

37 Inoue M, Chang L, Hwang J, Chiang SH, Saltiel AR. The exocyst complex is required for targeting of Glut4 to the plasma membrane by insulin. *Nature* 2003; **422**:629–633.

38 Boulton TG, Nye SH, Robbins DJ, Ip NY, Radziejewska E, Morgenbesser SD, *et al.* ERKs: a family of protein-serine/threonine kinases that are activated and tyrosine phosphorylated in response to insulin and NGF. *Cell* 1991; **65**:663–675.

39 Frodin M, Gammeltoft S. Role and regulation of 90 kDa ribosomal S6 kinase (RSK) in signal transduction. *Mol Cell Endocrinol* 1999; **151**:65–77.

40 Lazar DF, Wiese RJ, Brady MJ, Mastick CC, Waters SB, Yamauchi K, *et al.* Mitogen-activated protein kinase kinase inhibition does not block the stimulation of glucose utilization by insulin. *J Biol Chem* 1995; **270**:20801–20807.

41 Puig O, Tjian R. Transcriptional feedback control of insulin receptor by dFOXO/FOXO1. *Genes Dev* 2005; **19**:2435–2446.

42 Frittitta L, Spampinato D, Solini A, Nosadini R, Goldfine ID, Vigneri R, *et al.* Elevated PC-1 content in cultured skin fibroblasts correlates with decreased *in vivo* and *in vitro* insulin action in nondiabetic subjects: evidence that PC-1 may be an intrinsic factor in impaired insulin receptor signaling. *Diabetes* 1998; **47**:1095–1100.

43 Meyre D, Bouatia-Naji N, Tounian A, Samson C, Lecoeur C, Vatin V, *et al.* Variants of ENPP1 are associated with childhood and adult obesity and increase the risk of glucose intolerance and type 2 diabetes. *Nat Genet* 2005; **37**:863–867.

44 Holt LJ, Siddle K. Grb10 and Grb14: enigmatic regulators of insulin action – and more? *Biochem J* 2005; **388**:393–406.

45 Wick KR, Werner ED, Langlais P, Ramos FJ, Dong LQ, Shoelson SE, *et al.* Grb10 inhibits insulin-stimulated insulin receptor substrate (IRS)-phosphatidylinositol 3-kinase/Akt signaling pathway by disrupting the association of IRS-1/IRS-2 with the insulin receptor. *J Biol Chem* 2003; **278**:8460–8467.

46 Elchebly M, Payette P, Michaliszyn E, Cromlish W, Collins S, Lov AL, *et al.* Increased insulin sensitivity and obesity resistance in mice lacking the protein tyrosine phosphatase-1B gene. *Science* 1999; **283**:1544–1548.

47 Asante-Appiah E, Kennedy BP. Protein tyrosine phosphatases: the quest for negative regulators of insulin action. *Am J Physiol Endocrinol Metab* 2003; **284**:E663–670.

48 Ahmad F, Considine RV, Bauer TL, Ohannesian JP, Marco CC, Goldstein BJ. Improved sensitivity to insulin in obese subjects following weight loss is accompanied by reduced protein-tyrosine phosphatases in adipose tissue. *Metabolism* 1997; **46**:1140–1145.

49 Ahmad F, Goldstein BJ. Increased abundance of specific skeletal muscle protein-tyrosine phosphatases in a genetic model of insulin-resistant obesity and diabetes mellitus. *Metabolism* 1995; **44**:1175–1184.

50 Leitges M, Plomann M, Standaert ML, Bandyopadhyay G, Sajan MP, Kanoh Y, *et al.* Knockout of PKC alpha enhances insulin signaling through PI3K. *Mol Endocrinol* 2002; **16**:847–858.

51 Liu YF, Herschkovitz A, Boura-Halfon S, Ronen D, Paz K, Leroith D, *et al.* Serine phosphorylation proximal to its phosphotyrosine binding domain inhibits insulin receptor substrate 1 function and promotes insulin resistance. *Mol Cell Biol* 2004; **24**:9668–9681.

52 Saghizadeh M, Ong JM, Garvey WT, Henry RR, Kern PA. The expression of TNF alpha by human muscle: relationship to insulin resistance. *J Clin Invest* 1996; **97**:1111–1116.

53 Kanety H, Feinstein R, Papa MZ, Hemi R, Karasik A. Tumor necrosis factor alpha-induced phosphorylation of insulin receptor substrate-1 (IRS-1): possible mechanism for suppression of insulin-stimulated tyrosine phosphorylation of IRS-1. *J Biol Chem* 1995; **270**:23780–23784.

54 Miller BS, Shankavaram UT, Horney MJ, Gore AC, Kurtz DT, Rosenzweig SA. Activation of cJun NH2-terminal kinase/stress-activated protein kinase by insulin. *Biochemistry* 1996; **35**:8769–8775.

55 Hirosumi J, Tuncman G, Chang L, Görgün CZ, Uysal KT, Maeda K, *et al.* A central role for JNK in obesity and insulin resistance. *Nature* 2002; **420**:333–336.

56 Cai D, Yuan M, Frantz DF, Melendez PA, Hansen L, Lee J, *et al.* Local and systemic insulin resistance resulting from hepatic activation of IKK-beta and NF-kappaB. *Nat Med* 2005; **11**:183–190.

57 Verma IM, Stevenson JK, Schwarz EM, Van Antwerp D, Miyamoto S. Rel/NF-kappa B/I kappa B family: intimate tales of association and dissociation. *Genes Dev* 1995; **9**:2723–2735.

58 Chung HY, Cesari M, Anton S, Marzetti E, Giovannini S, Seo AY, *et al.* Molecular inflammation: underpinnings of aging and age-related diseases. *Ageing Res Rev* 2009; **8**:18–30.

59 Kim JK, Kim YJ, Fillmore JJ, Chen Y, Moore I, Lee J, *et al.* Prevention of fat-induced insulin resistance by salicylate. *J Clin Invest* 2001; **108**:437–446.

60 Yuan M, Konstantopoulos N, Lee J, Hansen L, Li ZW, Karin M, *et al.* Reversal of obesity- and diet-induced insulin resistance with salicylates or targeted disruption of Ikkbeta. *Science* 2001; **293**:1673–1677.

61 Rohl M, Pasparakis M, Baudler S, Baumgartl J, Gautam D, Huth M, *et al.* Conditional disruption of IkappaB kinase 2 fails to prevent obesity-induced insulin resistance. *J Clin Invest* 2004; **113**:474–481.

62 Shoelson SE, Lee J, Yuan M. Inflammation and the IKK beta/I kappa B/NF-kappa B axis in obesity- and diet-induced insulin resistance. *Int J Obes Relat Metab Disord* 2003; **27**(Suppl 3):S49–52.

63 Nakashima N, Sharma PM, Imamura T, Bookstein R, Olefsky JM. The tumor suppressor PTEN negatively regulates insulin signaling in 3T3-L1 adipocytes. *J Biol Chem* 2000; **275**:12889–12895.

64 Mooney RA, Senn J, Cameron S, Inamdar N, Boivin LM, Shang Y, *et al.* Suppressors of cytokine signaling-1 and -6 associate with and inhibit the insulin receptor: a potential mechanism for cytokine-mediated insulin resistance. *J Biol Chem* 2001; **276**:25889–25893.

65 Du K, Herzig S, Kulkarni RN, Montminy M. TRB3: a tribbles homolog that inhibits Akt/PKB activation by insulin in liver. *Science* 2003; **300**:1574–1577.

66 Koo SH, Satoh H, Herzig S, Lee CH, Hedrick S, Kulkarni R, *et al.* PGC-1 promotes insulin resistance in liver through PPAR-alpha-dependent induction of TRB-3. *Nat Med* 2004; **10**:530–534.

67 Blot V, McGraw TE. GLUT4 is internalized by a cholesterol-dependent nystatin-sensitive mechanism inhibited by insulin. *Embo J* 2006; **25**:5648–5658.

68 Ros-Baro A, Lopez-Iglesias C, Peiro S, Bellido D, Palacin M, Zorzano A, *et al.* Lipid rafts are required for GLUT4 internalization in adipose cells. *Proc Natl Acad Sci U S A* 2001; **98**:12050–12055.

69 Thong FS, Bilan PJ, Klip A. The Rab GTPase-activating protein AS160 integrates Akt, protein kinase C, and AMP-activated protein kinase signals regulating GLUT4 traffic. *Diabetes* 2007; **56**:414–423.

70 Jiang L, Fan J, Bai L, Wang Y, Chen Y, Yang L, *et al.* Direct quantification of fusion rate reveals a distal role for AS160 in insulin-stimulated fusion of GLUT4 storage vesicles. *J Biol Chem* 2008; **283**: 8508–8516.

71 Santos JM, Ribeiro SB, Gaya AR, Appell HJ, Duarte JA. Skeletal muscle pathways of contraction-enhanced glucose uptake. *Int J Sports Med* 2008; **29**:785–794.

72 Goodyear LJ. AMP-activated protein kinase: a critical signaling intermediary for exercise-stimulated glucose transport? *Exerc Sport Sci Rev* 2000; **28**:113–116.

73 Mu J, Brozinick JT Jr, Valladares O, Bucan M, Birnbaum MJ. A role for AMP-activated protein kinase in contraction- and hypoxia-regulated glucose transport in skeletal muscle. *Mol Cell* 2001; **7**: 1085–1094.

74 Azzout-Marniche D, Becard D, Guichard C, Foretz M, Ferre P, Foufelle F. Insulin effects on sterol regulatory-element-binding protein-1c (SREBP-1c) transcriptional activity in rat hepatocytes. *Biochem J* 2000; **350**:389–393.

75 Shimano H, Yahagi N, Amemiya-Kudo M, Hasty AH, Osuga J, Tamura Y, *et al.* Sterol regulatory element-binding protein-1 as a key transcription factor for nutritional induction of lipogenic enzyme genes. *J Biol Chem* 1999; **274**:35832–35839.

76 Londos C, Brasaemle DL, Schultz CJ, Adler-Wailes DC, Levin DM, Kimmel AR, *et al.* On the control of lipolysis in adipocytes. *Ann N Y Acad Sci* 1999; **892**:155–168.

77 Holm C. Molecular mechanisms regulating hormone-sensitive lipase and lipolysis. *Biochem Soc Trans* 2003; **31**:1120–1124.

78 Yeaman SJ. Hormone-sensitive lipase: new roles for an old enzyme. *Biochem J* 2004; **379**:11–22.

79 Blanchette-Mackie EJ, Dwyer NK, Barber T, Coxey RA, Takeda T, Rondinone CM, *et al.* Perilipin is located on the surface layer of intracellular lipid droplets in adipocytes. *J Lipid Res* 1995; **36**:1211–1226.

80 Fricke K, Heitland A, Maronde E. Cooperative activation of lipolysis by protein kinase A and protein kinase C pathways in 3T3-L1 adipocytes. *Endocrinology* 2004; **145**:4940–4947.

81 Tansey JT, Sztalryd C, Gruia-Gray J, Roush DL, Zee JV, Gavrilova O, *et al.* Perilipin ablation results in a lean mouse with aberrant adipocyte lipolysis, enhanced leptin production, and resistance to diet-induced obesity. *Proc Natl Acad Sci U S A* 2001; **98**:6494–6499.

82 Arimura N, Horiba T, Imagawa M, Shimizu M, Sato R. The peroxisome proliferator-activated receptor gamma regulates expression of the perilipin gene in adipocytes. *J Biol Chem* 2004; **279**:10070–10076.

83 Fernandez-Novell JM, Bellido D, Vilaro S, Guinovart JJ. Glucose induces the translocation of glycogen synthase to the cell cortex in rat hepatocytes. *Biochem J* 1997; **321**:227–231.

84 Summers SA, Kao AW, Kohn AD, Backus GS, Roth RA, Pessin JE, *et al.* The role of glycogen synthase kinase 3beta in insulin-stimulated glucose metabolism. *J Biol Chem* 1999; **274**:17934–17940.

85 Shrago E, Lardy HA, Nordlie RC, Foster DO. Metabolic and hormonal control of phosphoenolpyruvate carboxykinase and malic enzyme in rat liver. *J Biol Chem* 1963; **238**:3188–3192.

86 Samson SL, Wong NC. Role of Sp1 in insulin regulation of gene expression. *J Mol Endocrinol* 2002; **29**:265–279.

87 Rena G, Woods YL, Prescott AR, Peggie M, Unterman TG, Williams MR, *et al.* Two novel phosphorylation sites on FKHR that are critical for its nuclear exclusion. *Embo J* 2002; **21**:2263–2271.

88 Obsil T, Ghirlando R, Anderson DE, Hickman AB, Dyda F. Two 14-3-3 binding motifs are required for stable association of Forkhead transcription factor FOXO4 with 14-3-3 proteins and inhibition of DNA binding. *Biochemistry* 2003; **42**:15264–15272.

89 Tang ED, Nunez G, Barr FG, Guan KL. Negative regulation of the forkhead transcription factor FKHR by Akt. *J Biol Chem* 1999; **274**:16741–16746.

90 Hall RK, Yamasaki T, Kucera T, Waltner-Law M, O'Brien R, Granner DK. Regulation of phosphoenolpyruvate carboxykinase and insulin-like growth factor-binding protein-1 gene expression by insulin: the role of winged helix/forkhead proteins. *J Biol Chem* 2000; **275**: 30169–30175.

91 Daitoku H, Hatta M, Matsuzaki H, Aratani S, Ohshima T, Miyagishi M, *et al.* Silent information regulator 2 potentiates Foxo1-mediated transcription through its deacetylase activity. *Proc Natl Acad Sci U S A* 2004; **101**:10042–10047.

92 Nakae J, Kitamura T, Kitamura Y, Biggs WH 3rd, Arden KC, Accili D. The forkhead transcription factor Foxo1 regulates adipocyte differentiation. *Dev Cell* 2003; **4**:119–129.

93 Puigserver P, Rhee J, Donovan J, Walkey CJ, Yoon JC, Oriente F, *et al.* Insulin-regulated hepatic gluconeogenesis through FOXO1-PGC-1alpha interaction. *Nature* 2003; **423**:550–555.

94 Raghow R, Yellaturu C, Deng X, Park EA, Elam MB. SREBPs: the crossroads of physiological and pathological lipid homeostasis. *Trends Endocrinol Metab* 2008; **19**:65–73.

95 Matsumoto M, Ogawa W, Teshigawara K, Inoue H, Miyake K, Sakaue H, *et al.* Role of the insulin receptor substrate 1 and phosphatidylinositol 3-kinase signaling pathway in insulin-induced expression of sterol regulatory element binding protein 1c and glucokinase genes in rat hepatocytes. *Diabetes* 2002; **51**:1672–1680.

96 Cao G, Liang Y, Broderick CL, Oldham BA, Beyer TP, Schmidt RJ, *et al.* Antidiabetic action of a liver x receptor agonist mediated by inhibition of hepatic gluconeogenesis. *J Biol Chem* 2003; **278**:1131–1136.

97 Zitzer H, Wente W, Brenner MB, Sewing S, Buschard K, Gromada J, *et al.* Sterol regulatory element-binding protein 1 mediates liver X receptor-beta-induced increases in insulin secretion and insulin messenger ribonucleic acid levels. *Endocrinology* 2006; **147**:3898–3905.

98 Yoon JC, Puigserver P, Chen G, Donovan J, Wu Z, Rhee J, *et al.* Control of hepatic gluconeogenesis through the transcriptional coactivator PGC-1. *Nature* 2001; **413**:131–138.

99 Yeagley D, Guo S, Unterman T, Quinn PG. Gene- and activation-specific mechanisms for insulin inhibition of basal and glucocorticoid-induced insulin-like growth factor binding protein-1 and phosphoenolpyruvate carboxykinase transcription: roles of forkhead and insulin response sequences. *J Biol Chem* 2001; **276**:33705–33710.

100 Garvey WT, Olefsky JM, Griffin J, Hamman RF, Kolterman OG. The effect of insulin treatment on insulin secretion and insulin action in type II diabetes mellitus. *Diabetes* 1985; **34**:222–234.

101 Rossetti L, Giaccari A, DeFronzo RA. Glucose toxicity. *Diabetes Care* 1990; **13**:610–630.

102 Marshall S. Role of insulin, adipocyte hormones, and nutrient-sensing pathways in regulating fuel metabolism and energy homeostasis:

a nutritional perspective of diabetes, obesity, and cancer. *Sci STKE* 2006; 2006: re7.

103 Kadowaki T, Yamauchi T. Adiponectin and adiponectin receptors. *Endocr Rev* 2005; **26**:439–451.

104 Cooksey RC, Hebert LF Jr, Zhu JH, Wofford P, Garvey WT, McClain DA. Mechanism of hexosamine-induced insulin resistance in transgenic mice overexpressing glutamine:fructose-6-phosphate amidotransferase: decreased glucose transporter GLUT4 translocation and reversal by treatment with thiazolidinedione. *Endocrinology* 1999; **140**:1151–1157.

105 D'Alessandris C, Andreozzi F, Federici M, Cardellini M, Brunetti A, Ranalli M, *et al.* Increased O-glycosylation of insulin signaling proteins results in their impaired activation and enhanced susceptibility to apoptosis in pancreatic beta-cells. *Faseb J* 2004; **18**:959–961.

106 Fingar DC, Richardson CJ, Tee AR, Cheatham L, Tsou C, Blenis J. mTOR controls cell cycle progression through its cell growth effectors S6K1 and 4E-BP1/eukaryotic translation initiation factor 4E. *Mol Cell Biol* 2004; **24**:200–216.

107 Burnett PE, Barrow RK, Cohen NA, Snyder SH, Sabatini DM. RAFT1 phosphorylation of the translational regulators p70 S6 kinase and 4E-BP1. *Proc Natl Acad Sci U S A* 1998; **95**:1432–1437.

108 Sarbassov DD, Guertin DA, Ali SM, Sabatini DM. Phosphorylation and regulation of Akt/PKB by the rictor-mTOR complex. *Science* 2005; **307**:1098–1101.

109 Shah OJ, Wang Z, Hunter T. Inappropriate activation of the TSC/Rheb/mTOR/S6K cassette induces IRS1/2 depletion, insulin resistance, and cell survival deficiencies. *Curr Biol* 2004; **14**:1650–1656.

110 Kim DH, Sarbassov DD, Ali SM, King JE, Latek RR, Erdjument-Bromage H, *et al.* mTOR interacts with raptor to form a nutrient-sensitive complex that signals to the cell growth machinery. *Cell* 2002; **110**:163–175.

111 Um SH, Frigerio F, Watanabe M, Picard E, Joaquim M, Sticker M, *et al.* Absence of S6K1 protects against age- and diet-induced obesity while enhancing insulin sensitivity. *Nature* 2004; **431**:200–205.

112 Nobukuni T, Joaquin M, Roccio M, Dann SG, Kim SY, Gulati P, *et al.* Amino acids mediate mTOR/raptor signaling through activation of class 3 phosphatidylinositol 3OH-kinase. *Proc Natl Acad Sci U S A* 2005; **102**:14238–14243.

113 Krebs M, Brunmair B, Brehm A, Artwohl M, Szendroedi J, Nowotny P, *et al.* The Mammalian target of rapamycin pathway regulates nutrient-sensitive glucose uptake in man. *Diabetes* 2007; **56**:1600–1607.

114 Hardie DG. Roles of the AMP-activated/SNF1 protein kinase family in the response to cellular stress. *Biochem Soc Symp* 1999; **64**:13–27.

115 Leclerc I, Kahn A, Doiron B. The 5′-AMP-activated protein kinase inhibits the transcriptional stimulation by glucose in liver cells, acting through the glucose response complex. *FEBS Lett* 1998; **431**:180–184.

116 Yang J, Craddock L, Hong S, Liu ZM. AMP-activated protein kinase suppresses LXR-dependent sterol regulatory element-binding protein-1c transcription in rat hepatoma McA-RH7777 cells. *J Cell Biochem* 2009; **106**:414–426.

117 Nourooz-Zadeh J, Rahimi A, Tajaddini-Sarmadi J, Tritschler H, Rosen P, Halliwell B, *et al.* Relationships between plasma measures of oxidative stress and metabolic control in NIDDM. *Diabetologia* 1997; **40**:647–653.

118 Nathan C. Specificity of a third kind: reactive oxygen and nitrogen intermediates in cell signaling. *J Clin Invest* 2003; **111**:769–778.

119 Dinarello CA. Interleukin-1beta. *Crit Care Med* 2005; **33**:S460–462.

120 Somm E, Cettour-Rose P, Asensio C, Charollais A, Klein M, Theander-Carrillo C, *et al.* Interleukin-1 receptor antagonist is upregulated during diet-induced obesity and regulates insulin sensitivity in rodents. *Diabetologia* 2006; **49**:387–393.

121 Ozcan L, Ergin AS, Lu A, Chung J, Sarkar S, Nie D, *et al.* Endoplasmic reticulum stress plays a central role in development of leptin resistance. *Cell Metab* 2009; **9**:35–51.

122 Scheuner D, Kaufman RJ. The unfolded protein response: a pathway that links insulin demand with beta-cell failure and diabetes. *Endocr Rev* 2008; **29**:317–333.

8 Control of Weight: How Do We Get Fat?

George A. Bray

Pennington Biomedical Research Center, Baton Rouge, LA, USA

Keypoints

- Positive energy balance is the essential ingredient required to store body fat and become overweight.
- It is what the energy balance concept does not tell us that is important; for example, it does not explain genetic factors, gender differences in fatness, or effects of age or medications.
- An epidemiologic model for developing overweight in response to the environment identified food, reductions in energy expenditure, viruses, toxins, and drugs as contributing mechanisms.
- Cost of food has an important role in food choices.
- A homeostatic model for control of food intake and energy expenditure helps isolate the specific mechanisms that can be targeted for understanding and treating the problem.

Introduction

Research over the past two decades has provided an unprecedented expansion of our knowledge about the physiologic and molecular mechanisms regulating body weight and body fat [1]. One great step was the cloning of genes corresponding to five types of obesity in experimental animals that were due to single genes – so-called monogenic obesity syndromes – and the ensuing characterization of the human counterparts to these syndromes [2,3]. Subsequent research has added a number of other genes with lesser effects to the list of genes modifying obesity [4]. Extensive molecular and reverse genetic studies (mouse knockouts) have helped to identify critical pathways regulating body fat and food intake, and have validated or refuted the importance of previously identified pathways [2].

This chapter reviews this rapidly expanding literature from two perspectives. The first is an epidemiologic approach, considering environmental agents that affect the human being. The second views body weight regulation from a "set-point" or homeostatic approach by considering the way in which one part of the metabolic system communicates with another and how this system may be "overridden" by hedonic or pleasure centers.

Textbook of Diabetes, 4th edition. Edited by R. Holt, C. Cockram, A. Flyvbjerg and B. Goldstein.

Genetic factors

The epidemic of overweight is occurring on a genetic background that does not change as fast as the epidemic has been exploding. It is nonetheless clear that genetic factors have an important role in its development [2,4]. One analogy for the role of genes in overweight is that "genes load the gun and a permissive or toxic environment pulls the trigger."

Identification of genetic factors involved in the development of obesity increases yearly. From the time of the early twin and adoption studies more than 10 years ago [2], the focus has been on evaluating large groups of individuals for genetic defects related to the development of overweight [3,4]. These genetic factors can be divided into two groups: the rare genes that produce excess body fat and a group of more common genes that underlie susceptibility to becoming overweight – the so-called 'susceptibility' genes [2,4]. The field of genetic factors has been given a recent boost from genome-wide association studies, in which variants in large populations of tens of thousands of people are examined [4]. Using this genome-wide association strategy, 17 genes are now known that account for a small fraction of the variance in human body weight [5]. The most important of these is the FTO gene, which accounts for half of this effect. All of these genes are thought to affect the regulation of food intake.

Underlying the following discussion is the reality that genetic responses to the environment differ between individuals and affect the magnitude of the weight changes. Several genes have such potent effects that they produce overweight in almost any environment where food is available. Leptin deficiency is one of them [3]. Most other genes that affect the way body weight and body fat vary under different environmental influences have only a small effect. That these small differences exist and differ between individuals accounts for much of the variability in the response to diet that we see.

Epigenetic and intrauterine imprinting

Over the past decade it has become clear that infants who are small for their age are at higher risk for metabolic diseases later in life. This idea was originally proposed by Professor David Barker and is often called the Barker or Developmental Origins of Health and Disease hypothesis [6]. Several examples illustrate its role in human obesity. The first was the Dutch winter famine of 1944, in which the calories available to the residents of the city of Amsterdam were severely reduced by the Nazi occupation [7]. During this famine, intrauterine exposure occurred during all parts of the pregnancy; caloric restriction during the first trimester increased the subsequent risk of overweight in the offspring [7].

Two other examples that fall into the category of fetal imprinting are the increased risk of obesity in offspring of mothers with diabetes [8] and in the offspring of mothers who smoked during the individual's intrauterine period [9,10]. In a study of infants born to Pima Indian women before and after the onset of maternal diabetes, Dabelea *et al.* [8] noted that the infants born after diabetes developed were heavier than those born to the same mother before diabetes developed [11,12]. The risk for overweight at age 3 years was predicted by smoking at first prenatal visit with an odds ratio (OR) of 2.16 (95% confidence interval [CI] 1.05–4.47). Despite being smaller at birth, these infants more than caught up by age 3 years [11,12].

Smoking during pregnancy increases the risk of overweight at entry to school from just under 10% to over 15% if smoking continued throughout pregnancy and to nearly 15% if it was discontinued after the first trimester, indicating that most of the effect is in the early part of pregnancy [13,14].

Environmental agents and overweight: an epidemiologic approach

One way to view the etiology of increased body fat is from the epidemiologic or environmental perspective. Food, medications, viruses, toxins and sedentary lifestyle can each act on the host to produce increased fatness. We need to remember, however, that for each of these agents there are genetic components.

Food is an environmental agent for obesity

We obtain all of our energy from the foods we eat and the beverages we drink. Thus, without food there could be no life, let alone excess stores of fat. The cost of this food is an important determinant of food choices. In addition to cost and total quantity, food styles of eating and specific food components may be important in determining whether or not we become fat.

Costs of food

Economic factors may have an etiologic role in explaining the basis for the intake of a small number of "excess calories" over time that leads to overweight [1]. What we consume is influenced by the price we have to pay for it. In the recent past, particularly since the beginning of the 1970s, the prices of foods that are high in energy density (fat and sugar-rich) have fallen relative to other items. The Consumer Price Index rose by 3.8% per year from 1980 to 2000 [15] compared with the rise in food prices, which rose by 3.4% per year. In the period 1960–1980, when there was only a small increase in the prevalence of overweight, food prices rose at a rate of 5.5% per year – slightly faster than the Consumer Price Index, which grew at a rate of 5.3% per year. The relative prices of foods high in sugar and fat have decreased since the early 1980s compared with those of fruits and vegetables. By comparison, Finkelstein *et al.* [15] note that between 1985 and 2000, the prices of fresh fruits and vegetables rose 118%, fish 77% and dairy 56%, compared with sugar and sweets, which rose only 46%, fats and oils 35% and carbonated beverages only 20%. Is it any wonder that people with limited income eat more sugar and fat-containing foods?

Quantity of food eaten

Eating more food energy over time than we need for our daily energy requirements produces extra fat. In the current epidemic the increase in body weight is on average 0.5–1 kg/year. The amount of net energy storage required by an adult to produce 1 kg of added body weight, 75% of which is fat, can be calculated by using a few assumptions. One kilogram of adipose tissue contains about 7000 kcal (29.4 mJ) of energy. If the efficiency of energy storage were 50%, with the other 50% being used by the synthetic and storage processes, we would need to ingest 14 000 kcal (58.8 mJ) of food energy. As there are 365 days in the year this would be an extra 20 kcal/day (40 kcal/day × 365 day/year = 14 600 kcal) [16]. For simplicity we can round this to 50 kcal/day or the equivalent of 10 teaspoons of sugar.

Has the intake of energy increased? The energy intake (kcal/day) was relatively stable during the first 80 years of the 20th century. During the last 20 years, however, there was a clear rise from about 2300 kcal/day to about 2600 kcal/day, or an increase of 300 kcal/day. This is more than enough to account for the 50 kcal/day net (100 kcal gross) required to produce the 1 kg weight gain each year [17].

Portion size

Portion sizes have dramatically increased in the past 40 years [18] and now need reduction. One consequence of the larger portion sizes is more food and more calories [17]. The US Department of Agriculture (USDA) estimates that between 1984 and 1994 daily calorie intake increased by 340 kcal/day or 14.7%. Refined grains provided 6.2% of this increase, fats and oils 3.4%, but fruits and vegetables only 1.4% and meats and dairy products only 0.3%. Calorically sweetened beverages that contain 10% high-fructose corn syrup (HFCS) are made from these grain products. These beverages are available in containers of 12, 20 or 32 oz, which provide 150, 250 or 400 kcal if all is consumed. Many foods list the calories per serving, but the package often contains more than one serving. In 1954, the burger served by Burger King weighed 2.8 oz and had 202 kcal. By 2004, the size had grown to 4.3 oz and 310 kcal. In 1955, McDonald's served French fries weighing 2.4 oz and having 210 kcal. By 2004, this had increased to 7 oz and 610 kcal. Popcorn served at movie theaters has grown from 3 cups containing 174 kcal in 1950 to 21 cups with 1700 kcal in 2004 [19]. Nielsen & Popkin [18] have examined the portion sizes consumed by Americans and have shown the increased energy intake associated with the larger portions of essentially all items examined. Guidance for intake of beverages suggests intake of more water, tea, coffee and low-fat dairy products with lesser consumption of beverages that contain primarily water and caloric sweeteners [20]. The importance of drinking water as an alternative to consuming calories is suggested in a recent study. There was an inverse relationship between water intake expressed per unit of food and beverage intake and total energy intake. When the water intake was less than 20 g/gram of food + beverages, energy intake was 2485 kcal/day. At the highest quartile, when water intake was at or above 90 g/gram of food + beverage, energy intake had fallen to 1791 kcal/day. Thus, drinking water may be one strategy for lowering overall energy intake [21].

Energy density

Energy density interacts with portion size to affect how much is eaten. Energy density refers to the amount of energy in a given weight of food (kcal/g). Energy density of foods is increased by dehydrating them or by adding fat. Conversely, lower energy density is produced by adding water or removing fat. When energy density of meals was varied and all meals were provided for 2 days, the participants ate the same amount of food, but as a result obtained more energy when the foods were higher in energy density. In this experiment, they obtained about 30% less energy when the meals had low rather than high energy density [22,23]. When energy density and portion size were varied, Kral *et al.* [24] showed that both factors influence the amount that is eaten. The meals with low energy density and small portion sizes provided the fewest calories (398 kcal vs 620 kcal) [24].

Styles of eating

Breastfeeding is a case in which the style of eating can be associated with later weight gain. In infants, breast milk is their first food, and for many infants their sole food for several months. There are now a number of studies showing that breastfeeding for more than 3 months significantly reduces the risk of being overweight at entry into school and in adolescence when compared with infants who are breastfed for less than 3 months [25]. This may be an example of "infant imprinting" [26,27].

Restaurants and fast-food establishments

Eating outside the home has increased significantly over the past 30 years. There are now more fast-food restaurants (277 208) than churches in the USA [28]. The number of fast-food restaurants has risen since 1980 from 1 per 2000 people to 1 per 1000 Americans. Of the 206 meals per capita eaten out in 2002, fast-food restaurants served 74% of them. Other important figures are that Americans spent $100 billion on fast food in 2001, compared to $6 billion in 1970. An average of three orders of French-fried potatoes are ordered per person per week, and French-fried potatoes have become the most widely consumed vegetable. More than 100 000 new food products were introduced between 1990 and 1998. Eating outside the home has become easier over the last four decades as the number of restaurants has increased, and the percent of meals eaten outside the home reflects this. In 1962, less than 10% of meals were eaten outside the home. By 1992 this had risen to nearly 35%, where it has remained. In a telephone survey of body mass index (BMI) in relation to proximity to fast-food restaurants in Minnesota, however, Jeffrey *et al.* [29] found that eating at a fast-food restaurant was associated with having children, with eating a high-fat diet and having a high BMI, but not with proximity to the restaurant.

Eating in a fast-food restaurant also changes the foods consumed [30,31]. Paeratakul *et al.* [30] compared a day in which individuals ate at a fast-food restaurant with a day when they did not. On the day when food was eaten in the fast-food restaurant, less cereal, milk and vegetables were consumed, but more soft drinks and French-fried potatoes were eaten. Similar findings were reported by Bowman *et al.* [31], who reported in addition that on any given day, over 30% of the total sample group consumed fast food. In this national survey, several other features were also associated with eating at fast-food restaurants, including being male, having a higher household income and residing in the US South. Children who ate at fast-food restaurants consumed more energy, more fat and added sugars, and more sweetened beverages than children who did not eat at fast-food restaurants.

Night-eating syndrome

The original description of the night-eating syndrome was published in a classic paper by Stunkard in 1955 and updated recently [32]. Recent studies have refined this syndrome. It consists of individuals who eat more than 50% of their daily energy intake during the nighttime [1].

Frequency of food intake

Frequency of eating may increase the risk of obesity. Crawley & Summerbell [33] showed that among males, but not females, the number of meal-eating events per day was inversely related to BMI. Males with a BMI of 20–25 ate just over 6 times per day compared to less than 6 times for those with a BMI >25 kg/m^2.

Eating breakfast is associated with eating more frequently, and there are data showing that eating breakfast is associated with lower body weight. Eating breakfast cereal has been related to decreased BMI in adolescent girls. Using longitudinal data on adolescent girls, Barton *et al.* [34] showed that as cereal intake per week increased from 0 to 3 times per week, there was a small, but significant, decrease in BMI.

Calorically sweetened soft drinks

One of the consequences of the lower farm prices in the 1970s was a drop in the price of corn, which made inexpensive the production of corn starch which is converted to HFCS. With the development of the isomerase technology in the late 1960s which could convert starch into the highly sweet molecule, fructose, manufacture of soft drinks entered a new era [35]. From the early 1970s through the mid-1990s, HFCS gradually replaced sugar in many manufactured products, and almost entirely replaced sugar in soft drinks manufactured in the USA. In addition to being cheap, HFCS is very sweet. We have argued that this "sweetness" in liquid form is one factor driving the consumption of increased calories which are needed to fuel the current epidemic of obesity.

The relationship of soft-drink consumption to calorie intake, to body weight and to the intake of other dietary components has been examined in both cross-sectional and longitudinal studies [36]. Of the 11 cross-sectional studies examining the relation of caloric intake and soft-drink consumption, nine found a moderately positive association. Among the four longitudinal studies, the strength of the association was slightly stronger. The authors conclude that when humans consume soft drinks there is little caloric compensation. That is, the soft drinks are "added" calories and do not lower the intake of energy in other forms. The strengths of these relationships were stronger in women and in adults. Not surprisingly, they found that studies funded by the food industry had weaker associations than those funded by independent sources.

Several studies on the consumption of calorically sweetened beverages in relation to the epidemic of overweight have received significant attention [35]. Ludwig *et al.* [37] reported that the intake of soft drinks was a predictor of initial BMI in children in the Planet Health Study. They went on to show that higher soft-drink consumption also predicted the increase in BMI during nearly 2 years of follow-up. Those with the highest soft-drink consumption at baseline had the highest increase in BMI. In one of the few randomized well-controlled intervention studies, Danish investigators [38] showed that individuals consuming calorically sweetened beverages during 10 weeks gained weight, whereas subjects drinking the same amount of artificially sweetened beverages lost weight. Equally important, drinking sugar-sweetened beverages was associated with a small, but significant, increase in blood pressure. Women in the Nurses' Health Study [39] also showed that changes in the consumption of soft drinks predicted changes in body weight over several years of follow-up. In children, a study focusing on reducing intake of "fizzy" drinks and replacing them with water showed slower weight gain than for those not advised to reduce the intake of fizzy drinks [40].

Fructose consumption, either in beverages or food, may have an additional detrimental effect. It has been linked to the development of cardiometabolic risk factors and the metabolic syndrome in participants in the Framingham Study [41]. Cross-sectionally, individuals consuming ≥1 soft drink per day had a higher prevalence of the metabolic syndrome (OR 1.48; 95% CI 1.30–1.69) and an increased risk of developing the metabolic syndrome over 4 years of follow-up. It may also increase the risk of gout [42] and diabetes [43].

Dietary fat

Dietary fat is another component of the diet that may be important in the current obesity epidemic [44–46]. In epidemiologic studies, dietary fat intake is related to the fraction of the population that is overweight [45]. In an 8-year follow-up of the Nurses' Health Study, Field *et al.* [47] found a weak overall association of percent fat and a stronger effect of animal fat, saturated fat and *trans* fat on fatness. In experimental animals, high-fat diets generally produce fat storage. In humans, the relationship of dietary fat to the development of overweight is controversial. It is certainly clear that ingesting too many calories is essential for the increase in body fat. Because the storage capacity for carbohydrate is very limited, it must be oxidized first. Thus, when people overeat, they oxidize carbohydrate and store fat. When fat is a large component of a diet, the foods tend to be "energy dense" and thus overconsumption is easy to achieve.

Low levels of physical activity

Epidemiologic data show that low levels of physical activity and watching more television predict higher body weight [48]. Recent studies suggest that individuals in US cities where they had to walk more than people in other cities tended to weigh less [49]. Low levels of physical activity also increase the risk of early mortality [50]. Using normal weight, physically active women as the comparison group, Hu *et al.* [51] found that the relative risk of mortality increased from 1.00 to 1.55 (55%) in inactive lean women compared with active lean ones, to 1.92 in active overweight women, and to 2.42 in women who are overweight and physically inactive. It is thus better to be thin than fat and to be physically active rather than inactive.

Television has been one culprit blamed for the reduced levels of physical activity, particularly in children. The first suggestion that TV viewing was associated with overweight was published by Gortmaker and Dietz. Using data from the National Health Examination Survey [52] and the National Longitudinal Study of Youth [53], they found a linear gradient from 11–12% overweight in children watching 0–2 hours/day to over 20–30% when watching more than 5 hours/day. Since that time a number of studies have shown that in both children and adults, those who watch TV more are more overweight. By one estimate about 100 kcal of extra food energy is ingested for each hour of TV viewing. In studies focusing on reducing sedentary activity, which largely means decreasing TV viewing, there was a significant decrease in energy intake with increased activity [54]. In the Early

Childhood Longitudinal Study, investigators found that between kindergarten and third grade, children watching more TV (OR 1.02) and eating fewer family meals together (OR 1.08) predicted a modest increase in weight [55].

Effect of sleep time and environmental light

Sleep time declines from an average of 14.2 ± 1.9 (mean ± SD) hours/day in infancy (11.0 ± 1.1 hours/day by 1 year of age) to 8.1 ± 0.8 hours/day at 16 years of age [56]. Sleep time declined across the cohorts from 1974 to 1993 due largely to later bedtime, but similar arising time. Nine epidemiologic studies have been published that relate shortness of sleep time with overweight. Six of these studies are cross-sectional in design, and three are longitudinal. The earliest of these studies was only published in 1992, but most were published after 2002. They include both children and adults. In a small case–control study involving 327 short-sleepers compared with 704 controls, Locard *et al.* [57] found that short-sleepers were heavier than the controls.

In two large cross-sectional studies in children, Sekine *et al.* [58] and von Kries *et al.* [59] found that there was a dose-dependent relationship between the amount of sleep and the weight of children when they entered school. Von Kries *et al.* [59] studied 6862 children aged 5–6 years whose sleeping time was reported in 1999–2000 by the parent, and followed-up in 2001–2002. Overweight in this study was defined as a weight for height greater than the 97th percentile. Children with reported sleeping time of less than 10 hours had a prevalence of overweight of 5.4% (95% CI 4.1–7.0), those who slept 10.5–11.0 hours per night had a prevalence of 2.8% (95% CI 2.3–3.3) and those who slept more than 11.5 hours had a prevalence of overweight of 2.1% (95% CI 1.5–2.9). Among the 8274 children from the Toyama Birth Cohort in Japan [58], there was a graded increase in the risk of overweight, defined as a BMI above 25 kg/m^2, as sleep time decreased. If the children who were reported to sleep more than 10 hours at age 3 had an OR of 1.0, those who slept 9–10 hours had an OR of 1.49, those with 8–9 hours sleep an OR of 1.89, and those children who were reported to sleep less than 8 hours had an OR for overweight of 2.87.

Another setting in which lighting has a role in the development of weight gain is seasonal affective depressive syndrome (SADS). For some people, the shortening of the daylight hours with the onset of winter is associated with depression and weight gain. When the days begin to lengthen in the spring this symptom complex is reversed. Current evidence suggests that it is related to changing activity of the serotonin system and can be treated with exposure to light or by manipulating brain levels of serotonin pharmacologically.

Medications that produce weight gain

Several drugs can cause weight gain, including a variety of hormones and psychoactive agents [1,60]. The degree of weight gain is generally less than 10 kg and not sufficient to cause substantial overweight. These drugs may also increase the risk of future type 2 diabetes mellitus.

Toxins

Smoking

The rise of smoking from 1900 to 1970 and its decline during the last 30 years of the 20th century has been tracked by the Centers for Disease Control. Weight gain after stopping smoking is gender-dependent, with men gaining an average of 3.8 kg and women 2.8 kg [61]. In a more recent analysis, men were found to gain 4.4 kg and women 5.0 kg [62] and it was calculated that this gain could account for about one-quarter to one-sixth of the increased prevalence of overweight. Several factors predict the weight gain, including younger age, lower socioeconomic status, heavier smoking and genetic factors [63]. Economists have calculated that a 10% increase in the price of cigarettes could increase BMI by 0.0251 kg/m^2 as a result of the decrease in smoking [64]. Snacks are the major component of food intake that rises when people stop smoking.

Organochlorines

In human beings, we know that body fat stores many "toxic" chemicals and that they are mobilized with weight loss. Backman first showed in 1970s that organochlorines in the body decreased after bariatric surgery. The metabolic rate can be reduced by organochlorine molecules [65], and conceivably prolonged exposure to many chlorinated chemicals in our environment has affected metabolic pathways and energy metabolism. Under these conditions, thyroid hormone synthesis is decreased, plasma T3 and T4 are decreased, thyroid hormone clearance is increased, and mitochondrial oxidation is reduced in skeletal muscle.

Monosodium glutamate

Food additives are another class of chemicals that are widely distributed and may be involved in the current epidemic of overweight. In experimental animals, exposure during the neonatal period to monosodium glutamate, a common flavoring ingredient in food, produces fatness [66].

Viruses as environmental agents

Several viruses produce weight gain in animals and the possibility that they do this in human beings needs more study. (This subject is ably reviewed by Atkinson [67].) It has been known for many years that the injection of several viruses into the central nervous system could produce fatness in mice. The list of viruses now includes canine distemper virus, RAV-7 virus, Borna disease virus, scrapie virus, SMAM-1 virus and three adenoviruses (types 5, 24 and 36). These observations were generally assumed to be pathologic in nature and not relevant to overweight humans. However, the recent finding that antibodies to one of the adenoviruses (AM-36) appear in larger amounts in some overweight humans than in controls challenges this view. This viral syndrome, resulting from AM-36, can be replicated in the ferret, a non-human primate. The features of the syndrome are modest increase in weight and a low cholesterol concentration in the circulation. Further studies are needed to establish that a syndrome of weight loss associated with low concentrations of cholesterol clearly exists in human beings. If so, this would enhance the value of the epidemiologic model.

Regulation of body fat as a problem of homeostatic energy regulation with a hedonic override

A defect in the way the body responds to feedback signals is another way to view the problem of overweight. Such a system has four parts. The control center in the brain is analogous to the thermostat in a heating system. It receives information about the state of the animal or human, transduces this information into neurochemical signals, and activates pathways that lead to or inhibit feeding and the search for food. The signals that the brain receives come from the environment through sense organs and from the body through neural, nutrient or hormonal signals. The response the brain makes includes both the activation and inhibition of motor systems and the modulation of the autonomic nervous system or hormonal control system. Outside of the brain is the so-called controlled system and, for the purpose of this discussion, includes the digestive tract, which ingests, digests and absorbs food; the metabolic systems in liver, muscle and kidney, which transform nutrients; and the adipose tissue, which both stores and releases fatty acids and acts as a secretory endocrine organ [1].

Digestion, metabolism and fat storage

The controlled system consists of the gastrointestinal tract, liver, muscles, fat tissues, cardiovascular–pulmonary–renal system and supporting bone tissue. The ingestion, digestion and absorption of food provide nutrients to the body and also provide signals from these nutrients to the vagus nerve, which provides the major neural control of gastrointestinal function, and from hormones released by the gastrointestinal tract. The nutrients that are absorbed can be metabolized to provide energy, or they can be stored as glycogen in liver, as protein in muscle or as fat in adipose tissue.

The largest part of the energy we expend each day is for "resting" metabolism, which includes the metabolism of food, the transport of sodium, potassium and other ions across cell membranes, repair of DNA, synthesis of protein, the beating of the heart and functioning of the brain, liver and kidneys. Energy expenditure is most strongly associated with fat-free body mass.

We conclude that day-to-day energy balance is either positive or negative. We do not achieve meal-to-meal or day-to-day energy balance. Rather, if we are to avoid weight gain, we must achieve this over a longer time interval.

If we are to maintain a stable body weight, the metabolic mix of carbohydrate, fat and protein that is oxidized by the body must equal the amounts of these nutrients taken in as food. That is, to maintain energy balance requires that the mix of foods we eat be completely metabolized or oxidized. The capacity for storage of carbohydrate as glycogen is very limited and the capacity to store protein is also restricted. Only the fat stores can readily expand to accommodate increasing levels of energy intake above those required for daily energy needs. Several studies now show that a high rate of carbohydrate oxidation, as measured by a high respiratory quotient, predicts future weight gain [68]. One explanation for this is that when carbohydrate oxidation is higher than the intake of carbohydrate, carbohydrate stores are depleted. To replace this carbohydrate, an individual must eat more carbohydrate or reduce the oxidation of carbohydrate by the body, because the body cannot convert fatty acids to carbohydrate and the conversion of amino acids to carbohydrate mobilizes important body proteins [69]. Obese individuals who have lost weight are less effective in increasing fat oxidation in the presence of a high-fat diet than normal weight individuals, and this may be one reason why they are so susceptible to regaining weight that has been lost.

Physical activity gradually declines with age. If we are to avoid becoming overweight as we age, we must gradually reduce our food intake or we must maintain a regular exercise program. A moderate level of exercise is beneficial in two ways. First, it reduces risk of cardiovascular disease and type 2 diabetes, and second, it facilitates the oxidation of fat in the diet [70]. Maintaining an exercise program, however, is difficult for many people, particularly as they get older.

The concept of "energy wasting" through uncoupling proteins is one of the expanding basic science aspects of obesity. The original uncoupling protein-1 (UCP1) found in brown fat has a well-established role in helping newborn infants maintain body temperature. Increased expression and/or activation of this protein uncouples oxidation from phosphorylation by enhancing a leak of protons from the inner mitochondrial space, resulting in the conversion of energy to heat without storing the energy in ATP molecules. The UCP1 molecule is important in human infants, but its importance in adults, because of the very low levels of brown fat (and hence UCP1 expression) in adult humans, has been questioned until recently [71]. This new evidence for active brown adipose tissue in adult humans comes from the use of sophisticated techniques combining glucose uptake in tissues (using the ^{18}fluoro-deoxy-glucose) measured by positron emission tomography and computed tomography. Deposits of brown adipose tissue were demonstrated in the supraclavicular region, along the cervical vertebrae and along thoracic vertebrae. This activity can be blocked by propranolol, a broad-based beta-adrenergic-blocking drug, indicating that this glucose uptake is under control of the sympathetic nervous system. Activity can also be modulated by environmental temperature, with higher temperatures eliminating the uptake and lower temperatures increasing the uptake of labeled glucose. Whether the activity of this tissue can be enhanced by continued stimulation remains to be demonstrated.

The fat cell

The fat cells in adipose tissue serve two major functions. First, they are the cells that store and release fatty acids ingested in the food we eat or synthesized in the liver or fat cell. Second, fat cells are a major endocrine cell, secreting many important metabolic and hormonal molecules [1].

Before fat cells can undertake these functions, however, they must be converted from precursor mesenchymal cells to mature fat cells. *In vitro* studies have shown a two-stage process – proliferation followed by differentiation. The proliferative phase is initiated by hormonal stimulation with insulin and glucocorticoids. After the cells begin to grow they enter a state of differentiation where they acquire the genetic state of mature fat cells that can store fatty acids, break down triglycerides, and make and release the many hormones that characterize the mature fat cell. Most of the fatty acids that are stored in human fat cells are derived from the diet, although these cells maintain the capacity for *de novo* synthesis of fatty acids [72].

The discovery of leptin catapulted the fat cell into the arena of endocrine cells [73]. The finding of a peptide released from adipose tissue that acts at a distance has refocused interest in the fat cell from primarily a cell that stores fatty acids to a cell with endocrine and paracrine functions. In addition to leptin, the fat cell secretes a variety of peptides, including lipoprotein lipase, adipsin (complement D), complement C, adiponectin, tumor necrosis factor-α (TNF-α), interleukin-6 (IL-6), plasminogen activator inhibitor-1 (PAI-1), angiotensinogen, bradykinin and resistin, in addition to other metabolites such as lactate, fatty acids, glycerol and prostacyclin formed from arachidonic acid. This important endocrine tissue has thus greatly expanded its role. Adiponectin and resistin are recent additions to the growing list.

Messages to the brain from the environment and from the body

The brain receives a continuous stream of information from both the external and internal environments that have a role in the control of feeding. The external information provided by sight, sound and smell are all distant signals for identifying food. Taste and texture of foods are proximate signals generated when food enters the mouth. The classic tastes are sweet, sour, bitter and salty as well as "umami," a fifth taste. In nature most "sweet" foods also have vitamins and minerals, because they come from fruits. Sour and particularly bitter foods often contain unwanted chemical compounds. The extreme example of this is "bait shyness" or "taste aversion," the property that some items have that produces a permanent rejection of future food with the same taste. This is a "hard-wired" response in the brain that overrides the usual "feedback" signals.

A taste for fats, specifically unsaturated fatty acids, may be a sixth taste. Receptors on the tongue can identify certain fatty acids. The discovery of taste and smell receptors for polyunsaturated fatty acids on the taste bud that involves a potassium rectifier channel offers an opening into modifying taste inputs into the food-intake system [74]. An important advance was showing that the CD-36 receptor, which binds fatty acids, is the receptor for these fatty acids. These receptors are located on the lingual papillae of the tongue. Mice that do not have the CD36 receptor do not prefer solutions enriched with long-chain fatty acids or a high-fat diet. These receptors are in close proximity to Ebner glands, a source of lingual lipase, which cleaves triglycerides into fatty acids that can activate the CD36 receptor. When this receptor is activated, there is a rise in pancreatic secretions and an increase in their content [75].

Several gastrointestinal peptides have been studied as potential regulators of food intake. Most of these peptides, including cholecystokinin, gastrin-releasing peptide, oxyntomodulin, neuromedin B and polypeptide YY3-36 [76] reduce food intake. Cholecystokinin (CCK) was the first peptide shown to reduce food intake in animals and humans alike [77]. Investigation of the growth hormone secretagogue receptor has led to the identification of a new gastrointestinal hormone involved with the control of feeding. This peptide, ghrelin, is produced in oxyntic cells of the gastric fundus. It is a 28 amino acid peptide with an n-octanoyl residue on the serine in the 3-position. It is encoded by a gene with the symbol GHRL (OMIM 506353, chromosome 3p26-p25), and is derived from a 117 amino acid precursor. It stimulates food intake and reduces energy expenditure by acting on NPY/Agrp neurons that in turn inhibit anorexigenic neuromodulators that function through melanocortin and MC4R and works in animals and human beings when given systemically or into the brain. The level is low in overweight people, suggesting that it may have a role in controlling appetite and weight gain [78–80].

Pancreatic peptides, including amylin, glucagon-like peptide-1 (GLP-1), and enterostatin, also modulate feeding. Amylin is produced in the beta cell of the pancreas along with insulin and is co-secreted. In experimental studies, amylin has been shown to reduce food intake by acting on the amylin (calcitonin-like gene product) receptor. The major locations for this receptor are in the hind-brain and hypothalamus [81]. Pramlintide is a commercial analog of amylin which is currently used to treat diabetes. Both glucagon and its 629 amino acid derivative, GLP-1, reduce food intake in animals and humans. GLP-1 works in the brain and after peripheral administration. Exenatide is a GLP-1-like peptide isolated from the salivary glands of the Gila monster. It has been approved for the treatment of diabetes.

Nutrients may also be afferent signals to reduce food intake. A dip in the circulating level of glucose precedes the onset of eating in more than 50% of the meals in animals and human beings [82]. When this dip is blocked, food intake is delayed. The pattern recognized by this dip is independent of the level from which the drop in glucose begins. The small drop in glucose continues even when food is not available. The dip follows a small rise in insulin, suggesting a relationship of these two signals [1,77].

The brain and food intake

The brain plays the central role as receiver, transducer and transmitter of information from the peripheral organs [83]. This control is accomplished through sensory organs and internal signals that are integrated through central neurotransmitters that in turn activate neural, hormonal and motor efferent pathways.

Function of the right prefrontal cortex (PFC) may be particularly important. Brain diseases that affect the PFC have suggested that this area is involved in cognitive processes relevant for food intake and physical activity, and dysfunction of this area may represent a central event in the etiology of human obesity [84]. Weight gain and overeating were common side effects of frontal leucotomy performed in the mid-1900s for psychosis. Damage to the right frontal lobe can cause the gourmand syndrome, a passion for eating and a specific preference for fine food. Hyperphagia correlates positively with right frontal atrophy and negatively with left frontal atrophy in degenerative dementia. Hypoperfusion of the right frontal lobe using single photon emission computed tomography (SPECT) can be demonstrated in overeating conditions such as Kleine–Levin syndrome. In contrast, hyperactivity of the right PFC can lead to anorexia-like symptoms.

Monoamines, such as norepinephrine, serotonin, dopamine and histamine, as well as certain amino acids and neuropeptides, are involved in the regulation of food intake. The serotonin system has been one of the most extensively studied of the monoamine pathways [1,77]. Its receptors modulate both the quantity of food eaten and macronutrient selection. Stimulation of the serotonin receptors in the paraventricular nucleus reduces fat intake with little or no effect on the intake of protein or carbohydrate. This reduction in fat intake is probably mediated through 5-HT_{2C} receptors, because its effect is attenuated in mice that cannot express the 5-HT_{2C} receptor.

Stimulation of α_1-noradrenergic receptors also reduces food intake [1,77]. Phenylpropanolamine is an agonist acting on this receptor that has a modest inhibition of food intake. Some of the antagonists to the α_1 receptors that are used to treat hypertension produce weight gain, indicating that this receptor is also clinically important.

Stimulation of α_2 receptors increases food intake in experimental animals, and a polymorphism in the α_{2a}-adrenoceptor has been associated with reduced metabolic rate in humans. The activation of β_2 receptors in the brain, however, reduces food intake. These receptors can be activated by agonist drugs (beta-blockers), by releasing norepinephrine in the vicinity of these receptors, or by blocking the reuptake of norepinephrine.

Histamine receptors can also modulate feeding. Stimulation of the H_1 receptor in the central nervous system reduces feeding. Experimentally this has been utilized by modulating the H_3 autoreceptor, which controls histamine release. When the autoreceptor is stimulated, histamine secretion is reduced and food intake increases. Blockade of this H_3 autoreceptor decreases food intake. The histamine system is important in control of feeding because drugs that modulate histamine receptors may produce weight gain.

In animals, seasonally variable dopamine transmission in the suprachiasmatic nucleus appears to drive the storage of food at the appropriate time of year in anticipation of hibernation or migration. Loss-of-function mutations in the D_2 receptor gene are associated with overweight in human beings, and dopamine antagonists can induce obesity in humans. One suggestion is that this is through modulation of nutrient partitioning, with obesity in humans or fat storage in migratory and hibernating species as the results [85].

The opioid receptors were the first group of peptide receptors shown to modulate feeding. They also modulate fat intake [86]. Both the mu and kappa opioid receptors can stimulate feeding. Stimulation of the mu-opioid receptors increases the intake of dietary fat in experimental animals. Corticotropin releasing hormone (CRH) and the closely related urocortin reduce food intake and body weight in experimental animals.

The endocannabinoid system is a most recent addition to the central controllers of feeding [87]. Tetrahydrocannbinol, isolated from the marijuana plant, stimulates food intake. Isolation of the cannabinoid receptor was followed by identification of two fatty acids, anandamide and 2-arachidonoylglycerol, which are endogenous ligands in the brain for this receptor. Infusion of anandamide or 2-arachidonoylglycerol into the brain stimulates food intake. The cannabinoid-1 (CB-1) receptor is a preganglionic receptor, meaning that its activation inhibits synaptic transmission. Antagonists to this receptor have been shown to reduce food intake and lead to weight loss. There is also a peripheral ligand, oleylethanolamide, which inhibits food intake.

The discovery of leptin in 1994 opened a new window on the control of food intake and body weight [1,77,88]. This peptide is produced primarily in adipose tissue, but can also be produced in the placenta and stomach. As a placental hormone it can be used as an indicator of trophoblastic activity in patients with trophoblastic tumors (hydatidiform moles or choriocarcinoma). Leptin is secreted into the circulation and acts on a number of tissues, with the brain being one of its most important targets. The response of leptin-deficient children to leptin indicates the critical role that this peptide has in the control of energy balance.

To act on leptin receptors in the brain, leptin must enter brain tissue, probably by transport across the blood–brain barrier [86]. Leptin acts on receptors in the arcuate nucleus near the base of the brain to regulate, in a reciprocal fashion, the production and release of at least four peptides. Leptin inhibits the production of neuropeptide Y (NPY) and agouti-related peptide (AGRP) while enhancing the production of pro-opiomelanocortin (POMC), the source of α-melanocyte stimulating hormone (α-MSH) and cocaine and amphetamine-related transcript (CART) [86]. NPY is one of the most potent stimulators of food intake. It produces these effects through interaction with either the Y-1 or the Y-5 receptor. Mice that do not make NPY have no disturbances (phenotype) in food intake or body weight.

AGRP is the second peptide that is co-secreted with NPY into the paraventricular nucleus (PVN). This peptide antagonizes the inhibitory effect of α-MSH on food intake. Animals that overexpress AGRP overeat because the inhibitory effects of α-MSH are blocked.

The third peptide of interest in the arcuate nucleus is POMC, which is the precursor for several peptides, including α-MSH. α-MSH acts on the melanocortin-3 and melanocortin-4 (MC4) receptors in the medial hypothalamus to reduce feeding. When these receptors are knocked out by genetic engineering, the mice become grossly overweight. In recent human studies, genetic defects in the melanocortin receptors are associated with significant excess of body weight. Many genetic alterations have been identified in the MC4 receptor, some of which are in the coding region of the gene and others in the regulatory components [89]. Some of these genetic changes profoundly affect feeding, whereas others have little or no effect.

Another important peptide in the arcuate nucleus is CART. This peptide is co-localized with POMC and, like α-MSH, inhibits feeding. Antagonists to these peptides or drugs that prevent them from being degraded would make sense as potential treatment strategies.

Two other peptide systems with neurons located in the lateral hypothalamus in the brain have also been linked to the control of feeding. The first of these is melanin-concentrating hormone (MCH) [90]. This peptide increases food intake when injected into the ventricular system of the brain. It is found almost exclusively in the lateral hypothalamus. Animals that overexpress this peptide gain weight and animals that cannot produce this peptide are lean. These observations suggest an important physiologic function for MCH.

The second peptide is orexin A (also called hypocretin). This peptide was identified in a search of G-protein linked peptides that affect food intake. It increases food intake, but its effects are less robust than those described above. However, it does seem to have a role in sleep.

Another recent addition to the list of peptides involved in feeding is the arginine-phenylalanine-amide group (RFa). The first of these peptides to be isolated from a mollusk had only four amino acids. The structure of the RFa peptides is highly conserved, with nearly 80% homology between the frog, rat, cow and humans [91]. In mammals there are five genes and five receptors for these peptides. The 26 and 43 amino acid members of the RFa peptide family stimulate feeding in mammals and are the ligands for two orphan G-protein coupled receptors located in the lateral hypothalamus and the ventromedial nucleus. This family of peptides has been involved in feeding from early phylogetic times including *Caenorhabdis elegans*. Their role in human beings is not yet established.

Neural and hormonal control of metabolism

The motor system for acquisition of food and the endocrine and autonomic nervous systems provide the major information for control of the major efferent systems involved with acquiring food and regulating body fat stores. Among the endocrine controls are growth hormone, thyroid hormone, gonadal steroids (testosterone and estrogens), glucocorticoids and insulin.

During growth, growth hormone and thyroid hormone work together to increase the growth of the body. At puberty, gonadal steroids enter the picture and lead to shifts in the relationship of body fat to lean body mass in boys and girls. A distinctive role for growth hormone has been suggested from studies with transgenic mice overexpressing growth hormone in the central nervous system. These mice are hyperphagic and obese, and show increased expression of NPY and agouti-related protein as well as marked hyperinsulinemia and peripheral insulin resistance [92]. Testosterone increases lean mass relative to fat and reduces visceral fat. Estrogen has the opposite effect. Testosterone levels fall as human males grow older, and there is a corresponding increase in visceral and total body fat and a decrease in lean body mass in older men. This may be compounded by the decline in growth hormone that is also associated with an increase in fat relative to lean mass, particularly visceral fat.

One recent finding suggests that the activity of the enzyme 11-β-hydroxysteroid dehydrogenase type 1, which reversibly converts cortisone to cortisol, may be important in determining the quantity of visceral adipose tissue. Changes in this enzyme may contribute to the risk of women of developing more visceral fat after menopause. A high level of this enzyme keeps the quantity of cortisol in visceral fat high and provides a fertile ground for developing new fat cells.

The sympathetic nervous system is an important link between the brain and peripheral metabolism. It appears to be involved in the oscillation of fatty acids in visceral fat that accompanies the increased fat as dogs overeat a high-fat diet [93]. Using genetic homologous recombination (knockout) mice lacking the β1, β2 and β3 receptor have been produced. These animals show a normophagic obesity with cold intolerance. They have higher circulating levels of free fatty acids. Thus sympathetic nervous system function is essential to prevent obesity and to resist cold [94–96].

Conclusions

This chapter aims to provide a snapshot of our understanding of the regulatory systems for factors that are etiologic in obesity. Both epidemiologic and metabolic feedback models are reviewed in assembling this information. We have not reached the end of the story. It is clear, however, that we have a much better glimpse into its operation – one that can provide us a better framework for thinking about both the etiology of obesity and its possible treatments.

References

1 Bray GA. *The Metabolic Syndrome and Obesity*. Totawa, NJ: Humana Press, 2007.

2 Pérusse L, Rankinen T, Zuberi A, Chagnon YC, Weisnagel SJ, Argyropoulos G, *et al.* The human obesity gene map: the 2004 update. *Obes Res* 2005; **13**:381–490.

3 Farooqi IS, O'Rahilly S. Genetic evaluation of obese patients. In: Bray GA, Bouchard C, eds. *Handbook of Obesity, Clinical Applications*, 3rd edn. New York: Informa, 2008: 45–54.

4 Willer CJ, Speliotes EK, Loos RJ, Li S, Lindgren CM, Heid IM, *et al.* for the GIANT Consortium. Six new loci associated with body mass

index highlight a neuronal influence on body weight regulation. *Nat Genet* 2009; **41**:25–31.

5 Meyre D, Delplanque J, Chèvre JC, Lecoeur C, Lobbens S, Gallina S, *et al.* Genome-wide association study for early-onset and morbid adult obesity identifies three new risk loci in European populations. *Nat Genet* 2009; **41**:157–159.

6 Barker DJ, Hales CN, Fall CH, Osmond C, Phipps K, Clark PM. Type 2 (non-insulin-dependent) diabetes mellitus, hypertension and hyperlipidaemia (syndrome X): relation to reduced fetal growth. *Diabetologia* 1993; **36**:62–67.

7 Ravelli AC, van Der Meulen JH, Osmond C, Barker DJ, Bleker OP. Obesity at the age of 50 years in men and women exposed to famine prenatally. *Am J Clin Nutr* 1999; **70**:811–816.

8 Dabelea D, Pettitt DJ, Hanson RL, Imperatore G, Bennett PH, Knowler WC. Birth weight, type 2 diabetes, and insulin resistance in Pima Indian children and young adults. *Diabetes Care* 1999; **22**:944–950.

9 Power C, Jefferis BJ. Fetal environment and subsequent obesity: a study of maternal smoking. *Int J Epidemiol* 2002; **31**:413–419.

10 Leary SD, Smith GD, Rogers IS, Reilly JJ, Wells JCK, Ness AR. Smoking during pregnancy and offspring fat and lean mass in childhood. *Obesity* 2006; **14**:2284–2293.

11 Fetita L-A, Sobngwi E, Serradas P, Calvo F, Gautier J-F. Review: Consequences of fetal exposure to material diabetes in offspring. *J Clin Endocrinol Metab* 2006; **91**:3718–3724.

12 Adams, AK, Harvey HE, Prince RJ. Association of material smoking with overweight at age 3 in American Indian Children. *Am J Clin Nutr* 2005; **82**:393–398.

13 Toschke AM, Ehlin AG, von Kries R, Ekbom A, Montgomery SM. Maternal smoking during pregnancy and appetite control in offspring. *J Perinat Med* 2003; **31**:251–256.

14 Arenz S, Rückerl R, Koletzko B, von Kries R. Breast-feeding and childhood obesity: a systematic review. *Int J Obes Relat Metab Disord* 2004; **28**:1247–1256.

15 Finkelstein EA, Ruhm CJ, Kosa KM. Economic causes and consequences of obesity. *Annu Rev Public Health* 2005; **26**:239–257.

16 Hill JO, Peters JC. Environmental contributions to the obesity epidemic. *Science* 1998; **280**:1371–1374.

17 Putnam J, Allshouse JE. *Food Consumption, Prices and Expenditures, 1970–97*. US Department of Agriculture Economic Research Service, 1999.

18 Nielsen SJ, Popkin BM. Patterns and trends in food portion sizes, 1977–1998. *JAMA* 2003; **289**:450–453.

19 Newman C. Why are we so fat? The heavy cost of fat. *Natl Geogr Mag* 2004; **206**:46–61.

20 Popkin BM, Armstrong LE, Bray GM, Caballero B, Frei B, Willett WC. A new proposed guidance system for beverage consumption in the United States. *Am J Clin Nutr* 2006; **83**:529–542. Erratum in: *Am J Clin Nutr* 2007; **86**:525.

21 Stookey JD, Barclay D, Arieff A, Popkin BM. The altered fluid distribution in obesity may reflect plasma hypertonicity. *Eur J Clin Nutr* 2007; **61**:190–199.

22 Bell EA, Castellanos VH, Pelkman CL, Thorwart ML, Rolls BJ. Energy density of foods affects energy intake in normal-weight women. *Am J Clin Nutr* 1998; **67**:412–420.

23 Stubbs RJ, Johnstone AM, Harbron CG, Reid C. Covert manipulation of energy density of high carbohydrate diets in 'pseudo free-living' humans. *Int J Obes Relat Metab Disord* 1998; **22**:885–892.

24 Kral TV, Roe LS, Rolls BJ. Combined effects of energy density and portion size on energy intake in women. *Am J Clin Nutr* 2004; **79**:962–968.

25 Rogers I; EURO-BLCS Study Group. The influence of birthweight and intrauterine environment on adiposity and fat distribution in later life. *Int J Obes Relat Metab Disord* 2003; **27**:755–777.

26 Harder T, Bergmann R, Kallischnigg G, Plagemann A. Duration of breastfeeding and risk of overweight: a meta-analysis. *Am J Epidemiol* 2005; **162**:397–403.

27 Gillman MW, Rifas-Shiman SL, Berkey CS, Frazier AL, Rockett HR, Camargo CA Jr, *et al.* Breast-feeding and overweight in adolescence: within-family analysis [corrected]. *Epidemiology* 2006; **17**:112–114. Erratum in: *Epidemiology* 2007; **18**:506.

28 Tillotson JE. Wal-Mart and our food. *Nutr Today* 2005; **40**:234–237.

29 Jeffery RW, Baxter J, McGuire M, Linde J. Are fast food restaurants an environmental risk factor for obesity? *Int J Behav Nutr Phys Act* 2006; **25**:2.

30 Paeratakul S, Ferdinand DP, Champagne CM, Ryan DH, Bray GA. Fast-food consumption among US adults and children: dietary and nutrient intake profile. *J Am Diet Assoc* 2003; **103**:1332–1338.

31 Bowman SA, Gortmaker SL, Ebbeling CB, Pereira MA, Ludwig DS. Effects of fast-food consumption on energy intake and diet quality among children in a national household survey. *Pediatrics* 2004; **113**:112–118.

32 Allison KC, Engel SG, Crosby RD, de Zwaan M, O'Reardon JP, Wonderlich SA, *et al.* Evaluation of diagnostic criteria for night eating syndrome using item response theory analysis. *Eat Behav* 2008; **9**:398–407.

33 Crawley H, Summerbell C. Feeding frequency and BMI among teenagers aged 16–17 years. *Int J Obes Relat Metab Disord* 1997; **21**:159–161.

34 Barton BA, Eldridge AL, Thompson D, Affenito SG, Striegel-Moore RH, Franko DL, *et al.* The relationship of breakfast and cereal consumption to nutrient intake and body mass index: the National Heart, Lung, and Blood Institute Growth and Health Study. *J Am Diet Assoc* 2005; **105**:1383–1389.

35 Bray GA, Nielsen SJ, Popkin BM. Consumption of high-fructose corn syrup in beverages may play a role in the epidemic of obesity. *Am J Clin Nutr* 2004; **79**:537–543. Erratum in: *Am J Clin Nutr* 2004; **80**:1090.

36 Vartanian LR, Schwartz MB, Brownell KD. Effects of soft drink consumption on nutrition and health: a systematic review and meta-analysis. *Am J Public Health* 2007; **97**:667–675.

37 Ludwig DS, Peterson KE, Gortmaker SL. Relation between consumption of sugar-sweetened drinks and childhood obesity: a prospective, observational analysis. *Lancet* 2001; **357**:505–508.

38 Raben A, Agerholm-Larsen L, Flint A, Holst JJ, Astrup A. Meals with similar energy densities but rich in protein, fat, carbohydrate, or alcohol have different effects on energy expenditure and substrate metabolism but not on appetite and energy intake. *Am J Clin Nutr* 2003; **77**:91–100.

39 Schulze MB, Manson JE, Ludwig DS, Colditz GA, Stampfer MJ, Willett WC, *et al.* Sugar-sweetened beverages, weight gain, and incidence of type 2 diabetes in young and middle-aged women. *JAMA* 2004; **292**:927–934.

40 James J, Thomas P, Cavan D, Kerr D. Preventing childhood obesity by reducing consumption of carbonated drinks: cluster randomised controlled trial. *BMJ* 2004; **328**:1237. Erratum in: *BMJ* 2004; **328**:1236.

41 Dhingra R, Sullivan L, Jacques RF, Wang TJ, Fox CS, Meigs JB, *et al.* Soft drink consumption and risk of developing cardiometabolic risk factors and the metabolic syndrome in middle-aged adults in the community. *Circulation* 2007; **116**:480–488. Erratum in: *Circulation* 2007; **116**:e557.
42 Choi HK, Curhan G. Soft drinks, fructose consumption, and the risk of gout in men: prospective cohort study. *BMJ* 2008; **336**:309–312.
43 Johnson RJ, Perez-Pozo SE, Sautin YY, Manitius J, Sanchez-Lozada LG, Feig DI, *et al.* Hypothesis: could excessive fructose intake and uric acid cause type 2 diabetes? *Endocr Rev* 2009; **30**:96–116.
44 Astrup A, Grunwald GK, Melanson EL, Saris WH, Hill JO. The role of low-fat diets in body weight control: a meta-analysis of ad libitum dietary intervention studies. *Int J Obes Relat Metab Disord* 2000; **24**:1545–1552.
45 Bray GA, Popkin BM. Dietary fat intake does affect obesity! *Am J Clin Nutr* 1998; **68**:1157–1173.
46 Bray GA, Flatt JP, Volaufova J, Delany JP, Champagne CM. Corrective responses in human food intake identified from an analysis of 7-day food-intake records. *Am J Clin Nutr* 2008; **88**:1504–1510.
47 Field AE, Willet WC, Lissner L, Colditz GA. Dietary fat and weight gain among women in the Nurses' Health Study. *Obesity* 2007; **15**: 967–976.
48 Hancox RJ, Milne BJ, Poulton R. Association between child and adolescent television viewing and adult health: a longitudinal birth cohort study. *Lancet* 2004; **364**:257–262.
49 Saelens BE, Sallis JF, Black JB, Chen D. Neighborhood-based differences in physical activity: an environment scale evaluation. *Am J Public Health* 2003; **93**:1552–1558.
50 Blair SN, Brodney S. Effects of physical inactivity and obesity on morbidity and mortality: current evidence and research issues. *Med Sci Sports Exerc* 1999; **31**(11 Suppl):S646–662.
51 Hu FB, Willett WC, Li T, Stampfer MJ, Colditz GA, Manson JE. Adiposity as compared with physical activity in predicting mortality among women. *N Engl J Med* 2004; **351**:2694–2703.
52 Dietz WH Jr, Gortmaker SL. Do we fatten our children at the television set? Obesity and television viewing in children and adolescents. *Pediatrics* 1985; **75**:807–812.
53 Gortmaker SL, Must A, Sobol AM, Peterson K, Colditz GA, Dietz WH. Television viewing as a cause of increasing obesity among children in the United States, 1986–1990. *Arch Pediatr Adolesc Med* 1996; **150**:356–362.
54 Epstein LH, Roemmich JN, Paluch RA, Raynor HA. Influence of changes in sedentary behavior on energy and macronutrient intake in youth. *Am J Clin Nutr* 2005; **81**:361–366.
55 Gable S, Change Y, Kruss JL. Television watching and frequency of family meals are predictive of overweight onset and persistence in a national sample of school-aged children. *J Am Diet Assoc* 2007; **107**: 53–61.
56 Iglowinski I, Jenni OG, Molinari L, Largo RH. Sleep duration from infancy to adolescence: reference values and generational trends. *Pediatrics* 2003; **111**:302–307.
57 Locard E, Mamelle N, Billette A, Miginiac M, Munoz F, Rey S. Risk factors of obesity in a five year old population: parental versus environmental factors. *Int J Obes Relat Metab Disord* 1992; **16**:721–729.
58 Sekine M, Yamagami T, Handa K, Saito T, Nanri S, Kawaminami K, *et al.* A dose–response relationship between short sleeping hours and childhood obesity: results of the Toyama Birth Cohort Study. *Child Care Health Dev* 2002; **28**:163–170.
59 von Kries R, Toschke AM, Wurmser H, Sauerwald T, Koletzko B. Reduced risk for overweight and obesity in 5- and 6-year-old children by duration of sleep: a cross-sectional study. *Int J Obes Relat Metab Disord* 2002; **26**:710–716.
60 Allison DB, Mentore JL, Heo M, Chandler LP, Cappelleri JC, Infante MC, *et al.* Antipsychotic-induced weight gain: a comprehensive research synthesis. *Am J Psychiatry* 1999; **156**:1686–1696.
61 Williamson DF, Madans J, Anda RF, Kleinman JC, Giovino GA, Byers T. Smoking cessation and severity of weight gain in a national cohort. *N Engl J Med* 1991; **324**:739–745.
62 Flegal KM, Troiano RP, Pamuk ER, Kuczmarski RJ, Campbell SM. The influence of smoking cessation on the prevalence of overweight in the United States. *N Engl J Med* 1995; **333**:1165–1170.
63 Filizof C, Fernandez Pinilla MC, Fernandez-Crus A. Smoking cessation and weight gain. *Obes Rev* 2004; **5**:95–103.
64 Cutler DM, Glaeser EL, Shapiro JM. Why have Americans become more obese? *J Econ Perspect* 2003; **17**:93–118.
65 Tremblay A, Pelletier C, Doucet E, Imbeault P. Thermogenesis and weight loss in obese individuals: a primary association with organochlorine pollution. *Int J Obes Relat Metab Disord* 2004; **28**:936–939.
66 Olney JW. Brain lesions, obesity, and other disturbances in mice treated with monosodium glutamate. *Science* 1969; **164**:719–721.
67 Atkinson RL. Viruses as an etiology of obesity. *Proc Mayo Clin* 2007; **82**:1192–1198.
68 Zurlo F, Lillioja S, Esposito-Del Puente A, Nyomba BL, Raz I, Saad MF, *et al.* Low ratio of fat to carbohydrate oxidation as predictor of weight gain: study of 24-h RQ. *Am J Physiol* 1990; **259**:E650–657.
69 Flatt JP. Use and storage of carbohydrate and fat. *Am J Clin Nutr* 1995; **61**(Suppl):952S–959S.
70 Smith SR, de Jonge L, Zachwieja JJ, Roy H, Nguyen T, Rood JC, *et al.* Fat and carbohydrate balances during adaptation to a high-fat. *Am J Clin Nutr* 2000; **71**:450–457.
71 Nedergaard J, Bengtsson T, Cannon B. Unexpected evidence for active brown adipose tissue in adult humans. *Am J Physiol* 2007; **293**:E444–E452.
72 Hellerstein MK, Neese RA, Schwarz JM. Model for measuring absolute rates of hepatic *de novo* lipogenesis and reesterification of free fatty acids. *Am J Physiol* 1993; **265**:E814–820.
73 Zhang Y, Proenca R, Maffei M, Barone M, Leopold L, Friedman JM. Positional cloning of the mouse obese gene and its human homologue. *Nature* 1994; **372**:425–432. Erratum in: *Nature* 1995; **374**:479.
74 Gilbertson TA, Liu L, Kim I, Burks CA, Hansen DR. Fatty acid responses in taste cells from obesity-prone and -resistant rats. *Physiol Behav* 2005; **86**:681–690.
75 Laugerette F, Passilly-Degrace P, Patris B, Niot I, Febbraio M, Montmayeur JP, *et al.* CD36 involvement in orosensory detection of dietary lipids, spontaneous fat preference, and digestive secretions. *J Clin Invest* 2005; **115**:3177–3184.
76 Beglinger C, Degen L. Gastrointestinal satiety signals in humans: physiologic roles for GLP-1 and PYY? *Physiol Behav* 2006; **89**:460–464.
77 Bray GA, Greenway FL. Current and potential drugs for treatment of obesity. *Endocr Rev* 1999; **20**:805–875.
78 Cummings DE. Ghrelin and the short-and long-term regulation of appetite and body weight. *Physiol Behav* 2006; **89**:71–84.
79 Abizaid A, Liu ZW, Andrews ZB, Shanabrough M, Borok E, Elsworth JD, *et al.* Ghrelin modulates the activity and synaptic input organiza-

tion of midbrain dopamine neurons while promotong appetite. *J Clin Invest* 2006; **116**:3229–3239.

80 Theander-Carrillo C, Wiedmer P, Cettour-Rose P, Nogueiras R, Perez-Tilve D, Pfluger P, *et al.* Ghrelin action in the brain controls adipocyte metabolism *J Clin Invest* 2006; **116**:1983–1993.

81 Barth SW, Riediger T, Lutz TA, Rechkemmer G. Peripheral amylin activates circumventricular organs expressing calcitonin receptor a/b subtypes and receptor-activity modifying proteins in the rat. *Brain Res* 2004; **997**:97–102.

82 Campfield LA, Smith FJ. Blood glucose dynamics and control of meal initiation: a pattern detection and recognition theory. *Physiol Rev* 2003; **83**:25–58.

83 Berthoud HR, Morrison C. The brain, appetite, and obesity. *Annu Rev Psychol* 2008; **59**:55–92.

84 Alonso-Alonso M, Pascual-Leone A. The right brain hypothesis for obesity. *JAMA* 2007; **297**:1819–1822.

85 Pijl H. Reduced dopaminergic tone in hypothalamic neural circuits: expression of a "thrifty" genotype underlying the metabolic syndrome? *Eur J Pharmacol* 2003; **480**:125–131.

86 Cowley MA, Pronchuk N, Fan W, Dinulescu DM, Colmers WF, Cone RD. Integration of NPY, AGRP, and melanocortin signals in the hypothalamic paraventricular nucleus: evidence of a cellular basis for the adipostat. *Neuron* 1999; **24**:155–163.

87 Pagotto U, Marsicano G, Cota D, Lutz B, Pasquali R. The emerging role of the endocannabinoid system in endocrine regulation and energy balance. *Endocr Rev* 2006; **27**:73–100.

88 Hida K, Wada J, Eguchi J, Zhang H, Baba M, Seida A, *et al.* Visceral adipose tissue-derived serine protease inhibitor: a unique insulin-sensitizing adipocytokine in obesity. *Proc Natl Acad Sci U S A* 2005; **102**:10610–10615.

89 Farooqi IS, Keogh JM, Yeo GS, Lank EJ, Cheetham T, O'Rahilly S. Clinical spectrum of obesity and mutations in the melanocortin 4 receptor gene. *N Engl J Med* 2003; **348**:1085–1095.

90 Ludwig DS, Tritos NA, Mastaitis JW, Kulkarni R, Kokkotou E, Elmquist J, *et al.* Melanin-concentrating hormone overexpression in transgenic mice leads to obesity and insulin resistance. *J Clin Invest* 2001; **107**:379–386.

91 Dockray GJ. The expanding family of -RFamide peptides and their effects on feeding behaviour. *Exp Physiol* 2004; **89**:229–235.

92 Bohlooly-YM, Olsson B, Bruder CE, Lindén D, Sjögren K, Bjursell M, *et al.* Growth hormone overexpression in the central nervous system results in hyperphagia-induced obesity associated with insulin resistance and dyslipidemia. *Diabetes* 2005; **54**:51–62. Erratum in: *Diabetes* 2005; **54**:1249.

93 Hücking K, Hamilton-Wessler M, Ellmerer M, Bergman RN. Burst-like control of lipolysis by the sympathetic nervous system *in vivo. J Clin Invest* 2003; **111**:257–264.

94 Himenez M, Leger B, Canola K, Lehr L, Arboit P, Seydoux J, *et al.* B1/B2/B3 adrenoceptor knockout mice are obese and cold-sensitive but have normal lipolytic responses to fasting. *FEBS Lett* 2002; **530**:37–40.

95 Travernier G, Jimenez M, Giacobino J-P, Hulo N, Lafontan M, Muzzin P, *et al.* Norepinephrine induces lipolysis in B1/B2/B2 adrenoceptor knockout mice. *Mol Pharmacol* 2005; **68**:793–799.

96 Soloveva V, Graves RA, Rasenick MM, Spiegelman BM, Ross SR. Transgenic mice overexpressing the b1 adrenergic receptor in adipose tissue are resistant to obesity. *Mol Endocrinol* 1997; **11**:27–38.

3 Pathogenesis of Diabetes

9 Type 1 Diabetes

Autoimmune Type 1 Diabetes

Ahmed J. Delli, Helena Elding Larsson, Sten-A. Ivarsson & Åke Lernmark
Department of Clinical Sciences, University Hospital MAS, Malmö, Sweden

Other Disorders with Type 1 Phenotype

Alice P.S. Kong & Juliana C.N. Chan
Department of Medicine and Therapeutics, The Chinese University of Hong Kong and The Prince of Wales Hospital, Hong Kong

Autoimmune type 1 diabetes

Ahmed J. Delli, Helena Elding Larsson, Sten-A. Ivarsson & Åke Lernmark

Keypoints

- The pathophysiologic mechanisms in type 1 diabetes (T1DM) involve loss of islet β-cell secretory function caused by selective killing of these cells primarily by aggressive autoimmune responses involving both cellular and humoral immune pathways.
- Inflammatory cells heavily infiltrate pancreatic islets leading to insulitis where $CD8^+$ T lymphocytes are thought to be responsible for selective and specific killing of β-cells.
- The complex etiology of T1DM involves a strong genetic predisposition, mainly human leukocyte antigen class II genes, and several putative environmental factors, which are thought to trigger autoimmunity or progression to clinical T1DM.
- A preclinical prodrome in T1DM may vary in duration in which one or more islet autoantibodies may precede insulitis and predict the disease at the early stages of pathologic insult.
- In genetically susceptible individuals with islet autoantibodies, metabolic indicators such as insulin release abnormalities and insulin resistance may best predict T1DM especially near clinical onset.
- Based on the improving understanding of the etiopathogenesis of T1DM, several clinical trials have been launched aiming at halting the autoimmunity responses, retarding disease progression or preserving remaining β-cell function after clinical onset.

Introduction

The differentiation between the two main forms of diabetes mellitus – type 1 (previously known as insulin dependent or juvenile onset) and type 2 diabetes (non-insulin dependent or adult onset) – has been possible for almost 50 years. In 1965, insulitis was rediscovered [1], supporting the view that autoimmune islet inflammation was associated with the etiopathology in type 1 diabetes mellitus (T1DM), a phenomenon absent in type 2 diabetes mellitus (T2DM) [2].The evidence for islet autoimmunity was further supported during the last decade by the identification of cellular reactivity with islet antigens [3] and the association between T1DM and other organ-specific autoimmune disorders [4]. More importantly, the long sought after antibodies against islet cells (ICA) were finally detected in sera of patients with concomitant T1DM and autoimmune polyendocrine syndrome [5]. At the same time, T1DM was found to be strongly associated

Textbook of Diabetes, 4th edition. Edited by R. Holt, C. Cockram, A. Flyvbjerg and B. Goldstein.

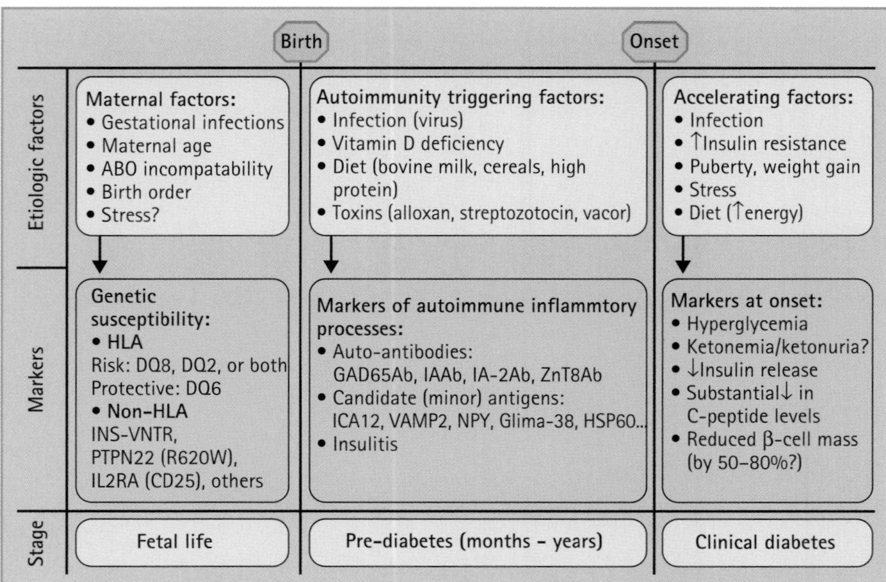

Figure 9.1 Schematic presentation of the natural history of type 1 diabetes (T1DM) showing possible etiopathologic factors and disease markers.

with the human leukocyte antigen (HLA) [6]. It was also noted, however, that around 10% of adult patients classified as having T2DM were positive for ICA, a group of patients now commonly known as having latent autoimmune diabetes of adults (LADA) [7]. Several genetic and autoimmune similarities are found between childhood T1DM and LADA; nevertheless, these two entities differ in other genetic and autoimmune processes [8].

T1DM results from an almost complete loss of insulin brought about by selective autoimmune destruction of the pancreatic islets β-cells, which manifests clinically as hyperglycemia-related symptoms and signs. Among non-Hispanic Caucasian populations, more than 90% of T1DM is immune-mediated (also known as T1ADM), in which HLA association is documented and one or more islet cell autoantibodies are detectable at time of diagnosis [2]. The remaining 10%, often termed "idiopathic" (also known as T1BDM as discussed later in this chapter), is highly inheritable but has neither HLA associations nor detectable islet cell autoantibodies [2]. The latter subgroup is found among non-Caucasian ethnic groups such as Asians [9], African-Americans and Hispanic-Americans and is thought to be related to viral infections [2,10]. Clinically, the two forms have similar clinical manifestations and diabetic ketoacidosis may develop in both.

The pathophysiologic mechanisms in T1DM include two distinct stages in genetically susceptible individuals:

1 Triggering of autoimmunity resulting in one or multiple islet cell autoantibodies associated with gradual β-cell killing; and

2 Loss of β-cell secretory function manifested by the loss of first-phase insulin release (FPIR), reduced C peptide levels, then glucose intolerance and finally hyperglycemia (Figure 9.1).

The autoimmune process with mononuclear infiltration of inflammatory cells (insulitis) including autoreactive $CD8^+$ T lymphocytes selectively destroys the β-cells. Both the humoral and cellular pathways of immunity are involved in the disease process; however, the role of B lymphocytes is evident in laboratory animals such as the non-obese diabetic (NOD) mice but not in humans [11]. Islet autoantibodies, however, may be present before insulitis [12] and therefore may not be a direct consequence of insulitis but rather markers of ensuing islet autoimmunity. The induction of islet autoimmunity in genetically susceptible individuals and the appearance of autoantibodies against specific islet cells autoantigens may precede the clinical syndrome by months to several years (Figure 9.2) [13]. During

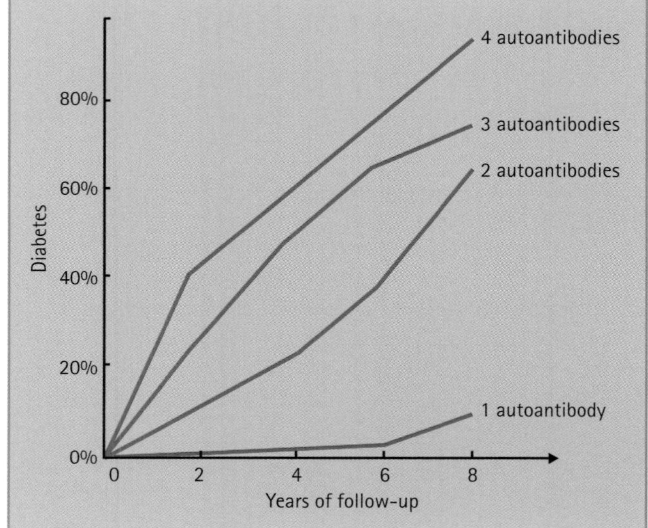

Figure 9.2 Diagrammatic presentation showing the effects of multiple islet autoantibodies on the risk of type 1 diabetes (T1DM) in the Diabetes Prevention Trial Type 1 (DTP-1). Courtesy of Jay Skyler.

this autoimmunity period the number of islet autoantibodies may reflect how β-cells are gradually destroyed. It is proposed that clinical manifestations became overt after loss of more than 80% of viable β-cell mass [14], although there may be variable degrees of both cellular regeneration and insulin sensitivity (Figure 9.3) [15].

The continuing progress in the understanding of the natural history of T1DM will be dependent on several longitudinal studies aiming at detecting factors that predict the disease and to implement both prevention and intervention trials.

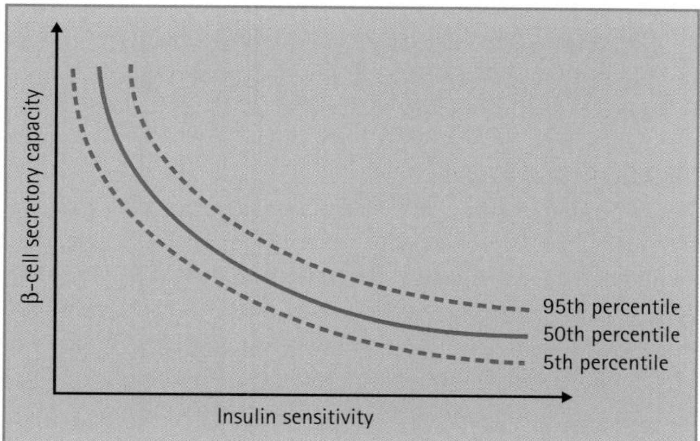

Figure 9.3 The relation between β-cell secretory capacity and insulin sensitivity. Courtesy of Carla Greenbaum, after Kahn *et al.* [15].

Etiology

The etiology of T1DM is multifaceted and may be divided into genetic and environmental etiology and possible gene–environment interactions. Genetic susceptibility increases predisposition for triggering islet autoimmune responses (Figure 9.1). Genetic factors may also help to accelerate the failure of β-cell secretion in response to exogenous environmental factors such as obesity.

Genetics

The concordance rate of T1DM among monozygotic twins ranges from 30–50% up to 70% [16], depending on follow-up duration, compared to only 10–19% among dizygotic twins [17]. This variability highlights the complexity of etiologic components of T1DM that involves the interaction of multiple genetic factors with a variety of environmental factors. Although more than 85% of T1DM occurs in individuals with no previous first-degree family history, the risk among first-degree relatives is about 15 times higher than the general population [18]. An affected father confers a 6–9% risk of T1DM to his offspring compared to 2–4% if the mother is affected and up to 30% risk if both parents are affected [18,19].

The genetics of T1DM has been studied extensively despite the fact that the mode of inheritance remains uncertain. Recent genome-wide association studies have confirmed the strong associations between T1DM and HLA; however, at least 47 non-HLA genetic factors are thought to contribute. The most prominent genetic factors are listed in Table 9.1.

Table 9.1 The most important genetic factors associated with the risk of type 1 diabetes mellitus (T1DM).

Genetic factor	Location	Description		Odds ratio
HLA genes*	Chr.6p21	Highest risk *Genotype*	*DR3-DQ2/DR4-DQ8*	18.7
HLA class II		Highest risk *Haplotypes*	*DR4-DQ8 (DRB1*04‡-DQA1*0301-B1*0302)*	2.0–11.4
			*DR3-DQ2 (DRB1*03-DQA1*0501-B1*0201)*	2.5–5.0
		Most protective *Haplotypes*	*DR15-DQ6 (DRB1*15-DQA1*0102-B1*0602)*	0.03–0.2
			*DR14-DQ5 (DRB1*14-DQA1*0101-B1*0503)*	0.02
Non-HLA genes†				
INS-VNTR	Chr.11p15	Insulin II: Regulate central tolerance to insulin		2.25
PTPN22	Chr.1p13	PTPN8, LYP. Protein tyrosine phosphatase non-receptor type 22		1.95
IL2RA (CD25)	Chr.10p15	Interleukin-2 receptor, alfa chain		1.70
C12orf30	Chr.12q24	Shares similarity with KIAA0614 protein		1.33
ERBB3	Chr.12p13	v-erb-b2 erythroblastic leukemia viral oncogene homolog 3		1.25
PTPN2	Chr.18p11	Protein tyrosine phosphatase non-receptor type 2		1.22
CLEC16A	Chr.16p13	KIAA0350: C-type lectine domain family 16, member A		1.22
CTLA-4	Chr.2q33	Cytotoxic T-lymphocyte-associated protein-4		1.20
IFH1 (MDA5)	Chr.2q24	Interferon induced with helicase C domain 1		1.15

HLA, human leukocyte antigen.
*The odds ratio (OR) varies and ranges shown represent high-risk populations. Data from [24,26].
† OR, odds ratio at 95% confidence interval. Data from [27].
‡ Not *DRB1*0403*.

The major histocompatibility complex (MHC) of the short arm of chromosome 6 harbors the main loci involved in the genetic susceptibility of T1DM as well as many other autoimmune diseases [20]. The HLA genes represent almost 50% of the familial risk of T1DM. Certain alleles of the HLA region, such as the HLA class II DR and DQ alleles, are mainly present in specific association with each other, a phenomenon known as linkage disequilibrium. The HLA association of T1DM (Table 9.1) is therefore often described by haplotype or genotype of the individual [21].

The genotype that confers the highest risk of T1DM is the heterozygosity of the two high-risk HLA class II haplotypes: DR3-DQ2 (*DRB1*03-DQA1*0501-B1*0201*) and DR4-DQ8 (*DRB1*04-DQA1*0301-B1*0302*) (Table 9.1) [21,22]. One or both of these haplotypes were found in more than 95% of people with T1DM younger than 30 years but also in approximately 40–50% of the general population [23]. The concomitant inheritance of high-risk alleles and haplotypes appears to increase the risk of T1DM significantly through synergistic association of their single risks. For example, in patients with T1DM, DQ8 (*DQA1*0301-B1*0302*) is mostly inherited with certain variants of *DRB1*04* especially *DRB1*0401*, *DRB1*0404*, *DRB1*0402* but not *DRB1*0403* which has negative association (Table 9.1). DQ2 (*DQA1*0501-B1*0201*), however, is mostly inherited with *DRB1*03* [21,24]. While certain alleles confer higher risk, such as *DQB1*0302*, *DRB1*03* and *DRB1*0401*, which possesses an independent risk, others confer protection and may "neutralize" high-risk alleles when they are inherited together [25]. The most common protective haplotypes are DQ6 (*DQA1*0102-B1*0602* and *DQA1*0102-B1*0603*), also *DQA1*0101-B1*0503* and *DQA1*0202-B1*0303* [21,26]. Furthermore, other HLA class II (such as DPB1) and class I alleles have also been associated with T1DM risk and the search for new associations is continuing (for review see [24]).

Using a candidate gene approach, several other non-HLA genes were found to be associated with increased risk of T1DM, but their contribution is less than the HLA haplotype associations (for references see http://www.t1dbase.org/page/Welcome/display or the T1D Genome Consortium website: https://www.t1dgc.org/home.cfm). The most important genes are *INS-VNTR* on chromosome 11, *PTPN22* (*LYP*) on chromosome 1, *IL2RA* (*CD25*) on chromosome 10 (Table 9.1) [27].

Environmental factors

The concordance rate of 50–70% among identical twins [16], the seasonality of diabetes incidence and time of birth [28], the association of diabetes with viral infections [29] and the fact that only 10% of HLA-susceptible individuals develop T1DM [28] are among several observations that indicate a possible etiologic role of environmental factors (Figure 9.1).

Table 9.2 The main putative environmental risk factors associated with type 1 diabetes mellitus (T1DM).

Factor	Proposed effect mechanisms	Examples
Maternal factors	Triggering autoimmune response	Gestational infections
	Unknown	Higher maternal age
	Unknown	Higher birth order
	Unknown	ABO blood group incompatibility
Virus infections	Direct β-cell killing (cytolysis)	Mumps virus
	Mimicry of β-cell autoantigens	Rubella virus
	Autoreactive T-cell activation and subsequent β-cell killing	Enterovirus/Coxsackie B virus Rotavirus
	Inhibition of insulin production through inducing expression of HLA genes and interferon	Cytomegalovirus Epstein–Barr virus
Dietary factors	Triggering autoimmune response	Bovine milk/short breastfeeding
	Triggering autoimmune response	Cereals
	Unknown	High protein content
	Lack of possible protective effect of vitamin D	Vitamin D deficiency
Factors related to insulin sensitivity and/or resistance	Stressing β-cells with excess demands "accelerator hypothesis"	Puberty High energy food
	Increase insulin resistance	Weight gain
Psychologic stress	Affect hypothalamic-pituitary-adrenal axis leading to disturbance in autonomic nervous system and autoimmune dysregulation	Stress during pregnancy Child–parent separation Behavioral deviances Difficult adaptation
Toxic substances	Direct damage to β-cells	Alloxan Streptozocin Vacor

The most prominent environmental factors (Table 9.2) include maternal factors [30], viral infections [29], dietary [31,32], high birth weight and growth rate [33], psychologic stress [34] and toxic substances [35]. The concurrent association of islet autoimmunity and factors increasing insulin resistance such as obesity and accelerated growth may boost the autoimmune destruction of β-cells [36]. The hygiene hypothesis proposes that better sanitation created a pathogen-free environment reducing the exposure to pathogens and their products. According to this hypothesis, the immune systems of children tend to be underdeveloped and therefore prone to autoimmune reactions. Additionally, it was also proposed that younger children received low-level antibodies from their mothers and, when exposed to infections such as enterovirus, it increased their T1DM risk [29].

Pathogenesis

Autoimmune T1DM results from loss of immunologic tolerance to β-cells and environmental factors are thought to be involved in initiation or promotion of autoimmunity or both [28]. The selective destruction of β-cells implies specific mechanisms targeting β-cells by autoimmune reactions, which involve infiltration of pancreatic islets by $CD4^+$ and $CD8^+$ T lymphocytes and macrophages leading to insulitis [1]. During the period preceding the clinical onset, autoantibodies targeting specific islet autoantigens such as insulin, glutamic acid decarboxylase (GAD65), islet antigen-2 (IA-2) and zinc transporter (ZnT8) may be detectable for months up to years before hyperglycemia becomes overt [11]. It has been assumed that the occurrence and number of islet autoantibodies such as GAD65Ab and IA-2Ab were associated with insulitis [37]. A recent study, however, detected islet autoantibodies among 62 (4%) individuals out of 1507 pancreatic donors aged 25–60 years [12]. Although those 62 individuals also had HLA susceptibility, only two of them showed insulitis, indicating that the presence of islet autoantibodies is not necessarily a marker of insulitis. The exact role of these autoantibodies is therefore not understood and it needs to be established to what extent they are markers of β-cell destruction by cellular autoimmunity [38].

The intensity and duration of β-cell destruction varies and seems to be related to the presence of high-risk HLA haplotypes especially DR3-DQ2, DR4-DQ8, or both [39]. The HLA class II family molecules are expressed on the surface of antigen-presenting cells (APC) such as dendritic cells and macrophages but also on activated B and T lymphocytes or even activated endothelial cells. High-risk HLA molecules on APC are likely to facilitate activation of $CD8^+$ T lymphocytes by $CD4^+$ T lymphocytes. This activation is indirectly exemplified in T1DM siblings who developed the disease by the age of 12 years because T1DM occurred in 55% of siblings sharing the high-risk HLA DR3-DQ2/DR4-DQ8 genotype compared with only 5% of those who shared zero or one haplotype [40].

It has been widely claimed, based on autopsy studies, that around 80–90% of β-cells are already lost at clinical onset [14,41]. Recent reanalysis of patients who died soon after diagnosis, however, revealed that the level of β-cell loss required for hyperglycemia was age-dependent, being about 40% in subjects aged 20 years [42]. Additionally, there are suggestions that β-cell regeneration may have taken place, contributing to the approximately 50% of viable β-cells present at diagnosis [43]. The progressive destruction of β-cells is likely to vary in intensity and duration depending on the age at diagnosis [44]. It is a major drawback, however, that direct and precise assessments of β-cell loss before and after diagnosis are not available in humans. Much of the current knowledge of β-cell function prior to the clinical onset has been derived from laboratory animals such as NOD mice and bio-breeding rats [45]. The β-cell destruction in humans may be estimated indirectly by assessing insulin secretion during intravenous glucose tolerance tests (IVGTT). In particular, FPIR measured by insulin or C peptide is thought to reflect loss of β-cells and to predict T1DM [46]. Data from the Diabetes Prevention Trial Type 1 showed that post-challenge C peptide levels were remarkably reduced 6 months before clinical onset [47].

Cellular autoimmunity

The genetic susceptibility of T1DM predisposing to loss of immunologic tolerance and eventual autoimmune killing of β-cells may be explained by a disordered antigen presenting mechanism [43]. The HLA class II molecules are heterodimers that regulate the immune response and are expressed on the surface of APC such as macrophages. The heterodimer binds peptides generated intracellularly either from self-proteins or from exogenous antigens taken up by phagocytosis. The resulting trimolecular complex represents the ligand for the T-cell receptor (TCR). The interaction between the trimolecular complex and the TCR activates the T lymphocyte. The HLA class II molecules on APC are responsible for antigen presentation to T-helper lymphocytes ($CD4^+$). Upon non-antigenic stimulation, macrophages from people with T1DM and the high-risk HLA DQB1*0201/*0302 genotype showed excessive secretion of proinflammatory cytokines and prostaglandin E_2 [48]. Cytokines may damage β-cells directly or indirectly by activating other cells such as T and B lymphocytes [49]. The APC presenting β-cell autoantigens may thus be actively involved in the anti-self autoimmune response that may result from failure to sustain self-recognition or from promoting an anti-self response. APC, $CD4^+$ and $CD8^+$ T lymphocytes were all detected in pancreatic autopsies of subjects who died shortly after onset [50], indicating their role in insulitis. Autoreactive $CD8^+$ T lymphocytes may have the most significant role in autoimmune destruction of β-cells [51]. Natural killer cells (NK) may also be found with abnormal activity and count [52]. The detection of autoreactive T lymphocytes in insulitis and in the circulation at the time of diagnosis, in addition to the notion that immunosuppressive drugs such as cyclosporine or anti-CD3 monoclonal antibodies can temporarily abort disease progression, are all considered to support the role of cellular immunity in β-cell destruction [53].

The mechanism involved in β-cell destruction is not yet fully clear. One possible scenario is that β-cells are first destroyed by an environmental factor such as virus. The dying or dead β-cell is next phagocytozed by local dendritic cells (APC), which are then activated and migrate through the lymphatics to a pancreatic draining lymph node. The antigen presentation to and activation of $CD4^+$ T lymphocytes takes place in the lymph node to include activation of $CD8^+$ T lymphocytes specific for islet autoantigens. These islet autoantigen-specific $CD8^+$ T lymphocytes return to the blood circulation, eventually ending up in islets to destroy β-cells. The β-cell killing will generate a new cycle of islet autoantigen presentation known as epitope spreading [49,54]. $CD4^+CD25^+$ regulatory T lymphocytes are also thought to have an important role in pathogenesis of T1DM as they may inhibit islet autoantigen specific $CD4^+$ T lymphocytes [54,55]. These cells express FOXp3 from the X chromosome and are important in development of peripheral tolerance.

The identification of islet autoantigen-specific T lymphocytes has been challenging and the development of standardized assays of T lymphocytes specific to islet autoantigens (insulin, GAD65 and IA-2) is still difficult to achieve [53,55]. Soluble HLA class II tetramer assays to assess autoantigen-specific T lymphocytes [56] and ELISPOT (enzyme-linked immunospot) [57] assays to measure cytokines of each T lymphocytes are tests to assess anti-islet autoantigen T-lymphocyte reactivity. During islet autoimmunity prior to the clinical onset these autoantigen-specific T lymphocytes may not be found in peripheral circulation, rather they may accumulate in islets and are therefore hard to detect [58].

Humoral autoimmunity

Islet cell autoantibodies

The identification in 1974 of ICA was achieved using frozen pancreatic sections and indirect immunofluorescence [5]. Four years later, islet surface antibodies (ICSA) were identified [59] and complement-dependent antibody-mediated islet cell cytotoxicity was described in 1980 [60]. Because ICA assays showed wide variations among ICA-positive sera [61], assays specific to individual autoantigens were later developed to detect autoantibodies against GAD65, IA-2 [62], insulin [63] and recently ZnT8 (Table 9.3) [64]. Islet autoimmunity (single or multiple autoantibodies persistent for 3–6 months) proved to be useful in differentiating T1DM from other forms of diabetes [11]. Multiple islet autoantibodies (≥2) usually appear within 6–12 months following the appearance of the first autoantibody (Figure 9.2) [65]. Nevertheless, some individuals develop transient islet autoantibodies but they are usually solitary and associated with lower risk [66], possibly because of the presence of protective genes such as HLA DR15–DQ6 [25]. One or more of these autoantibodies can be detected months up to years before clinical onset in more than 95% of newly diagnosed patients with T1DM, even as early as in the perinatal period [67]. Moreover, the detection

Table 9.3 Characteristics of islet autoantigenes and autoantibodies.

	GAD65	IA-2	Insulin	ZnT8
Chromosome	10p11	IA-2: 2q35-36 IA-2β: 7q36	11p15	8q24
Molecular weight (kD)	64	IA-2: 40 IA-2β: 37	5.8	67
Tissue specificity	Pancreas, neuron, ovary, testis, kidney	Neuroendocrine cells (pancreas, brain, pituitary)	β-cell specific	β-cell specific
Function	GABA production (an inhibitory neurotransmitter)	Not clear (lack enzymatic activity)	Regulates glucose metabolism	Zn^{2+} transport and accumulation in β-cell vesicles
Genetic association	DR3-DQ2 DR4-DQ8	DRB1*0401	INS-VNTR, DR4	SLC30A8
Antibody abbreviation	GAD65Ab	IA-2Ab	IAA	ZnT8Ab
Standardized assay	RBA, ELISA	RBA	RBA	RBA
Sensitivity (%)	RBA: 80 ELISA: 89	RBA: 70 ELISA: 65	RBA: >60	RBA: 50 (C terminal)
Specificity (%)	RBA: 96 ELISA: 98	RBA: 99 ELISA: 99	RBA: 95	RBA: 98 (C terminal)
Variation with age	Higher detection with increase age	Less with increasing age	Higher predictivity in children	Increasing predictivity with age
Variation with gender	Female preference if onset <10 years	Male preference	None	None

ELISA, enzyme linked immunosorbent assay; RBA, radiobinding assay.
Workshop sensitivity and specificity for GAD65Ab and IA-2Ab were from the Diabetes Antibody Standardization Program [62].
Diagnostic sensitivity at 95% diagnostic specificity for insulin autoantibodies (IAA) were from [63].

of the four main autoantibodies may predict the disease by as much as 98% (Figure 9.2) [68].

Glutamic acid decarboxylase autoantibodies

The enzyme glutamic acid decarboxylase (GAD) is found in neurons and islet β-cells and produces γ-aminobutyric acid (GABA), which is a major inhibitory neurotransmitter. The 64K protein identified as GAD after immunoprecipitation of human islet [69] was found to represent GAD65, not the previously known GAD67 isoform, which shares 65% of the GAD65 amino acid sequence [70]. Unlike GAD67, GAD65, which is encoded by a gene on chromosome 10p11, is expressed mainly in pancreatic islets (Table 9.3) [70].

Autoantibodies against GAD are most commonly to the GAD65 isoform (GAD65Ab), which were found in 70–80% of children with new onset T1DM, 8% of T1DM first-degree relatives but also in about 1% of general population [71]. Unlike ICA, GAD65Ab remain detectable for many years even after considerable loss of β-cell function [72]. Additionally, GAD65Ab detection rate rises with age in new onset T1DM. If the onset was before 10 years of age, some gender differences with female preference is observed. Because GAD65Ab levels are persistent, more prevalent and correlated well with plasma levels of C peptide [38], they are currently considered as good markers for both prediction and follow-up of β-cell dysfunction among individuals at risk.

GAD65Ab were found to be associated with the high-risk HLA haplotypes DR4-DQ8 (*DRB1*04-DQA1*0301-B1*0302*) and DR3-DQ2 (*DRB1*03-DQA1*0501-B1*0201*) [73] but more often with the latter [72]. Recently, anti-idiotypic GAD65Ab were found to be markers that have lower frequency in T1DM and their absence was more predictive than the presence of GAD65Ab [74]. GAD65Ab can be detected with both radiobinding assays and enzyme-linked immunosorbent assay (ELISA) and these assays have been assessed and standardized in the latest Diabetes Antibody Standardization Program (DASP) [62]. The high and improved performance of these assays emphasizes the value of these autoantibodies in prediction and classification of T1DM and also their value as screening tools in individuals at risk (Table 9.3).

Islet antigen-2 autoantibodies IA-2Ab and IA-2βAb

This autoantigen is a member of the plasma membrane protein tyrosine phosphatase family [75]. Its composed of two isoforms: IA-2 (formerly known as ICA512) which is a 40K protein encoded on chromosome 2, and IA-2β (phogrin) which is a 37K protein encoded on chromosome 7 (Table 9.3) [76]. The two isoforms share many common epitopes and are present in several neuroendocrine tissues in addition to pancreatic islets with no clear function because they lack enzymatic activity.

The autoantibody reactivity of IA-2Ab is directed to the cytoplasmic portion of the autoantigen and the immuno-reactivity in T1DM is directed against the C-terminal region of IA-2 [77]. IA-2Ab is detected in about 60–70% of patients with new-onset T1DM [78] and in less than 1% of the general population [79]. IA-2Ab are often preceded by IAA, GAD65Ab and ICA, respectively [65], and the frequency decreases with increased age of onset [80]. This indicates that the predictive and screening abilities of IA-2Ab are more useful for younger children especially when combined with GAD65Ab and other markers.

Using radiobinding assays to determine epitope-specific IA-2Ab/IA-2βAb among healthy siblings of children with T1DM [81], it was found that progression to T1DM was more common with autoantibodies to the juxtamembrane region of IA-2 (IA-2-JM-Ab) while IgE-IA-2Ab conferred protection even when IA-2-JM-Ab were positive. Higher frequencies of IA-2Ab were found in association with *DRB1*0401* rather than with DQ8 [72]. Furthermore, patients with DQ2 [82] had less association with IA-2Ab indicating a role for additional mechanisms related to the HLA genetic component.

Assays to identify IA-2Ab were developed and standardized using radiobinding tests that can precipitate IA-2Ab, IA-2βAb along with GAD65Ab. These assays have high levels of sensitivity and specificity and were improved in subsequent DASP workshops [62]. Similarly, ELISA assays combining IA-2Ab and GAD65Ab using biotin-labeled preparations were also standardized and the latest evaluation showed progress in performance of these assays (Table 9.3) [62].

Insulin autoantibodies

The most highly specific autoantigens of β-cells are insulin and its precursor proinsulin because they are expressed only in β-cells. In 1983, using radioligand-binding assays, insulin autoantibodies (IAA) were first identified in 50% of patients with newly diagnosed diabetes before initiating treatment with exogenous insulin [83]. IAA, which are able to react with both insulin and proinsulin, tend to be the earliest marker of islet autoimmunity [65] but their levels are often fluctuating and present in low titers. The predictive value for T1DM using IAA alone appears to be related to age; it is higher among younger children, possibly related to a higher rate of β-cell destruction. IAA were detectable in 90% of children who progress to T1DM before the age of 5 years compared with only 40–50% of adolescents older than 15 years (Table 9.3) [84].

DR4 is associated with a higher frequency of IAA, which may be related to the linkage disequilibrium with the high-risk DQ8 haplotype [85]. IAA were also associated with the insulin gene on chromosome 11p15 [86] where the number of tandem repeats (VNTR) were found to be associated with T1DM whether IAA were present or not.

Antibodies against exogenous insulin showed no correlation with IAA levels detected at clinical onset of T1DM and appear to be independent of autoimmunity [87]; however, they do share some similar binding features [88]. Unlike IAA, antibodies against exogenous insulin shows higher specificity, therefore they may be detected using the ELISA test, which does not predict T1DM [89]. The IAA fluid-phase radioimmunoassay shows high sensitivity and specificity to detect T1DM and has been modified to use less serum volume (25 μL instead of 600 μL) in a new assay known as "micro-IAA" (Table 9.3) [90]. Nevertheless, poor inter-laboratory concordance remains a problem that has delayed standardization of IAA [63].

ZnT8 Transporter (SLC30A8) autoantibodies ZnT8Ab

The zinc transporter (ZnT8 isoform-8 transporter) has recently been described as a second novel β-cell-specific autoantigen, in addition to insulin [64]. A polymorphism in the gene encoding this autoantigen, SLC30A8, is also associated with the risk of T2DM [91]. ZnT8 is important for zinc-insulin crystallization and insulin secretion. It facilitates transport and accumulation of cytoplasmic zinc into the secretory vesicles of β-cells. Inside these vesicles, insulin molecules are co-crystallized with two Zn^{2+} ions to form solid hexamers.

Nearly 60–80% of patients with new onset T1DM react positively to ZnT8Ab [91], which were detected in around 26% of patients who were negative for the conventional islet autoantibodies (GAD65Ab, IA-2Ab and IAA) [68]. By contrast, ZnT8Ab were detected in only 2% of controls and less than 3% of T2DM [68,91]. Additionally, ZnT8Ab were also detected in 30% of patients with other autoimmune diseases associated with T1DM [64]. Being a target of humoral immunity in T1DM, the high β-cell specificity of ZnT8 is seen as an advantage over other non-specific β-cell autoantigens such as GAD65 and IA-2. This high specificity and independence from other islet autoimmune markers, in addition to the fact that ZnT8Ab titers increase with age, all emphasize the value of ZnT8Ab in predicting T1DM, especially among older children.

The polymorphic *SLC30A8* gene located on chromosome 8 encodes the ZnT8 [91]. This locus and other chromosome 8 loci have not been associated with T1DM risk as such but were associated with the risk of ZnT8Ab [92]. ZnT8Ab were found to react with the C-terminal of the autoantigen and variation at amino acid position 325 determines two important susceptibility markers of ZnT8Ab, which can either be arginine (ZnT8-R) or tryptophan (ZnT8-W) [92]. Immunoprecipitation assays for ZnT8Ab were developed and fluid phase radioassays for the C-terminal of ZnT8Ab were standardized and validated in the DASP workshop (Table 9.3).

Candidate (minor) autoantigens

Several studies have reported associations of a group of molecules and substances with T1DM. This group included a wide variety of minor or candidate autoantigens that are thought to be associated with T1DM, autoimmunity or both; examples are, ICA12/SOX13 [93], glima-38 [94], vesicle-associated membrane protein-2 (VAMP2) [95], neuropeptide Y [95], carboxypeptidase H [96], GLUT-2 [97], heat shock protein 60 [98], imogen 38 [99], ICA69 [100] and others (Table 9.4).

Conclusions

Considerable progress has been made in the understanding of T1DM pathogenesis as it relates to the appearance of islet autoimmunity prior to the clinical onset of the disease. The development

Table 9.4 The main candidate (minor) islet autoantigens.

Autoantigen	Molecular weight (kD)	Description	Autoantibody frequency
ICA12 (SOX13)	–	SOX family protein present in pancreas, kidney and placenta. Anti-SOX-13-Ab found more in children	T1DM: 10–30% T2DM: 6–9% Healthy controls: 2–4%
Glima-38	38	Amphiphilic glycated β-cell membrane protein. Specific expression on islet and neuron cells	New onset T1DM: 19% Prediabetes phase: 14% Healthy controls: missing
VAMP2	12.6	β-cell secretory vesicles-related protein	T1DM: 21% Healthy controls: 4%
NPY	10.9	β-cell secretory vesicles-related protein	T1DM: 9% Healthy controls: 2%
CPH	43.4	Carboxypeptidase B-like glycoprotein present in islets and brain. Related to cleavage of insulin from proinsulin	ICA^+ relatives: 20% Healthy controls: missing
GLUT-2	55	Glucose transporter type 2 of β-cells	New onset T1DM: 32–80% Healthy controls: 6.6%
HSP 60	60	A "stress" protein which is thought to be produced and upregulated in response to cellular stress	T1DM: 15% Rheumatoid arthritis: 20% Healthy controls: 1.2%
Imogen 38	38	A protein found in β-cell mitochondria and to a lesser extent in α-cells	No antibodies found
ICA 69	69	A peptide mainly present in islets and neuroendocrine, but also brain, kidney and lung	New onset T1DM: 5–30% Healthy controls: 6% Rheumatoid arthritis 20%

of standardized islet autoantibody tests (GAD65Ab, IA-2Ab, ZnT8Ab) has made it possible to begin screening for subjects at risk to be included in clinical trials aimed at preserving residual β-cell function. Analyses of cell-mediated immunity need further development and standardization to be useful in clinical trials. HLA-DQ on chromosome 6 remains the most important genetic factor for T1DM risk. It is well-established that these HLA class II heterodimeric proteins are necessary but not sufficient for disease. Recent genome-wide association studies have provided a smorgasbord of candidate factors to be explored for T1DM risk. We are still at a loss as to which environmental factor(s) may be responsible for triggering islet autoimmunity and studies such as The Environmental Determinants of Diabetes in the Young (TEDDY) [101] are needed to test fully the multitude of candidate triggers.

References

1 Gepts W. Pathologic anatomy of the pancreas in juvenile diabetes mellitus. *Diabetes* 1965; **14**:619–633.

2 American Diabetes Association. Diagnosis and classification of diabetes mellitus. *Diabetes Care* 2007; **30**(Suppl 1):S42–S47.

3 Nerup J, Andersen OO, Bendixen G, Egeberg J, Gunnarsson R, Kromann H, *et al.* Cell-mediated immunity in diabetes mellitus. *Proc R Soc Med* 1974; **67**:506–513.

4 Nerup J, Binder C. Thyroid, gastric and adrenal auto-immunity in diabetes mellitus. *Acta Endocrinol (Copenh)* 1973; **72**:279–286.

5 Bottazzo GF, Florin-Christensen A, Doniach D. Islet-cell antibodies in diabetes mellitus with autoimmune polyendocrine deficiencies. *Lancet* 1974; **2**:1279–1283.

6 Nerup J, Platz P, Andersen OO, Christy M, Lyngsoe J, Poulsen JE, *et al.* HL-A antigens and diabetes mellitus. *Lancet* 1974; **2**:864–866.

7 Irvine WJ, McCallum CJ, Gray RS, Duncan LJ. Clinical and pathogenic significance of pancreatic-islet-cell antibodies in diabetics treated with oral hypoglycaemic agents. *Lancet* 1977; **1**:1025–1027.

8 Palmer JP, Hampe CS, Chiu H, Goel A, Brooks-Worrell BM. Is latent autoimmune diabetes in adults distinct from type 1 diabetes or just type 1 diabetes at an older age? *Diabetes* 2005; **54**(Suppl 2):S62–S67.

9 Imagawa A, Hanafusa T. Pathogenesis of fulminant type 1 diabetes. *Rev Diabet Stud* 2006; **3**:169–177.

10 Umpierrez GE, Casals MM, Gebhart SP, Mixon PS, Clark WS, Phillips LS. Diabetic ketoacidosis in obese African-Americans. *Diabetes* 1995; **44**:790–795.

11 Miao D, Yu L, Eisenbarth GS. Role of autoantibodies in type 1 diabetes. *Front Biosci* 2007; **12**:1889–1898.

12 In't Veld P, Lievens D, De Grijse J, Ling Z, Van der Auwera B, Pipeleers-Marichal M, *et al.* Screening for insulitis in adult autoantibody-positive organ donors. *Diabetes* 2007; **56**:2400–2404.

13 Pihoker C, Gilliam LK, Hampe CS, Lernmark A. Autoantibodies in diabetes. *Diabetes* 2005; **54**(Suppl 2):S52–S61.

14 Butler AE, Galasso R, Meier JJ, Basu R, Rizza RA, Butler PC. Modestly increased beta cell apoptosis but no increased beta cell replication in recent-onset type 1 diabetic patients who died of diabetic ketoacidosis. *Diabetologia* 2007; **50**:2323–2331.

15 Kahn SE, Prigeon RL, McCulloch DK, Boyko EJ, Bergman RN, Schwartz MW, *et al.* Quantification of the relationship between insulin sensitivity and beta-cell function in human subjects: evidence for a hyperbolic function. *Diabetes* 1993; **42**:1663–1672.

16 Redondo MJ, Yu L, Hawa M, Mackenzie T, Pyke DA, Eisenbarth GS, *et al.* Heterogeneity of type I diabetes: analysis of monozygotic twins in Great Britain and the United States. *Diabetologia* 2001; **44**:354–362.

17 Kumar D, Gemayel NS, Deapen D, Kapadia D, Yamashita PH, Lee M, *et al.* North-American twins with IDDM. Genetic, etiological, and clinical significance of disease concordance according to age, zygosity, and the interval after diagnosis in first twin. *Diabetes* 1993; **42**:1351–1363.

18 Todd JA, Farrall M. Panning for gold: genome-wide scanning for linkage in type 1 diabetes. *Hum Mol Genet* 1996; **5**:1443–1448.

19 Akesson K, Nystrom L, Farnkvist L, Ostman J, Lernmark A, Kockum I. Increased risk of diabetes among relatives of female insulin-treated patients diagnosed at 15–34 years of age. *Diabet Med* 2005; **22**:1551–1557.

20 Schranz DB, Lernmark A. Immunology in diabetes: an update. *Diabetes Metab Rev* 1998; **14**:3–29.

21 Thomson G, Valdes AM, Noble JA, Kockum I, Grote MN, Najman J, *et al.* Relative predispositional effects of HLA class II DRB1-DQB1 haplotypes and genotypes on type 1 diabetes: a meta-analysis. *Tissue Antigens* 2007; **70**:110–127.

22 Hermann R, Bartsocas CS, Soltesz G, Vazeou A, Paschou P, Bozas E, *et al.* Genetic screening for individuals at high risk for type 1 diabetes in the general population using HLA Class II alleles as disease markers: a comparison between three European populations with variable rates of disease incidence. *Diabetes Metab Res Rev* 2004; **20**:322–329.

23 Notkins AL, Lernmark A. Autoimmune type 1 diabetes: resolved and unresolved issues. *J Clin Invest* 2001; **108**:1247–1252.

24 Pociot F, McDermott MF. Genetics of type 1 diabetes mellitus. *Genes Immun* 2002; **3**:235–249.

25 Redondo MJ, Fain PR, Eisenbarth GS. Genetics of type 1A diabetes. *Recent Prog Horm Res* 2001; **56**:69–89.

26 Erlich H, Valdes AM, Noble J, Carlson JA, Varney M, Concannon P, *et al.* HLA DR-DQ haplotypes and genotypes and type 1 diabetes risk: analysis of the type 1 diabetes genetics consortium families. *Diabetes* 2008; **57**:1084–1092.

27 Todd JA, Walker NM, Cooper JD, Smyth DJ, Downes K, Plagnol V, *et al.* Robust associations of four new chromosome regions from genome-wide analyses of type 1 diabetes. *Nat Genet* 2007; **39**:857–864.

28 Knip M, Veijola R, Virtanen SM, Hyoty H, Vaarala O, Akerblom HK. Environmental triggers and determinants of type 1 diabetes. *Diabetes* 2005; **54**(Suppl 2):S125–S136.

29 van der Werf N, Kroese FG, Rozing J, Hillebrands JL. Viral infections as potential triggers of type 1 diabetes. *Diabetes Metab Res Rev* 2007; **23**:169–183.

30 Hawa MI, Leslie RD. Early induction of type 1 diabetes. *Clin Exp Immunol* 2001; **126**:181–183.

31 Gerstein HC. Cow's milk exposure and type 1 diabetes mellitus: a critical overview of the clinical literature. *Diabetes Care* 1994; **17**: 13–19.

32 Vaarala O. Environmental causes: dietary causes. *Endocrinol Metab Clin North Am* 2004; **33**:17–26, vii.

33 Hypponen E, Kenward MG, Virtanen SM, Piitulainen A, Virta-Autio P, Tuomilehto J, *et al.* Infant feeding, early weight gain, and

risk of type 1 diabetes. Childhood Diabetes in Finland (DiMe) Study Group. *Diabetes Care* 1999; **22**:1961–1965.

34 Sepa A, Ludvigsson J. Psychological stress and the risk of diabetes-related autoimmunity: a review article. *Neuroimmunomodulation* 2006; **13**:301–308.

35 Myers MA, Mackay IR, Zimmet PZ. Toxic type 1 diabetes. *Rev Endocr Metab Disord* 2003; **4**:225–231.

36 Bingley PJ, Mahon JL, Gale EA. Insulin resistance and progression to type 1 diabetes in the European Nicotinamide Diabetes Intervention Trial (ENDIT). *Diabetes Care* 2008; **31**:146–150.

37 Imagawa A, Hanafusa T, Tamura S, Moriwaki M, Itoh N, Yamamoto K, *et al.* Pancreatic biopsy as a procedure for detecting in situ autoimmune phenomena in type 1 diabetes: close correlation between serological markers and histological evidence of cellular autoimmunity. *Diabetes* 2001; **50**:1269–1273.

38 Scholin A, Bjorklund L, Borg H, Arnqvist H, Bjork E, Blohme G, *et al.* Islet antibodies and remaining beta-cell function 8 years after diagnosis of diabetes in young adults: a prospective follow-up of the nationwide Diabetes Incidence Study in Sweden. *J Intern Med* 2004; **255**:384–391.

39 Knip M, Ilonen J, Mustonen A, Akerblom HK. Evidence of an accelerated B-cell destruction in HLA-Dw3/Dw4 heterozygous children with type 1 (insulin-dependent) diabetes. *Diabetologia* 1986; **29**:347–351.

40 Aly TA, Ide A, Jahromi MM, Barker JM, Fernando MS, Babu SR, *et al.* Extreme genetic risk for type 1A diabetes. *Proc Natl Acad Sci U S A* 2006; **103**:14074–14079.

41 Gepts W, De Mey J. Islet cell survival determined by morphology: an immunocytochemical study of the islets of Langerhans in juvenile diabetes mellitus. *Diabetes* 1978; **27**(Suppl 1):251–261.

42 Klinke DJ 2nd. Extent of beta cell destruction is important but insufficient to predict the onset of type 1 diabetes mellitus. *PLoS ONE* 2008; **3**:e1374.

43 Haller MJ, Atkinson MA, Schatz D. Type 1 diabetes mellitus: etiology, presentation, and management. *Pediatr Clin North Am* 2005; **52**:1553–1578.

44 Wallensteen M, Dahlquist G, Persson B, Landin-Olsson M, Lernmark A, Sundkvist G, *et al.* Factors influencing the magnitude, duration, and rate of fall of B-cell function in type 1 (insulin-dependent) diabetic children followed for two years from their clinical diagnosis. *Diabetologia* 1988; **31**:664–669.

45 Akirav E, Kushner JA, Herold KC. Beta-cell mass and type 1 diabetes: going, going, gone? *Diabetes* 2008; **57**:2883–2888.

46 Keskinen P, Korhonen S, Kupila A, Veijola R, Erkkila S, Savolainen H, *et al.* First-phase insulin response in young healthy children at genetic and immunological risk for type 1 diabetes. *Diabetologia* 2002; **45**:1639–1648.

47 Sosenko JM, Palmer JP, Rafkin-Mervis L, Krischer JP, Cuthbertson D, Matheson D, et al. Glucose and C-peptide changes in the perionset period of type 1 diabetes in the Diabetes Prevention Trial-Type 1. *Diabetes Care* 2008; **31**:2188–2192.

48 Plesner A, Greenbaum CJ, Gaur LK, Ernst RK, Lernmark A. Macrophages from high-risk HLA-DQB1*0201/*0302 type 1 diabetes mellitus patients are hypersensitive to lipopolysaccharide stimulation. *Scand J Immunol* 2002; **56**:522–529.

49 Morran MP, McInerney MF, Pietropaolo M. Innate and adaptive autoimmunity in type 1 diabetes. *Pediatr Diabetes* 2008; **9**:152–161.

50 Bottazzo GF, Dean BM, McNally JM, MacKay EH, Swift PG, Gamble DR. *In situ* characterization of autoimmune phenomena and expression of HLA molecules in the pancreas in diabetic insulitis. *N Engl J Med* 1985; **313**:353–360.

51 Pinkse GG, Tysma OH, Bergen CA, Kester MG, Ossendorp F, van Veelen PA, *et al.* Autoreactive CD8 T cells associated with beta cell destruction in type 1 diabetes. *Proc Natl Acad Sci U S A* 2005; **102**: 18425–18430.

52 Rodacki M, Milech A, de Oliveira JE. NK cells and type 1 diabetes. *Clin Dev Immunol* 2006; **13**:101–107.

53 Roep BO. The role of T-cells in the pathogenesis of type 1 diabetes: from cause to cure. *Diabetologia* 2003; **46**:305–321.

54 Knip M, Siljander H. Autoimmune mechanisms in type 1 diabetes. *Autoimmun Rev* 2008; **7**:550–557.

55 Tree TI, Roep BO, Peakman M. A mini meta-analysis of studies on $CD4^{+}CD25^{+}$ T cells in human type 1 diabetes: report of the Immunology of Diabetes Society T Cell Workshop. *Ann N Y Acad Sci* 2006; **1079**:9–18.

56 Reijonen H, Novak EJ, Kochik S, Heninger A, Liu AW, Kwok WW, *et al.* Detection of GAD65-specific T-cells by major histocompatibility complex class II tetramers in type 1 diabetic patients and at-risk subjects. *Diabetes* 2002; **51**:1375–1382.

57 Schloot NC, Meierhoff G, Karlsson Faresjo M, Ott P, Putnam A, Lehmann P, *et al.* Comparison of cytokine ELISpot assay formats for the detection of islet antigen autoreactive T cells. Report of the Third Immunology and Diabetes Society T-cell Workshop. *J Autoimmun* 2003; **21**:365–376.

58 Lohmann T, Hawa M, Leslie RD, Lane R, Picard J, Londei M. Immune reactivity to glutamic acid decarboxylase 65 in stiffman syndrome and type 1 diabetes mellitus. *Lancet* 2000; **356**:31–35.

59 Lernmark A, Freedman ZR, Hofmann C, Rubenstein AH, Steiner DF, Jackson RL, *et al.* Islet-cell-surface antibodies in juvenile diabetes mellitus. *N Engl J Med* 1978; **299**:375–380.

60 Dobersen MJ, Scharff JE, Ginsberg-Fellner F, Notkins AL. Cytotoxic autoantibodies to beta cells in the serum of patients with insulin-dependent diabetes mellitus. *N Engl J Med* 1980; **303**:1493–1498.

61 Boitard C, Bonifacio E, Bottazzo GF, Gleichmann H, Molenaar J. Immunology and Diabetes Workshop: report on the Third International (Stage 3) Workshop on the Standardisation of Cytoplasmic Islet Cell Antibodies. Held in New York, NY, October 1987. *Diabetologia* 1988; **31**:451–452.

62 Torn C, Mueller PW, Schlosser M, Bonifacio E, Bingley PJ. Diabetes Antibody Standardization Program: evaluation of assays for autoantibodies to glutamic acid decarboxylase and islet antigen-2. *Diabetologia* 2008; **51**:846–852.

63 Achenbach P, Schlosser M, Williams AJ, Yu L, Mueller PW, Bingley PJ, *et al.* Combined testing of antibody titer and affinity improves insulin autoantibody measurement: Diabetes Antibody Standardization Program. *Clin Immunol* 2007; **122**:85–90.

64 Wenzlau JM, Juhl K, Yu L, Moua O, Sarkar SA, Gottlieb P, *et al.* The cation efflux transporter ZnT8 (Slc30A8) is a major autoantigen in human type 1 diabetes. *Proc Natl Acad Sci U S A* 2007; **104**:17040–17045.

65 Kupila A, Keskinen P, Simell T, Erkkila S, Arvilommi P, Korhonen S, *et al.* Genetic risk determines the emergence of diabetes-associated autoantibodies in young children. *Diabetes* 2002; **51**:646–651.

66 Barker JM, Barriga KJ, Yu L, Miao D, Erlich HA, Norris JM, *et al.* Prediction of autoantibody positivity and progression to type 1 dia-

betes: Diabetes Autoimmunity Study in the Young (DAISY). *J Clin Endocrinol Metab* 2004; **89**:3896–38902.

67 Lynch KF, Lernmark B, Merlo J, Cilio CM, Ivarsson SA, Lernmark A. Cord blood islet autoantibodies and seasonal association with the type 1 diabetes high-risk genotype. *J Perinatol* 2008; **28**:211–217.

68 Eisenbarth GS, Jeffrey J. The natural history of type 1A diabetes. *Arq Bras Endocrinol Metabol* 2008; **52**:146–155.

69 Baekkeskov S, Aanstoot HJ, Christgau S, Reetz A, Solimena M, Cascalho M, *et al.* Identification of the 64K autoantigen in insulin-dependent diabetes as the GABA-synthesizing enzyme glutamic acid decarboxylase. *Nature* 1990; **347**:151–156.

70 Karlsen AE, Hagopian WA, Grubin CE, Dube S, Disteche CM, Adler DA, *et al.* Cloning and primary structure of a human islet isoform of glutamic acid decarboxylase from chromosome 10. *Proc Natl Acad Sci U S A* 1991; **88**:8337–8341.

71 Bonifacio E, Genovese S, Braghi S, Bazzigaluppi E, Lampasona V, Bingley PJ, *et al.* Islet autoantibody markers in IDDM: risk assessment strategies yielding high sensitivity. *Diabetologia* 1995; **38**:816–822.

72 Sanjeevi CB, Hagopian WA, Landin-Olsson M, Kockum I, Woo W, Palmer JP, *et al.* Association between autoantibody markers and subtypes of DR4 and DR4-DQ in Swedish children with insulin-dependent diabetes reveals closer association of tyrosine pyrophosphatase autoimmunity with DR4 than DQ8. *Tissue Antigens* 1998; **51**:281–286.

73 Serjeantson SW, Kohonen-Corish MR, Rowley MJ, Mackay IR, Knowles W, Zimmet P. Antibodies to glutamic acid decarboxylase are associated with HLA-DR genotypes in both Australians and Asians with type 1 (insulin-dependent) diabetes mellitus. *Diabetologia* 1992; **35**:996–1001.

74 Oak S, Gilliam LK, Landin-Olsson M, Torn C, Kockum I, Pennington CR, *et al.* The lack of anti-idiotypic antibodies, not the presence of the corresponding autoantibodies to glutamate decarboxylase, defines type 1 diabetes. *Proc Natl Acad Sci U S A* 2008; **105**:5471–5476.

75 Lu J, Li Q, Xie H, Chen ZJ, Borovitskaya AE, Maclaren NK, *et al.* Identification of a second transmembrane protein tyrosine phosphatase, IA-2beta, as an autoantigen in insulin-dependent diabetes mellitus: precursor of the 37-kDa tryptic fragment. *Proc Natl Acad Sci U S A* 1996; **93**:2307–2311.

76 Bonifacio E, Lampasona V, Genovese S, Ferrari M, Bosi E. Identification of protein tyrosine phosphatase-like IA2 (islet cell antigen 512) as the insulin-dependent diabetes-related 37/40K autoantigen and a target of islet-cell antibodies. *J Immunol* 1995; **155**:5419–5426.

77 Payton MA, Hawkes CJ, Christie MR. Relationship of the 37,000- and 40,000-M(r) tryptic fragments of islet antigens in insulin-dependent diabetes to the protein tyrosine phosphatase-like molecule IA-2 (ICA512). *J Clin Invest* 1995; **96**:1506–1511.

78 Graham J, Hagopian WA, Kockum I, Li LS, Sanjeevi CB, Lowe RM, *et al.* Genetic effects on age-dependent onset and islet cell autoantibody markers in type 1 diabetes. *Diabetes* 2002; **51**:1346–1355.

79 Palmer JP, Hirsch IB. What's in a name: latent autoimmune diabetes of adults, type 1.5, adult-onset, and type 1 diabetes. *Diabetes Care* 2003; **26**:536–538.

80 Solimena M, Dirkx R Jr, Hermel JM, Pleasic-Williams S, Shapiro JA, Caron L, *et al.* ICA 512, an autoantigen of type I diabetes, is an intrinsic membrane protein of neurosecretory granules. *EMBO J* 1996; **15**:2102–2114.

81 Hoppu S, Harkonen T, Ronkainen MS, Simell S, Hekkala A, Toivonen A, *et al.* IA-2 antibody isotypes and epitope specificity during the prediabetic process in children with HLA-conferred susceptibility to type 1 diabetes. *Clin Exp Immunol* 2006; **144**:59–66.

82 Graham J, Kockum I, Sanjeevi CB, Landin-Olsson M, Nystrom L, Sundkvist G, *et al.* Negative association between type 1 diabetes and HLA DQB1*0602-DQA1*0102 is attenuated with age at onset. Swedish Childhood Diabetes Study Group. *Eur J Immunogenet* 1999; **26**:117–127.

83 Palmer JP, Asplin CM, Clemons P, Lyen K, Tatpati O, Raghu PK, *et al.* Insulin antibodies in insulin-dependent diabetics before insulin treatment. *Science* 1983; **222**:1337–1339.

84 Vardi P, Ziegler AG, Mathews JH, Dib S, Keller RJ, Ricker AT, *et al.* Concentration of insulin autoantibodies at onset of type 1 diabetes: inverse log-linear correlation with age. *Diabetes Care* 1988; **11**:736–739.

85 Castano L, Ziegler AG, Ziegler R, Shoelson S, Eisenbarth GS. Characterization of insulin autoantibodies in relatives of patients with type 1 diabetes. *Diabetes* 1993; **42**:1202–1209.

86 Undlien DE, Bennett ST, Todd JA, Akselsen HE, Ikaheimo I, Reijonen H, *et al.* Insulin gene region-encoded susceptibility to IDDM maps upstream of the insulin gene. *Diabetes* 1995; **44**:620–625.

87 Karjalainen J, Knip M, Mustonen A, Akerblom HK. Insulin autoantibodies at the clinical manifestation of type 1 (insulin-dependent) diabetes: a poor predictor of clinical course and antibody response to exogenous insulin. *Diabetologia* 1988; **31**:129–133.

88 Arslanian SA, Becker DJ, Rabin B, Atchison R, Eberhardt M, Cavender D, *et al.* Correlates of insulin antibodies in newly diagnosed children with insulin-dependent diabetes before insulin therapy. *Diabetes* 1985; **34**:926–930.

89 Gianani R, Eisenbarth GS. The stages of type 1A diabetes: 2005. *Immunol Rev* 2005; **204**:232–249.

90 Williams AJ, Bingley PJ, Bonifacio E, Palmer JP, Gale EA. A novel micro-assay for insulin autoantibodies. *J Autoimmun* 1997; **10**:473–478.

91 Wenzlau JM, Hutton JC, Davidson HW. New antigenic targets in type 1 diabetes. *Curr Opin Endocrinol Diabetes Obes* 2008; **15**:315–320.

92 Wenzlau JM, Liu Y, Yu L, Moua O, Fowler KT, Rangasamy S, *et al.* A common nonsynonymous single nucleotide polymorphism in the SLC30A8 gene determines ZnT8 autoantibody specificity in type 1 diabetes. *Diabetes* 2008; **57**:2693–2697.

93 Kasimiotis H, Fida S, Rowley MJ, Mackay IR, Zimmet PZ, Gleason S, *et al.* Antibodies to SOX13 (ICA12) are associated with type 1 diabetes. *Autoimmunity* 2001; **33**:95–101.

94 Aanstoot HJ, Kang SM, Kim J, Lindsay LA, Roll U, Knip M, *et al.* Identification and characterization of glima 38, a glycosylated islet cell membrane antigen, which together with GAD65 and IA2 marks the early phases of autoimmune response in type 1 diabetes. *J Clin Invest* 1996; **97**:2772–2783.

95 Hirai H, Miura J, Hu Y, Larsson H, Larsson K, Lernmark A, *et al.* Selective screening of secretory vesicle-associated proteins for autoantigens in type 1 diabetes: VAMP2 and NPY are new minor autoantigens. *Clin Immunol* 2008; **127**:366–374.

96 Castano L, Russo E, Zhou L, Lipes MA, Eisenbarth GS. Identification and cloning of a granule autoantigen (carboxypeptidase-H) associated with type 1 diabetes. *J Clin Endocrinol Metab* 1991; **73**:1197–1201.

97 Inman LR, McAllister CT, Chen L, Hughes S, Newgard CB, Kettman JR, *et al.* Autoantibodies to the GLUT-2 glucose transporter of beta cells in insulin-dependent diabetes mellitus of recent onset. *Proc Natl Acad Sci U S A* 1993; **90**:1281–1284.

98 Ozawa Y, Kasuga A, Nomaguchi H, Maruyama T, Kasatani T, Shimada A, *et al.* Detection of autoantibodies to the pancreatic islet heat shock protein 60 in insulin-dependent diabetes mellitus. *J Autoimmun* 1996; **9**:517–524.

99 Arden SD, Roep BO, Neophytou PI, Usac EF, Duinkerken G, de Vries RR, *et al.* Imogen 38: a novel 38-kD islet mitochondrial autoantigen recognized by T cells from a newly diagnosed type 1 diabetic patient. *J Clin Invest* 1996; **97**:551–561.

100 Martin S, Kardorf J, Schulte B, Lampeter EF, Gries FA, Melchers I, *et al.* Autoantibodies to the islet antigen ICA69 occur in IDDM and in rheumatoid arthritis. *Diabetologia* 1995; **38**:351–355.

101 The Environmental Determinants of Diabetes in the Young (TEDDY) Study. *Ann N Y Acad Sci* 2008; **1150**:1–13.

Other Disorders with Type 1 Phenotype

Alice P.S. Kong & Juliana C.N. Chan

Keypoints

- Patients with type 1 diabetes classically present early, require continuous insulin treatment and carry autoimmune markers such as antibodies to glutamic acid decarboxylase (GAD).
- There are other types of diabetes with type 1 phenotype secondary to heterogeneous etiologies including: maturity-onset diabetes of the young (MODY) and other forms of monogenic diabetes caused by mutations of mitochondria, amylin or pathways implicated in pancreatic β-cell function; latent autoimmune diabetes of adults (LADA); fulminant type 1 diabetes presenting with diabetic ketoacidosis after viral infections and another form which reverts to a clinical course resembling type 2 diabetes after the initial ketotic presentation.
- The correct diagnosis of these disorders with type 1 phenotype is clinically important because of their different clinical course, prognosis and management.

Introduction

Classic type 1 diabetes mellitus (T1DM) is considered an autoimmune disease with pancreatic β-cell destruction. Affected subjects typically have onset of their disease at a young age with an acute presentation including diabetic ketoacidosis requiring continuous insulin treatment [1]. With a better understanding of the epidemiology and molecular mechanism of diabetes, however, clinical features such as the younger age of onset (e.g. less than 35 years old) or dependence on insulin treatment cannot adequately define the etiology of patients presenting with hyperglycemia.

Furthermore, there are major ethnic differences in disease pattern in terms of presentation and natural progression. In Caucasians, over 90% of patients with diabetes diagnosed before the age of 35 years have type 1 disease [1]. By contrast, autoimmune T1DM is uncommon in non-Caucasian populations [2–5]. Using Hong Kong as an example, which has a relatively homogenous southern Chinese population leading an affluent lifestyle, less than 10% of adults presenting with diabetic ketoacidosis have autoimmune markers. Similarly, only 10% of Hong Kong Chinese patients with young onset of disease had a type 1 presentation or antibodies to glutamic acid decarboxylase (GAD) [6]. Similar epidemiologic findings have also been reported in other Asian populations from India, Malaysia, Singapore and Mainland China [7]. In most case series, 60–80% of Caucasian people with T1DM have autoimmune markers such as autoantibodies to GAD and/or islet cell antigens (e.g. ICA-512). Conversely, 5–20% of young Asian patients with a non-ketotic presentation have autoimmune markers with a wide range of insulin reserve. These findings suggest that latent autoimmune diabetes in adults (LADA) is not uncommon in young patients with diabetes, especially those of Asian ethnicity, and there is considerable overlap between type 1 and 2 diabetes phenotypes (Figure 9.4) [6,8].

Our current understanding of the molecular pathways involved in the neogenesis, differentiation and maturation of pancreatic β-cells as well as the intracellular signaling mechanisms leading to insulin secretion are summarized in Figure 9.5. This large body of knowledge has provided the basis for the discovery and description of subtypes of diabetes with predominant β-cell failure from causes other than autoimmunity, such as monogenic diabetes. Patients with monogenic diabetes often have young onset of disease and lean body mass (see Chapter 15). They may also have delayed presentation with complications brought about by the insidious nature of their symptoms [9,10]. With the rising prevalence of young onset diabetes especially in low and middle income countries [11], there is a need for health care providers to be aware of these non-classic presentations of T1DM, because they have important implications on clinical management and family screening.

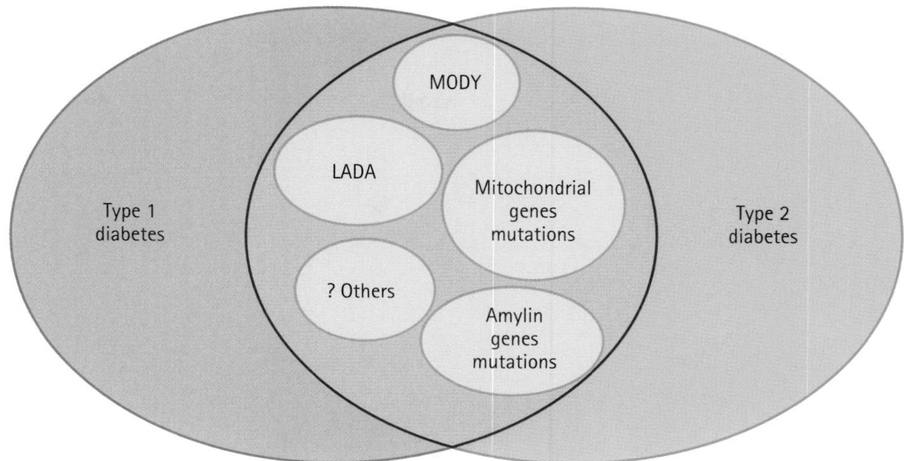

Figure 9.4 There are considerable overlaps between the phenotypes of type 1 and type 2 diabetes because of the heterogeneous genetic and autoimmune etiologies. These include maturity-onset diabetes of the young (MODY), latent autoimmune diabetes in adult (LADA) and genetic variants affecting the insulin, amylin and mitochondrial pathways. Other rare causes include fibrocalculous pancreatic diabetes and fulminant type 1 diabetes.

Atypical diabetes: heterogeneous etiologies of young-onset diabetes

In 1980, Winter *et al.* [12] first described a cohort of 129 African-American youths with acute ketotic presentation, of whom 12 patients subsequently did not require insulin and followed a clinical course resembling type 2 diabetes (T2DM). Since then, a number of reports have shown that there is a poor correlation between the mode of presentation of hyperglycemia, clinical course, need for insulin treatment and autoimmune status in different ethnic groups including Asians [13–15]. Many of these patients did not have HLA genotypes or autoantibodies typical of autoimmune T1DM. Some patients were obese, with insulin resistance and glucotoxicity contributing to the initial ketotic presentation [16].

Monogenic diabetes caused by genetic mutations encoding pathways implicated in insulin synthesis and secretion may lead to young-onset diabetes with atypical presentation. In young Chinese patients with diabetes, there is a higher prevalence of parental history of diabetes (32–47%), particularly maternal history, compared with those having a late onset of disease (12–19%) [10,17,18]. A progressively earlier age of onset of disease in successive generations has also been reported in some of these affected families [19]. These patients may exhibit a mixed phenotype, including young age of diagnosis, insulinopenia and normal body weight (as in type 1), with a non-ketotic state typical of T2DM, despite lack of insulin resistance and metabolic syndrome [20].

Monogenic diabetes

Maturity-onset diabetes of the young

Patients with maturity-onset diabetes of the young (MODY) typically present before the age of 25 years with a strong family history suggestive of autosomal dominant inheritance (see Chapter 15). Despite a non-ketotic mode of presentation, these patients often have features of abnormal pancreatic β-cell function. Some patients with MODY have a rapid deterioration in glycemic control after initial presentation while others experience mild hyperglycemia and do not require insulin despite having a long duration of disease.

To date, several subtypes of MODY have been reported. These include mutations of transcription factors: *MODY 1*: hepatic nuclear factor 4α (HNF-4α); *MODY 3*: HNF-1α or transcription factor 1 (TCF1); *MODY 4*: insulin promotion factor 1 (IPF-1); *MODY 5*: HNF-1β or transcription factor 2 (TCF-2); *MODY 6*: neurogenic differentiation 1 (NeuroD1) and *MODY 7*: carboxyl ester lipase (CEL) and glucokinase which is the glucose-sensor of the pancreatic β-cells (*MODY 2*). Transcription factors have key roles in pancreatic development including differentiation and proliferation of β-cells (Figure 9.4b). While genetic mutations in transcription factors typically cause significant insulin insufficiency and hyperglycemia, common polymorphisms of some of these transcription factors (e.g. HNF-1α [21], HNF-4α [22] and HNF-1β [23]) have also been shown to be associated with increased risk of diabetes or metabolic traits which may interact with other genetic or environmental and/or lifestyle factors to give rise to overt diabetes.

Over 80% of Caucasian patients with classic MODY (i.e. age of onset less than 25 years with autosomal pattern of inheritance) have been reported to have mutations in HNF-1α or glucokinase, while other MODY subtypes (HNF-4α, HNF-1β and IPF-1 mutations) were less common [24]. The frequencies of HNF-1α mutations ranged 25–50% in French [25], 36% in German [26], 13–18% in British [27], 8% in Japanese [28] and 5% in Chinese patients [9]. In unrelated young Chinese patients with diabetes, 5–10% were found to have glucokinase or HNF-1α mutations [13,29,30].

Although patients with some forms of MODY (e.g. *MODY 2*) have mild clinical course and rarely develop complications, other forms of MODY may be associated with severe insulin insufficiency and complications often brought about by the late pres-

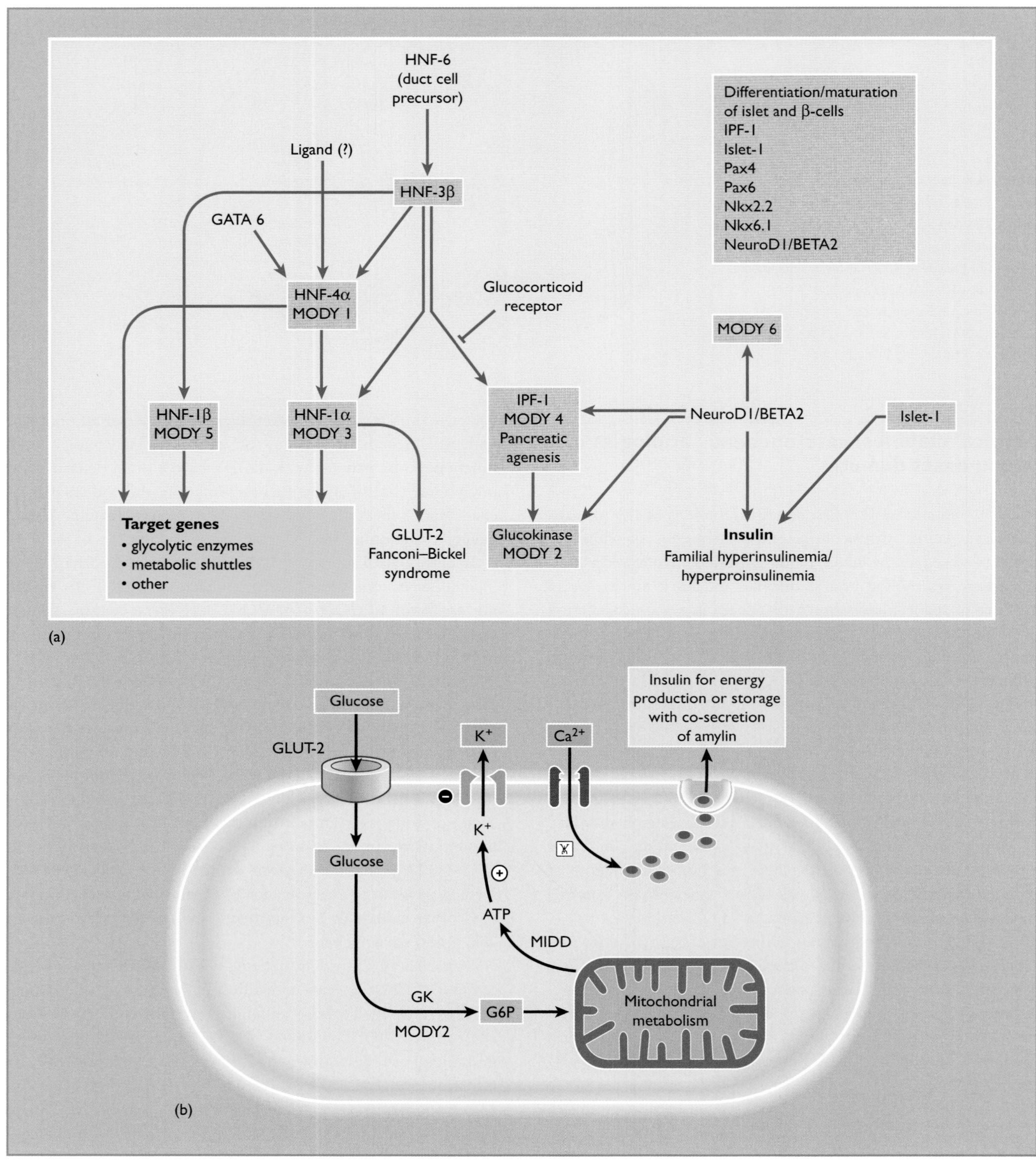
HNF-6
(duct cell
precursor)
Differentiation/maturation
of islet and β-cells
IPF-1
Islet-1
Pax4
Pax6
Nkx2.2
Nkx6.1
NeuroD1/BETA2
Ligand (?)
HNF-3β
GATA 6
HNF-4α
MODY 1
Glucocorticoid
receptor
MODY 6
HNF-1β
MODY 5
HNF-1α
MODY 3
IPF-1
MODY 4
Pancreatic
agenesis
NeuroD1/BETA2
Islet-1
Target genes
• glycolytic enzymes
• metabolic shuttles
• other
GLUT-2
Fanconi–Bickel
syndrome
Glucokinase
MODY 2
Insulin
Familial hyperinsulinemia/
hyperproinsulinemia
(a)
Glucose
GLUT-2
K+
Ca2+
Insulin for energy
production or storage
with co-secretion
of amylin
K+
Glucose
ATP
MIDD
GK
G6P
MODY2
Mitochondrial
metabolism
(b)

entation and/or delayed use of insulin [10]. In light of the potential long duration of disease, young patients with diabetes are more prone to develop microvascular complications than those with late onset of disease [31], thus emphasizing the importance of family screening.

Furthermore, heterogeneous mutations in these transcription factors can be expressed sequentially in renal tubules with possible roles in various stages of the development of renal tubules [32]. Thus, patients with MODY may have heterogeneous phenotypes with metabolic and renal manifestations. Patients with *MODY 3* from mutations in HNF-1α were found to have a low renal threshold for glucose [33] while patients with *MODY 5* from mutations in HNF-1β may have mild diabetes but increased susceptibility to severe renal disease and other urogenital malformations [34]. In a consecutive unrelated cohort consisting of 74 young Chinese patients with T2DM and nephropathy, a novel missense genetic variant in exon 3 (E260D, GAG→GAC) of the HNF-1β gene was identified. Extended family analysis revealed four other siblings carrying this variant with heterogeneity in clinical presentation that included one member with uncomplicated diabetes, one with impaired glucose tolerance and one with microalbuminuria with normal glucose tolerance. A silent polymorphism Q378Q was identified in another unrelated subject in this study. While these findings will need replication in independent and larger cohorts, the phenotypic heterogeneity associated with these genetic variants is noteworthy [35].

Mitochondrial gene mutations

Mitochondria are important intracellular organelles in the maintenance of glucose homeostasis and energy balance. Mitochondria have their own genome and unlike nuclear DNA which is protected by histones, mitochondrial DNA is more vulnerable to oxidative stress and environmental toxins. Superoxide radicals generated by the mitochondrial respiratory chain are a major source of damage to mitochondrial DNA. Aged patients with a positive family history of diabetes have a high frequency of mitochondrial mutations [36]. Because of its maternal inheritance, mitochondrial DNA is a well-known cause of a subtype of maternally inherited diabetes mellitus [37].

In 1992, an A3243G mutation in the mitochondrial DNA coding for $tRNA^{Leu(UUR)}$ (mt3243) was first reported. This form of diabetes was found in patients with both type 1 and type 2 diabetes and was characterized by maternal inheritance and deafness [38]. In a random cohort of Chinese patients with diabetes, 1–3% had this mutation with either type 1 or type 2 clinical course [39–41]. Other point mutations associated with increased risk of diabetes include sites at 3316, 3394 and 14577 as well as deletion and rearrangement in mitochondrial DNA [36].

In keeping with its candidacy as a "thrifty gene," the frequency of a common polymorphism of the mitochondrial DNA (T16189C) is higher in Chinese subjects with metabolic syndrome than those without (44% vs 33%), after adjustment for age and body mass index (BMI) [42]. In a meta-analysis, Asian subjects without diabetes had a higher frequency of the 16189C variant than their European counterparts (31.0% vs 9.2%) [43]. Despite negative reports in European populations [43], there are consistent data showing the risk association of the 16189C variant with T2DM in Asians [44,45].

Amylin gene mutations

Amylin, a 37 amino acid polypeptide, is co-secreted with insulin by pancreatic β-cells. It is the principal constituent of the amyloid deposits in the islets of Langerhans in T2DM [46,47]. In autopsy series, pancreatic amyloidosis was associated with β-cell loss in both Caucasian and Chinese subjects [48–50]. It is now evident that formation of intracellular islet amyloid polypeptide (IAPP) oligomers may contribute to pancreatic β-cell loss and progressive hyperglycemia [47]. Changes in metabolic milieu or genetic variants encoding proteins involved in amylin metabolism may lead to structural changes of amylin and increased oligomerization with β-cell death [51].

A S20G variant of the amylin gene has been shown to enhance cytotoxicity in transfected COS-1 cells and amyloidogenicity *in vitro* [52,53]. This genetic variant is found in 2–3% of Japanese, Chinese and Pacific Islanders with diabetes [9,52,54–57]. In Taiwanese Chinese, normoglycemic carriers of the S20G variant had reduced early phase insulin secretion [58]. Co-segregation findings in family studies of S20G variant, however, are incon-

Figure 9.5 (a) The cascade of transcription factors involved in pancreatic development as well as neogenesis, differentiation and maturation of pancreatic β-cells. Maturity-onset diabetes of the young (MODY) includes subtypes with mutations in transcription factors, namely MODY 1 with mutations of hepatic nuclear factor (HNF-4α); MODY 3: HNF-1α; MODY 4: insulin promotion factor (IPF-1); MODY 5: HNF-1β; MODY 6: NeuroD1: neurogenic differentiation 1 and MODY 7: carboxyl ester lipase (CEL) as well as glucokinase (GK) which is the glucose-sensor of the pancreatic β-cells (MODY 2). There are also interactions of glucose transporter 2 (GLUT 2) and endodermal factor, including GATA and various important genes and transcription factors governing the differentiation and maturation of pancreatic islet and beta cells. These include Pax genes family and genes encoding the homeodomain transcription factor Nkx 2.2 and Nkx 6.1. In South Asian Indian population, interaction of the NeuroD1, neurogenin-3 (NEUROG3) and HNF-1α genes has been observed to have combined effect in controlling islet cell development and insulin secretion, thus contributing to the overall glucose tolerance [93]. (b) The multiple steps involved in regulation of insulin secretion commencing with sensing of ambient blood glucose level by GLUT-2, glycolysis by GK, and ATP production by mitochondria. The generated ATP particles then close the potassium channel leading to membrane depolarization and opening of calcium channels. The intracellular calcium influx is associated with translocation of insulin and amylin containing vesicles to the cellular surface for extracytosis. During these processes, transcription factors are also activated resulting in insulin gene transcription and production to replenish the insulin containing vesicles and maintain continuous insulin secretion. GLUT, glucose transporter; MIDD, maternal inherited diabetes and deafness; MODY, maturity-onset diabetes of the young.

clusive, suggesting that it is likely to be a risk-modifying factor rather than a major diabetes gene [9,52,58].

Other genetic mutations affecting pancreatic β-cell function

Genetic variants of transcription factors implicated in pancreatic β-cell development, structure and function such as Pax6, Nkx2-2, Nkx6-1, NEUROG3 have also been reported in patients with type 1 or type 2 diabetes [59]. The pancreatic β-cell ATP-sensitive K^+ channels (K_{ATP} channels) comprises of two subunits, the inwardly rectifying potassium channel Kir6.2 and the sulfonylurea receptor SUR1. This transmembrane channel has an important regulatory role in insulin secretion (Figure 9.5b). Genetic variants encoding the K_{ATP} channels subunits Kir6.2 (KCNJ11) and SUR1 (ABCC8) are associated with reduced insulin secretion and diabetes in different ethnic populations [60–65] including Asians [59]. In the recent genome-wide association studies, polymorphisms encoding components of these K_{ATP} channels such as KCNJ11 and KCNQ1 have also been found to be associated with 20–30% increased risk of diabetes in Caucasian and Asian populations [66,67].

Autoimmune diabetes in adults

Autoantibodies to GAD are suggested to be sensitive markers of T1DM in Caucasians [13] although they can also be detected in patients with T2DM such as those with autoimmune diabetes in adults (LADA). In the UK Prospective Diabetes Study (UKPDS), approximately 10% of patients with T2DM had anti-GAD antibodies, the majority of whom eventually progressed to insulin dependency [68,69]. Reports from different ethnic groups suggest an estimated 10% prevalence of LADA in diabetic populations [68–70]. In Asians, 10–50% of patients with diabetes and acute or early onset of disease had anti-GAD antibodies depending on selection criteria and assay methodologies [2,6,13,71].

LADA is a slowly progressive form of autoimmune disease causing diabetes and is characterized by the presence of serum autoantibodies to pancreatic antigens [72,73]. Similar to T1DM, patients with LADA often carry other autoantibodies associated with celiac disease, adrenal and thyroid disorders [74,75]. Thus, it is plausible that LADA represents one end of a continuum of autoimmune diabetes with classic T1DM occupying the other end of the spectrum [76].

The nomenclature for this subtype of diabetes have been confusing, including T2DM with islet autoantibodies, slowly progressive insulin-dependent diabetes mellitus [77], type one-and-a-half diabetes [78,79], latent autoimmune diabetes in children (LADC) [80], latent autoimmune diabetes in the young (LADY) [81], autoimmune diabetes [82] and autoimmune diabetes in adults with slowly progressive β-cell failure (ADASP) [70], although LADA remains the most commonly used term. The World Health Organization (WHO) and American Diabetes Association (ADA) acknowledged LADA as a slowly progressive form of T1DM [83,84].

The correct diagnosis of LADA is clinically important because early use of insulin instead of sulphonylurea may prevent or reduce the rate of deterioration of β-cell function in these young patients with diabetes [85]. In patients with LADA, impaired β-cell response is evident at diagnosis and early use of insulin may reduce the adverse effects of glucotoxicity on β-cells [70,82]. Apart from high clinical suspicion, HLA studies may distinguish LADA from classic T1DM. In Caucasian populations, LADA is associated with HLA DQA1-DQB1*0102(3)-*0602(3)/X which is uncommon in patients with typical T1DM [86].

Other subtypes of diabetes with type 1 phenotype

In Japan and Korea, uncommon cases of fulminant T1DM presenting with diabetic ketoacidosis (often after a viral infection) have been reported in both young and old patients. These cases were characterized by absence of insulitis, negative autoantibodies, low C peptide levels, elevated pancreatic enzyme concentrations and association with HLA haplotypes [87,88].

In India, T2DM in youth often overlaps with monogenic forms of diabetes, fibrocalculous pancreatic diabetes and diabetes associated with malnourishment, all of which are ketosis-resistant forms of youth-onset diabetes [89]. In Indian patients with tropical calcific pancreatitis, the loss of endocrine function accompanying the exocrine damage may be an additional factor contributing to the clinical manifestation of diabetes in the presence of other stressors [90]. Using pancreatic specimens, Asian researchers have reported significant correlations between BMI and relatively low volume of β-cells [91] with amyloidosis, inflammation and fibrosis as common pathologic features [92].

Conclusions

Until recently, autoimmune T1DM was considered to be the predominant form of diabetes in children and young adults. With a better understanding of the pathogenesis of diabetes, it is now recognized that genetic or acquired factors that affect the pancreatic β-cell structure and function as well as associated mechanisms such as amylin deposition and mitochondrial damage may give rise to a broad range of clinical manifestations with considerable overlap between type 1 and type 2 phenotypes. Detailed medical history-taking (e.g. family history of diabetes, mode of presentation and exposure to infection), a complete physical examination (e.g. body leanness, microvascular complications, metabolic syndrome and associated cardiovascular risk factors) and the use of appropriate laboratory testing (e.g. autoantibodies against pancreatic antigens and genetic markers) may help clinicians refine the diagnosis. This will help to guide the treatment of these patients who often present at a young and have a long duration of diabetes ahead of them, this makes them eopecially at risk for the long-term chronic complications of diabetes.

References

1 Laakso M, Pyorala K. Age of onset and type of diabetes. *Diabetes Care* 1985; **8**:114–117.

2 Zimmet PZ, Rowley MJ, Mackay IR, Knowles WJ, Chen QY, Chapman LH, *et al*. The ethnic distribution of antibodies to glutamic acid decarboxylase: presence and levels in insulin-dependent diabetes mellitus in Europoid and Asian subjects. *J Diabet Complications* 1993; **7**:1–7.

3 Tajiman N, La Porte RE, Hibi I, Kitagawa T, Fujita H, Drash AL. A comparison of the epidemiology of youth-onset insulin-dependent diabetes mellitus between Japan and the United States (Allegheny County, Pennsylvania). *Diabetes Care* 1985; **8**(Suppl 1):17–23.

4 Huen KF, Low LC, Wong GW, Tse WW, Yu AC, Lam YY, *et al*. Epidemiology of diabetes mellitus in children in Hong Kong: the Hong Kong childhood diabetes register. *J Pediatr Endocrinol Metab* 2000; **13**:297–302.

5 Wong GWK, Leung SSF, Opphenheimer SJ. Epidemiology of IDDM in southern Chinese children in Hong Kong. *Diabetes Care* 1993; **16**:926–928.

6 Ko GTC, Chan JCN, Yeung VTF, Chow CC, Li JKY, Lau MSW, *et al*. Antibodies to glutamic acid decarboxylase in young Chinese diabetic patients. *Ann Clin Biochem* 1998; **35**:761–767.

7 Thai AC, Mohan V, Khalid BA, Cockram CS, Pan CY, Zimmet P, *et al*. Islet autoimmunity status in Asians with young-onset diabetes (12–40 years): association with clinical characteristics, beta cell function and cardio-metabolic risk factors. *Diabetes Res Clin Pract* 2008; **80**:224–230.

8 Thai AC, Ng WY, Loke KY, Lee WR, Lui KF, Cheah JS. Anti-GAD antibodies in Chinese patients with youth and adult-onset IDDM and NIDDM. *Diabetologia* 1997; **40**:1425–1430.

9 Ng MCY, Lee SC, Ko GTC, Li JKY, So WY, Hashim Y, *et al*. Familial early onset type 2 diabetes in Chinese: the more significant roles of obesity and genetics than autoimmunity. *Diabetes Care* 2001; **24**:667–671.

10 Ng MCY, Li JKY, So WY, Critchley JAJH, Cockram CS, Bell GI, *et al*. Nature or nuture: an insightful illustration from a Chinese family with hepatocyte nuclear factor 1-alpha diabetes (MODY3). *Diabetologia* 2000; **43**:816–818.

11 Roglic G, Unwin N, Bennett PH, Mathers C, Tuomilehto J, Nag S, *et al*. The burden of mortality attributable to diabetes: realistic estimates for the year 2000. *Diabetes Care* 2005; **28**:2130–2135.

12 Winter WE, Maclaren NK, Riley WJ, Clarke DW, Kappy MS, Spillar RP. Maturity-onset diabetes of youth in black Americans. *N Engl J Med* 1987; **316**:285–291.

13 Chan JC, Yeung VT, Chow CC, Ko GT, Mackay IR, Rowley MJ, *et al*. Pancreatic beta cell function and antibodies to glutamic acid decarboxylase (anti-GAD) in Chinese patients with clinical diagnosis of insulin-dependent diabetes mellitus. *Diabetes Res Clin Pract* 1996; **32**:27–34.

14 Tan KCB, Mackay IR, Zimmet PZ, Hawkins BR, Lam KSL. Metabolic and immunologic features of Chinese patients with atypical diabetes mellitus. *Diabetes Care* 2000; **23**:353–338.

15 Li JKY, Chan JCN, Zimmet PZ, Rowley MJ, Mackay IR, Cockram CS. Young Chinese adults with new onset of diabetic ketoacidosis: clinical course, autoimmune status and progression of pancreatic beta cell function. *Diabetic Med* 2000; **17**:295–298.

16 Banerji MA, Chaiken RL, Huey H, Tuomi T, Norin AJ, Mackay IR, *et al*. GAD antibody negative NIDDM in adult Black subjects with diabetic ketoacidosis and increased frequency of human leukocyte antigen DR3 and DR4. Flatbush Diabetes. *Diabetes* 1994; **43**:741–745.

17 Chan JCN, Cheung CK, Swaminathan R, Nicholls MG, Cockram CS. Obesity, albuminuria and hypertension among Hong Kong Chinese with non-insulin-dependent diabetes mellitus (NIDDM). *Postgrad Med J* 1993; **69**:204–210.

18 Lee SC, Ko GTC, Li JKY, Chow CC, Yeung VTF, Critchley JAJH, *et al*. Factors predicting the age at diagnosis of type 2 diabetes in Hong Kong Chinese. *Diabetes Care* 2001; **24**:646–649.

19 Chan JCN, Ng MCY. Lessons learned from young onset diabetes in China. *Curr Diab Rep* 2003; **3**:101–107.

20 Moller AM, Dalgaard LT, Pociot F, Nerup J, Hansen T, Pedersen O. Mutations in the hepatocyte nuclear factor-1alpha gene in Caucasian families originally classified as having Type I diabetes. *Diabetologia* 1998; **41**:1528–1531.

21 Armendariz AD, Krauss RM. Hepatic nuclear factor 1-alpha: inflammation, genetics, and atherosclerosis. *Curr Opin Lipidol* 2009; **20**:106–111.

22 Ghosh S, Watanabe RM, Hauser ER, Valle T, Magnuson VL, Erdos MR, *et al*. Type 2 diabetes: evidence for linkage on chromosome 20 in 716 Finnish affected sib pairs. *Proc Natl Acad Sci U S A* 1999; **96**:2198–2203.

23 Wang C, Hu C, Zhang R, Bao Y, Ma X, Lu J, *et al*. Common variants of hepatocyte nuclear factor 1β are associated with type 2 diabetes in a Chinese population. *Diabetes* 2009; **58**:1023–1027.

24 Fajans SS, Bell GI, Polonsky KS. Molecular mechanisms and clinical pathophysiology of maturity onset diabetes of the young. *N Engl J Med* 2001; **345**:971–980.

25 Vaxillaire M, Rouard M, Yamagata K, Oda N, Kaisaki PJ, Boriraj VV, *et al*. Identification of nine novel mutations in the hepatocyte nuclear factor 1 alpha gene associated with maturity-onset diabetes of the young (MODY3). *Hum Mol Genet* 1997; **6**:583–586.

26 Kaisaki PJ, Menzel S, Lindner T, Oda N, Rjasanowski I, Sahm J, *et al*. Mutations in the hepatocyte nuclear factor-1alpha gene in MODY and early-onset NIDDM: evidence for a mutational hotspot in exon 4. *Diabetes* 1997; **46**:528–535.

27 Frayling TM, Bulman MP, Appleton M, Hattersley AT, Ellard S. A rapid screening method for hepatocyte nuclear factor 1 alpha frameshift mutations; prevalence in maturity-onset diabetes of the young and late-onset non-insulin dependent diabetes. *Hum Genet* 1997; **101**:351–354.

28 Iwasaki N, Oda N, Ogata M, Hara M, Hinokio Y, Oda Y, *et al*. Mutations in the hepatocyte nuclear factor-1alpha/MODY3 gene in Japanese subjects with early- and late-onset NIDDM. *Diabetes* 1997; **46**:1504–1508.

29 Xu JY, Chan V, Zhang WY, Wat NM, Lam KS. Mutations in the hepatocyte nuclear factor-1alpha gene in Chinese MODY families: prevalence and functional analysis. *Diabetologia* 2002; **45**: 744–746.

30 Xu JY, Dan QH, Chan V, Wat NM, Tam S, Tiu SC, *et al*. Genetic and clinical characteristics of maturity-onset diabetes of the young in Chinese patients. *Eur J Hum Genet* 2005; **13**:422–427.

31 Lee ET, Lu M, Bennett PH, Keen H. Vascular disease in younger-onset diabetes: comparison of European, Asian and American Indian cohorts of the WHO Multinational Study of Vascular Disease in Diabetes. *Diabetologia* 2001; **44**(Suppl 2):S78–S81.

32 Cereghini S, Ott MO, Power S, Maury M. Expression patterns of vHNF1 and HNF1 homeoproteins in early postimplantation embryos

suggest distinct and sequential developmental roles. *Development* 1992; **116**:783–797.
33 Menzel R, Kaisaki PJ, Rjasanowski I, Heinke P, Kerner W, Menzel S. A low renal threshold for glucose in diabetic patients with a mutation in the hepatocyte nuclear factor-1alpha (HNF-1alpha) gene. *Diabet Med* 1998; **15**:816–820.
34 Horikawa Y, Iwasaki N, Hara M, Furuta H, Hinokio Y, Cockburn BN, *et al.* Mutation in hepatocyte nuclear factor-1 beta gene (TCF2) associated with MODY. *Nat Genet* 1997; **17**:384–385.
35 So WY, Ng MC, Horikawa Y, Njolstad PR, Li JK, Ma RC, *et al.* Genetic variants of hepatocyte nuclear factor-1beta in Chinese young-onset diabetic patients with nephropathy. *J Diabet Complications* 2003; **17**:369–373.
36 Li MZ, Yu DM, Yu P, Liu DM, Wang K, Tang XZ. Mitochondrial gene mutations and type 2 diabetes in Chinese families. *Chin Med J (Engl)* 2008; **121**:682–686.
37 Maassen JA, LM TH, Van Essen E, Heine RJ, Nijpels G, Jahangir Tafrechi RS, *et al.* Mitochondrial diabetes: molecular mechanisms and clinical presentation. *Diabetes* 2004; **53**(Suppl 1):S103–S109.
38 van den Ouweland JM, Lemkes HH, Ruitenbeek W, Sandkuijl LA, de Vijlder MF, Struyvenberg PA, *et al.* Mutation in mitochondrial tRNA(Leu)(UUR) gene in a large pedigree with maternally transmitted type II diabetes mellitus and deafness. *Nat Genet* 1992; **1**:368–371.
39 Ng MCY, Yeung VTF, Chow CC, Li JKY, Smith PR, Mijovic CH, *et al.* Mitochondrial DNA A3243G mutation in patients with early or late onset Type 2 diabetes mellitus in Hong Kong Chinese. *J Endocrinol* 2000; **52**:557–564.
40 Ji L, Hou X, Han X. Prevalence and clinical characteristics of mitochondrial tRNA leu(UUR) mt 3243 A→G and ND-1 gene mt 3316 G→A mutations in Chinese patients with type 2 diabetes. *Chin Med J (Engl)* 2001; **114**:1205–1207.
41 Xiang K, Wang Y, Wu S, Lu H, Zheng T, Sun D, *et al.* Mitochondrial tRNA(Leu(UUR)) gene mutation diabetes mellitus in Chinese. *Chin Med J (Engl)* 1997; **110**:372–378.
42 Weng SW, Liou CW, Lin TK, Wei YH, Lee CF, Eng HL, *et al.* Association of mitochondrial deoxyribonucleic acid 16189 variant (T→C transition) with metabolic syndrome in Chinese adults. *J Clin Endocrinol Metab* 2005; **90**:5037–5040.
43 Chinnery PF, Elliott HR, Patel S, Lambert C, Keers SM, Durham SE, *et al.* Role of the mitochondrial DNA 16184-16193 poly-C tract in type 2 diabetes. *Lancet* 2005; **366**:1650–1651.
44 Liou CW, Lin TK, Huei Weng H, Lee CF, Chen TL, Wei YH, *et al.* A common mitochondrial DNA variant and increased body mass index as associated factors for development of type 2 diabetes: additive effects of genetic and environmental factors. *J Clin Endocrinol Metab* 2007; **92**:235–239.
45 Park KS, Chan JC, Chuang LM, Suzuki S, Araki E, Nanjo K, *et al.* A mitochondrial DNA variant at position 16189 is associated with type 2 diabetes mellitus in Asians. *Diabetologia* 2008; **51**:602–608.
46 Lorenzo A, Razzaboni B, Weir GC, Yankner BA. Pancreatic islet cell toxicity of amylin associated with type-2 diabetes mellitus. *Nature* 1994; **368**:756–760.
47 Haataja L, Gurlo T, Huang CJ, Butler PC. Islet amyloid in type 2 diabetes, and the toxic oligomer hypothesis. *Endocr Rev* 2008; **29**:303–316.
48 Zhao H, Lai F, Tong P, Zhong D, Yang D, Tomlinson B, *et al.* Prevalence and clinicopathological characteristics of islet amyloid in Chinese patients with type 2 diabetes. *Diabetes* 2003; **52**:2759–2766.
49 Clark A, Nilsson MR. Islet amyloid: a complication of islet dysfunction or an aetiological factor in Type 2 diabetes? *Diabetologia* 2004; **47**:157–169.
50 Clark A, Wells CA, Buley ID, Cruickshank JK, Vanhegan RI, Matthews DR, *et al.* Islet amyloid, increased A-cells, reduced B-cells and exocrine fibrosis: quantitative changes in the pancreas in type 2 diabetes. *Diabetes Res* 1988; **9**:151–159.
51 Hayden MR, Tyagi SC, Kerklo MM, Nicolls MR. Type 2 diabetes mellitus as a conformational disease. *JOP* 2005; **6**:287–302.
52 Sakagashira S, Sanke T, Hanabusa T, Shimomura H, Ohagi S, Kumagaye KY, *et al.* Missense mutation of amylin gene (S20G) in Japanese NIDDM patients. *Diabetes* 1996; **45**:1279–1281.
53 Sakagashira S, Hiddinga HJ, Tateishi K, Sanke T, Hanabusa T, Nanjo K, *et al.* S20G mutant amylin exhibits increased in vitro amyloidogenicity and increased intracellular cytotoxicity compared to wild-type amylin. *Am J Pathol* 2000; **157**:2101–2109.
54 Poa NR, Cooper GJ, Edgar PF. Amylin gene promoter mutations predispose to Type 2 diabetes in New Zealand Maori. *Diabetologia* 2003; **46**:574–578.
55 Lee SC, Hashim Y, Li JKY, Ko GTC, Critchley JAJH, Cockram CS, *et al.* The islet amyloid polypeptide (amylin) gene S20G mutation in Chinese subjects: evidence for associations with type 2 diabetes and cholesterol levels. *J Endocrinol* 2001; **54**:541–546.
56 Seino S. S20G mutation of the amylin gene is associated with Type II diabetes in Japanese. Study Group of Comprehensive Analysis of Genetic Factors in Diabetes Mellitus. *Diabetologia* 2001; **44**:906–909.
57 Ma Z, Westermark GT, Sakagashira S, Sanke T, Gustavsson A, Sakamoto H, *et al.* Enhanced *in vitro* production of amyloid-like fibrils from mutant (S20G) islet amyloid polypeptide. *Amyloid* 2001; **8**:242–249.
58 Chuang LM, Lee KC, Huang CN, Wu HP, Tai TY, Lin BJ. Role of S20G mutation of amylin gene in insulin secretion, insulin sensitivity, and type II diabetes mellitus in Taiwanese patients. *Diabetologia* 1998; **41**:1250–1251.
59 Yokoi N, Kanamori M, Horikawa Y, Takeda J, Sanke T, Furuta H, *et al.* Association studies of variants in the genes involved in pancreatic beta-cell function in type 2 diabetes in Japanese subjects. *Diabetes* 2006; **55**:2379–2386.
60 Inoue H, Ferrer J, Welling CM, Elbein SC, Hoffman M, Mayorga R, *et al.* Sequence variants in the sulfonylurea receptor (SUR) gene are associated with NIDDM in Caucasians. *Diabetes* 1996; **45**:825–831.
61 Hani EH, Clement K, Velho G, Vionnet N, Hager J, Philippi A, *et al.* Genetic studies of the sulfonylurea receptor gene locus in NIDDM and in morbid obesity among French Caucasians. *Diabetes* 1997; **46**:688–694.
62 Nielsen LB, Ploug KB, Swift P, Orskov C, Jansen-Olesen I, Chiarelli F, *et al.* Co-localisation of the Kir6.2/SUR1 channel complex with glucagon-like peptide-1 and glucose-dependent insulinotrophic polypeptide expression in human ileal cells and implications for glycaemic control in new onset type 1 diabetes. *Eur J Endocrinol* 2007; **156**:663–671.
63 van Tilburg JH, Rozeman LB, van Someren H, Rigters-Aris CA, Freriks JP, Pearson PL, *et al.* The exon 16-3t variant of the sulphonylurea receptor gene is not a risk factor for Type II diabetes mellitus in the Dutch Breda cohort. *Diabetologia* 2000; **43**:681–682.
64 Gloyn AL, Hashim Y, Ashcroft SJ, Ashfield R, Wiltshire S, Turner RC. Association studies of variants in promoter and coding regions of beta-cell ATP-sensitive K-channel genes SUR1 and Kir6.2 with Type 2 diabetes mellitus (UKPDS 53). *Diabet Med* 2001; **18**:206–212.

65 van Dam RM, Hoebee B, Seidell JC, Schaap MM, de Bruin TW, Feskens EJ. Common variants in the ATP-sensitive K^+ channel genes KCNJ11 (Kir6.2) and ABCC8 (SUR1) in relation to glucose intolerance: population-based studies and meta-analyses. *Diabet Med* 2005; **22**:590–598.

66 Laukkanen O, Pihlajamaki J, Lindstrom J, Eriksson J, Valle TT, Hamalainen H, *et al.* Polymorphisms of the SUR1 (ABCC8) and Kir6.2 (KCNJ11) genes predict the conversion from impaired glucose tolerance to type 2 diabetes. The Finnish Diabetes Prevention Study. *J Clin Endocrinol Metab* 2004; **89**:6286–6290.

67 Yasuda K, Miyake K, Horikawa Y, Hara K, Osawa H, Furuta H, *et al.* Variants in KCNQ1 are associated with susceptibility to type 2 diabetes mellitus. *Nat Genet* 2008; **40**:1092–1097.

68 Turner RC, Stratton I, Horton V, Manley S, Zimmet P, Mackay IR, *et al.* UKPDS 25: autoantibodies to islet-cell cytoplasm and glutamic acid decarboxylase for prediction of insulin requirement in type 2 diabetes. UK Prospective Diabetes Study Group. *Lancet* 1997; **350**:1288–1293.

69 Owen KR, Stride A, Ellard S, Hattersley AT. Etiological investigation of diabetes in young adults presenting with apparent type 2 diabetes. *Diabetes Care* 2003; **26**:2088–2093.

70 Stenstrom G, Gottsater A, Bakhtadze E, Berger B, Sundkvist G. Latent autoimmune diabetes in adults: definition, prevalence, beta-cell function, and treatment. *Diabetes* 2005; **54**(Suppl 2):S68–S72.

71 Tuomi T, Zimmet P, Rowley MJ, Min HK, Vichayanrat A, Lee HK, *et al.* Differing frequency of autoantibodies to glutamic acid decarboxylase among Koreans, Thais, and Australians with diabetes mellitus. *Clin Immunol Immunopathol* 1995; **74**:202–206.

72 Fielding AM, Brophy S, Davies H, Williams R. Latent autoimmune diabetes in adults: increased awareness will aid diagnosis. *Ann Clin Biochem* 2007; **44**:321–323.

73 van Deutekom AW, Heine RJ, Simsek S. The islet autoantibody titres: their clinical relevance in latent autoimmune diabetes in adults (LADA) and the classification of diabetes mellitus. *Diabet Med* 2008; **25**:117–125.

74 Kucera P, Novakova D, Behanova M, Novak J, Tlaskalova-Hogenova H, Andel M. Gliadin, endomysial and thyroid antibodies in patients with latent autoimmune diabetes of adults (LADA). *Clin Exp Immunol* 2003; **133**:139–143.

75 Gambelunghe G, Forini F, Laureti S, Murdolo G, Toraldo G, Santeusanio F, *et al.* Increased risk for endocrine autoimmunity in Italian type 2 diabetic patients with GAD65 autoantibodies. *Clin Endocrinol (Oxf)* 2000; **52**:565–573.

76 Leslie RD, Williams R, Pozzilli P. Clinical review: Type 1 diabetes and latent autoimmune diabetes in adults – one end of the rainbow. *J Clin Endocrinol Metab* 2006; **91**:1654–1659.

77 Kobayashi T, Maruyama T, Shimada A, Kasuga A, Kanatsuka A, Takei I, *et al.* Insulin intervention to preserve beta cells in slowly progressive insulin-dependent (type 1) diabetes mellitus. *Ann N Y Acad Sci* 2002; **958**:117–130.

78 Juneja R, Palmer JP. Type 1 1/2 diabetes: myth or reality? *Autoimmunity* 1999; **29**:65–83.

79 Palmer JP, Hirsch IB. What's in a name: latent autoimmune diabetes of adults, type 1.5, adult-onset, and type 1 diabetes. *Diabetes Care* 2003; **26**:536–538.

80 Aycan Z, Berberoglu M, Adiyaman P, Ergur AT, Ensari A, Evliyaoglu O, *et al.* Latent autoimmune diabetes mellitus in children (LADC) with autoimmune thyroiditis and celiac disease. *J Pediatr Endocrinol Metab* 2004; **17**:1565–1569.

81 Lohmann T, Nietzschmann U, Kiess W. "Lady-like": is there a latent autoimmune diabetes in the young? *Diabetes Care* 2000; **23**:1707–1708.

82 Fourlanos S, Dotta F, Greenbaum CJ, Palmer JP, Rolandsson O, Colman PG, *et al.* Latent autoimmune diabetes in adults (LADA) should be less latent. *Diabetologia* 2005; **48**:2206–2212.

83 Diagnosis and classification of diabetes mellitus. *Diabetes Care* 2009; **32**(Suppl 1):S62–S67.

84 Alberti KGMM, Zimmet PZ. Definition, diagnosis and classification of diabetes mellitus and its complications. Part 1: Diagnosis and classification of diabetes mellitus provisional report of a WHO consultation. *Diabetic Med* 1998; **15**:539–553.

85 Kobayashi T, Nakanishi K, Murase T, Kosaka K. Small doses of subcutaneous insulin as a strategy for preventing slowly progressive beta-cell failure in islet cell antibody-positive patients with clinical features of NIDDM. *Diabetes* 1996; **45**:622–626.

86 Stenstrom G, Berger B, Borg H, Fernlund P, Dorman JS, Sundkvist G. HLA-DQ genotypes in classic type 1 diabetes and in latent autoimmune diabetes of the adult. *Am J Epidemiol* 2002; **156**:787–796.

87 Imagawa A, Hanafusa T. Fulminant type 1 diabetes-is it an Asian-oriented disease? *Intern Med* 2005; **44**:913–914.

88 Cho YM, Kim JT, Ko KS, Koo BK, Yang SW, Park MH, *et al.* Fulminant type 1 diabetes in Korea: high prevalence among patients with adult-onset type 1 diabetes. *Diabetologia* 2007; **50**:2276–2279.

89 Mohan V, Jaydip R, Deepa R. Type 2 diabetes in Asian Indian youth. *Pediatr Diabetes* 2007; **8**(Suppl 9):28–34.

90 Yajnik CS, Sahasrabudhe RA, Naik SS, Katrak A, Shelgikar KM, Kanitkar SV, *et al.* Exocrine pancreatic function (serum immunoreactive trypsin, fecal chymotrypsin, and pancreatic isoamylase) in Indian diabetics. *Pancreas* 1990; **5**:631–638.

91 Yoon KH, Ko SH, Cho JH, Lee JM, Ahn YB, Song KH, *et al.* Selective beta-cell loss and alpha-cell expansion in patients with type 2 diabetes mellitus in Korea. *J Clin Endocrinol Metab* 2003; **88**:2300–2308.

92 Zhao HL, Sui Y, Guan J, He L, Lai FM, Zhong DR, *et al.* Higher islet amyloid load in men than in women with type 2 diabetes mellitus. *Pancreas* 2008; **37**:e68–73.

93 Jackson AE, Cassell PG, North BV, Vijayaraghavan S, Gelding SV, Ramachandran A, *et al.* Polymorphic variations in the neurogenic differentiation-1, neurogenin-3, and hepatocyte nuclear factor-1alpha genes contribute to glucose intolerance in a South Indian population. *Diabetes* 2004; **53**:2122–2125.

10 Abnormalities of Insulin Secretion and β-Cell Defects in Type 2 Diabetes

Mazen Alsahli & John E. Gerich

University of Rochester School of Medicine, Rochester, NY, USA

Keypoints

- Type 2 diabetes mellitus (T2DM) is a heterogeneous disorder caused by a combination of genetic and environmental factors which adversely affect β-cell function and tissue insulin sensitivity.
- About 10% of patients with phenotypic T2DM actually have a late-onset form of autoimmune diabetes while up to another 5% have autosomal dominantly inherited forms such as maturity-onset diabetes of the young and mitochondrial diabetes. The remaining 85% of patients have "garden variety" T2DM which is a polygenic disorder.
- The preponderance of available information indicate that genetic factors primarily affect β-cell function whereas acquired factors (obesity, physical inactivity, glucose and lipid toxicity) are mainly responsible for the insulin resistance seen in this condition. Impaired β-cell function can be detected in genetically predisposed individuals (i.e. the monozygotic twin or first-degree relative of someone who has T2DM) at a time when they have normal glucose tolerance and normal tissue insulin sensitivity.
- T2DM develops because of a progressive deterioration in β-cell function coupled with the addition of acquired insulin resistance for which the β-cell cannot compensate. At time of diagnosis, β-cell function is already reduced about 50% and most of the defects demonstrable in people with T2DM are already present in individuals with impaired glucose tolerance and those genetically predisposed to develop T2DM.
- Commonly found insulin secretion abnormalities include: absent first-phase and diminished second-phase release. Responses to ingestion of mixed meals and to non-glucose stimuli are reduced with a decrease in maximal secretory capacity. The secretory pulses, both rapid and ultradian, are smaller and less regular. The ratio of proinsulin to insulin release is also elevated.
- Normally there is a curvilinear hyperbolic relationship between β-cell function and tissue insulin sensitivity so that as tissue insulin sensitivity decreases (as in obesity and pregnancy), β-cell function increases in a compensatory fashion to maintain normal glucose tolerance. Prospective longitudinal studies have shown that people who have impaired glucose tolerance and progress to T2DM fall off this curve because of an inability of the β-cell to compensate for insulin resistance.
- Acquired factors also adversely affect β-cell function and contribute to the development of T2DM. These include adverse effects of hyperglycemia and increased plasma free fatty acids, respectively termed glucotoxicity and lipotoxicity, alterations in incretins (GLP-1, GIP) and malnutrition *in utero* and in early life which may affect programing of the β-cell with respect to glucose sensing, apoptosis, regeneration and the ability to compensate for insulin resistance. Endoplasmic reticulum stress-induced apoptosis and the effect interleukin-1β has on β-cell function and life cycle are recently receiving more attention for their role in the pathogenesis of T2DM.
- A pathologic feature present in 90% of patients with T2DM is the abnormal extracellular deposits of islet amyloid. It is composed of insoluble fibrils formed from the protein islet amyloid polypeptide (IAPP). Other histologic changes include a 30–50% decrease in islet mass and an alteration in the relative proportion of the islet cell population.
- The IAPP and its amyloid deposits have not been clearly found to be cytotoxic to β-cell and recent evidence from animal studies suggests that the formation of intracellular smaller IAPP oligomers is possibly the cytotoxic form associated with increased β-cell apoptosis.

Type 2 diabetes (T2DM) is a heterogeneous disorder, phenotypically, genotypically and pathogenetically. Approximately 10% of patients have a late-onset form of autoimmune diabetes which may represent a hybrid of type 1 and type 2 diabetes (see Chapter 9) [1]; up to another 5% of patients have one of the autosomally dominant inherited forms of maturity-onset diabetes of youth (MODY); another 1% may have rare genetic mutations involving insulin receptors and elements of the insulin signaling pathway (see Chapter 15). The remaining 85% of patients have "garden variety" T2DM which is the subject of this chapter.

Textbook of Diabetes, 4th edition. Edited by R. Holt, C. Cockram, A. Flyvbjerg and B. Goldstein.

Impaired β-cell function vs insulin resistance

The common variety of T2DM results from a combination of genetic and acquired factors which adversely affect β-cell function and tissue insulin sensitivity (see Chapter 11) [2,3]. For many years it was controversial whether impaired β-cell function or tissue insulin resistance was the underlying pathogenetic element. Until recently, it was generally thought that insulin resistance preceded β-cell dysfunction and was the primary genetic factor, while β-cell dysfunction was a late phenomenon brought about by exhaustion after years of compensatory hypersecretion [4–6]. During the past several years, however, the accumulation of evidence from sophisticated studies examining β-cell function and tissue insulin sensitivity, both cross-sectionally and longitudinally, have swung the pendulum over to the concept that impaired β-cell function is the primary underlying, probably genetic, defect [2,7–9].

The idea that insulin resistance could be the primary defect can be traced back to the classic studies of Himsworth & Kerr [10] more than 60 years ago, in which it was demonstrated that lean patients with early-onset diabetes were sensitive to exogenous injection of insulin, whereas obese patients with late-onset diabetes were resistant. Twenty-one years later, the first measurement of plasma insulin levels in patients with T2DM [11] found that they had greater than normal values in the fasting and postprandial state, providing further evidence for insulin resistance. Over the following 40 years, numerous studies (summarized in [4,5,12]) reported that patients with T2DM, people with impaired glucose tolerance (IGT), and first-degree relatives of individuals with T2DM who subsequently developed T2DM were hyperinsulinemic and insulin resistant [13,14].

The problem with interpretation of the results of these studies is that they failed to take the following into consideration:

- Importance of the dynamics of insulin secretion.
- Appropriateness of the plasma insulin level for the prevailing stimulus for insulin secretion (i.e. plasma glucose level).
- Relation of β-cell function to insulin resistance.

Importance of the dynamics of insulin secretion

Although the finding was originally described by Yalow & Berson in 1960, it was not well appreciated until 1967 that, during oral glucose tolerance tests, the elevated 2-hour post-challenge plasma insulin levels in people with T2DM were accompanied by reduced early (30 minute) insulin responses [15]. These decreases in early insulin release are evident even in individuals with mild IGT (Figure 10.1). This reduction in early insulin response has been shown to diminish suppression of endogenous glucose production after glucose ingestion [16]; the resultant hyperglycemia provides a greater stimulus to the β-cell, explaining the late (2 hour) hyperinsulinemia. The latter had often been erroneously interpreted to be the result of insulin resistance [4–6]. Studies in normal volunteers, however, in whom early insulin responses were diminished by infusion of somatostatin so as to simulate the situation in people with IGT and T2DM produced late hyperinsulinemia [17]. Moreover, restoration of early insulin responses either by insulin or an insulin secretogogue reduces late hyperinsulinemia [18,19].

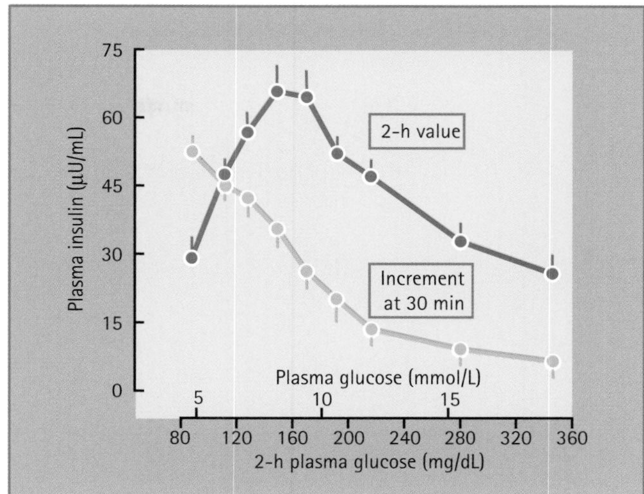

Figure 10.1 Relationship between early (30 minutes) and late (2 hour) plasma insulin levels and 2-hour plasma glucose levels during oral glucose tolerance tests (n = 294, mean ± SEM). Reproduced from Gerich [2], with permission from The Endocrine Society.

Appropriateness of the plasma insulin level for the prevailing glucose level

The major factor acutely regulating insulin is the plasma glucose concentration. In addition to glucose, increases in circulating amino acid, free fatty acid (FFA), gastrointestinal hormones (incretins: glucagon-like peptide [GLP-1], glucose-dependent insulinotropic peptide [GIP]) augment insulin secretion whereas increases in other factors such as catecholamines, cortisol, growth hormone, leptin, and tumor necrosis factor α (TNF-α) can reduce β-cell responses (see Chapter 6).

As glucose is the predominant stimulus for insulin secretion, the prevailing plasma glucose concentration must be taken into consideration in judging whether the plasma insulin concentration is appropriate. For example, the plasma insulin level in an individual with diabetes whose plasma glucose concentration is 180 mg/dL (10 mmol/L) may be twice as great as that of an individual without diabetes with a plasma glucose concentration of 90 mg/dL (5 mmol/L), but is clearly inappropriate because the non-diabetic individual would have a plasma insulin level four times as great at the same hyperglycemia [20]. Such evaluation is difficult with data from oral glucose tolerance tests (OGTT). Although equations exist that relate OGTT responses to those of hyperglycemic clamps [21], the latter are considered to be the gold standard for assessing β-cell function, because with this technique an identical stimulus for insulin release is used and both phases of insulin release can be evaluated.

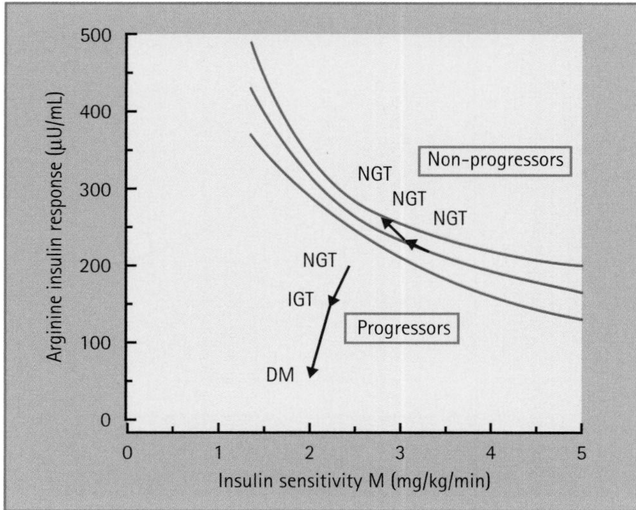

Figure 10.2 Curvilinear relationship between β-cell function (represented by the acute insulin response to intravenous arginine) and insulin sensitivity (represented by the glucose infusion rate necessary to maintain euglycemia [M] during a hyperinsulinemic clamp). People who maintained normal glucose tolerance (NGT) stayed on the curvilinear line. People whose glucose tolerance deteriorated to impaired glucose tolerance (IGT) and to type 2 diabetes (DM) fell below the line, demonstrating inadequate β-cell compensation for insulin resistance. Reproduced from Weyer *et al.* [22], with permission from the American Society for Clinical Investigation.

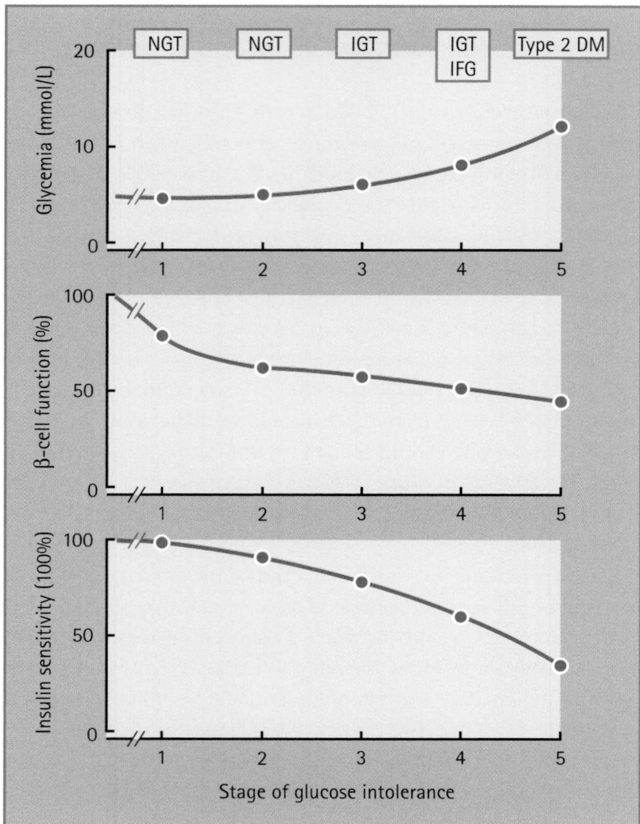

Figure 10.3 The stages of glucose tolerance and associated β-cell function and insulin sensitivity, from normal glucose tolerance (NGT) through impaired glucose tolerance (IGT), with or without impaired fasting glucose (IFG), and finally type 2 diabetes mellitus (DM).

Relation of β-cell function to insulin resistance

Obesity and other acquired factors that cause insulin resistance result in an adaptation of the β-cell so as to maintain normal glucose homeostasis [7,22]. This adaptation, first demonstrated in the case of obesity in 1974, results in an increase in the β-cell sensitivity to glucose [23]. The hyperbolic relationship between β-cell function and tissue insulin sensitivity, first demonstrated by Bergman *et al.* [24] in 1981 and subsequently confirmed in numerous other studies [7,22,25], exists in such a way that as tissue insulin sensitivity decreases, β-cell function increases to maintain normal glucose homeostasis (Figure 10.2). Thus, in addition to the prevailing stimulus for insulin secretion (e.g. plasma glucose concentration) the status of an individual's insulin sensitivity must be taken into consideration in order to assess the appropriateness of β-cell function [7,8].

Role of β-cell defects in the natural history of type 2 diabetes

Longitudinal and cross-sectional studies indicate that most individuals destined to develop T2DM pass through five stages (Figure 10.3) [7,8,26]. The first stage begins at birth, when glucose homeostasis is normal but individuals are at risk for T2DM because of genetic polymorphisms (diabetogenic genes) or an *in utero* environment predisposing them to become obese and limiting the ability of their pancreatic β-cells to compensate for insulin resistance. In genetically predisposed individuals with normal glucose tolerance, impaired β-cell function is demonstratable even when no insulin resistance is apparent [27–29]. During stage 2, decreases in insulin sensitivity emerge usually as a result of unhealthy lifestyles (environmental), and these, at least initially, are compensated for by an increase in β-cell secretion so that glucose tolerance remains normal. Nevertheless, despite this increase in insulin secretion, a reduction in β-cell function can be demonstrated even when individuals' plasma glucose levels are in the normal range [27–31]. During stage 3, β-cell function deteriorates further to the point that when challenged, as during a glucose tolerance test or a standardized meal, postprandial glucose tolerance becomes abnormal. At this point, β-cell function is clearly abnormal but sufficient to maintain normal fasting plasma glucose concentrations. In stage 4, there is further deterioration in β-cell function noted at least in part from glucose toxicity as a result of postprandial hyperglycemia. This also can reduce insulin sensitivity. Fasting plasma glucose concentrations increase in this stage because of an increase in basal endogenous glucose production. Finally, in stage 5, as a result of further deterioration in β-cell function, both fasting and postprandial glucose levels reach levels diagnostic of diabetes.

Insulin secretion normally decreases with age. The decline rate has been shown to be about 0.7–1% per year for basal and glucose-stimulated insulin secretion during adult human life in individuals with normal glucose tolerance [32–36]. The rate of decline is about twofold greater in people with IGT [33] and reaches approximately 6% per year in patients with T2DM [37,38]. Insulin sensitivity does not decrease per se with aging and decreases in insulin sensitivity when observed are most likely related to other factors such as changes in body composition and physical fitness.

Insulin secretion in type 2 diabetes, in IGT and in genetically predisposed individuals with normal glucose tolerance

Overview of insulin secretion in healthy individuals

Proinsulin, the insulin precursor, is converted to insulin and C peptide within the β-cell secretory granule. The conversion process requires the sequential action of three peptidase enzymes (prohormone convertases 2 and 3, and carboxypeptidase H) and produces four proinsulin conversion intermediates (32,33-split, 65,66-split, des-31,32-split, and des-64,65-split proinsulins) before ultimately yielding insulin and C peptide (see Figure 6.5). Normally, a small amount of intact proinsulin and its conversion intermediates, mostly the des-31,32-split proinsulin, are released into the circulation along with insulin and C peptide. They are estimated to constitute 10–20 % of total immunoreactive insulin measured in the circulation during the basal state [39,40].

The events that lead to release of insulin from β-cells are complex (see Chapter 6). In response to an acute square wave of hyperglycemia such as that used in hyperglycemic clamp experiments in humans or in studies of perfused rat pancreas, insulin release is biphasic (Figure 10.4). It is characterized by an acute increase in insulin release lasting approximately 10 minutes, termed first-phase release, followed by a slowly increasing second phase of insulin release that is more sustained and typically persists as long as glucose is elevated. The first-phase release has been related to insulin-secretory granules located close to the β-cell plasma membrane (immediate releasable pool). In response to an increase in extracellular glucose, islet ATP and cyclic adenosine monophosphate (cAMP) levels increase, causing closure of ATP-sensitive potassium channels; this causes depolarization of the β-cell membrane and an influx of calcium through voltage-sensitive calcium channels; the resultant increase in intracellular calcium leads to movement of insulin-containing granules toward the β-cell membrane, where they merge/incorporate/melt into the membrane with release of the granules' contents. The second-phase insulin release involves synthesis of new insulin molecules as well as ATP-dependent mobilization of granules from a storage pool into the rapidly releasable pool (see Chapter 6). Thus, the normal β-cell response to an increase in glucose concentration is

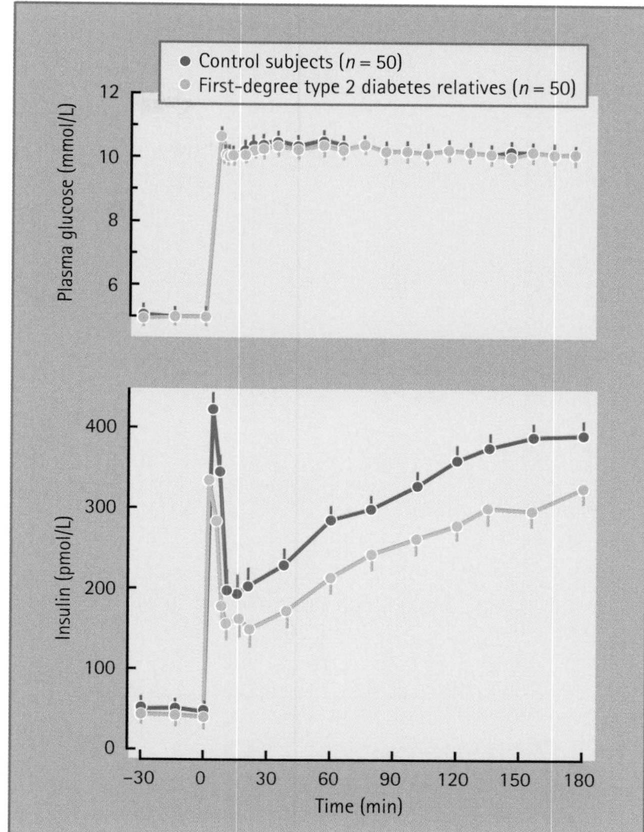

Figure 10.4 Biphasic plasma insulin responses during a square wave hyperglycemic clamp in normal volunteers with and without a first-degree relative with type 2 diabetes. Reproduced from Pimenta *et al.* [29], with permission from the American Medical Association.

dependent upon glucose entry in the β-cell and its metabolism, synthesis of insulin and insulin granules, cytochemical structures (microfilaments/microtubules) and other proteins necessary for moving granules toward the β-cell membrane and facilitating their melting into the membrane so that their contents can be released.

The insulin secretion pattern throughout the day is more complicated than that seen during acute square wave of hyperglycemia in hyperglycemic clamp experiments. *In vivo* insulin secretion was found to be pulsatile, undergoing short (rapid) and long (ultradian) oscillations. The basis for these is still poorly understood, but there is evidence that the integrity of these responses is necessary for maintenance of normal glucose homeostasis [41]. The rapid oscillations correspond to serial secretory insulin bursts (Figure 10.5). These high frequency bursts occur every 5–15 minutes and account for the majority of insulin secreted in humans [42–44]. Additionally, enhanced insulin secretion following stimulation with GLP-1, sulfonylureas, or oral glucose can be accounted for by increase in the amplitude of these secretory pulses [45–48]. By contrast, inhibition of insulin

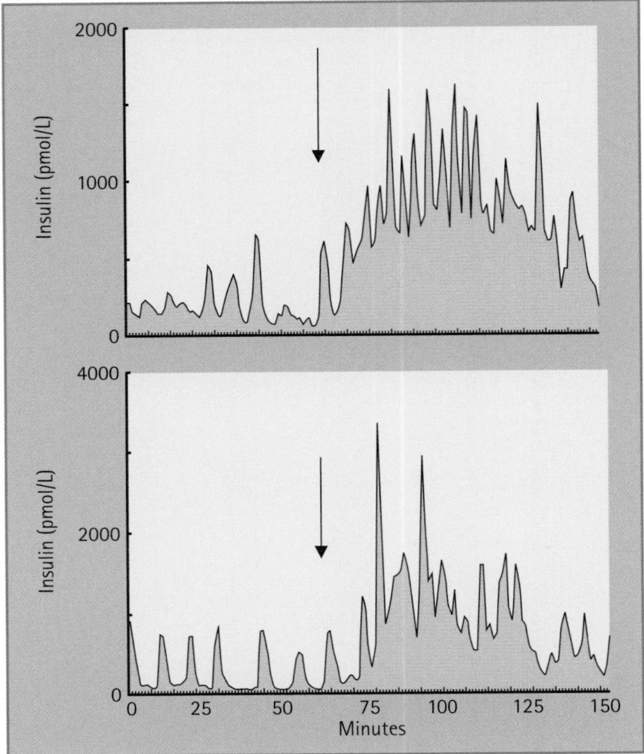

Figure 10.5 Insulin concentration profile in a canine portal vein illustrating the rapid secretory oscillations before and after glucose ingestion. There is a marked increase in pulse amplitude after glucose ingestion (arrow). Reproduced from Porksen *et al.* [47], with permission from the American Diabetes Association.

secretion by somatostatin or insulin-like growth factor 1 (IGF-1) is accomplished by a decrease in the amplitude of these pulses [49,50]. These rapid oscillations are superimposed on slower and larger ultradian oscillations (Figure 10.6) which occur every 80–150 minutes. The ultradian oscillations are present during basal conditions and have clear amplification after meals. They also tend to closely follow similar oscillations of plasma glucose [51,52].

Abnormalities in type 2 diabetes

Defects in β-cell function are quite obvious by the time T2DM is diagnosed. For example, in the UK Prospective Diabetes Study, evaluation of β-cell function using the homeostasis model assessment (HOMA) indicated that β-cell function was at diagnosis already reduced by 50% and that there was subsequent further deterioration, regardless of therapy (Figure 10.7) [37]. Commonly found abnormalities include absent first-phase and diminished second-phase release in response to hyperglycemia in hyperglycemic clamp experiments [53–55]. Responses to ingestion of mixed meals (Figure 10.8) and to non-glucose stimuli are delayed or blunted with a decrease in maximal secretory capacity [55–58]. Abnormal oscillatory pattern is also observed. The pulses, both rapid and ultradian, are smaller and less regular. The ultradian pulses are less amplified after meals and less likely to follow plasma glucose oscillations [42,59].

The ratio of proinsulin and its conversion intermediates to insulin in the circulation is at least twice as high in patients with T2DM than population norms. The increased ratio is noted in the basal and stimulated insulin secretion states and indicates less successful proinsulin to insulin conversion within β-cell secretory granules [39,40,60].

Abnormalities in patients with IGT and in genetically predisposed individuals

Most of the above abnormalities are also found in individuals with IGT, although at a lesser intensity. These include reduced first and second-phase responses to intravenous glucose (Figure 10.9) [61], reduced early insulin response to oral glucose [16], decreased responses to non-glucose stimuli [62], reduced ability of the β-cell to compensate for insulin resistance [7,22], alterations in rapid and ultradian oscillations of insulin secretion [63,64] as well as increased proinsulin : insulin ratio [65].

Perhaps the most convincing evidence that impaired β-cell function is the primary genetic defect comes from studies of first-degree relatives of individuals with T2DM who still have normal glucose tolerance but have reduced insulin responses in the absence of insulin resistance [2,61], especially studies of monozygotic twins [31,66–68].

Other than hyperinsulinemia to compensate for the increased insulin resistance, obese patients have insulin secretion pattern similar to non-obese subjects, and most of the above abnormalities are not present in obesity in the absence of comorbid diabetes or IGT conditions [51,69].

Possible mechanisms

Genetic causes

β-Cell dysfunction in T2DM results from a combination of genetic and acquired factors. Unlike MODY, "garden variety" T2DM is a polygenic disorder; this means that multiple genes (i.e. polymorphisms), each insufficient in themselves, must be present with or without acquired abnormalities in order to cause diabetes [70,71]. Such genes may affect β-cell apoptosis, regeneration, glucose sensing, glucose metabolism, ion channels, energy transduction, microtubules/microfilaments and other islet proteins necessary for the synthesis, packaging, movement and release of secretory granules [72,73]. To date, only a few polymorphisms have been identified as risk factors with confidence (see Chapter 12): one involves an amino acid polymorphism (Pro12Ala) in the peroxisome proliferator-activated receptor-γ (PPARγ), which is expressed in insulin target tissues and β-cells [74]; this apparently conveys susceptibility to adverse effects of FFA on insulin release. A second involves the gene encoding calpain-10, a cysteine protease that modulates insulin release as well as insulin effects on muscle and adipose tissue [75]. A third is the E23K variant of the *KIR6.2* gene (potassium inwardly-rectifying channel J11 gene),

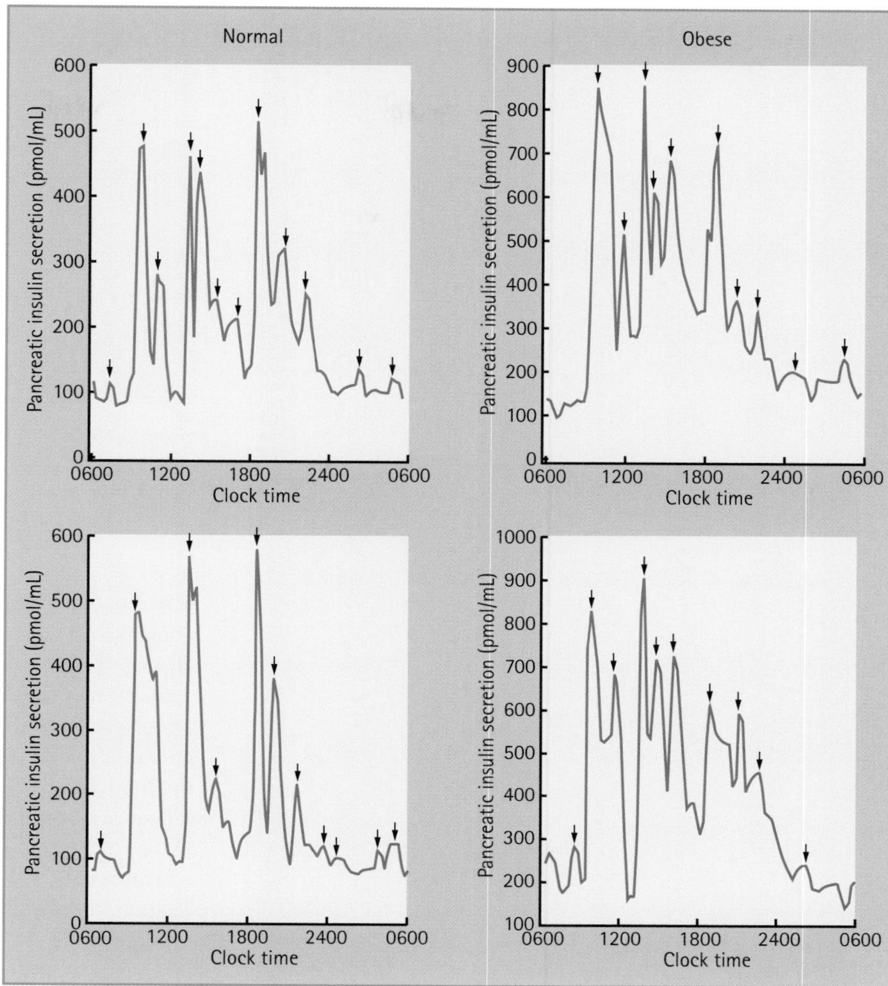

Figure 10.6 Twenty-four hour insulin secretory profile showing ultradian oscillations in a normal weight subject. Meals were consumed at 0900, 1300 and 1800. Statistically significant pulses of secretion are shown by the arrows. Reproduced from Polonsky *et al.* [51], with permission from the American Society for Clinical Investigation.

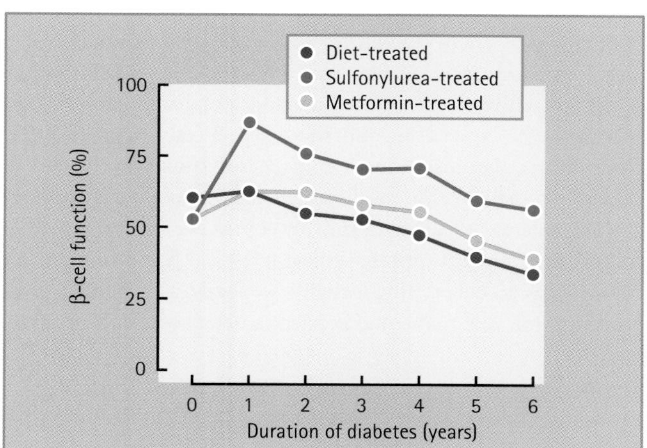

Figure 10.7 β-Cell function as measured by the homeostasis model assessment (HOMA) method in patients with type 2 diabetes from the UK Prospective Diabetes Study (UKPDS). β-Cell function is already reduced to 50% at diagnosis and declines thereafter, despite therapy. Adapted from UK Prospective Diabetes Study Group [37].

which has been shown in a large association study to increase the risk of T2DM presumably through its effect on β-cells' potassium channel and, in turn, on insulin secretion [76,77].

More recently, variants of the transcription factor 7-like 2 gene (*TCF7L2*) were found to be associated with increased risk of T2DM [78–80]. Insulin secretion is decreased in carriers of the at-risk alleles [78]. This is thought to be a result of impaired expression of GLP-1, a peptide encoded by the human glucagon gene (*GCG*) whose expression in gut endocrine cells is regulated by *TCF7L2* [81].

Use of knockout techniques in mice has identified several elements of the insulin signaling cascade that might be potential sites where genetic polymorphisms may affect β-cell function, but to date none of these has been found to occur in people with T2DM [82].

Acquired factors

Several acquired and/or environment factors have been identified that may increase the risk for developing T2DM by impairing β-cell function.

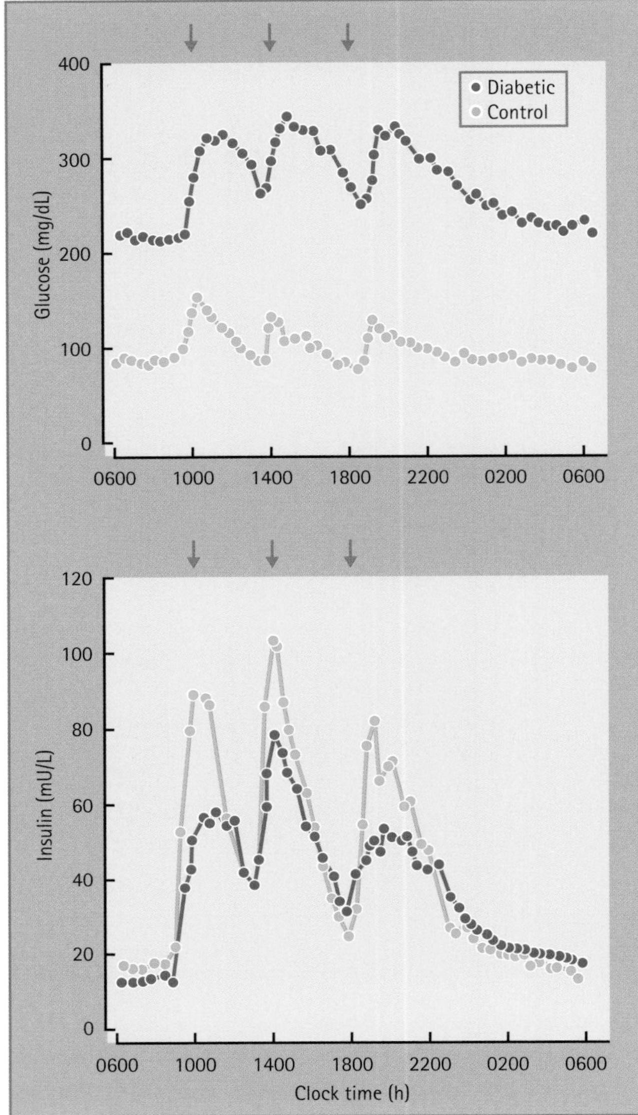

Figure 10.8 Plasma concentrations of glucose and insulin in subjects with type 2 diabetes and non-diabetic control subjects in response to mixed meals. Adapted from Polonsky *et al.* [165].

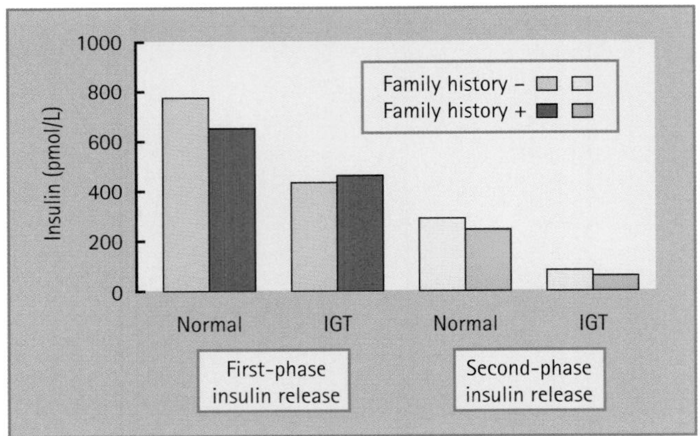

Figure 10.9 β-Cell function in individuals with normal glucose tolerance and impaired glucose tolerance (IGT), with or without a family history of diabetes. Data from Van Haeften *et al.* [61].

Malnutrition *in utero* and early childhood

Animal experiments and retrospective studies in humans have provided evidence that malnutrition *in utero* and early childhood, as well as *in utero* exposure to hyperglycemia, is associated with an increased risk to develop T2DM later in life. Hales *et al.* [83,84] demonstrated an inverse relationship between weight at birth and at 1 year and the development of T2DM in adult life. It was proposed that malnutrition *in utero* and during the first few months of life may damage β-cell development; it is also possible that nutritional deficiency at this stage may program the β-cell so as to limit its subsequent ability to adapt to overnutrition. The latter possibility is supported by the fact that the strongest link was between those who were born thin and subsequently became obese. Recall that one of the hallmarks of individuals destined to develop T2DM is their failure to increase their insulin release appropriately to compensate for their acquired insulin resistance [85]. Nevertheless, because not all individuals with early life malnutrition subsequently develop T2DM if they become obese, this situation must be viewed as one risk factor among many that influence susceptibility.

Glucotoxicity

There is abundant evidence that both prolonged [86] and acute hyperglycemia [87] can adversely affect β-cell function. Moreover, improving glycemic control with the use of secretogogues, insulin sensitizers and even insulin will improve β-cell function in patients with T2DM [88–91]. The mechanisms by which hyperglycemia exerts its adverse effects on β-cells are complex and multifactorial. There is evidence that these mechanisms involve increased production of reactive oxygen species (ROS) within β-cells, oxidative stress-induced alteration of genes transcription and proteins expression, and increased β-cell apoptosis [92]. Nevertheless, because impaired β-cell dysfunction is clearly evident in genetically predisposed individuals with normal glucose tolerance [2] and because optimization of glycemic control does not completely reverse impaired β-cell function in T2DM, this so-called glucotoxicity is clearly a secondary phenomenon but one that could accelerate deterioration over time.

Lipotoxicity

In addition to elevated levels of plasma glucose, individuals with T2DM have increased circulating levels of FFA as do people who are obese [93]. Obese individuals have greater plasma FFA levels primarily because of their greater fat mass [94]. Obese people with T2DM have somewhat greater circulating FFA levels than obese people without T2DM, not because of greater release of FFA into the circulation, but because of decreased FFA clearance

[95]. A number of *in vitro* and animal studies have demonstrated that prolonged elevation of plasma FFA impairs β-cell function [96,97]. Evidence suggests that fatty acids inhibit glucose stimulated insulin secretion, impair insulin gene expression and, more importantly, promote β-cell apoptosis [92]. One proposed mechanism involves the uncoupling protein-2 (UCP-2), a mitochondrial carrier protein that uncouples substrate oxidation from ATP synthesis [98]. FFA increase UCP-2 activity in β-cells. This impairs ATP generation from glucose metabolism and consequently decreases glucose stimulated insulin secretion [99,100]. FFA impair insulin gene expression by increasing ceramide generation which reduces the binding activity of pancreas-duodenum homeobox-1 (Pdx-1) and MafA, two transcription factors essential for regulation of multiple islet-associated genes including insulin gene [101]. In healthy human volunteers, however, it has not been possible to demonstrate consistently a deleterious effect of acute elevation of plasma FFA on β-cell function. Moreover, the effect of chronic elevation of plasma FFA on β-cell function has not been studied in humans [102,103]. Some animal and *in vitro* studies suggest that FFA exert their adverse effects on β-cell function only in the presence of hyperglycemia, hence the suggestion to use the term glucolipotoxicity instead of lipotoxicity [92]. It is clear that increased plasma FFA is not a primary cause of T2DM, but it is possible that a certain genetic background may prevent some individuals from responding to the adverse effects of FFA on β-cell function and thus increase their risk for developing T2DM.

Obesity

Obesity is associated with insulin resistance and is the most predictive acquired risk factor for development of T2DM (see Chapter 14) [104]. This may be mediated by a variety of factors released from adipose tissue that can adversely affect β-cell function, including elevated levels of FFA, TNF-α [105], resistin [106], leptin [107], adipsin [108] and amylin [109], as well as tissue accumulation of lipid [110,111]. Most obese individuals, however, compensate for their insulin resistance with an appropriate increase in insulin release and do not develop diabetes.

Inadequate stimulation by incretins

Incretins are hormones released by the gut in response to food ingestion, which augment insulin release in what is known as the incretin effect (i.e. more insulin responses after oral than intravenous glucose despite comparable glycemia). Two major incretins are GLP-1 and GIP (see Chapters 6 and 30). In addition to promoting the biosynthesis and secretion of insulin [112], they increase β-cell replication and inhibit its apoptosis *in vitro* and were found, in rodent model, to increase β-cell mass [113–116].

Patients with T2DM have higher plasma GIP levels after meal ingestion when compared with healthy subjects [114,117]. Results are conflicting in regard to GLP-1 and, if found, the differences in levels between patients with T2DM and healthy subjects have been generally modest [118–120]. The incretin effect, nevertheless, is impaired in T2DM [121,122]. Insulin responses to both GLP-1 [123] and GIP [124] are reduced. It is not clear whether the defective incretin effect is merely a manifestation of a generalized reduction in β-cell function as is the reduced insulin response to arginine [56,57,121,125]. Antidiabetic drugs, however, that enhance incretins activity or level (GLP-1 analogues and dipeptidyl peptidase-IV inhibitors) have proven to be effective in lowering glucose in T2DM [126].

Islet amyloid

A characteristic feature present in over 90% of patients with T2DM is the deposition of islet amyloid (see below). Amyloid is composed of insoluble fibrils formed from a protein called amylin or islet amyloid polypeptide (IAPP) [127,128]. Normally, IAPP is co-secreted with insulin from β-cells at the molar ratio of 1 : 10–50 [129]. Although the mature form of human IAPP has been reported to impair insulin release and to be β-cell cytotoxic [130], it is unlikely to have a primary role in the pathogenesis of T2DM because it is not present in all patients with T2DM and is actually found in up to 20% of islets in elderly individuals with normal glucose tolerance [131]. Moreover, most obese individuals who hypersecrete insulin do not develop T2DM even though IAPP is co-secreted with insulin.

Recent evidence from *in vitro* and animal studies suggests that small membrane permeant oligomers, but not the mature IAPP fibrils, are the cytotoxic form of IAPP. These oligomers form and act inside the β-cell, possibly causing endoplasmic reticulum stress-induced apoptosis [132,133]. In human, there is still no evidence that patients with T2DM have these toxic oligomers present in their pancreatic islets. However, the S20G mutation of the IAPP gene that increases the susceptibility of IAPP to form oligomers is linked to a rare familial form of T2DM [134–136].

Cytokines

β-Cell function and life cycle are known to be influenced by cytokines especially the proinflammatory cytokine interleukin-1β (IL-1β). IL-1β is known for its cytokine-meditated β-cell destruction in type 1 diabetes [137,138] but, more recently, it has received attention for its role in the pathogenesis of T2DM. *In vitro* studies have shown that β-cells are capable of producing IL-1β in response to high glucose and leptin levels [139,140]. IL-1β expressing β-cells were found in pancreatic sections of patients with T2DM but not in healthy subjects [140]. At low concentrations, IL-1β enhances human β-cell proliferation and decreases its apoptosis, whereas at higher concentration it impairs β-cell insulin release and increases its apoptosis [140–142]. Apoptosis here is thought to be mediated by Fas, a member of the tumor necrosis factor receptor family that triggers apoptotic cell death independent of TNF-α. IL-1β upregulates Fas expression within β-cells, ultimately enabling Fas-induced apoptosis [142,143]. An IL-1 receptor antagonist (IL-1Ra), which protected human β-cell from IL-1β adverse effects *in vitro* [140], improved glycemic control in patients with T2DM through enhanced β-cell secretory function in a preliminary study [144].

Other inflammatory changes and immunologic abnormalities have been reported in patients with IGT and T2DM. In addition to increased systemic cytokines, these abnormalities involve acute-phase proteins and mediators associated with endothelial cell activation [145]. Most of these changes are small and their contribution to β-cell failure is unclear.

Islet and islet cell changes in type 2 diabetes

Pancreatic islets represent 3–5% of the adult normal pancreas and β-cells comprise 60–80% of the islet cell population (see Chapter 6).

Histology of islets in type 2 diabetes

A pathologic feature present in 90% of patients with T2DM is the abnormal extracellular deposits of islet amyloid (Figures 10.10 and 10.11). These deposits are localized in the pancreas and are not part of a systemic amyloidosis disorder. The islet amyloid is formed from IAPP or amylin, a 37 amino acid peptide [127,128]. IAPP is normally produced by the β-cell, stored along with insulin in its secretory granules, and then co-secreted with insulin following β-cell stimulation [129,146]. IAPP has no known physiologic function in human. In patients with T2DM, the soluble IAPP peptides assume a β-sheet structure and oligomerize to form insoluble amyloid deposits [147,148]. It is still not clear what triggers this process and whether this simply reflects islet cell deterioration and destruction. Similar deposits, nevertheless, can be found in a minority of people without diabetes, especially with aging [131]. The IAPP and its amyloid deposits have not been clearly found to be cytotoxic to β-cells and recent evidence suggests that the formation of intracellular smaller IAPP oligomers is possibly the cytotoxic form associated with increased β-cell apoptosis in animal studies [132,133].

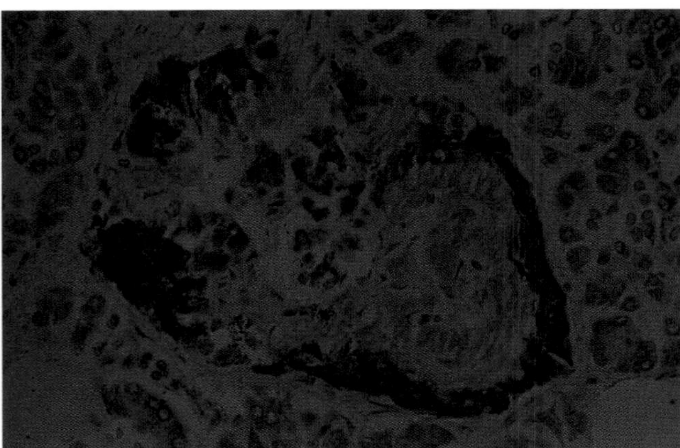

Figure 10.10 Amyloid deposition in islets of a patient with type 2 diabetes. Amyloid formed from islet amyloid polypeptide (IAPP; stained pink with Congo red) occupies more than 50% of the islet mass and is largely in the centre of the islet. Insulin-containing β-cells (labeled brown with immunoperoxidase) are clustered towards the periphery of the islet and are very reduced in number. Original magnification ×400.

Other histologic changes include a decreased islet mass, an alteration in the relative proportion of the islet cell population (see below), and variable degrees of fibrosis of islets and endocrine tissue [131,149–151].

β-Cell changes

It is generally agreed that β-cell mass in T2DM is reduced by about 30–50% compared with that of weight-matched individuals with normal glucose tolerance [131,150–159]. β-Cell mass has also been reported to be decreased in people with impaired fasting glucose [154]. Reduction in β-cell secretory granules amount has also been reported [160]. The decline in β-cell mass is caused by a decrease in the number of cells rather than the volume of individual cells. A several-fold increase in β-cell apoptosis without an adequate compensatory increase in replication or neogenesis rate is responsible for the reduction in cell numbers

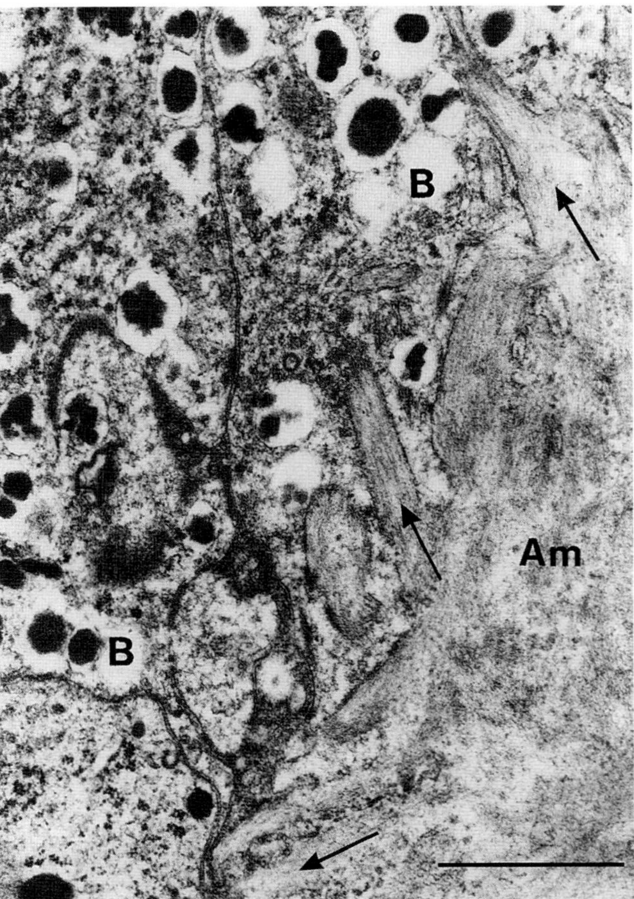

Figure 10.11 Electron-micrographic appearances of islet amyloid deposits in type 2 diabetes. In a patient with type 2 diabetes, amyloid (Am) fibrils closely surround the β-cells (B) and deeply invaginate the distorted cell membrane. Scale bar, 1 μm.

[154,160]. The reduced β-cell mass is usually insufficient by itself to explain the decrease in insulin secretory capacity in patients with T2DM [55,58], suggesting additional functional, therefore potentially reversible, defects.

α-Cell and glucagon changes

The α-cell mass is either unchanged or slightly increased [131,151]; this would result in a relative increase in α-cells because β-cell mass decreases. Abnormal α-cell function in people with IGT and T2DM include: impaired suppression by hyperglycemia, excessive responses to amino acid or mixed meals and diminished responses to hypoglycemia [161]. This has been correlated with reduced β-cell function and could therefore be a secondary phenomenon involving glucose toxicity, lipotoxicity and resistance to insulin.

Absolute or relative hyperglucagonemia is a hallmark of both T1DM and T2DM. Although this exacerbates the consequences of impaired insulin release on hepatic glucose production [16], it is likely to be a secondary phenomenon, because it is readily correctable by physiologic insulin replacement [161].

δ-Cell and somatostatin changes

δ-Cells of the islets release somatostatin, an inhibitor of insulin and glucagon secretion. Relatively little is known of alterations in δ-cell population and function in people with T2DM. Studies have reported δ-cell mass to be either increased [162] or with no significant change [151,152]. Somatostatin secretion is found to be increased in animal models [163,164]. Given the above findings, it is unlikely that alterations in δ-cell mass and release of somatostatin to be a primary cause for the reduced insulin secretion and the relatively excessive glucagon release found in T2DM.

Conclusions

Type 2 diabetes is a disorder involving both inheritable and acquired abnormalities that adversely affect β-cell function and mass and tissue responses to insulin. Current evidence favors the concept that the predominant genetic impact involves impaired insulin secretion whereas additional acquired elements, and thus potentially preventable factors, also adversely affect β-cell function and tissue responses to insulin. Much of the research focus in recent years is directed toward understanding the molecular and genetic basis of the disease. Being a polygenic disorder, multiple different polymorphisms that diminish β-cell function are likely to be identified. New therapies that preserve β-cell function and eventually reverse the defects may be developed in the future.

References

1 Wroblewski M, Gottsater A, Lindgarde F, Fernlund P, Sundkvist G. Gender, autoantibodies, and obesity in newly diagnosed diabetic patients aged 40–75 years. *Diabetes Care* 1998; **21**:250–255.

2 Gerich J. The genetic basis of type 2 diabetes mellitus: impaired insulin secretion versus impaired insulin sensitivity. *Endocr Rev* 1998; **19**:491–503.

3 Hamman R. Genetic and environmental determinants of noninsulin dependent diabetes mellitus (NIDDM). *Diabetes Metab Rev* 1992; **8**:287–338.

4 Reaven G. Pathophysiology of insulin resistance in human disease. *Physiol Rev* 1995; **75**:473–486.

5 DeFronzo R. The triumvirate: B-cell, muscle, and liver: a collusion responsible for NIDDM. *Diabetes* 1988; **37**:667–687.

6 Olefsky J, Nolan J. Insulin resistance and non-insulin-dependent diabetes mellitus: cellular and molecular mechanisms. *Am J Clin Nutr* 1995; **61**(Suppl):980S–986S.

7 Kahn S. The importance of β-cell failure in the development and progression of type 2 diabetes. *J Clin Endocrinol Metab* 2001; **86**: 4047–4058.

8 Pratley R, Weyer C. The role of impaired early insulin secretion in the pathogenesis of type II diabetes mellitus. *Diabetologia* 2001; **44**:929–945.

9 Polonsky K, Sturis J, Bell G. Noninsulin-dependent diabetes mellitus: a genetically programmed failure of the beta cell to compensate for insulin resistance. *N Engl J Med* 1996; **334**:777–783.

10 Himsworth H, Kerr R. Insulin-sensitive and insulin-insensitive types of diabetes mellitus. *Clin Sci* 1939; **4**:119–152.

11 Yalow R, Berson S. Immunoassay of endogenous plasma insulin in man. *J Clin Invest* 1960; **39**:1157–1175.

12 DeFronzo R, Bonadonna R, Ferrannini E. Pathogenesis of NIDDM: a balanced overview. *Diabetes Care* 1992; **15**:318–368.

13 Warram J, Martin B, Krolewski A, Soeldener S, Kahn C. Slow glucose removal rate and hyperinsulinemia precede the development of type II diabetes in the offspring of diabetic parents. *Ann Intern Med* 1990; **113**:909–915.

14 Lillioja S, Mott D, Howard B, Bennet P, Yki-Jarvinen H, Freymond D, *et al.* Impaired glucose tolerance as a disorder of insulin action: longitudinal and cross-sectional studies in Pima Indians. *N Engl J Med* 1988; **318**:1217–1225.

15 Seltzer H, Allen E, Herror A, Brennan M. Insulin response to glycemic stimulus: relation of delayed initial release to carbohydrate intolerance in mild diabetes. *J Clin Invest* 1967; **46**: 323–335.

16 Mitrakou A, Kelley D, Mokan M, Veneman T, Pangburn T, Reilly J, *et al.* Role of reduced suppression of glucose production and diminished early insulin release in impaired glucose tolerance. *N Engl J Med* 1992; **326**:22–29.

17 Calles-Escandon J, Robbins, D. Loss of early phase of insulin release in humans impairs glucose tolerance and blunts thermic effect of glucose. *Diabetes* 1987; **36**:1167–1172.

18 Luzi L, DeFronzo R. Effect of loss of first-phase insulin secretion on hepatic glucose production and tissue glucose disposal in humans. *Am J Physiol* 1989; **257**:E241–E246.

19 Hollander P, Schwartz S, Gatlin M, Haas S, Zheng H, Foley J, *et al.* Importance of early insulin secretion: comparison of nateglinide and glyburide in previously diet-treated patients with type 2 diabetes. *Diabetes Care* 2001; **24**:983–988.

20 Perley J, Kipnis D. Plasma insulin responses to oral and intravenous glucose: studies in normal and diabetic subjects. *J Clin Invest* 1967; **46**:1954–1962.

21 Stumvoll M, Mitrakou A, Pimenta W, Jenssen T, Yki-Järvinen H, Van Haeften T, *et al.* Use of the oral glucose tolerance test to assess

insulin release and insulin sensitivity. *Diabetes Care* 2000; **23**:295–301.

22 Weyer C, Bogardus C, Mott D, Pratley R. The natural history of insulin secretory dysfunction and insulin resistance in the pathogenesis of type 2 diabetes mellitus. *J Clin Invest* 1999; **104**:787–794.

23 Karam J, Grodsky G, Ching K, Schmid F, Burrill K, Forsham P. "Staircase" glucose stimulation of insulin secretion in obesity: measure of beta-cell sensitivity and capacity. *Diabetes* 1974; **23**:763–770.

24 Bergman R, Phillips J, Cobelli C. Physiologic evaluation of factors controlling glucose tolerance in man: measurement of insulin sensitivity and B-cell glucose sensitivity from the response to intravenous glucose. *J Clin Invest* 1981; **68**:1456–1467.

25 Buchanan T. Pancreatic B-cell defects in gestational diabetes: implications for the pathogenesis and prevention of type 2 diabetes. *J Clin Endocrinol Metab* 2001; **86**:989–993.

26 Borch-Johnson K, Nissen H, Hendriksen E, Kreiner S, Salling N, Deckert T, *et al.* The natural history of insulin-dependent diabetes mellitus in Denmark: long term survival with and without diabetic complications. *Diabet Med* 1987; **4**:201–210.

27 Vaag A, Henriksen J, Madsbad S, Holm N. Insulin secretion, insulin action, and hepatic glucose production in identical twins discordant for non-insulin-dependent diabetes mellitus. *J Clin Invest* 1995; **95**:690–698.

28 Johnston C, Ward K, Beard C, McKnight B, Porte D. Islet function and insulin sensitivity in the nondiabetic offspring of conjugal type II diabetic patients. *Diabetic Med* 1990; **7**:119–125.

29 Pimenta W, Kortytkowski M, Mitrakou A, Jenssen T, Yki-Jarvinen H, Evron W, *et al.* Pancreatic beta-cell dysfunction as the primary genetic lesion in NIDDM: evidence from studies in normal glucose-tolerant individuals with a first-degree NIDDM relative. *JAMA* 1995; **273**:1855–1861.

30 Ferrannini E, Gastaldelli A, Miyazaki Y, Matsuda M, Mari A, DeFronzo RA. Beta-cell function in subjects spanning the range from normal glucose tolerance to overt diabetes: a new analysis. *J Clin Endocrinol Metab* 2005; **90**:493–500.

31 Vaag A, Alford F, Beck-Nielsen H. Intracellular glucose and fat metabolism in identical twins discordant for non-insulin-dependent diabetes mellitus (NIDDM): acquired versus genetic metabolic defects. *Diabetic Med* 1996; **13**:806–815.

32 Chiu KC, Lee NP, Cohan P, Chuang LM. Beta cell function declines with age in glucose tolerant Caucasians. *Clin Endocrinol (Oxf)* 2000; **53**:569–575.

33 Szoke E, Shrayyef MZ, Messing S, Woerle HJ, van Haeften TW, Meyer C, *et al.* Effect of aging on glucose homeostasis: accelerated deterioration of beta-cell function in individuals with impaired glucose tolerance. *Diabetes Care* 2008; **31**:539–543.

34 Iozzo P, Beck-Nielsen H, Laakso M, Smith U, Yki-Jarvinen H, Ferrannini E. Independent influence of age on basal insulin secretion in nondiabetic humans. European Group for the Study of Insulin Resistance. *J Clin Endocrinol Metab* 1999; **84**:863–868.

35 Fritsche A, Madaus A, Stefan N, Tschritter O, Maerker E, Teigeler A, *et al.* Relationships among age, proinsulin conversion, and beta-cell function in nondiabetic humans. *Diabetes* 2002; **51**(Suppl 1):S234–S239.

36 Utzschneider KM, Carr DB, Hull RL, Kodama K, Shofer JB, Retzlaff BM, *et al.* Impact of intra-abdominal fat and age on insulin sensitivity and beta-cell function. *Diabetes* 2004; **53**:2867–2872.

37 UK Prospective Diabetes Study Group. UK Prospective Diabetes study 16. Overview of 6 years' therapy of type II diabetes: a progressive disease. *Diabetes* 1995; **44**:1249–1258.

38 Kahn SE, Haffner SM, Heise MA, Herman WH, Holman RR, Jones NP, *et al.* Glycemic durability of rosiglitazone, metformin, or glyburide monotherapy. *N Engl J Med* 2006; **355**:2427–2443.

39 Kahn SE, Halban PA. Release of incompletely processed proinsulin is the cause of the disproportionate proinsulinemia of NIDDM. *Diabetes* 1997; **46**:1725–1732.

40 Ward WK, LaCava EC, Paquette TL, Beard JC, Wallum BJ, Porte D Jr. Disproportionate elevation of immunoreactive proinsulin in type 2 (non-insulin-dependent) diabetes mellitus and in experimental insulin resistance. *Diabetologia* 1987; **30**:698–702.

41 Matthews D. Physiological implications of pulsatile hormone secretion. *Ann N Y Acad Sci* 1991; **618**:28–37.

42 Porksen N, Hollingdal M, Juhl C, Butler P, Veldhuis JD, Schmitz O. Pulsatile insulin secretion: detection, regulation, and role in diabetes. *Diabetes* 2002; **51**(Suppl 1):S245–S254.

43 Porksen N, Nyholm B, Veldhuis JD, Butler PC, Schmitz O. In humans at least 75% of insulin secretion arises from punctuated insulin secretory bursts. *Am J Physiol* 1997; **273**:E908–E914.

44 Porksen N, Munn S, Steers J, Vore S, Veldhuis J, Butler P. Pulsatile insulin secretion accounts for 70% of total insulin secretion during fasting. *Am J Physiol* 1995; **269**:E478–E488.

45 Porksen N, Grofte B, Nyholm B, Holst JJ, Pincus SM, Veldhuis JD, *et al.* Glucagon-like peptide 1 increases mass but not frequency or orderliness of pulsatile insulin secretion. *Diabetes* 1998; **47**:45–49.

46 Porksen NK, Munn SR, Steers JL, Schmitz O, Veldhuis JD, Butler PC. Mechanisms of sulfonylurea's stimulation of insulin secretion *in vivo*: selective amplification of insulin secretory burst mass. *Diabetes* 1996; **45**:1792–1797.

47 Porksen N, Munn S, Steers J, Veldhuis JD, Butler PC. Effects of glucose ingestion versus infusion on pulsatile insulin secretion: the incretin effect is achieved by amplification of insulin secretory burst mass. *Diabetes* 1996; **45**:1317–1323.

48 Ritzel R, Schulte M, Porksen N, Nauck MS, Holst JJ, Juhl C, *et al.* Glucagon-like peptide 1 increases secretory burst mass of pulsatile insulin secretion in patients with type 2 diabetes and impaired glucose tolerance. *Diabetes* 2001; **50**:776–784.

49 Porksen N, Munn SR, Steers JL, Veldhuis JD, Butler PC. Effects of somatostatin on pulsatile insulin secretion: elective inhibition of insulin burst mass. *Am J Physiol* 1996; **270**:E1043–E1049.

50 Porksen N, Hussain MA, Bianda TL, Nyholm B, Christiansen JS, Butler PC, *et al.* IGF-1 inhibits burst mass of pulsatile insulin secretion at supraphysiological and low IGF-1 infusion rates. *Am J Physiol* 1997; **272**:E352–E358.

51 Polonsky KS, Given BD, Van Cauter E. Twenty-four-hour profiles and pulsatile patterns of insulin secretion in normal and obese subjects. *J Clin Invest* 1988; **81**:442–448.

52 Sturis J, Van Cauter E, Blackman JD, Polonsky KS. Entrainment of pulsatile insulin secretion by oscillatory glucose infusion. *J Clin Invest* 1991; **87**:439–445.

53 Ferner RE, Ashworth L, Tronier B, Alberti KG. Effects of short-term hyperglycemia on insulin secretion in normal humans. *Am J Physiol* 1986; **250**:E655–E661.

54 VanHaeften T, Voetberg G, Gerich J, Van der Veen E. Dose–response characteristics for arginine-stimulated insulin secretion in man and influence of hyperglycemia. *J Clin Endocrinol Metab* 1989; **69**:1059–1064.

55 VanHaeften T, VAn Maarschalkerveerd W, Gerich J, Van der Veen E. Decreased insulin secretory capacity and normal pancreatic B- cell glucose sensitivity in non-obese patients with NIDDM. *Eur J Clin Invest* 1991; **21**:168–174.

56 Dimitriadis G, Pehling G, Gerich J. Abnormal glucose modulation of islet A- and B-cell responses to arginine in non-insulin-dependent diabetes mellitus. *Diabetes* 1985; **34**:541–547.

57 Hollander P, Asplin C, Palmer J. Glucose modulation of insulin and glucagon secretion in nondiabetic and diabetic man. *Diabetes* 1982; **31**:489–495.

58 Ward W, Bolgiano D, McKnight B, Halter J, Porte D. Diminished β-cell secretory capacity in patients with noninsulin-dependent diabetes mellitus. *J Clin Invest* 1984; **74**:1318–1328.

59 Sturis J, Polonsky KS, Shapiro ET, Blackman JD, O'Meara NM, Van Cauter E. Abnormalities in the ultradian oscillations of insulin secretion and glucose levels in type 2 (non-insulin-dependent) diabetic patients. *Diabetologia* 1992; **35**:681–689.

60 Yoshioka N, Kuzuya T, Matsuda A, Taniguchi M, Iwamoto Y. Serum proinsulin levels at fasting and after oral glucose load in patients with type 2 (non-insulin-dependent) diabetes mellitus. *Diabetologia* 1988; **31**:355–360.

61 Van Haeften T, Pimenta W, Mitrakou A, Korytkowski M, Jenssen T, Yki-Järvinen H, *et al.* Relative contributions of β-cell function and tissue insulin sensitivity to fasting and postglucose-load glycemia. *Metabolism* 2000; **49**:1318–1325.

62 Larsson H, Berglund G, Ahren B. Glucose modulation of insulin and glucagon secretion is altered in impaired glucose tolerance. *J Clin Endocrinol Metab* 1995; **80**:1778–1782.

63 O'Meara N, Sturis J, VanCouter E, Polonsky K. Lack of control by glucose of ultradian insulin secretory oscillations in impaired glucose tolerance and in non-insulin-dependent diabetes mellitus. *J Clin Invest* 1993; **92**:262–271.

64 O'Rahilly S, Turner R, Matthews D. Impaired pulsatile secretion of insulin in relatives of patients with noninsulin-dependent diabetes. *N Engl J Med* 1988; **318**:1225–1230.

65 Larsson H, Ahren B. Relative hyperproinsulinemia as a sign of islet dysfunction in women with impaired glucose tolerance. *J Clin Endocrinol Metab* 1999; **84**:2068–2074.

66 Cerasi E, Luft R. Insulin response to glucose infusion in diabetic and nondiabetic monozygotic twin pairs: genetic control of insulin response. *Acta Endocrinol* 1967; **55**:330–345.

67 Barnett A, Spiliopoulos A, Pyke D, Stubbs W, Burrin J, Alberti K. Metabolic studies in unaffected co-twins of noninsulin dependent diabetics. *Br Med J* 1981; **282**:1656–1658.

68 Pyke D, Taylor K. Glucose tolerance and serum insulin in unaffected identical twins of diabetics. *Br Med J* 1967; **4**:21–22.

69 Polonsky K, Given B, Hirsch L, Shapiro E, Tillil H, Beebe C, *et al.* Quantitative study of insulin secretion and clearance in normal and obese subjects. *J Clin Invest* 1988; **81**:435–441.

70 Bell G, Polonsky K. Diabetes mellitus and genetically programmed defects in β-cell function. *Nature* 2001; **414**:788–791.

71 Busch C, Hegele R. Genetic determinants of type 2 diabetes mellitus. *Clin Genet* 2001; **60**:243–254.

72 Edlund H. Factors controlling pancreatic cell differentiation and function. *Diabetologia* 2001; **44**:1071–1079.

73 Stumvoll M, Goldstein BJ, van Haeften TW. Pathogenesis of type 2 diabetes. *Endocr Res* 2007; **32**:19–37.

74 Stefan N, Fritsche A, Haring H, Stumvoll M. Effect of experimental elevation of free fatty acids on insulin secretion and insulin sensitivity in healthy carriers of the Pro12Ala polymorphism of the peroxisome proliferator-activated receptor-gamma2 gene. *Diabetes* 2001; **50**:1143–1148.

75 Horikawa Y, Oda N, Cox N, Li X, Orho-Melander M, Hara M, *et al.* Genetic variation in the gene encoding calpain-10 is associated with type 2 diabetes mellitus. *Nat Genet* 2000; **26**:163–175.

76 Gloyn AL, Weedon MN, Owen KR, Turner MJ, Knight BA, Hitman G, *et al.* Large-scale association studies of variants in genes encoding the pancreatic beta-cell KATP channel subunits Kir6.2 (KCNJ11) and SUR1 (ABCC8) confirm that the KCNJ11 E23K variant is associated with type 2 diabetes. *Diabetes* 2003; **52**:568–572.

77 Florez JC, Jablonski KA, Kahn SE, Franks PW, Dabelea D, Hamman RF, *et al.* Type 2 diabetes-associated missense polymorphisms KCNJ11 E23K and ABCC8 A1369S influence progression to diabetes and response to interventions in the Diabetes Prevention Program. *Diabetes* 2007; **56**:531–536.

78 Florez JC, Jablonski KA, Bayley N, Pollin TI, de Bakker PI, Shuldiner AR, *et al.* TCF7L2 polymorphisms and progression to diabetes in the Diabetes Prevention Program. *N Engl J Med* 2006; **355**:241–250.

79 Zhang C, Qi L, Hunter DJ, Meigs JB, Manson JE, van Dam RM, Hu FB. Variant of transcription factor 7-like 2 (TCF7L2) gene and the risk of type 2 diabetes in large cohorts of US women and men. *Diabetes* 2006; **55**:2645–2648.

80 Grant SF, Thorleifsson G, Reynisdottir I, Benediktsson R, Manolescu A, Sainz J, *et al.* Variant of transcription factor 7-like 2 (TCF7L2) gene confers risk of type 2 diabetes. *Nat Genet* 2006; **38**: 320–323.

81 Yi F, Brubaker PL, Jin T. TCF-4 mediates cell type-specific regulation of proglucagon gene expression by beta-catenin and glycogen synthase kinase-3beta. *J Biol Chem* 2005; **280**:1457–1464.

82 Saltiel A, Kahn C. Insulin signalling and the regulation of glucose and lipid metabolism. *Nature* 2001; **414**:799–806.

83 Hales C, Barker D, Clark P, Cox L, Fall C, Osmond C, *et al.* Fetal and infant growth and impaired glucose tolerance at age 64. *Br Med J* 1991; **303**:1019–1022.

84 Hales C, Barker D. Type 2 (non-insulin-dependent) diabetes mellitus: the thrifty phenotype hypothesis. *Diabetologia* 1992; **35**:595–601.

85 Weyer C, Pratley R, Tataranni PA. Role of insulin resistance and insulin secretory dysfunction in the pathogenesis of type 2 diabetes mellitus: lessons from cross-sectional, prospective, and longitudinal studies in Pima Indians. *Curr Opin Endocrinol Diabetes Obes* 2002; **9**:130–138.

86 Yki-Järvinen H. Glucose toxicity. *Endocr Rev* 1992; **13**:415–431.

87 Meyer J, Sturis J, Katschinski M, Arnold R, Goke B, Byrne M. Acute hyperglycemia alters the ability of the normal beta-cell to sense and respond to glucose. *Am J Physiol Endocrinol Metab* 2002; **282**:E917–E922.

88 Kosaka K, Kuzuya T, Hagura R. Increase in insulin response after treatment of overt maturity-onset diabetes is independent of the mode of treatment. *Diabetologia* 1980; **18**:23–28.

89 Garvey W, Olefsky J, Griffin J, Hamman R, Kolterman O. The effect of insulin treatment on insulin secretion and insulin action in type II diabetes mellitus. *Diabetes* 1985; **34**:222–234.

90 Andrews W, Vasquez B, Nagulesparan M, Klimes I, Foley J, Unger R, *et al.* Insulin therapy in obese non-insulin-dependent diabetes induces improvements in insulin action and secretion that are maintained for two weeks after insulin withdrawal. *Diabetes* 1984; **33**:634–642.

91 Yki-Jarvinen H. Thiazolidinediones. *N Engl J Med* 2004; **351**:1106–1118.

92 Poitout V, Robertson RP. Glucolipotoxicity: fuel excess and beta-cell dysfunction. *Endocr Rev* 2008; **29**:351–366.

93 Perriello G, Mitrakou A, Gumbiner B, Gerich J. Non-esterified fatty acids in non-insulin-dependent diabetes: a critical update. *Diabetes Ann* 1995; 91–106.

94 Jansson PA, Larrson A, Smith V, Lonroth P. Glycerol production in subcutaneous adipose tissue in lean and obese humans. *J Clin Invest* 1992; **89**:1610–1617.

95 Taskinen M, Bogardus C, Kennedy A, Howard B. Multiple disturbances of free fatty acid metabolism in noninsulin dependent diabetes. *J Clin Invest* 1985; **76**:637–644.

96 Poitout V, Robertson R. Minireview: Secondary beta-cell failure in type 2 diabetes: a convergence of glucotoxicity and lipotoxicity. *Endocrinology* 2002; **143**:339–342.

97 Poitout V. Lipid partitioning in the pancreatic β-cell: physiologic and pathophysiologic implications. *Curr Opin Endocrinol Diabetes Obes* 2002; **9**:152–159.

98 Fleury C, Sanchis D. The mitochondrial uncoupling protein-2: current status. *Int J Biochem Cell Biol* 1999; **31**:1261–1278.

99 Chan CB, MacDonald PE, Saleh MC, Johns DC, Marban E, Wheeler MB. Overexpression of uncoupling protein 2 inhibits glucose-stimulated insulin secretion from rat islets. *Diabetes* 1999; **48**:1482–1486.

100 Medvedev AV, Robidoux J, Bai X, Cao W, Floering LM, Daniel KW, *et al.* Regulation of the uncoupling protein-2 gene in INS-1 beta-cells by oleic acid. *J Biol Chem* 2002; **277**:42639–42644.

101 Hagman DK, Hays LB, Parazzoli SD, Poitout V. Palmitate inhibits insulin gene expression by altering PDX-1 nuclear localization and reducing MafA expression in isolated rat islets of Langerhans. *J Biol Chem* 2005; **280**:32413–32418.

102 Carpentier A, Mittelman SD, Bergman RN, Giacca A, Lewis GF. Prolonged elevation of plasma free fatty acids impairs pancreatic beta-cell function in obese nondiabetic humans but not in individuals with type 2 diabetes. *Diabetes* 2000; **49**:399–408.

103 Boden G. Role of fatty acids in the pathogenesis of insulin resistance and NIDDM. *Diabetes* 1997; **46**:3–10.

104 Choi B, Shi F. Risk factors for diabetes mellitus by age and sex: results of the national population health survey. *Diabetologia* 2001; **44**:1221–1231.

105 Hotamisligil G, Spiegelman B. Tumor necrosis factor α: a key component of the obesity–diabetes link. *Diabetes* 1994; **43**:1271–1278.

106 Steppan C, Bailey S, Bhat S, Brown E, Banerjee R, Wright C, *et al.* The hormone resistin links obesity to diabetes. *Nature* 2001; **409**: 307–312.

107 Ahima R, Flier J. Leptin. *Annu Rev Physiol* 2000; **62**:413–437.

108 Ahima R, Flier J. Adipose tissue as an endocrine organ. *Trends Endocrinol Metab* 2000;**11**:327–332.

109 Sanke T, Hanabusa T, Nakano Y, Oki C, Okai K, Nishimura S, *et al.* Plasma islet amyloid polypeptide (amylin) levels and their responses to oral glucose in type 2 (non-insulin-dependent) diabetic patients. *Diabetologia* 1991; **34**:129–132.

110 Kelley D, Goodposter B. Skeletal muscle triglyceride: an aspect of regional adiposity and insulin resistance. *Diabetes Care* 2001; **24**:933–941.

111 Virkamaki A, Korsheninnikova E, Seppala-Lindroos A, Vehkavaara S, Goto T, Halavaara J, *et al.* Intramyocellular lipid is associated with resistance to *in vivo* insulin actions on glucose uptake, antilipolysis, and early insulin signaling pathways in human skeletal muscle. *Diabetes* 2001; **50**:2337–2343.

112 Creutzfeldt W, Nauck M. Gut hormones and diabetes mellitus. *Diabetes Metab Rev* 1992; **8**:149–177.

113 Xu G, Stoffers DA, Habener JF, Bonner-Weir S. Exendin-4 stimulates both beta-cell replication and neogenesis, resulting in increased beta-cell mass and improved glucose tolerance in diabetic rats. *Diabetes* 1999; **48**:2270–2276.

114 Salehi M, Aulinger BA, D'Alessio DA. Targeting beta-cell mass in type 2 diabetes: promise and limitations of new drugs based on incretins. *Endocr Rev* 2008; **29**:367–379.

115 Wang Q, Brubaker PL. Glucagon-like peptide-1 treatment delays the onset of diabetes in 8 week-old db/db mice. *Diabetologia* 2002; **45**:1263–1273.

116 Trumper A, Trumper K, Trusheim H, Arnold R, Goke B, Horsch D. Glucose-dependent insulinotropic polypeptide is a growth factor for beta (INS-1) cells by pleiotropic signaling. *Mol Endocrinol* 2001; **15**:1559–1570.

117 Krarup T. Immunoreactive gastric inhibitory polypeptide. *Endocr Rev* 1988; **9**:122–134.

118 Orskov C, Jeppesen J, Madsbad S, Holst JJ. Proglucagon products in plasma of noninsulin-dependent diabetics and nondiabetic controls in the fasting state and after oral glucose and intravenous arginine. *J Clin Invest* 1991; **87**:415–423.

119 Vilsboll T, Krarup T, Sonne J, Madsbad S, Volund A, Juul AG, *et al.* Incretin secretion in relation to meal size and body weight in healthy subjects and people with type 1 and type 2 diabetes mellitus. *J Clin Endocrinol Metab* 2003; **88**:2706–2713.

120 O'Donovan DG, Doran S, Feinle-Bisset C, Jones KL, Meyer JH, Wishart JM, *et al.* Effect of variations in small intestinal glucose delivery on plasma glucose, insulin, and incretin hormones in healthy subjects and type 2 diabetes. *J Clin Endocrinol Metab* 2004; **89**:3431–3435.

121 Knop FK, Vilsboll T, Hojberg PV, Larsen S, Madsbad S, Volund A, *et al.* Reduced incretin effect in type 2 diabetes: cause or consequence of the diabetic state? *Diabetes* 2007; **56**:1951–1959.

122 Nauck M, Stockmann F, Ebert R, Creutzfeldt W. Reduced incretin effect in type 2 (non-insulin-dependent) diabetes. *Diabetologia* 1986; **29**:46–52.

123 Kjems LL, Holst JJ, Volund A, Madsbad S. The influence of GLP-1 on glucose-stimulated insulin secretion: effects on beta-cell sensitivity in type 2 and nondiabetic subjects. *Diabetes* 2003; **52**: 380–386.

124 Vilsboll T, Krarup T, Madsbad S, Holst JJ. Defective amplification of the late phase insulin response to glucose by GIP in obese type II diabetic patients. *Diabetologia* 2002; **45**:1111–1119.

125 Nauck MA, El Ouaghlidi A, Gabrys B, Hucking K, Holst JJ, Deacon CF, *et al.* Secretion of incretin hormones (GIP and GLP-1) and incretin effect after oral glucose in first-degree relatives of patients with type 2 diabetes. *Regul Pept* 2004; **122**:209–217.

126 Amori RE, Lau J, Pittas AG. Efficacy and safety of incretin therapy in type 2 diabetes: systematic review and meta-analysis. *JAMA* 2007; **298**:194–206.

127 Cooper GJ, Willis AC, Clark A, Turner RC, Sim RB, Reid KB. Purification and characterization of a peptide from amyloid-rich pancreases of type 2 diabetic patients. *Proc Natl Acad Sci U S A* 1987; **84**:8628–8632.

128 Westermark P, Wernstedt C, O'Brien TD, Hayden DW, Johnson KH. Islet amyloid in type 2 human diabetes mellitus and adult dia-

betic cats contains a novel putative polypeptide hormone. *Am J Pathol* 1987; **127**:414–417.

129 Cooper G. Amylin compared with calcitonin gene-related peptide: structure, biology, and relevance to metabolic disease. *Endocr Rev* 1994; **15**:163–201.

130 Lorenzo A, Razzaboni B, Weir G, Yankner B. Pancreatic islet cell toxicity of amylin associated with type-2 diabetes mellitus. *Nature* 1994; **368**:756–760.

131 Clark A, Wells C, Buley I, Cruickshank J, Vanhegan R, Matthews D, *et al.* Islet amyloid, increased alpha-cells, reduced beta-cells and exocrine fibrosis: quantitative changes in the pancreas in type 2 diabetes. *Diabetes Res* 1988; **9**:151–159.

132 Haataja L, Gurlo T, Huang CJ, Butler PC. Islet amyloid in type 2 diabetes, and the toxic oligomer hypothesis. *Endocr Rev* 2008; **29**:303–316.

133 Meier JJ, Kayed R, Lin CY, Gurlo T, Haataja L, Jayasinghe S, *et al.* Inhibition of human IAPP fibril formation does not prevent beta-cell death: evidence for distinct actions of oligomers and fibrils of human IAPP. *Am J Physiol Endocrinol Metab* 2006; **291**:E1317–E1324.

134 Seino S. S20G mutation of the amylin gene is associated with type II diabetes in Japanese. Study Group of Comprehensive Analysis of Genetic Factors in Diabetes Mellitus. *Diabetologia* 2001; **44**:906–909.

135 Ma Z, Westermark GT, Sakagashira S, Sanke T, Gustavsson A, Sakamoto H, *et al.* Enhanced *in vitro* production of amyloid-like fibrils from mutant (S20G) islet amyloid polypeptide. *Amyloid* 2001; **8**:242–249.

136 Eizirik DL, Cardozo AK, Cnop M. The role for endoplasmic reticulum stress in diabetes mellitus. *Endocr Rev* 2008; **29**:42–61.

137 Loweth AC, Williams GT, James RF, Scarpello JH, Morgan NG. Human islets of Langerhans express Fas ligand and undergo apoptosis in response to interleukin-1β and Fas ligation. *Diabetes* 1998; **47**:727–732.

138 Mandrup-Poulsen T. The role of interleukin-1 in the pathogenesis of IDDM. *Diabetologia* 1996; **39**:1005–1029.

139 Maedler K, Sergeev P, Ehses JA, Mathe Z, Bosco D, Berney T, *et al.* Leptin modulates beta cell expression of IL-1 receptor antagonist and release of IL-1beta in human islets. *Proc Natl Acad Sci U S A* 2004; **101**:8138–8143.

140 Maedler K, Sergeev P, Ris F, Oberholzer J, Joller-Jemelka HI, Spinas GA, *et al.* Glucose-induced beta cell production of IL-1beta contributes to glucotoxicity in human pancreatic islets. *J Clin Invest* 2002; **110**:851–860.

141 Maedler K, Schumann DM, Sauter N, Ellingsgaard H, Bosco D, Baertschiger R, *et al.* Low concentration of interleukin-1beta induces FLICE-inhibitory protein-mediated beta-cell proliferation in human pancreatic islets. *Diabetes* 2006; **55**:2713–2722.

142 Donath MY, Storling J, Berchtold LA, Billestrup N, Mandrup-Poulsen T. Cytokines and beta-cell biology: from concept to clinical translation. *Endocr Rev* 2008; **29**:334–350.

143 Maedler K, Spinas GA, Lehmann R, Sergeev P, Weber M, Fontana A, *et al.* Glucose induces beta-cell apoptosis via upregulation of the Fas receptor in human islets. *Diabetes* 2001; **50**:1683–1690.

144 Larsen CM, Faulenbach M, Vaag A, Volund A, Ehses JA, Seifert B, *et al.* Interleukin-1-receptor antagonist in type 2 diabetes mellitus. *N Engl J Med* 2007; **356**:1517–1526.

145 Kolb H, Mandrup-Poulsen T. An immune origin of type 2 diabetes? *Diabetologia* 2005; **48**:1038–1050.

146 Kahn SE, D'Alessio DA, Schwartz MW, Fujimoto WY, Ensinck JW, Taborsky GJ Jr, *et al.* Evidence of cosecretion of islet amyloid polypeptide and insulin by beta-cells. *Diabetes* 1990; **39**:634–638.

147 Hull RL, Westermark GT, Westermark P, Kahn SE. Islet amyloid: a critical entity in the pathogenesis of type 2 diabetes. *J Clin Endocrinol Metab* 2004; **89**:3629–3643.

148 Hoppener JW, Ahren B, Lips CJ. Islet amyloid and type 2 diabetes mellitus. *N Engl J Med* 2000; **343**:411–419.

149 Saito K, Iwama N, Takahashi T. Morphometrical analysis on topographical difference in size distribution, number and volume of islets in the human pancreas. *Tohoku J Exp Med* 1978; **124**:177–186.

150 Sakuraba H, Mizukami H, Yagihashi N, Wada R, Hanyu C, Yagihashi S. Reduced beta-cell mass and expression of oxidative stress-related DNA damage in the islet of Japanese type II diabetic patients. *Diabetologia* 2002; **45**:85–96.

151 Rahier J, Goebbels R, Henquin J. Cellular composition of the human diabetic pancreas. *Diabetologia* 1983; **24**:366–371.

152 Del Guerra S, Lupi R, Marselli L, Masini M, Bugliani M, Sbrana S, *et al.* Functional and molecular defects of pancreatic islets in human type 2 diabetes. *Diabetes* 2005; **54**:727–735.

153 Kloppel G, Lohr M, Habich K, Oberholzer M, Heitz P. Islet pathology and the pathogenesis of type 1 and type 2 diabetes mellitus revisited. *Surv Synth Pathol Res* 1985; **4**:110–125.

154 Butler AE, Janson J, Bonner-Weir S, Ritzel R, Rizza RA, Butler PC. Beta-cell deficit and increased beta-cell apoptosis in humans with type 2 diabetes. *Diabetes* 2003; **52**:102–110.

155 Stefan Y, Orci L, Malaisse-Lagae F, Perrelet A, Patel Y, Unger RH. Quantitation of endocrine cell content in the pancreas of nondiabetic and diabetic humans. *Diabetes* 1982; **31**:694–700.

156 Gepts W. [Contribution to the morphological study of the islands of Langerhans in diabetes; study of the quantitative variations of the different insular constituents.] *Ann Soc R Sci Med Nat Brux* 1957; **10**:5–108.

157 Saito K, Yaginuma N, Takahashi T. Differential volumetry of A, B, and D cells in the pancreatic islets of diabetic and nondiabetic subjects. *Tohoku J Exp Med* 1979; **129**:273–283.

158 Westermark P, Wilander E. The influence of amyloid deposits on the islet volume in maturity onset diabetes mellitus. *Diabetologia* 1978; **15**:417–421.

159 Rahier J, Guiot Y, Goebbels RM, Sempoux C, Henquin JC. Pancreatic beta-cell mass in European subjects with type 2 diabetes. *Diabetes Obes Metab* 2008;**10**(Suppl 4):32–42.

160 Marchetti P, Del Guerra S, Marselli L, Lupi R, Masini M, Pollera M, *et al.* Pancreatic islets from type 2 diabetic patients have functional defects and increased apoptosis that are ameliorated by metformin. *J Clin Endocrinol Metab* 2004; **89**:5535–5541.

161 Dunning BE, Gerich JE. The role of alpha-cell dysregulation in fasting and postprandial hyperglycemia in type 2 diabetes and therapeutic implications. *Endocr Rev* 2007; **28**:253–283.

162 Iki K, Pour PM. Distribution of pancreatic endocrine cells including IAPP-expressing cells in non-diabetic and type 2 diabetic cases. *J Histochem Cytochem* 2007; **55**:111–118.

163 Gerich J. Somatostatin and diabetes. *Am J Med* 1981; **70**:619–626.

164 Basabe J, Karabatas L, Arata M, Pivetta O, Cresto J. Secretion and effect of somatostatin in early stages of the diabetic syndrome in C57BL/KsJ-mdb mice. *Diabetologia* 1986; **29**:485–488.

165 Polonsky KS, Given BD, Hirsch LJ, Tillil H, Shapiro ET, Beebe C, *et al.* Abnormal patterns of insulin secretion in non-insulin-dependent diabetes mellitus. *N Engl J Med* 1988; **318**:1231–1239.

11 Insulin Resistance in Type 2 Diabetes

Hannele Yki-Järvinen
Department of Medicine, Division of Diabetes, University of Helsinki, Helsinki, Finland

Keypoints

- Insulin resistance both precedes and predicts type 2 diabetes mellitus (T2DM). The insulin resistance preceding T2DM is commonly referred to as the metabolic syndrome. Development of T2DM (i.e. overt hyperglycemia), however, also requires the presence of a relative defect in insulin secretion (see Chapter 10).
- Although obesity and physical inactivity have precipitated the epidemic of T2DM, these factors are poorer predictors of cardiovascular disease than a combination of risk factors that define the metabolic syndrome. Diagnosis of the metabolic syndrome requires measurement of waist circumference, glucose, triglycerides and high density lipoprotein cholesterol and blood pressure. These features are not observed in all obese people and can occur even in normal weight individuals. Subjects who develop the metabolic syndrome commonly have excess fat deposited in ectopic locations, especially in the liver. Non-alcoholic fatty liver disease (NAFLD) is defined as excess fat in the liver in the absence of excess alcohol abuse or other known causes of liver disease. The amount of fat in the liver is closely correlated with all features of the metabolic syndrome independent of obesity. Thus, NAFLD frequently coexists in subjects with the metabolic syndrome and may indeed be regarded as another defining feature of the metabolic syndrome. As the metabolic syndrome, NAFLD also predicts both T2DM and cardiovascular disease independent of obesity.
- In the liver, insulin resistance of glucose metabolism in patients with T2DM is characterized by an impaired ability of insulin to inhibit hepatic glucose production leading to mild hyperglycemia and stimulation of insulin secretion. Hepatic insulin resistance is also manifested by failure of insulin suppression of very low density lipoprotein production, which leads to hypertriglyceridemia. High density lipoprotein levels decrease because of increased exchange of cholesterol esters for triglyceride, mediated by cholesterol ester transfer protein. Small, dense, low density lipoprotein particles also predominate in insulin-resistant states, and are highly atherogenic. Hepatic insulin resistance is directly proportional to the amount of fat in the liver, although the molecular mechanisms underlying this association in humans are unclear. Liver fat is increased in obesity but the relationship is weak, implying that many other factors regulate liver fat. These include genetic and dietary factors.
- Insulin resistance in adipose tissue is characterized by inflammation, decreased production of the insulin-sensitizing hormone adiponectin and by an impaired ability of insulin to suppress lipolysis. Raised non-esterified fatty acid (NEFA) levels are the most important source of intrahepatocellular triglyceride both under fasting and post-prandial conditions. Adiponectin deficiency may also contribute to fat accumulation in the liver.
- Insulin stimulation of glucose uptake in skeletal muscle is decreased in patients with T2DM compared with subjects without diabetes if measured under similar conditions of hyperinsulinemia and glycemia. At the molecular level, insulin resistance in muscle is associated with by defects at multiple post-receptor sites, including impairment of insulin receptor substrate 1 tyrosine phosphorylation, phosphoinositide 3′ (PI_3) kinase activation and the glucose transporter 4 translocation, which mediates insulin-stimulated glucose uptake; glycogen synthesis is also decreased. Raised NEFA levels also interfere with glucose utilization and uptake by muscle.
- Chronic hyperglycemia per se reduces insulin sensitivity (glucose toxicity) and could at least partly explain why insulin resistance is more severe in patients with established T2DM than in equally obese subjects without diabetes.

Insulin resistance – definitions and role in the natural history of type 2 diabetes

Insulin resistance can be defined as the inability of insulin to produce its usual biologic actions at circulating concentrations that are effective in normal subjects. Insulin resistance in the context of glucose metabolism leads to impaired suppression of endogenous glucose production – under basal conditions as well as after eating (when the physiologic rise in insulin in response to glucose entry from the gut normally shuts down glucose production by the liver) – and to reduced peripheral uptake of glucose. Resistance to the ability of insulin to suppress very low density lipoprotein (VLDL) cholesterol production increases circulating serum triglycerides, while resistance in adipose tissue increases the flux of non-esterified fatty acid (NEFA) both to the

Textbook of Diabetes, 4th edition. Edited by R. Holt, C. Cockram, A. Flyvbjerg and B. Goldstein.

liver and skeletal muscle and impairs the action of insulin on glucose metabolism in these tissues (see Chapters 7 and 13). Resistance to other actions of insulin, such as its vasodilatator and antiplatelet aggregation effects, also characterize insulin resistance in patients with T2DM. Insulin resistance may also become more severe in patients with T2DM brought about by any factor causing insulin resistance. Such factors are listed in Table 11.1.

There has been much debate as to whether insulin resistance is the primary defect that precedes β-cell failure in the evolution of hyperglycemia in T2DM, or vice versa. There is a linear decrease in both first-phase insulin release and insulin sensitivity in individuals who progress from normal to impaired glucose tolerance [1]. Once the plasma glucose concentration 2 hours after an oral glucose challenge (75 g) reaches the upper limit for impaired glucose tolerance (11.1 mmol/L, 200 mg/dL), post-glucose insulin concentrations fall and glucose then rises into the diabetic range (Figure 11.1). A similar picture has been observed in prospective studies. Thus, low insulin sensitivity and impaired first-phase insulin release both predict the onset of T2DM [1]. These data imply that development of overt hyperglycemia requires a relative decrease in insulin secretion as depicted in Figure 11.1.

The following sections describe the pathogenesis and significance of the cluster of clinical features of insulin resistance called the metabolic syndrome, which characterizes most patients with the common form of T2DM [2]. The metabolic syndrome shares

Table 11.1 Causes of variation in insulin action in patients with type 2 diabetes. Genetic forms of insulin resistance are discussed in Chapters 12 and 15.

Factor	Change in insulin sensitivity	Reference
Physiologic variations		
Physical training, increased muscle mass*	↑	[110]
Increased fat mass, fat distribution	↓	[97]
Puberty	↓	[154]
Pregnancy	↓	[155]
Gender	Female > male	[156]
Menstrual cycle	No effect	
Diet-induced changes		
Overfeeding	↓	[157]
Starvation	↓	[158]
Alcohol	↓	[159]
Saturated vs monounsaturated fat	↓	[160]
Metabolite and electrolyte disturbances		
High free fatty acid concentrations	↓	[83]
Chronic hyperglycemia	↓	[111]
Hypoglycemia	↓	[161]
Acidosis	↓	[162]
Hyperosmolality	↓	[163]
Hypophosphatemia	↓	[164]
Other causes		
Excessive secretion of counter-regulatory hormones	↓	[165–168]
• Conditions associated with physical or mental stress	↑	
• Acromegaly, Cushing disease, pheochromocytoma, growth hormone deficiency	↓	
Hypothyroidism and hyperthyroidism	↓	[169,170]
Non-alcoholic fatty liver	↓	[3]
Uremia	↓	[171]
Many infections	↓	[172]

*Aerobic training increases glucose uptake per unit muscle mass; resistive training does not increase glucose uptake per unit muscle but increases muscle bulk.

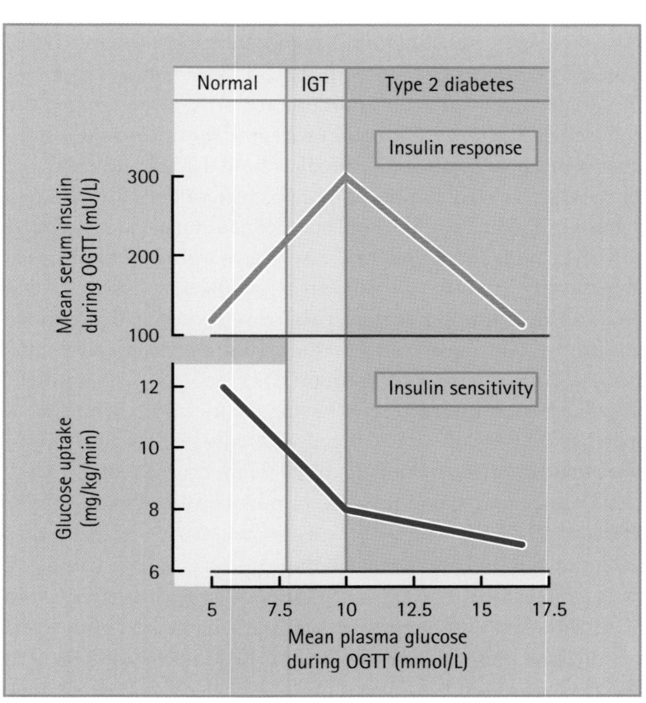

Figure 11.1 Natural history of type 2 diabetes (T2DM). Upper panel: the relationship between mean glucose and mean insulin concentrations during an oral glucose tolerance test (OGTT), in individuals with normal (NGT), impaired glucose tolerance (IGT) and diabetes (T2DM). There is a linear positive correlation between glucose and insulin concentrations during an OGTT in individuals with NGT and IGT. By contrast, T2DM is characterized by worsening relative insulin deficiency (i.e. insulin concentrations decline with rising glucose concentrations). Bottom panel: the relationship between glucose concentrations during the OGTT and insulin sensitivity (determined by the euglycemic clamp technique). Insulin sensitivity decreases linearly as glucose tolerance worsens and, in patients with T2DM, insulin sensitivity worsens as glucose concentrations increase. This could be caused by effects of chronic hyperglycemia per se on glucose uptake, or of relative insulin deficiency coupled with increases in NEFA concentrations. These data are from cross-sectional studies [173] but longitudinal studies [1] yield similar findings.

many features in common with non-alcoholic fatty liver disease (NAFLD), which is therefore also briefly described [3]. This is followed by a characterization of features of insulin resistance in individual tissues: the liver, adipose tissue, skeletal muscle and additional sites. The underlying causes are also discussed, focusing on acquired factors. Genetics of T2DM is discussed in Chapter 12. This chapter focuses on the sites, causes and consequences of "insulin resistance" in the common form of T2DM. Certain conditions that may resemble T2DM are discussed in detail in other chapters (see Chapters 2, 15, and 19).

Metabolic syndrome and non-alcoholic fatty liver disease

Definitions and significance

Metabolic syndrome

Insulin resistance in various tissues leads to hyperglycemia, hypertriglyceridemia and low high-density liporotein (HDL) cholesterol. Most patients with T2DM have these features of insulin resistance and, in addition, are often hypertensive and abdominally obese. Although each of the causes and consequences of insulin resistance predicts both T2DM and increased cardiovascular risk, identification of a cluster of abnormalities in a given individual confers a substantial additional cardiovascular risk over and above the risk associated with each individual abnormality [2]. A number of expert groups have developed criteria for identification of such a risk cluster called the metabolic syndrome. The most recent is the definition proposed by the International Diabetes Federation (IDF). According to this definition, a person is identified as having the metabolic syndrome if they have central obesity (defined with ethnicity specific values) plus any two of the following: raised triglycerides; reduced HDL cholesterol; raised blood pressure; or raised fasting plasma glucose (Tables 11.2 and 11.3). Using these criteria, 20–25% of the world's adult population have the metabolic syndrome. This risk of death from cardiovascular disease is increased approximately twofold in subjects with the metabolic syndrome compared with those not meeting these criteria (see Part 8). In addition, subjects with the metabolic syndrome have a fivefold greater risk of developing T2DM [2].

Non-alcoholic fatty liver disease

Subjects with metabolic syndrome who are abdominally obese, have an increase in fat accumulation in the liver and hepatic insulin resistance independent of their obesity and body fat distribution [4,5]. This increase in liver fat associated with insulin resistance is called non-alcoholic fatty liver disease (NAFLD). NAFLD is defined as excess fat in the liver (>5–10% fat histologically) which is not brought about by excess alcohol use (over 20 g/day), effects of other toxins, autoimmune, viral or other causes of steatosis [4]. NAFLD has been shown to predict both T2DM and cardiovascular disease in multiple prospective studies independent of obesity [3].

Table 11.2 The International Diabetes Federation (IDF) definition of the metabolic syndrome.

According to the new IDF definition, for a person to be defined as having the metabolic syndrome they must have:

Central obesity (defined as waist circumference ≥94 cm for Europid men and ≥80 cm for Europid women, with ethnicity specific values for other groups; see Table 11.3; below) plus any two of the following four factors:

1 Raised triglyceride level: ≥150 mg/dL (1.7 mmol/L), or specific treatment for this lipid abnormality

2 Reduced HDL cholesterol: <40 mg/dL (1.0 mmol/L) in males and <50 mg/dL (1.3 mmol/L) in females, or specific treatment for this lipid abnormality

3 Raised blood pressure: systolic BP ≥130 or diastolic BP ≥85 mmHg, or treatment of previously diagnosed hypertension

4 Raised fasting plasma glucose ≥100 mg/dL (5.6 mmol/L), or previously diagnosed type 2 diabetes. If above 5.6 mmol/L (100 mg/dL), an oral glucose tolerance test is strongly recommended but is not necessary to define presence of the syndrome

If BMI is >30 kg/m^2, central obesity can be assumed and waist circumference does not need to be measured

Table 11.3 Ethnic specific values for waist circumference.

Country/ethnic group	Waist circumference (cm)
Europids In the USA, the ATP III values (102 cm male; 88 cm female) are likely to continue to be used for clinical purposes	Male ≥94 Female ≥80
South Asians Based on a Chinese, Malay and Asian-Indian population	Male ≥90 Female ≥80
Chinese	Male ≥90 Female ≥80
Japanese	Male ≥85 Female ≥90
Ethnic South and Central Americans	Use South Asian recommendations until more specific data are available
Sub-Saharan Africans and Eastern Mediterranean and Middle East (Arab) populations	Use European data until more specific data are available

NAFLD covers a spectrum of liver disease including not only steatosis but also non-alcoholic steatohepatitis (NASH) and cirrhosis (Figure 11.2) [4]. The reasons why the liver develops inflammatory changes, as in NASH, in some individuals is unclear. In addition to the epidemic of obesity, T2DM and cardiovascular disease, the incidence of serious liver damage brought about by NAFLD is increasing. It has even been predicted that NASH will become the number one cause of orthotopic liver transplantation by the year 2020 [6].

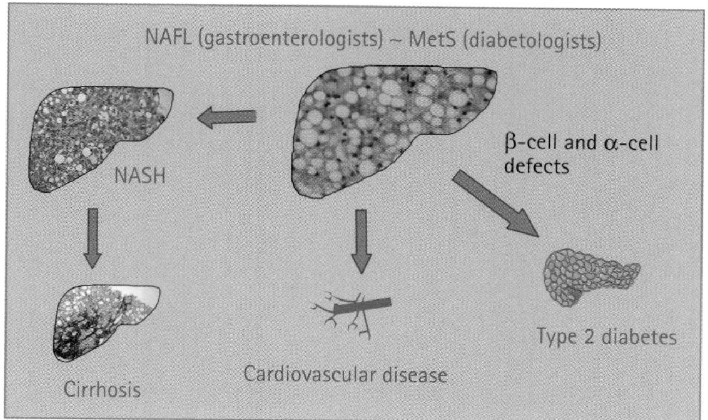

Figure 11.2 Overview of the relationship between non-alcoholic fatty liver (NAFL), metabolic syndrome (MetS), non-alcoholic steatohepatitis (NASH), type 2 diabetes and cardiovascular disease.

Insulin resistance in the liver

Characteristics

Insulin action on glucose metabolism in the fasting state

After an overnight fast, insulin restrains endogenous glucose production (see Chapter 7). Isotopic measurements of glucose production under truly steady-state conditions show a significant relationship between endogenous glucose production and fasting plasma glucose concentration in patients with T2DM [7]. This relationship is observed despite hyperglycemia and normoinsulinemia or hyperinsulinemia, and demonstrates that insulin resistance contributes to the increase in basal endogenous glucose production. This hepatic insulin resistance is associated with excess fat accumulation in the liver. After an overnight fast, when glucose uptake is largely insulin-independent and driven by the mass-action effect of hyperglycemia, the absolute rate of glucose utilization is normal or even increased (Figure 11.3). The clinical implications of these findings are that strategies designed to lower fasting glucose should aim at inhibiting overproduction of glucose from the liver rather than further increasing glucose uptake in T2DM [8].

Insulin action on glucose metabolism in the post-prandial state

After a meal, increases in insulin and glucose concentrations and a concomitant decrease in glucagon almost completely suppress endogenous glucose production under normal conditions. In patients with T2DM, this suppression is incomplete both because of hepatic insulin resistance, deficient insulin and excessive glucagon secretion [9–11]. Hepatic insulin resistance has been documented by direct measurement of a reduced effect of insulin to decrease hepatic glucose production [11]. This defect correlates closely with liver fat content (Figure 11.4) [12,13]. The pathogenesis and causes of this hepatic insulin resistance are discussed below. Persistent hepatic glucose production after eating is the main reason for sustained maintenance of post-meal hyperglycemia [9]. Under post-prandial conditions, approximately one-third of glucose is utilized in skeletal muscle, one-third is oxidized in the brain and the remaining third is stored in the liver [14]. In patients with T2DM, the ability of the liver to store glucose during a meal appears intact or is only slightly diminished [9,15]. In absolute terms, the overall rate of glucose utilization is also quantitatively normal, because hyperglycemia per se, via the mass action effect of glucose, acts to compensate for impaired insulin stimulation of glucose uptake into peripheral tissues [16]. Finally, the brain utilizes similar amounts of glucose in both normal subjects and patients with T2DM. Thus, post-prandial hyperglycemia must be caused by the incomplete suppression of endogenous glucose production.

Lipoprotein metabolism

Evidence from both *in vitro* [17,18] and *in vivo* [19] studies has suggested that insulin normally suppresses the production of VLDL, especially VLDL1 apoB particles from the liver (see Chapter 40). This effect is brought about not only by decreases in NEFA availability following inhibition of lipolysis in fat tissue, but also by a direct hepatic effect of insulin, inhibiting the assembly and production of VLDL particles [19]. In contrast to normal subjects, insulin fails to suppress VLDL apoB production in those with T2DM, even though it profoundly suppresses NEFA concentrations [20]. Overproduction of VLDL [21] and the defect in insulin suppression of VLDL production [22] correlates with the amount of fat in the liver and appears to be one major contributory mechanism underlying the increase in serum triglycerides in patients with insulin-resistant T2DM (Figure 11.3) [23].

HDL levels are reduced in insulin-resistant patients with high serum triglycerides. Under hypertriglyceridemic conditions, there is excessive exchange of cholesterol esters and triglycerides between HDL and the expanded pool of triglyceride-rich lipoproteins, mediated by cholesterol ester transfer protein (CETP) [24]. HDL particles become enriched with triglycerides (predominantly separating in the lighter HDL_3 density range), rendering them as a good substrate for hepatic lipase which removes HDL particles form the circulation at an accelerated rate. Subnormal activity of LPL may further decrease levels of HDL cholesterol by decreasing the conversion of HDL_3 to HDL_2 particles [24]. Elevated concentrations of VLDL particles in the serum of patients with T2DM also increase the CETP-mediated exchange of cholesterol ester and triglyceride between VLDL and low density lipoprotein (LDL) cholesterol particles [25]. This increases the triglyceride content of LDL particles and makes them a better substrate for hepatic lipase [26], which hydrolyzes triglycerides in the LDL particles and increases their density. This sequence of events at least partly explains why patients with T2DM have smaller and more dense LDL particles than individuals without diabetes [27,28]. The small dense LDL particles are known to be highly atherogenic and provide a plausible link between insulin resistance and cardiovascular disease [29–32].

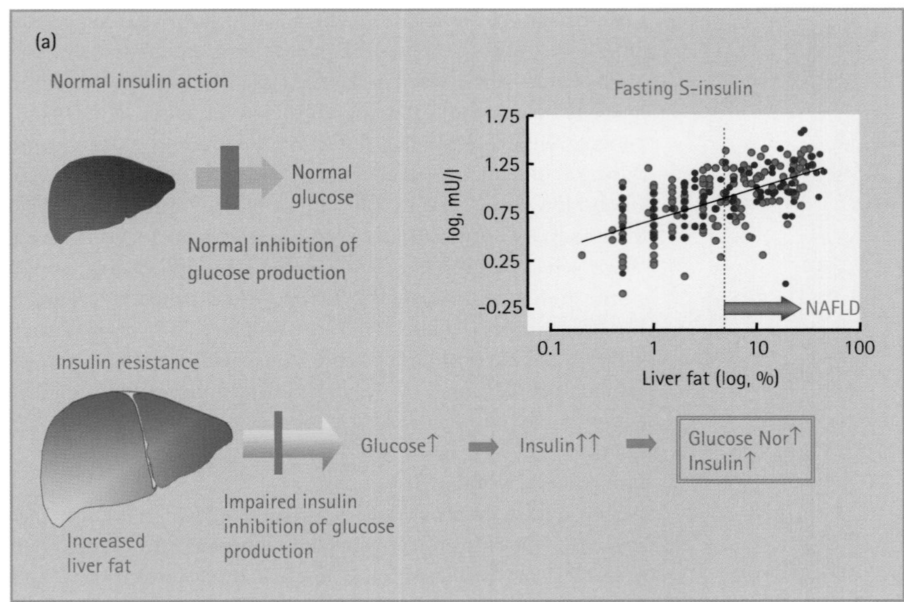

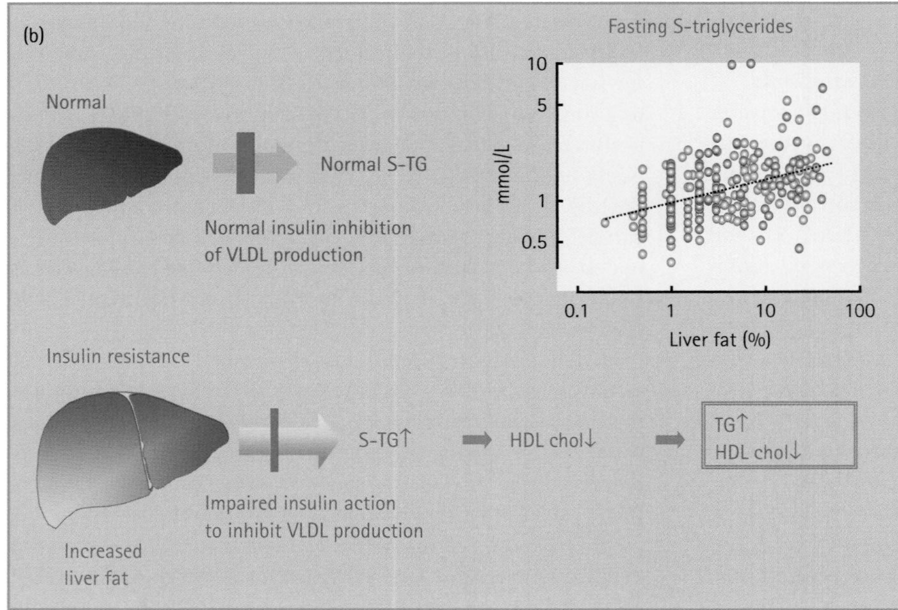

Figure 11.3 Role of the fatty liver in the pathogenesis of hyperglycemia and (a) hyperinsulinemia and (b) hypertriglyceridemia. (a) Insulin normally restrains hepatic glucose production, which maintains glucose at normal levels. Once the liver is fatty and insulin-resistant, this action of insulin is impaired, leading to hyperglycemia and stimulation of insulin secretion. This results in the combination of near-normal glucose levels and hyperinsulinemia, as long as panreatic insulin secretion is intact. The insert in (a) denotes the relationship between liver fat and fasting serum insulin. Pink circles, female; blue circles, male. Data from Kotronen *et al.* [5]. If liver fat exceeds 5–10% as a result of non-alcoholic causes, this is defined as non-alcoholic fatty liver disease (NAFLD). (b) Insulin normally inhibits production of very low density lipoprotein (VLDL) cholesterol from the liver. If the liver is fatty and and insulin resistant, this ability of insulin is impaired. This results in hypertriglyceridemia and this in turn is the main reason for lowering of high density lipoprotein (HDL) cholesterol. The insert in (b) depicts the relationship between liver fat and fasting serum triglycerides. Pink circles, female; blue circles, male. Data from Kotronen *et al.* [5].

Pathogenesis of hepatic insulin resistance and the fatty liver

It is not ethically possible to sample human liver for research purposes, and therefore data on the pathogenesis of hepatic insulin resistance in humans are mainly based on *in vivo* studies using stable isotope and hepatic venous catheterization techniques.

Sources of intrahepatocellular triglyceride

The fatty acids in intrahepatocellular triglycerides can be derived from dietary chylomicron remnants, NEFAs released from adipose tissue, or from post-prandial lipolysis of chylomicrons, which can occur at a rate in excess of what can be taken up by tissues (spillover), and from *de novo* lipogenesis [33]. *In vivo* studies using stable isotope techniques have shown that after an overnight fast, the majority of hepatic fatty acids originate from adipose tissue lipolysis [34]. The contribution of splanchnic lipolysis to hepatic free fatty acid (FFA) delivery averages 5–10% in normal weight subjects and increases to 30% in men and women with visceral obesity [35]. Thus, subcutaneous adipose tissue provides the majority of hepatic FFA delivery. In the post-prandial state, the contribution of the spillover pathway and uptake of

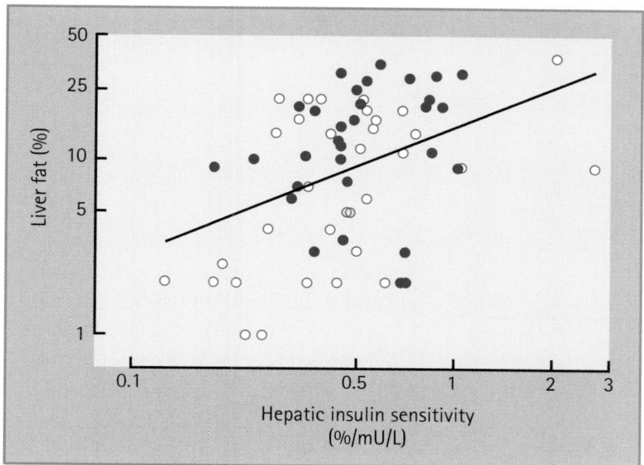

Figure 11.4 Relationship between hepatic insulin sensitivity (measured by the ability of insulin to suppress hepatic glucose production by insulin) and liver fat in normal subjects (open circles) and in patients with type 2 diabetes (closed circles). Data from Kotronen *et al.* [174].

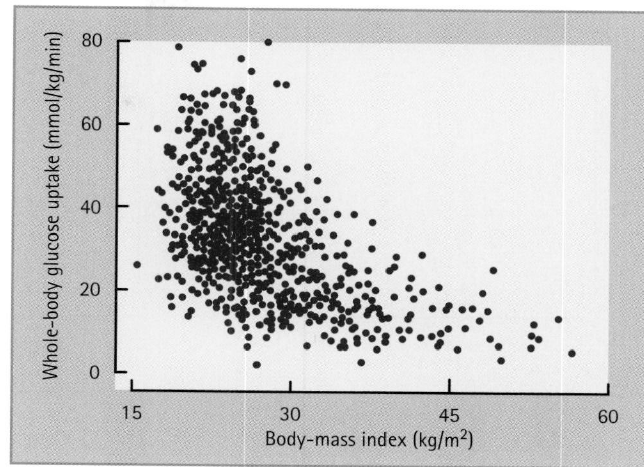

Figure 11.5 The relationship between body mass index and insulin sensitivity of glucose metabolism as determined by the euglycemic clamp technique in subjects without diabetes. Data from the European Group for the Study of Insulin Resistance (EGIR) (kindly provided by Professor Eleuterio Ferrannini).

chylomicron remnants increase and can account for up to half of the fatty acids secreted as VLDL triglyceride. *De novo* lipogenesis accounts for less than 5% in normal subjects post-prandially [36]; however, in subjects with fatty liver, rates of *de novo* lipogenesis appear to be significantly elevated [34,37]. This may result from excess carbohydrate intake [38]. An impaired ability of insulin-resistant subjects to store carbohydrate as glycogen in muscle could also contribute to excess *de novo* lipogenesis in the liver [39].

The fatty acid composition of intrahepatocellular triglyceride changes as a function of the amount of liver fat present. The fatty liver contains increased amounts of saturated fatty acids and decreased amounts of polyunsaturated fatty acids [40]. Whether the increase in saturated fatty acids is caused by *de novo* lipogenesis, which produces saturated fatty acids [41], or other sources is unclear.

Cellular mechanism of hepatic insulin resistance

Triglycerides themselves are inert and cannot explain hepatic insulin resistance. Data from animal studies suggest at least two lipid mediators, ceramides and diacylglycerols, which could cause insulin resistance. Ceramides are sphingolipids, with a sphingoid backbone that relies on the availability of saturated fatty acids [42]. Ceramides appear to be required for insulin resistance induced by saturated, but not unsaturated, fatty acids in rat soleus muscle [43]. Ceramides accumulate in the liver during tristearin (18:0) – but not triolein (18:1 n-9) enriched diets [44]. Ceramides are upregulated in skeletal muscle [45] and adipose tissue [46] of insulin-resistant subjects, but data are sparse on the ceramide content of human fatty liver [40]. Diacylglycerols, which are immediate precursors of triacylglycerols, activate protein kinase Cε (PKCε) in the liver, which binds to and inactivates the insulin receptor tyrosine kinase and decreases insulin receptor substrate 2 (IRS-2) tyrosine phosphorylation. In downstream signaling, this leads to reduced insulin activation of PI_3-kinase, AKT2, glygogen synthase kinase 3 (GSK-3) and FOXO phosphorylation, which decreases hepatic glycogen synthesis and reduces inhibition of hepatic gluconeogenesis [47]. In the human liver, diacylglycerol concentrations are increased in proportion to increases in intrahepatocellular triglyceride [40]. PKCε activity has been shown to be increased in the liver of patients with T2DM [48].

Acquired causes of variation in hepatic insulin sensitivity and liver fat content

Body weight

Obesity is related to insulin resistance, although at any given body mass index (BMI), insulin sensitivity, measured as the amount of glucose required to maintain normoglycemia during hyperinsulinemia (a measure of whole body insulin resistance, which could be both hepatic and peripheral), varies considerably (Figure 11.5). Obesity impairs both insulin stimulation of glucose uptake and insulin inhibition of endogenous glucose production [11,49]. Liver fat content and hepatic insulin resistance are related to BMI and waist circumference; however, the variation at any given BMI is large (Figure 11.6).

Weight loss induces rapid and substantial changes in liver fat content and hepatic insulin sensitivity [50,51]. In a study where obese women lost 8% of their body weight over 18 weeks, liver fat content and total body fat mass decreased by 39% and 14%, respectively [52]. In another study, 7% weight loss decreased liver fat content by approximately 40% over 7 weeks [53]. In this study, a 30% decrease in liver fat was observed as early as after 2 days of a low carbohydrate diet (~1000 kcal, approximately 10% carbohydrate). In both of these studies, there was a marked

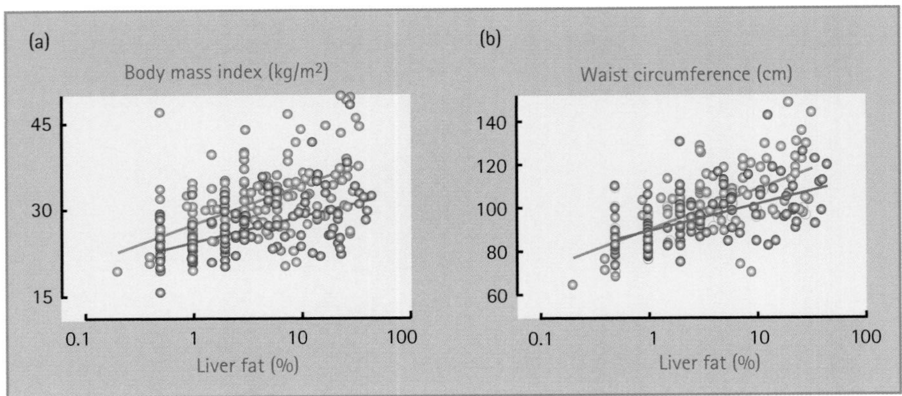

Figure 11.6 The relationship between liver fat and body mass index (a), and liver fat and waist circumference (b) in 271 non-diabetic subjects (red circles denote women and blue circles men). Data from Kotronen *et al.* [5].

improvement in directly measured hepatic insulin sensitivity [52,53]. Weight gain increases liver fat. In an overfeeding study of healthy volunteers, 9.5% weight gain over 4 weeks was associated with a 2.5-fold increase in liver fat content, hyperinsulinemia and a 4.4-fold increase in serum alanine aminotransferase (ALT) activity [54].

Fat distribution

Over 50 years ago, Vague [55] classified obese subjects according to the degree of "masculine differentiation" into those with "gynoid" and those with "android" obesity. Gynoid obesity was characterized by lower body deposition of fat (around the thighs and buttocks) and relative underdevelopment of the musculature, while android obesity defined upper body (truncal) adiposity, greater overall muscular development and a tendency to develop hypertension, diabetes, atherosclerosis and gout. These phenotypic observations have subsequently been confirmed in prospective studies [56–58].

The mechanisms linking upper body obesity to features of insulin resistance are poorly understood. Regarding hepatic insulin resistance and liver fat, it has been suggested that truncal obesity is harmful because it is accompanied by visceral fat accumulation within the abdomen, and because this fat depot is more metabolically active than subcutaneous adipose tissue. Omental and mesenteric adipocytes have a higher rate of lipolysis than subcutaneous, and could liberate excessive amounts of NEFA into the portal vein, thus causing the liver to become insulin resistant. This "portal theory", however, lacks firm supporting evidence from *in vivo* studies [59]. Limited data suggest that concentrations of NEFA and glycerol in the portal vein are close to those in arterial plasma, and tracer studies have shown that NEFA released within the splanchnic (visceral) bed contribute only about 10% of total NEFA delivery to the liver [60]. Furthermore, although the turnover rate of NEFA is higher in women with upper, compared to those with lower body obesity, the excess NEFA have been found to originate from subcutaneous fat in the upper body rather than from the splanchnic bed [61]. Visceral fat also has been proposed to release more inflammatory cytokines such as interleukin 6 (IL-6) than subcutaneous adipose tissue, but such data do not prove cause and effect [62,63]. Thus, visceral fat could be an innocent bystander as well as a culprit [59].

Diet composition

Very few human data are available regarding the effects of changes in diet composition on hepatic insulin sensitivity and liver fat content. Cross-sectional data have suggested that the relative amount of fat, especially saturated fat in the diet, is directly correlated with liver fat [52,64] and that the percentage of dietary saturated fat intake is increased in NAFLD compared with controls [65]. A small intervention study suggested that a high fat (56% of kcal) low carbohydrate diet may increase liver fat compared to a low fat (16% of kcal) high carbohydrate diet [66]. The dietary carbohydrate content, however, may also be important. A cross-sectional study in 247 healthy subjects showed that a high glycemic index diet is associated with high liver fat independent of carbohydrate, fiber, protein and fat intake [67], but there are no intervention studies to confirm this finding.

Genetic causes regulating liver fat and hepatic insulin sensitivity

Twin studies suggest that 35–60% of the variation in the levels of circulating liver enzymes in serum of subjects not using excess alcohol and who have no known liver disease is genetically determined [68,69]. Recently, a genome-wide association scan of non-synonymous sequence variations in a population comprising Hispanic, African-American and European-American individuals identified an allele in the *PNPLA3* (adiponutrin) gene to be strongly associated with increased liver fat [70]. The finding that hepatic fat content is more than twofold higher in *PNPLA3* rs738409[G] homozygotes than in non-carriers has been confirmed in multiple studies [70,71]. The missense mutation I148M in adiponectin promotes triglyceride accumulation by inhibiting triglyceride hydrolysis [72].

Insulin resistance in adipose tissue

Adipose tissue is not merely a depot for excess energy but an active endocrine organ, which releases hormones such as adiponectin and leptin to the circulation (see Chapter 8). In addition, it has recently been shown that in obese subjects [73] and in subjects with a fatty liver independent of obesity [46], adipose tissue is inflamed. This inflammation is characterized by macrophage infiltration and increased expression of proinflammatory molecules such as tumor necrosis factor α (TNF-α) and IL-6, and of chemokines such as MCP-1 [73–76]. The initial trigger of the inflammatory changes is unknown.

Cinti *et al.* [77] showed that in both obese (db/db) mice and humans >90% of the macrophages surround dead adipocytes, and the number of macrophages correlated positively with adipocyte size [73,77]. An increased number of macrophages surrounding dead adipocytes also characterized subjects with a fatty liver compared to equally obese subjects with normal liver fat content [46]. The inflammation in adipose tissue may cause insulin resistance, not only in adipose tissue, but possibly also in other tissues such as the liver. Although it is in general difficult to prove cause and effect in human studies, it is likely that increases in NEFA from the insulin resistance of antilipolysis and the decrease in the concentration of adiponectin are likely mediators of systemic, mainly hepatic, insulin resistance as a consequence of changes occurring in adipose tissue. Macrophage accumulation in human adipose tissue is at least in part reversible as weight loss can reduce both macrophage infiltration and expression of genes involved in macrophage recruitment [78].

Resistance to the antilipolytic action of insulin

Lipolysis in adipose tissue is exquisitely insulin sensitive: in normal subjects, rates of glycerol production are half-maximally suppressed at a plasma insulin concentration of 13 mU/L [79,80]. Triglyceride breakdown is increased and plasma NEFA concentrations are higher in patients with T2DM than in normal subjects studied at comparable insulin levels, suggesting that adipose tissue is also affected by insulin resistance [81,82]. Unrestrained lipolysis to a degree that could lead to ketoacidosis, however, does not occur spontaneously in T2DM, because insulin deficiency is not sufficiently profound.

Increased NEFA concentrations may contribute to worsening of hyperglycemia because of multiple interactions between NEFA and glucose metabolism. A large increase in plasma NEFA concentrations can decrease insulin-stimulated glucose uptake [83] and NEFA may be deposited as triglycerides in skeletal muscle [84,85]. Second, the increased concentration of NEFA reflects increased NEFA turnover, which increases delivery to the liver, where NEFA can be deposited as triglycerides. In the liver, NEFA also stimulate glucose production, especially via gluconeogenesis. The biochemical mechanisms through which NEFA might interfere with insulin action are discussed in Chapter 13.

Adiponectin deficiency

Adiponectin is a hormone produced in adipose tissue. Based on animal studies, its main target is the liver, where it has both anti-inflammatory and insulin-sensitizing effects and decreases liver fat content [86]. The marked increase in serum adiponectin observed during treatment with peroxisome proliferator-activated receptor γ (PPAR-γ) agonists and the close correlation between changes in liver fat and serum adiponectin concentrations [87] support the possibility that adiponectin regulates liver fat content in humans. Serum adiponectin levels are decreased in obese compared to non-obese subjects and in subjects with the metabolic syndrome compared to those without the syndrome.

Insulin resistance in skeletal muscle

There is abundant evidence that the ability of insulin to stimulate *in vivo* glucose disposal is decreased in skeletal muscle of patients with T2DM when measured under similar conditions in age, gender and weight-matched subjects without diabetes [88–90]. Under real-life conditions, however, hyperglycemia compensates for the defect in insulin-stimulated glucose uptake, and maintains the rate of absolute glucose utilization at a normal level in patients with T2DM compared with subjects without diabetes [16].

Mechanisms of insulin resistance in muscle

Multiple defects in the insulin signaling cascade have been identified. There do not appear to be any major disturbances in insulin-receptor binding, and the minor decreases in the tyrosine kinase activity of the receptor β-subunit appear to be secondary to the metabolic disturbances, because they are reversible with weight loss [91].

The abnormality must therefore lie at a post-receptor level. Defects in insulin signaling in human skeletal muscle have been demonstrated in early signaling events such as activation by tyrosine phosphorylation of IRS-1 – a substrate of the insulin receptor's tyrosine kinase – and in the activation of PI_3 kinase [92], which is required for insulin's stimulation of glucose transport and glycogen synthesis (see Chapter 7). Insulin-enhanced glucose uptake, mediated by translocation of the glucose transporter 4 (GLUT-4) protein to the cell surface, and stimulation of glucose phosphorylation via hexokinase II are also diminished [93,94].

The defects in insulin action in skeletal muscle are generally more severe than in equally obese, non-diabetic subjects of the same age, gender and body fat distribution. This suggests that there is an additional genetic defect (see Chapter 12) or that metabolic disturbances such as chronic hyperglycemia (glucose toxicity), or extracellular NEFA or lipid accumulation within the myocytes (lipotoxicity) could be responsible. Indeed, intramyocellular lipid content is higher in patients with T2DM than in equally obese non-diabetic subjects [95] or in lean subjects without diabetes [96].

Causes of insulin resistance in muscle

Obesity

Obesity decreases insulin-stimulated glucose uptake in skeletal muscle independently of changes in physical fitness (see Chapter 14). This decrease could be partly caused by increased NEFA produced by adipose tissue and fat accumulation in myocytes [84,85].

Abdominal obesity

Insulin resistance in skeletal muscle is more severe in subjects with android than those with gynoid obesity [97]. Histologically, abdominally obese subjects have a decreased capillary density and an insulin-resistant fiber type in their skeletal muscles [98,99].

Physical inactivity

The sedentary lifestyle that characterizes Westernized societies is an important contributor to obesity and to T2DM (see Chapters 4 and 23). Data from several prospective epidemiologic studies such the Nurse's Health Study [100] have shown an inverse association between physical activity and the incidence of T2DM [101–103].

Insulin sensitivity of glucose uptake by skeletal muscle is directly proportional to physical fitness measured by maximal oxygen consumption ($\dot{V}O_{2max}$) [104]. Decreased physical fitness (maximal aerobic power) in muscle in patients with T2DM is characterized by decreased capillary density and impaired mitochondrial oxidative phosphorylation [105]. Glucose tolerance and insulin-stimulated glucose uptake are also enhanced by resistive training, which increases total muscle mass without influencing glucose uptake per unit muscle mass [104].

Insulin and exercise stimulate glucose uptake through independent mechanisms. While insulin enhances glucose uptake in skeletal muscle via the classic insulin signaling pathway (see Chapter 7), exercise has no effect on tyrosine phosphorylation of the insulin receptor or of IRS-1 [106]. The mechanism of contraction-stimulated glucose uptake involves adenosine 5′ monophosphate-activated protein kinase (AMPK) [107]. AMPK, especially its $\alpha 2$ isoform, is activated by muscle contraction in human skeletal muscle, and this results in GLUT-4 translocation to the cell membrane and an increase in inward glucose transport [107].

In insulin-resistant patients with T2DM, the ability of insulin to stimulate tyrosine phosphorylation of the insulin receptor and of IRS-1, IRS-1 associated PI_3 kinase activity [92] and translocation of GLUT-4 [108] are all subnormal. Aerobic training, however, has been shown to increase the GLUT-4 content in skeletal muscle [109] and the expression and activity of glycogen synthase [110] to a comparable degree to normal subjects. Thus, the signaling pathways through which exercise enhances glucose uptake may be intact in patients with T2DM. This has the practical implication that the glycemic response to exercise is not blunted by insulin resistance.

Chronic hyperglycemia

Hyperglycemia itself, independent of insulin, NEFA or counter-regulatory hormones, can induce insulin resistance in human skeletal muscle [111]. This "glucose toxicity" induced insulin resistance could contribute to the lower rates of insulin-stimulated glucose uptake in patients with T2DM compared with weight, age and gender-matched subjects without diabetes and measured during maintenance of similar levels of glycemia and insulinemia. Although chronic hyperglycemia induces insulin resistance, however, glucose utilization is stimulated acutely via the mass action effects of glucose even in patients with diabetes. This effect explains why hyperglycemic patients with T2DM are able to utilize as much glucose as normal subjects at normoglycemia, in spite of the insulin resistance in the subjects with diabetes [111,112].

The degree of insulin resistance in patients with T2DM is directly proportional to the severity of hyperglycemia [111]. Thus, insulin resistance induced by the hexosamine pathway in hyperglycemic patients with T2DM could be viewed as a compensatory mechanism that protects muscles against excessive uptake of glucose. Consistent with this, in isolated skeletal muscle from patients with T2DM [112], insulin-stimulated glucose transport in muscles of hyperglycemic patients with T2DM was similar to that in normoglycemic subjects but impaired when measured after short-term exposure to normoglycemia. Prolonged exposure to normoglycemia completely normalized the defect in insulin-stimulated glucose transport [112]. Clinically, the ability of hyperglycemia to induce insulin resistance in patients with T2DM may explain why any treatment, such as sulfonylureas, which improves glycemic control may also improve insulin sensitivity even if the primary site of action is not in insulin-sensitive tissues [111].

The hexosamine pathway was discovered in 1991, by Marshall *et al.* [113], who found that it mediated glucose-induced insulin resistance in primary cultured rat adipocytes. Downregulation of the insulin-responsive glucose transport system was observed to require three components: glucose, insulin and glutamine. Inactivation of the glutamine-requiring enzyme, glutamine:fructose-6-amidotransferase (GFA), the rate-limiting enzyme of the hexosamine pathway, by glutamine analogs, prevented glucose-induced desensitization of glucose transport [113]. GFA catalyzes the interconversion of glutamine and fructose-6-phosphate to form glucosamine-6-phosphate (GlcN-6-P) and glutamate [114]. GFA is expressed in insulin target tissues such as skeletal muscle, where its activity is increased in patients with T2DM [115]. The end-product of the pathway, UDP-*N*-acetyl-glucosamine (UDP-*N*AcGln) is attached to the OH-group of threonine and serine residues of proteins (these same residues can also be phosphorylated), which results in O-glycation of proteins. These include multiple proteins involved in glucose-responsive and insulin-dependent transcription and signaling events [114].

Resistance to other actions of insulin

Vascular effects of insulin

At physiologic concentrations and within a physiologic time-frame, insulin decreases the stiffness of large arteries [116]. This effect is blunted in obesity [117]. These data are consistent with epidemiologic data that indicate that insulin resistance and arterial stiffness are independently associated in subjects without diabetes. Patients with T2DM have stiffer arteries than age and weight-matched healthy subjects [118,119].

Another vascular effect of insulin is vasodilatation of peripheral resistance vessels [120], mediated at least in part by enhanced nitric oxide (NO) production by the endothelium [121]. Because this effect requires prolonged or high doses of insulin, its physiologic significance has thus been questioned [120]. In patients with T2DM, defects in insulin action on blood flow have not been observed when tested at insulin concentrations within the physiologic range, but have been observed at grossly supraphysiologic insulin levels (600 mU/L) [120].

Insulin stimulates NO production in endothelial cells [122], and acutely increases endothelium-dependent but not endothelium-independent vasodilatation in normal subjects [121]. Endothelium-dependent vasodilatation is known to be impaired in T2DM and other insulin-resistant states [123,124]. Whether this defect is caused by insulin resistance at the level of endothelial cells [125] or to indirect causes of endothelial dysfunction such as chronic hyperglycemia [126] or dyslipidemia [124] cannot be determined from cross-sectional human data.

Effects of insulin on autonomic nervous tone

Another of the many actions of insulin is its effect on the autonomic nervous system. Insulin can enter the hypothalamus and other parts of the brain, where insulin receptors are expressed at high levels, and it acts centrally to stimulate the sympathetic nervous system. Manifestations include increases in muscle sympathetic nervous activity [127] and in norepinephrine spillover rate (a measure of norepinephrine release from sympathetic nerve endings in the tissues) [128]. Insulin also regulates the autonomic control of heart rate, decreasing vagal tone and increasing sympathetic drive [129]. In insulin-resistant obese subjects, basal sympathetic tone is increased and the subsequent response to insulin blunted [130]. This defect is also observed in non-obese but insulin-resistant subjects [129], and in patients with T2DM [131]. Enhanced central effects of the associated hyperinsulinemia may contribute.

Insulin resistance, hemostasis and coagulation

Insulin normally inhibits platelet aggregation [132], and this action is blunted both *in vitro* [132] and *in vivo* [133] in insulin-resistant obese subjects without diabetes and those with T2DM.

Plasminogen activator inhibitor 1 (PAI-1) is an inhibitor of fibrinolysis, and raised plasma levels predict increased risk of a coronary event [134]. Procoagulant changes, such as impaired fibrinolysis and increased levels of PAI-1, and defects in platelet function are frequently associated with insulin resistance, especially in obese patients with T2DM. These abnormalities predispose to atherothrombotic vascular disease (see Part 8).

Effects of insulin on uric acid metabolism

In normal subjects, insulin acutely reduces the renal clearance of both sodium and uric acid [135]. These actions are preserved in insulin-resistant states such as obesity, diabetes and essential hypertension, and so provide a potential mechanistic link for the clustering of hyperinsulinemia with hyperuricemia and hypertension [136,137].

Other effects of insulin

Insulin acutely lowers serum potassium concentrations by stimulating potassium uptake into skeletal muscle and the splanchnic bed [138]. It also attenuates agonist-induced intracellular increases in Ca^{2+} concentrations in vascular smooth muscle cells [139] and inhibits sodium, potassium and phosphate excretion by the kidney [138]. The hypokalemic antinatriuretic actions of insulin are both preserved in patients with insulin resistance affecting glucose metabolism and essential hypertension [140,141] and in those with T2DM [142].

Relationship of insulin resistance to hypertension

Of the putative components of the "insulin resistance syndrome," the association between insulin resistance and hypertension is perhaps the most controversial. Hypertension and insulin resistance have been shown to be linked, independently of confounding factors such as obesity [143], but the relationship appears inconsistent [144–146]. Numerous mechanisms have been postulated to explain this association, but it is currently unclear which – if any – are relevant. In insulin-resistant patients with essential hypertension, basal intracellular Ca^{2+} levels have been shown to be elevated, and the normal ability of insulin to attenuate angiotensin II induced increases in intracellular Ca^{2+} is blunted in skin fibroblasts [139]; however, there are no data in patients with T2DM. The renal action of insulin to reabsorb sodium is similar in normotensive and hypertensive insulin-resistant subjects and in patients with T2DM [142], which implies that changes in the antinatriuretic effect of insulin cannot explain the increased prevalence of hypertension in insulin-resistant individuals or those with T2DM. The suggestion that insulin sensitivity influences salt sensitivity is controversial [147–151]. Insulin resistance has consistently been found to correlate with high sodium–lithium counter-transport in erythrocyte membranes; this is thought to parallel increased activity of the Na^+–H^+ pump in the cell membrane of other tissues, which could raise intracellular Na^+ and Ca^{2+} concentrations and enhance vascular smooth muscle contractility. Such defects may contribute to the development of hypertension in both insulin-resistant subjects without diabetes and in patients with T2DM (see Chapter 40).

In theory, an increase in peripheral vascular resistance (which would raise diastolic blood pressure) could also be a consequence of impaired insulin-induced vasodilatation. Such defects, however, have not been documented under physiologic conditions [120]. It is also unclear whether the defects in endothelium-dependent vasorelaxation observed at very high insulin concentrations are specific to insulin or are a consequence of a more generalized defect in endothelial or smooth-muscle function, or of structural changes in arteries secondary to hypertension. Increased systolic blood pressure is, in most hypertensive individuals, a consequence of increased arterial stiffness [152]. Resistance to the normal ability of insulin to decrease stiffness could therefore increase systolic blood pressure [117].

Conclusions

Insulin resistance, even when present in individuals without diabetes, is characterized not only by abnormalities in glucose homeostasis, but also by defects in insulin regulation of lipid and uric acid metabolism, vascular function, hemostasis and coagulation. These consequences of insulin resistance (normal or impaired glucose tolerance, hypertriglyceridemia, a low HDL cholesterol concentration, small LDL size, hypertension, increases in uric acid and PAI-1 concentrations) and fasting hyperinsulinemia were called "syndrome X" by Reaven [153] to emphasize that insulin resistance comprises a cluster of abnormalities.

This syndrome, now called the metabolic syndrome (Table 11.2) rather than syndrome X, is important to recognize clinically as it is associated with many components that can potentially be modified to prevent premature atherosclerosis and cardiovascular disease, the main cause of excessive mortality in those with T2DM. Various mechanisms have been proposed to explain how insulin resistance and/or the accompanying hyperinsulinemia could cause these abnormalities. Accumulation of fat in the liver appears to occur in those individuals who develop the metabolic syndrome, independent of obesity. The liver, once fatty, is insulin

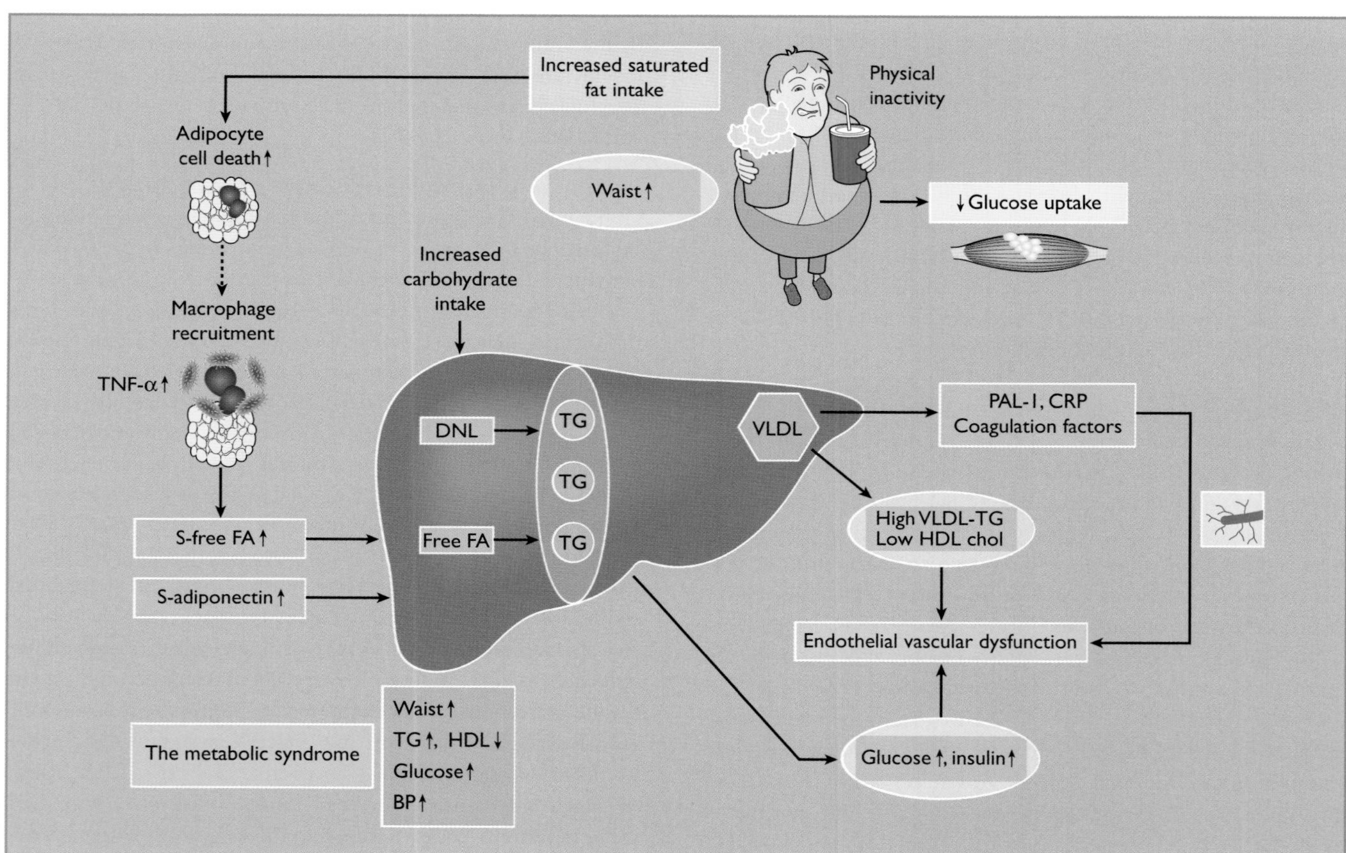

Figure 11.7 Causes and consequences of insulin resistance and pathogenesis of the metabolic syndrome. Overeating and inactivity are common and important causes of obesity. In many obese but also sometimes in non-obese subjects, fat accumulates in the liver. Saturated fat and high refined carbohydrate intake may be particularly harmful. Genetic predisposition also has a role, at least in fat accumulation in the liver. In obese subjects with a fatty liver, adipose tissue is inflamed. This inflammation is characterized by increased expression of cytokines such as tumor necrosis factor α (TNF-α), and increased macrophage infiltration around dead adipocytes. The cause of the inflammation poorly understood. Inflamed adipose tissue is insulin-resistant and overproduces free fatty acids (FFA) which contribute to excess triglyceride storage (TG) in the liver. Adiponectin deficiency also characterizes inflamed adipose tissue and decreases insulin sensitivity. Once fatty the liver overproduces glucose and VLDL as depicted in Figure 11.3, and also other factors such as plasminogen activator 1 (PAI-1) and coagulation factors. Excess refined carbohydrate may increase *de novo* lipogenesis in the liver (DNL), thus increasing intrahepatocellular triglyceride. Overeating and inactivity are also characterized by insulin resistance of glucose uptake by skeletal muscle.

resistant and overproduces glucose, VLDL, PAI-1, C-reactive protein and coagulation factors, which could all contribute to increased cardiovascular risk (Figure 11.7). The exact causes of why fat accumulates in the liver of some but not others are unknown but appear to involve genetic factors (adiponutrin polymorphism) and acquired factors (use of refined carbohydrates, high saturated fat untake, weight gain). Insulin resistance and inflammation characteize adipose tissue of those who have a fatty liver. In patients with T2DM, insulin resistance is further worsened by chronic hyperglycemia, which itself causes insulin resistance.

References

1 Lillioja S, Mott DM, Spraul M, Ferraro R, Foley JE, Ravussin E, *et al.* Insulin resistance and insulin secretory dysfunction as precursors of non-insulin-dependent diabetes mellitus. *N Engl J Med* 1993; **329**:1988–1992.

2 International Diabetes Federation (IDF). *The IDF Consensus Worldwide Definition of the Metabolic Syndrome.* International Diabetes Federation, 2006.

3 Kotronen A, Yki-Jarvinen H. Fatty liver: a novel component of the metabolic syndrome. *Arterioscler Thromb Vasc Biol* 2008; **28**:27–38.

4 Neuschwander-Tetri B, Caldwell S. Nonalcoholic steatohepatitis: summary of an AASLD single topic conference. *Hepatology* 2003; **37**:1202–1219.

5 Kotronen A, Westerbacka J, Bergholm R, Pietilainen KH, Yki-Jarvinen H. Liver fat in the metabolic syndrome. *J Clin Endocrinol Metab* 2007; **92**:3490–3497.

6 Charlton M. Nonalcoholic fatty liver disease: a review of current understanding and future impact. *Clin Gastroenterol Hepatol* 2004; **2**:1048–1058.

7 Jeng CY, Sheu WH, Fuh MM, Chen YD, Reaven GM. Relationship between hepatic glucose production and fasting plasma glucose concentration in patients with NIDDM. *Diabetes* 1994; **43**:1440–1444.

8 Gerich JE, Mitrakou A, Kelley D, Mandarino L, Nurjhan N, Reilly J, *et al.* Contribution of impaired muscle glucose clearance to reduced postabsorptive systemic glucose clearance in NIDDM. *Diabetes* 1990; **39**:211–216.

9 Mitrakou A, Kelley D, Veneman T, Jenssen T, Pangburn T, Reilly J, *et al.* Contribution of abnormal muscle and liver metabolism to postprandial hyperglycemia in NIDDM. *Diabetes* 1990; **39**:1381–1390.

10 Campbell PJ, Mandarino LJ, Gerich JE. Quantification of the relative impairment in actions of insulin on hepatic glucose production and peripheral glucose uptake in non-insulin-dependent diabetes mellitus. *Metabolism* 1988; **37**:15–21.

11 Kolterman OG, Gray RS, Griffin J, Burstein P, Insel J, Scarlett JA, *et al.* Receptor and postreceptor defects contribute to the insulin resistance in noninsulin-dependent diabetes mellitus. *J Clin Invest* 1981; **68**:957–969.

12 Ryysy L, Häkkinen AM, Goto T, Vehkavaara S, Westerbacka J, Halavaara J, *et al.* Hepatic fat content and insulin action on free fatty acids and glucose metabolism rather than insulin absorption are associated with insulin requirements during insulin therapy in type 2 diabetic patients. *Diabetes* 2000; **49**:749–758.

13 Seppala-Lindroos A, Vehkavaara S, Hakkinen AM, Goto T, Westerbacka J, Sovijärvi A, *et al.* Fat accumulation in the liver is associated with defects in insulin suppression of glucose production and serum free fatty acids independent of obesity in normal men. *J Clin Endocrinol Metab* 2002; **87**:3023–3028.

14 Kelley D, Mitrakou A, Marsh H, Schwenk F, Benn J, Sonnenberg G, *et al.* Skeletal muscle glycolysis, oxidation, and storage of an oral glucose load. *J Clin Invest* 1988; **81**:1563–1571.

15 Basu A, Basu R, Shah P, Vella A, Johnson CM, Jensen M, *et al.* Type 2 diabetes impairs splanchnic uptake of glucose but does not alter intestinal glucose absorption during enteral glucose feeding: additional evidence for a defect in hepatic glucokinase activity. *Diabetes* 2001; **50**:1351–1362.

16 Yki-Järvinen H. Acute and chronic effects of hyperglycemia on glucose metabolism. *Diabetologia* 1990; **33**:579–585.

17 Sparks JD, Sparks CE. Insulin modulation of hepatic synthesis and secretion of apolipoprotein B by rat hepatocytes. *J Biol Chem* 1990; **265**:8854–8862.

18 Durrington PN, Newton RS, Weinstein DB, Steinberg D. Effects of insulin and glucose on very low density lipoprotein triglyceride secretion by cultured rat hepatocytes. *J Clin Invest* 1982; **70**:63–73.

19 Malmström R, Packard CJ, Caslake M, Bedford D, Stewart P, Yki-Järvinen H, *et al.* Defective regulation of triglyceride metabolism by insulin in the liver in NIDDM. *Diabetologia* 1997; **40**:454–462.

20 Malmström R, Packard CJ, Caslake M, Bedford D, Stewart P, Yki-Järvinen H, *et al.* Effects of insulin and acipimox on VLDL1 and VLDL2 apolipoprotein B production in normal subjects. *Diabetes* 1998; **47**:779–787.

21 Adiels M, Taskinen MR, Packard C, Caslake MJ, Soro-Paavonen A, Westerbacka J, *et al.* Overproduction of large VLDL particles is driven by increased liver fat content in man. *Diabetologia* 2006; **49**:755–765.

22 Adiels M, Westerbacka J, Soro-Paavonen A, Häkkinen AM, Vehkavaara S, Caslake MJ, *et al.* Acute suppression of VLDL1 secretion rate by insulin is associated with hepatic fat content and insulin resistance. *Diabetologia* 2007; **50**:2356–2365.

23 Adiels M, Olofsson SO, Taskinen MR, Boren J. Overproduction of very low-density lipoproteins is the hallmark of the dyslipidemia in the metabolic syndrome. *Arterioscler Thromb Vasc Biol* 2008; **28**:1225–1236.

24 Eisenberg S. High-density lipoprotein metabolism. In: Betteridge DJ, Illingworth DR, Shepherd J, eds. *Lipoproteins in Health and Disease*, 1st edn. London: Arnold, 1999: 71–85.

25 Deckelbaum RJ, Granot E, Oschry Y, Rose L, Eisenberg S. Plasma triglyceride determines structure-composition in low and high density lipoproteins. *Arteriosclerosis* 1984; **4**:225–231.

26 Zambon A, Austin MA, Brown BG, Hokanson JE, Brunzell JD. Effect of hepatic lipase on LDL in normal men and those with coronary artery disease. *Arterioscler Thromb* 1993; **13**:147–153.

27 Lahdenpera S, Syvanne M, Kahri J, Taskinen M-R. Regulation of low-density lipoprotein particle size distribution in NIDDM and coronary disease: importance of serum triglycerides. *Diabetologia* 1996; **39**:453–461.

28 Gray RS, Robbins DC, Wang W, Yeh JL, Fabsitz RR, Cowan LD, *et al.* Relation of LDL size to the insulin resistance syndrome and coronary heart disease in American Indians: The Strong Heart Study. *Arterioscler Thromb Vasc Biol* 1997; **17**:2713–2720.

29 Austin MA, Rodriguez BL, McKnight B, McNeely MJ, Edwards KL, Curb JD, *et al.* Low-density lipoprotein particle size, triglycerides,

and high-density lipoprotein cholesterol as risk factors for coronary heart disease in older Japanese-American men. *Am J Cardiol* 2000; **86**:412–416.

30 Coresh J, Kwiterovich POJ, Smith HH, Bachorik PS. Association of plasma triglyceride concentration and LDL particle diameter, density, and chemical composition with premature coronary artery disease in men and women. *J Lipid Res* 1993; **34**:1687–1697.

31 Gardner CD, Fortmann SP, Krauss RM. Association of small low-density lipoprotein particles with the incidence of coronary artery disease in men and women. *JAMA* 1996; **276**:875–881.

32 Austin MA, Mykkanen L, Kuusisto J, Edwards KL, Nelson C, Haffner SM, *et al.* Prospective study of small LDLs as a risk factor for non-insulin dependent diabetes mellitus in elderly men and women. *Circulation* 1995; **92**:1770–1778.

33 Parks EJ, Hellerstein MK. Thematic review series: patient-oriented research: recent advances in liver triacylglycerol and fatty acid metabolism using stable isotope labeling techniques. *J Lipid Res* 2006; **47**:1651–1660.

34 Donnelly KL, Smith CI, Schwarzenberg SJ, Jessurun J, Boldt MD, Parks EJ. Sources of fatty acids stored in liver and secreted via lipoproteins in patients with nonalcoholic fatty liver disease. *J Clin Invest* 2005; **115**:1343–1351.

35 Nielsen S, Guo Z, Johnson CM, Hensrud DD, Jensen MD. Splanchnic lipolysis in human obesity. *J Clin Invest* 2004; **113**:1582–1588.

36 Parks EJ. Dietary carbohydrate's effects on lipogenesis and the relationship of lipogenesis to blood insulin and glucose concentrations. *Br J Nutr* 2002; **87**(Suppl 2):S247–S253.

37 Diraison F, Moulin P, Beylot M. Contribution of hepatic *de novo* lipogenesis and reesterification of plasma non-esterified fatty acids to plasma triglyceride synthesis during non-alcoholic fatty liver disease. *Diabetes Metab* 2003; **29**:478–485.

38 Chong MF, Hodson L, Bickerton AS, Roberts R, Neville M, Karpe F, *et al.* Parallel activation of *de novo* lipogenesis and stearoyl-CoA desaturase activity after 3 d of high-carbohydrate feeding. *Am J Clin Nutr* 2008; **87**:817–823.

39 Petersen KF, Dufour S, Savage DB, Bilz S, Solomon G, Yonemitsu S, *et al.* The role of skeletal muscle insulin resistance in the pathogenesis of the metabolic syndrome. *Proc Natl Acad Sci U S A* 2007; **104**:12587–12594.

40 Kotronen A, Seppanen-Laakso T, Westerbacka J, Kiviluoto T, Arola J, Ruskeepää AL, *et al.* Hepatic stearoyl-CoA desaturase (SCD)-1 activity and diacylglycerol but not ceramide concentrations are increased in the nonalcoholic human fatty liver. *Diabetes* 2009; **58**:203–208.

41 Aarsland A, Wolfe RR. Hepatic secretion of VLDL fatty acids during stimulated lipogenesis in men. *J Lipid Res* 1998; **39**:1280–1286.

42 Summers SA. Ceramides in insulin resistance and lipotoxicity. *Prog Lipid Res* 2006; **45**:42–72.

43 Holland WL, Brozinick JT, Wang LP, Hawkins ED, Sargent KM, Liu Y, *et al.* Inhibition of ceramide synthesis ameliorates glucocorticoid-, saturated-fat-, and obesity-induced insulin resistance. *Cell Metab* 2007; **5**:167–179.

44 Miyazaki M, Flowers MT, Sampath H, Chu K, Otzelberger C, Liu X, *et al.* Hepatic stearoyl-CoA desaturase-1 deficiency protects mice from carbohydrate-induced adiposity and hepatic steatosis. *Cell Metab* 2007; **6**:484–496.

45 Adams JM 2nd, Pratipanawatr T, Berria R, Wang E, DeFronzo RA, Sullards MC, *et al.* Ceramide content is increased in skeletal muscle from obese insulin-resistant humans. *Diabetes* 2004; **53**:25–31.

46 Kolak M, Westerbacka J, Velagapudi VR, Wågsäter D, Yetukuri L, Makkonen J, *et al.* Adipose tissue inflammation and increased ceramide content characterize subjects with high liver fat content independent of obesity. *Diabetes* 2007; **56**:1960–1968.

47 Savage DB, Petersen KF, Shulman GI. Disordered lipid metabolism and the pathogenesis of insulin resistance. *Physiol Rev* 2007; **87**:507–520.

48 Considine RV, Nyce MR, Allen LE, Morales LM, Triester S, Serrano J, *et al.* Protein kinase C is increased in the liver of humans and rats with non-insulin dependent diabetes mellitus: an alteration not due to hyperglycemia. *J Clin Invest* 1995; **95**:2938–2944.

49 Bonadonna RC, Groop L, Kraemer N, Ferrannini E, Del Prato S, DeFronzo RA. Obesity and insulin resistance in humans: a dose–response study. *Metabolism* 1990; **39**:452–459.

50 Luyckx FH, Lefebvre PJ, Scheen AJ. Non-alcoholic steatohepatitis: association with obesity and insulin resistance, and influence of weight loss. *Diabetes Metab* 2000; **26**:98–106.

51 Hollingsworth KG, Abubacker MZ, Joubert I, Allison ME, Lomas DJ. Low-carbohydrate diet induced reduction of hepatic lipid content observed with a rapid non-invasive MRI technique. *Br J Radiol* 2006; **79**:712–715.

52 Tiikkainen M, Bergholm R, Vehkavaara S, Rissanen A, Häkkinen AM, Tamminen M, *et al.* Effects of identical weight loss on body composition and features of insulin resistance in obese women with high and low liver fat content. *Diabetes* 2003; **52**:701–707.

53 Kirk E, Reeds DN, Finck BN, Mayurranjan MS, Klein S. Dietary fat and carbohydrates differentially alter insulin sensitivity during caloric restriction. *Gastroenterology* 2009; **136**:1552–1560.

54 Kechagias S, Ernersson A, Dahlqvist O, Lundberg P, Lindstrom T, Nystrom FH. Fast-food-based hyper-alimentation can induce rapid and profound elevation of serum alanine aminotransferase in healthy subjects. *Gut* 2008; **57**:649–654.

55 Vague J. La differentiation sexuelle: facteur determinant des formes de l'obesite. *Presse Med* 1947; **55**:339.

56 Fontbonne A, Thibult N, Eschwege E, Ducimetiere P. Body fat distribution and coronary heart disease mortality in subjects with impaired glucose tolerance or diabetes mellitus: the Paris Prospective Study, 15-year follow-up. *Diabetologia* 1992; **35**:464–468.

57 Folsom AR, Kaye SA, Sellers TA, Hong CP, Cerhan JR, Potter JD, *et al.* Body fat distribution and 5-year risk of death in older women. *JAMA* 1993; **269**:483–487.

58 Kalmijn S, Curb JD, Rodriguez BL, Yano K, Abbott RD. The association of body weight and anthropometry with mortality in elderly men: the Honolulu Heart Program. *Int J Obes Relat Metab Disord* 1999; **23**:395–402.

59 Frayn KN. Visceral fat and insulin resistance: causative or correlative? *Br J Nutr* 2000; **83**(Suppl 1):S71–S77.

60 Havel RJ, Kane JP, Balasse EO, Segel N, Basso LV. Splanchnic metabolism of free fatty acids and production of triglyserides of very low density lipoproteins in normotriglyceridemic and hypertriglyceridemic humans. *J Clin Invest* 1970; **49**:2017–2035.

61 Martin ML, Jensen MD. Effects of body fat distribution on regional lipolysis in obesity. *J Clin Invest* 1991; **88**:609–613.

62 Rasouli N, Kern PA. Adipocytokines and the metabolic complications of obesity. *J Clin Endocrinol Metab* 2008; **93**:S64–S73.

63 Jensen MD. Role of body fat distribution and the metabolic complications of obesity. *J Clin Endocrinol Metab* 2008; **93**:S57–S63.

64 Pietiläinen KH, Rissanen A, Kaprio J, Mäkimattila S, Häkkinen AM, Westerbacka J, *et al.* Acquired obesity is associated with increased

liver fat, intra-abdominal fat, and insulin resistance in young adult monozygotic twins. *Am J Physiol Endocrinol Metab* 2005; **288**: E768–E774.

65 Musso G, Gambino R, De Michieli F, Cassader M, Rizzetto M, Durazzo M, *et al.* Dietary habits and their relations to insulin resistance and postprandial lipemia in nonalcoholic steatohepatitis. *Hepatology* 2003; **37**:909–916.

66 Westerbacka J, Lammi K, Häkkinen AM, Rissanen A, Salminen I, Aro A, *et al.* Dietary fat content modifies liver fat in overweight nondiabetic subjects. *J Clin Endocrinol Metab* 2005; **90**:2804–2809.

67 Valtuena S, Pellegrini N, Ardigo D, Del Rio D, Numeroso F, Scazzina F, *et al.* Dietary glycemic index and liver steatosis. *Am J Clin Nutr* 2006; **84**:136–142.

68 Bathum L, Petersen HC, Rosholm JU, Hyltoft PP, Vaupel J, Christensen K. Evidence for a substantial genetic influence on biochemical liver function tests: results from a population-based Danish twin study. *Clin Chem* 2001; **47**:81–87.

69 Makkonen JJ, Pietiläinen KH, Rissanen A, Kaprio J, Yki-Järvinen H. Genetic factors contribute to variation in serum alanine aminotransferase activity independent of obesity and alcohol: a study in monozygotic and dizygotic twins. *J Hepatol* 2009; **50**:1035–1042.

70 Romeo S, Kozlitina J, Xing C, Pertsemlidis A, Cox D, Pennacchio LA, *et al.* Genetic variation in PNPLA3 confers susceptibility to nonalcoholic fatty liver disease. *Nat Genet* 2008; **40**:1461–1465.

71 Kotronen A, Johansson LE, Johansson LM, Roos C, Westerbacka J, Hamsten A, *et al.* A common variant in PNPLA3, which encodes adiponutrin, is associated with liver fat content in humans. *Diabetologia* 2009; **52**:1056–1060.

72 He S, McPhaul C, Zhong Li J, Garuti R, Kinch L, Grishin W, Cohen JC, Hobbs HH. A sequence variation (I148M) in PNPLA3 associated with nonalcoholic fatty liver disease disrupts triglyceride hydrolysis. *J Biol Chem*; in press. E-pub ahead of print Dec 23, 2009.

73 Weisberg SP, McCann D, Desai M, Rosenbaum M, Leibel RL, Ferrante AW Jr. Obesity is associated with macrophage accumulation in adipose tissue. *J Clin Invest* 2003; **112**:1796–1808.

74 Xu H, Barnes GT, Yang Q, Tan G, Yang D, Chou CJ, *et al.* Chronic inflammation in fat plays a crucial role in the development of obesity-related insulin resistance. *J Clin Invest* 2003; **112**:1821–1830.

75 Di Gregorio GB, Yao-Borengasser A, Rasouli N, Varma V, Lu T, Miles LM, *et al.* Expression of CD68 and macrophage chemoattractant protein-1 genes in human adipose and muscle tissues: association with cytokine expression, insulin resistance, and reduction by pioglitazone. *Diabetes* 2005; **54**:2305–2313.

76 Cancello R, Tordjman J, Poitou C, Tordjman J, Lacasa D, Guerre-Millo M, *et al.* Increased infiltration of macrophages in omental adipose tissue is associated with marked hepatic lesions in morbid human obesity. *Diabetes* 2006; **55**:1554–1561.

77 Cinti S, Mitchell G, Barbatelli G, Murano I, Ceresi E, Faloia E, *et al.* Adipocyte death defines macrophage localization and function in adipose tissue of obese mice and humans. *J Lipid Res* 2005; **46**:2347–2355.

78 Cancello R, Heregar C, Viguerie N, Taleb S, Poitou C, Rouault C *et al.* Reduction of Macrophage infiltration and chemoattractant gene expression changes white adipose tissue of morbidly obese subjects after surgery-induced weight loss. *Diabetes* 2005;**54**:2277–2286.

79 Howard BV, Savage PJ, Nagulesparan M, Bennion LJ, Unger RH, Bennet PH. Evidence for marked sensitivity to the antilipolytic action of insulin in obese maturity-onset diabetes. *Metab Clin Exp* 1979; **28**:744–750.

80 Nurjhan N, Campbell PJ, Kennedy FP, Miles JM, Gerich JE. Insulin dose–response charateristics for suppression of glycerol release and conversion to glucose in humans. *Diabetes* 1986; **35**:1326–1331.

81 Groop LC, Bonadonna RC, DelPrato S, Ratheiser K, Zyck K, Ferrannini E, *et al.* Glucose and free fatty acid metabolism in non-insulin-dependent diabetes mellitus: evidence of multiple sites of insulin resistance. *J Clin Invest* 1989; **84**:205–213.

82 Fraze E, Donner CC, Swislocki AL, Chiou YA, Chen YD, Reaven GM. Ambient plasma free fatty acid concentrations in noninsulin-dependent diabetes mellitus: evidence for insulin resistance. *J Clin Endocrinol Metab* 1985; **61**:807–811.

83 Ferrannini E, Barrett EJ, Bevilacqua S, DeFronzo RA. Effect of fatty acids on glucose production and utilization in man. *J Clin Invest* 1983; **72**:1737–1747.

84 Pan DA, Lillioja S, Kriketos AD, Milner MR, Baur LA, Bogardus C, *et al.* Skeletal muscle triglyceride levels are inversely related to insulin action. *Diabetes* 1997; **46**:983–988.

85 Krssak M, Falk PK, Dresner A, DiPietro L, Vogel SM, Rothman DL, *et al.* Intramyocellular lipid concentrations are correlated with insulin sensitivity in humans: a 1H NMR spectroscopy study. *Diabetologia* 1999; **42**:113–116.

86 Kadowaki T, Yamauchi T. Adiponectin and adiponectin receptors. *Endocr Rev* 2005; **26**:439–451.

87 Yki-Jarvinen H, Westerbacka J. The fatty liver and insulin resistance. *Curr Mol Med* 2005; **5**:287–295.

88 Ginsberg H, Kimmerling G, Olefsky JM, Reaven GM. Demonstration of insulin resistance in untreated adult onset diabetic subjects with fasting hyperglycemia. *J Clin Invest* 1975; **55**:454–461.

89 Shen S-W, Reaven GM, Farquhar JW. Comparison of impedance to insulin-mediated glucose uptake in normal subjects and subjects with latent diabetes. *J Clin Invest* 1970; **49**:2151–2160.

90 DeFronzo RA, Gunnarson R, Björkman O, Olsson M, Wahren J. Effects of insulin on peripheral and splanchnic glucose metabolism in noninsulin-dependent (type II) diabetes mellitus. *J Clin Invest* 1985; **76**:149–155.

91 Freidenberg GR, Reichart D, Olefsky JM, Henry RR. Reversibility of defective adipocyte insulin receptor kinase activity in non-insulin-dependent diabetic subjects. *J Clin Invest* 1988; **82**:1398–1406.

92 Cusi K, Maezono K, Osman A, Pendergrass M, Patti ME, Pratipanawatr T, *et al.* Insulin resistance differentially affects the PI 3-kinase- and MAP kinase-mediated signaling in human muscle. *J Clin Invest* 2000; **105**:311–320.

93 Pendergrass M, Koval J, Vogt C, Yki-Jarvinen H, Iozzo P, Pipek R, *et al.* Insulin-induced hexokinase II expression is reduced in obesity and NIDDM. *Diabetes* 1998; **47**:394.

94 Zierath JR, Krook A, Wallberg-Henriksson H. Insulin action in skeletal muscle from patients with NIDDM. *Mol Cell Biochem* 1998; **182**:153–160.

95 Levin K, Daa SH, Alford FP, Beck-Nielsen H. Morphometric documentation of abnormal intramyocellular fat storage and reduced glycogen in obese patients with type II diabetes. *Diabetologia* 2001; **44**:824–833.

96 He J, Watkins S, Kelley DE. Skeletal muscle lipid content and oxidative enzyme activity in relation to muscle fiber type in type 2 diabetes and obesity. *Diabetes* 2001; **50**:817–823.

97 Krotkiewski M, Bjorntorp P, Sjostrom L, Smith U. Impact of obesity on metabolism in men and women: importance of regional adipose tissue distribution. *J Clin Invest* 1983; **72**:1150–1162.

98 Lillioja S, Young AA, Culter CL, Ivy JL, Abbott WG, Zawadzki JK, *et al.* Skeletal muscle capillary density and fiber type are possible determinants of *in vivo* insulin resistance in man. *J Clin Invest* 1987; **80**:415–424.

99 Lithell H, Lundqvist G, Nygaard E, Vessby B, Saltin B. Body weight, skeletal muscle morphology, and enzyme activities in relation to fasting seum insulin concentration and glucose tolerance in 48-year-old men. *Diabetes* 1981; **30**:19–25.

100 Hu FB, Sigal RJ, Rich-Edwards JW, Colditz GA, Solomon CG, Willett WC, *et al.* Walking compared with vigorous physical activity and risk of type 2 diabetes in women: a prospective study. *JAMA* 1999; **282**:1433–1439.

101 Helmrich SP, Ragland DR, Leung RW, Paffenbarger RS. Physical activity and reduced occurrence of non-insulin-dependent diabetes mellitus. *N Engl J Med* 1991; **325**:147–152.

102 Manson JE, Nathan DM, Krolewski AS, Stapfer MJ, Willett WC, Hennekens CH. A prospective study of exercise and incidence of diabetes among US male physicians. *JAMA* 1992; **268**: 63–67.

103 Manson J, Rimm EB, Stampfer MJ, *et al.* Physical activity and incidence of non-insulin-dependent diabetes mellitus in women. *Lancet* 1991; **338**:774–778.

104 Yki-Järvinen H, Koivisto VA. Effect of body composition on insulin sensitivity. *Diabetes* 1983; **32**:965–969.

105 Mootha VK, Lindgren CM, Eriksson KF, Subramanian A, Sihaq S, Lehar J, *et al.* PGC-1alpha-responsive genes involved in oxidative phosphorylation are coordinately downregulated in human diabetes. *Nat Genet* 2003; **34**:267–273.

106 Koval JA, Maezono K, Patti ME, Pendergrass M, DeFronzo RA, Mandarino LJ. Effects of exercise and insulin on insulin signaling proteins in human skeletal muscle. *Med Sci Sports Exerc* 1999; **31**:998–1004.

107 Winder WW, Hardie DG. AMP-activated protein kinase, a metabolic master switch: possible roles in type 2 diabetes. *Am J Physiol* 1999; **277**:E1–E19.

108 Guma A, Zierath JR, Wallberg-Henriksson H, Klip A. Insulin induces translocation of GLUT4 glucose transporters in human skeletal muscle. *Am J Physiol* 1995; **268**:E613–E622.

109 Dela F, Ploug T, Handberg A, Petersen LN, Larsen JJ, Mikines KJ, *et al.* Physical training increases muscle GLUT4 protein and mRNA in patients with NIDDM. *Diabetes* 1994; **43**:862–865.

110 Dela F, Larsen JJ, Mikines KJ, Ploug T, Petersen LN, Galbo H. Insulin-stimulated muscle glucose clearance in patients with NIDDM: effects of one-legged physical training. *Diabetes* 1995; **44**:1010–1020.

111 Yki-Järvinen H. Glucose toxicity. *Endocr Rev* 1992; **13**:415–431.

112 Zierath JR, Galuska D, Nolte LA, Thörne A, Smedegaard Kristensen J, Wallberg-Henriksson H. Effect of glycaemia on glucose transport in isolated skeletal muscle from patients with NIDDM: *in vitro* reversal of muscular insulin resistance. *Diabetologia* 1994; **37**:270–277.

113 Marshall S, Bacote V, Traxinger RR. Discovery of a metabolic pathway mediating glucose-induced desensitization of the glucose transport system: role of hexosamine biosynthesis in the induction of insulin resistance. *J Biol Chem* 1991; **266**:4706–4712.

114 Copeland MJ, Bullen JW, Hart GW. Cross-talk between GLcNAcylation and phosphorylation: roles in insulin resistance and glucose toxicity. *Am J Physiol Endocrinol Metab* 2008; **295**:E17–E28.

115 Yki-Järvinen H, Daniels MC, Virkamäki A, Mäkimattila S, DeFronzo RA, McClain D. Increased glutamine: fructose-6-phosphate amidotransferase activity in skeletal muscle of patients with NIDDM. *Diabetes* 1996; **45**:302–307.

116 Westerbacka J, Wilkinson I, Cockcroft J, Utriainen T, Vehkavaara S, Yki-Järvinen H. Diminished wave reflection in the aorta: a novel physiological action of insulin on large blood vessels. *Hypertension* 1999; **33**:1118–1122.

117 Westerbacka J, Vehkavaara S, Bergholm R, Wilkinson I, Cockcroft J, Yki-Järvinen H. Marked resistance of the ability of insulin to decrease arterial stiffness characterizes human obesity. *Diabetes* 1999; **48**:821–827.

118 Taniwaki H, Kawagishi T, Emoto M, Shoji T, Kanda H, Maekawa K, *et al.* Correlation between the intima-media thickness of the carotid artery and aortic pulse-wave velocity in patients with type 2 diabetes: vessel wall properties in type 2 diabetes. *Diabetes Care* 1999; **22**:1851–1857.

119 Devereux RB, Roman MJ, Paranicas M, O'Grady MJ, Lee ET, Welty TK, *et al.* Impact of diabetes on cardiac structure and function: the strong heart study. *Circulation* 2000; **101**:2271–2276.

120 Yki-Järvinen H, Utriainen T. Insulin-induced vasodilatation: physiology or pharmacology? *Diabetologia* 1998; **41**:369–379.

121 Westerbacka J, Bergholm R, Tiikkainen M, Yki-Jarvinen H. Glargine and regular human insulin similarly acutely enhance endothelium-dependent vasodilatation in normal subjects. *Arterioscler Thromb Vasc Biol* 2004; **24**:320–324.

122 Zeng G, Quon MJ. Insulin-stimulated production of nitric oxide is inhibited by Wortmannin: direct measurement in vascular endothelial cells. *J Clin Invest* 1996; **98**:894–898.

123 Vehkavaara S, Yki-Jarvinen H. 3.5 years of insulin therapy with insulin glargine improves *in vivo* endothelial function in type 2 diabetes. *Arterioscler Thromb Vasc Biol* 2004; **24**:325–330.

124 Vakkilainen J, Mäkimattila S, Seppälä-Lindroos A, Vehkavaara S, Lahdenperä S, Groop PH, *et al.* Endothelial dysfunction in men with small LDL particles. *Circulation* 2000; **102**:716–721.

125 Jiang ZY, Lin YW, Clemont A, Feener EP, Hein KD, Igarashi M, *et al.* Characterization of selective resistance to insulin signaling in the vasculature of obese Zucker (fa/fa) rats. *J Clin Invest* 1999; **104**:447–457.

126 Du XL, Edelstein D, Dimmeler S, Ju Q, Sui C, Brownlee M. Hyperglycemia inhibits endothelial nitric oxide synthase activity by posttranslational modification at the Akt site. *J Clin Invest* 2001; **108**:1341–1348.

127 Berne C, Fagius J, Pollare T, Hjemdahl P. The sympathetic response to euglycemic hyperinsulinaemia. *Diabetologia* 1992; **35**:873–879.

128 Lembo G, Napoli R, Capaldo B, Rendina V, Iaccarino G, Volpe M, *et al.* Abnormal sympathetic overactivity evoked by insulin in the skeletal muscle of patients with essential hypertension. *J Clin Invest* 1992; **90**:24–29.

129 Bergholm R, Westerbacka J, Vehkavaara S, Seppala-Lindroos A, Goto T, Yki-Jarvinen H. Insulin sensitivity regulates autonomic control of heart rate variation independent of body weight in normal subjects. *J Clin Endocrinol Metab* 2001; **86**:1403–1409.

130 Vollenweider P, Randin D, Tappy L, Jequier E, Nicod P, Scherrer U. Impaired insulin-induced sympathetic neural activation and vasodilatation in skeletal muscle in obese humans. *J Clin Invest* 1994; **93**:2365–2371.

131 Paolisso G, Manzella D, Rizzo MR, Barbieri M, Varricchio G, Gambardella A, *et al.* Effects of insulin on the cardiac autonomic

nervous system in insulin-resistant states. *Clin Sci (Colch)* 2000; **98**:129–136.

132 Anfossi G, Mularoni EM, Burzacca S, Ponziani MC, Massucco P, Mattiello L, *et al.* Platelet resistance to nitrates in obesity and obese NIDDM, and normal platelet sensitivity to both insulin and nitrates in lean NIDDM. *Diabetes Care* 1998; **21**:121–126.

133 Westerbacka J, Yki-Järvinen H, Turpeinen A, Rissanen A, Vehkavaara S, Syrjälä M, *et al.* Inhibition of platelet-collagen interaction: a novel *in vivo* action of insulin abolished by insulin resistance in obesity. *Arterioscler Thromb Vasc Biol* 2002; **22**:167–172.

134 Juhan-Vague I, Alessi MC, Vague P. Thrombogenic and fibrinolytic factors and cardiovascular risk in non-insulin-dependent diabetes mellitus. *Ann Med* 1996; **28**:371–380.

135 Quiñones GA, Natali A, Baldi S, Frascerra S, Sanna G, Ciociaro D, *et al.* Effect of insulin on uric acid excretion in humans. *Am J Physiol* 1995; **268**:E1–E5.

136 Vuorinen-Markkola H, Yki-Järvinen H. Hyperuricemia and insulin resistance. *J Clin Endocrinol Metab* 1994; **78**:25–28.

137 Quinones-Galvan A, Ferrannini E. Renal effects of insulin in man. *J Nephrol* 1997; **10**:188–191.

138 DeFronzo RA, Cooke CR, Andres R, Faloona GR, Davis PJ. The effect of insulin on renal handling of sodium, potassium, calcium, and phosphate in man. *J Clin Invest* 1975; **55**:845–855.

139 Ceolotto G, Valente R, Baritono E, Reato S, Iori E, Monari A, *et al.* Effect of insulin and angiotensin II on cell calcium in human skin fibroblasts. *Hypertension* 2001; **37**:1486–1491.

140 Natali A, Santoro D, Palombo C, Cerri M, Ghione M, Ferrannini E. Impaired insulin action on skeletal muscle metabolism in essential hypertension. *Hypertension* 1991; **17**:170–178.

141 Ferrannini E, Taddei S, Santoro D, Natali A, Boni C, Del Chiaro D, *et al.* Independent stimulation of glucose metabolism and Na^+-K^+ exchange by insulin in the human forearm. *Am J Physiol* 1988; **255**:E953–E958.

142 Skott P, Vaag A, Bruun NE, Hother-Nielsen O, Gall MA, Beck-Nielsen H, *et al.* Effect of insulin on renal sodium handling in hyperinsulinaemic type 2 (non-insulin-dependent) diabetic patients with peripheral insulin resistance. *Diabetologia* 1991; **34**:275–281.

143 Ferrannini E, Buzzigoli G, Bonadonna R, Giorico MA, Oleggini M, Graziadei L, *et al.* Insulin resistance in essential hypertension. *N Engl J Med* 1987; **317**:350–357.

144 Dowse GK, Collins VR, Alberti KG, Zimmet PZ, Tuomilehto J, Chitson P, *et al.* Insulin and blood pressure levels are not independently related in Mauritians of Asian Indian, Creole or Chinese origin. The Mauritius Non-Communicable Disease Study Group. *J Hypertens* 1993; **11**:297–307.

145 Modan M, Halkin H. Hyperinsulinemia or increased sympathetic drive as links for obesity and hypertension. *Diabetes Care* 1991; **14**:470–487.

146 Liese AD, Mayer-Davis EJ, Chambless LE, Folsom AR, Sharrett AR, Brancati FL, *et al.* Elevated fasting insulin predicts incident hypertension: the ARIC study. Atherosclerosis Risk in Communities Study Investigators. *J Hypertens* 1999; **17**:1169–1177.

147 Sarafidis PA, Bakris GL. The antinatriuretic effect of insulin: an unappreciated mechanism for hypertension associated with insulin resistance? *Am J Nephrol* 2007; **27**:44–54.

148 Dengel DR, Hogikyan RV, Brown MD, Glickman SG, Supiano MA. Insulin sensitivity is associated with blood pressure response to sodium in older hypertensives. *Am J Physiol* 1998; **274**:E403–E409.

149 Lind L, Lithell H, Gustafsson IB, Pollare T, Ljunghall S. Metabolic cardiovascular risk factors and sodium sensitivity in hypertensive subjects. *Am J Hypertens* 1992; **5**:502–505.

150 Fuenmayor N, Moreira E, Cubeddu LX. Salt sensitivity is associated with insulin resistance in essential hypertension. *Am J Hypertens* 1998; **11**:397–402.

151 Galletti F, Strazzullo P, Ferrara I, Annuzzi G, Rivellese AA, Gatto S, *et al.* NaCl sensitivity of essential hypertensive patients is related to insulin resistance. *J Hypertens* 1997; **15**:1485–1491.

152 Franklin SS, Gustin W, Wong ND, Larson MG, Weber MA, Kannel WB, *et al.* Hemodynamic patterns of age-related changes in blood pressure. The Framingham Heart Study. *Circulation* 1997; **96**:308–315.

153 Reaven G. Banting lecture 1988: role of insulin resistance in human disease. *Diabetes* 1988; **37**:1595–1607.

154 Amiel SA, Sherwin RS, Simonson DC, Lauritano AA, Tamborlane WV. Impaired insulin action in puberty: a contributing factor to poor glycemic control in adolescents with diabetes. *N Engl J Med* 1986; **315**:215–219.

155 Kautzky-Willer A, Prager R, Waldhausl W, Pacini G, Thomaseth K, Wagner OF, *et al.* Pronounced insulin resistance and inadequate beta-cell secretion characterize lean gestational diabetes during and after pregnancy. *Diabetes Care* 1997; **20**:1717–1723.

156 Yki-Järvinen H. Sex and insulin sensitivity. *Metabolism* 1984; **33**:1011–1015.

157 Mott DM, Lillioja S, Bogardus C. Overnutrition induced changes decrease in insulin action for glucose storage: *in vivo* and *in vitro* in man. *Metab Clin Exp* 1986; **35**:160–165.

158 DeFronzo RA, Soman V, Sherwin R, Hendler R, Felig P. Insulin binding to monocytes and insulin action in human obesity, starvation and refeeding. *J Clin Invest* 1978; **62**:204–213.

159 Yki-Järvinen H, Nikkilä EA. Ethanol decreases glucose utilization in healthy man. *J Clin Endocrinol Metab* 1985; **61**:941–945.

160 Vessby B, Uusitupa M, Hermansen K, *et al.* Substituting dietary saturated for monounsaturated fat impairs insulin sensitivity in helathy men and women: the KANWU study. *Diabetologia* 2001; **44**:312–319.

161 De Feo P, Perriello G, De Cosmo S, Ventura MM, Campbell PJ, Brunetti P, *et al.* Comparison of glucose counterregulation during short-term and prolonged hypoglycemia in normal humans. *Diabetes* 1986; **35**:563–569.

162 DeFronzo RA, Beckles AD. Glucose metabolism following chronic metabolic acidosis in man. *Am J Physiol* 1979; **236**:E328–E334.

163 Bratusch-Marrain PR, DeFronzo RA. Impairment of insulin mediated glucose metabolism by hyperosmolality in man. *Diabetes* 1983; **32**:1028–1034.

164 DeFronzo RA, Lang R. Hypophosphatemia and glucose intolerance: evidence for tissue insensitivity to insulin. *N Engl J Med* 1980; **303**:1259–1263.

165 Brandi LS, Santoro D, Natali A, Altomonte F, Baldi S, Frascerra S, *et al.* Insulin resistance of stress: sites and mechanisms. *Clin Sci (Colch)* 1993; **85**:525–535.

166 Moller N, Schmitz O, Joorgensen JO, Astrup J, Bak JF, Christensen SE, *et al.* Basal- and insulin-stimulated substrate metabolism in patients with active acromegaly before and after adenomectomy. *J Clin Endocrinol Metab* 1992; **74**:1012–1019.

167 Nosadini R, Del Prato S, Tiengo A, Valerio A, Muggeo M, Opocher G, *et al.* Insulin resistance in Cushing's syndrome. *J Clin Endocrinol Metab* 1983; **57**:529–536.

168 Hwu CM, Kwok CF, Lai TY, *et al.* Growth hormone (GH) replacement reduces total body fat and normalizes insulin sensitivity in GH-deficient adults: a report of one-year clinical experience. *J Clin Endocrinol Metab* 1997; **82**:3285–3292.

169 Pedersen O, Richelsen B, Bak J, Arnfred J, Weeke J, Schmitz O. Characterization of the insulin resistance of glucose utilization in adipocytes from patients with hyper- and hypothyroidism. *Acta Endocrinol (Copenh)* 1988; **119**:228–234.

170 Raboudi N, Arem R, Jones RH, Chap Z, Pena J, Chou J, *et al.* Fasting and postabsorptive hepatic glucose and insulin metabolism in hyperthyroidism. *Am J Physiol* 1989; **256**:E159–E166.

171 DeFronzo RA, Alvestrand A, Smith D, Hendler R, Hendler E, Wahren J. Insulin resistance in uremia. *J Clin Invest* 1981; **67**:563–568.

172 Yki-Järvinen H, Sammalkorpi K, Koivisto VA, Nikkilä EA. Severity, duration and mechanisms of insulin resistance during acute infections. *J Clin Endocrinol Metab* 1989; **69**:317–323.

173 Lillioja S, Mott DM, Howard BV, Bennett PH, Yki-Järvinen H, Freymond D, *et al.* Impaired glucose tolerance as a disorder of insulin action: longitudinal and cross-sectional studies in Pima indians. *N Engl J Med* 1988; **318**:1217–1225.

174 Kotronen A, Juurinen L, Tiikkainen M, Vehkavaara S, Yki-Jarvinen H. Increased liver fat, impaired insulin clearance, and hepatic and adipose tissue insulin resistance in type 2 diabetes. *Gastroenterology* 2008; **135**:122–130.

12 The Genetics of Type 2 Diabetes: From Candidate Gene Biology to Genome-wide Studies

Martine Vaxillaire[1] & Philippe Froguel[1,2]

[1] CNRS-8090 Unit, Pasteur Institute, Lille, France

[2] Section of Genomic Medicine, Imperial College London, London, UK

Keypoints

- Type 2 diabetes (T2DM) is a multifactorial heterogeneous disease with a complex interplay of genetic and environmental factors influencing intermediate traits such as β-cell mass and development, insulin secretion and action, and fat distribution.
- Three general approaches to identifying genetic susceptibility factors are used: the study of candidate genes selected as having a plausible role in glucose homeostasis; a genome-wide scan to detect chromosomal regions with linkage in nuclear families; a genome-wide scan for association with common variants (single nucleotide polymorphisms and copy number variant); and the study of spontaneous, bred or transgenic animal models of T2DM.
- Common T2DM shows familial clustering, but does not segregate in a classic Mendelian fashion. It is thought to be polygenic and probably multigenic (many different gene combinations among people with diabetes). Only a small fraction of the genetic risk for common adult T2DM is known.
- Common nucleotide variants within or near the genes implicated in monogenic forms of diabetes (e.g. *GCK*, *HNF4A* or *HNF1B/TCF2* in maturity-onset diabetes of the young [MODY], or *WFS1* in Wolfram syndrome) may contribute to T2DM with modest risk effects.
- Candidate genes identified as having an association with common polygenic T2DM include the insulin promoter, class III alleles of the variable region upstream of the insulin gene, the peroxisome proliferator-activated receptor γ (*PPARG*), *KCNJ11* encoding the pore forming Kir6.2 subunit of the β-cell inwardly rectifying K_{ATP} channel. Minor susceptibility might operate in some populations from other genes, including insulin receptor substrate 1 (*IRS-1*), adiponectin (*ACDC*) or ectonucleotide pyrophosphatase/phosphodiesterase 1 enzyme (*ENPP1*) in a context of obesity or diabesity.
- In genome scans of diabetic families, loci for T2DM have been found at several sites, including chromosomes 1q, 2q (*NIDDM1*), 2p, 3q, 12q, 11q, 10q and 20. *NIDDM1* has been identified as coding for calpain 10, a non-lysosomal cysteine protease with actions at the mitochondria and plasma membrane, and also in pancreatic β-cell apoptosis.
- In 2007, five large genome-wide association studies in European descent populations have identified new potential T2DM genes, including the Wnt signaling related transcription factors *TCF7L2* and *HHEX*, the zinc transporter ZnT8 (*SLC30A8*), the CDK5 regulatory subunit-associated protein 1-like 1 (*CDKAL1*) and a regulatory protein for IGF2 (*IGF2BP2*). A consensus of close to 20 confirmed T2DM-susceptibility loci to date provided novel insights into the biology of T2DM and glucose homeostasis, but individually with a relatively small genetic effect. Importantly, these genes implicate several pathways involved in β-cell development and function.
- Compared with clinical risk factors alone, the inclusion of common genetic variants (at least those identified to date) associated with the risk of T2DM has a small effect on the ability to predict future development of T2DM. At the individual level, however, a combined genotype score based on 15 risk alleles confers a 5–8 fold increased risk of developing T2DM. Identifying the subgroups of individuals at higher risk is important to target these subjects with more effective preventative measures.

Genetic architecture of type 2 diabetes: a complex interaction of genetic susceptibility and environmental exposures

Type 2 diabetes mellitus (T2DM) is a heterogeneous metabolic disease resulting from defects of both insulin secretion and action [1,2]. The prevalence of diabetes has been estimated as 12.3% of the population of the USA, and worldwide to affect 285 million people with a projection to increase to 435 million by 2030 [3]; the vast majority of these individuals have T2DM. The disease affects various groups differently; minority racial groups including Hispanics, African-Americans, Native Americans or people living in the Middle East are affected at a higher rate than white individuals.

The etiology of T2DM is multifactorial, including genetic as well as prenatal and postnatal factors that influence several

Textbook of Diabetes, 4th edition. Edited by R. Holt, C. Cockram, A. Flyvbjerg and B. Goldstein. © 2010 Blackwell Publishing.

different defects of glucose homeostasis, primarily in β-cell function and also in muscle and liver. It is generally accepted that T2DM results from a complex interplay of genetic and environmental factors influencing a number of intermediate traits of relevance to the diabetic phenotype (β-cell mass, insulin secretion, insulin action, fat distribution and obesity) [3]. Quantitative phenotypes related to glucose homeostasis are also known to be heritable, with a greater relative impact of genetic components on *in vivo* insulin secretion [4].

Although several monogenic forms of diabetes have been identified (see Chapter 15), such as maturity-onset diabetes of the young (MODY) and maternally inherited diabetes and deafness (MIDD) [5,6], diabetes in adulthood seems to be a polygenic disorder in the majority of cases. T2DM shows a clear familial aggregation, with a risk for people with familial diabetes that is increased by a factor of 2–6 compared with those without familial diabetes; it does not segregate in a classical Mendelian fashion, and appears to result from several combined gene defects, or from the simultaneous action of several susceptibility alleles, or else from combinations of frequent variants at several loci that may have deleterious effects when predisposing environmental factors are present [3,7]. T2DM is probably also multigenic, meaning that many different combinations of gene defects may exist among subgroups of people with diabetes. Whereas the current worldwide epidemic of T2DM is greatly driven by lifestyle and dietary changes, a combination of these environmental factors and susceptible genetic determinants contribute to the development of T2DM [7].

The primary biochemical events leading to common diabetes in adulthood are still largely unknown in most cases, even if new genetic and biologic insights into T2DM etiology have recently arisen from the completion of genome-wide association (GWA) studies in several European descent populations [3,7]. Genetic and environmental factors may affect both insulin secretion and insulin action [1], and a variety of environmental factors can be implicated in the clinical expression of T2DM (see Chapter 4), such as the degree and type of obesity, sedentary lifestyle, malnutrition in fetal and perinatal periods, lifestyle and different kinds of drugs such as steroids, diuretics and antihypertensive agents (see Chapter 16). It is noteworthy that obesity, which is one of the so-called risk factors of T2DM, is also clearly under genetic control. Both disorders are frequently associated and share many metabolic abnormalities, which suggests that they might also share susceptibility genes [8,9]. Moreover, retrospective studies have shown that low birth weight is associated with insulin resistance and T2DM in adulthood [10,11]. It has been proposed that this association results from a metabolic adaptation to poor fetal nutrition [12]. The identification of gene variants that contribute both to variation in fetal growth and to the susceptibility to T2DM, however, suggests that this metabolic "programming" could also be partly genetically determined [13].

These complex interactions between genes and environment complicate the task of identifying any single genetic susceptibility factor for T2DM. Three general approaches have been adopted to search for genes underlying complex traits such as T2DM [6], as described in Table 12.1.

Table 12.1 Genetic and genomic approaches used for the study of type 2 diabetes genes.

Family-based studies
Linkage studies (genome-wide scan with microsatellite markers)
Transmission disequilibrium test (in sibships or nuclear families)
Study of monogenic diabetes (extreme phenotypes, syndromic diseases)
Population-based studies
Survey of candidate genes and targeted genomic regions (~100 SNPs)
Genome-wide association study (HapMap-based SNPs choice, 500K–1M SNPs)
Other types of genetic markers (rare variants, CNVs, insertion/deletion)
Study of general populations and prospective cohorts (epidemiology-based data)
Functional genomic approaches
Gene expression profiling, transcriptomics (microarray gene expression data in human and animal models)
Molecular and cellular analyses (*in vitro* and *in vivo* model systems)
Expressed quantitative trait linkage (in human and animal models)
Epigenetics (in humans, and animal models)

CNV, copy number variant; SNP, single nucleotide polymorphism.

The first approach was to focus on candidate genes, that is, genes selected as having a plausible role in the control of glucose homeostasis and/or insulin secretion, on the basis of their known or presumed biologic functions. Although this approach has led to the identification of several susceptibility genes with small effects (see below), no genes with a moderate or major effect on the polygenic forms of diabetes have been found. Possible explanations for this failure to identify genes with a major effect include the possibility that they do not exist, or our incomplete knowledge of the pathophysiologic mechanisms of T2DM and the genes that control them, has obscured the choice of candidates.

The second approach is to perform genome-wide scans for linkage in collections of nuclear families or sib-pairs with T2DM [14], or for GWA in large case–control samples, as was performed in recent years [15]. These "hypothesis-free" approaches require no presumptions as to the function of the susceptibility loci. Although a large number of genomic regions with presumed linkage have been mapped [11–14], identification of the susceptibility genes and causal variants within these regions has proceeded at a very slow pace. In contrast, the recently completed GWA studies from several independent European case–control cohorts have released at least a dozen of confirmed at-risk loci, with unexpected susceptibility genes for T2DM and a number of at-risk variants having been replicated in most of the European populations investigated [6,15,16].

A third approach has used microarray gene expression analysis in attempt to define genetic alterations in T2DM. Through such analysis, a defect in skeletal muscle of people with diabetes was discovered and characterized by a coordinated decrease in the expression of nuclear-encoded genes involved in mitochondrial oxidative phosphorylation [17]. This defect appears to be secondary to reduced expression of the transcriptional coactivators PGC-1α and PGC-1β. Similar changes in expression have been observed in some cohorts of first-degree relatives of individuals with diabetes, suggesting that these may be heritable traits [18]. A second potential gene is the transcription factor ARNT/HIF1β, which was identified using islets isolated from individuals with T2DM compared with normal glucose-tolerant controls. Reduced ARNT levels in human diabetic islets were associated with altered β-cell expression of other genes involved in glucose sensing, insulin signaling and transcriptional control [19], suggesting an important role for ARNT in the impaired islet function of human T2DM.

Another complementary approach to identifying diabetes genes is to study spontaneous (such as the Zucker diabetic fatty rats or fat/fat mice, [20]), bred (like the GK rats, [21]) or transgenic (using β-cell-specific gene inactivation, [22–24]) animal models of T2DM. The genes responsible for diabetes in these models may not necessarily be major players in typical T2DM in humans, but such studies provide the most direct way of improving the overall understanding of the molecular circuitry that maintains glucose homeostasis. Nevertheless, despite the evidence of a strong genetic background in T2DM, very little is yet known about the genetic risk factors for T2DM. By far the most striking results in defining etiologic genes have been obtained by studying the highly familial MODY form of young-onset diabetes or other rare forms of monogenic diabetes.

Genes involved in monogenic diabetes and their relevance to adult-onset T2DM

Some of the most compelling evidence that inherited gene defects can cause glycemic dysregulation comes from the clinical and genetic description of monogenic forms of diabetes, including MODY characterized by an autosomal dominant inheritance of young-onset diabetes, neonatal or early infancy diabetes, or diabetes with extrapancreatic features (see Chapter 15) [4,6]. Although rare, these monogenic forms of diabetes provide a paradigm for understanding and investigating some of the genetic components of more complex forms of diabetes in adults.

The well-defined mode of inheritance of MODY, with a high penetrance and early-onset diabetes, allows the collection of multigenerational pedigrees, making MODY an attractive model for genetic studies. MODY usually develops in thin young adults (usually before 25 years of age; in childhood, adolescence or young adulthood), and is associated with primary insulin-secretion defects [4,5]. The prevalence of MODY is estimated to be less than 1–2% of patients with T2DM, although it could represent as many as 5% of European cases of diabetes [4,25]. MODY is not a single entity, but involves genetic, metabolic and clinical heterogeneity. So far, heterozygous mutations or chromosome rearrangements in seven genes have been identified as responsible for the disease (Table 12.2). These genes encode the enzyme glucokinase (*GCK*, MODY type 2) [26–28], the transcription factors hepatocyte nuclear factor 4α (HNF-4α//*HNF4A*, MODY type 1) [29], hepatocyte nuclear factor 1α (HNF-1α/*HNF1A*,

Table 12.2 The different subtypes of maturity-onset diabetes of the young (MODY).

MODY type	Gene locus	Gene name	Year of discovery	Distribution	Onset of diabetes	Primary defect	Severity of diabetes	Complications	OMIM
MODY1	20q	*HNF4A* (*TCF14*)	1996	Rare (2–3%)	Adolescence/ early adulthood	Pancreas/other	Severe	Frequent	600281
MODY2	7p	*GCK*	1992	20–60%*	Early childhood/ life-long	Pancreas/liver	Mild IFG	Rare	138079
MODY3	12q	*TCF1* (*HNF1A*)	1996	15–60%*	Adolescence/ early adulthood	Pancreas/kidney other	Severe	Frequent	142410
MODY4	13q	*IPF-1*	1997	Rare (<1%)	Early adulthood	Pancreas/other	Severe	Unknown; pancreas agenesis and NDM in homozygote (rare)	600733
MODY5	17q	*TCF2* (*HNF1B*)	1997	Rare (2%)	Early adulthood	Kidney/pancreas	Severe	Kidney disease (RCAD); pancreas agenesis and NDM in homozygote (rare)	189907
MODY6	2q32	*NEUROD1*	1999	Rare (<1%)	Early adulthood	Pancreas	Severe	Unknown; NDM in homozygote (rare)	601724
MODY7	11p15.5	*INS*	2008	Rare (<1%)	Early childhood/ early adulthood	Pancreas	Mild to severe	Rare	176730

IFG, impaired fasting glycemia; NDM, neonatal diabetes mellitus; RCAD, renal cysts and diabetes syndrome.
* Different distributions in different populations.

MODY type 3) [30,31], insulin promoter factor 1 (IPF-1, MODY type 4) [32,33], hepatocyte nuclear factor 1β (HNF-1β/*TCF2*, MODY type 5) [34] and NEUROD1/β2 (MODY type 6) [35], and the preproinsulin (*INS*) (MODY type 7) [6]. Moreover, additional unknown genes (MODY-X) related to the MODY phenotype remain to be discovered from families in which early-onset diabetes cosegregates with genetic markers outside the known *MODY* loci [36–38].

The relative prevalence of the different subtypes of MODY has been shown to vary greatly in studies of British, French, German and Spanish family cohorts [39–42]. These contrasting results may be caused by differences in the genetic background of these populations, or else may reflect, at least partly, ascertainment bias in the recruitment of families. Altogether, mutations in *GCK* and *HNF1A* are the cause of the two most prevalent MODY2 and MODY3 subtypes, accounting for around 50–60% of all MODY cases. Mutations in *HNF4A* and *TCF2*/Hnf-1β were identified in many dozens of families and the other defects caused by mutations in *PDX1* and *NEUROD1* are rarer disorders [43,44].

Recent challenging studies have tried to identify a connection between monogenic diabetes genes and common T2DM, that is to test whether common but less severe variants might have a role in the pathogenesis of common multifactorial forms of the disease. Indeed, if major mutations (i.e. causing a substantial functional defect and normally rare or absent in the general population) lead to a highly penetrant form of diabetes, it seems plausible that more subtle genetic changes affecting the structure or expression of the gene product might have a role in determining (minor) susceptibility to T2DM. Our current understanding of genetic variants influencing T2DM supports this hypothesis [3,4,6], but common variants (also referred as single nucleotide polymorphisms [SNPs]) in the known MODY genes seem to contribute very modestly to the common forms of T2DM, as recently assessed in a staged case–control study from multiple clinical samples [45]. In this study, the strongest effects were found for an intronic variant of *TCF2*/HNF-1β and for the −30 G/A variant of *GCK*. The −30 G/A polymorphism in the β-cell specific promoter of glucokinase was found to modulate diabetes risk, with the (−30) A-allele being associated with an increased risk) [45]. A similar genetic association was observed with a stronger effect in a French prospective study of a middle-aged general population, along with a significant impact on the modulation of fasting glycemia and insulin secretion HOMA-B index [46]. Furthermore, a meta-analysis of previously reported association results for *GCK* (−30A) with T2DM showed a modest overall effect on disease risk of 1.08 ($P = 0.004$) in European populations [45].

Mutations in *HNF1α* were identified in African-Americans and Japanese subjects with atypical non-autoimmune diabetes with acute onset [47,48]. In the Oji-Cree native Canadian population the G319S mutation in *HNF1A*, found in approximately 40% of patients with diabetes, accelerates the onset of T2DM by 7 years [49]. Such findings show that *HNF1A* mutations can be associated with typical adult-onset insulin-resistant obesity-related diabetes in addition to MODY.

A population-based study in Swedish and Finnish cohorts using both *in vitro* and *in vivo* experiments has shown that common variants in and upstream of the *HNF1A* gene influence transcriptional activity and insulin secretion *in vivo* [50]. Some of these variants are associated with a modestly higher risk of diabetes in subsets of elderly overweight individuals. Mutations in *HNF4A* and *IPF1* genes were also identified in a number of families with late-onset T2DM [51]. IPF-1/Pdx-1 has a dosage-dependent regulatory effect on the expression of β-cell-specific genes and therefore assists in the maintenance of euglycemia. As a consequence, frequent variants in the regulatory sequences controlling IPF-1/Pdx-1 expression in the β-cell, or in genes coding for transcription factors known to regulate IPF-1, could contribute to common T2DM susceptibility. Two independent studies, from the Ashkenazim [52] and Finnish [53] populations, have reported significant associations between common variants adjacent to the *HNF4A* P2 promoter and T2DM. Interestingly, some of the diabetes-associated variants account for most of the evidence of linkage to chromosome 20q13 reported in these two populations. Consistent with these results, genetic variation near the P2 region of *HNF4A* is associated with T2DM in other Danish and UK populations, but not in French and other Caucasian populations [54] which argues for genetic heterogeneity in *HNF4A* variants susceptibility [55].

Recent studies have evaluated the genotype–phenotype correlation between the MODY genes and the common form of T2DM and have reported that several common variants (MAF >0.05) in *TCF2/HNF1β* may contribute to T2DM risk but with modest effects (allelic odds ratio [OR] <1.25); the strongest effect was found for an intronic variant with corrected *P* values <0.01 and OR of 1.13 [45]. Independently, a GWA scan performed to search for sequence variants conferring risk of prostate cancer demonstrated with replication from eight case–control groups that two intronic variants located in the first and second intron of *TCF2* gene confer protection against T2DM (OR 0.91, $P \sim 10^{-7}$) in individuals of European, African and Asian descent [56]. Several epidemiologic studies have reported an inverse relationship between T2DM and the risk of prostate cancer, and a recent meta-analysis estimated the relative risk of prostate cancer to be 0.84 (95% CI 0.71–0.92) among patients with diabetes [57]. Previous explanations of this inverse relationship between T2DM and prostate cancer have centered on the impact of the metabolic and hormonal environment in men. The protective effect of the *TCF2* SNPs against T2DM is too modest to explain their impact on prostate cancer risk by a consequence of an effect on diabetes. The primary functional impact of *TCF2* variants may lie within one or more metabolic or hormonal pathway, and incidentally may modulate the risk of developing prostate cancer and T2DM throughout life.

Genetic variation in the *WFS1* gene, which encodes a 890-amino-acid polypeptide named wolframin, a transmembrane protein located in the endoplasmic reticulum (ER), which serves as an calcium channel, not only results in the rare Wolfram syndrome (known as DIDMOAD and characterized by early-onset non-autoimmune diabetes mellitus, diabetes insipidus, optic atrophy and deafness) [58,59] but is also associated with susceptibility to adult T2DM [60]. In a pooled case–control analysis comprising >20 000 individuals, several SNPs in *WFS1* (including a non-synonymous SNP, R611H) were shown to modulate diabetes risk (OR ~0.92 for a minor allele frequency of ~40% [60]), with a population attributable fraction of 9%, which could explain 0.3% of the excess familial risk. This study provides further evidence that wolframin has an essential role in the ER stress response in insulin-producing pancreatic β-cells, and contributes to the risk of common T2DM.

Search for T2DM genes in the pre-GWA era

Before the completion of GWA studies in early 2007, numerous focused candidate gene studies, driven by biologic or functional hypotheses, and the hypothesis-free linkage approach, have delivered a small number of validated T2DM susceptibility genes which effects the disease process (both insulin secretion and insulin sensitivity), although contributing at the individual level with a modest risk effect.

Candidate gene approach

The molecular screening of candidate genes to search for genetic variants (either rare when the allele frequency is <0.01, or common in the population tested) potentially associated with diabetes status (i.e. more frequent in individuals with T2DM) has so far been the most frequently used approach to tackle the genetic determinants of T2DM [61]. There are many reasons why specific genes may be candidates:

- A gene may have a known or presumed biologic function in glucose homeostasis or energy balance in humans.
- It may be implicated in subtypes of diabetes, such as MODY or neonatal diabetes.
- It may be associated with diabetes or associated traits in animal models.
- It may be responsible for an inherited disease that includes diabetes (e.g. mitochondrial cytopathies, Wolfram syndrome).
- The gene products may be differentially expressed in diabetic and normal tissues.

For obvious reasons, the insulin gene was among the first genes to be studied. Apart the more recent identification of rare mutations in the sequence of the preproinsulin gene responsible for neonatal and non-autoimmune early infancy diabetes [5,6], mutations in the coding regions of the insulin gene have been reported to be associated with familial hyperinsulinemia in less than 10 families, but are not consistently associated with T2DM [62]. Mutations in the promoter region, however, could affect the regulation of the insulin gene, leading to absolute or relative hypoinsulinemia. A variant allele of the promoter has been observed in about 5% of African-Americans with T2DM, and shown to be associated with decreased transcriptional activity [63]. An association between T2DM and paternally transmitted class III alleles of the variable number tandem repeat (VNTR) region upstream of the insulin gene (*INS-VNTR*) was observed in British families [64]. Interestingly, class III alleles (one of the two main classes of *INS-VNTR* allele length, with 141–209 repeats) were also found to be associated with increased length and weight at birth [65] and with a dominant protection against type 1 diabetes [66] compared with type I alleles.

Key components of the insulin signaling pathways have also been tested. They were at first thought to be important players in the context of the insulin resistance of T2DM. Several of these genes are also expressed in pancreatic β-cells, and several studies from knockout animals have demonstrated that they may also have an important role in the mechanisms of insulin secretion [23,24]. More than 50 different mutations have been found in the coding regions of the insulin receptor gene on chromosome 19p (see Chapter 15) [67]; patients with these mutations seldom present with the common form of T2DM [68], but rather with a syndrome of severe insulin resistance associated with leprechaunism, or with acanthosis nigricans, hirsutism and major hyperinsulinemia [69]. Missense variants in the gene encoding the first substrate for the insulin receptor kinase (*IRS1*) on chromosome 2q have been detected in several populations [70–73] but an association of these variants with diabetes was not observed in all studies [74,75].

Similarly, an association between polymorphisms of the muscle glycogen synthase gene (*GYS1*) on chromosome 19q and T2DM has been observed in Finnish [76] and in Japanese [77] subjects, but not in French subjects [78]. Taken together, these results suggest that the *IRS1* and *GYS1* genes may act in some populations as minor susceptibility genes, which are neither necessary nor sufficient for disease expression, but may nevertheless modulate the phenotype in the patients. This is important in the light of more recent data obtained from combined and meta-analyses conducted by GWA follow-up studies, which report a significant effect of common variants at the *IRS1* locus on T2DM risk in European descent populations (unpublished results).

Functionally significant polymorphisms have also been identified in other proteins involved in insulin action, such as the phosphatidylinositol 3 kinase [79] and the ectonucleotide pyrophosphatase/phosphodiesterase 1 enzyme (ENPP1 or PC-1), a transmembrane glycoprotein that downregulates insulin signaling by inhibiting insulin-receptor tyrosine kinase activity [80]. ENPP1 is expressed in multiple tissues including three targets of insulin action: adipose tissue, muscle and liver. A missense variation in its gene *ENPP1*, in which lysine 121 is replaced by glutamine (K121Q, rs1044498), results in a gain-of-function mutation leading to greater inhibition of the insulin receptor and clinical insulin resistance [81]. Pizutti *et al.* [82] first identified the association while studying healthy non-obese non-diabetic Sicilian subjects. *ENPP1* K121Q is also associated with an earlier onset of T2DM in Europeans and obese children, suggesting that the variant may accelerate disease onset in predisposing individuals. Not all studies have replicated these results, and some studies have reported that high body mass index (BMI) exacerbates, or in some cases is a prerequisite for, the deleterious role of *ENPP1* K121Q on insulin resistance-related phenotypes and T2DM [83,84]. Meyre *et al.* [85] reported an effect of the Q121 variant on the risk of both morbid obesity and hyperglycemia in large samples of French children and adults, as observed in children from Germany [86] and British adults [87]. Given the major role of obesity in deteriorating glucose homeostasis, the different effect of the Q121 variant on BMI in different samples may be, at least partly, responsible for the non-homogeneous results so far reported on the risk of across different studies. A recent large meta-analysis performed on published case–control studies has shown that, although results are not homogeneous across all samples, individuals carrying the variant have an approximately 20% increased risk of T2DM [88].

Another biologic candidate gene that was extensively studied is the peroxisome proliferator-activated receptor γ gene (*PPARG*), where mutations that severely decrease the transactivation potential were found to cosegregate with extreme insulin resistance, diabetes and hypertension in two families, with autosomal-dominant inheritance [89]. A common amino-acid polymorphism (Pro12Ala) in *PPARG* has been associated with T2DM; homozygous carriers of the Pro12 allele are more insulin resistant than those having one Ala12 allele and have a 1.25-fold increased risk of developing diabetes [90]. This common polymorphism has a modest, yet extensively replicated effect on the risk of T2DM. There is also evidence for interaction between this polymorphism and the insulin secretion in response to fatty acids [91], and BMI [92]; the protective effect of the alanine allele was lost in subjects with a BMI greater than $35\,kg/m^2$. A widespread Gly482Ser polymorphism of PGC1-α (known as *PPARGC1*), a transcriptional coactivator of a series of nuclear receptors including *PPARG*, has been associated with a 1.34 genotype relative risk of T2DM [93]. In this study, a test for interaction with the Pro12Ala variant in *PPARG* gave no indication for additive effects on diabetes status.

Other genes have been shown to be implicated in the genetic susceptibility to insulin resistance. Although they do not appear to be directly linked or associated with T2DM, they may also modulate the disease expression. A common and widespread polymorphism at codon 905 in the gene encoding the glycogen associated regulatory subunit of protein phosphatase 1 (PP1), which is expressed in skeletal muscle and plays a crucial part in muscle tissue glycogen synthesis and breakdown, has been shown to be associated with insulin resistance and hypersecretion of insulin in Danish subjects with T2DM [94]. A missense mutation in the intestinal fatty acid binding protein 2 (*FABP2*) gene on chromosome 4q has been found to be associated with increased fatty acid binding, increased fat oxidation and insulin resistance in the Pima Indians of Arizona [95], an ethnic group with the highest reported prevalence of T2DM and insulin resistance in the world. A rare P387L variant in protein tyrosine phosphatase-1B (PTP-1B), a negative regulator for insulin and leptin signaling, has been described to be associated with a 3.7 genotype-relative risk of T2DM in a Danish Caucasian population, resulting in impaired *in vitro* serine phosphorylation of the PTP-1B protein [96]. In an extensive analysis of the *PTPN1* gene locus, Bento *et al.* [97] found convincing associations between multiple SNPs and T2DM in two independent Caucasian American case–control samples. A modest effect of *PTPN1* gene variants on disease risk was observed in the French population, whereas consistent associations with metabolic variables reflecting insulin resistance and dyslipidemia were found for two intronic SNPs, thereby influencing susceptibility to metabolic diseases [98].

Mutations in transcription factors have also been reported to contribute to the genetic risk for T2DM through various mechanisms: dysregulation of target genes involved in glucose or lipid metabolism (HNFs, *PPARG, IPF-1, IB1, TIEG2/KLF11*), impaired β-cell development and differentiation (*IPF-1, NEUROD1*/β2, *TIEG2/KLF11*), and increased β-cell apoptosis (*IB1/MAPK8IP1*). Deleterious mutations that significantly impair the transactivation activity of these transcription factors can be responsible in some families for monogenic-like forms of diabetes with late age of onset, which may represent an intermediary phenotype between MODY and the most common forms of T2DM. This is the case for the *TIEG2/KLF11* gene encoding the Krüppel-like factor 11 (KLF11), an SP1-like pancreas expressed transcription factor that is induced by the transforming growth factor β (TGF-β) and regulates cell growth in the exocrine pancreas. A common polymorphism (Q62R) in *KLF11* was reported to be associated with polygenic T2DM developing in adulthood and to affect the function of KLF11 *in vitro* [99]. Insulin levels were found to be lower in carriers of the minor allele at Q62R [99] but attempts of replication in other populations only found a minor, or no detectable effect of the Q62R common variant on diabetes risk [100]. Sequencing of *KLF11* gene in families enriched for early-onset T2DM uncovered two missense mutations which segregated with diabetes in three pedigrees [99], but proof of their causality was only based on *in vitro* experiments. These findings suggest a role for the TGF-β signaling pathway in pancreatic diseases affecting endocrine islets (diabetes) or exocrine cells (cancer) [101].

Another example is the identification of a mutation in islet brain 1 (*IB1, MAPK8IP1*) found to be associated with diabetes in one family [102]. *IB1* is a homologue of the c-*jun* amino-terminal kinase interacting protein 1 (JIP-1), which has a role in the modulation of apoptosis [103]. *IB1* is also a transactivator of the islet glucose transporter GLUT-2. The mutant *IB1* was found to be unable to prevent apoptosis *in vitro* [102]. It is thus possible that the abnormal function of this mutant *IB1* may render the β-cells more susceptible to apoptotic stimuli, thus decreasing β-cell mass. As glucotoxicity and lipotoxicity are known to induce both apoptosis and transcription factor down regulation in pancreatic β-cells, inherited or acquired defects in *IB1* activity could have deleterious effects in β-cell function.

Other genes encoding key components of insulin secretion pathways have also been tested as potential candidates for a role in the genetic susceptibility of T2DM. The pancreatic β-cell ATP-sensitive potassium channel (IKATP) has a central role in glucose-induced insulin secretion by linking signals derived from glucose metabolism to cell-membrane depolarization and insulin exocytosis (see Chapter 6) [104]. IKATP is composed of two distinct subunits: an inwardly rectifying ion channel forming the pore (Kir6.2), and a regulatory subunit, which is a sulfonylurea receptor (SUR1) belonging to the ATP-binding cassette (ABC) superfamily [105]; both subunits are expressed in neuroendocrine cells. The *KCNJ11* and *ABCC8* genes encoding these two subunits are located 4.5 kb apart on human chromosome 11p15.1. Inactivating mutations in each of these genes may result in familial persistent hyperinsulinemic hypoglycemia in infancy, and gain-of-function mutations are responsible of the opposite phenotype of neonatal diabetes (either permanent or transient forms of the disease with distinct distributions of mutations in each gene), demonstrating their role in the regulation of insulin secretion (see Chapter 15) [106]. Studies in various populations with different ethnic backgrounds have provided evidence for associations of SNPs in these genes with T2DM [107–112]. In particular, a common variant, E23K, of *KCNJ11*/K_{IR}6.2 has now been convincingly associated with an increased risk of T2DM and decreased insulin secretion in glucose-tolerant subjects [113,114]. Large-scale studies and meta-analyses have consistently associated the lysine variant with T2DM, with an OR of 1.15 [115].

Increasing evidence from more recent studies also suggested that inflammatory processes may have a pivotal role in metabolic diseases: prospective studies have shown that high plasma interleukin 6 (IL-6) levels increased T2DM risk [116], but conflicting associations were found between a promoter polymorphism (G-174C) in *IL6* and T2DM [117,118]. In a large joint analysis of 21 case–control studies, representing >20 000 participants in one of the largest association studies addressing the role of a candidate gene in T2DM susceptibility, the *IL6* promoter variant was found to be associated with a lower risk (OR 0.91, $P = 0.037$) [119]. In addition, association between T2DM and *IL6R*-D358A was reported in Danish white people [120], and with *TNF* G-308A promoter SNP in the Finnish Diabetes Prevention Study [118]. The effects of both *IL6* and *IL6R* variants on developing T2DM risk in interaction with age have been reported in a prospective study of a general French population [46].

Hypothesis-free genome-wide approach and positional cloning of T2DM genes

The second approach used in the years 1995–2005 for identifying genes underlying common polygenic T2DM, the so-called genome-wide familial linkage (GWL) studies, was based on genome-wide scans to detect chromosomal regions showing linkage with diabetes in large collections of nuclear families or sib-pairs. This strategy required no assumptions regarding the function of genes at the susceptibility loci, because it attempted to map genes purely by position. Genotyping of approximately 400 multiallelic markers (short tandem repeats or microsatellites, with a density of ~1 marker/10 cmol) allows identification of polymorphic markers showing strong allele identity by descent in diabetic family members (i.e. allele sharing in sibships is significantly higher than 50%). Once identified, such susceptibility genes for diabetes may then be positionally cloned in the intervals of linkage.

This total genome approach has been used for some time in other multifactorial diseases such as type 1 diabetes [121] and obesity [5]. More than 20 genome scans for T2DM have been completed, involving thousands of pedigrees from different populations and ethnic groups. One of the limitations of the genome-scan approach is the relatively low power of the method, which is unable to detect a weak linkage signal because of the low relative risk for diabetes in siblings (about a three- to fivefold increase in comparison with the general population). Working on very large family collections (>500 sib-pairs), in more homogeneous ethnic groups (e.g. island populations), or in large pedigrees using quantitative intermediary traits instead of the dichotomous diabetes status, has improved the effectiveness of this approach in detecting linkage. Indeed, intermediary phenotypes were shown to have greater heritability than the dichotomous endpoint. To avoid bias brought about by the effect of chronic hyperglycemia on many traits, other strategies have been proposed to analyze the general population [122] or to collect sibships of the offspring of subjects with diabetes who are not yet diabetic but are at high risk of developing the disease [123]. False-positive results are likely to occur. Thus, stringent criteria for linkage (in the magnitude of $P < 10^{-5}$) need to be used to minimize bias brought about by multiple testing. Indeed, a level of statistical significance at the genome-wide level (i.e. giving a less than 5% chance that a linked locus is false) implies a multipoint lod score higher than 3.6 at a given chromosomal region. This value is not a rigid one; each case is different, and sophisticated simulations are needed to provide an empirical *P* value, and therefore to assess the robustness of the data obtained. Indeed, the validation (or the absence of validation) of a linked locus has strong implications for further research, and careful examination is necessary. For this reason, another criterion for a true locus has been the replication of the findings by others. Although less stringent *P* values are required (10^{-3}), replication is difficult, because genetic heterogeneity, ascertainment biases and phenotypic differences across studies may mask a confirmatory linkage. Furthermore, genotyping errors have a substantial effect on linkage analyses.

Since 1996, the results of several genome scans in families with diabetes have been published [123]. A summary of the best T2DM linkage replication results is presented in Table 12.3. A locus for T2DM on chromosome 2q (*NIDDM1*) was initially found in Mexican Americans [14], and it was shown that an interaction between this locus and a locus on chromosome 15 further increases the susceptibility to diabetes in this population [124]. A region of replicated linkage between diabetes and

Table 12.3 Genomic locations of best type 2 diabetes linkage replications.

Chromosome location	LOD ≥ 3.0*	LOD ≥ 3.6*	Ethnic contribution†	Phenotypes‡ in the interval	Potential or validated candidate genes
1q21-q25.3	6	4	Af(1)CJ(2)Eu(9)MA(4)	10D6Q	*PKLR, USF1, DUSP12, APOA2, RXRG*
2q24.1-q31.1	2	1	Eu(4)MA(2)Yc(3)	4D5Q	
2q35-q37.3	3	1	Af(1)CJ(2)Eu(6)MA(1)Yc(3)	8D5Q	*CAPN10*
3q27-q29	3	1	Eu(4)MA(1)Yc(1)	2D4Q	*ACDC, IGF2BP2*
6q23.1-q24.1	3	2	CJ(3)Eu(6)MA(2)Yc(1)	8D4Q	*ENPP1*
8p23.3-p12	3	2	Af(1)CJ(1)Eu(7)MA(4)Yc(2)	9D6Q	
9q21.11-q21.31	2	1	CJ(4)Eu(2)MA(1)	4D3Q	
10q25.1-q26.3	2	0	Af(2)CJ(1)Eu(5)MA(4)	4D8Q	*TCF7L2*
14q11.2-q21.1	1	0	CJ(2)Eu(7)MA(1)Yc(1)	7D4Q	
17p13.3-q11.2	3	1	Af(1)CJ(1)Eu(7)MA(1)Yc(3)	5D8Q	
18p11.32-p11.21	2	1	Af(1)CJ(1)Eu(7)Yc(1)	6D4Q	
19p13.3-p13.12	1	1	Af(2)Eu(5)MA(3)	4D6Q	
19q13.32-q13.43	2	0	Af(1)Eu(6)MA(1)Yc(1)	1D8Q	
20q11-q13.32	2	1	Af(1)CJ(5)Eu(5)MA(1)	9D3Q	*HNF4A, PTPN1*
22q11.1-q12.3	2	0	Af(1)CJ(1)Eu(5)MA(3)	5D5Q	

*The data on the number of LOD scores in each interval that met the threshold criteria are adapted from the study by Lillioja & Wilton [206].

†Ethnic origins of the populations showing a genetic linkage in each interval (Af, African; CJ, Chinese/Japanese; Eu, European; MA, Mexican American; Yc, other/combined data) followed in parentheses by the number of such results.

‡Phenotypes in each interval (D, type 2 diabetes; Q, quantitative trait) and the number of each type of result.

chromosome 1q21-25 was reported in different populations of European origin and in Pima Indians [123]. Linkages with diabetes and with the age at onset of diabetes were found on chromosome 3q27 [125–127], and in a region on chromosome 10q in Mexican American families from San Antonio, Texas [128]. Linkage was found at a locus near *TCF1* on chromosome 12q in Finnish T2DM families, characterized by a predominant insulin secretion defect [13]. Evidence for an obesity–diabetes locus on chromosome 11q23-q25 [129] and linkage of several chromosomal regions with prediabetic traits [14] were observed in Pima Indians from Arizona, an ethnic group with a high prevalence of diabetes and obesity. Evidence for the presence of one or more diabetes loci on chromosome 20 was found in different populations [130,131]. In these and other studies, a large number of loci showing only suggestive or weak indication of linkage with diabetes-related traits have also been reported, several of which fall in overlapping regions.

Some concerns have therefore been raised about the heterogeneity and reliability of genetic data in multifactorial diseases in general (e.g. the lack of replication), and in T2DM in particular. A new series of genome scans published in 2000 and later [125–127], however, has surprisingly shown that results obtained from T2DM families may be reproducible, despite differences in ethnicity and in environmental factors. It is likely that progress both in automated genotyping and statistical analyses of larger sample sets have improved the quality of the data. A meta-analysis of the data obtained from all European studies has confirmed findings on 1q, 2p and 12q, and also revealed a new locus on 17p linked to the metabolic syndrome in the US population [132,133]. These data provide a strong basis for believing that some important genetic contributors to common T2DM exist.

Although genome-wide scans have mapped T2DM loci, each hit represents 10–20 million nucleotides. The challenge was to identify the diabetes-related genes within these intervals, knowing that hundreds of genes may be present. To identify the true etiologic gene variants associated with an enhanced risk for T2DM, one first positional cloning approach was to refine the chromosomal regions of linkage using a dense map of biallelic SNPs as markers for the detection of linkage disequilibrium (LD) mapping [134–136]. DNA polymorphisms located away from the true functional variant may be associated with the disease, or with the variation of a diabetes-associated trait. The strength of LD is quite variable within the genome, ranging from 10 to 300 kb or more. It has been postulated that working in a so-called "isolated" population should significantly enhance results with LD, but even research in Finns or in Icelanders may not resolve the problems [137].

The identification of the *NIDDM1/CAPN10* gene (coding for calpain-10, a non-lysosomal cysteine protease) on 2q37 confirmed that LD mapping may be a successful strategy for unravelling other polygenic diseases [138]. This work, however, also showed the complexity of the search, because in this case an intronic polymorphism (UCSNP-43) was associated with T2DM in Mexican Americans. In fact, three non-coding polymorphisms, including SNP-43, SNP-44 and SNP-63, have been identified as defining an at-risk haplotype [138]. In other ethnic groups, such as French Caucasians, the rarity of this high-risk haplotype made it difficult to achieve a definite answer concerning the role of calpain-10 in T2DM. Nonetheless, recent pooled and meta-analyses as well as the LD and haplotype diversity studies suggest a role for genetic variation in *CAPN10* affecting risk of T2DM in Europeans [139]. *CAPN10* was thus the first diabetes gene to be identified through a genome-wide scan approach. Many investigators, but not all, have subsequently found associations between *CAPN10* polymorphism(s) and T2DM as well as insulin action, insulin secretion, aspects of adipocyte biology and microvascular functions. This has not always been with the same SNP or haplotype or the same phenotype, suggesting that there might be more than one disease-associated *CAPN10* variant and that these might vary between ethnic groups and the phenotype under study. Indeed, both genetic and functional data indicated that calpain-10 has an important role in insulin resistance and intermediate phenotypes, including those associated with the adipocyte [140]. In this regard, emerging evidence would suggest that calpain-10 facilitates GLUT-4 translocation and acts in the reorganization of the cytoskeleton. Interestingly, calpain-10 is also an important molecule in the β-cell. It is likely to be a determinant of fuel sensing and insulin exocytosis, with actions at the mitochondria and plasma membrane, respectively, and also of pancreatic β-cell apoptosis [141].

Only a few other chromosomal regions have shown highly significant lod scores in several populations. The best example is probably the chromosome 1q21-25 region (in particular the 30 Mb stretch adjacent to the centromere), which ranks alongside the regions on chromosomes 10 and 20 as amongst the strongest in terms of the replicated evidence for GWL to T2DM. Linkage has been reported in samples of European (UK, French, Amish, Utah), East Asian (Chinese, Hong Kong) and Native American (Pima) origin (summarized in [123]). The homologous region has also emerged as a diabetes-susceptibility locus from mapping efforts in several well-characterized rodent models [142]. The human region concerned is gene-rich and contains a disproportionate share of excellent biologic candidates, and genetic variation in a number of them has already been investigated with details in the populations showing 1q21-linkage (e.g. the genes *USF1* encoding the upstream stimulatory factor 1, *LMNA1* encoding Lamin A/C, *PBX1* encoding a TALE-homeodomain transcription factor that has a role in pancreatic development and is an important cofactor of Pdx1, the "master regulator" of pancreatic development and function, *ATF6* encoding activating transcription factor 6, or *DUSP12* encoding the glucokinase-associated, dual-specificity phosphatase 12). These studies have been conducted by an international consortium, which represent a coordinated effort by the groups with the strongest evidence for 1q linkage, by using a high-density, custom LD mapping approach applied to a well-powered set of multi-ethnic samples to identify variants causal for that signal [143]. Detection of low-frequency susceptibility variants also requires new approaches and the future plans of the 1q consortium include deep resequencing of the 1q region of interest, focusing at least initially on exons and conserved sequence.

Linkage with chromosome 20 has been also found in several ethnic groups, from Finns to Japanese subjects [147], but the linked region is rather large, raising the issue of whether there may be several susceptibility genes. While common variants upstream of *HNF4A* that maps to chromosome 20q13 have been reported to explain the linkage signals seen in Finns and Ashkenazim [144,145], these associations have proved difficult to replicate in many other populations [146].

Loci overlapping between T2DM, obesity and the metabolic syndrome have appeared on chromosome 2p [125,147] and on chromosome 3q27 [125,126,127]. Several candidate genes map to the 3q27 region, including the *APM1/ACDC* gene encoding the differentiated adipocyte-secreted protein, adipocyte complement-related protein 30 (Acrp30/adiponectin), which is an adipokine abundantly present in plasma. The purified C-terminal domain of adiponectin has been reported to protect mice on a high-fat diet from obesity, and to rescue obese or lipoatrophic mice models from severe insulin resistance, by decreasing levels of plasma free fatty acids (FFAs) and enhancing lipid oxidization in muscle [148]. Moreover, plasma levels of adiponectin have been shown to be decreased in obese subjects with diabetes and to correlate with insulin sensitivity [149], which makes *ACDC/ACRP30* an attractive candidate gene for fat-induced metabolic syndrome and T2DM.

Both common and rare variants of *ACDC/ACRP30* were found to be associated with T2DM in numerous obese populations, but do not contribute to the 3q27 linkage in the French families, suggesting that other genes may be involved. Common variants in and upstream of *EIF4A2* (encoding the eukaryotic translation initiation factor 4 α2) have been shown to contribute to both age of onset of diabetes and linkage in the French families studied [150].

One notable exception is the identification of *TCF7L2* as a T2DM gene with the largest risk effect of intronic variants of any diabetes gene identified to date. In early 2006, common intronic variants of the *TCF7L2* gene encoding the transcription factor 7-like 2 (TCF7L2) were identified to be strongly associated with T2DM risk in the Icelandic population by DeCODE Genetics (Reykjavik, Iceland) during a follow-up positional cloning study from a modest linkage signal on chromosome 10q [151]; but it turned out that despite not explaining this linkage signal, multiple intronic SNPs also showed strong association in US and Danish samples [151]. This initial study was rapidly followed by widespread replications in different ethnic backgrounds from white Europeans, West Africans, Mexican Americans, Indian and Japanese populations [152], confirming that *TCF7L2* variants have the largest risk effect of any of the known T2DM susceptibility loci. As shown in a meta-analysis from >20 studies in diverse ethnicities, the estimated risk of rs7903146 T allele (the most T2DM-associated variant) was 1.46 ($P = 5.4 \times 10^{-140}$) [153].

At the individual level, carrying one *TCF7L2* risk allele may increase diabetes risk by 40%–60% [152]. As a marked variation in *TCF7L2* rs7903146 T allele frequency exists between individuals from different ethnic groups, this implies a variable impact in the respective general populations. In European general populations, rs7903146 T allele has been estimated to contribute to 10–25% of all cases of diabetes in lean individuals [152]. In Eastern Asians, the population attributable risk fraction was assessed at 18.7% for other specific risk alleles [154]. The rs7903146 variant has been shown to influence progression to diabetes (with a hazard ratio of 1.81 for the homozygote TT group in the participants from the Diabetes Prevention Program) [155].

In the French and UK populations, rs7903146 T allele was associated with lower BMI in individuals with T2DM and with a higher risk for T2DM in non-obese subjects [152], but it is not a risk factor for obesity in European populations, whereas its effect on T2DM risk was found to be modulated by adiposity [156]. Watanabe *et al.* [157] suggested that an interaction between TCF7L2 and adiposity may be caused by a better β-cell compensation in obese individuals.

TCF7L2 is a member of the T-cell specific high mobility group (HMG) box containing family of transcription factors which, upon binding β-catenin, transduces signals generated by Wnt receptors at the cell surface to modify expression of multiple genes, many of which are associated with the cell cycle. Mutations in *TCF7L2* are also implicated in certain types of cancer [158], but rare *TCF7L2* mutations are not contributing to monogenic forms of diabetes such as MODY and neonatal diabetes [159]. One mechanism whereby *TCF7L2* variants increase diabetes risk might involve an impairment of incretin effects (i.e. GLP-1) on islet functions [160,161]. Indeed, variants of *TCF7L2* specifically impair GLP-1-induced insulin secretion [162], and the stimulation of β-cell proliferation by GLP-1 is TCF7L2 dependent [163]. TCF7L2 is also required to maintain glucose-stimulated insulin secretion and β-cell survival because its deletion in human islets reduces insulin secretion and increased apoptosis [164]. Furthermore, the overexpression of TCF7L2 protects β-cells from glucose and cytokine-induced apoptosis [164]. Clinical studies have demonstrated that the at-risk SNP is associated with defects in β-cell function and insulin release. The study by Lyssenko *et al.* [161] suggested that pancreatic islets from subjects with T2DM bearing the at-risk TT genotype have increased TCF7L2 RNA levels, indicating that excessive TCF7L2 expression may be associated with the reported insulin secretory defects. Expression studies carried out by Elbein *et al.* [165] on adipose tissue and muscle, however, showed that TCF7L2 expression was not altered by genotype and did not correlate with insulin sensitivity or BMI. As the most associated SNP rs7903146 is found in an intronic region, a potential mechanism through which it may confer an increased risk of diabetes is by altering TCF7L2 expression levels, but the functional mechanisms through which TCF7L2 modulates glucose sensing and insulin release in pancreatic β-cells remain to be clarified. A recent study showed that *TCF7L2* silencing in primary mouse islets as well as in clonal MIN6 and INS-1(832/13) cells decreases both basal and glucose-stimulated insulin secretion [166]. *TCF7L2* silencing also abolished the stimulatory effects of GLP-1 on secretion, whilst having little impact on glucose-induced changes in intracellular ATP or free Ca^{2+} concentrations. The study by da Silva Xavier *et al.* [166] showed that TCF7L2 controls the expression of genes involved in insulin granule fusion at the plasma membrane (notably syntaxin 1A and Munc 18-1 which may be direct targets for regulation by TCF7L2). Thus, defective insulin exocytosis may underlie increased diabetes incidence in carriers of the at-risk *TCF7L2* alleles.

The era of GWA studies improved knowledge of T2DM susceptibility genes

New discoveries in the genetic etiology of T2DM

Important advances in T2DM genetics have been made with the completion of GWA studies based on HapMap-selected common SNPs. This has become reality with the outstanding breakthroughs made in the knowledge and assessment of human genome variations, their mapping and their links with the genetic background of common diseases [167], and in the development and accessibility to very high throughput genotyping techniques based on microarray technology and to biostatistical tools for large cohort data analyses.

Within only few months of 2007, five independent GWA screens for T2DM, based on the Illumina 300K or Affymetrix 500K genotyping arrays both capturing about 80% of common variants present in the human genome of Caucasian individuals, identified dozens of potential candidates; at least 15 new loci emerged as being most consistently associated with risk of T2DM across multiple studies (Table 12.4). These include variants within or near *SLC30A8*, *HHEX*, *CDKAL1*, *CDKN2A/2B*, *IGF2BP2* and *JAZF1* [15]. Three of the associated loci correspond to genes that had already been implicated in T2DM (*TCF7L2*, *KCNJ11*, *PPARG*). These studies also confirmed that *TCF7L2* was the highest genetic risk factor for T2DM in populations of European descent. The next strongest SNP is in a 33-kb LD block within the coding region of *SLC30A8* encoding a zinc membrane transporter (ZnT8) which is highly expressed in pancreatic islets [168]. Interestingly, the overexpression of ZnT8 in the HeLa cell line is associated with an accumulation of zinc in intracellular vesicles [168]. In the INS-1E β-cell line, which overexpresses ZnT8, the intracellular zinc level is increased and the insulin secretion is stimulated [169]. Furthermore, overexpressing ZnT8 does not sensitize the cells to toxic doses of zinc but confers a resistance to apoptosis after zinc depletion [169]. The non-synonymous polymorphism showing an increased risk of T2DM (OR per risk allele: 1.18) corresponds to an arginine to tryptophan substitution at position 325, and the at-risk C-allele is associated with impaired β-cell function *in vivo*. An impaired transporter function may decrease the amount of zinc available for co-crystallization with insulin in the secretory vesicles of

Table 12.4 Validated type 2 diabetes susceptibility genes in the post genome-wide association era.

Chromosome location	Representative SNP	Gene symbol	Predicted disease mechanism	Approximate effect size for T2DM risk	Year of major publication (key references)
3p25	rs1801282	*PPARG*	Insulin resistance/muscle/adipocyte	1.23	2000 [90]
2q37	rs2975760	*CAPN10*	Glucose transport/insulin resistance/β-cell dysfunction	1.18	2003 [139]
11p15	rs5219	*KCNJ11*	β-cell dysfunction (K_{ATP} channel)	1.15	2003 [115]
20q12	Multiple SNPs at P2 site	*HNF4A*	β-cell dysfunction/other	1.05–1.70*	2004 [52,53,55]
6q23	rs1044498	*ENPP1*	Insulin resistance/muscle/adipocyte	1.38†	2005 [83,85,88]
10q25	rs7903146	*TCF7L2*	β-cell dysfunction/β-cell mass/incretin effect	1.47	2006 [15,153]
8q24	rs13266634	*SLC30A8*	β-cell dysfunction/Zn transport	1.15	2007 [16]
10q23-q25	rs1111875	*HHEX-IDE*	Pancreatic development	1.15	2007 [15,16]
6p22	rs10946398	*CDKAL1*	β-cell dysfunction/β-cell mass	1.16	2007 [15,172]
9p21	rs10811661	*CDKN2A/2B*	β-cell dysfunction/cell cycle regulation	1.20	2007 [15]
3q28	rs4402960	*IGF2BP2*	mRNA processing in the β-cell	1.14	2007 [15]
4p16	rs10010131	*WFS1*	β-cell dysfunction/ER stress/other	1.11	2007 [15,60]
17q21	rs4430796	*TCF2*	β-cell dysfunction/development	1.10	2007 [45,56]
1p12	rs10923931	*NOTCH2*	Pancreatic development	1.13	2008 [174]
3p14	rs4607103	*ADAMTS9*	Metalloprotease/cell–cell interactions; insulin resistance	1.09	2008 [174]
2p21	rs7578597	*THADA*	β-cell dysfunction/apoptosis	1.15	2008 [174]
1p12	rs2641348	*ADAM30*	Metalloprotease/cell–cell interactions	1.10	2008 [174]
12q21	rs7961581	*TSPAN8-LGR5*	Cell surface glycoprotein	1.09	2008 [174]
10p13-p14	rs12779790	*CDC123-CAMK1D*	Cell cycle regulation in the β-cell	1.11	2008 [174]
7p15	rs864745	*JAZF1*	Transcriptional regulation in the β-cell	1.10	2008 [174]
11p15	rs2237892	*KCNQ1*	β-cell dysfunction (K^+ channel)	1.40	2008 [207,208]
11q21	rs10830963	*MTNR1B*	β-cell dysfunction (melatonin signaling)/ other	1.09	2009 [181–183]

* Difference in effect size for T2DM risk between populations (the strongest effect was found in the Ashkenazim [55]).
† Under a recessive model of inheritance in white populations (according to the meta-analysis by McAteer *et al.* [88]).

β-cells. *SLC30A8*/ZnT-8 has also recently been identified as an autoantigen in human type 1 diabetes [170].

A locus on 10q23 ranked third for association with T2DM in the French GWA study was then independently replicated in the other large studies, but with a combined OR of only 1.13. SNPs at this locus have been found to be associated with measures of insulin secretion in a large multicentric study from Europe and in the Diabetes Prevention Program (DPP) study [171]. The association signal lies in a 295-kb block of LD that includes at least three potential T2DM genes: *HHEX* (a homeobox transcription factor); *KIF11* (a kinesin interacting factor); and *IDE* (an insulin degrading enzyme).

Another well-replicated association signal maps to 6q22 within a 15-kb LD block in the intron 5 of the *CDKAL1* gene coding for CDK5 regulatory subunit-associated protein 1-like 1, with the strongest association observed in the DeCODE study [172]. CDK5 itself has been shown to blunt insulin secretion in response to glucose and to have a permissive role in the decrease of insulin gene expression that results from glucotoxicity. Thus, it is speculated that reduced expression of *CDKAL1* would result in enhanced activity of CDK5 in β-cells, and lead to decreased insulin secretion; in agreement, variants at this locus were significantly associated with small decreases in insulin response to a glucose load [171,173].

A meta-analysis of three GWA scans followed by a large-scale replication (Diagram consortium including more than 50 000 individuals in total) has identified additional susceptibility loci for T2DM, with OR ranging from 1.09 to 1.15, near six genes: *JAZF1*, *CDC123-CAMK1D*, *TSPAN8-LGR5*, *THADA*, *ADAMTS9* and *NOTCH2* [174]. Variants at *JAZF1*, *CDC123-CAMK1D* and *TSPAN8-LGR5* are associated with small alterations in insulin secretion, whereas the mechanisms linking the other loci to T2DM remain to be clarified [175]. In each GWA scan, other loci showed significant associations with T2DM, but were not fol-

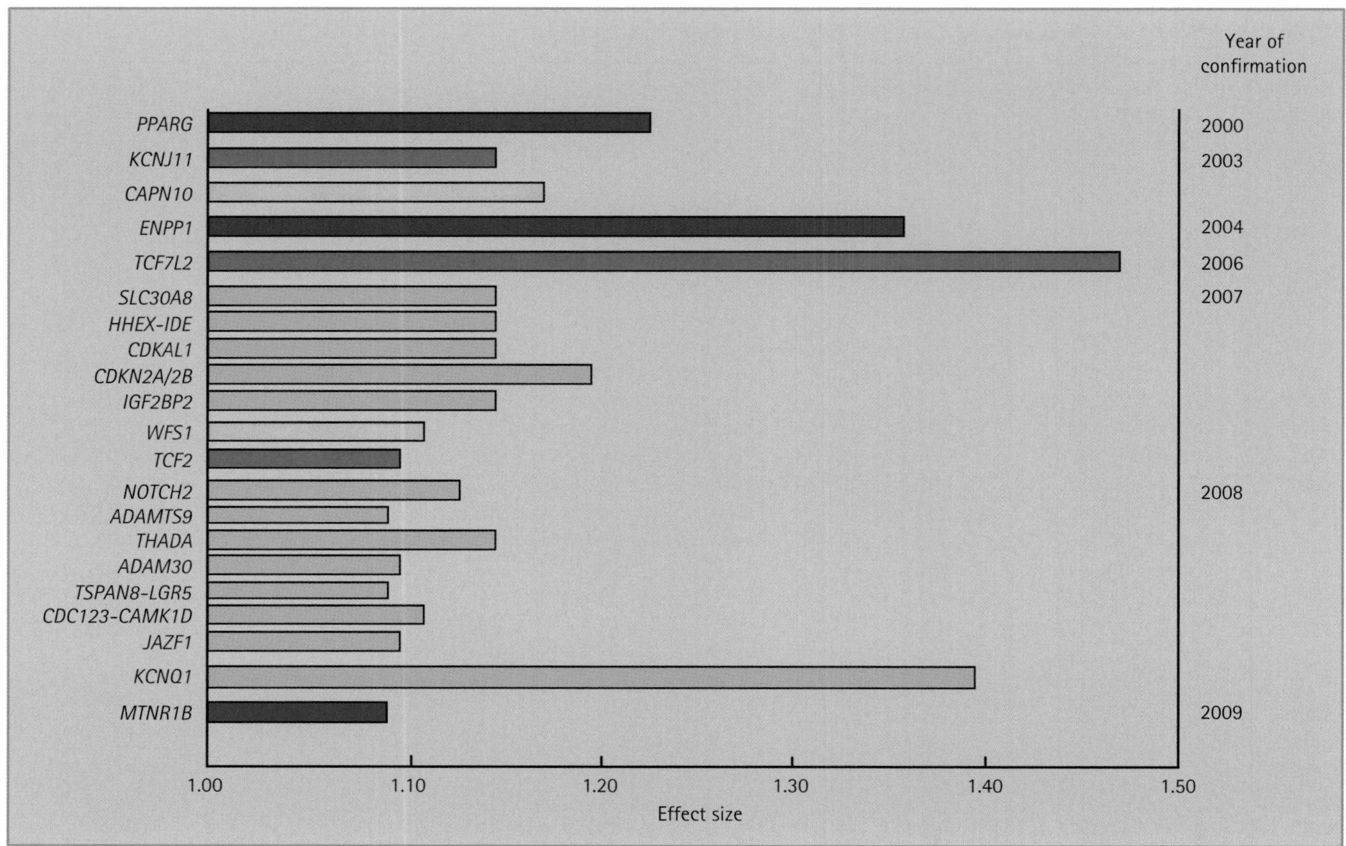

Figure 12.1 Chronology in the discovery of the genetic loci associated with type 2 diabetes. Validated type 2 diabetes-associated genes are plotted by year of publication and approximate effect size. Allelic effect sizes (OR value) are derived from major publications of definitive associations (as indicated in Table 12.4). Color code: purple indicates candidate genes with a biologic effect on insulin sensitivity at different sites; red with an effect on pancreatic islet function and insulin secretion; yellow with effects on both insulin secretion and sensitivity; red with pink lines indicates genes uncovered via genome-wide association studies, for which common variants increase disease risk through impaired β-cell function (for most of them); blue for one gene modulating fasting plasma glucose and type 2 diabetes risk through impaired β-cell function and other mechanism(s).

lowed up because of lack of replication across multiple studies. A larger meta-analysis study including almost all GWA studies for T2DM performed in European populations will extend the list of potentially at-risk alleles and genes (Figure 12.1).

These GWA results suggest that T2DM may be more heterogeneous and more polygenic than previously believed, and thereby represents a large number of different disorders which might also differ at a clinical level. The second finding is the relatively high frequency of each of the risk variants in the population (ranging from 0.26 for *TCF7L2* to 0.90 for *THADA*), together with a small risk of disease conferred by each allele translating into a very large number of individuals who carry several of the susceptibility variants but do not develop T2DM. Such low penetrance is consistent with the mild effect of the risk variants, requiring the presence of other factors, presumably environmental for the development of hyperglycemia, and may also be explained by the fact that most of these variants are in noncoding regions of the gene, where they may produce only subtle differences in regulation of expression. This is in contrast with Mendelian forms of diabetes, such as MODY, which are caused by rare mutations in the coding sequence resulting in significant amino acid substitutions or truncated proteins, leading to hyperglycemia even in the absence of other diabetogenic exposures.

It is also worthy of note that the loci identified to date appear to explain only a small proportion of the familial clustering of T2DM, and thus are just the tip of the iceberg. Indeed, there is a discrepancy between the linkage and GWA studies, and this may be explained by the presence of multiple, uncommon, mildly deleterious polymorphisms scattered throughout the regulatory and coding regions of genes for T2DM.

The current genetic models of how genes interact with each other and with the environment may be too simplistic, and probably clouded by our underestimation of the role of genetic imprinting and/or epigenetics on gene expression and disease.

These new discoveries lead to the proposal of new etiologic mechanisms for T2DM, and would suggest that the genetic components to T2DM risk act preferentially through β-cell

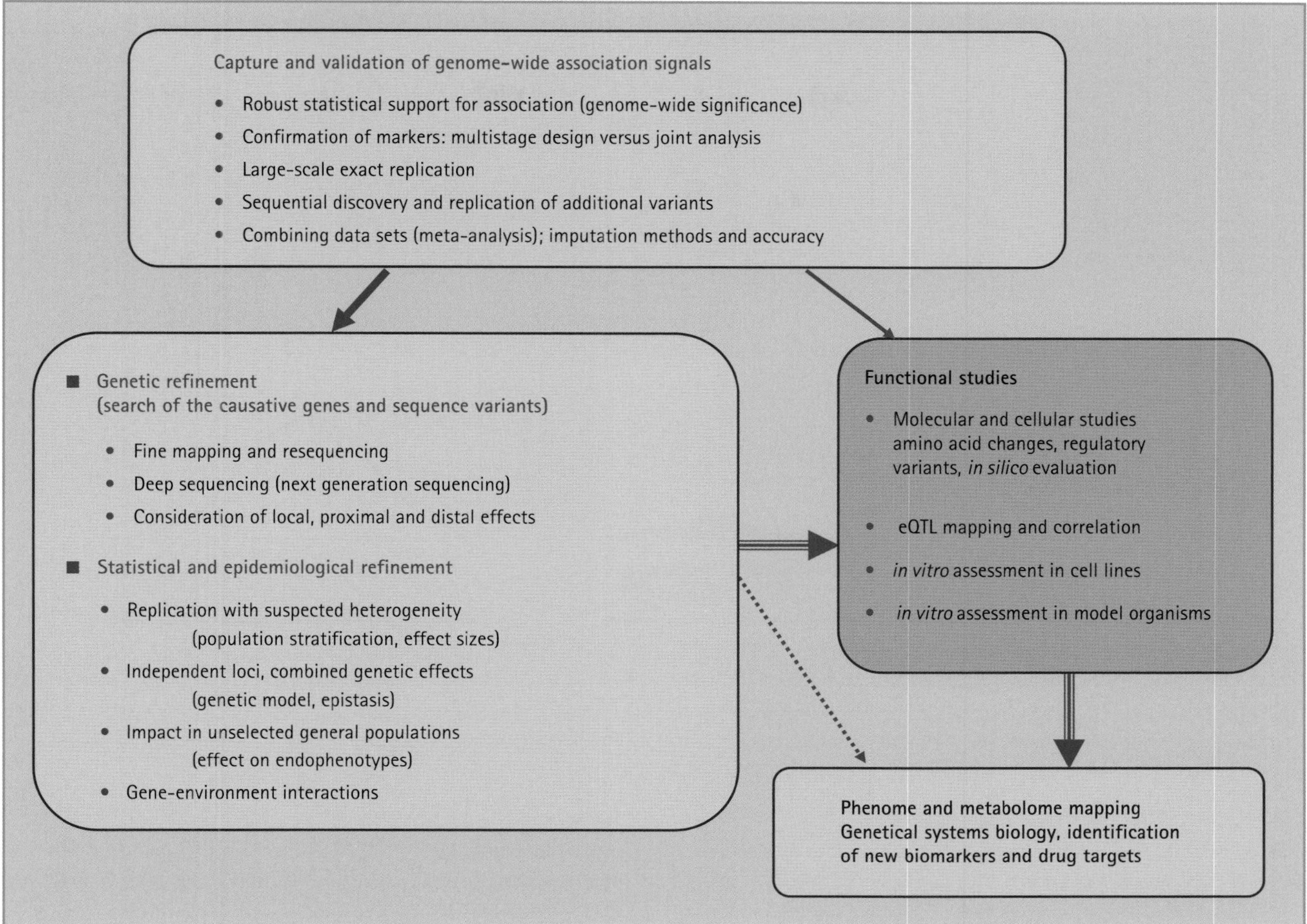

Figure 12.2 From the capture of genomic information to phenome and metabolome mapping. Flow chart of the research approaches and methods required to document, refine and validate genome-wide association signals. These steps have a rationale sequence, but this can also be modulated by the availability of resources and data, and the specific challenges that arise in each field.

defects, given that several of the genes placed in the proximity of GWA signals are expressed in β-cells and risk alleles at many of these loci alter insulin secretion capacity of the β-cells. Variants predisposing to diabetes through effects on insulin sensitivity, however, may be more difficult to track down because of strong environment–gene interactions for insulin resistance with body weight, physical activity, nutrient intake and other factors, compared with the potentially purer genetic control on insulin secretion. More generally, exploring these novel association data and truly causative DNA sequences as well as functional mechanisms requires pursuing other research efforts (Figure 12.2).

A concept emerging from these new discoveries is that there is a genetic overlap between T2DM and prostate cancer. Common variants in the T2DM susceptibility genes *TCF2* and *JAZF1* also influence prostate cancer risk [176]. For *TCF2*, the risk allele for T2DM has a protective effect on prostate cancer susceptibility, whereas two variants in *JAZF1* predispose to the two diseases, which are not correlated with each other [174,177]. The mechanisms by which these genes influence disease are unknown; however, they are thought to be involved in cell-cycle control.

Additional loci associated with quantitative metabolic traits

Analyses of quantitative traits among the non-diabetic controls in GWA studies have also identified common variants that modulate fasting glycemia, although these effects do not always appear to translate into an increased risk of T2DM (Figure 12.3).

Fasting plasma glucose (FPG) levels are tightly regulated within a narrow physiologic range by a feedback mechanism that targets a particular fasting glucose setpoint for each individual. Disruption of normal glucose homeostasis and substantial elevations of FPG are hallmarks of T2DM and typically result from sustained reduction in pancreatic β-cell function and insulin secretion [178,179]. Elevated FPG levels within the normal range are an independent risk factor for T2DM and are associated with increased risk of mortality in prospective studies [178].

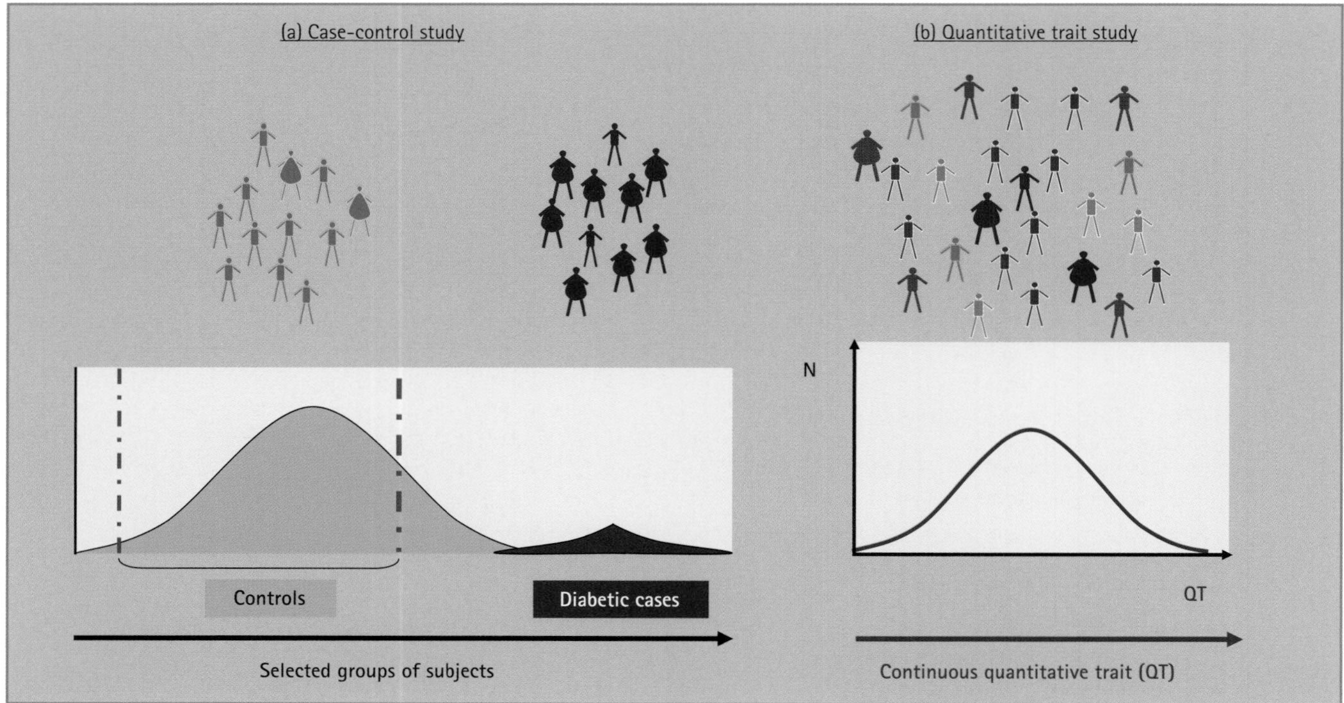

Figure 12.3 Schematic representation of the two major study designs used in the genetic mapping of complex traits and complex diseases. (a) Case–control study to search for genes and gene variants associated with disease risk. (b) Quantitative trait study to correlate genotype effects with modulation of continuous quantitative variables (i.e. values of a biologic measure, measured or calculated metabolic variables).

Even within the healthy non-diabetic population, however, there is substantial variation in fasting glucose levels; around one-third of this variation is genetic. There is growing evidence to suggest that common variants contributing to variation in FPG are largely distinct from those associated with major disruptions of β-cell function that predispose to established T2DM. Common sequence variants in the *GCK* (glucokinase) promoter and around genes encoding glucokinase regulatory protein (*GCKR*) and the islet-specific glucose-6-phosphatase (*G6PC2*) [180] have been associated with individual variation in FPG, whereas weak effects on T2DM risk were found. Three large independent studies in European populations, however, have recently demonstrated that non-coding variants in *MTNR1B* (encoding melatonin receptor 1B) are consistently associated with increased FPG levels (0.07 mmol/L per G-allele of rs10830963, the strongest signal observed at the locus), reduced β-cell function as measured by the homeostasis model assessment (HOMA-B index) and increased T2DM risk (OR of 1.09 for the same G-allele) [181–183], and with impairment of early insulin response to both oral and intravenous glucose and with faster deterioration of insulin secretion over time [183,184]. *MTNR1B* encodes one of the two known melatonin receptors and, as well as being highly expressed in the brain (mainly in the suprachiasmatic nucleus that controls the circadian rhythm) and retina, MT2 is also transcribed in human islets and sorted β-cells [181,185]. The study by Lyssenko *et al.* [183] showed an increased expression of MT2 in islets of individuals without diabetes carrying the risk allele and of individuals with T2DM, and that insulin released from clonal β-cells in response to glucose was inhibited in the presence of melatonin. These data support a direct role of MT2 in mediating the inhibitory effect of melatonin on insulin secretion, and that the circulating hormone melatonin, which is released from the pineal gland in the brain to regulate the circadian rhythm by translating photoperiodic information from the eyes to the brain, is involved in the pathogenesis of T2DM. These pathogenic effects are likely to be exerted via a direct inhibitory effect on β-cells. In view of these results, blocking the melatonin ligand-receptor system could be a therapeutic option in T2DM.

The total variance in FPG attributable to these four signals is approximately 1.5%, indicating that additional loci remain to be found. The ongoing MAGIC (Meta-Analyses of Glucose and Insulin-related traits Consortium) transnational study group, which represents a collaborative effort to combine data from multiple GWAs to identify additional loci that affect glycemic and metabolic traits, and other studies from the Northern Finland Birth Cohorts, the ENGAGE consortium (including 20 000 individuals in multiple European cohorts and family studies) or other large cohorts, case–control studies and clinical trials from Europe and the USA, will continue to deliver novel association signals in additional loci, which may highlight novel pathways involved in regulation of common metabolic traits.

One recent study has reported a novel association between glycated hemoglobin (HbA_{1c}) levels and intronic variants of *HK1* encoding the hexokinase type 1 isoform predominantly found in erythrocytes, although it is also expressed in other human tissues that depend strongly on glucose utilization for their physiologic functioning such as brain and muscle [186]. Three other loci – *GCK*, *G6PC2* and *SLC30A8* – have been identified in this study as being significantly associated with HbA_{1c} levels in individuals without diabetes. While genetic variants of *GCK* and *G6PC2* are known to influence FPG levels in people without diabetes, the association with the diabetes gene *SLC30A8* has not been previously identified. Because intra-erythrocyte glucose concentration is thought to be the main determinant of HbA_{1c} rate and HK1 is the initial and rate-limiting enzymatic step in erythrocyte glucose metabolism after glucose transporter mediated-diffusion, it is likely that variation in HK1 activity would affect glycation. Alternatively, genetic variations at HK1 might modulate systemic glucose metabolism, raising the possibility that these variations are associated with the risk of incident diabetes. Indeed, HK1 is expressed in muscle, an insulin-sensitive tissue recognized for its importance in glucose metabolism. Whether the differences in hemoglobin glycation associated with genetic polymorphisms are paralleled by differences in glycation in other tissues that are thought to underlie long-term complications of diabetes remains an open question.

Serum lipids are important determinants of cardiovascular diseases and are related to morbidity [187]. The high heritability of circulating lipid levels is well established, and earlier studies of individuals with extreme lipid values or families with Mendelian forms of dyslipidemias have reported the involvement of numerous genes and respective proteins in lipid metabolism [188]. Recent GWA studies mostly carried out in samples enriched for T2DM cases have implicated a total of 19 loci controlling serum high density lipoprotein (HDL) cholesterol, low density lipoprotein (LDL) cholesterol and triglycerides (TG). The loci include the genes encoding *ABCA1*, *APOB*, *CELSR2*, *CETP*, *DOCK7*, *GALNT2*, *GCKR*, *HMGCR*, *LDLR*, *LIPC*, *LIPG*, *LPL*, *MLXIPL*, *NCAN*, *PCSK9* and *TRIB1*, and three genomic regions with multiple associated genes including *MVK-MMAB*, *APOA5-APOA4-APOC3-APOA1* and *APOE-APOC1-APOC4-APOC2* [188,189].

Many of these have also been consistently associated with lipid levels in candidate gene studies reported over the past 30 years; many of the same loci with common variants have already been shown to lead to monogenic lipid disorders in humans and/or mice, suggesting that a spectrum of common and rare alleles at each validated locus contributes to blood lipid concentrations [188].

More recently, larger scale GWA studies have identified additional loci for lipid levels [190,191], and sequencing of these loci should pinpoint all associated alleles. For three loci (*HMGCR* encoding HMGCoA, the drug target for statins, *NCAN* and *LPL*) effect sizes differed significantly by sex (i.e. gene–sex interactions) [190]. The construction of genetic risk profiles suggests that the cumulative effect of multiple common variants contributes to polygenic dyslipidemia [191].

With a full catalog of DNA polymorphisms in hand, a panel of lipid-related variants can be studied to provide clinical risk stratification and targeting of therapeutic interventions.

Combined genetic effects of multiple susceptibility gene variants and clinical implications

GWA studies have dramatically increased the number of common genetic variants that are robustly associated with T2DM. A possible clinical use of this novel information is to identify individuals at high risk of developing the disease in the general population, so that preventative measures may be more effectively targeted (Figure 12.4).

A first study in a UK population showed that individuals combining T2DM risk alleles in *TCF7L2*, *PPARG* and *KCNJ11* had an OR of 5.71-fold compared with those with no risk alleles to develop the disease [192]. Then, using a similar case–control design, a second study in a French population reported that after adjustment for age, BMI and gender, subjects with at least 18 risk alleles (representing 14.5% of French subjects with T2DM) had

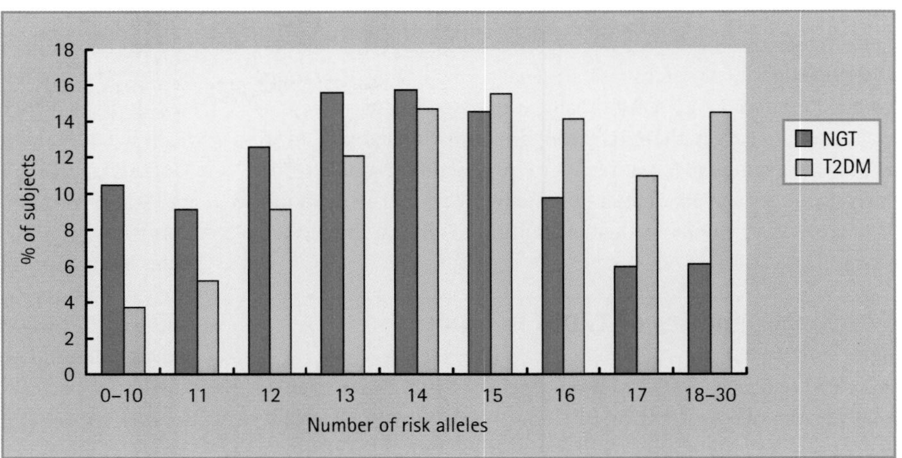

Figure 12.4 Additive effects of common genetic variants (i.e. SNPs) on T2DM risk in the population. The distribution of normoglucose-tolerant (NGT, indicated by red bars) individuals and individuals, with diabetes (T2DM, indicated by yellow bars) is shown according to the number of at-risk alleles in each class (for a total of 15 single nucleotide polymorphisms genotyped in each individual, from the best replicated variants following the results of genome-wide association studies). The study was performed in 4232 patients with diabetes and 4595 normoglycemic adult subjects. Adapted from Cauchi *et al.* [193].

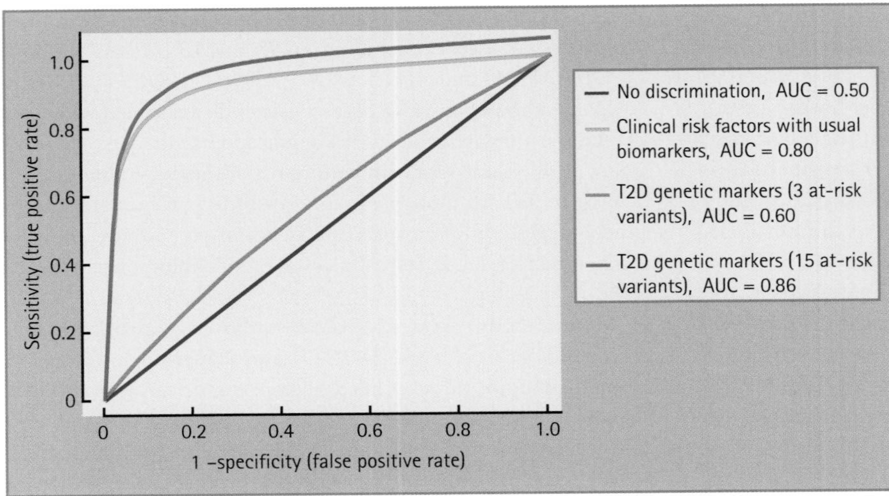

Figure 12.5 The predictive value of type 2 diabetes gene variants. Examples of receiver operator characteristic (ROC) curves for a test including classic clinical risk factors (in green) or three genetic variants at-risk for T2DM (in orange) or 15 genetic variants at-risk for T2DM (in red). The area under the ROC curve (AUC) is a measure of the discriminatory power of the test evaluating the predictive power of defined clinical factors or genetic variants (a test with no discriminatory power would have an AUC of 0.50). For details see [46,192–196].

approximately ninefold higher risk of developing T2DM compared with the reference group (with an area under the receiver operator characteristic (ROC) curve, a measure of discriminative accuracy, of 0.86; Figure 12.5) [193].

Two more recent population-based studies using a longitudinal design with prospectively investigated cohorts have examined the predictive value of a genotype score in addition to common risk factors for prediction of T2DM [194,195]. Meigs *et al.* [194] reported that a genotype score based on 18 risk alleles predicted new cases of diabetes in the community but provided only a slightly better prediction of risk than knowledge of common clinical risk factors alone [195]. A similar conclusion was drawn in the paper by Lyssenko *et al.* [196], along with an improved value of genetic factors with an increasing duration of follow-up, suggesting that assessment of genetic risk factors is clinically more meaningful the earlier in life they are measured. They also showed that β-cell function adjusted for insulin resistance (using the disposition index) was the strongest predictor of future diabetes, although subjects in the prediabetic stage presented with many features of insulin resistance. It is also noteworthy that many of the variants that were genotyped appear to influence β-cell function. The addition of DNA data to the clinical model improved not only the discriminatory power, but also the reclassification of the subjects into different risk strategies. Identifying subgroups of the population at substantially different risk of disease is important to target these subgroups of individuals with more effective preventative measures. As more genetic variants are now identified, tests with better predictive performance should become available with a valuable addition to clinical practice.

Pharmacogenetics of T2DM in adults

An early focus of T2DM pharmacogenetic studies has been to examine the effect of *PPARG* P12A on the response to thiazolidinediones, because the nuclear receptor PPAR-γ is the known drug target of thiazolidinedione medications. In the TRIPOD study, one-third of subjects showed no increase in insulin sensitivity in response to troglitazone (400 mg/day); however, the P12A variant did not explain this failure [197]. Similarly, in the DPP study, no effect of *PPARG* P12A or five other polymorphisms was observed on response to troglitazone therapy in 340 participants randomized to this thiazolidinedione [198]. Knowledge of allelic variation at this locus does not seem to offer a rationale for therapeutic choices. The impact of the *KCNJ11*/ genetic variant (E23K) on the effectiveness of sulfonylurea therapy is also unclear. In the study by Sesti *et al.* [199], which genotyped the E23K variant in 525 white patients with T2DM, carriers of the 23K allele have a relative risk of failure (defined as FPG >300 mg/dL) of 1.45 compared with E23E homozygotes, and the risk allele was also associated with an earlier onset of diabetes and worse metabolic control in non-responders. These results stand in contrast to those of the UK Prospective Diabetes Study (UKPDS), in which no significant association was found between the E23K variant and response to sulfonylurea therapy in 364 patients with newly diagnosed T2DM [200]. Interestingly, in the DPP study, metformin was effective in lowering the risk of diabetes for the E23E homozygotes, but failed to protect carriers of the risk K-allele. In addition, K23K homozygotes randomized to metformin did not show the expected improvement in insulin sensitivity at 1 year [201].

In regard to a possible drug–*TCF7L2* genotype interaction, the GoDARTs study genotyped 6516 UK participants for the rs7903146 variant and found that the TT homozygote case and control subjects had a higher HbA_{1c}, with the TT cases with diabetes being more likely to require oral medication or insulin than the CC homozygotes [202]. This suggests that *TCF7L2* risk variants may be associated with increased disease severity and therapeutic failure. The same group reported the effect of *TCF7L2* genotypes on therapeutic response in 901 patients with diabetes treated with sulfonylurea and 945 patients treated with metformin. Carriers of the risk *TCF7L2* variants were more likely not to respond to sulfonylurea but to respond to metformin therapy as measured by a HbA_{1c} >7% within 3–12 months after treatment initiation [203]. This finding further supports the hypothesis that *TCF7L2* variation is important in β-cell function. The DPP study reported that the lifestyle intervention was effective in reducing the genetic risk conferred by the high-risk homozygous genotype in the participants with impaired glucose tolerance and elevated fasting glucose [204].

Another example in which genetic variability may have a significant impact on therapy response is the organic cation transporter 1 (*OCT1*), which participates in the hepatic uptake of metformin, a widely used biguanide, and was shown to be highly polymorphic in humans. A clinical study by Shu *et al.* [205] reported that genetic variation in *OCT1* affects the metformin therapeutic action and the response to the drug.

Conclusions and perspectives

Our knowledge of the genetic architecture of T2DM has greatly improved with the new GWA findings, and this will have promising implications on new diagnostics and therapeutics for T2DM. It is likely, however, that other yet unidentified genes may contribute to the genetic risk of T2DM, because only a part of the inheritance of T2DM in families has so far been explained. It should be emphasized that the current GWA studies are based on the "common disease/common variant" hypothesis, whereas the alternative "allelic heterogeneity" hypothesis holding that susceptibility to common disorders may result from a large number of rare variants, each having a relatively large effect, still has to be tested. Identification of such rare variants, if they exist, will require deep resequencing of T2DM loci (those already established, and novel) in cases of diabetes and in normoglycemic individuals, which is becoming more realistic with the ongoing development of new powerful sequencing methods. Likewise, the contribution of structural variants, such as copy number variants, insertions, deletions and duplications, could also contribute to genetic susceptibility not explained by single nucleotide substitutions. Further more novel approaches looking at epigenetic sites, multitissue genome expression related to genetic traits, metabonomics and metagenomics should bring even more knowledge in the near future.

Together, these discoveries will continue to improve our understanding of the biologic mechanisms that maintain glucose homeostasis, and of still hidden molecular defects leading to chronic hyperglycemia, and could also lead to the development of more specifically targeted antidiabetic drugs or even gene-based therapies. Moreover, pharmacogenetic testing might then be used to predict, for each patient, the therapeutic response to different classes of drugs. The identification of T2DM genes will also provide the tools for the timely identification of high-risk individuals who may benefit from early behavioral or medical intervention to prevent the development of diabetes. An important reduction in diabetes-related morbidity and mortality could be then expected, along with a reduction in the costs of the treatment of diabetes and its complications.

References

1 Stumvoll M, Goldstein BJ, van Haeften TW. Type 2 diabetes: principles of pathogenesis and therapy. *Lancet* 2005; **365**:1333–1346.

2 Bonadonna RC. Alterations of glucose metabolism in T2D mellitus: an overview. *Rev Endocr Metab Disord* 2004; **5**:89–97.

3 International Diabetes Federation. *Diabetes Facts and Figures*. Available from: www.diabetesatlas.org/content/diabetes-and-impaired-glucose-tolerance. Accessed on 18 December, 2009.

4 Poulsen P, Levin K, Petersen I, Christensen K, Beck-Nielsen H, Vaag A. Heritability of insulin secretion, peripheral and hepatic insulin action, and intracellular glucose partitioning in young and old Danish twins. *Diabetes* 2005; **54**:275–283.

5 Vaxillaire M, Froguel P. Genetic basis of maturity-onset diabetes of the young. *Endocrinol Metab Clin North Am* 2006; **35**:371–384.

6 McCarthy MI, Hattersley AT. Learning from molecular genetics: novel insights arising from the definition of genes for monogenic and type 2 diabetes. *Diabetes* 2008; **57**:2889–2898.

7 Doria A, Patti ME, Kahn CR. The emerging genetic architecture of type 2 diabetes. *Cell Metab* 2008; **8**:186–200.

8 Carmelli D, Carmelli D, Cardon LR, Fabsitz R. Clustering of hypertension, diabetes, and obesity in adult male twins: same genes or same environments? *Am J Hum Genet* 1994; **55**:566–573.

9 Prudente S, Trischitta V. The pleiotropic effect of the ENPP1 (PC-1) gene on insulin resistance, obesity, and type 2 diabetes. *J Clin Endocrinol Metab* 2006; **91**:4767–4768.

10 Hales CN, Barker DJ, Clark PM, Cox LJ, Fall C, Osmond C, *et al.* Fetal and infant growth and impaired glucose tolerance at age 64. *Br Med J* 1991; **303**:1019–1022.

11 Lithell HO, McKeigue PM, Berglund L, Mohsen R, Lithell UB, Leon DA. Relation of size at birth to non-insulin dependent diabetes and insulin concentrations in men aged 50–60 years. *Br Med J* 1996; **312**:406–410.

12 Barker DJ. The fetal and infant origins of disease. *Eur J Clin Invest* 1995; **25**:457–463.

13 Hattersley AT, Tooke JE. The fetal insulin hypothesis: an alternative explanation of the association of low birthweight with diabetes and vascular disease. *Lancet* 1999; **353**:1789–1792.

14 Hanis CL, Boerwinkle E, Chakraborty R, Ellsworth DL, Concannon P, Stirling B, *et al.* A genome-wide search for human non-insulin-dependent (type 2) diabetes genes reveals a major susceptibility locus on chromosome 2. *Nat Genet* 1996; **13**:161–166.

15 Frayling TM. Genome-wide association studies provide new insights into T2D aetiology. *Nat Rev Genet* 2007; **8**:657–662.

16 Sladek R, Rocheleau G, Rung J, Dina C, Shen L, Serre D, *et al.* A genome-wide association study identifies novel risk loci for type 2 diabetes. *Nature* 2007; **445**:881–885.

17 Mootha VK, Lindgren CM, Eriksson KF, Subramanian A, Sihaq S, Lehar J, *et al.* PGC-1alpha-responsive genes involved in oxidative phosphorylation are coordinately downregulated in human diabetes. *Nat Genet* 2003; **34**:267–273.

18 Patti ME, Butte AJ, Crunkhorn S, Cusi K, Berria R, Kashyap S, *et al.* Coordinated reduction of genes of oxidative metabolism in humans with insulin resistance and diabetes: potential role of PGC1 and NRF1. *Proc Natl Acad Sci U S A* 2003; **100**:8466–8471.

19 Gunton JE, Kulkarni RN, Yim S, Okada T, Hawthorne WJ, Tseng YH, *et al.* Loss of ARNT/HIF1beta mediates altered gene expression and pancreatic-islet dysfunction in human type 2 diabetes. *Cell* 2005; **122**:337–349.

20 Naggert JK, Fricker LD, Varlamov O, Nishina PM, Rouille Y, Steiner DF, *et al.* Hyperproinsulinaemia in obese fat/fat mice associated with a carboxypeptidase E mutation which reduces enzyme activity. *Nat Genet* 1995; **10**:135–142.

21 Gauguier D, Froguel P, Parent V, Bernard C, Bihoreau MT, Portha B, *et al.* Chromosomal mapping of genetic loci associated with non-insulin dependent diabetes in the GK rat. *Nat Genet* 1996; **12**:38–43.

22 Ahlgren U, Jonsson J, Jonsson L, Simu K, Edlund H. Beta-cell-specific inactivation of the mouse IPF-1/Pdx1 gene results in loss of the beta-cell phenotype and maturity onset diabetes. *Genes Dev* 1998; **12**:1763–1768.

23 Withers DJ, Gutierrez JS, Towery H, Burks DJ, Ren JM, Previs S, *et al.* Disruption of IRS-2 causes T2D in mice. *Nature* 1998; **391**:900–904.

24 Kulkarni RN, Bruning JC, Winnay JN, Postic C, Magnuson MA, Kahn CR. Tissue-specific knockout of the insulin receptor in pancreatic beta cells creates an insulin secretory defect similar to that in T2D. *Cell* 1999; **96**:329–339.

25 Ledermann HM. Is maturity onset diabetes at young age (MODY) more common in Europe than previously assumed? *Lancet* 1995; **345**:648.

26 Froguel P, Vaxillaire M, Sun F, Velho G, Zouali H, Butel MO, *et al.* Close linkage of glucokinase locus on chromosome 7p to early-onset non-insulin-dependent diabetes mellitus. *Nature* 1992; **356**:162–164.

27 Froguel P, Zouali H, Vionnet N, Velho G, Vaxillaire M, Sun F, *et al.* Familial hyperglycaemia due to mutations in glucokinase: definition of a subtype of diabetes mellitus. *N Engl J Med* 1993; **328**:697–702.

28 Velho G, Blanche H, Vaxillaire M, Bellanne-Chantelot C, Pardini VC, Timsit J, *et al.* Identification of 14 new glucokinase mutations and description of the clinical profile of 42 MODY-2 families. *Diabetologia* 1997; **40**:217–224.

29 Yamagata K, Furuta H, Oda N, Kaisaki PJ, Menzel S, Cox NJ, *et al.* Mutations in the hepatocyte nuclear factor-4a gene in maturity-onset diabetes of the young (MODY1). *Nature* 1996; **384**:458–460.

30 Vaxillaire M, Boccio V, Philippi A, Vigouroux C, Terwilliger J, Passa P, *et al.* A gene for maturity onset diabetes of the young (MODY) maps to chromosome 12q. *Nat Genet* 1995; **9**:418–423.

31 Yamagata K, Oda N, Kaisaki PJ, Menzel S, Furuta H, Vaxillaire M, *et al.* Mutations in the hepatocyte nuclear factor-1α gene in maturity-onset diabetes of the young (MODY3). *Nature* 1996; **384**:455–458.

32 Stoffers DA, Ferrer J, Clarke WL, Habener JF. Early-onset type-II diabetes mellitus (MODY4) linked to IPF-1. *Nat Genet* 1997; **17**:138–139.

33 Stoffers DA, Zinkin NT, Stanojevic V, Clarke WL, Habener JF. Pancreatic agenesis attributable to a single nucleotide deletion in the human IPF-1 gene coding sequence. *Nat Genet* 1997; **15**:106–110.

34 Horikawa Y, Iwasaki N, Hara M, Furuta H, Hinokio Y, Cockburn BN, *et al.* Mutation in hepatocyte nuclear factor-1 beta gene (TCF2) associated with MODY. *Nat Genet* 1997; **17**:384–385.

35 Malecki MT, Jhala US, Antonellis A, Fields L, Doria A, Orban T, *et al.* Mutations in NEUROD1 are associated with the development of T2D mellitus. *Nat Genet* 1999; **23**:323–328.

36 Chevre JC, Hani EH, Boutin P, Vaxillaire M, Blanche H, Vionnet N, *et al.* Mutation screening in 18 Caucasian families suggest the existence of other MODY genes. *Diabetologia* 1998; **41**:1017–1023.

37 Frayling TM, Lindgren CM, Chevre JC, Menzel S, Wishart M, Benmezroua Y, *et al.* A genome-wide scan in families with maturity-onset diabetes of the young: evidence for further genetic heterogeneity. *Diabetes* 2003; **52**:872–881.

38 Kim SH, Ma X, Weremowicz S, Ercolino T, Pwers C, Mlynarski W, *et al.* Identification of a locus for maturity-onset diabetes of the young on chromosome 8p23. *Diabetes* 2004; **53**:1375–1384.

39 Frayling TM, Bulamn MP, Ellard S, Appleton M, Dronsfield MJ, Mackie AD, *et al.* Mutations in the hepatocyte nuclear factor-1a gene are a common cause of maturity-onset diabetes of the young in the UK. *Diabetes* 1997; **46**:720–725.

40 Chèvre JC, Hani EH, Boutin P, *et al.* Mutation screening of the hepatocyte nuclear factor-1a and -4a genes in MODY families: suggestion of the existence of at least a fourth MODY gene. *Diabetologia* 1997; **40**(Suppl 1):612, A157.

41 Lindner TH, Cockburn BN, Bell GI. Molecular genetics of MODY in Germany. *Diabetologia* 1999; **42**:121–123.

42 Costa A, Bescos M, Velho G, Chevre J, Vidal J, Sesmilo G, *et al.* Genetic and clinical characterisation of maturity-onset diabetes of the young in Spanish families. *Eur J Endocrinol* 2000; **142**:380–386.

43 Matschinsky FM. Glucokinase, glucose homeostasis, and diabetes mellitus. *Curr Diab Rep* 2005; **5**:171–176.

44 Pearson ER, Pruhova S, Tack CJ, Johansen A, Castleden HA, Lumb PJ, *et al.* Molecular genetics and phenotypic characteristics of MODY caused by hepatocyte nuclear factor 4alpha mutations in a large European collection. *Diabetologia* 2005; **48**:878–885.

45 Winckler W, Weedon MN, Graham RR, McCarroll SA, Purcell S, Almgren P, *et al.* Evaluation of common variants in the six known maturity-onset diabetes of the young (MODY) genes for association with T2D. *Diabetes* 2007; **56**:685–693.

46 Vaxillaire M, Veslot J, Dina C, Proenca C, Cauchi S, Charpentier G, *et al.* Impact of common T2D risk polymorphisms in the DESIR Prospective Study. *Diabetes* 2008; **57**:244–254.

47 Boutin P, Gresh L, Cisse A, Hara M, Bell G, Babu S, *et al.* Missense mutation Gly574Ser in the transcription factor HNF-1alpha is a marker of atypical diabetes mellitus in African-American children. *Diabetologia* 1999; **42**:380–381.

48 Iwasaki N, Oda N, Ogata M, Hara M, Hinokio Y, Oda Y, *et al.* Mutations in the hepatocyte nuclear factor-1a/MODY3 gene in Japanese subjects with early- and late-onset NIDDM. *Diabetes* 1997; **46**:1504–1508.

49 Triggs-Raine BL, Kirkpatrick RD, Kelly SL, Norquay LD, Cattini PA, Yamagata K, *et al.* HNF-1alpha G319S, a transactivation-deficient mutant, is associated with altered dynamics of diabetes onset in an Oji-Cree community. *Proc Natl Acad Sci U S A* 2002; **99**:4614–4619.

50 Holmkvist J, Cervin C, Lyssenko V, Winckler W, Anevski D, Cilio C, *et al.* Common variants in HNF-1 alpha and risk of T2D. *Diabetologia* 2006; **49**:2882–2891.

51 Hani EH, Stoffers DA, Chevre JC, Durand E, Stanojevic V, Dina C, *et al.* Defective mutations in the insulin promoter factor-1 (IPF-1) gene in late-onset T2D mellitus. *J Clin Invest* 1999; **104**:R41–48.

52 Love-Gregory LD, Wasson J, Ma J, Jin CH, Glaser B, Suarez BK, *et al.* A common polymorphism in the upstream promoter region of the hepatocyte nuclear factor-4α gene on chromosome 20q is associated with T2D and appears to contribute to the evidence for

linkage in an Ashkenazi Jewish population. *Diabetes* 2004; **53**:1134–1140.

53 Silander K, Mohlke KL, Scott LJ, Peck EC, Hollstein P, Skol AD, *et al.* Genetic variation near the hepatocyte nuclear factor-4alpha gene predicts susceptibility to T2D. *Diabetes* 2004; **53**:1141–1149.

54 Vaxillaire M, Dina C, Lobbens S, Dechaume A, Vasseur-Delannoy V, Helbecque N, *et al.* Effect of common polymorphisms in the HNF4α promoter on T2D susceptibility in the French Caucasian population. *Diabetologia* 2005; **48**:440–444.

55 Barroso I, Luan J, Wheeler E, Whittaker P, Wasson J, Zeggini E, *et al.* Population-specific risk of type 2 diabetes conferred by HNF4A P2 promoter variants: a lesson for replication studies. *Diabetes* 2008; **57**:3161–3165.

56 Gudmundsson J, Sulem P, Steinthorsdottir V, Bergthorsson JT, Thorleifsson G, Manolescu A, *et al.* Two variants on chromosome 17 confer prostate cancer risk, and the one in TCF2 protects against T2D. *Nat Genet* 2007; **39**:977–983.

57 Kasper JS, Giovannucci E. A meta-analysis of diabetes mellitus and the risk of prostate cancer. *Cancer Epidemiol Biomarkers Prev* 2006; **15**:2056–2062.

58 Domenech E, Gomez-Zaera M, Nunes V. Wolfram/DIDMOAD syndrome, a heterogenic and molecularly complex neurodegenerative disease. *Pediatr Endocrinol Rev* 2006; **3**:249–257.

59 Sparsø T, Andersen G, Albrechtsen A, Jorgensen T, Borch-Johnsen K, Sandbaek A, *et al.* Impact of polymorphisms in WFS1 on prediabetic phenotypes in a population-based sample of middle-aged people with normal and abnormal glucose regulation. *Diabetologia* 2008; **51**:1646–1652.

60 Sandhu MS, Weedon MN, Fawcett KA, Wasson J, Debenham SL, Daly A, *et al.* Common variants in WFS1 confer risk of T2D. *Nat Genet* 2007; **39**:951–953.

61 Hansen L, Pedersen O. Genetics of type 2 diabetes mellitus: status and perspectives. *Diabetes Obes Metab* 2005; **7**:122–135.

62 Haneda M, Polonsky KS, Bergenstal RM, Jaspan JB, Shoelson SE, Blix PM, *et al.* Familial hyperinsulinemia due to a structurally abnormal insulin: definition of an emerging new clinical syndrome. *N Engl J Med* 1984; **310**:1288–1294.

63 Olansky L, Welling C, Giddings S, Adler S, Bourey R, Dowse G, *et al.* A variant insulin promoter in non-insulin-dependent diabetes mellitus. *J Clin Invest* 1992; **89**:1596–1602.

64 Huxtable SJ, Saker PJ, Haddad L, Walker M, Frayling TM, Levy JC, *et al.* Analysis of parent–offspring trios provides evidence for linkage and association between the insulin gene and T2D mediated exclusively through paternally transmitted class III variable number tandem repeat alleles. *Diabetes* 2000; **49**:126–130.

65 Dunger DB, Ong KK, Huxtable SJ, Sherriff A, Woods KA, Ahmed ML, *et al.* Association of the INS VNTR with size at birth. ALSPAC Study Team. Avon Longitudinal Study of Pregnancy and Childhood. *Nat Genet* 1998; **19**:98–100.

66 Bennett ST, Lucassen AM, Gough SC, Powell EE, Undlien DE, Pritchard LE, *et al.* Susceptibility to human type 1 diabetes at IDDM2 is determined by tandem repeat variation at the insulin gene minisatellite locus. *Nat Genet* 1995; **9**:284–292.

67 Taylor SI. Lilly Lecture: Molecular mechanisms of insulin resistance: lessons from patients with mutations in the insulin-receptor gene. *Diabetes* 1992; **41**:1473–1490.

68 Kan M, Kanai F, Iida M, Jinnouchi H, Todaka M, Imanaka T, *et al.* Frequency of mutations of insulin receptor gene in Japanese patients with NIDDM. *Diabetes* 1995; **44**:1081–1086.

69 Flier JS. Lilly Lecture: Syndromes of insulin resistance: from patient to gene and back again. *Diabetes* 1992; **41**:1207–1219.

70 Almind K, Bjorbaek C, Vestergaard H, Hansen T, Echwald S, Pedersen O. Aminoacid polymorphisms of insulin receptor substrate-1 in non-insulin-dependent diabetes mellitus. *Lancet* 1993; **342**:828–832.

71 Hager J, Zouali H, Velho G, Froguel P. Insulin receptor substrate (*IRS-1*) gene polymorphisms in French NIDDM families. *Lancet* 1993; **342**:1430.

72 Hitman GA, Hawrami K, McCarthy MI, Viswanathan M, Snehalatha C, Ramachandran A, *et al.* Insulin receptor substrate-1 gene mutations in NIDDM: implications for the study of polygenic disease. *Diabetologia* 1995; **38**:481–486.

73 Ura S, Araki E, Kishikawa H, Shirotani T, Todaka M, Isami S, *et al.* Molecular scanning of the insulin receptor substrate-1 (*IRS-1*) gene in Japanese patients with NIDDM: identification of five novel polymorphisms. *Diabetologia* 1996; **39**:600–608.

74 Zeggini E, Parkinson J, Halford S, Owen KR, Frayling TM, Walker M, *et al.* Association studies of insulin receptor substrate 1 gene (*IRS1*) variants in type 2 diabetes samples enriched for family history and early age of onset. *Diabetes* 2004; **53**:3319–3322.

75 Florez JC, Sjögren M, Agapakis CM, Burtt NP, Almgren P, Lindblad U, *et al.* Association testing of common variants in the insulin receptor substrate-1 gene (*IRS1*) with type 2 diabetes. *Diabetologia* 2007; **50**:1209–1217.

76 Groop LC, Kankuri M, Schalin-Jantti C, Ekstrand A, Nikula-Ijäs P, Widén E, *et al.* Association between polymorphism of the glycogen synthase gene and non-insulin-dependent diabetes mellitus. *N Engl J Med* 1993; **328**:10–14.

77 Kuroyama H, Sanke T, Ohagi S, Furuta M, Furuta H, Nanjo K. Simple tandem repeat DNA polymorphism in the human glycogen synthase gene is associated with NIDDM in Japanese subjects. *Diabetologia* 1994; **37**:536–539.

78 Zouali H, Velho G, Froguel P. Polymorphism of the glycogen synthase gene and non-insulin-dependent diabetes mellitus. *N Engl J Med* 1993; **328**:1568.

79 Daimon M, Sato H, Oizumi T, Toriyama S, Saito T, Karasawa S, *et al.* Association of the PIK3C2G gene polymorphisms with type 2 DM in a Japanese population. *Biochem Biophys Res Commun* 2008; **365**:466–471.

80 Maddux BA, Sbraccia P, Kumakura S, Sasson S, Youngren J, Fisher A, *et al.* Membrane glycoprotein PC-1 and insulin resistance in non-insulin-dependent diabetes mellitus. *Nature* 1995; **373**:448–451.

81 Costanzo BV, Trischitta V, Di Paola R, Spampinato D, Pizzuti A, Vignere R, *et al.* The Q allele variant (GLN121) of membrane glycoprotein PC-1 interacts with the insulin receptor and inhibits insulin signaling more effectively than the common K allele variant (LYS121). *Diabetes* 2001; **50**:831–836.

82 Pizzuti A, Frittitta L, Argiolas A, Baratta R, Goldfine ID, Bozzali M, *et al.* A polymorphism (K121Q) of the human glycoprotein PC-1 gene coding region is strongly associated with insulin resistance. *Diabetes* 1999; **48**:1881–1884.

83 Bacci S, Ludovico O, Prudente S, Zhang YY, Di Paola R, Mangiacotti D, *et al.* The K121Q polymorphism of the ENPP1/PC-1 gene is associated with insulin resistance/atherogenic phenotypes, including earlier onset of type 2 diabetes and myocardial infarction. *Diabetes* 2005; **54**:3021–3025.

84 Bochenski J, Placha G, Wanic K, Malecki M, Sieradzki J, Warram JH, *et al.* New polymorphism of ENPP1 (PC-1) is associated with

increased risk of type 2 diabetes among obese individuals. *Diabetes* 2006; **55**:2626–2630.

85 Meyre D, Bouatia-Naji N, Tounian A, Samson C, Lecoeur C, Vatin V, *et al.* Variants of ENPP1 are associated with childhood and adult obesity and increase the risk of glucose intolerance and type 2 diabetes. *Nat Genet* 2005; **37**:863–867.

86 Böttcher Y, Körner A, Reinehr T, Enigk B, Kiess W, Stumvoll M, *et al.* ENPP1 variants and haplotypes predispose to early onset obesity and impaired glucose and insulin metabolism in German obese children. *J Clin Endocrinol Metab* 2006; **91**:4948–9852.

87 Barroso I, Luan J, Middelberg RP, Franks PW, Jakes RW, Clayton D, *et al.* Candidate gene association study in type 2 diabetes indicates a role for genes involved in beta-cell function as well as insulin action. *PLoS Biol* 2003; **1**:E20.

88 McAteer JB, Prudente S, Bacci S, Lyon HN, Hirschhorn JN, Trischitta V, *et al.* The ENPP1 K121Q polymorphism is associated with type 2 diabetes in European populations: evidence from an updated meta-analysis in 42,042 subjects. *Diabetes* 2008; **57**:1125–1130.

89 Barroso I, Gurnell M, Crowley VE, Agostini M, Schwabe JW, Soos MA, *et al.* Dominant negative mutations in human PPARγ associated with severe insulin resistance, diabetes mellitus and hypertension. *Nature* 1999; **402**:880–883.

90 Altshuler D, Hirschhorn JN, Klannemark M, Lindgren CM, Vohl MC, Nemesh J, *et al.* The common PPARγ Pro12Ala polymorphism is associated with decreased risk of T2D. *Nat Genet* 2000; **26**:76–80.

91 Stefan N, Fritsche A, Haring H, Stumvoll M. Effect of experimental elevation of free fatty acids on insulin secretion and insulin sensitivity in healthy carriers of the Pro12Ala polymorphism of the peroxisome proliferator-activated receptor-γ2 gene. *Diabetes* 2001; **50**:1143–1148.

92 Florez JC, Jablonski KA, Sun MW, Bayley N, Kahn SE, Shamoon H, *et al.* Effects of the type 2 diabetes-associated PPARG P12A polymorphism on progression to diabetes and response to troglitazone. *J Clin Endocrinol Metab* 2007; **92**:1502–1509.

93 Ek J, Andersen G, Urhammer SA, Gaede PH, Drivsholm T, Borch-Johnsen K, *et al.* Mutation analysis of peroxisome proliferator-activated receptor-gamma coactivator-1 (PGC-1) and relationships of identified amino acid polymorphisms to type II diabetes mellitus. *Diabetologia* 2001; **44**:2220–2226.

94 Hansen L, Hansen T, Vestergaard H, Bjorbaek C, Echwald SM, Clausen JO, *et al.* A widespread amino acid polymorphism at codon 905 of the glycogen-associated regulatory subunit of protein phosphatase-1 is associated with insulin resistance and hypersecretion of insulin. *Hum Mol Genet* 1995; **4**:1313–1320.

95 Baier LJ, Sacchettini JC, Knowler WC, Eads J, Paolisso G, Tataranni PA, *et al.* An amino acid substitution in the human intestinal fatty acid binding protein is associated with increased fatty acid binding, increased fat oxidation, and insulin resistance. *J Clin Invest* 1995; **95**:1281–1287.

96 Echwald SM, Bach H, Vestergaard H, Richelsen B, Kristensen K, Drivsholm T, *et al.* A P387L variant in protein tyrosine phosphatase-1B (PTP-1B) is associated with T2D and impaired serine phosphorylation of PTP-1B *in vitro*. *Diabetes* 2002; **51**:1–6.

97 Bento JL, Palmer ND, Mychaleckyj JC, Langefeld CD, Campbell JK, Norris JM, *et al.* Association of protein tyrosine phosphatase 1B gene polymorphisms with T2D. *Diabetes* 2004; **53**:3007–3012.

98 Cheyssac C, Lecoeur C, Dechaume A, Bibi A, Charpentier G, Balkau B, *et al.* Analysis of common PTPN1 gene variants in type 2 diabetes, obesity and associated phenotypes in the French population. *BMC Med Genet* 2006; **7**:44.

99 Neve B, Fernandez-Zapico ME, Ashkenazi-Katalan V, Dina C, Hamid YH, Joly E, *et al.* Role of transcription factor KLF11 and its diabetes-associated gene variants in pancreatic beta cell function. *Proc Natl Acad Sci U S A* 2005; **102**:4807–4812.

100 Florez JC, Saxena R, Winckler W, Burtt NP, Almgren P, Bengtsson Boström K, *et al.* The Krüppel-like factor 11 (KLF11) Q62R polymorphism is not associated with type 2 diabetes in 8,676 people. *Diabetes* 2006; **55**:3620–3624.

101 Rane SG, Lee JH, Lin HM. Transforming growth factor-beta pathway: role in pancreas development and pancreatic disease. *Cytokine Growth Factor Rev* 2006; **17**:107–119.

102 Waeber G, Delplanque J, Bonny C, Mooser V, Steinmann M, Widmann C, *et al.* The gene MAPK8IP1, encoding islet-brain-1, is a candidate for T2D. *Nat Genet* 2000; **24**:291–295.

103 Ling Z, Van de Casteele M, Dong J, Heimberg H, Haeflinger JA, Waeber G, *et al.* Variations in IB1/JIP1 expression regulate susceptibility of beta-cells to cytokine-induced apoptosis irrespective of C-Jun NH2-terminal kinase signaling. *Diabetes* 2003; **52**:2497–2502.

104 Dukes ID, Philipson LH. K channels: generating excitement in pancreatic beta-cells. *Diabetes* 1996; **45**:845–853.

105 Inagaki N, Gonoi T, Clement JP, Namba N, Inazawa J, Gonzalez G, *et al.* Reconstitution of IKATP. an inward rectifier subunit plus the sulfonylurea receptor. *Science* 1995; **270**:1166–1170.

106 Ashcroft FM, Gribble FM. ATP-sensitive K channels and insulin secretion: their role in health and disease. *Diabetologia* 1999; **42**:903–919.

107 Inoue H, Ferrer J, Welling CM, Elbein SC, Hoffman M, Mayorga R, *et al.* Sequence variants in the sulfonylurea receptor (SUR) gene are associated with NIDDM in Caucasians. *Diabetes* 1996; **45**:825–831.

108 Hani EH, Clement K, Velho G, Vionnet N, Hager J, Philippi A, *et al.* Genetic studies of the sulfonylurea receptor gene locus in NIDDM and in morbid obesity among French Caucasians. *Diabetes* 1997; **46**:688–694.

109 Hani EH, Boutin P, Durand E, Inoue H, Permutt MA, Velho G, *et al.* Missense mutations in the pancreatic islet beta cell inwardly rectifying K^+ channel gene (KIR6.2/BIR): a meta-analysis suggests a role in the polygenic basis of type II diabetes mellitus in Caucasians. *Diabetologia* 1998; **41**:1511–1515.

110 Hansen T, Echwald SM, Hansen L, Moller AM, Almind K, Clausen JO, *et al.* Decreased tolbutamide-stimulated insulin secretion in healthy subjects with sequence variants in the high-affinity sulfonylurea receptor gene. *Diabetes* 1998; **47**:598–605.

111 Ohta Y, Tanizawa Y, Inoue H, Hosaka T, Ueda K, Matsutani A, *et al.* Identification and functional analysis of sulfonylurea receptor 1 variants in Japanese patients with NIDDM. *Diabetes* 1998; **47**:476–481.

112 Hart LM, de Knijff P, Dekker JM, Stolk RP, Nijpels G, van der Does FE, *et al.* Variants in the sulphonylurea receptor gene: association of the exon 16–3t variant with type II diabetes mellitus in Dutch Caucasians. *Diabetologia* 1999; **42**:617–620.

113 Riedel MJ, Steckley DC, Light PE. Current status of the E23K Kir6.2 polymorphism: implications for type-2 diabetes. *Hum Genet* 2005; **116**:133–145.

114 Nielsen EM, Hansen L, Carstensen B, Echwald SM, Drivsholm T, Glümer C, *et al.* The E23K variant of Kir6.2 associates with impaired

post-OGTT serum insulin response and increased risk of T2D. *Diabetes* 2003; **52**:573–577.

115 van Dam RM, Hoebee B, Seidell JC, Schaap MM, de Bruin TW, Feskens EJ. Common variants in the ATP-sensitive K+ channel genes KCNJ11 (Kir6.2) and ABCC8 (SUR1) in relation to glucose intolerance: population-based studies and meta-analyses. *Diabet Med* 2005; **22**:590–598.

116 Spranger J, Kroke A, Mohlig M, Hoffmann K, Bergmann MM, Ristow M, *et al.* Inflammatory cytokines and the risk to develop type 2 diabetes: results of the prospective population-based European Prospective Investigation into Cancer and Nutrition (EPIC)-Potsdam Study. *Diabetes* 2003; **52**:812–817.

117 Vozarova B, Fernandez-Real JM, Knowler WC, Gallart L, Hanson RL, Gruber JD, *et al.* The interleukin-6 (-174) G/C promoter polymorphism is associated with type-2 diabetes mellitus in Native Americans and Caucasians. *Hum Genet* 2003; **112**:409–413.

118 Kubaszek A, Pihlajamaki J, Komarovski V, Lindi V, Lindström J, Eriksson J, *et al.* Promoter polymorphisms of the TNF-alpha (G-308A) and IL-6 (C-174G) genes predict the conversion from impaired glucose tolerance to type 2 diabetes: the Finnish Diabetes Prevention Study. *Diabetes* 2003; **52**:1872–1876.

119 Huth C, Heid IM, Vollmert C, Gieger C, Grallert H, Wolford JK, *et al.* IL6 gene promoter polymorphisms and type 2 diabetes: joint analysis of individual participants' data from 21 studies. *Diabetes* 2006; **55**:2915–2921.

120 Hamid YH, Urhammer SA, Jensen DP, Glümer C, Borch-Johnsen K, Jorgensen T, *et al.* Variation in the interleukin-6 receptor gene associates with type 2 diabetes in Danish whites. *Diabetes* 2004; **53**:3342–3345.

121 Davies JL, Kawaguchi Y, Bennett ST, Copeman JB, Cordell HJ, Pritchard LE, *et al.* A genome-wide search for human type 1 diabetes susceptibility genes. *Nature* 1994; **371**:130–136.

122 Duggirala R, Blangero J, Almasy L, Arya R, Dyer TD, Williams KL, *et al.* A major locus for fasting insulin concentrations and insulin resistance on chromosome 6q with strong pleiotropic effects on obesity-related phenotypes in nondiabetic Mexican Americans. *Am J Hum Genet* 2001; **68**:1149–1164.

123 McCarthy MI. Growing evidence for diabetes susceptibility genes from genome scan data. *Curr Diab Rep* 2003; **3**:159–167.

124 Cox NJ, Frigge M, Nicolae DL, Concannon P, Hanis CL, Bell GI, *et al.* Loci on chromosomes 2 (NIDDM1) and 15 interact to increase susceptibility to diabetes in Mexican Americans. *Nat Genet* 1999; **21**:213–215.

125 Vionnet N, Hani EH, Dupont S, Gallina S, Francke S, Dotte S, *et al.* Genomewide search for T2D-susceptibility genes in French whites: evidence for a novel susceptibility locus for early-onset diabetes on chromosome 3q27-qter and independant replication of a type 2-diabetes locus on chromosome 1q21-q24. *Am J Hum Genet* 2000; **67**:1470–1480.

126 Kissebah AH, Sonnenberg GE, Myklebust J, Goldstein M, Broman K, James RG, *et al.* Quantitative trait loci on chromosomes 3 and 17 influence phenotypes of the metabolic syndrome. *Proc Natl Acad Sci U S A* 2000; **97**:14478–1483.

127 Mori Y, Otabe S, Dina C, Yasuda K, Populaire C, Lecoeur C, *et al.* Genome-wide search for T2D in Japanese affected sib-pairs confirms susceptibility genes on 3q, 15q, and 20q and identifies two new candidate loci on 7p and 11p. *Diabetes* 2002; **51**:1247–1255.

128 Duggirala R, Blangero J, Almasy L, Dyer TD, Williams KL, Leach RJ, *et al.* Linkage of T2D mellitus and of age at onset to a genetic location on chromosome 10q in Mexican Americans. *Am J Hum Genet* 1999; **64**:1127–1140.

129 Norman RA, Tataranni PA, Pratley R, Thompson DB, Hanson RL, Prochazka M, *et al.* Autosomal genomic scan for loci linked to obesity and energy metabolism in Pima Indians. *Am J Hum Genet* 1998; **62**:659–668.

130 Ji L, Malecki M, Warram JH, Yang Y, Rich SS, Krolewski AS. New susceptibility locus for NIDDM is localized to human chromosome 20q. *Diabetes* 1997; **46**:876–881.

131 Zouali H, Hani EH, Philippi A, Vionnet N, Beckmann JS, Demenais F, *et al.* A susceptibility locus for early-onset non-insulin dependent (type 2) diabetes mellitus maps to chromosome 20q, proximal to the phosphoenolpyruvate carboxykinase gene. *Hum Mol Genet* 1997; **6**:1401–1408.

132 Kissebah AH, Sonnenberg GE, Myklebust J, Goldstein M, Broman K, James RG, *et al.* Quantitative trait loci on chromosomes 3 and 17 influence phenotypes of the metabolic syndrome. *Proc Natl Acad Sci U S A* 2000; **97**:14478–14483.

133 Demenais F, Kanninen T, Lindgren CM, Wiltshire S, Gaget S, Dandrieux C, *et al.* A meta-analysis of four European genome screens (GIFT Consortium) shows evidence for a novel region on chromosome 17p11.2-q22 linked to T2D. *Hum Mol Genet* 2003; **12**:1865–1873.

134 Terwilliger JD, Weiss KM. Linkage disequilibrium mapping of complex disease: fantasy or reality? *Curr Opin Biotechnol* 1998; **9**:578–594.

135 Zollner S, Von Haeseler A. A coalescent approach to study linkage disequilibrium between single-nucleotide polymorphisms. *Am J Hum Genet* 2000; **66**:615–628.

136 Abecasis GR, Noguchi E, Heinzmann A, Traherne JA, Bhattacharyya S, Leaves NI, *et al.* Extent and distribution of linkage disequilibrium in three genomic regions. *Am J Hum Genet* 2001; **68**:191–197.

137 Eaves IA, Merriman TR, Barber RA, Nutland S, Tuomilehto-Wolf E, Tuomilehto J, *et al.* The genetically isolated populations of Finland and Sardinia may not be a panacea for linkage disequilibrium mapping of common disease genes. *Nat Genet* 2000; **25**:320–323.

138 Horikawa Y, Oda N, Cox NJ, Li X, Orho-Melander M, Hara M, *et al.* Genetic variation in the gene encoding calpain-10 is associated with T2D mellitus. *Nat Genet* 2000; **26**:163–175.

139 Tsuchiya T, Schwarz PE, Bosque-Plata LD, Geoffrey Haynes M, Dina C, Froquel P, *et al.* Association of the calpain-10 gene with T2D in Europeans: results of pooled and meta-analyses. *Mol Genet Metab* 2006; **89**:174–184.

140 Turner MD, Cassell PG, Hitman GA. Calpain-10: from genome search to function. *Diabetes Metab Res Rev* 2005; **21**:505–514.

141 Marshall C, Hitman GA, Partridge CJ, Clark A, Ma H, Shearer TR, *et al.* Evidence that an isoform of calpain-10 is a regulator of exocytosis in pancreatic beta-cells. *Mol Endocrinol.* 2005; **19**:213–224.

142 Wallace KJ, Wallis RH, Collins SC, Argoud K, Laisaki PJ, Kyorza A, *et al.* Quantitative trait locus dissection in congenic strains of the Goto-Kakizaki rat identifies a region conserved with diabetes loci in human chromosome 1q. *Physiol Genomics* 2004; **19**:1–10.

143 Zeggini E, Damcott CM, Hanson RL, Karim MA, Rayner NW, Groves CJ, *et al.* Variation within the gene encoding the upstream stimulatory factor 1 does not influence susceptibility to type 2 diabetes in samples from populations with replicated evidence of linkage to chromosome 1q. *Diabetes* 2006; **55**:2541–2548.

144 Silander K, Mohlke KL, Scott LJ, Peck EC, Hollstein P, Skol AD, *et al.* Genetic variation near the hepatocyte nuclear factor-4 alpha

gene predicts susceptibility to type 2 diabetes. *Diabetes* 2004; **53**:1141–1149.

145 Love-Gregory LD, Wasson J, Ma J, Jin CH, Glaser B, Suarez BK, *et al.* A common polymorphism in the upstream promoter region of the hepatocyte nuclear factor-4α gene on chromosome 20q is associated with T2D and appears to contribute to the evidence for linkage in an Ashkenazi Jewish population. *Diabetes* 2004; **53**:1134–1140.

146 Barroso I, Luan J, Wheeler E, Whittaker P, Wasson J, Zeggini E, *et al.* Population-specific risk of T2D conferred by HNF4A P2 promoter variants: a lesson for replication studies. *Diabetes* 2008; **57**:3161–3165.

147 Comuzzie AG, Hixson JE, Almasy L, Mitchell BD, Mahaney MC, Dyer TD, *et al.* A major quantitative trait locus determining serum leptin levels and fat mass is located on human chromosome 2. *Nat Genet* 1997; **15**:273–276.

148 Fruebis J, Tsao T, Javorschi S, Ebbets-Reed D, Erickson MR, Yen FT, *et al.* Proteolytic cleavage product of 30-kDa adipocyte complement-related protein increases fatty acid oxidation in muscle and causes weight loss in mice. *Proc Natl Acad Sci U S A* 2001; **98**:2005–2010.

149 Arita Y, Kihara S, Ouchi N, Takahashi M, Maede K, Miyagawa J, *et al.* Paradoxical decrease of an adipose-specific protein, adiponectin, in obesity. *Biochem Biophys Res Commun* 1999; **257**:79–83.

150 Cheyssac C, Dina C, Leprêtre F, Vasseur-Delannov V, Dechaume A, Lobbens S, *et al.* EIF4A2 is a positional candidate gene at the 3q27 locus linked to type 2 diabetes in French families. *Diabetes* 2006; **55**:1171–1176.

151 Grant SF, Thorleifsson G, Reynisdottir I, Benediktsson R, Manolescu A, Sainz J, *et al.* Variant of transcription factor 7-like 2 (TCF7L2) gene confers risk of type 2 diabetes. *Nat Genet* 2006; **38**:320–323.

152 Cauchi S, Froguel P. TCF7L2 genetic defect and type 2 diabetes. *Curr Diab Rep* 2008; **8**:149–155.

153 Cauchi S, El Achhab Y, Choquet H, Dina C, Krempler F, Weitgasser R, *et al.* TCF7L2 is reproducibly associated with type 2 diabetes in various ethnic groups: a global meta-analysis. *J Mol Med* 2007; **85**:777–782.

154 Chang YC, Chang TJ, Jiang YD, Kuo SS, Lee KC, Chiu KC, *et al.* Association study of the genetic polymorphisms of the transcription factor 7-like 2 (TCF7L2) gene and type 2 diabetes in the Chinese population. *Diabetes* 2007; **56**:2631–2637.

155 Florez JC, Jablonski KA, Bayley N, Pollin TI, de Bakker PI, Shuldiner AR, *et al.* TCF7L2 polymorphisms and progression to diabetes in the Diabetes Prevention Program. *N Engl J Med* 2006; **355**:241–250.

156 Cauchi S, Choquet H, Gutiérrez-Aguilar R, Capel F, Grau K, Proenca C, *et al.* Effects of TCF7L2 polymorphisms on obesity in European populations. *Obesity* 2008; **16**:476–482.

157 Watanabe RM, Allayee H, Xiang AH, Trigo E, Hartiala J, Lawrence JM, *et al.* Transcription factor 7-like 2 (TCF7L2) is associated with gestational diabetes mellitus and interacts with adiposity to alter insulin secretion in Mexican Americans. *Diabetes* 2007; **56**:1481–1485.

158 Slattery ML, Folsom AR, Wolff R, Herrick J, Caan BJ, Potter JD. Transcription factor 7-like 2 polymorphism and colon cancer. *Cancer Epidemiol Biomarkers Prev* 2008; **17**:978–982.

159 Cauchi S, Vaxillaire M, Choquet H, Durand E, Duval A, Polak M, *et al.* No major contribution of TCF7L2 sequence variants to maturity onset of diabetes of the young (MODY) or neonatal diabetes mellitus in French white subjects. *Diabetologia* 2007; **50**:214–216.

160 Yi F, Brubaker PL, Jin T. TCF-4 mediates cell type-specific regulation of proglucagon gene expression by beta-catenin and glycogen synthase kinase-3beta. *J Biol Chem* 2005; **280**:1457–1464.

161 Lyssenko V, Lupi R, Marchetti P, Del Guerra S, Orho-Melander M, Almgren P, *et al.* Mechanisms by which common variants in the TCF7L2 gene increase risk of type 2 diabetes. *J Clin Invest* 2007; **117**:2155–2163.

162 Schafer SA, Tschritter O, Machicao F, Thamer C, Stefan N, Gallwitz B, *et al.* Impaired glucagon-like peptide-1-induced insulin secretion in carriers of transcription factor 7-like 2 (TCF7L2) gene polymorphisms. *Diabetologia* 2007; **50**:2443–2450.

163 Liu Z, Habener JF. Glucagon-like peptide-1 activation of TCF7L2-dependent Wnt signaling enhances pancreatic beta cell proliferation. *J Biol Chem* 2008; **283**:8723–8735.

164 Shu L, Sauter NS, Schulthess FT, Matveyenko AV, Oberholzer J, Maedler K. Transcription factor 7-like 2 regulates beta-cell survival and function in human pancreatic islets. *Diabetes* 2008; **57**:645–653.

165 Elbein SC, Chu WS, Das SK, Yao-Borengasser A, Hasstedt SJ, Wang H, *et al.* Transcription factor 7-like 2 polymorphisms and type 2 diabetes, glucose homeostasis traits and gene expression in US participants of European and African descent. *Diabetologia* 2007; **50**:1621–1630.

166 da Silva Xavier G, Loder MK, McDonald A, Tarasov AI, Carzaniga R, Kronenberger K, *et al.* TCF7L2 regulates late events in insulin secretion from pancreatic islet β-cells. *Diabetes* 2009; **58**:894–905.

167 Manolio TA, Brooks LD, Collins FS. A HapMap harvest of insights into the genetics of common disease. *J Clin Invest* 2008; **118**:1590–1605.

168 Chimienti F, Devergnas S, Favier A, Seve M. Identification and cloning of a beta-cell-specific zinc transporter, ZnT-8, localized into insulin secretory granules. *Diabetes* 2004; **53**:2330–2337.

169 Chimienti F, Devergnas S, Pattou F, Schuit F, Garcia-Cuenca R, Vandewalle B, *et al.* *In vivo* expression and functional characterization of the zinc transporter ZnT8 in glucose-induced insulin secretion. *J Cell Sci* 2006; **119**:4199–4206.

170 Wenzlau JM, Moua O, Sarkar SA, Yu L, Rewers M, Eisenbarth GS, *et al.* SlC30A8 is a major target of humoral autoimmunity in type 1 diabetes and a predictive marker in prediabetes. *Ann N Y Acad Sci* 2008; **1150**:256–259.

171 Pascoe L, Tura A, Patel SK, Ibrahim IM, Ferrannini E, Zeggini E, *et al.* Common variants of the novel type 2 diabetes genes CDKAL1 and HHEX/IDE are associated with decreased pancreatic beta-cell function. *Diabetes* 2007; **56**:3101–3104.

172 Steinthorsdottir V, Thorleifsson G, Reynisdottir I, Benediktsson R, Jonsdottir T, Walters GB, *et al.* A variant in CDKAL1 influences insulin response and risk of type 2 diabetes. *Nat Genet* 2007; **39**:770–775.

173 Palmer ND, Goodarzi MO, Langefeld CD, Ziegler J, Norris JM, Haffner SM, *et al.* Quantitative trait analysis of type 2 diabetes susceptibility loci identified from whole genome association studies in the Insulin Resistance Atherosclerosis Family Study. *Diabetes* 2008; **57**:1093–1100.

174 Zeggini E, Scott LJ, Saxena R, Voight BF, Marchini JL, Hu T, *et al.* Meta-analysis of genome-wide association data and large-scale replication identifies additional susceptibility loci for type 2 diabetes. *Nat Genet* 2008; **40**:638–645.

175 Krarup N, Andersen G, Krarup NT, Albrechtsen A, Schmitz O, Jørgensen T, *et al.* Association testing of novel type 2 diabetes risk

alleles in the JAZF1, CDC123/CAMK1D, TSPAN8, THADA, ADAMTS9, and NOTCH2 loci with insulin release, insulin sensitivity, and obesity in a population-based sample of 4,516 glucose-tolerant middle-aged Danes. *Diabetes* 2008; **57**:2534–2540.

176 Frayling TM, Colhoun H, Florez JC. A genetic link between type 2 diabetes and prostate cancer. *Diabetologia* 2008; **51**:1757–1760.

177 Thomas G, Jacobs KB, Yeager M, Kraft P, Wacholder S, Orr N, *et al.* Multiple loci identified in a genome-wide association study of prostate cancer. *Nat Genet* 2008, **40**:310–315.

178 Tirosh A, Shai I, Tekes-Manova D, Pereg D, Shochat T, Kochba I, *et al.* Normal fasting plasma glucose levels and type 2 diabetes in young men. *N Engl J Med* 2005; **353**:1454–1462.

179 Mason CC, Hanson RL, Knowler WC. Progression to type 2 diabetes characterized by moderate then rapid glucose increases. *Diabetes* 2007; **56**:2054–2061.

180 Bouatia-Naji N, Rocheleau G, Van Lommel L, Lemaire K, Schuit F, Cavalcanti-Proenca C, *et al.* A polymorphism within the G6PC2 gene is associated with fasting plasma glucose levels. *Science* 2008; **320**:1085–1088.

181 Bouatia-Naji N, Bonnefond A, Cavalcanti-Proenca C, Sparsø T, Holmkvist J, Marchand M, *et al.* A variant near MTNR1B is associated with increased fasting plasma glucose levels and type 2 diabetes risk. *Nat Genet* 2009; **41**:89–94.

182 Prokopenko I, Langenberg C, Florez JC, Saxena R, Soranzo N, Thorleifsson G, *et al.* Variants in MTNR1B influence fasting glucose levels. *Nat Genet* 2009; **41**:77–81.

183 Lyssenko V, Nagorny CL, Erdos MR, Wierup N, Jonsson A, Spégel P, *et al.* Common variant in MTNR1B associated with increased risk of type 2 diabetes and impaired early insulin secretion. *Nat Genet* 2009; **41**:82–88.

184 Staiger H, Machicao F, Schäfer SA, Kirchhoff K, Kantartzis K, Guthoff M, *et al.* Polymorphisms within the novel type 2 diabetes risk locus MTNR1B determine beta-cell function. *PLoS ONE* 2008; **3**:e3962.

185 Ramracheya RD, Muller DS, Squires PE, Brereton H, Sugden D, Huang GC, *et al.* Function and expression of melatonin receptors on human pancreatic islets. *J Pineal Res* 2008; **44**:273–279.

186 Paré G, Chasman DI, Parker AN, Nathan DM, Miletich JP, Zee RY, *et al.* Novel association of HK1 with glycated hemoglobin in a non-diabetic population: a genome-wide evaluation of 14,618 participants in the Women's Genome Health Study. *PLoS Genet* 2008; **4**:e1000312.

187 Pilia G, Chen WM, Scuteri A, Orru M, Albai G, Dei M, *et al.* Heritability of cardiovascular and personality traits in 6148 Sardinians. *PLoS Genet* 2006; **2**:e132.

188 Kathiresan S, Musunuru K, Orho-Melander M. Defining the spectrum of alleles that contribute to blood lipid concentrations in humans. *Curr Opin Lipidol* 2008; **19**:122–127.

189 Kathiresan S, Melander O, Guiducci C, Surti A, Burtt NP, Rieder MJ, *et al.* Six new loci associated with blood low-density lipoprotein cholesterol, high-density lipoprotein cholesterol or triglycerides in humans. *Nat Genet* 2008; **40**:189–197.

190 Aulchenko YS, Ripatti S, Lindqvist I, Boomsma D, Heid IM, Pramstaller PP, *et al.* Loci influencing lipid levels and coronary heart disease risk in 16 European population cohorts. *Nat Genet* 2009; **41**:47–55.

191 Kathiresan S, Willer CJ, Peloso GM, Demissie S, Musunuru K, Schadt EE, *et al.* Common variants at 30 loci contribute to polygenic dyslipidemia. *Nat Genet* 2009; **41**:56–65.

192 Weedon MN, McCarthy MI, Hitman G, Walker M, Groves CJ, Zeggini E, *et al.* Combining information from common type 2 diabetes risk polymorphisms improves disease prediction. *PLoS Med* 2006; **3**:e374.

193 Cauchi S, Meyre D, Durand E, Proença C, Marre M, Hadjadj S, *et al.* Post genome-wide association studies of novel genes associated with type 2 diabetes show gene–gene interaction and high predictive value. *PlosOne* 2008; **3**:e2031.

194 Meigs JB, Shrader P, Sullivan LM, McAteer JB, Fox CS, Dupuis J, *et al.* Genotype score in addition to common risk factors for prediction of type 2 diabetes. *N Engl J Med* 2008; **359**:2208–2219.

195 Balkau B, Lange C, Fezeu L, Tichet J, de Lauzon-Guillain B, Czernichow S, *et al.* Predicting diabetes: clinical, biological, and genetic approaches: data from the Epidemiological Study on the Insulin Resistance Syndrome (DESIR). *Diabetes Care* 2008; **31**:2056–2061.

196 Lyssenko V, Jonsson A, Almgren P, Pulizzi N, Isomaa B, Tuomi T, *et al.* Clinical risk factors, DNA variants, and the development of type 2 diabetes. *N Engl J Med* 2008; **359**:2220–2232.

197 Snitker S, Watanabe RM, Ani I, Xiang AH, Marroquin A, Ochoa C, *et al.* Changes in insulin sensitivity in response to troglitazone do not differ between subjects with and without the common, functional Pro12Ala peroxisome proliferator-activated receptor-gamma2 gene variant: results from the Troglitazone in Prevention of Diabetes (TRIPOD) study. *Diabetes Care* 2004; **27**:1365–1368.

198 Florez JC, Jablonski KA, Sun MW, Bayley N, Kahn SE, Shamoon H, *et al.* Effects of the type 2 diabetes-associated PPARG P12A polymorphism on progression to diabetes and response to troglitazone. *J Clin Endocrinol Metab* 2007; **92**:1502–1509.

199 Sesti G, Laratta E, Cardellini M, Andreozzi F, Del Guerra S, Irace C, *et al.* The E23K variant of KCNJ11 encoding the pancreatic beta-cell adenosine 5′-triphosphate-sensitive potassium channel subunit Kir6.2 is associated with an increased risk of secondary failure to sulfonylurea in patients with type 2 diabetes. *J Clin Endocrinol Metab* 2006; **91**:2334–2339.

200 Gloyn AL, Hashim Y, Ashcroft SJ, Ashfield R, Wiltshire S, Turner RC, *et al.* Association studies of variants in promoter and coding regions of beta-cell ATP-sensitive K-channel genes SUR1 and Kir6.2 with type 2 diabetes mellitus (UKPDS 53). *Diabetes Med* 2001; **18**:206–212.

201 Florez JC, Jablonski KA, Kahn SE, Franks PW, Dabelea D, Hamman RF, *et al.* Type 2 diabetes-associated missense polymorphisms KCNJ11 E23K and ABCC8 A1369S influence progression to diabetes and response to interventions in the Diabetes Prevention Program. *Diabetes* 2007; **56**:531–536.

202 Kimber CH, Doney AS, Pearson ER, McCarthy MI, Hattersley AT, Leese GP, *et al.* TCF7L2 in the Go-DARTS study: evidence for a gene dose effect on both diabetes susceptibility and control of glucose levels. *Diabetologia* 2007; **50**:1186–1191.

203 Pearson ER, Donnelly LA, Kimber C, Whitley A, Doney AS, McCarthy MI, *et al.* Variation in TCF7L2 influences therapeutic response to sulfonylureas: a GoDARTs study. *Diabetes* 2007; **56**:2178–2182.

204 Florez JC, Jablonski KA, Bayley N, Pollin TI, de Bakker PI, Shuldiner AR, *et al.* TCF7L2 polymorphisms and progression to diabetes in the Diabetes Prevention Program. *N Engl J Med* 2006; **355**:241–250.

205 Shu Y, Sheardown SA, Brown C, Owen RP, Zhang S, Castro RA, *et al.* Effect of genetic variation in the organic cation transporter 1 (OCT1) on metformin action. *J Clin Invest* 2007; **117**:1422–1431.

206 Lillioja S, Wilton A. Agreement among type 2 diabetes linkage studies but a poor correlation with results from genome-wide association studies. *Diabetologia* 2009; **52**:1061–1074.

207 Yasuda K, Miyake K, Horikawa Y, Hara K, Osawa H, Furuta H, *et al.* Variants in KCNQ1 are associated with susceptibility to type 2 diabetes mellitus. *Nat Genet* 2008; **40**:1092–1097.

208 Unoki H, Takahashi A, Kawaguchi T, Hara K, Horikoshi M, Andersen G, *et al.* SNPs in KCNQ1 are associated with susceptibility to type 2 diabetes in East Asian and European populations. *Nat Genet* 2008; **40**:1098–1102.

13 Metabolic Disturbances in Diabetes

Adrian Vella & Robert A. Rizza

Department of Internal Medicine, Division of Diabetes, Nutrition, Endocrinology & Metabolism, Mayo Clinic, Rochester, MN, USA

Keypoints

- Type 1 diabetes is an immune-mediated disorder that leads to destruction of the islets of Langerhans causing profound insulin deficiency.
- Metabolic changes observed in type 1 diabetes are secondary to insulin deficiency interacting with environmental influences such as diet and exercise.
- The pathogenesis of type 2 diabetes mellitus is complex and incompletely understood. It appears to be caused by an interaction of genetic and environmental factors that lead to defects in insulin secretion, insulin action and glucose effectiveness.

Introduction

Hyperglycemia, for better or for worse [1], is the metabolic abnormality that has been used to define the presence of, and characterize, diabetes. Diabetes comprises a heterogeneous group of disorders characterized by fasting and/or post-prandial hyperglycemia. The underlying abnormalities that lead to the development of hyperglycemia, however, differ amongst subgroups. Conventionally, diabetes has been categorized into two subgroups that, from a metabolic standpoint, differ in the degree of insulin deficiency present. This broad dichotomy is simplistic as a given patient may exhibit metabolic abnormalities previously considered unique to each category [2].

Type 1 (T1DM), or immune-mediated diabetes, is characterized by evidence of immune-mediated destruction of the insulin-secreting β-cells in the islets of Langerhans. Usually this leads to absolute insulin deficiency, which is insufficient to prevent unrestrained lipolysis during systemic illness or severe physical stress. In type 2 diabetes (T2DM), however, although the endocrine pancreas can produce insulin, secretion and circulating concentrations of insulin are inappropriate for the prevailing glucose concentrations. T2DM has traditionally been considered a disorder of insulin signaling (exacerbated by poor diet, obesity and lack of physical activity) rather than a deficiency of insulin.

It is important to remember that obese patients with T1DM can behave in a fashion similar to patients with long-standing T2DM and that metabolic differences between the two categories may be more imagined than real.

Textbook of Diabetes, 4th edition. Edited by R. Holt, C. Cockram, A. Flyvbjerg and B. Goldstein.

Carbohydrate metabolism

In the fasting state, glucose appearance is determined by the rate of endogenous glucose release from the liver and to a lesser extent the kidney. This is collectively referred to as endogenous glucose production. Glucose concentrations increase when glucose appearance exceeds glucose disappearance and continues to increase until these rates are equal. In humans without diabetes, glucose concentrations average 4.5–5.5 mmol/L following a 6–12-hour overnight fast.

Gluconeogenesis is responsible for approximately 50–60% of endogenous glucose production following an overnight fast, with the proportion increasing with increasing duration of the fast [3]. Gluconeogenesis utilizes three-carbon precursors such as lactate, alanine and glycerol to synthesize glucose molecules.

Following an overnight fast, approximately 80% of glucose disposal is insulin independent and occurs in the brain, splanchnic tissues and erythrocytes [4]. The majority of insulin-mediated glucose disposal occurs in muscle [5]. Because insulin levels are low in the post-absorptive state, muscle predominantly uses free fatty acids (FFA) for fuel [6]. In the presence of low insulin concentrations, glucose taken up by tissues predominantly is oxidized or undergoes glycolysis to release alanine and lactate which can be re-utilized by the liver for gluconeogenesis [7].

Sensitivity to insulin varies amongst tissues. Low concentrations of insulin limit lipolysis and prevent unrestrained breakdown of fat. The insulin concentrations sufficient to prevent lipolysis are insufficient to stimulate significant muscle glucose uptake. Whereas maximal suppression of endogenous glucose production occurs at insulin concentrations of approximately 250 pmol/L, these concentrations result in only half maximal stimulation of glucose uptake (Figure 13.1) [8].

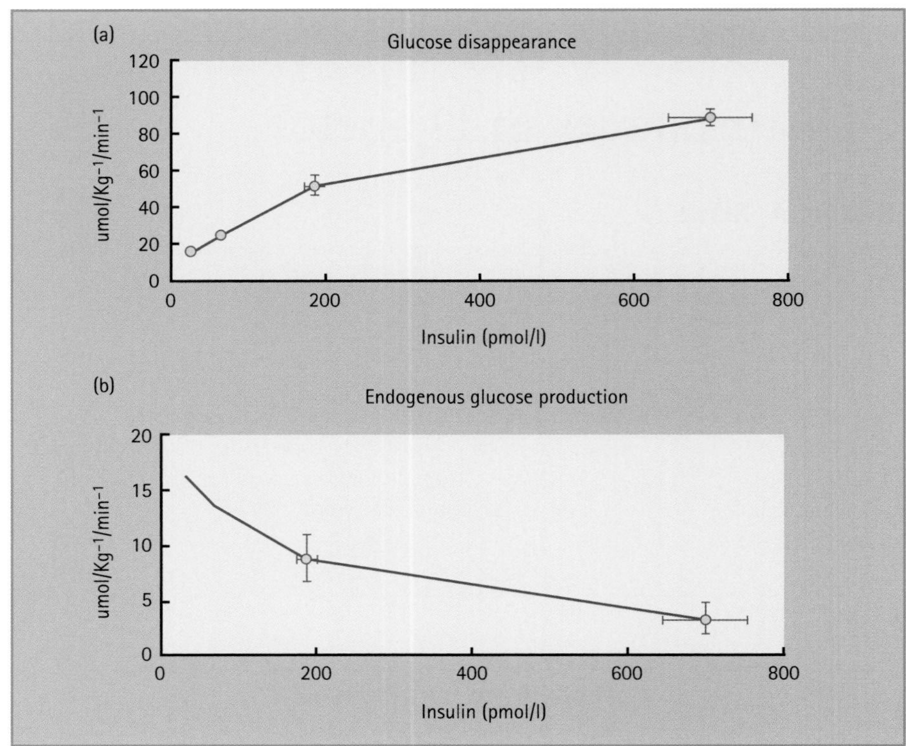

Figure 13.1 Insulin dose–response curves for glucose production and utilization in non-diabetic subjects. Adapted from Vella A. *Diabetologia* 2002; **45**:1410–1415, with permission from Springer-Verlag.

Increases in plasma glucose, which occur within 5–10 minutes after eating stimulate insulin secretion and suppress glucagon secretion. The reciprocal changes in hepatic sinusoidal insulin and glucagon concentrations in concert with the elevated glucose concentrations enhance hepatic glucose uptake and suppress hepatic glucose production [9,10]. The splanchnic tissues initially extract 10–25% of ingested glucose and eventually dispose of approximately 40% of ingested glucose, with muscle accounting for most of the remainder [11]. These coordinated changes in hepatic and extrahepatic glucose metabolism generally limit the post-prandial rise in glucose to 7–8 mmol/L. Late post-prandial hypoglycemia is avoided by a smooth increase in hepatic glucose output to rates that closely approximate glucose uptake.

In the transition from normal glucose metabolism to overt diabetes, the relative contribution of alterations in glucose disappearance or appearance is uncertain. Most [12–15] but not all [16] epidemiologic studies that have attempted to elucidate the pathogenesis of impaired fasting glucose (IFG; defined as a fasting glucose of 5.8–6.9 mmol/L) have reported that insulin action is decreased in individuals with IFG. Weyer *et al.* [15] reported that fasting endogenous glucose production was increased in people with IFG. Bock *et al.* [17] subsequently established that insulin-induced suppression of endogenous glucose production and gluconeogenesis are impaired in people with IFG indicating hepatic insulin resistance. Epidemiologic studies have shown that 20–30% of people with IFG will develop frank diabetes within 5–10 years [18,19]. Indeed, subjects with a fasting glucose between 5.3 and 5.7 mmol/L have an 8% risk of developing diabetes within the next 10 years.

Regulation of glucose concentrations after meal ingestion is more complex. The pattern of change of post-prandial plasma glucose concentrations is determined by the extent to which glucose entering the systemic circulation (equal to the sum of endogenous glucose production and the systemic appearance of ingested glucose) exceeds or is exceeded by the rate at which glucose leaves the systemic circulation (glucose disappearance). Therefore, differences in post-prandial glucose concentrations could theoretically arise because of differences, alone or in combination, in rates of meal glucose appearance, suppression of endogenous glucose production or stimulation of glucose uptake [20,21].

Post-prandial hyperglycemia is primarily caused by reduced post-prandial glucose disappearance because suppression of endogenous glucose production and the rate of appearance of ingested glucose do not differ in people with IFG and normal fasting glucose [17]. The insulin secretion in response to higher post-prandial glucose concentrations is impaired in the subjects with IFG with accompanying defects in glucose disappearance and consequent post-prandial hyperglycemia. A further reduction in insulin secretion eventually results in overt T2DM [17].

Endogenous glucose production is regulated (inhibited) by insulin which increases hepatic glucose uptake by stimulating glucokinase activity and decreases hepatic glucose release by decreasing the conversion of glucose-6-phosphate to glucose.

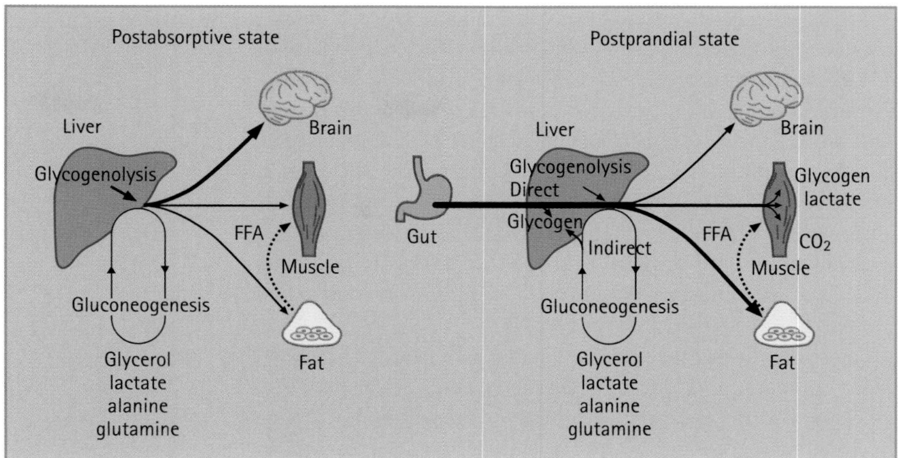

Figure 13.2 Major sites of glucose metabolism in the post-absorptive and post-prandial states. After meal ingestion, the primary site of glucose uptake shifts from insulin-independent organs to insulin-dependent tissues. Gluconeogenic substrates are derived predominantly from peripheral tissues. Hepatic glycogen synthesis may occur via the direct or indirect (gluconeogenesis) pathways. Adapted from Dinneen *et al.* [21]. Copyright © 1992 Massachusetts Medical Society. All rights reserved.

This latter step is regulated by glucose-6-phosphatase. Insulin can also stimulate glycogen synthesis, inhibit glycogen breakdown and suppress gluconeogenesis. Post-prandial hyperglycemia and hyperinsulinemia stimulate hepatic glycogen synthesis thereby replenishing hepatic glycogen stores. Hepatic glycogen synthesis occurs via both the direct (i.e. glycogen synthesis utilizing glucose-6-phosphate derived directly from extracellular glucose) or indirect pathway (i.e. glycogen synthesis utilizing glucose-6-phosphate derived from gluconeogenesis). The relative contribution of these two pathways appears to be determined by multiple factors including the duration of fast, composition of the meal and the prevailing insulin and glucagon concentrations [22,23].

In the presence of euglycemia, rising hepatic sinusoidal concentrations of insulin suppress endogenous glucose production by decreasing glycogenolysis. Insulin concentrations within the physiologic range in healthy humans do not appreciably suppress gluconeogenesis and direct glucose-6-phosphate (derived from gluconeogenesis) into glycogen (Figure 13.2) [24].

Carbohydrate metabolism in type 1 diabetes

T1DM is characterized by insulin deficiency as a result of autoimmune destruction of the pancreatic β-cells. Fasting hyperglycemia does not develop until most (>80%) of β-cells are lost to the underlying autoimmune process. Defects in insulin secretion, however, are evident years before the development of diabetes in asymptomatic affected individuals. For example, siblings of people with T1DM who are islet antibody positive (a group at high risk for the development of T1DM) frequently exhibit a decreased first-phase of insulin secretion in response to intravenous glucose injection [25,26]. This usually occurs at a time when the response to other stimuli such as oral glucose or mixed meal ingestion is intact, suggesting that incretins and other secretagogues are capable of compensating for decreased islet cell mass.

Impaired insulin secretion is frequently accompanied by impaired insulin action [27,28]. The severity of insulin resistance is related to the degree of glycemic control. People with poorly controlled T1DM may exhibit the same degree of insulin resistance as people with T2DM [28,29]. In people with T1DM, the defect in insulin action is tissue-specific; for example, glucose uptake in cardiac muscle, as opposed to skeletal muscle, is normal [30]. Glucose oxidation and non-oxidative storage in people with T1DM is decreased in proportion to glucose uptake, suggesting that glucose transport and/or phosphorylation (after transport across the membrane) are the sites of defective insulin action [31]. In contrast, insulin-induced suppression of glucose production is not impaired and may in fact be increased in people with T1DM [32,33].

Insulin binding and action has been reported to be decreased in adipocytes [34,35] but normal in fibroblasts [36,37] of people with T1DM. This may be explained by the fact that insulin binding in adipocytes is measured immediately after biopsy while insulin binding to fibroblasts is measured following several days of culture. Decreased insulin binding in the former but not the latter suggests an effect of abnormal metabolic milieu rather than an intrinsic defect of insulin action. This is supported by several observations that improved chronic glycemic control is accompanied by improved whole-body insulin action [38,39]. It should be noted that when insulin action is measured by means of a hyperglycemic hyperinsulinemic clamp, hyperglycemia may compensate for small defects in insulin action by means of its ability (glucose) to stimulate its own uptake and suppress its own release (glucose effectiveness) [33].

Because insulin is typically delivered via the subcutaneous, rather than the intraportal route, treatment with insulin leads to systemic hyperinsulinemia which has been shown to impair insulin action in humans without diabetes [40]. The improved insulin action observed in people with T1DM following treatment with insulin, however, suggests that any negative effects of systemic hyperinsulinemia on insulin action are more than offset by the lowering of glucose concentrations and the reversal of glucose toxicity.

In the absence of insulin-stimulated muscle glucose uptake, substantial glucose disappearance in insulin-deficient people with T1DM occurs by glucose excretion in the urine and by glucose uptake via non-insulin-mediated pathways [41]. Food ingestion does not result in a rise in insulin or a reciprocal decrease in glucagon concentration [42]. Because of this, the increase in splanchnic glucose uptake and the decrease in endogenous glucose production are not appropriate for the prevailing glucose concentration. Post-prandial glycogen synthesis is markedly decreased, with most of the glycogen being synthesized by the indirect gluconeogenic pathway [43,44].

Consequently, because of abnormal hepatic glucose handling, excessive amounts of glucose reach the systemic circulation. The excessive rise in post-prandial glucose concentrations is compounded by the low insulin concentrations and defective insulin action present in people with poorly controlled T1DM [41,45]. In contrast, the ability of glucose to stimulate its own uptake and suppress its own release (glucose effectiveness) is normal in T1DM and most post-prandial glucose disposal occurs predominantly via non-insulin mediated pathways and by glucose excretion in the urine [46].

Post-prandial glucose metabolism in the splanchnic and extra-splanchnic tissues can be almost completely normalized by insulin administration which increases circulating insulin concentrations and prevents the excessive rise in counter-regulatory hormones that accompanies insulin deficiency. Insulin administration also restores post-prandial suppression of glucose production and stimulation of glucose uptake to rates similar to those observed in subjects without diabetes [41,47].

Animal studies have shown diabetes to be associated with hypertrophy of the intestinal mucosa and increased intestinal glucose transport [48,49]. By contrast, when glucose, insulin and glucagon concentrations are matched in individuals with T1DM and age- and weight-matched controls, initial splanchnic glucose extraction and uridine diphosphate (UDP)-glucose flux (an index of hepatic glycogen synthesis) do not differ between groups. This demonstrates that relative insulin deficiency, glucagon excess or both, rather than an intrinsic defect in splanchnic glucose metabolism are the primary causes of post-prandial hyperglycemia in people with poorly controlled T1DM (Figure 13.3) [33].

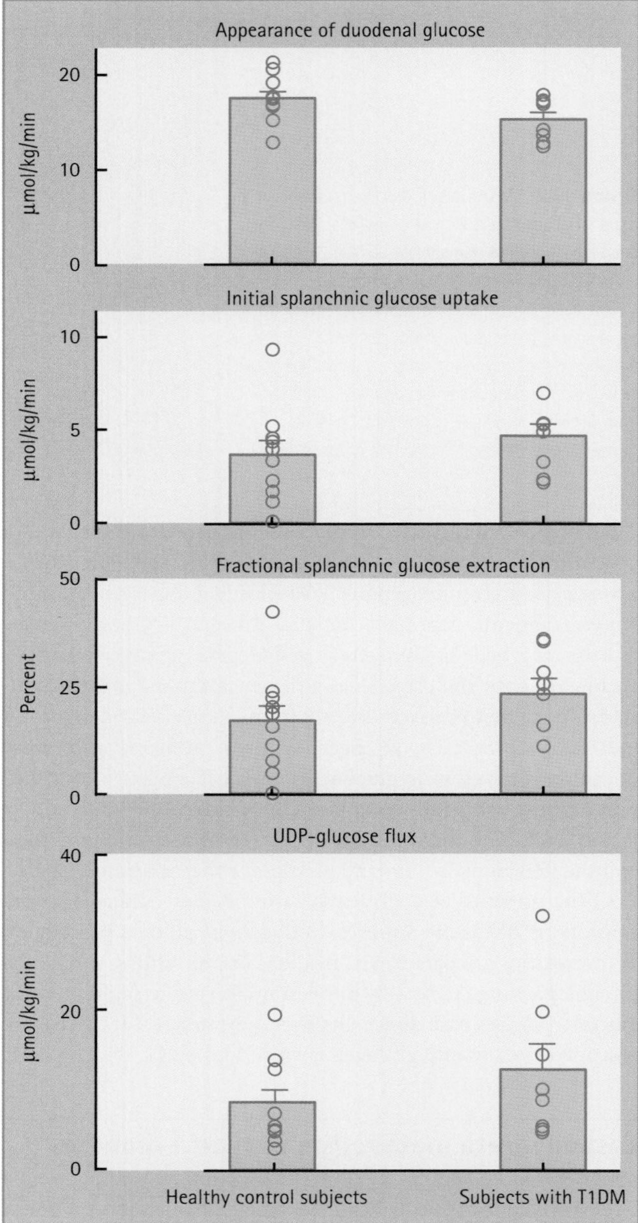

Figure 13.3 In the presence of matched glucose, insulin and glucagon concentrations initial splanchnic glucose extraction and UDP-glucose flux do not differ in individuals with type 1 diabetes and age- and weight-matched controls. FFA, free fatty acids; UDP-glucose, uridine diphosphate glucose. Adapted from Vella *et al.* [33].

Carbohydrate metabolism in type 2 diabetes

People with T2DM have elevated fasting glucose levels and excessive glycemic excursions following carbohydrate ingestion. Insulin secretion in those with T2DM is typically decreased and delayed following food ingestion [9,21]. Defects in insulin secretion are observed early in the evolution of T2DM. In fact, alterations in both the timing and amount of insulin secreted have been reported in relatives of patients with T2DM prior to the development of hyperglycemia [50,51].

Chronic hyperglycemia alone or in combination with elevated FFA impairs insulin secretion. Abnormalities in glucose sensing, insulin processing or intracellular signaling can alter insulin secretion [52]. In addition, β-cell mass decreases with increasing duration of diabetes [53,54]. Alterations in β-cell morphology occur in most people with T2DM with extensive intra-islet deposition of amylin commonly being observed [55,56].

Prolonged elevations in glucose concentration following ingestion of a carbohydrate-containing meal occur because post-prandial glucose appearance exceeds disappearance. The more significant the defects in insulin secretion and action, the higher glucose concentrations have to rise to balance glucose appearance and disappearance [57]. Glucose appearance is elevated because of failure to suppress hepatic glucose production because the systemic rate of appearance of ingested glucose does not differ from that observed in individuals without diabetes [9,11,17,58]. Although glucose disappearance is commonly higher in people with diabetes than in individuals without diabetes following a meal, this is in large part is accounted for by elevated rates of urinary glucose excretion. Furthermore, although elevated, the rates of glucose disappearance are not appropriate for the prevailing glucose concentrations [59,60].

Defects in insulin secretion and action both contribute to post-prandial hyperglycemia. A delay in the early rise in insulin concentrations causes a delay in suppression of glucose production, which in turn results in an excessive glycemic excursion. In contrast, a decrease in insulin action results in sustained hyperglycemia but has minimal effect of peak glucose concentrations. Whereas an isolated alteration in either hepatic or extrahepatic insulin action impairs glucose tolerance, a defect in both results in severe hyperglycemia [57].

Glucose is also an important regulator of its own metabolism. In the presence of basal insulin concentrations, an increase in plasma glucose stimulates glucose uptake and suppresses glucose production. The ability of glucose to regulate its own metabolism is impaired in T2DM. This is commonly referred to as a defect in "glucose effectiveness." Whereas intravenous infusion of 35 g glucose in individuals without diabetes whose insulin concentrations are clamped at basal levels produces only a modest rise in plasma glucose concentration, infusion of the same amount of glucose results in severe hyperglycemia in people with T2DM [61]. The excessive rise in glucose is caused by impaired glucose induced stimulation of glucose uptake because glucose induced suppression of glucose production is normal [61,62].

Inhibition of glucagon secretion lowers both fasting glucose and post-prandial glucose concentrations. Failure to suppress glucagon secretion appropriately, however, has minimal effect on glucose production and glucose tolerance when insulin secretion is intact [63,64]. In contrast, it causes marked hyperglycemia when insulin secretion is decreased and delayed, as is typical of T2DM. Taken together, these data suggest that agents that simultaneously improve insulin secretion, insulin action, glucose effectiveness as well glucagon secretion are likely to have a profound effect on glucose metabolism in people with T2DM (Figure 13.4) [64,65].

Amylin is a 37 amino acid polypeptide that is co-secreted with insulin by the pancreatic β-cells in response to nutrient stimuli and other secretagogues. Human studies have shown that the plasma concentrations of amylin and insulin rise and fall in parallel in both the fasted and fed states [66]. Because amylin is potentially toxic to β-cells, it has been suggested that excessive amylin secretion may contribute to β-cell destruction in T2DM [67,68].

The secretion of incretins such as glucagon-like peptide 1 (GLP-1), in response to meal ingestion is decreased in T2DM [69–71]. Supraphysiologic concentrations of GLP-1, achieved by either intravenous infusion or subcutaneous injection, lower both fasting and post-prandial glucose concentrations in people with T2DM. GLP-1 does so by increasing insulin secretion, inhibiting glucagon secretion and delaying gastric emptying [72–75]. By contrast, GLP-1 does not appear to alter insulin action or glucose effectiveness in T2DM [76].

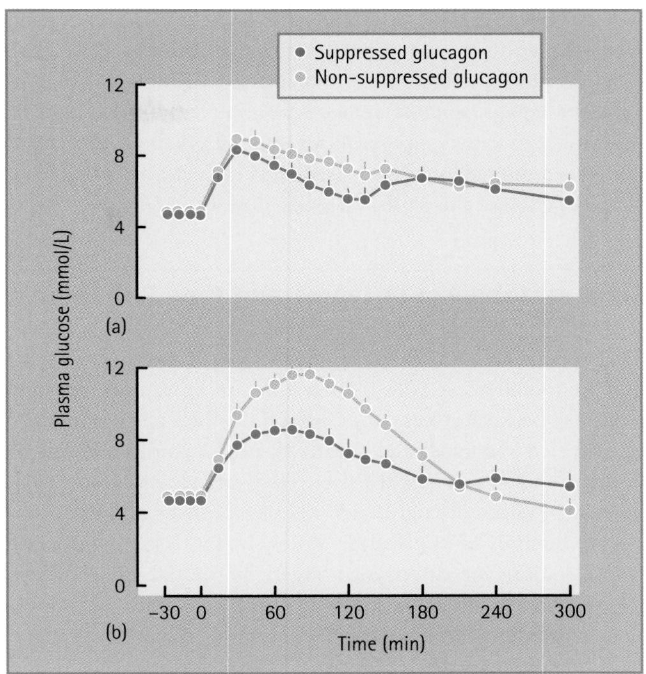

Figure 13.4 Healthy subjects received a non-diabetic (a) or a diabetic (b) insulin profile on two occasions. On one occasion glucagon was infused in a manner that replicated the fall in glucagon concentrations that normally occurs after meal ingestion. On the other occasion glucagon was infused constantly to replicate the lack of glucagon suppression observed in type 2 diabetes in response to meal ingestion. Glycemic excursion was significantly higher in the absence of glucagon suppression in subjects receiving an insulin profile similar to that observed in patients with type 2 diabetes. Adapted from Shah *et al.* [64], with permission from the American Physiological Society.

In addition to defects in insulin secretion, people with T2DM commonly exhibit defects in insulin action. Numerous studies have shown that insulin-induced stimulation of glucose uptake in muscle and adipose tissues as well as insulin-induced suppression of glucose production are impaired in T2DM [77,78]. The severity of insulin resistance is influenced by multiple factors including exercise, obesity and diet as well as genetic factors. Insulin resistance increases with increasing severity of diabetes and improves but is not normalized by improved glycemic control [79]. Defects in the ability of insulin to regulate muscle and fat glucose metabolism are evident in normoglycemic relatives of people with T2DM strongly implying a genetic basis for at least some degree of insulin resistance [50,80].

Both glucose production and the contribution of gluconeogenesis to glucose production are increased in people with "mild" as well as "severe" T2DM [81]. The increase in glucose production is correlated with the severity of hyperglycemia [21,58,82]. Insulin-induced stimulation of splanchnic (and therefore presumably hepatic) glucose uptake is also impaired in T2DM. The lower rates of hepatic uptake in subjects with diabetes are almost entirely accounted for by decreased uptake of extracellular glucose suggesting lower glucokinase activity [83,84].

Lipid metabolism in type 1 and type 2 diabetes

Triglycerides are an important energy source (and storage form) and are mobilized as FFA. Plasma FFA concentrations represent a balance between release and disposal. FFA are taken up by and re-esterified in adipose and hepatic tissues, or oxidized in muscle (cardiac and skeletal) or the liver. They are released from intravascular lipolysis of triglyceride-rich lipoproteins and intra-adipocyte lipolysis of triglyceride stores. In the fasting state, FFA concentrations are determined largely by the rate of entry into the circulation while in the post-prandial period the rate of uptake by adipose and hepatic tissue is also a major determinant in FFA concentrations [85].

Hormone-sensitive lipase is the principal regulator of FFA release from adipose and is exquisitely sensitive to insulin. Insulin is the main hormonal regulator of lipolysis. Increasing plasma glucose concentrations (e.g. after a meal) normally leads to increased insulin secretion which inhibits lipolysis [86]. Rising insulin concentrations suppress lipolysis leading to a fall in FFA concentrations. This insulin-induced suppression of FFA concentrations enhances insulin-dependent glucose disposal and insulin-induced suppression of endogenous glucose production [87].

Conversely, in individuals without diabetes, falling blood glucose concentrations increase lipolysis because of suppression of insulin secretion [88]. The resulting rise in FFA will stabilize or raise glucose concentrations. Hypoglycemia caused by exogenous hyperinsulinism will also suppress lipolysis and impair counter-regulation.

Absolute or relative insulin deficiency is responsible for most of the excess FFA available for oxidation in T1DM. Elevated FFA directly impair peripheral glucose uptake [89] and, at least acutely, stimulate endogenous glucose production [90]. Another consequence of elevated FFA flux is increased ketogenesis, a precursor to ketoacidosis [91]. Insulin is able to counteract the lipolytic effects of other hormones so that growth hormone or cortisol have little effect on lipolysis unless insulin availability is reduced [92]. Similarly, the lipolytic effect of catecholamines is blunted by hyperinsulinemia and accentuated by hypoinsulinemia [93]. Although glucagon has no effect on systemic FFA availability, increased concentrations, as seen in uncontrolled diabetes, may drive hepatic metabolism towards ketogenesis [91].

Moderate intensity exercise is normally accompanied by a fall in insulin and a rise in catecholamine concentrations which increases FFA availability and fatty acid oxidation [94]. Plasma insulin concentrations do not decrease with exercise in T1DM and, depending on the timing of exercise in relation to insulin administration, may not allow the normal increase in FFA that accompanies exercise [95]. In these instances, people with T1DM become dependent on the catecholamine response to exercise to mobilize FFA, a response that may be impaired in individuals with long-standing diabetes [96]. In people with fasting hyperglycemia, low insulin concentrations and, consequently, elevated resting FFA flux, exercise will increase FFA flux further [97]. This combined with the high glucagon concentrations commonly present in these situations will result in high rates of ketone body production.

FFA concentrations commonly are increased in the post-absorptive and post-prandial state in people with T2DM [77,98]. The ability of insulin to suppress lipolysis is impaired likely because of decreased sensitivity of hormone-sensitive lipase to insulin [99]. Insulin also promotes FFA disposal, however, by stimulating re-esterification in adipocytes to form triglyceride. This process is dependent on the provision of glycerol-3-phosphate derived from glucose uptake (also insulin-driven) and intra-adipocyte glycolysis. It is unknown, however, whether defects in adipose FFA esterification contribute to the FFA elevation observed in diabetes [85].

Circulating plasma triglycerides are dependent on the activity of lipoprotein lipase (LPL) to deliver FFA to the adipocyte. Insulin and glucose preferentially stimulate adipose LPL and inhibit muscle LPL thereby partitioning triglyceride and lipoprotein-derived fatty acids away from muscle and into adipose tissue [100]. By contrast, in T2DM, insulin-induced activation of adipose LPL is delayed while skeletal muscle LPL is activated [101]. Given that elevated FFA decrease muscle glucose uptake, this is especially of consequence in patients with already diminished insulin action. FFA decrease muscle glucose uptake by inhibiting glucose transport, glucose phosphorylation and muscle glycogen synthase [102].

Although elevated FFA concentrations have been reported to decrease hepatic insulin metabolism in animals, direct measurement of splanchnic insulin clearance suggest that this may not be the case in humans [103]. Elevated FFA stimulate both hepatic gluconeogenesis and triglyceride synthesis. Acute increases in FFA stimulate insulin secretion whereas chronic elevations inhibit insulin secretion [104]. Thus, elevated FFA have been implicated in many, but not all, of the metabolic abnormalities associated with T2DM.

Protein metabolism in type 1 and type 2 diabetes

Substrate availability and the hormonal milieu regulate protein synthesis and breakdown at any given time. Insulin is an important hormone in this regard and profound changes in body composition occur after the initiation of therapy in people with T1DM, especially if insulin deficiency has been severe and prolonged [105]. Urinary nitrogen excretion, a marker of protein catabolism, increases during insulin deprivation. If this is sufficiently prolonged, cachexia and a loss of muscle mass occurs [106,107]. Insulin deprivation increases the concentration of circulating amino acids because of the net increase in protein breakdown with an accompanying decline in amino acid disposal (utilization in protein synthesis or amino acid oxidation) [108,109].

Glucagon secretion is enhanced by ingestion of protein and facilitates disposal of glucogenic amino acids such as alanine or glutamine. The elevated glucagon concentrations present in poorly controlled T1DM stimulate alanine and glutamine uptake, resulting in normal or low concentrations despite increased appearance from protein breakdown from insulin deprivation [110]. Concentrations of branched chain amino acids are elevated in these situations but are rapidly lowered to non-diabetic levels by treatment with insulin [108,111].

In contrast, the effect of T2DM on protein metabolism is less clear-cut with some studies showing no evidence of increased catabolism [112,113] while others have reported increased protein turnover and/or amino acid catabolism [114–117]. The difference in protein metabolism between T1DM and T2DM likely occurs because people with T2DM have sufficient residual insulin secretion to limit protein catabolism and preserve lean body mass. Nevertheless, whole body nitrogen flux, protein synthesis and breakdown are increased in people with poorly controlled diabetes. These defects are restored to normal when glycemic control is improved by treatment with either oral agents or insulin [114,115]. Of interest, whereas T2DM impairs the ability of insulin to regulate glucose and fat metabolism, the effects of insulin on whole body protein synthesis and breakdown appear to be preserved [113].

Relatively few studies have examined regional protein dynamics in T2DM. Increased 3-methylhistidine excretion, an index of myofibrillar protein breakdown, has been demonstrated in subjects with poorly controlled T2DM when compared with healthy and obese subjects without diabetes [114]. Improved glycemic control reduced 3-methylhistidine excretion. People with T2DM and/or insulin resistance have been noted to have elevated circulating concentrations of certain clotting factors such as tissue plasminogen activator and plasminogen activator inhibitor 1 (PAI-1). This would imply that the synthesis of certain proteins by the liver and endothelium is clearly abnormal [118]. Preliminary evidence suggests that agents that improve the ability of insulin to regulate muscle and hepatic glucose metabolism (e.g. thiazolidinediones) will also restore concentrations, and possibly the activity, of these proteins to normal [119,120].

Counter-regulatory hormones

In humans without diabetes, insulin and glucagon exhibit coordinated and reciprocal changes in concentration in response to glucose ingestion [21]. In people with T1DM, however, carbohydrate ingestion fails to suppress glucagon [121,122], while protein ingestion commonly results in an excessive rise in glucagon concentrations [123]. The cause of these abnormalities in glucagon secretion is thought to be intra-islet insulin deficiency as insulin infusion inhibits glucagon secretion [124] and neutralization of intra-islet insulin with anti-insulin antibodies stimulates glucagon secretion [125]. Treatment with exogenous insulin rapidly lowers glucagon concentrations in people with T1DM but does not restore hypoglycemia-induced glucagon secretion [126].

Glucagon excess exacerbates hyperglycemia by increasing hepatic glucose release and decreasing hepatic glucose uptake [127,128]. In humans without diabetes, any increase in glucose concentrations is promptly accompanied by an increase in insulin secretion which antagonizes the effects of glucagon on the liver. By contrast, in people with diabetes who cannot increase insulin secretion (and consequently glucose disposal) to compensate for the increase in glucagon concentrations, increased hepatic glucose release is accompanied by further increases in glucose concentration [127].

Fasting epinephrine and norepinephrine concentrations may be elevated in individuals with poorly controlled diabetes [129,130] and may cause further deterioration in glycemic control by impairing insulin action at the hepatic and extrahepatic tissues [131]. Epinephrine also stimulates glucagon secretion leading to further increases in endogenous glucose production [132]. In the absence of circulating insulin, catecholamines will enhance lipolysis thereby increasing FFA concentrations and increased production of ketone bodies [133].

In the presence of severe defects in endogenous insulin secretion, as usually encountered in people with T1DM, the normal diurnal variation in plasma cortisol concentrations can adversely affect glycemic control [134]. Cortisol increases endogenous glucose production while decreasing tissue glucose uptake. The nocturnal rise in cortisol also increases ketone body concentrations, gluconeogenesis and lipolysis [134,135].

Growth hormone release increases in both amplitude and frequency in people with poorly controlled diabetes [136,137]. Growth hormone stimulates gluconeogenesis, proteolysis and lipolysis while impairing insulin-induced suppression of endogenous glucose production and stimulation of glucose uptake [138]. This is likely to occur in situations where insulin secretion cannot rise to match the increased insulin requirements because of excessive growth hormone secretion.

Diabetic ketoacidosis

Insulin deficiency to a degree sufficient to allow unrestrained lipolysis and hepatic ketogenesis is a necessary condition for the development of diabetic ketoacidosis [139]. Because of this, ketoacidosis is more commonly encountered in patients with T1DM than in people with T2DM because the latter generally have some degree of residual insulin secretion. Although insulin deficiency is a necessary condition for the development of ketoacidosis, the condition is often triggered by physical stress such as infection or surgery.

Glucagon concentrations rise in the presence of insulin deficiency and during physical stress. A decrease in effective circulating volume may also increase glucagon concentrations because glucagon is cleared by the kidneys. The concentrations of other counter-regulatory hormones also rise, which in turn further increase lipolysis [140].

Ketone bodies and glucose produce an osmotic diuresis that exacerbates the hypovolemia and electrolyte disturbances caused by metabolic acidosis. Furthermore, ketone bodies can induce vomiting, causing electrolyte and fluid losses. These losses also can directly contribute to metabolic acidosis. Cardiovascular collapse can occur if acidosis is sufficiently severe. Intracellular metabolic acidosis interferes with the activity of several enzymatic processes, which exacerbates the consequences of circulatory failure. Death is often caused by underlying comorbidities, the physical illness that precipitated ketoacidosis – myocardial infarction, pneumonia – or a direct consequence of severe metabolic acidosis [141].

References

1 McGarry JD. What if Minkowski had been ageusic? An alternative angle on diabetes. *Science* 1992; **258**:766–770.

2 Gale EA. Declassifying diabetes. *Diabetologia* 2006; **49**:1989–1995.

3 Rothman DL, Magnusson I, Katz LD, Shulman RG, Shulman GI. Quantitation of hepatic glycogenolysis and gluconeogenesis in fasting humans with 13C NMR. *Science* 1991; **254**:573–576.

4 Ferrannini E, Groop LC. Hepatic glucose production in insulin-resistant states. *Diabetes Metab Rev* 1989; **5**:711–726.

5 Andres R, Cader G, Zierler KL. The quantitatively minor role of carbohydrate in oxidative metabolism by skeletal muscle in intact man in the basal state: measurements of oxygen and glucose uptake and carbon dioxide and lactate production in the forearm. *J Clin Invest* 1956; **35**:671–682.

6 Dagenais GR, Tancredi RG, Zierler KL. Free fatty acid oxidation by forearm muscle at rest, and evidence for an intramuscular lipid pool in the human forearm. *J Clin Invest* 1976; **58**:421–431.

7 Consoli A, Nurjhan N, Reilly JJ, Jr., Bier DM, Gerich JE. Contribution of liver and skeletal muscle to alanine and lactate metabolism in humans. *Am J Physiol* 1990; **259**:E677–684.

8 Rizza RA, Mandarino LJ, Gerich JE. Dose–response characteristics for effects of insulin on production and utilization of glucose in man. *Am J Physiol* 1981; **240**:E630–639.

9 Butler PC, Rizza RA. Contribution to postprandial hyperglycemia and effect on initial splanchnic glucose clearance of hepatic glucose cycling in glucose-intolerant or NIDDM patients. *Diabetes* 1991; **40**:73–81.

10 Radziuk J, Norwich KH, Vranic M. Experimental validation of measurements of glucose turnover in nonsteady state. *Am J Physiol* 1978; **234**:E84–93.

11 Ferrannini E, Bjorkman O, Reichard GA Jr, Pilo A, Olsson M, Wahren J, *et al.* The disposal of an oral glucose load in healthy subjects: a quantitative study. *Diabetes* 1985; **34**:580–588.

12 Tripathy D, Carlsson M, Almgren P, Isomaa B, Taskinen MR, Tuomi T, *et al.* Insulin secretion and insulin sensitivity in relation to glucose tolerance: lessons from the Botnia Study. *Diabetes* 2000; **49**:975–980.

13 Li CL, Tsai ST, Chou P. Relative role of insulin resistance and beta-cell dysfunction in the progression to type 2 diabetes: the Kinmen Study. *Diabetes Res Clin Pract* 2003; **59**:225–232.

14 Jensen CC, Cnop M, Hull RL, Fujimoto WY, Kahn SE. Beta-cell function is a major contributor to oral glucose tolerance in high-risk relatives of four ethnic groups in the US. *Diabetes* 2002; **51**:2170–2178.

15 Weyer C, Bogardus C, Pratley RE. Metabolic characteristics of individuals with impaired fasting glucose and/or impaired glucose tolerance. *Diabetes* 1999; **48**:2197–2203.

16 Kim DJ, Lee MS, Kim KW, Lee MK. Insulin secretory dysfunction and insulin resistance in the pathogenesis of Korean type 2 diabetes mellitus. *Metabolism* 2001; **50**:590–593.

17 Bock G, Dalla Man C, Campioni M, Chittilapilly E, Basu R, Toffolo G, *et al.* Pathogenesis of pre-diabetes: mechanisms of fasting and postprandial hyperglycemia in people with impaired fasting glucose and/or impaired glucose tolerance. *Diabetes* 2006; **55**:3536–3549.

18 Tirosh A, Shai I, Tekes-Manova D, Israeli E, Pereg D, Shochat T, *et al.* Normal fasting plasma glucose levels and type 2 diabetes in young men. *N Engl J Med* 2005; **353**:1454–1462.

19 Dinneen SF, Maldonado D 3rd, Leibson CL, Klee GG, Li H, Melton LJ 3rd, *et al.* Effects of changing diagnostic criteria on the risk of developing diabetes. *Diabetes Care* 1998; **21**:1408–1413.

20 Dinneen SF. Mechanism of postprandial hyperglycaemia in diabetes mellitus. *Eur J Gastroenterol Hepatol* 1995; **7**:724–729.

21 Dinneen S, Gerich J, Rizza R. Carbohydrate metabolism in non-insulin-dependent diabetes mellitus. *N Engl J Med* 1992; **327**:707–713.

22 Moore MC, Cherrington AD, Cline G, Pagliassotti MJ, Jones EM, Neal DW, *et al.* Sources of carbon for hepatic glycogen synthesis in the conscious dog. *J Clin Invest* 1991; **88**:578–587.

23 Youn JH, Bergman RN. Enhancement of hepatic glycogen by gluconeogenic precursors: substrate flux or metabolic control? *Am J Physiol* 1990; **258**:E899–906.

24 Adkins A, Basu R, Persson M, Dicke B, Shah P, Vella A, *et al.* Higher insulin concentrations are required to suppress gluconeogenesis than glycogenolysis in nondiabetic humans. *Diabetes* 2003; **52**:2213–2220.

25 Vardi P, Crisa L, Jackson RA. Predictive value of intravenous glucose tolerance test insulin secretion less than or greater than the first percentile in islet cell antibody positive relatives of type 1 (insulin-dependent) diabetic patients. *Diabetologia* 1991; **34**:93–102.

26 Vialettes B, Mattei-Zevaco C, Badier C, Ramahandridona G, Lassmann-Vague V, Vague P. Low acute insulin response to intravenous glucose: a sensitive but non-specific marker of early stages of type 1 (insulin-dependent) diabetes. *Diabetologia* 1988; **31**:592–596.

27 Yki-Jarvinen H, Koivisto VA. Natural course of insulin resistance in type I diabetes. *N Engl J Med* 1986; **315**:224–230.

28 Yki-Jarvinen H, Koivisto VA. Insulin sensitivity in newly diagnosed type 1 diabetics after ketoacidosis and after three months of insulin therapy. *J Clin Endocrinol Metab* 1984; **59**:371–378.

29 DeFronzo RA, Simonson D, Ferrannini E. Hepatic and peripheral insulin resistance: a common feature of type 2 (non-insulin-

dependent) and type 1 (insulin-dependent) diabetes mellitus. *Diabetologia* 1982; **23**:313–319.
30 Nuutila P, Knuuti J, Ruotsalainen U, Koivisto VA, Eronen E, Teras M, *et al.* Insulin resistance is localized to skeletal but not heart muscle in type 1 diabetes. *Am J Physiol* 1993; **264**:E756–762.
31 Yki-Jarvinen H, Sahlin K, Ren JM, Koivisto VA. Localization of rate-limiting defect for glucose disposal in skeletal muscle of insulin-resistant type 1 diabetic patients. *Diabetes* 1990; **39**:157–167.
32 Hother-Nielsen O, Schmitz O, Bak J, Beck-Nielsen H. Enhanced hepatic insulin sensitivity, but peripheral insulin resistance in patients with type 1 (insulin-dependent) diabetes. *Diabetologia* 1987; **30**:834–840.
33 Vella A, Shah P, Basu R, Basu A, Camilleri M, Schwenk WF, *et al.* Type I diabetes mellitus does not alter initial splanchnic glucose extraction or hepatic UDP-glucose flux during enteral glucose administration. *Diabetologia* 2001; **44**:729–737.
34 Hjollund E, Pedersen O, Richelsen B, Beck-Nielsen H, Sorensen NS. Glucose transport and metabolism in adipocytes from newly diagnosed untreated insulin-dependent diabetics: severely impaired basal and postinsulin binding activities. *J Clin Invest* 1985; **76**: 2091–2096.
35 Pedersen O, Hjollund E. Insulin receptor binding to fat and blood cells and insulin action in fat cells from insulin-dependent diabetics. *Diabetes* 1982; **31**:706–715.
36 Podskalny JM, Kahn CR. Insulin binding and activation of glycogen synthase in fibroblasts from type 1 (insulin-dependent) diabetic patients. *Diabetologia* 1982; **23**:431–435.
37 Eckel RH, Fujimoto WY. Insulin-stimulated glucose uptake, leucine incorporation into protein, and uridine incorporation into RNA in skin fibroblast cultures from patients with diabetes mellitus. *Diabetologia* 1981; **20**:186–189.
38 Yki-Jarvinen H, Koivisto VA. Continuous subcutaneous insulin infusion therapy decreases insulin resistance in type 1 diabetes. *J Clin Endocrinol Metab* 1984; **58**:659–666.
39 Lager I, Lonnroth P, von Schenck H, Smith U. Reversal of insulin resistance in type 1 diabetes after treatment with continuous subcutaneous insulin infusion. *Br Med J (Clin Res Ed)* 1983; **287**:1661–1664.
40 Rizza RA, Mandarino LJ, Genest J, Baker BA, Gerich JE. Production of insulin resistance by hyperinsulinaemia in man. *Diabetologia* 1985; **28**:70–75.
41 Pehling G, Tessari P, Gerich JE, Haymond MW, Service FJ, Rizza RA. Abnormal meal carbohydrate disposition in insulin-dependent diabetes: relative contributions of endogenous glucose production and initial splanchnic uptake and effect of intensive insulin therapy. *J Clin Invest* 1984; **74**:985–991.
42 Gerich JE, Lorenzi M, Karam JH, Schneider V, Forsham PH. Abnormal pancreatic glucagon secretion and postprandial hyperglycemia in diabetes mellitus. *JAMA* 1975; **234**:159–155.
43 Hwang JH, Perseghin G, Rothman DL, Cline GW, Magnusson I, Petersen KF, *et al.* Impaired net hepatic glycogen synthesis in insulin-dependent diabetic subjects during mixed meal ingestion: a 13C nuclear magnetic resonance spectroscopy study. *J Clin Invest* 1995; **95**:783–787.
44 Cline GW, Rothman DL, Magnusson I, Katz LD, Shulman GI. 13C-nuclear magnetic resonance spectroscopy studies of hepatic glucose metabolism in normal subjects and subjects with insulin-dependent diabetes mellitus. *J Clin Invest* 1994; **94**:2369–2376.
45 Yki-Jarvinen H, Helve E, Koivisto VA. Relationship between oral glucose tolerance and insulin sensitivity in healthy man and type 1 diabetic patients. *Acta Endocrinol (Copenh)* 1986; **112**:355–360.
46 Hansen IL, Cryer PE, Rizza RA. Comparison of insulin-mediated and glucose-mediated glucose disposal in patients with insulin-dependent diabetes mellitus and in nondiabetic subjects. *Diabetes* 1985; **34**:751–755.
47 Benn JJ, Bozzard SJ, Kelley D, Mitrakou A, Aoki T, Sorensen J, *et al.* Persistent abnormalities of the metabolism of an oral glucose load in insulin-treated type I diabetics. *Metabolism* 1989; **38**:1047–1055.
48 Fujita Y, Kojima H, Hidaka H, Fujimiya M, Kashiwagi A, Kikkawa R. Increased intestinal glucose absorption and postprandial hyperglycaemia at the early step of glucose intolerance in Otsuka Long-Evans Tokushima Fatty rats. *Diabetologia* 1998; **41**:1459–1466.
49 Burant CF, Flink S, DePaoli AM, Chen J, Lee WS, Hediger MA, *et al.* Small intestine hexose transport in experimental diabetes: increased transporter mRNA and protein expression in enterocytes. *J Clin Invest* 1994; **93**:578–585.
50 Vauhkonen I, Niskanen L, Vanninen E, Kainulainen S, Uusitupa M, Laakso M. Defects in insulin secretion and insulin action in non-insulin-dependent diabetes mellitus are inherited: metabolic studies on offspring of diabetic probands. *J Clin Invest* 1998; **101**:86–96.
51 O'Rahilly S, Turner RC, Matthews DR. Impaired pulsatile secretion of insulin in relatives of patients with non-insulin-dependent diabetes. *N Engl J Med* 1988; **318**:1225–1230.
52 Fajans SS, Bell GI, Polonsky KS. Molecular mechanisms and clinical pathophysiology of maturity-onset diabetes of the young. *N Engl J Med* 2001; **345**:971–980.
53 Weyer C, Bogardus C, Mott DM, Pratley RE. The natural history of insulin secretory dysfunction and insulin resistance in the pathogenesis of type 2 diabetes mellitus. *J Clin Invest* 1999; **104**:787–794.
54 Leahy JL. Natural history of beta-cell dysfunction in NIDDM. *Diabetes Care* 1990; **13**:992–1010.
55 Johnson KH, O'Brien TD, Betsholtz C, Westermark P. Islet amyloid polypeptide: mechanisms of amyloidogenesis in the pancreatic islets and potential roles in diabetes mellitus. Laboratory investigation: a journal of technical methods and pathology. 1992; **66**:522–535.
56 Kawanishi H, Akazawa Y, Machii B. Islets of Langerhans in normal and diabetic humans: ultrastructure and histochemistry, with special reference to hyalinosis. *Acta Pathol Jpn* 1966; **16**:177–197.
57 Basu A, Alzaid A, Dinneen S, Caumo A, Cobelli C, Rizza RA. Effects of a change in the pattern of insulin delivery on carbohydrate tolerance in diabetic and nondiabetic humans in the presence of differing degrees of insulin resistance. *J Clin Invest* 1996; **97**:2351–2361.
58 McMahon M, Marsh HM, Rizza RA. Effects of basal insulin supplementation on disposition of mixed meal in obese patients with NIDDM. *Diabetes.* 1989; **38**:291–303.
59 Schirra J, Kuwert P, Wank U, Leicht P, Arnold R, Goke B, *et al.* Differential effects of subcutaneous GLP-1 on gastric emptying, antroduodenal motility, and pancreatic function in men. *Proc Assoc Am Physicians* 1997; **109**:84–97.
60 Mitrakou A, Kelley D, Veneman T, Jenssen T, Pangburn T, Reilly J, *et al.* Contribution of abnormal muscle and liver glucose metabolism to postprandial hyperglycemia in NIDDM. *Diabetes* 1990; **39**:1381–1390.
61 Basu A, Caumo A, Bettini F, Gelisio A, Alzaid A, Cobelli C, *et al.* Impaired basal glucose effectiveness in NIDDM: contribution of defects in glucose disappearance and production, measured using an

optimized minimal model independent protocol. *Diabetes* 1997; **46**:421–432.

62 Nielsen MF, Basu R, Wise S, Caumo A, Cobelli C, Rizza RA. Normal glucose-induced suppression of glucose production but impaired stimulation of glucose disposal in type 2 diabetes: evidence for a concentration-dependent defect in uptake. *Diabetes* 1998; **47**:1735–1747.

63 Frank JW, Camilleri M, Thomforde GM, Dinneen SF, Rizza RA. Effects of glucagon on postprandial carbohydrate metabolism in nondiabetic humans. *Metabolism* 1998; **47**:7–12.

64 Shah P, Basu A, Basu R, Rizza R. Impact of lack of suppression of glucagon on glucose tolerance in humans. *Am J Physiol* 1999; **277**:E283–290.

65 Shah P, Vella A, Basu A, Basu R, Schwenk WF, Rizza RA. Lack of suppression of glucagon contributes to postprandial hyperglycemia in subjects with type 2 diabetes mellitus. *J Clin Endocrinol Metab* 2000; **85**:4053–4059.

66 Hartter E, Svoboda T, Ludvik B, Schuller M, Lell B, Kuenburg E, *et al.* Basal and stimulated plasma levels of pancreatic amylin indicate its co-secretion with insulin in humans. *Diabetologia* 1991; **34**:52–54.

67 Hiddinga HJ, Eberhardt NL. Intracellular amyloidogenesis by human islet amyloid polypeptide induces apoptosis in COS-1 cells. *Am J Pathol* 1999; **154**:1077–1088.

68 O'Brien TD, Butler PC, Kreutter DK, Kane LA, Eberhardt NL. Human islet amyloid polypeptide expression in COS-1 cells: a model of intracellular amyloidogenesis. *Am J Pathol* 1995; **147**:609–616.

69 Lugari R, Dell'Anna C, Ugolotti D, Dei Cas A, Barilli AL, Zandomeneghi R, *et al.* Effect of nutrient ingestion on glucagon-like peptide 1 (7-36 amide) secretion in human type 1 and type 2 diabetes. *Horm Metab Res* 2000; **32**:424–428.

70 Vilsboll T, Krarup T, Deacon CF, Madsbad S, Holst JJ. Reduced postprandial concentrations of intact biologically active glucagon-like peptide 1 in type 2 diabetic patients. *Diabetes* 2001; **50**:609–613.

71 Mannucci E, Ognibene A, Cremasco F, Bardini G, Mencucci A, Pierazzuoli E, *et al.* Glucagon-like peptide (GLP)-1 and leptin concentrations in obese patients with type 2 diabetes mellitus. *Diabet Med* 2000; **17**:713–719.

72 Nauck MA, Wollschlager D, Werner J, Holst JJ, Orskov C, Creutzfeldt W, *et al.* Effects of subcutaneous glucagon-like peptide 1 (GLP-1 [7-36 amide]) in patients with NIDDM. *Diabetologia* 1996; **39**:1546–1553.

73 Gutniak M, Orskov C, Holst JJ, Ahren B, Efendic S. Antidiabetogenic effect of glucagon-like peptide-1 (7-36) amide in normal subjects and patients with diabetes mellitus. *N Engl J Med* 1992; **326**:1316–1322.

74 Gutniak MK, Linde B, Holst JJ, Efendic S. Subcutaneous injection of the incretin hormone glucagon-like peptide 1 abolishes postprandial glycemia in NIDDM. *Diabetes Care* 1994; **17**:1039–1044.

75 Naslund E, Gutniak M, Skogar S, Rossner S, Hellstrom PM. Glucagon-like peptide 1 increases the period of postprandial satiety and slows gastric emptying in obese men. *Am J Clin Nutr* 1998; **68**:525–530.

76 Vella A, Shah P, Basu R, Basu A, Holst JJ, Rizza RA. Effect of glucagon-like peptide 1 (7-36) amide on glucose effectiveness and insulin action in people with type 2 diabetes. *Diabetes* 2000; **49**:611–617.

77 Groop LC, Bonadonna RC, DelPrato S, Ratheiser K, Zyck K, Ferrannini E, *et al.* Glucose and free fatty acid metabolism in non-insulin-dependent diabetes mellitus: evidence for multiple sites of insulin resistance. *J Clin Invest* 1989; **84**:205–213.

78 Firth R, Bell P, Rizza R. Insulin action in non-insulin-dependent diabetes mellitus: the relationship between hepatic and extrahepatic insulin resistance and obesity. *Metabolism* 1987; **36**:1091–1095.

79 Ferrannini E. Insulin resistance versus insulin deficiency in non-insulin-dependent diabetes mellitus: problems and prospects. *Endocr Rev* 1998; **19**:477–490.

80 Eriksson J, Franssila-Kallunki A, Ekstrand A, Saloranta C, Widen E, Schalin C, *et al.* Early metabolic defects in persons at increased risk for non-insulin-dependent diabetes mellitus. *N Engl J Med* 1989; **321**:337–343.

81 Basu R, Schwenk WF, Rizza RA. Both fasting glucose production and disappearance are abnormal in people with "mild" and "severe" type 2 diabetes. *Am J Physiol Endocrinol Metab* 2004; **287**: E55–62.

82 Firth RG, Bell PM, Marsh HM, Hansen I, Rizza RA. Postprandial hyperglycemia in patients with noninsulin-dependent diabetes mellitus: role of hepatic and extrahepatic tissues. *J Clin Invest* 1986; **77**:1525–1532.

83 Basu A, Basu R, Shah P, Vella A, Johnson CM, Jensen M, *et al.* Type 2 diabetes impairs splanchnic uptake of glucose but does not alter intestinal glucose absorption during enteral glucose feeding: additional evidence for a defect in hepatic glucokinase activity. *Diabetes* 2001; **50**:1351–1362.

84 Basu A, Basu R, Shah P, Vella A, Johnson CM, Nair KS, *et al.* Effects of type 2 diabetes on the ability of insulin and glucose to regulate splanchnic and muscle glucose metabolism: evidence for a defect in hepatic glucokinase activity. *Diabetes* 2000; **49**:272–283.

85 Lewis GF, Carpentier A, Adeli K, Giacca A. Disordered fat storage and mobilization in the pathogenesis of insulin resistance and type 2 diabetes. *Endocr Rev* 2002; **23**:201–229.

86 Roust LR, Jensen MD. Postprandial free fatty acid kinetics are abnormal in upper body obesity. *Diabetes* 1993; **42**:1567–1573.

87 Saloranta C, Franssila-Kallunki A, Ekstrand A, Taskinen MR, Groop L. Modulation of hepatic glucose production by non-esterified fatty acids in type 2 (non-insulin-dependent) diabetes mellitus. *Diabetologia* 1991; **34**:409–415.

88 Klein S, Wolfe RR. Carbohydrate restriction regulates the adaptive response to fasting. *Am J Physiol* 1992; **262**:E631–636.

89 Kelley DE, Mokan M, Simoneau JA, Mandarino LJ. Interaction between glucose and free fatty acid metabolism in human skeletal muscle. *J Clin Invest* 1993; **92**:91–98.

90 Ferrannini E, Barrett EJ, Bevilacqua S, DeFronzo RA. Effect of fatty acids on glucose production and utilization in man. *J Clin Invest* 1983; **72**:1737–1747.

91 Miles JM, Haymond MW, Nissen SL, Gerich JE. Effects of free fatty acid availability, glucagon excess, and insulin deficiency on ketone body production in postabsorptive man. *J Clin Invest* 1983; **71**:1554–1561.

92 Dinneen S, Alzaid A, Turk D, Rizza R. Failure of glucagon suppression contributes to postprandial hyperglycaemia in IDDM. *Diabetologia* 1995; **38**:337–343.

93 Jensen MD, Haymond MW, Gerich JE, Cryer PE, Miles JM. Lipolysis during fasting: decreased suppression by insulin and increased stimulation by epinephrine. *J Clin Invest* 1987; **79**:207–213.

94 Kanaley JA, Haymond MW, Jensen MD. Effects of exercise and weight loss on leucine turnover in different types of obesity. *Am J Physiol* 1993; **264**:E687–692.

95 Ruegemer JJ, Squires RW, Marsh HM, Haymond MW, Cryer PE, Rizza RA, *et al.* Differences between prebreakfast and late afternoon glycemic responses to exercise in IDDM patients. *Diabetes Care* 1990; **13**:104–110.

96 Schneider SH, Vitug A, Ananthakrishnan R, Khachadurian AK. Impaired adrenergic response to prolonged exercise in type 1 diabetes. *Metabolism* 1991; **40**:1219–1225.

97 Wahren J, Sato Y, Ostman J, Hagenfeldt L, Felig P. Turnover and splanchnic metabolism of free fatty acids and ketones in insulin-dependent diabetics at rest and in response to exercise. *J Clin Invest* 1984; **73**:1367–1376.

98 Reaven GM, Hollenbeck C, Jeng CY, Wu MS, Chen YD. Measurement of plasma glucose, free fatty acid, lactate, and insulin for 24 h in patients with NIDDM. *Diabetes* 1988; **37**:1020–1024.

99 Coppack SW, Evans RD, Fisher RM, Frayn KN, Gibbons GF, Humphreys SM, *et al.* Adipose tissue metabolism in obesity: lipase action *in vivo* before and after a mixed meal. *Metabolism* 1992; **41**:264–272.

100 Campbell PJ, Carlson MG, Nurjhan N. Fat metabolism in human obesity. *Am J Physiol* 1994; **266**:E600–605.

101 Nurjhan N, Campbell PJ, Kennedy FP, Miles JM, Gerich JE. Insulin dose–response characteristics for suppression of glycerol release and conversion to glucose in humans. *Diabetes* 1986; **35**:1326–1331.

102 Roden M, Price TB, Perseghin G, Petersen KF, Rothman DL, Cline GW, *et al.* Mechanism of free fatty acid-induced insulin resistance in humans. *J Clin Invest* 1996; **97**:2859–2865.

103 Shah P, Vella A, Basu A, Basu R, Adkins A, Schwenk WF, *et al.* Effects of free fatty acids and glycerol on splanchnic glucose metabolism and insulin extraction in nondiabetic humans. *Diabetes* 2002; **51**:301–310.

104 Boden G. Role of fatty acids in the pathogenesis of insulin resistance and NIDDM. *Diabetes* 1997; **46**:3–10.

105 Moller N, Nair KS. Diabetes and protein metabolism. *Diabetes* 2008; **57**:3–4.

106 Walsh CH, Soler NG, James H, Harvey TC, Thomas BJ, Fremlin JH, *et al.* Studies in whole body potassium and whole body nitrogen in newly diagnosed diabetics. *Q J Med* 1976; **45**:295–301.

107 Atchley DW, Loeb RF, Richards DW, Benedict EM, Driscoll ME. On diabetic acidosis: a detailed study of electrolyte balances following the withdrawal and reestablishment of insulin therapy. *J Clin Invest* 1933; **12**:297–326.

108 Felig P, Wahren J, Sherwin R, Palaiologos G. Amino acid and protein metabolism in diabetes mellitus. *Arch Intern Med* 1977; **137**: 507–513.

109 Nair KS, Garrow JS, Ford C, Mahler RF, Halliday D. Effect of poor diabetic control and obesity on whole body protein metabolism in man. *Diabetologia* 1983; **25**:400–403.

110 Charlton MR, Adey DB, Nair KS. Evidence for a catabolic role of glucagon during an amino acid load. *J Clin Invest* 1996; **98**:90–99.

111 Nair KS, Ford GC, Ekberg K, Fernqvist-Forbes E, Wahren J. Protein dynamics in whole body and in splanchnic and leg tissues in type 1 diabetic patients. *J Clin Invest* 1995; **95**:2926–2937.

112 Halvatsiotis PG, Turk D, Alzaid A, Dinneen S, Rizza RA, Nair KS. Insulin effect on leucine kinetics in type 2 diabetes mellitus. *Diabetes Nutr Metab* 2002; **15**:136–142.

113 Luzi L, Petrides AS, De Fronzo RA. Different sensitivity of glucose and amino acid metabolism to insulin in NIDDM. *Diabetes* 1993; **42**:1868–1877.

114 Gougeon R, Marliss EB, Jones PJ, Pencharz PB, Morais JA. Effect of exogenous insulin on protein metabolism with differing nonprotein energy intakes in type 2 diabetes mellitus. *Int J Obes Relat Metab Disord* 1998; **22**:250–261.

115 Gougeon R, Styhler K, Morais JA, Jones PJ, Marliss EB. Effects of oral hypoglycemic agents and diet on protein metabolism in type 2 diabetes. *Diabetes Care* 2000; **23**:1–8.

116 Gougeon R, Morais JA, Chevalier S, Pereira S, Lamarche M, Marliss EB. Determinants of whole-body protein metabolism in subjects with and without type 2 diabetes. *Diabetes Care* 2008; **31**:128–133.

117 Pereira S, Marliss EB, Morais JA, Chevalier S, Gougeon R. Insulin resistance of protein metabolism in type 2 diabetes. *Diabetes* 2008; **57**:56–63.

118 Hughes K, Choo M, Kuperan P, Ong CN, Aw TC. Cardiovascular risk factors in non-insulin-dependent diabetics compared to non-diabetic controls: a population-based survey among Asians in Singapore. *Atherosclerosis* 1998; **136**:25–31.

119 Kruszynska YT, Yu JG, Olefsky JM, Sobel BE. Effects of troglitazone on blood concentrations of plasminogen activator inhibitor 1 in patients with type 2 diabetes and in lean and obese normal subjects. *Diabetes* 2000; **49**:633–639.

120 Yu JG, Javorschi S, Hevener AL, Kruszynska YT, Norman RA, Sinha M, *et al.* The effect of thiazolidinediones on plasma adiponectin levels in normal, obese, and type 2 diabetic subjects. *Diabetes* 2002; **51**:2968–2974.

121 Seino Y, Ikeda M, Kurahachi H, Taminato T, Sakurai H, Goto Y, *et al.* Failure of suppress plasma glucagon concentrations by orally administered glucose in diabetic patients after treatment. *Diabetes* 1978; **27**:1145–1150.

122 Gerich JE, Lorenzi M, Bier DM, Schneider V, Tsalikian E, Karam JH, *et al.* Prevention of human diabetic ketoacidosis by somatostatin: evidence for an essential role of glucagon. *N Engl J Med* 1975; **292**:985–989.

123 Muller WA, Faloona GR, Aguilar-Parada E, Unger RH. Abnormal alpha-cell function in diabetes: response to carbohydrate and protein ingestion. *N Engl J Med* 1970; **283**:109–115.

124 Raskin P, Unger RH. Effect of insulin therapy on the profiles of plasma immunoreactive glucagon in juvenile-type and adult-type diabetics. *Diabetes* 1978; **27**:411–419.

125 Stagner JI, Samols E, Koerker DJ, Goodner CJ. Perfusion with anti-insulin gamma globulin indicates a B to A to D cellular perfusion sequence in the pancreas of the rhesus monkey, *Macaca mulatta*. *Pancreas* 1992; **7**:26–29.

126 Dagogo-Jack S, Rattarasarn C, Cryer PE. Reversal of hypoglycemia unawareness, but not defective glucose counterregulation, in IDDM. *Diabetes* 1994; **43**:1426–1434.

127 Rizza R, Verdonk C, Miles J, Service FJ, Gerich J. Effect of intermittent endogenous hyperglucagonemia on glucose homeostasis in normal and diabetic man. *J Clin Invest* 1979; **63**:1119–1123.

128 Cherrington AD, Williams PE, Shulman GI, Lacy WW. Differential time course of glucagon's effect on glycogenolysis and gluconeogenesis in the conscious dog. *Diabetes* 1981; **30**:180–187.

129 Bolli G, De Feo P, De Cosmo S, Perriello G, Angeletti G, Ventura MR, *et al.* Effects of long-term optimization and short-term deterioration of glycemic control on glucose counterregulation in type 1 diabetes mellitus. *Diabetes* 1984; **33**:394–400.

130 Bolli G, Cartechini MG, Compagnucci P, Malvicini S, De Feo P, Santeusanio F, *et al.* Effect of metabolic control on urinary excretion

and plasma levels of catecholamines in diabetics. *Horm Metab Res* 1979; **11**:493–497.

131 Rizza RA, Cryer PE, Haymond MW, Gerich JE. Adrenergic mechanisms for the effects of epinephrine on glucose production and clearance in man. *J Clin Invest* 1980; **65**:682–689.

132 Gerich JE, Lorenzi M, Tsalikian E, Karam JH. Studies on the mechanism of epinephrine-induced hyperglycemia in man: evidence for participation of pancreatic glucagon secretion. *Diabetes* 1976; **25**:65–71.

133 Avogaro A, Valerio A, Gnudi L, Maran A, Miola M, Duner E, *et al.* The effects of different plasma insulin concentrations on lipolytic and ketogenic responses to epinephrine in normal and type 1 (insulin-dependent) diabetic humans. *Diabetologia* 1992; **35**:129–138.

134 Dinneen S, Alzaid A, Miles J, Rizza R. Effects of the normal nocturnal rise in cortisol on carbohydrate and fat metabolism in IDDM. *Am J Physiol* 1995; **268**:E595–603.

135 Schade DS, Eaton RP, Standefer J. Modulation of basal ketone body concentration by cortisol in diabetic man. *J Clin Endocrinol Metab* 1978; **47**:519–528.

136 Hayford JT, Danney MM, Hendrix JA, Thompson RG. Integrated concentration of growth hormone in juvenile-onset diabetes. *Diabetes* 1980; **29**:391–398.

137 Hansen AP. Effect of insulin on growth-hormone secretion in juvenile diabetics. *Lancet* 1972; **2**:432–433.

138 Press M, Tamborlane WV, Sherwin RS. Importance of raised growth hormone levels in mediating the metabolic derangements of diabetes. *N Engl J Med* 1984; **310**:810–815.

139 Miles JM, Rizza RA, Haymond MW, Gerich JE. Effects of acute insulin deficiency on glucose and ketone body turnover in man: evidence for the primacy of overproduction of glucose and ketone bodies in the genesis of diabetic ketoacidosis. *Diabetes* 1980; **29**:926–930.

140 Cryer PE, White NH, Santiago JV. The relevance of glucose counterregulatory systems to patients with insulin-dependent diabetes mellitus. *Endocr Rev* 1986; **7**:131–139.

141 Butkiewicz EK, Leibson CL, O'Brien PC, Palumbo PJ, Rizza RA. Insulin therapy for diabetic ketoacidosis: bolus insulin injection versus continuous insulin infusion. *Diabetes Care* 1995; **18**:1187–1190.

14 Obesity and Diabetes

Hans Hauner

Else Kröner-Fresenius-Center for Nutritional Medicine, Technical University of Munich, Munich, Germany

Keypoints

- Obesity is characterized by an excess of body fat mass and is defined by a body mass index equal to or greater than 30 kg/m^2. Its prevalence has increased considerably over the past decades in all parts of the world and currently affects 15–30% of the adult populations in Western countries.
- Overweight and/or obesity represents by far the most important modifiable risk factor for type 2 diabetes mellitus (T2DM). An abdominal type of body fat distribution is also closely associated with T2DM, particularly in the lower body mass index categories.
- Both obesity and T2DM have a strong genetic background. The known susceptibility genes for obesity mainly affect central pathways of food intake, whereas most risk genes for T2DM compromise β-cell function.
- Important environmental factors contributing to the development of obesity include energy-dense diets including large portion sizes and permanent availability of foods, lack of physical activity and low socioeconomic status.
- An expanded adipose tissue impairs insulin action and causes insulin resistance in muscle, adipose tissue, liver and possibly other organs.
- Obesity is also characterized by subacute chronic inflammation in adipose tissue because of an impaired paracrine–endocrine function of adipose tissue, but also by mitochondrial dysfunction, local hypoxia and other still poorly understood disturbances at the cellular level.
- Weight loss in obese individuals is followed by rapid amelioration of all metabolic disturbances including chronic inflammation and insulin resistance. These improvements are brought about by caloric restriction rather than the macronutrient composition of the dietary intervention.
- Bariatric surgery is the most powerful approach to treat morbid obesity and may lead to a marked improvement of the metabolic disturbances if not the resolution of T2DM.

Introduction

Obesity is defined as a common chronic disorder of excessive body fat and has become a global epidemic which is present not only in the industrialized world but also in many developing and even in underdeveloped countries. At present, the prevalence of obesity (defined as body mass index [BMI] ≥30 kg/m^2) is in the range 15–30% in the adult populations in Europe, North America and in many Arabic countries, with an unequivocal trend for further increases [1]. This condition increases the risk of developing a variety of adverse consequences to human health ranging from metabolic disturbances including type 2 diabetes mellitus (T2DM) and cardiovascular complications to disorders of the locomotor system and many types of cancer [2]. In addition, obesity impairs the subjective quality of life in affected people and can reduce life expectancy [3]. Although there is a very specific close relationship between excessive body weight and the risk of diabetes, the presence of obesity may induce many other disturbances that may aggravate the diabetic state.

Textbook of Diabetes, 4th edition. Edited by R. Holt, C. Cockram, A. Flyvbjerg and B. Goldstein.

Definition of obesity and the body fat distribution pattern

The diagnosis and classification of obesity is usually based on the BMI. This simple anthropometric index can be calculated from body weight and height, is independent of body height and correlates reasonably well with body fat mass (r = 0.4–0.7). The current classification of body weight according to the World Health Organization (WHO) is presented in Table 14.1. A BMI greater than 30 kg/m^2 is considered to be the central formal criterion for the definition of obesity which is further subdivided into three classes depending on the severity of excessive body fat. The BMI range of 25–29.9 kg/m^2 represents the category of overweight or pre-obesity which requires additional criteria to assess the concomitant health risks. In Western countries, 30–50% of the population fall into the category of overweight [1].

Not only the extent of excessive body fat mass, but also the anatomic location of the body fat mass determines the risk for metabolic and cardiovascular complications. This is particularly

Table 14.1 Classification of human obesity based on body mass index (BMI) classification (kg/m^2). Reproduced from World Health Organization [1] with permission.

Classification	kg/m^2
Underweight	<18.5
Normal weight	18.5–24.9
Overweight	≥25.0
Obesity	
grade I	30–34.9
grade II	35–39.9
grade III	≥40

Table 14.2 Classification of fat distribution pattern, threshold values for the moderately and markedly elevated risk for metabolic and cardiovascular diseases.

	Waist circumference (cm)	
	Elevated metabolic and cardiovascular risk	
	Moderately	Markedly
Men	>94	>102
Women	>80	>88

important for the category of moderate overweight and even in the upper normal range of BMI. At a defined BMI, the pattern of fat distribution can vary substantially. This has been most impressively shown using computed tomography (CT) or magnetic resonance imaging (MRI) scans which are the only imaging techniques to provide a direct assessment of the size of the intra-abdominal visceral adipose tissue. For practical means, waist circumference measured mid way between the lower rib margin and the upper iliac crest is used as a simple anthropometric measure to assess the fat distribution pattern. This variable has been used in many cross-sectional and longitudinal studies; therefore, the threshold levels demonstrated in Table 14.2 are now well based on human data sets concerning associated health risks. The waist circumference is closely correlated with BMI but cannot discriminate between subcutaneous and intra-abdominal fat depots.

Obesity is the most potent risk factor for type 2 diabetes

A large body of clinical data consistently demonstrates a close relationship between body fat mass and the risk of diabetes. It is noteworthy that in contrast to other obesity-associated metabolic disturbances, the diabetes risk already increases in the upper normal range of BMI. This has been shown for both men and women. In the prospective Nurses' Health Study, women in the upper normal range with a BMI of 23.0–24.9 kg/m^2 had a four- to fivefold increased risk of developing diabetes over a 14-year observation period compared with women with a BMI of <22 kg/m^2. In women with a BMI of 29.0–30.9 kg/m^2 the risk of diabetes was 27.6-fold higher than in the lean reference group. Almost two-thirds of newly diagnosed women with T2DM were obese at the time of diagnosis [4]. Similar observations were made for males in the Health Professionals' Study [5]. Moreover, changes in body weight also predicted the risk of diabetes. Weight gain in women after the age of 18 of 11.0–19.9 kg, which is the average range of weight change between adolescence and menopause in industrialized countries, was found to be associated with a 5.5-fold higher risk of diabetes compared with weight-stable women, whereas weight reduction of the same extent reduced the risk of diabetes by about 80% [4]. Very similar data were reported for men [5]. A recent analysis of the EPIC Potsdam cohort revealed that a weight gain of 1 BMI unit between the age of 25 and 40 years increased the relative risk of T2DM by 25% and had a greater effect than the same weight gain between 40 and 55 years of age [6]. It is also important to note that the duration of obesity has a strong impact on the risk of developing T2DM.

In a recent analysis of the relative contributions of different levels of overweight and obesity to the prevalence of diabetes between 1976–1980 and 2000–2004 in the USA it was found that the increase in total diabetes prevalence from 5.08% to 8.83% was largely caused by the increase in obesity. Of the increased number, 81% was attributed to the different classes of obesity (Figure 14.1). The authors concluded that the increase in diabetes prevalence over recent decades has disproportionately included persons with extreme levels of obesity [7]. Thus, obesity appears to be the main environmental driving force for the manifestation of T2DM.

In addition to the level and the duration of obesity, the risk of developing diabetes is also potently influenced by the fat distribution pattern. In an early study in humans, an abdominal pattern of fat distribution was found to be an independent risk factor for T2DM [8]. Subsequent studies confirmed this observation in many age groups and ethnic populations. Particularly at low degrees of overweight, and even in the upper normal range, the fat distribution pattern strongly predicts the risk for diabetes and the metabolic syndrome. Therefore, waist circumference should be routinely assessed when estimating the risk of diabetes even in normal-weight subjects. In the clinical setting, it is striking to observe that the majority of subjects with diabetes, particularly those of middle age, show a visible preferential truncal accumulation of excess body fat. It is also interesting to note that similar observations were made for the association between BMI and cardiovascular disease. Among overweight and obese subjects, only those with an abdominal type of fat distribution are at increased risk of coronary heart disease as recently documented in the INTERHEART study [9].

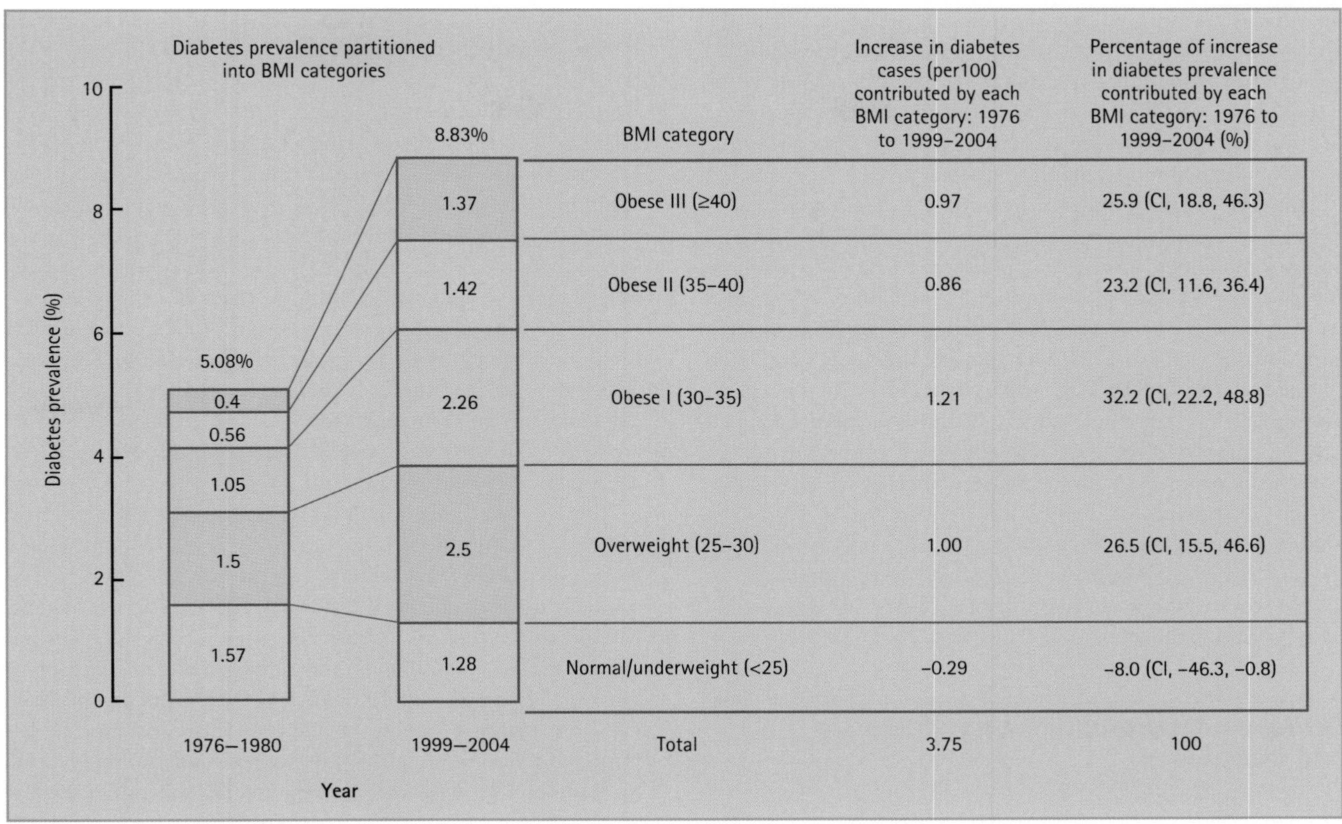

Figure 14.1 Contribution of five body mass index (BMI) categories to the overall prevalence of diabetes. National Health and Nutrition Examination Survey (NHANES) samples of 1976–1980 and 1999–2004 were compared. Reproduced from Gregg *et al.* [7], with permission from Elsevier.

Genetic predisposition for obesity and type 2 diabetes

It is well known from family, adoption and twin studies that obesity, like T2DM, has a strong genetic basis. In the classic adoption study by Stunkard *et al.* [10] there was no resemblance between the adult BMI of adopted Danish children and the BMI of the adopting parents, but a significant correlation to the BMI of the biologic parents, especially to the BMI class of the biologic mother. In a twin study of obesity, concordance rates for different degrees of overweight were twice as high for monozygotic twins as for dizygotic twins. This high heritability for BMI was seen at the age of 20 years and to a similar extent at a 25-year follow-up, suggesting that body fatness is under substantial genetic control [11]. There is also a very close correlation in monozygotic twins who were reared apart, also indicating a high heritability of the BMI trait. In a recent study of 5092 twins living in the London area, the authors estimated the heritability of BMI and waist circumference as 0.77, further supporting the strong effect of the genetic components irrespective of the force of the obesogenic environment [12].

During the last decade, a number of monogenic disorders that result in human obesity have been uncovered. These genetic disorders were only found in rare cases, however, usually children and adolescents with early onset of obesity. At present, a variety of homozygous and compound heterozygous mutations have been described in the leptin–melanocortin signaling pathway, some of them with functional consequences resulting in human obesity. Functional mutations in the melanocortin-4-receptor gene are considered to be the most frequent cause of monogenic obesity in children with a frequency of 2–4% of all obese cases. It is striking that these defects affect genes that are involved in the central control of food intake [13].

Recent genome-wide association (GWA) studies in large cohorts with BMI as phenotype reported common genetic variants on various chromosomes. These polymorphisms predisposing to obesity at the population level are also largely related to central pathways of food intake [14–16]. Thus, human obesity may represent a heritable neurobehavioral disorder that is highly sensitive to environmental conditions, especially an energy-dense palatable foods which are abundantly available in many societies [13]. Despite these remarkable advances in our understanding of the genetic factors related to obesity, the effect size of most of the novel "obesity genes" is rather modest. Only individuals who are homozygous for the high-risk allele of the *FTO* gene weigh on average 3 kg more than individuals with two low-risk alleles [14]. The gene is encoding a 2-oxoglutarate-dependent nucleic acid demethylase which is mainly expressed in the brain and in the arcuate nucleus of the hypothalamus [17]. Among the almost 20 gene variants found in GWA studies so far, variants near to the *FTO* and the *MC4R* gene appear to have the strongest effect size on body weight. All other recently discovered gene polymorphisms influence body weight by far less than 1 kg.

Thus, it is apparent from recent work that obesity represents a rather heterogeneous disorder in terms of genetic background and susceptibility to etiologic environmental factors. In addition, the risk for developing co-morbidities including T2DM may strongly depend on the individual genetic predisposition towards such diseases. In the case of T2DM, the lifetime risk of developing this disease is about 30% in the white North American population and similar in other ethnic groups [18]. It is currently assumed that only those obese subjects who exhibit a genetic failure of the pancreas to compensate for insulin resistance, which is a characteristic consequence of obesity, will develop T2DM [19]; even among severely obese subjects (BMI $\geq 40\,kg/m^2$) only 30–40% will develop diabetes throughout life. Thus, the development of T2DM requires the presence of "diabetes genes" which probably limit β-cell function.

Developmental programming of obesity and diabetes

A new component that may have a major role in the development of obesity and T2DM is the modification of gene expression by epigenetic mechanisms during fetal life. Although this is still a poorly defined phenomenon and it is rather unclear which mechanisms may underlie this association, there is some clue that epigenetics may also operate in this context. Observational studies suggest that infants of mothers with gestational diabetes are at increased risk of developing childhood obesity [20]. In another study, siblings born after the mother had developed gestational diabetes (i.e. exposed to diabetes *in utero*) have a much greater risk of T2DM in young adulthood than siblings not exposed to diabetes *in utero* (odds ratio 3.7; $P = 0.02$) [21].

Another interesting clinical observation is that excessive weight gain during pregnancy, independent of initial BMI, may also increase the risk of early development of obesity in the offspring [22,23]. It is speculated that both hyperglycemia and chronic overnutrition during pregnancy may cause fetal hyperinsulinemia, hypercortisolemia and hyperleptinemia. These hormonal changes may result in a persisting malprogramming of hypothalamic centers controlling energy homeostasis and metabolism, thereby increasing the lifetime risk for obesity and T2DM and possibly the risk for other adverse long-term health consequences [24]. The mechanisms mediating these effects are largely elusive, but it is speculated that epigenetic processes such as DNA methylation, histone modification and changes of the microRNA pattern are involved. Animal experiments suggest that this imprinting process may mainly affect central neuroendocrine pathways which may finally modify appetite regulation [24].

Pathophysiology of obesity

Irrespective of the strong genetic influence on body weight, there is also no doubt that the evolving worldwide epidemic of obesity is primarily a consequence of substantial changes in the environment and lifestyle (see Chapter 8). It is rather new to mankind that food is abundant in many countries and that physical activity is no longer a prerequisite for survival. These dramatic changes in environment and the subsequent changes in lifestyle have occurred within a few decades, a period probably too short to result in adaptations of the genetic background and biologic systems to optimize survival. To date, the relative contributions of the various environmental factors to the epidemic of obesity are hard to quantify in detail and there exist considerable differences between populations.

Humans, like other mammals, are characterized by a tight control of energy homeostasis allowing a stable body weight to be maintained. This setpoint of body weight can vary substantially among individuals and may also vary across lifetime. A complex regulatory system controls energy homeostasis which involves central pathways and peripheral components such as the size of adipose tissue which is sensed to the brain via the secretion of leptin. In addition, gut hormones, signals from the gastrointestinal nervous system and nutrients signal to the brain and induce a complex central integration according to the dietary intake and nutrient requirements of the organism. Central pathways are the anorexigenic leptin–melanocortin link and the orexigenic NPY–AgRP pathway. Many other factors such as insulin modify these signaling processes and thereby influence energy balance [25]. This complex and potent homeostatic system also serves to defend body weight against a critical energy deficiency but also against chronic overnutrition. Several adaptive systems are known to restore the initial body weight under such fluctuations of energy intake and expenditure. This may explain why obese humans exhibit a strong tendency to regain weight after intentional dietary weight reduction. The same tendency to return to initial body weight is observed after experimental overfeeding.

The role of energy homeostasis in the development of obesity has been elaborated by previous studies using indirect calorimetry to investigate the contribution of the resting metabolic rate (RMR) to the risk of obesity. In a study of Pima Indians, RMR was found to be a familial trait and to vary considerably across families [26]. In prospective studies in American Indians, a reduced rate of energy expenditure assessed in a respiratory chamber turned out to predict body weight gain over a 2-year follow-up period. This finding was confirmed in another group over a 4-year-follow-up period in the same paper, indicating that a low rate of energy expenditure may contribute to the aggregation of obesity in families [27]. At present, the genetic components for these differences in energy metabolism are still unknown.

Environmental factors promoting obesity and type 2 diabetes

It is now established that a complex gene–environment interaction determines the individual risk to develop obesity (Table 14.3). Even in societies with an abundance of affordable, highly palatable food there is a high variation in body weight across the populations ranging from lean individuals to extremely obese persons. Many other factors such as physical activity, education and socioeconomic status may also act as strong modifiers of body weight. After two to three decades of modern lifestyle the trend towards obesity appears to reach a plateau, as suggested by recent data from the USA and other Western countries. This observation also supports the concept that genetic and biologic factors contribute substantially to the susceptibility to develop obesity.

Despite the genetic predisposition it is widely accepted that the current worldwide epidemic of obesity is largely a consequence of dramatic changes in lifestyle and environment which emerged over the past 30–50 years. A dramatic change in eating habits and food selection took place, whereas physical activity decreased remarkably because of technologic development concerning transportation and workplaces. Although dietary abundance and sedentary lifestyles have multiple origins, both may equally contribute to a chronic positive energy balance which may result in energy storage in adipose tissue.

A rather novel phenomenon is the expansion of the fast-food culture characterized by high-fat, low-starch foods together with a high intake of sugar-sweetened beverages. In addition to having a high energy density, fast-food menus have large portion sizes. This combination has led to the assumption that frequent fast-food consumption is linked to body weight gain and maintenance of overweight and obesity in the population. Despite this popular explanation, there is rather limited evidence for this association in the scientific literature. Nevertheless, a recent systematic review of six cross-sectional and seven prospective cohort studies concluded that sufficient evidence exists, at least for the adult population [28]. In addition, a high intake of sugar-sweetened beverages is another part of the global fast-food culture. Another systematic review clearly concluded that a high intake of calorically sweetened beverages can be regarded as a determinant of obesity, although there was no support that this association is mediated via increased energy intake, suggesting that alternative biologic explanations should be also explored [29]. In view of the expansive growth of the fast-food industry in many countries this is a critical issue and may require more intense public discussion on the health consequences of this policy. According to a recent survey, people from the USA obtain one-third of their daily caloric intake from restaurant meals, and one-third of customers of chain restaurants in New York purchased meals containing more than 1000 calories [30]. Thus, there is a growing need to develop new public health policies to limit fast-food consumption and to facilitate a healthier food selection.

Table 14.3 Environmental factors promoting the development of obesity.

Ready availability of food
High palatability of food
High energy density
Relatively low cost of foods
High consumption of sugar-sweetened beverages
Aggressive commercial food promotion
Low physical activity

Another aspect in the context of high fast-food consumption which may further explain the elevated risk of obesity is the energy density of modern foods. There is convincing evidence that energy density of foods is a key determinant of caloric intake. From an evolutionary point of view, the human regulatory system for energy intake is adapted to starchy foods with low caloric content which requires large volumes to obtain sufficient energy. Today, most fast-foods have a high energy density which may favor a passive overconsumption of calories. A recent study showed that the average energy density of fast-food menus is approximately 1100 kJ/100 g, which is 65% higher than the average British diet (approximately 670 kJ/100 g) and more than twice the energy density of recommended healthy diets (approximately 525 kJ/100 g). It is 145% higher than in traditional African diets (approximately 450 kJ/100 g) which represent the levels against which human weight regulatory mechanisms have evolved. The authors concluded that the high energy density of many fast foods challenges human appetite control systems with conditions for which they were never developed [31].

Another determinant of the obesity epidemic may be the persistent trend over the last decades towards increasing portion sizes. A study from the USA demonstrated that the average portion size for many food items increased markedly between 1977 and 1998, with greatest increases for food consumed at fast-food restaurants and at home [32]. Similar trends have been documented in other countries. Experimental human studies have clearly established that both increasing the portion size and the energy density of food is associated with an increase in caloric intake and, in the long run, may therefore promote weight gain and obesity [33].

Finally, socioeconomic status is a strong determinant of obesity and of T2DM. In most countries there is a gradient between education and household income and the prevalence of obesity. A low socioeconomic status is associated with an unfavorable lifestyle including poor nutrition, low leisure-time physical activity and low health consciousness. This gradient is usually greater in females than males. Thus, the association between low household income and obesity may be mediated by the low costs of energy-dense foods, whereas prudent healthy diets based on lean meats, fish, vegetables and fruit may be less affordable for those of lower socioeconomic status [34].

Pathophysiologic links between obesity and type 2 diabetes

T2DM is characterized by an impaired insulin action or a defective secretion of insulin or both. Both defects are thought to be required for the manifestation of the disease and both are present many years before the clinical onset of the disease. To date, the mechanisms by which obesity increases the risk of developing T2DM are only partly understood and the evolving picture is getting more and more complex. The main adverse effect of obesity is on the action of insulin, particularly in liver, muscle and adipose tissue, but obesity also affects insulin secretion. Substantial advances have been made over recent years in our understanding how an excessive fat mass, but also chronic overnutrition, may cause metabolic disturbances resulting in overt T2DM in those with a genetic predisposition for the disease.

Lipids and insulin resistance

The earliest hypothesis to explain the relationship between obesity and T2DM is the "glucose–fatty acid cycle" which is based on the observation of a competition between glucose and fatty acid oxidation in the heart muscle and was introduced by Randle *et al.* [35]. The increased supply of non-esterified fatty acids from expanded adipose tissue depots competes with glucose utilization, particularly in muscle, which represents the organ that oxidizes the largest proportion of glucose. The proposed mechanism is an inhibition of the glycolytic enzymes pyruvate dehydrogenase, phosphofructokinase and hexokinase. As a consequence, the rate of glucose oxidation is reduced and glucose concentrations rise. The concomitant increased fatty acid turnover is accompanied by an increased release of glycerol from adipose tissue which is reutilized for hepatic glucose production, further augmenting the imbalance of glucose metabolism. Increased hepatic glucose output is another early disturbance contributing to glucose intolerance.

In addition, it was reported that elevated free fatty acids can directly impair insulin action. Recent studies suggested that obese subjects and those with T2DM have a high intramyocellular lipid accumulation which is an important feature of the insulin-resistant state. Exposure of skeletal muscle to an excessive lipid supply may lead to intramuscular accumulation, not only of neutral fatty acids, but also of lipid-derived metabolites such as ceramide, diacylglycerol and fatty acyl coenzyme A (CoA). This lipid accumulation is associated with coincident disturbances in insulin action mediated by an activation of a serine–threonine kinase cascade leading to serine–threonine phosphorylation of insulin receptor substrate 1 (IRS-1) and IRS-2 which may cause an impairment of insulin signaling including an impaired activation of phosphoinositol-3 kinase and other downstream elements [36]. This condition is also caused and exacerbated by chronic overnutrition with a high dietary fat intake. Thus, the increased availability of fatty acids may be the single most critical factor in disturbing insulin action in obesity.

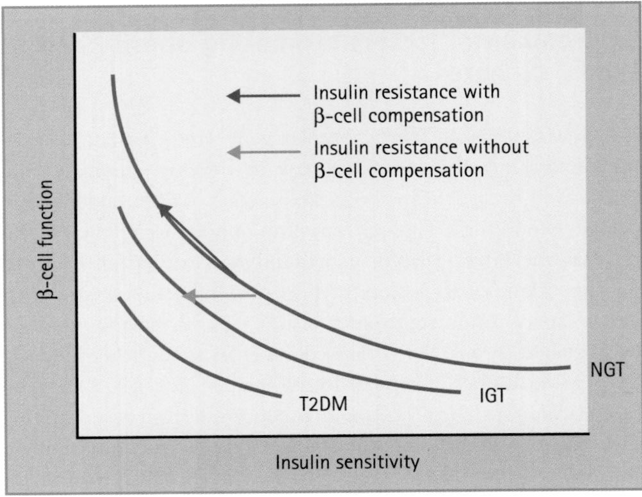

Figure 14.2 Hyperbolic relation between β-cell function and insulin sensitivity. IGT, impaired glucose tolerance; NGT, normal glucose tolerance; T2DM, type 2 diabetes mellitus. Reproduced from Stumvoll M, Goldstein BJ, van Haeften TW. Type 2 diabetes: principles of pathogenesis and therapy. *Lancet* 2005; **365**:1333–1346, with permission from Elsevier.

Lipids and β-cell function

Obesity is characterized by an elevated insulin secretion and a decreased hepatic insulin clearance. Human studies suggested that the β-cell volume is increased by about 50% in healthy obese subjects, probably because of hypertrophy of existing β-cells. Insulin release and insulin sensitivity are closely reciprocally related in a non-linear manner (Figure 14.2). Failure of this feedback system is known to result in a progressive decline in β-cell function and to underlie the development of T2DM. In addition to glucose, long-chain fatty acids may also exert a stimulatory effect on insulin secretion from the pancreatic β-cells via generation of fatty acyl CoA and activation of protein kinase C [36]. Another effect of fatty acids on insulin secretion is via binding to the G-protein-coupled receptor GPR 40 on the β-cell membrane which may result in a subsequent increase in intracellular calcium and secretory granule exocytosis [37]. Although fatty acids are critical for normal insulin secretion, a chronic exposure of β-cells to excessive fatty acids is associated with marked impairment of glucose-stimulated insulin secretion and decrease in insulin biosynthesis [38]. Another mechanism by which elevated fatty acids may impair insulin secretion in response to glucose is via an increased expression of uncoupling protein 2 (UCP-2) in β-cells. UCP-2 was found to be upregulated under glucolipotoxic conditions and mitochondrial superoxide has been identified as a post-translational negative regulator of UCP-2 activity in islets [39].

Glucose sensing of the pancreatic β-cells requires an intact oxidative mitochondrial metabolism to generate ATP. The resulting high ATP:ADP ratio is a prerequisite for normal insulin secretion. Studies in humans suggest that insulin resistance may

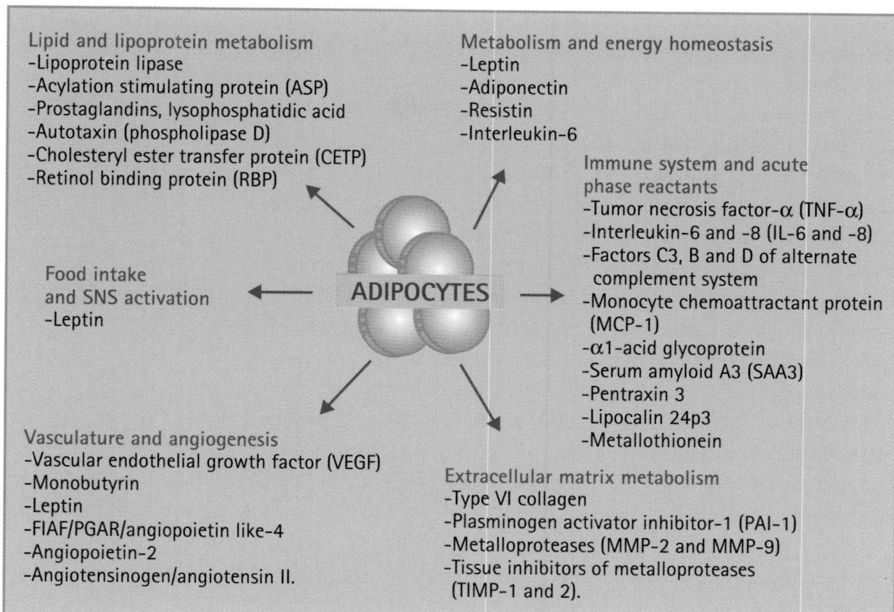

Figure 14.3 Secretory products from adipose tissue and functional relationship. Reproduced from Lafontan M. Fat cells: afferent and efferent messages define new approaches to treat obesity. *Annu Rev Pharmacol Toxicol* 2005; **45**:119–146, with permission from *Annual Reviews*.

also arise from defects in mitochondrial fatty acid oxidation which may lead to increased intracellular fatty acid metabolites (fatty acid CoA, diacylglycerol). It was recently shown that young insulin-resistant offspring of parents with T2DM have features of impaired mitochondrial function [40]. Furthermore, it was reported that obese individuals have smaller mitochondria with reduced bioenergetic capacity than lean controls [41]. Although studies on this topic are still limited, there is growing evidence that a defective mitochondrial function could be a prominent feature of disturbances in both insulin secretion and action [42].

Adipose tissue as a secretory organ

Another hypothesis that may explain the association between obesity and T2DM is the observation that adipose tissue is a secretory organ that produces and releases a variety of factors that may contribute to the development of insulin resistance and other health risks (Figure 14.3; Table 14.4). Among these factors most data have been collected for a mediator role of tumor necrosis factor α (TNF-α). TNF-α is a multifunctional cytokine which was the first found to be expressed in adipose tissue [43]. It was subsequently shown that TNF-α exerts a variety of catabolic effects in adipose tissue. In addition to TNF-α, it was reported that its two receptor subtypes are overexpressed in adipose tissue from obese subjects [44–46]. The upregulated TNF-α system induces multiple adverse effects at the local organ level such as inhibition of glucose uptake because of an impairment of insulin signaling and suppression of GLUT 4 expression, a reduction of lipoprotein lipase expression and activity, and an increase in lipolysis [47]. Moreover, TNF-α activates the NF-κB pathway in adipose tissue which leads to an increased expression of many proinflammatory proteins such as interleukin 6 (IL-6), IL-8 and monocyte chemotactic protein 1 (MCP-1) among others. Finally, TNF-α was demonstrated to reduce the expression of adiponectin, a protein that is abundantly expressed in fat cells and exerts direct antidiabetic and anti-atherosclerotic actions. A key mechanism by which TNF-α causes insulin resistance may be that this cytokine stimulates the phosphorylation of IRS-1 at the serine residue 307 which inhibits the transduction of the insulin signal to downstream elements [48].

Table 14.4 Secretory function of adipose tissue in obesity and potential clinical consequences.

Product	Secretion	Consequence
Free fatty acids	↑	Dyslipidemia (TG ↑), insulin resistance
TNF-α, IL-6, MCP-1 and other cytokines/chemokines	↑	Insulin resistance, type 2 diabetes
Angiotensinogen, angiotensin II and other vasoactive factors	↑	Hypertension
PAI-1	↑	Thrombembolic complications
CETP	↑	Low HDL cholesterol
Adiponectin	↓	Insulin resistance, atherosclerosis
Estrogens	↑	Endometrial and breast cancer

CETP, cholesterol ester transfer protein; HDL, high density lipoprotein; IL, interleukin; MCP, monocyte chemotactic protein; PAI, plasminogen activator inhibitor; TG, triglycerides; TNF, tumor necrosis factor.

Using an *in vitro* co-culture model of human adipocytes and muscle cells it was recently demonstrated that other fat cell secretory products, in addition to TNF-α, are also involved in the development of muscle insulin resistance [49]. Thus, it is likely that the negative effect on muscle insulin action is brought about by a combination of adipokines. Although we have currently little information on the nature and the complex interplay of such proinflammatory and anti-inflammatory factors, a few relevant players have been identified. One such element may be MCP-1 [50]. Other potential candidates with a prodiabetic action may include plasminogen activator inhibitor 1 (PAI-1), but also lipid metabolites such as ceramide. Retinol-binding protein 4 (RBP-4) was also shown to contribute to insulin resistance via reduced PI_3 kinase signaling and enhanced hepatic expression of the gluconeogenic enzyme phosphoenolpyruvate carboxykinase. An interesting observation in this context is that adiponectin may be able to antagonize the insulin resistance-promoting activity of proinflammatory cytokines released from adipose tissue in an autocrine fashion [51].

Adipocytes are also able to release products with anti-inflammatory properties including factors such as adiponectin, IL-1 receptor antagonist and IL-10. By far the most interesting component is adiponectin, which is the most abundantly expressed protein in adipose tissue. It was shown in a number of clinical studies that circulating adiponectin levels are inversely associated with BMI and that low concentrations predict the development of T2DM [52,53]. Adiponectin is now known to exert a variety of antidiabetic and anti-atherosclerotic effects (e.g. adiponectin stimulates fatty acid oxidation in an AMP-activated protein kinase-dependent manner) [54].

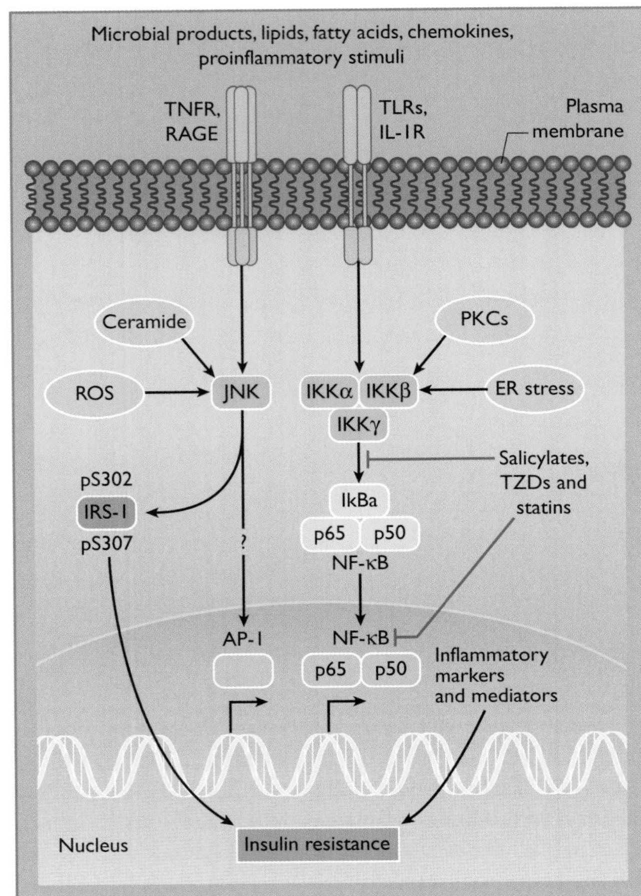

Figure 14.4 Potential cellular mechanisms for inflammation and development of insulin resistance. AP-1, activator protein 1; ER, endoplasmic reticulum; IKK, Iκ kinase; IL, interleukin; IRS, insulin receptor substrate; JNK, c-Jun N-terminal kinase; NF-κB, nuclear transcription factor κB; PKC, protein kinase C; ROS, reactive oxygen species; TLR, toll-like receptor; TNFR, tumor necrosis factor receptor; TZD, thiazolidinedione. Reproduced from Shoelson SE, Lee J, Goldfine AB. Inflammation and insulin resistance. *J Clin Invest* 2006; **116**:1793–801, with permission from the American Society for Clinical Investigation.

Signaling pathways of inflammation in adipose tissue

Current research has shown that the inflammatory response in human obesity is mediated via activation of the c-Jun N-terminal kinase (JNK) and IKKβ–NF-κB pathways. Both pathways are simultaneously stimulated by cytokines such as TNF-α and IL-6, but also by lipids. It has been convincingly demonstrated in experimental studies that genetic or chemical inhibition of these pathways can reduce inflammation and improve insulin resistance (for review see [55]) (Figure 14.4). In obesity, JNK activity is elevated not only in adipose tissue, but also in liver and muscle. Loss of JNK1 prevents the development of insulin resistance and diabetes in both genetic and dietary mouse models of obesity [56]. IKKβ can act on insulin signaling through at least two pathways. First, it can directly phosphorylate IRS-1 on serine residues and, second, it can phosphorylate the inhibitor of NF-κB (IκB) thus activating NK-κB, a transcription factor that stimulates the production of many proinflammatory mediators including TNF-α and IL-6 [57]. Mice heterozygous for IKKβ are partially protected against insulin resistance caused by lipid infusion, high-fat diet or genetic obesity [58]. Both the JNK and the IKKβ–NF-κB pathways are activated via pattern recognition receptors that function as membrane receptors for a variety of external signals. It is interesting to note that endogenous lipids and lipid conjugates were found to activate toll-like receptors (TLRs) in obesity. It was recently reported that saturated fatty acids bind and activate TLR-4 on adipocytes, thereby suggesting a direct link between exogenous nutrients that are redundant in the obese state and inflammation [59]. Mice with a loss-of-function mutation of TLR-4 were found to be protected from diet-induced obesity and insulin resistance. These mice also showed a reduced NF-κB and JNK activity under a high-fat diet compared to wild-type control mice [60]. In a similar model, markedly lower circulating levels of MCP-1 were measured. TLR-4 deficiency, however, did not attenuate the induction of TNF-α and IL-6 expression [61].

It is noteworthy that most proteins released from adipose tissue are not produced by fat cells but rather by pre-adipocytes and invading immune cells such as activated macrophages. While leptin and adiponectin are true adipokines which are almost exclusively produced by adipocytes, TNF-α, IL-6, IL-8, MCP-1, visfatin, PAI-1 and others are mainly expressed by pre-adipocytes, macrophages resident in adipose tissue and possibly other cells. The relative contributions of the various cellular components in adipose tissue to the secretion of these products remains unknown and may vary substantially according to depot and model. Nevertheless, all these locally secreted factors appear to participate in the induction and maintenance of the subacute inflammatory state associated with obesity. It is also important to mention that the invading macrophages release factors that substantially augment adipocyte inflammation and insulin resistance [62]. Another interesting observation in this context is that pre-adipocytes and macrophages share many common features [57].

The regulation and biologic functions of the secretory products are diverse and only poorly understood. In addition to the direct effects of fatty acids and their intracellular products, other factors may also contribute to the chronic inflammatory state in adipose tissue. It was recently shown that fat cell size may be a critical determinant of the production of proinflammatory and anti-inflammatory factors. Enlarged hypertrophic fat cells are characterized by a shift towards a proinflammatory state [63], thereby promoting insulin resistance. This is in agreement with clinical data showing that fat cell hypertrophy is associated with an increased risk of developing T2DM [64].

Obesity and endoplasmic reticulum stress

A recent observation suggests that obesity and chronic overnutrition overload the functional capacity of the endoplasmic reticulum (ER) and that the resulting ER stress contributes to the activation of the inflammatory signaling pathways including the JNK pathway. In both high-fat diet induced and genetic obesity models, obesity was shown to cause ER stress with inositol-requiring kinase-1α (IRE-1α) having a crucial role in insulin receptor signaling as a mediator of JNK activation [65]. In a mouse model of type 2 diabetes, systemic overexpression of 150-kDa oxygen-regulated protein (ORP150), a molecular chaperone located in the ER, improved insulin intolerance and enhanced glucose uptake indicating that this chaperone has an important role in insulin sensitivity and is a potential target for the treatment of T2DM [66].

Obesity and oxidative stress

A study from Japan demonstrated that fat accumulation is associated with systemic oxidative stress in humans and mice [67]. There was a selective production of reactive oxygen species (ROS) in adipose tissue of obese mice, accompanied by an increased expression of NADPH oxidase and a decreased expression of anti-oxidative enzymes. The authors also showed that fatty acids increased oxidative stress in cultured adipocytes via NADPH oxidase activation which was followed by dysregulated production of adipokines such as adiponectin, PAI-1, IL-6 and MCP-1. In addition, treatment with an NADPH oxidase inhibitor reduced ROS production, restored the dysregulation of adipokines in adipose tissue and improved diabetes, dyslipidemia and hepatic steatosis, indicating that the redox status in adipose tissue is a critical factor in the development of the metabolic syndrome [67].

Adipose tissue hypoxia

An expansion of the adipose tissue mass leads to fat cell hypertrophy and subsequent hypoxia of the tissue. Recent studies convincingly support the concept that hypoxia has an important if not central role in the development of chronic inflammation, macrophage infiltration, impaired adipokine secretion, ER stress and mitochondrial dysfunction in white adipose tissue in obesity [68,69]. These consequences are also accompanied by an inhibition of adipogenesis and triglyceride synthesis and elevated circulating free fatty acid concentrations. Measurement of the interstitial partial oxygen pressure (PO_2) in adipose tissue showed a reduction of up to 70% leading to oxygen levels of about 2% in obese animals compared to lean controls [69]. This observation was further substantiated by the determination of hypoxia response genes such as hypoxia-inducible factor 1α (HIF-1α), vascular endothelial growth factor (VEGF), heme oxygenase 1 (HO-1) and others. The low oxygen pressure may also contribute to a reduced mitochondrial respiration with a consecutive increase in lactate production. In humans, HIF-1α was also shown to be increased in white adipose tissue of obese patients and its expression was reduced after surgery-induced weight loss [70]. Hypoxia was also demonstrated to decrease adiponectin expression in adipocytes [71].

The physiologic basis of adipose tissue hypoxia may be related to a reduction in adipose tissue blood flow and capillary density which has been reported in both obese humans and animals. Although the hypoxic state leads to an increased production and release of pro-angiogenic factors from adipose tissue such as VEGF and others, this compensatory mechanism may not be sufficient to keep the PO_2 at a normal level as the free diffusion of oxygen in the adipose tissue may be limited [69].

Accumulation of immune cells

Leptin, TNF-α, MCP-1 and other chemokines have an essential role in the recruitment of macrophages to adipose tissue. The secretory profile of both pre-adipocytes and adipocytes includes a variety of chemoattractants for immune cells. It was recently reported that the attraction of T-lymphocytes possibly caused by stromal cell-derived factor 1 (SDF-1) represents the initial step which subsequently leads to the invasion and activation of circulating monocytes–macrophages resembling the scheme originally described for atherosclerosis [72]. Such accumulation of immune cells and inflammation of adipose tissue has been shown in obese humans [73] and appears to be more pronounced in omental than subcutaneous adipose tissue [74], which would also fit with the concept that the amount of visceral fat is the culprit for the metabolic and cardiovascular complications of obesity.

Role of body fat distribution pattern

Another important issue in this context is the distribution of body fat. It has long been known from early clinical studies that

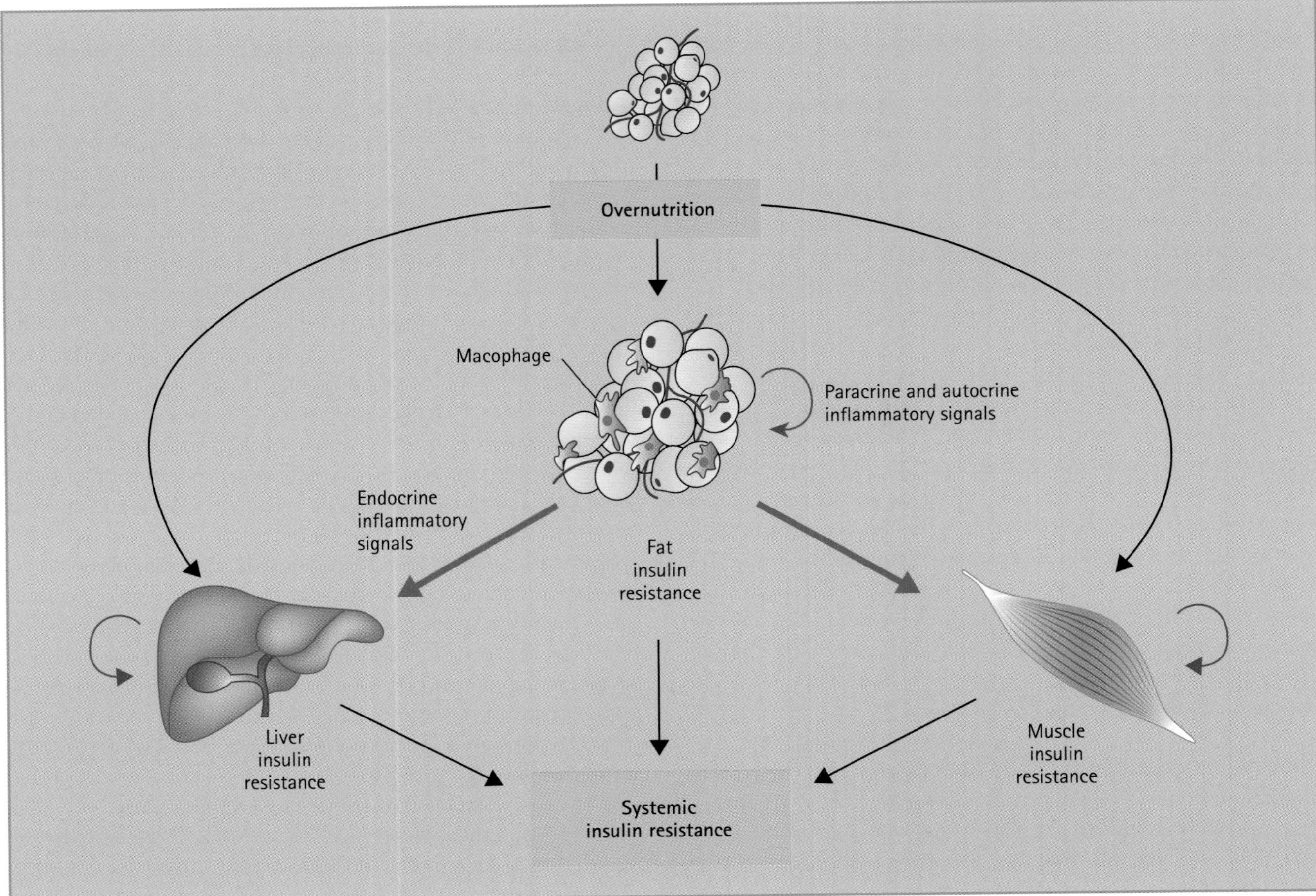

Figure 14.5 Nutrition and obesity-induced inflammation and development of systemic insulin resistance. Reproduced from De Luca C, Olefsky JM. Stressed out about obesity and insulin resistance. *Nat Med* 2006; **12**:41–42, with permission from Nature Publishing Group.

subjects with a more abdominal type of body fat distribution are at increased risk of developing T2DM and other metabolic and cardiovascular complications [75–77]; however, the underlying cause has only recently become evident. Intra-abdominal fat cells exhibit a differing expression profile and are lipolytically more active than subcutaneous adipocytes. Moreover, they show a greater accumulation of lymphocytes and macrophages, indicating greater proinflammatory activity. Visceral adipose tissue also has a much higher blood vessel and nerve density leading to a much greater metabolic activity. Visceral adipose tissue drains into the portal vein and thus the liver is directly exposed to fatty acids and proteins released from this active fat depot promoting insulin resistance in the liver. Thus, the inflammatory process is detected, not only at the level of adipose tissue, but may also affect the liver and possibly other organs. As enlarged visceral fat depots are frequently associated with fat accumulation in the liver, it was also hypothesized that secretory products from the visceral adipose tissue may directly cause hepatic insulin resistance.

In summary, a variety of data suggests that chronic overnutrition with a high-fat, high-sugar diet and as a consequence an accumulation of body fat is the primary cause of chronic inflammation in obesity and may promote the development of systemic insulin resistance which affects many tissue including liver, muscle and the brain (Figure 14.5). It should not be neglected that apart from an unhealthy diet, other lifestyle factors such as lack of physical activity may substantially contribute to these pathologic processes.

Treatment of obesity in the context of the metabolic syndrome and type 2 diabetes

The fact that obesity is the most powerful driving force for the development of T2DM provides the rationale to consider weight management as the most important initial treatment step. Numerous studies have consistently shown that weight loss is not only an effective means to prevent the development of T2DM in those at increased risk, but may also improve the metabolic disturbances and associated risk factors in those with overt T2DM. In addition, weight reduction facilitates reaching the primary treatment goal of a metabolic control close to normal. Interestingly, almost all disturbances mentioned above are potentially reversible by weight loss. This was particularly demonstrated for elevated circulating adipokines. A modest to moderate weight reduction was found to reduce significantly the concentrations of circulating factors such as leptin, C-reactive protein, PAI-1, IL-6, IL-8, MCP-1 and others by 10–50%. By contrast, adiponectin levels are known to rise in relation to weight reduction. In a recent study in surgically treated morbidly obese subjects a significant reduction in macrophage infiltration was documented in adipose tissue samples after a mean weight loss of 22 kg within 3 months [70].

Management of obesity in subjects with type 2 diabetes

For the reasons outlined, management of obesity should represent a central component in the treatment strategy for T2DM. Although currently available weight reduction programs for patients with diabetes have only limited success rates, particularly in the long run, in contrast to previous beliefs, recent studies show that obese subjects with T2DM can achieve clinically significant weight loss. In the prospective Look AHEAD study, the average weight loss in obese subjects with T2DM in the intensive lifestyle intervention group after 1 year of treatment was 8.6% of the initial body weight and was accompanied by substantial improvements of all weight-associated risk factors. Mean HbA_{1c} fell from 7.3% (56 mmol/mol) to 6.2% (44 mmol/mol) despite reductions in the dosage of glucose-lowering agents [78].

Despite this positive development, treatment of obese subjects with T2DM is usually considered to be more difficult than treating obese subjects without diabetes for several reasons. People with T2DM are usually older than obese subjects without diabetes, which may mean a smaller weight loss as energy expenditure decreases with age. Another reason is that subjects with diabetes focus more on blood glucose control which could result in neglecting other health problems. Finally, the effect of various antidiabetic agents to increase weight or prevent weight loss has to be considered [79].

Dietary approaches

The cornerstones of a weight reduction program for obese patients with diabetes include a moderately hypocaloric diet, an increase in physical activity and behavior modification, very similar to the recommendations for obese subjects without diabetes. Numerous studies have applied and examined such concepts and have been critically evaluated in reviews [80–82].

The gold standard in the dietary treatment of obese patients with T2DM is a balanced moderately energy-restricted diet with an energy deficit of at least 500 kcal/day (see Chapter 22). The most important single measure is the reduction in fat intake, particularly in saturated fatty acids. A low-fat, high carbohydrate diet is generally recommended. As shown recently, a diet rich in fiber and complex carbohydrates has some beneficial effects on measures of glucose and lipid metabolism but these effects may be small and possibly of limited clinical importance [83]. The concept of a high-carbohydrate, low-fat diet was challenged by clinical studies showing that replacement of saturated fat by monounsaturated fat compared to high-carbohydrate intake is equally favorable or even has advantages with regard to glycemic response and lipids [84]. More importantly, recent studies using a low-carbohydrate, high-protein diet were at least equally effective. In a recent meta-analysis of such studies, HbA_{1c}, fasting glucose and some lipid fractions improved with lower carbohydrate content diets [85]. In a study from Israel, a Mediterranean type of weight loss diet showed small advantages in comparison to the classic low-fat, low-carbohydrate diet in a subgroup of overweight participants with diabetes [86]. The message from this and other studies [87,88] is that the macronutrient composition of the diet is secondary for weight reduction. In patients with nephropathy, however, protein intake remains a critical issue and should be limited in accordance with current recommendations [89].

From a practical point of view it is extremely important to assess the habitual diet of patients with T2DM and to focus counseling on timely changes of their eating habits in order to approach current dietary recommendations [89]. It should be stressed that all efforts for dietary changes should be made as simple as possible for patients as they may also be burdened by many requirements to manage their diabetes. For obese subjects with T2DM the frequent recommendation to distribute their allowed calories over 5–6 meals is difficult to meet and may even hinder weight loss without being of any advantage for metabolic control [90]. Therefore, in patients without insulin, three meals a day may be more appropriate and advantageous to reach the individual dietary and weight goals.

Another possible dietary approach is the use of a very low calorie diet (VLCD) for initial weight loss. This option may be particularly valuable for patients with poor metabolic control. Dietary restriction is known to be associated with a rapid improvement of insulin resistance and glycemic control after even short periods of VLCD. There is also evidence that the pattern of adipokines and macrophage-associated gene expression can change dramatically under such conditions [91]. This approach, however, can only be applied for a limited period of time and requires intensive medical surveillance. The long-term results of VLCD are moderately better than those of conventional diets, although there is considerable weight regain under the former [92]. Therefore, there is need for new sophisticated solutions such as intermittent VLCD in combination with conventional hypocaloric diets to obtain better long-term results [93]. Another possibility is to change the pattern of nutrient intake to modify adipose tissue inflammation. To date, there is little practical information available to indicate whether specific effects of single components in the diet can ameliorate adipose tissue inflammation independent of calorie restriction. There is no doubt that more research is urgently required to explore the potential of dietary components and to develop novel strategies that may help to provide better dietary solutions for the management of obesity.

Antidiabetic drugs and body weight

It has long been recognized that antidiabetic drugs can promote weight gain in subjects with T2DM (see Chapters 27 and 29). The strongest weight-promoting effect is exerted by insulin. In the Diabetes Control and Complications Trial (DCCT), intensified insulin treatment was associated with substantial weight gain that resulted in unfavorable changes of lipid levels and blood pressure similar to those seen in the insulin resistance syndrome [94]. In the UK Prospective Diabetes Study (UKPDS), insulin treatment caused a mean weight gain of approximately 7 kg over 12 years of treatment in newly diagnosed subjects with T2DM [95]. In addition, sulfonylureas are known to promote weight gain because of their action to promote insulin secretion. In the UKPDS, the average weight gain under glibenclamide treatment amounted to about 5 kg [95].

Administration of glitazones, a relatively new class of PPAR-γ agonists with insulin sensitizing activity, leads to substantial weight gain of 4–5 kg on average. There is growing evidence, however, that weight gain under glitazone treatment occurs mainly in subcutaneous depots, not in the visceral depot, which should have less deleterious metabolic consequences. Furthermore, weight gain under administration of glitazones is not only caused by an increase in fat mass, but also by enhanced fluid retention. In contrast, metformin and α-glucosidase inhibitors have a modest weight lowering potential [79].

Recent data for the DPP-4 inhibitors show that these new drugs are weight neutral, whereas the administration of GLP-1 mimetics, such as exenatide, results in a substantial weight loss in a high proportion of patients [96].

Weight lowering drugs

Another component in the treatment of obesity is the adjunct administration of weight lowering drugs. As the efficacy of currently approved drugs is limited, drug treatment is only recommended if the non-pharmacologic treatment program is not sufficiently successful and if the benefit : risk ratio justifies drug administration [97]. At present, only two compounds are available that have demonstrated efficacy and safety in obese subjects with and without T2DM.

Orlistat is a gastric and pancreatic lipase inhibitor that impairs the intestinal absorption of ingested fat. In a recent systematic review of clinical studies over at least 12 weeks in obese subjects with T2DM, orlistat treatment produced a greater weight loss than placebo treatment by 2.0 kg on average, associated with a small improvement in HbA_{1c} compared with controls [98]. Furthermore, orlistat moderately decreases low density lipoprotein (LDL) cholesterol concentrations.

Sibutramine is a selective serotonin and noradrenaline reuptake inhibitor that enhances satiety and slightly increases thermogenesis.* The same systematic review showed an average weight loss of 5.1 kg in obese patients with T2DM, also accompanied by improvements of glycemic and lipid measures [98]. As sibutramine is known to activate the sympathetic nervous system, this drug should not be used in patients with diabetes and poorly controlled hypertension or coronary artery disease.

*The marketing authorization for sibutramine has recently been withdrawn in Europe following the publication of the SCOUT trial. In this trial which included 9,800 overweight or obese individuals at high risk of CVD events, treatment with sibutramine was associated with a 16% increased risk of non-fatal MI, non-fatal stroke, resuscitated cardiac arrest or CVD death. This result was driven by an increased incidence of non-fatal MI and stroke.

Bariatric surgery

Bariatric surgery is now an established method to reduce body weight in subjects with extreme obesity (≥40 kg/m^2), but there is growing consensus that this method can also be applied in subjects with T2DM at a BMI ≥35 kg/m^2. In this group of patients surgery is by far the most effective treatment mode with excellent long-term results compared to all other methods. In the Swedish Obese Subjects study, a large prospective trial comparing bariatric surgery with conventional dietary treatment, sustained weight loss ≥20 kg was achieved in the surgically treated subjects with practically no significant weight change in the control group. The surgical intervention not only reduced the incidence of T2DM, but also significantly reduced total mortality [99]. A recent meta-analysis of studies on the effect of bariatric surgery in obese patients with T2DM demonstrated that 78% had a complete remission of diabetes. Weight loss and diabetes resolution was greatest in patients undergoing combined restrictive and malabsorptive surgical methods [100]. The majority of insulin-treated patients can stop insulin treatment within a few months after surgery and all other medications for diabetes and other cardiovascular risk factors can be considerably reduced or discontinued. There are also many studies indicating how rapidly most circulating adipokines are normalized in relation to the degree of weight loss in these patients.

Conclusions

There is now growing information on how obesity is increasing the risk of developing T2DM. It is apparent that an excess of body fat promotes insulin resistance and impairs insulin secretion. As most patients with T2DM are overweight or obese, weight management must be a central component of any treatment strategy, as weight loss has been convincingly shown to provide a marked improvement in metabolic control. In parallel, most if not all underlying disturbances benefit from weight loss or dietary interventions. As conventional concepts combining an energy-reduced diet and an increase in physical activity frequently have poor long-term results, however, more effective weight loss strategies should be developed and evaluated.

References

1 World Health Organization. Obesity: preventing and managing the global epidemic. Report of a WHO consultation. *WHO Technical Report Series 894*. Geneva: World Health Organization, 2000.

2 Kopelman P. Obesity as a medical problem. *Nature* 2000; **404**:635–643.

3 Prospective Studies Collaboration. Body-mass index and cause-specific mortality in 900 000 adults: collaborative analyses of 57 prospective studies. *Lancet* 2009; **373**:1083–1096.

4 Colditz GA, Willett WC, Rotnitzky A, Manson JE. Weight gain as a risk factor for clinical diabetes in women. *Ann Intern Med* 1995; **122**:481–486.

5 Chan JM, Rimm EB, Colditz GA, Stampfer MJ, Willett WC. Obesity, fat distribution, and weight gain as risk factors for clinical diabetes in men. *Diabetes Care* 1994; **17**:961–969.

6 Schienkiewitz A, Schulze MB, Hoffmann K, Kroke A, Boeing H. Body mass index history and risk of type 2 diabetes: results from the European Prospective Investigation into Cancer and Nutrition (EPIC) – Potsdam study. *Am J Clin Nutr* 2006; **84**:427–433.

7 Gregg EW, Cheng YJ, Narayan V, Thompson TJ, Williamson DF. The relative contributions of different levels of overweight and obesity to the increased prevalence of diabetes in the United States: 1976–2004. *Prev Med* 2007; **45**:348–352.

8 Ohlson LO, Larsson B, Svärdsudd K, Welin L, Eriksson H, Wilhelmsen L, *et al.* The influence of body fat distribution on the incidence of diabetes mellitus: 13.5 years of follow-up of the participants in the study of men born in 1913. *Diabetes* 1985; **34**:1055–1058.

9 Yusuf S, Hawken S, Ounpuu S, Bautista L, Franzosi MG, Commerford P, *et al.*; INTERHEART Study Investigators. Obesity and the risk of myocardial infarction in 27 000 participants from 52 countries: a case–control study. *Lancet* 2005; **366**:1640–1649.

10 Stunkard AJ, Sorensen TI, Hanis C, Teasdale TW, Chakraborty R, Schull WJ, *et al.* An adoption study of human obesity. *N Engl J Med* 1986; **314**:193–198.

11 Stunkard AJ, Foch TT, Hrubec Z. A twin study of human obesity. *JAMA* 1986; **256**:51–54.

12 Wardle J, Carnell S, Haworth CM, Plomin R. Evidence for a strong genetic influence on childhood obesity despite the force of the obesogenic environment. *Am J Clin Nutr* 2008; **87**:398–404.

13 O'Rahilly S, Farooqi IS. Human obesity: a heritable neurobehavioral disorder that is highly sensitive to environmental conditions. *Diabetes* 2008; **57**:2905–2910.

14 Frayling TM, Timpson NJ, Weedon MN, Zeggini E, Freathy RM, Lindgren CM, *et al.* A common variant in the FTO gene is associated with body mass index and predisposes to childhood and adult obesity. *Science* 2007; **316**:889–894.

15 Willer CJ, Speliotes EK, Loos RJ, Li S, Lindgren CM, Heid IM, *et al.* Six new loci associated with body mass index highlight a neuronal influence on body weight regulation. *Nat Genet* 2009; **41**:25–34.

16 Thorleifsson G, Walters GB, Gudbjartsson DF, Steinthorsdottir V, Sulem P, Helgadottir A, *et al.* Genome-wide association yields new sequence variants at seven loci that associate with measures of obesity. *Nat Genet* 2009; **41**:18–24.

17 Gerken T, Girard CA, Tung YC, Webby CJ, Saudek V, Hewitson KS, *et al.* The obesity-associated FTO gene encodes a 2-oxoglutarate-dependent nucleic acid demethylase. *Science* 2007; **318**:1469–1472.

18 Narayan KM, Boyle JP, Thompson TJ, Sorensen SW, Williamson DF. Lifetime risk for diabetes mellitus in the United States. *JAMA* 2003; **290**:1884–1890.

19 Polonsky KS, Sturis SJ, Bell GI. Non-insulin-dependent diabetes mellitus: a genetically programmed failure of the beta cell to compensate for insulin resistance. *N Engl J Med* 1996; **334**:777–783.

20 Pettitt DJ, Baird HR, Aleck KA, Bennett PH, Knowler WC. Excessive obesity in offspring of Pima Indian women with diabetes during pregnancy. *N Engl J Med* 1983; **308**:242–245.

21 Dabelea D, Hanson RL, Lindsay RS, Pettitt DJ, Imperatore G, Gabir MM, *et al.* Intrauterine exposure to diabetes conveys risks for type 2 diabetes and obesity: a study of discordant sibships. *Diabetes* 2000; **49**:2208–2211.

22 Moreira P, Padez C, Mourao-Carvalhal I, Rosado V. Maternal weight gain during pregnancy and overweight in Portuguese children. *Int J Obes Relat Metab Disord* 2007; **31**:608–614.

23 Wrotniak BH, Shults J, Butts S, Stettler N. Gestational weight gain and risk of overweight in the offspring at age 7 y in a multicenter, multiethnic cohort study. *Am J Clin Nutr* 2008; **87**:1818–1824.

24 Plagemann A. Perinatal nutrition and hormone-dependent programming of food intake. *Horm Res* 2006; **65**(Suppl. 3):83–89.

25 Badman MK, Flier JS. The gut and energy balance: visceral allies in the obesity war. *Science* 2005; **307**:1909–1914.

26 Bogardus C, Lillioja S, Ravussin E, Abbott W, Zawadzki JK, Young A, *et al.* Familial dependence of the resting metabolic rate. *N Engl J Med* 1986; **315**:96–100.

27 Ravussin E, Lillioja S, Knowler WC, Christin L, Freymond D, Abbott WG, *et al.* Reduced rate of energy expenditure as a risk factor for body weight gain. *N Engl J Med* 1988; **318**:467–472.

28 Rosenheck R. Fast food consumption and increased caloric intake: a systematic review of a trajectory towards weight gain and obesity risk. *Obes Rev* 2008; **9**:535–547.

29 Olsen NJ, Heitmann BL. Intake of calorically sweetened beverages and obesity. *Obes Rev* 2008; **10**:68–75.

30 Mello MM. New York City's war on fat. *N Engl J Med* 2009; **360**:2015–2020.

31 Prentice AM, Jebb SA. Fast foods, energy density and obesity: a possible mechanistic link. *Obes Rev* 2003; **4**:187–194.

32 Nielsen SJ, Popkin BM. Patterns and trends in food portion size, 1977–1998. *JAMA* 2003; **289**:450–453.

33 Ello-Martin JA, Ledikwe JH, Rolls BJ. The influence of food portion size and energy density on energy intake: implications for weight maintenance. *Am J Clin Nutr* 2005; **82**(Suppl. 1):236S–41S.

34 Drewnowski A, Specter SE. Poverty and obesity: the role of energy density and energy costs. *Am J Clin Nutr* 2004; **79**:6–16.

35 Randle P, Garland P, Hales C, Newsholme E. The glucose–fatty acid cycle: its role in insulin sensitivity and the metabolic disturbances of diabetes mellitus. *Lancet* 1963; **i**:785–789.

36 Kahn SE, Hull RL, Utzschneider KM. Mechanisms linking obesity to insulin resistance and type 2 diabetes. *Nature* 2006; **444**:840–846.

37 Itoh Y, Kawamata Y, Harada M, Kobayashi M, Fujii R, Fukusumi S, *et al.* Free fatty acids regulate insulin secretion from pancreatic β cells through GPR40. *Nature* 2003; **422**:173–176.

38 Carpentier A, Mittelman SD, Lamarche B, Bergman RN, Giacca A, Lewis GE. Acute enhancement of insulin secretion by FFA in humans is lost with prolonged FFA elevation. *Am J Physiol* 1999; **276**:E1055–E1066.

39 Chan CB, Saleh MC, Koshkin V, Wheeler MB. Uncoupling protein 2 and islet function. *Diabetes* 2004; **53**(Suppl. 1):S136–S1342.

40 Petersen KF, Dufour S, Befroy D, Mason GF, de Graaf RA, Rothman DL, *et al.* Impaired mitochondrial activity in the insulin-resistant offspring of patients with type 2 diabetes. *N Engl J Med* 2004; **350**:664–671.

41 Kelley DE, He J, Menshikowa EV, Ritov VB. Dysfunction of mitochondria in human skeletal muscle in type 2 diabetes. *Diabetes* 2002; **51**:2944–2950.

42 Lowell BB, Shulman GI. Mitochondrial dysfunction and type 2 diabetes. *Science* 2005; **307**:384–387.

43 Hotamisligil GS, Shargill NS, Spiegelman BM. Adipose expression of tumor necrosis factor-alpha: direct role in obesity-linked insulin resistance. *Science* 1993; **259**:87–91.
44 Hotamisligil GS, Arner P, Caro JF, Atkinson RL, Spiegelman BM. Increased adipose tissue expression of tumor necrosis factor-α in human obesity and insulin resistance. *J Clin Invest* 1995; **95**:2409–2415.
45 Kern PA, Saghizadeh M, Ong JM, Bosch RJ, Deem R, Simsolo RB. The expression of tumor necrosis factor in human adipose tissue: regulation by obesity, weight loss and relationship to lipoprotein lipase. *J Clin Invest* 1995; **95**:2111–2119.
46 Hube F, Birgel M, Lee Y-M, Hauner H. Expression pattern of tumour necrosis factor receptors in subcutaneous and omental human adipose tissue: role of obesity and non-insulin-dependent diabetes mellitus. *Eur J Clin Invest* 1999; **29**:672–678.
47 Hauner H, Petruschke T, Russ M, Röhrig K, Eckel J. Effects of tumor necrosis factor-alpha (TNF) on glucose transport and lipid metabolism of newly differentiated human fat cells in culture. *Diabetologia* 1995; **38**:764–771.
48 Hotamisligil GS, Peraldi P, Budavari A, *et al.* IRS-1-mediated inhibition of insulin receptor tyrosine kinase activity in TNF-α- and obesity-induced insulin resistance. *Science* 1996; **271**:665–668.
49 Dietze D, Koenen M, Röhrig K, Horikoshi H, Hauner H, Eckel J. Impairment of insulin signaling in human skeletal muscle by co-culture with human adipocytes. *Diabetes* 2002; **51**:2369–2376.
50 Sell H, Dietze-Schröder D, Kaiser U, Eckel J. Monocyte chemotactic protein-1 is a potential player in the negative crosstalk between adipose tissue and skeletal muscle. *Endocrinology* 2006; **147**:2458–2467.
51 Dietze-Schröder D, Sell H, Uhlig M, Koenen M, Eckel J. Autocrine action of adiponectin on human fat cells prevents the release of insulin resistance inducing factors. *Diabetes* 2005; **54**:2003–2011.
52 Lindsay RS, Funahashi T, Hanson RL, Matsuzawa Y, Tanaka S, Tataranni PA, *et al.* Adiponectin and development of type 2 diabetes in the Pima Indian population. *Lancet* 2002; **360**:57–58.
53 Spranger J, Kroke A, Möhlig M, Bergmann MM, Ristow M, Boeing H, *et al.* Adiponectin and protection against type 2 diabetes mellitus. *Lancet* 2003; **361**:226–228.
54 Kadowaki T, Yamauchi T, Kubota N, Hara K, Ueki K, Tobe K. Adiponectin and adiponectin receptors in insulin resistance, diabetes, and the metabolic syndrome. *J Clin Invest* 2006; **116**:1784–1792.
55 Shoelsen SE, Lee J, Goldfine AB. Inflammation and insulin resistance. *J Clin Invest* 2006; **116**:1793–801.
56 Hirosumi J, Tuncman G, Chang L, Görgün CZ, Uysal KT, Maeda K, *et al.* A central role for JNK in obesity and insulin resistance. *Nature* 2002; **420**:333–336.
57 Wellen KE, Hotamisligil GS. Inflammation, stress, and diabetes. *J Clin Invest* 2005; **115**:111–119.
58 Yuan M, Konstantopoulos N, Lee J, Hansen L, Li ZW, Karin M, *et al.* Reversal of obesity- and diet-induced insulin resistance with salicylates or targeted disruption of IKK beta. *Science* 2001; **293**:1673–1677.
59 Lee JY, Sohn KH, Rhee SH, Hwang D. Saturated fatty acids, but not unsaturated fatty acids, induce the expression of cyclooxygenase-2 mediated through Toll-like receptor 4. *J Biol Chem* 2001; **276**:16683–16689.
60 Tsukumo DM, Carvalho-Filho MA, Carvalheira JB, Prada PO, Hirabara SM, Schenka AA, *et al.* Loss-of-function mutation in Toll-like receptor 4 prevents diet-induced obesity and insulin resistance. *Diabetes* 2007; **56**:1986–1998.
61 Davis JE, Gabler NK, Walker-Daniels J, Spurlock ME. TLR-4 deficiency selectively protects against obesity induced by diets high in saturated fat. *Obesity* 2008; **16**:1248–1255.
62 Permana PA, Menge C, Reaven PD. Macrophage-secreted factors induce adipocyte inflammation and insulin resistance. *Biochem Biophys Res Comm* 2006; **341**:507–514.
63 Skurk T, Alberti-Huber C, Herder C, Hauner H. Relationship between adipocyte size and adipokine expression and secretion. *J Clin Endocrinol Metab* 2007; **92**:1023–1033.
64 Weyer C, Foley JE, Bogardus C, Tataranni PA, Pratley RE. Enlarged subcutaneous abdominal adipocyte size, but not obesity itself predicts type II diabetes independent of insulin resistance. *Diabetologia* 2000; **43**:1498–1506.
65 Özcan U, Cao Q, Yilmaz E, Lee AH, Iwakoshi NN, Ozdelen E, *et al.* Endoplasmatic reticulum stress links obesity, insulin action, and type 2 diabetes. *Science* 2004; **306**:457–461.
66 Ozawa K, Miyazaki M, Matsuhisa M, Takano K, Nakatani Y, Hatazaki M, *et al.* The endoplasmic reticulum stress improves insulin resistance in type 2 diabetes. *Diabetes* 2005; **54**:657–663.
67 Furukawa S, Fujita T, Shimabukuro M, Iwaki M, Yamada Y, Nakajima Y, *et al.* Increased oxidative stress in obesity and its impact on metabolic syndrome. *J Clin Invest* 2004; **114**:1752–1761.
68 Trayhurn P, Wang B, Wood IS. Hypoxia in adipose tissue: a basis for the dysregulation of white adipose tissue. *Br J Nutr* 2008; **100**:227–235.
69 Ye J. Emerging role of adipose tissue hypoxia in obesity and insulin resistance. *Int J Obes Relat Metab Disord* 2009; **33**:54–66.
70 Cancello R, Henegar C, Viguerie N, Taleb S, Poitou C, Rouault C, *et al.* Reduction of macrophage infiltration and chemoattractant gene expression in white adipose tissue of morbidly obese subjects after surgery-induced weight loss. *Diabetes* 2005; **54**:2277–2286.
71 Ye J, Gao Z, Yin J, He H. Hypoxia is a potential risk factor for chronic inflammation and adiponectin reduction in adipose tissue of ob/ob and dietary obese mice. *Am J Physiol Endocrinol Metab* 2007; **293**:E1118–E1128.
72 Kintscher U, Hartge M, Hess K, Foryst-Ludwig A, Clemenz M, Wabitsch M, *et al.* T-lymphocyte infiltration in visceral adipose tissue: a primary event in adipose tissue inflammation and the development of obesity-mediated insulin resistance. *Arterioscler Thromb Vasc Biol* 2008; **28**:1304–1310.
73 Weisberg SP, McCann D, Desai M, Rosenbaum M, Leibel RL, Ferrante AW Jr. Obesity is associated with macrophage accumulation in adipose tissue. *J Clin Invest* 2003; **112**:1785–1808.
74 Bornstein SR, Abu-Asab M, Glasow A, Päth G, Hauner H, Tsokos M, *et al.* Immunohistochemical and ultrastructural localization of leptin and leptin receptor in human white adipose tissue and differentiating human adipose cells in primary culture. *Diabetes* 2000; **49**:532–538.
75 Vague J. The degree of masculine differentiation of obesities: a factor determining predisposition to diabetes, atherosclerosis, gout and uric calculous disease. *Am J Clin Nutr* 1956; **4**:20–34.
76 Krotkiewski M, Björntorp P, Sjöström L, Smith U. Impact of obesity on metabolism in men and women: importance of regional adipose tissue distribution. *J Clin Invest* 1983; **72**:1150–1162.
77 Kissebah AH, Krakower GR. Regional adiposity and morbidity. *Physiol Rev* 1994; **74**:761–811.

78 Look AHEAD Research Group. Reduction in weight and cardiovascular risk factors in individuals with type 2 diabetes: one-year results of the Look AHEAD trial. *Diabetes Care* 2007; **30**:1374–1383.

79 Hauner H. Managing type 2 diabetes mellitus in patients with obesity. *Treat Endocrinol* 2004; **3**:223–232.

80 Brown SA, Upchurch S, Anding R, Winter M, Ramirez G. Promoting weight loss in type II diabetes. *Diabetes Care* 1996; **19**:613–624.

81 Nield L, Moore HJ, Hooper L, Cruickshank JK, Vyas A, Whittaker V, *et al.* Dietary advice for treatment of type 2 diabetes in adults. *Cochrane Database Syst Rev* 2007; **3**:CD004097.

82 Magkos F, Yannakoulia M, Chan JL, Mantzoros CS. Management of the metabolic syndrome and type 2 diabetes through lifestyle modification. *Annu Rev Nutr* 2009; **29**:223–256.

83 Chandalia M, Grag A, Lutjohann D, von Bergmann K, Grundy SM, Brinkley LJ. Beneficial effects of high fiber intake in patients with type 2 diabetes mellitus. *N Engl J Med* 2000; **342**:1392–1398.

84 Garg A, Bonanome A, Grundy SM, Zhang ZJ, Unger RH. Comparison of a high-carbohydrate diet with high-monounsaturated-fat diet in patients with non-insulin-dependent diabetes mellitus. *N Engl J Med* 1988; **319**:829–834.

85 Kirk JK, Graves DE, Craven TE, Lipkin EW, Austin M, Margolis KL. Restricted-carbohydrate diets in patients with type 2 diabetes: a meta-analysis. *J Am Diet Assoc* 2008; **108**:91–100.

86 Shai I, Schwarzfuchs D, Henkin Y, Shahar DR, Witkow S, Greenberg I, *et al.* Weight loss with a low-carbohydrate, Mediterranean, or low-fat diet. *N Engl J Med* 2008; **359**:229–241.

87 Wolever TM, Gibbs AL, Mehling C, Chiasson JL, Connelly PW, Josse RG, *et al.* The Canadian Trial of Carbohydrates in Diabetes (CCD), a 1-y controlled trial of low-glycemic-index dietary carbohydrates in type 2 diabetes: no effect on glycated haemoglobin but reduction C-reactive protein. *Am J Clin Nutr* 2008; **87**:114–125.

88 Sacks FM, Bray GA, Carey VJ, Smith SR, Ryan DH, Anton SD, *et al.* Comparison of weight-loss diets with different compositions of fat, protein, and carbohydrate. *N Engl J Med* 2009; **360**:859–873.

89 American Diabetes Association. Nutrition recommendations and interventions for diabetes. *Diabetes Care* 2008; **31**(Suppl. 1):S61–S78.

90 Arnold L, Mann JI, Ball MJ. Metabolic effects of alterations in meal frequency in type 2 diabetes. *Diabetes Care* 1997; **20**:1651–1654.

91 Capel F, Klimcakova E, Viguerie N, Roussel B, Vítková M, Kovácikовá M, *et al.* Macrophages and adipocytes in human obesity: adipose tissue gene expression and insulin sensitivity during calorie restriction and weight stabilization. *Diabetes* 2009; **58**:1558–1567.

92 Anderson JW, Konz EC, Frederich RC, Wood CL. Long-term weight-loss maintenance: a meta-analysis of US studies. *Am J Clin Nutr* 2001; **74**:579–584.

93 Williams KV, Mullen ML, Kelley DE, Wing RR. The effect of short periods of caloric restriction on weight loss and glycemic control in type 2 diabetes. *Diabetes Care* 1998; **21**:2–8.

94 Purnell JQ, Hokanson JE, Marcovina SM, Steffes MW, Cleary PA, Brunzell JD. Effect of excessive weight gain with intensive therapy of type 1 diabetes on lipid levels and blood pressure: results from the DCCT. *JAMA* 1998; **280**:140–146.

95 UKPDS. Intensive blood-glucose control with sulphonylureas or insulin compared with conventional treatment and risk of complications in patients with type 2 diabetes (UKPDS 33). *Lancet* 1998; **12**:837–852.

96 Drucker DJ, Nauck MA. The incretin system: glucagon-like-peptide-1 receptor agonists and dipeptidyl pepdidase-4 inhibitors in type 2 diabetes. *Lancet* 2006; **368**:1696–1705.

97 National Task Force on the Prevention and Treatment of Obesity. Long-term pharmacotherapy in the management of obesity. *JAMA* 1996; **276**:1907–1915.

98 Norris SL, Zhang X, Avenell A, Gregg E, Schmid CH, Lau J. Pharmacotherapy for weight loss in adults with type 2 diabetes mellitus. *Cochrane Database Syst Rev* 2005; **1**:CD004096.

99 Sjöström L, Narbro K, Sjöström CD, Karason K, Larsson B, Wedel H, *et al.* Effects of bariatric surgery on mortality in Swedish obese subjects. *N Engl J Med* 2007; **357**:741–752.

100 Buchwald H, Estok R, Fahrbach K, Banel D, Jensen MD, Pories WJ, *et al.* Weight and type 2 diabetes after bariatric surgery: systematic review and meta-analysis. *Am J Med* 2009; **122**:248–256.

4 Other Types of Diabetes

15 Monogenic Causes of Diabetes

Angus Jones & Andrew T. Hattersley
Diabetes and Vascular Medicine, Peninsula Medical School, Exeter, Devon, UK

Keypoints

- Monogenic diabetes results from single-gene mutations that cause β-cell dysfunction or, less commonly, insulin resistance.
- Approximately 1–2% of diabetes is monogenic, but this is frequently misdiagnosed.
- Monogenic diabetes should be suspected where: presentation is atypical for type 1 or 2 diabetes; there is an autosomal dominant (or maternally inherited in mitochondrial disorders) family history; there are characteristic associated features such as deafness in mitochondrial diabetes or fat loss in lipodystrophy; or diabetes has been diagnosed within the first 6 months of life.
- Mutations in the glucokinase gene, which is important in "sensing" blood glucose levels in the pancreas, result in resetting of fasting glucose to a higher level (5.5–8.0 mmol/L). Patients have dominantly inherited mild fasting hyperglycemia with only modest changes in glycated hemoglobin. Complications are rare and no treatment is needed.
- Mutations in the transcription factor genes *HNF1A* and *HNF4A* result in dominantly inherited progressive hyperglycemia with symptomatic diabetes in adolescence or young adulthood. Patients with *HNF1A* or *HNF4A* diabetes are very sensitive to sulfonylurea treatment and may not require insulin until middle or old age.
- Mitochondrial mutations can result in maternally inherited diabetes often with sensorineural hearing loss and a range of other disorders.
- Diabetes diagnosed before 6 months is unlikely to be type 1 diabetes and a genetic cause should be sought even where the patient is now an adult. High dose sulfonylurea treatment is often more effective than insulin where mutations affecting Kir6.2 and SUR1 subunits of the β-cell potassium channel are identified.
- Acanthosis nigricans is the key feature of insulin resistance and a genetic cause should be considered where this is seen in non-obese patients. Partial lipodystrophy results in thin muscular limbs with hypertriglyceridemia and insulin resistance and suggests a mutation in *LMNA* or *PPARG*. In the absence of lipodystrophy an insulin receptor mutation is the most common cause.

Introduction

Monogenic diabetes results from inheritance of one or more mutations in a single gene and accounts for 1–2% of diabetes cases. Mutations may be inherited in a dominant or recessive fashion. The majority (90%) of monogenic diabetes cases are initially misdiagnosed as type 1 (T1DM) or type 2 diabetes (T2DM).

Correct genetic diagnosis is important to predict clinical course, explain other associated clinical features, enable genetic counseling and diagnose family members, and most importantly guide appropriate treatment.

Monogenic diabetes where the primary disorder affects the β-cell has four main clinical presentations: familial mild fasting hyperglycemia (glucokinase maturity-onset diabetes of the young [MODY]), familial young-onset diabetes (transcription factor MODY), neonatal diabetes and diabetes with extrapancreatic features. Clinical and biochemical features that help differentiate the common forms of monogenic diabetes that result in β-cell dysfunction from T1DM and T2DM are summarized in Table 15.1. Clinical features and management of monogenic diabetes without extrapancreatic features are further summarized in Figure 15.1. Single-gene mutations may also cause diabetes through insulin resistance as occurs in the inherited lipodystrophies and insulin receptor mutations. A number of monogenic multisystem diseases (e.g. hemochromatosis and cystic fibrosis) may cause diabetes; these are beyond the scope of this chapter and are discussed elsewhere (see Chapter 18).

Maturity-onset diabetes of the young

Maturity-onset diabetes of the young (MODY) is autosomal dominantly inherited diabetes that, despite a young age of onset, is not insulin dependent [1,2]. It results from β-cell dysfunction rather than insulin resistance [1]. The underlying genetic etiology has now been defined that allows MODY to be subclassified according to the gene involved [3,4]. Mutations in at least eight genes have been linked to MODY [5,6]. These include mutations

Textbook of Diabetes, 4th edition. Edited by R. Holt, C. Cockram, A. Flyvbjerg and B. Goldstein.

Table 15.1 Differentiating β-cell monogenic diabetes from type 1 and 2 diabetes.

Features	Type 1 diabetes	Young type 2	*GCK* MODY	*HNF1A* MODY	MIDD	K_{ATP} PNDM
Insulin dependent	Yes	No	No	No	+/–	Yes
Parent affected	2–4%	Usually	Yes	Yes	Mother	15%
Typical age of onset	6 months – young adult	Adolescent and young adult	Birth (may be diagnosed at any age)	Teens – young adult	Young adult	Under 6 months
Obesity	Pop freq	Yes	Pop freq	Pop freq	Rare	Pop freq
Acanthosis nigricans	No	Yes	No	No	No	No
Glycemia	High	Variable	Mild	High	Variable	High
β-Cell autoantibodies	Usually	Sometimes	No	No	No	No
Typical C peptide (pmol/L)	<200 Outside honeymoon period	500–>1000	100–900	100–700	<100–700	<200

DM, diabetes; GCK, glucokinase; *HNF1A*, hepatocyte nuclear factor 1A (*HNF4A* is similar); MIDD, maternally inherited diabetes and deafness; PNDM, permanent neonatal diabetes; Pop freq, population frequency (frequency of obesity seen in the general population).

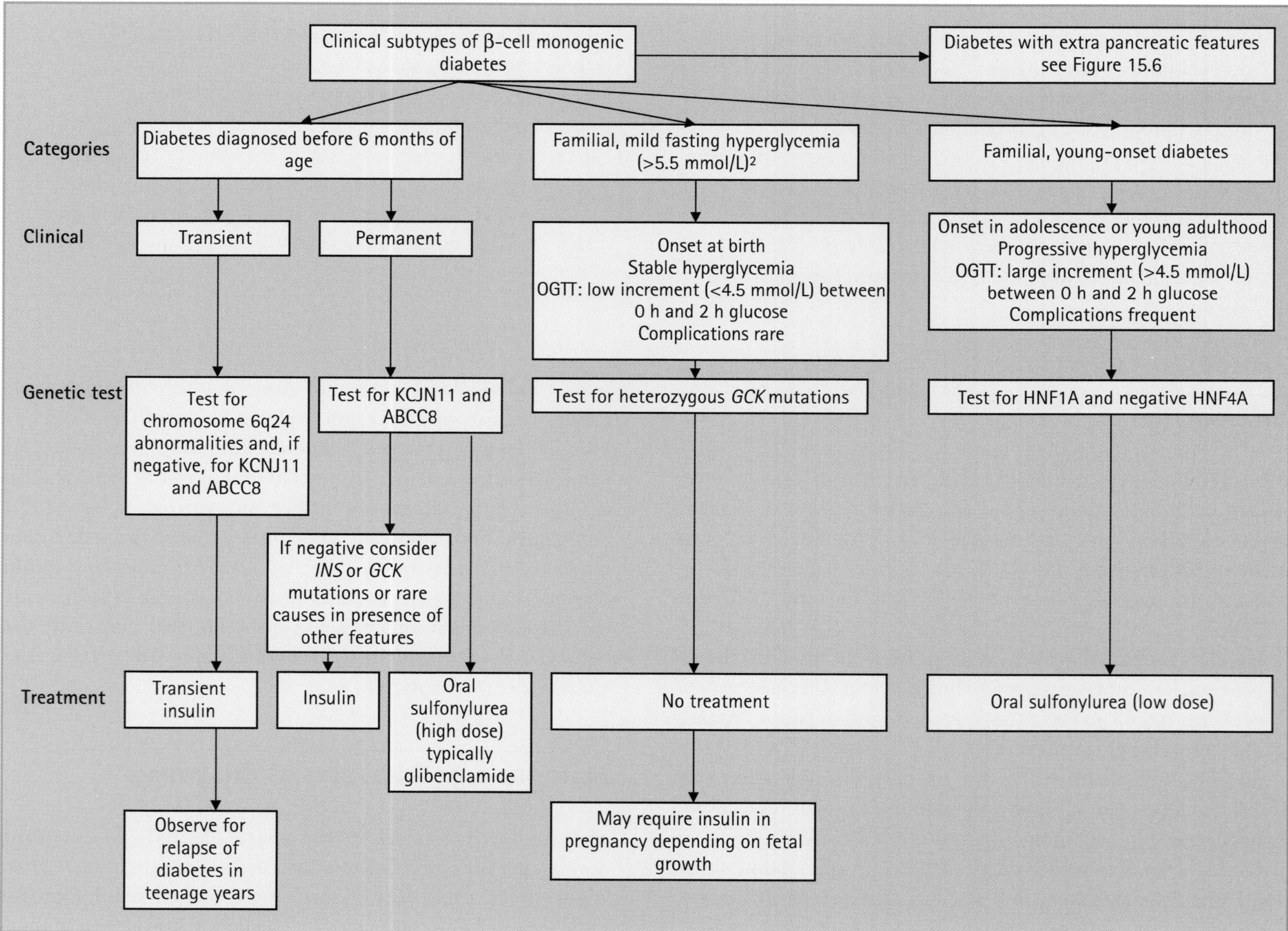

Figure 15.1 Clinical subtypes and management of monogenic β-cell diabetes without extrapancreatic features. To convert plasma glucose measurements to mg/dL multiple by 18. ABCC8, ATB binding cassette subfamily C; *GCK*, glucokinase gene; HNF, hepatocyte nuclear factor; *INS*, insulin gene; *KCNJ11*, potassium inwardly rectifying channel, subfamily J, member 11 gene; OGTT, oral glucose tolerance test.

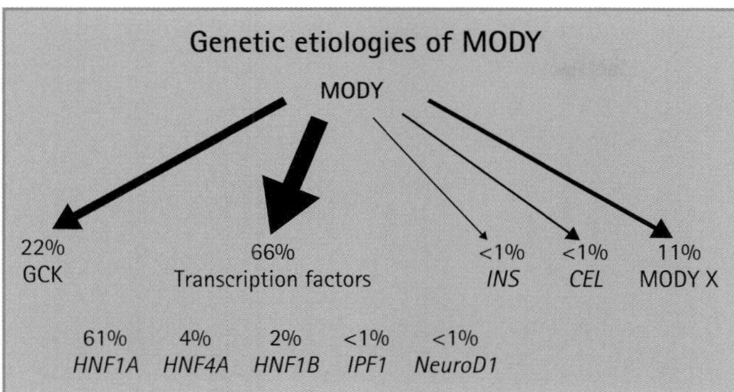

Figure 15.2 The different genetic etiology in a UK maturity-onset diabetes of the young (MODY) series. MODY X denotes dominantly inherited young-onset non-insulin dependent diabetes fitting clinical criteria for maturity-onset diabetes of the young where mutations in known MODY genes have not been identified. Adapted from McCarthy & Hattersley [6].

in the gene encoding the glucose sensing enzyme glucokinase (*GCK*) and mutations in several transcription factors that affect β-cell development and function, the frequencies of which are summarized in Figure 15.2. Clinical presentation varies greatly depending on the underlying genetic mutation. Table 15.2 summarizes the clinical features of glucokinase and transcription factor diabetes. The strikingly different subtypes of MODY mean it is important to define the underlying genetic etiology. We recommend the use of clinical categories based on underlying genetic cause – familial mild fasting hyperglycemia resulting from glucokinase gene mutations (*GCK* MODY), familial young-onset progressive diabetes resulting from *HNF1A* and *HNF4A* mutations (transcription factor MODY) and renal cysts and diabetes syndrome (RCAD) resulting from *HNF1B* mutations.

Mutations in the genes associated with MODY should be sought in patients with diabetes diagnosed under 25 years of age, who do not fully fit the phenotypes of T1DM or T2DM and who have a strong family history of diabetes (Table 15.1). Differentiating from apparent T1DM is particularly important as these patients can often be most effectively treated without the use of injected insulin.

Glucokinase MODY

Glucokinase catalyzes the phosphorylation of glucose to glucose-6-phosphate, the first and rate-limiting step in intracellular glucose metabolism in both β-cells and hepatocytes (Figure 15.3). Owing to the unique catalytic properties of the enzyme, the rate of glucose phosphorylation is proportional to the glucose concentration, thus allowing β-cells and hepatocytes to respond to changes in glycemia. In the β-cell, glucokinase acts as a glucose sensor ensuring insulin release is appropriate to the glucose concentration [7]. Heterozygous loss-of-function mutations in *GCK* result in a shift of the dose–response curve to the right [8].

Table 15.2 Comparison of the clinical characteristics of glucokinase and transcription factor maturity-onset diabetes of the young (MODY).

	Glucokinase MODY	Transcription factor MODY
Onset of hyperglycemia	Birth	Adolescence/early adulthood
Presentation	Usually asymptomatic, detected by screening or on routine testing	Usually symptomatic
Nature of hyperglycemia	Minimal increase in glycemia with age Mild (FPG usually 5.5–8 mmol/L) HbA_{1c} usually close or just above upper limit of normal	Progressive deterioration of glycemia with age May be severe (FPG frequently >14 mmol/L off treatment) HbA_{1c} variable depending on age and treatment, may be high
Pattern in an oral glucose tolerance test	FPG >5.5 mmol/L (2 hour – FPG) usually <3.5 mmol/L	FPG often <5.5 mmol/L (2 hour – FPG) usually >3.5 mmol/L
Microvascular complications	Rare	Frequent
Pathophysiology	β-Cell defect (glucose sensing defect)	β-Cell defect (initially insulin secretion maintained at normal glucose values but not increased in hyperglycemia)
Extrapancreatic manifestations	Reduced birth weight	See Table 15.3
Treatment	Pharmacologic treatment rarely needed	Sensitive to sulfonylurea treatment May progress to require insulin

FPG, fasting plasma glucose.

Glycemia is therefore regulated at a higher setpoint but remains tightly controlled. Subjects are still able to stimulate their β-cells maximally [8]. Glucokinase is also present in the liver and as a result patients have reduced hepatic glycogen synthesis [9].

Over 200 loss-of-function mutations in *GCK* have been identified, all causing a similar clinical picture. Homozygous loss-of-function glucokinase mutations are a rare cause of insulin-requiring diabetes presenting in the neonatal period [10]. Gain-of-function mutations cause congenital hyperinsulinism [11].

Clinical features

Patients have mild fasting hyperglycemia from birth, usually 5.5–8.0 mmol/L. There is only minor deterioration in fasting glucose with age (Figure 15.4) [12]. Patients do not have symptoms of hyperglycemia. Post meal glucose values are only mildly raised and there is frequently only a small increase (<3 mmol/L in 70% of patients) seen at 2 hours on an oral glucose tolerance test [13] which may explain the near normal HbA_{1c} and rarity of complications [14]. Glycated hemoglobin values above 7.5% would be suggestive of an alternative diagnosis. Marked worsen-

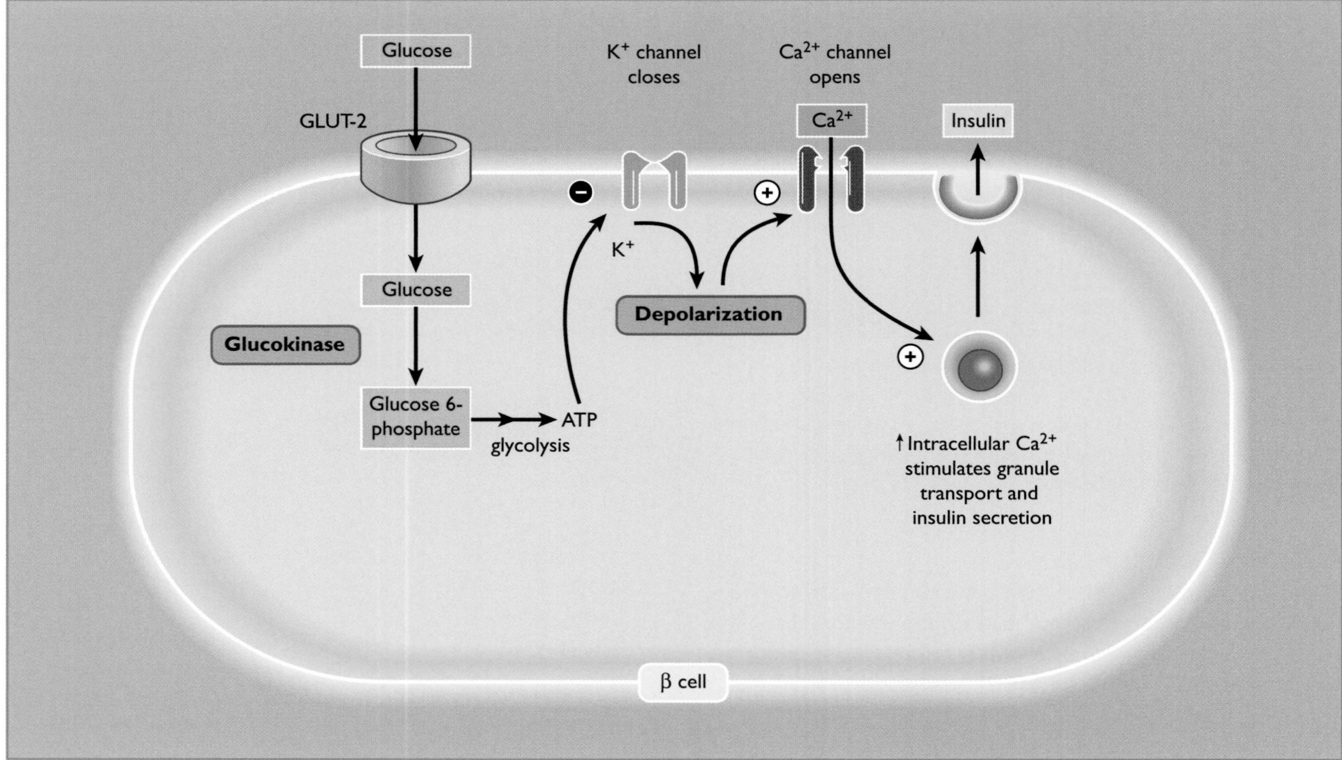

Figure 15.3 Glucokinase and its role within the β-cell. Glucokinase is the rate determining step in glucose metabolism, and therefore in the rate of production of ATP, which leads ultimately to insulin secretion.

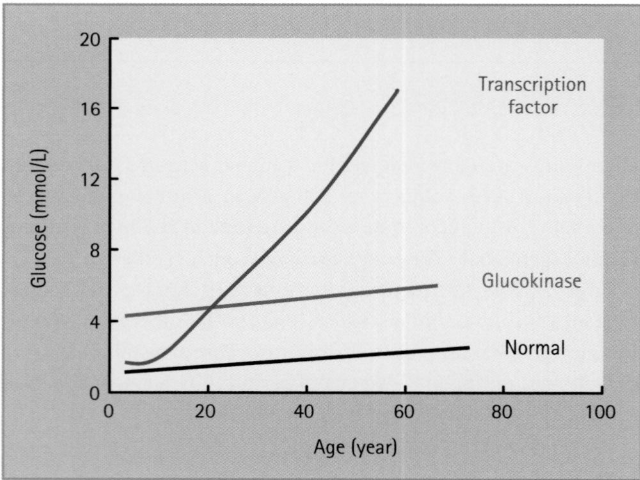

Figure 15.4 Variation of blood glucose concentration with age in patients with glucokinase and transcription factor MODY.

ing of the glycemia suggests that the patient has developed T1DM or T2DM in additon to their *GCK* mutation. Microvascular and macrovascular complications are rare even when no treatment is given [14]. Glucokinase MODY is asymptomatic and, although it is autosomal dominantly inherited, there may be no known family history of diabetes. Testing of apparently unaffected parents can reveal that one parent has mildly raised fasting plasma glucose.

Differentiating from type 1 and 2 diabetes

Diagnosis of glucokinase MODY is most important in young patients who may otherwise be thought to have T1DM and treated with insulin [15]. Unlike T1DM, hyperglycemia remains mild, β-cell antibodies are usually negative and (if tested) one parent is likely to have mild hyperglycemia. Fasting C-peptide will remain detectable and the post meal rise in glucose concentration will be far less than in T1DM. Differentiating glucokinase MODY from T2DM can be more difficult as both conditions can cause mild hyperglycemia with a strong family history. Lack of obesity and features of insulin resistance, a small increment on oral glucose tolerance testing and non-progression all suggest glucokinase MODY.

Management

Outside of pregnancy, hypoglycemic medication is not recommended as hyperglycemia is mild, complications are rare and medication appears to have minimal effect because the regulation of glycemia is preserved [16]. Once diagnosis is confirmed, treatment can usually be discontinued; however, this should be done with caution as it is possible for T1DM or T2DM to coexist with a *GCK* mutation.

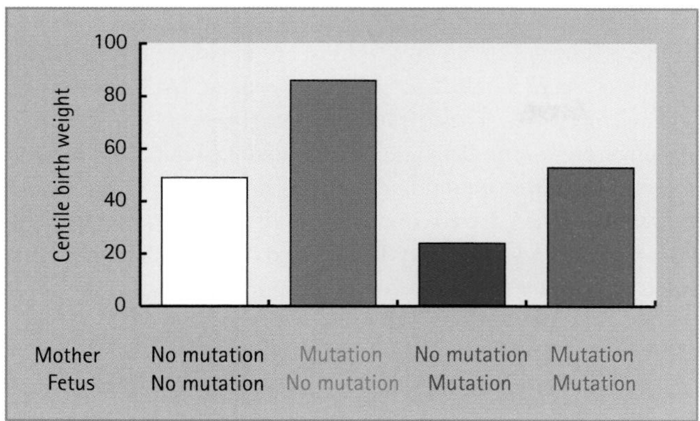

Figure 15.5 The centile birth weight of children in families with glucokinase mutations. The weight is increased by the presence of a maternal mutation and decreased by the presence of a fetal mutation. Data from Hattersley *et al.* [18].

Glucokinase MODY and pregnancy

Clinical features

Patients with *GCK* mutations are frequently found to have hyperglycemia during screening in pregnancy and represent approximately 3% of Caucasian patients with gestational diabetes [17]. Their identification is important because they have a different clinical course, both within and outside pregnancy, than other subjects with gestational diabetes. The birth weight of the newborn infant will depend on the mutation status of both the mother and the fetus (Figure 15.5). Where only the mother carries the mutation, maternal hyperglycemia may result in increased fetal insulin secretion and growth causing the fetus to be large for gestational age [18]. If the fetus inherits the mutation from the father, however, birth weight is reduced by approximately 500 g as a result of reduced fetal insulin secretion and insulin-mediated fetal growth [18]. If both mother and fetus have the *GCK* mutation the two opposing effects are cancelled out and the newborn infant is of normal weight.

Genetic testing for *GCK* mutations in pregnancy

We recommend testing for *GCK* mutations when a pregnant patient is found to have persistently raised fasting plasma glucose 5.5–8 mmol/L and an increment of <4.6 mmol/L on at least one oral glucose tolerance test (either during or outside pregnancy). An absence of family history should not exclude the diagnosis as asymptomatic hyperglycemia in a parent may not have been detected.

Management

Patients with hyperglycemia resulting from glucokinase mutations are often treated with insulin during pregnancy in an attempt to correct the fasting hyperglycemia. Fetal genotype, however, is a far greater determinant of fetal birth weight than treatment of the mother and insulin treatment appears to have little effect on fetal growth [19]. This probably reflects the difficulty in lowering the blood glucose in glucokinase patients because of increased counter-regulation [20]. Patients stop producing their own insulin and produce counter-regulatory hormones if blood glucose is reduced to normal levels, making successful control of blood glucose with insulin difficult. This results in frequent hypoglycemic symptoms at non-hypoglycemic blood sugar levels and means that large doses of insulin may be required to reduce fasting hyperglycemia to normal levels [20,21]. In some cases where the fetus has inherited the mutation, intensive insulin treatment has resulted in a low birth weight child [21]. This is to be expected as a small baby is seen when the fetus inherits a mutation from the father and is born to a normoglycemic mother [18,22]. Testing fetal genotype *in utero* is not without risk. Treatment decisions in glucokinase gestational diabetes should therefore be related to fetal growth as shown by scans rather than being made solely on maternal glycemia [21]. If the abdominal circumference is greater than the 75th centile insulin may be used but early delivery is the most successful strategy.

HNF1A and *HNF4A* (transcription factor MODY)

Transcription factors are proteins that bind to DNA and form part of a complex regulatory network controlling gene expression. The majority of patients with MODY have a heterozygous mutation in a transcription factor gene, by far the most common being mutations in the hepatic nuclear factors 1A and 4A (*HNF1A* and *HNF4A*). Diabetes resulting from mutations in other transcription factor encoding genes including *HNF1B*, insulin promoter factor 1 (IPF-1) and *NEUROD1* are discussed elsewhere in this chapter.

Transcription factor mutations alter insulin secretion in the mature β-cell as well as altering β-cell development, proliferation and cell death. Mutations in the hepatic nuclear factors appear to alter levels of proteins critical in metabolism including the GLUT-2 glucose transporter and key enzymes in the mitochondrial metabolism of glucose [23–25]. Reduced β-cell proliferation and preserved or increased apoptosis could explain the progressive deterioration in β-cell function seen in these patients [25–28].

Mutations in *HNF1A* account for up to 70% of cases of MODY with nearly 200 different mutations reported. *HNF4A*, the next most common, accounts for approximately 3% of cases [29].

Clinical features

Heterozygous transcription factor mutations cause autosomal dominant diabetes presenting in adolescence or early adulthood resulting from progressive failure of insulin secretion. While diabetes is similar in *HNF1A* and *HNF4A* mutation carriers as a result of a common pattern of β-cell dysfunction, a number of differences in extrapancreatic features occur (Table 15.3).

Diabetes

Patients are usually born with normal glucose tolerance and then show progressive β-cell dysfunction until they develop diabetes,

Table 15.3 Extrapancreatic features assisting in the differential diagnosis of transcription factor maturity-onset diabetes of the young (MODY).

Transcription factor	Extrapancreatic clinical features
HNF1A	Low renal glucose threshold (glycosuria) Raised HDL Raised cardiovascular risk (in excess of type 2 diabetes)
HNF4A	Increased birth weight/macrosomia Low HDL, low lipoprotein A1 and A2, raised LDL
HNF1B	Renal cysts and renal development disorders and multiple others. See Table 15.5
NeuroD1	None described

HDL, high density lipoprotein cholesterol; LDL, low density lipoprotein cholesterol.

usually between 10 and 30 years of age (Figure 15.4). Sixty-three percent of *HNF1A* carriers are diagnosed with diabetes by the age of 25 years and 79% by the age of 35 years; the age of diagnosis is partly related to the location of the underlying mutation within the gene [30–32]. Patients show deteriorating glycemia with age and require pharmacologic treatment. In the oral glucose tolerance test, in contrast to patients with glucokinase mutations, the fasting glucose is often normal initially but there is marked elevation of glycemia at 2 hours and consequently a large 2-hour increment (>5.0 mmol/L) [13]. This occurs because insulin secretion rates in early *HNF1A* MODY remain appropriate, with blood glucose values less than 8.0 mmol/L but are reduced significantly in comparison to non-diabetic non-mutation carriers above this level [33]. Microvascular complications are frequent particularly when hyperglycemia is inadequately treated [34]. Patients tend to be lean and insulin-sensitive. Obesity occurs at similar levels to the normal population.

Extrapancreatic clinical features

These are summarized in Table 15.3 and discussed in more detail below.

HNF1A

Patients with *HNF1A* mutations have elevated levels of high density lipoprotein cholesterol (HDL) which contrasts with the reduced HDL levels seen in T2DM [35]. Despite this they appear to have a greater risk of coronary heart disease than patients with T1DM [34]. Frequency of microvascular complications is similar to that seen in T1DM and T2DM and relates to degree of glycemic control [34]. Patients have a reduced renal threshold for glucose. Mutation carriers without diabetes may develop glycosuria after a glucose challenge even if glycemia remains within normal limits [36].

HNF4A

HNF4A mutations are associated with an 800 g increase in birth weight compared with non-mutation carrying siblings [37]. This means the offspring of *HNF4A* mutation carrying fathers, as well as the offspring of *HNF4A* mothers, are at risk of marked macrosomia. There is also an increased risk of hypoglycemia in affected neonates. These features appear to relate to increased insulin secretion *in utero* and in early infancy which evolves into reduced insulin secretion and diabetes in later life [37]. *HNF4A* mutation carriers have reduced levels of HDL (and lipoprotein A1 and A2) and frequently have raised LDL, while triglyceride levels are similar to population norms [38].

Differentiating from type 1 diabetes

These patients are usually diagnosed as having T1DM as they have symptomatic diabetes occurring in adolescence or young adulthood. We recommend genetic testing for *HNF1A* mutations in any young adult with apparent T1DM, a parent with diabetes, and who is antibody-negative at diagnosis. Evidence of non-insulin dependence increases the likelihood of a positive result; this would include no ketosis in the absence of insulin treatment, good glycemic control on low doses of insulin, or detectable C peptide with plasma glucose >8 mmol/L 3–5 years after diagnosis (outside the honeymoon period) [39]. While glutamine acid decarboxylase (GAD) antibodies are usually negative, positive GAD antibodies may be expected in up to 1–2% of the non-diabetic normal population, and therefore positive antibodies (particularly at low titer) may not exclude monogenic diabetes; testing should be considered where clinical suspicion is high [40,41]. *HNF4A* testing should be performed in any patient with a high suspicion of having *HNF1A* who tests negative for *HNF1A* mutations, particularly where there is evidence of increased birth weight and/or neonatal hypoglycemia.

Differentiating from type 2 diabetes

HNF1A should be suspected and mutation screening performed in patients otherwise suspected to be have T2DM where the following features are present ([39] and www.diabetesgenes.org):

1 Young-onset diabetes – typically before 25 years old in at least one family member;

2 Family history of diabetes – at least two generations and ideally two individuals diagnosed in their twenties or thirties), particularly where affected individuals are non-obese;

3 Absence of obesity, acanthosis nigricans or other evidence of insulin resistance.

In addition, a large increment in the glucose tolerance test (>5 mmol/L), presence of glycosuria with blood glucose less than 10 mmol/L, marked sensitivity to sulfonylureas and a lipid profile showing normal or raised HDL and normal or low triglycerides (atypical for T2DM) would all be supportive of a diagnosis of *HNF1A* instead of T2DM [35]. *HNF4A* should be suspected and tested in those patients who are suspected to have *HNF1A* mutations but test negative on *HNF1A* screening. These patients have a normal renal glucose threshold and frequently have a personal and/or family history of high birth weights and/or neonatal hypoglycemia.

Management

Patients with both *HNF1A* and *HNF4A* mutations are sensitive to sulfonylurea therapy which we recommend as first line treatment [38,42]. Glycemic control with sulfonylureas is often better than with insulin and the fasting glucose lowering effect is 4 times greater than that seen in T2DM [42,43]. Transfer to sulfonylurea treatment is successful in the majority of patients although insulin therapy may be required as diabetes progresses [44]. Even very low sulfonylurea doses may cause hypoglycemia. The starting dose should therefore be low – we use a starting dose of 40 mg/day gliclazide or 2.5 mg/day glibenclamide in adults. If there is hypoglycemia with low doses of standard agents, a short-acting agent such as nateglinide may be appropriate [45]. Because of the apparent increased risk of cardiovascular disease in *HNF1A*, statin therapy should be considered and we suggest it for all patients aged over 40 years.

Management in pregnancy

Evidence to support management strategies for *HNF1A* and *HNF4A* in pregnancy is very limited. Our current practice is to continue sulfonylureas if glycemic control is good before pregnancy but otherwise institute treatment with insulin. Consideration should be given to switching to glibenclamide in the prepregnancy period as this sulfonylurea has the most evidence for safety in pregnancy [46,47]. If a fetus carries *HNF4A*, the risk of macrosomia and neonatal hypoglycemia is high whether the mutation comes from the mother or father [37]. If either parent is known to carry a *HNF4A* mutation, we recommend:

1 Very tight glucose control in mothers with diabetes to attempt to minimize macrosomia;
2 Serial antenatal ultrasound scans to look for macrosomia with early delivery if this is marked; and
3 Early measurement of neonatal glucose and consideration of diazoxide treatment if hypoglycemia persists.

Other transcription factor MODY

Other transcription factor mutations causing autosomal dominant β-cell diabetes have been identified in the genes *IPF1*, *NEUROD1*, *KLF11* and *PAX 4* but all are very rare [48–53].

Neonatal diabetes and diabetes diagnosed within 6 months of life

Children diagnosed with diabetes within the first 6 months of life (referred to as neonatal diabetes) are likely to have monogenic diabetes and not T1DM [54–57]. These patients commonly present with ketoacidosis and absent C-peptide. Neonatal diabetes is rare, affecting 1 in 100 000–200 000 live births [58]. Approximately half of cases remit spontaneously and are therefore termed transient neonatal diabetes mellitus (TNDM) as opposed to permanent neonatal diabetes mellitus (PNDM) where diabetes persists. TNDM often recurs in later life [59]. Neonatal diabetes results from mutations of key genes involved in β-cell development or function. Table 15.4 summarizes the known genetic causes of neonatal diabetes.

Table 15.4 Causes of neonatal diabetes.

Pancreatic pathophysiology	Protein, chromosome or gene affected	Prevalence	Inheritance	Features in addition to neonatal diabetes and low birth weight
Reduced β-cell function	K_{ATP} channel (*KCNJ11* and *ABCC8*)	50% of permanent neonatal diabetes, 25% of transient neonatal diabetes	85% spontaneous. Remainder autosomal dominant or recessive	Developmental delay and epilepsy. Sulfonylurea responsive
	Chromosome 6q24	70% of transient neonatal diabetes	Variable	Macroglossia and umbilical hernia
	Glucokinase (homozygous for mutation)	Rare	Autosomal recessive	Both parents have heterozygous glucokinase associated hyperglycemia
	SLC2A2	Rare	Autosomal dominant	Hypergalactosemia, hepatic failure
	GLIS3	Rare	Autosomal recessive	Congenital hypothyroidism, glaucoma, liver fibrosis and cystic kidney disease
Reduced pancreatic mass	*PTF1A*	Rare	Autosomal recessive	Pancreatic and cerebellar agenesis
	PDX1	Rare	Autosomal recessive	Pancreatic agenesis
	HNF1B	Rare	Autosomal dominant	Exocrine pancreas insufficiency and renal cysts
Increased β-cell destruction	*EIF2AK3*	Rare	Autosomal recessive	Spondyloepiphyseal dysplasia, renal failure, recurrent hepatitis and mental retardation
	FOXP3	Rare	X-linked	Immune dysregulation, intractable diarrhoea, eczematous skin rash and elevated IgE
	INS	12% of permanent neonatal diabetes	Autosomal dominant	None

Permanent neonatal diabetes

Approximately half of PNDM is caused by mutations in the genes *KCNJ11* and *ABCC8* which encode the Kir6.2 and SUR1 subunits, respectively, of the β-cell ATP-sensitive potassium channel (K_{ATP} channel) [60–63]. This channel is constitutively open and regulates insulin secretion by closing in response to the raised intracellular ATP levels that occur as a consequence of hyperglycemia. Channel closure triggers depolarization of the β-cell membrane which leads to insulin secretion. Activating mutations in *KCNJ11* and *ABCC8* prevent closure of the potassium channel in response to increased ATP so the β-cell remains hyperpolarized and unable to secrete insulin [64]. Sulfonylureas close the β-cell K_{ATP} channel by an ATP independent route and they have been used successfully in the management of the majority of patients with neonatal diabetes resulting from *KCNJ11* and *ABCC8* mutations [65]. The K_{ATP} channel is also present in the brain, nerves and muscles. Reflecting this distribution of channels, 20% of patients with *KCNJ11* mutations (and occasional patients with *ABCC8* mutations) have associated neurologic features [57,60,61,64].

Heterozygous mutations in the insulin gene (*INS*) have been identified in 12% of cases of isolated PNDM and insulin treatment is required [66,67]. A number of other genetic causes have been found which all appear to be relatively rare [58] as outlined in Table 15.4.

The majority (85%) of PNDM resulting from K_{ATP} channel mutations arise spontaneously from *de novo* heterozygous mutations, with the remainder being familial and inherited mainly in an autosomal dominant pattern. About 40% of neonatal diabetes resulting from *ABCC8* mutations, however, are inherited in an autosomal recessive fashion [63].

Clinical features

Diabetes caused by *KCNJ11* mutations typically present in the first 26 weeks of life (median 4–6 weeks) with marked hyperglycemia often accompanied by ketosis. C-peptide is usually undetectable and islet cell antibodies negative [60]. As with all neonatal diabetes subtypes, infants are often small for gestational age as a result of reduced fetal insulin secretion with consequent decreased insulin mediated growth. About 20% of patients with PNDM and *KCNJ11* mutations have neurologic features, the most common being developmental delay, sometimes with muscle weakness and/or epilepsy. The most severe form where neonatal diabetes is accompanied by developmental delay and epilepsy has been named developmental delay, epilepsy and neonatal diabetes (DEND). "Intermediate DEND" refers to neonatal diabetes with less severe developmental delay and no epilepsy. The severity of the clinical condition relates closely to the underlying mutation and its effect on K_{ATP} channel ATP sensitivity [64,68].

Neonatal diabetes caused by *ABCC8* mutation has a similar phenotype but leads to transient neonatal diabetes more commonly than PNDM and has associated neurologic features only rarely [61–63]. Patients with neonatal diabetes and *INS* mutations present at a median age of 9 weeks and are also often small for gestational age but do not have extrapancreatic features [66].

Management

Although insulin therapy is commonly used in the initial period after diagnosis, the majority of patients with *KCNJ11* and *ABCC8* mutations can successfully transfer from insulin to sulfonylurea therapy, usually with significant improvements in glycemic control [62,65]. Ninety percent of those with *KCNJ11* mutations are able to discontinue insulin, while HbA_{1c} appears to improve in all patients with a mean drop from 65 to 46 mmol/mol (8.1 to 6.4%) after 12 weeks [65]. Glibenclamide was initially selected as it is non-selective and widely available; it has been used in the majority of cases and may be more effective than other sulfonylurea agents [69]. The doses needed are often higher than those needed for the treatment of T2DM: a median dose of 0.45 mg/kg/day is required with doses up to 1.5 mg/kg/day needed in some cases [65,70]. Diarrhoea is a possible side effect but this usually only lasts 1–3 days [71]. Sulfonylurea therapy may result in some improvement in neurologic features even where they are commenced in adulthood [69,72,73]. Further information on transferring patients from insulin to sulfonylureas can be found at www.diabetesgenes.org.

Neonatal diabetes resulting from *INS* mutations requires insulin treatment [66]. Affected individuals with a heterozygous *KCNJ11* mutation contemplating parenthood should be counseled that they have a 50% chance of passing on the mutation to their offspring. Where unaffected parents whose child is affected by a heterozygous mutation are planning further pregnancies, the risk of further affected children is low because of the possibility of a germline mutation is approximately 5–10% [74]. Where parents have a child with neonatal diabetes caused by a recessive *ABCC8* mutation, there is a 25% chance of each further offspring being affected but the risk is low for subsequent generations.

Transient neonatal diabetes

The genetic etiology of more than 90% of transient neonatal diabetes has been established. The majority (70%) of cases result from abnormalities the q24 region of chromosome 6 (6q24) affecting imprinted genes [58,75]. Genetic imprinting occurs when only the maternal or paternally inherited allele of a gene is expressed. In TNDM paternal uniparental disomy, paternal duplication of 6q24 or abnormal methylation of the maternal copy of the chromosome causes overexpression of the paternal copies of the genes *PLAGL1* (also known as *ZAC*) and *HYMAI* [75,76]. Paternal duplication of 6q24 can be inherited, therefore this abnormality causes the majority of inherited TNDM cases. Uniparental disomy causes sporadic TNDM; cases resulting from abnormal methylation of the maternal copy of chromosome 6 may be sporadic or inherited [75,76]. The majority (90%) of TNDM not associated with 6q24 abnormalities are caused by mutations in *KCNJ11* and *ABCC8* [57,59,62,77–81].

Clinical features

6q24 diabetes usually presents in the first week of life often with severe hyperglycemia and dehydration but usually without ketosis

[75]. Islet cell antibodies are usually negative and C-peptide is low or negligible [75]. Low birth weight is common (mean birth weight 2.1 kg), and there may be associated macroglossia and/or umbilical hernia. Insulin treatment is required for a median of 12 weeks before the patient goes into remission. Diabetes recurs later in life in 50–60% of patients as a result of β-cell dysfunction. The average age of recurrence is 14 years. In some cases hyperglycemia may be intermittent and seen only at times of stress [75,82]. Where TNDM is caused by *KCNJ11* and *ABCC8* mutations, diabetes tends to present later (median 4 weeks), takes longer to remit and is associated with less intrauterine growth restriction (median birth weight 2.6 kg) [59].

Management

Insulin is required in the neonatal period whereas treatment requirements following relapse vary from diet to oral hypoglycemics or insulin [82]. In TNDM cases resulting from *KCNJ11* and *ABCC8* mutations, diabetes may be successfully managed with sulfonylureas [59,62].

Genetic counseling depends on the underlying genetic etiology. Cases caused by uniparental disomy are sporadic and therefore have low risk of occurrence in either siblings or offspring of the affected child. Methylation defects often result from homozygous mutations in the transcription factor gene *ZFP57* and therefore may be inherited in an autosomal recessive manner [76]. Offspring of males with 6q24 duplication have a 50% chance of developing TNDM whereas if the abnormality is inherited from the mother they will not be affected but the TNDM may occur in the following generation [82].

Genetic testing in neonatal diabetes

At the time of diagnosis of neonatal diabetes it is not known whether the diabetes will be transient or permanent. We recommend testing for 6q24 abnormalities, *KCNJ11*, *ABCC8* and *INS* mutations at diagnosis in all diabetes diagnosed before 6 months. Identifying mutations in these genes is important as it will influence treatment. An early diagnosis and very low birth weight make 6q24 most likely. A genetic cause (*KCNJ11* or *INS*) can be established in approximately 7% of diabetes diagnosed between 6 months and 1 year of age so consideration should be given to testing this age group, especially where autoantibody tests are negative [56].

Diabetes with extrapancreatic features

A number of monogenic causes of diabetes are associated with distinct features occurring outside the pancreas. In many cases extrapancreatic disease may be the presenting feature, for example in cystic fibrosis and hemochromatosis (see Chapter 18). Clinical subtypes and management of monogenic β-cell diabetes that have extrapancreatic features are summarized in Figure 15.6.

Maternally inherited diabetes and deafness

Maternally inherited diabetes and deafness (MIDD) results from a mutation in mitochondrial DNA and causes maternally inherited diabetes with sensorineural deafness that may be accompanied by a wide range of other features. It affects up to 1% of patients with diabetes but is frequently undiagnosed [83].

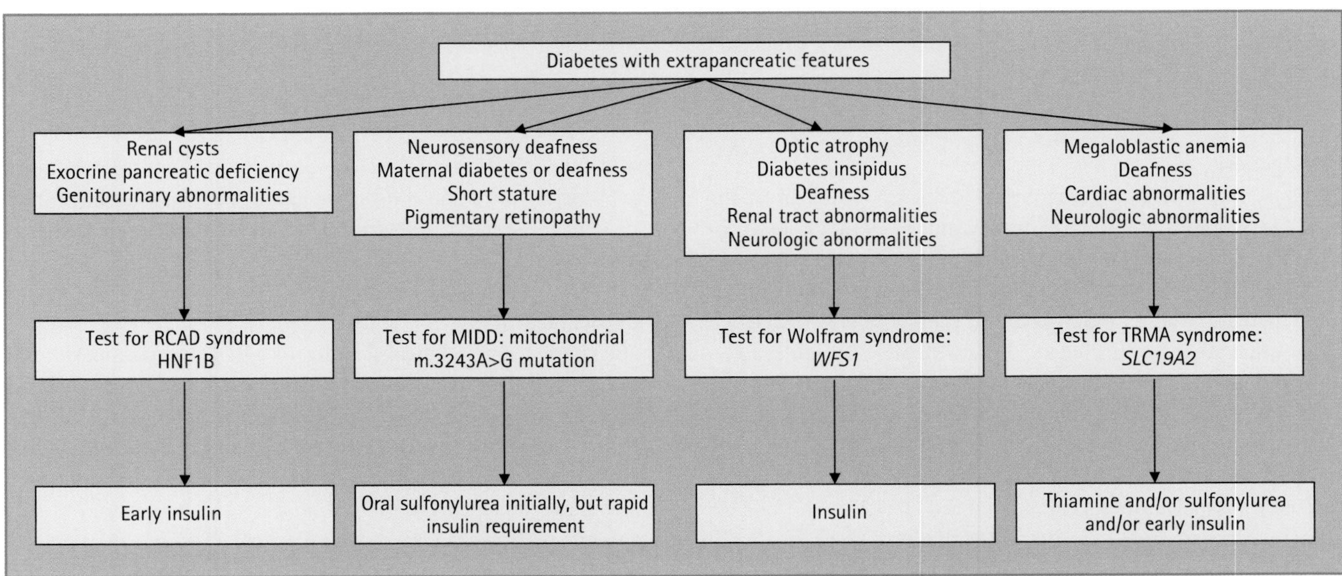

Figure 15.6 Clinical subtypes and management of monogenic β-cell diabetes that has extrapancreatic features. *HNF1B*, hepatocyte nuclear factor 1B; MIDD, maternally inherited diabetes and deafness; RCAD, renal cysts and diabetes; *SLC19A2*, solute carrier family 19, member 2 gene; TRMA, thiamine responsive megaloblastic anemia; *WFS1*, Wolfram syndrome 1 gene.

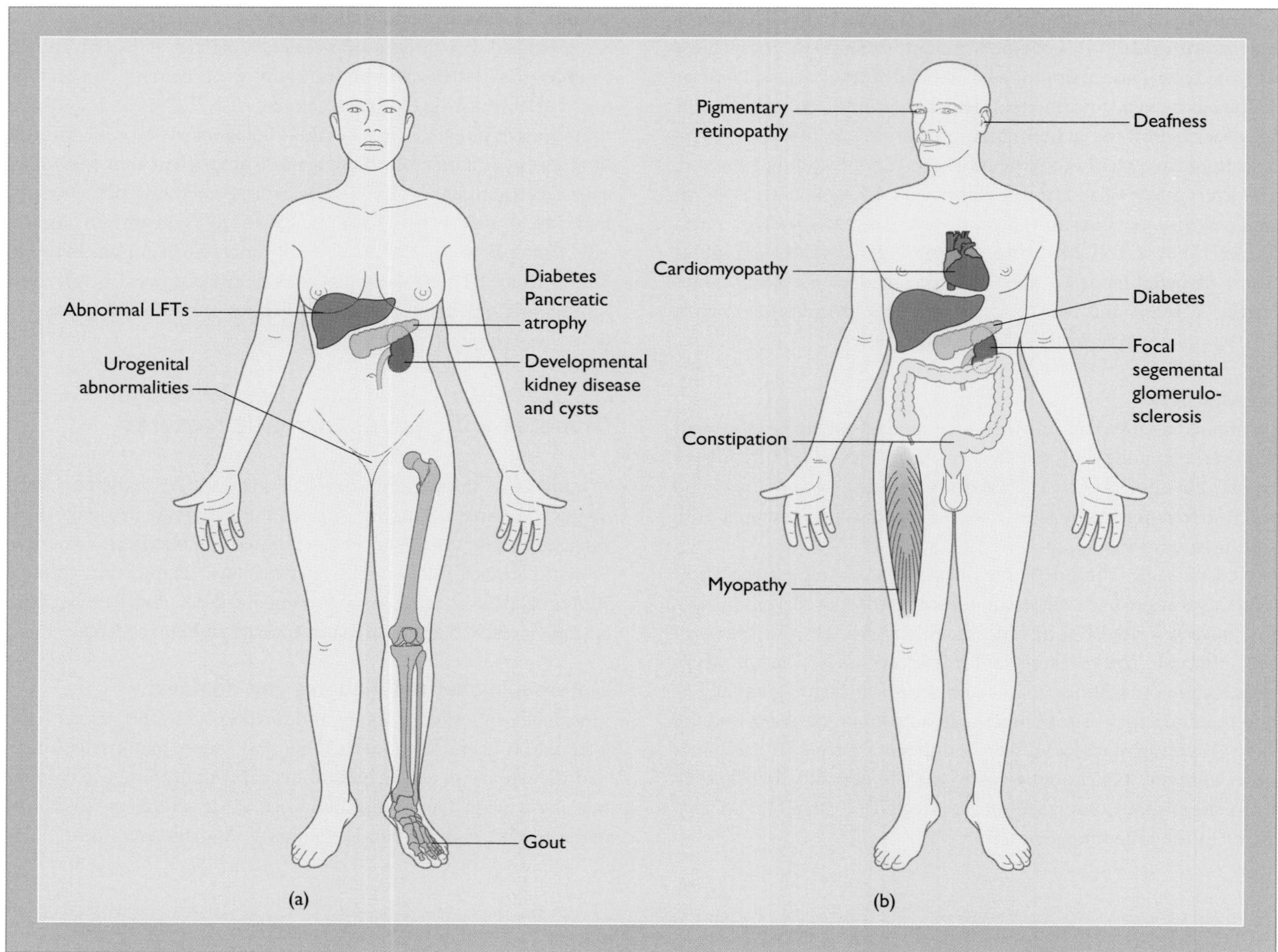

Figure 15.7 Phenotypes of: (a) renal cysts and diabetes syndrome due to *HNF1B* mutation or deletion; (b) maternally inherited diabetes and deafness caused by mitochondrial m.3243A>G mutation. Adapted from Murphy *et al.* [181].

Pathogenesis

The vast majority of mitochondrial diabetes results from the m.3243A>G point mutation in mitochondrial DNA. Other mitochondrial DNA mutations have been implicated but are rare [84].

The m.3243A>G mutation affects the mitochondrial respiratory chain and therefore may result in cellular energy deficiency. Organs that are most affected are those with high metabolic activity which include the endocrine pancreas, cochlea and in some cases the retina, muscle, kidney and brain. Mitochondrial dysfunction in pancreatic islets results in abnormal β-cell function, loss of β-cell mass and insulin deficiency while insulin sensitivity is usually normal although can be reduced (reviewed in [83]). As mitochondria are only inherited from the mother, the maternal line in a family is affected, and children of a male patient are not at risk. Although all children of an affected female are likely to carry the mutation, phenotype can vary widely in the same family because of heteroplasmy. Offspring inherit a mix of mutant and wild-type mitochondrial DNA – the proportion of mitochondria carrying the mutation will vary in offspring of an affected mother as will subsequent segregation of mitochondria to different tissues.

Clinical features

The characteristic clinical features of MIDD are summarized in Figure 15.7. The majority of mutation carriers develop diabetes (over 85%) and sensorineural hearing loss (over 75%) [85–88]. There is usually a family history of diabetes and/or hearing loss in maternal relatives but clinical features can vary greatly even within the same pedigree [89]. Diabetes is progressive and usually presents with insidious onset similar to T2DM but may present acutely, with ketoacidosis occurring in approximately 8% of cases [85,86,90]. Mean age at diagnosis of diabetes is 37 years but age of diagnosis can range from early adolescence to old age [86,90,91].

Hearing loss typically develops in early adulthood but again may occur in children as well as the elderly; it is more common and often more severe in men [86,88]. Patients with the m.3243A>G mutation have a high prevalence of renal failure with focal segmental glomerular sclerosis (FSGS) found more frequently than diabetic nephropathy on renal biopsy [86,92]. Diabetic retinopathy may be less prevalent than in other forms of diabetes; macular retinal dystrophy is frequent but rarely causes visual symptoms [83,86,92]. Cardiac abnormalities include left ventricular hypertrophy, heart failure (which can progress rapidly), cardiac autonomic neuropathy and cardiac arrhythmias [93–97]. Other possible clinical manifestations of the m.3243A>G mutation include short stature, MELAS (mitochondrial encephalomyopathy, lactic acidosis and stroke-like episodes), psychiatric disorders, proximal myopathy and gastrointestinal symptoms [83].

Differentiating from type 1 and 2 diabetes

Diabetes caused by the m.3243A>G mutation may present like T1DM or T2DM [85,86,90]. GAD antibodies are usually but not always negative [98–100]. The presence of deafness in the patient or clustering of diabetes and/or deafness in maternal relatives should prompt investigation for the m.3243A>G mutation. Short stature, early-onset cardiomyopathy, myopathy, early-onset stroke or macular retinal dystrophy on retinal screening may all raise suspicion of MIDD [83].

If there is clinical suspicion of MIDD, the diagnosis can be confirmed by testing for the m.3243A>G mutation, usually in blood leukocytes. In rare cases the result may be negative on blood-derived DNA testing despite the presence of the mutation in other tissues as a result of heteroplasmy. Testing of other samples (e.g. urine or mouthwash) may be more appropriate than blood [83].

Management

Diabetes usually requires early insulin treatment (mean 2 years post diagnosis) [85,86,90,100]. There is a theoretical basis for avoiding metformin in view of the risk of lactic acidosis [83,85]. There may be some benefit in co-enzyme Q10 supplementation although randomized double-blind control trials have yet to be performed [101,102]. Monitoring for cardiac manifestations should be considered from a young age, particularly if there are clinical features or family history of early cardiomyopathy. Aggressive blood pressure management and early angiotensin-converting enzyme (ACE) inhibitor treatment may be appropriate in view of the high risk of renal complications. Renal biopsy to exclude FSGS may be necessary in those who develop renal failure [83]. Management of hearing loss involves avoidance of exacerbating factors, prompt treatment of ear infections, hearing aids if necessary and consideration of cochlear implants where there is profound hearing loss [83,103,104].

Maternal relatives of affected patients and children of female patients should be assumed to carry the m.3243A>G mutation. Therefore, periodic screening for the features and complications of MIDD may be advisable. In contrast, paternal relatives and children of an affected male are not at risk of carrying the mutation.

Renal cysts and diabetes (*HNF1B* MODY)

HNF1B is a transcription factor with a role in regulating gene expression in a number of tissues including the pancreas, kidneys, liver genital tract and gut [105]. Heterozygous deletions or mutations in *HNF1B* can cause developmental abnormalities in all these organs although the most common phenotypes are renal abnormalities and diabetes. *HNF1B* abnormalities may show autosomal dominant inheritance, although 32–58% of cases arise spontaneously and there is a wide variation in phenotype even with identical mutations [106–110].

Clinical features

The clinical features are summarized in Table 15.5 and Figure 15.7. Developmental renal disease is the most consistent feature with renal cysts being the most common manifestation [106]. Other possible renal abnormalities include glomerulocystic kidney disease, cystic renal dysplasia and morphologic abnormalities such as horseshoe kidney. Renal function can range from

Table 15.5 Features of patients with *HNF1B* mutations causing RCAD (renal cysts and diabetes) in a UK cohort. Adapted from Bingham & Hattersley [108].

Clinical features	Subjects with *HNF1B* mutations and details (%)
Renal phenotype	
Renal cysts	66%
Renal impairment	86% (15% dialysis/transplantation)
Morphologic renal abnormalities	Horseshoe kidney
	Single kidney
Renal histology (includes)	Glomerulocystic kidney disease
	Cystic renal dysplasia
	Oligomeganephronia
Diabetes	58%
	Mean age of diagnosis 26 years, range 10–61 years
	Insulin treatment common
Other features	
Hypomagnesemia	40%
Short stature	20% <2 SD below mean height
Hyperuricemia and gout	20% (clinical gout)
Uterine abnormalities	17%
Hypospadias	17%
Joint laxity	Rare
Hearing loss	Rare
Prognathism	Rare
Pyloric stenosis	Rare
Learning difficulties	Rare
Chromophobe renal cell carcinoma	Rare

normal to dialysis dependent [111,112]. Half of *HNF1B* mutations carriers have early-onset diabetes caused by both insulin deficiency as a result of reduced β-cell number and increased hepatic insulin resistance. The sensitivity to sulfonylureas found with *HNF1A* and *HNF4A* mutations is absent [113]. Diabetes is usually associated with pancreatic hypoplasia and may be associated with exocrine dysfunction although this is rarely symptomatic [114–116]. Low birth weight is common and transient neonatal diabetes may occur [115]. Other clinical manifestations include abnormal liver function tests, genital tract malformations, hypomagnesemia, hyperuricemia and familial hyperuricemic nephropathy [114,117]. An association with chromophobe renal cell carcinoma has been reported reflecting a probable role for *HNF1B* as a tumour suppressor gene [118,119].

Differentiating from type 1 and 2 diabetes

Approximately 50% of *HNF1B* mutations and deletions are spontaneous and so patients may not have a family history. Testing for *HNF1B* abnormalities should be considered where there is unexplained cystic renal disease, glomerulocystic disease or other renal developmental abnormalities with or without a past medical or family history of diabetes. It should also be considered in individuals with genital tract abnormalities associated with renal abnormalities. Both simple renal cysts and diabetes are common in the general population and should not lead to testing for *HNF1B* abnormalities. Testing for *HNF1B* should always include dosage analysis to detect gene deletions as these are common and will be missed if the laboratory performs sequencing only [120].

Management

Early insulin therapy is usually required for management of diabetes. The sulfonylurea sensitivity seen in other transcription factor diabetes is not seen in *HNF1B*. Renal management is similar to management of other chronic progressive renal diseases. Our recommendation is to repeat renal ultrasound imaging every 2 years in view of the possible increased risk of chromophobe renal carcinoma and to screen for diabetes yearly in non-diabetic mutation carriers.

Other monogenic β-cell diabetes with extrapancreatic features

Wolfram syndrome

Wolfram syndrome (also known as DIDMOAD [diabetes insipidus, diabetes mellitus, optic atrophy and deafness]) is a rare recessive neurodegenerative disorder characterized by diabetes insipidus, diabetes mellitus, optic atrophy deafness and a variety of central nervous system abnormalities. Consideration should be given to this diagnosis where there is a combination of diabetes and optic atrophy [121,122].

Thiamine responsive megaloblastic anemia

Thiamine responsive megaloblastic anemia is a rare autosomal recessive condition characterized by megaloblastic anemia (which may be mild), non-autoimmune diabetes mellitus and sensorineural hearing loss. Treatment with high dose thiamine can improve some features including diabetes [123].

Wolcott–Rallison syndrome

Wolcott–Rallison syndrome is a rare autosomal recessive condition characterized by early-onset diabetes, spondyloepiphyseal dysplasia, acute hepatic failure, renal impairment and developmental delay. Diabetes usually presents in infancy and requires insulin treatment [124].

Monogenic diabetes with pancreatic exocrine dysfunction

Mutations in the carboxyl ester lipase (*CEL*) gene have recently been identified as a rare cause of monogenic diabetes with pancreatic exocrine dysfunction [125].

Insulin resistance

Monogenic causes of diabetes resulting from insulin resistance include the inherited lipodystrophies, mutations affecting the insulin receptor or post receptor signaling and other monogenic syndromes associated with insulin resistance where abnormalities of insulin action are not the primary disorder. There can be considerable clinical overlap in clinical presentation between these conditions [126]. The presence of acanthosis (Figure 15.8) in a thin patient with diabetes should prompt consideration of underlying monogenic causes of insulin resistance.

Insulin receptor gene mutations

Insulin exerts its effects through binding to a transmembrane receptor, consisting of two alfa and two beta subunits, present on the surface of target cells. Binding of insulin to the alfa subunit activates beta subunit tyrosine kinase activity triggering protein

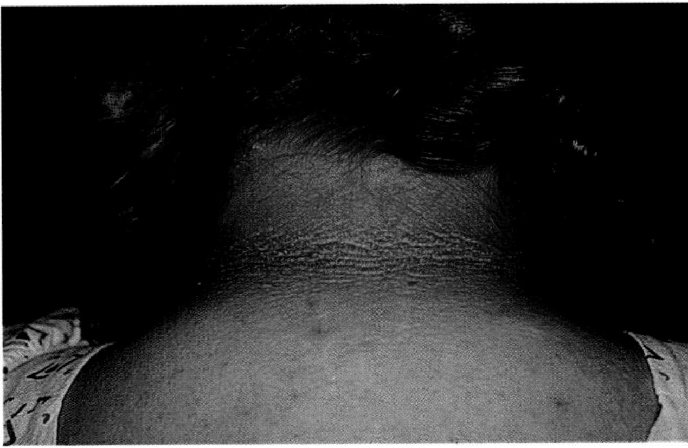

Figure 15.8 Acanthosis nigricans affecting the neck of a 26-year-old woman with severe insulin resistance. Reproduced from Moller & O'Rahilly [182] with permission.

activation cascades which lead to insulin's intracellular effects [127,128]. Mutations in the insulin receptor gene lead to inherited insulin resistance syndromes. The severity of the resulting clinical phenotype depends on the extent of impairment of signal transduction resulting from the underlying mutation [129].

Clinical features

Individuals with severe insulin resistance resulting from insulin receptor mutations may have a number of common features including hyperinsulinemia, acanthosis nigricans, ovarian hyperandrogenism and disturbances of glucose homeostasis which can include hypoglycemia as well as impaired glucose tolerance and diabetes [129]. Three main syndromes resulting from insulin receptor mutations resulting in severe insulin resistance have been described: Type A insulin resistance syndrome, Rabson–Mendenhall syndrome and leprechaunism (Donohue syndrome). There may be considerable clinical overlap and these syndromes may simply represent varying clinical features from a continuum of severity of receptor dysfunction rather than completely distinct syndromes [129]. Many patients with insulin receptor defects and severe insulin resistance (adult males in particular) may not fit into the syndromic descriptions below.

Features of the Type A insulin resistance syndrome include severe insulin resistance, acanthosis nigricans, polycystic ovarian disease, hirsutism and signs of virilization occurring in young females (often termed HAIR-AN syndrome). The patients with an underlying insulin receptor mutation are usually slim [130,131]. The most severe syndrome seen with insulin receptor mutations is leprechaunism (Donohue syndrome), a rare autosomal recessive disorder in which patients have low birth weight, growth restriction, disordered glucose homeostasis, characteristic dysmorphic features and usually do not survive infancy [131,132].

Rabson–Mendenhall syndrome is an autosomal recessive disorder that is between leprechaunism and Type A insulin resistance in terms of the severity of insulin resistance. Patients present in childhood with acanthosis nigricans, extreme growth retardation, dysplastic dentition, coarse facial features, lack of subcutaneous fat and pineal hyperplasia [131,133,135]. Reported renal abnormalities include medullary sponge kidney and nephrocalcinosis [133,135]. Patients may have paradoxical fasting hypoglycemia at diagnosis but develop frank diabetes (occasionally with ketoacidosis) in later years [134]. Life expectancy is markedly reduced, early death often occurring from complications of diabetes or intractable ketoacidosis.

Differentiating from type 1 and 2 diabetes

The presence of features of insulin resistance in a thin but not an obese individual is suggestive of an underlying insulin receptor gene mutation. Serum adiponectin levels are typically high in patients with insulin receptor mutations whereas they are low in other forms of insulin resistance. It has been suggested that adiponectin levels could be used as a screening test with sequencing of the insulin receptor gene reserved for those case where adiponectin levels are raised [126,136,137].

Unlike T2DM and the lipodystrophies, triglyceride levels in patients with insulin resistance caused by insulin receptor mutations are typically normal [131].

Management

While insulin sensitizers such as metformin and the thiazolidinediones may have a role in management their effect is often limited and insulin therapy is required as β-cell function declines [131]. Glycemic control is often poor despite very high doses of insulin (doses in excess of 500 units/kg/day have been reported). U500 insulin has a role in reducing the insulin volumes required [131,138]. Insulin-like growth factor I (IGF-I) is capable of stimulating glucose uptake and glycogen storage *in vivo* and has therefore been used in treatment of diabetes caused by insulin receptor mutations. Side effects were frequent in early studies but tolerability may be increased by combining IGF-I with its principal binding protein IGFBP-3 [139].

Inherited lipodystrophies

Lipodystrophies are clinically heterogenous disorders that are characterized by the selective loss of adipose tissue. They are associated with insulin resistance and other features such as diabetes mellitus, acanthosis, dyslipidemia, hepatic steatosis and (in female patients) hyperandrogenism, oligomenorrhoea and polycystic ovaries [140]. Lipodystrophies may be inherited or acquired. The inherited subtypes (all of which are rare) are described below.

Famililial partial lipodystrophy

Familial partial lipodystrophies are autosomal dominant disorders associated with the loss of peripheral subcutaneous fat. The two main subtypes result from mutations in *LMNA* and *PPARG*.

Familial partial lipodystrophy associated with *LMNA* mutations (also known as Dunnigan lipodystrophy) results in gradual peripheral subcutaneous fat loss from puberty. This, and the associated muscle hypertrophy, gives a muscular appearance of the arms and legs (Figure 15.9). There may be fat loss from the anterior abdomen and chest and excess fat deposition in the face, neck and intrabdominally [141,142]. Diabetes is common, particularly in female patients [143]. Hypertriglyceridemia may be marked and associated with pancreatitis. Acanthosis and polycystic ovarian syndrome are relatively uncommon. Although hepatic steatosis may develop cirrhosis appears rare [144,145]. Cardiovascular mortality is high.

Familial partial lipodystrophy associated with *PPARG* mutations appears to be phenotypically similar to that caused by *LMNA* mutations although hypertension is more common [146–155].

Diagnosis may be obvious in women but more difficult in males where a muscular appearance of limbs is more common. Early-onset diabetes in a non-obese patient with hypertriglyceridemia should raise suspicion of lipodystrophy particularly if there is marked peripheral fat loss [156].

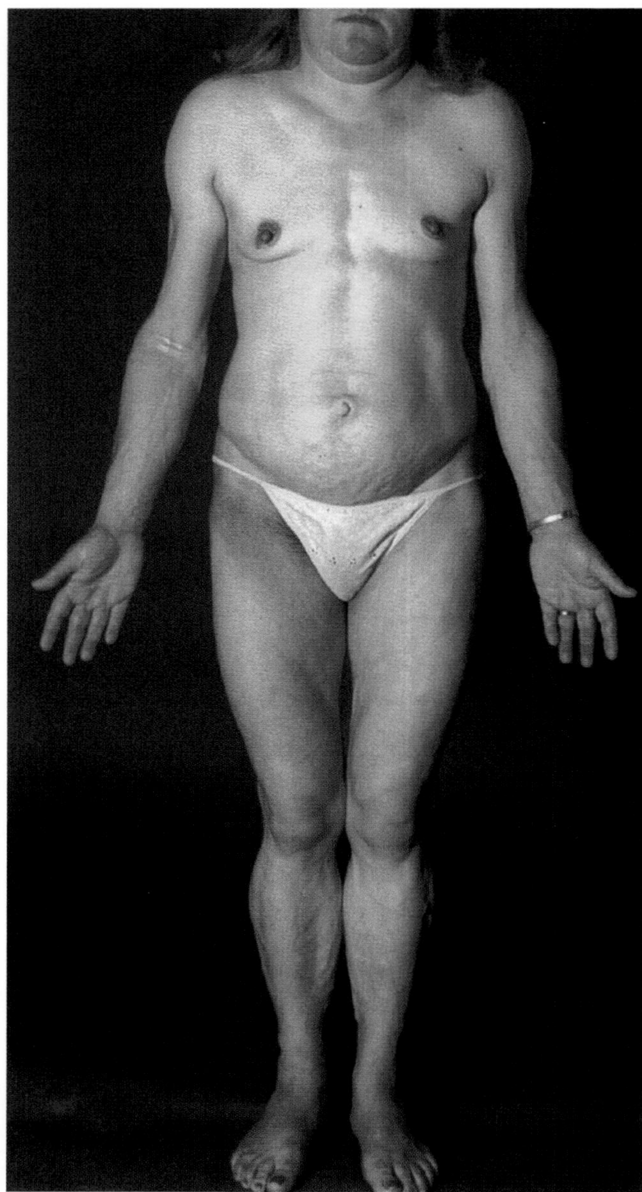

Figure 15.9 Familial partial lipodystrophy in a 46-year-old woman. There is truncal and limb lipodystrophy, preserved facial and neck adipose tissue, muscle hypertrophy and acanthosis apparent in the groin regions.

Congenital generalized lipodystrophy (Berardinelli–Seip syndrome)

This is a rare (estimated prevalence 1 in 10 million) autosomal recessive disorder characterized by a near complete absence of subcutaneous fat from birth, giving a muscular appearance [140]. Because of the absence of functioning adipocytes, lipids are stored in metabolically active tissues. Those affected have features of severe insulin resistance including often widespread acanthosis, hypertriglyceridemia and low HDL cholesterol [157]. Hepatic steatosis occurs early and may lead to cirrhosis; hepatomegaly is seen frequently [158–160]. Childhood growth is accelerated and bone age advanced. Diabetes commonly develops during adolescence [160]. Other associated features include acromegaloid features, hypertrophic cardiomyopathy, skeletal muscle hypertrophy, bone cysts and intellectual impairment [160]. Serum leptin and adiponectin levels are markedly reduced [161].

Three molecularly distinct forms have been identified: congenital generalized lipodystrophy types 1, 2 and 3 resulting from mutations in 1-acylglycerol 3-phosphate-O-acyltransferase 2 (*AGPAT2*), Berardinelli–Seip congenital lipodystrophy 2 (*BSCL2*) and Caveolin-1 (*CAV1*). *AGPAT2* and *BSCL2* account for the majority of cases and have some difference in phenotype. Some patients with this phenotype do not have mutations in any of these genes and so it is likely there are further genetic etiologies to be discovered [140,162,163].

Other inherited forms of lipodystrophy

Rare subtypes of lipodystrophy associated with dysmorphic features include mandibuloacral dysplasia (lipodystrophy with characteristic skeletal abnormalities), SHORT syndrome (short stature, hyperextensibility of joints, ocular depression, Reiger anomaly, teething delay) and neonatal progeroid syndrome [156].

Management of lipodystrophy

Management should address insulin resistance and the main causes of morbidity and mortality in lipodystrophy which include diabetes and its complications, cardiovascular and cerebrovascular disease, recurrent pancreatitis (as a result of severe hypertriglyceridemia), cirrhosis and psychologic distress related to appearance [140].

Lifestyle changes are important and should include an extremely low fat diet (<15% total energy from fat) and increased physical activity [140]. Hypertriglyceridemia that does not respond to lifestyle changes and control of hyperglycemia may require treatment with fibrates and high doses of fish oils. Estrogen replacement including contraceptive pills may exacerbate hypertriglyceridemia and is best avoided.

Glycemic control requires a combination of oral treatments and high dose insulin in the majority of patients. Metformin is commonly used to improve insulin sensitivity although there are no available trial data in inherited lipodystrophies [156]. Response to thiazolidinediones appears to vary with significant improvements in glycemic control and insulin resistance in some but not in all reported cases [155,164–169]. Where insulin is required dose requirements may be very high and U500 insulin appropriate [138,140]. Where proteinuric renal disease develops the threshold for renal biopsy should be low as non-diabetic renal disease (e.g. membranoproliferative glomerulonephritis and focal segmental glomerulosclerosis) appears to be more common than diabetic nephropathy [170].

Levels of the adipocytokine leptin are markedly reduced in severe lipodystrophies. Leptin replacement has been associated with marked improvements in glycemic control and hypertriglyceridemia in a number of cases of both generalized and partial inherited lipodystrophy [171–177] and may also improve hepatic steatosis [178,179].

Other monogenic conditions associated with insulin resistance

Other monogenic conditions associated with insulin resistance either have marked obesity (e.g. Alström and Bardet–Biedl syndromes); neurologic disease including myotonic dystrophy and Friedreich ataxia or rapid aging (e.g. Werner syndrome) [180].

Use of diagnostic and predictive molecular testing in monogenic diabetes

Diagnostic testing for the major causes of monogenic diabetes is now widely available. Specific recommendations for the different forms of monogenic diabetes are discussed in the relevant sections of this chapter. As molecular testing remains relatively expensive and time-consuming it is recommended that testing is restricted to those individuals with a moderate to high possibility of a positive result. The molecular genetic testing performed should be guided by the clinical phenotype and also the relative prevalence of mutations within that population. As many of these conditions are familial, the characteristics of other family members should also be considered. There should be some caution, however, as monogenic diabetes can occur in families that also have T1DM or T2DM. For similar reasons the results of molecular testing should be interpreted in the context of the clinical findings. For example, a patient with glucokinase diabetes could also develop T1DM or T2DM.

Where a family member has a confirmed genetic diagnosis, phenotypically unaffected relatives should be tested to assess whether they will be at risk of developing diabetes in the future. Where the main mutation phenotype is diabetes, regular urine or blood testing may be preferable as there is little clear extra benefit from prospective testing. Where families do request predictive testing, they should receive full counseling on the potential benefits and disadvantages and be allowed to make their own decisions on this.

Conclusions

Monogenic diabetes results from single gene changes that affect β-cell function or insulin sensitivity. Correct diagnosis can help define prognosis and the best treatment and allow screening of family members. Diagnostic testing is now widely available and should be considered where presentation is atypical for T1DM or T2DM, where there is an autosomal dominant family history, where there are characteristic associated features and in all cases where diabetes has been diagnosed within the first 6 months of life.

References

1 Tattersall RB. Mild familial diabetes with dominant inheritance. *Q J Med* 1974; **43**:339–357.

2 Tattersall R. Maturity-onset diabetes of the young: a clinical history. *Diabet Med* 1998; **15**:11–14.

3 WHO Study Group, Report of a WHO Consultation. *Part 1: Diagnosis and Classification of Diabetes Mellitus.* Geneva: World Health Organization, 1999.

4 American Diabetes Association. Diagnosis and classification of diabetes mellitus. *Diabetes Care* 2008; **31**(Suppl 1):S55–S60.

5 Fajans SS, Bell GI, Polonsky KS. Molecular mechanisms and clinical pathophysiology of maturity-onset diabetes of the young. *N Engl J Med* 2001; **345**:971–980.

6 McCarthy MI, Hattersley AT. Learning from molecular genetics: novel insights arising from the definition of genes for monogenic and type 2 diabetes. *Diabetes* 2008; **57**:2889–2898.

7 Matschinsky F, Liang Y, Kesavan P, Wang L, Froguel P, Velho G, *et al.* Glucokinase as pancreatic beta cell glucose sensor and diabetes gene. *J Clin Invest* 1993; **92**:2092–2098.

8 Byrne MM, Sturis J, Clement K, Vionnet N, Pueyo ME, Stoffel M, *et al.* Insulin secretory abnormalities in subjects with hyperglycemia due to glucokinase mutations. *J Clin Invest* 1994; **93**:1120–1130.

9 Velho G, Petersen KF, Perseghin G, Hwang JH, Rothman DL, Pueyo ME, *et al.* Impaired hepatic glycogen synthesis in glucokinase-deficient (MODY-2) subjects. *J Clin Invest* 1996; **98**:1755–1761.

10 Njolstad PR, Sagen JV, Bjorkhaug L, Odili S, Shehadeh N, Bakry D, *et al.* Permanent neonatal diabetes caused by glucokinase deficiency: inborn error of the glucose-insulin signaling pathway. *Diabetes* 2003; **52**:2854–2860.

11 Glaser B, Kesavan P, Heyman M, Davis E, Cuesta A, Buchs A, *et al.* Familial hyperinsulinism caused by an activating glucokinase mutation. *N Engl J Med* 1998; **338**:226–230.

12 Hattersley AT. Maturity-onset diabetes of the young: clinical heterogeneity explained by genetic heterogeneity. *Diabet Med* 1998; **15**:15–24.

13 Stride A, Vaxillaire M, Tuomi T, Barbetti F, Njolstad PR, Hansen T, *et al.* The genetic abnormality in the beta cell determines the response to an oral glucose load. *Diabetologia* 2002; **45**:427–435.

14 Velho G, Blanche H, Vaxillaire M, Bellanne-Chantelot C, Pardini VC, Timsit J, *et al.* Identification of 14 new glucokinase mutations and description of the clinical profile of 42 MODY-2 families. *Diabetologia* 1997; **40**:217–224.

15 Schnyder S, Mullis PE, Ellard S, Hattersley AT, Fluck CE. Genetic testing for glucokinase mutations in clinically selected patients with MODY: a worthwhile investment. *Swiss Med Wkly* 2005; **135**:352–356.

16 Gill-Carey O SB, Colclough K, Ellard S, Hattersley AT. Finding a glucokinase mutation alters patient treatment. *Diabet Med* 2007; **24**(Suppl 1):6.

17 Ellard S, Beards F, Allen LI, Shepherd M, Ballantyne E, Harvey R, *et al.* A high prevalence of glucokinase mutations in gestational diabetic subjects selected by clinical criteria. *Diabetologia* 2000; **43**:250–253.

18 Hattersley AT, Beards F, Ballantyne E, Appleton M, Harvey R, Ellard S. Mutations in the glucokinase gene of the fetus result in reduced birth weight. *Nat Genet* 1998; **19**:268–270.

19 Spyer G, Macleod KM, Shepherd M, Ellard S, Hattersley AT. Pregnancy outcome in patients with raised blood glucose due to a heterozygous glucokinase gene mutation. *Diabet Med* 2009; **26**:14–18.

20 Guenat E, Seematter G, Philippe J, Temler E, Jequier E, Tappy L. Counterregulatory responses to hypoglycemia in patients with glucokinase gene mutations. *Diabetes Metab* 2000; **26**:377–384.

21 Spyer G, Hattersley AT, Sykes JE, Sturley RH, MacLeod KM. Influence of maternal and fetal glucokinase mutations in gestational diabetes. *Am J Obstet Gynecol* 2001; **185**:240–241.

22 Velho G, Hattersley AT, Froguel P. Maternal diabetes alters birth weight in glucokinase-deficient (MODY2) kindred but has no influence on adult weight, height, insulin secretion or insulin sensitivity. *Diabetologia* 2000; **43**:1060–1063.

23 Wang H, Maechler P, Hagenfeldt KA, Wollheim CB. Dominant-negative suppression of HNF-1alpha function results in defective insulin gene transcription and impaired metabolism-secretion coupling in a pancreatic beta-cell line. *EMBO J* 1998; **17**:6701–6713.

24 Wang H, Antinozzi PA, Hagenfeldt KA, Maechler P, Wollheim CB. Molecular targets of a human HNF1 alpha mutation responsible for pancreatic beta-cell dysfunction. *EMBO J* 2000; **19**:4257–4264.

25 Shih DQ, Screenan S, Munoz KN, Philipson L, Pontoglio M, Yaniv M, *et al.* Loss of HNF-1alpha function in mice leads to abnormal expression of genes involved in pancreatic islet development and metabolism. *Diabetes* 2001; **50**:2472–2480.

26 Hagenfeldt-Johansson KA, Herrera PL, Wang H, Gjinovci A, Ishihara H, Wollheim CB. Beta-cell-targeted expression of a dominant-negative hepatocyte nuclear factor-1 alpha induces a maturity-onset diabetes of the young (MODY)3-like phenotype in transgenic mice. *Endocrinology* 2001; **142**:5311–5320.

27 Wobser H, Dussmann H, Kogel D, Wang H, Reimertz C, Wollheim CB, *et al.* Dominant-negative suppression of HNF-1 alpha results in mitochondrial dysfunction, INS-1 cell apoptosis, and increased sensitivity to ceramide, but not to high glucose-induced cell death. *J Biol Chem* 2002; **277**:6413–6421.

28 Yamagata K, Nammo T, Moriwaki M, Ihara A, Iizuka K, Yang Q, *et al.* Overexpression of dominant-negative mutant hepatocyte nuclear factor-1 alpha in pancreatic beta-cells causes abnormal islet architecture with decreased expression of E-cadherin, reduced beta-cell proliferation, and diabetes. *Diabetes* 2002; **51**:114–123.

29 Frayling TM, Evans JC, Bulman MP, Pearson E, Allen L, Owen K, *et al.* Beta-cell genes and diabetes: molecular and clinical characterization of mutations in transcription factors. *Diabetes* 2001; **50**(Suppl 1):S94–S100.

30 Shepherd M, Sparkes AC, Hattersley A. Genetic testing in maturity onset diabetes of the young (MODY): a new challenge for the diabetic clinic. *Pract Diabet Int* 2001; **18**:16–21.

31 Harries LW, Ellard S, Stride A, Morgan NG, Hattersley AT. Isomers of the TCF1 gene encoding hepatocyte nuclear factor-1 alpha show differential expression in the pancreas and define the relationship between mutation position and clinical phenotype in monogenic diabetes. *Hum Mol Genet* 2006; **15**:2216–2224.

32 Bellanne-Chantelot C, Carette C, Riveline JP, Valero R, Gautier JF, Larger E, *et al.* The type and the position of HNF1A mutation modulate age at diagnosis of diabetes in patients with maturity-onset diabetes of the young (MODY)-3. *Diabetes* 2008; **57**:503–508.

33 Byrne MM, Sturis J, Menzel S, Yamagata K, Fajans SS, Dronsfield MJ, *et al.* Altered insulin secretory responses to glucose in diabetic and nondiabetic subjects with mutations in the diabetes susceptibility gene MODY3 on chromosome 12. *Diabetes* 1996; **45**:1503–1510.

34 Isomaa B, Henricsson M, Lehto M, Forsblom C, Karanko S, Sarelin L, *et al.* Chronic diabetic complications in patients with MODY3 diabetes. *Diabetologia* 1998; **41**:467–473.

35 Pearson E, McEneny J, Young I, Hattersley A. HDL-cholesterol: differentiating between HNF-1alpha MODY and type 2 diabetes. *Diabet Med* 2003; **20**(Suppl 2):15.

36 Stride A, Ellard S, Clark P, Shakespeare L, Salzmann MB, Shepherd M, *et al.* Beta-cell dysfunction, insulin sensitivity, and glycosuria precede diabetes in hepatocyte nuclear factor-1alpha mutation carriers. *Diabetes Care* 2005; **28**:1751–1756.

37 Pearson ER, Boj SF, Steele AM, Barrett T, Stals K, Shield JP, *et al.* Macrosomia and hyperinsulinaemic hypoglycaemia in patients with heterozygous mutations in the HNF4A gene. *PLoS Med* 2007; **4**:e118.

38 Pearson ER, Pruhova S, Tack CJ, Johansen A, Castleden HA, Lumb PJ, *et al.* Molecular genetics and phenotypic characteristics of MODY caused by hepatocyte nuclear factor 4alpha mutations in a large European collection. *Diabetologia* 2005; **48**:878–885.

39 Ellard S, Bellanne-Chantelot C, Hattersley AT. Best practice guidelines for the molecular genetic diagnosis of maturity-onset diabetes of the young. *Diabetologia* 2008; **51**:546–553.

40 Levy-Marchal C, Tichet J, Fajardy I, Gu XF, Dubois F, Czernichow P. Islet cell antibodies in normal French schoolchildren. *Diabetologia* 1992; **35**:577–582.

41 LaGasse JM, Brantley MS, Leech NJ, Rowe RE, Monks S, Palmer JP, *et al.* Successful prospective prediction of type 1 diabetes in schoolchildren through multiple defined autoantibodies: an 8-year follow-up of the Washington State Diabetes Prediction Study. *Diabetes Care* 2002; **25**:505–511.

42 Pearson ER, Starkey BJ, Powell RJ, Gribble FM, Clark PM, Hattersley AT. Genetic cause of hyperglycaemia and response to treatment in diabetes. *Lancet* 2003; **362**:1275–1281.

43 Pearson ER, Liddell WG, Shepherd M, Corrall RJ, Hattersley AT. Sensitivity to sulphonylureas in patients with hepatocyte nuclear factor-1alpha gene mutations: evidence for pharmacogenetics in diabetes. *Diabet Med* 2000; **17**:543–545.

44 Shepherd M, Shields B, Ellard S, Rubio-Cabezas O, Hattersley AT. A genetic diagnosis of HNF1A diabetes alters treatment and improves glycaemic control in the majority of insulin-treated patients. *Diabet Med* 2009; **26**:437–441.

45 Tuomi T, Honkanen EH, Isomaa B, Sarelin L, Groop LC. Improved prandial glucose control with lower risk of hypoglycemia with nateglinide than with glibenclamide in patients with maturity-onset diabetes of the young type 3. *Diabetes Care* 2006; **29**:189–194.

46 Moretti ME, Rezvani M, Koren G. Safety of glyburide for gestational diabetes: a meta-analysis of pregnancy outcomes. *Ann Pharmacother* 2008; **42**:483–490.

47 Moore TR. Glyburide for the treatment of gestational diabetes: a critical appraisal. *Diabetes Care* 2007; **30**(Suppl 2):S209–S213.

48 Stoffers DA, Stanojevic V, Habener JF. Insulin promoter factor-1 gene mutation linked to early-onset type 2 diabetes mellitus directs expression of a dominant negative isoprotein. *J Clin Invest* 1998; **102**:232–241.

49 Kristinsson SY, Thorolfsdottir ET, Talseth B, Steingrimsson E, Thorsson AV, Helgason T, *et al.* MODY in Iceland is associated with mutations in HNF-1alpha and a novel mutation in NeuroD1. *Diabetologia* 2001; **44**:2098–2103.

50 Liu L, Furuta H, Minami A, Zheng T, Jia W, Nanjo K, *et al.* A novel mutation, Ser159Pro in the NeuroD1/BETA2 gene contributes to the development of diabetes in a Chinese potential MODY family. *Mol Cell Biochem* 2007; **303**:115–120.

51 Malecki MT, Jhala US, Antonellis A, Fields L, Doria A, Orban T, *et al.* Mutations in NEUROD1 are associated with the development of type 2 diabetes mellitus. *Nat Genet* 1999; **23**:323–328.

52 Plengvidhya N, Kooptiwut S, Songtawee N, Doi A, Furuta H, Nishi M, *et al.* PAX4 mutations in Thais with maturity onset diabetes of the young. *J Clin Endocrinol Metab* 2007; **92**:2821–2826.

53 Neve B, Fernandez-Zapico ME, Ashkenazi-Katalan V, Dina C, Hamid YH, Joly E, *et al.* Role of transcription factor KLF11 and its diabetes-associated gene variants in pancreatic beta cell function. *Proc Natl Acad Sci U S A* 2005; **102**:4807–4812.

54 Iafusco D, Stazi MA, Cotichini R, Cotellessa M, Martinucci ME, Mazzella M, *et al.* Permanent diabetes mellitus in the first year of life. *Diabetologia* 2002; **45**:798–804.

55 Edghill EL, Dix RJ, Flanagan SE, Bingley PJ, Hattersley AT, Ellard S, *et al.* HLA genotyping supports a nonautoimmune etiology in patients diagnosed with diabetes under the age of 6 months. *Diabetes* 2006; **55**:1895–1898.

56 Stoy J, Greeley SA, Paz VP, Ye H, Pastore AN, Skowron KB, *et al.* Diagnosis and treatment of neonatal diabetes: a United States experience. *Pediatr Diabetes* 2008; **9**:450–459.

57 Flanagan SE, Edghill EL, Gloyn AL, Ellard S, Hattersley AT. Mutations in KCNJ11, which encodes Kir6.2, are a common cause of diabetes diagnosed in the first 6 months of life, with the phenotype determined by genotype. *Diabetologia* 2006; **49**:1190–1197.

58 Aguilar-Bryan L, Bryan J. Neonatal diabetes mellitus. *Endocr Rev* 2008; **29**:265–291.

59 Flanagan SE, Patch AM, Mackay DJ, Edghill EL, Gloyn AL, Robinson D, *et al.* Mutations in ATP-sensitive K^+ channel genes cause transient neonatal diabetes and permanent diabetes in childhood or adulthood. *Diabetes* 2007; **56**:1930–1937.

60 Gloyn AL, Pearson ER, Antcliff JF, Proks P, Bruining GJ, Slingerland AS, *et al.* Activating mutations in the gene encoding the ATP-sensitive potassium-channel subunit Kir6.2 and permanent neonatal diabetes. *N Engl J Med* 2004; **350**:1838–1849.

61 Proks P, Arnold AL, Bruining J, Girard C, Flanagan SE, Larkin B, *et al.* A heterozygous activating mutation in the sulphonylurea receptor SUR1 (ABCC8) causes neonatal diabetes. *Hum Mol Genet* 2006; **15**:1793–1800.

62 Babenko AP, Polak M, Cave H, Busiah K, Czernichow P, Scharfmann R, *et al.* Activating mutations in the ABCC8 gene in neonatal diabetes mellitus. *N Engl J Med* 2006; **355**:456–466.

63 Ellard S, Flanagan SE, Girard CA, Patch AM, Harries LW, Parrish A, *et al.* Permanent neonatal diabetes caused by dominant, recessive, or compound heterozygous SUR1 mutations with opposite functional effects. *Am J Hum Genet* 2007; **81**:375–382.

64 Hattersley AT, Ashcroft FM. Activating mutations in Kir6.2 and neonatal diabetes: new clinical syndromes, new scientific insights, and new therapy. *Diabetes* 2005; **54**:2503–2513.

65 Pearson ER, Flechtner I, Njolstad PR, Malecki MT, Flanagan SE, Larkin B, *et al.* Switching from insulin to oral sulfonylureas in patients with diabetes due to Kir6.2 mutations. *N Engl J Med* 2006; **355**:467–477.

66 Stoy J, Edghill EL, Flanagan SE, Ye H, Paz VP, Pluzhnikov A, *et al.* Insulin gene mutations as a cause of permanent neonatal diabetes. *Proc Natl Acad Sci U S A* 2007; **104**:15040–15044.

67 Edghill EL, Flanagan SE, Patch AM, Boustred C, Parrish A, Shields B, *et al.* Insulin mutation screening in 1,044 patients with diabetes: mutations in the INS gene are a common cause of neonatal diabetes but a rare cause of diabetes diagnosed in childhood or adulthood. *Diabetes* 2008; **57**:1034–1042.

68 Proks P, Antcliff JF, Lippiat J, Gloyn AL, Hattersley AT, Ashcroft FM. Molecular basis of Kir6.2 mutations associated with neonatal diabetes or neonatal diabetes plus neurological features. *Proc Natl Acad Sci U S A* 2004; **101**:17539–17544.

69 Koster JC, Cadario F, Peruzzi C, Colombo C, Nichols CG, Barbetti F. The G53D mutation in Kir6.2 (KCNJ11) is associated with neonatal diabetes and motor dysfunction in adulthood that is improved with sulfonylurea therapy. *J Clin Endocrinol Metab* 2008; **93**:1054–1061.

70 Sagen JV, Raeder H, Hathout E, Shehadeh N, Gudmundsson K, Baevre H, *et al.* Permanent neonatal diabetes due to mutations in KCNJ11 encoding Kir6.2: patient characteristics and initial response to sulfonylurea therapy. *Diabetes* 2004; **53**:2713–2718.

71 Codner E, Flanagan S, Ellard S, Garcia H, Hattersley AT. High-dose glibenclamide can replace insulin therapy despite transitory diarrhea in early-onset diabetes caused by a novel R201L Kir6.2 mutation. *Diabetes Care* 2005; **28**:758–759.

72 Slingerland AS, Hurkx W, Noordam K, Flanagan SE, Jukema JW, Meiners LC, *et al.* Sulphonylurea therapy improves cognition in a patient with the V59M KCNJ11 mutation. *Diabet Med* 2008; **25**:277–281.

73 Mlynarski W, Tarasov AI, Gach A, Girard CA, Pietrzak I, Zubcevic L, *et al.* Sulfonylurea improves CNS function in a case of intermediate DEND syndrome caused by a mutation in KCNJ11. *Nat Clin Pract Neurol* 2007; **3**:640–645.

74 Edghill EL, Gloyn AL, Goriely A, Harries LW, Flanagan SE, Rankin J, *et al.* Origin of de novo KCNJ11 mutations and risk of neonatal diabetes for subsequent siblings. *J Clin Endocrinol Metab* 2007; **92**:1773–1777.

75 Temple IK, Gardner RJ, Mackay DJ, Barber JC, Robinson DO, Shield JP. Transient neonatal diabetes: widening the understanding of the etiopathogenesis of diabetes. *Diabetes* 2000; **49**:1359–1366.

76 Mackay DJ, Callaway JL, Marks SM, White HE, Acerini CL, Boonen SE, *et al.* Hypomethylation of multiple imprinted loci in individuals with transient neonatal diabetes is associated with mutations in ZFP57. *Nat Genet* 2008; **40**:949–951.

77 Gloyn AL, Reimann F, Girard C, Edghill EL, Proks P, Pearson ER, *et al.* Relapsing diabetes can result from moderately activating mutations in KCNJ11. *Hum Mol Genet* 2005; **14**:925–934.

78 Yorifuji T, Nagashima K, Kurokawa K, Kawai M, Oishi M, Akazawa Y, *et al.* The C42R mutation in the Kir6.2 (KCNJ11) gene as a cause of transient neonatal diabetes, childhood diabetes, or later-onset, apparently type 2 diabetes mellitus. *J Clin Endocrinol Metab* 2005; **90**:3174–3178.

79 Colombo C, Delvecchio M, Zecchino C, Faienza MF, Cavallo L, Barbetti F. Transient neonatal diabetes mellitus is associated with a recurrent (R201H) KCNJ11 (KIR6.2) mutation. *Diabetologia* 2005; **48**:2439–2441.

80 de Wet H, Proks P, Lafond M, Aittoniemi J, Sansom MS, Flanagan SE, *et al.* A mutation (R826W) in nucleotide-binding domain 1 of ABCC8 reduces ATPase activity and causes transient neonatal diabetes. *EMBO Rep* 2008; **9**:648–654.

81 Patch AM, Flanagan SE, Boustred C, Hattersley AT, Ellard S. Mutations in the ABCC8 gene encoding the SUR1 subunit of the

KATP channel cause transient neonatal diabetes, permanent neonatal diabetes or permanent diabetes diagnosed outside the neonatal period. *Diabetes Obes Metab* 2007; **9**(Suppl 2):28–39.

82 Temple IK, Shield JP. Transient neonatal diabetes, a disorder of imprinting. *J Med Genet* 2002; **39**:872–875.

83 Murphy R, Turnbull DM, Walker M, Hattersley AT. Clinical features, diagnosis and management of maternally inherited diabetes and deafness (MIDD) associated with the 3243A>G mitochondrial point mutation. *Diabet Med* 2008; **25**:383–399.

84 Maassen JA, Janssen GM, 'T Hart LM. Molecular mechanisms of mitochondrial diabetes (MIDD). *Ann Med* 2005; **37**:213–221.

85 Maassen JA, 'T Hart LM, Van Essen E, Heine RJ, Nijpels G, Jahangir Tafrechi RS, *et al.* Mitochondrial diabetes: molecular mechanisms and clinical presentation. *Diabetes* 2004; **53**(Suppl 1):S103–S109.

86 Guillausseau PJ, Massin P, Dubois-LaForgue D, Timsit J, Virally M, Gin H, *et al.* Maternally inherited diabetes and deafness: a multicenter study. *Ann Intern Med* 2001; **134**:721–728.

87 Suzuki S, Hinokio Y, Hirai S, Onoda M, Matsumoto M, Ohtomo M, *et al.* Pancreatic beta-cell secretory defect associated with mitochondrial point mutation of the tRNA(LEU(UUR)) gene: a study in seven families with mitochondrial encephalomyopathy, lactic acidosis and stroke-like episodes (MELAS). *Diabetologia* 1994; **37**:818–825.

88 Uimonen S, Moilanen JS, Sorri M, Hassinen IE, Majamaa K. Hearing impairment in patients with 3243A–>G mtDNA mutation: phenotype and rate of progression. *Hum Genet* 2001; **108**:284–289.

89 Remes AM, Majamaa K, Herva R, Hassinen IE. Adult-onset diabetes mellitus and neurosensory hearing loss in maternal relatives of MELAS patients in a family with the tRNA(Leu(UUR)) mutation. *Neurology* 1993; **43**:1015–1020.

90 Guillausseau PJ, Dubois-Laforgue D, Massin P, Laloi-Michelin M, Bellanne-Chantelot C, Gin H, *et al.* Heterogeneity of diabetes phenotype in patients with 3243 bp mutation of mitochondrial DNA (Maternally Inherited Diabetes and Deafness or MIDD). *Diabetes Metab* 2004; **30**:181–186.

91 Oka Y, Katagiri H, Ishihara H, Asano T, Kobayashi T, Kikuchi M. Beta-cell loss and glucose induced signalling defects in diabetes mellitus caused by mitochondrial tRNALeu(UUR) gene mutation. *Diabet Med* 1996; **13**(Suppl 6):S98–S102.

92 Massin P, Dubois-Laforgue D, Meas T, Laloi-Michelin M, Gin H, Bauduceau B, *et al.* Retinal and renal complications in patients with a mutation of mitochondrial DNA at position 3,243 (maternally inherited diabetes and deafness): a case–control study. *Diabetologia* 2008; **51**:1664–1670.

93 Silveiro SP, Canani LH, Maia AL, Butany JW, Gross JL. Myocardial dysfunction in maternally inherited diabetes and deafness. *Diabetes Care* 2003; **26**:1323–1324.

94 Nan DN, Fernandez-Ayala M, Infante J, Matorras P, Gonzalez-Macias J. Progressive cardiomyopathy as manifestation of mitochondrial disease. *Postgrad Med J* 2002; **78**:298–299.

95 Yoshida R, Ishida Y, Hozumi T, Ueno H, Kishimoto M, Kasuga M, *et al.* Congestive heart failure in mitochondrial diabetes mellitus. *Lancet* 1994; **344**:1375.

96 Momiyama Y, Suzuki Y, Ohtomo M, Atsumi Y, Matsuoka K, Ohsuzu F, *et al.* Cardiac autonomic nervous dysfunction in diabetic patients with a mitochondrial DNA mutation: assessment by heart rate variability. *Diabetes Care* 2002; **25**:2308–2313.

97 Majamaa-Voltti K, Peuhkurinen K, Kortelainen ML, Hassinen IE, Majamaa K. Cardiac abnormalities in patients with mitochondrial DNA mutation 3243A>G. *BMC Cardiovasc Disord* 2002; **2**:12.

98 Suzuki Y, Kobayashi T, Taniyama M, Astumi Y, Oka Y, Kadowaki T, *et al.* Islet cell antibody in mitochondrial diabetes. *Diabetes Res Clin Pract* 1997; **35**:163–165.

99 Kobayashi T, Oka Y, Katagiri H, Falorni A, Kasuga A, Takei I, *et al.* Association between HLA and islet cell antibodies in diabetic patients with a mitochondrial DNA mutation at base pair 3243. *Diabetologia* 1996; **39**:1196–1200.

100 Oka Y, Katagiri H, Yazaki Y, Murase T, Kobayashi T. Mitochondrial gene mutation in islet-cell-antibody-positive patients who were initially non-insulin-dependent diabetics. *Lancet* 1993; **342**:527–528.

101 Suzuki S, Hinokio Y, Ohtomo M, Hirai M, Hirai A, Chiba M, *et al.* The effects of coenzyme Q10 treatment on maternally inherited diabetes mellitus and deafness, and mitochondrial DNA 3243 (A to G) mutation. *Diabetologia* 1998; **41**:584–588.

102 Donovan LE, Severin NE. Maternally inherited diabetes and deafness in a North American kindred: tips for making the diagnosis and review of unique management issues. *J Clin Endocrinol Metab* 2006; **91**:4737–4742.

103 Edmonds JL, Kirse DJ, Kearns D, Deutsch R, Spruijt L, Naviaux RK. The otolaryngological manifestations of mitochondrial disease and the risk of neurodegeneration with infection. *Arch Otolaryngol Head Neck Surg* 2002; **128**:355–362.

104 Sinnathuray AR, Raut V, Awa A, Magee A, Toner JG. A review of cochlear implantation in mitochondrial sensorineural hearing loss. *Otol Neurotol* 2003; **24**:418–426.

105 Coffinier C, Barra J, Babinet C, Yaniv M. Expression of the vHNF1/HNF1beta homeoprotein gene during mouse organogenesis. *Mech Dev* 1999; **89**:211–213.

106 Edghill EL, Bingham C, Ellard S, Hattersley AT. Mutations in hepatocyte nuclear factor-1beta and their related phenotypes. *J Med Genet* 2006; **43**:84–90.

107 Decramer S, Parant O, Beaufils S, Clauin S, Guillou C, Kessler S, *et al.* Anomalies of the TCF2 gene are the main cause of fetal bilateral hyperechogenic kidneys. *J Am Soc Nephrol* 2007; **18**:923–933.

108 Bingham C, Hattersley AT. Renal cysts and diabetes syndrome resulting from mutations in hepatocyte nuclear factor-1beta. *Nephrol Dial Transplant* 2004; **19**:2703–2708.

109 Ulinski T, Lescure S, Beaufils S, Guigonis V, Decramer S, Morin D, *et al.* Renal phenotypes related to hepatocyte nuclear factor-1beta (TCF2) mutations in a pediatric cohort. *J Am Soc Nephrol* 2006; **17**:497–503.

110 Yorifuji T, Kurokawa K, Mamada M, Imai T, Kawai M, Nishi Y, *et al.* Neonatal diabetes mellitus and neonatal polycystic, dysplastic kidneys: phenotypically discordant recurrence of a mutation in the hepatocyte nuclear factor-1beta gene due to germline mosaicism. *J Clin Endocrinol Metab* 2004; **89**:2905–2908.

111 Bingham C, Ellard S, Allen L, Bulman M, Shepherd M, Frayling T, *et al.* Abnormal nephron development associated with a frameshift mutation in the transcription factor hepatocyte nuclear factor-1 beta. *Kidney Int* 2000; **57**:898–907.

112 Edghill EL, Oram RA, Owens M, Stals KL, Harries LW, Hattersley AT, *et al.* Hepatocyte nuclear factor-1beta gene deletions: a common cause of renal disease. *Nephrol Dial Transplant* 2008; **23**:627–635.

113 Pearson ER, Badman MK, Lockwood CR, Clark PM, Ellard S, Bingham C, *et al.* Contrasting diabetes phenotypes associated with hepatocyte nuclear factor-1alpha and -1beta mutations. *Diabetes Care* 2004; **27**:1102–1107.

114 Bellanne-Chantelot C, Chauveau D, Gautier JF, Dubois-Laforgue D, Clauin S, Beaufils S, *et al.* Clinical spectrum associated with hepato-

cyte nuclear factor-1beta mutations. *Ann Intern Med* 2004; **140**:510–517.

115 Edghill EL, Bingham C, Slingerland AS, Minton JA, Noordam C, Ellard S, *et al.* Hepatocyte nuclear factor-1 beta mutations cause neonatal diabetes and intrauterine growth retardation: support for a critical role of HNF-1beta in human pancreatic development. *Diabet Med* 2006; **23**:1301–1306.

116 Haldorsen IS, Vesterhus M, Raeder H, Jensen DK, Sovik O, Molven A, *et al.* Lack of pancreatic body and tail in HNF1B mutation carriers. *Diabet Med* 2008; **25**:782–787.

117 Horikawa Y, Iwasaki N, Hara M, Furuta H, Hinokio Y, Cockburn BN, *et al.* Mutation in hepatocyte nuclear factor-1 beta gene (TCF2) associated with MODY. *Nat Genet* 1997; **17**:384–385.

118 Lebrun G, Vasiliu V, Bellanne-Chantelot C, Bensman A, Ulinski T, Chretien Y, *et al.* Cystic kidney disease, chromophobe renal cell carcinoma and TCF2 (HNF1 beta) mutations. *Nat Clin Pract Nephrol* 2005; **1**:115–119.

119 Rebouissou S, Vasiliu V, Thomas C, Bellanne-Chantelot C, Bui H, Chretien Y, *et al.* Germline hepatocyte nuclear factor 1alpha and 1beta mutations in renal cell carcinomas. *Hum Mol Genet* 2005; **14**:603–614.

120 Bellanne-Chantelot C, Clauin S, Chauveau D, Collin P, Daumont M, Douillard C, *et al.* Large genomic rearrangements in the hepatocyte nuclear factor-1β (TCF2) gene are the most frequent cause of maturity-onset diabetes of the young type 5. *Diabetes* 2005; **54**:3126–3132.

121 d'Annunzio G, Minuto N, D'Amato E, de Toni T, Lombardo F, Pasquali L, *et al.* Wolfram syndrome (diabetes insipidus, diabetes, optic atrophy, and deafness): clinical and genetic study. *Diabetes Care* 2008; **31**:1743–1745.

122 Viswanathan V, Medempudi S, Kadiri M. Wolfram syndrome. *J Assoc Physicians India* 2008; **56**:197–199.

123 Olsen BS, Hahnemann JM, Schwartz M, Ostergaard E. Thiamine-responsive megaloblastic anaemia: a cause of syndromic diabetes in childhood. *Pediatr Diabetes* 2007; **8**:239–241.

124 Iyer S, Korada M, Rainbow L, Kirk J, Brown RM, Shaw N, *et al.* Wolcott–Rallison syndrome: a clinical and genetic study of three children, novel mutation in EIF2AK3 and a review of the literature. *Acta Paediatr* 2004; **93**:1195–1201.

125 Raeder H, Johansson S, Holm PI, Haldorsen IS, Mas E, Sbarra V, *et al.* Mutations in the CEL VNTR cause a syndrome of diabetes and pancreatic exocrine dysfunction. *Nat Genet* 2006; **38**:54–62.

126 Savage DB, Semple RK, Chatterjee VK, Wales JK, Ross RJ, O'Rahilly S. A clinical approach to severe insulin resistance. *Endocr Dev* 2007; **11**:122–132.

127 Ullrich A, Bell JR, Chen EY, Herrera R, Petruzzelli LM, Dull TJ, *et al.* Human insulin receptor and its relationship to the tyrosine kinase family of oncogenes. *Nature* 1985; **313**:756–761.

128 White MF, Kahn CR. The insulin signaling system. *J Biol Chem* 1994; **269**:1–4.

129 Krook A, O'Rahilly S. Mutant insulin receptors in syndromes of insulin resistance. *Baillieres Clin Endocrinol Metab* 1996; **10**:97–122.

130 Kahn CR, Flier JS, Bar RS, Archer JA, Gorden P, Martin MM, *et al.* The syndromes of insulin resistance and acanthosis nigricans: insulin-receptor disorders in man. *N Engl J Med* 1976; **294**:739–745.

131 Musso C, Cochran E, Moran SA, Skarulis MC, Oral EA, Taylor S, *et al.* Clinical course of genetic diseases of the insulin receptor (type A and Rabson–Mendenhall syndromes): a 30-year prospective. *Medicine (Baltimore)* 2004; **83**:209–222.

132 Donohue WL, Uchida I. Leprechaunism: a euphemism for a rare familial disorder. *J Pediatr* 1954; **45**:505–519.

133 Kumar S, Tullu MS, Muranjan MN, Kamat JR. Rabson–Mendenhall syndrome. *Indian J Med Sci* 2005; **59**:70–73.

134 Longo N, Wang Y, Pasquali M. Progressive decline in insulin levels in Rabson–Mendenhall syndrome. *J Clin Endocrinol Metab* 1999; **84**:2623–2629.

135 Harris AM, Hall B, Kriss VM, Fowlkes JL, Kiessling SG. Rabson–Mendenhall syndrome: medullary sponge kidney, a new component. *Pediatr Nephrol* 2007; **22**:2141–2144.

136 Semple RK, Soos MA, Luan J, Mitchell S, Wilson JC, Gurnell M, *et al.* Elevated plasma adiponectin in humans with genetically defective insulin receptors. *J Clin Endocrinol Metab* 2006; **91**:3219–3223.

137 Semple RK, Halberg NH, Burling K, Soos MA, Schraw T, Luan J, *et al.* Paradoxical elevation of high-molecular weight adiponectin in acquired extreme insulin resistance due to insulin receptor antibodies. *Diabetes* 2007; **56**:1712–1717.

138 Cochran E, Musso C, Gorden P. The use of U-500 in patients with extreme insulin resistance. *Diabetes Care* 2005; **28**:1240–1244.

139 McDonald A, Williams RM, Regan FM, Semple RK, Dunger DB. IGF-1 treatment of insulin resistance. *Eur J Endocrinol* 2007; **157**(Suppl 1):S51–S56.

140 Garg A. Acquired and inherited lipodystrophies. *N Engl J Med* 2004; **350**:1220–1234.

141 Dunnigan MG, Cochrane MA, Kelly A, Scott JW. Familial lipoatrophic diabetes with dominant transmission: a new syndrome. *Q J Med* 1974; **43**:33–48.

142 Garg A, Peshock RM, Fleckenstein JL. Adipose tissue distribution pattern in patients with familial partial lipodystrophy (Dunnigan variety). *J Clin Endocrinol Metab* 1999; **84**:170–174.

143 Haque WA, Oral EA, Dietz K, Bowcock AM, Agarwal AK, Garg A. Risk factors for diabetes in familial partial lipodystrophy, Dunnigan variety. *Diabetes Care* 2003; **26**:1350–1355.

144 Garg A. Gender differences in the prevalence of metabolic complications in familial partial lipodystrophy (Dunnigan variety). *J Clin Endocrinol Metab* 2000; **85**:1776–1782.

145 Haque WA, Vuitch F, Garg A. Post-mortem findings in familial partial lipodystrophy, Dunnigan variety. *Diabet Med* 2002; **19**:1022–1025.

146 Barroso I, Gurnell M, Crowley VE, Agostini M, Schwabe JW, Soos MA, *et al.* Dominant negative mutations in human PPARgamma associated with severe insulin resistance, diabetes mellitus and hypertension. *Nature* 1999; **402**:880–883.

147 Agarwal AK, Garg A. A novel heterozygous mutation in peroxisome proliferator-activated receptor-gamma gene in a patient with familial partial lipodystrophy. *J Clin Endocrinol Metab* 2002; **87**:408–411.

148 Hegele RA, Cao H, Frankowski C, Mathews ST, Leff T. PPARG F388L, a transactivation-deficient mutant, in familial partial lipodystrophy. *Diabetes* 2002; **51**:3586–3590.

149 Al-Shali K, Cao H, Knoers N, Hermus AR, Tack CJ, Hegele RA. A single-base mutation in the peroxisome proliferator-activated receptor gamma4 promoter associated with altered *in vitro* expression and partial lipodystrophy. *J Clin Endocrinol Metab* 2004; **89**:5655–5660.

150 Agostini M, Schoenmakers E, Mitchell C, Szatmari I, Savage D, Smith A, *et al.* Non-DNA binding, dominant-negative, human

PPARgamma mutations cause lipodystrophic insulin resistance. *Cell Metab* 2006; **4**:303–311.

151 Francis GA, Li G, Casey R, Wang J, Cao H, Leff T, *et al.* Peroxisomal proliferator activated receptor-gamma deficiency in a Canadian kindred with familial partial lipodystrophy type 3 (FPLD3). *BMC Med Genet* 2006; **7**:3.

152 Hegele RA, Ur E, Ransom TP, Cao H. A frameshift mutation in peroxisome-proliferator-activated receptor-gamma in familial partial lipodystrophy subtype 3 (FPLD3; MIM 604367). *Clin Genet* 2006; **70**:360–362.

153 Monajemi H, Zhang L, Li G, Jeninga EH, Cao H, Maas M, *et al.* Familial partial lipodystrophy phenotype resulting from a single-base mutation in deoxyribonucleic acid-binding domain of peroxisome proliferator-activated receptor-gamma. *J Clin Endocrinol Metab* 2007; **92**:1606–1612.

154 Ludtke A, Buettner J, Wu W, Muchir A, Schroeter A, Zinn-Justin S, *et al.* Peroxisome proliferator-activated receptor-gamma C190S mutation causes partial lipodystrophy. *J Clin Endocrinol Metab* 2007; **92**:2248–2255.

155 Ludtke A, Buettner J, Schmidt HH, Worman HJ. New PPARG mutation leads to lipodystrophy and loss of protein function that is partially restored by a synthetic ligand. *J Med Genet* 2007; **44**:e88.

156 Agarwal AK, Garg A. Genetic basis of lipodystrophies and management of metabolic complications. *Annu Rev Med* 2006; **57**:297–311.

157 Agarwal AK, Simha V, Oral EA, Moran SA, Gorden P, O'Rahilly S, *et al.* Phenotypic and genetic heterogeneity in congenital generalized lipodystrophy. *J Clin Endocrinol Metab* 2003; **88**:4840–4847.

158 Chandalia M, Garg A, Vuitch F, Nizzi F. Postmortem findings in congenital generalized lipodystrophy. *J Clin Endocrinol Metab* 1995; **80**:3077–3081.

159 Case records of the Massachusetts General Hospital. Weekly clinicopathological exercises. Case 1-1975. *N Engl J Med* 1975; **292**:35–41.

160 Van Maldergem L, Magre J, Khallouf TE, Gedde-Dahl T Jr, Delepine M, Trygstad O, *et al.* Genotype–phenotype relationships in Berardinelli–Seip congenital lipodystrophy. *J Med Genet* 2002; **39**:722–733.

161 Haque WA, Shimomura I, Matsuzawa Y, Garg A. Serum adiponectin and leptin levels in patients with lipodystrophies. *J Clin Endocrinol Metab* 2002; **87**:2395.

162 Kim CA, Delepine M, Boutet E, El Mourabit H, Le Lay S, Meier M, *et al.* Association of a homozygous nonsense caveolin-1 mutation with Berardinelli–Seip congenital lipodystrophy. *J Clin Endocrinol Metab* 2008; **93**:1129–1134.

163 Simha V, Agarwal AK, Aronin PA, Iannaccone ST, Garg A. Novel subtype of congenital generalized lipodystrophy associated with muscular weakness and cervical spine instability. *Am J Med Genet A* 2008; **146A**:2318–2326.

164 Gambineri A, Semple RK, Forlani G, Genghini S, Grassi I, Hyden CS, *et al.* Monogenic polycystic ovary syndrome due to a mutation in the lamin A/C gene is sensitive to thiazolidinediones but not to metformin. *Eur J Endocrinol* 2008; **159**:347–353.

165 Sleilati GG, Leff T, Bonnett JW, Hegele RA. Efficacy and safety of pioglitazone in treatment of a patient with an atypical partial lipodystrophy syndrome. *Endocr Pract* 2007; **13**:656–661.

166 Moreau F, Boullu-Sanchis S, Vigouroux C, Lucescu C, Lascols O, Sapin R, *et al.* Efficacy of pioglitazone in familial partial lipodystrophy of the Dunnigan type: a case report. *Diabetes Metab* 2007; **33**:385–389.

167 Ludtke A, Heck K, Genschel J, Mehnert H, Spuler S, Worman HJ, *et al.* Long-term treatment experience in a subject with Dunnigan-type familial partial lipodystrophy: efficacy of rosiglitazone. *Diabet Med* 2005; **22**:1611–1613.

168 Owen KR, Donohoe M, Ellard S, Hattersley AT. Response to treatment with rosiglitazone in familial partial lipodystrophy due to a mutation in the LMNA gene. *Diabet Med* 2003; **20**:823–827.

169 Savage DB, Tan GD, Acerini CL, Jebb SA, Agostini M, Gurnell M, *et al.* Human metabolic syndrome resulting from dominant-negative mutations in the nuclear receptor peroxisome proliferator-activated receptor-gamma. *Diabetes* 2003; **52**:910–917.

170 Musso C, Javor E, Cochran E, Balow JE, Gorden P. Spectrum of renal diseases associated with extreme forms of insulin resistance. *Clin J Am Soc Nephrol* 2006; **1**:616–622.

171 Oral EA, Simha V, Ruiz E, Andewelt A, Premkumar A, Snell P, *et al.* Leptin-replacement therapy for lipodystrophy. *N Engl J Med* 2002; **346**:570–578.

172 Javor ED, Cochran EK, Musso C, Young JR, Depaoli AM, Gorden P. Long-term efficacy of leptin replacement in patients with generalized lipodystrophy. *Diabetes* 2005; **54**:1994–2002.

173 Musso C, Cochran E, Javor E, Young J, Depaoli AM, Gorden P. The long-term effect of recombinant methionyl human leptin therapy on hyperandrogenism and menstrual function in female and pituitary function in male and female hypoleptinemic lipodystrophic patients. *Metabolism* 2005; **54**:255–263.

174 Guettier JM, Park JY, Cochran EK, Poitou C, Basdevant A, Meier M, *et al.* Leptin therapy for partial lipodystrophy linked to a PPAR-gamma mutation. *Clin Endocrinol* 2008; **68**:547–554.

175 Beltrand J, Beregszaszi M, Chevenne D, Sebag G, De Kerdanet M, Huet F, *et al.* Metabolic correction induced by leptin replacement treatment in young children with Berardinelli–Seip congenital lipoatrophy. *Pediatrics* 2007; **120**:e291–e296.

176 Park JY, Javor ED, Cochran EK, DePaoli AM, Gorden P. Long-term efficacy of leptin replacement in patients with Dunnigan-type familial partial lipodystrophy. *Metabolism* 2007; **56**:508–516.

177 Ebihara K, Kusakabe T, Hirata M, Masuzaki H, Miyanaga F, Kobayashi N, *et al.* Efficacy and safety of leptin-replacement therapy and possible mechanisms of leptin actions in patients with generalized lipodystrophy. *J Clin Endocrinol Metab* 2007; **92**:532–541.

178 Simha V, Szczepaniak LS, Wagner AJ, DePaoli AM, Garg A. Effect of leptin replacement on intrahepatic and intramyocellular lipid content in patients with generalized lipodystrophy. *Diabetes Care* 2003; **26**:30–35.

179 Petersen KF, Oral EA, Dufour S, Befroy D, Ariyan C, Yu C, *et al.* Leptin reverses insulin resistance and hepatic steatosis in patients with severe lipodystrophy. *J Clin Invest* 2002; **109**:1345–1350.

180 Krentz AJ. Insulin resistance. *Br Med J* 1996; **313**:1385–1389.

181 Murphy R, Ellard S, Hattersley AT. Clinical implications of a molecular genetic classification of monogenic beta-cell diabetes. *Nat Clin Pract Endocrinol Metab* 2008; **4**:200–213.

182 Moller DE, O'Rahilly S. Syndromes of severe insulin resistance. In: Moller DE, ed. *Insulin Resistance*. Chiches.

16 Drug-Induced Diabetes

Neil J.L. Gittoes[1], John Ayuk[1] & Robin E. Ferner[2]

[1] Centre for Endocrinology, Diabetes and Metabolism, University of Birmingham, Birmingham, UK
[2] West Midlands Centre for Adverse Drug Reaction Reporting, City Hospital, Birmingham, UK

Keypoints

- Many commonly used drugs interfere with glucose homeostasis and can provoke hyperglycemia in subjects without diabetes or worsen glycemic control in patients with diabetes.
- Glucocorticoids act on post insulin-receptor mechanisms to induce dose-dependent insensitivity to insulin in its target tissues.
- Glucocorticoid-induced diabetes often requires treatment with oral hypoglycemic agents or insulin while glucocorticoid treatment continues.
- Oral contraceptive pills rarely cause hyperglycemia, although it can occur with combined pills that contain high-dose estrogen or the progesterone levonorgestrel, and in women with a history of gestational diabetes.
- Estrogen replacement therapy in postmenopausal women does not affect glycemic control.
- Thiazide diuretics impair insulin secretion when given at high dosages. Impairment of insulin secretion is related to potassium depletion.
- Loop diuretics such as furosemide (frusemide) are less likely to cause hyperglycemia.
- Non-selective β-adrenoceptor antagonists inhibit insulin secretion and can impair glucose tolerance. Cardioselective β_1-adrenoceptor blockers have much less pronounced effects.
- Other drugs that can precipitate or aggravate hyperglycemia include:
  Streptozocin (streptozotocin), pentamidine and ciclosporin (cyclosporine) via β-cell toxicity;
  Diazoxide via inhibition of insulin secretion;
  β_2-Receptor agonists (salbutamol and ritodrine), which increase hepatic glucose production;
  Growth hormone in supraphysiologic doses;
  Protease inhibitors (indinavir, nelfinavir, ritonavir, saquinavir) by inducing insulin resistance; and
  Antipsychotics via weight gain and insulin resistance.

Many drugs can cause or worsen pre-existing hyperglycemia – a problem recently recognized by the World Health Organization (WHO) and the American Diabetes Association (ADA) with the identification of drug-induced diabetes as a separate etiologic category (see Chapter 2). The diabetogenic properties of drugs are important for two main reasons. First, polypharmacy is an unfortunate but common necessity in managing patients with diabetes; clear understanding of the potential hyperglycemic effects of drugs is therefore helpful in anticipating and avoiding deterioration in glycemic control. Secondly, various drugs can induce diabetes in previously normoglycemic individuals; this state is usually reversible and not insulin-dependent, but can become permanent.

Drugs can raise blood glucose concentrations through two broad mechanisms: by reducing insulin biosynthesis or secretion, or by reducing tissue sensitivity to insulin (Figure 16.1). Some important examples are listed in Table 16.1. Of particular note are the glucocorticoids, which are used in many diseases, and certain commonly used antihypertensive drugs [1–7]. Hypertension commonly accompanies diabetes, and most patients require more than one antihypertensive agent to meet the increasingly stringent targets for blood pressure control (see the first part of Chapter 40).

This chapter describes the drugs that can induce or aggravate hyperglycemia, together with a strategy for managing patients with drug-induced diabetes.

Glucocorticoids

Glucocorticoids were named for their hyperglycemic effects [8] and have by far the most powerful adverse effect on glycemic control of all the commonly prescribed drugs. During the 1930s, it became apparent that diabetic symptoms improved following either adrenalectomy [9] or hypophysectomy [10], indicating that glucocorticoids have important influences on glucose homeostasis. This fact was recognized in clinical practice [11–15], soon after the landmark discovery in 1949 by Hench *et al.* [16] that glucocorticoids had potent anti-inflammatory effects. Since then,

Textbook of Diabetes, 4th edition. Edited by R. Holt, C. Cockram, A. Flyvbjerg and B. Goldstein.

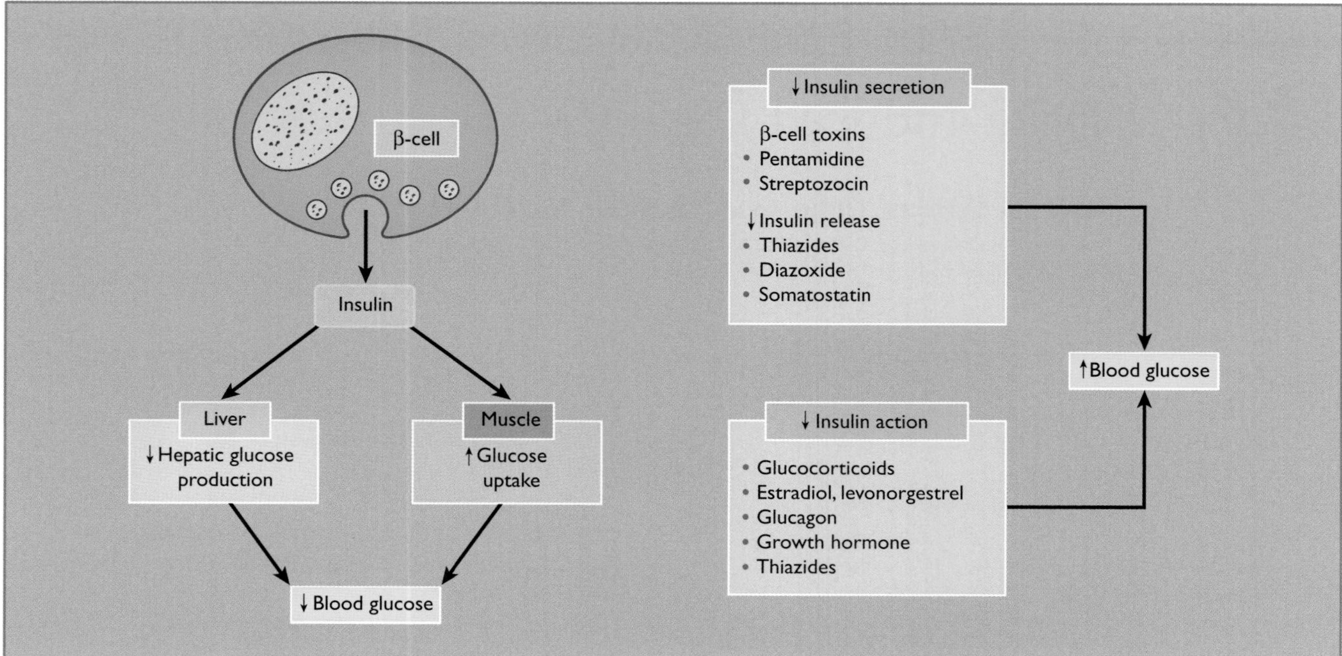

Figure 16.1 Mechanisms of drug-induced hyperglycemia.

therapeutic use of these agents has escalated; recent data from the General Practice Research Database suggest that nearly 1% of the UK population may be using oral glucocorticoids at any time, increasing to 2.5% in subjects aged 70–79 years [17]. Inhaled corticosteroid use is even more widespread, with more than 6% of the UK population currently using an inhaled corticosteroid [18].

Glucocorticoids worsen hyperglycemia in patients with diabetes, but can also cause significant increases in blood glucose (and insulin) concentrations in previously normoglycemic individuals when given in high doses (i.e. equivalent to 30 mg/day or more of prednisolone) [19]. Impaired glucose tolerance or diabetes mellitus have been reported in 14–28% of subjects receiving long-term glucocorticoids [20,21], and subjects who have an intrinsically low insulin response (e.g. in response to glucose loading) are particularly susceptible [22]. These subjects are thought to be at greater risk of developing type 2 diabetes (T2DM) in the future, compared to the general population [23]. Using data from the Health Improvement Network, Gulliford *et al.* [24] found that in a large primary care population, drawn from 114 family practices, orally administered glucocorticoids were associated with up to 2% of incident cases of diabetes mellitus.

Glucocorticoids reduce hepatic and peripheral tissue sensitivity to insulin through post-receptor mechanisms (Fig. 16.1). In adipocytes, dexamethasone inhibits the expression of the insulin-signaling intermediate protein, insulin receptor substrate 1 (IRS-1) [25], and this may contribute to insulin resistance (see Chapter 7). These effects may be partly offset by glucose-independent stimulation of insulin secretion [26].

All glucocorticoids cause dose-dependent insulin resistance at dosages greater than the equivalent of 7.5 mg/day prednisolone [21]. The duration of exposure to glucocorticoids does not appear to be important, and hyperglycemia is generally reversible on withdrawing the drug.

Most problems have been reported with oral glucocorticoids, but those administered topically can also induce severe hyperglycemia, especially if given at high dosage over large areas of damaged skin and under occlusive dressings [27]. This is more likely to occur in children because of their higher ratio of total body surface area to body weight [28]. Although inhaled corticosteroids do not cause significant hyperglycemia, there has been a single case report of deteriorating glycemic control in a patient with T2DM who was prescribed high-dose fluticasone propionate [29]. The hyperglycemic potency of glucocorticoids does not follow the hierarchy of their anti-inflammatory or immunosuppressive activities. For example, deflazacort, which has similar immunomodulating effects to other glucocorticoids, produces less hyperglycemia than prednisone or dexamethasone [30].

Other commonly encountered adverse effects of glucocorticoids are hypertension and sodium and water retention. Thiazide diuretics should not be used to treat these complications, as their own hyperglycemic action synergizes with that of glucocorticoids [31].

Corticotropin (adrenocorticotropic hormone [ACTH]) or tetracosactide (tetracosactrin), previously given as an alternative to glucocorticoid therapy (e.g. in exacerbations of multiple sclerosis), is no longer recommended for therapeutic use. It can cause hyperglycemia and hyperinsulinemia in rodents [32,33].

Table 16.1 Drugs that cause or exacerbate hyperglycemia.

Potentially potent effects	Minor or no effects
Glucocorticoids	Oral contraceptives
Oral contraceptives	Progestogen-only pills
High-dose estrogen	Levonorgestrel in combination pills
Thiazide diuretics (especially high dosages)*	Loop diuretics
Non-selective β-adrenoceptor antagonists	Calcium-channel blockers
β_2-adrenoceptor agonists	α_1-adrenoceptor antagonists
Salbutamol	Growth hormone (physiologic doses)
Ritodrine	Somatostatin analogs†
Antipsychotics	Androgen deprivation therapy for prostate cancer
HIV protease inhibitors	Selective serotonin reuptake inhibitors
Indinavir, nelfinavir, ritonavir and others	Nicotinic acid
	Lamivudine
	Isoniazid
Others	
Pentamidine	
Gatifloxacin	
Streptozocin (streptozotocin)	
Diazoxide	
Ciclosporin (cyclosporine)	
Tacrolimus	
Temsirolimus	
Interferon-α	
L-asparaginase	

HIV, human immunodeficiency virus.
* "High" dosages of thiazides correspond to ≥5 mg/day bendroflumethiazide.
† Somatostatin analogs may induce hyperglycemia in type 2 but not type 1 diabetes.

The metabolic adverse effects of glucocorticoids have stimulated the development of selective glucocorticoid receptor ligands with similar anti-inflammatory efficacy to glucocorticoids currently in use but with fewer adverse effects. A number of these compounds have been developed and shown in animal studies not to induce hyperglycemia [34]. These agents are likely to be tested clinically in humans in the near future.

Oral contraceptive pills and estrogen replacement therapy

Estrogens and some progestogens used in contraceptive agents are potentially diabetogenic. This is not surprising, as endogenous sex steroids have been shown to affect glucose homeostasis in women without diabetes: insulin sensitivity rises during the follicular phase of the menstrual cycle and falls during the luteal phase [35]. As with glucocorticoids, post-receptor insulin resistance appears to be responsible; *in vivo* studies have demonstrated a decrease in insulin sensitivity in women without diabetes taking certain contraceptive pills [36,37], and a number of implantable hormonal contraceptives have been linked to alterations in carbohydrate metabolism, including impaired glucose tolerance and increased insulin resistance [38,39]. The tendency to cause hyperglycemia was particularly marked with the early pills, which had a relatively high estrogen content; the overall risk of developing impaired glucose tolerance was 35% [40], and even greater in women with a history of diabetes during pregnancy [41,42]. Impaired glucose tolerance during pregnancy remains a potent risk factor, even with the newer oral contraceptives; these women are three times more likely to develop diabetes with a progestogen-only pill than with a low-dose combined pill [43].

Most currently available combined oral contraceptives contain low estrogen dosage (25–50 μg/day). In 1992, Rimm *et al.* [44] reported the metabolic effects of oral contraceptives in a large prospective survey of healthy volunteers, and found transient rises in serum insulin concentrations and impairment of glucose tolerance with all formulations. Consistent with this, metabolic studies have demonstrated fasting hyperinsulinemia and reduced insulin sensitivity [36,37,45]. Reassuringly, however, recent studies, including a massive prospective follow-up of almost 99 000 non-diabetic participants [46], found no appreciable increase in the incidence of diabetes among users of current oral contraceptives [46,47]. The authors of a recent Cochrane review [48] concluded that hormonal contraceptives have little clinical impact on carbohydrate metabolism. Low-dose combined oral contraceptives are safe in younger women with uncomplicated well-controlled diabetes [49].

In contrast to the older high-estrogen pills, the effect on glucose homeostasis of low-estrogen combination pills is determined mainly by the type and dosage of progestogen, with monophasic levonorgestrel combinations having the most deleterious effect. Oral progestogen-only formulations cause only minor hyperglycemia in healthy subjects, although diabetes may develop in women who had hyperglycemia during previous pregnancies [43]. The long-acting progestogens, such as depot medroxyprogesterone (Depo-Provera) and sustained-release low-dose levonorgestrel, cause a statistically but not clinically significant deterioration in glucose tolerance in healthy women [39,50]. There is little evidence, however, to suggest that this translates into clinical harm, and the WHO medical eligibility criteria for contraceptive use do not restrict the use of progestogen-only contraceptives in women with diabetes unless diabetes has been present for over 20 years or complications are present [51]. A primary care study in the UK found that progestogen-only methods of contraception, including the injectable contraceptive Depo-Provera and progestogen-only pills, are significantly more likely to be prescribed for women with diabetes than for those without diabetes [52]. There is no convincing evidence that the Mirena coil is associated with any change in glucose metabolism.

Hyperglycemia induced by hormonal contraceptives is usually reversible on withdrawal of the contraceptive pill. The current low-dosage contraceptive pills do not apparently predispose to the subsequent development of T2DM, although there is some evidence that this is a hazard in patients previously exposed to high-dosage pills [53].

Estrogen replacement therapy in women with diabetes

A number of observational studies of hormone replacement therapy (HRT) use in T2DM have demonstrated an association between HRT use and reduced cardiovascular risk [54,55]. This is in contrast to the general population, where HRT is not associated with a reduction in the incidence of cardiovascular disease in postmenopausal women [56]. HRT preparations differ with regard to type and dose of estrogen, type of combination progestogen and route of administration, and it is likely that these differences may be important in determining the overall balance of cardiovascular risk and benefit in specific patient subgroups such as those with diabetes. One placebo-controlled randomized study in 25 postmenopausal women with T2DM found that conjugated equine estrogen therapy (0.625 mg/day) had beneficial effects on blood glucose and lipid profiles [57]. A further study in 28 postmenopausal women with T2DM using continuous oral 17β estradiol (1 mg) and norethisterone (0.5 mg) had similar findings [58]. In the Women's Health Initiative study, involving over 160 000 postmenopausal women aged 50–79 years, those randomized to HRT had a lower incidence of self-reported diabetes than those randomized to placebo. This was true both for women taking conjugated equine estrogen alone and those taking a combination of conjugated equine estrogen plus medroxyprogesterone acetate [59,60]. The results of these studies, along with the findings of a meta-analysis quantifying the effect of HRT on components of the metabolic syndrome in postmenopausal women [61], provide some reassurance that postmenopausal estrogen replacement therapy can be offered to patients with diabetes.

Antihypertensive and cardiovascular agents

Thiazide diuretics

Hyperglycemia was recognized as an adverse effect of chlorothiazide (the first marketed thiazide diuretic) within a year of its introduction in 1957 [62]. Thiazides can induce adverse biochemical changes, including hyperglycemia, hypokalemia and dyslipidemia [63–68]. The overall frequency of impaired glucose tolerance is around 3–6 cases per 1000 patient-years when high dosages of thiazides (≥5 mg/day bendroflumethiazide (bendrofluazide) are used. With low dosages (≤2.5 mg/day bendroflumethiazide) and the correction of any fall in plasma potassium concentration, the problem is far less common [69–74].

Long-term studies show that impaired glucose tolerance usually develops slowly, with a lag period of 2 years after starting the thiazide [66,67]. The precise mechanism by which thiazide diuretics impair glucose tolerance has not been elucidated. It was previously thought to be secondary to both reduced glucose-stimulated insulin release and to insulin resistance (Figure 16.1), but some recent evidence suggests the mechanism involves reduced pancreatic insulin release alone and not reduced insulin sensitivity [75]. The severity of glucose intolerance is strongly correlated with the degree of hypokalemia [67]; the impairment of insulin secretion is secondary to potassium depletion, which appears to inhibit the cleavage of proinsulin to insulin and is reversible on restoring normokalemia [73,76,77]. The result is post-prandial hyperglycemia, with elevated proinsulin concentrations between meals that may downregulate insulin receptors in peripheral tissues. This phenomenon affects people without diabetes and those with T2DM, but not patients with type 1 diabetes (T1DM) receiving exogenous insulin replacement.

β-Adrenoceptor antagonists

β-Adrenoceptors modulate glucose homeostasis at several different points (Figure 16.2). Long-term studies suggest that β-adrenoceptor antagonists induce insulin resistance, possibly partly through weight gain [78]. This diabetogenic effect is amplified if high-dose thiazides are also given [79]. The authors of a recent meta-analysis of 94 492 patients with hypertension concluded that treatment with β-adrenoceptor antagonists is associated with a 22% increased risk for new-onset diabetes [80]. The risk was greater in patients with higher baseline body mass indexes and higher baseline fasting glucose concentrations.

β-Adrenoceptor antagonists differ in their diabetogenic potential; in the meta-analysis, the risk for new-onset diabetes was 30% greater for atenolol and 34% greater with metoprolol than other agents [80]. In contrast, there was no increase in the risk for new-onset diabetes with propranolol compared with placebo. In fact, in the GEMINI trial, carvedilol stabilized glycated hemoglobin and improved insulin resistance in patients with diabetes and hypertension [81].

The possible importance of β-adrenoceptor antagonists in masking hypoglycemic symptoms is discussed in Chapter 26.

Calcium-channel blockers

In vitro and *in vivo* studies have demonstrated that calcium-channel blockers can impair glucose metabolism. Very few cases of clinically significant hyperglycemia have been reported, however, [82–88], and most were associated with excessive dosage of these drugs. Verapamil inhibits the second phase of glucose-stimulated insulin release by blocking the uptake of calcium into the cytosol of β-cells [89]; it also inhibits sulfonylurea and glucagon-induced insulin secretion [90]. Hyperglycemia and metabolic acidosis are well described in verapamil poisoning, and *in vivo* animal studies suggest that hyperglycemia may be caused by a combination of impaired insulin release and insulin resistance, causing a fall in insulin-mediated glucose clearance, together with increased action of circulating catecholamines [91]. Serum glucose concentrations have been found to correlate directly with the severity of the calcium-channel blocker intoxica-

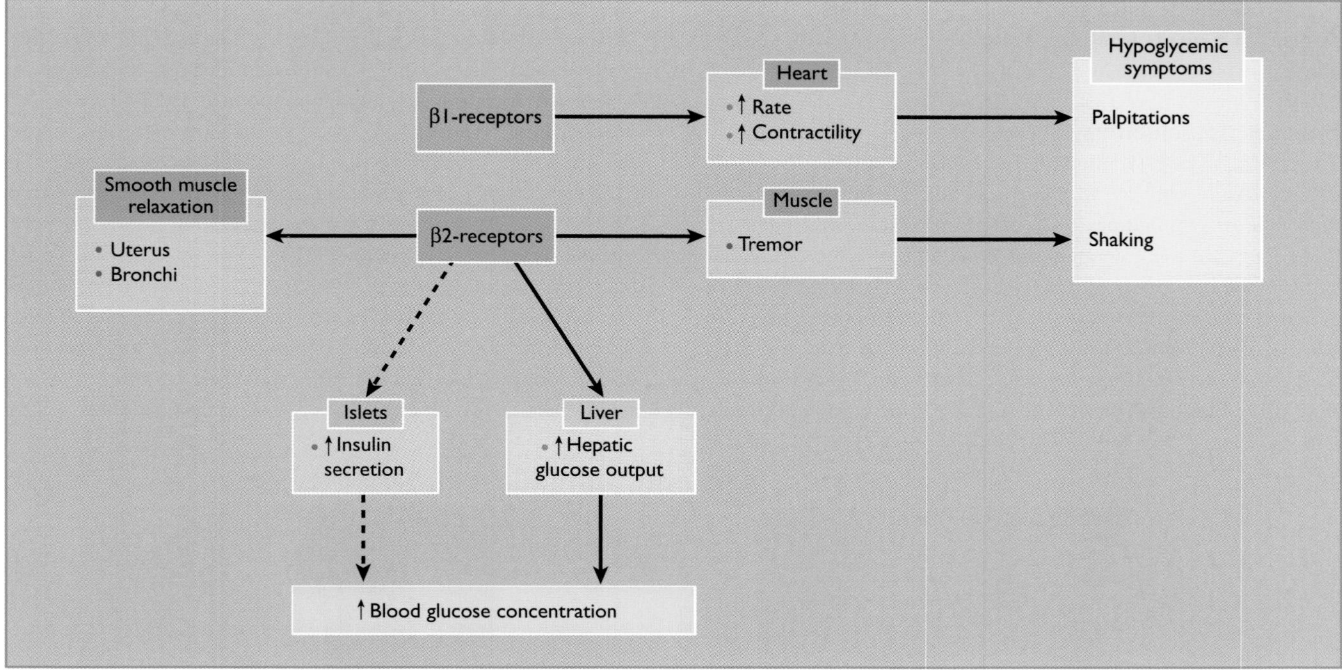

Figure 16.2 Effects mediated by β_1- and β_2-adrenoceptors.

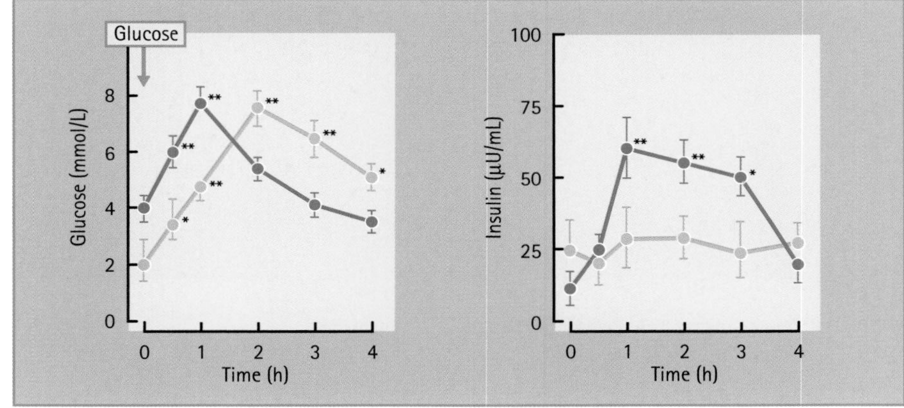

Figure 16.3 Plasma glucose and insulin concentrations during an oral glucose tolerance test, in 20 healthy controls (red) and in four dysglycemic subjects treated with intravenous pentamidine (yellow). Data are mean ± SEM. * $P < 0.05$, ** $P < 0.01$ vs baseline. Reproduced from Assan *et al.* [100] with permission from the American Diabetes Association.

tion [92]. Nonetheless, calcium-channel blockers used appropriately can be regarded as safe in patients with diabetes [82,93–96].

Other drugs

β-Cell toxins

A few drugs act directly as β-cell toxins and can cause permanent diabetes, often insulin-dependent. A classic example is the nitrosourea, streptozocin (streptozotocin), which has long been used to induce experimental insulin-dependent diabetes in rodents; in humans, it is employed as chemotherapy for inoperable or metastatic insulinoma.

Pentamidine, used to treat *Pneumocystis jirovecii* infection in patients with AIDS [97], is closely related to another experimental diabetogenic drug, alloxan. It causes destruction of β-cells and may initially induce insulin release and transient hypoglycemia [98], followed subsequently by diabetes [99]. This effect is predominantly seen when pentamidine is given intravenously (Figure 16.3), but can also follow inhalation of an aerosol [100]. In one series of 128 patients with AIDS treated with pentamidine for *Pneumocystis jirovecii* infection, nearly 40% developed significant abnormalities of glucose homeostasis: hypoglycemia (5%), hypoglycemia followed by diabetes (15%) and diabetes alone (18%) [100]. Higher doses of pentamidine, higher plasma creatinine concentration and more severe anoxia were risk factors for the development of these glucose abnormalities.

The rodenticide pyriminil (Vacor) has also caused irreversible diabetes in humans when ingested accidentally or with suicidal intent.

HIV protease inhibitors

The treatment of HIV infection has evolved dramatically during the last decade, with the wide introduction of protease inhibitors such as indinavir, nelfinavir, ritonavir and saquinavir. In general, these drugs are well tolerated, but worsening of pre-existing diabetes or the new onset of T2DM has been reported in 2–6% of patients receiving them [101–103]. Transient elevations in glucose concentrations are common in these patients, and there is a fivefold increase in the incidence of sustained glucose intolerance [101]. Because of similarities to the pathogenesis and clinical presentation of T2DM, it has been advised that treatment of protease inhibitor-associated hyperinsulinemia and hyperglycemia should follow the recommendations of the American Diabetes Association for the management of T2DM [104].

A striking syndrome of peripheral lipodystrophy, hyperlipidemia and insulin resistance has also been described in patients receiving HIV protease inhibitors, especially long term (Figure 16.4). This suggests that the underlying cause of hyperglycemia is insulin resistance [103]. The mechanism is not fully understood; Carr *et al.* [103] propose that protease inhibitors may bind to as yet uncharacterized target proteins that regulate lipid metabolism, leading to elevated circulating fatty acids that could interfere with insulin signaling or enter the fatty acid cycle and compete with glucose cycle intermediates. Recent

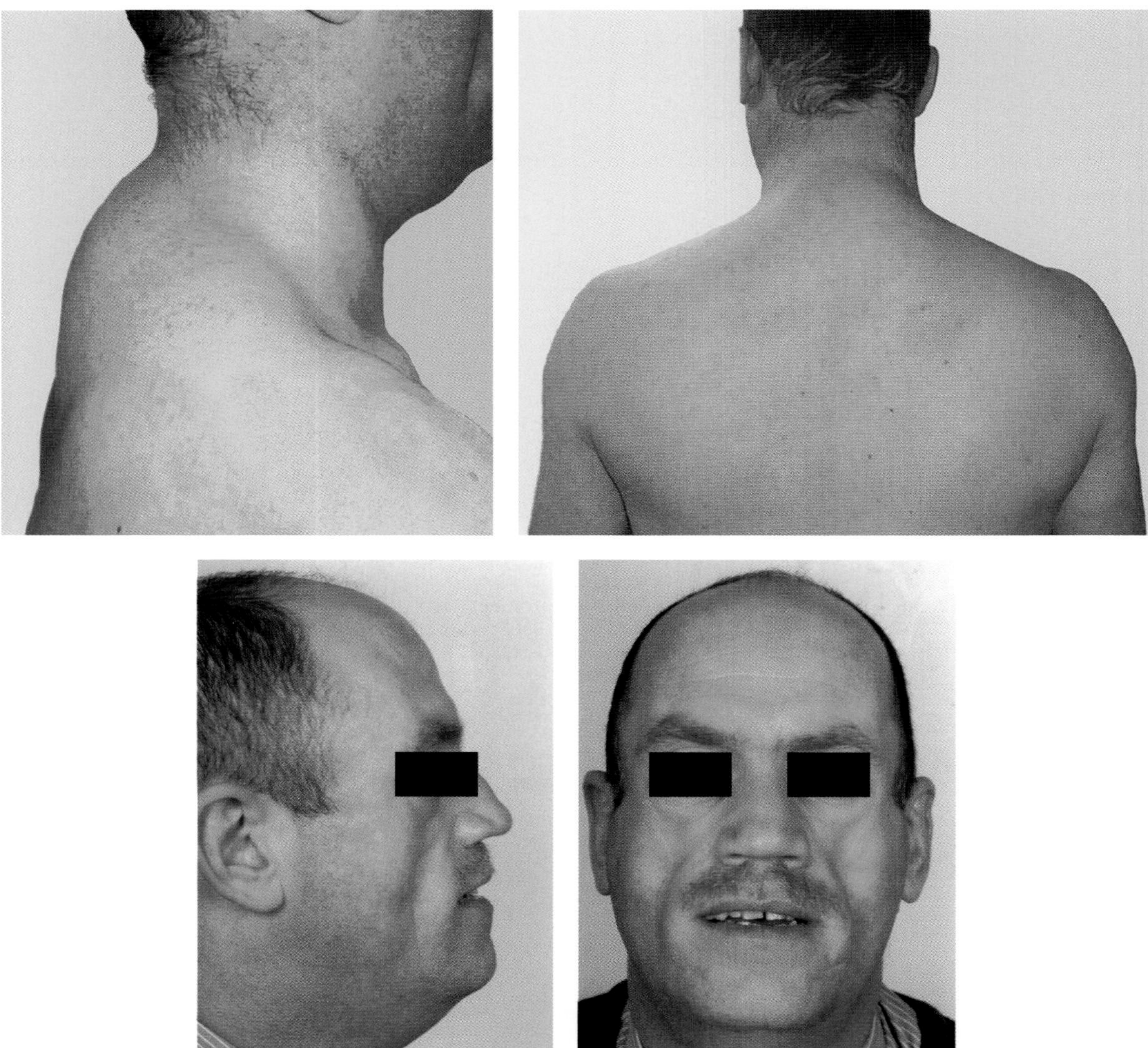

Figure 16.4 Protease inhibitor-induced lipodystrophy. (a,b) "Buffalo hump" caused by nuchal fat deposition. (c,d) Facial fat atrophy. Courtesy of Professor Munir Pirmohamed, University of Liverpool, UK.

studies indicate that these drugs have direct effects on adipocytes, including resistance to insulin's actions in promoting glucose uptake and inhibiting lipolysis [105], as well as impairment of differentiation from pre-adipocytes to mature fat cells [106].

β_2-Adrenoceptor agonists

β_2-Adrenoceptor agonists stimulate insulin secretion, but this effect is overwhelmed by increased hepatic glucose output, and the usual net effect is hyperglycemia (Figure 16.2). High dosage of β_2-agonist drugs (e.g. salbutamol, ritodrine and terbutaline) is commonly used to treat asthma and premature labor. Hyperglycemia often results [107], and diabetic ketoacidosis has even been induced in previously non-diabetic pregnant women [108]. Continuous nebulization of β_2-agonist drugs for status asthmaticus can also result in hyperglycemia [109]. The effects of β_2-agonists are most pronounced in patients with T1DM. When dexamethasone is administered together with a β_2-agonist, as in the treatment of preterm labor, the resulting hyperglycemia can be severe, even in previously normoglycemic patients. In view of this, current guidance from the National Institute for Health and Clinical Excellence (NICE) recommends that when tocolysis is indicated in women with diabetes, an alternative to β_2-adrenoceptor agonists should be used to avoid hyperglycemia and ketoacidosis [110].

Epinephrine (adrenaline) [111], dopamine [112] and theophylline can also cause hyperglycemia through similar mechanisms.

Diazoxide

Diazoxide is a non-diuretic benzothiadiazine derivative with potent vasodilator properties, which was previously used to treat hypertensive crises; it is now rarely used for this indication, but is sometimes helpful in cases of inoperable insulinoma and to treat profound hypoglycemia following sulfonylurea overdose. The dose used for treatment of patients with insulinoma ranges between 100 and 600 mg/day, often in divided doses [113]. It acts on the β-cell membrane to open the ATP-dependent potassium channel, thus hyperpolarizing the membrane and inhibiting insulin secretion (see Chapter 6). Diazoxide can cause hyperglycemia after only two or three doses.

Somatostatin analogs

Somatostatin suppresses insulin secretion but also inhibits the release of the counter-regulatory hormones, growth hormone and glucagon; the net effect in subjects without diabetes is usually to maintain euglycemia. Octreotide, a somatostatin analog used to treat neuroendocrine tumors, has different metabolic effects in T1DM and T2DM [114]. In patients with T1DM treated with exogenous insulin, suppression of glucagon and growth hormone decreases hepatic glucose production and can lower blood glucose and/or insulin requirements. In patients with T2DM, inhibition of endogenous insulin can predominate, leading to hyperglycemia. There is some evidence that treatment with octreotide, lanreotide and the long-acting preparations of both drugs can impair glucose tolerance and occasionally cause diabetes, notably in people with acromegaly whose glucose homeostasis is already impaired (see Chapter 17) [115–117]. The effect of long-acting somatostatin analogs on glucose metabolism in patients with acromegaly is complex; they reduce the insulin resistance caused by elevated growth hormone concentrations, but also suppress insulin secretion from islet β-cells. The net balance between the two effects determines whether long-acting somatostatin analogs improve or worsen glucose metabolism [118]. These effects are inconsistent and unpredictable, with worsening glucose metabolism occasionally seen in the presence of improving growth hormone concentrations [119].

Utilizing its suppressive effect on insulin release, octreotide has been used effectively to manage refractory hypoglycemia caused by acute sulfonylurea poisoning or quinine treatment [120–123].

Recombinant human growth hormone

Biosynthetic growth hormone (GH), now widely used to treat growth failure, is an insulin antagonist that can cause reversible mild glucose intolerance [124]. A recent large study of over 23 000 children treated with human recombinant human growth hormone (hGH) showed a sixfold higher frequency of T2DM than expected [125], although the incidence of T1DM was not increased. These data from a young cohort suggest that GH probably accelerates the development of the disease in individuals who may have a genetic predisposition to T2DM.

Increasingly, hGH has become accepted as long-term therapy in adults with GH deficiency (GHD) (see Chapter 17); as yet, no significant adverse effects on glycemic control have been reported. Fasting plasma glucose and glycated hemoglobin usually increase, but remain within the reference range, in subjects without diabetes during prolonged hGH replacement; in subjects with pre-existing impaired glucose tolerance, they tend not to rise further above pretreatment baseline values [126]. This probably reflects the complex interaction between hGH, insulin-like growth factor I (IGF-I) and body composition. Many people with adult GHD have abnormal body composition with central adiposity and decreased lean body mass. In the short term, rhGH acts as an insulin antagonist but in the longer term leads to increases in IGF-I and decreased fat mass, which tend to improve insulin sensitivity (see Chapter 17). It is recommended, however, that overdosing be avoided and glycemic control be monitored [127].

New-onset diabetes mellitus has been described in patients with the HIV wasting syndrome (AIDS cachexia) treated with hGH in supraphysiological doses [128].

Antirejection drugs

Post-transplantation diabetes mellitus (PTDM) has been reported in non-diabetic adult transplant recipients taking ciclosporin (cyclosporine) [129,130]. Animal studies have implicated reversible β-cell damage [131], causing reduced insulin secretion [132–

134]. In addition, pancreas allograft biopsies from transplant patients receiving ciclosporin show histologic changes compatible with islet cell damage, including cytoplasmic swelling, vacuolization and apoptosis [135]. Recent studies suggest that the risk of PTDM increases progressively with time after transplantation. Newer preparations of ciclosporin which are better absorbed from the gastrointestinal tract achieve higher blood concentrations and thus higher cumulative exposure, and increase the incidence of diabetes [136].

PTDM is also commonly observed in up to 28% of adults receiving tacrolimus (FK506), a newer and more potent immunosuppressive agent [137–139]. More recent trials, however, suggest the risk of developing PTDM can be reduced by the use of low-dose tacrolimus (0.15–0.2 mg/kg/day) [140]. Altered insulin and glucagon responses to arginine in patients treated with these drugs suggest a defect in the β-cell–α-cell axis within the islet (see Chapter 6) [141]. The diabetogenic effects of both ciclosporin and tacrolimus are largely reversible with appropriate reductions in the drug dosage.

Recently developed immunosuppression protocols aiming to minimize the use of steroids and nephrotoxic immunosuppressants have resulted in the extensive use of potent non-nephrotoxic immunosuppressants, such as mycophenolate mofetil and sirolimus. The incidence of PTDM associated with these agents is uncertain. Study results with sirolimus have been inconsistent, with some suggesting an increased risk of developing PTDM [142,143] and others not [144].

α-Interferon therapy has been associated with the development of both T1DM and T2DM, sometimes with ketoacidosis; autoimmune mechanisms have been implicated [145].

Drugs used in psychiatric disorders

Antipsychotic agents

Hyperglycemia occurs occasionally with conventional antipsychotic drugs, but the use of the newer atypical antipsychotics, especially clozapine and olanzapine, have been widely reported to be associated with the development of *de novo* diabetes mellitus and exacerbation of pre-existing diabetes [146–148]. A causative relationship between antipsychotic and diabetes has not been established beyond doubt because many patients receiving these drugs who develop diabetes have traditional risk factors for diabetes. Indeed, the rates of diabetes in people with severe mental illness were reported to be higher in the pre-antipsychotic era (see Chapter 55). Possible underlying mechanisms linking antipsychotics and the development of diabetes include hepatic dysregulation caused by antagonism of hepatic serotonergic mechanisms [149]. Weight gain, associated with fasting hyperglycemia and hyperinsulinemia, point to insulin resistance as the underlying mechanism although some *in vitro* studies suggest that the antipsychotics may have a direct effect on insulin secretion. In a few cases, blood glucose concentrations may return to normal once the drug is discontinued. Despite a wealth of evidence from a number of sources (anecdotal case reports, drug safety studies, pharmacoepidemiologic studies, prospective studies) linking glucose intolerance to the use of atypical antipsychotics, one estimate of the attributable risk of diabetes associated with atypical antipsychotics ranged from 0.05% for risperidone to 2.03% for clozapine, suggesting that the absolute excess risk associated with atypical antipsychotics is probably low [150]. Consequently, most individuals receiving antipsychotics will not develop diabetes and for those who do, the cause is unlikely to be related to their treatment. When prescribing atypical antipsychotic medication, however, baseline screening and follow-up monitoring is recommended.

Antidepressants

Depression is an important problem among people with diabetes (see Chapter 55), and various antidepressant drugs can affect plasma glucose and insulin concentrations [151,152]. The tricyclic antidepressant, nortriptyline, worsens glycemic control [153], and has been shown to reduce insulin concentrations in animal studies [152]. There is also a single case report in the literature of another tricyclic agent, clomipramine, causing significant symptomatic hyperglycemia which resolved when the drug was discontinued and recurred when the patient was rechallenged with the drug [154]. The selective serotonin reuptake inhibitors (SSRIs), fluoxetine and fluvoxamine, cause hyperglycemia in mice, apparently because increased serotonergic neurotransmission enhances catecholamine release from the adrenal medulla while suppressing insulin release [151]. This does not, however, appear to be a significant problem in humans; indeed, various antidepressant drugs, including SSRIs, have been shown to improve glycemic control in patients with diabetes by decreasing appetite while relieving depression and helping to improve compliance with antidiabetic treatment [155].

Other drugs

- *Asparaginase* (crisantaspase), an anticancer drug used to treat acute lymphoblastic leukemia, causes predictable impairment of glucose tolerance which is secondary to insulin resistance. In one trial in children, 10% of cases developed hyperglycemia, and all showed glycosuria [156].
- *Oxymetholone* and *danazol*, certain synthetic steroid derivatives with androgenic properties, impair glucose tolerance, probably by inducing insulin resistance at a post-receptor site [157]; stimulation of glucagon secretion may also contribute [158].
- *Nicotinic acid*, used to treat dyslipidemia, is reported to cause hyperglycemia which is occasionally severe [118,159], although no such deleterious effect was observed in a recent trial in people with diabetes [160]. Its analog, acipimox, does not have adverse effects on glycemic control in people with diabetes [161].
- *Phenytoin* can cause hyperosmolar hyperglycemic syndrome or overt diabetes by interfering with calcium ion entry into β-cells, thus inhibiting insulin secretion [162].
- *Gatifloxacin* is a broad-spectrum 8-methoxyfluoroquinolone antibacterial agent previously used to treat a variety of infections. There have been several postmarketing reports of dysglycemia, both hypoglycemia and hyperglycemia, associated with the use of

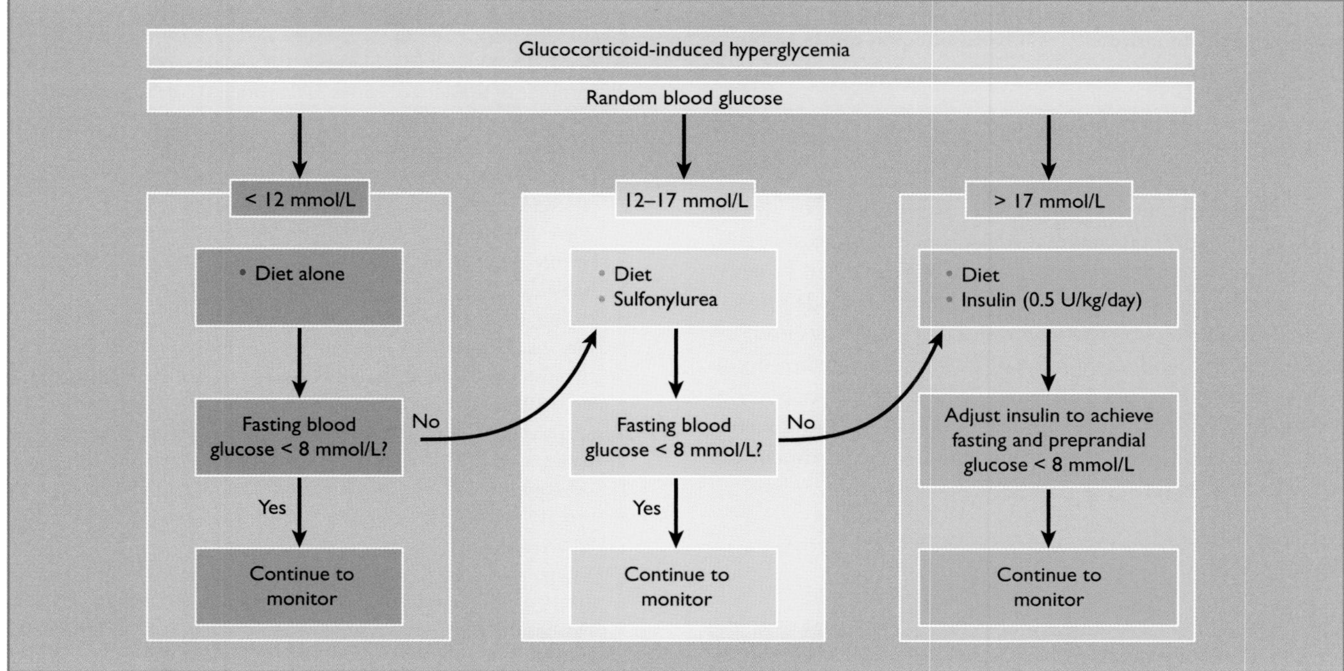

Figure 16.5 Treatment algorithm for glucocorticoid-induced hyperglycemia.

gatifloxacin [163,164]. The incidence of gatifloxacin-induced hyperglycemia is estimated at around 1%, and reported cases have involved both new-onset diabetes and worsening of glycemic control in patients with existing diabetes. The exact underlying mechanism is unknown, but data from animal studies point towards possible inhibition of insulin secretion [164] or increased secretion of epinephrine [165].

Transient hyperglycemia has been described following treatment or overdose with a number of commonly prescribed drugs such as non-steroidal anti-inflammatory drugs [166] and isoniazid. There are also anecdotal reports of drug-induced hyperglycemia associated with nalidixic acid [167], carbamazepine [168], encainide [169], benzodiazepines [170] and mianserin [171].

Treatment of drug-induced hyperglycemia

Clinically relevant hyperglycemia occurs most commonly with high doses of glucocorticoids. If hyperglycemia occurs during thiazide treatment, the need for the drug should be reassessed. If a diuretic is required, then a small dose of furosemide or bumetanide may be substituted. If an antihypertensive agent is needed, it may be possible to reduce the dosage of bendroflumethiazide (e.g. to 2.5 mg/day), or to replace it with another class of drug.

Steroid-induced diabetes

It may not be possible to withdraw glucocorticoid therapy, although "steroid-sparing" immunosuppressive drugs such as azathioprine can sometimes be introduced for certain indications. Other measures are often needed to control hyperglycemia. Management depends primarily upon the severity of hyperglycemia (Figure 16.5). Random blood glucose measurements provide only an approximate guide, and therapy should be adjusted by frequent blood glucose monitoring; simple relief of symptoms alone is inadequate. A target fasting blood glucose concentration of <8 mmol/L may be suitable in the short term, and the usual criteria for good control should be applied if long-term glucocorticoid therapy is undertaken (see Chapter 20).

If significant hyperglycemia develops with high-dose glucocorticoid therapy (e.g. prednisolone 40 mg/day or more), insulin therapy may be started at 0.5 U/kg bodyweight per day, divided between morning and evening doses of short- and intermediate-acting insulin. This dosage is unlikely to produce hypoglycemia and indeed may need to be increased progressively, as dictated by blood glucose monitoring. If the patient presents as a hyperglycemic emergency, standard therapy with intravenous insulin should be started; because steroids induce insulin resistance, insulin delivery rates of 6–8 U/hour may be required initially (see Chapter 34).

Patients with diabetes who are to begin high-dosage glucocorticoid therapy must be warned that their glycemic control will worsen, and treatment for their diabetes should be adjusted prospectively. Those with T2DM treated by diet alone and whose fasting blood glucose concentration is 7–10 mmol/L will require addition of a sulfonylurea or insulin, while those poorly controlled with high dosages of oral agent will need insulin therapy. For patients already taking insulin, the dosage may need to be increased by 50% initially, starting on the same day as steroid therapy. Further adjustments will be based upon results of blood glucose monitoring.

Conclusions

Many drugs can cause hyperglycemia and diabetes, or worsen blood glucose control in patients with diabetes. The possible contribution of diabetogenic drugs should be considered in newly diagnosed patients with diabetes, or if hyperglycemia develops in subjects with previously well-controlled diabetes. Drug effects are often reversible and there are often alternative treatments to achieve the same therapeutic goals. Where the prescription of diabetogenic drugs is inevitable, careful monitoring of glycemic control and prudent use of suitable antidiabetic treatment can mitigate their effects.

References

1 Lithell H. Insulin resistance and cardiovascular drugs. *Clin Exp Hypertens* 1992; **14**:151–162.
2 Lithell H. Effect of antihypertensive drugs on insulin, glucose, and lipid metabolism. *Diabetes Care* 1991; **14**:203–209.
3 Mancini M, Ferrara A, Strazzullo P, Marotta T. Metabolic disturbances and antihypertensive therapy. *J Hypertens* 1991; **9**(Suppl): S47–S50.
4 Pool P, Seagren S, Salel A. Metabolic consequences of treating hypertension. *Am J Hypertens* 1991; **4**:494S–502S.
5 Berne C, Pollare T, Lithell H. Effects of antihypertensive treatment on insulin sensitivity with special reference to ACE inhibitors. *Diabetes Care* 1991; **14**(Suppl. 4):39–47.
6 Skarfors E, Selinus K, Lithell H. Risk factors for developing non-insulin dependent diabetes: a 10 year follow up of men in Uppsala. *Br Med J* 1991; **303**:755–760.
7 Bengtsson C. Incidence of diabetes during antihypertensive treatment. *Horm Metab Res* 1990; **22**(Suppl):38–42.
8 Selye H. *Textbook of Endocrinology*. Montreal: Acta Endocrinologica, 1947.
9 Long CNH, Lukens FDW. The effects of adrenalectomy and hypophysectomy upon experimental diabetes in the cat. *J Exp Med* 1936; **63**:465–490.
10 Ingle DJ. The production of glycosuria in the normal rat by means of 17-hydroxy-11-dehydrocorticosterone. *Endocrinology* 1941; **29**:649–652.
11 Conn J, Fajans S. Symposium on the influence of adrenal cortical steroids on carbohydrate metabolism in man. *Metab Clin Exp* 1956; **5**:114–121.
12 Issekutz C, Allen M. Effect of catecholamines and methylprednisolone on carbohydrate metabolism in dogs. *Metab Clin Exp* 1972; **21**:48–51.
13 Kahn C, Megyesi R, Bar R, *et al.* Receptors for peptide hormones: new insights into the pathophysiology of disease states in man. *Ann Intern Med* 1977; **86**: 205–211.
14 Munck A. Glucocorticoid inhibition of glucose uptake by peripheral tissues: old and new evidence, molecular mechanisms, and physiological significance. *Perspect Biol Med* 1971; **14**:265–271.
15 Owen O, Cahill G. Metabolic effects of exogenous glucocorticoids in fasted man. *J Clin Invest* 1973; **52**:2596–2600.
16 Hench PS, Kendall EC, Slocumb CH, Polley HF. The effect of a hormone of the adrenal cortex (17-hydroxy-11-dehydrocorticosterone: compound E) and of pituitary adrenocorticotropic hormone on rheumatoid arthritis. *Proc Mayo Clin* 1949; **24**:181–197.
17 van Staa TP, Leufkens HGM, Abenhaim L, *et al.* Use of oral corticosteroids in the United Kingdom. *Q J Med* 2000; **93**:105–111.
18 Office for National Statistics. *Key Health Statistics from General Practice 1996* (Series MB6 No. 1). London: Office for National Statistics, 1998.
19 Pagano G, Caballo-Perin P, Cassader M, Bruno A, Ozzello A, Masciola P, *et al.* An *in vivo* and *in vitro* study of the mechanism of prednisolone-induced insulin resistance in healthy subjects. *J Clin Invest* 1983; **72**:1814–1820.
20 Schubert G, Schulz H. Contribution to the clinical picture of steroid diabetes. *Dtsch Med Wochenschr* 1963; **8**:1175–1188.
21 Lieberman P, Patterson R, Kunske R. Complications of long-term steroid therapy for asthma. *J Allergy Clin Immunol* 1972; **49**:329–336.
22 Wajngot A, Giacca A, Grill V, Vranic M, Efendic S. The diabetogenic effects of glucocorticoids are more pronounced in low- than in high-insulin responders. *Proc Natl Acad Sci U S A* 1992; **89**:6035–6039.
23 Efendic S, Luft R, Wajngot A. Aspects of the pathogenesis of type 2 diabetes. *Endocr Rev* 1984; **5**:395–410.
24 Gulliford MC, Charlton J, Latinovic R. Risk of diabetes associated with prescribed glucocorticoids in a large population. *Diabetes Care* 2006; **29**:2728–2729.
25 Turnbow M, Keller S, Rice K, Garner CW. Dexamethasone down-regulation of insulin receptor substrate-1 in 3T3-L1 adipocytes. *J Biol Chem* 1994; **269**:2516–2520.
26 Hosker JP, Burnett MA, Matthews DR, Turner RC. Prednisolone enhances beta-cell function independently of ambient glycemic levels in type II diabetes. *Metabolism* 1993; **42**:1116–1120.
27 Gomez E, Frost P. Induction of glycosuria and hyperglycaemia by topical corticosteroid therapy. *Arch Dermatol* 1976; **112**:1559–1562.
28 Hengge UR, Ruzicka T, Schwartz RA, Cork MJ. Adverse effects of topical glucocorticosteroids. *J Am Acad Dermatol* 2006; **54**:1–15.
29 Faul JL, Tormey V, Burke C. High dose corticosteroids and dose dependent loss of diabetic control. *Br Med J* 1998; **317**:1491.
30 Gobbi M, Scudeletti M. Deflazacort in the treatment of haematologic disorders. *Eur J Clin Pharmacol* 1993; **45**(Suppl. 1):S25–S28.
31 Atef M, Hanafy M, Arbid M. Enhanced diabetogenic effects of combined treatment with hydrochlorothiazide and prednisolone in adjuvant arthritic rats. *Pharmacology* 1991; **42**:177–180.
32 Bailey CJ, Flatt PR. Insulin releasing effects of adrenocorticotropin (ACTH 1–39) and ACTH fragments (1–24 and 18–39) in lean and genetically obese hyperglycaemic (ob/ob) mice. *Int J Obes* 1987; **11**:175–181.
33 Knudtzon J. Acute *in vivo* effects of adrenocorticotrophin on plasma levels of glucagon, insulin, glucose and free fatty acids in rabbits: involvement of the alpha-adrenergic nervous system. *J Endocrinol* 1984; **100**:345–352.
34 Schacke H, Berger M, Rehwinkel H, Asadullah K. Selective glucocorticoid receptor agonists (SEGRAs): novel ligands with an improved therapeutic index. *Mol Cell Endocrinol* 2007; **275**:109–117.

35 Escalante Pulido JM, Alpizar Salazar M. Changes in insulin sensitivity, secretion and glucose effectiveness during menstrual cycle. *Arch Med Res* 1999; **30**:19–22.

36 Kojima T, Lindheim SR, Duffy DM, Vijod MA, Stanczyk FZ, Lobo RA. Insulin sensitivity is decreased in normal women by doses of ethinyl estradiol used in oral contraceptives. *Am J Obstet Gynecol* 1993; **169**:1540–1544.

37 Petersen KR, Christiansen E, Madsbad S, Skouby SO, Andersen LF, Jespersen J. Metabolic and fibrinolytic response to changed insulin sensitivity in users of oral contraceptives. *Contraception* 1999; **60**:337–344.

38 Dorflinger LJ. Metabolic effects of implantable steroid contraceptives for women. *Contraception* 2002; **65**:47–62.

39 Kahn HS, Curtis KM, Marchbanks PA. Effects of injectable or implantable progestin-only contraceptives on insulin-glucose metabolism and diabetes risk. *Diabetes Care* 2003; **26**:216–225.

40 Spellacy W. A review of carbohydrate metabolism and the oral contraceptives. *Am J Obstet Gynecol* 1969; **104**:448–460.

41 Szabo A, Cole H, Grimaldi R. Glucose tolerance in gestational diabetic women during and after treatment with a combination-type oral contraceptive. *N Engl J Med* 1970; **282**:646–650.

42 Beck P, Wells S. Comparison of the mechanisms underlying carbohydrate intolerance in subclinical diabetic women during pregnancy and during post-partum oral contraceptive steroid treatment. *J Clin Endocrinol Metab* 1969; **29**:107–118.

43 Kjos SL, Peters RK, Xiang A, Thomas D, Schaefer U, Buchanan TA. Contraception and the risk of type 2 diabetes mellitus in Latina women with prior gestational diabetes mellitus. *JAMA* 1998; **280**:533–538.

44 Rimm E, Manson J, Stampfer M, Colditz GA, Willett WC, Rosner B, *et al*. Oral contraceptive use and the risk of type 2 (non-insulin-dependent) diabetes mellitus in a large prospective study of women. *Diabetologia* 1992; **35**:967–972.

45 Crook D, Godsland IF, Worthington M, Felton CV, Proudler AJ, Stevenson JC. A comparative metabolic study of two low-estrogen-dose oral contraceptives containing desogestrel or gestodene progestins. *Am J Obstet Gynecol* 1993; **169**:1183–1189.

46 Chasan-Taber L, Willett WC, Stampfer MJ, Hunter DJ, Colditz GA, Spiegelman D, *et al.* A prospective study of oral contraceptives and NIDDM among US women. *Diabetes Care* 1997; **20**:330–335.

47 Petersen KR, Skouby SO, Jespersen J. Contraception guidance in women with pre-existing disturbances in carbohydrate metabolism. *Eur J Contracept Reprod Health Care* 1996; **1**:53–59.

48 Lopez LM, Grimes DA, Shulz KF. Steroidal contraceptives: effect on carbohydrate metabolism in women without diabetes mellitus. *Cochrane Database Syst Rev* 2007; CD006133.

49 Girling JDE, Swiet M. Contraception for women with diabetes or hypertension. *Trends Urol Gynaecol Sexual Health* 1997; **2**:23–34.

50 Kjos SL. Contraception in diabetic women. *Obstet Gynecol Clin North Am* 1996; **23**:243–258.

51 World Health Organization (WHO). Improving access to quality care in family planning; medical eligibility criteria for contraceptive use. 2004. http://www.who.int/reproductive-health/publications/mec/

52 Shawe J, Mulnier H, Nicholls P, Lawrenson R. Use of hormonal contraceptive methods by women with diabetes. *Prim Care Diabetes* 2008; **2**:195–199.

53 Gaspard U, Lefebone P. Clinical aspects of the relationship between oral contraceptive pills, abnormalities in carbohydrate metabolism, and the development of cardiovascular disease. *Am J Obstet Gynecol* 1990; **163**:334–343.

54 Kaplan RC, Heckbert SR, Weiss NS, Wahl PW, Smith NL, Newton KM, *et al.* Postmenopausal estrogens and risk of myocardial infarction in diabetic women. *Diabetes Care* 1998; **21**:1117–1121.

55 Newton KM, LaCroix AZ, Heckbert SR, Abraham L, McCulloch D, Barlow W. Estrogen therapy and risk of cardiovascular events among women with type 2 diabetes. *Diabetes Care* 2003; **26**:2810–2816.

56 Anderson GL, Limacher M, Assaf AR, Bassford T, Beresford SA, Black H, *et al.* Effects of conjugated equine estrogen in postmenopausal women with hysterectomy: the Women's Health Initiative randomized controlled trial. *JAMA* 2004; **291**:1701–1712.

57 Friday KE, Dong C, Fontenot RU. Conjugated equine estrogen improves glycemic control and blood lipoproteins in post-menopausal women with type 2 diabetes. *J Clin Endocrinol Metab* 2001; **86**:48–52.

58 Kernohan AF, Sattar N, Hilditch T, Cleland SJ, Small M, Lumsden MA, *et al.* Effects of low-dose continuous combined hormone replacement therapy on glucose homeostasis and markers of cardiovascular risk in women with type 2 diabetes. *Clin Endocrinol (Oxf)* 2007; **66**:27–34.

59 Margolis KL, Bonds DE, Rodabough RJ, Tinker L, Phillips LS, Allen C, *et al.* Effect of oestrogen plus progestin on the incidence of diabetes in postmenopausal women: results from the Women's Health Initiative Hormone Trial. *Diabetologia* 2004; **47**:1175–1187.

60 Bonds DE, Lasser N, Qi L, Brzyski R, Caan B, Heiss G, *et al.* The effect of conjugated equine oestrogen on diabetes incidence: the Women's Health Initiative randomised trial. *Diabetologia* 2006; **49**:459–468.

61 Salpeter SR, Walsh JM, Ormiston TM, Greyber E, Buckley NS, Salpeter EE. Meta-analysis: effect of hormone-replacement therapy on components of the metabolic syndrome in postmenopausal women. *Diabetes Obes Metab* 2006; **8**:538–554.

62 Wilkins R. New drugs for the treatment of hypertension. *Ann Intern Med* 1959; **50**:1–10.

63 Duke M. Thiazide-induced hypokalemia: association with acute myocardial infarction and ventricular fibrillation. *JAMA* 1978; **239**:43–49.

64 Goldner M, Zurkowitz H, Akgun S. Hyperglycemia and glycosuria due to thiazide derivatives administered in diabetes mellitus. *N Engl J Med* 1960; **262**:403–405.

65 Shapiro A, Benedek T, Small J. Effect of thiazides on carbohydrate metabolism in patients with hypertension. *N Engl J Med* 1961; **265**:1028–1033.

66 Lewis P, Kohner E, Petrie A, Dollery CT. Deterioration of glucose tolerance in hypertensive patients on prolonged diuretic treatment. *Lancet* 1976; **i**:564–566.

67 Murphy M, Lewis P, Kohner E, Schumer B, Dollery CT. Glucose intolerance in hypertensive patients treated with diuretics: 14 year follow-up. *Lancet* 1982; **ii**:1293–1295.

68 Amery A, Wasir H, Bulpitt C, Conway J, Fagard R, Lijnen P, *et al.* Glucose intolerance during diuretic therapy: results of trial by the European Working Party on Hypertension in the Elderly. *Lancet* 1978; **i**:681–683.

69 Nguyen K. Are thiazides diabetogenic? *Tidsskr Nor Laegeforen* 1993; **113**:2587–2589.

70 Freis D. Adverse effects of diuretics. *Drug Saf* 1992; **7**:364–373.

71 Anderson O, Gudbrandsson T, Jamerson K. Metabolic adverse effects of thiazide diuretics: the importance of normokalaemia. *J Intern Med* 1991; **735**(Suppl.):89–96.

72 Sagild U, Andersen V, Andreasen P. Glucose tolerance and insulin responsiveness in experimental potassium depletion. *Acta Med Scand* 1961; **169**:243–251.

73 Helderman J, Elahi D, Andersen D, Raizes GS, Tobin JD, Shocken D, *et al.* Prevention of the glucose intolerance of thiazide diuretics by maintenance of body potassium. *Diabetes* 1983; **32**:106–111.

74 Berglund G, Andersson O, Widgren B. Low dose anti-hypertensive treatment with a thiazide diuretic is not diabetogenic. *Acta Med Scand* 1986; **220**:419–424.

75 Cutler JA. Thiazide-associated glucose abnormalities: prognosis, etiology, and prevention: is potassium balance the key? *Hypertension* 2006; **48**:198–200.

76 Rapoport M, Hurd H. Thiazide-induced glucose intolerance treated with potassium. *Arch Intern Med* 1964; **113**:405–408.

77 Zillich AJ, Garg J, Basu S, Bakris GL, Carter BL. Thiazide diuretics, potassium, and the development of diabetes: a quantitative review. *Hypertension* 2006; **48**:219–224.

78 Jacob S, Rett K, Henriksen EJ. Antihypertensive therapy and insulin sensitivity: do we have to redefine the role of beta-blocking agents? *Am J Hypertens* 1998; **11**:1258–1265.

79 Helgeland A, Leren P, Foss OP, Hjermann I, Holme I, Lund-Larse, PG. Serum glucose levels during long-term observation of treated and untreated men with mild hypertension: the Oslo study. *Am J Med* 1984; **76**:802–805.

80 Bangalore S, Parkar S, Grossman E, Messerli FH. A meta-analysis of 94,492 patients with hypertension treated with beta blockers to determine the risk of new-onset diabetes mellitus. *Am J Cardiol* 2007; **100**:1254–1262.

81 Bakris GL, Fonseca V, Katholi RE, McGill JB, Messerli FH, Phillips RA, *et al.* Metabolic effects of carvedilol vs metoprolol in patients with type 2 diabetes mellitus and hypertension: a randomized controlled trial. *JAMA* 2004; **292**:2227–2236.

82 Trost B, Weidmann P. Effects of calcium antagonists on glucose homeostasis and serum lipids in non-diabetic and diabetic subjects: a review. *J Hypertens* 1987; **5**(Suppl. 4):S81–S104.

83 Charles S, Ketelslegers J, Buysschaert M, Lambert AE. Hyperglycaemic effect of nifedipine. *Br Med J* 1981; **283**:19–20.

84 Leonetti G, Pasotti C, Ferrari G, Zanchetti A. Double-blind comparison of the antihypertensive effects of verapamil and propranolol. In: Zanchetti A, Krikler D, eds. *Calcium Antagonism in Cardiovascular Therapy: Experience with Verapamil.* Amsterdam: Excerpta Medica, 1981: pp. 260–269.

85 De Marinis L, Barbarino A. Calcium antagonists and hormone release, 1: effects of verapamil on insulin release in normal subjects and patients with islet-cell tumour. *Metabolism* 1980; **29**:599–604.

86 Sando H, Katagiri H, Okada M, *et al.* The effect of nifedipine and nicardipine on glucose tolerance, insulin and C-peptide. *Diabetes* 1983; **32**(Suppl. 1):66A.

87 Deedwania P, Shah J, Robison C, *et al.* Effects of nifedipine on glucose tolerance and insulin release in man. *J Am Cardiol* 1984; **3**:577.

88 Bhatnagar SK, Amin MM, Al-Yusuf A. Diabetogenic effects of nifedipine. *Br Med J* 1984; **289**:19.

89 Barbarino A, De Marinis L, Mancini A, Calabró F, Massari M, D'Amico C, *et al.* Calcium antagonists and hormone release, 6: effects of a calcium antagonist (verapamil) on the biphasic insulin release *in vivo*. *Diabetes Res* 1988; **8**: 21–24.

90 De Marinis L, Barbarino A. Calcium antagonists and hormone release, 1: effects of verapamil on insulin release in normal subjects and patients with islet-cell tumor. *Metabolism* 1980; **29**:599–604.

91 Kline JA, Raymond RM, Schroeder JD, Watts JA. The diabetogenic effects of acute verapamil poisoning. *Toxicol Appl Pharmacol* 1997; **145**:357–362.

92 Levine M, Boyer EW, Pozner CN, Geib AJ, Thomsen T, Mick N, *et al.* Assessment of hyperglycemia after calcium channel blocker overdoses involving diltiazem or verapamil. *Crit Care Med* 2007; **35**:2071–2075.

93 Buhler F. The case for calcium antagonists as first-line treatment of hypertension. *J Hypertens* 1992; **10**(Suppl):S17–S20.

94 Klauser R, Prager R, Gaube S, Gisinger C, Schnack C, Küenburg E, *et al.* Metabolic effects of isradipine versus hydrochlorothiazide in diabetes mellitus. *Hypertension* 1991; **17**:15–21.

95 Andronico G, Piazza G, Mangano M, Mule G, Carone MB, Cerasola G. Nifedipine vs. enalapril in treatment of hypertensive patients with glucose intolerance. *J Cardiovasc Pharmacol* 1991; **18**(Suppl. 10):S52–S54.

96 Hedner T, Samuelsson O, Lindholm L. Effects of antihypertensive therapy on glucose tolerance: focus on calcium antagonists. *J Intern Med* 1991; **735**(Suppl):101–111.

97 Grinspoon S, Bilezikian J. HIV disease and the endocrine system. *N Engl J Med* 1992; **327**:1360–1365.

98 Waskin H, Stehr-Green J, Helmick C, Sattler FR. Risk factors for hypoglycemia associated with pentamidine therapy for *Pneumocystis* pneumonia. *JAMA* 1988; **260**: 345–347.

99 Perronne C, Bricaire F, Leport C, Assan D, Vilde JL, Assan R. Hypoglycaemia and diabetes following parenteral pentamidine mesylate treatment in AIDS patients. *Diabet Med* 1990; **7**:585–589.

100 Assan R, Perronne C, Assan D, Chotard L, Mayaud C, Matheron S, *et al.* Pentamidine-induced derangements of glucose homeostasis: determinant roles of renal failure and drug accumulation. *Diabetes Care* 1995; **18**:47–55.

101 Tsiodras S, Mantzoros C, Hammer S, Samore M. Effects of protease inhibitors on hyperglycemia, hyperlipidemia, and lipodystrophy: a 5-year cohort study. *Arch Intern Med* 2000; **160**:2050–2056.

102 Dever LL, Oruwari PA, Figueroa WE, O'Donovan CA, Eng RH. Hyperglycemia associated with protease inhibitors in an urban HIV-infected minority patient population. *Ann Pharmacother* 2000; **34**:580–584.

103 Carr A, Samaras K, Burton S, Law M, Freund J, Chisolm DJ, Cooper DA. A syndrome of peripheral lipodystrophy, hyperlipidaemia and insulin resistance in patients receiving HIV protease inhibitors. *AIDS* 1998; **12**:F51–F58.

104 Calza L, Manfredi R, Chiodo F. Insulin resistance and diabetes mellitus in HIV-infected patients receiving antiretroviral therapy. *Metab Syndr Relat Disord* 2004; **2**:241–250.

105 Rudich A, Vanounou S, Riesenberg K, Porat M, Tirosh A, Harman-Boehm I, *et al.* The HIV protease inhibitor nelfinavir induces insulin resistance and increases basal lipolysis in 3T3-L1 adipocytes. *Diabetes* 2001; **50**:1425–1431.

106 Caron M, Auclair R, Vigoroux C, Glorian M, Forest C, Capeau J. The HIV protease inhibitor indinavir impairs sterol regulatory element-binding protein-1 intranuclear localization, inhibits preadipocyte differentiation, and induces insulin resistance. *Diabetes* 2001; **50**:1378–1388.

107 Gundogdu A, Brown P, Juul S, Sachs L, Sönksen PH. Comparison of hormonal and metabolic effects of salbutamol infusion in normal subjects and insulin-requiring diabetics. *Lancet* 1979; **ii**:1317–1321.

108 Thomas DJB, Goldberg R, Taylor MW, Imura H, Potter DE. Salbutamol-induced diabetic ketoacidosis. *Br Med J* 1977; **2**:438–440.

109 Portnoy J, Nadel G, Amado M, Willsie-Ediger S. Continuous nebulization for status asthmaticus. *Ann Allergy* 1992; **69**:71–79.

110 NICE Guidance. Diabetes in pregnancy: management of diabetes and its complications from preconception to the postnatal period. 2008. http://www.nice.org.uk/nicemedia/pdf/DiabetesFullGuidelineRevisedJULY2008.pdf.

111 Hamburg S, Hendler R, Sherwin R. Influence of small increments of epinephrine on glucose tolerance in normal humans. *Ann Intern Med* 1980; **93**:566–568.

112 Svedjeholm R, Hallhagen S, Ekroth R, Joachimsson PO, Ronquist G. Dopamine and high-dose insulin infusion (glucose–insulin–potassium) after a cardiac operation: effects on myocardial metabolism. *Ann Thorac Surg* 1991; **52**:262–270.

113 Gill GV, Rauf O, MacFarlane IA. Diazoxide treatment for insulinoma: a national UK survey. *Postgrad Med J* 1997; **73**:640–641.

114 Lunetta M, Di Mauro M, Le Moli R, Nicoletti F. Effects of octreotide on glycaemic control, glucose disposal, hepatic glucose production and counter-regulatory hormones secretion in type 1 and type 2 insulin treated diabetic patients. *Diabetes Res Clin Pract* 1997; **38**:81–89.

115 Verschoor L, Lamberts SW, Uitterlinden P, Del Pozo E. Glucose tolerance during long term treatment with a somatostatin analogue. *Br Med J* 1986; **293**:1327–1328.

116 Giusti M, Gussoni G, Cuttica CM, Giordano G. Effectiveness and tolerability of slow release lanreotide treatment in active acromegaly: six-month report on an Italian multicenter study. Italian Multicenter Slow Release Lanreotide Study Group. *J Clin Endocrinol Metab* 1996; **81**:2089–2097.

117 Attanasio R, Lanzi R, Losa M, Valentini F, Grimaldi F, De Menis E, *et al.* Effects of lanreotide Autogel on growth hormone, insulinlike growth factor 1, and tumor size in acromegaly: a 1-year prospective multicenter study. *Endocr Pract* 2008; **14**:846–855.

118 Ben Shlomo A, Melmed S. Somatostatin agonists for treatment of acromegaly. *Mol Cell Endocrinol* 2008; **286**:192–198.

119 Ayuk J, Stewart SE, Stewart PM, Sheppard MC. Long-term safety and efficacy of depot long-acting somatostatin analogs for the treatment of acromegaly. *J Clin Endocrinol Metab* 2002; **87**:4142–4146.

120 Chan JC, Cockram CS, Critchley JA. Drug-induced disorders of glucose metabolism: mechanisms and management. *Drug Saf* 1996; **15**:135–157.

121 Moore DF, Wood DF, Volans GN. Features, prevention and management of acute overdose due to antidiabetic drugs. *Drug Saf* 1993; **9**:218–229.

122 Phillips RE, Looareesuwran S, Molyneux ME, Hatz C, Warrell DA. Hypoglycaemia and counterregulatory hormone responses in severe falciparum malaria: treatment with Sandostatin. *Q J Med* 1993; **86**:233–240.

123 Fasano CJ, O'Malley G, Dominici P, Aguilera E, Latta DR. Comparison of octreotide and standard therapy versus standard therapy alone for the treatment of sulfonylurea-induced hypoglycemia. *Ann Emerg Med* 2008; **51**:400–406.

124 Wilson DM. Clinical actions of growth hormone. *Endocrinol Metab Clin N Am* 1992; **21**:519–537.

125 Cutfield WS, Wilton P, Benmarker H, Albertsson-Wikland K, Chatelain P, Ranke MB, *et al.* Incidence of diabetes mellitus and impaired glucose tolerance in children and adolescents receiving growth-hormone treatment. *Lancet* 2000; **355**:610–613.

126 Monson JP. Long-term experience with GH replacement therapy: efficacy and safety. *Eur J Endocrinol* 2003; **148**(Suppl 2):S9–S14.

127 Jorgensen JO, Moller L, Krag M, Billestrup N, Christiansen JS. Effects of growth hormone on glucose and fat metabolism in human subjects. *Endocrinol Metab Clin North Am* 2007; **36**:75–87.

128 Schauster AC, Geletko SM, Mikolich DJ. Diabetes mellitus associated with recombinant human growth hormone for HIV wasting syndrome. *Pharmacotherapy* 2000; **20**:1129–1134.

129 Jindal RM, Popescu I, Schwartz ME, Emre S, Boccagni P, Miller CM. Diabetogenicity of FK506 versus cyclosporine in liver transplant recipients. *Transplantation* 1994; **58**:370–372.

130 Roth D, Milgrom M, Esquenazi V, Fuller L, Burke G, Miller J. Posttransplant hyperglycaemia-increased incidence in cyclosporin-treated renal allograft recipients. *Transplantation* 1989; **47**:278–281.

131 Helmchen U, Schmidt W, Siegel E, Creutzfeldt W. Morphological and functional changes of pancreatic B cells in cyclosporin A-treated rats. *Diabetologia* 1984; **27**:416–418.

132 Robertson R. Cyclosporin-induced inhibition of insulin secretion in isolated rat islets and HIT cells. *Diabetes* 1986; **35**:1016–1019.

133 Yale J, Roy R, Grose M, Seemayer TA, Murphy GF, Marliss EB. Effects of cyclosporine on glucose tolerance in the rat. *Diabetes* 1985; **34**:1309–1313.

134 Penfornis A, Kury-Paulin S. Immunosuppressive drug-induced diabetes. *Diabetes Metab* 2006; **32**:539–546.

135 Drachenberg CB, Klassen DK, Weir MR, Wiland A, Fink JC, Bartlett ST, *et al.* Islet cell damage associated with tacrolimus and cyclosporine: morphological features in pancreas allograft biopsies and clinical correlation. *Transplantation* 1999; **68**:396–402.

136 Cosio FG, Pesavento TE, Osei K, Henry ML, Ferguson RM. Post-transplant diabetes mellitus: increasing incidence in renal allograft recipients transplanted in recent years. *Kidney Int* 2001; **59**:732–737.

137 Ericzon B, Groth C, Bismuth H, Calne R, McMaster P, Neuhaus P, *et al.* Glucose metabolism in liver transplant recipients treated with FK 506 or cyclosporin in the European multicentre study. *Transplant Int* 1994; **7**(Suppl. 1):S11–S14.

138 Shapiro R, Scantlebury VP, Jordan ML, Vivas C, Ellis D, Lombardozzi-Lane S, *et al.* Pediatric renal transplantation under tacrolimus-based immunosuppression. *Transplantation* 1999; **67**:299–303.

139 Furth S, Neu A, Colombani P, Plotnick L, Turner ME, Fivush B. Diabetes as a complication of tacrolimus (FK506) in pediatric renal transplant patients. *Pediatr Nephrol* 1996; **10**:64–66.

140 Backman LA. Post-transplant diabetes mellitus: the last 10 years with tacrolimus. *Nephrol Dial Transplant* 2004; **19**(Suppl 6):13–16.

141 Fernandez LA, Lehmann R, Luzi L, Battezzati A, Angelico MC, Ricordi C, *et al.* The effects of maintenance doses of FK506 versus cyclosporin A on glucose and lipid metabolism after orthotopic liver transplantation. *Transplantation* 1999; **68**:1532–1541.

142 Romagnoli J, Citterio F, Nanni G, Favi E, Tondolo V, Spagnoletti G, *et al.* Incidence of posttransplant diabetes mellitus in kidney transplant recipients immunosuppressed with sirolimus in combination with cyclosporine. *Transplant Proc* 2006; **38**:1034–1036.

143 Shaffer D, Kizilisik AT, Feurer I, Nylander WA, Helderman JH, Langone AJ, *et al.* Calcineurin inhibitor avoidance versus steroid

avoidance following kidney transplantation: postoperative complications. *Transplant Proc* 2006; **38**:3464–3465.

144 Veroux M, Corona D, Giuffrida G, Gagliano M, Sorbello M, Virgilio C, *et al.* New-onset diabetes mellitus after kidney transplantation: the role of immunosuppression. *Transplant Proc* 2008; **40**:1885–1887.

145 Bhatti A, McGarrity TJ, Gabbay R. Diabetic ketoacidosis induced by alpha interferon and ribavirin treatment in a patient with hepatitis C. *Am J Gastroenterol* 2001; **96**:604–605.

146 Gatta B, Rigalleau V, Gin H. Diabetic ketoacidosis with olanzapine treatment. *Diabetes Care* 1999; **22**:1002–1003.

147 Colli A, Cocciolo M, Francobandiera F, Rogantin F, Cattalini N. Diabetic ketoacidosis associated with clozapine treatment. *Diabetes Care* 1999; **22**:176–177.

148 Henderson DC, Cagliero E, Gray C, Nasrallah RA, Hayden DL, Schoenfeld DA, *et al.* Clozapine, diabetes mellitus, weight gain, and lipid abnormalities: a five-year naturalistic study. *Am J Psychiatry* 2000; **157**:975–981.

149 Hampson LJ, Mackin P, Agius L. Stimulation of glycogen synthesis and inactivation of phosphorylase in hepatocytes by serotonergic mechanisms, and counter-regulation by atypical antipsychotic drugs. *Diabetologia* 2007; **50**:1743–1751.

150 Leslie DL, Rosenheck RA. Incidence of newly diagnosed diabetes attributable to atypical antipsychotic medications. *Am J Psychiatry* 2004; **161**:1709–1711.

151 Yamada J, Sugimoto Y, Inoue K. Selective serotonin reuptake inhibitors fluoxetine and fluvoxamine induce hyperglycemia by different mechanisms. *Eur J Pharmacol* 1999; **382**:211–215.

152 Erenmemisoglu A, Ozdogan UK, Saraymen R, Tutus A. Effect of some antidepressants on glycaemia and insulin levels of normoglycaemic and alloxan-induced hyperglycaemic mice. *J Pharm Pharmacol* 1999; **51**:741–743.

153 Lustman PJ, Griffith LS, Clouse RE, Freedland KE, Eisen SA, Rubin EH, *et al.* Effects of nortriptyline on depression and glycaemic control in diabetes: results of a double-blind placebo-controlled trial. *Psychosom Med* 1997; **59**:241–250.

154 Mumoli N, Cei M. Clomipramine-induced diabetes. *Ann Intern Med* 2008; **149**:595–596.

155 Lustman PJ, Freedland KE, Griffith LS, Clouse RE. Fluoxetine for depression in diabetes: a randomized double-blind placebo-controlled trial. *Diabetes Care* 2000; **23**:618–623.

156 Pui C, Burghen G, Bowman W, Aur RJ. Risk factors for hyperglycemia in children with leukemia necessitating L-asparaginase and prednisolone. *J Pediatr* 1981; **99**:46.

157 Wynn V. Metabolic effects of danazol. *J Intern Med Res* 1977; **5**(Suppl. 3):25–35.

158 Williams G, Lofts F, Füessl H, Bloom S. Treatment with danazol and plasma glucagon concentration. *Br Med J* 1985; **291**:1155–1156.

159 Schwartz M. Severe reversible hyperglycaemia as a consequence of niacin therapy. *Arch Intern Med* 1993; **153**:2050–2052.

160 Elam MB, Hunninghake DB, Davis KB, Garg R, Johnson C, Egan D, *et al.* Effect of niacin on lipid and lipoprotein levels and glycemic control in patients with diabetes and peripheral arterial disease: the ADMIT study: a randomized trial. Arterial Disease Multiple Intervention Trial. *JAMA* 2000; **284**:1263–1270.

161 Dean JD, McCarthy S, Betteridge DJ, Whately-Smith C, Powell J, Owens DR. The effect of acipimox in patients with type 2 diabetes and persistent hyperlipidaemia. *Diabet Med* 1992; **9**:611–615.

162 Carter B, Small R, Mande M, *et al.* Phenytoin-induced hyperglycemia. *Am J Hosp Pharm* 1981; **38**:1508.

163 Park-Wyllie LY, Juurlink DN, Kopp A, Shah BR, Stukel TA, Stumpo C, *et al.* Outpatient gatifloxacin therapy and dysglycemia in older adults. *N Engl J Med* 2006; **354**:1352–1361.

164 Yip C, Lee AJ. Gatifloxacin-induced hyperglycemia: a case report and summary of the current literature. *Clin Ther* 2006; **28**:1857–1866.

165 Ishiwata Y, Sanada Y, Yasuhara M. Effects of gatifloxacin on serum glucose concentration in normal and diabetic rats. *Biol Pharm Bull* 2006; **29**:527–531.

166 Tkach J, Bozeman M. Indomethacin induced hyperglycaemia. *J Am Acad Dermatol* 1982; **7**:802.

167 Islam M, Sneedharan T. Convulsions, hyperglycemia and glycosuria from overdose of nalidixic acid. *JAMA* 1965; **192**:1100.

168 Seymour J. Carbamazepine overdose: feature of 33 cases. *Drug Saf* 1993; **8**:81–88.

169 Winter W. Encainide-induced diabetes: analysis of islet cell function. *Res Commun Chem Pathol Pharmacol* 1992; **76**:259–268.

170 Najim R, Clor K. Role of endorphins in benzodiazepine-induced hyperglycaemia in mice. *Pharmacol Biochem Behav* 1993; **46**:995–997.

171 Marley J, Rohan A. Mianserin-induced hyperglycaemia. *Lancet* 1993; **342**:1430–1431.

17 Endocrine Disorders that Cause Diabetes

Neil A. Hanley
Endocrine Sciences Research Group, University of Manchester, Manchester, UK

Keypoints

- Endocrine causes of diabetes are mainly a result of an excess of hormones that are counter-regulatory to insulin, and act by inhibiting insulin secretion and/or action.
- Acromegaly is almost always secondary to growth hormone-secreting adenomas of the anterior pituitary somatotrophs and disturbs glucose homeostasis in up to approximately 50% of patients.
- Cushing syndrome is caused by excessive levels of glucocorticoids and disturbs glucose homeostasis to some degree in over 50% of cases.
- Pheochromocytoma is a tumor of the chromaffin cells, which in 90% of cases is located in the adrenal medulla and causes hyperglycemia in approximately 50% of cases.
- Glucagonoma and somatostatinoma are rare islet cell tumors that produce hormones that inhibit the secretion and action of insulin.
- Thyrotoxicosis commonly causes mild glucose intolerance, but overt diabetes only occurs in a tiny minority.
- Other endocrinopathies such as primary aldosteronism and primary hyperparathyroidism can disturb glucose homeostasis.
- Polycystic ovarian syndrome occurs in 5–10% of women of reproductive age and associates with some degree of glucose intolerance or diabetes resulting from insulin resistance in approximately 50% of cases.

Introduction

The primary focus of this chapter is on those endocrine disorders that cause hyperglycemia and where effective treatment of the endocrinopathy can be expected to normalize the blood glucose concentration. These conditions mostly reflect excessive secretion of "counter-regulatory" hormones, the metabolic actions of which oppose those of insulin by inhibiting its secretion, action, or both.

Acromegaly

Etiology, incidence and clinical features of acromegaly

Acromegaly comprises a constellation of symptoms and signs caused by excessive growth hormone (GH) secretion that leads to bony and soft tissue overgrowth accompanied by cardiovascular and metabolic pathology (Figure 17.1a; Table 17.1) [1]. It affects approximately 60 people per million [2] and, in 99% of cases, is caused by a pituitary adenoma, most commonly larger than 1 cm in diameter (a "macroadenoma"; Figure 17.1b). A tiny minority of cases are caused by excessive secretion of GH-releasing hormone (GHRH) from a hypothalamic gangliocytoma or a carcinoid tumor of the lung or pancreas [1]. A small percentage of acromegaly occurs within the wider endocrine syndrome of multiple endocrine neoplasia type 1 (MEN1) caused by mutations in the tumor suppressor gene, *MENIN* [3]. MEN1 can also include glucagonomas and somatostatinomas, both of which are separately capable of causing secondary diabetes. Commonly, acromegaly has been present for a decade prior to diagnosis [4]. This long-standing hypersecretion of GH provides the time necessary for the characteristic external features of the disorder to develop (Figure 17.1a; Table 17.1).

Features of disturbance to glucose tolerance in acromegaly

Glucose intolerance or overt diabetes is common in acromegaly because of the direct hyperglycemic effects of GH excess (Figure 17.2). Overt diabetes has been reported in a range of 19–56% of patients with acromegaly, while impaired glucose intolerance (IGT) affects 16–46% [5–8]. Diabetes is most frequent in patients with higher GH levels [9,10]. There is also a correlation between serum insulin-like growth factor I (IGF-I), and both fasting and post-prandial glucose. In fact, placing age-adjusted IGF-I values into rising quartiles correlated very accurately to decreasing insulin sensitivity such that serum IGF-I levels could predict insulin sensitivity more accurately than either random GH levels or the nadir value following glucose tolerance testing [11].

Clinically, diabetes in acromegaly usually resembles the type 2 form (T2DM), with most patients not needing insulin therapy but being maintained with oral hypoglycemic agents or diet alone

Textbook of Diabetes, 4th edition. Edited by R. Holt, C. Cockram, A. Flyvbjerg and B. Goldstein.

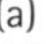

(a)

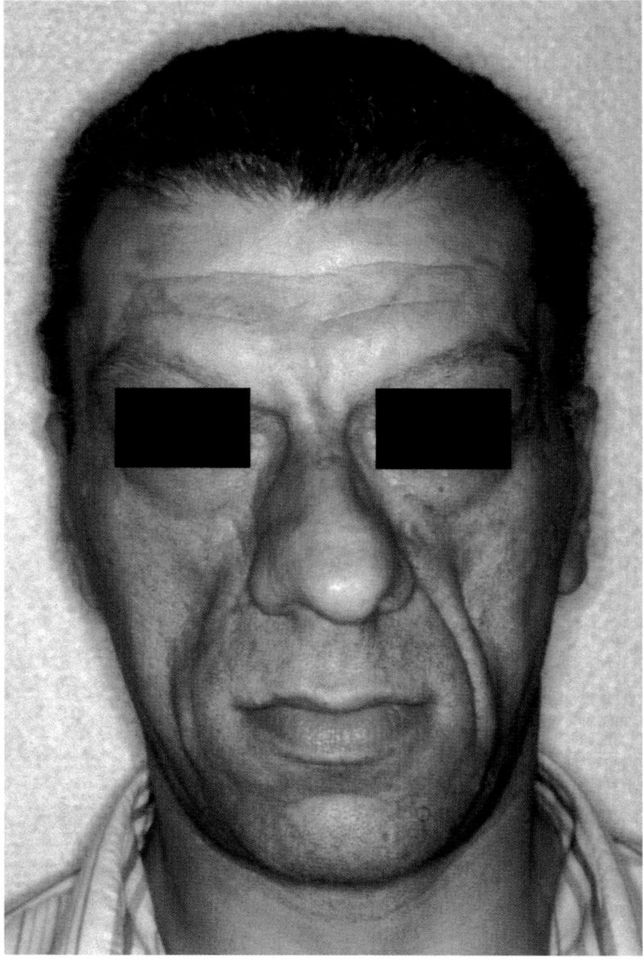

(b)

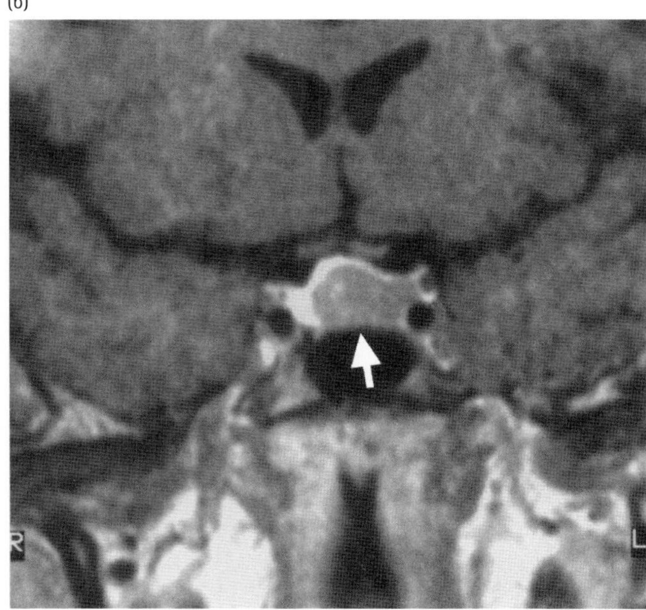

Figure 17.1 Acromegaly in a patient found to have a random blood glucose level of 13 mmol/L during preparation for sinus surgery. Features included: (a) the characteristic facial appearance; (b) a large adenoma (arrow) extending up to but not in contact with the optic chiasm demonstrated by magnetic resonance imaging (R, right; L, left). Following successful trans-sphenoidal removal of the tumor, glucose tolerance returned to normal.

[9]. GH can induce insulin resistance when infused into normal subjects [12,13], and insulin resistance is a consistent feature of people with acromegaly [14,15]. Insulin action is impaired in both the liver and extrahepatic tissues, with decreases in both the suppression of hepatic glucose production and in insulin-dependent glucose disposal [13,15]. For instance, impairment of insulin-mediated activation of glycogen synthase has been demonstrated in skeletal muscle [16–18]. Insulin resistance may also be exacerbated by the lipolytic action of GH, generating non-esterified fatty acids (NEFAs) which act on the liver to increase glucose production and in muscle to inhibit glucose utilization (via the "glucose–fatty acid" cycle) (Figure 17.2). Where pancreatic compensation is adequate, an exaggerated insulin secretory response creating hyperinsulinemia can counterbalance the insulin resistance and maintain euglycemia. Similar to the natural history of deteriorating blood glucose control in T2DM, eventually β-cell compensation fails, the insulin response is impaired and hypergylcemia ensues [14]. This has been termed the Starling curve of the pancreas (see Figure 11.1).

Diagnosis and treatment of acromegaly

GH release is normally pulsatile with intervening periods of low level or undetectable hormone, whereas secretion from pituitary adenomas is autonomous. Therefore, the diagnosis can be deduced from a series of random serum measurements where GH is consistently detected. An alternative, better diagnostic test takes advantage of the negative feedback on GH secretion by glucose. A failure of serum GH to suppress to below 2 mU/L (approximately 1 μg/L) within 3 hours of 75 g oral glucose is diagnostic of acromegaly. A further option, particularly suited as the initial screening test of outpatients, is measurement of serum IGF-I, which if raised above sex- and age-matched controls is diagnostic of acromegaly, unless there is a possibility of GH abuse [1]. It is noteworthy that the diagnosis of acromegaly can be difficult in patients with type 1 diabetes mellitus (T1DM) where GH hypersecretion is observed. Whereas this might compromise the use of serum GH as a diagnostic biomarker of a somatotroph adenoma, IGF-I values tend to be low in poorly controlled T1DM indicative of the state of GH resistance. Thus, raised serum IGF-I values

Table 17.1 Clinical features of acromegaly.

Musculoskeletal
Protruding mandible (prognathia) with lower teeth separation
Big tongue (macroglossia)
Enlarged forehead (frontal bossing)
Large hands and feet (carpal tunnel syndrome, tight rings, increasing shoe size)
Osteoarthritis from abnormal joint loading
Increased stature (gigantism; if GH excess occurs prior to epiphyseal closure)
Skin
Irritating, thickened, greasy (increased sebum production)
Excessive sweating
Cardiovascular
Dilated cardiomyopathy causing cardiomegaly and cardiac failure
Hypertension
Metabolic
Impaired glucose tolerance or potentially diabetes
General
Headaches
Tiredness, often very disabling and lowers quality of life/ability to work
Local tumor effects
Compression of the optic chiasm (superior tumor growth) or cranial nerves III, IV and/ or VI (lateral tumor growth into cavernous sinus)

GH, growth hormone.

remain a confident predictor for a diagnosis of acromegaly in people with T1DM. Having diagnosed acromegaly, magnetic resonance imaging (MRI) of the anterior pituitary defines the extent of the adenoma (Figure 17.1b).

Based on this investigation, symptoms, patient wishes and co-morbidity, and GH levels, treatment can be either surgical, medical or radiotherapy (Table 17.2) [1,19]. When the tumor is a macroadenoma, especially if it extends beyond the pituitary fossa, curative surgery becomes unlikely or impossible; however, surgery can be useful for "debulking" and rapid lowering of serum GH levels in patients who are highly symptomatic, or where the tumor has encroached upon the optic chiasm and affected visual fields. The standard approach is trans-sphenoidal, either via the nostril or from behind the upper lip. Once the sphenoid sinus has been traversed and midline access to the sella turcica gained, tumor is removed from the anteroinferior aspect causing the residual tissue to drop back down into or towards the pituitary fossa. Tumor beyond the fossa, in locations such as the cavernous sinus, cannot be approached directly, hence the reason why surgery for large tumors is not anticipated to be curative [19]. Conversely, cure can be commonly achieved for over 50% of microadenomas (<1 cm diameter). The reported ranges vary widely according to expertise.

Medical therapy, most commonly using somatostatin analogs, is effective at both lowering GH levels and shrinking the tumor volume [1,20,21]. Approximately 60% of patients respond to somatostatin analogs because of the presence of predominantly

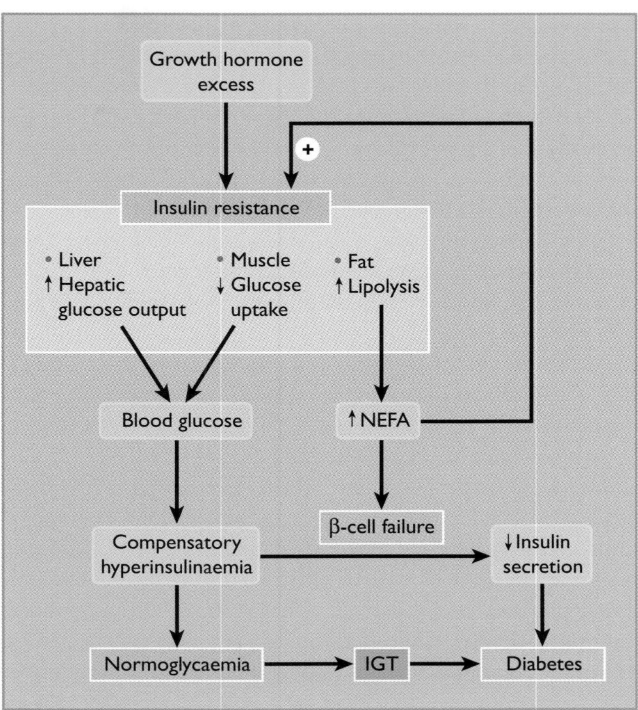

Figure 17.2 Mechanisms of hyperglycemia and diabetes in acromegaly. Diabetes develops if β-cells fail to compensate for the increased demand for insulin. IGT, impaired glucose tolerance; NEFA, non-esterified fatty acid.

Table 17.2 Treatment of acromegaly (Adapted from Holt and Hanley [130].)

Advantages	Disadvantages
Trans-sphenoidal surgery	
Rapid effect	Invasive and requires general anesthetic
Can restore vision in optic nerve compression	Non-curative for large extrasellar tumors
Might be curative if complete resection	
Somatostatin analog drugs	
Non-invasive	Monthly intramuscular injection
May shrink tumor	Expensive
Decreases GH in ~60% of patients	Gastrointestinal side effects (commonly diarrhea)
	Unlikely to be curative (i.e. continuous therapy needed)
Pegvisomant	
Non-invasive	Expensive
Blocks GH action	GH concentrations remain elevated
Radiotherapy	
Non-invasive	Slow to act – may take up to 10 years
Likely to shrink tumor	Standard external three-beam radiotherapy likely to cause hypopituitarism by destroying other pituitary cell types
Likely to reduce GH levels	
Might be curative	

GH, growth hormone.

type 2 and type 5 somatostatin receptors on the tumor cell surface [1,21]. The analogs can be administered subcutaneously; however, once it is clear that they are tolerated, the most common formulation is month-long intramuscular depot preparations. They can be used either prior to surgery, with the goal of operating on a shrunken tumor, on a long-term basis in place of surgery or post-surgery where GH levels have not been normalized.

Some GH-secreting adenomas co-express dopamine receptors more characteristic of prolactinomas [21]. Indeed, 25% of cases of acromegaly show raised levels of both prolactin and GH possibly indicating a tumor cell phenotype more consistent with the somatomammotroph from which it is thought that somatotrophs (GH secretion) and lactotrophs (prolactin secretion) terminally differentiate. In these instances, dopamine agonists, as used in hyperprolactinemia, can be useful, especially as they can be administered orally, and allow reduction in dosage of the more expensive intramuscular depot somatostatin analogs. This opportunity to use lower doses of somatostatin analogs may also lessen their side-effects, such as gastrointestinal disturbance (most commonly diarrhea) and gallstones. It has recently been questioned, however, whether commonly used ergot alkaloid derived dopamine agonists, such as cabergoline, cause fibrotic side-effects, especially involving heart valves [22,23]. Despite concerns from regulatory agencies, the prevailing view from endocrinologists is that the doses of these agents used to treat endocrine disorders (compared with the therapeutic regimens in Parkinson disease) are not problematic. In any case, alternative non-ergot derived agents, such as quinagolide, are available. Bromocriptine is less commonly used because of the almost inevitable side-effects of nausea. Responsiveness to both dopamine and somatostatin analog therapy can be easily assessed at the start of treatment by hourly measurement of serum GH over 8 hours following the administration of a test dose of each agent given sequentially on two consecutive days.

The last decade has seen the appearance of a new clinical agent that blocks GH action. GH induces signal transduction via binding to its receptor as a dimer. Pegvisomant has been developed as a GH antagonist by preventing this dimerization and thus inhibiting GH action. This leaves elevated GH levels from the somatotroph adenoma but, nevertheless, pegvisomant is effective at reversing the clinical features of acromegaly [1,24]. The major problem with its use in many countries has been its prohibitive cost. Concern over tumor growth because of loss of negative feedback (a scenario akin to Nelson syndrome following bilateral adrenalectomy in Cushing disease) seems unfounded [1,24].

Radiation therapy is most commonly administered as conventional three-field external beam radiotherapy [1]. It is effective at lowering GH and IGF-I levels [25]. This approach delivers approximately 4500 Gy to the pituitary region with the total dose calculated such that the optic chiasm receives less than 8 Gy. An alternative is stereotactic radiotherapy (also known as γ-knife therapy or radiosurgery), which by using more sources can focus a higher concentration of radiation to a defined area of tumor. Whereas the latter modality allows greater preservation of adjacent normal pituitary tissue, the former approach is a more all-encompassing strategy to ensure tumor destruction, albeit with a higher post-therapy incidence of hypopituitarism. The choice is important as there is evidence that pituitary radiotherapy is associated with increased morbidity and mortality from subsequent cerebrovascular disease meaning that repeat therapy is not undertaken lightly [26].

Outcome of acromegaly and disturbance to glucose tolerance

Unless there are cogent reasons against, attempts should be made to normalize GH excess in acromegaly to decrease the morbidity and mortality associated with the disorder [1,26]. Curative treatment is best defined by a nadir serum GH of less than 2 mU/L upon 75 g oral glucose challenge. Glucose tolerance improves and insulin levels decrease after successful treatment by pituitary surgery and irradiation [27,28]. Hyperglycemia may worsen in a few patients, presumably those with a stronger underlying tendency to T2DM, when treated with somatostatin analogs because these drugs also suppress insulin secretion [29,30]. In the longer term, somatostatin analogs tend to improve glucose tolerance [31,32]. Insulin sensitivity is also improved with pegvisomant therapy in patients with both glucose intolerance and diabetes [33–36]. If hyperglycemia persists after serum GH levels have been normalized then the patient should be considered as having T2DM. One caveat to this is the possibility of GH deficiency as part of hypopituitarism post-surgery or radiotherapy [14]. GH deficiency causes centripetal fat deposition, which would itself cause or accentuate insulin resistance and potential loss of euglycemia.

Generally, diabetic complications are considered rare in acromegaly. Nevertheless, it is worth considering GH action in the context of both macrovascular and microvascular diabetic complications. Untreated GH excess increases cardiovascular morbidity and mortality and, potentially, abnormalities of glucose metabolism occurring in acromegaly could contribute to hypertension which affects over 50% of patients with acromegaly [5]. GH has been linked to proliferative diabetic retinopathy ever since resolution of diabetic retinopathy was noted in a woman who developed rapid-onset pan-hypopituitarism [37,38], so much so that hypophysectomy was used as treatment prior to the advent of laser photocoagulation [38]. This view is supported by the observations that patients with diabetes who are GH-deficient rarely develop retinopathy [39], and an experimental study in mice demonstrated that inhibition of GH secretion ameliorated diabetic retinopathy [40]. Patients with diabetes who are acromegalic, however, do not show an increased incidence of diabetic retinopathy [41,42]. Data on the progression of diabetic retinopathy treated with either pegvisomant or somatostatin analog are contradictory, and the outcome of larger trials are awaited [38].

Effects of diabetes on GH–IGF-I axis

Dysregulation of the GH–IGF-I axis has been well documented in T1DM. The main disturbances include increased GH secretion (Figure 17.3), paradoxically associated with decreased serum

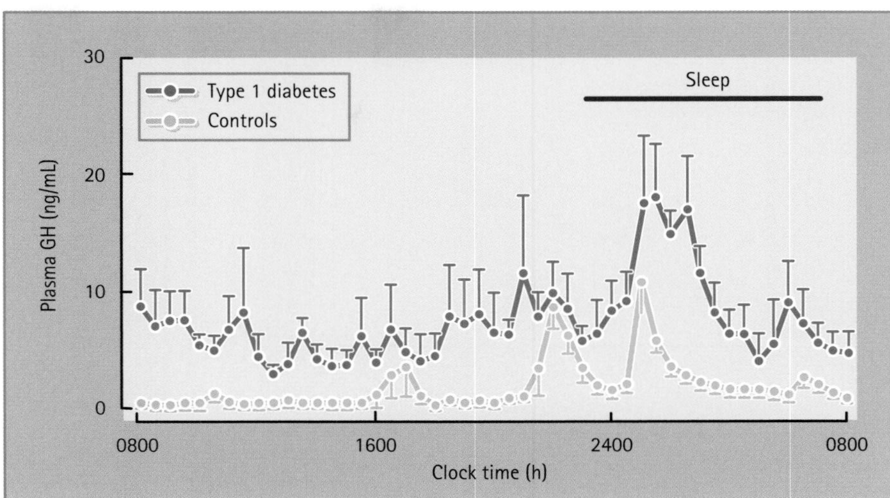

Figure 17.3 Increased growth hormone (GH) secretion in type 1 diabetes. Note the marked hypersecretion during sleep in the early hours of the morning. Reproduced from Hansen *et al.* [127], with permission from Wiley-Blackwell.

IGF-I levels [43]. GH secretory pulses are larger and more frequent and total 24 hour serum and urinary GH levels are elevated. High circulating GH levels are most obvious during periods of poor diabetic control, and return towards normal with improved control. Pulses of GH secretion during sleep in the early hours of the morning lead to insulin resistance, which manifests itself before breakfast and is largely responsible for the "dawn phenomenon" of fasting hyperglycemia [44]. This physiologic effect, along with that caused by exercise and GHRH, is exaggerated in patients with T1DM, especially those who are poorly controlled. GH secretion accounts for much of the decreased insulin sensitivity observed during normal puberty, as well as the deterioration in glycemic control at this time in adolescents with T1DM. Despite GH hypersecretion, levels of IGF-I – the principal mediator of GH activity – are inappropriately low, indicating a state of GH resistance (Figure 17.4). Hepatic resistance to GH has been attributed both to decreased number of GH receptors and to post-receptor defects [43]. Circulating levels of GH-binding protein (GHBP) are also decreased in T1DM. Administration of recombinant human IGF-I (rhIGF-I) as an adjunct to insulin has been demonstrated to reverse GH hypersecretion and improve glycemic control, while reducing insulin requirements. Co-administration of IGF-binding protein 3 (IGFBP-3) with IGF-I has similar beneficial effects on carbohydrate metabolism, and also avoids side effects of IGF-I, notably edema, headache, retinal edema and jaw pain [45]. Recombinant IGF-I has also been used to treat states of severe insulin resistance in which the insulin receptor is functionally impaired, such as the spectrum from Donohue to Rabson–Mendenhall syndrome (see Chapter 15) [46]. In such patients, rhIGF-I can be used to treat ketoacidosis, which is the major cause of death and may fail to respond even to massive doses of insulin.

Abnormalities of IGFBP may also alter the regulation of the GH–IGF-I axis in diabetes (Figure 17.4). Six IGFBPs have been identified in humans, the two most relevant being IGFBP-1 (molecular weight 25 kDa), whose synthesis by hepatocytes is inhibited by insulin but independently of GH, and IGFBP-3 (molecular weight 44 kDa), which is GH-dependent [47]. IGFBP-1 levels are increased in T1DM as a result of portal and hepatic insulin deficiency (Figure 17.4) [43], and increase with worsening insulin deficiency and rising HbA_{1c} concentrations (Figure 17.5). Increased IGFBP-1 levels have been shown to inhibit IGF-I bioactivity. Portal insulin deficiency in T1DM can thus account for

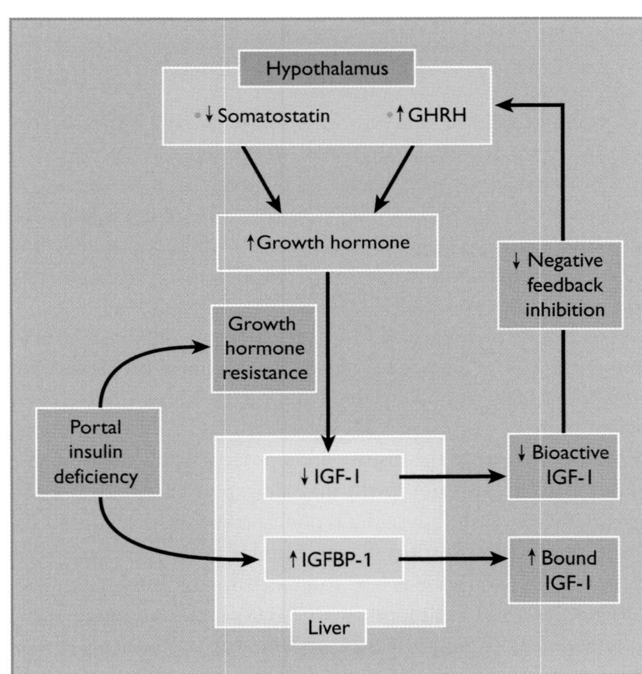

Figure 17.4 Mechanisms of growth hormone (GH) hypersecretion in diabetes. Insulin-like growth factor 1 binding protein 1 (IGFBP-1) binds and reduces the bioavailability of insulin-like growth factor I (IGF-I), which normally decreases GH secretion by negative feedback inhibition on the hypothalamus and pituitary; IGFBP-1 expression is inhibited by insulin.

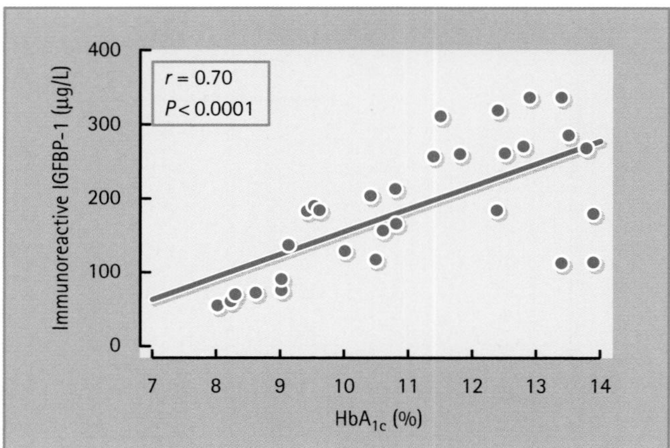

Figure 17.5 Correlation between serum immunoreactive insulin-like growth factor 1 binding protein 1 (IGFBP-1) and glycated hemoglobin (HbA_{1c}) concentrations in 48 patients with type 1 diabetes mellitus. Reproduced from Langford and Miell [128], with permission from the *European Journal of Clinical Investigation*.

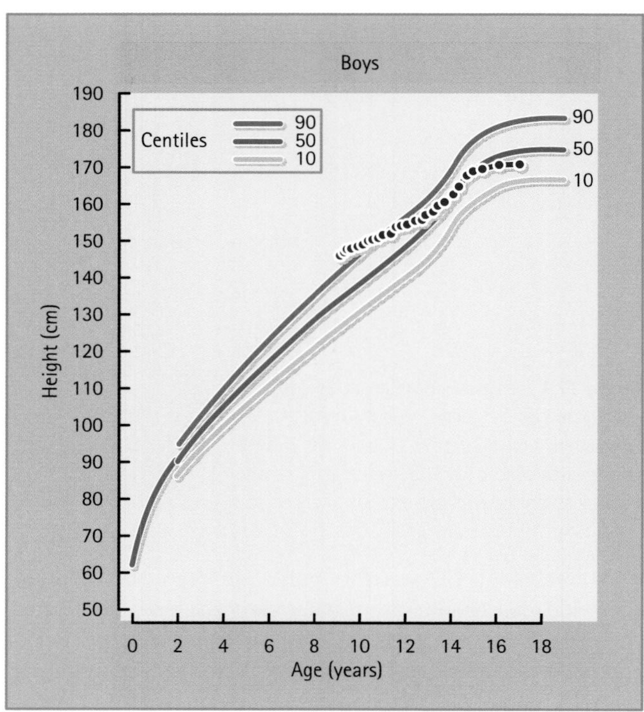

Figure 17.6 Growth failure in a boy with diabetes. Height fell progressively below the centiles (97th centile at diagnosis) and the pubertal growth spurt was delayed, resulting in a lower final height than predicted.

GH resistance, through downregulation of hepatic GH receptors and increased IGFBP-1 levels, both reducing IGF-I production and bioactivity [48]. Decreased IGF-I levels in turn cause GH hypersecretion via reduced negative feedback at the hypothalamus and pituitary, and this exacerbates insulin resistance, thus establishing a vicious circle of raised GH and poor glycemic control (Figures 17.2 and 17.3).

Another consequence of IGF-I deficiency is impaired growth at puberty [48]. Paradoxically, children with new-onset diabetes tend to be taller, especially if the disease develops several years before puberty; increased GH and insulin levels during the preclinical evolution of the disease are a possible explanation. Once diabetes is established, growth may slow, particularly before the age of 10 years and if glycemia is poorly controlled (Figure 17.6). The pubertal growth spurt may be blunted and/or delayed, especially in girls, and this may lead to a reduction in final height [48]. Growth failure in adolescents with T1DM is rare nowadays, possibly because of improved management and monitoring of diabetes. Indeed, intensified insulin treatment has been shown to raise IGF-I levels, in parallel with an increase in growth velocity [48]. Finally, growth failure may be associated with truncal obesity, hepatomegaly (secondary to glycogen and/or triglyceride deposition) and sexual infantilism in the Mauriac syndrome [49]. This condition was reported in children with poor glycemic control and excessively high insulin dosages, but is now rare.

Table 17.3 Clinical features of Cushing syndrome.

Clinical features
Easily bruised, thin skin; poor wound healing
Striae (purple or "violaceous" rather than white)
Thin (osteoporotic) bones that easily fracture
Glucose intolerance/diabetes mellitus
Central obesity, characteristic rounded facies, "buffalo" hump
Susceptibility to infection
Predisposition to gastric ulcer
Hypertension
Disturbance of menstrual cycle; symptoms overlap with PCOS
Mood disturbance (depression, psychosis)

PCOS, polycystic ovarian syndrome.

Cushing syndrome

Etiology, incidence and clinical features of Cushing syndrome

Cushing syndrome comprises a constellation of symptoms and signs caused by excessive levels of glucocorticoid that leads to a characteristic appearance accompanied by metabolic and cardiovascular pathology (Figure 17.7; Table 17.3) [50–52]. It occurs most commonly as a side effect of synthetic glucocorticoids administered exogenously for conditions such as rheumatoid arthritis or reversible airways disease. Endogenous Cushing syndrome arises in approximately two-thirds of cases from adrenocorticotropin (ACTH) secreting corticotroph adenomas of the anterior pituitary which affect 5–10 individuals per million. In one-fifth of cases, the cause is a glucocorticoid-secreting tumor of the adrenal cortex and in one-tenth of cases is secondary to syndromes of ectopic ACTH secretion, most commonly from small cell carcinoma of the lung or, more rarely, carcinoid tumors [50–52]. Cushing syndrome is more common in women than

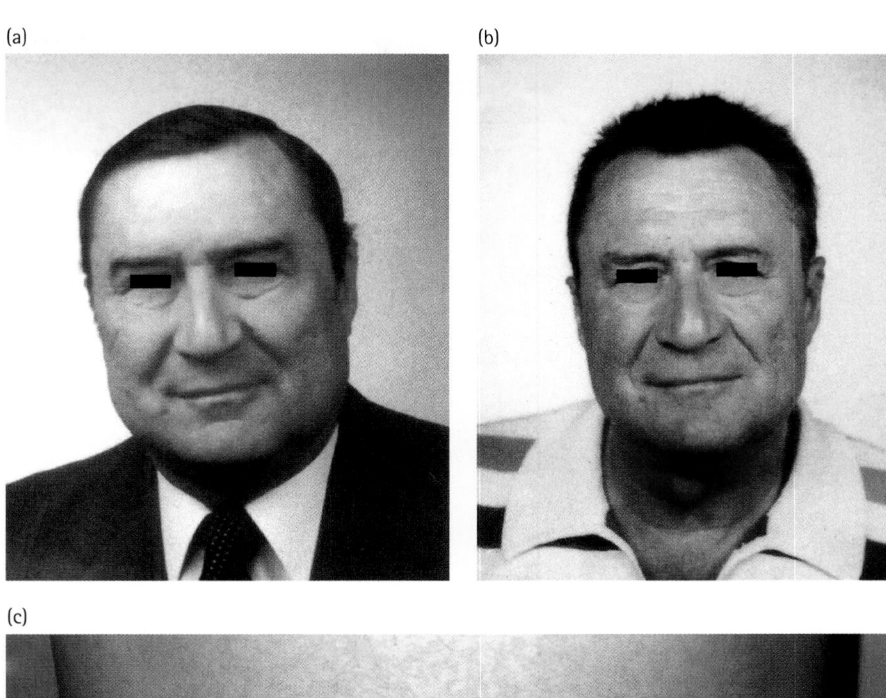

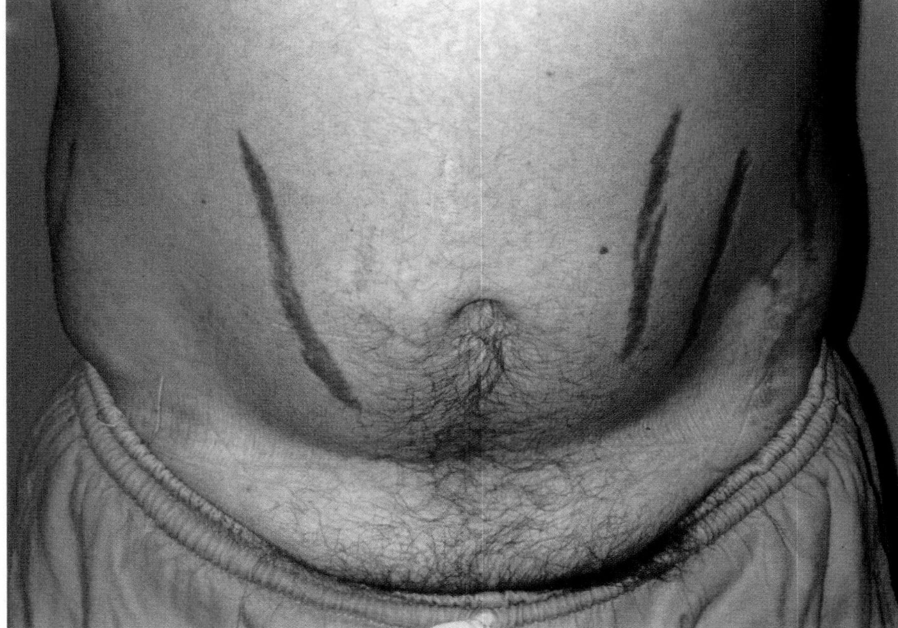

Figure 17.7 Cushing syndrome in a 53-year-old hypertensive man presenting with diabetes that required insulin to control hyperglycemia. Features included back pain from osteoporotic vertebral collapse, proximal myopathy that prevented him from climbing stairs, characteristic rounded facies (a) and truncal obesity with violaceous striae (c). After removal of the 10-mm corticotroph pituitary adenoma, his facial appearance returned to normal (b), as did blood pressure and blood glucose.

men, with a greater predilection for corticotroph adenomas as the underlying pathology. Prolonged excessive levels of cortisol, the major glucocorticoid in humans, either directly from an adrenocortical tumor or from excessive ACTH causing bilateral hyperfunctional adrenal cortices, causes the characteristic external features of the disorder to develop and results in excess cardiovascular morbidity and mortality (Fig. 17.7a; Table 17.3) [50–52].

Features of disturbance to glucose tolerance in Cushing syndrome

Impairment of glucose tolerance is observed in 30–60% of cases [7,50,53]. Overt diabetes occurs in 20–50%, arguably in patients predisposed to diabetes (e.g. those with a family history of the disorder) [7,50,53]. It resembles T2DM because glucocorticoid excess causes hyperglycemia primarily by inducing insulin resistance, reflected by hyperinsulinemia [53]. Insulin-stimulated glucose uptake and utilization by peripheral tissues are both reduced, while hepatic glucose production is greatly increased through stimulation of gluconeogenesis [50,54]. This results from the direct activation of hepatic gluconeogenic enzymes such as phosphoenolpyruvate carboxykinase (PEPCK), and an increasing supply of glucogenic substrates (amino acids and glycerol) generated by muscle proteolysis and peripheral adipose tissue lipolysis (Figure 17.8) [55]. Glucocorticoids also have permissive effects on the gluconeogenesis induced by epinephrine (adrena-

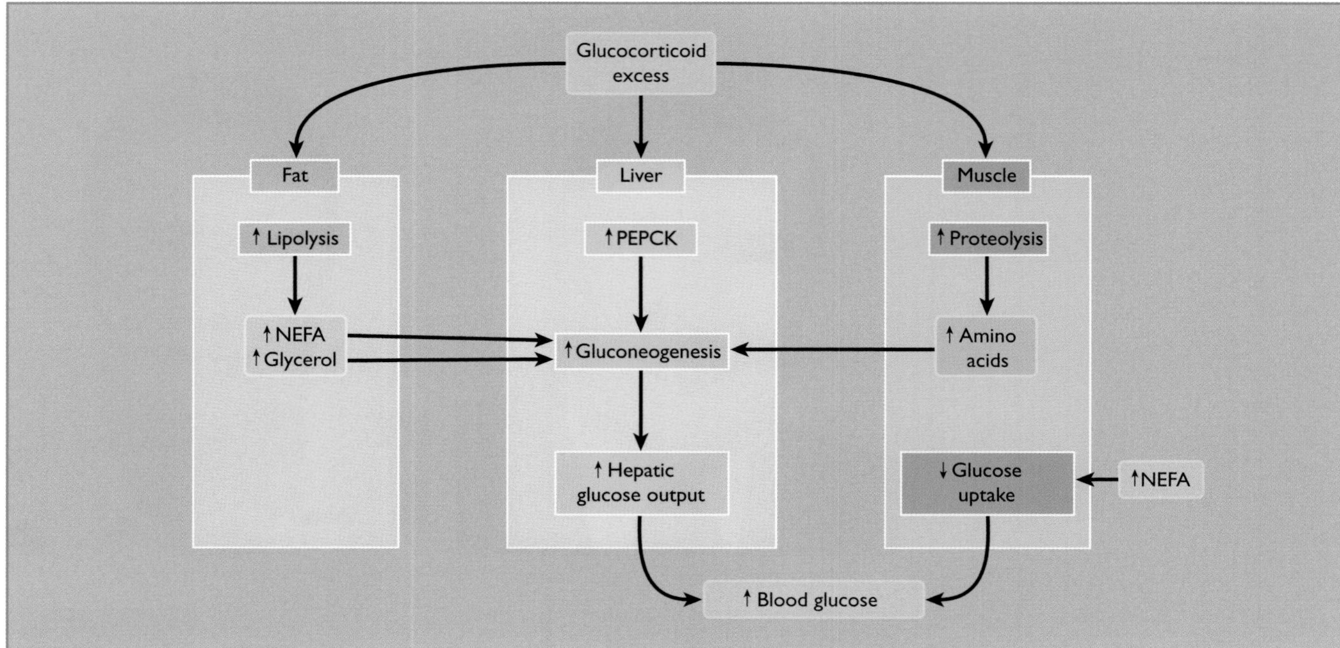

Figure 17.8 Mechanisms of hyperglycemia and diabetes in Cushing syndrome. NEFA, non-esterified fatty acids; PEPCK, phosphoenolpyruvate carboxykinase.

line) and glucagon. Besides enhancing hepatic gluconeogenesis, glucocorticoids also increase hepatic glycogen storage [55].

With endogenous causes of Cushing syndrome, the hyperglycemia can sometimes be effectively treated with sulfonylureas, but many cases require insulin therapy [56]. For Cushing syndrome caused by exogeneous drugs, treatment can be tailored from knowledge of the timing and half-life of the glucocorticoid drug as a predictable period of hyperglycemia follows. For instance, prednisolone administered for reversible airways disease at breakfast will generate elevated glucocorticoid levels throughout the remainder of the day with levels falling in the evening. This profile makes the choice of an intermediate acting insulin administered at breakfast appropriate (see Chapter 27).

Diagnosis and treatment of Cushing syndrome

For exogenously administered glucocorticoids, the diagnosis and treatment of Cushing syndrome are straightforward: wherever possible remove or reduce the offending medication. The major challenge in diagnosing Cushing syndrome resulting from endogenous causes is frequently one of simply considering the condition as the underlying cause of otherwise very common symptoms such as tiredness and weight gain. Avoiding this pitfall is aided by thorough clinical examination when more specific signs may be detected, for instance violaceous stretch marks (called "striae"; Figure 17.7c) or proximal myopathy [50–52]. This issue may be particularly pertinent to the T2DM clinic, with some evidence that occult Cushing syndrome may affect 2% of patients [57].

The first goal is to establish the presence of either autonomous secretion or excessive levels of cortisol [50–52]. Several screening tests with high sensitivity have been designed (Table 17.4). Circulating cortisol is relatively high during the day and low at bedtime. Maintained daytime levels at night indicate excess. This can be tested by measuring midnight serum cortisol, although this requires prior acclimatization of inpatients for at least 24 hours and quiet surroundings as cortisol levels rise with minimal stress. Where assays have been validated, bedtime salivary cortisol measurement can be very useful as patients can post samples to the laboratory from home. Levels are approximately 10% of those in serum so care must be taken to avoid contamination with blood (e.g. from brushing teeth). The "low dose" dexamethasone suppression tests interrogate the potential loss of physiologic negative feedback at the corticotroph leading to autonomous ACTH secretion. The formal 48-hour test is marginally more specific [51]; however, it is also more inconvenient to perform in the outpatient setting compared with the overnight 1 mg suppression test. Caution needs to be exercised in patients where dexamethasone metabolism is enhanced (e.g. by antiepileptic medication) as this can lead to false-positive results. An alternative screening test examines total excretion of cortisol in a 24-hour urine collection, commonly on several occasions, as an integrated assessment of one day's adrenocortical function. It is usual for endocrinologists to apply more than one of these various screening tests, which, if failed, provides proof of excess glucocorticoids and a diagnosis of Cushing syndrome.

Several endocrine tests have been developed to differentiate the various etiologies of endogenous Cushing syndrome (Table 17.4) [50–52]. Undetectable serum ACTH indicates an adrenocortical

Table 17.4 Diagnosis of Cushing syndrome from endogenous causes.

Test	Interpretation
Screening tests to diagnose Cushing syndrome	
Midnight serum cortisol measurement or bedtime salivary cortisol assay	Maintained daytime levels at night-time indicates autonomous cortisol production of Cushing syndrome
1 mg overnight DST. Oral dexamethasone taken at midnight	Serum cortisol >50 nmol/L at following 9 AM consistent with Cushing syndrome
Formal low-dose DST (0.5 mg × 8 doses 6-hourly ending at 3AM)	Serum cortisol >50 nmol/L at following 9 AM consistent with Cushing syndrome
24-hour urinary free cortisol measurement	Elevated values support diagnosis of Cushing syndrome
Tests to localize cause of cortisol excess	
Serum ACTH measurement	If suppressed, indicates autonomous adrenocortical overproduction of cortisol (e.g. an adrenocortical adenoma)
If serum ACTH detectable:	
High dose dexamethasone suppression test (2 mg × 8 doses 6-hourly ending at 3 AM)	>50% suppression of 9 AM serum cortisol from pre- to post-test indicates anterior pituitary source; <50% suppression indicates extrapituitary "ectopic" source of ACTH
Bilateral IPS sampling	Gradient from IPS to periphery of >2:1 supports anterior pituitary source (test can also incorporate CRH administration; see text)
MRI (can include gadolinium enhancement)	Should only be considered once biochemical evidence of pituitary source obtained. Helpful for surgeon in planning trans-sphenoidal surgery

ACTH, adenocorticotropic hormone; CRH, corticotropin releasing hormone; DST, dexamethasone suppression test; IPS, inferior petrosal sinus; MRI, magnetic resonance imaging.

source of excessive cortisol causing suppression of ACTH secretion by the anterior pituitary. It can be particularly challenging to distinguish between anterior pituitary and ectopic sources of ACTH causing Cushing syndrome. Corticotroph adenomas, especially intrasellar ones, usually retain a partial capacity for negative feedback; the "high dose" dexamethasone suppression test, administered as eight 2-mg doses every 6 hours, can be expected to reduce cortisol levels by at least 50%. As this cause underlies the original description of the disorder by Harvey Cushing in 1912, pituitary-driven glucocorticoid excess is called Cushing disease. Extrapituitary tumors secreting ectopic ACTH less commonly display this degree of negative feedback such that ACTH levels and consequently cortisol levels are likely to be higher. Although these tumors may be relatively indolent carcinoids, more commonly they are aggressive carcinomas of the bronchus characterized by a rapid onset of symptoms within a few months, marked hypokalemia and weight loss. The high level of *POMC* gene expression and dysregulated post-translational processing also leads to significant melanocyte stimulating hormone (MSH) secretion resulting in skin pigmentation. Venous sampling of the bilateral inferior petrosal sinuses can distinguish between ectopic or anterior pituitary sources of excessive ACTH. For pituitary sources, a gradient in ACTH levels of at least 2:1 (or 3:1 after the injection of 100 μg corticotropin releasing hormone [CRH] intravenously) should be found between central and peripheral samples. Although it can be very useful, bilateral inferior petrosal sinus sampling (BIPSS) also carries the risk of thrombosis in approximately 1% of cases, meaning that its use by endocrinologists is not always considered warranted. This is especially true where preceding biochemical tests have been conclusive and MRI shows clear radiologic evidence for a tumor. Where biochemistry is supportive of a pituitary source of ACTH excess, but the MRI is equivocal, even after gadolinium enhancement, BIPSS can help to lateralize a corticotroph adenoma by detecting a clear gradient between the right and left sinuses or vice versa. Sources of ectopic ACTH, most commonly in the chest, can be imaged with fine cut computerized tomography (CT), MRI or by using isotope-labeled scintigraphy to detect somatostatin receptors present on approximately two-thirds of ectopic ACTH-secreting carcinoid tumors. Autonomous cortisol-secreting tumors of the adrenal cortex can be imaged satisfactorily by CT or MRI when it can be possible to make assessment of functionality according to lipid content; features of high lipid content implying a tumor with active steroidogenesis.

Wherever possible, curative approaches are undertaken to normalize cortisol secretion as Cushing syndrome carries a high morbidity and markedly increases mortality from cardiovascular causes [50–52,58]. For adrenocortical sources, unilateral adrenalectomy is performed. For ectopic ACTH-secreting tumors, excision of carcinoids is potentially curative, whereas the natural history of carcinoma of the bronchus with ectopic hormone secretion usually makes palliative care more appropriate. Medical therapy to treat corticotroph adenomas remains disappointing. Some excitement was gained for high dose peroxisome proliferator-activated receptor γ (PPAR-γ) agonists but larger trials have been disappointing. Pituitary tumors are treated by either trans-sphenoidal surgery or radiotherapy when the indications and complications are largely the same as for those described in the section on acromegaly. The fact that ACTH-secreting adenomas are commonly microadenomas can increase the chances of curative surgery, although this remains heavily operator-dependent. If surgery is delayed, suppressants of adrenocortical steroidogenesis such as ketoconazole or metyrapone can be used temporarily where patients are highly symptomatic [50–52]. In extremis, bilateral adrenalectomy provides a rapid resolution of excessive cortisol secretion, although the total loss of negative feedback to a corticotroph adenoma can result in dangerous pituitary tumor growth that becomes refractory to further treatment, a scenario called Nelson syndrome. In patients where ACTH levels continue to rise, concomitant radiotherapy to the anterior pituitary can help reduce the risk of this problem arising.

Outcome of Cushing syndrome and disturbance to glucose tolerance

After successful surgery, the patient is reliant on external glucocorticoid administered as oral hydrocortisone, but a return of cortisol secretion from the adrenal gland(s) can be anticipated over ensuing weeks. Commonly, a physiologic return of diurnal rhythm is never achieved postoperatively [59]. For some, the extensiveness of anterior pituitary surgery, or the long-term suppression either of normal corticotrophs (pituitary or ectopic ACTH secreting tumors) or normal adrenocortical cells (cortisol-secreting tumors) causes a permanent state of hypocortisolism because of underactivity of remaining tissue. This can require continued hydrocortisone administration as for patients with Addison disease, except that mineralocorticoid replacement should not be required.

With successful treatment of Cushing syndrome (Figure 17.7), glucose intolerance may resolve. In such instances, when the patient might be entirely dependent on replacement doses of hydrocortisone, care needs to be taken not to cause hypoglycemia by continued antidiabetes medication. By contrast, persisting abnormalities are relatively common, most likely associated with persistent visceral obesity and metabolic syndrome [59]. On close analysis in one case series, there was a marked persistence of visceral obesity and glucose intolerance in approximately 60% of patients who fulfilled criteria for remission of Cushing syndrome [60].

Effects of diabetes on hypothalamic–anterior pituitary–adrenal cortex axis

Evidence of overactivity of the hypothalamic–pituitary–adrenal (HPA) axis has been reported in children, adolescents and adults with diabetes, including moderate increases in urinary free cortisol excretion, plasma cortisol and ACTH concentrations [61–64]. These abnormalities have been related to the duration of diabetes [62,63] and to the presence of diabetic neuropathy [64]. Serum cortisol levels fall as metabolic control improves [65].

Pheochromocytoma

Etiology, incidence and clinical features of pheochromocytoma

Pheochromocytomas are catecholamine-secreting tumors arising from the chromaffin cells of the adrenal medulla (Figure 17.9) [66,67]. Approximately 10% lie in extra-adrenal sites (paragangliomas) along the sympathetic chain in para-aortic or chest regions and approximately 10% are bilateral. Although most pheochromocytomas are sporadic, advances in molecular genetics have demonstrated that a hereditary basis underlies approximately one-fifth to one-quarter of diagnoses, not just in well-known syndromes, such as MEN2, von Recklinghausen neurofibromatosis and von Hippel–Lindau disease [66]. Such advances have also associated particular genetic defects to tumor type. For instance, succinate dehydrogenase subunit B (*SDHB*) and succinate dehydrogenase subunit D (*SDHD*) mutations are more frequent in extra-adrenal tumors [66]. Mutations in *SDHB* are more commonly associated with a malignant phenotype [68]. The risk of malignancy also increases with tumor size [68].

The clinical manifestations of pheochromocytoma are largely caused by hypersecretion of catecholamines, classically as a triad of symptoms: headaches, sweating and tachycardia [69]. Hypertension is the most common clinical finding and occurs in 80–90% of cases. It can be paroxysmal or sustained, the latter occurring especially in children and in noradrenaline-secreting tumors [66]. Other symptoms may be secondary to the co-secretion of various other peptide hormones such as vasoactive intestinal peptide (VIP), substance P, atrial natriuretic factor, endothelin-1, CRH and GHRH [70]. The normal adrenal medulla predominantly secretes epinephrine, converted from norepinephrine by methylation. This reaction is governed by the enzyme phenylethanolamine-*N*-methyltransferase (PNMT), the expression of which is dependent on high concentrations of cortisol draining centripetally from the outer adrenal cortex towards the adrenal vein [69]. For this reason, larger tumors with more marked disturbance of the normal anatomy or extra-adrenal pheochromocytomas are notable for predominantly secreting norepinephrine as conversion to epinephrine is compromised.

Features of disturbance to glucose tolerance in pheochromocytoma

Hyperglycemia occurs in up to approximately 50% of patients with pheochromocytoma. The prevalence of diabetes is approximately 35% [71]. Its presence in a young hypertensive person of normal body weight should raise suspicion of pheochromocytoma. The predominant mechanism is catecholamine-mediated reduction in insulin sensitivity and insulin secretion, predominantly caused by epinephrine rather than norepinephrine (Figure 17.10) [72,73]. Epinephrine inhibits β-cell insulin secretion via stimulation of α_2-adrenergic receptors [74]. In the liver, epinephrine activates β_2-adrenoceptors to enhance glycogenolysis transiently and gluconeogenesis in a more sustained fashion [75–77]. This hepatic gluconeogenesis is fueled by the precursors, lactate, alanine and glycerol, generated by β_2-adrenergic stimulation of muscle glycolysis and adipose tissue lipolysis. Lipolysis in adipose tissue is also stimulated via the β_1- and β_3-adrenoceptors. In addition, epinephrine can impair glucose utilization in muscle through direct β_2-adrenergic effects. The predominance of these β_2-adrenergic effects probably explains why epinephrine, with its higher affinity for β_2-receptors, is more potent than norepinephrine in producing hyperglycemia [75,77]. All these effects are potent mechanisms that raise blood glucose, explaining why epinephrine release is an important component in correcting hypoglycemia after inhibition of insulin and increased glucagon secretion in the hierarchy of counter-regulatory responses (see Chapter 33).

(a)

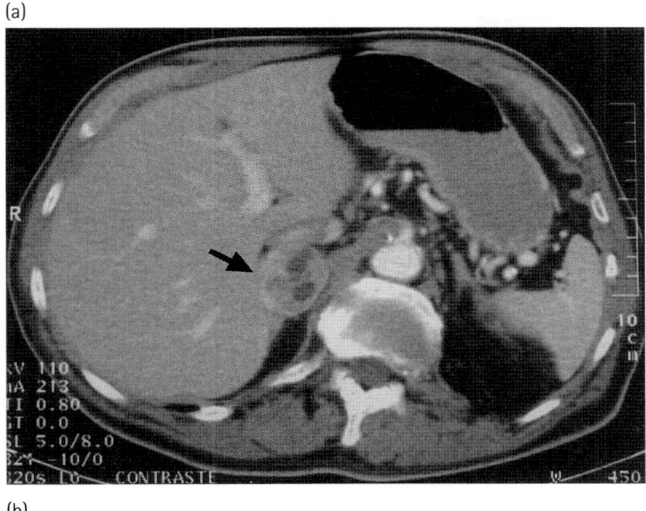

(b)

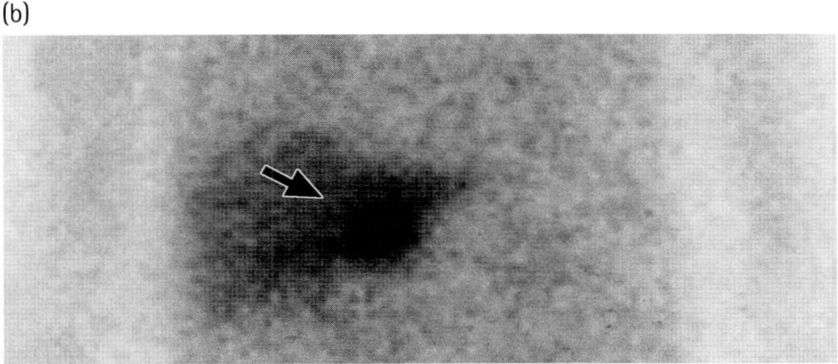

(c)

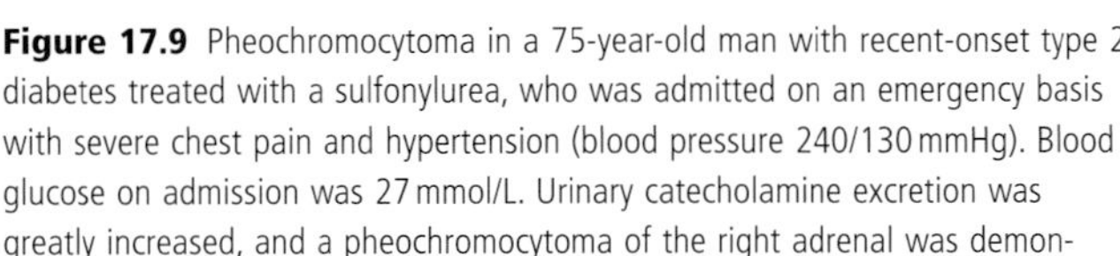

Figure 17.9 Pheochromocytoma in a 75-year-old man with recent-onset type 2 diabetes treated with a sulfonylurea, who was admitted on an emergency basis with severe chest pain and hypertension (blood pressure 240/130 mmHg). Blood glucose on admission was 27 mmol/L. Urinary catecholamine excretion was greatly increased, and a pheochromocytoma of the right adrenal was demonstrated by: (a) computed tomography; (b) scanning with ^{131}I-metaiodobenzylguanidine, which is taken up by catecholamine-synthesizing tissues; and (c) positron emission tomography with ^{18}F-fluorodeoxyglucose. After laparoscopic removal of the tumor, diabetes and hypertension both resolved.

Diagnosis and treatment of pheochromocytoma

Pheochromocytomas are diagnosed by demonstrating an excess of circulating catecholamines [66–68]. As a proxy marker, this can be achieved by several 24-hour urine collections measuring catecholamines, such as epinephrine, norepinephrine and their metabolites. Assessment of the metabolite vanylmandelic acid is inadequate as it has a high false-negative rate [66]. Where specific circumstances dictate, for instance in screening those with a genetic predisposition to pheochromocytoma, or where urinary results are equivocal, serum measurement of normetanephrine and metanephrine are very sensitive and specific markers of pheochromocytoma (normetanephrine is the more sensitive) [67]. Imaging the tumor can be performed by either MRI or CT. Treatment is surgical removal of the tumor as an adrenalectomy, increasingly performed laparoscopically unless malignancy is suspected [66–68]. Preoperative preparation must be meticulous to prevent both a hypertensive crisis during manipulation of the tumor and cardiovascular collapse after its removal. This is achieved by initial α-receptor blockade followed by beta-blocker. The order of implementation is important to prevent a hypertensive crisis from unopposed α-adrenoceptor stimulation. The preoperative α-adrenergic blockade often controls hypertension, but has less effect on glucose intolerance [75,78]. In malignant pheochromocytoma where surgery is not possible, adrenolytic drugs, such as mitotane, can be used palliatively.

Outcome of pheochromocytoma and disturbance to glucose tolerance

Removal of the tumor corrects the metabolic abnormalities. If presentation, diagnosis and treatment have occurred without undue delay, it also resolves the hypertension [56,75,78,79].

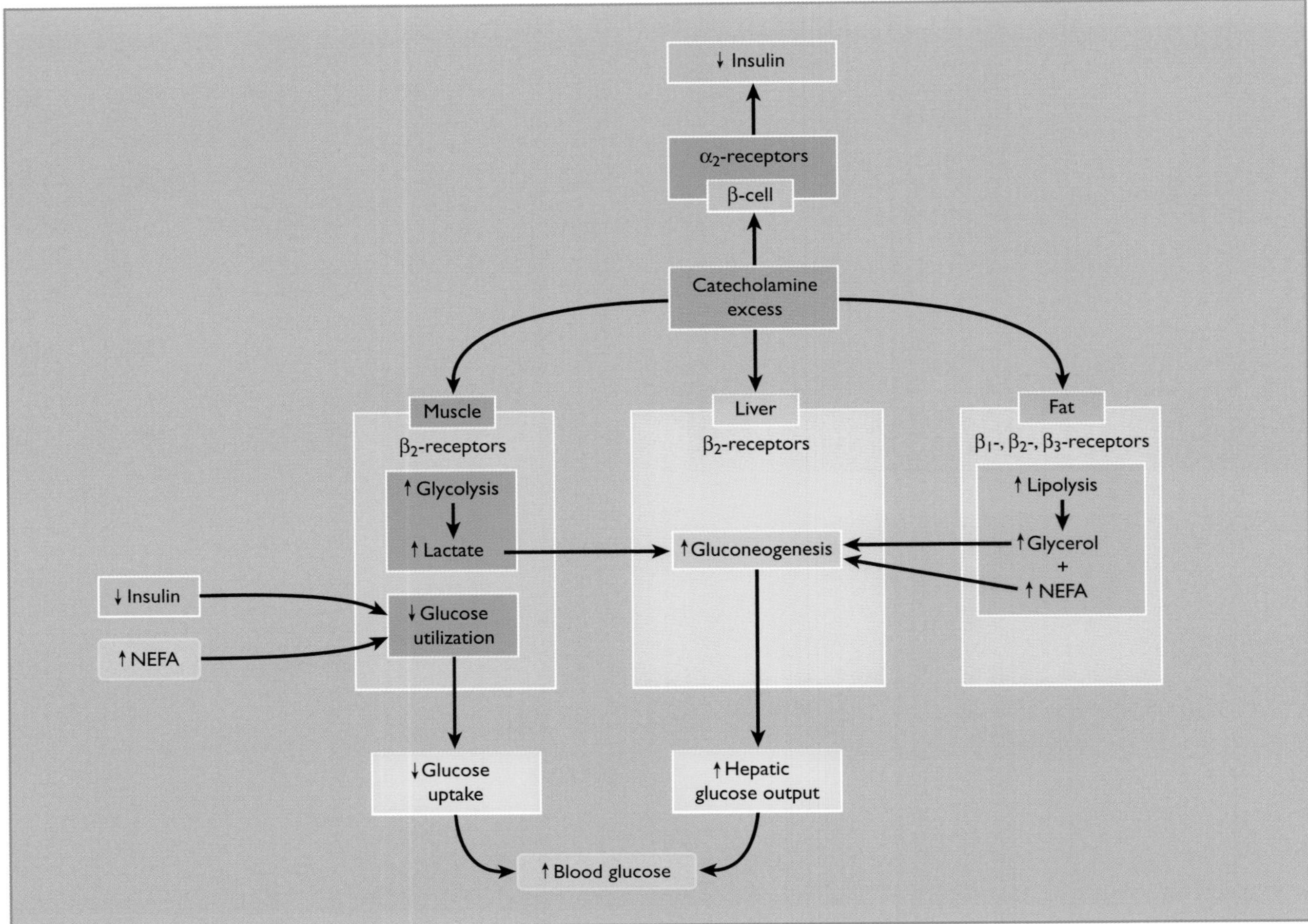

Figure 17.10 Mechanisms of hyperglycemia in pheochromocytoma. NEFA, non-esterified fatty acid.

Although practice varies, greater understanding of the molecular genetics of pheochromocytoma makes clinical genetics input advisable; some laboratories now undertake germline mutation analyses in seemingly isolated tumors [66]. It is also straightforward to exclude hyperparathyroidism by measuring serum calcium as this simple test, if normal, goes a long way to excluding MEN1. Some clinics offer annual follow-up screening for pheochromocytoma by 24-hour urine collection. Patients with pheochromocytomas caused by identified genetic disorders should be followed up at least annually in dedicated clinical genetics endocrinology clinics.

Effects of diabetes on adrenal medulla function

Function of the adrenal medulla may be selectively impaired in patients with long-standing diabetes and hypoglycemia unawareness; attenuation of the epinephrine response to hypoglycemia can delay the restoration of normal serum glucose levels. Epinephrine responses can remain normal to other stimuli, indicating failure of sympathetic activation at a specific, possibly hypothalamic, level (see Chapter 33).

Other endocrine conditions causing disturbance of glucose tolerance

Glucagonoma

Glucagonoma is a rare tumor of the α-cell of the pancreatic islet. The first clear-cut case was reported in 1942, but the "glucagonoma syndrome" (in a series of nine patients with similar symptoms) was not described until 1974 [80,81]. It may form part of MEN1 caused by mutations in the tumor suppressor gene, *MENIN* [82]. In a series of 21 patients [83], the syndrome's most striking clinical features were weight loss (71%), necrolytic migratory erythema (67%) (Figure 17.11a), diabetes (38%), cheilosis or stomatitis (29%) and diarrhea (29%). In this report, patients with the combination of necrolytic migratory erythema and diabetes mellitus were diagnosed more rapidly (after a mean of 7 months), but some cases remain undetected for years. Glucagonoma should always be considered in patients with diabetes and unexplained weight loss or a chronic skin rash.

(a)

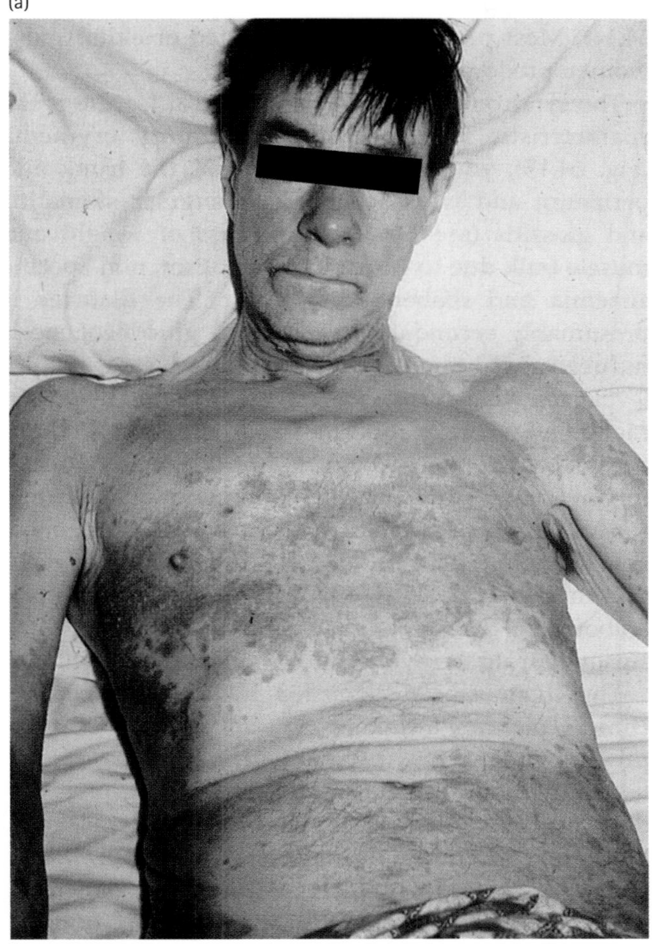

(b)

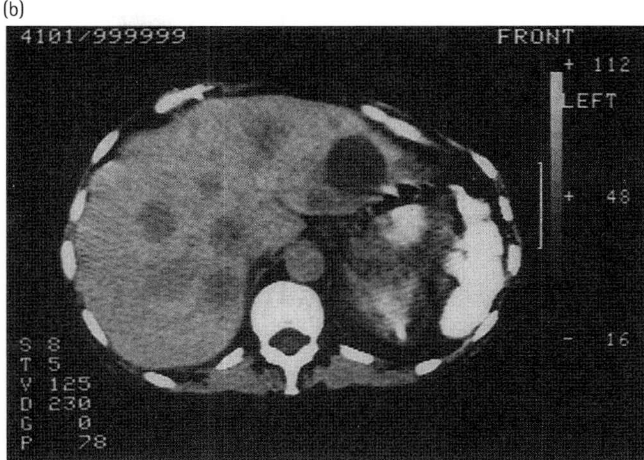

Figure 17.11 Glucagonoma showing characteristic necrolytic migratory erythema (a) and multiple hepatic metastases (b). This patient had non-ketotic diabetes, controlled with low dosages of insulin; the rash recurred many times despite treatment with somatostatin analog. He died from pulmonary embolus. Courtesy of Professor Stephen Bloom, Imperial College School of Medicine, London.

Necrolytic migratory erythema (Figure 17.11a) is described in full in Chapter 47. It usually involves the buttocks, groin, thighs and distal extremities, and characteristically remits and relapses [80,81]. Hyperglucagonemia may contribute to the rash, as may hypoaminoacidemia through glucagon's enhancement of amino acid uptake by the liver and zinc deficiency [81]. The glucagonoma syndrome is also characterized by a normochromic normocytic anemia, a tendency to thrombosis (pulmonary embolism is a common cause of death) and neuropsychiatric disturbances [80]. Reporting of the prevalence of diabetes in glucagonoma has been variable but it probably affects approximately three-quarters of individuals [80]. In cohorts with this detection rate, the hyperglycemia has most commonly been mild and may respond to oral hypoglycemic agents. In studies with lower rates of diagnosis, 75% of patients required insulin [80]. The hyperglycemia is largely brought about by the effects of glucagon on stimulating hepatic gluconeogenesis and, in adequately fed individuals, glycogenolysis [81].

The diagnosis is suggested by finding a pancreatic mass and high fasting plasma glucagon concentration in the absence of other causes of hyperglucagonemia (e.g. severe stress, hepatic and renal failure, poorly controlled diabetes, small-bowel malabsorption and synthetic androgenic drugs) [80,81]. Surgical removal of the tumor is the treatment of choice, but 50% of tumors have metastasized to the liver by the time of diagnosis (Figure 17.11b) [83]. Treatment can then be completed by hepatic artery embolization and/or chemotherapy; somatostatin analogs can also suppress glucagon secretion. The rash may respond to normalization of glucagon levels following removal of the tumor or the use of somatostatin analogs; the administration of zinc, a high-protein diet and control of the diabetes with insulin may also help [80,81,83].

Somatostatinoma

Somatostatinomas are extremely rare tumors arising in 1 in 40 million individuals from δ-cells of the pancreatic islet or enteroendocrine cells of the duodenum and ampulla of Vater [84]. They may be sporadic or as part of genetic syndromes, such as MEN1 [84]. The first two somatostatinomas were found incidentally during cholecystectomy [85,86], but a subsequent case was diagnosed preoperatively and extensively investigated [87]. The diagnosis was suggested by the triad of diabetes, steatorrhea and gallstones, associated with a tumor of the duodenum [87]. These features, together with hypochlorhydria, are attributable to the widespread inhibitory effects of somatostatin on endocrine and exocrine secretions [84]. Consistent with inhibition of both insulin and glucagon by somatostatin, hyperglycemia is mild, non-ketotic and satisfactorily controlled without insulin [87].

Diagnosis is made by clinical presentation, measuring elevated fasting levels of circulating somatostatin and imaging by CT or MRI. Octreotide scintigraphy can also be used to localize the tumor. Surgical resection is the treatment of choice and can be curative. Where tumors are large and malignant with metastases at the time of diagnosis, debulking, embolization and chemotherapy (including radiolabeled somatostatin analogs) are appropriate [84].

VIPoma

The first VIP-secreting tumor was recognized by Verner and Morrison in 1958 [88]. Classic features are caused by elevated circulating VIP levels and include watery diarrhea (pancreatic cholera), hypokalemia and achlorhydria [89]. Hypercalcemia and glucose intolerance occur in half of the patients, but overt diabetes is unusual; hyperglycemia is probably secondary to the glycogenolytic effect of VIP and/or to hypokalemia, which can impair both insulin secretion and insulin sensitivity. Diagnosis is aided by serum assay for fasting VIP levels. The tumors are usually large and have metastasized from the pancreatic tail by the time of diagnosis. Debulking surgery forms the mainstay of treatment and 10-year survival is approximately 40% [89].

Hyperthyroidism

Hyperthyroidism is defined by overproduction of thyroid hormones. Hyperthyroidism leads to thyrotoxicosis; the manifestations of increased circulating thyroid hormones (Table 17.5) [90]. Ignoring the association of autoimmune hyperthyroidism (Graves disease) with T1DM, thyrotoxicosis per se can disturb glucose tolerance in approximately one-third of individuals, with diabetes occurring in a further 8% of patients [91]. There is evidence for insulin resistance as the primary defect [90,91], especially in those who are overweight [92], although insulin secretion may also be impaired [91,93]. Glucose production and expression of the hepatocyte glucose transporter 2 (GLUT-2) protein are enhanced by thyroid hormone excess [94,95]. The insulin resistance is improved with restoration of euthyroidism even if body mass index (BMI) rises [91]. When hyperthyroidism develops in insulin-treated patients with diabetes, glucose control deteriorates and insulin requirements increase in approximately half the patients; these changes are reversed following treatment of hyperthyroidism [96]. In addition to these alterations in insulin secretion and action, the response to oral glucose tolerance testing is also altered in hyperthyroidism because of faster intestinal absorption [97].

Table 17.5 Clinical features of thyrotoxicosis plus features associated with Graves disease.

Clinical features of thyrotoxicosis
Weight loss despite full, possibly increased, appetite
Tremor
Heat intolerance and sweating
Agitation and nervousness
Palpitations, shortness of breath/tachycardia ± atrial fibrillation
Glucose intolerance
Amenorrhea/oligomenorrhea and consequent subfertility
Diarrhea
Hair loss
Easy fatigability, muscle weakness and loss of muscle mass
Rapid growth rate and accelerated bone maturation (children)
Specific features associated with Graves disease
Bruit in a diffuse, firm goiter
Thyroid eye disease, also called Graves orbitopathy
Pretibial myxoedema – thickened skin over the lower tibia
Thyroid acropachy (clubbing of the fingers)
Other autoimmune features (e.g. vitiligo)

Primary hyperaldosteronism

Primary hyperaldosteronism was originally described by Conn in 1955 in a patient with hypertension, hypokalemia and neuromuscular symptoms associated with an adrenocortical adenoma secreting aldosterone [69]. A benign adenoma is the most common primary cause (65%) with bilateral hyperplasia accounting for 30% of cases. A handful of cases are brought about by a genetic recombination event between the genes encoding two closely related steroidogenic enzymes. This causes aldosterone secretion under the regulation of ACTH, which is suppressible by glucocorticoids [69]. Although debate is active over whether more subtle normokalemic aldosterone excess is a wider cause of hypertension, the relevance of primary hyperaldosteronism to glucose tolerance relies largely on the hypokalemia, which is part of the classic Conn syndrome as low serum potassium impairs insulin secretion [56,69]. Others have questioned whether aldosterone might exert other diabetogenic effects on glucose metabolism, although this remains unclear [98]. Glucose intolerance has been reported in approximately 50% of patients [99]. This is generally mild and overt diabetes is unusual. Defective insulin release has been implicated with delayed or reduced insulin responses following oral glucose challenge. Removal of the aldosteronoma or potassium loading can correct these defects [99].

Primary hyperparathyroidism

Primary hyperparathyroidism is secondary to hypersecretion of parathyroid hormone (PTH), usually by a parathyroid adenoma and less commonly by parathyroid hyperplasia [100]. The prevalence of diabetes in primary hyperparathyroidism is approximately threefold higher than in the general population [101–103], with some cases requiring insulin therapy. Insulin resistance with hyperinsulinemia is generally held responsible, with raised intracellular calcium limiting cellular glucose uptake [103]. It has been debated whether parathyroidectomy for primary hyperparathyroidism improves glucose homeostasis: some reports argue that it is beneficial for both diabetes and impaired glucose tolerance [104,105] while others find less effect [106,107]. Possibly this relates to duration and severity of the calcium disturbance. With the widespread availability of serum biochemistry, hyperparathyroidism is shifting from a symptomatic disorder to an asymptomatic one where serum calcium tends to be only marginally elevated. In the latter scenario, glucose tolerance appears less affected [108].

Hypopituitarism with growth hormone deficiency

In children, lack of GH increases insulin sensitivity such that young GH-deficient children tend to develop fasting and readily provoked hypoglycemia [109,110]. Using insulin tolerance tests, GH-deficient children were more insulin-sensitive than short children with normal GH secretion [109]. This exaggerated insulin sensitivity attenuates with age and puberty, possibly following increased gonadal steroid production [109] such that adults with GH deficiency demonstrate insulin resistance [12]. Given that GH excess is diabetogenic and acute GH administration raises fasting glucose and fasting insulin levels, and reduces insulin sensitivity [14,17], the value of GH replacement to improve glucose tolerance is likely to be related to whether it can be administered physiologically.

Given this challenge, it is not surprising that the long-term results of GH replacement are somewhat conflicting [12]: a 30-month study showed a deterioration in glucose tolerance and insulin sensitivity despite an increase in lean body tissue and a reduction of fat mass [111]; another study of 6 months' duration found rises in fasting glucose and HbA_{1c} without effects on peripheral or hepatic sensitivity [112]; however, a 5-year trial concluded that GH replacement decreased HbA_{1c} levels [113]. Another study, evaluating the impact of GH therapy in GH-deficient patients during transition from childhood to adulthood, showed that the beneficial effects of chronic treatment on body composition did not overcome the direct antagonistic effects on insulin action [114]. Insulin secretion may also deteriorate during GH administration [111]. Thus, the replacement of GH in hypopituitary patients with diabetes is contentious: long-term treatment with GH may improve insulin sensitivity via improvements in body composition; however, such patients need to be monitored regularly and overtreatment that might lead to the development of diabetes should be avoided [12,115].

Endocrine disorders that associate with diabetes

Several endocrine disorders that are associated with T1DM because of a common etiology and similar pathology (e.g. autoimmune adrenalitis [Addison disease] or autoimmune thyroid disease). Attention in these disorders is warranted for the onset of new autoimmune pathologies. In patients with T1DM, screening can be justified to exclude hyperthyroidism or hypothyroidism by measuring serum thyroid stimulating hormone (TSH) annually. The development of Addison disease in patients with T1DM markedly increases sensitivity to insulin such that unanticipated hypoglycemic reactions occur as dose requirements fall. Even in the absence of diabetes and insulin therapy, Addison disease can cause hypoglycemia, especially in children. Rare conditions resembling T1DM with associated endocrinopathies, such as the autoimmune polyglandular syndromes or POEMS syndrome may occur. Monogenic causes of diabetes that affect other endocrine organs are covered in Chapter 15. Examples (and their respective endocrine disorder) include the various types of hemochromatosis (primary hypogonadism), Wolfram syndrome (diabetes insipidus) and Kearns–Sayre syndrome (hypoparathyroidism, hypogonadism and hypopituitarism). Here, polycystic ovarian syndrome (PCOS) is addressed as a complex endocrine disorder that includes insulin resistance. The hormonal alterations in PCOS share relevance with some of the mechanisms underlying glucose homeostasis in pregnancy and obesity, covered in Chapters 53 and 14, respectively.

Polycystic ovarian syndrome

PCOS is defined as clinical or biochemical hyperandrogenism with oligo- or anovulation where other definable causes have been excluded [116–120]. Some definitions incorporate the detection of multiple ovarian cysts into the diagnosis [119,120], although these occur in approximately half of patients with Cushing syndrome and are non-discriminatory (Figure 17.12) [121,122]. PCOS occurs in 5–10% of women of reproductive age and is characterized primarily by insulin resistance although there is also evidence of β-cell dysfunction [123,124]. Impaired glucose tolerance and T2DM are present in nearly 40% and 7.5–10%, respectively, of women with PCOS, with the former having a tendency to progress to T2DM and being associated with an approximate threefold higher risk of gestational diabetes [123,124]. These data are confounded to some degree by the effect of obesity, but the incidence of PCOS remains increased across ethnicities whereas obesity rates vary [124]. Indeed, it can be argued that PCOS in women with normal BMI represents the most severe form of the disorder where genetic screening programs are most likely to identify PCOS susceptibility genes.

The source of the androgens is both the adrenal cortex and the ovary [124]. The raised insulin levels can stimulate androgen production by the ovary and interfere with other aspects of ovarian function. Within the adrenal cortex, where insulin receptors are expressed in the zona fasciculata of the adrenal cortex [125], there is some evidence that insulin can influence glucocorticoid versus sex steroid precursor production [124].

The diagnosis of PCOS is one of exclusion, meaning that clinical and biochemical findings are only supportive of the condition

(a) (b)

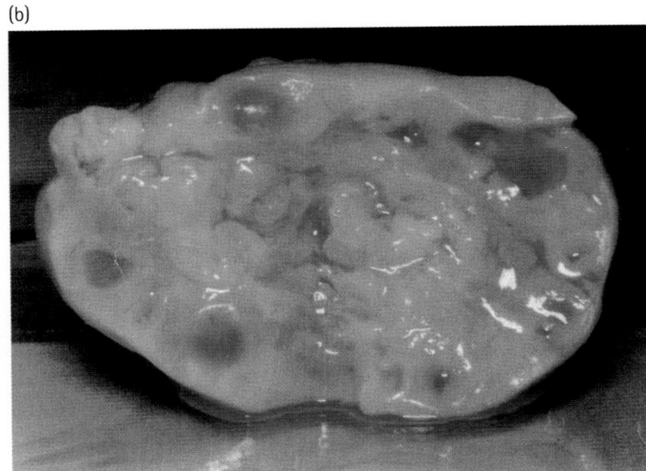

Figure 17.12 Polycystic ovary syndrome, showing (a) characteristic ultrasonographic appearance of large, mainly peripheral cysts (asterisks) and (b) the cut surface of a polycystic ovary. From Franks [129], with permission from *New England Journal of Medicine*. Courtesy of (a) Dr D. Kiddy and (b) Professor Steve Franks, Imperial College School of Medicine, London, UK.

[116,121]. Serum estradiol is detectable and usually >200 pmol/L. Endocrine abnormalities include increases in serum luteinizing hormone (LH) leading to a raised LH : FSH (follicle stimulating hormone) ratio, androstenedione and testosterone concentrations. Serum sex hormone-binding globulin (SHBG) levels are commonly low. Ovarian ultrasound is useful to help exclude the presence of a tumor underlying the androgen excess [121].

Further evidence that the condition is caused by insulin resistance comes from its amelioration with exercise and agents that improve insulin sensitivity such as metformin or thiazolidinediones [126]. As well as lowering blood glucose, these agents improve menstrual regularity and increase the chance of ovulatory cycles [126].

References

1 Melmed S. Medical progress: acromegaly. *N Engl J Med* 2006; **355**:2558–2573.

2 Holdaway IM, Rajasoorya C. Epidemiology of acromegaly. *Pituitary* 1999; **2**:29–41.

3 Horvath A, Stratakis CA. Clinical and molecular genetics of acromegaly: MEN1, Carney complex, McCune–Albright syndrome, familial acromegaly and genetic defects in sporadic tumors. *Rev Endocr Metab Disord* 2008; **9**:1–11.

4 Rajasoorya C, Holdaway IM, Wrightson P, Scott DJ, Ibbertson HK. Determinants of clinical outcome and survival in acromegaly. *Clin Endocrinol (Oxf)* 1994; **41**:95–102.

5 Colao A, Auriemma RS, Pivonello R, Galdiero M, Lombardi G. Medical consequences of acromegaly: what are the effects of biochemical control? *Rev Endocr Metab Disord* 2008; **9**:21–31.

6 Kreze A, Kreze-Spirova E, Mikulecky M. Risk factors for glucose intolerance in active acromegaly. *Braz J Med Biol Res* 2001; **34**:1429–1433.

7 Biering H, Knappe G, Gerl H, Lochs H. Prevalence of diabetes in acromegaly and Cushing syndrome. *Acta Med Austriaca* 2000; **27**:27–31.

8 Kasayama S, Otsuki M, Takagi M, Saito H, Sumitani S, Kouhara H, *et al.* Impaired beta-cell function in the presence of reduced insulin sensitivity determines glucose tolerance status in acromegalic patients. *Clin Endocrinol (Oxf)* 2000; **52**:549–555.

9 Nabarro JD. Acromegaly. *Clin Endocrinol (Oxf)* 1987; **26**:481–512.

10 Jadresic A, Banks LM, Child DF, Diamant L, Doyle FH, Fraser TR, *et al.* The acromegaly syndrome: relation between clinical features, growth hormone values and radiological characteristics of the pituitary tumours. *Q J Med* 1982; **51**:189–204.

11 Puder JJ, Nilavar S, Post KD, Freda PU. Relationship between disease-related morbidity and biochemical markers of activity in patients with acromegaly. *J Clin Endocrinol Metab* 2005; **90**:1972–1978.

12 Jorgensen JO, Norrelund H, Conceicao F, Moller N, Christiansen JS. Somatropin and glucose homeostasis: considerations for patient management. *Treat Endocrinol* 2002; **1**:229–234.

13 Moller N, Jorgensen JO, Abildgard N, Orskov L, Schmitz O, Christiansen JS. Effects of growth hormone on glucose metabolism. *Horm Res* 1991; **36**(Suppl 1):32–35.

14 Jorgensen JO, Krag M, Jessen N, Norrelund H, Vestergaard ET, Moller N, *et al.* Growth hormone and glucose homeostasis. *Horm Res* 2004; **62**(Suppl 3):51–55.

15 Hansen I, Tsalikian E, Beaufrere B, Gerich J, Haymond M, Rizza R. Insulin resistance in acromegaly: defects in both hepatic and extrahepatic insulin action. *Am J Physiol* 1986; **250**:E269–E273.

16 Fowelin J, Attvall S, von Schenck H, Smith U, Lager I. Characterization of the insulin-antagonistic effect of growth hormone in man. *Diabetologia* 1991; **34**:500–506.

17 Fowelin J, Attvall S, von Schenck H, Smith U, Lager I. Characterization of the insulin-antagonistic effect of growth hormone in insulin-dependent diabetes mellitus. *Diabet Med* 1995; **12**:990–996.

18 Bak JF, Moller N, Schmitz O. Effects of growth hormone on fuel utilization and muscle glycogen synthase activity in normal humans. *Am J Physiol* 1991; **260**:E736–E742.

19 Ben-Shlomo A, Melmed S. Acromegaly. *Endocrinol Metab Clin North Am* 2008; **37**:101–122, viii.

20 Bush ZM, Vance ML. Management of acromegaly: is there a role for primary medical therapy? *Rev Endocr Metab Disord* 2008; **9**:83–94.

21 Carmichael JD, Bonert VS. Medical therapy: options and uses. *Rev Endocr Metab Disord* 2008; **9**:71–81.

22 Schade R, Andersohn F, Suissa S, Haverkamp W, Garbe E. Dopamine agonists and the risk of cardiac-valve regurgitation. *N Engl J Med* 2007; **356**:29–38.

23 Roth BL. Drugs and valvular heart disease. *N Engl J Med* 2007; **356**:6–9.

24 Higham CE, Trainer PJ. Growth hormone excess and the development of growth hormone receptor antagonists. *Exp Physiol* 2008; **93**:1157–1169.

25 Jenkins PJ, Bates P, Carson MN, Stewart PM, Wass JA. Conventional pituitary irradiation is effective in lowering serum growth hormone and insulin-like growth factor-1 in patients with acromegaly. *J Clin Endocrinol Metab* 2006; **91**:1239–1245.

26 Ayuk J, Clayton RN, Holder G, Sheppard MC, Stewart PM, Bates AS. Growth hormone and pituitary radiotherapy, but not serum insulin-like growth factor-1 concentrations, predict excess mortality in patients with acromegaly. *J Clin Endocrinol Metab* 2004; **89**:1613–1617.

27 Moller N, Schmitz O, Joorgensen JO, Astrup J, Bak JF, Christensen SE, *et al.* Basal- and insulin-stimulated substrate metabolism in patients with active acromegaly before and after adenomectomy. *J Clin Endocrinol Metab* 1992; **74**:1012–1019.

28 Wass JA, Cudworth AG, Bottazzo GF, Woodrow JC, Besser GM. An assessment of glucose intolerance in acromegaly and its response to medical treatment. *Clin Endocrinol (Oxf)* 1980; **12**:53–59.

29 Tolis G, Angelopoulos NG, Katounda E, Rombopoulos G, Kaltzidou V, Kaltsas D, *et al.* Medical treatment of acromegaly: comorbidities and their reversibility by somatostatin analogs. *Neuroendocrinology* 2006; **83**:249–257.

30 Ho KK, Jenkins AB, Furler SM, Borkman M, Chisholm DJ. Impact of octreotide, a long-acting somatostatin analogue, on glucose tolerance and insulin sensitivity in acromegaly. *Clin Endocrinol (Oxf)* 1992; **36**:271–279.

31 Colao A, Ferone D, Marzullo P, Cappabianca P, Cirillo S, Boerlin V, *et al.* Long-term effects of depot long-acting somatostatin analog octreotide on hormone levels and tumor mass in acromegaly. *J Clin Endocrinol Metab* 2001; **86**:2779–2786.

32 Ferone D, Colao A, van der Lely AJ, Lamberts SW. Pharmacotherapy or surgery as primary treatment for acromegaly? *Drugs Aging* 2000; **17**:81–92.

33 Colao A, Pivonello R, Auriemma RS, De Martino MC, Bidlingmaier M, Briganti F, *et al.* Efficacy of 12-month treatment with the GH receptor antagonist pegvisomant in patients with acromegaly resistant to long-term, high-dose somatostatin analog treatment: effect on IGF-I levels, tumor mass, hypertension and glucose tolerance. *Eur J Endocrinol* 2006; **154**:467–477.

34 Barkan AL, Burman P, Clemmons DR, Drake WM, Gagel RF, Harris PE, *et al.* Glucose homeostasis and safety in patients with acromegaly converted from long-acting octreotide to pegvisomant. *J Clin Endocrinol Metab* 2005; **90**:5684–5691.

35 Drake WM, Rowles SV, Roberts ME, Fode FK, Besser GM, Monson JP, *et al.* Insulin sensitivity and glucose tolerance improve in patients with acromegaly converted from depot octreotide to pegvisomant. *Eur J Endocrinol* 2003; **149**:521–527.

36 Lindberg-Larsen R, Moller N, Schmitz O, Nielsen S, Andersen M, Orskov H, *et al.* The impact of pegvisomant treatment on substrate metabolism and insulin sensitivity in patients with acromegaly. *J Clin Endocrinol Metab* 2007; **92**:1724–1728.

37 Poulsen JE. Recovery from retinopathy in a case of diabetes with Simmonds' disease. *Diabetes* 1953; **2**:7–12.

38. Frank RN. Diabetic retinopathy. *N Engl J Med* 2004; **350**:48–58.

39 Merimee TJ. A follow-up study of vascular disease in growth-hormone-deficient dwarfs with diabetes. *N Engl J Med* 1978; **298**:1217–1222.

40 Smith LE, Kopchick JJ, Chen W, Knapp J, Kinose F, Daley D, *et al.* Essential role of growth hormone in ischemia-induced retinal neovascularization. *Science* 1997; **276**:1706–1709.

41 Janssen JA, Lamberts SW. Circulating IGF-1 and its protective role in the pathogenesis of diabetic angiopathy. *Clin Endocrinol (Oxf)* 2000; **52**:1–9.

42 Moller N, Orskov H. Growth hormone, IGF-1 and diabetic angiopathy revisited. *Clin Endocrinol (Oxf)* 2000; **52**:11–12.

43 Bereket A, Lang CH, Wilson TA. Alterations in the growth hormone-insulin-like growth factor axis in insulin dependent diabetes mellitus. *Horm Metab Res* 1999; **31**:172–181.

44 Carroll MF, Schade DS. The dawn phenomenon revisited: implications for diabetes therapy. *Endocr Pract* 2005; **11**:55–64.

45 Clemmons DR, Moses AC, McKay MJ, Sommer A, Rosen DM, Ruckle J. The combination of insulin-like growth factor I and insulin-like growth factor-binding protein-3 reduces insulin requirements in insulin-dependent type 1 diabetes: evidence for *in vivo* biological activity. *J Clin Endocrinol Metab* 2000; **85**:1518–1524.

46 McDonald A, Williams RM, Regan FM, Semple RK, Dunger DB. IGF-1 treatment of insulin resistance. *Eur J Endocrinol* 2007; **157**(Suppl 1):S51–S56.

47 Le Roith D. The insulin-like growth factor system. *Exp Diabesity Res* 2003; **4**:205–212.

48 Chiarelli F, Giannini C, Mohn A. Growth, growth factors and diabetes. *Eur J Endocrinol* 2004; **151**(Suppl 3):U109–U117.

49 Kim MS, Quintos JB. Mauriac syndrome: growth failure and type 1 diabetes mellitus. *Pediatr Endocrinol Rev* 2008; **5**(Suppl 4):989–993.

50 Arnaldi G, Angeli A, Atkinson AB, Bertagna X, Cavagnini F, Chrousos GP, *et al.* Diagnosis and complications of Cushing's syndrome: a consensus statement. *J Clin Endocrinol Metab* 2003; **88**:5593–5602.

51 Newell-Price J, Bertagna X, Grossman AB, Nieman LK. Cushing's syndrome. *Lancet* 2006; **367**:1605–1617.

52 Nieman LK, Ilias I. Evaluation and treatment of Cushing's syndrome. *Am J Med* 2005; **118**:1340–1346.

53 Arnaldi G, Mancini T, Polenta B, Boscaro M. Cardiovascular risk in Cushing's syndrome. *Pituitary* 2004; **7**:253–256.

54 Rizza RA, Mandarino LJ, Gerich JE. Cortisol-induced insulin resistance in man: impaired suppression of glucose production and stimulation of glucose utilization due to a postreceptor detect of insulin action. *J Clin Endocrinol Metab* 1982; **54**:131–138.

55 Stewart PM. The adrenal cortex. In: Kronenberg HM, Melmed S, Polonsky KS, Larsen PR, eds. *Williams Textbook of Endocrinology*, 11th edn. Saunders Elsevier, 2008:445–503.

56 Nestler JE, McClanahan MA. Diabetes and adrenal disease. *Baillieres Clin Endocrinol Metab* 1992; **6**:829–847.

57 Catargi B, Rigalleau V, Poussin A, Ronci-Chaix N, Bex V, Vergnot V, *et al.* Occult Cushing's syndrome in type 2 diabetes. *J Clin Endocrinol Metab* 2003; **88**:5808–5813.

58 Lindholm J, Juul S, Jorgensen JO, Astrup J, Bjerre P, Feldt-Rasmussen U, *et al.* Incidence and late prognosis of Cushing's syndrome: a population-based study. *J Clin Endocrinol Metab* 2001; **86**:117–123.

59 Pivonello R, De Martino MC, De Leo M, Tauchmanova L, Faggiano A, Lombardi G, *et al.* Cushing's syndrome: aftermath of the cure. *Arq Bras Endocrinol Metabol* 2007; **51**:1381–1391.

60 Faggiano A, Pivonello R, Spiezia S, De Martino MC, Filippella M, Di Somma C, *et al.* Cardiovascular risk factors and common carotid artery caliber and stiffness in patients with Cushing's disease during active disease and 1 year after disease remission. *J Clin Endocrinol Metab* 2003; **88**:2527–2533.

61 Radetti G, Paganini C, Gentili L, Barbin F, Pasquino B, Zachmann M. Altered adrenal and thyroid function in children with insulin-dependent diabetes mellitus. *Acta Diabetol* 1994; **31**:138–140.

62 Dacou-Voutetakis C, Peppa-Patrikiou M, Dracopoulou M. Urinary free cortisol and its nyctohemeral variation in adolescents and young adults with IDDM: relation to endothelin 1 and indices of diabetic angiopathy. *J Pediatr Endocrinol Metab* 1998; **11**:437–445.

63 Roy MS, Roy A, Brown S. Increased urinary-free cortisol outputs in diabetic patients. *J Diabetes Complications* 1998; **12**:24–27.

64 Tsigos C, Young RJ, White A. Diabetic neuropathy is associated with increased activity of the hypothalamic–pituitary–adrenal axis. *J Clin Endocrinol Metab* 1993; **76**:554–558.

65 Wurzburger MI, Prelevic GM, Sonksen PH, Peric LA, Till S, Morris RW. The effects of improved blood glucose on growth hormone and cortisol secretion in insulin-dependent diabetes mellitus. *Clin Endocrinol (Oxf)* 1990; **32**:787–797.

66 Karagiannis A, Mikhailidis DP, Athyros VG, Harsoulis F. Pheochromocytoma: an update on genetics and management. *Endocr Relat Cancer* 2007; **14**:935–956.

67 Eisenhofer G, Siegert G, Kotzerke J, Bornstein SR, Pacak K. Current progress and future challenges in the biochemical diagnosis and treatment of pheochromocytomas and paragangliomas. *Horm Metab Res* 2008; **40**:329–337.

68 Chrisoulidou A, Kaltsas G, Ilias I, Grossman AB. The diagnosis and management of malignant phaeochromocytoma and paraganglioma. *Endocr Relat Cancer* 2007; **14**:569–585.

69 Young W. Endocrine hypertension. In: Kronenberg HM, Melmed S, Polonsky KS, Larsen PR, eds. *Williams Textbook of Endocrinology*, 11th edn. Saunders Elsevier, 2008:505–537.

70 Kaltsas GA, Papadogias D, Grossman AB. The clinical presentation (symptoms and signs) of sporadic and familial chromaffin cell tumours (phaeochromocytomas and paragangliomas). *Front Horm Res* 2004; **31**:61–75.

71. La Batide-Alanore A, Chatellier G, Plouin PF. Diabetes as a marker of pheochromocytoma in hypertensive patients. *J Hypertens* 2003; **21**:1703–1707.

72 Bluher M, Windgassen M, Paschke R. Improvement of insulin sensitivity after adrenalectomy in patients with pheochromocytoma. *Diabetes Care* 2000; **23**:1591–1592.

73 Turnbull DM, Johnston DG, Alberti KG, Hall R. Hormonal and metabolic studies in a patient with a pheochromocytoma. *J Clin Endocrinol Metab* 1980; **51**:930–933.

74 Porte D Jr. A receptor mechanism for the inhibition of insulin release by adrenaline in man. *J Clin Invest* 1967; **46**:86–94.

75 Clutter WE, Rizza RA, Gerich JE, Cryer PE. Regulation of glucose metabolism by sympathochromaffin catecholamines. *Diabetes Metab Rev* 1988; **4**:1–15.

76 Deibert DC, DeFronzo RA. Adrenaline-induced insulin resistance in man. *J Clin Invest* 1980; **65**:717–721.

77 Sacca L, Vigorito C, Cicala M, Corso G, Sherwin RS. Role of gluconeogenesis in adrenaline-stimulated hepatic glucose production in humans. *Am J Physiol* 1983; **245**:E294–E302.

78 Vance JE, Buchanan KD, O'Hara D, Williams RH, Porte D Jr. Insulin and glucagon responses in subjects with pheochromocytoma: effect of alpha adrenergic blockade. *J Clin Endocrinol Metab* 1969; **29**:911–916.

79 Martin JF, Martin LN, Yugar-Toledo JC, Loureiro AA, Cury PM, Junior HM. Coronary emergency and diabetes as manifestations of pheochromocytoma. *Int J Cardiol* 2008; e-pub.

80 Chastain MA. The glucagonoma syndrome: a review of its features and discussion of new perspectives. *Am J Med Sci* 2001; **321**:306–320.

81 van Beek AP, de Haas ER, van Vloten WA, Lips CJ, Roijers JF, Canninga-van Dijk MR. The glucagonoma syndrome and necrolytic migratory erythema: a clinical review. *Eur J Endocrinol* 2004; **151**:531–537.

82 Oberg K, Eriksson B. Endocrine tumours of the pancreas. *Best Pract Res Clin Gastroenterol* 2005; **19**:753–781.

83 Wermers RA, Fatourechi V, Wynne AG, Kvols LK, Lloyd RV. The glucagonoma syndrome: clinical and pathologic features in 21 patients. *Medicine (Baltimore)* 1996; **75**:53–63.

84 Nesi G, Marcucci T, Rubio CA, Brandi ML, Tonelli F. Somatostatinoma: clinico-pathological features of three cases and literature reviewed. *J Gastroenterol Hepatol* 2008; **23**:521–526.

85 Larsson LI, Hirsch MA, Holst JJ, Ingemansson S, Kuhl C, Jensen SL, *et al.* Pancreatic somatostatinoma: clinical features and physiological implications. *Lancet* 1977; **1**:666–668.

86 Ganda OP, Weir GC, Soeldner JS, Legg MA, Chick WL, Patel YC, *et al.* "Somatostatinoma": a somatostatin-containing tumor of the endocrine pancreas. *N Engl J Med* 1977; **296**:963–967.

87 Krejs GJ, Orci L, Conlon JM, Ravazzola M, Davis GR, Raskin P, *et al.* Somatostatinoma syndrome: biochemical, morphologic and clinical features. *N Engl J Med* 1979; **301**:285–292.

88 Verner JV, Morrison AB. Islet cell tumor and a syndrome of refractory watery diarrhea and hypokalemia. *Am J Med* 1958; **25**:374–380.

89 Akerstrom G, Hellman P. Surgery on neuroendocrine tumours. *Best Pract Res Clin Endocrinol Metab* 2007; **21**:87–109.

90 Davies TF, Larsen PR. Thyrotoxicosis. In: *Williams Textbook of Endocrinology*, 11th edn. Kronenberg HM, Melmed S, Polonsky KS, Larsen PR, eds. Saunders Elsevier, 2008:333–375.

91 Roubsanthisuk W, Watanakejorn P, Tunlakit M, Sriussadaporn S. Hyperthyroidism induces glucose intolerance by lowering both insulin secretion and peripheral insulin sensitivity. *J Med Assoc Thai* 2006; **89**(Suppl 5):S133–S140.

92 Gonzalo MA, Grant C, Moreno I, Garcia FJ, Suarez AI, Herrera-Pombo JL, *et al.* Glucose tolerance, insulin secretion, insulin sensitivity and glucose effectiveness in normal and overweight hyperthyroid women. *Clin Endocrinol (Oxf)* 1996; **45**:689–697.

93 Fukuchi M, Shimabukuro M, Shimajiri Y, Oshiro Y, Higa M, Akamine H, *et al.* Evidence for a deficient pancreatic beta-cell response in a rat model of hyperthyroidism. *Life Sci* 2002; **71**:1059–1070.

94 Mokuno T, Uchimura K, Hayashi R, Hayakawa N, Makino M, Nagata M, *et al.* Glucose transporter 2 concentrations in hyper- and hypothyroid rat livers. *J Endocrinol* 1999; **160**:285–289.

95 Karlander SG, Khan A, Wajngot A, Torring O, Vranic M, Efendic S. Glucose turnover in hyperthyroid patients with normal glucose tolerance. *J Clin Endocrinol Metab* 1989; **68**:780–786.

96 Cooppan R, Kozak GP. Hyperthyroidism and diabetes mellitus: an analysis of 70 patients. *Arch Intern Med* 1980; **140**:370–373.

97 Resmini E, Minuto F, Colao A, Ferone D. Secondary diabetes associated with principal endocrinopathies: the impact of new treatment modalities. *Acta Diabetol* 2009; **46**:85–95.

98 Corry DB, Tuck ML. The effect of aldosterone on glucose metabolism. *Curr Hypertens Rep* 2003; **5**:106–109.

99 Conn JW. Hypertension, the potassium ion and impaired carbohydrate tolerance. *N Engl J Med* 1965; **273**:1135–1143.

100 Bringhurst F, Demay M, Kronenberg HM. Hormones and disorders of mineral metabolism. In: *Williams Textbook of Endocrinology*, 11th edn. Kronenberg HM, Melmed S, Polonsky KS, Larsen PR, eds. Saunders Elsevier, 2008:1203–1268.

101 Ljunghall S, Palmer M, Akerstrom G, Wide L. Diabetes mellitus, glucose tolerance and insulin response to glucose in patients with primary hyperparathyroidism before and after parathyroidectomy. *Eur J Clin Invest* 1983; **13**:373–377.

102 Taylor WH. The prevalence of diabetes mellitus in patients with primary hyperparathyroidism and among their relatives. *Diabet Med* 1991; **8**:683–687.

103 Taylor WH, Khaleeli AA. Coincident diabetes mellitus and primary hyperparathyroidism. *Diabetes Metab Res Rev* 2001; **17**:175–180.

104 Khaleeli AA, Johnson JN, Taylor WH. Prevalence of glucose intolerance in primary hyperparathyroidism and the benefit of parathyroidectomy. *Diabetes Metab Res Rev* 2007; **23**:43–48.

105 Akgun S, Ertel NH. Hyperparathyroidism and coexisting diabetes mellitus: altered carbohydrate metabolism. *Arch Intern Med* 1978; **138**:1500–1502.

106 Kautzky-Willer A, Pacini G, Niederle B, Schernthaner G, Prager R. Insulin secretion, insulin sensitivity and hepatic insulin extraction in primary hyperparathyroidism before and after surgery. *Clin Endocrinol (Oxf)* 1992; **37**:147–155.

107 Bannon MP, van Heerden JA, Palumbo PJ, Ilstrup DM. The relationship between primary hyperparathyroidism and diabetes mellitus. *Ann Surg* 1988; **207**:430–433.

108 Ayturk S, Gursoy A, Bascil Tutuncu N, Ertugrul DT, Guvener Demirag N. Changes in insulin sensitivity and glucose and bone metabolism over time in patients with asymptomatic primary hyperparathyroidism. *J Clin Endocrinol Metab* 2006; **91**:4260–4263.

109 Husbands S, Ong KK, Gilbert J, Wass JA, Dunger DB. Increased insulin sensitivity in young, growth hormone deficient children. *Clin Endocrinol (Oxf)* 2001; **55**:87–92.

110 Bougneres PF, Artavia-Loria E, Ferre P, Chaussain JL, Job JC. Effects of hypopituitarism and growth hormone replacement therapy on the production and utilization of glucose in childhood. *J Clin Endocrinol Metab* 1985; **61**:1152–1157.

111 Rosenfalck AM, Maghsoudi S, Fisker S, Jorgensen JO, Christiansen JS, Hilsted J, *et al.* The effect of 30 months of low-dose replacement therapy with recombinant human growth hormone (rhGH) on insulin and C-peptide kinetics, insulin secretion, insulin sensitivity, glucose effectiveness, and body composition in GH-deficient adults. *J Clin Endocrinol Metab* 2000; **85**:4173–4181.

112 McConnell EM, Atkinson AB, Ennis C, Hadden DR, McCance DR, Sheridan B, *et al.* The effects on insulin action in adult hypopituitarism of recombinant human GH therapy individually titrated for six months. *J Clin Endocrinol Metab* 2001; **86**:5342–5347.

113 Gotherstrom G, Svensson J, Koranyi J, Alpsten M, Bosaeus I, Bengtsson B, *et al.* A prospective study of 5 years of GH replacement therapy in GH-deficient adults: sustained effects on body composition, bone mass, and metabolic indices. *J Clin Endocrinol Metab* 2001; **86**:4657–4665.

114 Norrelund H, Moller N, Nair KS, Christiansen JS, Jorgensen JO. Continuation of growth hormone (GH) substitution during fasting in GH-deficient patients decreases urea excretion and conserves protein synthesis. *J Clin Endocrinol Metab* 2001; **86**:3120–3129.

115 Jeffcoate W. Can growth hormone therapy cause diabetes? *Lancet* 2000; **355**:589–590.

116 Azziz R. Diagnostic criteria for polycystic ovary syndrome: a reappraisal. *Fertil Steril* 2005; **83**:1343–1346.

117 Azziz R. Controversy in clinical endocrinology: diagnosis of polycystic ovarian syndrome: the Rotterdam criteria are premature. *J Clin Endocrinol Metab* 2006; **91**(3):781–785.

118 Franks, S. Diagnosis of polycystic ovary syndrome: in defence of the Rotterdam criteria. *J Clin Endocrinol Metab* 2006; **91**:786–789.

119 The Rotterdam ESHRE/ASRM-Sponsored PCOS Consensus Workshop Group. Revised 2003 consensus on diagnostic criteria and long-term health risks related to polycystic ovary syndrome (PCOS). *Hum Reprod* 2004; **19**:41–47.

120 The Rotterdam ESHRE/ASRM-Sponsored PCOS Consensus Workshop Group. Revised 2003 consensus on diagnostic criteria and long-term health risks related to polycystic ovary syndrome. *Fertil Steril* 2004; **81**:19–25.

121 Kaltsas GA, Isidori AM, Besser GM, Grossman AB. Secondary forms of polycystic ovary syndrome. *Trends Endocrinol Metab* 2004; **15**:204–210.

122 Fegan PG, Sandeman DD, Krone N, Bosman D, Wood PJ, Stewart PM, *et al.* Cushing's syndrome in women with polycystic ovaries and hyperandrogenism. *Nat Clin Pract Endocrinol Metab* 2007; **3**:778–783.

123 Creatsas G, Deligeoroglou E. Polycystic ovarian syndrome in adolescents. *Curr Opin Obstet Gynecol* 2007; **19**:420–426.

124 Dunaif A. Insulin resistance and the polycystic ovary syndrome: mechanism and implications for pathogenesis. *Endocr Rev* 1997; **18**:774–800.

125 Penhoat A, Chatelain PG, Jaillard C, Saez JM. Characterization of insulin-like growth factor 1 and insulin receptors on cultured bovine adrenal fasciculata cells: role of these peptides on adrenal cell function. *Endocrinology* 1988; **122**:2518–2526.

126 Cussons AJ, Stuckey BG, Walsh JP, Burke V, Norman RJ. Polycystic ovarian syndrome: marked differences between endocrinologists and gynaecologists in diagnosis and management. *Clin Endocrinol (Oxf)* 2005; **62**:289–295.

127 Hansen AP, Ledet T, Lundbaek K. Growth hormone and diabetes. In: Brownlee M, ed. *Handbook of Diabetes Mellitus*, vol. 4: *Biochemical Pathology*. Chichester: Wiley, 1981; 231–279.

128 Langford KS, Miell JP. The insulin-like growth factor-1/binding protein axis: physiology, pathophysiology and therapeutic manipulation. *Eur J Clin Invest* 1993; **23**:503–516.

129 Franks S. Polycystic ovary syndrome. *N Engl J Med* 1995; **333**:853–861.

130 Holt RIG, Hanley NA. *Essential Endocrinology and Diabetes*, 5th edn. Oxford: Blackwell, 2006.

18 Pancreatic Diseases and Diabetes

Ranjit Unnikrishnan & Viswanathan Mohan

Dr. Mohan's Diabetes Specialities Centre, Madras Diabetes Research Foundation (WHO Collaborating Centre for Non-communicable Diseases Prevention and Control & IDF Centre of Education), Chennai, India

Keypoints

- Pancreatic disease is a rare cause of diabetes.
- Acute pancreatitis is associated with transient hyperglycemia which rarely persists.
- Chronic pancreatitis secondary to any cause can lead to permanent diabetes which is typically difficult to control; imaging studies reveal dilated ducts and pancreatic calculi.
- Tropical calcific pancreatitis is a disease of unknown etiology found in low and middle income countries associated with large pancreatic calculi and diabetes (fibrocalculous pancreatic diabetes).
- Hereditary hemochromatosis is an inherited disorder that produces diabetes secondary to iron deposition in the pancreatic islets and subsequent islet cell damage.
- Pancreatic carcinoma may complicate type 2 diabetes, diabetes secondary to chronic pancreatitis and, most commonly, with fibrocalculous pancreatic diabetes. It is important to suspect malignancy in any patient who complains of back pain, jaundice or weight loss in spite of good glycemic control.
- Pancreatic surgery can lead to diabetes that is insulin-requiring and often difficult to control.
- Cystic fibrosis is a relatively common genetic disorder affecting the lung, pancreas and other organs. Up to 75% of adults with cystic fibrosis have some degree of glucose intolerance.

Introduction

Pancreatic disease is a rare cause of diabetes, accounting for less than 0.5% of all cases of diabetes. A number of disease processes affecting the pancreas can lead to diabetes; some of these are listed in Table 18.1.

Most of these conditions damage the exocrine as well as endocrine components of the pancreas. The exocrine parenchyma and islet tissue lie in intimate contact with each other and are functionally related. This may explain why parenchymal disease can readily impair β-cell function [1].

Acute pancreatitis

Acute pancreatitis varies considerably in its impact on the gland and its metabolism. Pathologic findings vary from mild edema to hemorrhagic necrosis, and the clinical presentation spans a wide spectrum from mild to fulminating or fatal illness.

The most common causes of acute pancreatitis are alcoholism and gallstone disease. Table 18.2 sets out the causes of acute pancreatitis. Classically, the disease presents with sudden onset of epigastric pain, associated with nausea and vomiting, aggravated by food and partially relieved by sitting up and leaning forward. Physical examination reveals low grade fever, tachycardia and hypotension. Jaundice may also be found infrequently. Cullen sign (periumbilical discoloration) and Grey Turner sign (flank discoloration) indicate severe necrotizing pancreatitis.

Commonly found metabolic abnormalities include hyperglycemia, hypocalcemia, hyperlipidemia, hypoalbuminemia and coagulation disorders [2]. Serum levels of amylase and lipase are elevated, but these are neither sensitive nor specific. Computed tomography (CT) or magnetic resonance imaging (MRI) shows edema of the pancreas. Loss of the normal enhancement on dynamic CT scanning indicates pancreatic necrosis.

Most patients with acute pancreatitis develop transient hyperglycemia, which mostly results from a rise in glucagon levels rather than from β-cell injury [3]. Hyperglycemia is usually mild and resolves within days to weeks without needing insulin treatment. Permanent diabetes is rare and occurs mostly in cases with fulminant disease and multiorgan failure, in whom the incidence approaches 25% [4]. Blood glucose levels exceeding 11.1 mmol/L (200 mg/dL) during the first 24 hours indicate a poor prognosis [5].

Non-specific elevations of serum amylase and lipase may also be found in diabetic ketoacidosis [6]. Acute pancreatitis, however,

Textbook of Diabetes, 4th edition. Edited by R. Holt, C. Cockram, A. Flyvbjerg and B. Goldstein.

Table 18.1 Pancreatic diseases associated with glucose intolerance and diabetes.

Inflammatory
Acute
Chronic, including fibrocalculous pancreatic diabetes
Infiltration
Hereditary hemochromatosis
Secondary hemochromatosis
Very rare causes: sarcoidosis, amyloidosis, cystinosis
Neoplasia
Adenocarcinoma of the pancreas
Glucagonoma
Surgical resection or trauma
Cystic fibrosis

may affect up to 11% of patients with ketoacidosis, usually with mild or even no abdominal pain [5].

Chronic pancreatitis

This condition is characterized by progressive and irreversible destruction of the exocrine pancreatic tissue, leading to exocrine pancreatic insufficiency and varying degrees of glucose intolerance which often require insulin. The causes of chronic pancreatitis vary according to the geographic location (Table 18.3).

Alcohol abuse accounts for most of the cases (>85%) in Western populations. Alcohol alters the composition of pancreatic secretions, leading to the formation of proteinaceous plugs that block the ducts and act as foci for calculi formation. Tropical pancreatitis is a distinct form of the disease that is not associated with excessive alcohol intake and is prevalent in the developing world [7].

Hereditary chronic pancreatitis is a rare entity, inherited in an autosomal dominant fashion. Mutations in a number of genes have been implicated including *PRSS1* (encoding cationic trypsinogen), *SPINK1* (serine protease inhibitor, Kazal type 1) and *CFTR* (cystic fibrosis transmembrane conductance regulator) [8–11].

Obstructive chronic pancreatitis is a rare condition that follows occlusion of pancreatic ducts by tumors, scarring, pseudocysts or congenital anomalies. Stones are not seen. Surgery or endoscopic dilatation may occasionally be curative.

Idiopathic pancreatitis, which accounts for 10–20% of all cases, affects two distinct age groups, one with onset at 15–25 years and the other at 55–65 years [12]. Cigarette smoking is a risk factor and mutations in specific genes have also been postulated [11,13,14].

Epidemiology

Chronic pancreatitis is prevalent worldwide. In Western countries, the incidence is about 4 cases per year per 100 000 population [15,16]. Tropical chronic pancreatitis is confined to tropical and subtropical regions of the world.

Table 18.2 Causes of acute pancreatitis.

Common (75% of cases)	Uncommon
Alcohol abuse	**Drugs**
Gallstone disease	Sulfonamides
Idiopathic	Tetracyclines
	Valproate
	Didanosine
	Estrogens
	Exenatide
	Metabolic disorders
	Hypertriglyceridemia
	Hypercalcemia
	Diabetic ketoacidosis
	Infections
	Mumps, Coxsackie and HIV viruses
	Mycoplasma pneumoniae
	Trauma
	Abdominal injury
	Surgery, including ERCP
	Miscellaneous
	Hereditary relapsing pancreatitis
	Pancreatic cancer
	Connective tissue diseases
	Pancreas divisum

ERCP, endoscopic retrograde cholangiopancreatography.

Table 18.3 Causes of chronic pancreatitis.

Common (90% of cases)	Rare
Alcohol abuse	Hereditary relapsing pancreatitis
Idiopathic	Obstructive chronic pancreatitis
Tropical calcific pancreatitis	

Pathologic features

The term chronic calcific pancreatitis accurately describes the pathologic changes in over 95% of cases of chronic pancreatitis in Western countries. The ductal and acinar lumina are filled with proteinaceous plugs which later calcify, forming small stones composed chiefly of calcium carbonate or calcite. Huge stones can occur but are more characteristic of tropical pancreatitis. The stones are found diffusely throughout the affected organ. Microscopically, there is atrophy of the ductal epithelium and stenosis of the ducts, associated with patchy fibrosis. There may also be foci of necrosis, with infiltration by lymphocytes, plasma cells and histiocytes [17]. Ultimately, the pancreas shrivels and develops an opaque capsule that may adhere to surrounding organs.

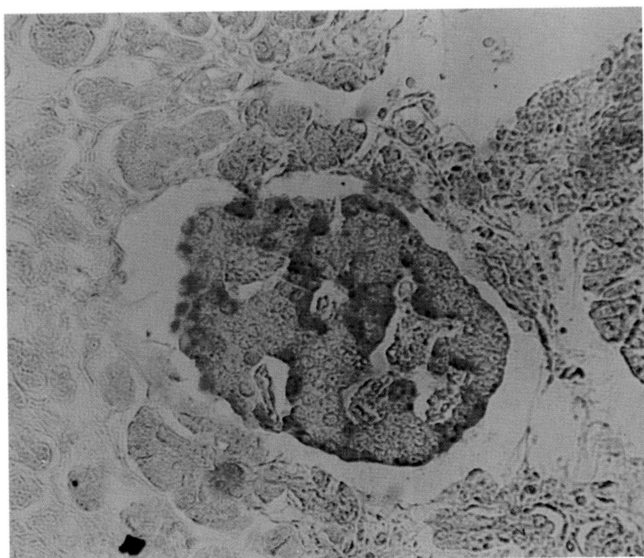

Figure 18.1 Nesidioblastosis, from a case of fibrocalculous pancreatic diabetes, showing islet tissue arising from ductal remnants. Stain aminoethylcarbazole; magnification ×40.

Table 18.4 Islet cell changes in chronic pancreatitis [25].

Cell type	Changes observed
β-cells	Decreased numbers (40% below controls)
α-cells	Increased numbers
β-cell : α-cell ratio	0.6–2.5 (controls, 3.0–3.5)
PP cells	Increased numbers
δ (D) cells	Unchanged

As fibrosis progresses, the acini atrophy and eventually disappear, leaving clusters of islets surrounded by sclerosed parenchyma. Neoformation of islet cells from ductal tissue can occur (nesidioblastosis) (Figure 18.1). Immunohistochemistry studies reveal generalized decrease in the number of islets, accompanied by overall reduction in β-cell density and insulin immunoreactivity which correspond to disease duration and C-peptide levels (Figure 18.2; Table 18.4) [18,19].

Clinical features and diagnosis

Abdominal pain is the predominant symptom and the usual reason for seeking medical care. The pain is usually steady, boring and agonizing and located in the epigastrium or left hypochondrium with radiation to the dorsal spine or the left shoulder. Bending forward or assuming the knee–chest position relieves the pain. The cause of the pain is unknown, but may relate to increased intrapancreatic or intraductal pressure, or to ischemia of the pancreas. It tends to remit and relapse and follows an unpredictable course. The development of end-stage pancreatic disease is associated with disappearance of the pain in many cases.

(a)

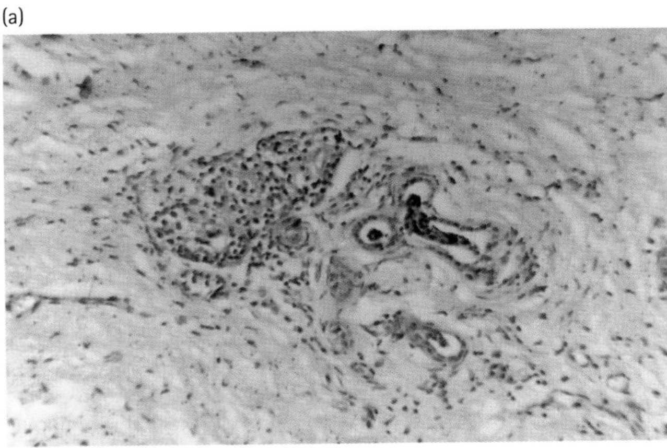

(b)

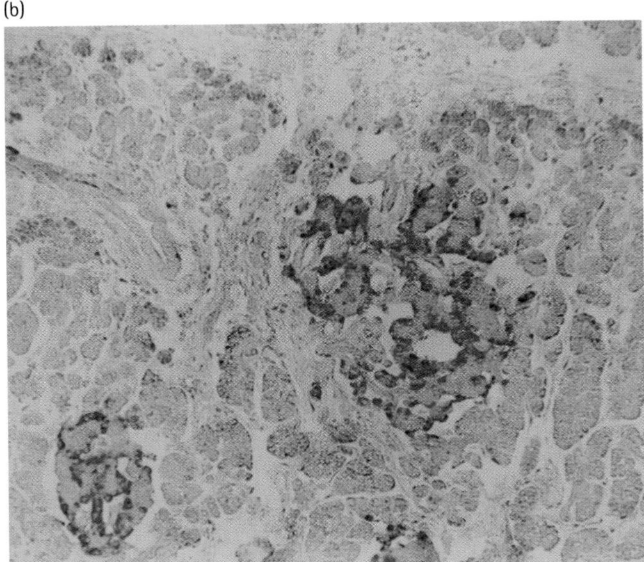

Figure 18.2 Histologic features of chronic pancreatitis, from cases of fibrocalculous pancreatic diabetes. (a) Exocrine tissue is entirely replaced by dense fibrosis that spares the islets. Hematoxylin and eosin stain; magnification ×40. (b) A hyperplastic islet. Section immunostained for insulin; magnification ×40.

Exocrine pancreatic insufficiency may manifest with steatorrhea and features of fat-soluble vitamin deficiency. Steatorrhea may not be apparent on a low-fat diet. The combination of oily and greasy stools with diabetes should raise the suspicion of chronic pancreatitis.

Investigations

Demonstration of pancreatic calculi on a plain X-ray of the abdomen is diagnostic (Figure 18.3). In cases where obvious calculi cannot be found, ultrasonography, CT scanning or endoscopic retrograde cholangiopancreatography (ERCP) will help to confirm the diagnosis. ERCP is considered the gold standard and usually reveals irregular dilatation of the pancreatic ducts with filling defects caused by stones (Figure 18.4). CT scanning shows patchy increases in parenchymal density and, ultimately, atrophy of the gland.

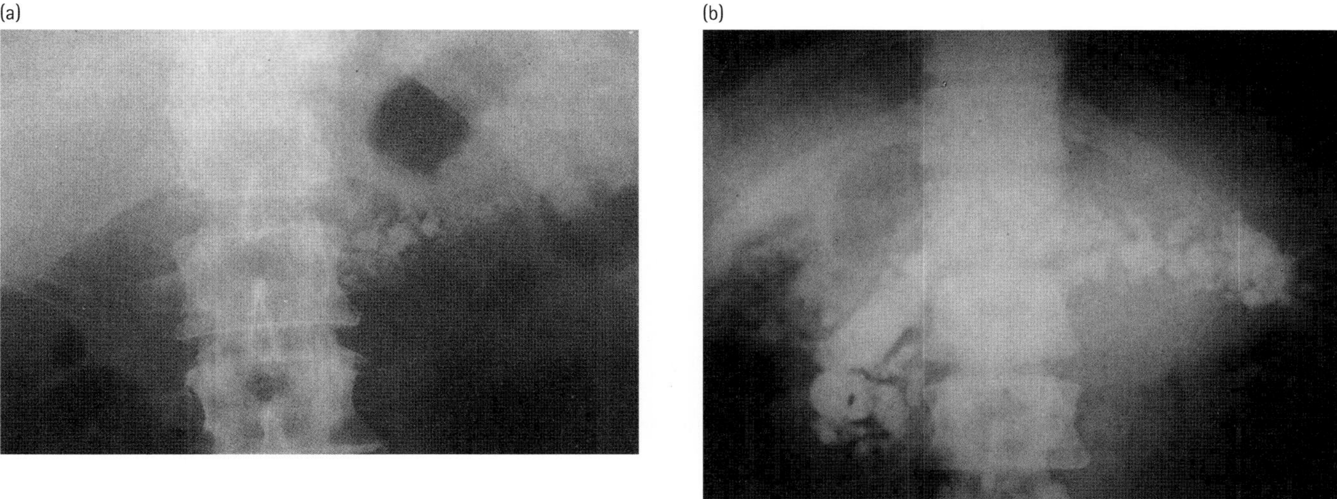

Figure 18.3 Pancreatic calculi, showing characteristic patterns in (a) alcoholic chronic pancreatitis, and (b) fibrocalculous pancreatic diabetes.

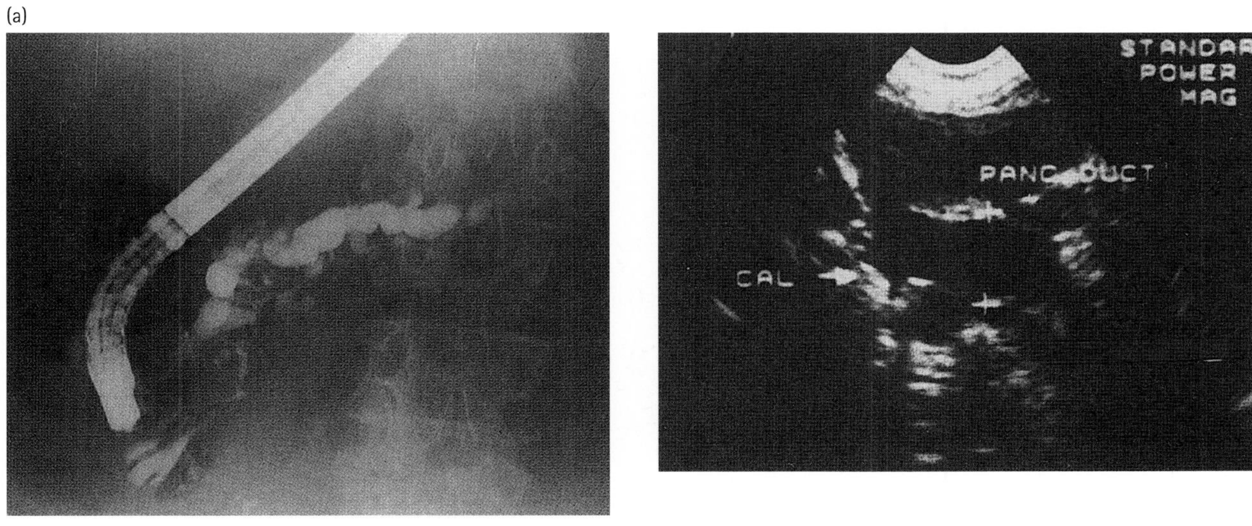

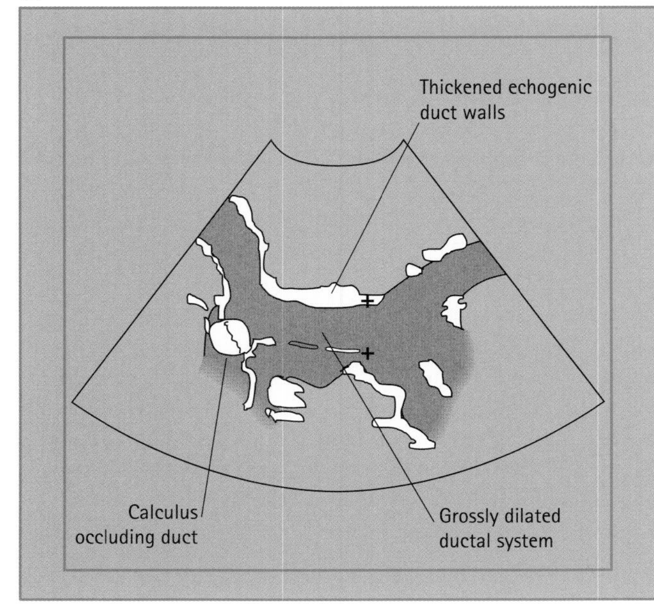

Figure 18.4 Investigations in chronic pancreatitis. (a) Endoscopic retrograde cholangiopancreatogram, showing dilatation and irregularity of the pancreatic ductal system in a patient with alcoholic chronic pancreatitis. Courtesy of Professor Jonathan Rhodes, Liverpool. (b) Ultrasound scan of the pancreas from a patient with fibrocalculous pancrdeatic diabetes, demonstrating highly echogenic parenchyma and duct walls (fibrosis), grossly dilated ducts and calculi. Courtesy of Dr. S. Suresh, Chennai, India.

Exocrine pancreatic function can be assessed by measuring the urinary excretion of compounds that are liberated in the gut by pancreatic enzyme action on orally ingested precursors such as NBT-PABA (para-aminobenzoic acid) or fluorescein dilaurate (pancreolauryl). Screening tests of pancreatic enzymes (fecal chymotrypsin, fecal elastase) are also used as they are simpler to perform but are less specific. Measurement of pancreatic output (via a tube placed in the duodenum) following ingestion of the Lundh test meal may also be helpful. Serum amylase is usually normal, except during acute attacks.

Diabetes in chronic pancreatitis

Abnormal glucose tolerance and diabetes complicate around 40–50% of cases of chronic pancreatitis. Unlike acute pancreatitis, the cause here is damage to the β-cells, owing to loss of trophic signals from the exocrine tissue [1,20]. The diabetes is of insidious onset and usually occurs several years after the onset of pain. The prevalence has been assessed at 60% after 20 years [21]. Half or more of patients require insulin for optimal glycemic control [22,23], but ketoacidosis is rare, even if insulin is withdrawn. Possible explanations include better preservation of β-cell function (compared with type 1 diabetes; T1DM) [24], reduced glucagon secretion and lower body stores of triglyceride, the major substrate for ketogenesis [24,25]. On account of the lower glucagon reserve, these patients are also prone to severe and prolonged hypoglycemia, and often diabetes is difficult to control with wide fluctuations of blood glucose levels.

Chronic diabetic complications

It was originally thought that patients with pancreatic diabetes were not at increased risk of microvascular complications. It has now been shown that retinopathy [26], nephropathy [27] and neuropathy [28] occur in these patients at frequencies similar to those with type 2 diabetes (T2DM). The risks of macrovascular complications, however, are relatively low. This may partly be explained by the low blood lipid levels that often accompany the malnutrition commonly seen in these patients [29].

Management of diabetes in chronic pancreatitis

Removal of obvious causes such as alcohol and hypertriglyceridemia will help to prevent progression of the damage to the gland.

Pain can be very difficult to manage. Measures include total abstinence from alcohol, dietary modification (small frequent meals with low fat content), analgesics and the somatostatin analogue, octreotide, which suppresses pancreatic exocrine secretion. In a subgroup of patients, massive doses of non-enteric-coated preparations of pancreatic enzymes have been shown to reduce pain. Surgical interventions include sphincterotomy, internal drainage of pancreatic cysts, endoscopic removal of calculi (via ERCP), insertion of duct stents and denervation procedures. Total resection of the pancreas followed by whole pancreas or islet cell transplantation may be an option for intractable cases.

Malabsorption can be effectively treated with a low fat diet with pancreatic enzyme supplements (along with histamine H_2 blocker or proton pump inhibitor to block gastric acid secretion) taken at meal times.

Diabetes can be managed along conventional lines, with a few caveats. High carbohydrate and protein intakes are encouraged along with fat restriction in order to prevent steatorrhea. Over 80% of patients require insulin; however, the required doses are typically low, around 30–40 units/day [22,23]. Diabetic control is often difficult to achieve, with frequent and severe hypoglycemia; reduced glucagon secretion may be responsible.

Tropical calcific pancreatitis

This is a distinct variety of chronic pancreatitis seen predominantly in low and middle income countries in the tropical and subtropical regions of the world [30,31]. This entity was first reported in 1959 by Zuidema [31] in patients from Indonesia. Later on, the disease was reported from several countries in Africa and Asia. The highest prevalence appears to be in Southern India, particularly in the states of Kerala and Tamil Nadu [32].

The disease usually starts in childhood with recurrent abdominal pain and during adolescence progresses to large pancreatic calculi and ductal dilatation (Figures 18.3 and 18.5). By adulthood, frank diabetes is found in more than 90% of patients [33]. Nevertheless, it remains a rare cause of diabetes, constituting less than 1% of all cases of diabetes even in regions where it is most prevalent [34]. A recent study in urban southern India reported a prevalence of 0.36% among subjects with self-reported diabetes and 0.019% among the general population [35].

The term tropical calcific pancreatitis is used to denote the prediabetic stage of the disease whereas the term fibrocalculous pancreatic diabetes (FCPD) is used to describe the clinical picture once diabetes has supervened (Figure 18.6).

The etiology of this condition remains unknown. Poor nutrition has been implicated as a possible factor; however, this may be the consequence rather than a cause of the pancreatopathy. The condition can also affect well-nourished individuals [36]. In the past, attention was also focused on the role of dietary toxins

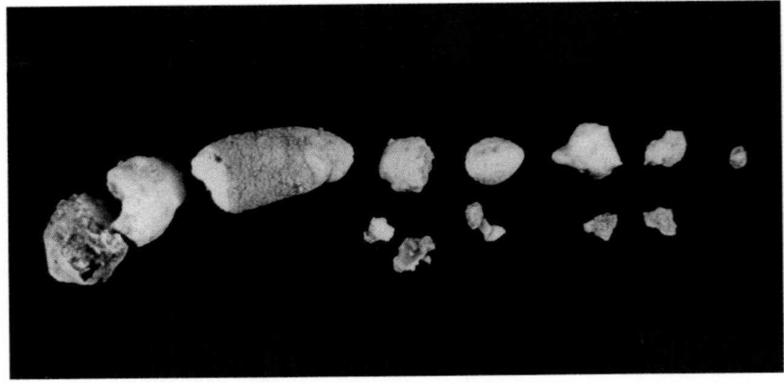

Figure 18.5 Calcite stones of various sizes removed from the pancreas of a patient with fibrocalcuous pancreatic diabetes.

such as cyanogens (found in cassava), but this link has not been substantiated. Cases have been found to cluster in families, which may suggest a genetic etiology for the disease [37–40]. A number of studies have reported an association between the *SPINK1* gene and tropical calcific pancreatitis [41–47]. A role has also been suggested for oxidant stress and free radical-mediated injury but this has not been proven conclusively [48].

Salient differences between alcoholic chronic pancreatitis and tropical calcific pancreatitis are summarized in the Table 18.5. The classic clinical triad of tropical calcific pancreatitis consists of abdominal pain, steatorrhea and eventually diabetes. The disease often progresses steadily from euglycemia through impaired glucose tolerance to frank diabetes. Most patients require insulin but are generally not prone to ketosis; some can be managed with oral antidiabetic agents (Figure 18.7). Studies have shown that the risk of developing pancreatic carcinoma in tropical calcific pancreatitis is 100-fold greater than in those without the disease and is much higher than in other forms of chronic pancreatitis [49]. Pancreatic malignancy should be suspected in individuals with tropical calcific pancreatitis if they complain of intractable pain or significant weight loss even after attaining good glycemic control.

Management of tropical calcific pancreatitis and FCPD is similar to that outlined for chronic pancreatitis.

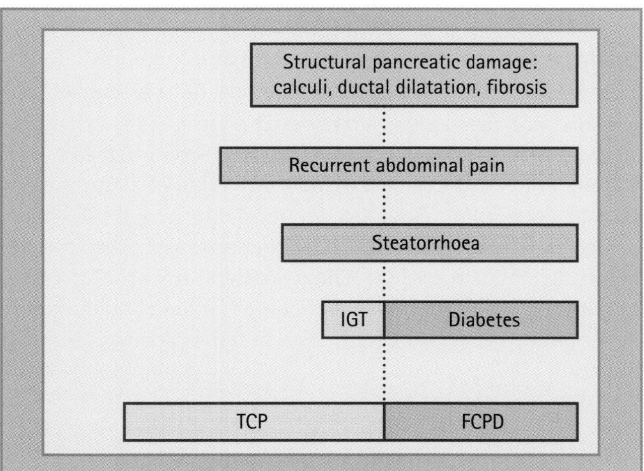

Figure 18.6 Natural history of tropical calcific pancreatitis and fibrocalculous pancreatic diabetes.

Hereditary hemochromatosis

This condition, also called idiopathic or primary hemochromatosis, is the most common autosomal recessive genetic disorder in Caucasians, with a prevalence of 4–5 per 1000 [50,51]. The classic triad of diabetes, cirrhosis and bronzed hyperpigmenta-

Table 18.5 Differences between tropical calcific pancreatitis and alcoholic chronic pancreatitis.

	Tropical calcific pancreatitis	Alcoholic chronic pancreatitis
Demographic features		
Male : female	70 : 30	90 : 10
Peak age at onset (years)	20–30	30–50
Socioeconomic status	Poor > affluent	All groups
Alcohol abuse	Absent	Present
Pancreatic morphology		
Prevalence of calculi	>90%	50–60%
Features of calculi	Large; in large ducts	Small, speckled; in small ducts
Ductal dilatation	Usually marked	Usually moderate
Fibrosis	Heavy	Variable
Risk of pancreatic cancer	Markedly increased	Increased
Diabetes		
Prevalence	>90%	50%
Time course	Faster evolution	Slower evolution

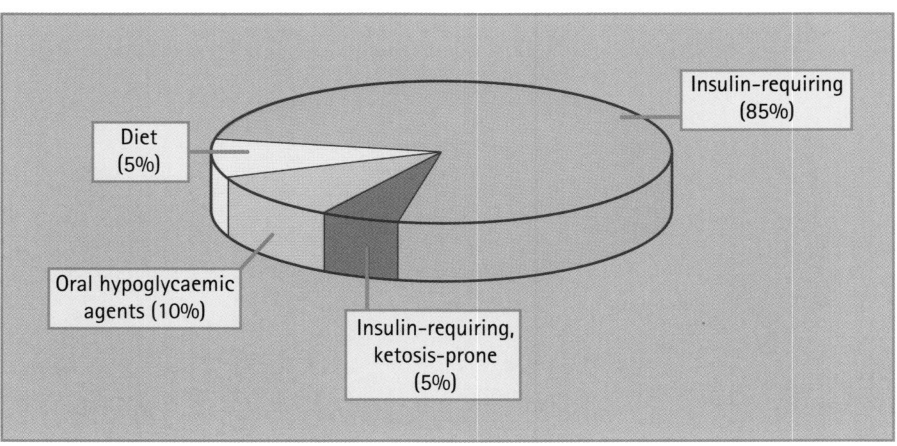

Figure 18.7 The spectrum of diabetes in fibrocalculous pancreatic diabetes. Data from Mohan *et al.* [29].

tion of the skin was first described by Trousseau in 1865 and called "hemochromatosis" by von Recklinghausen in 1889 [52].

Etiology and pathology

Genetic basis

Most cases of primary hemochromatosis arise from mutations in the hemochromatosis gene (*HFE*), located on the short arm of chromosome 6, close to the major histocompatibility complex (MHC), which explains the linkage with HLA A3 [53]. The HFE protein encoded by this gene is expressed on the cell surface of various tissues, including the enterocytes of the duodenal brush border, where iron is chiefly absorbed. The *HFE* gene modulates iron absorption by binding to the transferrin receptor. In two-thirds of cases, a C282Y mutation (substitution of cysteine by tyrosine at position 282) in the *HFE* gene is responsible [50]. Another mutation, H63D, seems to act synergistically with C282Y [54]. These mutations inhibit the binding of HFE to transferrin, leading to excessive and inappropriate increase in intestinal iron absorption and greatly increased body iron stores. Non-*HFE* mutations are also rarely found to be responsible in some cases.

Pathophysiology

The primary defect is excessive iron absorption across the mucosa of the proximal small intestine, which continues even in the setting of greatly increased total body iron stores (often 15–20 g: cf. normal adult iron stores of 1–2 g). Excess iron is deposited preferentially in the liver, pancreas (exocrine tissue as well as islets), pituitary, heart and parathyroids (Figure 18.8). Tissue injury is postulated to occur as a result of rupture of iron-laden lysosomes, generation of free radicals (by the Fenton reaction) and by the stimulation of collagen synthesis by activated stellate cells.

Clinical features

The classic clinical features are hepatic cirrhosis, diabetes and skin hyperpigmentation ("bronzed diabetes") (Figure 18.9). Hepatic fibrosis and cirrhosis usually only develop after age 40 years, unless other factors such as alcoholism are present. Portal hypertension, hepatic failure and hepatocellular carcinoma (in 15% of cases) are late sequelae [55]. Bronzing of the skin, which occurs in 70% of cases but may be less evident in darker-skinned races, is caused by both iron deposition in the subcutaneous tissue and increased melanin in the basal dermis. Hypopituitarism, hypogonadism, hypoparathyroidism and chondrocalcinosis with pseudogout are less common features.

Presenting symptoms include weakness, weight loss, diabetic symptoms, arthralgia, erectile dysfunction and skin pigmentation. Signs include hepatosplenomegaly, heart failure, skin pigmentation, testicular atrophy, arthropathy, hypogonadism and occasionally hypothyroidism. Many patients with hemochromatosis, however, are asymptomatic and may be detected during investigation for unrelated reasons.

Diabetes in primary hemochromatosis

The prevalence of diabetes depends on the severity of iron overload and presence of cirrhosis [56]. Up to 50% of patients have glucose intolerance and 25% have overt diabetes [57], although the disease is an extremely rare cause of diabetes in the general population. Both insulin resistance and β-cell failure contribute to the development of diabetes, and most patients eventually require insulin. These patients are prone to both microvascular and macrovascular complications [58], the risk of nephropathy being particularly high in those carrying the H63D mutation [59].

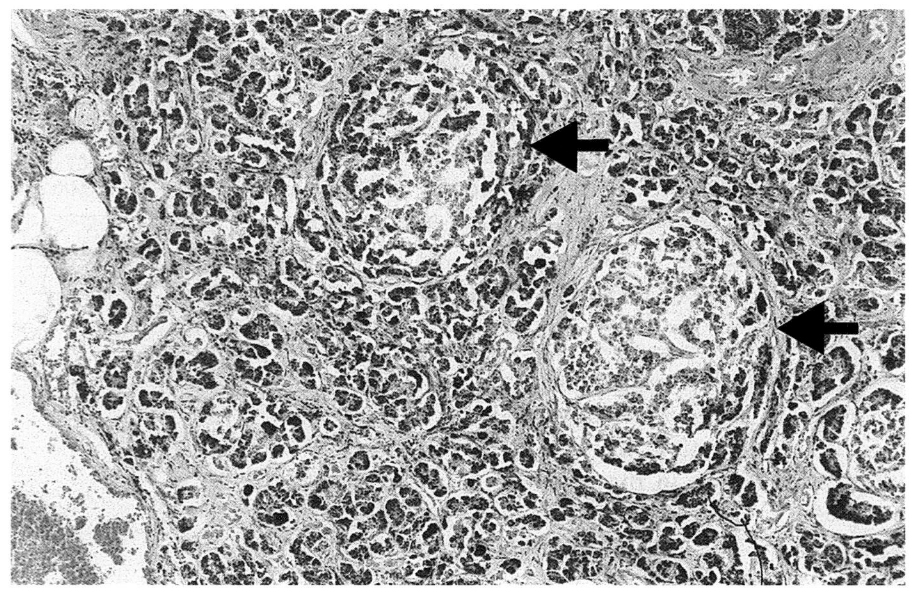

Figure 18.8 Hereditary hemochromatosis. Perls stain shows heavy iron deposition (blue) in exocrine and islet tissue in the pancreas (arrows). Original magnification ×375. Courtesy of Dr. A. Clark, Wirral Hospital, UK.

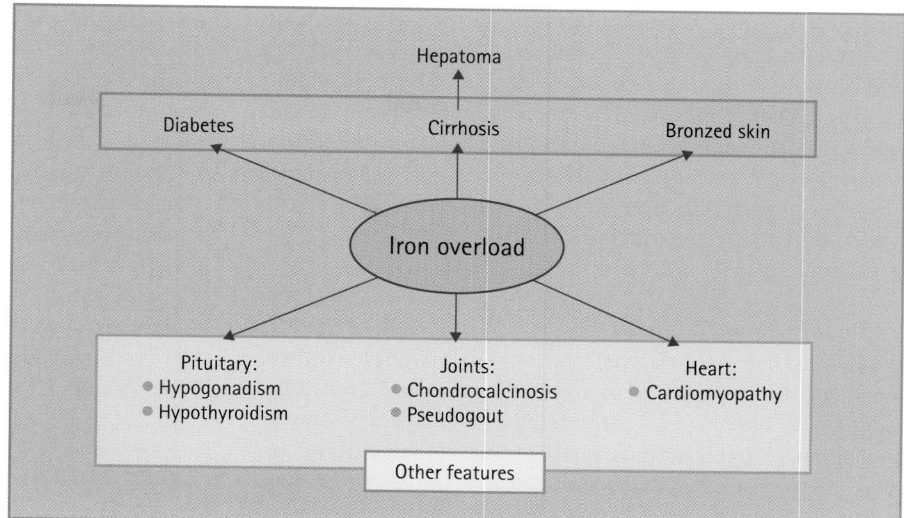

Figure 18.9 Clinical features of hereditary hemochromatosis. The classic triad comprises diabetes, cirrhosis and hyperpigmentation of the skin ("bronzed diabetes").

Investigations and diagnosis

The diagnosis should be suspected in any patient with diabetes, hepatomegaly or liver disease, skin pigmentation, arthritis and hypogonadism. A high index of suspicion is required to make an early diagnosis, because significant iron overload can exist with few or none of these clinical manifestations.

The total-body iron stores can be assessed using measurement of serum ferritin and percent saturation of transferrin. Serum ferritin is a useful screening test for relatives of affected individuals, but because ferritin is an acute phase reactant whose levels can be elevated in inflammatory states, abnormally high results should be confirmed by other tests (Table 18.6) [60]. Serum iron and percent saturation of transferrin are elevated early in the course of the disease, but lack specificity. A combined measurement of the percent transferrin saturation and serum ferritin levels provide a simple and reliable screening test for hemochromatosis. A positive test mandates genetic testing.

The role of liver biopsy in diagnosis and management of hemochromatosis has significantly diminished following the development of genetic testing for the C282Y mutation. The major role of liver biopsy at the present time is in excluding the presence of cirrhosis, which is a major risk factor in the development of hepatocellular carcinoma. Hepatic iron overload can also be detected using imaging techniques such as CT or MRI scanning.

All first-degree adult relatives of a patient with hemochromatosis should be tested for C282Y and H63D mutations, in an attempt to detect disease in the early precirrhotic phase at which stage treatment can prevent further progression.

Treatment

Treatment of hereditary hemochromatosis is by repeated venesection, which must be started as early as possible. Removal of excess iron by venesection prevents diabetes and cirrhosis and prolongs survival (Figure 18.10). Chelating agents such as desfer-

Table 18.6 Diagnostic tests in hereditary hemochromatosis [60].

	Hemochromatosis	Normal
Serum iron (μg/dL)	180–300	50–150
Transferrin saturation	80–100	20–50
Total iron-binding capacity (μg/dL)	200–300	250–370
Serum ferritin (μg/dL)		
Men	500–6000	20–300
Women	500–6000	15–250
Hepatic iron concentration (μg/g dry weight)	10 000–30 000	300–1800

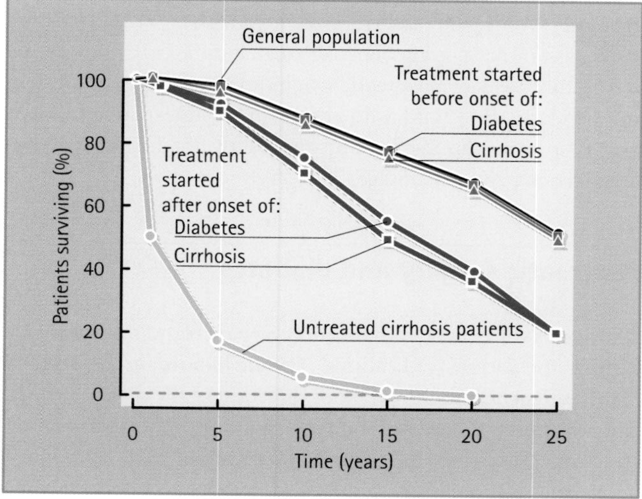

Figure 18.10 Venesection treatment in hereditary hemochromatosis. When treatment is started before the onset of cirrhosis or diabetes, life expectancy is normalized. Adapted from Dymock *et al.* [58].

rioxamine are more expensive, less safe and less effective than venesection. Diabetes may be improved by venesection, but usually requires insulin treatment. Management is often complicated by hypoglycemia caused by concomitant α-cell damage and glucagon deficiency. Hepatic transplantation for hereditary hemochromatosis were previously associated with a poor prognosis, but survival rates have improved of late. Diabetes tends to worsen after transplantation because of the use of immunosuppressant drugs [61].

Secondary hemochromatosis

Conditions such as thalassemia major, which require frequent blood transfusion, may lead to massive iron overload. Pancreatic damage and diabetes frequently result. The duration of disease and number of transfusions correlate well with the degree of glucose intolerance. It has been postulated that iron overload may induce autoimmune attack against the β-cells, thereby contributing to development of diabetes [62].

Pancreatic neoplasia

Adenocarcinoma of the pancreas is the fifth most common cause of cancer death and is increasing in its incidence [63]. It has a poor prognosis, with a 5-year survival rate of less than 3%.

Although diabetes has long been associated with pancreatic adenocarcinoma, the nature and strength of the association remain controversial. A meta-analysis of 20 epidemiologic studies showed a twofold increased risk of pancreatic cancer among people with diabetes of more than 5 years' duration [64], suggesting that diabetes is a risk factor for the neoplasm. Other studies, however, have concluded that the cancer preceded and caused the diabetes [65], a view supported by observations that diabetes may improve after resection of the tumor. Some studies have even suggested that diabetes protects against pancreatic cancer [66]. Tropical chronic pancreatitis is associated with a 100-fold increase in the risk of developing pancreatic carcinoma [50].

The diagnosis of pancreatic carcinoma must be suspected in any patient with T2DM who complains of unexplained weight loss (despite insulin therapy and apparently good control of diabetes), back pain or jaundice.

Pancreatic surgery and diabetes

Diabetes is a frequent complication of pancreatic resection performed for various indications. The incidence and severity of diabetes depends on the extent of resection of the distal segment, where the islets are most abundant. In one study, diabetes developed in 56% of cases following distal resection [67].

Diabetes is more likely to follow subtotal pancreatectomy than procedures such as lateral pancreaticojejunostomy and pancreaticoduodenoctomy (Whipple procedure). Diabetes is obviously inevitable following total pancreatectomy.

Management of diabetes caused by pancreatic surgery

The diabetes is usually difficult to control, with wide excursions in blood glucose levels. Patients are exquisitely insulin-sensitive and prone to hypoglycemia as a result of the loss of glucagon function. Frequent small meals and multiple small doses of insulin can minimize these problems to an extent. Use of a subcutaneous insulin infusion pump may be beneficial in some cases. Patients with diabetes following pancreatectomy are ideal candidates for whole pancreas or islet cell transplantation.

Associated exocrine pancreatic insufficiency should also be addressed. Meals should be low in fat and high in carbohydrate and protein. Pancreatic enzyme therapy will help in controlling steatorrhea and stabilizing blood glucose [68].

Cystic fibrosis

Cystic fibrosis is a multisystem disease characterized by recurrent airway infection leading to bronchiectasis, pancreatic insufficiency, abnormal sweat gland function and urogenital dysfunction. It is an autosomal recessive disorder caused by mutations in the *CFTR* gene located on chromosome 7q22. This gene encodes a protein, cystic fibrosis transmembrane conductance regulator (CFTR), which regulates the chloride secretion across epithelial surfaces. Various mutations have been described of which deletion of the phenylalanine residue at position 508 (Δ508) is the most common [69,76]. The defect produces unusually viscid secretions which lead to pancreatic ductular obstruction, dilatation and pancreatic insufficiency. The incidence is 1 in 2500 live births in Caucasian populations, but the disease is much less common in Africans and Asians [70].

The most common clinical features are steatorrhea, failure to thrive and growth retardation, recurrent lung infections, hepatobiliary complications and symptoms of fat-soluble vitamin deficiency such as night blindness. The diagnosis is confirmed by the presence of an elevated sweat chloride concentration in excess of 60 mmol/L.

Diabetes in cystic fibrosis

The incidence of diabetes in children with cystic fibrosis is 2–3% (about 20 times higher than in the general population). The incidence rises steadily through adolescence, with up to 25% of patients in their twenties developing diabetes and a further 50% having glucose intolerance [71].

As the treatment of the lung disease in cystic fibrosis has improved, more and more patients are surviving into adulthood. This has led to an increase in the prevalence of diabetes in cystic fibrosis.

The major factor in the pathogenesis of diabetes is damage to the pancreatic β-cells secondary to exocrine pancreatic degeneration. Other postulated mechanisms include enhanced absorption of glucose [72] and autoimmune attack against the β-cell, which may explain why T1DM is more common in relatives of patients with cystic fibrosis [73]. The physiologic insulin resistance of normal puberty may also contribute. Interestingly, diabetes develops more commonly in patients homozygous for Δ508 than in heterozygotes [74].

Diabetes is usually insidious in onset and characterized by a delayed, flattened and prolonged insulin secretory response to glucose [75]. Ketoacidosis is rare, although insulin treatment is usually required. As patients now survive longer [69], chronic microvascular complications are also frequently seen.

Management

Although some patients initially respond to sulfonylureas, most ultimately need insulin [76]. In addition to controlling diabetes, insulin also improves body weight and pulmonary and pancreatic function [71,77,78]. Starting from adolescence, all patients with cystic fibrosis should be regularly screened for diabetes using the oral glucose tolerance test or serial measurements of HbA_{1c} [78].

Dietary modification in patients with cystic fibrosis who also have diabetes presents much the same difficulties as in patients with chronic pancreatitis. A diet rich in carbohydrates and protein but restricted in fat is recommended. Oral pancreatic enzyme therapy helps to improve nutrient digestion and absorption. Enteric-coated preparations of lipase can control steatorrhea. Fibrosing colonopathy is a concern in patients receiving higher strengths of lipase [79].

Conclusions

Although rare, diabetes secondary to pancreatic disease is potentially important. The underlying pancreatic disease may need treatment in its own right, while disorders with a genetic basis must be identified so that other family members can be screened. Diagnosis of pancreatic diabetes requires a high index of suspicion. Suggestive symptoms include features of pancreatic disease (steatorrhea, unexplained weight loss or back pain) and severe and brittle diabetes in the absence of a family history of diabetes.

Acknowledgments

The authors acknowledge the contributions of C.S. Pitchumoni and G. Premalatha to this chapter in the previous edition of this textbook.

References

1 Williams JA, Goldfine ID. The insulin–pancreatic acinar axis. *Diabetes* 1985; **34**:980–986.

2 Agarwal N, Pitchumoni CS. Acute pancreatitis: a multisystem disease. *Gastroenterologist* 1993; **1**:115–128.

3 Gorelick FS. Diabetes mellitus and the exocrine pancreas. *Yale J Biol Med* 1983; **56**:271–275.

4 Scuro LA, Angelini G, Cavallini G, Vantini I. The late outcome of acute pancreatitis. In: Gyr KL, Singer MV, Sarles H, eds. *Pancreatitis: Concepts and Classification.* Amsterdam: Excerpta Medica, 1984: 403–408.

5 Agarwal N, Pitchumoni CS. Assessment of severity in acute pancreatitis. *Am J Gastroenterol* 1991; **86**:1385–1391.

6 Vantyghem MC, Haye S, Balduyck M, Hober C, Degand PM, Lefebvre J. Changes in serum amylase, lipase and leukocyte elastase during diabetic ketoacidosis and poorly controlled diabetes. *Acta Diabetol* 1999; **36**:39–44.

7 Mohan V, Chari S, Viswanathan M, Madanagopalan N. Tropical calcific pancreatitis in southern India. *Proc R Coll Phys Edinb* 1990: **20**:34–42.

8 Witt H, Sahin-Tóth M, Landt O, Chen JM, Kähne T, Drenth JP, *et al.* A degradation-sensitive anionic trypsinogen (*PRSS2*) variant protects against chronic pancreatitis. *Nat Genet* 2006; **38**:668–673.

9 Witt H, Luck W, Hennies HC, Classen M, Kage A, Lass U, *et al.* Mutations in the gene encoding the serine protease inhibitor, Kazal type 1 are associated with chronic pancreatitis. *Nat Genet* 2000; **25**:213–216.

10 Sharer N, Schwarz M, Malone G, Howarth A, Painter J, Super M, *et al.* Mutations of the cystic fibrosis gene in patients with chronic pancreatitis. *N Engl J Med* 1998; **339**:645–652.

11 Cohn JA, Friedman KJ, Noone PG, Knowles MR, Silverman LM, Jowell PS. Relation between mutations of the cystic fibrosis gene and idiopathic pancreatitis. *N Engl J Med* 1998; **339**:653–658.

12 Layer P, Yamamoto H, Kalthoff L, Clain JE, Bakken LJ, DiMagno EP. The different courses of early- and late-onset idiopathic and alcoholic chronic pancreatitis. *Gastroenterology* 1994; **107**:1481–1487.

13 Pitchumoni CS. Does cigarette smoking cause chronic pancreatitis? *J Clin Gastroenterol* 2000; **31**:274–275.

14 Matozaki T, Sakamoto C, Suzuki T, Chujo S, Matsuda K, Wada K, *et al.* Idiopathic chronic calcifying pancreatitis with diabetes mellitus: analysis of pancreatic stone protein gene. *Dig Dis Sci* 1993; **38**:963–967.

15 O'Sullivan JN, Nobrega FT, Morlock CG, Brown AL Jr, Bartholomew LG. Acute and chronic pancreatitis in Rochester, Minnesota, 1940 to 1969. *Gastroenterology* 1972; **62**:373–379.

16 Copenhagen Pancreatitis Study. An interim report from a prospective epidemiological multi-center study. *Scand J Gastroenterol* 1981: **16**:305–312.

17 Nagalotimath SJ. Pancreatic pathology in pancreatic calcification with diabetes. In: Viswanathan M, Podolsky S, eds. *Secondary Diabetes: the Spectrum of the Diabetic Syndrome.* New York: Raven Press, 1980: 117–145.

18 Govindarajan M, Mohan V, Deepa R, Ashok S, Pitchumoni CS. Histopathology and immunohistochemistry of pancreatic islets in fibrocalculous pancreatic diabetes. *Diabetes Res Clin Pract* 2001; **51**:29–38.

19 Klöppel G, Bommer G, Commandeur G, Heitz P. The endocrine pancreas in chronic pancreatitis: immunocytochemical and ultrastructural studies. *Virchows Arch A Pathol Anat Histol* 1978; **377**:157–174.

20 Kang SY, Go VL. Pancreatic exocrine–endocrine interrelationship: clinical implications. *Gastroenterol Clin North Am* 1999; **28**:551–569.

21 Bank S, Marks IN, Vinik AI. Clinical and hormonal aspects of pancreatic diabetes. *Am J Gastroenterol* 1975; **64**:13–22.

22 Mohan V, Mohan R, Susheela L, Snehalatha C, Bharani G, Mahajan VK, *et al.* Tropical pancreatic diabetes in South India: heterogeneity in clinical and biochemical profile. *Diabetologia* 1985; **28**:229–232.

23 Mohan V, Pitchumoni CS. Tropical chronic pancreatitis. In: Beger HG, Warshaw AL, Buchler MW, *et al.*, eds. *The Pancreas.* Vol 1. Oxford: Blackwell Science, 1998: 668–697.

24 Mohan V, Snehalatha C, Ramachandran A, Chari S, Madanagopalan N, Viswanathan M. Plasma glucagon responses in tropical fibrocalculous pancreatic diabetes. *Diabetes Res Clin Pract* 1990; **9**:97–101.

25 Yajnik CS, Shelgikar KM, Naik SS, Kanitkar SV, Orskov H, Alberti KG, *et al.* The ketosis-resistance in fibro-calculous-pancreatic-diabetes. 1. Clinical observations and endocrine-metabolic measurements during oral glucose tolerance test. *Diabetes Res Clin Pract* 1992; **15**:149–156.

26 Mohan R, Rajendran B, Mohan V, Ramachandran A, Viswanathan M, Kohner EM. Retinopathy in tropical pancreatic diabetes. *Arch Ophthalmol* 1985; **103**:1487–1489.

27 Shelgikar KM, Yajnik CS, Mohan V. Complications in fibrocalculous pancreatic diabetes: the Pune Madras Experience. *Int J Diabetes Dev Countries* 1995; **15**:70–75.

28 Ramachandran A, Mohan V, Kumaravel TS, Velmurugendran CU, Snehalatha C, Chinnikrishnudu M, *et al.* Peripheral neuropathy in tropical pancreatic diabetes. *Acta Diabetol Lat* 1986; **23**:135–140.

29 Mohan V, Ramachandran A, Viswanathan M. Two case reports of macrovascular complications in fibrocalculous pancreatic diabetes. *Acta Diabetol Lat* 1989; **26**:345–349.

30 Nair S, Yadav D, Pitchumoni CS. Association of diabetic ketoacidosis and acute pancreatitis: observations in 100 consecutive episodes of DKA. *Am J Gastroenterol* 2000; **95**:2795–2800.

31 Zuidema PJ. Cirrhosis and disseminated calcification of the pancreas in patients with malnutrition. *Trop Geogr Med* 1959; **11**:70–74.

32 Geevarghese PJ. *Calcific Pancreatitis.* Bombay: Varghese, 1985.

33 Geevarghese PJ. *Pancreatic Diabetes.* Bombay: Popular Prakashan, 1968: 110–115.

34 Mohan V, Premalatha G. Fibrocalculous pancreatic disease. *Int J Diabetes* 1995; **23**:71–82.

35 Mohan V, Farooq S, Deepa M. Prevalence of fibrocalculous pancreatic diabetes in Chennai in South India. *JOP* 2008; **9**:489–492.

36 Mohan V, Nagalotimath SJ, Yajnik CS, Tripathy BB. Fibrocalculous pancreatic diabetes. *Diabetes Metab Rev* 1998; **14**:153–170.

37 Sood R, Ahuja MMS, Karmarkar MG. Serum C-peptide levels in young ketosis resistant diabetics. *Indian J Med Res* 1983; **78**:661–664.

38 Pitchumoni CS. Familial pancreatitis. In: Pai KN, Soman CR, Varghese R, eds. *Pancreatic Diabetes.* Trivandrum: Geo Printers, 1970: 46–48.

39 Mohan V, Chari S, Hitman GA, Suresh S, Madanagopalan N, Ramachandran A, *et al.* Familial aggregation in tropical firbrocalculous pancreatic diabetes. *Pancreas* 1989; **4**:690–693.

40 Kambo PK, Hitman GA, Mohan V, Ramachandran A, Snehalatha C, Suresh S, *et al.* The genetic predisposition to fibrocalculous pancreatic diabetes. *Diabetologia* 1989; **32**:45–51.

41 Consensus statement. International workshop on types of diabetes peculiar to the tropics, 17–19 October 1995, Cuttack, India. *Acta Diabetol Lat* 1996; **33**:62–64.

42 Anonymous. Report of the expert committee on the diagnosis of diabetes mellitus. *Diabetes Care* 1997; **20**:1183–1197.

43 Hassan Z, Mohan V, Ali L, Allotey R, Barakat K, Farunque MO, *et al.* SPINK1 is a major gene for susceptibility to fibrocalculous pancreatic diabetes in subjects from southern Indian subcontinent. *Am J Hum Genet* 2002; **71**:964–968.

44 Chandak GR, Idris MM, Reddy DN, Bhaskar S, Srinam PV, Singh L. Mutations in the pancreatic secretory trypsin inhibitor gene (PSTI/SPINK1) rather than the cationic trypsinogen gene (PRSS1) are significantly associated with tropical calcific pancreatitis. *J Med Genet* 2002; **39**:347–351.

45 Suman A, Schneider A, Rossi L, Barmada MM, Beglinger C, Parvin S, *et al.* SPINK1 mutations in tropical pancreatitis and diabetes patients from Bangladesh. *Pancreas* 2001; **23**:462–467.

46 Bhatia E, Choudhuri G, Sikora SS, Landt O, Kage A, Becker M, *et al.* Tropical calcific pancreatitis: strong association with SPINK1 trypsin inhibitor mutation. *Gastroenterology* 2002; **123**:1020–1025.

47 Schneider A, Suman A, Rossi L, Barmada MM, Beglinger C, Parvin S, *et al.* SPINK 1/PSTI 1 mutation are associated with tropical pancreatitis and type 2 diabetes in Bangladesh. *Gastroenterology* 2002; **123**:1026–1030.

48 Braganza JM, Sherry J, Indira P, *et al.* Xenobiotics and tropical chronic pancreatitis. *Int J Pancreatol* 1990: 222–245.

49 Chari ST, Mohan V, Pitchumoni CS, Viswanathan M, Madanagopalan N, Lowenfels AB. Risk of pancreatic carcinoma in tropical calcific pancreatitis. *Pancreas* 1993; **9**:62–66.

50 Tavill AS. Clinical implications of the hemochromatosis gene. *N Engl J Med* 1999; **341**:755–757.

51 Merryweather-Clarke AT, Pointon JJ, Shearman JD, Robson KJ. Global prevalence of putative haemochromatosis mutations. *J Med Genet* 1997; **34**:275–278.

52 von Recklinghausen FD. Uber Hamochromatose. *Berlin Klin Wochenschr* 1889; **26**:925.

53 Simon M, Bourel M, Fauchet R, Genetet B. Association of HLA-A3 and HLA-B14 antigens with idiopathic haemochromatosis. *Gut* 1976; **17**:332–334.

54 Pietrangelo A, Montosi G, Totaro A, Garuti C, Conte D, Cassanelli S, *et al.* Hereditary hemochromatosis in adults without pathogenic mutations in the hemochromatosis gene. *N Engl J Med* 1999; **341**:725–732.

55 Dymock IW, Cassar J, Pyke DA, Oakley WG, Williams R. Observations on the pathogenesis, complications and treatment of diabetes in 115 cases of haemochromatosis. *Am J Med* 1972; **52**:203–210.

56 Niederau C. Diabetes mellitus in hemochromatosis. *Z Gastroenterol* 1999; **1**(Suppl):22–32.

57 Adams PC, Kertesz AE, Valberg LS. Clinical presentation of hemochromatosis: a changing scene. *Am J Med* 1991; **90**:445–449.

58 Dymock IW, Cassar J, Pyke DA, Oakley WG, Williams R. Observations on the pathogenesis, complications and treatment of diabetes in 115 cases of haemochromatosis. *Am J Med* 1972; **52**:203–210.

59 Moczulski DK, Grzeszczak W, Gawlik B. Role of hemochromatosis C282Y and H63D mutations in HFE gene in development of type 2 diabetes and diabetic nephropathy. *Diabetes Care* 2001; **24**:1187–1191.

60 Fried Hagedorn CH. Inherited disorders causing cirrhosis. In: Stein SF, Kokko JP, eds. *The Emory University Comprehensive Board Review in Internal Medicine.* New York: Mc-Graw-Hill Health Professions Division, 2000: 533–534.

61 Yu L, Ioannou GN. Survival of liver transplant recipients with hemochromatosis in the United States. *Gastroenterlogy* 2007; **133**:489–495.

62 Monge L, Pinach S, Caramellino L, Bertero MT, Dall'omo A, Carta Q. The possible role of autoimmunity in the pathogenesis of

diabetes in B-thalassemia major. *Diabetes Metab* 2001; **27**:149–154.

63 Rosewicz S, Wiedenmann B. Pancreatic carcinoma. *Lancet* 1997; **349**:485–489.

64 Everhart J, Wright D. Diabetes mellitus as a risk factor for pancreatic cancer: a meta-analysis. *JAMA* 1995; **273**:1605–1609.

65 Gullo L. Diabetes and the risk of pancreatic cancer. *Ann Oncol* 1999; **4**(Suppl):79–81.

66 Permert J, Larsson J, Ihse I, Pour PM. Diagnosis of pancreatic cancer: alteration of glucose metabolism. *Int J Pancreatol* 1991; **9**:113–117.

67 Buhler L, Schmidlin F, de Perot M, Borst F, Mentha G, Morel P. Long-term results after surgery for chronic pancreatitis. *Hepatogastroenterology* 1999: **46**:1986–1999.

68 Mohan V, Poongothai S, Pitchumoni CS. Oral pancreatic enzyme therapy in the control of diabetes mellitus in tropical calculous pancreatitis. *Int J Pancreatol* 1998; **24**:19–22.

69 Gaskin K. Exocrine pancreatic dysfunction in cystic fibrosis. In: Walker J, Durie P, Hamilton R, Walker-Smith J, Walkins J, eds. *Pediatric Gastrointestinal Disease*. Hamilton, BC: Decker, 2000: 1353–1370.

70 Dodge JA, Goodall J, Geddes D. Cystic fibrosis in the United Kingdom 1977–85: an improving picture. British Pediatric Association Working Party on Cystic Fibriosis. *Br Med J* 1988; **297**:1599–1602.

71 Robert JJ, Mosnier-Pudar H. Diagnosis and treatment of diabetes in adult patients with cystic fibrosis. *Rev Mal Respir* 2000; **17**:798–801.

72 Frase LL, Strickland AD, Kachel GW, Krejs GJ. Enhanced glucose absorption in the jejunum of patients with cystic fibrosis. *Gastroenterology* 1985; **88**:478–484.

73 Stutchfield PR, O'Halloran SM, Smith CS, Woodrow JC, Bottazzo GF, Heaf D. HLA type, islet cell antibodies, and glucose intolerance in cystic fibrosis. *Arch Dis Child* 1988; **63**:1234–1239.

74 Hamdi I, Payne SJ, Barton DE, McMahon R, Green M, Shneerson JM, Hales CN. Genotype analysis in cystic fibrosis in relation to the occurrence of diabetes mellitus. *Clin Genet* 1993; **43**:186–189.

75 Hartling SG, Garne S, Binder C, Heilmann C, Petersen W, Petersen KE, *et al.* Proinsulin, insulin, and C-peptide in cystic fibrosis after an oral glucose tolerance test. *Diabetes Res* 1988; **7**:165–169.

76 Hodson ME. Diabetes mellitus and cystic fibrosis. *Baillieres Clin Endocrinol Metab* 1992; **6**:797–805.

77 Lanng S, Thorsteinsson B, Nerup J, Koch C. Diabetes mellitus in cystic fibrosis: effect of insulin therapy on lung function and infections. *Acta Paediatr* 1994; **83**:849–853.

78 Nousia-Arvanitakis S, Galli-Tsinopoulou A, Karamouzis M. Insulin improves clinical status of patients with cystic-fibrosis-related diabetes mellitus. *Acta Paediatr* 2001; **90**:515–519.

79 Stevens JC, Maguiness KM, Hollingsworth J, Heilman DK, Chong SK. Pancreatic enzyme supplementation in cystic fibrosis patients before and after fibrosing colonopathy. *J Pediatr Gastroenterol Nutr* 1998; **26**:80–84.

5 Managing the Patient with Diabetes

19 Clinical Presentations of Diabetes

Ee Lin Lim & Roy Taylor

Diabetes Research Group, Institute of Cellular Medicine, Newcastle University, Newcastle upon Tyne, UK

Keypoints

- Patients with type 1 diabetes usually present with classic symptoms and occasionally diabetic ketoacidosis.
- Patients with type 2 diabetes mellitus (T2DM) may be asymptomatic or present with classic symptoms.
- With advancing age, the renal threshold for glucose increases and thirst perception diminishes.
- T2DM may present with complications of diabetes which may be either microvascular or macrovascular.
- Initial diagnosis of T2DM during acute myocardial infarction or stroke is common.
- Presentation may be asymptomatic and discovered on routine examination or laboratory test.

Introduction

Diabetes has long since taken over from syphilis as the great imitator, and nowhere is this more apparent than in the wide variation of possible modes of initial presentation. The classic triad of thirst, polydipsia and polyuria accounts for only a modest proportion of new diagnoses of diabetes. The relatively acute onset of such symptoms associated with loss of weight is the hallmark of type 1 diabetes mellitus (T1DM). Ketoacidosis and hyperosmolar hyperglycemic syndrome may precipitate a dramatic presentation to emergency services. Non-specific symptoms including tiredness, general malaise and repeated or persistent skin infections may lead to a biochemical diagnosis of diabetes. Screening of at-risk groups or individuals allows early diagnosis. Regrettably, the nature of the condition is such as to allow it to remain asymptomatic for years, allowing the clinical presentation to be a long-term complication of diabetes. This could be in the form of macrovascular disease (myocardial infarction, stroke, black toe) or in the form of microvascular disease (loss of visual acuity, neuropathy). Pregnancy may cause gestational diabetes (GDM), which although may remit after delivery, does indicate a high risk for future type 2 diabetes mellitus (T2DM).

Clinical considerations at presentation

At the heart of any consultation involving the presentation of diabetes there is a patient. Depending upon prior knowledge, "diabetes" may be associated in their mind with blindness and amputation, disability and premature death. Alternatively, it may be associated with vague concepts of malaise along with lumbago or fibrositis. The patient's beliefs and thoughts on diabetes need to be established if the diagnostic consultation is to be a therapeutic consultation. In an era of medicine by numbers, often traduced as "evidence-based medicine," it is easy to overlook the impact of the consultation itself upon the person who will live with diabetes. "Where were you when JFK was shot?" "What was it like when you were told you have diabetes?" The moment is likely to be memorable and influential.

The therapeutic consultation will involve listening, a process that need not be unduly time consuming. "Do you know of anyone with diabetes?" "What do you know of diabetes just now?" The information received will allow the patient's likely type of diabetes and immediate prognosis to be put into perspective. Together with other aspects of sound clinical history-taking, it will also transform that person's view of the consultation. Patients list "listening" as the most valued attribute of a doctor. Although others may listen too, this cannot be delegated to the health care team.

At what stage of diabetes is the person in front of you? The implications for the individual who was identified on routine screening are quite different from those for the person presenting with a black toe. The former is likely to be at an early stage of a long process with good chance of modifying disease progression, whereas the latter is likely to have other tissue complications already established. Clearly, genetic susceptibility to develop complications plays a part as well as natural history time course. The former patient may never develop more than microaneurysms in the eye and be resistant to diabetic nephropathy. Even if they are to be susceptible to complications, these are amenable to intervention over a period of many years. The latter patient, however, requires clear explanation of what can be done and how

Textbook of Diabetes, 4th edition. Edited by R. Holt, C. Cockram, A. Flyvbjerg and B. Goldstein.

future trouble can be avoided. Hippocrates summed it up nicely: "Cure sometimes, relieve often, comfort always."

The possibility of cure should not be overlooked. Diabetes has long been regarded as incurable. However, this is not always true. At the beginning of the 21st century and with further advances in our understanding, the number of circumstances where diabetes can be cured will increase. Look out for the slatey grey person with large liver and hemoglobin level of 19 gm/dL. Hemochromatosis is rare as a cause of diabetes but it is treatable and therefore important (see Chapter 18). The person taking a combination of thiazide diuretic and beta-blocker will be pleased to have hyperglycemia at least ameliorated by use of alternative agents (see Chapter 16). Cushing syndrome may include curable diabetes (see Chapter 17). Few people on systemic steroid therapy can be taken off treatment just because of development of diabetes, but knowledge is cheering that the diabetes will go away or become much more easily controllable when the steroid course finishes. Cure of T2DM by substantial and sustained weight loss coupled with increased daily physical activity is possible for those who have the determination and willpower to change long-standing behavior patterns. Bariatric surgery produces dramatic and long-term cure of T2DM in the early years of the condition [1].

Types of diabetes

The classification of diabetes will remain the cause of much debate until the exact etiology of each subtype has been established. Currently, the paradigm is to group together those people who appear to have primary β-cell destruction as T1DM, and those who are not slim and who can be controlled at least in the early years with diet and oral agents as T2DM. The monogenic causes of diabetes are capable of precise genetic description and are clearly separate (see Chapter 15). Similarly, pancreatic disease such as chronic pancreatitis, pancreatic carcinoma and hemochromatosis is capable of precise diagnosis (see Chapter 18). T2DM, however, is a term used to describe all those conditions that do not fit into the other, more easily described categories. It is clear that more subtypes will be identified in due course.

The important practical question at the initial presentation of a person with diabetes is whether insulin therapy is necessary. In some circumstances there is no doubt, such as diabetic ketoacidosis or severe weight loss with ketonuria and glycosuria in a child (Figure 19.1). More usually in adult practice the question must be asked. Table 19.1 lays out the common and distinguishing features from the clinical history, examination and urinalysis to help the clinician come to the answer. The subsequent sections consider the separate features in context.

Thirst, polydipsia and polyuria

These symptoms result from an osmotic diuresis as a consequence of hyperglycemia. The symptoms are common to all types of diabetes although the time course is likely to be shorter and the symptoms more severe in T1DM. Not infrequently, sugar-containing carbonated drinks are selected to slake thirst with resulting worsening of symptoms. A careful history documenting the time course of symptoms and any change in intake of specific drinks is important. Remembering how many times per day urine is passed is not easy, but nocturia is more clear-cut and the number of times urine is passed at night should be quantified. "Do you need to drink water when you get up at night?" is a reasonably objective measure of thirst.

For glucose to escape into the urine, plasma glucose concentration must exceed the renal threshold for tubular reabsorption of glucose and the absolute amount of glucose delivered to the renal tubules must exceed the maximum absorptive capacity. The renal threshold averages 11 mmol/L but displays a wide individual variation of around 6–14 mmol/L [2]. Additionally, the maximum absorptive capacity varies with age such that older people exhibit glycosuria at higher plasma glucose levels [3].

The rise in maximum renal tubular absorptive capacity with increasing age is clinically significant as older people will only develop osmotic symptoms at higher plasma glucose levels. Conversely, a negative urine test is even less likely to exclude a diagnosis of diabetes than in younger people. In addition to the need for higher plasma glucose levels in older people to produce osmotic symptoms, the threshold for triggering the sensation of thirst rises with advancing years [4]. This is important because, once the maximum renal absorptive capacity has been exceeded, dehydration will become considerably more advanced before thirst is sensed. These age-related changes are highly relevant to development of severe hyperosmolar states.

The presence of chronic hyperglycemia itself changes the renal sensitivity to vasopressin such that thirst is not appreciated despite rising plasma osmolarity [5]. Hence, the combination of undiagnosed diabetes and advanced age is particularly potent in delaying appropriate action to increase oral fluid intake as dehydration progresses. The clinical features identified from the history at presentation will vary in relation to the above factors. In older people, thirst may be experienced despite an osmotic diuresis and polydipsia will be absent. The most reliably quantitated feature of an osmotic presentation is therefore frequency of nocturia, and specifically an increase from habitual levels.

In children, enuresis may be the first symptom of polyuria. Sudden onset of enuresis should always prompt testing of urine for glucose. It must be noted that a urine test is entirely appropriate as an initial screen in this situation, as the absence of glucose from the urine absolutely excludes hyperglycemia as a potential cause of polyuria.

Weight loss

Establishing whether significant weight loss has occurred is the most important aspect of history-taking in those with newly presenting diabetes. Unless secondary to concurrent disease, the

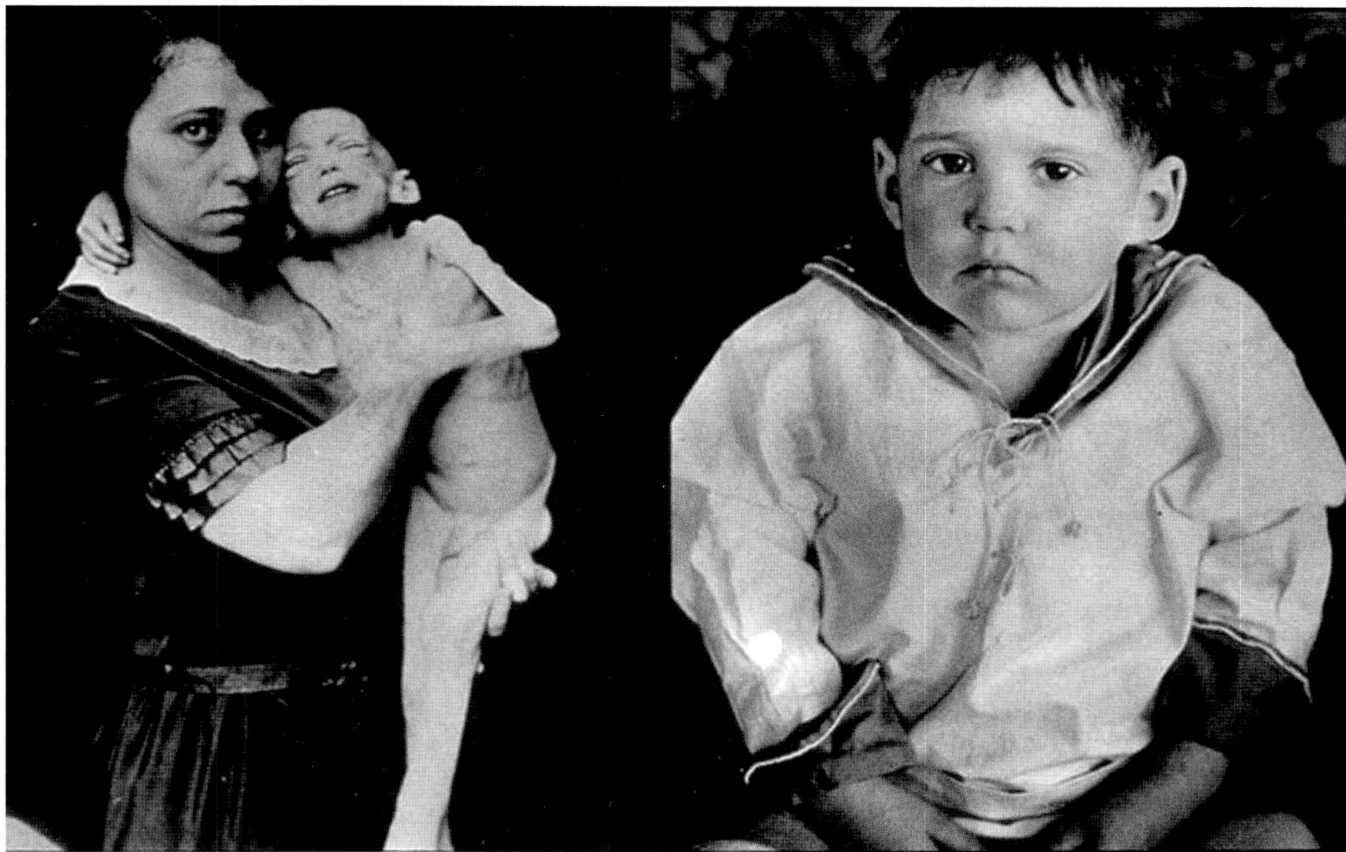

Figure 19.1 A 3-year-old boy before and after 3 months of insulin therapy (1922). The severe wasting of muscle and adipose tissue due to the insulin deficiency of type 1 diabetes is painfully evident in the left-hand panel. There is no more dramatic reminder of weight loss as a prominent presenting feature of type 1 diabetes especially if presentation is delayed. The speed of restoration of body mass on replacing insulin (right-hand panel) is impressive. Reproduced with permission from Eli Lilly & Co.

Table 19.1 Clinical features at presentation of type 1, type 2 and monogenic diabetes. This is a diagnostic guide with exceptions because of specific circumstances. It is not exhaustive and does not include rarer forms of diabetes, including syndromic diabetes.

	Type 1	Type 2	Monogenic	Pancreatic
Weight loss	Yes (not essential e.g. in slow onset T1DM)	Usually, no	No	Possible. If marked consider pancreatic carcinoma
Ketonuria	Yes (not essential in slow onset T1DM)	No unless recent fasting	No unless recent fasting	Yes, but not necessary for diagnosis
Time course of symptoms	Weeks or days	Months	Months	Weeks or months
Severity of symptoms (e.g. nocturia >3)	Can be marked	Variable but not usually extreme unless fueled by sugary drinks to assuage thirst	Not usually severe	Depends on clinical situation
Family history	Possibly of insulin dependence at a young age	Present in 30% with onset in adult life	Present in almost all with onset in childhood or adult life	Only by chance except in association with hemochromatosis
Age	Peak age in preschool and teenage years but can present at any age	Typically after the age of 20 years	Childhood, adolescence or adult	Usually middle aged and older

symptom strongly suggests insulin deficiency and hence newly presenting T1DM. Its absence does not exclude T1DM as the speed of onset of insulin deficiency and the presence of intercurrent illness, which may have exacerbated osmotic symptoms, may mean that weight loss has not yet commenced.

Weight loss at presentation of T2DM may occur as a result of dietary restriction often undertaken because of suspicion of impending health problems. Such deliberate changes in eating habit are readily established from the history. Typically, weight does not change, or even continues to rise, prior to the symptomatic onset of T2DM.

The weight loss reflects mainly the relative loss of the anabolic actions of insulin. Muscle wasting may be prominent, especially in young men. Associated loss of muscle strength may be reported. As an anabolic hormone, insulin acts principally to inhibit protein degradation [6]. Its relative absence allows the balance between continuous protein synthesis and breakdown to be disturbed. There is an additional effect of insulin deficiency in the failure of normal promotion of lipogenesis and inhibition of lipolysis. Excess non-esterified fatty acids accumulate in plasma, forming substrate for ketogenesis. If the clinical presentation of diabetes is acute, a component of the weight loss will reflect the loss of both intracellular and extracellular water.

Blurred vision

Major changes in plasma glucose will be followed over a period of days and weeks by blurring of vision. The symptom is typically present after a relatively acute change, usually in the context of presentation of T1DM or in the specific circumstance of a hyperosmolar presentation of T2DM. It is most important to explain to the patient that the visual blurring will become worse following the relatively rapid correction of gross hyperglycemia. This explanation is vital to avoid the supposition that diabetic blindness is already progressing with consequent unnecessary worry. It is also important to prevent the unnecessary purchase of spectacles that will be redundant after the hyperglycemia is treated.

It is reasonably assumed that shifts in osmotic pressure between plasma and inside the eyeball accounts for the visual change. Certainly, this provides a practical and immediately understandable explanation. Detailed tests, however, have not to date tied down any identifiable refractive change [7].

Infections

Exposure of leukocytes to glucose concentrations above 11 mmol/L produces paralysis of phagocytic and other functions [8]. This effect, together with other possible effects upon immune function, explains the impaired ability to fight off bacterial and fungal infections. Susceptibility to viral infections appears to be little changed although clear data are lacking.

Recurrent or refractory yeast infections may draw attention to previously undiagnosed diabetes. Most frequently this involves vaginal candidiasis in women or balanitis in men. Initial control of blood glucose levels will permit clearance of the infection with continued antifungal application. Staphylococcal pustules, boils and carbuncles may be present at the diagnosis of diabetes, especially T1DM. This clinical observation was supported by a prospective study of 482 patients with skin or mucous membrane sepsis presenting to an accident and emergency department who were found to have over a threefold increased incidence of capillary blood glucose >7.8 mmol/L compared with a background population [9].

Very rare but serious infective presentations of diabetes must be considered. Necrotizing fasciitis is considerably more common in people with diagnosed and undiagnosed diabetes [10]. Fournier gangrene (gangrene of the perineum and genitalia) is associated with diabetes in almost 50% of cases [11]. The rare and often fatal facial and/or maxillary sinus fungal infection mucormycosis is most often associated with diabetes [12].

Diabetic ketoacidosis

Diabetic ketoacidosis (DKA) occurs as a result of marked insulin deficiency associated with an increase in circulating levels of counter-regulatory hormones. It is characterized by hyperglycemia, acidosis and ketonuria. It mainly occurs in patients with T1DM, but it is not uncommon in some patients with T2DM. There is a wide geographic variation in the reported incidence of DKA. For example, EURODIAB, a cross-sectional survey of 3250 people with T1DM in 29 centers in Europe, reported that 8.6% of patients had been admitted with a diagnosis of DKA in the previous 12 months [13]. In 25% of cases, DKA is the presenting feature of T1DM [14]. The overall mortality rate from DKA ranges 2–5%, but is higher in the elderly.

DKA typically presents with the symptoms of hyperglycemia (i.e. thirst, polyuria and polydipsia). Patients may also complain of malaise or lethargy and muscle cramps. Abdominal pain and vomiting may be sufficiently severe as to mimic an acute surgical problem. It is critically important to recognize this, as the administration of an anesthetic is almost invariable fatal. All doctors dealing with emergencies should be aware of the potential pitfall of missing this telltale sign of DKA.

Clinical signs include dehydration, deep, sighing respirations (air hunger or Kussmaul respiration) and a sweet-smelling fetor (like nail varnish remover) caused by the ketones on the breath. As the ability to detect the smell of ketones is genetically determined, and approximately one-third of people are unable to do this, it is important that individual doctors are aware if they are not equipped with this additional diagnostic tool. Consciousness may be clouded. If the condition has progressed to the stage of coma, the associated signs of dehydration must lead to urgent checking of blood glucose, urinary ketones and arterial blood pH in order to expedite definitive treatment.

The marked deficiency or absence of insulin in this condition means that insulin-mediated glucose uptake into tissues such as muscle, fat and liver cannot occur. In the meantime, the dysregulated secretion of counter-regulatory hormones (glucagon, growth hormone and catecholamines) enhances the breakdown of triglyceride into free fatty acids and increases the rate of gluconeogenesis, which is the main cause for the high blood glucose level in diabetic ketoacidosis. Beta-oxidation of these free fatty acids leads to formation of ketone bodies (β-hydroxybutyrate, acetoacetate and acetone). Acetone is volatile and is released from the lungs, giving the characteristic sweet smell to the breath. Metabolic acidosis ensues when the ketone bodies are released into circulation and deplete the acid buffers.

The hyperglycemia-induced osmotic diuresis further depletes sodium, potassium, phosphates and water. Patients are often profoundly dehydrated and have a significantly depleted total body potassium at presentation. Sometimes, a normal or even elevated serum potassium level is seen as a result of the extracellular shift of potassium with severe acidosis. Great care must be taken to monitor serum potassium levels repeatedly once insulin treatment is started as the concentration can drop precipitously.

Hyperosmolar hyperglycemic syndrome

Hyperosmolar hyperglycemic syndrome (HSS) occurs exclusively in patients with T2DM. Often there is a history of several days of ill health. The principal clinical feature is profound dehydration. Confusion is usual, and focal neurologic symptoms such as weakness on one side or hemi-sensory abnormalities may develop and be easily confused with stroke. HSS was previously termed hyperosmolar non-ketotic coma. This terminology has been changed as coma is a relatively rare feature (<10%) and mild ketosis may be present at diagnosis.

HSS shares many features in common with DKA, the major exceptions being the absence of significant ketoacidosis. This is likely because of the residual low level insulin secretion, which suppresses lipolysis sufficiently to avert ketogenesis but not sufficient to prevent hyperglycemia. Additionally, hyperosmolarity itself may decrease lipolysis, limiting the amount of free fatty acids available for ketogenesis. HSS accounts for 10–30% of hyperglycemic emergencies. As the prevalence of T2DM rises inexorably, it is becoming an increasingly common hospital admission. Up to two-thirds of those affected have not previously been diagnosed as having diabetes.

Macrovascular presentations

Acute myocardial infarction

As the risk of ischemic heart disease is linearly related to fasting and post-prandial blood glucose concentrations, it is not surprising that both impaired glucose tolerance (IGT) and diabetes are over-represented in populations presenting with acute myocardial infarction (AMI) [15]. Consequently, T2DM frequently presents for the first time at hospitalization for AMI.

This presentation is complicated by stress hyperglycemia resulting from the catecholamine and cortisol elevations. Although this may cause problems for the purist wishing to evaluate an effect of diabetes per se, from the perspective of the patient with a life-threatening condition exacerbated by dysglycemia, exact definitions of diabetes are not relevant. Stress hyperglycemia and established diabetes have similarly increased mortality from AMI. In a New York municipal hospital cohort of patients with AMI, 3-year mortality was 52% in those with stress hyperglycemia (defined as admission blood glucose >7.0 mmol/L) compared with 42% in those with diabetes [16]. The 3-year death rate in those with normal glucose levels was 24% in the same study. A meta-analysis has confirmed this effect, with a 3.9-fold increase risk of death associated with stress hyperglycemia compared with a 1.7-fold increased risk of death associated with established diabetes [17]. In this context, one of the most important findings of the DIGAMI study is often overlooked. The effect of reasonable glycemic management (blood glucose <10 mmol/L) for those with no prior insulin therapy and stratified as having low coronary risk factors produced a 52% improvement in mortality [18]. This group would have included those with stress hyperglycemia. In contrast, the DIGAMI study showed no significant benefit of acute blood glucose control for individuals previously treated with insulin.

Estimates of the incidence of stress hyperglycemia at presentation of AMI range 10–16% [19,20]. This compares with estimates of prevalence of diabetes at presentation of AMI of 25–32% [19,21,22]. Variation in these figures is likely to reflect the background prevalence of IGT and T2DM in the population, as well as increased awareness and effective screening processes to identify previously undiagnosed T2DM.

Good clinical practice demands measurement of plasma glucose on diagnosis of an acute coronary syndrome. If plasma glucose is raised (7 mmol/L may be quoted, but in the individual case interpretation depends upon time since last meal), then both fasting plasma glucose and HbA_{1c} should be measured. Raised plasma glucose should indicate a need for particular attention to adequate glucose control during the acute event. Given that the HbA_{1c} result is unlikely to be available immediately, hyperglycemia indicates a need for rapid control in the acute situation when the first few hours are critical. A fasting plasma glucose of >5.6 mmol/L during the acute admission and/or admission plasma glucose of >7.8 mmol/L yielded a sensitivity of almost 90% and a positive predictive value of 44% for detecting diabetes [23].

Where there is diagnostic uncertainty, targeted screening in the post-acute setting with a standard 75 g oral glucose tolerance test (OGTT) is acceptable. But when is the optimal time to perform this test? In a group of AMI patients with no previous diagnosis of diabetes, both pre-discharge and 6 weeks post-discharge OGTTs were performed and correlation with pre-discharge OGTT was good [24]. There was 49% concordance between classifications to which each patient was assigned in both OGTTs. The best predictor of abnormal glucose handling (IGT or diabetes) being diagnosed at 3 months was observed to be the 60-minute blood glucose level during the pre-discharge OGTT.

Acute stroke

The prevalence of previously diagnosed diabetes in patients with acute stroke is 8–28% but an additional 6–42% have unrecognized pre-existing dysglycemia [25]. Plasma glucose at presentation is a major prognostic factor. One series of 86 patients with acute stroke demonstrated that full functional recovery at 4 weeks was restricted to those with presenting blood glucose levels <8 mmol/L [26]. None of the individuals with a raised presenting plasma glucose regained full function by 4 weeks. The extent to which this reflects the metabolic stress response in proportion to the severity of the cerebrovascular insult as opposed to hyperglycemia itself impairing subsequent recovery from ischemic damage cannot be ascertained from these observational data.

The observations on poorer outcome in those who had stress hyperglycemia following AMI have been reproduced in respect of acute stroke disease. In a systematic review of observational studies examining the prognostic significance of hyperglycemia in acute stroke, the unadjusted relative risk of in-hospital or 30-day mortality was 3.07 (95% CI 2.50–3.79) in non-diabetic patients with admission plasma glucose level >6–8 mmol/L and 1.30 (95% CI 0.49–3.43) in those with known diabetes [27]. The relative risk of poor functional outcome in hyperglycemic non-diabetic patients was 1.41 (95% CI 1.16–1.73). It appears that sudden increase in plasma glucose levels impair tissue function more in those individuals who have not been habituated to hyperglycemia.

Persistent hyperglycemia (defined as blood glucose >7.0 mmol/L) in the 72 hours after acute stroke was found to be associated with an increase in infarct size, measured using magnetic resonance imaging, and worse stroke outcome [28]. Nonetheless, there are currently no satisfactory outcome studies of control of plasma glucose upon the outcome of stroke [29]. The largest study to date, which included 993 patients, failed to achieve control of plasma glucose at 24 hours [30]. Importantly, no assessment has yet been conducted of plasma glucose control during the first few hours after presentation with acute stroke, and it is likely that it is in this window of time that this particular presentation of hyperglycemia may most beneficially be managed.

Microvascular presentations

Eye presentations

Symptomatic loss of vision may occasionally be the presenting feature of T2DM, where hyperglycemia has been present for an uncertain number of years, silently causing tissue damage and retinopathy. Loss of vision as a diagnostic event is most often a consequence of macula edema but may also be secondary to vitreous hemorrhage. Central or branch retinal vein occlusion is more common in diabetes and may also cause symptomatic presentation of the condition.

Around the time of diagnosis of T2DM, marked retinopathy with cotton wool spots or intraretinal microvascular abnormalities (IRMA) was found to be present in 8% of men and 4% of women in the UK Prospective Diabetes Study (UKPDS) [31]. The critical importance of arranging full retinal examination, preferably by digital retinal imaging, is illustrated in Figure 19.2. Approximately 1% of individuals presenting with symptomatic T2DM have sight-threatening retinopathy at that time. Very early recognition is essential as the initial treatment of the diabetes will decrease blood glucose levels, cause retinal blood flow to return acutely to normal levels and may result in marked worsening of the retinopathy.

In the UKPDS, the severity of retinopathy was found to be related to higher fasting plasma glucose levels. In addition, in men, increased alcohol consumption was related to increased

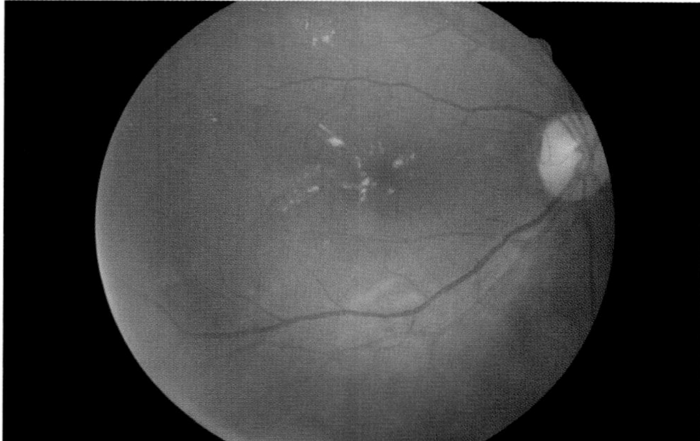

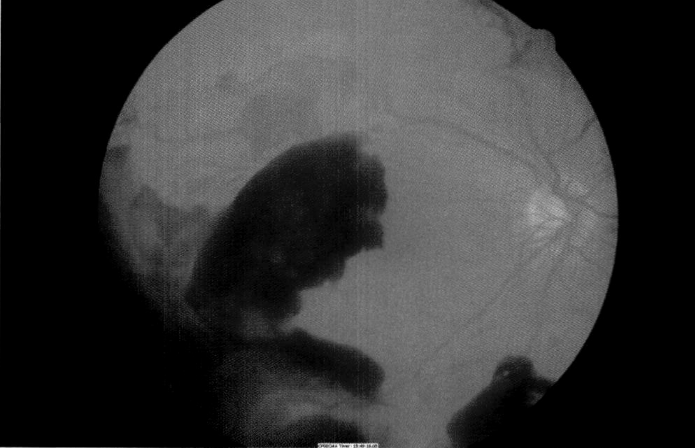

Figure 19.2 Upper panel: immediate laser therapy was required for the macular edema associated with the severe exudative maculopathy present at the time of diagnosis. Lower panel: new vessels are present both arising from the optic disk and from the peripheral retina. Bleeding from the latter caused the prominent pre-retinal hemorrhages which obscure the fovea and in this case caused presentation because of loss of visual acuity.

severity of retinopathy, while leaner women had more severe eye lesions. Visual acuity was normal in most patients, but in men there was a trend for those with more severe retinal lesions to have worse visual acuity.

The potential severity of diabetic retinopathy at the time of diagnosis of T2DM is illustrated by the observation that 15% of those with moderate background retinopathy progress to require photocoagulation therapy within 3 years [32]. The specific reason for photocoagulation therapy was maculopathy alone in 72% and proliferative retinopathy in 11% in this group of individuals with T2DM.

Neuropathic syndromes

Although any of the neuropathic syndromes of diabetes may precipitate the initial presentation, symmetrical distal sensory neuropathy, mononeuropathies and amyotrophy are the most likely candidates. The possibility of diabetes underlying most presentations of neurologic symptoms must be considered.

Diffuse symmetrical sensory neuropathy is the most common neuropathy. A precise estimate of the true prevalence of this neuropathy has been difficult to ascertain, and reports vary from 7 to 60% in people with diabetes, depending on the criteria and methods used to define the neuropathy [33,34]. The prevalence increases with both age and duration of diabetes. At 12-year follow-up in the UKPDS, 64% of men and 44% of women who were free of neuropathy at baseline developed at least one neuropathic abnormality [35].

Any nerve may be affected by an acute diabetic mononeuropathy, but palsy of cranial nerves III, IV, VI and VII present most often. It is a rare mode of presentation of T2DM, but not T1DM.

Diabetic amyotrophy may present as weight loss, and unless pain in the thighs is prominent the clinical picture may resemble that of malignant disease. Weakness of quadriceps, with visible wasting and absence of the knee tendon reflex, should allow recognition and lead to the measurement of plasma glucose. Such presentation is likely to be associated with T2DM but again is rare.

A foot lesion can be a presenting sign of diabetes, and it is estimated that the lifetime risk of developing a foot ulcer in people with diabetes may be as high as 25% [36]. Presentation with a black toe is associated with T2DM particularly. Peripheral neuropathy leads to sensory motor and autonomic dysfunction, with loss of the protective pain sensation, dry skin and callus formation. Loss of pain sensation in the feet is usually unnoticed and subsequent trauma does not come to attention until obvious injury is apparent. In approximately half of these patients with foot ulcers, concomitant peripheral arterial disease (PAD) is present [37]. In the EURODIALE study, foot ulcers with presence of PAD were associated with considerably lower healing rates, higher major amputation and mortality rates [38].

Pregnancy

The time course of presentation of GDM may be predicted from knowledge of its pathogenesis. The key variable is the physiologic insulin resistance that develops during pregnancy. Although several necessarily small studies have quantitated this, it is most clearly illustrated by an observation of the change in exogenous insulin requirements during pregnancy in T1DM. During steady glycemic control and food intake, insulin requirements do not change until around 18 weeks' gestation, whereafter there is a linear increase until around 28 weeks' gestation [39]. The extent of change varies in individual pregnancies from none to over threefold increase, with an average increase in daily insulin dose of 40% [40]. The range is assumed to be a function of the placenta (fetal-derived tissue) as considerable variation is exhibited between successive pregnancies in the same woman.

In the light of this information, it can be understood why the elevated blood glucose levels of GDM are not seen in the first half of pregnancy. Screening for GDM will be most sensitive later in pregnancy but this sensitivity must be balanced with the opportunities to intervene. Current guidelines therefore recommend testing at 24–28 weeks' gestation. Predisposed women cannot mount an adequate β-cell response if the degree of insulin resistance becomes too great. Following one pregnancy complicated by GDM, although increased, the risk of recurrence in a subsequent pregnancy is far from certain, reflecting the variation in insulin resistance in successive pregnancies. Higher rates have been reported in South Asian and Hispanic populations, as would be expected from the higher background prevalence of T2DM (52–69%) [41]. The importance of detection and treatment of GDM is reflected by the data shown in Figure 19.3. The rate of intrauterine growth is as rapid in GDM as it is in T1DM and T2DM [42]. Early diagnosis of GDM carries major advantages for mother and child. The risk of developing subsequent diabetes in those with GDM ranges from 2.6 to 70% over periods from 6 weeks to 28 years [43]. Current NICE guidelines (March 2008) for "Diabetes in Pregnancy" recommend that fasting plasma glucose should be performed at 6 weeks as well as repeated annually for those patients with GDM. This will miss a proportion of women with normal fasting plasma glucose and IGT, but it should be noted that the occurrence of GDM should be the trigger to advise vigorous lifestyle change and weight loss in particular.

Mild degrees of elevation of plasma glucose may be sufficient to be deleterious to the fetus, and these are far less than those that could produce osmotic symptoms [44]. Screening for GDM is therefore essential. Symptomatic presentation of GDM is unusual in the context of a health care system that provides universal screening for GDM. Where osmotic symptoms and superficial fungal infections are part of the clinical presentation, however, it is important to ask whether this is new onset T1DM or T2DM. The former tends to be associated with higher plasma glucose levels and ketonuria. Both are associated with clearly elevated

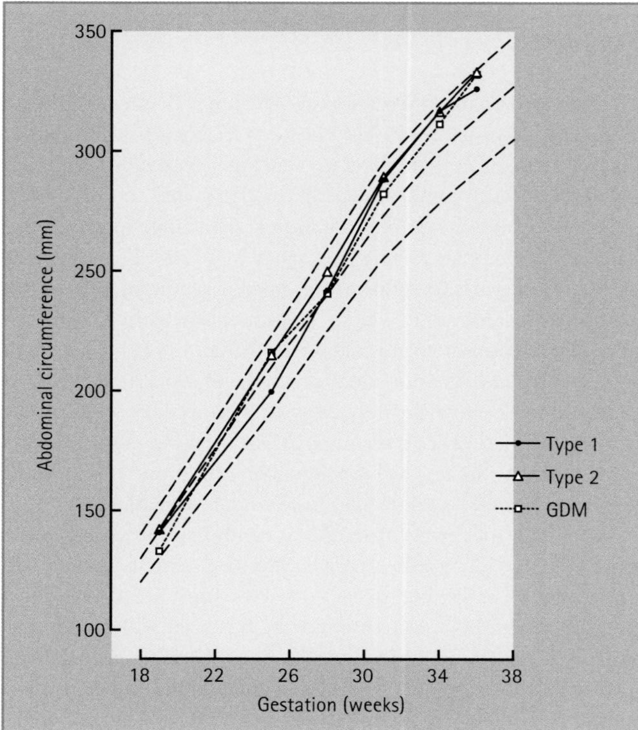

Figure 19.3 Similar rates of increase in fetal abdominal circumference in gestational diabetes (GDM) and pre-gestational diabetes as measured by ultrasound. Reproduced from Lim *et al.* [42], with permission from RSM Journals.

HbA_{1c} levels as the hyperglycemia has been present for several weeks or months. If the presentation is in the first half of pregnancy, it is likely that it will not remit after delivery. If the presentation is in the first half of pregnancy and is associated with raised HbA_{1c}, then a diagnosis of non-GDM may confidently be made and discussed with the patient [42].

Screening

It has been estimated from the 2002 NHANES survey that one-third of the 13.3 million US adults with diabetes remained undiagnosed [45]. A similar estimate has been made for the UK [46]. Universal screening has not been implemented in the UK, however, as criteria for cost-effective and clinically effective screening are not met [47]. It is recommended that screening of high-risk groups (obese, strong family history of diabetes, South Asian or other high-risk ethnicity) should be undertaken.

Fasting glucose, 2-hour post-challenge glucose and HbA_{1c} all equally well predict the future microvascular complications of diabetes and can be considered diagnostic as well as screening tests [48]. The use of the concept of "impaired fasting glucose" with a cutoff of 5.5 mmol/L offers a simple way of excluding or demonstrating dysglycemia [49]. Urinalysis for glycosuria has a high specificity (96–100%) but a low sensitivity (16–43%). Testing random blood glucose is specific but insensitive [50].

The population of individuals with early T2DM who are identified by any screening procedure differs considerably from those who present symptomatically. They are less likely to have established microvascular or macrovascular complications of diabetes. Attitudes to health may differ. The diagnosis will be less welcome as it does not point the way to relief of discomfort and may not be accepted as important for future health. Compliance with therapeutic advice concerning weight, diet and physical activity may not be as good as following a symptomatic presentation. For these reasons, a more careful approach to discussing the need for future action is required with appropriately sensitive follow-up by the diabetes team.

Other presentations

Ants clustering around urine is a classic description of diabetes, although it is not clear how often this comprises the presenting complaint today. Periodontal disease, especially aggressive periodontitis, is more common in those with diabetes and may occasionally be the presenting complaint [51]. Cataracts typically develop 10 years earlier in people with diabetes [52]. Altered taste or excess production of saliva have been reported as presenting features of diabetes [53].

Conclusions

The mode of presentation is enormously varied. Especially as the incidence of diabetes is rising in all age groups, both in the UK and worldwide [54], the onus is upon health care professionals to diagnose the condition effectively. Failure to recognize presenting features of diabetes can be costly for the patient.

References

1 Taylor R. Pathogenesis of type 2 diabetes: tracing the reverse route from cure to cause. *Diabetologia* 2008; **51**:1781–1789.
2 Johansen K, Svendsen PA, Lorup B. Variations in renal threshold for glucose in type 1 (insulin-dependent) diabetes mellitus. *Diabetologia* 1984; **26**:180–182.
3 Butterfield WJ, Keen H, Whichelow MJ. Renal glucose threshold variations with age. *Br Med J* 1967; **4**:505–507.
4 Baylis PH, Thompson CJ. Osmoregulation of vasopressin secretion and thirst in health and disease. *Clin Endocrinol (Oxf)* 1988; **29**:549–576.
5 Agha A, Smith D, Finucane F, Sherlock M, Morris A, Baylis P, *et al.* Attenuation of vasopressin-induced antidiuresis in poorly controlled type 2 diabetes. *Am J Physiol Endocrinol Metab* 2004; **287**:E1100–1106.
6 Liu Z, Long W, Fryburg DA, Barrett EJ. The regulation of body and skeletal muscle protein metabolism by hormones and amino acids. *J Nutr* 2006; **136**(Suppl):212–217.

7 Wiemer NG, Dubbelman M, Ringens PJ, Polak BC. Measuring the refractive properties of the diabetic eye during blurred vision and hyperglycaemia using aberrometry and Scheimpflug imaging. *Acta Ophthalmol* 2009; **87**:176–182.

8 Turina M, Fry DE, Polk HC Jr. Acute hyperglycemia and the innate immune system: clinical, cellular, and molecular aspects. *Crit Care Med* 2005; **33**:1624–1633.

9 Baynes C, Caplan S, Hames P, Swift R, Poole S, Wadsworth J, *et al.* The value of screening for diabetes in patients with skin sepsis. *J R Soc Med* 1993; **86**:148–151.

10 Dworkin MS, Westercamp MD, Park L, McIntyre A. The epidemiology of necrotizing fasciitis including factors associated with death and amputation. *Epidemiol Infect* 2009; **137**:1609–1614.

11 Yanar H, Taviloglu K, Ertekin C, Guloglu R, Zorba U, Cabioglu N, *et al.* Fournier's gangrene: risk factors and strategies for management. *World J Surg* 2006; **30**:1750–1754.

12 Haliloglu NU, Yesilirmak Z, Erden A, Erden I. Rhino-orbito-cerebral mucormycosis: report of two cases and review of the literature. *Dentomaxillofac Radiol* 2008; **37**:161–166.

13 Levy-Marchal C, Patterson CC, Green A. Geographical variation of presentation at diagnosis of type I diabetes in children: the EURODIAB study. *Diabetologia* 2001; **44**(Suppl 3):B75–80.

14 Westphal SA. The occurrence of diabetic ketoacidosis in non-insulin-dependent diabetes and newly diagnosed diabetic adults. *Am J Med* 1996; **101**:19–24.

15 Jarrett RJ, McCartney P, Keen H. The Bedford survey: ten year mortality rates in newly diagnosed diabetics, borderline diabetics and normoglycaemic controls and risk indices for coronary heart disease in borderline diabetics. *Diabetologia* 1982; **22**:79–84.

16 Nordin C, Amiruddin R, Rucker L, Choi J, Kohli A, Marantz PR. Diabetes and stress hyperglycemia associated with myocardial infarctions at an urban municipal hospital: prevalence and effect on mortality. *Cardiol Rev* 2005; **13**:223–230.

17 Capes SE, Hunt D, Malmberg K, Gerstein HC. Stress hyperglycaemia and increased risk of death after myocardial infarction in patients with and without diabetes: a systematic overview. *Lancet* 2000; **355**:773–778.

18 Malmberg K, Rydén L, Efendic S, Herlitz J, Nicol P, Waldenstrom A, *et al.* Randomized trial of insulin-glucose infusion followed by subcutaneous insulin treatment in diabetic patients with acute myocardial infarction (DIGAMI study): effects on mortality at 1 year. *J Am Coll Cardiol* 1995; **26**:57–65.

19 Tenerz A, Lonnberg I, Berne C, Nilsson G, Leppert J. Myocardial infarction and prevalence of diabetes mellitus: is increased casual blood glucose at admission a reliable criterion for the diagnosis of diabetes? *Eur Heart J* 2001; **22**:1102–1110.

20 Weston C, Walker L, Birkhead J. Early impact of insulin treatment on mortality for hyperglycaemic patients without known diabetes who present with an acute coronary syndrome. *Heart* 2007; **93**:1542–1546.

21 Aguilar D, Solomon SD, Kober L, Rouleau JL, Skali H, McMurray JJ, *et al.* Newly diagnosed and previously known diabetes mellitus and 1-year outcomes of acute myocardial infarction: the VALsartan In Acute myocardial iNfarcTion (VALIANT) trial. *Circulation* 2004; **110**:1572–1578.

22 Lankisch M, Futh R, Gulker H, Lapp H, Bufe A, Haastert B, *et al.* Screening for undiagnosed diabetes in patients with acute myocardial infarction. *Clin Res Cardiol* 2008; **97**:753–759.

23 Okosieme OE, Peter R, Usman M, Bolusani H, Suruliram P, George L, *et al.* Can admission and fasting glucose reliably identify undiagnosed diabetes in patients with acute coronary syndrome? *Diabetes Care* 2008; **31**:1955–1959.

24 Tenerz A, Norhammar A, Silveira A, Hamsten A, Nilsson G, Ryden L, *et al.* Diabetes, insulin resistance, and the metabolic syndrome in patients with acute myocardial infarction without previously known diabetes. *Diabetes Care* 2003; **26**:2770–2776.

25 Oppenheimer SM, Hoffbrand BI, Oswald GA, Yudkin JS. Diabetes mellitus and early mortality from stroke. *Br Med J (Clin Res Ed)* 1985; **291**:1014–1015.

26 Gray CS, Taylor R, French JM, Alberti KG, Venables GS, James OF, *et al.* The prognostic value of stress hyperglycaemia and previously unrecognized diabetes in acute stroke. *Diabet Med* 1987; **4**:237–240.

27 Capes SE, Hunt D, Malmberg K, Pathak P, Gerstein HC. Stress hyperglycemia and prognosis of stroke in nondiabetic and diabetic patients: a systematic overview. *Stroke* 2001; **32**:2426–2432.

28 Baird TA, Parsons MW, Phanh T, Butcher KS, Desmond PM, Tress BM, *et al.* Persistent poststroke hyperglycemia is independently associated with infarct expansion and worse clinical outcome. *Stroke* 2003; **34**:2208–2214.

29 McCormick MT, Muir KW, Gray CS, Walters MR. Management of hyperglycemia in acute stroke: how, when, and for whom? *Stroke* 2008; **39**:2177–2185.

30 Gray CS, Hildreth AJ, Sandercock PA, O'Connell JE, Johnston DE, Cartlidge NEF, *et al.* Glucose-potassium-insulin infusions in the management of post-stroke hyperglycaemia: the UK Glucose Insulin in Stroke Trial (GIST-UK). *Lancet Neurol* 2007; **6**:397–406.

31 Kohner EM, Aldington SJ, Stratton IM, Manley SE, Holman RR, Matthews DR, *et al.* United Kingdom Prospective Diabetes Study, 30: diabetic retinopathy at diagnosis of non-insulin-dependent diabetes mellitus and associated risk factors. *Arch Ophthalmol* 1998; **116**:297–303.

32 Kohner EM, Stratton IM, Aldington SJ, Holman RR, Matthews DR. Relationship between the severity of retinopathy and progression to photocoagulation in patients with type 2 diabetes mellitus in the UKPDS (UKPDS 52). *Diabet Med* 2001; **18**:178–184.

33 Young MJ, Boulton AJ, MacLeod AF, Williams DR, Sonksen PH. A multicentre study of the prevalence of diabetic peripheral neuropathy in the United Kingdom hospital clinic population. *Diabetologia* 1993; **36**:150–154.

34 Tapp RJ, Shaw JE, de Courten MP, Dunstan DW, Welborn TA, Zimmet PZ. Foot complications in type 2 diabetes: an Australian population-based study. *Diabet Med* 2003; **20**:105–113.

35 Stratton IM, Holman RR, Boulton AJ. Risk factors for neuropathy in UKPDS. Presented at the 40th Annual Meeting of the European Association for the Study of Diabetes. 2004 September 5–9.

36 Singh N, Armstrong DG, Lipsky BA. Preventing foot ulcers in patients with diabetes. *JAMA* 2005; **293**:217–228.

37 Prompers L, Huijberts M, Apelqvist J, Jude E, Piaggesi A, Bakker K, *et al.* High prevalence of ischaemia, infection and serious comorbidity in patients with diabetic foot disease in Europe: baseline results from the EURODIALE study. *Diabetologia* 2007; **50**:18–25.

38 Prompers L, Schaper N, Apelqvist J, Edmonds M, Jude E, Mauricio D, *et al.* Prediction of outcome in individuals with diabetic foot ulcers: focus on the differences between individuals with and without peripheral arterial disease.: the EURODIALE Study. *Diabetologia* 2008; **51**:747–755.

39 Taylor R, Lee C, Kyne-Grzebalski D, Marshall SM, Davison JM. Clinical outcomes of pregnancy in women with type 1 diabetes. *Obstet Gynecol* 2002; **99**:537–541.

40 Taylor R, Davison JM. Type 1 diabetes and pregnancy. *Br Med J* 2007; **334**:742–745.

41 Kim C, Berger DK, Chamany S. Recurrence of gestational diabetes mellitus: a systematic review. *Diabetes Care* 2007; **30**:1314–1319.

42 Lim EL, Burden T, Marshall SM, Davison JM, Blott MJ, Waugh JSJ, *et al.* Intrauterine growth rate in pregnancies complicated by type 1, type 2 and gestational diabetes. *Obstetric Med* 2009; **2**:21–25.

43 Kim C, Newton KM, Knopp RH. Gestational diabetes and the incidence of type 2 diabetes: a systematic review. *Diabetes Care* 2002; **25**:1862–1868.

44 Metzger BE, Lowe LP, Dyer AR, Trimble ER, Chaovarindr U, Coustan DR, *et al.* Hyperglycemia and adverse pregnancy outcomes. *N Engl J Med* 2008; **358**:1991–2002.

45 Cowie CC, Rust KF, Byrd-Holt DD, Eberhardt MS, Flegal KM, Engelgau MM, *et al.* Prevalence of diabetes and impaired fasting glucose in adults in the US population: National Health And Nutrition Examination Survey 1999–2002. *Diabetes Care* 2006; **29**:1263–1268.

46 Holt TA, Stables D, Hippisley-Cox J, O'Hanlon S, Majeed A. Identifying undiagnosed diabetes: cross-sectional survey of 3.6 million patients' electronic records. *Br J Gen Pract* 2008; **58**:192–196.

47 National Screening Committee policy – diabetes screening (in adults). National Screening Committee, UK; 2006 [updated 2006; cited]; Available from: http://www.library.nhs.uk/screening/ViewResource.aspx?resID=60981

48 McCance DR, Hanson RL, Charles MA, Jacobsson LT, Pettitt DJ, Bennett PH, *et al.* Comparison of tests for glycated haemoglobin and fasting and two hour plasma glucose concentrations as diagnostic methods for diabetes. *Br Med J* 1994; **308**:1323–1328.

49 Report of the expert committee on the diagnosis and classification of diabetes mellitus. *Diabetes Care* 2003; **26**(Suppl 1):S5–20.

50 Andersson DK, Lundblad E, Svardsudd K. A model for early diagnosis of type 2 diabetes mellitus in primary health care. *Diabet Med* 1993; **10**:167–173.

51 Borrell LN, Kunzel C, Lamster I, Lalla E. Diabetes in the dental office: using NHANES III to estimate the probability of undiagnosed disease. *J Periodontal Res* 2007; **42**:559–565.

52 Klein BE, Klein R, Lee KE. Diabetes, cardiovascular disease, selected cardiovascular disease risk factors, and the 5-year incidence of age-related cataract and progression of lens opacities: the Beaver Dam Eye Study. *Am J Ophthalmol* 1998; **126**:782–790.

53 Gibson J, Lamey PJ, Lewis M, Frier B. Oral manifestations of previously undiagnosed non-insulin dependent diabetes mellitus. *J Oral Pathol Med* 1990; **19**:284–287.

54 Wild S, Roglic G, Green A, Sicree R, King H. Global prevalence of diabetes: estimates for the year 2000 and projections for 2030. *Diabetes Care* 2004; **27**:1047–1053.

20 The Aims of Diabetes Care

Richard I.G. Holt[1] & Barry J. Goldstein[2]

[1] Institute of Developmental Sciences, University of Southampton, Southampton, UK
[2] Clinical Research, Metabolism, Merck Research Laboratories, Rahway, NJ, USA

Keypoints

- People with diabetes should be seen as individuals with a condition that has medical, personal and social consequences, instead of being passive recipients of health care.
- The optimal management of diabetes occurs when the multidisciplinary diabetes care team actively involves the person with diabetes as an equal partner in their care.
- Life-threatening diabetes emergencies, such as diabetic ketoacidosis, should be effectively managed, and attention paid to prevention.
- Acute symptoms of hyperglycemia need to be addressed by careful lifestyle and pharmacologic management.
- Much of diabetes management is focused on reducing the risk of long-term complications through screening and supporting achievement of improved glycemic control and cardiovascular risk factor management.
- The time of diagnosis is a key milestone in the management of diabetes, when education, support and treatment are needed.
- Regular lifelong contact between the person with diabetes and their health care team is essential in order to support them to cope with the demands of a complex condition which changes throughout life.
- Diabetic complications should be managed effectively, if and when they present, to reduce morbidity.

Introduction

Diabetes is a lifelong condition that is, for the majority, currently incurable. It is associated with premature mortality and morbidity from an increased prevalence of cardiovascular disease and microvascular complications affecting the kidney, nerve and eye [1,2]. High-quality randomized trials have shown that improving glycemic control is associated with a reduction in microvascular complications [3–5] while a multifaceted approach to cardiovascular risk factors will reduce cardiovascular morbidity and mortality [6].

The person living with diabetes will spend the vast majority of their time managing their diabetes and only an estimated 1% of their time in contact with health care professionals. Therefore, the person with diabetes needs to be supported to take upon themselves much of the responsibility for the management of their diabetes. Given the central role of the person with diabetes and the relatively little contact with health care professionals, it is important that the purposes of the consultation or other contacts with the diabetes health care team are well defined and their aims are made clear so that the patient derives the maximum benefit from the time spent with their diabetes health care team, whether this is in a hospital or primary care setting. As well as the clinic visit, diabetes care may also be through phone or email contact or through educational sessions outside a traditional clinic setting.

This chapter provides an overview of the aims and philosophy of diabetes care. Separate aspects of care are covered in greater detail in subsequent chapters. The aims of diabetes care and management are fourfold. Life-threatening diabetes emergencies, such as diabetic ketoacidosis or severe hypoglycemia, should be managed effectively including preventative measures. The acute manifestations of hyperglycemia, such as polyuria and polydipsia, need to be addressed. In practice, these occupy only a minority of the work undertaken by diabetes health care professionals. Much of the focus of care is therefore directed towards minimizing the long-term complications through screening and working together with the person with diabetes to support improved glycemic control and cardiovascular risk factor management. This provides a challenge for the diabetes team because people often have no symptoms at the time of care and yet are asked to make lifestyle changes and take medications that may place a considerable burden on that individual. It is also important that clinicians bear in mind the fourth aim of care which is to avoid iatrogenic side effects, such as hypoglycemia. Involvement of the person with diabetes in this care planning is paramount to success.

Textbook of Diabetes, 4th edition. Edited by R. Holt, C. Cockram, A. Flyvbjerg and B. Goldstein.

St. Vincent's Declaration

During the 1980s, there was a transformation in the widely held perceptions of the roles of people with diabetes and philosophy of care. Instead of being viewed as passive recipients of health care, there was an increasing recognition that people with diabetes were individuals with a condition that has medical, personal and social consequences. During this time, there was an increasing awareness and acceptance of the concept that each person with diabetes should accept part of the responsibility for their treatment and act as equal partners with health care professionals. In response to this paradigm shift, representatives of government health departments and diabetes organizations from all European countries met with diabetes experts under the auspices of the Regional Offices of the World Health Organization (WHO) and the International Diabetes Federation (IDF) in the hillside town of St. Vincent, Italy, October 10–12, 1989. They unanimously agreed upon a series of recommendations for diabetes care and urged that action should be taken in all countries throughout Europe to implement them [7]. Since this time, this philosophy of partnership between people with diabetes and health care professionals has been adopted within individual nation's strategies to improve the quality of diabetes care.

The diabetes care team

The diabetes care team involves a multidisciplinary group of health care professionals who are available to support the person with diabetes (Figure 20.1). A key component of diabetes care is to ensure that the individual with diabetes is at the center of the provision of care. This means that the person with diabetes should work together with the health care professionals as an equal member of the diabetes care team. This relationship should provide the information, advice, and education to support the

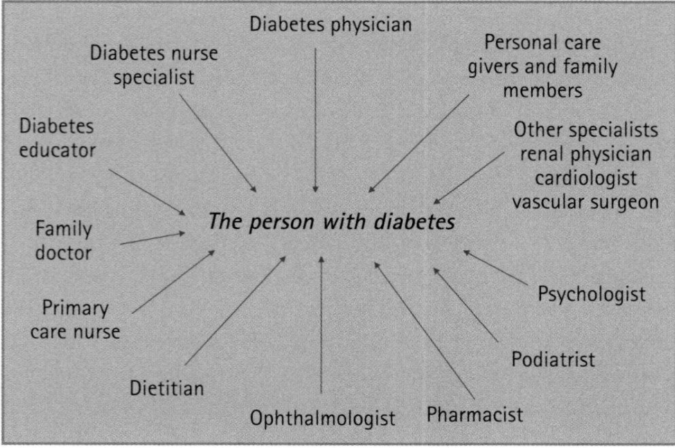

Figure 20.1 The multidisciplinary group of health care professionals who are available to support the person with diabetes.

Box 20.1 St. Vincent's Declaration [7]

- Elaborate, initiate and evaluate comprehensive programs for detection and control of diabetes and of its complications with self-care and community support as major components
- Raise awareness in the population and among health care professionals of the present opportunities and the future needs for prevention of the complications of diabetes and of diabetes itself
- Organize training and teaching in diabetes management and care for people of all ages with diabetes, for their families, friends and working associates and for the health care team
- Ensure that care for children with diabetes is provided by individuals and teams specialized both in the management of diabetes and of children, and that families with a child with diabetes obtain the necessary social, economic and emotional support
- Reinforce existing centres of excellence in diabetes care, education and research
- Create new centers where the need and potential exist
- Promote independence, equity and self-sufficiency for all people with diabetes, children, adolescents, those in the working years of life and the elderly
- Remove hindrances to the fullest possible integration of people with diabetes into society
- Implement effective measures for the prevention of costly complications:
  - Reduce new blindness caused by diabetes by one-third or more
  - Reduce numbers of people entering end-stage renal failure by at least one-third
  - Reduce by half the rate of limb amputations
  - Cut morbidity and mortality from coronary heart disease by vigorous programs of risk factor reduction
  - Achieve pregnancy outcomes in women with diabetes that approximate that of women without diabetes
- Establish monitoring and control systems using state-of-the-art information technology for quality assurance of diabetes health care provision and for laboratory and technical procedures in diabetes diagnosis, treatment and self-management
- Promote European and international collaboration in programs of diabetes research and development through national, regional and World Health Organization (WHO) agencies and in active partnership with the person with diabetes and diabetes organizations
- Take urgent action in the spirit of the WHO program, "Health for All," to establish joint machinery between WHO and International Diabetes Federation European Region to initiate, accelerate and facilitate the implementation of these recommendations

empowerment of the individual with diabetes to enable them to take control of their condition and ensures that care offered is made appropriate for the individual and their circumstances.

The large number of health professionals involved in the diabetes care team means that the roles and responsibilities of all must be clearly presented and agreed. It is often helpful for the person with diabetes if the key members of the diabetes care team are identified, as they will have more contact with some health care staff than others.

Most routine diabetes care takes place in a primary care setting but some people with diabetes with additional or complex needs will require management and support in a specialist setting for some or all of their care [8]. The diabetes physician usually takes the overall responsibility for the diabetes medical care but other specialists may be involved, for example an ophthalmologist may be needed to examine the eyes carefully and treat diabetic retinopathy if present. Diabetes care is multidisciplinary, involving doctors, nurses and many allied health care professionals whose responsibility is to support the person living with diabetes in the management of their condition. A close collaboration between primary and secondary health care professionals and among specialists is needed to ensure that all involved are aware of the issues that are relevant to the individual with diabetes and that care is integrated and coordinated across the wide range of disciplines involved. Placing the person with diabetes at the center of care is likely to facilitate collaboration.

Given the chronic nature of diabetes, continuity of care is essential. Ideally, this should be provided by the same doctors and nurses at each visit, but where this is not possible, the health care team should have access to previous records so that they are fully aware of the medical history and background of the person with diabetes. In some low and middle income countries, where medical records are focused on the acute care of infectious diseases, this is particularly challenging [9].

With the involvement of the person with diabetes in the diabetes team come a number of responsibilities for that individual. The task of implementing the day-to-day management plan lies with the person with diabetes and sometimes it can be difficult for health care professionals to accept this. It must be understood that managing diabetes is challenging, but the diabetes care team should be there to support the person through their experiences with their condition. Adolescence can be particularly challenging as this period of the person's life coincides with a time of change when experimentation and adaptation by the adolescent are to be expected (see Chapter 52).

Improving the outcome of the consultation

The time that a person with diabetes spends with a health care professional is limited and should be used as effectively as possible. It is important that both the person with diabetes and the health care professional prepare for the clinic visit. In the UK, the Department of Health has provided literature entitled *Questions to Ask*, which provides guidance about the questions a person with diabetes should ask during a consultation to maximize the benefit from the visit to their health care team [10].

Box 20.2 Top tips for people with diabetes to achieve a successful consultation [10]

Before your appointment
Write down your two or three most important questions
List or bring all your medicines and pills – including vitamins and supplements
Write down details of your symptoms, including when they started and what makes them better or worse
Ask your hospital or surgery for an interpreter or communication support if needed
Ask a friend or family member to come with you, if you like

During your appointment
Don't be afraid to ask if you don't understand. For example, "Can you say that again? I still don't understand"
If you don't understand any words, ask for them to be written down and explained
Write things down, or ask a family member or friend to take notes

Before you leave your appointment check that:
You've covered everything on your list
You understand, for example "Can I just check I understood what you said?"
You know what should happen next – and when. Write it down
Ask who to contact if you have any more problems or questions
Ask about support groups and where to go for reliable information
Ask for copies of letters written about you – you are entitled to see these

After your appointment, don't forget to:
Write down what you discussed and what happens next. Keep your notes
Book any tests that you can and put the dates in your diary
Ask what will happen if you are not sent your appointment details
"Can I have the results of any tests?" (If you don't get the results when you expect – ask for them.) Ask what the results mean

The consultation or education program should lead the person with diabetes to gain a clear understanding of their condition. This can only be achieved effectively when professionals and people with diabetes are enabled to work together. The interaction should not be seen as an opportunity for the health care profession to "give care" to the patient, but an opportunity for equal involvement in decision-making and care.

People with diabetes should be encouraged to ask questions to check knowledge and further explanation and literature may be needed. It is good practice to provide the person with diabetes with copies of any letters written about them [11,12]. Questions about their treatment should be encouraged and they should be aware of what will happen next, including any requirement for further investigation. Regular review of management plans through joint dialogue, listening, discussion and decision-making between the person with diabetes and health care professional, sometimes known as care planning, is the key to enhancing relationships and partnership working [13]. Contact details should be made available so the individual with diabetes knows where to seek help if further questions arise.

Following diagnosis

The period following the diagnosis of diabetes is crucial for the long-term management of diabetes. A huge amount of information and skills need to be assimilated by the person with diabetes at a time when they may be in denial or angry with the diagnosis [14]. Considerable skill is therefore needed to support them at this time. The diabetes team should perform a medical examination (usually the physician) and develop a program of care with the person with diabetes. It is important that this is individualized so that it suits the particular person with diabetes and should include treatment-oriented goals.

Issues relating to diagnosis

The diagnosis of diabetes is based on the finding of one or more glucose values above internationally agreed values (see Chapter 2) [15]. Usually, a diagnosis has been made prior to referral to the diabetes clinic but this is not always the case. In the absence of symptoms, individuals should have two values above the diagnostic criteria. Where there is diagnostic doubt, the 75-g oral glucose tolerance test is the investigation of choice but there is ongoing discussion about the use of glycated hemoglobin as a diagnostic test [16].

While the diagnosis of diabetes has frequently been made prior to referral, advice may be required to determine the type of diabetes as the distinction is not always as clear as may be expected. When a young preschool child develops weight loss, polyuria, polydipsia and ketoacidosis over a short period of time, the diagnosis is obviously type 1 diabetes mellitus (T1DM). In contrast, if an asymptomatic elderly overweight individual is found to be hyperglycemic, the diagnosis is type 2 diabetes (T2DM) (see Chapter 19). These presentations lie at two ends of a spectrum, and the diagnosis of the type of diabetes may be less clear when the onset occurs in the thirties in an overweight adult who is found to have islet cell antibodies. Diabetes health care professionals should also be alert to the possibility of monogenic causes of diabetes (see Chapter 15).

Although a precise diagnosis may not be needed from the outset, an early decision should be made about the necessity for insulin therapy (see Chapter 19). While there are clinical features that suggest the type of diabetes, time is often a useful diagnostic tool to determine whether the person with diabetes requires insulin.

Diabetes education

A key component of the empowerment of the person with diabetes is the provision of diabetes education (see Chapter 21) [17]. This information should be provided in a patient-centered manner as it is retained more effectively when delivered in this way. Education may be provided individually or in a group setting.

It is essential that the person with diabetes understands their diabetes and develops the skills and competencies required to take control of their condition as well as possible if they are going to be an effective partner in the diabetes care team.

People with newly diagnosed diabetes should have the chance to speak with a diabetes specialist nurse (or practice nurse) who can explain what diabetes is [18]. This will provide an opportunity to discuss the treatment and goals as well as providing a practical demonstration of any equipment required to manage the diabetes such as blood glucose meters or insulin devices. The importance of ketones testing for those with T1DM should be explained. When self-monitoring of blood glucose has been advocated, it is essential that the person with diabetes knows how to interpret the results and what action is required in response to the treatment.

A qualified dietitian should provide advice about how to manage the relationships between food, activity and treatment (see Chapter 22). Where necessary, they should explain about the links between diabetes and diet and the benefits of a healthy diet, exercise and good diabetes control. As an essential member of an effective clinical care team, a diabetes specialist nurse or practice nurse often has a role in providing dietary advice together with relevant literature [18].

The social effects of diabetes should be discussed, as they may relate to employment, insurance or driving (see Chapter 24). Some countries require individuals with diabetes to inform the appropriate licensing authorities. Advice about diabetes and foot care should also be given (see Chapter 44).

Although education is essential following diagnosis, it is important to appreciate that this is a lifelong process that should take into account recent advances in medical science and changes in circumstances of the person with diabetes [17].

The best measure of successful education may not be simply that someone knows more, but rather that they behave differently. The simple provision of knowledge by itself is often insufficient to influence behavioral change. This can be a particular challenge for the person with T2DM who may have been asymptomatic prior to diagnosis. High demands are placed on the person with diabetes regardless of the type of diabetes, especially when the benefits are not immediate, may only accrue with time and even then may not be appreciated. The individual with diabetes needs to gain an understanding that improved glycemic control can help in preventing the complications of diabetes, such as a myocardial infarction or proliferative retinopathy, even though they may have never experienced these conditions.

The diagnosis of diabetes may provoke a grief reaction and support is needed from the diabetes team to help person with diabetes through this. Engagement is needed to help the person with diabetes come to terms with their diabetes and take control rather than being left with the feeling that their diabetes or their health care team is taking control of them. For some it may take a very long time to accept their diabetes and the demands this places on their life. Therefore, emotional and psychological support and techniques need to be available in the long term.

People with newly diagnosed diabetes often want to speak with others who have diabetes who have had similar experiences while developing diabetes. Many countries have diabetes-related charities that can provide this support and it is therefore important that the information given includes local centers or patient support groups.

The clinic visit

The diabetes team needs to work to together with the person with diabetes to review the program of care including the management goals and targets at each visit [19]. It is important that the person with diabetes shares in any decisions about treatment or care as this improves the chance of jointly agreed goals being adopted following the consultation. A family member, friend or carer should be encouraged to attend the clinic to help them stay abreast of developments in diabetes care and help the person with diabetes make informed judgments about diabetes care.

An important goal of diabetes management is to prevent the microvascular and macrovascular complications of diabetes without inducing iatrogenic side effects. This involves active management of hyperglycemia together with a multifaceted approach targeting other cardiovascular risk factors.

Glycemic management

Enquiries and discussions should be made about hyperglycemic symptoms, problems with medications, including issues relating to injections, hypoglycemia and self-monitoring of blood glucose.

Hyperglycemic symptoms

Symptoms relating to hyperglycemia usually occur when the blood glucose rises above the renal threshold leading to an osmotic diuresis. Polyuria, particularly at night, polydipsia and tiredness may ensure. General malaise may also occur and is not always ascribed to the hyperglycemia.

Medications

The diabetes care team is responsible for ensuring that the person with diabetes has access to the medication and equipment necessary for diabetes control. In many countries this is available free or at a reduced rate; many people with diabetes may be unaware of this and timely advice may alleviate some of the anxieties about the cost of diabetes.

Oral hypoglycemic drugs

Each of the oral hypoglycemic drugs has its strengths and profile of side effects (see Chapter 29) and these should be discussed. Strategies should be devised to maximize the tolerability of diabetes medications. For example, the timing of metformin in relationship to meals, or the use of long-acting preparations, may reduce the risk of gastrointestinal upset. Where treatments are not being tolerated, these may need to be changed in order to facilitate improved concordance with the regimen. Another example is the need to discuss the risks of hypoglycemia with sulfonylureas.

Insulin

Insulin therapy is complex: it must be given by self-injection or pump and there is considerable variation in the doses, regimens and devices available. It is important that during the clinic visit the individual has an opportunity to discuss injection technique and any difficulties with injection sites, which should be examined at least annually. Information about the appropriate storage of insulin and safe disposal of sharps (needles) is needed.

The most common side effects of insulin are hypoglycemia and weight gain (see Chapter 27). In addition to these, there are a number of other issues that should be addressed including injection site problems, such as lipohypertrophy, and device problems.

Assessment of glucose control

Supporting the person with diabetes to achieve excellent glycemic control is an essential component of diabetes care. The methods of assessing glucose control essentially involve short-term measures such as self-monitoring of blood glucose and long-term measures such as glycated hemoglobin (see Chapter 25). Not all those with diabetes will undertake self-monitoring of blood glucose, but when they do it is incumbent on the health care professional to discuss the findings with the person with diabetes and how these will affect future management. The glycated hemoglobin provides a further measure of the adequacy of glycemic control and sometimes there may be a discrepancy between this measure and self-monitored blood glucose. It is important to explore the reasons that underlie the differences, which may range from biologic issues such as genetically determined rates of glycation, through to inappropriately timed glucose readings to fabricated results. A pristine sheet (with no blood stains from fingersticks) and with the use of a single pen color may be a clue to the latter. The use of computers and the ability to download results may help to observe patterns of hyperglycemia, although it is important to make sure that the meter has not been shared.

It is clearly important that people with diabetes are encouraged to tell the truth. Sometimes clinicians can appear judgmental which may result in people with diabetes falsifying their results because they are scared. They can feel as if some clinicians are headteachers and they do not want to be reprimanded. It is understandable why someone would not put themselves through that if they did not have to. It is better to break down these barriers and to build a relationship whereby the person with diabetes feels that it does not benefit them to lie, and that the health care professional is there to support, not to judge.

Table 20.1 Glycemic and cardiovascular risk factor targets [20–22,38].

	Glycated hemoglobin	Blood pressure (mmHg)	Lipid profile
ADA	<53 mmol/mol (<7.0%)	<140/90	LDL < 100 mg/dL HDL > 40 mg/dL for men >5.0 mg/dL for women Triglycerides < 150 mg/dL
EASD	<53 mmol/mol (<7.0%)	<130/80	LDL < 1.8 mmol/L (<70 mg/dL) HDL > 1.0 mmol/L (>40 mg/dL) for men >1.2 mmol/L (>46 mg/dL) for women Triglycerides < 1.7 mmol/L (<150 mg/dL)
IDF	<48 mmol/mol (<6.5%)	<130/80	LDL < 2.5 mmol/L (<95 mg/dL) Triglycerides < 2.3 mmol/L (<200 mg/dL) HDL > 1.0 mmol/L (>39 mg/dL)
NICE	<48 mmol/mol (<6.5%)	<130/80	Total cholesterol 4.0 mmol/L LDL cholesterol 2.0 mmol/L

ADA, American Diabetes Association; EASD, European Association for the Study of Diabetes; HDL, high density lipoprotein cholesterol; IDF, International Diabetes Federation; LDL, low density lipoprotein cholesterol; NICE, National Institute for Health and Clinical Excellence.

The Diabetes Control and Complications Trial and the UK Prospective Diabetes Study (UKPDS) have clearly established that lower levels of glycemia are associated with a reduced risk of long-term microvascular complications in T1DM and T2DM, respectively [3–5]. For this reason, learned societies such as the American Diabetes Association (ADA) and European Association for the Study of Diabetes (EASD), and government bodies such as the National Institute for Health and Clinical Excellence have set tight glycemic targets to minimize the risk of complications for person with diabetes (Table 20.1) [20–22]. Despite these targets, many people with diabetes are unable to achieve this level of control. It is important for the health care professional to explore the reasons with the person with diabetes why the control is not ideal. Advice about adjustment of treatment or further education may be needed.

A common limiting factor in the ability to achieve good control is hypoglycemia which is one of the most uncomfortable, inconvenient and feared side effects of diabetes medication (see Chapter 33). The frequency and severity of hypoglycemic episodes should be discussed. An exploration of the underlying causes and advice about prevention are required for the future.

When a person with diabetes is treated with insulin, it is important to ensure that they carry a readily accessible source of glucose such as glucose tablets. Concentrated glucose solution and glucagon should also be made available for use in more severe hypoglycemia. As these treatments may only be used infrequently, it is worth checking whether they are in date. Furthermore, as they need to be administered by another individual, it is important to ensure that the friends and relatives of the person with diabetes know how to administer them before they are needed.

In some instances, the only way of avoiding disabling hypoglycemia is to accept a lesser degree of glycemic control. This recalibration of glycemic goals should be decided with the person with diabetes and an individual target appropriate for the circumstances should be agreed. As well as the risk of hypoglycemia, other factors should be considered when discussing the target including the overall clinical situation and risk of complications affecting the individual.

The natural history of the development of complications is long and in some situations may be longer than the life expectancy of the person with diabetes. It would be a poor trade to insist on switching a frail complication-free 90-year-old person to insulin if they subsequently fell and broke their hip and died as a result of insulin-induced hypoglycemia. Less melodramatic but still important is the consideration about dietary and lifestyle change in people with low risk of disabling complications: is it really necessary to deny an elderly person with diabetes a piece of birthday cake if this is one of the few pleasures in their life? A more sensible approach would be to advise a limit to portion size, rather than insist on severe dietary limitations.

Although there is a clinical emphasis on glycemic targets, the results of the Action to Control Cardiovascular risk in Diabetes (ACCORD) trial [23], the Action in Diabetes and Vascular disease: Preteraz and diamicron MR controlled evaluation (ADVANCE) trial [24] and Veterans Affairs Diabetes Trial (VA-DT) have led to a note of caution [25]. These trials have shown that tight glycemic control in people with a longer duration of diabetes did not prolong life. In the case of the ACCORD trial, increased cardiovascular mortality was seen in those receiving intensive glycemic control [23]. The underlying reasons for these findings are discussed in Part 8, but again their findings highlight the need for individualized targets.

Assessment of cardiovascular risk

The most common cause of death in people with diabetes is cardiovascular disease (CVD) and much effort has been expended to develop strategies that will reduce its morbidity and mortality [26].

Cardiovascular risk should be assessed at least once a year for people with diabetes. This should include a history of cardiovascular risk factors, such as family history, smoking, an examination to include weight, waist circumference and blood pressure as well as investigations such as a lipid profile. The results of this assessment can be used to calculate cardiovascular risk using the various risk engines available. Some, such as the UKPDS risk engines for coronary heart disease and stroke, were designed specifically for use in people with diabetes [27,28].

Because the risk of myocardial infarction is as high in people with diabetes as in non-diabetic people with pre-existing CVD, the diabetes itself is widely considered to be a major risk factor for CVD [29]. This has influenced prescribing guidelines which now recommend that specific pharmacologic interventions are required to reduce the incidence of CVD in people with diabetes regardless of risk assessment. Large randomized controlled trials have shown the effectiveness of these interventions and are discussed in greater detail in Chapter 40 [30].

Although physicians may appreciate the close connection between diabetes and CVD, many people with diabetes have never been told about this increased risk, and the importance of blood pressure and lipid control in diabetes. Thus, many individuals are not taking appropriate drugs for cardiovascular prevention or if they are then the doses may be inadequate to bring the individuals to the recommended targets (Table 20.1). When working with someone with diabetes, it is important that strategies to reduce CVD and the need for preventative drugs are discussed. In addition, the increased vascular damage promoted by smoking in the setting of diabetes may not be appreciated.

The main classes of drugs used are lipid-lowering drugs, predominantly statins, antihypertensives, particularly drugs acting on the renin-angiotensin system and aspirin. Antihypertensives are also important in the prevention of microvascular complications.

While each individual intervention for various risk factors is important in the prevention of macrovascular disease, the Steno II study has demonstrated that a coordinated approach to the management of cardiovascular risk can be successful [6]. In this study, the clinic setting and protocol-driven approach to overall cardiovascular risk led to improved mortality compared with routine care.

Microvascular complications

Around 80% of individuals will have developed microvascular complications by the time they have had diabetes for 20 years [31]. Many complications will remain asymptomatic until they have catastrophic consequences. The management of microvascular complications involves measures to prevent, detect and treat. General measures such as optimal glycemic and blood pressure control lead to a reduction in the incidence and progression of microvascular complications but specific preventative measures are also needed and are discussed below [3–5,32].

Eyes

Diabetic retinopathy is the most common cause of blindness in people of working age (see Chapter 36). It is almost invariably asymptomatic until there is a catastrophic sight-threatening hemorrhage. For this reason it is important to screen regularly for retinopathy to allow treatment before hemorrhage and visual loss occur. Traditionally, this has been performed by examination of the visual acuity and fundoscopy within the diabetes clinic at least on an annual basis. Alternatively, in many countries, dilated ophthalmologic examinations are regularly performed by a specialist.

The gold standard for screening now is digital retinal photography, which may be undertaken in several different settings. When this is performed outside the traditional diabetes clinic, communication between the screener and diabetes team is essential if other aspects of diabetes care are to take account of the development of retinopathy. Where retinopathy is detected within the clinic, it is the responsibility of the clinic to ensure that the patient is referred for specialist ophthalmologic attention in a timely fashion.

Neuropathy

Distal symmetrical polyneuropathy is the most common form of neuropathy seen in diabetes and is addressed in the following section on the diabetic foot. Autonomic neuropathy may affect the person with diabetes in a number of ways (e.g. gustatory sweating, postural hypotension or bloating) (see Chapter 38). Health care professionals should be alert to this possibility if symptoms suggestive of these conditions are raised.

Diabetic foot

Diabetes is the most common cause of non-traumatic lower limb amputation in the developed world (see Chapter 44). Around 10–15% of all people with diabetes develop a foot ulcer as a result of the combination of peripheral neuropathy and vascular insufficiency to the foot.

Prevention of ulceration is an important goal and requires education of the person with diabetes so that they are aware of this possibility. It is important to inform people that they should not delay obtaining professional help if problems ensue.

An assessment of the risk of foot ulceration is needed at least annually, and more frequently when neuropathy or vascular disease is present. The assessment should include a history of previous ulceration and trauma as well as an examination of the skin, vascular supply and sensation. Opportunistic foot screening should also be performed if an individual with diabetes is admitted to hospital.

In patients with numbness, close attention to discovering unsuspected foot lesions, including examination of the sole of the foot using a small mirror, must be performed by the patient on a regular basis. This can lead to a rapid intervention and prevent an early infection from progressing, potentially averting such devastating consequences as osteomyelitis and gangrene.

Prompt referral to the podiatrist and foot clinic should be arranged by the diabetes clinic if needed.

Kidneys

Diabetic nephropathy is characterized by a progressive increase in urinary albumin excretion which is accompanied by increasing blood pressure and decline in glomerular filtration rate, ultimately culminating in end-stage renal disease (ESRD). It is also associated with a marked increase in the rate of CVD.

Microalbuminuria, the earliest stage of nephropathy, affects around 50% of people with diabetes after 30 years while frank proteinuria affects one-quarter of people with T1DM after 25 years. Diabetic nephropathy is a common reason for the initiation of renal replacement therapy. Although it appears that with modern treatments of diabetes, the percentage of people with diabetes developing ESRD appears to be falling, the absolute numbers requiring renal replacement therapy is increasing in line with the increased prevalence of diabetes worldwide.

Diabetic nephropathy is asymptomatic and so screening is required annually. This is usually achieved by measurement of urinary albumin excretion. The most common method is a single urinary albumin:creatinine ratio (ACR) measurement which should be repeated 2–3 times if abnormal. An estimation of glomerular filtration rate should be obtained annually.

The primary prevention of nephropathy relies on excellent glycemic control as well as tight blood pressure control. Once nephropathy is present, blood pressure management is the mainstay as there is little evidence that glycemic control at this stage slows the rate of progression. The antihypertensive drugs of choice are angiotensin-converting enzyme (ACE) inhibitors of the renin-angiotensin system (ACE inhibitors or angiotensin-2 receptor antagonists) as they have specific effects on renal blood flow [33,34].

There has been some debate about the value of undertaking urinary ACR measurements in people with T2DM, the argument being that tight blood pressure control (often including an ACE inhibitor or angiotensin-2 receptor antagonist) together with good glycemic control should form part of the general management of cardiovascular risk reduction.

It is important that the person with diabetes understands the need for screening and then treatment if nephropathy develops. Timely referral to the nephrology team is needed to ensure that the management of renal disease is managed promptly in patients with abnormal renal function.

Diabetes emergencies

Diabetic ketoacidosis and hyperosmolar hyperglycemic syndrome

Diabetic ketoacidosis and hyperosmolar hyperglycemic syndrome are potentially life-threatening emergencies (see Chapter 34). It is important that the person with diabetes is educated about the risk of these and discusses strategies to prevent them. If a person with diabetes has been admitted with diabetic ketoacidosis or hyperosmolar hyperglycemic syndrome, the opportunity should be taken to explore the reasons why this episode occurred and to identify what might be changed to prevent this from happening in future. The most common causes of hyperglycemic emergencies in those with pre-existing diabetes are infections and insulin omission and errors. It is particularly important that people with diabetes understand the "sick day" rules: insulin should never be discontinued and indeed doses may need to be increased, even when appetite is diminished.

Hypoglycemia

Hypoglycemia is a much more common diabetic emergency, affecting around 10% of people with T1DM and 2.4% of insulin-treated people with T2DM (see Chapter 33). Hypoglycemia can have a major adverse effect on quality of life and is the most important limiting factor in the achievement of good glycemic control.

Box 20.3 Causes of hypoglycemia

Excessive insulin administration:
- Person with diabetes, doctor or pharmacist error
- Deliberate overdose during a suicide or parasuicide attempt

Excessive sulfonylurea administration

Unpredictable insulin absorption:
- Insulin is absorbed more rapidly from the abdomen
- Lipohypertophy

Altered clearance of insulin:
- Decreased insulin clearance in renal failure

Decreased insulin requirement:
- Missed, small or delayed meals
- Alcohol: inhibits hepatic glucose output
- Vomiting: may occur with gastroparesis, a long-term complication of diabetes
- Exercise
  - Promotes glucose uptake into muscle
  - Increases rate of insulin absorption

Recurrent hypoglycemia and unawareness

It is important that the person with diabetes is educated about the symptoms of hypoglycemia and the actions to be taken to prevent and treat this. Friends and family members should be invited to learn about hypoglycemia and its management in order to intervene where necessary, for example providing glucagon treatment if the person with diabetes is unconscious. If hypoglycemia becomes disabling or recurrent it is important to explore underlying causes.

Lifestyle issues

Diabetes has a number of social, as well as medical, consequences and one aspect of diabetes care is to discuss how diabetes is affecting issues such as driving, education and employment (see Chapter 24). The health care professional may need to act as an advocate for the person where discrimination is occurring. Some aspects of lifestyle also affect diabetes care, such as diet, exercise, smoking and alcohol. These issues should be discussed carefully and sensitively in order to help the person with diabetes understand how their lifestyle affects their diabetes and general health. Support should be given to help and encourage a person with diabetes to make changes to their lifestyle.

Psychologic issues

The diagnosis of diabetes can provoke a number of psychologic reactions, such as anger and sadness in the individual which may be akin to a bereavement reaction (see Chapter 49). More serious mental health problems such as depression are common in people with diabetes and these can impede the person's ability to achieve good glycemic control (see Chapter 55) [35].

It is important for those working in diabetes care to explore with the person with diabetes whether they are experiencing psychologic problems as there may be reticence in raising this in the consultation. While all members of the diabetes team should be able to recognize and address basic psychologic issues, the psychologist is an important team member to address more complex needs, such as eating disorders. Despite the importance of psychologic issues, this need is frequently unmet because of a lack of trained health care professionals.

Sexual health

Sexual dysfunction

Sexual dysfunction is more common in both men and women with diabetes than the general population. This can affect the person's quality of life considerably. Many people are reluctant to discuss this aspect of their lives because of embarrassment and so it is the responsibility of the health care professional to enquire about this. There are now effective treatments for erectile dysfunction and failure to ask about this can deny the person with diabetes the opportunity to receive treatment.

Pregnancy planning

Starting a family is an important milestone for many and the presence of diabetes can make this decision more difficult for the woman or man with diabetes (see Chapter 53). People are often worried about the effects that diabetes will have on their pregnancy and vice versa. The implications for the long-term risk of diabetes in the offspring are also of concern.

Planning for a pregnancy by a woman with diabetes can dramatically improve the outcome, reducing the risk of miscarriage, congenital malformations and macrosomia, with its attendant risks of shoulder dystocia, and neonatal hypoglycemia [36]. Some oral medications should not be used in pregnancy and the treatment regimen may need to be altered as part of the planning process.

Despite this, women frequently enter pregnancy without adequate preparation or pre-conception care. It is therefore incumbent on the health care professional to discuss pregnancy with all women of childbearing age, including adolescents, to ascertain their plans regarding pregnancy. The answers are often not black and white; women may state that they are not actively planning to become pregnant despite being sexually active and not using effective contraception. Contraceptive advice is needed and where a pregnancy is being planned, women should be referred to a dedicated pre-conception clinic as these have been shown to improve the outcomes of diabetic pregnancies.

With an increasing number of women with T2DM of childbearing age, it is important that pre-conception is not solely focused towards those with T1DM. This is particularly relevant as some women with T2DM are not seen in specialist centers.

Prompt referral to a joint diabetes antenatal clinic is necessary once a woman becomes pregnant.

Inpatient diabetes care

It is estimated that around 10–15% of people in hospital have diabetes (see Chapter 32). In many instances, the diabetes is coincidental to the admission and the person with diabetes remains capable of managing their own diabetes, often with greater skill than the health care professionals around them. Good diabetes control remains an important goal as this improves the rate of recovery and may lead to an earlier discharge.

Admission to hospital is a worrying time but much of the fear can be alleviated if a full explanation of the treatment in hospital is given along with an opportunity to discuss any particular concerns. Being given the opportunity to discuss the management of diabetes is reassuring. Where possible, the person with diabetes should be allowed to continue to self-manage their diabetes. The individual should be encouraged to bring in their own insulin supplies where admissions are planned. There should be access to their regular diabetes health care team where possible as the admission may provide an occasion to check techniques and results. Ready access to carbohydrate and appropriate coordination of mealtimes, snacks and medication should obviate the need for more dramatic treatment of hypoglycemia.

There will be times when the person with diabetes is unable to manage their diabetes themselves. In these instances, the responsibility will fall entirely on the health care team, for example during surgery when the person with diabetes is unconscious and requires intravenous insulin and dextrose.

Following discharge, clear communication with the primary care team and diabetes clinic is essential so that any changes in management or medication are made known to those involved in the individual's care.

Involving people with diabetes in the planning of health care and service development

Involving people with diabetes and their carers in the planning and decision-making of local health services allows these to be built around the needs of those who use the service, rather than the needs of the system [37]. An open dialogue is needed and service users should feel that their views are listened to. This will improve the accountability and legitimacy for any decisions made and is likely to improve clinical and care outcomes. People with diabetes should be encouraged to express their views and concerns about their services as better feedback about service provision which should help to improve and shape future provision of care.

Conclusions

The aim of diabetes care is to improve the lives of those with diabetes. This can only be achieved through a partnership between the person with diabetes and a multifunctional health care team that should be in place to support the person with diabetes.

Acknowledgments

The authors acknowledge Bridget Turner of Diabetes UK and June James, Consultant Nurse, University Hospitals of Leicester Trust, UK, for their helpful comments on this chapter.

References

1 DECODE Study Group. Glucose tolerance and mortality: comparison of WHO and American Diabetes Association diagnostic criteria. The DECODE study group. European Diabetes Epidemiology Group. Diabetes Epidemiology: Collaborative analysis Of Diagnostic criteria in Europe. *Lancet* 1999; **354**:617–621.

2 DECODE Study Group. Glucose tolerance and cardiovascular mortality: comparison of fasting and 2-hour diagnostic criteria. *Arch Intern Med* 2001; **161**:397–405.

3 Diabetes Control and Complications Trial Research Group. The effect of intensive treatment of diabetes on the development and progression of long-term complications in insulin-dependent diabetes mellitus. *N Engl J Med* 1993; **329**:977–986.

4 Holman RR, Paul SK, Bethel MA, Matthews DR, Neil HA. 10-year follow-up of intensive glucose control in type 2 diabetes. *N Engl J Med* 2008; **359**:1577–1589.

5 UK Prospective Diabetes Study (UKPDS) Group. Intensive blood-glucose control with sulphonylureas or insulin compared with conventional treatment and risk of complications in patients with type 2 diabetes (UKPDS 33). *Lancet* 1998; **352**:837–853.

6 Gaede P, Lund-Andersen H, Parving HH, Pedersen O. Effect of a multifactorial intervention on mortality in type 2 diabetes. *N Engl J Med* 2008; **358**:580–591.

7 WHO/IDF St. Vincent Declaration Working Group. Diabetes mellitus in Europe: a problem at all ages in all countries – a model for prevention and self care. *Acta Diabetol* 1990; **27**:181–183.

8 Ensuring access to high quality care for people with diabetes. Available from: http://www.diabetes.org.uk/About_us/Our_Views/Position_statements/Ensuring_access_to_high_quality_care_for_people_with_diabetes. Accessed on 21 August, 2009.

9 Yudkin JS, Holt RI, Silva-Matos C, Beran D. Twinning for better diabetes care: a model for improving healthcare for non-communicable diseases in resource-poor countries. *Postgrad Med J* 2009; **85**:1–2.

10 Department of Health. *Questions to Ask*. London: Department of Health, 2007.

11 Lloyd BW. A randomised controlled trial of dictating the clinic letter in front of the patient. *Br Med J* 1997; **314**:347–348.

12 Treacy K, Elborn JS, Rendall J, Bradley JM. Copying letters to patients with cystic fibrosis (CF): letter content and patient perceptions of benefit. *J Cyst Fibros* 2008; **7**:511–514.

13 Department of Health. *Care Planning in Diabetes: Report from the Joint Department of Health and Diabetes UK Care Planning Working Group*. London: Department of Health, 2006.

14 Garay-Sevilla ME, Malacara JM, Gutierrez-Roa A, Gonzalez E. Denial of disease in type 2 diabetes mellitus: its influence on metabolic control and associated factors. *Diabet Med* 1999; **16**:238–244.

15 World Health Organization. *Definition, Diagnosis and Classification of Diabetes Mellitus and its Complications: Report of a WHO Consultation*. WHO/NCD/NCS/99.2. Geneva: World Health Organization, 1999.

16 International Expert Committee report on the role of the A1C assay in the diagnosis of diabetes. *Diabetes Care* 2009; **32**:1327–1334.

17 Funnell MM, Brown TL, Childs BP, Haas LB, Hosey GM, Jensen B, *et al.* National standards for diabetes self-management education. *Diabetes Care* 2009; **32**(Suppl 1):87–94.

18 Diabetes UK. What to expect when you have just been diagnosed. Available from: http://www.diabetes.org.uk/Guide-to-diabetes/What_care_to_expect/From_your_healthcare_team/What_to_expect_when_you_have_just_been_diagnosed. Accessed on 21 August, 2009.

19 Diabetes UK. What to expect on a regular basis. Available from: http://www.diabetes.org.uk/Guide-to-diabetes/What_care_to_expect/From_your_healthcare_team/What_to_expect_on_a_regular_basis. Accessed on 21 August, 2009.

20 Nathan DM, Buse JB, Davidson MB, Ferrannini E, Holman RR, Sherwin R *et al.* Medical management of hyperglycaemia in type 2 diabetes mellitus: a consensus algorithm for the initiation and adjustment of therapy. Consensus statement from the American Diabetes Association and the European Association for the Study of Diabetes. *Diabetologia* 2009; **52**:17–30.

21 National Institute for Clinical Excellence (NICE). *Diabetes Type 2 (update): NICE guidance*. NICE, 2008.

22 National Institute for Clinical Excellence (NICE). *Type 1 Diabetes in Adults: NICE guidance*. NICE, 2008.

23 Gerstein HC, Miller ME, Byington RP, Goff DC Jr, Bigger JT, Buse JB, *et al.* Effects of intensive glucose lowering in type 2 diabetes. *N Engl J Med* 2008; **358**:2545–2559.

24 Patel A, MacMahon S, Chalmers J, Neal B, Billot L, Woodward M, *et al.* Intensive blood glucose control and vascular outcomes in patients with type 2 diabetes. *N Engl J Med* 2008; **358**:2560–2572.

25 Duckworth W, Abraira C, Moritz T, Reda D, Emanuele N, Reaven PD, *et al.* Glucose control and vascular complications in veterans with type 2 diabetes. *N Engl J Med* 2009; **360**:129–139.

26 Roper NA, Bilous RW, Kelly WF, Unwin NC, Connolly VM. Cause-specific mortality in a population with diabetes: South Tees Diabetes Mortality Study. *Diabetes Care* 2002; **25**:43–48.

27 Kothari V, Stevens RJ, Adler AI, Stratton IM, Manley SE, Neil HA, *et al.* UKPDS 60: risk of stroke in type 2 diabetes estimated by the UK Prospective Diabetes Study risk engine. *Stroke* 2002; **33**:1776–1781.

28 Stevens RJ, Kothari V, Adler AI, Stratton IM. The UKPDS risk engine: a model for the risk of coronary heart disease in type II diabetes (UKPDS 56). *Clin Sci (Lond)* 2001; **101**:671–679.

29 Haffner SM, Lehto S, Ronnemaa T, Pyorala K, Laakso M. Mortality from coronary heart disease in subjects with type 2 diabetes and in nondiabetic subjects with and without prior myocardial infarction. *N Engl J Med* 1998; **339**:229–234.

30 Collins R, Armitage J, Parish S, Sleigh P, Peto R. MRC/BHF Heart Protection Study of cholesterol-lowering with simvastatin in 5963 people with diabetes: a randomised placebo-controlled trial. *Lancet* 2003; **361**:2005–2016.

31 Klein R, Knudtson MD, Lee KE, Gangnon R, Klein BE. The Wisconsin Epidemiologic Study of Diabetic Retinopathy: XXII the twenty-five-year progression of retinopathy in persons with type 1 diabetes. *Ophthalmology* 2008; **115**:1859–1868.

32 UK Prospective Diabetes Study Group. Tight blood pressure control and risk of macrovascular and microvascular complications in type 2 diabetes: UKPDS 38. *Br Med J* 1998; **317**:703–713.

33 EUCLID Study Group. Randomised placebo-controlled trial of lisinopril in normotensive patients with insulin-dependent diabetes and normoalbuminuria or microalbuminuria. *Lancet* 1997; **349**:1787–1792.

34 Parving HH, Lehnert H, Brochner-Mortensen J, Gomis R, Andersen S, Arner P. The effect of irbesartan on the development of diabetic nephropathy in patients with type 2 diabetes. *N Engl J Med* 2001; **345**:870–878.

35 Anderson RJ, Freedland KE, Clouse RE, Lustman PJ. The prevalence of comorbid depression in adults with diabetes: a meta-analysis. *Diabetes Care* 2001; **24**:1069–1078.

36 National Collaborating Centre for Women's and Children's Health. *Diabetes in Pregnancy: Management of Diabetes and its Complications from Pre-conception to the Postnatal Period.* London: National Institute for Health and Clinical Excellence, 2008.

37 Diabetes UK. Involving people with diabetes in health care planning and service development. Available from: http://www.diabetes.org.uk/About_us/Our_Views/Position_statements/Involving_people_-_with_diabetes_in_health_care_planning_and_service_development. Accessed on 21 August, 2009.

38 Ryden L, Standl E, Bartnik M, Van den Berghe G, Betteridge J, de Boer MJ, *et al.* Guidelines on diabetes, pre-diabetes, and cardiovascular diseases: executive summary: The Task Force on Diabetes and Cardiovascular Diseases of the European Society of Cardiology (ESC) and of the European Association for the Study of Diabetes (EASD). *Eur Heart J* 2007; **28**:88–136.

21 Educating the Patient with Diabetes

Carolé Mensing[1] & Barbara Eichorst[2]

[1] Joslin Diabetes Center, Boston, MA, USA
[2] Healthy Interactions, Chicago, IL, USA

Keypoints

- Diabetes education is an important cornerstone of diabetes care, and supports the philosophy of the chronic disease model.
- Diabetes education improves clinical outcomes, and requires periodic follow-up.
- Time spent with a diabetes educator is the best predictor for improvement in diabetes outcomes.
- Patients and physicians agree that diabetes education is a necessary part of care.
- Being prepared with a variety of educational delivery methods is beneficial and necessary to meet the variety of patient learning styles.
- Understanding educational theories builds a strong base for selecting appropriate approaches to meet the needs of individual patients.
- A written plan developed in collaboration with a patient and their educator and care provider offers more chance of achievement.

Introduction

Diabetes education continues to be cited as a cornerstone of effective diabetes care and supports the philosophy of chronic care models (Table 21.1) [1,2]. It is well established that the practice of diabetes self-management education (DSME) is critical to the care and management of people with diabetes, and that measurable behavior change is the unique outcome of working with a diabetes educator [3,4].

Now more than ever, diabetes educators are being held more accountable for their role in diabetes management. Over time it has become apparent that education standards and a system or framework describing self-care behavior could have an important role in supporting people with diabetes to consider behavior changes that might enhance their quality of life and support better management of their condition. The 2000 Standards for Diabetes Self-Management Education [5] and recent 2007 update [6], American Association of Diabetes Educators (AADE) Standards Development for Outcome Measure [3] and the outcomes model, the AADE7™ Self-Care Behaviors framework [7,8], now provide a common reference for establishing behavior change goals and establishing measurable outcomes. The seven self-care behaviors are: healthy eating; being active; monitoring; taking medicine; problem-solving; reducing risks; and healthy coping.

Textbook of Diabetes, 4th edition. Edited by R. Holt, C. Cockram, A. Flyvbjerg and B. Goldstein.

Background

Standards and educational practice guidelines

DSME is central to delivering desirable metabolic and clinical care in diabetes. DSME is a comprehensive patient education structure that involves a multidisciplinary team to help achieve the necessary metabolic outcomes and improve the lives of those living with diabetes [9,10]. Metabolic improvements such as glucose, lipids and blood pressure in type 2 diabetes (T2DM) care are best achieved with a healthy lifestyle and appropriate use of pharmacologic interventions.

In 2003, the AADE published Standards for Outcomes Measurement of Diabetes Self-Management Education [3], complementing the National Standards for DSME in 2000 [5]. This publication was subsequently updated and revised in 2007 [6]. These standards offer the educator a program framework, which is based on five evidence-based principles:

1 In the short term, diabetes education is effective for improving clinical outcomes and quality of life;
2 DSME has evolved to a more theoretically based empowerment model;
3 There is no one best approach;
4 Ongoing support is critical to sustain progress; and
5 Behavioral goal setting is an effective strategy to support self-management behaviors.

This publication clearly identified that behavior change was the unique measurable outcome of diabetes education [3]. In 2004, these self-care behaviors were adopted by AADE leadership, trademarked as the AADE Seven™ [7,8], and have been incorporated into a framework for educators, community leaders and

Table 21.1 Definitions.

Diabetes educator: a professional who provides education
Diabetes self-management education (DSME): the ongoing process of facilitating the knowledge, skill and ability necessary for diabetes self-care [7]
Education: a combination of interactive experiences
Instructional curriculum: a deliberate arrangement of conditions, written content, to promote actions towards an intentional goal [20]
Learning: An active goal-directed process, transforming skills, knowledge and application of values into new observable behavior
MNT: medical nutrition therapy
Teaching: a system of actions to bring about learning

medical professionals to advocate for diabetes self-care management. In addition, this framework provides the potential to be generalized to other chronic diseases and wellness care, and thrives on assessment and documentation.

Educators are guided by professional and discipline-specific scope of practice; these position papers, evidence-based research and standards for diabetes education practise the belief that behavior change can be effectively achieved by using these frameworks.

Three of the main components of DSME are an assessment, intervention and outcomes evaluation of the patient [9,11]. Ongoing collaboration and partnership between the patient and health care professionals is essential for effective DSME. The process involves interactive, collaborative and ongoing education that engages a person with diabetes in therapeutic decision-making [9]. DSME is available throughout the lifespan of the individual with diabetes and enables ongoing reassessment of self-management goals [9]. Diabetes is a progressive disease in which the clinical manifestations vary throughout the patient's lifespan [12]. Changes in stress, acute illness, aging and metabolic abnormalities can impact the clinical manifestations [12]. DSME approaches are typically adjusted as the patient's lifestyle changes and their condition progresses [9,11].

Also appreciated are the similarities and yet the variety of methodologies and delivery options to assist all people with diabetes and those affected by diabetes to achieve healthier outcomes, including adults, children, parents and older people. The purpose of this section is to introduce the concepts of how to acquire useful self-care information, and change concepts into behaviors that can be useful, measured and maintained over time. Although people with diabetes vary in age, type and duration of diabetes, the principles of education remain the same and are reflected in the following content.

Considering change

The provision of DSME is challenging in any setting, whether outpatient, private practice, community service areas or hospital settings, and is constantly changing. A paradigm shift has occurred in diabetes education. The learner is no longer the "patient," rather a "person with diabetes." DSME includes a circle of further learners, and others who are affected by diabetes, such as family members, work colleagues and neighbors. The health care team (nurse, dietitian, pharmacist, physician, other providers) are not just a deliverer of information, with a complacent learner; rather they are "educators" with learners involved in an active "interactive" (go-between) process. In this paradigm, the learners are both the educator and the people involved with diabetes. Each acquires a desire to learn based on need and consider all the alternatives available to them including information, treatment choices and equipment. Both attendee and educator are adjusting to new technologies, and the ever-changing techniques, approaches, settings and fiscal directives.

In addition, researchers on diabetes education programs have adequately demonstrated increased participant knowledge and corresponding improvements in glycemic control [13–16]. The optimal approaches in DSME delivery that are associated with better outcomes focus on behavioral strategies, encourage active engagement of patients, build self-efficacy, use cognitive reframing as a teaching method, are learner-centered and evidence-based where possible [10,17].

Diabetes education is a revered first step in preparing people with diabetes to make the necessary modifications to their lifestyle. Typically, health care professionals teach patients information that they believe is necessary. Evidence indicates, however, that most of the information shared by a health care professional with patients is forgotten soon after. Up to 80% of patients forget what their doctor tells them as soon as they leave the clinic and nearly 50% of what they remember is recalled incorrectly [18]. The Diabetes Attitudes, Wishes, and Needs (DAWN) study indicates that while 50% of persons with T2DM receive DSME, only 16.2% report adhering to the recommended self-management activities [19]. The DAWN study identified key goals that need to be achieved to improve outcomes: reducing barriers to therapy; promoting self-management; improving psychologic care and enhancing communication with health care providers, people with diabetes and their primary care providers that is consistent with educational standards (DSME) previously presented.

This said, the traditional lecture format, with its instructional knowledge-based content outlines, has also changed to involve and evolve using more interactive processes. The new standards for DSME [6] offer the format of "structure, process and outcome" directives for an established program to meet. These formats serve as an influence for third party reimbursement as well as offering the educator a structured evidence-based format for program development, implementation and evaluation. The standards also encourage new opportunities for alternative program involvement of educational options. The nine curricula (Table 21.2) offer the educator a written instructional topic-driven plan for education, and intentionally closely resemble the AADE7 self-management outcome behaviors (Table 21.3). The AADE7 then offers a template for behavior change identification,

Table 21.2 Nine content areas (DSME) [6].

1. Describing the diabetes disease process and treatment options
2. Incorporating nutritional management into lifestyle
3. Incorporating physical activity into lifestyle
4. Using medication(s) safely and for maximum therapeutic effectiveness
5. Monitoring blood glucose and other variables and interpreting and using results for self-management decision-making
6. Preventing, detecting and treating acute complications
7. Preventing, detecting and treating chronic complications
8. Developing personal strategies to address psychosocial issues and concerns
9. Developing personal strategies to promote health and behavior change

Table 21.3 The AADE7 self-management outcome behaviors. Data from AADE website (www.diabeteseducator.org/AADE7).

1. **Healthy eating** Making healthy food choices, understanding portion sizes and learning the best times to eat are central to managing diabetes. Diabetes education classes can assist people with diabetes in gaining knowledge, teaching food choice skills, and addressing related barriers
2. **Being active** Regular activity is important for overall fitness, weight management and blood glucose control. Collaboration between patients, providers and educators best addresses barriers, and helps develop an appropriate activity plan that balances food and medication with the activity level
3. **Monitoring** Daily self-monitoring of blood glucose provides people with diabetes the information they need to assess how food, physical activity and medications affect their blood glucose levels. Monitoring includes: blood pressure, urine ketones and weight. Education is offered about equipment choices, testing times, target values, and interpretation and use of results
4. **Taking medication** Diabetes is a progressive condition. The health care team will be able to determine which medications people with diabetes should be taking and help them understand how the medications work. Effective drug therapy in combination with healthy lifestyle choices, can lower blood glucose levels, reduce the risk for diabetes complications and produce other clinical benefits
5. **Problem-solving** Assistance to make rapid informed decisions about food, activity and medications, and develop coping strategies
6. **Reducing risks** Effective risk reduction behaviors such as smoking cessation, and regular eye, foot and dental examinations reduce diabetes complications and maximize health and quality of life, available preventive services. These include smoking cessation, foot inspections, blood pressure monitoring, self-monitoring of blood glucose, aspirin use and maintenance of personal care records
7. **Healthy coping** Health status and quality of life are affected by psychologic and social factors. Coping: a person's ability to self-manage their diabetes is related to their skills. Identifying the individual's motivation to change behavior, set achievable behavioral goals and provide support.

process for change and evaluation of outcome. New and less experienced providers of education may find adopting these existing formats useful, while experienced educators may reconstruct, adapt and create more unique options. All educators are encouraged to participate in the discovery of alternative and creative activities to engage the learner and provide excitement and variety to their educational delivery methods. Mensing and Norris [20] offer instructional tips and educational skills for both.

The purpose of this chapter is to offer the educator and their colleagues the ability to review current education practice and to acquire more in-depth knowledge of interventions focusing on self-care behaviors. These behaviors can then more strongly offer information and potential behavior change opportunities based on a set of practices, presented in a curriculum framework.

The new standards and AADE7 frameworks offer educators an approach that is holistic, empowering and opportunities for patients to strengthen their independence and quality of life. The approach also supports a more public health, patient-centered approach for the person with diabetes and the educator.

Patient-centered educational approaches

Patient-centered education, or learner-centered education, is now promoted by educators moving from provider-directed to "patient-centered" care and education in line with public health and chronic disease models of illness management. Diabetes educators were early proponents of this model and quickly incorporated strategies to meet the patients' agenda at each encounter [21].

This more patient-centered approach frees the educator to provide personalized (less didactic) information, encouraging lessons to be learned and then applied into patients' own lives thereby providing reinforcement and follow-up. As summarized by Funnell [7], patients are more successful if they hear consistent messages and the same single messages from all care providers, educators and team members.

Diabetes education is a first step in preparing patients to make necessary modifications to their lifestyle. As many patients forget much of what is said in clinic, educators and clinicians must recognize the need to involve patients in determining what they feel they need and address this first as a way to engage patients, and improve their retention of information.

The information sharing among health care professionals and retention of information by people with diabetes is not enough to help them to change their behavior. The quality and quantity of effective communication between health care professionals and people with diabetes is the most critical indicator of successful DSME. Increased contact time between health care professionals and patients has been associated with better regimen adherence and glucose reduction [15].

So what is the best way to teach people with diabetes? How do we know that they are learning? What is the evidence supporting the education methods we choose to utilize? A simple elementary school approach from Anna Devere Smith, which "thinks of education as a garden where questions grow," seems to describe the learner-centered approach applicable for adults with diabetes most aptly [73]. People with diabetes need an appropriate environment where they can share their challenges with their lives with diabetes, ask health care professionals for help with strategies and consequently concord with the prescribed regimen.

The principles of facilitation and patient-centered intervention have been recognized to be superior to a didactic and more passive teaching approach [9,10]. One of the DSME standards states that "there is no one best education program or approach; however, programs incorporating behavioral and psychosocial strategies demonstrate improved outcomes. Ongoing support is critical to sustain progress made by participants during the DSME program" [9]. There is strong evidence that goals generated by patients produce better outcomes than goals that are generated by health care professionals [9].

There are many educational approaches that are utilized by diabetes educators to help patients acquire knowledge, skills and commitment to self-care behaviors necessary for effective diabetes care [9]. Typically, individual adult T2DM education interventions allow the educator to tailor the approach to the patient's specific needs and consequently provide effective therapy. However, evidence indicates that group diabetes interventions can be more cost-effective, patient-centered and provide interactive learning with a high level of patient satisfaction compatible with individual interventions. The educational approaches and methods utilized in group education differ among diabetes educators. Therefore, further research is needed to determine which educational approach and method utilized by diabetes educators contributes to effective teaching that produces the best clinical outcomes in adults with T2DM. The existing best practices in group education indicate that the best outcomes are produced with an empowerment approach, which focuses on when and what patients want to learn. Problem-based, culturally tailored approaches that include psychosocial, behavioral and clinical issues relevant to the patients' needs and readiness to learn have resulted in improved outcomes [22].

DSME aligns with a chronic disease model that indicates that educational approaches should be non-complex, individualized to a patient's needs and lifestyle, reinforced over time, respectful to an individual's habits, and should incorporate social support [9,23,24]. Chronic disease care approaches use similar strategies to DSME as they focus on collaborative problem definition, goal-setting, continuum of self-management training and support services [9]. The general consensus on chronic disease interventions indicates that the most beneficial components of education are individualization, relevance, feedback, reinforcement and facilitation [23–25].

How do we provide learner-centered education in a group setting? How do we evaluate everyone's unique learning needs and provide individual attention they deserve? The complexity of the individual needs assessment and training in a group setting presents a challenge for effective self-management education. The challenge is to individualize the approaches similar to a typical one-on-one session but in a group session. Successfully individualizing the group session allows the patients to learn, retain their knowledge and be committed to the follow-up action plan. Traditional didactic education that focuses on teaching information through lectures without patients' engagement has been shown to be ineffective in helping patients change their lifestyle behaviors necessary to improve clinical outcomes [26–28]. Diabetes knowledge does not guarantee changes in behaviors that eventually lead to better outcomes. The learner-centered approach employs non-didactic and less passive strategies in an attempt to promote active engagement in the learning process. A patient-centered education reflects the best practices and theories that have been shown to promote patients' knowledge retention, commitment and improved self-care outcomes. These include facilitation, empowerment, motivational interviewing, behavioral goal-setting, behavioral and psychosocial strategies, and ongoing support [26–34]. The process allows for the patients to discuss their understanding of diabetes, internalize their commitment and determine their priorities. This process also allows for ongoing implementation of short and long-term goals, which can then be monitored for progress. Patients come up with their own solutions to their own diabetes challenges instead of being told what they should do by the educator. The expectation is that by identifying what is practical and achievable, patients ultimately own their own commitments and will be more likely to accomplish the requisite lifestyle changes [28,35,36].

Effective diabetes education aligns with the principles of adult learning as adults learn most effectively when information is simple, practical and relevant (i.e. directed by their interests), the learning builds on participants' experiences and there is a focus on application (i.e. when learning is applied to action) [37]. This process of learning involves cognition, emotions and environmental factors that impact knowledge level, skill acquisition and views [38].

Educational theory behind the practice: models and methods

The core foundation of the diabetes education philosophy is that patients are ultimately responsible for their own self-management. The assumption is that patients want to maximize the quality of their life and self-management education [39]. Health care professionals help patients identify ways to make changes necessary for a healthy way of life. Each person with diabetes differs and therefore requires unique lifestyle skill strategies that are applicable to his or her circumstances.

Traditional lecture-based didactic education approaches place the learner in the role of the recipient and the instructor in the role of the "knowledge-giver." It does not allow the learner to think critically and perceive their own personal and social reality, which are critical steps for adapting to chronic disease [30,31]. DSME allows patients to be part of the decision-making about their self-care and management [32]. Patients develop confidence in making informed decisions about their medical condition and can choose to act on it.

An additional approach that aligns with effective diabetes education methodology is motivational interviewing. This is closely linked with the empowerment theory as it focuses on creating opportunities for patients to come up with their own assessments and set their own goals [33]. Motivational interviewing is another example of a learner-centered intervention that is considered an effective approach to promote patients' knowledge retention, self-care commitment and improved self-care outcomes [24,33,34].

The proposed theoretical basis evident in a patient-centered diabetes education concept includes the Health Belief Model, the Trans-theoretical Model/Stages of Change, Common Sense Model, the Social Learning Theory and the Dual Processing Theory [40–43]. These commonly utilized theories in diabetes education allow for successful communication with patients through fostering effective listening, relationship building and creating an environment of respect and trust. These theories strengthen an educator's theoretical basis for an effective diabetes education technique. The theories also reflect on the approaches utilized to promote a meaningful dialogue with those involved in diabetes education. The theories help to integrate concepts better for a wider variety of individuals, regardless of age, gender or ethnicity.

Theory: the Health Belief Model

The Health Belief Model is a psychologic framework that outlines predictable health related behaviors [40]. People's life experiences and exposures to past events shape their perception of susceptibility, severity, barriers, benefits and cost of adhering to prescribed interventions. The process of diabetes education should allow for an effective discussion and exploration of beliefs which is needed to promote appropriate self-care. Without an adequate Health Belief Model patient assessment, patients may lack the necessary motivation to overcome their belief barriers.

Theory: the Stages of Change Model

Learning and making changes in one's lifestyle is a process of adjusting what can be done, when and how. The multiple interactions with patients allow diabetes educators to guide them to transition with their commitments to make the change. The Prochaska's Stages of Change Model [44] outlines the predicable process of change as patients not only learn what they are ready to learn, but also understand the reasons behind the need for change and strategies. The Stages of Change Model illustrates the five stages in a continuum of behavior change: pre-contemplation, contemplation, preparation, action, maintenance and relapse [44]. Each stage has an important role in supporting an evolutionary process whereby learners recognize the need for change, act, evaluate and react.

Diabetes educators can help patients to increase their realization of importance of change, confidence, and readiness by asking meaningful questions. Importance of change can be addressed by asking why? Is it worthwhile? Why should I? How will I benefit? What will change? At what cost? Do I really want to? Will it make a difference? By asking how and what diabetes educators can help patients to evaluate their confidence to change. Consider asking, can I? How will I do it? How will I cope with …? Will I succeed if …? What change …? When assessing readiness, start asking when? Should I do it now? How about other priorities? [45].

Theory: the Common Sense Model

The theoretical framework of the Common Sense Model is based on the balance of danger and fear control [40]. This theory implies that people will not self-regulate unless there is a significant and relevant understanding of the condition, cause, disease timeline, consequences, curability and controllability. The internal cognitive representation of the illness is balanced by emotions that require effective coping skills and appraisal.

The first component of the five assumptions in the theory is that patient identifies the condition. The second is the patient's perception on what actually caused the condition. The third consideration is of a timeline and how long the patient thinks that the condition is going to last. The fourth component of the Common Sense Model is the patient's understanding of the consequences of the disease and how it will affect their future. The fifth component relates to a patient's perception of treatment effectiveness [40]. The perceived vulnerability to diabetes complications is more significant among patients who have witnessed severe complications among people they know, such as family members or loved ones [46]. Witnessing and getting to know other patients in a group setting with varied levels of diabetes complications can allow people to internalize the necessary steps to control their condition more effectively.

Theory: the Social Learning Theory

The foundation of the group education session is a discussion among patients that allows them to learn from one other. The Social Learning Theory outlines the social context necessary for role modeling. It also asserts that the inspiration and support generated by group interaction helps patients change their behaviors [41]. Both social interactions and psychologic factors influence learning. According to Bandura [47]: "Learning skills is not enough, individuals should also develop confidence in the skills that they are learning. Success is not necessarily based on the possession of the necessary skills for performance; it also requires the confidence to use these skills effectively."

Theory: the Social Cognitive Theory

In the attempt to turn the Social Learning Theory into an observational behavior that the educator can witness, four categories can be derived from the Social Cognitive Theory [47]. In terms of the educator's role, these four categories can illuminate the behaviors seen within the group education session. The first characteristic is the role of the facilitator who creates an environment for a successful experience. The second is role modeling through various experiences whereby the educator observes others' performance. The third is verbal persuasion, where the facilitator skillfully summarizes the information, acknowledges the situation and participants' beliefs, indicating that the problem can be managed. The facilitator actively encourages people to be verbally explicit when elaborating on their management and future choices. The final aspect involves physical and affective state of identification of physical and emotional sources of symptoms. The facilitator acknowledges and/or responds to emotional utterances by the participants [47].

Theory: the Dual Processing Theory

The Dual Processing Theory relates to a patient's individual understanding of the medical condition by allowing the learner to discover his or her own solutions. The theory dictates the need to involve patients actively in the learning process [42]. The Dual Processing Theory has two actions, such as activation of a mental representation of an issue and its interpretation based on mental retrieval of events and feelings related to it [43]. The effective group education needs to allow a learner to discover his or her own solutions which increases the patient's understanding of their medical condition.

Effective diabetes group education approaches use facilitation instead of traditional didactic teaching to produce effective learning [26–28]. The health care professional is responsible for managing the group dynamics and the scope of the group's conversation. Participants are responsible for addressing issues of relevance to their diabetes management and developing strategies to care for themselves better.

Productive diabetes education strategies utilize the best in adult education methodology that allows for patient engagement. Learning theories demonstrate that adults learn best what is personally applicable and important to them [31]. Without a meaningful learning experience, they may ignore or dismiss the presented information. Also, adults learn best in social circumstances rather than classroom settings [32]. Adults prefer to learn from discussion, incorporation of life experiences and other interactive approaches over lecture, print, computer-based or audiovisual presentations [33,48]. Effective learning activities for adults should involve participants in the learning process, motivate, promote self-determination, meet the learning needs, allow the sharing of personal knowledge and experiences, promote competence, reinforce positive behaviors and help adults to identify consequences of behaviors [32,49].

Curriculum

There are many DSME curricula available for the diabetes educator to choose that can be integrated as a complementary tool to the existing DSME curriculum or can be used as a stand-alone approach. However, most of the curricula have not been validated with sound research and studies. Many of the available curricula utilize evidence-based approaches in diabetes self-management education but as an independent approach have not been validated.

An example of a reliable and valid curriculum has been carried out in a study by Kulzer *et al.* [26], which compared three diabetes educational methods and their effect on clinical indicators. The three educational approaches were:

1 A didactic method involving four sessions of 90 minutes in a group setting with a focus on knowledge acquisition, skill and information;

2 A group education with a non-didactic focus on self-management and empowerment that addressed the emotional side, the cognitive side and motivational interviewing to promote learning within 90 minutes over 12 sessions; and

3 The same empowerment focus as the second method but conducted as individual interventions for half of the 12 sessions and as a group for the other half.

The study included 181 patients with T2DM, non-insulin treated, body mass index (BMI) above 26.7 kg/m^2, no acute psychiatric illness and the ability to read and speak German. The results indicated no change in HbA_{1c} for the didactic group. There was a significant improvement in HbA_{1c} in the second group, which was the empowerment-based group. The third group intervention resulted in an initial improvement in HbA_{1c} that was not sustained for the duration of the study, indicating that individual intervention to deliver empowerment had no superior effect to group intervention. The results of this study build on the patient-centered educational assumptions that effectively facilitated group diabetes education produces superior clinical and behavioral outcomes than individual interventions. Also, patient-centered approaches and empowerment focused education produced better outcomes than a didactic curriculum. The applicable curriculum attempts to utilize the principles of the effective group-based empowerment education.

An example of a curriculum that is based on a collection of the evidence-based approaches but not validated as an independent strategy is the Diabetes Conversation Map™ program. In an effort to increase the availability of DSME to adults with T2DM, Healthy Interactions Inc. collaborated with the American Diabetes Association (ADA) to develop the US Diabetes Conversation Map® tools and on a global market with the International Diabetes Federation (IDF) to develop the Diabetes Conversations program [50]. The goal of the program is to engage patients more effectively through their interactions with health care professionals and to learn about diabetes and lifestyle modifications that can lead to improved diabetes self-management [51].

The Diabetes Conversation Map tools' content is based on current clinical practice guidelines that represent the best intervention approaches and national standards for DSME. The tools are designed to create meaningful discussions about diabetes between participants that are patient-focused and that help formulate behavior change goals. Patient-centered group interventions such as those used in the Conversation Map learning approach are intended to improve behavioral, clinical and metabolic markers [35,36,52–55]. A few other examples of curricula are: *Life with Diabetes: A Series of Teaching Outlines* by the Michigan DRTC (ADA); *Diabetes Education Curriculum: Guiding Patients to Successful Self-Management* (AADE); *Basics Diabetes Education Curricula*, International Diabetes Center products; and *On the Road* (USDA, Joslin Diabetes Center).

In 2003, the *Technology Appraisal 60* from the National Institute for Health and Clinical Excellence (NICE) in the UK defined diabetes patient structured education as: "a planned and graded programme that is comprehensive in scope, flexible in content, responsive to an individual's clinical and psychological needs, and adaptable to his or her educational and cultural background." In its review of the evidence, NICE identified some principles of good practice including that: "education should be provided by an appropriately trained multidisciplinary team to groups of people with diabetes, unless group work is considered unsuitable for an individual."

Further work published in 2005, *Structured Patient Education in Diabetes – Report from the Patient Education Working Group*, identified the criteria to be used when assessing whether diabetes structured education programs met the NICE guidance. In 2006, a self-assessment tool was developed for existing and future programs, which helped to make the criteria more explicit, and which gave programs a framework for developing an action plan so that the criteria could be met [56–58].

The key criteria for to meet NICE guidelines for structured education are that the programs must:

- Have a structured written curriculum;
- Have trained educators;
- Be quality assured; and
- Be audited.

The current status of Diabetes Structured Education in the UK includes several well-established national and local programs for both T1DM (DAFNE) and T2DM (DESMOND and X-PERT). In addition, there are a number of locally developed programs such as JIGSAW and BERTIE. Not all of these programs profess to meet the NICE guidance in its entirety, as elements of the criteria are still in various stages of development for different programs (e.g. audit, quality assurance). What is currently being expected of programs is that they are "seeking to fulfil the NICE criteria" or "working towards meeting the criteria for NICE guidance" and have development plans in place.

The main limiting factor in Diabetes Structured Education is that it does not include ongoing care and education. Once patients complete the program in its entirety they do not have a component of ongoing support to allow tailoring of the education to their changing lifestyle and diabetes care needs. The provided education becomes education for life and therefore conclusive, without opportunity for an information refresher or support mechanism needed to adjust to changes in perceived needs and preferences of people with diabetes. The lifelong process of diabetes self-management requires adjustments in knowledge, skills and motivation to assess the risks, to understand what there is to gain from changing the behavior or lifestyle and to act on that understanding by engaging in appropriate behaviors. Education should be a lifelong process, starting at the point of diagnosis and remaining as an essential component of diabetes care.

Despite availability and good access to Diabetes Structured Education in 55% of primary care trusts, less than 10% of people reported attending an education course on how to manage their diabetes. A total of 16–41% of people with diabetes who had not attended a course, however, reported that they would like to attend such a course [74]).

The DSME in the USA has a component of ongoing lifelong education where it is federally covered for the Medicare beneficiaries with diabetes. DSME is delivered for 10 hours initially during the first education program and 2 hours annually for subsequent education programs [59]. However, only 54.3% of people with diabetes who responded to a national survey in 2005 reported attending some type of DSME class [60]. The 2007 Diabetes Patient Market Study indicated that 26% of patients had seen a diabetes educator in the past 12 months [61]. The AADE analysis of the Center for Medicare and Medicaid Services reimbursement for DSME found that only about 1% of its applicable beneficiaries received DSME in 2004 and 2005 [62]. These results might suggest that patients with diabetes choose not to attend the DSME programs, do not know about their availability or have inadequate access. The existing trends in diabetes education rates indicates a strong probability that the Healthy People 2010 goal of increasing the DSME rate to 60% is unlikely to be achieved [63].

A systematic review of the clinical effectiveness of diabetes education models for type 2 diabetes indicates varied significance and inconsistent results in achieving desirable markers of success. The positive trends are attributable to longer term interventions with a shorter duration between the end of the intervention and the follow-up evaluation point with a multidisciplinary team approach. The inconsistencies in the markers of success and applicable approaches to measure them in the long-term constitute a barrier in their interpretation and practical applications. Also, it is unclear what is needed to prepare and support educators adequately to ensure that they can deliver programs successfully. The need for future research still exists on the comprehensive, ongoing and complex interventions education methods; this should include high quality, longer term studies with a careful consideration around the nature of any control group as well as factors and/or qualifications necessary among educators to ensure success and cost-effectiveness of education programs [64].

Patient education: engaging techniques

Education is initiated at the first encounter by asking what information the person wishes to obtain from this visit. To engage patients in the process and assess needs, a few simple techniques can be applied:

1 Ask "leading" questions, as people respond better to their own interests:

- For example, utilize the technique of open-ended enquiry stems: "Tell me about …," "What do you find the most challenging about …" or "How do you …?"
- Reflective listening stems are another source of assessment tools. The phrases "It sounds like …" or "Let me see if I understand you …" Allow for conversation, clarification, developing some of their own solutions and a chance for the patient to determine if you have the correct information and understand their situation. Encouraging them to tell their personal story helps open the door for a more personal collaborative relationship [65,66].

2 Encourage interaction leading to content discovery, determining the need for more information, improving accuracy and skill development. This technique is as useful for other group attendees, including family and friends who are also attending the visit with the patient.

3 Take more time to get the real story, not just yes or no answers to questions. As described by Anderson and Patrias [67]: "When patients fully describe their concerns and express their feelings, it is time to help them consider possible solutions."

- The use of a form with leading questions, completed while in the waiting room, pre visit, can set the stage for a more patient-centered directed visit [67].
- In addition, directing enquiry statements to focus towards the AADE7 healthy behaviors assists in crafting goals and targeting behaviors and action plans for the future.

Planning ahead: experiment, reframe, facilitate, evaluate

Difficulties sometimes arise when there are time constraints or a variety of learning styles (audio, visual, tactile). New diagnoses or an unexpected change in treatment plan may also be challenging for the individual. The learning environment and acquisition of knowledge and skills can be compromised. It is to the educator's advantage to plan ahead both for coping and problem-solving and to alter the curriculum to fit the situation. In times of stress, however, some educators may fall back on more traditional lectures, and the use of PowerPoint and pre-prepared handouts. Having a variety of core techniques, topics and alternative key delivery strategies can help to refocus back to the person, keeping the session patient-centered [20,21,65].

These core techniques help the educator regroup, and aid in planning for a variety of ways to deliver the same message.

Experiment

As you begin to understand the patient and their preferences and desires, think about experimenting with alternative ways to deliver the informational message, build skills, knowledge base and application in the real world. For example, to deliver a key message about the AADE7 domain of "healthy eating," consider using a local restaurant's menu to plan a festive holiday dinner instead of the didactic teaching of the number of "carbs" in a meal plan.

Reframe the information

Change your wording; for example, instead of "dieting" – use "meal planning." Another example in the domain of "being active" could be the reframing of "increasing activity." Think of using a phrase such as "decreasing inactivity" and "new activity planning."

Plan ahead

Identify at least two or three alternatives for the delivery of a concept; for example, appeal to each of the audio "Hear a message", visual "See the message in words or picture" and tactile/kinesthetic "Perform an activity" learning styles. In addition, the use of a variety of effective teaching learning strategies assists in moving concepts across the spectrum of age, culture and literacy.

Faciliate, don't teach

You already know the answer and so the key to facilitation is to determine what the patient knows and what information they have on hand to begin problem-solving (discovery learning). Your expertise is, of course, implied. Drawing out information and encouraging problem-solving from the patient directly helps them integrate and synthesize information that will support future thinking and confidence.

Trust

A relationship of trust between educator and patient is the basis for successful achievement, and the patient has a right to privacy.

Evaluate

It is important to plan to keep track of content items discussed and the behavior change goals that are set. Often, educators spend the majority of their time covering the same content, repeating concepts over and over again. This may be because of educator comfort level, and preplanned content, rather than establishing what the person with diabetes might prefer. This may occur in both DSME and during medical nutrition therapy sessions. When this happens, behavior outcome goals related to healthy coping and behavior change goal-setting are often the least addressed, whereas healthy eating, monitoring and being active are the most common behavior change goals identified. Thus, mutually identified healthy coping and problem-solving goals may improve targeted appropriate educational strategies to support patients in meeting their goals and finding resources from the outside world [68].

Whitlock reviewed self-management processes and described a model for educational counseling to assist with broadening the educational experience by focusing on patient needs versus educator goals for the session. This approach consists of 5 A's (Table 21.4): assessment, advise, agreement, assistance and arrangement. Another approach is the Mensing reference (Table 21.5) which

Table 21.4 Whitlock model.

1 **Assess** risks and readiness to change
2 **Advise** with clear personalized change advice
3 **Agree** by setting collaborative goals
4 **Assist** using behavior change techniques and social support
5 **Arrange** for follow-up

Table 21.5 Drafting a Written Plan. Adapted with permission from Mensing [65].

Assessment	View as critical to problem-solving – listen Tune into culture, uses new techniques
Developing a plan	Plan ahead, be practical, plan some problem-solving Keep a good pace, and include a behavioral action plan Better to cover fewer topics and select implementation plan Avoid overload
Implementation of diabetes education	Consider learning styles, readiness of learner and teacher Practice sensitivity and cultural awareness Help translate the science into everyday self-care practices Be flexible Education is ongoing, not just a one time event
Evaluate and document outcomes	Captures information, progress and fosters reinforcement Useful to patient progress, teaching strategies and process Assists with tracking educational content consistency Acknowledges potential behavior change goals, and comparisons with clinical care goals

offers a set of quick reminders, key elements and assessment, through follow-up and documentation [20,69].

Collaboration: drafting a written plan

A critical outcome of diabetes education is the patient's behavior change plan. Self-care behaviors as the key outcome of DSME have been established. A written plan is set up with indicators such as an overall goal and an identified outcome. The goal is defined as a general non-specific health outcome (e.g. to lose weight, or to feel better). The AADE7 domains are useful categories. The patient and educator collaboratively take this goal and set up very concrete, specific actions as a plan, which describes the steps to be taken to achieve this goal. The steps are written in very concrete terms, are measurable, realistic and mark progress over time. The action steps clearly describe exactly what the patient intends to do. Educators are encouraged to help the patient determine how convinced they are that this activity will happen, how confident they are. This is sometimes objectively identified on a scale of 0–10 (not confident to extremely confident) [8,65]. This technique offers clarity and discussion, while supporting the establishment of realistic action plans. Review of

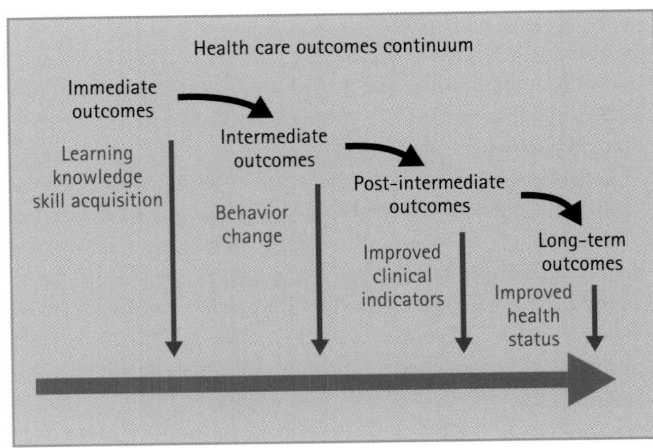

Figure 21.1 Diabetes self-management education (DSME) outcomes continuum. Reproduced from Peeples *et al.* [70], with permission from Sage Publications.

the plan at intervals assists the patient and the educator in evaluating progress towards the goal, if the goal is appropriate or if expectations and action steps need to be altered. The AADE outcomes system assists with identifying immediate outcomes (knowledge, skill) and sets the expectation for longer term outcomes, such as improved HbA_{1c}, lipids and general health status (Figure 21.1).

In addition, it has also evaluated progress, and has provided tools for data documentation, tabulation, configuration, aggregation, analysis and review. A number of data software systems are available to ease data recording. Zgibor *et al.* [68] identified that the domains of "healthy eating" and "physical activity" are the most frequently identified behaviors. Educators are encouraged to consider offering more time to identifying these problem-solving goals. Of note, patients seldom identified more than one goal, and clearly not more than one of substance, yet, as was referenced, the domains of healthy coping and problem-solving may be more useful in the long-term behavior changes that help patients toward successful accomplishments, rather than just the familiar food, activity, monitoring references [68].

In summary, educators should utilize of a wide variety of models and techniques that enhance the acquisition of information, and offer an interesting and creative educational, learning and empowering environment for all the learners, educators and patients alike.

Maintaining and promoting achievement

Measurable behavior change is the unique outcome of working with a diabetes educator. Healthy People 2010 has identified the need to increase the percentage of patients with diabetes receiving education, so that the current 40% would be increased to be at least 60% [68].

Adopting an outcomes framework, directing energy and time to developing educational plans following the guidance of the main existing frameworks, DSME and incorporating the AADE7 approach into everyday practice is just the beginning. The structure helps to assess current preferences and behaviors of the individual with diabetes, discuss potential benefits, barriers, problem-solving and set a mutually agreed upon plan of behavioral interventions.

Key to the process lies in the follow-up. Methods for setting up measurable indicators, monitoring schedules and documentation are needed for evaluation. Summary information is then available for the patient, health care team, and potentially for insurance and regulatory purposes.

Conclusions

In summary, as more and more systems and standardized educational frameworks such as the AADE7 are implemented, behaviors and clinical outcomes will be better linked and evidence-based benchmarks will become available. Behavior change and diabetes education have been shown to be effective for short-term outcomes [71,72]. Further investigation needs to be conducted to assess long-term outcomes. Clinician and educator time will be well spent by individualizing care plans, paying attention to the process of educational information delivery methods and offering patient-centered care.

References

1 Norris SL, Engelgau MM, Narayan KM. Effectiveness of self-management training in type 2 diabetes: systematic review of randomized controlled trials. *Diabetes Care* 2001; **24**:561–587.

2 Piatt GA, Orchard TJ, Emerson S, Simmons D, Songer TJ, Brooks MM, *et al.* Translating the chronic care model into community: results from a randomized controlled trial of a multifaceted diabetes care intervention. *Diabetes Care* 2006; **29**:811–827.

3 Mulcahy K, Maryniuk M, Peeples M, Peyrot M, Tomky D, Weaver T, *et al.* Diabetes self-management education core outcomes measures. *Diabetes Educ* 2003; **29**:804–816.

4 Austin MM. Importance of self-care behaviors in diabetes management: business briefing. *US Endocr Rev* 2005; 16–21.

5 Mensing CR, Boucher J, Cypress M, Weinger K, Mulcahy K, Barta P, *et al.* National standards for diabetes self-management education. *Diabetes Care* 2000; **23**:682–689.

6 Funnell MM, Brown TL, Childs BR, Haas LB, Hosey GM, Jensen B, *et al.* National standards for diabetes self-management education. *Diabetes Care* 2007; **30**:1630–1637.

7 Funnell MM. National Standards for diabetes self-management education: what do they mean for providers? *Rev Endocrinol* 2007; 51–53.

8 Peeples M, Tomky D, Mulcahy K, Peyrot M, Siminerio L, *et al.* Evolution of the American Association of Diabetes Educators' diabetes education outcomes project. *Diabetes Educ* 2007; **33**:794–817.

9 Funnell MM, Brown TL, Childs BP, Haas LB, Hosey GM, Jensen B, *et al.* National standards for diabetes self-management education. *Diabetes Care* 2009; **32**(Suppl. 1):S87–S94.

10 International Diabetes Federation (IDF). *International Standards for Diabetes Education.* Available from: www.idf.org/webdata/docs/International%20Standards.pdf. Accessed on 23 December, 2009.

11 International Diabetes Federation (IDF). *International Curriculum for Diabetes Health Professional Education.* Available from: www.idf.org/webdata/docs/Curriculum_final%20041108_EN.pdf. Accessed on 23 December, 2009.

12 American Diabetes Association. Standards of Medical Care in Diabetes, 2009. *Diabetes Care* 2009; **32**:S13–S61. Available from: http://care.diabetesjournals.org/content/vol32/Supplement_1/. Accessed on 10 January, 2009.

13 Gary TL, Genkinger JM, Guallar E, Peyrot M, Brancati FL. Meta-analysis of randomized educational and behavioral interventions in type 2 diabetes. *Diabetes Educ* 2003; **29**:488–501.

14 Ellis SE, Speroff T, Dittus RS, Brown A, Pichert JW, Elasy TA. Diabetes patient education: a meta-analysis and meta-regression. *Patient Educ Couns* 2004; **52**:97–105.

15 Norris SL, Nichols PJ, Caspersen CJ, Glasgow RE, Engelgau MM, Jack L, et al. The effectiveness of disease and case management for people with diabetes: a systematic review. *Am J Prev Med* 2002; **22**:15–38.

16 Gary TL, Genkinger JM, Guallar E, Peyrot M, Brancati FL. Meta-analysis of randomized educational and behavioral interventions in type 2 diabetes. *Diabetes Educ* 2003; **29**:488–501.

17 American Association of Diabetes Educators (AADE). *Guidelines for the Practice of Diabetes Self-Management Education and Training (DSME/T).* Chicago, IL: American Association of Diabetes Educators, 2009.

18 Kessels RP. Patients' memory for medical information. *J R Soc Med* 2003; **96**:219–222.

19 Funnell MM. The Diabetes Attitudes, Wishes, and Needs study (DAWN). *Diabetes Care.* 2006; **24**:154–155.

20 Mensing CR, Norris SL. Diabetes Spectr Group education in diabetes: effectiveness and implementation. 2003; **16**:96–103.

21 Funnell MM. *Patient-Centered Education: AADE in Practice.* 2007; **3**, 7.

22 Tang TS, Funnell MM, Anderson RM. Group education strategies for diabetes self-management. *Diabetes Spectrum* 2006; **19**:99–105.

23 Chodosh J, Morton SC, Mojica W, *et al.* Meta-analysis: chronic disease self-management programs for older adults. *Ann Intern Med* 2005; **143**:427–438.

24 Bodenheimer T, MacGregor K, Sharifi C. *Helping Patients Manage Their Chronic Conditions.* Oakland, CA: California Health Care Foundation, 2005.

25 Glasgow RE, Funnell MM, Bonomi AE, Davis C, Beckham V, Wagner EH. Self-management aspects of the improving chronic illness care breakthrough series: design and implementation with diabetes and heart failure teams. *Ann Behav Med* 2002; **24**:80–87.

26 Kulzer B, Hermanns N, Reinecker H, Haak T. Effects of self-management training in type 2 diabetes: a randomized, prospective trial. *Diabet Med* 2007; **24**:415–423.

27 Yamaoka K, Tango T. Efficacy of lifestyle education to prevent type 2 diabetes. a meta-analysis of randomized controlled trials. *Diabetes Care* 2005; **28**:2780–2786.

28 Funnell MM, Anderson RM. Patient empowerment: a look back, a look ahead. *Diabetes Educ* 2003; **29**:454–464.

29 Vég A, Rosenqvist U, Sarkadi A. Variation of patients' views on type 2 diabetes management over time. *Diabet Med* 2007; **24**:408–414.

30 Freire P. *The Politics of Education: Culture, Power, and Liberation.* South Hadley, MA: Bergin & Garvey, 1985.

31 Shor I, Freire P. *A Pedagogy for Liberation: Dialogues on Transforming Education*. South Hadley, MA: Bergin & Garvey, 1987.

32 Funnell MM, Anderson RM. Empowerment and self-management of diabetes. *Clin Diabetes* 2004; **22**:123–127.

33 Welch GR, Ernst D. Motivational interviewing and diabetes: what is it, how is it used, and does it work? *Diabetes Spectr* 2006; **19**:5–11.

34 Akimoto M, Fukunishi I, Kanno K, Oogai Y, Horikawa N, Yamazaki T, et al. Psychosocial predictors of relapse among diabetes patients: a 2-year follow-up after inpatient diabetes education. *Psychosomatics* 2004; **45**:343–349.

35 Mensing CR, Norris SL. Group education in diabetes: effectiveness and implementation. *Diabetes Spectr* 2003; **6**:96–103.

36 Trento MP, Passera E, Borgo M, Tomalino M, Bajardi F, Cavallo Porta M. A 5-year randomized controlled study of learning, problem solving ability, and quality of life modifications in people with type 2 diabetes managed by group care. *Diabetes Care* 2004; **27**:670–675.

37 How Adults Learn. Ageless Learner, 1997–2007. Available from: http://agelesslearner.com/intros/adultlearning.html. Accessed on 20 September, 2208.

38 Sheehan MJ. Learning and implementing group process facilitation: individual experiences. Doctoral thesis, Griffith University, 2000.

39 Huang ES, Brown SES, Ewigman BG, Foley EC, Meltzer DO. Patient perceptions of quality of life with diabetes-related complications and treatments. *Diabetes Care* 2007; **30**:2478–2483.

40 Leventhal H, Brissette I, Leventhal EA. The common-sense model of self-regulation of health and illness. In: Cameron LD, Leventhal H, eds. *The Self-Regulation of Health and Illness Behaviour*. London: Routledge, 2003: 42–65.

41 Bandura A. *Social Learning Theory*. New York: General Learning Press, 1977.

42 Chaiken S, Wood W, Eagly A. Principles of persuasion. In: Higgins ET, Kruglansksi AW, eds. *Social Psychology: Handbook of Basic Principles*. New York: Guilford Press, 1996: 702–744.

43 Parkin T, Skinner TC. Does patient perception of consultation concord with professional perception of consultation. *Diabet Med* 2002; **19**(Suppl. 2): A14.

44 Prochaska JO, DiClemente CC, Norcross JC. In search of how people change. *Am Psychol* 1992; **47**:1102–1104.

45 Rollnick S, Mason P, Butler CC. *Health Behavior Change: A Guide for Practitioners*. Churchill Livingstone, 1999.

46 Harrison TA, Hindorff LA, Kim H, Wines RC, Bowen DJ, McGrath BB, et al. Family history of diabetes as a potential public health tool. *Am J Prev Med* 2003; **24**:152–159.

47 Bandura A. Health promotion by social cognitive means. *Health Educ Behav* 2004; **31**:143–164.

48 Wlodkowski RJ. Strategies to enhance adult motivation to learn. In: Galbraith MW, ed. *Adult Learning Methods*, 2nd edn. Malabar, FL: Krieger Publishing Company, 1998: 91–111.

49 Long, HB. Understanding adult learners. In: Galbraith MW, ed. *Adult Learning Methods*, 2nd edn. Malabar, FL: Krieger Publishing Company, 1998: 21–35.

50 The Diabetes Conversation Map™ educational tools. Healthy Interactions Inc. (Healthyi). Available from: http://www.healthyinteractions.com. Accessed on 1 June, 2009.

51 Bio-Medicine. Press release from June 22–26, 2007. American Diabetes Association and Healthy Interactions announce a collaboration to transform diabetes education. Available from: http://www.bio-medicine.org/medicine-news-1/Healthy-Interactions-and-Merck-Announce-Further-Collaboration-to-Transform-Diabetes-Education-in-the-U-S-21134-1. Accessed on 10 March, 2009.

52 Deakin T, McShane CE, Cade JE, Williams RD. Group based training for self-management strategies in people with type 2 diabetes mellitus. *Cochrane Database Syst Rev* 2005; **2**:CD003417.

53 Rickheim PL, Weaver TW, Flader JL, Kendall DL. Assessment of group versus individual diabetes education: a randomized study. *Diabetes Care* 2002; **25**:269–274.

54 Smaldone A, Weinger K. Review: group based education in self-management strategies improves outcomes in type 2 diabetes mellitus. *Evid Based Nurs* 2005; **8**:111.

55 Sarkadi A, Rosenqvist U. Experience-based group education in type 2 diabetes a randomised controlled trial. *Patient Educ Couns* 2004; **53**:291–298.

56 Department of Health. *National Service Framework for Diabetes: Standards* (2001); Department of Health. *National Service Framework for Diabetes: Delivery Strategy* (2003). Available from: http://www.dh.gov.uk/PublicationsAndStatistics/Publications/PublicationsPolicyAndGuidance/PublicationsPolicyAndGuidanceArticle/fs/en?CONTENT_ID=4002951&chk=09Kkz1 and http://www.dh.gov.uk/PublicationsAndStatistics/Publications/PublicationsPolicyAndGuidance/PublicationsPolicyAndGuidanceArticle/fs/en?CONTENT_ID=4003246&chk=lKNg9r2. Accessed on 10 March, 2009.

57 National Institute for Health and Clinical Excellence. Diabetes (types 1 and 2): patient education models (No. 60). The clinical effectiveness and cost effectiveness of patient education models for diabetes (April 2003). Available from: http://www.nice.org.uk/page.aspx?o=TA060. Accessed on 10 March, 2009.

58 How to Assess Structured Diabetes Education: An improvement toolkit for commissioners and local diabetes communities. Available from: http://www.diabetes.nhs.uk/downloads/Patient_Education_Tools_Project/Patient_Education_Tools_Project_2006.pdf. Accessed on 10 March, 2009.

59 American Diabetes Association Recognition Programs. Available from: http://www.diabetes.org/for-health-professionals-and-scientists/recognition/edrecognition.jsp. Accessed on 10 January, 2009.

60 National diabetes self-management class attendance data. Diabetes Prevention and Control Programs. Available from: http://www.gov/diabetes/statistics/preventive/fy_class.htm. Accessed on 20 March, 2009.

61 Diabetes Education Fact Sheet. 2007 Roper US Diabetes Patient Market Study. Available from: http://www.diabeteseducator.org/export/sites/aade/_resources/pdf/Diabetes_Education_Fact_Sheet-DP.pdf. Accessed on 20 April, 2009.

62 Diabetes Education Fact Sheet. Available from: www.diabeteseducator.org/export/sites/aade/_resources/pdf/Diabetes_Education_Fact_Sheet-DP.pdf. Accessed on 20 March, 2009.

63 Healthy People 2010: Summary of Objectives. Available from: www.healthypeople.gov/document/HTML/Volume1/05Diabetes.htm. Accessed on 20 February, 2009.

64 Loveman E, Frampton GK, Clegg AJ. The clinical effectiveness of diabetes education models for type 2 diabetes: a systematic review. *Health Technol Assess* 2008; **12**:1–116.

65 Mensing C. *The Art and Science of Diabetes Education: A Reference Book for Health Professionals*. American Association of Diabetes Educators (AADE), 2006: 574–574.

66 Pearson TL. *Faciliating Behavior Change: Hear your Patient's Story*. AADE in Practice. 2007; **4**:6.

67 Anderson RM, Patrias R. Getting out ahead: the diabetes concerns assessment form. *Clin Diabetes* 2007; **25**:141–143.

68 Zgibor JC, Peyrot M, Ruppert K, Noullet W, Siminerio LM, Peeples M, et al. Using the American Association of Diabetes Educators outcomes system to identify patient behavior change goals and diabetes educator responses. *Diabetes Educ* 2007; **33**:839–842.

69 Whitlock EP, Orleans T, Pender N, Allan J. Evaluating primary care behavioral counseling interventions: an evidence based approach. *Am J Prev Med* 2002; **22**:267–284.

70 Peeples M, Tomky D, Mulcahy K, Peyrot M, Siminerio L. AADE Outcomes Project and AADE/UMPC Diabetes Education Outcomes Project. Evolution of the American Association of Diabetes Educators' Diabetes Education Outcomes Project. *Diabetes Educ* 2007; **33**:794–817.

71 Bodenheimer T, Davis C, Holman H. Practical Pointer: helping patients adopt healthy behaviors. *Clin Diabetes* 2007; **25**:66–70.

72 Norris SL, Nichols PJ, Caspersen CJ, Glasgow RE, Engelgau MM, Jack L, et al. The effectiveness of disease and case management for people with diabetes: a systematic review. *Am J Med* 2002; **22**(Suppl):15.

73 Available from: http://www.medialit.org/reading_room/article8.html.

74 *Managing Diabetes. Improving services for people with diabetes.* Commission for Healthcare Audit and Inspection 2007, London. Available from: http://www.cqc.org.uk/_db/_documents/Managing_Diabetes_1_200707300356.pdf. Accessed on 23 December, 2009.

22 Lifestyle Issues: Diet

Monika Toeller

German Diabetes Center, Heinrich Heine University Düsseldorf and Leibniz Center for Diabetes Research, Düsseldorf, Germany

Keypoints

- Lifestyle interventions to improve glucose, blood pressure and lipid levels, and to promote weight loss or at least to avoid weight gain remain the underlying strategy throughout the management of diabetes even when additional medications are needed.
- Metabolic variables, such as HbA_{1c}, post-prandial blood glucose concentrations, serum triglyceride and low density lipoprotein cholesterol levels, can be used to suggest the most appropriate intakes of carbohydrate-containing foods.
- Vegetables, legumes, fruits and wholegrain cereal-based foods should be part of the diet because they are rich in dietary fiber, low in glycemic index or load and provide a range of micronutrients.
- In those treated with insulin or oral hypoglycemic agents, the timing and dosage of medication should match the quantity and nature of carbohydrate to avoid hyperglycemia or hypoglycemia. Blood glucose self-monitoring may help to make appropriate choices.
- Saturated, trans-unsaturated fatty acids and dietary cholesterol should be restricted to reduce the risk for vascular disease, whereas oils rich in monounsaturated fatty acids as well as oily fish rich in n-3 polyunsaturated fatty acids are useful fat sources.
- In patients with type 1 or 2 diabetes without evidence of nephropathy, usual protein intake (up to 20% of the total energy intake) need not be modified. In those with established nephropathy, protein restriction to 0.8 g/kg normal body weight per day may be beneficial.
- Alcohol intake should be moderate.
- Foods naturally rich in dietary antioxidants, trace elements and other vitamins are encouraged. Routine supplementation and the use of so-called special diabetic foods are not recommended.
- Individual dietary advice by physicians and dietitians and structured nutritional training are an essential part in the continuing treatment and education process of people with type 1 and 2 diabetes.

Introduction

Nutritional management in diabetes aims to assist in optimizing metabolic control and reducing risk factors for chronic complications. This includes the achievement of blood glucose and glycosylated hemoglobin (HbA_{1c}) levels as close to normal as is safely possible and serum lipid concentrations as well as blood pressure values that may be expected to decrease the risk for macrovascular disease. Individual therapeutic needs and the quality of life of the person with diabetes have to be considered when nutritional objectives are defined [1,2].

Diabetes health care teams should use the best available scientific evidence while giving dietary advice to the individual patient with diabetes. During recent years, the development of evidence-based guidelines in the management of type 1 (T1DM) and type 2 diabetes (T2DM) has adopted a more formal approach to the evaluation of evidence underlying the guidance [3].

Currently available evidence-based nutritional recommendations for individuals with diabetes have involved a formal search of the literature using agreed sets of descriptors and relevant databases. The strength of evidence for the different nutritional recommendations is graded according to the type and quality of published studies as well as by statements from expert committees, which also take into account clinical experiences of respected authorities. Ideally, evidence-based guidelines are formulated from trials with fatal or non-fatal clinical endpoints; however, as this information is often not available, surrogate endpoints, such as glycemia, body composition, lipoprotein profile, blood pressure, insulin sensitivity and renal function, are frequently used to determine the potential of dietary modification to influence glycemic control and risk of acute and chronic complications of diabetes [1]. Tables 22.1–22.3 provide important dietary recommendations for people with T1DM and T2DM and the degree of evidence assigned to these recommendations by the Diabetes and Nutrition Study Group of the European Association for the Study of Diabetes (DNSG EASD) and the American Diabetes Association (ADA).

Energy balance and body weight

Controlling body weight to reduce risks related to diabetes is of great importance. When weight loss and increased levels of activ-

Textbook of Diabetes, 4th edition. Edited by R. Holt, C. Cockram, A. Flyvbjerg and B. Goldstein.

ity are achieved and maintained, in T2DM in particular, these interventions represent an established and effective therapeutic strategy for achieving target glycemic control [1,2,4]. Therefore, there is a consensus that such lifestyle interventions should be initiated as part of the treatment of new-onset T2DM [5–8]. Even modest weight loss, especially in abdominal fat, improves insulin sensitivity and glucose tolerance and reduces serum lipid concentrations and blood pressure. Weight loss may lead to greater benefit for cardiac risk factors in people with a high waist circumference [1,4]. Visceral body fat, as measured by waist circumference, is used in conjunction with body mass index (BMI) to assess the risk of diabetes and cardiovascular disease (CVD).

Overweight patients with T1DM may also become insulin resistant and weight reduction in these people may lead to a decrease of the insulin dose and improved glycemic control [1].

Prevention of weight regain is an important target in those who have lost some excess weight. Long-term restricted energy intake is necessary to sustain the metabolic improvements that can be achieved by weight reduction.

Losing weight is particularly difficult for those genetically predisposed to obesity. Nevertheless, the potential of structured weight loss programs should be exploited in overweight patients to achieve the possible beneficial effects [1,4,9]. Standard weight loss strategies plan 500–1000 fewer calories than estimated for weight maintenance. This may result in an initial loss of 0.5–1.0 kg body weight per week; however, many people regain the weight they have lost, and continued support by the health care team is needed to achieve long-term improvements of body weight and waist measurement. Advice concerning the reduction of high-fat and energy-dense foods, in particular those high in saturated fat and free sugars, will usually help to achieve weight loss. In addition, fiber intake should be encouraged. Regular physical activity should also be an important component of lifestyle approaches to the treatment of overweight. So far, the consensus by experts is that the use of very low energy diets, as an approach to promote initial weight loss, should be restricted to people with a BMI >35 kg/m^2 [1,2]. The evidence for recommendations regarding energy balance and body weight published by the ADA and by the DNSG EASD is summarized in Tables 22.1 and 22.3.

Table 22.1 Nutritional recommendations with the evidence grade A for persons with type 1 and type 2 diabetes. Evidence obtained from meta-analyses of randomized controlled trials or at least one randomized controlled trial [1,2].

	DNSG EASD	ADA
Energy balance and body weight	Energy reduction in overweight (BMI >25 kg/m^2) to move towards recommended BMI range Prevention of weight regain	Weight loss in overweight and obese individuals (improves insulin resistance) For weight loss low CHO or low fat calorie restricted diets may be effective in the short-term (up to 1 year)
CHO	Metabolic characteristics suggest the most appropriate intake: vegetables, legumes, fruits, wholegrain foods, naturally occurring foods rich in fiber Fiber intake should be ideally ≈20 g/1000 kcal/day Low glycemic index foods provided other attributes of these foods are appropriate Moderate amounts of free sugars (up to 50 g/day)	Monitoring carbohydrate by CHO counting, CHO exchanges or experience-based estimation of CHO remain a key strategy in achieving glycemic control Sucrose-containing foods can be substituted for other carbohydrate; if added should be covered with insulin or other glucose-lowering medication, excess intake should be avoided
Dietary fat	Saturated and trans-unsaturated fatty acids <10% total energy (<8% if LDL cholesterol is elevated) Dietary cholesterol <300 mg/day (further reduction if LDL is elevated)	Saturated fat <7% total energy
Protein	0.8 g/kg normal body weight in patients with type 1 diabetes and established nephropathy	Protein should not be used to treat or prevent nighttime hypoglycemia; it can increase insulin response without increasing plasma glucose in type 2 patients
Micronutrients	Salt intake should be <6 g/day; further reduction for patients with elevated blood pressure	No clear evidence of benefit from vitamin or mineral supplementation Routine supplementation (e.g. vitamins E, C and carotene) is not advised; because of concern related to long-term safety
Type 1 diabetes		Patients using rapid-acting insulin should adjust the meal and snack insulin based on the carbohydrate content of meals and snacks
CVD risk		Sodium intake (<2300 mg/day) Diet high in fruits, vegetables and low-fat dairy products in normotensive and hypertensive individuals
Hypoglycemia		15–20 g glucose is the preferred treatment (also other glucose-containing carbohydrate possible)

ADA, American Diabetes Association; BMI, body mass index; CHO, carbohydrate; DNSG EASD, Diabetes and Nutrition Study Group of the European Association for the Study of Diabetes; HDL, high density lipoprotein; LDL, low density lipoprotein.

Table 22.2 Nutritional recommendations with the evidence grade B for persons with type 1 and type 2 diabetes. Evidence obtained from at least one well designed and controlled study without randomization, well-designed quasi-experimental or non-experimental descriptive studies [1,2].

	DNSG EASD	ADA
CHO	There is no justification for the recommendation of very low carbohydrate diets in persons with diabetes Cereal-based foods should, whenever possible, be wholegrain and high in fiber	CHO from fruits, vegetables, whole grains, legumes and low fat milk is encouraged Consumption of a variety of fiber-containing foods is recommended The use of glycemic index and load may provide a modest additional benefit over that when total CHO is considered
Dietary fat	Oils rich in mono-unsaturated fatty acids are encouraged (10–20% total energy), total fat <35% total energy 2–3 servings of oily fish/week and plant sources of n-3-fatty acids (e.g. rapeseed oil, soybean oil, nuts) are recommended	2 or more servings of fish/week (n-3-poly-unsaturated fatty acids) are recommended
Protein	10–20% total energy in patients with no evidence of nephropathy	
Alcohol	Moderate use up to 10 g/day for women and up to 20 g/day for men is possible In patients treated with insulin or insulin secretagogues alcohol should be taken with carbohydrate to avoid hypoglycemia	Moderate intake (when ingested alone) has no acute effect on glucose and insulin, alcohol co-ingested with CHO may raise blood glucose
Microvascular complications		0.8–1 g protein/kg body weight/day in early stages of chronic kidney disease (microalbuminuria, decline in glomerular filtration) 0.8 g protein/kg body weight/day in later stages (macroalbuminuria) of kidney disease
CVD risk		HbA_{1c} to be kept as close to normal as possible without significant hypoglycemia
Acute illness		Adequate amounts of fluids and carbohydrate (glucose and ketone testing)
Long-term care facilities		Caution when prescribing weight loss diets in elderly; avoid undernutrition

ADA, American Diabetes Association; CHO, carbohydrate: CVD, cardiovascular disease; DNSG EASD, Diabetes and Nutrition Study Group of the European Association for the Study of Diabetes.

Macronutrient distribution in weight loss diets

The optimal macronutrient distribution of weight loss diets has not yet been established [2,10–12]. Low fat diets have been traditionally and effectively promoted for weight loss [1,13]; however, recently it has been demonstrated that low carbohydrate, higher fat diets may result in even greater weight loss over short periods of time, up to 6 months [2,10,14]. Although changes in serum triglycerides and high density lipoprotein (HDL) cholesterol were more favorable with low carbohydrate, higher fat diets than with high carbohydrate and lower fat diets in these trials, low density lipoprotein (LDL) cholesterol was significantly higher in patients on high fat, low carbohydrate diets [2]. However, long-term metabolic effects of low carbohydrate, high fat diets are unclear and no controlled long-term trials are available to prove their safety with regard to CVD. Such diets eliminate several foods that are important sources of fiber, vitamins and minerals. It has also been shown that it was difficult to substitute monounsaturated fatty acids (MUFA) as the favorable fat source for carbohydrate because foods providing appreciable amounts of MUFA are limited, and even in Mediterranean areas, nowadays, people tend to consume undesirably high amounts of saturated fat in high fat diets. The ADA has summarized the current recommendations for weight loss in diabetes as follows: "For weight loss either low-carbohydrate or low-fat calorie restricted diets may be effective in the short-term (up to 1 year)" [2]. After initial weight loss it is important to avoid regain of weight [1].

Weight loss in the prevention of diabetes

With regard to weight loss in the prevention of diabetes in individuals at high risk for developing T2DM, lifestyle changes that included a reduced energy and a reduced dietary fat intake, and an increased fiber consumption together with regular physical activity (e.g. 150 minutes/week) [15,16] have shown improvements in several vascular risk factors including dyslipidemia, hypertension and markers of inflammation in addition to the significant reduction of the development of T2DM. So far, clinical trials on the efficacy of low carbohydrate diets for primary prevention of T2DM are not available.

Carbohydrate and diabetes

It is important that the advice for carbohydrate intake is individualized, based on the patient's nutrition assessment, metabolic

Table 22.3 Nutritional recommendations for persons with type 1 and type 2 diabetes with lower grades (C–E) of evidence. Evidence obtained from expert committee reports or opinions and/or clinical experiences of respected authorities [1,2].

	DNSG EASD	ADA
Energy balance and body weight	Prevention of weight regain Avoidance of further weight gain Advise reduction of energy-dense foods high in saturated fat and free sugars	When low CHO diets are used for weight reduction monitor lipid profiles, renal function, protein intake (in those with nephropathy) and adjust hypoglycemic therapy
CHO, fiber, sucrose and other free sugars	Consider quantity, sources and distribution of CHO to facilitate near-normal long-term glycemic control Timing and dosage of insulin or hypoglycemic agents should match quantity and nature of CHO Daily consumption of 5 servings of fiber-rich vegetables or fruits and 4 servings of legumes per week help to achieve recommended fiber intake Total free sugars should not exceed 10% total energy	When fixed daily insulin doses are used CHO intake (time and amount) should be consistent For planned exercise extra CHO may be needed Blood glucose tests can be used to monitor appropriate adjustments There is no evidence to support prescribing diets such as "no concentrated sweets" or "no sugar added"
Dietary fat	Polyunsaturated fatty acids should not exceed 10% total daily energy Total fat intake should not exceed 35% total energy	Intake of trans-fats should be minimized (evidence grade B in the guidelines of 2009) Cholesterol below 200 mg/day
Protein	Insufficient evidence for recommendations about the preferred type of dietary protein For type 1 diabetes with incipient nephropathy and type 2 diabetes with incipient or established nephropathy no firm recommendations regarding protein restriction	For persons with diabetes and normal renal function insufficient evidence to modify usual protein intake (15–20% of energy) High protein diets are not recommended as a method for weight loss Long-term effects of protein >20% of calories on kidney function are unknown
Alcohol	Intake should be limited in overweight, hypertensive, hypertriglyceridemic individuals as well as during pregnancy and in advanced neuropathy	Daily intake should be limited to a moderate amount (1 drink for women, 2 drinks for men) Alcohol should be consumed with food in individuals treated with insulin or insulin secretagogues to reduce the risk of nocturnal hypoglycemia
Micronutrients	Foods naturally rich in dietary antioxidants, trace elements and other vitamins are encouraged: daily consumption of a range of vegetables and fruit, regular intake of wholegrain breads, cereals and oily fish	Benefit from chromium supplementation is not proven and therefore not recommended

ADA, American Diabetes Association; CHO, carbohydrate; DNSG EASD, Diabetes and Nutrition Study Group of the European Association for the Study of Diabetes.

results and treatment goals [1,2,17–19]. There is a broad range of possible carbohydrate intake in people with diabetes (e.g. 45–60% of total energy intake). This advice is mainly based on recommended restrictions for the intakes of fat and protein. In many European countries, the mean carbohydrate intake of people with diabetes is only around 42% of total energy intake (Table 22.4) [20,21]. In the EURODIAB Complications Study, which included 3250 people with T1DM coming from 31 different European centers, the mean carbohydrate intake did not show major changes at the 7-year follow-up investigation compared with these intakes at baseline. Similar relatively low proportions of carbohydrate consumption and high intakes of total and saturated fatty acids have also been demonstrated in people with T2DM from the Mediterranean area [22,23].

Usually, carbohydrate intake in people with diabetes is lower than recommended by nutrition associations for the general population who receive advice to consume around 50% of total energy intake as carbohydrate. Many people with diabetes tend to reduce their carbohydrate intake because they fear an increase in blood glucose concentrations after the ingestion of carbohydrate-containing foods. In affluent countries, lower carbohydrate diets are usually accompanied by high fat, predominantly an undesirable high saturated fat intake. With such a diet it is also difficult to achieve sufficient fiber intake to meet recommendations [1,24,25]. Having this in mind, it does not appear to be productive to overemphasize the present renaissance of low carbohydrate strategies in diabetes. Furthermore, several recent reports on this topic do not clearly define what is meant by "low" or "high" carbohydrate and whether a carbohydrate intake of around 40% of total energy, which is consumed by many people with diabetes, already corresponds to a low carbohydrate diet [26,27].

Glycemic effects of different carbohydrate

Not only the amount of carbohydrate, but also the quality of carbohydrate is important for individuals with diabetes. Vegetables, legumes, fresh fruit, wholegrain foods and low fat milk products should be part of a healthy diet [1,2]. These foods provide also a range of micronutrients and fiber.

Table 22.4 Nutritional intake and further life-style factors in persons with type 1 diabetes. Data are presented for the total EURODIAB cohort (31 centres, n = 3250) and different European regions [21].

	South (n = 1371)	East (n = 539)	Northwest (n = 1340)	All (n = 3250)	Center range
Total energy (kcal/day)[a]	2148	2352	2407	2288	1851–2786
Carbohydrate (% of energy)	43.0	41.9	42.3	42.5	36.7–48.1
Fiber (g/day)[a]	17.0	15.4	18.4	17.3	13.9–21.9
Total fat (% of energy)	36.5	39.7	38.6	37.9	30.3–45.1
Saturated fatty acids (% of energy)	12.5	14.8	15.1	14.0	9.4–17.2
Cholesterol (mg/day)[a]	286	415	342	328	232–487
Protein (% of energy)	18.3	17.8	16.9	17.6	15.2–21.1
Alcohol (g/day)[b]	0.8	0	1.5	0	0–4.2
Current smokers (n %)	31.2	39.0	30.5	32.2	21.9–46.4
Ex-smokers (n %)	16.6	15.5	20.1	17.9	1.6–28.6
Vigorous exercise ≥ once/week (n %)	13.6	11.1	15.1	13.8	2.4–26.3

Data are means or prevalences: a, geometric mean; b, median.
Southern European Centers (n = 12): Athens, Bari, Cagliary, Lisbon, Milan, Padua, Perugia, Pisa, Rome, Turin, Thessaloniki, Verona.
Eastern European Centers (n = 4): Bucharest, Budapest, Krakow, Zagreb.
Northwestern European Centers (n = 15): Cork, Düsseldorf (two centres), Gent, Helsinki, Leiden, London, Luxembourg, Manchester, Munich, Paris, Sheffield, Valenciennes, Vienna, Wolverhampton.

The amount of carbohydrate is an essential factor for post-prandial glucose results in people with T1DM and T2DM [28–30]. In the process of achieving desirable glycemic control, many individuals with diabetes use either carbohydrate counting, carbohydrate exchanges or experience-based estimation of carbohydrate intake as a helpful means to monitor their consumption of carbohydrate at meals or snacks [2]. Different carbohydrates have different glycemic effects. Besides the amount of carbohydrate, other factors including the nature of starch, the amount of dietary fiber and the type of sugar influence the glycemic response to carbohydrate-containing foods [31–34].

The glycemic index (GI) of a carbohydrate-containing food describes its post-prandial blood glucose response over 2 hours in the area under the blood glucose curve compared with a reference food with the same amount of carbohydrate, usually 50 g glucose (or white bread in some studies). Foods can be differentiated into high (GI: 70–100), average (GI: 55–70) or low (GI: <55) glycemic index foods; however, measured GIs are only available for a range of foods, with the data mainly coming from investigations in Canada and Australia. The glycemic load considers the amount as well as the quality of carbohydrate and is defined as gram of carbohydrate within the food multiplied with the GI of the food divided by 100.

It has been shown that the use of the GI or glycemic load of a food may confer moderate additional benefits – over that observed when only total carbohydrate is considered – not only for post-prandial glycemia, but also for the lipid profile [2,35]. Therefore, foods with known low GI (e.g. legumes, pasta, parboiled rice, wholegrain breads, oats, certain raw fruits) should be substituted when possible for those with a high GI (e.g. mashed potatoes, white rice, white bread, cookies, sugary drinks) [36–39]. For example, eating fresh fruits is superior to a fruit juice with the same amount of carbohydrate. Low GI foods are only favorable, however, provided other attributes of these foods are also in line with a healthy nutrition [1]. Some foods with a low GI are high in fat and energy. Chocolates are such an example, with low GI but a high content of saturated fat. Some products specifically advertised for people with diabetes have reduced the GI of usual foods by replacing sucrose with sugar alcohols or fructose. A substantial benefit from these expensive so-called "diabetic" preparations has not been proven. Therefore, special foods for people with diabetes are not recommended. Proper food labeling may help the person with diabetes to make healthy choices from available usual foods.

Potential of dietary fiber

In many countries, people with diabetes consume only few foods that are rich in dietary fiber and therefore total fiber intake is much lower than recommended (Figure 22.1). With the relatively low carbohydrate intake in people with diabetes it is not easy to meet recommended quantities of fiber. Total dietary fiber intake in the EURODIAB Complications Study was on average only 8.0 g/1000 kcal or 19.5 g/day [20,21]. People with diabetes should be encouraged to choose a variety of fiber-containing foods (vegetables, fruits, wholegrain products) to profit from the proven benefits for glycemic control, insulinemia and serum lipid concentrations [32–34,40]. Although total fiber intake was not high, epidemiologic data based on the EURODIAB Complications Study showed an inverse association between dietary fiber intake and HbA_{1c} independent of possible confounders [32], an inverse association between fiber and LDL cholesterol and a positive association between fiber and HDL cholesterol. In addition,

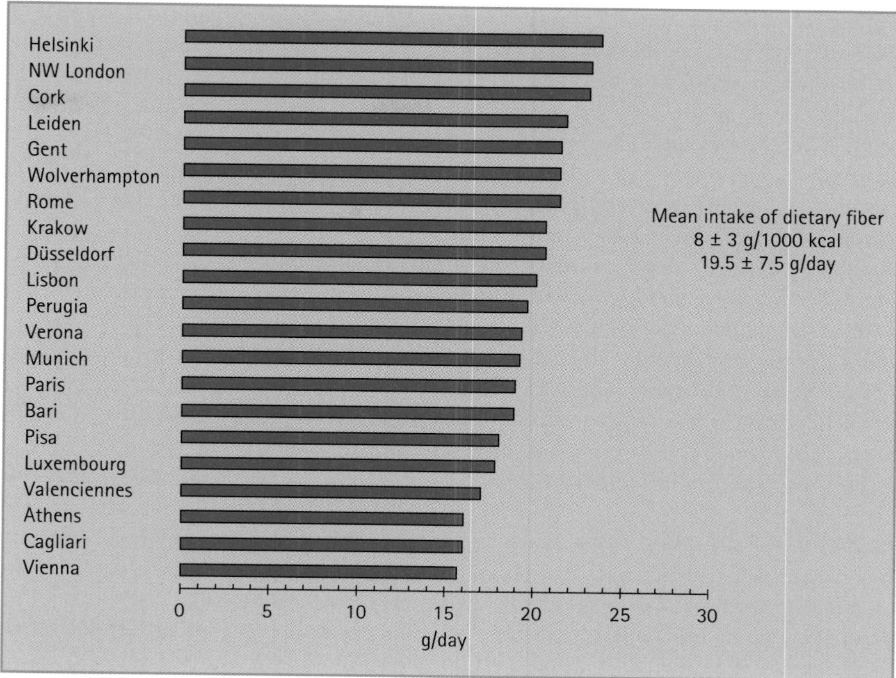

Figure 22.1 Fiber intake (g/day) in persons with type 1 diabetes (total n = 1102) from 21 centers in Europe. Data from EURODIAB Complications Study [20,21].

dietary fiber was inversely and significantly related to cardiovascular disease [34]. Dietary fiber was also associated with lower levels of BMI [26]. The degree of evidence for recommended carbohydrate and dietary fiber intakes is shown in Tables 22.1–22.3.

Sucrose and other sugars

Moderate intake of sucrose (<10% total energy) or other added sugars may be included in the diet of people with diabetes without worsening glycemic control [1,2,25,41]. Although fructose produces a reduction in post-prandial glycemia when it replaces sucrose, this potential benefit is tempered by the fact that fructose may adversely effect serum triglycerides as well as uric acid levels [1,8]. There is no reason to recommend that people with diabetes should avoid naturally occurring fructose (e.g. in fruits, vegetables or other foods) [1,2]; however, added fructose, added sugar alcohols or other nutritive sweeteners are energy sources that do not have substantial advantage over sucrose and therefore should not be encouraged. Higher quantities of sugar substitutes may promote undesirable gastrointestinal side effects. Furthermore, it is unlikely that energy-containing sugar substitutes such as sugar alcohols in the amounts likely to be consumed will contribute to an appreciable reduction in total energy intake although they are only partially absorbed from the small intestine [2,8].

Approved non-nutritive sweeteners may also be used by people with diabetes although a special long-term benefit in metabolic control has not been proven. Nevertheless, they are safe when acceptable daily intakes (ADI values) are followed [2,8].

Adjustment of insulin or insulin secretagogues to carbohydrate intake

For people who are treated with insulin or hypoglycemic agents, it is important to match the medication with the amount, type and time of carbohydrate intake to avoid hypoglycemia as well as excessive post-prandial hyperglycemia [1,2]. Individuals receiving intensive insulin treatment should adjust their premeal insulin dose based on the amount of carbohydrate in snacks or meals while considering also the GI of these foods [37,42,43]. This advice is now part of many nutrition education programs for people with diabetes who are treated with intensified insulin regimens [18,44]. Self-monitoring of blood glucose offers a helpful means of determining the most appropriate timing of food intake and to make optimal food choices [1]. Individual preferences and the needs of different treatment strategies remain the most important determinants of appropriate meal frequency, portion sizes and carbohydrate intake. Extra carbohydrate may be needed prior to exercise although adjustment of the insulin dosage in those on intensified insulin treatment is often an alternative and preferred choice. Structured training and continuing advice by the diabetes team is needed to enable the people with diabetes to adjust the insulin dosage while considering all three components: blood glucose results, amount and quality of carbohydrate intake as well as the degree of physical activity.

Dietary fat

The primary goal concerning dietary fat intake is to restrict the consumption of saturated fatty acids, trans-fats and dietary cholesterol to reduce the risk for vascular disease [1,2,45,46]. Compared with the non-diabetic population, people with diabetes have an increased risk of developing vascular disease. Fat modification in people with diabetes is an established principle to assist in achieving desirable serum lipid concentrations and to avoid vascular lesions in high-risk groups. Although most of this evidence is obtained from studies of people without diabetes, it seems that the recommendations are also relevant in the diabetic population as their risk for vascular disease is even higher than in the general population [1,47]. Even if statins are often needed to meet the treatment goals for serum lipid concentrations, possible lifestyle modifications should always be exploited, and remain the basic therapeutic approach to achieve a desirable lipid profile. The degree of evidence for the recommendations relating to the recommended amounts of fat intake or fat modification, respectively, is shown in Tables 22.1–22.3.

Reduction of saturated fatty acids

It is suggested that saturated fatty acids could be either replaced by carbohydrate foods rich in fiber or by unsaturated fatty acids, particularly by *cis*-monounsaturated fatty acids for people on a weight-maintaining diet. Such diets have been shown to achieve improvements in glycemia, insulin sensitivity and serum lipid values, compared to diets high in saturated fat [47–51].

Omega-3-fatty acids

Observational evidence supports the intake of n-3 polyunsaturated (omega-3) fatty acids as they have the potential to reduce serum triglycerides and have beneficial effects on platelet aggregation and thrombogenicity, thus offering cardioprotective effects [52]. A consumption of 2–3 servings of oily fish and plant sources such as rapeseed oil, soya bean oil and nuts will help to ensure an adequate intake of n-3 fatty acids [1,2,53,54].

Trans-fats and dietary cholesterol

Unfortunately, in most countries, the quantity of trans-unsaturated fatty acids is not well documented on many food products. The effects of trans-fats are similarly adverse as those of saturated fatty acids in raising LDL cholesterol. Therefore, their intake should be minimized [1,2]. Trans-fats are found in many manufactured products such as biscuits, cakes, confectionery, soups and some hard margarine. Food labeling informs whether hydrogenated fats and oils were added to a food product and the ranking of ingredients on the food label gives at least some information whether high quantities of trans-fats could have a role.

Data from healthy people and individuals with T1DM support the recommendation to restrict dietary cholesterol. With increasing intake, serum cholesterol levels may increase and contribute to the development of CVD [1,55].

Current fat intake in individuals with diabetes

Fat intake data of European people with T1DM from the EURODIAB Complications Study demonstrated that on average the current target to keep the intake of saturated fatty acids below 7% of total energy was not achieved (Table 22.4). In the whole cohort of this study, the mean intake of saturated fatty acids was 14% of total energy (twice as high as recommended by the ADA) (Figure 22.2) [20,21], and even patients from the Mediterranean area who traditionally consumed a favorable fat intake no longer reach the goal to remain below 7% of saturated fat consumption [22,23]. In conclusion, fat modification remains an important

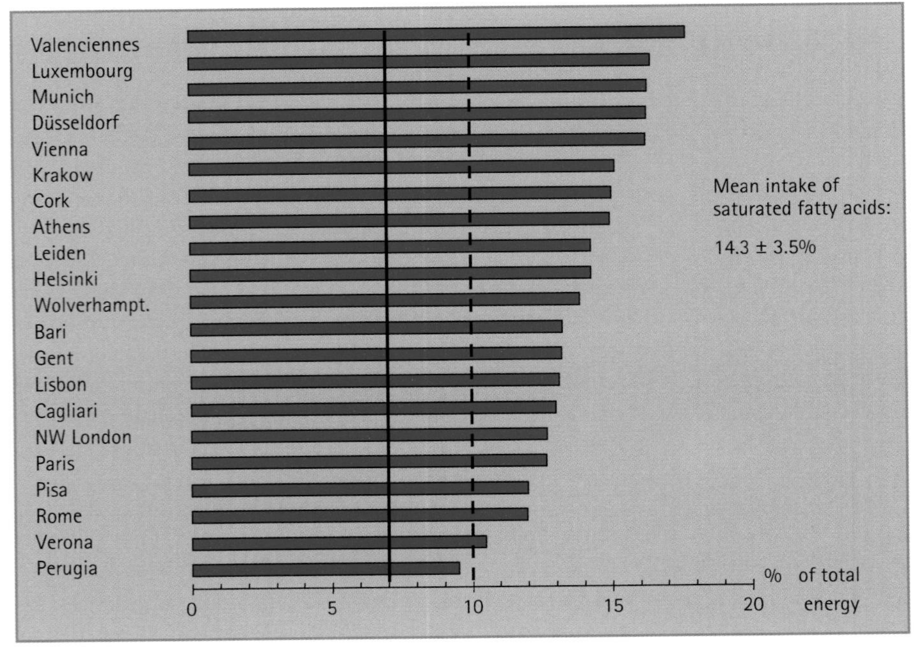

Figure 22.2 Intake of saturated fatty acids (% of energy) in persons with type 1 diabetes (total n = 1102) from 21 centers in Europe. The solid vertical line marks the currently recommended upper limit of intake for saturated fatty acids by the ADA (7% total energy) The dotted vertical line represents the limit of 10% total energy for saturated fatty acids recommended by Diabetes and Nutrition Study Group of the European Association for the Study of Diabetes (DNSG EASD) in 2004. Data from the EURODIAB Complications Study. [20,21].

target nutritional education topic to reduce the risk for vascular disease in people with both T1DM and T2DM.

Dietary protein

For individuals with diabetes and normal renal function, there is insufficient evidence that usual protein intake should be modified [1,2]. From nutrition intake data of different countries and patient groups, it is documented that there seems to be little concern that people with diabetes may develop protein deficiency (Table 22.4) [20–23]. However, it is unclear whether a long-term high protein intake above 20% of total energy would have untoward effects on renal function [2,56,57]. Although such diets may produce short-term weight loss and improved glycemia, it has not been established that these benefits are maintained long term. Therefore, high protein diets are not recommended as a method for weight loss at this time [2].

Protein restriction

Several studies have focused on protein restriction as a means to reverse or retard the progression of proteinuria in people with diabetes [58–60]. Progression of diabetes complications may be modified by improving glycemic control, lowering blood pressure and potentially reducing protein intake. Normal protein intake (15–20% of energy) does not appear to be associated with an increased risk of developing diabetic nephropathy [1,2]. In some studies of subjects, particularly with T1DM and macroalbuminuria, urinary albumin excretion rates and decline in glomerular filtration were favorably influenced by a reduction of protein intake to around 0.8 g/kg body weight/day [59]; however, there is insufficient evidence to make recommendations about the preferred type of dietary protein. The evidence for recommended protein intake in diabetes is summarized in Tables 22.1–22.3.

Micronutrients

Regular consumption of a variety of vegetables, fresh fruit, legumes, low fat milk products, vegetable oils, nuts, wholegrain breads and oily fish should be encouraged to ensure that recommended vitamin and mineral requirements are met [1]. Salt or sodium intake, respectively, should be limited particularly when elevated blood pressure is a problem [61,62]. Replacement of added salt intake using salt substitutes with potassium and magnesium in hypertensive people with T2DM has been shown to lead to a significant reduction in systolic but not in diastolic blood pressure. Such substitutes may be tried in selected patients but cannot generally be recommended to lower high blood pressure in people with diabetes.

People with diabetes may have increased oxidative stress and several studies have investigated the potential benefit of recommending the intake of antioxidant vitamins [63]. These trials have failed to show clear benefit from supplementation [64]. Therefore routine supplementation (e.g. of vitamins E, C and carotene) is not advised because of concern related to long-term safety [1,2]. Also, the role of folate supplementation in reducing cardiovascular events is not clear and still under further investigation. In the light of current evidence, diabetes associations do not offer recommendations regarding supplements or functional foods [1,2]. Most of the promoted fiber-enriched products, margarines which contain plant sterols or stanols, supplements containing various n-3 fatty acids, minerals, trace elements and herbs, some of which have been shown to have potentially relevant functional effects, have not been tested in long-term formal clinical trials. As long as there is insufficient evidence from randomized studies to demonstrate significant benefit without causing undesirable side effects they cannot be recommended [1,2,65]. Vitamin or mineral supplementation in pharmacologic dosages should be viewed as a therapeutic intervention and recommended only in cases of proven deficiencies [1]. Given the importance of vitamin D in bone metabolism and the bony consequences associated with diabetes, it appears that dietary vitamin D intake, sunshine exposure and vitamin D levels should be monitored. Nutrition education to promote healthy eating and to meet recommended intakes is important for people with T1DM and T2DM.

Alcohol

Alcohol may have both undesirable and beneficial effects [66–69] which exhibit a U-shaped relationship. The intake of moderate amounts (5–15 g/day) is associated with a decreased risk of coronary heart disease, while a strong association between excess habitual alcohol intake (>30–60 g/day) and undesirable raised blood pressure is found in both men and women. The amount of alcohol seems to be predictive whereas the type of alcohol-containing beverages consumed does not appear to be of major importance. If people with diabetes choose to drink alcohol, intake should be moderate, with no more than 10 g/day alcohol (1 drink) for females and no more than 20 g/day alcohol (2 drinks) for males [1,2]. These limits are also recommended to the healthy population by nutrition associations.

In studies where alcoholic beverages were consumed with carbohydrate-containing food by people with diabetes, no acute effects were seen on blood glucose. The recommendation, particularly to patients treated with insulin or insulin secretagogues, to consume carbohydrate when alcohol is taken is made because of the potential risk of alcohol-induced hypoglycemia [70,71]. The risk increases with the quantity of alcohol consumed and may last well into the following day. Abstention from alcohol is advised in women during pregnancy, people with a history of pancreatitis or alcohol abuse as well as in those with hypertriglyceridemia and advanced neuropathy. Alcohol may also be an important energy source which should be considered in people with overweight. High alcohol consumption is associated with greater waist : hip ratio independently of BMI. The evidence obtained from studies and expert reports concerning alcohol intake are shown in Table 22.2 and 22.3.

Diet in special circumstances

Diet in pregnancy

To avoid fetal and maternal complications it is essential to achieve blood glucose concentrations as close to normal as possible without inducing hypoglycemia [72]. Nutritional therapy should assist in achieving recommended fasting blood glucose values of 60–90 mg/dL (3.3–5.0 mmol/L) and post-prandial values below 120 mg/dL (6.7 mmol/L). To reach this goal, women with known T1DM as well as women who develop gestational diabetes during pregnancy need detailed dietary counseling as an essential part of therapy. Energy intake should be adequate to provide appropriate weight gain and nutrient intakes should consider special needs during pregnancy. In women with normal weight additional energy intake may be 70–240 kcal/day in the first and second trimester and 300 kcal in the third trimester of pregnancy. Additional calorie intake should be less in obese pregnant women; however, total daily energy should not be under 1600 kcal/day.

During pregnancy, hyperglycemia as well as ketonemia and starvation ketosis should be avoided. As in all pregnant women, folic acid supplementation is recommended to prevent neural tube defects. Several bodies (e.g. National Institute for Health and Clinical Excellence) have recommended using higher doses of folate supplementation (5.0 mg vs 400 μg) in women with diabetes because of the higher risk of neural tube defects in women with diabetes. Further individual supplementation with calcium, iron and iodine may be considered to avoid deficiencies (Table 22.5).

Table 22.5 Diet in pregnancy.

Food choices for adequate weight gain, normoglycemia and absence of ketones
Weight loss is not recommended
For overweight or obese women with gestational diabetes, modest energy and carbohydrate intake
Starvation ketosis should be avoided
Pregnant women on insulin therapy need individualized carbohydrate-controlled recommendations with consistency of times and amounts of food to avoid hypoglycemia
Insulin and meal plan adjustments should be guided by blood glucose self-monitoring
Consider changes in insulin sensitivity and the necessity to adjust the insulin dosage during the different trimesters of pregnancy
Consider special needs of protein (1.2–2 g/kg body weight), calcium (1300 mg/day), iron (30 mg/day), iodine (230 μg/day) and folate (600 μg/day) beginning in the second trimester of pregnancy

Diet in children with diabetes

Dietary recommendations should focus on achieving desirable blood glucose concentrations without severe hypoglycemia. As in all healthy children, energy and nutrient intakes should be adequate to ensure normal growth and development. Healthy nutrition may also contribute to maintaining normal serum lipid values and blood pressure goals. Individualized counseling is necessary to support adequate decision-making for food intake and flexible insulin doses based on blood glucose self-monitoring. Meal plans must be individualized to accommodate food preferences and the eating pattern of the family.

Planning carbohydrate intake and premeal insulin dosage are the main educational targets in the training of children with T1DM and their parents. As energy requirements change with age, growth rates have to be monitored and the evaluation of a meal plan has to be rechecked at least once a year. In a case where the child becomes overweight, calories should be restricted. The child with diabetes has also to learn that early signs of hypoglycemia must lead to taking rapidly available carbohydrate (glucose) and that unusual exercise needs blood glucose monitoring before and after physical activity, which should be used to guide potential extra carbohydrate or insulin dosage adjustments [73].

Nutritional training in individuals with T1DM and T2DM

Nutritional training must be an integral component of disease management in all individuals with diabetes [2,18,72–75]. It requires the use of currently available scientific evidence on the potential of diet to assist in achieving treatment goals. A knowledgeable diabetes care team including the individual with diabetes should work together to maintain the pleasure of eating and drinking, while only limiting food choices when this is indicated by scientific evidence (Table 22.6). A balance must be achieved between the demands of metabolic control, risk factor management and the patient's well-being and safety [76]. Furthermore, it has to be taken into account that the therapeutic needs of an individual person will change with time and special life events, and therefore nutritional assessment and continuing dietary advice must be provided.

Evaluation of outcome

All steps in the dietary management of the individual with diabetes should be documented in the patient's record forms. The outcome should be evaluated by important markers such as HbA_{1c}, fasting and post-prandial blood glucose concentrations, blood pressure, serum lipids, albumin excretion rate, body weight, waist circumference and well-being of the individual with T1DM and T2DM [18,77].

Table 22.6 Dietary advice and structured nutritional training for individuals with diabetes.

How often is nutritional advice needed?
- Always at diagnosis of diabetes mellitus
- At each consultation if metabolic control is insufficient or vascular risk factors are not well controlled
- Every year as a routine
- At the initiation of insulin therapy
- When special nutritional problems come up

What should be checked on a regular basis?
- Is healthy eating part of the individual's lifestyle?
- Is energy intake appropriate to achieve or maintain a desirable body weight?
- Is alcohol intake moderate or could it be undesirably influencing hyperlipidemia, hypertension or the risk of hypoglycemia?
- Does the person consume unnecessary special diabetic food products?
- Does the selection and distribution of meals reflect the glucose-lowering medication?
- Does raised blood pressure suggest a benefit from salt restriction?

Which advice is essential to achieve a healthy diet?
- Restrict the intake of saturated fatty acids and trans-fats
  Choose only small portions of fatty meat, sausages, cheese, spreads and fatty bakery
  Prefer lower fat products
  Chocolates, cakes, cookies, cream, chips and fatty fast food should be eaten in small servings only and not consumed on a daily basis
- Consider the quality of fat
  Prefer vegetable oils (e.g. olive oil, rapeseed oil, soybean oil), nuts, seeds
  Consume oily fish 2–3 times per week
- Consume foods rich in dietary fiber and micronutrients
  5 servings of fresh fruit and vegetables per day as well as the consumption of legumes and wholegrain products are recommended
- Sugar is not forbidden; however, excessive intake is not desirable.
  Non-caloric sweeteners are safe, when daily allowances are followed
- Alcoholic beverages should only be taken in moderation
  1–2 small glasses of wine or beer are tolerable when no specific contraindication must be considered; however, consider the caloric amounts and also the risk of hypoglycemia when consumed without food
- Special dietetic foods for persons with diabetes are unnecessary. Persons with diabetes can enjoy usual foods
- Meals, snacks and food choices should match individual therapeutic needs, preferences and culture

References

1 Mann J, De Leeuw I, Hermansen K, Karamanos B, Karlström B, Katsilambros N, *et al.* on behalf of the Diabetes and Nutrition Study Group (DNSG) of the European Association for the Study of Diabetes (EASD). Evidence-based nutritional approaches to the treatment and prevention of diabetes mellitus. *Nutr Metab Cardiovasc Dis* 2004; **14**:373–394.

2 American Diabetes Association. Nutrition recommendations and interventions for diabetes. A position statement of the American Diabetes Association. *Diabetes Care* 2008; **1**(Suppl.1):S61–S78.

3 Scottish Intercollegiate Guidelines Network (SIGN). SIGN Guidelines. An Introduction to SIGN methodology for the development of evidence-based clinical guidelines. 1999, www.show.scot.nhs.uk/sign/home.htm Neu: http://www.sign.ac.uk

4 Klein S, Sheard NF, Pi-Sunyer X, Daly A, Wylie-Rosett J, Kulkarni K, *et al.* Weight management through lifestyle modification for the prevention and management of type 2 diabetes: rationale and strategies: a statement of the American Diabetes Association, the North American Association for the Study of Obesity, and the American Society for Clinical Nutrition. *Diabetes Care* 2004; **27**:2067–2073.

5 Wolf AM, Conaway MR, Crowther JQ, Hazen KY, Nadler L, Oneida B, *et al.* Translating lifestyle intervention to practice in obese patients with type 2 diabetes: Improving Control with Activity and Nutrition (ICAN) study. *Diabetes Care* 2004; **27**:1570–1576.

6 Nathan DM, Buse JB, Davidson MB, Ferranini E, Holman RR, Sherwin R, *et al.* Management of hyperglycaemia in type 2 diabetes: a consensus algorithm fort he initiation and adjustment of therapy. A consensus statement from the American Diabetes Association and the European Association for the Study of Diabetes. *Diabetologia* 2006; **49**:1711–1721.

7 UKPDS Group. UK Prospective Diabetes Study 7: Response of fasting plasma glucose to diet therapy in newly presenting type II patients with diabetes. *Metabolism* 1990; **39**:905–912.

8 Mann J, Lean M, Toeller M, Slama G, Uusitupa M, Vessby B, on behalf of the Diabetes and Nutrition Study Group (DNSG) of the European Association for the Study of Diabetes (EASD). Recommendations for the nutritional management of patients with diabetes mellitus. *Eur J Clin Nutr* 2000; **54**:353–355.

9 Ryan DH, Espeland MA, Foster GD, Haffner SM, Hubbard VS, Johnson KC, *et al.* Look AHEAD (Action for Health in Diabetes): design and methods for a clinical trial of weight loss for the prevention of cardiovascular disease in type 2 diabetes. *Control Clinical Trials* 2003; **24**:610–628.

10 Nordmann AJ, Nordmann A, Briel M, Keller U, Yancy WS Jr, Brehm BJ. Effects of low-carbohydrate vs low-fat diets on weight loss and cardiovascular risk factors: a meta-analysis of randomized controlled trials. *Arch Intern Med* 2006; **166**:285–293.

11 Van der Laar FA, Akkermans RP, van der Binsbergen JJ. Limited evidence for effects of diet for type 2 diabetes from systematic reviews. *Eur J Clin Nutr* 2007; **61**:929–937.

12 Sawyer L, Gale EAM. Diet, delusion and diabetes: editorial. *Diabetologia* 2009; **52**:1–7.

13 Astrup A, Grunwald GK, Melanson EL, Saris WHM, Hill JO. The role of low-fat diets in body weight control: a meta-analysis of ad libitum dietary intervention studies. *Int J Obes Relat Metab Disord* 2000; **24**:1545–1552.

14 Gannon MC, Nuttall FQ. Effect of a high-protein, low-carbohydrate diet on blood glucose control in people with type 2 diabetes. *Diabetes* 2004; **53**:2375–2382.

15 Heilbronn LK, Noakes M, Clifton PM. Effect of energy restriction, weight loss, and diet composition on plasma lipids and glucose in patients with type 2 diabetes. *Diabetes Care* 1999; **22**:889–895.

16 Uusitupa M, Lindi V, Louheranta A, Salupuro T, Lindström J, Tuomilehto J, for the Finnish Diabetes Prevention Program Research Group. Long-term improvement in insulin sensitivity by changing lifestyles of people with impaired glucose tolerance: 4-year results from the Finnish Diabetes Prevention Study. *Diabetes* 2003; **52**:2532–2538.

17 Riccardi G, Rivellese AA. Dietary treatment of the metabolic syndrome: the optimal diet. *Br J Nutr* 2000; **83**(Suppl.1):143–148.
18 Toeller M, Mann JI. Nutrition in the etiolgy and management of type 2 diabetes. In: Goldstein BJ, Müller-Wieland D, eds. *Type 2 Diabetes. Principles and Practice*, 2nd edn. New York/London: Informa Healthcare, 2008: 59–71.
19 Garg A, Bantle JP, Henry RR, Coulston AM, Griver KA, Raatz SK, *et al.* Effects of varying carbohydrate content of diet in patients with non-insulin-dependent diabetes mellitus. *JAMA* 1994; **271**:1421–1428.
20 Toeller M, Klischan A, Heitkamp G, Schumacher W, Milne R, Buyken A, *et al.* and the EURODIAB IDDM Complications Study Group. Nutritional intake of 2868 IDDM patients from 30 centers in Europe. *Diabetologia* 1996; **39**:929–939.
21 Toeller M, Buyken AE, Heitkamp G, Berg G, Scherbaum WA, and the EURODIAB IDDM Complications Study Group. Prevalence of chronic complications, metabolic control and nutritional intake in type 1 diabetes: comparison between different European regions. *Horm Metab Res* 1999; **31**:680–685.
22 Thanopoulou A, Karamanos B, Angelico F, Assaad-Khalil S, Barbato A, Del Ben M, *et al.* Nutritional habits of subjects with type 2 diabetes mellitus in the Mediterranean Basin: comparison with the non-diabetic population and the dietary recommendations. Multi-Centre Study of the Mediterranean Group for the Study of Diabetes (MGSD). *Diabetologia* 2004; **47**:367–376.
23 Karamanos B, Thanopoulou A, Angelico F, Assaad-Khalil S, Barbato A, Del Ben M, *et al.* Nutritional habits in the Mediterranean Basin: the macronutrient composition of diet and its relation with the traditional Mediterranean diet. Multicentre study of the Mediterranean Group for the Study of Diabetes (MGSD). *Eur J Clin Nutr* 2002; **56**:983–991.
24 Wylie-Rosett J, Segal-Isaacson CJ, Segal-Isaacson A. Carbohydrates and increases in obesity: does the type of carbohydrate make a difference? *Obes Res* 2004; **12**(Suppl.2):124S–129S.
25 Buyken AE, Toeller M, Heitkamp G, Irsigler K, Holler C, Santeusanio F, *et al.* and the EURODIAB IDDM Complications Study Group. Carbohydrate sources and glycaemic control in type 1 diabetes mellitus. *Diabetic Medicine* 2000; **17**:351–359.
26 Toeller M, Buyken AE, Heitkamp G, Cathelineau G, Ferriss B, Michel G, and the EURODIAB IDDM Complications Study Group. Nutrient intakes as predictors of body weight in European people with type 1 diabetes. *Int J Obes* 2001; **25**:1815–1822.
27 Poppitt SD, Keogh GF, Prentice AM, Wiliams DE, Sonnemans HM, Valk EE, *et al.* Long-term effects of ad libitum low-fat, high-carbohydrate diets on body weight and serum lipids in overweight subjects with metabolic syndrome. *Am J Clin Nutr* 2002; **75**:11–20.
28 Sheard NF, Clark NG, Brand-Miller JC, Franz MJ, Pi-Sunyer FX, Mayer-Davis E, *et al.* Dietary carbohydrate (amount and type) in the prevention and management of diabetes. a statement of the American Diabetes Association. *Diabetes Care* 2004; **27**:2266–2271.
29 Mayer-Davis EJ, Dhawan A, Liese AD, Teff K, Schulz M. Towards understanding of glycaemic index and glycaemic load in habitual diet: associations with measures of glycaemia in the Insulin Resistance Atherosclerosis Study. *Br J Nutr* 2006; **95**:397–405.
30 Liese AD, Schulz M, Fang F, Wolever TM, D'Agostino RB Jr, Sparks KC, *et al.* Dietary glycemic index and glycemic load, carbohydrate and fiber intake, and measures of insulin sensitivity, secretion, and adiposity in the Insulin Resistance Atherosclerosis Study. *Diabetes Care* 2005; **28**:2832–2838.
31 Rizkalla SW, Taghrid L, Laromiguiere M, Huet D, Boillot J, Rigoir A, *et al.* Improved plasma glucose control, whole-body glucose utilization, and lipid profile on a low-glycemic index diet in type 2 diabetic men: a randomized controlled trial. *Diabetes Care* 2004; **27**:1866–1872.
32 Buyken A, Toeller M, Heitkamp G, Vitelli F, Stehle P, Scherbaum WA, *et al.* and the EURODIAB IDDM Complications Study Group. Relation of fibre intake to HbA1c and the prevalence of severe ketoacidosis and severe hypoglycaemia. *Diabetologia* 1998; **41**:882–890.
33 Giacco R, Parillo M, Rivellese AA, Lasorella G, Giacco A, D'Episcopo L, *et al.* Long-term dietary treatment with increased amounts of fiber-rich low glycemic index natural foods improves blood glucose control and reduces the number of hypoglycaemic events in type 1 diabetic patients. *Diabetes Care* 2000; **23**:1461–1466.
34 Toeller M, Buyken A, Heitkamp G, De Pergola G, Giorgino F, Fuller JH, and the EURODIAB IDDM Complications Study Group. Fiber intake, serum cholesterol levels and cardiovascular disease in European individuals with type 1 diabetes. *Diabetes Care* 1999; **22**(Suppl.2):B21–B28.
35 Buyken AE, Toeller M, Heitkamp G, Karamanos B, Rottiers R, Muggeo M, *et al.* and the EURODIAB IDDM Complications Study Group. Glycemic index in the diet of European outpatients with type 1 diabetes: relations to HbA1c and serum lipids. *Am J Clin Nutr* 2001; **73**:574–581.
36 Järvi AE, Karlström BK, Granfeldt YE, Björck IME, Asp N-G, Vessby BOH. Improved glycemic control and lipid profile and normalized fibrinolytic activity on a low glycemic index diet in type 2 diabetes mellitus patients. *Diabetes Care* 1999; **22**:10–18.
37 Gilbertson H, Brand-Miller J, Thorburn A, Evans S, Chondros P, Werther G. The effect of flexible low glycemic index dietary advice versus measured carbohydrate exchange diets on glycemic control in children with type 1 diabetes. *Diabetes Care* 2001; **24**:1137–1143.
38 Brand-Miller J, Hayne S, Petocz P, Colagiuri S. Low-glycemic index diets in the management of diabetes: a meta-analysis of randomized controlled trials. *Diabetes Care* 2003; **26**:2261–2267.
39 Mann J, Hermansen K, Vessby B, Toeller M. Evidence-based nutritional recommendations for the treatment and prevention of diabetes and related complications: a European perspective (letter). *Diabetes Care* 2002; **25**:1256–1258.
40 Chandalia M, Garg A, Lutjohann D, von Bergmann K, Grundy SM, Brinkley LJ. Beneficial effects of high dietary fiber intake in patients with type 2 diabetes. *N Engl J Med* 2000; **342**:1392–1398.
41 Tariq SH, Karcic E, Thomas DR, Thomson K, Philpot C, Chapel DL, *et al.* The use of no-concentrated-sweets diet in the management of type 2 diabetes in nursing homes. *J Am Diet Assoc* 2001; **101**:1463–1466.
42 DAFNE Study Group. Training in flexible, intensive insulin management to enable dietary freedom in people with type 1 diabetes. dose adjustment for normal eating (DAFNE) randomized controlled trial. *Br Med J* 2002; **325**:746–782.
43 Rabasa-Lhoret R, Garon J, Langelier H, Poisson D, Chiasson JL. Effects of meal carbohydrate content on insulin requirements in type 1 diabetic patients treated intensively with the basal-bolus (Ultralente-regular) insulin regimen. *Diabetes Care* 1999; **22**:667–673.
44 Franz MJ, Bantle JP, Beebe CA, Brunzell JD, Chiasson JL, Garg A, *et al.* Evidence-based nutrition principles and recommendations for the treatment and prevention of diabetes and related complications: technical review. *Diabetes Care* 2002; **25**:148–198.

45 Soinio M, Laakso M, Lehto S, Hakala P, Rönnemaa T. Dietary fat predicts coronary heart disease events in subjects with type 2 diabetes. *Diabetes Care* 2003; **26**:619–624.

46 Tanasescu M, Cho E, Manson JE, Hu FB. Dietary fat and cholesterol and the risk of cardiovascular disease among women with type 2 diabetes. *Am J Clin Nutr* 2004; **79**:999–1005.

47 Vessby B, Uusitupa M, Hermansen K, Riccardi G, Rivellese AA, Tapsell LC, *et al.* Substituting dietary saturated for monounsaturated fat impairs insulin sensitivity in healthy men and women: the KANWU Study. *Diabetologia* 2001; **44**:312–319.

48 Parker B, Noakes M, Luscombe N, Clifton P. Effect of a high-protein, high mono-unsaturated fat weight loss diet on glycemic control and lipid levels in type 2 diabetes. *Diabetes Care* 2002; **25**:425–430.

49 Summers LK, Fielding BA, Bradshaw HA, Ilic V, Beysen C, Clark ML, *et al.* Substituting dietary saturated fat with polyunsaturated fat changes abdominal fat distribution and improves insulin sensitivity. *Diabetologia* 2002; **45**:369–377.

50 Perez-Jimenez F, Lopez-Miranda J, Pinillos MD, Gomez P, Paz-Rojas E, Montilla P, *et al.* A mediterranean and a high-carbohydrate diet improve glucose metabolism in healthy young persons. *Diabetologia* 2001; **44**:2038–2043.

51 Strychar I, Ishac A, Rivard M, Lussier-Cacan S, Beauregard H, Aris-Jilwan N, *et al.* Impact of a high-monounsaturated fat diet on lipid profile in subjects with type 1 diabetes. *J Am Diet Assoc* 2003; **103**:467–474.

52 West SG, Hecker KD, Mustad VA, Nicholson S, Schoemer SL, Wagner P, *et al.* Acute effects of monounsaturated fatty acids with and without omega-3 fatty acids on vascular reactivity in individuals with type 2 diabetes. *Diabetologia* 2005; **48**:113–122.

53 Wang C, Harris WS, Chung M, Lichtenstein AH, Balk EM, Kupelnick B, *et al.* N-3 fatty acids from fish or fish-oil supplements, but not (alpha)-linolenic acid, benefit cardiovascular outcomes in primary- and secondary-prevention studies: a systematic review. *Am J Clin Nutr* 2006; **84**:5–17.

54 Kris-Etherton PM, Harris WS, Appell LJ. Fish consumption, fish oil, omega-3 fatty acids, and cardiovascular disease. *Circulation* 2002; **106**:2747–2757.

55 Toeller M, Buyken AE, Heitkamp G, Scherbaum WA, Krans HMJ, Fuller JH, and the EURODIAB IDDM Complications Study Group. Associations of fat and cholesterol intake with serum lipid levels and cardiovascular disease: The EURODIAB IDDM Complications Study. *Exp Clin Endocrinol Diabetes* 1999; **107**:512–521.

56 Toeller M, Buyken AE. Protein intake: a new evidence for its role in diabetic nephropathy. Editorial comment. *Nephrol Dialysis Transpl* 1998; **13**:1926–1927.

57 Toeller M, Buyken A, Heitkamp G, Brämswig S, Mann, J, Milne R, *et al.* and the EURODIAB IDDM Complications Study Group. Protein intake and urinary albumin excretion rates in the EURODIAB IDDM Complications Study. *Diabetologia* 1997; **40**:1219–1226.

58 Pijls LT, de Vries H, van Eijk JT, Donker AJ. Protein restriction, glomerular filtration rate and albuminuria in patients with type 2 diabetes mellitus: a randomized trial. *Eur J Clin Nutr* 2002; **56**:1200–1207.

59 Hansen HP, Tauber-Lassen E, Jensen BR, Parving HH. Effect of dietary protein restriction on prognosis in patients with diabetic nephropathy. *Kidney Int* 2002; **62**:220–228.

60 Meloni C, Morosetti M, Suraci C, Pennafina MG, Tozzo C, Taccone-Gallucci M, *et al.* Severe dietary protein restriction in overt diabetic nephropathy: benefits or risks? *J Ren Nutr* 2002; **12**:96–101.

61 Dodson PM, Beevers M, Hallworth R, Webberley MJ, Fletcher RF, Taylor KG. Sodium restriction and blood pressure in hypertensive type II diabetics: randomised blind controlled and crossover studies of moderate sodium restriction and sodium supplementation. *Br Med J* 1989; **289**:227–230.

62 Sacks FM, Svetkey LP, Vollmer WM, Appel LJ, Bray GA, Harsha D, *et al.* Effects on blood pressure of reduced dietary sodium and the Dietary Approaches to Stop Hypertension (DASH) diet: DASH-Sodium Collaborative Research Group. *N Engl J Med* 2001; **344**:3–10.

63 Hasanain B, Mooradian AD. Antioxidant vitamins and their influence in diabetes mellitus. *Curr Diab Rep* 2002; **2**:448–456.

64 Lonn E, Yusuf S, Hoogwerf B, Pogue J, Yi Q, Zinman B, *et al.* Effects of vitamin E on cardiovascular and microvascular outcomes in high-risk patients with diabetes: results of the HOPE study and MICRO-HOPE substudy. *Diabetes Care* 2002; **25**:1919–1927.

65 Yeh GY, Eisenberg DM, Kaptchuk TJ, Phillips RS. Systematic review of herbs and dietary supplements for glycemic control in diabetes. *Diabetes Care* 2003; **26**:1277–1294.

66 Howard AA, Arnsten JH, Gourevitch MN. Effect of alcohol consumption on diabetes mellitus: a systematic review. *Ann Intern Med* 2004; **140**:211–219.

67 Koppes LL, Dekker JM, Hendriks HF, Bouter LM, Heine RJ. Meta-analysis oft he relationship between alcohol consumption and coronary heart disease and mortality in type 2 diabetic patients. *Diabetologia* 2006; **49**:648–652.

68 Ajani UA, Gaziano JM, Lotufo PA, Liu S, Hennekens CH, Buring JE, *et al.* Alcohol consumption and risk of coronary heart disease by diabetes status. *Circulation* 2000; **102**:500–505.

69 Beulens JWJ, Kruidhof JS, Grobbee DE, Chaturvedi N, Fuller JH, Soedamah-Muthu SS. Alcohol consumption and risk of microvascular complications in type 1 diabetes patients: the EURODIAB Prospective Complications Study. *Diabetologia* 2008; **51**:1631–1638.

70 Turner BC, Jenkins E, Kerr D, Sherwin RS, Cavan DA. The effect of evening alcohol consumption on next-morning glucose control in type 1 diabetes. *Diabetes Care* 2001; **24**:1888–1893.

71 Cryer PE, Davis SN, Shamoon H. Hypoglycemia in diabetes. *Diabetes Care* 2003; **26**:1902–1912.

72 Crowther CA, Hiller JE, Moss JR, McPhee AJ, Jeffries WS, Robinson JS. Effect of treatment of gestational diabetes mellitus on pregnancy outcomes. *N Engl J Med* 2005; **352**:2477–2486.

73 Silverstein J, Klingensmith G, Copeland K, Plotnick L, Kaufman F, Laffel L, *et al.* Care of children and adolescents with type 1 diabetes mellitus: a statement of the American Diabetes Association. *Diabetes Care* 2005; **28**:186–212.

74 Brown AF, Mangione CM, Saliba D, Sarkisian CA. Guidelines for improving the care of the older person with diabetes mellitus. *J Am Geriatr Soc* 2003; **51**:S265–S280.

75 Clement S, Braithwaite SS, Magee MF, Ahmann A, Smith EP, Schafer RG, *et al.* for the American Diabetes Association Diabetes in Hospitals Writing Committee. Management of diabetes and hyperglycemia in hospitals. *Diabetes Care* 2004; **27**:553–591.

76 Horani MH, Mooradian AD. Management of obesity in the elderly: special considerations. *Treat Endocrinol* 2002; **1**:387–398.

77 Miller CK, Edwards L, Kissling G, Sanville L. Nutrition education improves metabolic outcomes among older adults with diabetes mellitus: results from a randomized controlled trial. *Prev Med* 2002; **34**:252–259.

23 Lifestyle Issues: Exercise

Jane E. Yardley[1,2], Angela Alberga[2], Glen P. Kenny[1,2] & Ronald J. Sigal[1,2,3]

[1] Ottawa Hospital Research Institute, University of Ottawa, Ottawa, Ontario, Canada
[2] Faculty of Health Sciences, University of Ottawa, Ottawa, Ontario, Canada
[3] Faculties of Medicine and Kinesiology, University of Calgary, Calgary, Alberta, Canada

Keypoints

- Regular exercise increases insulin sensitivity in both individuals with and without diabetes.
- In individuals without diabetes, plasma insulin levels decrease during low to moderate intensity exercise to compensate for increases in insulin sensitivity. Glucose production and glucose disposal increase in parallel in order to maintain blood glucose homeostasis.
- In individuals with type 1 diabetes (T1DM), low to moderate intensity exercise can result in hypoglycemia, as insulin levels cannot be regulated physiologically.
- During and after high intensity exercise, glucose production can exceed glucose disposal, causing hyperglycemia in individuals both with and without diabetes. In T1DM, hyperglycemia can be more marked and prolonged, as insulin cannot increase in response.
- It is recommended that individuals with T1DM adjust their insulin dose and carbohydrate consumption prior to, during and/or after exercise to accommodate the type, intensity and duration of exercise performed.
- While regular exercise has not conclusively been found to improve glycemic control in T1DM, it is associated with decreased long-term morbidity and mortality in this population.
- Structured supervised diet and exercise interventions can reduce the risk of developing type 2 diabetes mellitus (T2DM) by about 60% in individuals with impaired glucose tolerance.
- Regular exercise improves glycemic control significantly in T2DM.
- Individuals with T1DM and T2DM with moderate or high aerobic fitness have long-term mortality that is 50–60% lower than individuals with diabetes and low cardiorespiratory fitness.
- Resistance training is a safe and effective means of improving glycemic control in individuals with T2DM of all ages. To maximize the impact of lifestyle measures on glycemic control, combined aerobic and resistance exercise is more effective than either type of exercise alone.

Glossary of terms

The definitions in Table 23.1 are adapted from those found in the *Physical Activity Guidelines Advisory Committee Report, 2008* produced by the US Department of Health and Human Services [1].

Types of exercise training and their effects on healthy individuals

Aerobic exercise

Effects of regular aerobic exercise training

Regular aerobic training generally leads to improved lung function and cardiac output, allowing for the provision of more oxygen for working muscles. Higher plasma volume and greater capillary density in the muscles allow increased muscle blood flow during peak exercise. Eventually, a shift in the fuels being used to supply the energy demands of activity is seen as the oxidative metabolic system becomes more efficient. In general, changes become more noticeable when training is of higher volume and intensity.

Fuel metabolism during acute aerobic exercise

During the first 5–10 minutes of exercise, muscle glycogen is the main source of energy. As exercise continues, the bloodborne substrates, glucose and non-esterified fatty acids become increasingly important. If exercise of moderate intensity continues for several hours, the contribution of glucose diminishes and non-esterified fatty acids become the major fuel (Figure 23.1) [2]. During moderate intensity aerobic exercise, blood glucose levels remain virtually unchanged. Insulin secretion is reduced while the release of glucagon is promoted, encouraging a two- to four-fold increase in hepatic glucose production (controlled by the glucagon : insulin molar ratio at the portal vein) [3] to meet the needs of the exercising muscle. Glucose production and utilization fall rapidly and in parallel to baseline during the post-

Textbook of Diabetes, 4th edition. Edited by R. Holt, C. Cockram, A. Flyvbjerg and B. Goldstein.

Table 23.1 Glossary of terms.

Physical activity The expenditure of energy above that of resting by contraction of skeletal muscle to produce bodily movement

Exercise A type of physical activity that involves planned, structured and repetitive bodily movement performed for the purpose of improving or maintaining physical fitness

Cardiorespiratory fitness/cardiorespiratory endurance/aerobic fitness Refers to the circulatory and respiratory systems' ability to supply oxygen during sustained exercise

Aerobic exercise Exercise that uses primarily aerobic energy-producing systems and involves the repeated and continuous movement of the same large muscle groups for extended periods of time (at least 10 minutes at a time). If performed with sufficient intensity and frequency this type of exercise increases cardiorespiratory fitness. Aerobic activities include walking, cycling, jogging, swimming, etc.

Anaerobic exercise Short, high intensity exercise involving anaerobic energy-producing systems. If performed with sufficient intensity and frequency this type of exercise can increase the body's ability to tolerate acid-base imbalance during high intensity exercise

Intensity of aerobic exercise Generally described in relation to an individual's maximal aerobic capacity ($\dot{V}O_{2max}$), as measured using indirect calorimetry during a graded maximal exercise test. An activity level corresponding to 40–60% of $\dot{V}O_{2max}$ is generally considered to be "moderate" in intensity, while "vigorous" aerobic activities consist of those performed at greater than 60% of $\dot{V}O_{2max}$

Muscular fitness Includes the force a muscle can exert (strength) and the ability of the muscle to perform continuously without fatigue (endurance)

Resistance exercise Also known as strength training or weight training. Resistance exercise involves the use of muscular strength to work against a resistive load or move a weight. Examples include lifting free weights, or using weight machines. Regular resistance exercise at sufficient (moderate to high) intensity increases muscular fitness

Intensity of resistance exercise The intensity of resistance exercise is often considered "moderate" if the resistance provided is 50–74% of the maximum that can be lifted a single time (1 repetition maximum [1 RM]). High intensity resistance exercise involves resistance ≥75% of 1 RM

Repetition The number of times a resistance exercise is repeated during each set

Set A grouping of repetitions of a specific resistance exercise

exercise "recovery" phase, as insulin levels rise and glucagon secretion decreases. If moderate intensity aerobic exercise lasts for several hours without caloric intake, hepatic glucose production can no longer keep pace with increased utilization, and the blood glucose level begins to decline, eventually resulting in hypoglycemia [4].

Effects of regular training on fuel metabolism

Aerobically trained athletes without diabetes have low fasting plasma insulin levels and reduced insulin responses to a glucose challenge in the face of normal glucose tolerance, and increased insulin-mediated glucose uptake under glucose clamp conditions [5]. Physical training is also known to increase muscle and hepatic insulin sensitivity in previously untrained individuals [6]. Lipid and lipoprotein profiles become less atherogenic with regular training: serum high density lipoprotein (HDL) cholesterol levels may increase, while total and low density lipoprotein (LDL) cholesterol levels may remain unchanged or decline [7,8]. Some studies have found that serum triglyceride levels decline after training [7,8]. Even when LDL cholesterol concentrations remain unchanged with aerobic exercise training there is an increase in mean LDL particle diameter, reflecting more buoyant and less atherogenic LDL cholesterol particles [9].

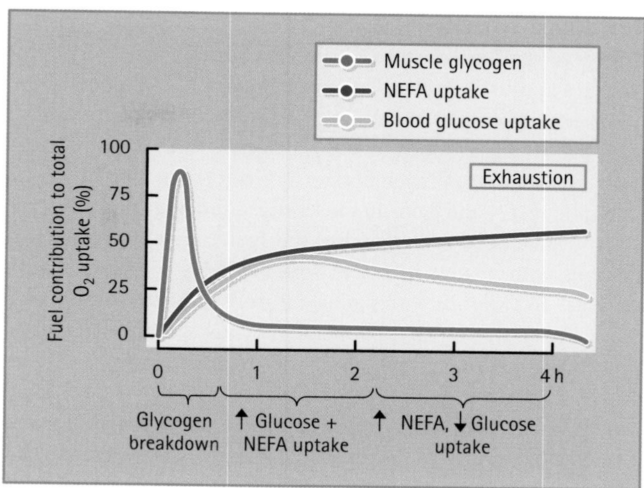

Figure 23.1 The relative contributions of muscle glycogen breakdown and uptake of blood-borne glucose and non-esterified fatty acids (NEFA) to fuel utilization at various stages of prolonged low-intensity exercise in a healthy individual. The exercise intensity corresponds to 30% of maximal. Data from Ahlborg *et al.* [2].

Anaerobic exercise

Effects of regular anaerobic exercise training

Regular anaerobic training improves the body's ability to provide the fuels necessary for the production of anaerobic power. Adenosine triphosphate (ATP) and phosphocreatine levels (the main fuels for short powerful bursts) increase within muscle tissue, allowing the individual to sustain higher absolute exercise intensities for longer periods of time.

Fuel metabolism during anaerobic activity

With very intense exercise (more than 80% of $\dot{V}O_{2max}$ – a level sustainable for no more than 15 minutes by most individuals), hepatic glucose production may exceed the rate of glucose utilization, leading to a 5- to 10-fold increase in blood glucose [10–12]. During recovery from very intense exercise, hyperglycemia often occurs in fit individuals without diabetes, as glucose utilization decreases more quickly than glucose production [10–12]. In response to the hyperglycemia, plasma insulin levels increase and glycemia is restored to baseline within about 45 minutes.

Resistance exercise

Effects of regular resistance exercise training

Declines in muscle strength of approximately 12–15% per decade have been reported after the age of 50 years [13,14], with muscle mass decreasing as much as 6% per decade [5,16]. With regular heavy resistance training, increases of greater than 30% in muscle strength [15,17] and gains in muscle mass ranging from 3 to 12% [18,19] have been found within the first couple of months of training, with relative increases typically being higher in elderly subjects [16,18]. Initial strength gains during the first 6 weeks are generally as a result of peripheral nervous system adaptations (improved muscle recruitment) and are not accompanied by muscle hypertrophy. Resistance training can be of additional benefit to older adults as improvements in postural stability and dynamic balance may decrease the risk of fall-related injuries [20].

When muscles are forced to perform for a given period of time at or near their maximal strength and endurance capacity (either by lifting weights or working against some other form of resistance), it will result in an increase in muscle strength, endurance and hypertrophy. Performing more repetitions (up to 2 minutes per set of each exercise) with lower resistance tends to increase endurance, while lifting heavier weights for fewer repetitions will favor strength gains [21].

Fuel metabolism during resistance exercise

High intensity, short duration resistance exercise is fueled by energy generated from the breakdown of stored intramuscular high-energy phosphates, ATP and phosphocreatine. During such exercise, adequate rest periods (2–5 minutes) between sets are necessary to allow regeneration of phosphocreatine stores. Glycolytic anaerobic energy production (with concomitant blood lactate accumulation) becomes more important as intensity decreases, the number of repetitions per set increases, and rest periods between sets become shorter [22]. This can result in local muscle lactate accumulation even after a single set. Where multiple sets are performed, longer sets and shorter rest periods between sets are associated with greater increases in blood lactate (which can reduce muscle contractility) and declines in muscle glycogen [23,24].

Metabolic and hormonal effects of exercise in diabetes

Type 1 diabetes

Higher amounts of habitual physical activity are associated with decreased incidence of diabetes-related complications and reduced mortality in individuals with type 1 diabetes mellitus (T1DM) [25]. In a prospective study, 548 patients with T1DM were followed for 7 years to ascertain the prevalence of complications and mortality [25]. The risk of microvascular complications varied inversely with self-reported activity levels at baseline. Sedentary male patients were three times more likely to die than

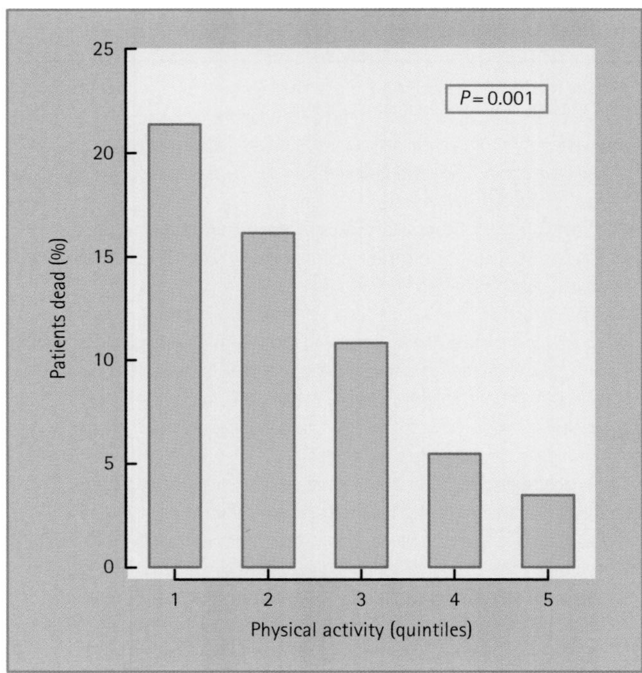

Figure 23.2 Proportion of men who died during a 7-year follow-up period among 548 patients with type 1 diabetes, stratified according to the physical activity quintile. Quintile cut-offs were <398; 398–1000; 1000–2230; 2230–4228 and >4228 kcal/week. The difference among groups is highly significant. Data from Moy *et al.* [25].

the active ones after adjusting for age, body mass index, smoking and diabetic complications (Figure 23.2) [25]. A similar, although statistically non-significant, relationship was also seen in females.

Studies have also shown an inverse association between physical activity and the severity of several complications in T1DM [26–29]. A longitudinal study of 1680 individuals with T1DM showed that self-reported leisure time physical activity levels were inversely correlated with measures of glycemic control and insulin sensitivity [29]. Women with diabetes in the study with low levels of leisure time physical activity tended to have poor glycemic control when compared with those with higher activity levels. Estimates of insulin sensitivity were also higher among more active men and women [29]. A follow-up study involving 1945 individuals with T1DM reported that those involved in either little leisure time physical activity or low intensity activity were more likely to have impaired renal function, a higher degree of proteinuria, as well as greater rates of retinopathy and cardiovascular disease when compared with more frequently and more vigorously active counterparts [28]. More recently, a randomized trial showed that the onset of diabetic peripheral neuropathy can be prevented and its progression delayed over a 4-year period by regular exercise [26].

General metabolic considerations

The intensity and duration of exercise, the patient's level of blood glucose control, the type, dose and site of pre-exercise insulin

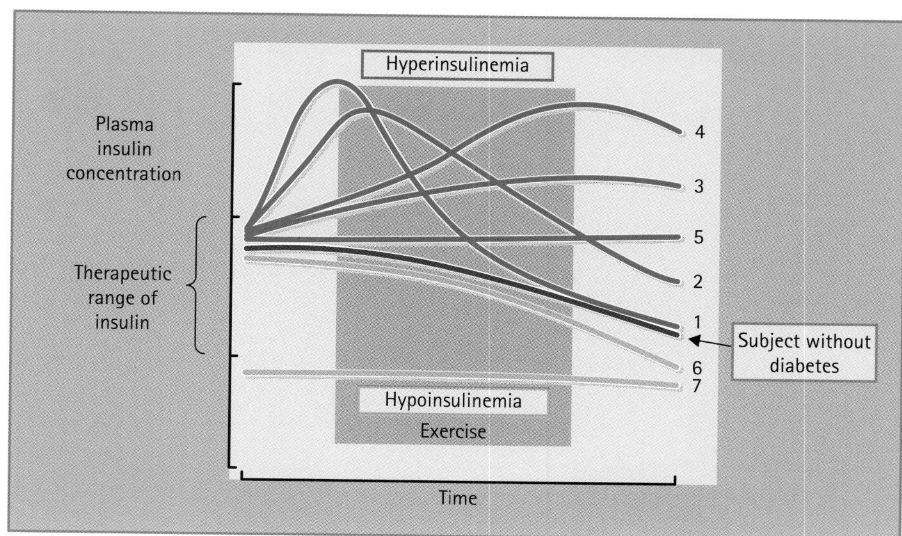

Figure 23.3 Plasma insulin levels may vary widely during exercise in patients with insulin-treated diabetes, whereas healthy subjects (as well as patients with type 2 diabetes) show a steady decline during moderate intensity aerobic exercise. Hyperinsulinemia and hypoglycemia may occur when the peak action of a short-acting insulin analog (1), conventional soluble (regular) insulin (2) or intermediate-acting insulin (3) occurs during exercise, or if exercise itself accelerates the absorption from the injection site (4). Steady-state but elevated plasma insulin concentrations may occur if intermediate or long-acting insulin has been injected a few hours before exercise, or if the patient is using an insulin pump (5). Declining levels (6) or hypoinsulinemia (7) occur when the previous injection depots are exhausted.

injections, and the timing of the previous insulin injection and meal relative to the exercise can all affect the response of an individual with diabetes to physical activity (Figure 23.3). Accordingly, blood glucose concentrations can decline (the most common response in moderate aerobic exercise), increase (particularly in very intense exercise) or remain unchanged (Table 23.2). Whereas insulin secretion declines during moderate intensity aerobic exercise in individuals without diabetes, compensating for exercise-induced increased muscle insulin sensitivity, this physiologic decline in insulinemia cannot occur in T1DM because all insulin is exogenous. Insulin attenuates the appropriate rise in hepatic glucose production and further accelerates the exercise-induced stimulation of glucose uptake into the contracting muscle.

Hyperinsulinemia may occur for several reasons (Figure 23.4). Regular insulin injected a few hours previously may exert its peak action during exercise. This effect is exaggerated if the previously injected limb is exercised, as insulin absorption is accelerated by exercise [30]. Moreover, the use of intermediate or long-acting insulin generally produces higher peripheral insulin levels than would be found in an individual without diabetes of similar body composition. The result is often hypoglycemia, unless the insulin dose prior to exercise is decreased or extra carbohydrate is consumed. Hyperinsulinemia can also prevent the normal increase in lipid mobilization during exercise, leading to reduced availability of non-esterified fatty acids as a fuel.

Conversely, if insulin levels are too low, the inhibitory effect of insulin on hepatic glucose production and its stimulatory effect on glucose uptake are both reduced. In addition, the counter-regulatory response (catecholamines, glucagon, growth hormone, cortisol) to exercise is higher than normal under conditions of insulin deficiency [30]. The overall result is markedly increased hepatic glucose production and diminished glucose utilization by the exercising muscle, thus leading to hyperglycemia.

Table 23.2 Factors determining the glycemic response to acute exercise in people with type 1 diabetes.

Blood glucose tends to decrease if:
- Hyperinsulinemia exists during moderate intensity aerobic exercise
- Exercise is prolonged (>30–60 minutes)
- No extra snacks are taken before or during moderate intensity exercise

Blood glucose generally remains unchanged if:
- Exercise is brief and mild to moderate in intensity
- Appropriate snacks are taken before and during moderate intensity exercise

Blood glucose tends to increase if:
- Hypoinsulinemia exists during exercise
- Exercise is very intense
- Excessive carbohydrate is taken before or during exercise

Aerobic exercise in type 1 diabetes

Effects of regular aerobic exercise training in type 1 diabetes

Insulin sensitivity is reduced to varying degrees in patients who have had T1DM for several years [31]. Participation in a regular exercise training program improves whole-body insulin sensitivity in these patients, as it does in those without diabetes, which may help to induce and prolong remission in newly presenting T1DM [32]. It has been difficult to ascertain whether or not regular aerobic exercise improves glycemic control in T1DM, as outcomes of exercise intervention have been inconsistent. While some studies have demonstrated improvements, albeit not statistically significant, in blood glucose control as measured by decreases in HbA_{1c} [33,34], most studies have either not shown any changes [35] or have produced increases in HbA_{1c} [36]. The main reason for this is probably excessive reductions of insulin dose or disproportionate carbohydrate consumption before exercise in an effort to avoid hypoglycemia. It is important to note

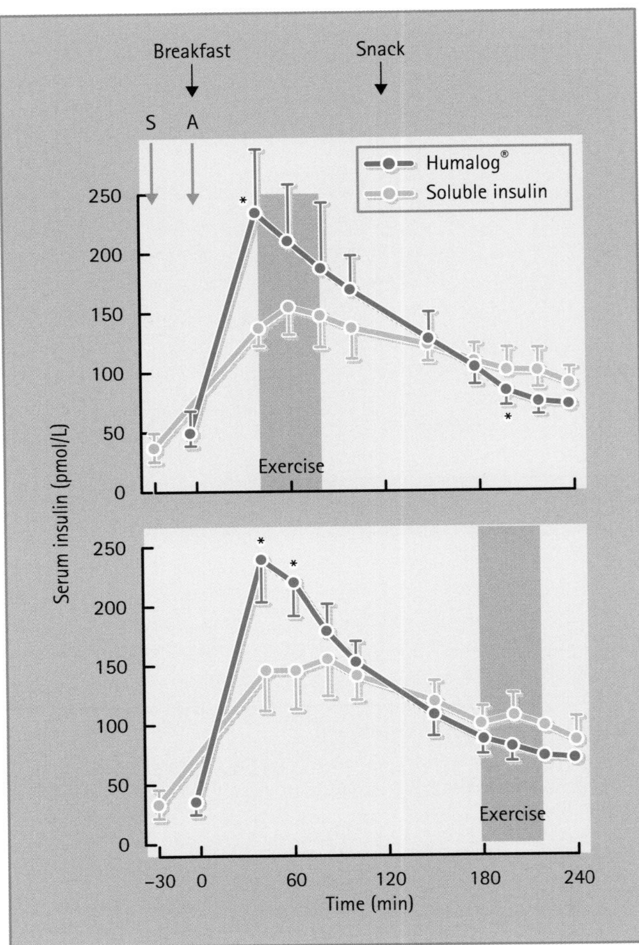

Figure 23.4 Insulin concentrations during exercise depend on the type of insulin and the time interval between the injection and exercise. Serum insulin concentrations during early exercise are higher after injection of the lispro (Humalog) insulin analog (A) than after conventional soluble insulin (S), whereas the opposite situation applies during delayed exercise. Soluble insulin was injected 30-min and lispro insulin 5-min after breakfast, and exercise was started either 40-min (early) or 180-min (late) after breakfast. $^{*}P < 0.05$. Data from Tuominen *et al.* [163].

that participants in several studies still experienced many exercise-related benefits including lower body fat percentage [34], improved muscle mass [37], increased aerobic capacity [34,36,37], improved lipid profiles [34,36,37] and greater insulin sensitivity (with a consequent lower need for exogenous insulin) [36].

Fuel metabolism during aerobic activity

Under ideal conditions of low insulin and euglycemia, fuel selection during mild to moderate exercise can be very similar in people with T1DM as those without diabetes, with a gradual shift towards lipid oxidation with increasing exercise duration [38]. Conversely, if the levels of circulating insulin are too high, muscle, adipose and hepatic cells will continue to take up glucose for storage rather than leaving it available for working muscles. While glucagon can still be produced in individuals with T1DM [39], the glucagon : insulin molar ratio at the portal vein may not reach the level necessary for adequate levels of hepatic glucose production to occur. Compared with individuals without diabetes, those with T1DM may demonstrate a lower reliance on hepatic glycogen stores during low intensity aerobic activity [40]. If the rate of glucose appearance in the system is not high enough to supply the demand, blood glucose levels will drop, thereby increasing the potential for hypoglycemia [39].

Levels of insulinemia and glycemia will also affect the fuels used during aerobic activity. Hyperinsulinemia can lead to a greater reliance on exogenous glucose utilization during moderate aerobic exercise, without sparing glycogen stores [41]. In a study where insulinemia was kept constant, the contribution of carbohydrates to overall energy metabolism during exercise was greater in hyperglycemia than in euglycemia [38]. The shift towards greater carbohydrate metabolism during exercise in hyperglycemia was accompanied by a blunted cortisol and growth hormone response. Insulin, glucagon and catecholamine levels were comparable between conditions [38]. Overall, individuals with T1DM seem to have a greater reliance on muscle glycogenolysis and gluconeogenesis to produce fuel during physical activity than their non-diabetic counterparts [40,42].

Despite the complexities of glucoregulation, well-motivated people with T1DM can successfully undertake several hours of exhaustive aerobic exercise if appropriate insulin and dietary adjustments are made [43–45]. After prolonged exercise, patients may be prone to hypoglycemia for many hours, even extending overnight and to the following day. This can be explained by persistently enhanced glucose uptake by the exercised muscles to replenish the depleted glycogen stores [43]; however, after certain types of prolonged exercise, such as a marathon run, increased lipid oxidation can persist, as occurs in healthy individuals [44]. In this case, the use of glucose as a fuel and insulin sensitivity are reduced after exercise, thereby decreasing the risk of post-exercise hypoglycemia [44]. It should also be noted that individuals who experience frequent bouts of hypoglycemia (whether exercise-related or not), may have further blunting of counter-regulatory responses to exercise, potentially creating a vicious cycle of hypoglycemic events [46–50].

Effects of regular anaerobic exercise training in type 1 diabetes

There is currently a gap in the literature as to how physical and metabolic adaptations to regular anaerobic training in individuals with T1DM differ from those of non-diabetic individuals. People with T1DM who participate in competitive sports may find that their glycemic control worsens, probably secondary to an irregular schedule of very vigorous exercise, insulin dose reduction and high carbohydrate consumption [51]. In spite of the elevation in physical fitness and $\dot{V}O_{2max}$, these individuals may not have increased insulin sensitivity, but instead show enhanced use of non-esterified fatty acids as a fuel [51]. It is likely that many individuals with T1DM will have to compromise some tightness of control to be able to participate effectively in competitive sports and high intensity activities, to avoid the fear of hypoglycemia during exercise. Whether or not this affects their physical and metabolic adaptations to these types of activities requires further research. More details on carbohydrate and insulin adjustments for exercise can be found later in this chapter.

Fuel selection during high intensity exercise

Extremely strenuous acute exercise may cause hyperglycemia even in the presence of normal or high insulin levels. High counter-regulatory hormone action (especially catecholamines) can stimulate glucose production beyond the limits of peripheral utilization [52–56]. In addition, in T1DM the normal physiologic doubling of insulin concentration after cessation of such intense exercise cannot occur, resulting in more prolonged hyperglycemia [52,55,56]. Augmented lipid mobilization and ketogenesis in the liver increase blood ketone-body concentrations; the hypoinsulinemic individuals may thus become hyperketonemic and ketonuric after exercise.

Several recent studies have shown that such high intensity exercise is effective in increasing blood glucose levels and thereby delaying or preventing hypoglycemia related to moderate exercise even when performed in extremely short bouts [57–61]. Bussau *et al.* [57,58] showed that a 10-second sprint performed either prior to [58] or at the completion of [57] 20 minutes of low intensity cycling significantly attenuated post-exercise drops in blood glucose, when compared with exercise sessions where no sprint was performed. Similar results were found by Guelfi *et al.* [59,60] where post-exercise blood glucose levels remained higher after cycling exercise sessions where 4-second sprints were performed every 2 minutes versus those where the participants cycled continuously at constant moderate intensity (Figure 23.5). The post-exercise window in these studies, however, was limited to 120 minutes. One small study using continuous glucose monitoring systems (CGMS) found a trend towards late onset post-exercise hypoglycemia after high intensity activity [62]; however, further studies with larger sample sizes will be necessary to confirm this.

Resistance exercise

Effects of regular resistance exercise training in type 1 diabetes

There is a paucity of information regarding the outcomes of training programs consisting of only resistance exercise in individuals with T1DM. The one study completed to date involved a cross-over design with 10 weeks of heavy resistance exercise three times a week followed by a 6-week period with no resistance training, or vice versa [63]. Mean HbA_{1c} was 6.9 ± 1.4% (52 ± 15 mmol/mol) at the end of the non-resistance exercise period and 5.8 ± 0.9% (40 ± 10 mmol/mol) at the end of the 10-week resistance exercise training period. Serum cholesterol and self-monitored glucose levels were also lower at the end of the resistance training period.

One study has compared the effects of 12 weeks of resistance training with those of a comparable period of aerobic training in individuals with T1DM [64]. While both groups showed decreases in waist circumference, reduced insulin dosage and lower self-monitored blood glucose after the training period, these variables only reached significance in the aerobically trained group. However, HbA_{1c} levels showed a statistically significant increase in the aerobic training group (from 8.7 ± 1.6 to 9.8 ± 1.8%; 72–84 mmol/mol), while a non-significant decrease (from 8.2 ± 2.9 to 7.6 ± 1.6%; 60–66 mmol/mol) was found in the resistance training group.

A handful of pre–post studies have also examined the effects of combined aerobic and resistance training programs in individuals with T1DM [65–67]. Outcomes of these studies were generally positive, with benefits including lower HbA_{1c} [65,67], decreased blood pressure [65,66], improved nerve conduction [65], higher cardiorespiratory fitness [67], greater muscular strength [67], higher lean body mass [65,67] and improvements in lipid profiles [67]. Nevertheless, it should be noted that the interpretation of these studies is limited by their lack of

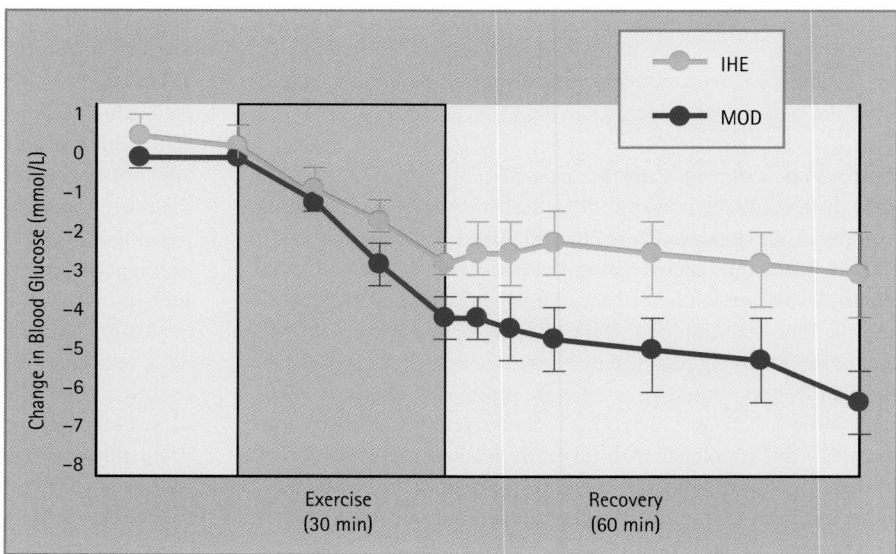

Figure 23.5 Effect of 30 min of intermittent high intensity exercise (IHE) or moderate continuous exercise (MOD) on normalized blood glucose levels. Data from Guelfi *et al.* [59].

Table 23.3 Clinical trials involving resistance exercise with people with type 1 diabetes mellitus.

Source	No. of participants (n)	Sessions/week, no of weeks	No. of exercises	No. of sets, rest interval and intensity of exercise	HbA_{1c} [mean (SD)]
Type 1 diabetes – resistance training only					
Durak *et al.* (1990) [63]	n = 8 (T1DM)	3 sessions/week; 10 weeks Training sessions after 5:00 PM Lunch time injections and food intake completed no later than 12:00 PM	5 lower body and 10 upper body exercises	3–7 sets (varied with exercise; 30 s to 2 min rest interval between sets, pyramid-type training routine used with 12 RM used for set 1, decreased with subsequent sets with addition of weight	6.9 (1.4) after 6 weeks with no resistance training and 5.8 (0.9)* after 10 weeks of resistance exercise training (cross-over design)
Type 1 diabetes – combined aerobic and resistance training					
Mosher *et al.* (1998) [67]	n = 10 (T1DM) n = 11 (control)	3 sessions/week; 12 weeks All training sessions performed between 1100 and 1200. Subjects consumed an evening meal supplemented by 5–10 g complex CHO ≈ 2 h before exercise	Aerobic and weight training circuit; circuit composed of 5 aerobic stations, each followed by 5 strength and callisthenic exercises	4–5 min of aerobic exercise (75–85% HR_{max}) followed by 5 strength and callisthenic exercises (upper and lower body strength exercises performed at 50% and 40% of 1-RM, respectively). Aerobic exercise followed by a 1-min recovery period. 5 successive 30-s strength and callisthenic exercises were then performed	Control group (without diabetes): 4.50 (0.45) to 4.47 (0.60) Intervention group (type 1 DM): 7.72 (1.26) to 6.76 (1.07)
Type 1 diabetes – comparison of aerobic training to resistance training					
Ramalho *et al.* (2006) [64]	n = 7 (aerobic) n = 6 (resistance)	3 sessions/week; 12 weeks All sessions supervised	Aerobic training: Treadmill walking or running Resistance training: 4 upper and 4 lower body exercises using weight machines	40 min walking/running with intensity increasing progressively every 2 weeks from 60–70% HR_{max} at week 0 to 70–90 HR_{max} at 12 weeks 10 min stretching and 30 min resistance exercise training. 3 sets of 8 to 12 reps progressing from 60 to 80% of 1-RM. 60-s rest between sets	Aerobic group: 8.7 (1.6) to 9.8 (1.8)* Resistance group: 8.2 (2.9) to 7.6 (1.6)

CHO, carbohydrate; DM, diabetes mellitus; HR_{max}, maximum heart rate; 1-RM, maximum weight that can be lifted once; T1DM, type 1 diabetes mellitus.
* Indicates significant difference from baseline at $P < 0.05$.
The following equation should be used to convert HbA_{1c} to IFCC Units: DCCT result (%) = (0.0915 × IFCC result in mmol/mol) +2.15.

concurrent diabetic control groups. All studies involving resistance exercise interventions in individuals with T1DM (alone or in combination with aerobic exercise) published by March 1, 2009 are outlined in Table 23.3.

Fuel selection during resistance exercise

Very little is known about the acute hormonal and resulting blood glucose responses to resistance exercise in individuals with T1DM. Resistance exercise in individuals without diabetes produces elevated epinephrine levels, which enhance hepatic glucose production, resulting in an increase in blood glucose levels [68]. As studies involving high intensity exercise demonstrate that catecholamine responses are similar in young fit individuals with and without T1DM [55,57,59], it is likely that resistance-type activities are associated with increases in blood glucose during and after exercise. However, the authors are unaware of any published research examining the glycemic response during and after this type of exercise in people with T1DM.

Type 2 diabetes

Exercise and type 2 diabetes prevention

In large prospective cohort studies, higher levels of physical activity and/or cardiorespiratory fitness have consistently been associated with reduced risk of developing T2DM [69–81]. After adjustment for confounding variables, participants who exercised the most had a 25–60% lower risk of subsequent diabetes compared to those who were most sedentary. This was true regardless of the presence or absence of additional risk factors for diabetes such as hypertension, parental history of diabetes and obesity in most studies. Comparable magnitudes of risk reduction are seen with walking compared to more vigorous activity when total energy expenditures are similar [77].

Several clinical trials have demonstrated that supervised structured physical activity programs, with or without concomitant dietary interventions, reduce the risk of developing T2DM in individuals with impaired glucose tolerance (IGT) [82–85]. In the non-randomized Malmö trial [82,86,87], 260 men aged 47–49 years with IGT were identified through population screening and were offered a 6–12-month intervention including supervised exercise programs and dietary counseling. Among those attending a 5-year follow-up examination, 21% of the control participants (those who had declined the intervention) had developed diabetes, compared to only 11% of those receiving the intervention. Over 12 years, mortality among the controls was 14.0 per 1000 person-years, but only 6.5 per 1000 person-years in the intervention group [87].

In the Da Qing IGT and Diabetes Study [83], 577 people with IGT from 33 clinics were cluster-randomized by clinic to diet only, exercise only, diet and exercise or control, and followed for 6 years. The cumulative incidence of T2DM was 68% in controls, but only 44%, 41% and 46% in the diet, exercise, and diet and exercise groups, respectively. Li *et al.* [88] recently published a follow-up paper to the Da Qing Study [83] assessing the long-term effect of the 6-year intervention on the risk of diabetes. They found that, 14 years after the end of the trial, incidence of diabetes remained significantly lower in those originally randomized to one of the intervention groups versus controls.

In the Finnish Diabetes Prevention Study [89], 523 Finnish adults with IGT were randomized to an exercise and diet intervention or control. Patients in the control group had one meeting per year with a physician and dietitian, at which they received standard advice on diet and exercise. The intervention group received individualized exercise plans, thrice-weekly supervised facility-based aerobic and resistance exercise, and seven 1-hour meetings with a dietitian focusing on weight reduction, reduced fat intake and reduced total caloric intake. At 4 years, 22% of the control group and only 10% of the intervention group had developed diabetes – a 58% risk reduction. Three years after the end of the study, participants originally randomized to the intervention group continued to have much higher levels of physical activity than those originally in the control group [90]. Incidence of diabetes in the individuals who were previously in the intervention group remained 43% lower than in those who were previously in the control group [90].

In the US-based Diabetes Prevention Program [85], 3234 American men and women with IGT were randomly assigned to placebo, metformin or a lifestyle modification program. The goals of the lifestyle modification program included a 7% weight loss and at least 150 minutes of exercise per week. The lifestyle intervention included 16 lessons in the first 24 weeks, covering diet, exercise and behavior modification (delivered one-on-one by a case manager). A minimum of two supervised exercise sessions per week and at least monthly contact with the study personnel were maintained thereafter. The study was ended after a mean of 2.8 years of follow-up, 1 year earlier than originally planned, because of clear-cut superiority of the lifestyle arm. Cumulative incidences of T2DM were 11.0 per 100 person-years in the placebo group, 7.8 per 100 person-years in the metformin group and only 4.8 per 100 person-years in the intensive lifestyle group. The risk of T2DM was 58% lower in the lifestyle group than in the placebo group, and 39% lower than in the metformin group. An epidemiologic analysis of the data by Hamman *et al.* determined that, after adjusting for changes in self-reported diet and physical activity, there was a 16% reduction in diabetes risk for every kilogram of weight loss among the lifestyle intervention participants [169]. Increased physical activity was a significant predictor of weight loss and had an important role in weight maintenance. In addition, participants who met the goal of more than 150 minutes of moderate exercise per week had a 46% reduction in diabetes risk.

Aerobic exercise in type 2 diabetes

Regular exercise is associated with reduced morbidity and mortality in T2DM. A 10-year follow-up of a large prospective cohort study including 347 individuals with diabetes and 1317 individuals without diabetes) found that the lowest aged-adjusted all-cause death rate was among those with diabetes who walked a mile or more daily [91]. Similarly, a prospective study of 1263 men with diabetes followed over 12 years found that, compared with the least fit men (bottom 20% as determined by maximal treadmill testing), those with moderate cardiorespiratory fitness had a 60% lower risk of cardiovascular and overall mortality [79]. The effect of fitness on mortality was considerably greater than the effect of body mass index. Further follow-up of this cohort confirmed these findings [92,93]. Greater habitual exercise was also associated with a lower subsequent risk of cardiovascular disease among women in the Nurses Health Study [94].

Effects of regular aerobic exercise training in type 2 diabetes

Exercise-induced stimulation of glucose uptake may involve many factors (Figure 23.6), as reviewed by Ivy *et al.* [95]. They include increased post-receptor insulin signaling [96], increased glucose transporter protein and mRNA [97], increased activity of glycogen synthase [98] and hexokinase [99], decreased release and increased clearance of free fatty acids [95], increased muscle glucose delivery as a result of increased muscle capillary density [99–101], changes in muscle composition favoring increased glucose disposal [99,102,103] and changes in adipose tissue mass and distribution [104]. Decreases in visceral fat result in decreased concentrations of tumor necrosis factor α [105] and free fatty acids [106], leading to decreased insulin resistance.

Inflammatory markers present in the bloodstream predict the onset of cardiovascular disease and related complications. Regular aerobic exercise training is generally associated with improvements in metabolic profile and results in anti-inflammatory effects in individuals with T2DM [107,108]. Exercise training in individuals with T2DM has been reported to produce anti-atherogenic blood lipid changes and to reduce other risk factors for coronary heart disease (hypertension, obesity, coagulation abnormalities) in some but not in all studies [109–115]. For instance, in elderly patients with relatively advanced atherosclerosis, exercise training may be less effective in retarding atherogenesis [113]. The prophylactic value of exercise against atherosclerosis might be greater in younger healthier individuals who have not yet developed disease.

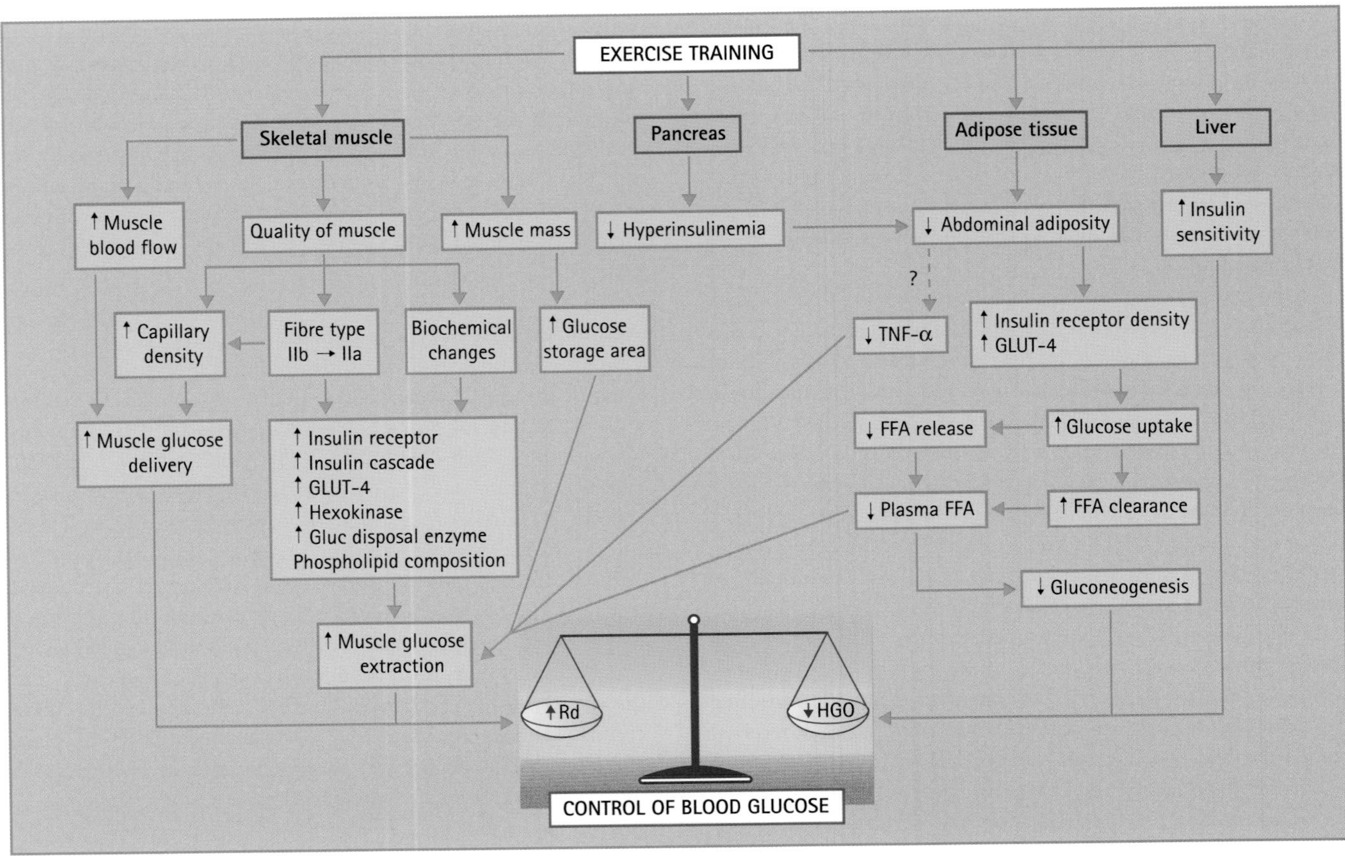

Figure 23.6 Mechanisms by which exercise training may improve insulin action and the control of blood glucose in type 2 diabetes. FFA, free fatty acid; GLUT, glucose transporter; HGO, hepatic glucose output; Rd, glucose uptake; TNF-α, tumour necrosis factor-α. Reproduced from Ivy *et al.* [95], with permission from Lippincott Williams & Wilkins.

Fuel metabolism during aerobic activity

Individuals with T2DM are characterized by both hepatic and peripheral insulin resistance and by hyperinsulinemia in the fasting state. During moderate intensity exercise, peripheral glucose uptake usually rises more than hepatic glucose production, and the blood glucose concentration tends to decline [116]. At the same time, plasma insulin levels fall, and the risk of exercise-induced hypoglycemia in individuals with T2DM not taking exogenous insulin is relatively small, even during prolonged exercise [117]. It has been shown that moderate intensity exercise decreases glycogen content similarly in individuals with and without diabetes [118]; however, glycogen and plasma glucose decreases more in obese individuals with diabetes compared with those without diabetes whether obese or lean [118]. The effects of moderate exercise on glucose tolerance and insulin sensitivity are similar whether the activity is performed in single versus multiple bouts of the same total duration [119]. Moderate aerobic exercise has also been shown to attenuate the increase in circulating triglyceride levels following ingestion of a high fat meal [120].

Anaerobic exercise in type 2 diabetes

Fuel metabolism during high intensity activity

If individuals with T2DM perform strenuous glycogen-depleting exercise, both peripheral and hepatic insulin sensitivity are increased and remain so for 12–16 hours thereafter [121]. Following maximal aerobic exercise (>85% $\dot{V}O_{2max}$), sedentary individuals with T2DM demonstrate higher levels of blood glucose compared with sedentary individuals without diabetes and active individuals with diabetes [122].

Resistance exercise

Effects of regular resistance exercise training in type 2 diabetes

The age-related decline of muscle mass may cause reduced insulin sensitivity. Resistance training can potentially counteract the age-associated decrease in muscle mass, and therefore warrants important consideration as an effective intervention in managing T2DM [95,123]. Resistance training has been shown to improve insulin sensitivity and glucose metabolism in both men and women [124–130] and has also been associated with modest improvements in lipid profiles [63,67,128]. In longitudinal studies involving healthy untrained adults, insulin responses to an oral glucose challenge are lower in both healthy younger [124,131] and older [131,132] individuals after resistance training. Resistance exercise, and its resulting increase in lean body mass, has also been associated with greater resting energy expenditure in older adults [133]. Whether or not this occurs in T2DM is still uncertain [134].

Studies published by Dunstan *et al.* [135] and Castaneda *et al.* [136], involving high intensity resistance training resulted in decreases in HbA_{1c} of 1.2% (13 mmol/mol) with a 26-week program, accompanied by a moderate energy restriction diet [135] and 1.0% (11 mmol/mol) with a 16-week program [136], respectively. Meta-analyses have confirmed that resistance training exercise effectively reduces HbA_{1c} in individuals with T2DM [137,138]. In a meta-analysis of clinical trials examining the effect of aerobic and resistance exercise interventions on glycemic control and body mass in T2DM (Figure 23.7), Boulé *et al.* [138] found no difference in HbA_{1c} between aerobic and resistance exercise. Overall, participants in exercise intervention groups had HbA_{1c} levels that were 0.66% (7 mmol/mol) lower post-intervention than those in control groups. Post-intervention body weight did not differ between exercise and control participants, suggesting that exercise is beneficial in its own right, not merely as an avenue to reduce body weight. Snowling & Hopkins [137] found in a more recent meta-analysis that the two types of exercise had similar effects on glucose control. An overview of clinical trials involving resistance exercise (both on its own and when combined with aerobic exercise training) in T2DM is provided in Table 23.4.

Fuel metabolism during resistance exercise in type 2 diabetes

The authors were unable to find any published research on fuel metabolism during resistance exercise in T2DM.

Combined aerobic and resistance exercise training

Snowling & Hopkins [137] reviewed controlled studies published in May 2006 or earlier that assessed the effects of aerobic training, resistance training or combined training on glucose control in T2DM. All three exercise modalities showed clinically significant reductions in HbA_{1c}, while the combined training showed an additive and large beneficial effect on insulin sensitivity. The HbA_{1c} meta-analyzed mean decreased by 0.8% (9 mmol/mol) in the combined exercise training studies compared to 0.7% (8 mmol/mol) and 0.5% (5 mmol/mol) for the aerobic and resistance training groups, respectively.

Three recent studies have investigated the combination of aerobic training and resistance training exercise on glycemic control [19,139,140] and one other study has examined the combined exercise effect on cardiac function in T2DM [114,115]. Study outcomes have been consistent, showing increases in aerobic fitness and muscular fitness [114,115,134] as well as improvements in body composition [139,140] and cardiovascular disease risk profile [19,114,115,139,140].

Balducci *et al.* [139] assessed the effects of a supervised facility-based combined aerobic and resistance exercise training program on glycemic control, cardiovascular disease (CVD) risk factors and body composition in previously sedentary individuals with T2DM. Participants (aged 60–70 years) were randomized into an exercising intervention group (three times per week) or a non-exercising control group for 1 year. The exercise group showed a significant decrease in body mass index, fasting glucose, HbA_{1c} and improved lipid profile. In addition, those in the exercise group using medication showed a decreasing trend in medication use whereas the control group showed an increasing trend. A study of shorter duration by Cauza *et al.* [140] also found improvements in HbA_{1c} and lipid profiles in a combined aerobic and resistance exercise intervention group in comparison to a sedentary control group.

In the Diabetes Aerobic and Resistance Exercise (DARE) trial [19], 251 previously sedentary individuals with T2DM were randomized into four arms: aerobic exercise training; resistance exercise training; combined aerobic and resistance exercise training; or a non-exercising control group. Intervention groups performed exercise three times per week for 6 months in community facilities, supervised by personal trainers. Improvements in glycemic control were found in all exercise groups, and the improvements in the combined aerobic and resistance exercise group were significantly greater than with either aerobic training or resistance training alone. In contrast to this, a smaller study with participants randomized to combined exercise, aerobic exercise or non-exercise control did not find significant differences between the two exercising groups [141]. In this smaller study, there was no provision to keep dietary intake and/or medication use the same among groups, and statistical power was far more limited than in the DARE trial.

In the Italian Diabetes and Exercise Study [142], 606 individuals with T2DM from 22 clinics in Italy were randomized to a full year of either exercise counseling alone or supervised facility-based combined aerobic and resistance exercise training twice weekly plus exercise counseling. The group receiving the combined aerobic and resistance exercise training had significantly more favorable results for glycemic control, lipids, body composition, blood pressure and estimated cardiovascular risk than the group receiving exercise counseling alone. This study provides compelling evidence for incremental benefits of supervised structured exercise over exercise counseling alone for people with T2DM.

Recommendations for exercise in diabetes

Most types of exercise can be recommended to both individuals with T1DM and T2DM. Exercise does not need to be strenuous, and even regular walking has beneficial effects [79,94]. Specific recommendations and guidelines for exercise in individuals with diabetes have been published by the American Diabetes Association [143,144] and the American College of Sports Medicine [145]. These and other guidelines are summarized in Tables 23.5–23.7. Advice should be tailored to individuals, taking

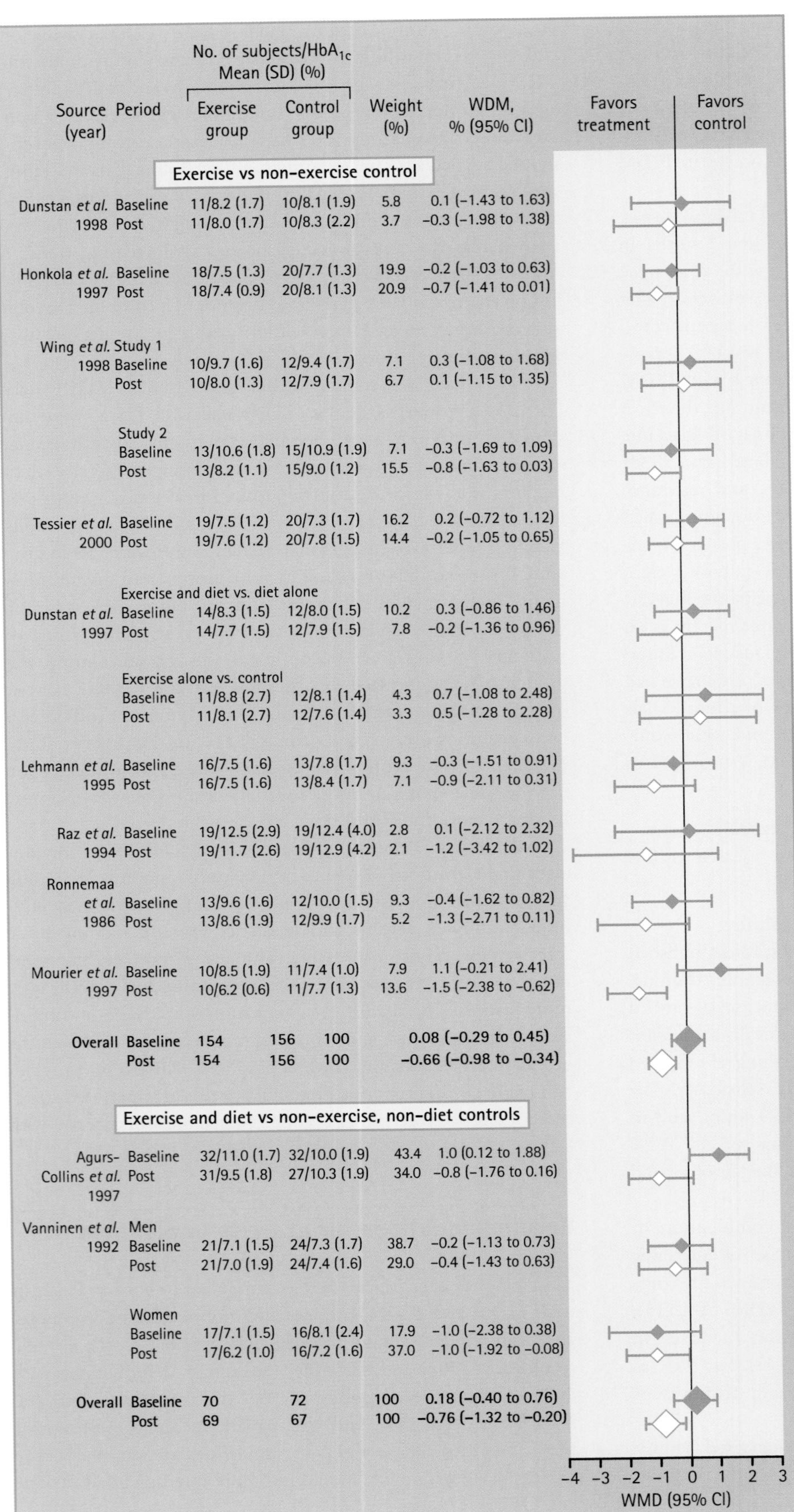

Figure 23.7 Meta-analysis of exercise interventions in type 2 diabetes and the effect of glycemic control, as measured by HbA_{1c}. CI, confidence interval; WMD, weighted mean difference. Studies are placed in ascending order of the intensity of the exercise intervention and represent the mean difference and the 95% CI for baseline and post-intervention measurements. Exercise vs. non-exercise control: baseline values, the chi-squared test for heterogeneity was 4.78 ($P = 0.91$) and the z score for overall effect was 0.45 ($P = 0.65$); post-intervention values, the chi-squared test for heterogeneity was 9.76 ($P = 0.46$) and the z score for overall effect was 4.01 ($P < 0.001$). Exercise and diet vs. control: baseline values, the chi-squared test for heterogeneity was 6.77 ($P = 0.03$) and the z score for overall effect was 0.60 ($P = 0.55$); post-intervention values, the chi-squared test for heterogeneity was 0.74 ($P = 0.69$) and the z score for overall effect was 2.66 ($P = 0\ 008$). The following equation should be used to convert HbA_{1c} to IFCC Units: DCCT result (%) = (0.0915 × IFCC result in mmol/mol) +2.15. Data from Boulé *et al.* [138].

Table 23.4 Clinical trials involving resistance exercise with people with type 2 diabetes mellitus.

Source	No. of Participants (n)	Sessions/week, no. of weeks	No. of exercises	No. of sets, rest interval and intensity of exercise	HbA_{1c} [Mean (SD)]
Type 2 diabetes – resistance training only					
Castaneda *et al.* (2002) [136]	n = 31 (resistance) n = 31 (control)	3 sessions/week; 16 weeks	3 lower and 2 upper body exercises	Control group: no exercise Intervention group: 3 sets of 8 reps at 60–80% 1RM	Control group: 8.4 (SE 0.3) to 8.3 (SE 0.5) Intervention group: 8.7 (SE 0.3) to 7.6 (SE 0.2)** (Note: all subjects were Hispanic-American)
Dunstan *et al.* (2002) [135]	n = 19 (resistance) n = 17 (control)	3 sessions/week; 26 weeks	1 core, 2 lower and 6 upper body exercises	Control group: 5 min cycling and 30 min of static stretching ("placebo exercise") Intervention group: 1) initial 3 sessions: 8–10 reps at 50–60% of 1-RM; 2) increased to 3 sets in the subsequent 3 sessions; and 3) 8–10 reps at 75–85% of 1-RM for the duration of the intervention	Control group (placebo exercise): decreased 0.4 (0.8) Intervention group (type 2 DM): decreased 1.2 (1.0)**† (Note: all subjects followed a moderate energy restriction diet)
Type 2 diabetes – combined aerobic and resistance exercise training					
Balducci *et al.* (2004) [139]	n = 62 (aerobic and resistance) n = 58 (control)	3 sessions/week; 52 wks	6 exercises for trunk, upper body and lower body for resistance exercise component	Control group: no exercise Intervention group: 30 minutes of aerobic activity at 40–80% HRR and 30 minutes of resistance exercise: 3 sets of 12 reps at 40–60% 1-RM	Control group: No significant change from baseline Intervention group: 8.31 (1.73) to 7.1 (1.16)‡
Cauza *et al.* (2006) [140]	n = 10 (aerobic and resistance) n = 10 (control)	3 sessions/week; 32 wks	1 core, 1 lower and 4 upper body exercises for resistance exercise component	Control: either aerobic or resistance exercise for the first 16 weeks, no exercise for the last 16 weeks Intervention group: either aerobic or resistance exercise for the first 16 weeks, combined exercise for the last 16 weeks Aerobic component consisted of 20–30 minutes of cycling (60% $\dot{V}O_{2peak}$). Resistance component consisted of 3 sets of 10–15 reps	Control group: Baseline: 8.1 (0.5) 16 wks: 7.5 (0.4) 32 wks: 8.7 (0.6)* Intervention group: Baseline: 8.1 (0.8) 16 weeks: 6.9 (0.4) 32 weeks: 6.2 (0.2)**

Continued on p. 370

Table 23.4 *Continued*

Source	No. of Participants (n)	Sessions/week, no. of weeks	No. of exercises	No. of sets, rest interval and intensity of exercise	HbA_{1c} [Mean (SD)]
Cuff *et al.* (2003) [166]	n = 10 (aerobic and resistance) n = 9 (aerobic only) n = 9 (control)	3 sessions/week; 16 wks	3 lower and 2 upper body exercises for resistance exercise component	Control group: no exercise Combined group: total duration of 75 min. Aerobic component: 60–75% HRR and resistance exercise component: 2 sets of 12 reps Aerobic group: 75 minutes at 60–75% HRR	Control group: decreased 0.03 Combined group: decreased 0.1 (0.22) Aerobic group: 0.1 (0.11)
Lambers *et al.* (2008) [141]	n = 17 (aerobic and resistance) n = 18 (aerobic) n = 11 (control)	3 sessions/week; 12 wks	Unavailable	Control group: no exercise Aerobic group: 60–85% HRR Combined group: aerobic component plus 3 sets of 10–15 reps at 60–85% of 1-RM for the resistance component	Control group: 6.7 (0.97) to 7.0 (0.88) Aerobic group: 7.4 (1.70) to 7.0 (1.61) Combined group: 7.4 (1.45) to 6.9 (1.20)*
Loimalaa *et al.* (2003) [115]	n = 24 (aerobic and resistance) n = 25 (control)	2 sessions/week; 12 months	8 for trunk, upper body and lower body exercises for resistance exercise component	Control group: no exercise Combined group: 3 sets of 10–12 reps at 70–80% of 1-RM for resistance component plus 65–75% $\dot{V}O_{2max}$ for aerobic exercise component	Control group: 8.0 (1.3) to 8.3 (1.4) Combined group: 8.2 (2.1) to 7.6 (1.4)**
Sigal *et al.* (2007) [19]	n = 64 (aerobic and resistance) n = 60 (aerobic) n = 64 (resistance) n = 63 (control)	3 sessions/week; 26 weeks	1 core, 2 lower and 4 upper body exercises for resistance exercise component	Control group: no exercise Aerobic group: 15–45 min at 60–75% HR_{max} Resistance group: 2–3 sets of 7–9 reps Combined group: aerobic component plus resistance training component	Control group: 7.44 (1.38) to 7.51 (1.47), significant difference of change $P < 0.05$ from aerobic group and resistance group Aerobic group: 7.41 (1.50) to 6.98 (1.50)**, significant difference of change $P < 0.05$ from combined group Resistance group: 7.48 (1.47) to 7.18 (1.52)**, significant difference of change $P = 0.001$ from combined group Combined group: 7.46 (1.48) to 6.56 (1.55)[†], significant difference of change $P < 0.05$ compared to aerobic training group and $P = 0.001$ compared to resistance training group

HR_{max}, maximum heart rate; HRR, heart rate reserve; $\dot{V}O_{2max}$, maximal oxygen uptake; 1-RM, maximum weight that can be lifted once.
* Indicates significant difference from baseline at $P < 0.05$.
** Indicates significant difference of change compared to control group at $P < 0.05$.
[†] Indicates significant difference from baseline at $P < 0.01$.
[‡] Indicates significant difference from baseline at $P < 0.0001$.
The following equation should be used to convert HbA_{1c} to IFCC Units: DCCT result (%) = (0.0915 × IFCC result in mmol/mol) +2.15.

Table 23.5 Exercise recommendations.

Aerobic training				Resistance training		
Reference	**Frequency**	**Intensity**	**Duration**	**Frequency**	**No. of exercises**	**Sets/Repetitions**
Healthy/sedentary adults						
2008 CDC Guidelines [1]	At least 3 days/ week	Moderate/vigorous	Accumulate 150 min/week of continuous moderate activity or 75 min/week of intense activity	At least 2 days/week	Involve all major muscle groups	At least 1 set of 8–12 reps, 2–3 sets preferable
2007 ACSM/AHA [146]	3–5 days/wk	Moderate/vigorous Start at lower intensity if initially unfit or sedentary	30–60 min of moderate aerobic activities or 20–30 min vigorous aerobic activity. Can be accumulated in bouts lasting >10 min	2 days/week (non-consecutive)	8–10 exercises involving major muscle groups	1 set, 8–12 reps
Elderly persons (65 or older)						
2007 ACSM/AHA Physical Activity Guidelines [147]	3–5 days/week	Moderate/vigorous	30–60 min of moderate aerobic activities or 20–30 minutes of vigorous aerobic activity Can be accumulated in bouts lasting >10 min	2 days/week (non-consecutive	8–10 exercises involving major muscle groups	1 set, 10–15 reps
Cardiac patients						
1995 AHA Exercise Standards [167]	Minimum 3–5 days/week	50–60% $\dot{V}O_{2max}$ or HRR	Minimum of 30 min of continuous physical activity	2–3 days/week	8–10 exercises involving major muscle groups	1 set, 10–15 reps
2006 AACVPR [168]	3–5 days/week	50–60% $\dot{V}O_{2max}$ or HRR	30–45 min of continuous or intermittent aerobic activity	2–3 days/week	Incorporate all major muscle groups	1 set, 10–15 reps
Individuals with type 2 diabetes						
2006 ADA Consensus Statement on Physical Activity/ Exercise and Type 2 Diabetes [144]	3–5 days/week No more than 2 consecutive days without exercise	50–70% HR_{max} (moderate) or >70% HR_{max} (vigorous)	at least 150 min/week of moderate aerobic exercise and/ or at least 90 min/week of vigorous aerobic exercise	3 days/week	Targeting all major muscle groups	Progressing to 3 sets of 8–10 reps

AACVPR, American Association of Cardiovascular and Pulmonary Rehabilitation; ACSM, American College of Sports Medicine, ADA, American Diabetes Association; AHA, American Heart Association; CDC, Centers for Disease Control.

Table 23.6 Precautions and advice regarding exercise in diabetes.

Relative contraindications

- If receiving insulin treatment: sports in which hypoglycemia would be dangerous (e.g. diving, climbing, single-handed sailing, motor racing). Individuals participating in this type of sport must test the capillary blood glucose concentration very frequently and take strict measures to avoid hypoglycemia. Whenever possible, another person should be close by and able to assist when needed. Note that the Amateur International Boxing Association prohibits people with insulin-requiring diabetes from participating in boxing
- With untreated proliferative retinopathy: very strenuous exercise, because of the risk of hemorrhage. However, a patient whose retinopathy has been adequately treated with laser therapy and is regularly followed by a retinal specialist can probably undertake strenuous exercise without undue risk

Cautions

Cardiovascular disease: there is a high prevalence of this in middle-aged and older people with diabetes. Middle aged and older individuals with diabetes wishing to undertake exercise more vigorous than brisk walking should probably first have a maximal exercise stress test with continuous electrocardiography monitoring. Patients with abnormal stress test results should be referred for additional cardiac investigations

Table 23.7 Guidelines for exercise diabetes mellitus.

General guidelines

- Exercise used to reduce weight should be combined with dietary measures
- Moderate intensity aerobic exercise should be part of the daily schedule if possible, accumulating 150 minutes each week. More vigorous exercise (≥70% of $\dot{V}O_{2max}$) undertaken 3–5 times per week will provide additional health benefits. Previously sedentary patients may have to build up exercise volume gradually, starting with as little as 5–10 min/day
- Multiple shorter exercise sessions lasting at least 10 min each in the course of a day are probably as useful as a single longer session of equivalent length and intensity
- Include low intensity warm-up and cool-down periods especially if vigorous exercise is undertaken
- Exercise should be appropriate to the person's general physical condition and lifestyle
- Resistance exercise performed 2–3 times per week will provide benefits over and above those of aerobic training. The studies reporting greatest impact of resistance exercise on HbA_{1c} have had subjects progress to 3 sets of approximately 8 resistance type exercises at relatively high intensity (8 repetitions performed at the maximum weight that can be lifted 8 times)
- Use proper footwear and, if appropriate, other protective equipment
- Avoid exercise in extreme heat or cold
- Inspect feet before and after exercise

Specific considerations for exercise in type 1 diabetes

Avoid hypoglycemia during exercise by:

- Avoiding heavy exercise during peak insulin action
- Using non-exercising sites for insulin injection
- If using multiple daily injections reducing pre-exercise insulin dosages by 20–50% or more if necessary. If using an insulin pump, decrease basal rate and/or amount of last bolus before exercise. These reductions should be individualized and based on blood glucose monitoring; not all individuals will require an insulin dose reduction
- Monitor glycemia before, during and after exercise as necessary
- Taking extra carbohydrate before and hourly during exercise. This amount should be individualized and based on blood glucose monitoring
- After prolonged exercise, monitor glycemia and take extra carbohydrate to avoid delayed hypoglycemia. The quantity required can be estimated using the semi-quantitative technique (1 g CHO/kg body weight/hour of activity) or by consulting tables of energy requirements for particular activities
- Use extra caution in monitoring glycemia if exercise is being performed within 24 hours of a hypoglycemic episode

Specific considerations for exercise in type 2 diabetes

- Hypoglycemia is less common during exercise than in type 1 diabetes, and extra carbohydrate is therefore usually unnecessary
- Patients taking insulin or sulfonylureas may need to reduce the doses of these medications during days when they exercise. Such adjustments should be guided by glucose monitoring

into account their interests, personal goals, levels of fitness, possible contraindications and available resources. If the patient is interested in sports or is even a professional athlete, diabetes should not interfere with his or her athletic career, and treatment should be adjusted according to the demands of the activity. For activities and competitions considered to be higher risk for individuals with insulin-treated diabetes (e.g. car racing, flying, boxing), individual governing bodies should be consulted regarding restrictions in competition. It is also important to note that insulin is considered a banned substance by the World Anti-Doping Agency, and that elite level athletes with diabetes will be required to apply for a Therapeutic Use Exemption certificate prior to competition.

Aerobic training

It is generally recommended that all individuals accumulate at least 150 minutes of moderate aerobic activity, and/or at least 90 minutes of vigorous aerobic exercise every week, and that this activity be spread over at least 3–5 days [143,146,147]. A day's activity need not occur in a single session, but may be accumulated in bouts of 10 or more minutes at a time, performed throughout the day. Performing progressively greater amounts of moderate activity (in excess of the minimum 150 minutes) is associated with progressively greater benefits. Studies have also shown that group exercise environments can provide motivation, social support and enjoyment for individuals starting and maintaining exercise training programs [148].

Resistance training

A recent meta-analysis showed that resistance exercise can be safe and effective even for vulnerable cardiac patients [149]. High intensity weightlifting in healthy older men (mean age 64 years) caused less circulatory stress than walking up 192 stairs [150]. Weightlifting was not associated with increased proliferative retinopathy risk in the Wisconsin Epidemiologic Study of Diabetic Retinopathy, although the statistical power of the study was limited [151]. When properly performed, resistance training can be safe and enjoyable while at the same time producing significant health benefits.

Resistance training programs should be progressive in nature. Previously sedentary individuals should always start with a low intensity workload. It is important that individuals receive proper instruction on lifting and breathing techniques used during resistance training in order to maximize the benefits of the exercise, while at the same time minimizing the risk of injury. The authors recommend that beginners use weight machines in the initial stages of a training program, before moving on to free-weight exercise once sufficient strength has been gained and appropriate lifting techniques have been mastered [21]. Warming up before each training session with low intensity aerobic activity or light sets of selected exercises is also thought to help minimize the risk of injury [21]. When multiple exercises are performed in a workout, exercises involving the use of large muscle groups (e.g. lunges or pull-downs) should be performed before exercises requiring the use of smaller muscle groups (e.g. calf raises or bicep curls). Multiple joint exercises such as squats, chest press or seated row should precede single joint exercises such as leg extensions or tricep extensions [21]. Although one set of each exercise may be sufficient to increase muscle strength [152], the resistance exercise studies with the greatest HbA_{1c} reductions [63,153,154] have used three or more sets of each exercise. The authors therefore suggest that three sets of each exercise be performed on three non-consecutive days per week (assuming the same muscle groups are being targeted) to ensure the best possible metabolic benefits [1,143,146,147].

Special considerations in people with long-term complications of diabetes

Some advanced long-term complications of diabetes may limit individuals' ability to perform certain types of exercise safely, but should not prevent them from becoming active at all. Where proliferative or severe non-proliferative retinopathy is present, it has been suggested that individuals may want to avoid vigorous activity (both aerobic and resistance) because of the possible increased risk of triggering vitreous hemorrhage or retinal detachment [155]. Mild to moderate activity can still be encouraged for these individuals. In individuals with peripheral neuropathy, weight-bearing activity could, in theory, increase the risk of skin breakdown and infection as well as Charcot joint destruction [156,157]; however, a recent study showed that the incidence of foot ulcers was no greater in individuals with diabetic neuropathy than in individuals without neuropathy after a 6-month walking intervention [158]. As exercise training is important in delaying the progression of peripheral neuropathy [26], it can be recommended that these individuals stay active by walking, swimming or bicycling. Before changing or adding activities for individuals with autonomic neuropathy, it is generally recommended that these individuals undergo cardiac investigation [159,160], as the risk of CVD in such individuals is high. Decreased cardiac responsiveness to exercise, postural hypotension, unpredictable carbohydrate delivery increasing the risk of hypoglycemia where gastroparesis is present and impaired thermoregulation have all been associated with autonomic neuropathy, warranting caution in the practice of certain activities in this population [157]. The authors know of no evidence justifying any specific exercise restrictions in nephropathy.

Insulin and oral hypoglycemic agent adjustments for exercise

In individuals with T1DM or T2DM treated with multiple insulin injections, the dosage of short-acting insulin taken before exercise can be reduced instead of using dietary adjustment. The amount of such reduction, if required, should be tailored to each individual, based on blood glucose monitoring results before, during and after exercise, at least until the pattern of glucose response to exercise for that individual is known. Depending on the intensity and duration of exercise, the reduction required can be as much as 75% of the usual dose [30], although dose reductions of 20–50% are more typical. The insulin formulation (short- or intermediate-acting) to be reduced is that which has its maximal action at the time of exercise. For brief, very intense exercise such as competitive hockey, weightlifting or sprinting, there may be no need to reduce insulin dose. If the blood glucose concentration increases during exercise, the insulin dosage may need to be slightly increased or the injection schedule changed in order to achieve higher plasma insulin concentrations during exercise. Use of an insulin pump may be advantageous for many physically active individuals, as circulating insulin levels can be more easily adjusted to accommodate meals, snacks and exercise [161]. The variability of glucose absorption is also generally decreased, lowering the risk of hypoglycemia [161]. Decreases in insulin for pump users may or may not need to be accompanied by carbohydrate supplementation [161].

In individuals with T2DM, exercise does not usually cause hypoglycemia, and in obese individuals it can be a valuable tool to improve glycemic control and assist with weight maintenance. For these reasons, carbohydrate supplementation is usually unnecessary with exercise (Table 23.7). If blood glucose declines rapidly during exercise, as may occur in individuals taking oral hypoglycemic agents or insulin, the dosage of the drug should be reduced or the drug withheld on exercising days.

Carbohydrate supplementation

There are few controlled studies regarding the appropriate type and amount of carbohydrates to be taken with exercise in people with T1DM. A reasonable starting point is to take approximately 15 g carbohydrate before and 15–40 g at 30–60-minute intervals during longer exercise sessions. Supplementation should be advised if pre-exercise blood glucose levels are <5.6 mmol/L. The amount of carbohydrate consumed should be adjusted according to blood glucose monitoring results; some individuals will not require any carbohydrate supplementation whereas some will require large amounts. During strenuous exercise, at least part of this can be taken as a sucrose-containing beverage. If exercise is performed post-prandially, there is less need for carbohydrate supplementation, whereas larger snacks should be taken if some hours have elapsed since the last meal. Also, the risk of hypoglycemia and subsequent need for exogenous carbohydrate supplementation decreases as the amount of time since the last insulin injection increases [162,163].

A recent review by Perkins & Riddell [161] describes several methods of carbohydrate supplementation. The goal is for the patient to consume a quantity of oral carbohydrate that matches the amount of glucose being used by the working muscles during activity. This can involve either a basic approach (where 15–30 g of carbohydrate is consumed for every 30–60 minutes of exercise), a semi-quantitative approach (consuming approximately 1 g glucose/kg body weight/hour of activity) or a quantitative method, based on standardized tables of energy requirements for specific activities, intensities and individual body weights [161]. The latter is referred to as "excarbs" (extra carbohydrates for exercise), developed originally by Walsh & Roberts [164]. However, it should be noted that only a finite amount of carbohydrate (40–60 g/hour) can be absorbed while the body is moderately or vigorously active [165], requiring that a certain amount of the carbohydrate be consumed prior to exercise or during recovery. Regular glucose monitoring is still recommended, especially where the participant is experimenting with new types, intensities or durations of exercise training.

Acknowledgments

The authors are grateful for the contributions of Veiko Koivisto to this chapter in previous editions of this textbook. Jane Yardley was supported by a Doctoral Student Award from the Canadian Diabetes Association and funds from the Ottawa Hospital Research Institute Research Chair in Lifestyle Research. Glen Kenny holds a University Research Chair from the University of Ottawa. Ronald Sigal is a Senior Health Scholar of the Alberta Heritage Foundation for Medical Research.

References

1 Physical Activity Guidelines Advisory Committee. *Physical Activity Guidelines Advisory Committee Report, 2008*. Washington, DC: US Department of Health and Human Services, 2008.

2 Ahlborg G, Felig P, Hagenfeldt L, Hendler R, Wahren J. Substrate turnover during prolonged exercise in man: splanchnic and leg metabolism of glucose, free fatty acids, and amino acids. *J Clin Invest* 1974; **53**:1080–1090.

3 Wasserman DH, Davis SN, Zinman B. Fuel metabolism during exercise in health and diabetes. In: Ruderman N, Devlin JT, Schneider SH, eds. *Handbook of Exercise in Diabetes*. Alexandria, VA: American Diabetes Association, 2002:63–99.

4 Felig P, Cherif A, Minagawa A, Wahren J. Hypoglycemia during prolonged exercise in normal men. *N Engl J Med* 1982; **306**:895–900.

5 Koivisto VA, Yki-Jarvinen H, DeFronzo RA. Physical training and insulin sensitivity. *Diabetes Metab Rev* 1986; **1**:445–481.

6 DeFronzo RA, Sherwin RS, Kraemer N. Effect of physical training on insulin action in obesity. *Diabetes* 1987; **36**:1379–1385.

7 Halbert JA, Silagy CA, Finucane P, Withers RT, Hamdorf PA. Exercise training and blood lipids in hyperlipidemic and normolipidemic adults: a meta-analysis of randomized, controlled trials. *Eur J Clin Nutr* 1999; **53**:514–522.

8 Miller TD, Balady GJ, Fletcher GF. Exercise and its role in the prevention and rehabilitation of cardiovascular disease. *Ann Behav Med* 1997; **19**:220–229.

9 Despres JP, Lamarche B. Low-intensity endurance exercise training, plasma lipoproteins and the risk of coronary heart disease. *J Intern Med* 1994; **236**:7–22.

10 Calles J, Cunningham JJ, Nelson L, Brown N, Nadel E, Sherwin RS, *et al.* Glucose turnover during recovery from intensive exercise. *Diabetes* 1983; **32**:734–738.

11 Kjaer M, Farrell PA, Christensen NJ, Galbo H. Increased epinephrine response and inaccurate glucoregulation in exercising athletes. *J Appl Physiol* 1986; **61**:1693–1700.

12 Marliss EB, Sigal RJ, Miles PDG, *et al.* Glucoregulation in intense exercise, and its implications for persons with diabetes mellitus. In: Kawamori R, Vranic M, Horton E, Kubota M, eds. *Glucose Fluxes, Exercise and Diabetes*. London: Smith Gordon/Nishimura, 1995:55–66.

13 Kamel HK. Sarcopenia and aging. *Nutr Rev* 2003; **61**:157–167.

14 Doherty TJ. The influence of aging and sex on skeletal muscle mass and strength. *Curr Opin Clin Nutr Metab Care* 2001; **4**:503–508.

15 Lynch NA, Metter EJ, Lindle RS, Fozard JL, Tobin JD, Roy TA, *et al.* Muscle quality. I. Age-associated differences between arm and leg muscle groups. *J Appl Physiol* 1999; **86**:188–194.

16 Kenny GP, Yardley JE, Martineau L, Jay O. Physical work capacity in older adults: implications for the aging worker. *Am J Ind Med* 2008; **51**:610–625.

17 Lemmer JT, Hurlbut DE, Martel GF, Tracy BL, Ivey FM, Metter EJ, *et al.* Age and gender responses to strength training and detraining. *Med Sci Sports Exerc* 2000; **32**:1505–1512.

18 Tracy BL, Ivey FM, Hurlbut D, Martel GF, Lemmer JT, Siegel EL, *et al.* Muscle quality. II. Effects Of strength training in 65- to 75-yr-old men and women. *J Appl Physiol* 1999; **86**:195–201.

19 Sigal RJ, Kenny GP, Boule NG, Wells GA, Prud'homme D, Fortier M, *et al.* Effects of aerobic training, resistance training, or both on glycemic control in type 2 diabetes: a randomized trial. *Ann Intern Med* 2007; **147**:357–369.

20 Bellew JW, Symons TB, Vandervoort AA. Geriatric fitness: effects of aging and recommendations for exercise in older adults. *Cardiopulm Phys Ther J* 2005; **16**:20–31.

21 American College of Sports Medicine position stand. Progression models in resistance training for healthy adults. *Med Sci Sports Exerc* 2009; **41**:687–708.

22 Jacobs I, Tesch PA, Bar-Or O, Karlsson J, Dotan R. Lactate in human skeletal muscle after 10 and 30 s of supramaximal exercise. *J Appl Physiol* 1983; **55**:365–367.

23 Vanhelder WP, Goode RC, Radomski MW. Effect of anaerobic and aerobic exercise of equal duration and work expenditure on plasma growth hormone levels. *Eur J Appl Physiol Occup Physiol* 1984; **52**:255–257.

24 Tesch PA, Colliander EB, Kaiser P. Muscle metabolism during intense, heavy-resistance exercise. *Eur J Appl Physiol Occup Physiol* 1986; **55**:362–366.

25 Moy CS, Songer TJ, LaPorte RE, Dorman JS, Kriska AM, Orchard TJ, *et al.* Insulin-dependent diabetes mellitus, physical activity, and death. *Am J Epidemiol* 1993; **137**:74–81.

26 Balducci S, Iacobellis G, Parisi L, Di Biase N, Calandriello E, Leonetti F, *et al.* Exercise training can modify the natural history of diabetic peripheral neuropathy. *J Diabetes Complications* 2006; **20**:216–223.

27 Kriska AM, LaPorte RE, Patrick SL, Kuller LH, Orchard TJ. The association of physical activity and diabetic complications in individuals with insulin-dependent diabetes mellitus: the Epidemiology of Diabetes Complications Study: VII. *J Clin Epidemiol* 1991; **44**:1207–1214.

28 Waden J, Forsblom C, Thorn LM, Saraheimo M, Rosengard-Barlund M, Heikkila O, *et al.* Physical activity and diabetes complications in patients with type 1 diabetes: the Finnish Diabetic Nephropathy (FinnDiane) Study. *Diabetes Care* 2008; **31**:230–232.

29 Waden J, Tikkanen H, Forsblom C, Fagerudd J, Pettersson-Fernholm K, Lakka T, *et al.* Leisure time physical activity is associated with poor glycemic control in type 1 diabetic women: the FinnDiane study. *Diabetes Care* 2005; **28**:777–782.

30 Rabasa-Lhoret R, Bourque J, Ducros F, Chiasson JL. Guidelines for premeal insulin dose reduction for postprandial exercise of different intensities and durations in type 1 diabetic subjects treated intensively with a basal-bolus insulin regimen (ultralente, lispro). *Diabetes Care* 2001; **24**:625–630.

31 Yki-Jarvinen H, Koivisto VA. Natural course of insulin resistance in type I diabetes. *N Engl J Med* 1986; **315**:224–230.
32 Koivisto VA, Leirisalo-Repo M, Ebeling P, Tuominen JA, Knip M, Turunen U, *et al.* Seven years of remission in a type I diabetic patient. *Diabetes Care* 1993; **16**:990–995.
33 Stratton R, Wilson DP, Endres RK, Goldstein DE. Improved glycemic control after supervised 8-wk exercise program in insulin-dependent diabetic adolescents. *Diabetes Care* 1987; **10**:589–593.
34 Laaksonen DE, Atalay M, Niskanen LK, Mustonen J, Sen CK, Lakka TA, *et al.* Aerobic exercise and the lipid profile in type 1 diabetic men: a randomized controlled trial. *Med Sci Sports Exerc* 2000; **32**:1541–1548.
35 Wallberg-Henriksson H, Gunnarsson R, Rossner S, Wahren J. Long-term physical training in female type 1 (insulin-dependent) diabetic patients: absence of significant effect on glycaemic control and lipoprotein levels. *Diabetologia* 1986; **29**:53–57.
36 Yki-Jarvinen H, DeFronzo RA, Koivisto VA. Normalization of insulin sensitivity in type I diabetic subjects by physical training during insulin pump therapy. *Diabetes Care* 1984; **7**:520–527.
37 Wallberg-Henriksson H, Gunnarsson R, Henriksson J, DeFronzo R, Felig P, Ostman J, *et al.* Increased peripheral insulin sensitivity and muscle mitochondrial enzymes but unchanged blood glucose control in type I diabetics after physical training. *Diabetes* 1982; **31**:1044–1050.
38 Jenni S, Oetliker C, Allemann S, Ith M, Tappy L, Wuerth S, *et al.* Fuel metabolism during exercise in euglycaemia and hyperglycaemia in patients with type 1 diabetes mellitus: a prospective single-blinded randomised crossover trial. *Diabetologia* 2008; **51**:1457–1465.
39 Shilo S, Sotsky M, Shamoon H. Islet hormonal regulation of glucose turnover during exercise in type 1 diabetes. *J Clin Endocrinol Metab* 1990; **70**:162–172.
40 Robitaille M, Dube MC, Weisnagel SJ, Prud'homme D, Massicotte D, Peronnet F, *et al.* Substrate source utilization during moderate intensity exercise with glucose ingestion in type 1 diabetic patients. *J Appl Physiol* 2007; **103**:119–124.
41 Chokkalingam K, Tsintzas K, Norton L, Jewell K, Macdonald IA, Mansell PI. Exercise under hyperinsulinaemic conditions increases whole-body glucose disposal without affecting muscle glycogen utilisation in type 1 diabetes. *Diabetologia* 2007; **50**:414–421.
42 Petersen KF, Price TB, Bergeron R. Regulation of net hepatic glycogenolysis and gluconeogenesis during exercise: impact of type 1 diabetes. *J Clin Endocrinol Metab* 2004; **89**:4656–4664.
43 Meinders AE, Willekens FL, Heere LP. Metabolic and hormonal changes in IDDM during long-distance run. *Diabetes Care* 1988; **11**:1–7.
44 Tuominen JA, Ebeling P, Vuorinen-Markkola H, Koivisto VA. Post-marathon paradox in IDDM: unchanged insulin sensitivity in spite of glycogen depletion. *Diabet Med* 1997; **14**:301–308.
45 Sane T, Helve E, Pelkonen R, Koivisto VA. The adjustment of diet and insulin dose during long-term endurance exercise in type 1 (insulin-dependent) diabetic men. *Diabetologia* 1988; **31**:35–40.
46 Sandoval DA, Guy DL, Richardson MA, Ertl AC, Davis SN. Acute, same-day effects of antecedent exercise on counterregulatory responses to subsequent hypoglycemia in type 1 diabetes mellitus. *Am J Physiol Endocrinol Metab* 2006; **290**:E1331–E1338.
47 Galassetti P, Tate D, Neill RA, Richardson A, Leu SY, Davis SN. Effect of differing antecedent hypoglycemia on counterregulatory responses to exercise in type 1 diabetes. *Am J Physiol Endocrinol Metab* 2006; **290**:E1109–E1117.
48 Davis SN, Galassetti P, Wasserman DH, Tate D. Effects of antecedent hypoglycemia on subsequent counterregulatory responses to exercise. *Diabetes* 2000; **49**:73–81.
49 Galassetti P, Tate D, Neill RA, Morrey S, Wasserman DH, Davis SN. Effect of antecedent hypoglycemia on counterregulatory responses to subsequent euglycemic exercise in type 1 diabetes. *Diabetes* 2003; **52**:1761–1769.
50 Sandoval DA, Guy DL, Richardson MA, Ertl AC, Davis SN. Effects of low and moderate antecedent exercise on counterregulatory responses to subsequent hypoglycemia in type 1 diabetes. *Diabetes* 2004; **53**:1798–1806.
51 Ebeling P, Tuominen JA, Bourey R, Koranyi L, Koivisto VA. Athletes with IDDM exhibit impaired metabolic control and increased lipid utilization with no increase in insulin sensitivity. *Diabetes* 1995; **44**:471–477.
52 Purdon C, Brousson M, Nyveen SL, Miles PD, Halter JB, Vranic M, *et al.* The roles of insulin and catecholamines in the glucoregulatory response during intense exercise and early recovery in insulin-dependent diabetic and control subjects. *J Clin Endocrinol Metab* 1993; **76**:566–573.
53 Sigal RJ, Fisher SJ, Manzon A, Morais JA, Halter JB, Vranic M, *et al.* Glucoregulation during and after intense exercise: effects of alpha-adrenergic blockade. *Metabolism* 2000; **49**:386–394.
54 Sigal RJ, Fisher S, Halter JB, Vranic M, Marliss EB. The roles of catecholamines in glucoregulation in intense exercise as defined by the islet cell clamp technique. *Diabetes* 1996; **45**:148–156.
55 Sigal RJ, Fisher SJ, Halter JB, Vranic M, Marliss EB. Glucoregulation during and after intense exercise: effects of beta-adrenergic blockade in subjects with type 1 diabetes mellitus. *J Clin Endocrinol Metab* 1999; **84**:3961–3971.
56 Sigal RJ, Purdon C, Fisher SJ, Halter JB, Vranic M, Marliss EB. Hyperinsulinemia prevents prolonged hyperglycemia after intense exercise in insulin-dependent diabetic subjects. *J Clin Endocrinol Metab* 1994; **79**:1049–1057.
57 Bussau VA, Ferreira LD, Jones TW, Fournier PA. The 10-s maximal sprint: a novel approach to counter an exercise-mediated fall in glycemia in individuals with type 1 diabetes. *Diabetes Care* 2006; **29**:601–606.
58 Bussau VA, Ferreira LD, Jones TW, Fournier PA. A 10-s sprint performed prior to moderate-intensity exercise prevents early post-exercise fall in glycaemia in individuals with type 1 diabetes. *Diabetologia* 2007; **50**:1815–1818.
59 Guelfi KJ, Jones TW, Fournier PA. The decline in blood glucose levels is less with intermittent high-intensity compared with moderate exercise in individuals with type 1 diabetes. *Diabetes Care* 2005; **28**:1289–1294.
60 Guelfi KJ, Jones TW, Fournier PA. Intermittent high-intensity exercise does not increase the risk of early postexercise hypoglycemia in individuals with type 1 diabetes. *Diabetes Care* 2005; **28**:416–418.
61 Guelfi KJ, Ratnam N, Smythe GA, Jones TW, Fournier PA. Effect of intermittent high-intensity compared with continuous moderate exercise on glucose production and utilization in individuals with type 1 diabetes. *Am J Physiol Endocrinol Metab* 2007; **292**:E865–E870.
62 Iscoe KE, Campbell JE, Jamnik V, Perkins BA, Riddell MC. Efficacy of continuous real-time blood glucose monitoring during and after prolonged high-intensity cycling exercise: spinning with a continuous glucose monitoring system. *Diabetes Technol Ther* 2006; **8**:627–635.

63 Durak EP, Jovanovic-Peterson L, Peterson CM. Randomized crossover study of effect of resistance training on glycemic control, muscular strength, and cholesterol in type I diabetic men. *Diabetes Care* 1990; **13**:1039–1043.
64 Ramalho AC, de Lourdes Lima M, Nunes F, Cambui Z, Barbosa C, Andrade A, *et al.* The effect of resistance versus aerobic training on metabolic control in patients with type 1 diabetes mellitus. *Diabetes Res Clin Pract* 2006; **72**:271–276.
65 Peterson CM, Jones RL, Dupuis A, Levine BS, Bernstein R, O'Shea M. Feasibility of improved blood glucose control in patients with insulin-dependent diabetes mellitus. *Diabetes Care* 1979; **2**:329–335.
66 Peterson CM, Jones RL, Esterly JA, Wantz GE, Jackson RL. Changes in basement membrane thickening and pulse volume concomitant with improved glucose control and exercise in patients with insulin-dependent diabetes mellitus. *Diabetes Care* 1980; **3**:586–589.
67 Mosher PE, Nash MS, Perry AC, LaPerriere AR, Goldberg RB. Aerobic circuit exercise training: effect on adolescents with well-controlled insulin-dependent diabetes mellitus. *Arch Phys Med Rehabil* 1998; **79**:652–657.
68 French DN, Kraemer WJ, Volek JS, Spiering BA, Judelson DA, Hoffman JR, *et al.* Anticipatory responses of catecholamines on muscle force production. *J Appl Physiol* 2007; **102**:94–102.
69 Helmrich SP, Ragland DR, Leung RW, Paffenbarger RS Jr. Physical activity and reduced occurrence of non-insulin-dependent diabetes mellitus. *N Engl J Med* 1991; **325**:147–152.
70 Manson JE, Rimm EB, Stampfer MJ, Colditz GA, Willett WC, Krolewski AS, *et al.* Physical activity and incidence of non-insulin-dependent diabetes mellitus in women. *Lancet* 1991; **338**:774–778.
71 Manson JE, Nathan DM, Krolewski AS, Stampfer MJ, Willett WC, Hennekens CH. A prospective study of exercise and incidence of diabetes among US male physicians. *JAMA* 1992; **268**:63–67.
72 Burchfiel CM, Sharp DS, Curb JD, Rodriguez BL, Hwang LJ, Marcus EB, *et al.* Physical activity and incidence of diabetes: the Honolulu Heart Program. *Am J Epidemiol* 1995; **141**:360–368.
73 Perry IJ, Wannamethee SG, Walker MK, Thomson AG, Whincup PH, Shaper AG. Prospective study of risk factors for development of non-insulin dependent diabetes in middle aged British men. *Br Med J* 1995; **310**:560–564.
74 Gurwitz JH, Field TS, Glynn RJ, Manson JE, Avorn J, Taylor JO, *et al.* Risk factors for non-insulin-dependent diabetes mellitus requiring treatment in the elderly. *J Am Geriatr Soc* 1994; **42**:1235–1240.
75 Schranz A, Tuomilehto J, Marti B, Jarrett RJ, Grabauskas V, Vassallo A. Low physical activity and worsening of glucose tolerance: results from a 2-year follow-up of a population sample in Malta. *Diabetes Res Clin Pract* 1991; **11**:127–136.
76 Lynch J, Helmrich SP, Lakka TA, Kaplan GA, Cohen RD, Salonen R, *et al.* Moderately intense physical activities and high levels of cardiorespiratory fitness reduce the risk of non-insulin-dependent diabetes mellitus in middle-aged men. *Arch Intern Med* 1996; **156**:1307–1314.
77 Hu FB, Sigal RJ, Rich-Edwards JW, Colditz GA, Solomon CG, Willett WC, *et al.* Walking compared with vigorous physical activity and risk of type 2 diabetes in women: a prospective study. *JAMA* 1999; **282**:1433–1439.
78 Wei M, Gibbons LW, Mitchell TL, Kampert JB, Lee CD, Blair SN. The association between cardiorespiratory fitness and impaired fasting glucose and type 2 diabetes mellitus in men. *Ann Intern Med* 1999; **130**:89–96. [Published erratum appears in *Ann Intern Med* 1999; 131:394.]
79 Wei M, Gibbons LW, Kampert JB, Nichaman MZ, Blair SN. Low cardiorespiratory fitness and physical inactivity as predictors of mortality in men with type 2 diabetes. *Ann Intern Med* 2000; **132**:605–611.
80 Villegas R, Shu XO, Li H, Yang G, Matthews CE, Leitzmann M, *et al.* Physical activity and the incidence of type 2 diabetes in the Shanghai women's health study. *Int J Epidemiol* 2006; **35**:1553–1562.
81 Krause MP, Hallage T, Gama MP, Goss FL, Robertson R, da Silva SG. Association of adiposity, cardiorespiratory fitness and exercise practice with the prevalence of type 2 diabetes in Brazilian elderly women. *Int J Med Sci* 2007; **4**:288–292.
82 Eriksson KF, Lindgarde F. Prevention of type 2 (non-insulin-dependent) diabetes mellitus by diet and physical exercise: the 6-year Malmo feasibility study. *Diabetologia* 1991; **34**:891–898.
83 Pan XR, Li GW, Hu YH, Wang JX, Yang WY, An ZX, *et al.* Effects of diet and exercise in preventing NIDDM in people with impaired glucose tolerance: the Da Qing IGT and Diabetes Study. *Diabetes Care* 1997; **20**:537–544.
84 Tuomilehto J, Lindstrom J, Eriksson JG, Valle TT, Hamalainen H, Ilanne-Parikka P, *et al.* Prevention of type 2 diabetes mellitus by changes in lifestyle among subjects with impaired glucose tolerance. *N Engl J Med* 2001; **344**:1343–1350.
85 Diabetes Prevention Program Research Group. Reduction in the incidence of type 2 diabetes with lifestyle intervention or metformin. *N Engl J Med* 2002; **346**:393–403.
86 Berglund G, Nilsson P, Eriksson KF, Nilsson JA, Hedblad B, Kristenson H, *et al.* Long-term outcome of the Malmo preventive project: mortality and cardiovascular morbidity. *J Intern Med* 2000; **247**:19–29.
87 Eriksson KF, Lindgarde F. No excess 12-year mortality in men with impaired glucose tolerance who participated in the Malmo Preventive Trial with diet and exercise. *Diabetologia* 1998; **41**:1010–1016.
88 Li G, Zhang P, Wang J, Gregg EW, Yang W, Gong Q, *et al.* The long-term effect of lifestyle interventions to prevent diabetes in the China Da Qing Diabetes Prevention Study: a 20-year follow-up study. *Lancet* 2008; **371**:1783–1789.
89 Tuomilehto J, Lindstrom J, Eriksson JG, Valle TT, Hamalainen H, Ilanne-Parikka P, *et al.* Prevention of type 2 diabetes mellitus by changes in lifestyle among subjects with impaired glucose tolerance. *N Engl J Med* 2001; **344**:1343–1350.
90 Lindstrom J, Ilanne-Parikka P, Peltonen M, Aunola S, Eriksson JG, Hemio K, *et al.* Sustained reduction in the incidence of type 2 diabetes by lifestyle intervention: follow-up of the Finnish Diabetes Prevention Study. *Lancet* 2006; **368**:1673–1679.
91 Smith TC, Wingard DL, Smith B, Kritz-Silverstein D, Barrett-Connor E. Walking decreased risk of cardiovascular disease mortality in older adults with diabetes. *J Clin Epidemiol* 2007; **60**:309–317.
92 Church TS, Cheng YJ, Earnest CP, Barlow CE, Gibbons LW, Priest EL, *et al.* Exercise capacity and body composition as predictors of mortality among men with diabetes. *Diabetes Care* 2004; **27**:83–88.
93 Church TS, LaMonte MJ, Barlow CE, Blair SN. Cardiorespiratory fitness and body mass index as predictors of cardiovascular disease mortality among men with diabetes. *Arch Intern Med* 2005; **165**:2114–2120.

94 Hu FB, Stampfer MJ, Solomon C, Liu S, Colditz GA, Speizer FE, *et al.* Physical activity and risk for cardiovascular events in diabetic women. *Ann Intern Med* 2001; **134**:96–105.

95 Ivy JL, Zderic TW, Fogt DL. Prevention and treatment of non-insulin-dependent diabetes mellitus. *Exerc Sport Sci Rev* 1999; **27**:1–35.

96 Dela F, Handberg A, Mikines KJ, Vinten J, Galbo H. GLUT4 and insulin receptor binding and kinase activity in trained human muscle. *J Physiol (Lond)* 1993; **469**:615–624.

97 Dela F, Ploug T, Handberg A, Petersen LN, Larsen JJ, Mikines KJ, *et al.* Physical training increases muscle GLUT4 protein and mRNA in patients with NIDDM. *Diabetes* 1994; **43**:862–865.

98 Ebeling P, Bourey R, Koranyi L, Tuominen JA, Groop LC, Henriksson J, *et al.* Mechanism of enhanced insulin sensitivity in athletes. Increased blood flow, muscle glucose transport protein (GLUT-4) concentration, and glycogen synthase activity. *J Clin Invest* 1993; **92**:1623–1631.

99 Coggan AR, Spina RJ, Kohrt WM, Holloszy JO. Effect of prolonged exercise on muscle citrate concentration before and after endurance training in men. *Am J Physiol* 1993; **264**:E215–E220.

100 Mandroukas K, Krotkiewski M, Hedberg M, Wroblewski Z, Bjorntorp P, Grimby G. Physical training in obese women: effects of muscle morphology, biochemistry and function. *Eur J Appl Physiol* 1984; **52**:355–361.

101 Saltin B, Henriksson J, Nygaard E, Andersen P, Jansson E. Fiber types and metabolic potentials of skeletal muscles in sedentary man and endurance runners. *Ann N Y Acad Sci* 1977; **301**:3–29.

102 Andersson A, Sjodin A, Olsson R, Vessby B. Effects of physical exercise on phospholipid fatty acid composition in skeletal muscle. *Am J Physiol* 1998; **274**:E432–E438.

103 Krotkiewski M, Bjorntorp P. Muscle tissue in obesity with different distribution of adipose tissue: effects of physical training. *Int J Obes* 1986; **10**:331–341.

104 Despres JP. Visceral obesity, insulin resistance, and dyslipidemia: contribution of endurance exercise training to the treatment of the plurimetabolic syndrome. *Exerc Sport Sci Rev* 1997; **25**:271–300.

105 Halle M, Berg A, Northoff H, Keul J. Importance of TNF-alpha and leptin in obesity and insulin resistance: a hypothesis on the impact of physical exercise. *Exerc Immunol Rev* 1998; **4**:77–94.

106 Busetto L. Visceral obesity and the metabolic syndrome: effects of weight loss. *Nutr Metab Cardiovasc Dis* 2001; **11**:195–204.

107 Kadoglou NP, Iliadis F, Angelopoulou N, Perrea D, Ampatzidis G, Liapis CD, *et al.* The anti-inflammatory effects of exercise training in patients with type 2 diabetes mellitus. *Eur J Cardiovasc Prev Rehabil* 2007; **14**:837–843.

108 Yates T, Davies M, Brady E, Webb D, Gorely T, Bull F, *et al.* Walking and inflammatory markers in individuals screened for type 2 diabetes. *Prev Med* 2008.

109 Ruderman NB, Schneider SH. Diabetes, exercise, and atherosclerosis. *Diabetes Care* 1992; **15**:1787–1793.

110 Schneider SH, Kim HC, Khachadurian AK, Ruderman NB. Impaired fibrinolytic response to exercise in type II diabetes: effects of exercise and physical training. *Metabolism* 1988; **37**:924–929.

111 Holloszy JO, Schultz J, Kusnierkiewicz J, Hagberg JM, Ehsani AA. Effects of exercise on glucose tolerance and insulin resistance: brief review and some preliminary results. *Acta Med Scand Suppl* 1986; **711**:55–65.

112 Dunstan DW, Mori TA, Puddey IB, Beilin LJ, Burke V, Morton AR, *et al.* A randomised, controlled study of the effects of aerobic exercise and dietary fish on coagulation and fibrinolytic factors in type 2 diabetics. *Thromb Haemost* 1999; **81**:367–372.

113 Skarfors ET, Wegener TA, Lithell H, Selinus I. Physical training as treatment for type 2 (non-insulin-dependent) diabetes in elderly men: a feasibility study over 2 years. *Diabetologia* 1987; **30**:930–933.

114 Loimaala A, Groundstroem K, Rinne M, Nenonen A, Huhtala H, Vuori I. Exercise training does not improve myocardial diastolic tissue velocities in type 2 diabetes. *Cardiovasc Ultrasound* 2007; **5**:32.

115 Loimaala A, Huikuri HV, Koobi T, Rinne M, Nenonen A, Vuori I. Exercise training improves baroreflex sensitivity in type 2 diabetes. *Diabetes* 2003; **52**:1837–1842.

116 Minuk HL, Vranic M, Marliss EB, Hanna AK, Albisser AM, Zinman B. Glucoregulatory and metabolic response to exercise in obese noninsulin-dependent diabetes. *Am J Physiol* 1981; **240**:E458–E464.

117 Koivisto VA, DeFronzo RA. Exercise in the treatment of type II diabetes. *Acta Endocrinol* 1984; **262**(Suppl.):1070111.

118 Sriwijitkamol A, Coletta DK, Wajcberg E, Balbontin GB, Reyna SM, Barrientes J, *et al.* Effect of acute exercise on AMPK signaling in skeletal muscle of subjects with type 2 diabetes: a time–course and dose–response study. *Diabetes* 2007; **56**:836–848.

119 Baynard T, Franklin RM, Goulopoulou S, Carhart R Jr, Kanaley JA. Effect of a single vs multiple bouts of exercise on glucose control in women with type 2 diabetes. *Metabolism* 2005; **54**:989–994.

120 Tobin LW, Kiens B, Galbo H. The effect of exercise on postprandial lipidemia in type 2 diabetic patients. *Eur J Appl Physiol* 2008; **102**:361–370.

121 Devlin JT, Hirshman M, Horton ED, Horton ES. Enhanced peripheral and splanchnic insulin sensitivity in NIDDM men after single bout of exercise. *Diabetes* 1987; **36**:434–439.

122 Villa-Caballero L, Nava-Ocampo AA, Frati-Munari AC, Rodriguez de Leon SM, Becerra-Perez AR, Ceja RM, *et al.* Hemodynamic and oxidative stress profile after exercise in type 2 diabetes. *Diabetes Res Clin Pract* 2007; **75**:285–291.

123 Ivy JL. Role of exercise training in the prevention and treatment of insulin resistance and non-insulin-dependent diabetes mellitus. *Sports Med* 1997; **24**:321–336.

124 Miller JP, Pratley RE, Goldberg AP, Gordon P, Rubin M, Treuth MS, *et al.* Strength training increases insulin action in healthy 50- to 65-yr-old men. *J Appl Physiol* 1994; **77**:1122–1127.

125 Smutok MA, Reece C, Kokkinos PF, Farmer C, Dawson P, Shulman R, *et al.* Aerobic versus strength training for risk factor intervention in middle-aged men at high risk for coronary heart disease. *Metabolism* 1993; **42**:177–184.

126 Fluckey JD, Hickey MS, Brambrink JK, Hart KK, Alexander K, Craig BW. Effects of resistance exercise on glucose tolerance in normal and glucose-intolerant subjects. *J Appl Physiol* 1994; **77**:1087–1092.

127 Dunstan DW, Puddey IB, Beilin LJ, Burke V, Morton AR, Stanton KG. Effects of a short-term circuit weight training program on glycaemic control in NIDDM. *Diabetes Res Clin Pract* 1998; **40**:53–61.

128 Honkola A, Forsen T, Eriksson J. Resistance training improves the metabolic profile in individuals with type 2 diabetes. *Acta Diabetol* 1997; **34**:245–248.

129 Ishii T, Yamakita T, Sato T, Tanaka S, Fujii S. Resistance training improves insulin sensitivity in NIDDM subjects without altering maximal oxygen uptake. *Diabetes Care* 1998; **21**:1353–1355.

130 Ryan AS, Hurlbut DE, Lott ME, Ivey FM, Fleg J, Hurley BF, *et al.* Insulin action after resistive training in insulin resistant older men and women. *J Am Geriatr Soc* 2001; **49**:247–253.

131 Craig BW, Everhart J, Brown R. The influence of high-resistance training on glucose tolerance in young and elderly subjects. *Mech Ageing Dev* 1989; **49**:147–157.

132 Hurley BF, Hagberg JM, Goldberg AP, Seals DR, Ehsani AA, Brennan RE, *et al.* Resistive training can reduce coronary risk factors without altering VO_{2max} or percent body fat. *Med Sci Sports Exerc* 1988; **20**:150–154.

133 American College of Sports Medicine. American College of Sports Medicine Position Stand: exercise and physical activity for older adults. *Med Sci Sports Exerc* 1998; **30**:992–1008.

134 Jennings A, Alberga A, Sigal R, Jay O, Boule NG, Kenny GP. The effects of exercise training on resting metabolic rate in type 2 diabetes mellitus. *Med Sci Sports Exerc* 2009; **41**:1558–1565.

135 Dunstan DW, Daly RM, Owen N, Jolley D, De Courten M, Shaw J, *et al.* High-intensity resistance training improves glycemic control in older patients with type 2 diabetes. *Diabetes Care* 2002; **25**:1729–1736.

136 Castaneda C, Layne JE, Munoz-Orians L, Gordon PL, Walsmith J, Foldvari M, *et al.* A randomized controlled trial of resistance exercise training to improve glycemic control in older adults with type 2 diabetes. *Diabetes Care* 2002; **25**:2335–2341.

137 Snowling NJ, Hopkins WG. Effects of different modes of exercise training on glucose control and risk factors for complications in type 2 diabetic patients: a meta-analysis. *Diabetes Care* 2006; **29**:2518–2527.

138 Boulé NG, Haddad E, Kenny GP, Wells GA, Sigal RJ. Effects of exercise on glycemic control and body mass in type 2 diabetes mellitus: a meta-analysis of controlled clinical trials. *JAMA* 2001; **286**:1218–1227.

139 Balducci S, Leonetti F, Di Mario U, Fallucca F. Is a long-term aerobic plus resistance training program feasible for and effective on metabolic profiles in type 2 diabetic patients? *Diabetes Care* 2004; **27**:841–842.

140 Cauza E, Hanusch-Enserer U, Strasser B, Kostner K, Dunky A, Haber P. The metabolic effects of long term exercise in type 2 diabetes patients. *Wien Med Wochenschr* 2006; **156**:515–519.

141 Lambers S, Van Laethem C, Van Acker K, Calders P. Influence of combined exercise training on indices of obesity, diabetes and cardiovascular risk in type 2 diabetes patients. *Clin Rehabil* 2008; **22**:483–492.

142 Balducci S, Zanuso S, Fernando F, Nicolucci A, Cardelli P, Cavallo S, *et al.* The Italian diabetes and exercise study. *Diabetes* **57**:A306–A307.

143 American Diabetes Association Position Statement. Standards of medical care in diabetes, 2008. *Diabetes Care* 2008; **31**(Suppl 1):S12–S54.

144 Sigal RJ, Kenny GP, Wasserman DH, Castaneda-Sceppa C, White RD. Physical activity/exercise and type 2 diabetes: a consensus statement from the American Diabetes Association. *Diabetes Care* 2006; **29**:1433–1438.

145 Albright A, Franz M, Hornsby G, Kriska A, Marrero D, Ullrich I, *et al.* American College of Sports Medicine position stand: exercise and type 2 diabetes. *Med Sci Sports Exerc* 2000; **32**:1345–1360.

146 Haskell WL, Lee IM, Pate RR, Powell KE, Blair SN, Franklin BA, *et al.* Physical activity and public health: updated recommendation for adults from the American College of Sports Medicine and the American Heart Association. *Med Sci Sports Exerc* 2007; **39**:1423–1434.

147 Nelson ME, Rejeski WJ, Blair SN, Duncan PW, Judge JO, King AC, *et al.* Physical activity and public health in older adults: recommendation from the American College of Sports Medicine and the American Heart Association. *Med Sci Sports Exerc* 2007; **39**:1435–1445.

148 Jolly K, Taylor R, Lip GY, Greenfield S, Raftery J, Mant J, *et al.* The Birmingham Rehabilitation Uptake Maximization Study (BRUM). Home-based compared with hospital-based cardiac rehabilitation in a multi-ethnic population: cost-effectiveness and patient adherence. *Health Technol Assess* 2007; **11**:1–118.

149 Braith RW, Beck DT. Resistance exercise: training adaptations and developing a safe exercise prescription. *Heart Fail Rev* 2008; **13**:69–79.

150 Benn SJ, McCartney N, McKelvie RS. Circulatory responses to weight lifting, walking, and stair climbing in older males. *J Am Geriatr Soc* 1996; **44**:121–125.

151 Cruickshanks KJ, Moss SE, Klein R, Klein BE. Physical activity and the risk of progression of retinopathy or the development of proliferative retinopathy. *Ophthalmology* 1995; **102**:1177–1182.

152 Carpinelli RN, Otto RM. Strength training: single versus multiple sets. *Sports Med* 1998; **26**:73–84.

153 Castaneda C, Munoz-Orians L, Layne J, Walsmith J, Foldvari M, Gordon P, *et al.* A randomized trial of progressive resistance training to improve glycemic control in Hispanic elders with diabetes. *Diabetes* 2001; **50**(Suppl 1):A906–A909.

154 Dunstan DW, Daly RM, Lekhtman E, Bauzon H, McConell K, Robinson L, *et al.* Effects of high-intensity resistance training and diet on glycemic control in older persons with type 2 diabetes. *Med Sci Sports Exerc* 2001; **33**(Suppl.):258.

155 Aiello LP, Wong J, Cavallerano JD, Bursell S-E, Aiello LM. Retinopathy. In: Ruderman N, Devlin JT, Schneider SH, Kriska A, eds. *Handbook of Exercise in Diabetes*, 2nd edn. Alexandria, VA: American Diabetes Association, 2002:401–413.

156 Levin ME. The diabetic foot. In: Ruderman N, Devlin JT, Schneider SH, Kriska A, eds. *Handbook of Exercise in Diabetes*, 2nd edn. Alexandria, VA: American Diabetes Association, 2002:385–399.

157 Vinik AI, Erbas T. Neuropathy. In: Ruderman N, Devlin JT, Schneider SH, Kriska A, eds. *Handbook of Exercise in Diabetes*, 2nd edn. Alexandria, VA: American Diabetes Association, 2002:463–496.

158 Lemaster JW, Mueller MJ, Reiber GE, Mehr DR, Madsen RW, Conn VS. Effect of weight-bearing activity on foot ulcer incidence in people with diabetic peripheral neuropathy: feet first randomized controlled trial. *Phys Ther* 2008; **88**:1385–1398.

159 Wackers FJ, Young LH, Inzucchi SE, Chyun DA, Davey JA, Barrett EJ, *et al.* Detection of silent myocardial ischemia in asymptomatic diabetic subjects: the DIAD study. *Diabetes Care* 2004; **27**:1954–1961.

160 Valensi P, Sachs RN, Harfouche B, Lormeau B, Paries J, Cosson E, *et al.* Predictive value of cardiac autonomic neuropathy in diabetic patients with or without silent myocardial ischemia. *Diabetes Care* 2001; **24**:339–343.

161 Perkins B, Riddell M. Type 1 diabetes and exercise: using the insulin pump to maximum advantage. *Can J Diabetes* 2006; **30**:72–79.

162 Francescato MP, Geat M, Fusi S, Stupar G, Noacco C, Cattin L. Carbohydrate requirement and insulin concentration during

moderate exercise in type 1 diabetic patients. *Metabolism* 2004; **53**:1126–1130.

163 Tuominen JA, Karonen SL, Melamies L, Bolli G, Koivisto VA. Exercise-induced hypoglycaemia in IDDM patients treated with a short-acting insulin analogue. *Diabetologia* 1995; **38**:106–111.

164 Walsh J, Roberts R. *Pumping Insulin*, 3rd edn. San Diego, CA: Torry Pines Press, 2000.

165 Jeukendrup AE. Carbohydrate intake during exercise and performance. *Nutrition* 2004; **20**:669–677.

166 Cuff DJ, Meneilly GS, Martin A, Ignaszewski A, Tildesley HD, Frohlich JJ. Effective exercise modality to reduce insulin resistance in women with type 2 diabetes. *Diabetes Care* 2003; **26**:2977–2982.

167 Fletcher GF, Balady G, Froelicher VF, Hartley LH, Haskell WL, Pollock ML. Exercise standards: a statement for healthcare professionals from the American Heart Association, Writing Group. *Circulation* 1995; **91**:580–615.

168 American Association of Cardiovascular and Pulmonary Rehabilitation. *Cardiac Rehabilitation Resource Manual*, 3rd edn. Champaign, IL: Human Kinetics, 2006.

169 Hamman RF, Wing RR, Edelstein SZ, Lachin JM, Bray GA, Delahanty L, *et al.* Effect of weight loss with lifestyle intervention on risk of diabetes. *Diabetes Care* 2006; **29**:2102–2107.

24 Social Aspects of Diabetes

Brian M. Frier[1] & Mark W.J. Strachan[2]

[1]Department of Diabetes, Royal Infirmary of Edinburgh, Edinburgh
[2]Metabolic Unit, Western General Hospital, Edinburgh

Keypoints

Driving

- Potential hazards facing the driver with diabetes include hypoglycemia, visual impairment, and disability from severe neuropathy or leg amputation.
- Hypoglycemia can severely disrupt driving skills by causing cognitive dysfunction and mood changes. Motor skills and judgment can become impaired when blood glucose falls below 3.8 mmol/L, often without inducing hypoglycemic symptoms. Impaired awareness of hypoglycemia is a relative contraindication to driving. Drivers with diabetes must take precautions to avoid hypoglycemia and know how to treat it if it occurs while driving.
- Corrected visual acuity that is worse than 6/12 in the better eye precludes driving in the general population. People with diabetes may fulfill this criterion, but still have significant visual impairment (e.g. field loss, poor night vision and perception of movement) secondary to retinopathy, laser treatment or cataracts.
- In many countries, drivers with diabetes are legally required to declare the diagnosis for their driving license and motor insurance. Failure to do this will invalidate insurance claims.
- Driving licenses are often issued for fixed terms and only renewed following satisfactory medical review. In many countries, insulin-treated drivers are barred from driving passenger-carrying vehicles and large goods vehicles.

Employment

- Diabetes is not a bar to most occupations, and people with diabetes are protected in many countries by legislation against discrimination on the grounds of disability.
- People with insulin-treated diabetes are barred from certain occupations because of the risk of hypoglycemia. These include the armed forces, emergency services, commercial pilots, prison and security services, and jobs in potentially dangerous areas (e.g. at heights, underwater and offshore).
- Severe hypoglycemia in the workplace is uncommon and shift work seldom compromises glycemic control. Depressive illness and poor glycemic control are associated with higher unemployment and sickness absence in people with diabetes.

Prison and custody

- Glycemic control may be suboptimal in prison because of restrictions in diet, exercise and blood glucose monitoring. Intercurrent illness and metabolic abnormalities may not be recognized or treated promptly.
- Input from a diabetes specialist may improve the quality of care. Knowledge of diabetes among prison officers and staff of short-term custodial units is often limited and may be improved by liaising with local diabetes specialist services.

Insurance

- Diabetes should be declared to insurers, who may impose higher premiums or limited coverage. Many insurers' decisions are based on outdated actuarial data or misconceptions about the current prognosis of diabetes. National diabetes organizations can provide details of insurance brokers who do not weight policies against people with diabetes.
- Life expectancy in type 1 diabetes can be modeled from age, sex and the presence of proliferative retinopathy and nephropathy. As the latter is a major determinant of survival, life insurance premiums should be reduced for all those who reach the age of 50 years without renal impairment.

Alcohol

- The association between excessive alcohol consumption, chronic pancreatitis and secondary diabetes is well established. Alcohol excess is also associated with central obesity and poor compliance with medication; both could increase the risk of type 2 diabetes and compromise control of established diabetes. Most epidemiologic studies, however, have demonstrated a U-shaped relationship between alcohol consumption and diabetes, with moderate intake being associated with a lower risk of diabetes.
- In type 2 diabetes, moderate alcohol consumption is associated with a 35% reduction in total mortality and lower risk of cardiovascular disease compared to abstinence. Excessive alcohol consumption is associated with hypertriglyceridemia and resistant hypertension; affected individuals have an increased vascular risk.

Textbook of Diabetes, 4th edition. Edited by R. Holt, C. Cockram, A. Flyvbjerg and B. Goldstein. © 2010 Blackwell Publishing.

- Ethanol inhibits hepatic gluconeogenesis and increases the risk, severity and duration of hypoglycemia. Alcohol obscures the ability, both of the individual and of observers, to recognize and treat hypoglycemia, and intoxication can simulate hypoglycemia.

Recreational drugs
- Approximately one-third of young people with diabetes use recreational drugs at some time. The most common class of drug taken is cannabis, but amfetamine-type stimulants (including 'ecstasy'), cocaine and opiates are also used.
- Recreational drug use is associated with a sixfold higher risk of death from acute metabolic complications of diabetes. Intravenous drug use is uncommon but is dangerous and is associated with omission of insulin therapy, frequent hospital admissions (usually with diabetic ketoacidosis) and high mortality.
- Cocaine and amfetamine-type stimulants can have profound hemodynamic effects through sympatho-adrenal activation. In addition to an increased risk of cardiac arrhythmias and myocardial ischemia, the sympathetic activation antagonizes the action of insulin and can precipitate diabetic ketoacidosis.

Travel
- Diabetes is not a bar to traveling, but changes in meals, physical activity and antidiabetic drug treatment *en route* and after arrival all need careful consideration. Important issues include travel insurance, medical identification, supplies and storage of medication and monitoring equipment and immunizations.
- During long flights, blood glucose should be monitored frequently and glycemic control relaxed to avoid hypoglycemia. Insulin injection schedules may require in-flight adjustment, especially if the time-shift exceeds 4 hours.

Leaving home
- In the Diabetes UK Cohort Study, "living alone" was associated with a more than fourfold increase in risk of death from acute metabolic complications of diabetes.
- Leaving home is potentially a period of high risk for young people with diabetes; particular concern has been expressed about the welfare of university students with type 1 diabetes.

Diabetes influences many aspects of daily life, principally through the effects of treatment and its potential side effects, particularly hypoglycemia. The development of diabetic complications, such as neuropathy and retinopathy, can also affect everyday activities, particularly when these are severe with clinical manifestations, or require time-consuming treatment such as dialysis for chronic renal failure.

Driving

Driving is an everyday activity that demands complex psychomotor skills, visuospatial coordination, vigilance and satisfactory judgment. Although motor accidents are common, medical disabilities are seldom responsible. Diabetes is designated a "prospective disability" for driving because of its potential to progress and cause complications, while side effects of treatment (principally hypoglycemia) can affect driving performance. In most countries, the duration of the license of a driver with diabetes is period-restricted by law, and its renewal is subject to review of medical fitness to drive. The problems associated with diabetes and driving and the limitations of relevant research data have been reviewed [1,2].

The main problems for the driver with diabetes are hypoglycemia and visual impairment resulting from cataract or retinopathy. Rarely, peripheral neuropathy, peripheral vascular disease and lower limb amputation can present mechanical difficulties with driving (Table 24.1), but these problems may be overcome by adapting the vehicle and using automatic transmission systems.

Despite these challenges, drivers with diabetes do not appear to be involved in more accidents than their non-diabetic counterparts [3]. Population studies have shown no excess in accident rates among drivers with diabetes in Northern Ireland [4], Scotland [5], England [6], Germany [7], Iceland [8] or Pittsburgh in the USA [9], while a large survey of over 30 000 drivers in Wisconsin, USA found only a modest increase [10]. In most surveys, however, incidents were self-reported and probably underestimated, while fatal accidents (in which a diabetes-related cause, such as hypoglycemia, could have had a role) were excluded. Accident rates may also have been lowered by regulatory authorities barring high-risk drivers and by drivers with advancing diabetic complications who voluntarily stop driving [4,5]. Practical advice for drivers with diabetes is given in Table 24.2.

Table 24.1 Reasons for drivers with diabetes to cease driving.

Newly diagnosed people with diabetes, especially insulin-treated, should not drive until glycemic control and vision are stable
Recurrent daytime hypoglycemia (particularly if severe)
Impaired awareness of hypoglycemia, if disabling
Reduced visual acuity in *both* eyes (worse than 6/12 on Snellen chart) – note use of mydriatics for eye examination will affect visual acuity
Severe sensorimotor peripheral neuropathy, especially with loss of proprioception
Severe peripheral vascular disease
Lower limb amputation

Hypoglycemia

Drivers with insulin-treated diabetes often experience hypoglycemia while driving [4,5,11] and this can interfere with driving

Table 24.2 Advice for drivers with diabetes.

Inform licensing authority* (statutory requirement) and motor insurer of diabetes and its treatment
Do not drive if eyesight deteriorates suddenly
Check blood glucose before driving (even on short journeys) and at intervals on longer journeys
Take frequent rests with snacks or meals; avoid alcohol
Keep a supply of fast-acting and longer-acting carbohydrate in the vehicle for emergency use
Carry personal identification to indicate that you have diabetes (and are prone to hypoglycemia)
If hypoglycemia develops, stop driving, switch off engine, leave the driver's seat and then treat
Do not resume driving for 45 minutes after blood glucose has returned to normal (delayed cognitive recovery)

* In the UK, the licensing authority is the Driver and Vehicle Licensing Agency (DVLA), Swansea, SA99 1TU, UK.

skills by causing cognitive dysfunction, even during relatively mild hypoglycemia that does not induce symptoms. Studies of subjects with type 1 diabetes (T1DM) using a driving simulator showed that driving performance often became impaired at blood glucose concentrations of 3.4–3.8 mmol/L, and deteriorated further at lower levels [12]. Problems included poor road positioning, driving too fast, inappropriate braking and causing "crashes" by stopping suddenly. Alarmingly, most did not experience hypoglycemic symptoms or doubt their competence to drive; only one-third treated the hypoglycemia, and only when blood glucose had fallen below 2.8 mmol/L [12]. In the UK, the Driver and Vehicle Licensing Agency (DVLA) does not distinguish between type of diabetes, and the restrictions are based on the use of insulin as therapy, as this can cause hypoglycemia in any person using this treatment. The risk of hypoglycemia in insulin-treated type 2 diabetes (T2DM) rises with duration of insulin therapy.

Judgement and insight become impaired during hypoglycemia, and some drivers with diabetes describe episodes of irrational and compulsive behavior while at the wheel [12]. Hypoglycemia also causes potentially dangerous mood changes, including irritability and anger [13]. In addition, asymptomatic hypoglycemia impairs visual information processing and contrast sensitivity, particularly in poor visibility [14,15], which may diminish driving performance.

Poor perception of hypoglycemia is also potentially dangerous. Many drivers with diabetes subjectively overestimate their current blood glucose level and feel competent to drive when they are actually hypoglycemic [16]. Impaired awareness of hypoglycemia, often associated with more frequent severe episodes, is particularly hazardous and is a common reason for revocation of the driving license. It is not an absolute contraindication to driving if it can be demonstrated, by frequent self-monitoring, that there is prolonged freedom from hypoglycemia [17].

Hypoglycemia is a recognized cause of road traffic accidents, but its true frequency and causal relationship to an accident are often difficult to ascertain. Blood glucose is seldom estimated immediately after a crash, and evidence for preceding hypoglycemia is often circumstantial. Hypoglycemia was the main cause of non-fatal motor accidents in the Diabetes Control and Complications Trial (DCCT); hypoglycemia was three times more common in the intensively treated patients, but the rate of major accidents was no higher, perhaps because of better precautionary advice [18]. Other studies found that the frequency of hypoglycemic episodes during driving correlates with the total number of accidents [4,5,19]. The frequency of hypoglycemia-related accidents is substantially lower than those caused by alcohol and drugs.

Avoiding and treating hypoglycemia while driving

General measures to avoid hypoglycemia are discussed in Chapter 33. All drivers with insulin-treated diabetes should keep some fast-acting carbohydrate in the vehicle: disturbingly, some do not [20,21]. Each car journey, no matter how short, should be planned in advance to anticipate possible risks for hypoglycemia, such as traffic delays. It is advisable to check blood glucose before and during long journeys, and to take frequent rest and meals. Unfortunately, this is seldom undertaken [22]. Driving expends energy and – as with other forms of exercise – prophylactic carbohydrate should be taken if the blood glucose is <5.0 mmol/L [23].

If hypoglycemia occurs during driving, the car should be stopped in a safe place, and the engine switched off before consuming some glucose. In the UK, the patient should vacate the driver's seat and remove the keys from the ignition, as a charge can be brought for driving while under the influence of a drug (insulin) even if the car is stationary. Driving should not be resumed for at least 45 minutes after blood glucose has returned to normal, because cognitive function is slow to recover after hypoglycemia [13].

Many features of hypoglycemia resemble alcohol intoxication, and semi-conscious hypoglycemic diabetic drivers are sometimes arrested on the assumption that they are drunk. Drivers with insulin-treated diabetes should therefore carry a card or identity bracelet stating the diagnosis. Individuals with newly diagnosed insulin-treated diabetes may have to stop driving temporarily until their glycemic control is stable.

Sulfonylureas is the only group of oral antidiabetic drugs that may cause hypoglycemia while driving, and people treated with these agents should be informed of this possibility. While GLP-1 agonists alone are not associated with a risk of hypoglycemia, this may be a problem when used in combination with a sulfonylurea. Blood glucose testing in relation to driving is not a requisite for drivers with group 1 licenses (see below), but may be required for holders of group 2 licenses who are taking this treatment combination.

Visual impairment

In the UK, monocular vision is accepted for driving, provided that the person meets the minimum legal requirement, i.e. is able

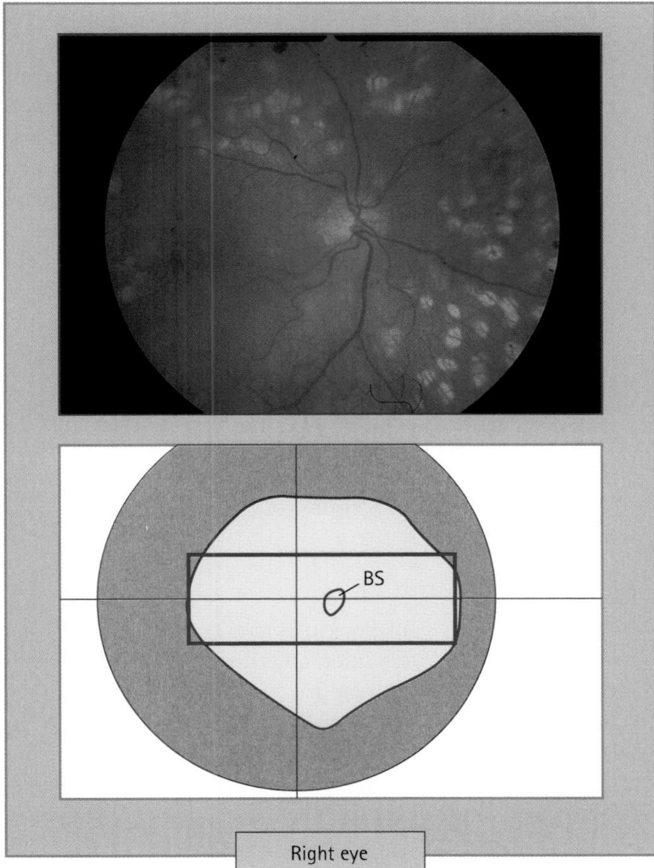

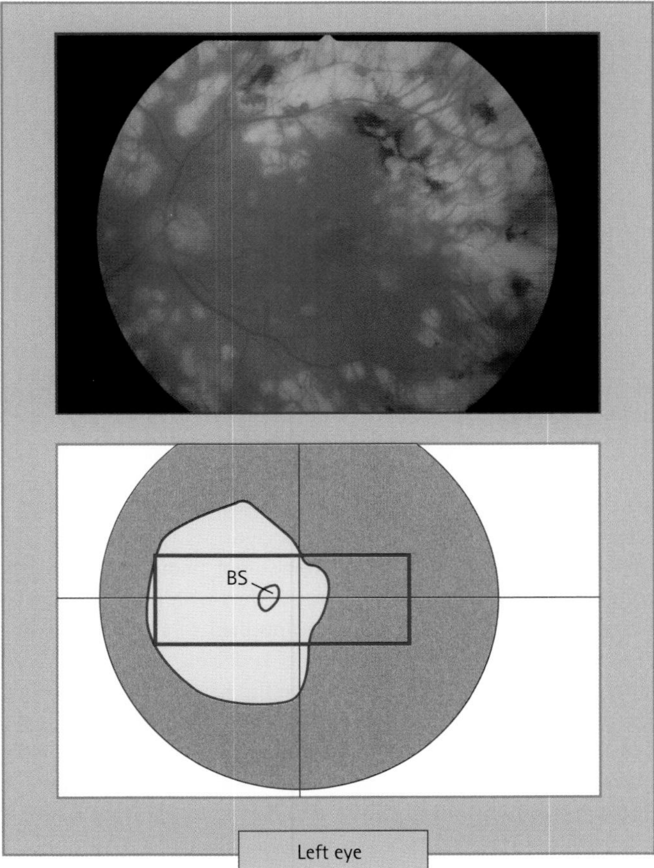

Figure 24.1 Visual field loss caused by photocoagulation. This 60-year-old man with diabetes needed heavy laser photocoagulation to the temporal retina of the left eye, causing nasal visual field loss which caused this eye to fail the standard test for driving. The right eye required less intensive laser treatment and the visual field was adequate for driving. BS, blind spot. Blue rectangle: minimum area recommended for safe driving. Courtesy of D. Flanagan, Addenbrooke's Hospital, Cambridge, UK.

to read a number plate with letters 8.9 cm (3.5 inches) high at a distance of 30 m (75 feet), wearing spectacles if necessary. This corresponds to a distance visual acuity of approximately 6/10 on the Snellen chart. The number plate test has deficiencies: it is poorly reproducible under clinical conditions and does not assess visual fields, night vision or the ability to see moving objects. All of these may be severely reduced by retinal ischemia in preproliferative retinopathy [24], while visual field loss can be caused by extensive laser photocoagulation for diabetic retinopathy [25,26] or macular edema (Figure 24.1) [27]; careful containment of laser burns may help to preserve vision [28]. Cataracts often accentuate glare from headlights, and in such cases driving in the dark should be avoided.

Previous surveys have identified very few drivers with diabetes who would fail the standard eyesight test. Impaired vision is an uncommon reason for the driving license to be refused or revoked [29], although many people stop driving voluntarily because their eyesight is deteriorating. Worsening vision from diabetic (or other) eye disease should be reported by the individual to the licensing authority.

Eye screening is a crucial part of assessing medical fitness to drive. Pupillary dilatation for fundoscopy or retinal photography temporarily reduces visual acuity, particularly if the usual binocular visual acuity is 6/9 or worse [30]. Patients should be told not to drive for at least 2 hours after the use of mydriatics. The driving regulatory authority may request perimetry to assess visual fields (Figure 24.1).

Statutory requirements for drivers with diabetes

In most developed countries, drivers with diabetes are required by law to declare their diabetes to the relevant regulatory authority (in the UK this is the DVLA). The statutory requirements for ordinary and vocational (professional) driving licenses vary considerably around the world; the national licensing authority should be contacted for details.

European driving licenses

Ordinary driving licenses (group 1)

The European Union (EU) States all use the same classification for driving licenses but this is not applicable to other areas. In the

UK, the DVLA must be informed when a person with diabetes applies for a driving license, or if diabetes develops subsequently. Failure to do this constitutes "concealment of a material fact," which can incur a fine [29], and can invalidate a claim to the motor insurers; professed ignorance of the law is not accepted as an excuse. The onus to declare rests with the individual driver, and doctors who provide diabetic care, including general practitioners, have a responsibility to inform patients of this legal requirement, and should offer practical advice (Table 24.2). Drivers with diabetes who are treated with diet alone or with antidiabetic medications do not have to notify the DVLA unless they have visual impairment or other diabetes-related problems that could affect medical fitness to drive. In the UK, a driving license is usually issued for a maximum of 3 years, and is renewed after completion of a medical questionnaire. The DVLA request further medical reports in a few cases, and always when an applicant reports a medical problem that may seriously affect driving (e.g. recurrent hypoglycemia). GLP-1 agonists (given by injection) can be used without restriction, other than when used in combination with a sulfonylurea for drivers with group 2 (vocational) licenses, when this must be notified to the DVLA and requires assessment of medical fitness to drive.

Although the member states of the EU have an agreed policy on restrictions on driving licenses for people with insulin-treated diabetes, considerable variations in policy and practical application exist between countries with respect to the implementation of the recommended regulations and how these are reviewed.

Vocational driving licenses (group 2)

It is extremely difficult to estimate the risk and likely outcome of a motor accident. In the absence of scientific evidence, risk and hazard are gauged by the size of vehicle being driven, which is perhaps not unreasonable, given the potential consequences of a hypoglycemic person losing control of a vehicle weighing several tons.

Most European countries restrict vocational (group 2) driving licenses for people with insulin-treated diabetes. These include category C licenses for large goods vehicles (LGV; previously called heavy goods vehicles) weighing over 7500 kg, and category D licenses for passenger-carrying vehicles (PCV; previously called public service vehicles), or those with more than 17 seats (including the driver's). In 1991, the then European Community (now the European Union) extended group 2 licenses to include small lorries and vans weighing 3500–7500 kg (category C1) and minibuses with 9–16 seats (category D1). Although all EU member states agreed to this policy (2nd European Council Directive on Driving Licences, 91/439/EEC), and presumably enacted appropriate legislation, considerable variations exist in the interpretation and imposition of these restrictions, and in some countries the EU Directive is openly disregarded. A few countries, such as the UK, Sweden and Spain, have robust systems in place to review medical fitness to drive at regular intervals. In the UK, C1 (but not D1) licenses are issued to drivers with insulin-treated diabetes as "exceptional cases" provided specific medical criteria are satisfied. A recent EU directive on driving has recommended individual assessment of all insulin-treated drivers with diabetes who apply for a Group 2 license, so medical fitness criteria will be modified in 2010.

Oral antidiabetic medication is not a bar to vocational driving licenses in the UK. In practice, however, many public transport companies restrict the employment of drivers with T2DM who take sulfonylureas; metformin or exenatide treatment is not a contraindication, but medical assessment is usually necessary. Progression to insulin therapy will terminate the employment of bus and train drivers. Taxi and ambulance drivers are not covered by the statutory regulations. In the UK, taxi licenses are issued by local authorities, which vary considerably in the assessment of medical fitness to drive [32,33], although many have now adopted group 2 licensing standards.

The European approach to vocational licensing has been criticized as being draconian and discriminatory against drivers with diabetes, showing how difficult it can be to balance the civil rights of the person with diabetes against the need to safeguard public safety.

Driving outside Europe

Outside Europe, the regulations in different countries range from a complete ban to no restriction other than a medical examination for prospective or current drivers who require insulin [31]. Differences in approach between countries are influenced by the level of economic development and the prevalence of insulin-treated diabetes; many low and middle income countries impose no restriction on vocational driving licenses for people with insulin-treated diabetes [31]. In the USA, the Federal Highways Administration (FHWA) prohibits drivers with insulin-treated diabetes from driving commercial motor vehicles across state borders [35]. Within most states, drivers with insulin-treated diabetes can drive commercial vehicles except for lorries transporting hazardous materials and passenger-carrying buses.

In most other countries, insulin treatment alone is targeted by legislation, even though hypoglycemia can occur with other diabetic drugs. Interestingly, a Canadian survey of crashes involving truck and commercial vehicle drivers with diabetes revealed an increased in risk for drivers with T2DM treated with sulfonylureas [34], the presumption being that unsuspected hypoglycemia is a causal factor.

Aircraft pilot licenses

The UK Civil Aviation Authority does not allow individuals with diabetes treated with insulin or sulfonylureas to fly commercial aircraft or to work as air traffic controllers. Private pilot licenses can be issued to individuals with diabetes taking sulfonylureas (provided that they have a safety license endorsement), but not insulin. The EU has discussed introducing common airworthiness regulations for pilots with medical disorders.

Employment

With a few provisos, people with diabetes can successfully undertake a wide range of employment. There remains some prejudice against people with diabetes, but employment prospects in the UK and many other countries have improved with the introduction of legislation that makes it unlawful to treat a disabled person less favorably.

The main concern when considering people with diabetes for employment is the risk to safety associated with the condition or its treatment. Employers often fail to make the crucial distinction between a "hazard" (something with the potential to cause harm) and a "risk" (the likelihood that such harm will occur). The potential problems of diabetes relevant to employment are the hazards of acute hypoglycemia related to insulin and sulfonylureas, poor control of diabetes and the development of serious diabetic complications that may affect ability to work or interfere with performance at work.

Employment is generally restricted where hypoglycemia could be hazardous to the worker with diabetes, their colleagues or the general public. Employment-related issues, however, are not confined to people with T1DM. The rising prevalence of T2DM in the population of working age, along with the increasing use of insulin, has become an issue for occupational health assessment. Access to employment may be limited through discriminatory employment practices and restrictions posed by companies (rather than by legislation) because of perceived problems associated with diabetes or to job-sensitive issues related to the potential risks of hypoglycemia or to visual impairment. Diabetes can also affect employment through increased sick leave and absenteeism and by adversely influencing productivity. Diabetes in general has a negative long-term influence on the economic productivity of the individual; health-related disabilities can cause work limitations, especially in older employees in whom early retirement is more common on medical grounds.

A prospective survey in Edinburgh of 243 people with insulin-treated diabetes in full-time employment found that hypoglycemia occurred uncommonly at work (14% of all severe episodes) and had few adverse effects [36]. The study cohort, however, may have been subject to selection bias in terms of occupational diversity and many had suboptimal glycemic control; surprisingly few participants had impaired awareness of hypoglycemia. For some occupations (e.g. commercial airline pilots or train drivers) any risk of hypoglycemia is obviously unacceptable. Elsewhere, the case for employment restrictions may be less clear-cut.

Jobs that restrict the employment of workers with insulin-treated diabetes are listed in Table 24.3. People treated with insulin are not usually permitted to work alone in isolated or dangerous areas, or at unprotected heights. Shift-work is not necessarily a contraindication: one study in a car assembly plant found no difference in glycemic control between day and night-shift workers with diabetes, although control deteriorated if shift rotas were changed frequently [37].

In one British survey, the prevalence of diabetes in the workforce was 7.5 per 1000, including a lower-than-anticipated rate of 2.6 per 1000 for people treated with insulin [38]. Employment is generally disbarred in the armed forces, emergency work such as fire-fighting, civil aviation, jobs in the off-shore oil industry and in many forms of commercial driving [38]. Workers with diabetes seldom conceal their medical condition from their employers, and any blanket policy that disbars workers with diabetes from a specific occupation may be inappropriate or even discriminatory. Individual assessment is crucial, as employment regulations may not differentiate between different types and treatments of diabetes. Some bureaucratic regulations have been successfully challenged on medical grounds: for example, active fire fighters in the UK and a US air traffic controller were reinstated following appeals against dismissal.

Table 24.3 Forms of employment from which insulin-treated people with diabetes are generally excluded in the UK. Data from Waclawski [38] and Waclawski & Gill [56].

Vocational driving
Large goods vehicles (LGV)
Passenger-carrying vehicles (PCV)
Locomotives and underground trains
Professional drivers (chauffeurs)
Taxi drivers (variable; depends on local authority)
Civil aviation
Commercial pilots and flight engineers
Aircrew
Air-traffic controllers
National and emergency services
Armed forces (army, navy, air force)
Police force
Fire brigade or rescue services
Merchant navy
Prison and security services
Dangerous areas for work
Offshore: oil-rigs, gas platforms
Moving machinery
Incinerators and hot-metal areas
Work on railway tracks
Coal mining
Heights: overhead lines, cranes, scaffolding

In some cases, entering or persevering with a specific occupation may not always be in the individual's long-term interests (e.g. with the advance of disabling complications). This is clearly a difficult issue, which may require sympathetic medical counseling because of possible repercussions on the individual's income, self-esteem, future quality of life and the financial support of dependants.

Unemployment, sickness and diabetes

According to a British survey, employers do not generally believe that diabetes *per se* limits employment prospects, because most workers with diabetes have few medical problems and can tackle a wide range of occupations [39]. Discrimination by employers, however, may affect hiring practices; a US study reported that job applicants who told prospective employers of their diabetes were more likely to be refused than their non-diabetic siblings or individuals who did not declare that they had diabetes [40].

Some British and Dutch surveys reported no apparent excess of unemployment among people with diabetes as compared with the general population [41–44], but other studies in the UK [45,46] found that relatively more people with diabetes were not earning because of inability to work, intercurrent illness, early retirement or by being housewives. Although in many cases there was no apparent reason why an individual with diabetes could not obtain employment [46], depressive illness is strongly associated with unemployment and difficulties with work performance [47]. Adolescents with diabetes appear more likely than their non-diabetic peers to lose jobs, or to fail to follow their desired occupation or cope with shift-work [48]. Reduced employment and income in workers with diabetes in North American have been related to disability, which was seven times more common than among a sibling control group, was mainly related to diabetic complications [49,50] and was associated with lower employment income [51,52]. Sickness absence rates among employees with diabetes are reportedly either similar to, or 1.5- to twofold higher than in non-diabetic workers [40,53–55]. Workers with insulin-treated diabetes and good glycemic control had fewer sickness absences than those with poor control [56]; poor control itself (86 mmol/mol [HbA_{1c} >10%]) is associated with a high rate of sickness absence [57].

Prison and custody

Imprisonment and short-term custody are unusual but troublesome life situations that can interfere with the management of diabetes. Hypoglycemia can occur if food is withheld after arrest, and may be confused with intoxication by alcohol or drugs. Diabetes is generally managed badly in prison because of the unsuitability of prison diets, lack of exercise and the practical difficulty of using some insulin regimens (e.g. basal bolus); also, self-monitoring may be prohibited, and glucose to treat hypoglycemia may be unavailable during long "lock-up" periods. Most prison medical personnel have no specialist knowledge of diabetes and there may be no access to specialist supervision during custody.

Some prisoners with diabetes deliberately manipulate their treatment (e.g. by omitting insulin to induce ketoacidosis to have themselves removed to hospital which arguably offers a more amenable environment [59]). By contrast, treatment of intercurrent illness may be delayed by prison staff, who think that the prisoner is "misbehaving."

In some cases, withdrawal of alcohol, better dietary compliance and weight loss may actually improve glycemic control while in prison, and structured diabetic care can be provided effectively by an attending specialist physician [60,61]. Facilities for people with diabetes in police custody are generally limited, with an inability to measure blood glucose, treat diabetic emergencies or to provide insulin and appropriate meals [62]. A Scottish liaison initiative between a specialist diabetes department and the local police force identified and successfully addressed deficiencies in their custody facilities, including the provision of glucose monitoring equipment and the training of police staff [62]; this has been assisted by the development of a forensic nursing service.

Insurance

In many societies, insurance is viewed as essential to protect individuals and their families from the financial risk of unexpected events or illness, and insurance is often necessary to secure a financial loan, as for house purchase. People with diabetes are sometimes refused insurance or have to accept higher premiums and limited coverage, because the disorder is associated with reduced life expectancy, the risk of complications and greater use of health care services. Several factors are important for insurance underwriting, including the severity and duration of the diabetes, the extent of diabetic complications and other concurrent medical disorders. It is reasonable for an insurer to be cautious in dealing with applicants who have poorly controlled long-standing diabetes and established complications.

There is wide variation in insurance terms and premiums among different European countries [63], in the USA [64] and even within the UK [65], which suggests that insurers work from assumptions about diabetes rather than using scientific evidence from actuarial studies. The presence of T1DM may be the only factor considered by insurers [64], and many still base potentially discriminatory decisions on outdated information that reflects the poor outcome of diabetes diagnosed and treated decades ago. There are no standardized guidelines, nor is there any uniformity in the approach to diabetes and insurance [65], although risk classifications for life insurance have been published [66]. Some companies do not accept applicants with diabetes, while others do so without financial penalty. People with diabetes seeking insurance cover should therefore request quotations from several companies, and should be supported by a medical assessment from a physician who is competent in the specialty. Many national patient organizations have negotiated favorable terms with insurance brokers and will provide details on request.

The prognosis of people with diabetes (particularly T1DM) has improved considerably during the last 50 years, and the impact of this on life insurance for people with T1DM has been analyzed in Scandinavia [67]. In the last 30–40 years, median life expectancy has increased by over 15 years, largely because of substantial reductions in diabetic nephropathy. It has therefore been suggested that life insurance in T1DM should focus entirely on the risk of developing diabetic nephropathy [68], and a model to calculate insurance terms has been proposed, based on current age, age at diagnosis, sex, presence of nephropathy or proliferative retinopathy and other pre-existing disease [67]. As the risk of nephropathy falls after 25 years of diabetes, all people who reach the age of 50 without nephropathy should have their insurance premium reduced. This approach has been adopted by most insurance companies in the Nordic countries, and by some in other European countries. To avoid penalizing people with diabetes, there must be regular updating of mortality and life expectancy data, and this information must be transmitted to actuarial advisers and insurance underwriters.

People with diabetes also face higher premiums for accident insurance, which is unjustified because there is no evidence that they have more accidents or permanent disability than the general population [69]. Neither is there any rationale for higher motor insurance premiums [64,65,70], particularly for those not treated with insulin, because no excess in road traffic accidents has been demonstrated (see above). A US study of the insurance cost of employees with diabetes showed that while health care expenditure was three times higher than all health care consumers, it was not more expensive than other chronic illnesses such as heart disease, asthma and cancer [71].

Diabetes must always be disclosed to the insurer: concealing the diagnosis constitutes the withholding of a material fact, which nullifies the contract with the insurer and thus the insurer's liability in the event of a claim.

Alcohol

Many people enjoy drinking alcohol and diabetes should not be a barrier to social drinking. Accumulating data suggest that moderate alcohol consumption not only reduces the risks of developing T2DM but improves metabolic control and restricts diabetic complications. By contrast, alcohol can promote hypoglycemia and chronic excessive consumption may be deleterious both to long-term diabetes management and general health.

Alcohol consumption and risk of diabetes

Chronic high consumption of alcohol can predispose to the development of secondary diabetes. Alcohol has a direct toxic effect on the pancreas resulting in both acute and chronic pancreatitis. Diabetes complicates about 45% of cases of chronic pancreatitis (see Chapter 18). Insulin treatment is usually required to control hyperglycemia in patients with chronic pancreatitis, although diabetic ketoacidosis is rare. This may be because the pancreatic damage also destroys the α-cells that secrete glucagon, which is an essential factor in ketogenesis (see Chapters 13 and 34). A heavy alcoholic binge, with concomitant low food intake, can result in alcoholic ketoacidosis.

By contrast, modest alcohol consumption appears to protect against T2DM, reducing risk by up to 30% [72,73]. A U-shaped relationship has been observed between alcohol consumption and risk of diabetes, such that heavier drinkers and those who abstain from alcohol share a similar risk of developing T2DM (Figure 24.2). In epidemiologic and clamp studies, moderate alcohol consumption is associated with enhanced insulin sensitivity, which in part may be a consequence of reduced central adiposity [74]. Such epidemiologic data, however, may not provide an accurate assessment of risk for very heavy drinkers who tend to be underrepresented in such studies.

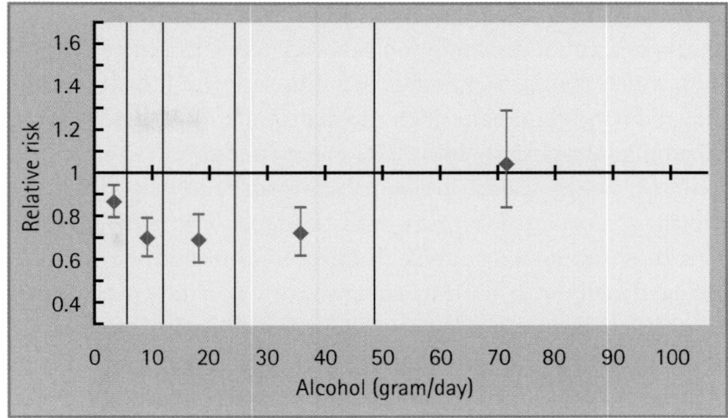

Figure 24.2 Pooled relative risk estimates for development of type 2 diabetes (with 95% confidence intervals) for five alcohol consumption categories (demarcated by the vertical lines) from 15 prospective studies. The categories are: ≤6 g/day; 6–12 g/day; 12–24 g/day; 24–48 g/day and ≥48 g/day. Reproduced from Koppes *et al.* [73], with permission from American Diabetes Association.

Alcohol and glycemic control

Hypoglycemia

Ethanol has marked metabolic effects on the liver, which metabolizes over 90% of an alcohol load. Gluconeogenesis is suppressed, even at blood alcohol levels that are not usually associated with intoxication [75–77], while the processes of recycling carbon as glucose and lactate between hepatic gluconeogenesis and muscle glycolysis [76] and fatty acid oxidation are also inhibited by alcohol. Thus, alcohol has the potential both to predispose to hypoglycemia and to inhibit glucose recovery. In non-diabetic individuals, total hepatic glucose production is not reduced by alcohol, despite the inhibition of gluconeogenesis [77], and alcohol-induced hypoglycemia only occurs if hepatic glycogen stores are already depleted; for example, by fasting for at least 36 hours [78].

In people with diabetes, alcohol consumption may impede recovery from insulin-induced hypoglycemia. This effect is often delayed, occurring up to 24 hours after alcohol ingestion and may occur during the night or the following day [79]. Those with a deficient glucagon response to hypoglycemia (see Chapter 33) may be at greater risk, because they are unable to increase hepatic gluconeogenesis. The signs of hypoglycemia may be missed or mistaken for those of alcohol intoxication by the individual or by observers and even moderate alcohol consumption increases the cognitive impairment that occurs during hypoglycemia [80]. People with insulin-treated diabetes should be advised not to drink *any* alcohol before driving.

Overall, alcohol is an important contributory factor to many episodes of hypoglycemia in people with diabetes – an estimated 20% in one study [81]. Hypoglycemia-induced brain damage is rare, but when it occurs, it is often preceded by excessive alcohol consumption, which presumably promotes protracted neuroglycopenia. Severe hypoglycemia caused permanent neurologic damage after binge drinking in five alcoholic patients with insulin-treated diabetes, two of whom died [82].

Hyperglycemia

Excessive alcohol consumption is associated with central obesity [83], which may be a consequence of the adverse lifestyle factors that tend to accompany high alcohol intake. It should also be noted that alcohol provides 7 kcal energy per gram (1 unit = 10 g alcohol) in an easily consumable form and can therefore provide a substantial caloric intake, particularly as beer and lager. This is a commonly overlooked source of calories in obese, middle-aged males with T2DM, who are having difficulty in achieving weight loss by dietary means. The caloric content of spirits is much lower but may be augmented by adding sugar-rich mixers to drinks. Low-carbohydrate beers and lagers (such as Pilsner) have been marketed as being suitable for patients with diabetes but should not be recommended because of their high alcohol content.

Heavy drinking has also been linked with poorer compliance with medications, outpatient follow-up and self blood glucose monitoring [84,85]. Despite this, and the association with increased central obesity, excessive alcohol consumption does not appear to be associated with poorer glycemic control. Indeed, in one large registry study, a linear inverse relationship was found between glycemic control and alcohol consumption [86]; however, the same caveat applies to these data with respect to very heavy consumption.

Alcohol and diabetic complications

Moderate alcohol consumption in people with T2DM is associated with a 35% reduction in total mortality compared with non-drinkers (i.e. a similar magnitude to the effect of moderate alcohol on the risk of developing T2DM) [87]. High alcohol consumption (more than 18 g/day) is not associated with any excess mortality, and indeed cardiovascular mortality and incident coronary heart disease are lower than in non-drinkers (Figure 24.3). These favorable effects of alcohol consumption

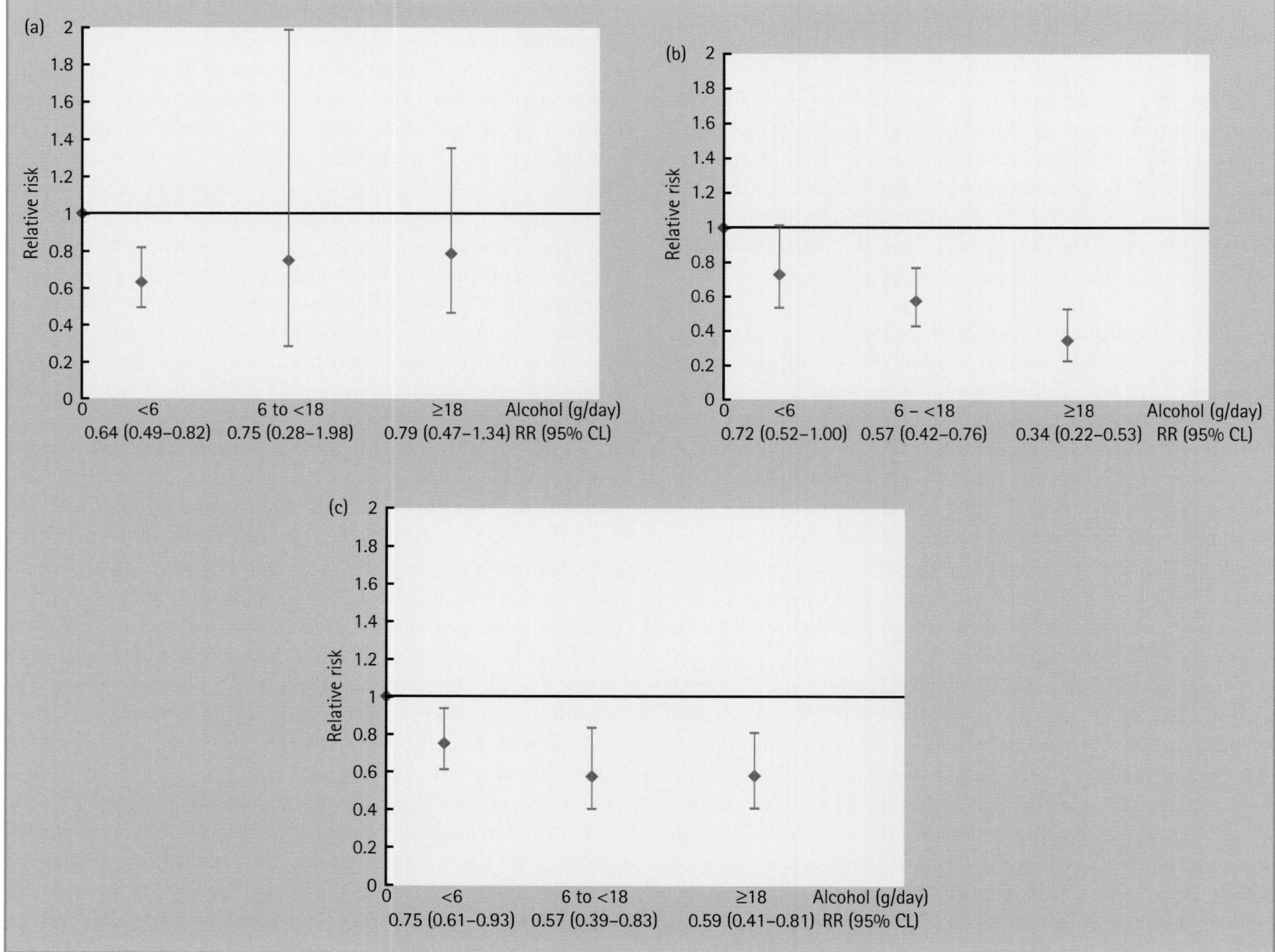

Figure 24.3 Pooled relative risk estimates (with 95% confidence intervals) of: (a) total mortality; (b) coronary heart disease mortality; and (c) coronary heart disease incidence for three alcohol consumption categories, with non-drinkers as the reference. Reproduced from Koppes *et al.* [87], with permission from Springer-Verlag.

may be a consequence of enhanced insulin sensitivity, lower blood pressure and favorable changes in lipids and hemostatic factors [74]. These observations do not include data on substantive numbers of very heavy drinkers and it is well established that excessive alcohol consumption increases serum triglyceride concentrations in susceptible individuals and raises blood pressure; excess alcohol consumption is an important cause of hypertension failing to respond to treatment (see Chapter 40). It might be anticipated in such individuals that cardiovascular risk would be higher [88].

With regard to microvascular complications, a U-shaped relationship is again observed between risk and alcohol consumption [89]. Moderate consumption (30–70 g/week) is associated with a 40% reduction in risk of proliferative retinopathy and neuropathy in T1DM, and over 60% reduction in risk for macroalbuminuria. Conversely, chronic excessive consumption of alcohol in people with diabetes is associated with peripheral neuropathy and exacerbation of neuropathic symptoms [90] and also with erectile dysfunction.

Recommended alcohol intake

Diabetes UK recommends that women with diabetes should drink no more than 2 units of alcohol per day and men no more than 3 units. Guidelines issued by comparable organizations in other countries are broadly similar. Although these limits have been chosen arbitrarily for the non-diabetic population, it seems reasonable to apply them to people with diabetes as well. The general advice given to people with diabetes regarding alcohol is summarized in Table 24.4.

Table 24.4 General advice on alcohol for people with diabetes. Reproduced with permission from Diabetes UK.

Moderate amounts of alcohol can be drunk shortly before, during or soon after a meal without affecting short-term blood glucose control and can be beneficial for the heart
Alcohol should never be drunk on an empty stomach as the alcohol will be absorbed too quickly
Alcoholic drinks should not be substituted for usual meals or snacks as this may cause hypoglycemia
Severe hypoglycemia can occur with larger quantities of alcohol, particularly when taken by people treated with insulin and especially if insufficient carbohydrate has been eaten
Hypoglycemia may occur up to 16 hours after heavy drinking
Observers may be less aware of hypoglycemic symptoms when a person with insulin-treated diabetes has been drinking; some form of diabetes identification should be worn. A hypoglycemic episode can be confused with drunkenness
Continuous heavy drinking can lead to raised blood pressure
All types of alcoholic drinks contain calories and may contribute to weight gain or failed dietary effort
Drinking alcohol can worsen neuropathy and aggravate associated symptoms
Drinking low carbohydrate beers and cider offer no benefit because of their higher alcohol content
Low alcohol wines are often higher in sugar than ordinary ones, so intake should be restricted
Mixer drinks should be "diet" or "sugar-free" such as diet tonic water and diet cola
Drinking and driving should be avoided.

Recreational drugs

Use of recreational (illicit) drugs is a serious problem in the general population, but can pose particular difficulties for people with diabetes [91]. The main classes of drugs involved are cannabis, amfetamine-type stimulants (including "ecstasy"), cocaine and opiates, with cannabis being the most commonly used drug by far.

Regulation

In the UK, drugs that are associated with dependence or misuse are regulated under the Misuse of Drugs Act, 1971. This Act grades drugs according to harm associated with misuse and specifies controls over manufacture, supply and possession (Table 24.5). The Misuse of Drugs Regulations, 2001 define the classes of individuals who are authorized to supply and possess controlled drugs and lay down the conditions under which these activities may be carried out. Drugs are classified under five schedules, which specify the requirements governing import, export, production, supply, possession, prescribing and record keeping. Cannabis and lysergide (LSD) classified as Schedule 1 as they have no medicinal use, while opiates, cocaine and amfetamine are

Table 24.5 Classification of controlled drugs. Data from UK Misuse of Drugs Act 1971.

Class A includes:*
Cocaine
Diamorphine (heroin)
Methadone
Methylenedioxymethamfetamine (MDMA, "ecstasy")
Morphine
Opium
Pethidine
Class B includes:
Oral amfetamines
Barbiturates
Codeine
Cannabis
Class C includes:
Most benzodiazepines
Ketamine
Zolpidem
Androgenic and anabolic steroids

* Includes Class B substances when prepared for injection.

classified as Schedule 2 and as such are subject to full controlled drug requirements.

Prevalence of recreational drug use

On a global scale, approximately 5% of adults aged 15–64 years (208 million people) use recreational drugs on at least an annual basis and 2.6% (112 million people) use such drugs on at least a monthly basis [92]. In the UK, drug abuse is more common in men and in people under 25 years of age [93]. Approximately one-third of adults have used recreational drugs at least once in their lifetime and approximately 10% over the previous year [93]. Trends in recreational drug use have changed in recent years with a decline in the use of LSD and solvents and an increase in the use of amfetamine-type drugs and ketamine, particularly associated with the night-club and "rave" culture.

Data specifically about the use of recreational drugs by people with diabetes are sparse. Two uncontrolled questionnaire surveys of young adults with T1DM, one from the USA and one from the UK, have reported a similar prevalence and pattern of recreational drug use to that observed in the general population [94,95]. In the UK survey, approximately 30% of respondents had used recreational drugs, with cannabis (28.2% of respondents), amfetamine-type stimulants (13%) and cocaine (12%) being used most commonly [95]. Many (15% of respondents) used more than one drug. A report from Chile has suggested that use of recreational drugs was lower in school-aged adolescents with T1DM than in the general population (9.6% vs 22.2%), although this difference disappeared during later years at school [96]. The prevalence of recreational drug use in people with T2DM is low, which reflects the pattern in adults of similar age in the general population [97].

Impact of recreational drug use on diabetes

In the Diabetes UK Cohort Study, acute metabolic complications (diabetic ketoacidosis and, to a lesser extent, severe hypoglycemia) were the most common causes of death in adults with T1DM under the age of 30 years, closely followed by accidents and violence [98]. In that study, a history of previous drug abuse was associated with a nearly sixfold increase risk of death from acute complications. Drug misuse has also been identified as a major cause of death in young people with T1DM [99]. Substance abuse co-occurring with mental illness is associated with a particularly high mortality [100].

Intravenous drug abuse

Recreational drug use often disrupts normal lifestyle and a person with diabetes may abandon the daily routine of regular meals and insulin injections. Recreational drug use may also be only one aspect of a chaotic lifestyle associated with other high-risk behaviors. This can result from the use of any recreational drug, but intravenous drug abuse (particularly of opiates, but also amfetamines) is particular damaging and is strongly associated with poor social support, criminality and mental illness. Intravenous drug use is uncommon in people with diabetes (as it is in the general population), but is associated with omission of insulin therapy, frequent admissions to hospital and high mortality, both from diabetic ketoacidosis and deliberate or accidental opiate overdose [101]. Unsurprisingly, intravenous drug abusers with diabetes may also present with complications related to the route of drug administration: deep venous thrombosis and abscesses at groin or limb injection sites. Intravenous drug abusers often default from outpatient clinic attendance (this may be associated with imprisonment) and maintaining contact with such individuals is usually difficult.

Cocaine and amfetamines

Cocaine and amfetamine-type stimulants can have dramatic effects on the cardiovascular system through activation of the sympathetic nervous system [102]. Cocaine is a sympathomimetic that inhibits reuptake of norepinephrine and dopamine at sympathetic nerve terminals. Amfetamine and ecstasy potentiate the release of norepinephrine, dopamine and serotonin from the central and autonomic nervous systems. Cocaine toxicity may be potentiated by cannabis, while amfetamine toxicity is enhanced by alcohol. Drug-induced sympathetic activation leads to tachycardia, vasoconstriction and hypertension. Myocardial ischemia and infarction, supraventricular and ventricular tachyarrhythmias, and severe hypotension can all occur. Prolonged use can result in a dilated cardiomyopathy. The sympathetic activation produced by these drugs antagonizes the action of insulin and cocaine use has been identified as an independent risk factor for diabetic ketoacidosis [103]. The risk of diabetic ketoacidosis may be increased by the omission of insulin before discos and parties to avoid the potential risk and embarrassment of hypoglycemia.

Ecstasy is also associated with severe hyponatremia, secondary to inappropriate secretion of antidiuretic hormone, which may complicate the management of diabetic ketoacidosis [95].

Cannabis

Cannabis is not known to affect glucose metabolism but its effects on the central nervous system may increase appetite and impair recognition of hypoglycemia. Use of cannabis in low doses is associated with sympathetic activation and tachycardia; at high doses, parasympathetic activation may predominate, resulting in bradycardia and hypotension. In the absence of any structural heart disease, these effects are usually well tolerated.

Hypoglycemia

While the association between recreational drug use and diabetic ketoacidosis is well established, there are few data suggesting any association with hypoglycemia. Such drugs, however, are often taken in conjunction with alcohol and may be associated with poor oral intake of carbohydrate both of which will increase the risk of hypoglycemia. Moreover, amfetamine-like stimulants can induce frenetic behavior at night clubs and raves which can induce hypoglycemia in people treated with insulin [104]. The hallucinatory, or central nervous system, depressant effects of recreational drugs may impair an individual's ability to recognize and treat hypoglycemia. Furthermore, the sympathomimetic effects of cocaine and amfetamine-type stimulants may mimic the autonomic signs and symptoms of hypoglycemia.

Advice on recreational drug use in diabetes

Illicit drugs cause significant morbidity and are hazardous for people with diabetes. Their dangers must be emphasized to people with T1DM (particularly teenagers and young adults), but advice must be given in a sensitive and non-judgmental manner. When exposed to recreational drugs and alcohol, modest reductions in insulin dosage and regular consumption of carbohydrate-based snacks or non-alcoholic sugary drinks are required, particularly if strenuous dancing is to be undertaken. In such situations, dehydration occurs and water should be drunk regularly.

Travel

Diabetes must not be regarded as a bar to short or long-distance travel, although careful planning may be required to avoid metabolic disturbances and other problems of diabetes that could have particularly serious consequences away from home. Diet and an adequate fluid intake may be disrupted while traveling or staying abroad, and local differences in climate, food, endemic diseases and medical facilities may compromise diabetes control. Blood glucose levels should be monitored frequently during travel and holidays, and people with diabetes must be able to take a pragmatic approach to deal with contingencies (e.g. loss of insulin, delays during travel) that could perturb their diabetes. Occasionally, specific diabetic complications or other medical disorders such as uncontrolled hypertension or ischemic heart disease can jeopardize health and safety during travel and periods away from home.

Preparation for travel

Personal identification

Travelers with diabetes should carry a doctor's letter stating the diagnosis and treatment, and ideally some other form of identification such as the "Medic Alert" bracelets or necklaces or "Medi-Tag" labels (these contain personalized medical information and are recognized worldwide). These should also allay the suspicions of airline security, immigration and customs officials who discover syringes and drugs in luggage. Many national diabetes associations provide an identification card that shows the patient's photograph, doctor's name and contact telephone number. Diabetes UK issues a card with the statement "I have type 1 diabetes" in five different languages.

If a prolonged stay abroad is intended, it is useful to carry a prescription letter listing all medications (with generic names, as brand names often vary between countries), insulin-injection devices and blood-testing items.

Insurance and medical care abroad

Comprehensive medical insurance is essential to cover accidents and illness that require medical assistance, and loss of medical equipment and drugs. The insurance policy must cover diabetes and other pre-existing medical conditions, as claims relating to these may otherwise be rejected. Most travel policies contain exclusions, which frequently include diabetes; a person with diabetes may not be covered for conditions such as a stroke or myocardial infarction for which diabetes is a recognized risk factor. When appropriate, insurance must be adequate to cover any dangerous sporting activities (when hypoglycemia could be particularly hazardous), and the costs of emergency air transport home in the event of a serious accident or illness.

Most countries in the EU provide emergency medical attention free or at reduced rates to visitors from other member states, although immediate payment for treatment may be demanded in some countries, such as France. Travelers from the EU can obtain a form (E111) in their home country, which confirms their entitlement to this scheme, although full medical travel insurance is still recommended. Those planning to stay in an EU country for over 6 months will require an E112 form. Some non-EU countries (e.g. Australia and Russia) offer free or reduced-rate medical care for EU members. Details are given in leaflet SA30, obtainable from travel agents and government departments. In the USA, emergency medical treatment can be extremely expensive, and insurance premiums are correspondingly high. A list of insurers who do not load premiums against people with diabetes can be obtained from national diabetes associations.

Irrespective of medical insurance cover, it should be appreciated that emergency medical care available in some countries is suboptimal or even potentially dangerous for a diabetes-related emergency. In some parts of the world, insulin is not readily obtainable and intravenous fluids are in short supply. These considerations may influence the choice of holiday destination for people with diabetes.

Drugs and equipment

Essential items for the diabetic traveller are listed in Table 24.6.

• *Immunization.* Routine recommendations should always be followed for the relevant destination. Occasionally, a severe reaction to a vaccine may cause a temporary rise in insulin requirements.

• *Medication.* Air travelers treated with insulin should carry an ample supply in their hand luggage. Preferably, another supply of medication should be carried by a relative or friend in case of loss or theft. When traveling by air, medication and blood monitoring equipment should not be consigned to the hold, because of the risk of losing luggage. During travel, insulin can be carried in an insulated cool bag or a pre-cooled vacuum flask. People on CSII should carry insulin pens as a back-up in case of pump failure and the contact details of the pump manufacturer so that a replacement can be ordered.

Table 24.6 Checklist of essential items for travelers with insulin-treated diabetes.

Documents
Diabetes identity card/bracelet
Document stating diagnosis and treatment
Blood glucose monitoring diary
Equipment
Insulin vials or cartridges
Syringes and needles/pens and spare pen needles
Flask or cool bag for insulin storage
Blood glucose meter; spare meter and batteries
Finger pricker and spare lancets; container for used needles
Blood glucose strips (visual reading)
Fluids
Glucose free drinks (screw-top container)
Bottled water (plastic container)
Hypoglycemia treatment
Quick-acting carbohydrate:
• Glucose drinks (screw-top container)
• Glucose tablets/confectionery
Slow-acting carbohydrate:
• Biscuits or cereal bars

• *Blood glucose monitoring.* Extremes of temperature and high altitude can disable some blood glucose meters and affect the accuracy of blood glucose test strips, although the cabin pressure of passenger aircraft (equivalent to an altitude of up to 8000 feet) should not pose problems [105]. While on holiday, it is sensible to carry a spare meter and/or visually read glucose strips in case the meter fails.

• *Other considerations.* Those prone to motion sickness should take an anti-emetic to prevent nausea and vomiting from disrupting glycemic control. Antidiarrhoeal agents and a broad-spectrum antibiotic should be carried, particularly if traveling to regions with a high risk of acquiring gastroenteritis. People with peripheral sensory neuropathy should take comfortable and appropriate footwear for travel and for holiday use, as foot ulceration may be caused by wearing ill-fitting sandals or walking barefoot across rocks or even hot sand.

Long flights and crossing time zones

These pose several potential problems, ranging from the timing and composition of airline meals to ensuring that insulin dosages will cover the flight and adjust to local time on arrival.

Meals

Times of serving in-flight meals after take-off can usually be obtained from the airline. Meals can either be regarded as snacks or as main meals, depending on the travel schedule. Some airlines provide so-called "diabetic" meals but these are mainly intended for people with T2DM and are small and low in carbohydrate [106], thus increasing the risk of hypoglycemia. Vegetarian meals may be more suitable for people with T1DM, as they often contain pasta-based dishes or rice. In-flight meals can be supplemented with the patient's own supply of suitable carbohydrate, but it is impractical to carry large quantities, not least because of the limits of what foods may be imported into many countries. Allowance may have to be made for delayed flights or long intervals between meals, while fatigue or travel sickness may blunt appetite.

Alcohol

Drinking alcohol before and during air travel is best avoided because of the risk of hypoglycemia; also, the diuretic effects of alcohol favor dehydration, which has been implicated in deep venous thrombosis and pulmonary embolism during long-haul flights (although diabetes does not appear to confer greater risk) [107]. Water or non-alcoholic sugar-free drinks should be drunk liberally.

Blood glucose

Blood glucose levels should be monitored frequently while in transit and when changing time zones. It is often safer to allow in-flight blood glucose values to be slightly higher than usual to avoid the risk of hypoglycemia.

Insulin treatment

There is no evidence-based information on how to adjust insulin dosages during flights that cross several time zones, and this probably accounts for the variability in the advice that is given [108]. Each case should be discussed individually with the patient, taking into account the duration of the flight and the change in time zone, the usual insulin preparations and dosages, the size and timing of meals, and the results of glucose monitoring. Some general guidelines are suggested in Table 24.7 and Fig. 24.4.

Guiding principles are:

• Do not aim for strict blood glucose control while flying. A few hours of mild or moderate hyperglycemia (e.g. 10–13 mmol/L) will do no harm and, as long as glucose levels are monitored regularly, it is safer to reduce usual insulin dose and use small additional insulin dosages rather than risk hypoglycemia.

• Blood glucose levels should be checked every 2–3 hours.

• Time changes of less than 4 hours in either direction usually need no major adjustment of the usual insulin schedule: simply give the next dose of insulin at its usual clock time, using the destination's time zone.

• Westward flights lengthen the "day." Give the next dose of delayed-acting or premixed insulin at its usual clock time (using the destination's time zone) or adjust the insulin infusion rate using an insulin pump. If this injection is delayed by more than 12 hours, then additional insulin with food will be needed in the interim. The most convenient way to do this is with small doses (usually a few units) of soluble insulin or a rapid-acting analogue,

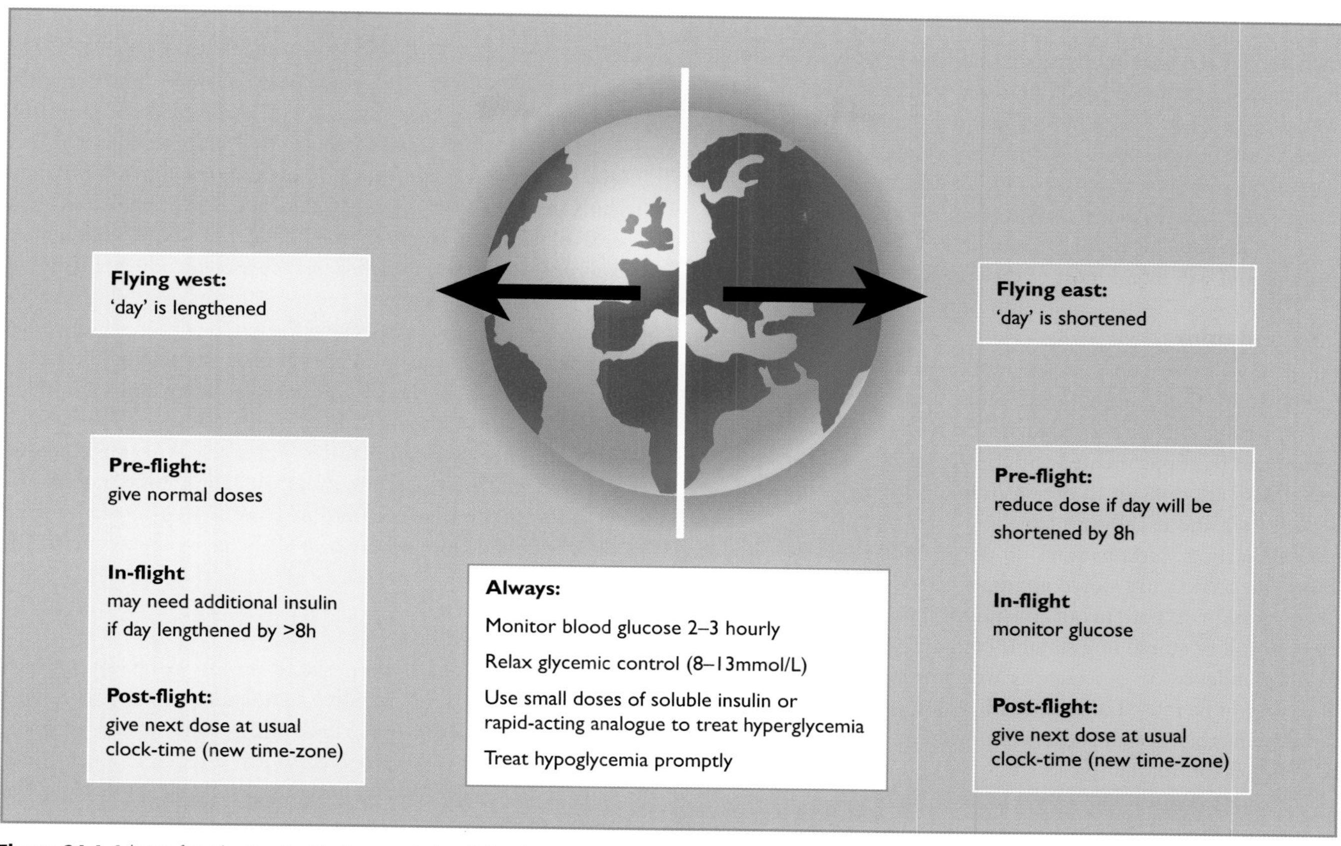

Figure 24.4 Scheme for adjusting insulin dosages during flights that cross time zones.

Table 24.7 Management of diabetes during long-distance air travel.

Obtain advice from the diabetes clinic before traveling
Obtain essential information, including the local time of departure, flight duration and local time of arrival
Inform the airline that you have diabetes, especially if treated with insulin
Carry extra supplies of carbohydrate
Anticipate that delays may occur
Time zone travel may necessitate two consecutive morning or evening insulin doses, before and after the flight
Ensure that you can monitor your blood glucose frequently during travel
Do not strive for meticulous control of blood glucose while traveling
Adjust insulin doses if necessary

injected every 4 hours or so on the basis of blood glucose measurements.

• Eastward flights shorten the "day." The next dose of delayed-acting or premixed insulin should again be given at its usual clock time (destination time zone), but because this injection will effectively be earlier than usual, the previous dose of delayed-action insulin should be reduced if the interval between the injections is less than 12 hours.

• Extremely long flights with a time shift of 12 hours or more may require two "morning" or two "evening" insulin dosages to be injected consecutively, before and after the flight.

• Any additional insulin needed to fill in long gaps between delayed-action injections or to correct hyperglycemia is best given as small doses of soluble or a rapid-acting analogue, ideally using a pen injection device.

Oral antidiabetic agents

Additional doses are not usually required to cover an extended day.

Insulin treatment in hot climates

A patient's insulin requirements may change markedly in different countries, the main factors being differences in diet and daily physical activity. Subcutaneous insulin absorption can be accelerated by high ambient temperatures, such as in a sauna (see Chapter 27), and this effect has variable clinical significance in very hot climates.

Modern formulations are quite stable, but sometimes denature if exposed to high temperatures and shaken; in this case, discolored particles or a granular appearance (distinct from the normal cloudiness of delayed-action preparations) may be seen when the insulin is resuspended. Sometimes, there are no visible changes, but the insulin appears to lose its effect, with the usual dosages failing to lower blood glucose. Particularly in hot countries, insulin is best stored in a refrigerator; if one is not available, insulin can be protected by a damp flannel or a porous clay pot containing some water or wet sand, placed in a cool part of the room. Even these measures may be unnecessary, as most insulin preparations can survive being kept at 25°C or more for up to 6 months, and will retain most of their biologic activity [109].

Food and drink

When traveling abroad, it is essential to know the basic form of carbohydrate that is eaten locally, and useful to learn to judge quantities of foods such as pasta or rice. Items selected from local menus can be supplemented with bread, biscuits or fruit. Sugar-free drinks are difficult to obtain in many countries but bottled water is safe and usually available.

Quick-acting carbohydrate to treat hypoglycemia should always be carried and stored appropriately: dextrose tablets may disintegrate or set hard in hot and humid climates unless wrapped in silver foil or stored in a suitable container, while the temperature-dependence of chocolate is well known. Cartons of fruit juice cannot be reused once opened; a plastic bottle with a screw top is preferable. Sealed packets of powdered glucose may be the best option for hot damp climates.

Traveling companions should carry a supply of quick-acting carbohydrate (and glucagon) for emergency use, and should know how to test the patient's blood glucose and how to treat hypoglycemia.

Intercurrent illness

Any intercurrent infection should be treated promptly and appropriately, with adequate replacement of fluids and carbohydrate in the form of drinks if possible. Insulin therapy must never be discontinued and dosage may have to be increased, and blood glucose should be checked every 3–4 hours, with testing for urinary ketones is possible. The "sick-day" rules described in Chapter 27 should be followed.

Recreational activities

The impact of physical exercise and sport on diabetes is discussed in Chapter 23. Patients need advice about strenuous and unaccustomed exercise during holidays, such as beach sports or prolonged and vigorous dancing. Swimming alone should be avoided. The risks of alcohol and recreational drugs have been described above.

Leaving home

As a child with diabetes grows up, inevitably parental input to the day-to-day management of diabetes is reduced with increasing autonomy of the adolescent. In teenage years this is often manifest by a deterioration in glycemic control (Chapter 52). Even in adolescence, parents or guardians still have a very important role with the provision of regular meals and in the recognition and treatment of hypoglycemia, particularly at night. Therefore, the eventual move away from the parental home can pose problems, especially if the individual with T1DM is living alone and if they move to another town. Social isolation may exist until new friends are made and access to alcohol and recreational drugs may increase, with the attendant risks that have been highlighted. Sexual activity may commence or increase, introducing issues of sexual health and pregnancy, and novel forms of exercise may be more readily available. On leaving the parental home, individuals often become removed from the familiar support of the health care professionals in their local diabetes centre and initially do not have the similar contact and immediate access to advice from doctors and nurses about diabetes – precisely at a time it may be most needed. It is a disturbing fact that "living alone" was associated with a more than fourfold increase risk of mortality from acute metabolic complications of diabetes in the Diabetes UK Cohort Study [98].

Students with diabetes

Particular emphasis has been placed on the welfare of students with T1DM who have left home to attend university or college. In part, this has been because of high-profile instances where individuals with T1DM have died shortly after commencing university [110]. Several surveys have suggested that students do find diabetes more difficult to manage, although this does not necessarily translate into a rise in glycated hemoglobin concentrations [111–116]. Barriers to diabetes control include fear of hypoglycemia, diet, irregular schedules, lack of parental involvement, limited finances, recreational drugs and alcohol. There is a natural desire for students with diabetes not to appear different from their peers and this may lead them to assign a lower priority to diabetes management than they would normally and to undertake potentially high risk activities.

Diabetes services need to be responsive to the needs of adolescents and young adults who are leaving home. Such individuals are often poorly informed about the inherent risks associated with, for example, alcohol and drugs [95,116] and these and other needs may not be addressed in the context of a routine diabetes consultation [115]. Before the individual leaves home, a formal re-education program should be offered in which alcohol, drugs, exercise, sex and sick-day management are discussed [117]. Individuals leaving home need to think about their mealtimes; it can be difficult for someone living alone to motivate themselves to prepare substantial meals and many adolescents have limited cooking skills. Regular meals are provided in university halls of residence, but the nature and content of the food, particularly the carbohydrate content, may not be ideal. Students should be advised to monitor blood glucose levels frequently during examination periods. Many students report that studying and undertaking examinations can cause marked fluctuations in glucose levels – this may partly be associated with stress or varying carbohydrate intake. Both acute hypoglycemia and hyperglycemia impair cognitive function and can cause mood changes and may affect examination performance adversely. Therefore, students should try to optimise glucose control during examinations and ensure that a supply of rapid-acting carbohydrate is available during an examination.

Many students may prefer to remain under the care of their "home" diabetes team, but it is important that they know how to contact local specialist diabetes services in the university town for advice or assistance. Medical practitioners in university health services have a duty to ensure that students with diabetes are offered regular diabetes follow-up. The student should be encouraged to confide at an early stage with a reliable friend or colleague about their diabetes and the potential problems that may arise [117]. This may cause embarrassment talking to recent acquaintances about having diabetes. University authorities have a pastoral responsibility for students with diabetes [111].

References

1 Stork ADM, Van Haeften TW, Veneman TF. Diabetes and driving: desired data, research methods and their pitfalls, current knowledge, and future research. *Diabetes Care* 2006; **29**:1942–1949.

2 Frier BM. Living with hypoglycaemia. In: Frier BM, Fisher M, eds. *Hypoglycaemia in Clinical Diabetes*, 2nd edn. Chichester: John Wiley & Sons, 2007: 309–332.

3 MacLeod KM. Diabetes and driving: towards equitable, evidence-based decision-making. *Diabet Med* 1999; **16**:282–290.

4 Stevens AB, Roberts M, McKane R, Atkinson AB, Bell PM, Hayes JR. Motor vehicle driving among diabetics taking insulin and non-diabetics. *Br Med J* 1989; **299**:591–595.

5 Eadington DW, Frier BM. Type 1 diabetes and driving experience: an eight year cohort study. *Diabet Med* 1989; **6**:137–141.

6 Lonnen KF, Powell RJ, Taylor D, Shore AC, MacLeod KM. Road traffic accidents and diabetes: insulin use does not determine risk. *Diabet Med* 2008; **25**:578–584.

7 Chantelau E, Danbeck S, Kimmerle R, Ross D. Zur Verkehrstüchtigkeit Insulin-behandelter Diabetiker. *Münsch Med Wschr* 1990; **132**:468–471.

8 Gislason T, Tomasson K, Reynisdottir H, Björnsson JK, Knistbjarnarson H. Medical risk factors amongst drivers in single-car accidents. *J Intern Med* 1997; **241**:213–219.

9 Songer TJ, LaPorte RE, Dorman JS, Orchard TJ, Cruickshanks KJ, Becker DJ, *et al.* Motor accidents and IDDM. *Diabetes Care* 1988; **11**:701–707.

10 Hansotia P, Broste SK. The effect of epilepsy or diabetes mellitus on the risk of automobile accidents. *N Engl J Med* 1991; **324**:22–26.

11 Frier BM, Matthews DM, Steel JM, Duncan LJP. Driving and insulin dependent diabetes. *Lancet* 1980; **i**:232–234.

12 Cox DJ, Gonder-Frederick LA, Kovatchev B, Julian DM, Clarke WL. Progressive hypoglycemia's impact on driving simulation performance. *Diabetes Care* 2000; **23**:163–170.

13 Deary IJ. Symptoms of hypoglycaemia and effects on mental performance and emotions. In: Frier BM, Fisher M, eds. *Hypoglycaemia in Clinical Diabetes*, 2nd edn. Chichester: John Wiley & Sons Ltd, 2007: 25–48.

14 McCrimmon RJ, Deary IJ, Huntly BJP, MacLeod KM, Frier BM. Visual information processing during controlled hypoglycaemia in humans. *Brain* 1996; **119**:1277–1287.

15 Ewing FME, Deary IJ, McCrimmon RJ, Strachan MWJ, Frier BM. Effect of acute hypoglycemia on visual information processing in adults with type 1 diabetes mellitus. *Physiol Behav* 1998; **64**:653–660.

16 Clarke WL, Cox DJ, Gonder-Frederick LA, Kovatchev B. Hypoglycemia and the decision to drive a motor vehicle by persons with diabetes. *JAMA* 1999; **282**:750–754.

17 Frier BM. Hypoglycemia and driving performance. *Diabetes Care* 2000; **23**:148–150.

18 Diabetes Control and Complications Trial Research Group. Adverse events and their association with treatment regimens in the Diabetes Control and Complications Trial. *Diabetes Care* 1995; **18**:1415–1427.

19 MacLeod KM, Hepburn DA, Frier BM. Frequency and morbidity of severe hypoglycaemia in insulin-treated diabetic patients. *Diabet Med* 1993; **10**:238–245.

20 Clarke B, Ward JD, Enoch BA. Hypoglycaemia in insulin dependent diabetic drivers. *Br Med J* 1980; **281**:647–650.

21 McNally PG, Maclver DH, Jowett NI, Hearnshaw JR. Hypoglycaemia in insulin dependent diabetics: is advice heeded? *Br Med J* 1987; **294**:1655–1656.

22 Graveling AJ, Warren RE, Frier BM. Hypoglycaemia and driving in people with insulin-treated diabetes: adherence to recommendations for avoidance. *Diabet Med* 2004; **21**:1014–1019.

23 Cox DJ, Gonder-Frederick LA, Kovatchev BP, Clarke WL. The metabolic demands of driving for drivers with type 1 diabetes mellitus. *Diabetes Metab Res Rev* 2002; **18**:381–385.

24 Chee CKL, Flanagan DW. Visual field loss with capillary non-perfusion in preproliferative and early proliferative diabetic retinopathy. *Br J Ophthalmol* 1993; **77**:726–730.

25 Williamson TH, George N, Flanagan DW, Norris V, Blamires T. Driving standard visual fields in diabetic patients after panretinal photocoagulation. *Vision in Vehicles III*. North Holland, 1991: 265–272.

26 Buckley SA, Jenkins L, Benjamin L. Fields, DVLC and panretinal photocoagulation. *Eye* 1992; **6**:623–625.

27 Hudson C, Flanagan JG, Turner GS, Chan HC, Young LB, McLeod D. Influence of laser photocoagulation for clinically significant diabetic macular oedema (DMO) on short-wavelength and conventional automated perimetry. *Diabetologia* 1998; **41**:1283–1292.

28 Hulbert MFG, Vernon SA. Passing the DVLC field regulations following pan-retinal photocoagulation in diabetics. *Eye* 1992; **6**:456–460.

29 Frier BM. Driving and diabetes. *Br Med J* 1992; **305**:1238–1239.

30 Jude EB, Ryan B, O'Leary BM, Gibson JM, Dodson PM. Pupillary dilatation and driving in diabetic patients. *Diabet Med* 1998; **15**:143–147.

31 DiaMond Project Group on Social Issues. Global regulations on diabetics treated with insulin and their operation of commercial motor vehicles. *Br Med J* 1993; **307**:250–253.

32 Jones GC, Frier BM. Medical assessment for licensing of taxi drivers by Scottish Local authorities. *Occup Med* 2000; **47**:40–44.

33 O'Neill S, Gill GV, and Driving and Employment Working Party of the British Diabetic Association. *Occup Med* 2000; **50**:19–21.

34 Laberge-Nadeau C, Dionne G, Ekoe J-M, Hamet P, Desjardins D, Messier S, *et al.* Impact of diabetes on crash risks of truck-permit holders and commerical drivers. *Diabetes Care* 2000; **23**:612–617.

35 Gower IF, Songer TJ, Hylton H, Thomas NL, Ekoe J-M, Lave LB, *et al*. Epidemiology of insulin-using commercial motor vehicle drivers. *Diabetes Care* 1992; **15**:1464–1467.
36 Leckie AM, Graham MK, Grant JB, Ritchie PJ, Frier BM. Frequency, severity and morbidity of hypoglycemia occurring in the workplace in people with insulin-treated diabetes. *Diabetes Care* 2005; **28**:1333–1338.
37 Poole C, Wright A, Nattrass M. Control of diabetes mellitus in shift workers. *Br J Indust Med* 1992; **49**:513–515.
38 Waclawski ER. Employment and diabetes: a survey of the prevalence of diabetic workers known by occupation physicians, and the restrictions placed on diabetic workers in employment. *Diabet Med* 1989; **6**:16–19.
39 Robinson N, Bush L, Protopapa LE, Yateman NA. Employers' attitudes to diabetes. *Diabet Med* 1989; **6**:692–697.
40 Pell S, D'Alonzo CA. Sickness absenteeism in employed diabetics. *Am J Public Health* 1967; **57**:253–258.
41 Hutchison SK, Kesson CM, Slater SD. Does diabetes affect employment prospects? *Br Med J* 1983; **287**:946–947.
42 Ardron M, MacFarlane I, Robinson C. Educational achievements, employment and social class of insulin dependent diabetics: a survey of a young adult clinic in Liverpool. *Diabet Med* 1987; **4**:546–548.
43 Lloyd CE, Robinson N, Fuller JH. Education and employment experiences in young adults with type 1 diabetes mellitus. *Diabet Med* 1992; **9**:661–666.
44 Bergers J, Nijhuis F, Janssen M, van der Horst F. Employment careers of young type 1 diabetic patients in the Netherlands. *J Occup Environ Med* 1999; **41**:1005–1010.
45 Robinson N, Yateman, NA, Protopapa LE, Bush L. Unemployment and diabetes. *Diabet Med* 1989; **6**:797–803.
46 Singh R, Press M. Employment in working age men with diabetes mellitus. *Pract Diab Int* 2007; **24**:75–77.
47 Von Korff M, Katon W, Lin EHB, Simon G, Ciechanowski P, Ludman E, *et al*. Work disability among individuals with diabetes. *Diabetes Care* 2005; **28**:1326–1332.
48 Robinson N, Stevens LK, Protopapa LE. Education and employment for young people with diabetes. *Diabet Med* 1993; **10**:983–989.
49 Songer TJ, LaPorte RE, Dorman JS, Orchard TJ, Becker DJ, Drash AL. Employment spectrum of IDDM. *Diabetes Care* 1989; **12**:615–622.
50 Mayfield JA, Deb P, Whitecotton L. Work disability and diabetes. *Diabetes Care* 1999; **22**:1105–1109.
51 Kraut A, Walld R, Tate R, Mustard C. Impact of diabetes on employment and income in Manitoba, Canada. *Diabetes Care* 2001; **24**:64–68.
52 Ng YC, Jacobs P, Johnson JA. Productivity losses associated with diabetes in the US. *Diabetes Care* 2001; **24**:257–261.
53 Welch RA. Employment of diabetics in a Post Office region. *J Soc Occup Med* 1986; **36**:80–85.
54 Waclawski ER. Sickness absence among insulin-treated diabetic employees. *Diabet Med* 1990; **7**:41–44.
55 Poole CJM, Gibbons D, Calver IA. Sickness absence in diabetic employees at a large engineering factory. *Occup Environ Med* 1994; **51**:299–301.
56 Waclawski ER, Gill GV. Diabetes mellitus and other endocrine disorders. In: Palmer KT, Cox RAF, Brown I, eds. *Fitness for Work: The Medical Aspects*, 4th edn. Oxford: Oxford University Press, 2007: 345–360.
57 Waclawski ER. Sickness absence and control of insulin treated diabetes as assessed by glycosylated haemoglobin. *J Soc Occup Med* 1991; **41**:119–120.
58 Tunceli K, Bradley CJ, Nerenz D, Williams LK, Pladevall M, Lafata, JE. The impact of diabetes on employment and work productivity. *Diabetes Care* 2007; **28**:2662–2667.
59 Gill GV, MacFarlane IA. Problems of diabetes in prison. *Br Med J* 1989; **298**:221–223.
60 MacFarlane IA, Gill GV, Masson E, Tucker NH. Diabetics in prison: can good diabetic care be achieved? *Br Med J* 1992; **304**:152–155.
61 Gill GV, MacFarlane IA, Tucker NH. Diabetes care in British prisons: existing problems and potential solutions. *Diabet Med* 1992; **9**:109–113.
62 Wright RJ, Barclay JIP, Plastow B, Frier BM. Management of diabetes in police custody: a liaison initiative between a diabetes specialist service and the police force. *Pract Diabetes Int* 2008; **25**:72–75.
63 Jervell J, Nilsson B. *Social rights of diabetic patients in Europe: a survey of European Regional Organisation of the International Diabetes Federation*. Aelvsjoe, Sweden: Swedish Diabetes Association, 1985.
64 Songer TJ, LaPorte RE, Dorman JS, Orchard TJ, Becker DJ, Drash AL. Health, life and automobile insurance characteristics in adults with IDDM. *Diabetes Care* 1991; **14**:318–324.
65 Frier BM, Sullivan FM, Stewart EJC. Diabetes and insurance: a survery of patient experience. *Diabet Med* 1984; **1**:127–130.
66 Cummins JD, Smith BD, Vance RN, VanDerhei JL. Underwriting medical impairments: diabetes mellitus. In: *Risk Classification in Life Insurance*. Boston: Kluwer-Nijhoff Publishing, 1983: 160–166.
67 Ramlau-Hansen H, Jespersen MCB, Andersen PK, Borch-Johnsen K, Deckert T. Life insurance for insulin-dependent diabetics. *Scand Actuar J* 1987: 19–36.
68 Borch-Johnsen K. Improving prognosis of type 1 diabetes mortality, accidents and impact on insurance. *Diabetes Care* 1999; **22**(Suppl 2):B1–B3.
69 Mathiesen B, Borch-Johnsen K. Diabetes and accident insurance: a 3 year follow-up of 7599 insured diabetic individuals. *Diabetes Care* 1997; **20**:1781–1784.
70 Jones KE, Gill GV. Insurance company attitudes to diabetes. *Pract Diabet* 1989; **6**:230–231.
71 Peele PB, Lave JR, Songer TJ. Diabetes in employer-sponsored health insurance. *Diabetes Care* 2002; **25**:1964–1968.
72 Carlsson S, Hammar N, Grill V. Alcohol consumption and type 2 diabetes: meta-analysis of epidemiological studies indicates a U-shaped relationship. *Diabetologia* 2005; **48**:1051–1054.
73 Koppes LLJ, Dekker JM, Hendriks HFJ, Bouter LM, Heine RJ. Moderate alcohol consumption lowers the risk of type 2 diabetes: a meta-analysis of prospective observational studies. *Diabetes Care* 2005; **28**:719–725.
74 van de Weil A. Diabetes mellitus and alcohol. *Diabetes Metab Res Rev* 2004; **20**:263–267.
75 Krebs HA, Freedland RA, Hems R, Stubbs M. Inhibition of hepatic gluconeogenesis by ethanol. *Biochem J* 1969; **112**:117–124.
76 Kreisberg RA, Siegal AM, Owen WC. Glucose-lactate interrelationships: effect of ethanol. *J Clin Invest* 1971; **50**:175–185.
77 Yki-Järvinen H, Koivisto VA, Ylikahri R, Taskinen MR. Acute effects of ethanol and acetate on glucose kinetics in normal subjects. *Am J Physiol* 1988; **254**:E175–E180.
78 Freinkel N, Singer DA, Arky RA, Bleicher SJ, Anderson JB, Silbert CK. Alcohol hypoglycemia 1. Carbohydrate metabolism of patients

with clinical alcohol hypoglycemia and the experimental reproduction of the syndrome with pure ethanol. *J Clin Invest* 1963; **42**:1112–1133.

79 Richardson T, Weiss M, Thomas P, Kerr D. Day after the night before: influence of evening alcohol on risk of hypoglycemia in patients with type 1 diabetes. *Diabetes Care* 2005; **28**:1801–1802.

80 Cheyne EH, Sherwin RS, Lunt MJ, Cavan DA, Thomas PW, Kerr D. Influence of alcohol on cognitive performance during mild hypoglycaemia: implications for type 1 diabetes. *Diabet Med* 2004; **21**:230–237.

81 Feher MD, Grout P, Kennedy A, Elkeles RS, Touquet R. Hypoglycaemia in an inner city accident and emergency department: a 12 month survey. *Arch Emerg Med* 1989; **6**:183–188.

82 Arky RA, Veverbrants E, Abramson EA. Irreversible hypoglycemia: a complication of alcohol and insulin. *JAMA* 1968; **206**:575–578.

83 Freiberg MS, Cabral HJ, Heeren TC, Vasan RS, Ellison RC. Alcohol consumption and the prevalence of the metabolic syndrome in the USA: a cross-sectional analysis of data from the Third National Health and Nutrition Examination Survey. *Diabetes Care* 2004; **27**:2954–2959.

84 Johnson KH, Bazargan M, Bing EG. Alcohol consumption and compliance among inner-city minority patients with type 2 diabetes mellitus. *Arch Fam Med* 2000; **9**:964–970.

85 Ahmed AT, Karter AJ, Liu J. Alcohol consumption is inversely associated with adherence to diabetes self-care behaviours. *Diabet Med* 2006; **23**:795–802.

86 Ahmed AT, Karter AJ, Warton EM, Doan JU, Weisner CM. The relationship between alcohol consumption and glycemic control among patients with diabetes: the Kaiser Permanente Northern Californian Diabetes Registry. *J Gen Intern Med* 2008; **23**:275–282.

87 Koppes LLJ, Dekker JM, Hendriks HFJ, Bouter LM, Heine RJ. Meta-analysis of the relationship between alcohol consumption and coronary heart disease and mortality in type 2 diabetic patients. *Diabetologia* 2006; **49**:648–652.

88 Pitsavos C, Makrilakis K, Panagiotakos DB, Chrysohoou C, Ioannidis I, Dimosthenopoulos C, *et al.* The J-shape effect of alcohol intake on the risk of developing acute coronary syndromes in diabetic subjects: the CARDIO200 II Study. *Diabetic Med* 2005; **22**:243–248.

89 Beulens JWJ, Kruidhof JS, Grobbee DE, Charturvedi N, Fuller JH, Soedamah-Muthu SS. Alcohol consumption and risk of microvascular complications in type 1 diabetes patients: the EURODIAB Prospective Complications Study. *Diabetologia* 2008; **51**:1631–1638.

90 McCulloch DK, Campbell IW, Prescott RJ, Clarke BF. Effect of alcohol intake on symptomatic peripheral neuropathy in diabetic men. *Diabetes Care* 1980; **3**:245–247.

91 Lee P, Nicoll AJ, McDonough M, Cloman PG. Substance abuse in young patients with type 1 diabetes: easily neglected in complex medical management. *Intern Med J* 2005; **35**: 359–361.

92 United Nations Office on Drugs and Crime. World Drug Report 2008. http://www.unodc.org/unodc/en/data-and-analysis/WDR-2008.html

93 Griffiths C, Romeri E, Brock A, Morgan O. Geographical variations in deaths related to drug misuse in England and Wales, 1993–2006. *Health Stat Q* 2008; **39**:14–21.

94 Glasgow AM, Tynan D, Scwartz R, Hicks JM, Tuek J, Driscol C, O'Donnell RM, Getson PR. Alcohol and drug use in teenagers with diabetes mellitus *J Adolesc Health* 1991; **12**:11–14.

95 Ng RSH, Darko DA, Hillson RM. Street drug use among young patients with Type 1 diabetes in the UK. *Diabet Med* 2004; **21**:295–296.

96 Martinez-Aguayo A, Aranenda JC, Fernandez D, Gleisner A, Perez V, Codner E. Tobacco, alcohol, and illicit drug use in adolescents with diabetes mellitus. *Paediatr Diabet* 2007; **8**:265–271.

97 Johnson KH, Bazargan M, Cherpitel CJ. Alcohol, tobacco, and drug use and the onset of type 2 diabetes among inner-city minority patients. *J Am Board Fam Pract* 2001; **14**:430–436.

98 Laing SP, Jones ME, Swerdlow AJ, Burden AC, Gatling W. Psychosocial and socioeconomic risk factors for premature death in young people with type 1 diabetes. *Diabetes Care* 2005; **28**:1618–1623.

99 Feltbower RG, Bodansky HJ, Patterson CC, Parslow RC, Stephenson CR, Reynolds C, *et al.* Acute complications and drug misuse are important causes of death for children and young adults with type 1 diabetes: results from the Yorkshire Register of diabetes in children and young adults. *Diabetes Care* 2008; **31**:922–926.

100 Jackson CT, Covell NH, Drake RE, Essock SM. Relationship between diabetes and mortality among persons with co-occurring psychotic and substance use disorders. *Psychiatr Serv* 2007; **58**:270–272.

101 Saunders SA, Democratis J, Martin J, Macfarlane IA. Intravenous drug abuse and type 1 diabetes: financial and healthcare implications. *Diabetic Med* 2004; **21**:1269–1273.

102 Ghuran A, Nolan J. Recreational drug misuse: issues for the cardiologist. *Heart* 2000; **83**:627–633.

103 Nyenwe EA, Loganathan RS, Blum S, Ezuteh DO, Erani DM, Wan JY, *et al.* Active use of cocaine: an independent risk factor for recurrent diabetic ketoacidosis in a city hospital. *Endocr Pract* 2007; **13**:22–29.

104 Jenks J, Watkinson M. Minimizing the risks of amphetamine use for young adults with diabetes. *J Diabet Nurs* 1998; **2**:179–182.

105 Gautier JP, Bigard AX, Douce P, Duvaller A, Cathelineau G. Influence of simulated altitudeon the performance of five blood glucose meters. *Diabetes Care* 1996; **19**:1430–1433.

106 Johnston RV, Neilly IJ, Lang JM, Frier BM. The high flying diabetic: dietary inadequacy of airline meals. *Diabet Med* 1986; **3**:580A.

107 Lapostelle F, Suget V, Borron SW, Desmaizieres M, Sordelet D, Lapandry C, *et al.* Severe pulmonary embolism associated with air travel. *N Engl J Med* 2001; **345**:779–783.

108 Gill GV, Redmond S. Insulin treatment, time-zones and air travel: a survey of current advice from British diabetic clinics. *Diabet Med* 1993; **10**:764–767.

109 Blakeman K. The characteristics and storage requirements of modern insulins. *Pharmaceut J* 1983; **253**:711–713.

110 Strachan MWJ, MacCuish AC, Frier BM. The care of students with insulin-treated diabetes mellitus living in university accommodation: scope for improvement? *Diabet Med* 2000; **17**:70–73.

111 Wdowik MJ, Kendall PA, Harris MA. College students with diabetes: using focus groups and interviews to determine psychosocial issues and barriers to control. *Diabetes Educ* 1997; **23**:558–562.

112 Ramchandani N, Cantey-Kiser JM, Alter CA, Brink SJ, Yeager SD, Tamborlane WV, *et al.* Self-reported factors that affect glycemic

control in college students with type 1 diabetes. *Diabetes Educ* 2000; **26**:656–666.

113 Eaton S, Williams R, Bodansky HJ. University students with diabetes. *Diabet Med* 2001; **18**:940–942.

114 Miller-Hagan RS, Janas BG. Drinking perceptions and management strategies of collage students with diabetes. *Diabetes Educ* 2002; **28**:233–244.

115 Geddes J, McGeough E, Frier BM. Young adults with type 1 diabetes in tertiary education: do students receive adequate specialist care? *Diabet Med* 2006; **23**:1155–1157.

116 Balfe M. Diets and discipline: the narratives of practice of university students with type 1 diabetes. *Sociol Health Illn* 2007; **29**:136–153.

117 Mellinger DC. Preparing students with diabetes for life at college. *Diabetes Care* 2003; **26**:2675–2678.

25 Monitoring Diabetes

Andrew J. Farmer
Department of Primary Health Care, University of Oxford, Oxford, UK

Keypoints

- Glycated hemoglobin (HbA_{1c}) levels will increasingly be presented using the International Federation of Clinical Chemistry standard expressed as mmol/mol of unglycated hemoglobin. The equivalent of the current HbA_{1c} levels of 6.5% and 7.5% are 48 mmol/mol and 59 mmol/mol.
- For patients with type 1 diabetes (T1DM), blood glucose control should be monitored with measurement of HbA_{1c} every 2–6 months depending on the level and stability of blood glucose control and change in therapy.
- Patients with T1DM should be encouraged to self-monitor blood glucose with capillary blood glucose meters. With treatment regimens intended to produce intensive glycemic control testing should be frequent (e.g. four or more times a day).
- For patients with type 2 diabetes (T2DM), blood glucose control should be monitored using high precision methods for measurement of HbA_{1c} every 2–6 months depending on the level and stability of blood glucose control and change in therapy.
- For non-insulin-treated patients with T2DM, self-monitoring of blood glucose is unlikely to be cost-effective for well-controlled patients and should therefore only be used when training and support is available and a clear purpose for use identified.

Why monitor?

> *"The overall goal of diabetes management is to achieve as near normal physiological or ideal values as possible, without detriment to quality of life and, for glucose control in particular, without causing significant hypoglycemia"* [1].

Diabetes is a disorder of glucose homeostasis. It currently affects 285 million people worldwide and is expected to affect 435 million by 2039 [2]. For people without diabetes, glucose levels are maintained in the range of 4–6 mmol/L (80–110 mg/dL). When blood glucose levels increase as a result of glycogen conversion or eating carbohydrate-containing food, insulin is released restoring homeostasis through hepatic conversion of glucose to glycogen, and uptake of glucose into muscle and fat cells. Conversely, if blood glucose levels fall too low as a result of exercise or lack of food, glucagon is released causing hepatic conversion of glycogen to glucose.

People with type 1 diabetes mellitus (T1DM) lack the normal homeostatic mechanism to control levels of blood glucose, while people with type 2 diabetes mellitus (T2DM) have an impaired or absent response. In addition to insulin, which is the most important of the regulatory mechanisms, growth hormone, thyroxine and catecholamines are also important counter-regulatory hormones and lead to increases in blood glucose levels. The aim of monitoring glycemic control is to diagnose the nature of any impairment of homeostatic mechanisms, allow patients to understand the nature of their disorder, determine optimum times for initiating therapeutic intervention; and guide the day-to-day adjustment of management regimens.

Glycated hemoglobin (HbA_{1c}) and blood glucose are the two most frequently used measures of glycemia in current practice. Glycated hemoglobin provides information about overall control of glucose levels in the previous 6–8 weeks allowing assessment of the need for therapy and therapeutic response with minimal within-person variation in measurement. Blood glucose concentrations provide information about the day-to-day level of control, variation in control and response to therapeutic intervention. Measurement and interpretation of blood glucose, however, may be difficult because of potentially wide within-person variations in measures other than when fasting. Prospective observational and intervention studies have confirmed that HbA_{1c} levels are related to long-term disease outcomes [3,4]. Both HbA_{1c} and blood glucose therefore, along with a number of other tests, including measurement of urinary glucose for those who do not intend to aim for intensive glucose control, remain an option for helping to identify poor glycemic control and to facilitate the adjustment of therapy to achieve optimal glucose levels.

Textbook of Diabetes, 4th edition. Edited by R. Holt, C. Cockram, A. Flyvbjerg and B. Goldstein.

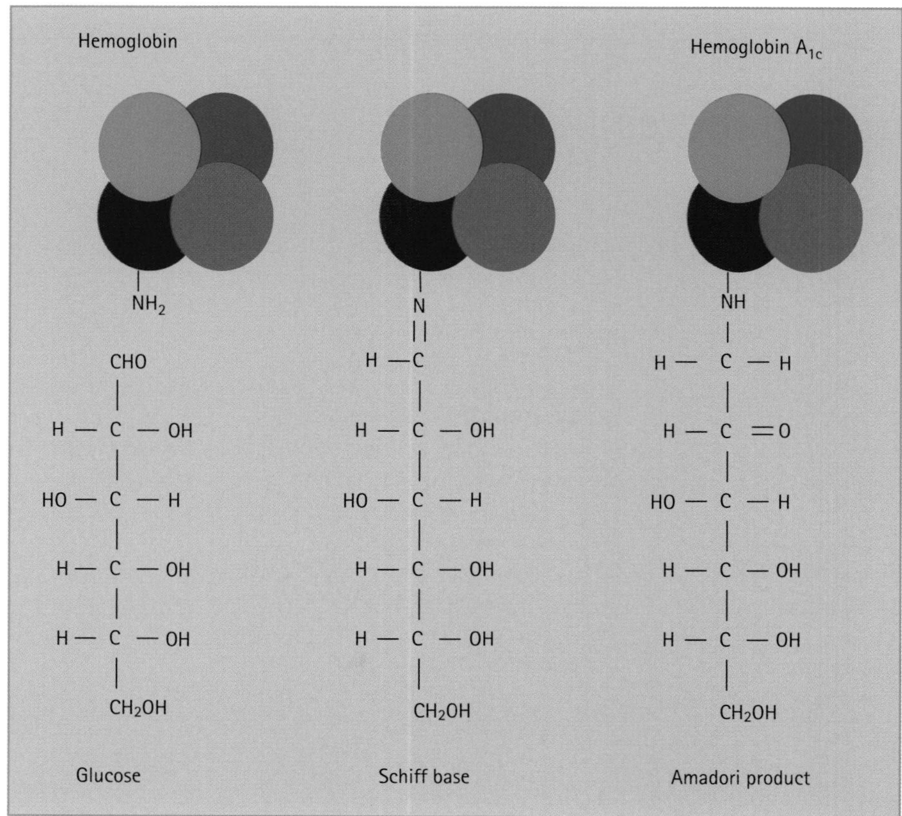

Figure 25.1 The Amadori reaction.

Tests and their characteristics

Glycated hemoglobin

Quality controlled HbA_{1c} measurement has a central role in the management of diabetes. Its pivotal role derives from its use in reports of the major outcome studies [5,6]; HbA_{1c} levels can be directly related to the risk of development of diabetic complications. Major national guidelines address this area and make recommendations about its use [5,7].

Hemoglobin reacts spontaneously with glucose to form glycated derivatives in a non-enzymatic manner. The process occurs slowly, with the extent of glycation determined by the concentration of glucose in blood. Human hemoglobin A undergoes such glycation to form HbA_{1c} from a reaction between the β-chain of hemoglobin A0 and glucose (Figure 25.1). Other compounds result from similar reactions on the α and β chains of hemoglobin and these can be measured as the total glycated hemoglobin.

Until the measurement of different glycated derivatives in the late 1990s, the difficulties of obtaining a common reference standard and the costs of the test made comparisons between laboratories difficult and availability limited. Many of these problems have been overcome, and the most common measured component, HbA_{1c}, is now widely accepted as a standard measurement of glycemic control.

Glycated hemoglobin can be affected by the presence of hemoglobin variants and uremia, but specific assays (e.g. high performance liquid chromatography rather than immunochemistry or affinity chromatography methods) can be used to obtain an accurate result. Vitamin C, hemolytic and iron deficiency anemia can also give abnormal results. Laboratories still differ in whether a result from a heterozygous patient with variant hemoglobin is reported as non-comparable to the Diabetes Control and Complications Trial/UK Prospective Diabetes Study (DCCT/UKPDS) standard, or whether it is not reported at all. Other conditions in which there is a rapid turnover of erythrocytes (e.g. polycythemia, anemia or blood transfusion) can also give inaccurate results (Table 25.1).

Table 25.1 Conditions that can affect the measurement of glycated hemoglobin.

Iron deficiency anemia
Hemoglobinopathies
Polycythemia
Blood transfusion
Hemolysis (hemolytic anemia)
Uremia caused by renal failure
High levels of vitamin C

Glycated hemoglobin serves as a retrospective indicator of the average glucose concentration over the previous 6–8 weeks. Approximately 50% of the variance in HbA_{1c} is determined by the average blood glucose concentration over the previous month, 25% by the concentration over 30–60 days, and the remaining 25% by the concentration from 60 to 120 days.

Alignment of assays for HbA_{1c}

New International Federation of Clinical Chemistry standard

Soon after glycated hemoglobin measurements were adopted into routine use, it became clear that there were significant differences between results from differing laboratories. The differences arose because of the range of assays used and lack of agreement over a common reference standard. With the publication of DCCT [5] in 1993 a number of countries developed national programs to standardize measurement, which included external quality assurance schemes to ensure that measurements between laboratories could be compared [8]. With the development of more advanced assays it became possible to propose a new reference method based on assaying a specific component of HbA_{1c} (the β-N-terminal hexapeptide).

Despite these efforts to standardize HbA_{1c} there are over 30 different methods in use for measurement. Manufacturers provide calibration factors for individual machines, and there is a global network of laboratories that maintain and monitor the relationship between the different standards.

The new reference standard, agreed by the International Federation of Clinical Chemistry and Laboratory Medicine (IFCC) was not initially viewed with enthusiasm because it would have lowered the reference range of HbA_{1c} by 1.5–2.0 percentage points, thus leading to confusion among both clinicians and patients and a potential deterioration in population glycemic control. A shift to the new reporting strategies, however, offers the opportunity for a global agreement about the requirements for manufacturers to supply equipment that can be standardized.

In Europe the new standard will be introduced to ensure laboratory and clinical practice is traceable to the IFCC reference method using units expressed as *mmol per mol* of unglycated hemoglobin. In addition, all results will be presented with both the DCCT aligned and the IFCC standard until at least June 2011. Thus, when HbA_{1c} results (DCCT aligned) are expressed as percent hemoglobin the equation deriving the relationship is:

$$\text{IFCC-HbA}_{1c}\ (\text{mmol/mol}) = [\text{DCCT-HbA}_{1c}\ (\%) - 2.15] \times 10.929$$

The conversion of integer HbA_{1c} (%) values to new units has an easy-to-remember numerical relationship known as "Kilpatrick's kludge" [9]. For example, for an HbA_{1c} of 7% subtract 2 = 5, and then subtract a further 2 = 3. Thus, a HbA_{1c} of 7% becomes 53 mmol/mol. For non-integer values the use of the formula or reference tables is required. The equivalent of the current HbA_{1c} targets of 6.5% and 7.5% are 48 mmol/mol and 59 mmol/mol in the new units (Table 25.2).

For both patients and clinicians, a shift to the new standard will reduce potential confusion between blood glucose levels and HbA_{1c} measurements. With current reference ranges it is relatively easy for confusion between a blood glucose value given in mmol/L to a value of a similar order to the HbA_{1c} (%) level but having different implications for clinical decision-making.

Table 25.2 IFCC aligned values for HbA_{1c}.

Current DCCT aligned HbA_{1c} (%)	IFCC HbA_{1c} (mmol/mol)
4.0	20
5.0	31
6.0	42
6.5	48
7.0	53
7.5	59
8.0	64
9.0	75
10.0	86

IFCC-HbA_{1c} (mmol/mol) = [DCCT-HbA_{1c} (%) − 2.15] × 10.929

Nevertheless, a considerable education initiative is needed to inform both patients and clinicians of the change.

Estimated average glucose measurements

As glycated hemoglobin levels are related to blood glucose concentrations and formulas, the American Diabetes Association (ADA) has proposed an alternative approach with the introduction of the estimated average glucose measurement (eAG).

Glycated hemoglobin provides information about the overall levels of glucose to which tissue is exposed. For a non-insulin-using patient with T2DM with regular fasting plasma glucose (FPG) levels of 6.5 mmol/L, an HbA_{1c} of around 53 mmol/mol (7%) would be expected, but prandial elevation of blood glucose makes an additional contribution to the rate of glycosylation, thus affecting individual results [10].

A large international study has recently established a strong correlation between continuous blood glucose monitoring results and HbA_{1c} ($r = 0.92$) in 507 Caucasian adults. The authors proposed a formula to derive eAG [11], and led to the recent ADA position statement recommending the use of the eAG measure [5]. Concerns about the extent to which the relationship between HbA_{1c} and eAG are generalizable, the limited information about applicability to all ethnic groups and the potential for patient confusion about the measurements have led to limited adoption outside the USA.

The extent to which eAG are related to diabetes complications is controversial. There are no long-term studies relating continuous blood glucose measurement to long-term diabetes outcomes. Instead, HbA_{1c} remains both a target of intervention in many trials, as well as a measure of success in improving glycemic control. This approach is based on the demonstrated relationships between HbA_{1c} and diabetes outcomes. There is therefore concern that the introduction of an eAG might lead patients and clinicians to place weight on measurement of blood glucose, while the assay is actually of HbA_{1c}.

Use of HbA_{1c} in the diagnosis of diabetes

Current guidance continues to recommend that the diagnosis of diabetes is based on at least two laboratory measurements of blood glucose ≥7 mmol/L or random samples of ≥11.1 mmol/L. In the event of uncertainty, an oral glucose tolerance test is proposed. HbA_{1c} offers a potentially easier, non-fasting and therefore more acceptable test. Furthermore, there appears to be less intra-individual variation with HbA_{1c} than glucose testing. Previously, there were concerns that despite the variation in results of oral glucose testing within the same person, the alternative of a single HbA_{1c} test would be unsatisfactory because the threshold for screening (usually identified as 53 mmol/mol [7%]) would miss a substantial number of people with diabetes. There is also considerable potential for confusion, because current guidance for people with diabetes is to aim, if possible, for HbA_{1c} levels of 48–59 mmol/mol (6.5–7.5%) [7]. One possible alternative to simplify diagnosis is the combined measurement of fasting blood glucose and HbA_{1c}, making use of an algorithm developed from studies in which the two measurements were compared against the results of an oral glucose tolerance test [12]. There are ongoing discussions about the use of HbA_{1c} of a diagnostic test and, at the time of writing, it has been proposed that an HbA_{1c} of 48 mmol/mol (6.5%) would be diagnostic of diabetes. This test will not replace the glucose criteria as in many parts of the world HbA_{1c} is not available.

Point of care HbA_{1c}

Point of care testing for HbA_{1c} is now possible with clinic-based analyzers and may allow timely decisions on therapy changes when needed. A recent study of their use, however, carried out in a clinic setting, does not yet provide sufficient information about the benefits to justify their widespread deployment [13,14].

Measurement of fructosamine

Albumin is the main component of plasma proteins. Albumin contains free amino groups which can react non-enzymatically with glucose to form fructosamine. Measurement of fructosamine reflects glucose levels over the previous 1–3 weeks. Fructosamine measurement is not appropriate for routine use because the assay is markedly affected by excessive turnover or excretion of albumin in, for example, renal disease. In addition, fructosamine assays are not standardized in the same way as HbA_{1c} assays. Fructosamine testing remains useful in a number of circumstances, for example in pregnancy where glucose requirements change rapidly, or in the preconception period where motivation to improve control is high and the changes can be evaluated at shorter intervals. With the lower cost and increased standardization of HbA_{1c}, however, it is possible that more frequent measurements of HbA_{1c} may be an alternative strategy, particularly if evaluating potentially large improvements in the blood glucose over the preceding 4–6 weeks contributing to a clinically important change from a previous HbA_{1c} result [15].

Blood glucose

Blood glucose (or the level of glucose to which the body's organs are exposed) is expressed as the plasma glucose concentration. Blood glucose was traditionally given as whole blood values, but plasma glucose levels are now measured and reported by most laboratories. Blood samples for analysis need to be taken under controlled conditions to allow accurate measurement of glucose levels. Red blood cells may continue to metabolize glucose after collection, continuing glycolysis, and thus leading to reductions in glucose levels. This should be avoided by rapid centrifugation, collection onto ice and storage in a refrigerator. If blood is to be transported at room temperature it should be collected into fluoride-containing tubes which inhibit further glucose metabolism. If a patient has an intravenous line *in situ*, blood should be drawn from the arm opposite to the one with the line to prevent contamination of the sample from any infusion.

Blood glucose measurement is a term that is frequently used without precise definition. Measurement of glucose levels is usually carried out either on capillary or venous samples of blood. Most laboratories measure the level of glucose in plasma, which again differs from measurements made on whole blood. Table 25.3 shows the equivalent measurements from the different sites and samples taken.

Blood glucose levels are expressed in SI (Systeme International) units as millimoles/liter (mmol/L). The traditional unit for measuring blood glucose is milligrams/decilitre (mg/dL), although use of these units is now largely confined to the USA. To convert mmol/L glucose to mg/dL, multiply by 18 (Table 25.4).

Sampling and preparation of the sample affect measurement. Whole blood glucose is also affected by the concentration of protein (mainly hemoglobin) in the sample. Whole blood concentrations are therefore 12–15% lower than plasma concentra-

Table 25.3 Values for diagnosis of diabetes mellitus.

Time of measurement	Glucose concentration (mmol/L)*			
	Plasma		Whole blood	
	Venous	Capillary	Venous	Capillary
Fasting	≥7.0	≥7.0	≥6.1	≥6.1
2 h after a glucose load	≥11.1	≥12.2	≥10.0	≥11.1

* 1 mmol/L = 18 mg/dL.

Table 25.4 Correlation of HbA_{1c} with average glucose.

HbA_{1c} (%)	Mean plasma glucose	
	mg/dL	mmol/L
6	126	7.0
7	154	8.6
8	183	10.2
9	212	11.8
10	240	13.4
11	269	14.9
12	298	16.5

tions. Venous blood glucose levels are normally similar to arterial and capillary levels when fasting. The arterial and capillary levels most closely reflect the glucose concentrations at the organ level. After meals, venous blood will have lower glucose concentrations than arterial blood and can be as much as 10% lower.

Analytical techniques and quality assurance

A range of analytical techniques are used for the laboratory measurement of blood glucose levels. Chemical oxidation/reduction methods have a low cost for reagents and, although less specific, are still valid. Enzymatic analysis of glucose is more specific, although more expensive. The enzymatic reference method for glucose is the hexokinase/G6PDH method. The glucose oxidase methods are comparable, although the presence of reducing substances may cause error. Glucose oxidase methods are frequently used because of their convenience and lower cost. Measurements are accurate and precise with measurement coefficient of variance of around 2%. Self-measurement of blood glucose is possible using capillary blood glucose meters with test strip systems. Specific issues associated with their use are considered in the next section.

Capillary blood glucose meters use test strips that release gluconic acid and hydrogen peroxide from a blood sample. The reaction is quantified by one of a range of methods to measure blood glucose. Most of the currently marketed handheld capillary blood glucose meters give results as an equivalent to venous plasma glucose but this is not always the case. The same type of handheld meter may be calibrated to report whole blood glucose in one country and plasma values in another. Until this issue is resolved, the calibration of a meter should be checked and the thresholds for action set accordingly.

In a hospital or "site-of-care" setting, capillary blood glucose measurement can be used to replace venepuncture, with greater comfort and more rapidly available results. Standards have been laid down to ensure that bedside glucose determinations can be made accurately and include the need for well-defined policies which include adequate training, quality control procedures and regular maintenance of equipment [16]. Blood glucose meters may require entry of a number or insertion of a coding chip to ensure calibration to the batch of testing strips used.

Accuracy of blood glucose meters

Although laboratory methods of blood glucose measurement are accurate, the convenience and rapidity of capillary blood glucose meters means that, despite their higher coefficient of variance compared to laboratory testing and the possibility of user error, they are in wide use. The majority conform to international standards (www.iso.org), with 95% of readings within 0.83 mmol/L for readings <4 mmol/L and within 20% for higher glucose readings. The newer meters have minimized the possibility of user error by requirement for smaller volumes of blood for measurement and automated calibration methods. Operator error, however, remains a significant source of error, including failure to calibrate meters (some newer meters do not require external calibration), poor handwashing technique and dirty meters [17].

Measurement error can be minimized by careful training and consistent technique in making measurements, incorporating an allowance for the possibility of error in the reading when calculating insulin dose, and undertaking regular testing to identify results that do not fit the usual pattern, with retesting as necessary.

Despite their imprecision, blood glucose meters remain helpful at higher blood glucose values, where, for example, it is of less importance to distinguish a plasma glucose of 11 mmol/L from one of 14 mmol/L. In such circumstances, the aim of management is to achieve a substantial reduction in plasma glucose. At lower plasma glucose levels, however, the consequences of an imprecision of 15% are much greater. For many well-controlled patients aiming to keep their glucose levels in the range 4–6 mmol/L, the majority of readings below 4 mmol/L will result from the variance of the measurement rather than reflecting a true "low" value.

Measurement of urinary glucose

Measurement of glucose in urine has limited arguments in favor of its use for routinely monitoring diabetes. It is rapid, inexpensive, non-invasive and can provide a quantitative result, however, it does not reflect the changing levels of hyperglycemia with any accuracy and so interpretation may be difficult if not impossible. In addition, the renal threshold varies between individuals and varies during pregnancy and with aging. In any case, glucose is not excreted renally at levels where blood glucose is significantly elevated above that which should be targeted to minimize diabetic complications.

Urine fraction should be analyzed immediately, preserved at pH <5 to inhibit bacterial metabolism or stored at 4 °C. The enzyme used is glucose oxidase/peroxidase which may lead to false-positive results with hydrogen peroxide and false-negative test results with the presence of ascorbic acid.

Urine testing should no longer be used in most health care settings because of the availability of alternative and more accurate tests. For the moment it may have a role in resource-poor settings where identification and treatment of individuals with poorly controlled diabetes is the highest priority.

Monitoring in clinical practice

Glycated hemoglobin measurement is recommended to assess the maintenance of glycemic control and should be measured with high precision methods. Results should be reported in IFCC units (mmol/mol) or eAG (mmol/L or mg/dL) alongside the DCCT aligned (%) units. In general, HbA_{1c} measurements should be performed at least twice a year in patients meeting treatment targets and with stable glycemic control. An interval of 3 months between tests is usually recommended following changes in therapy or when levels are unstable, although a test after 2 months may provide some additional information [18].

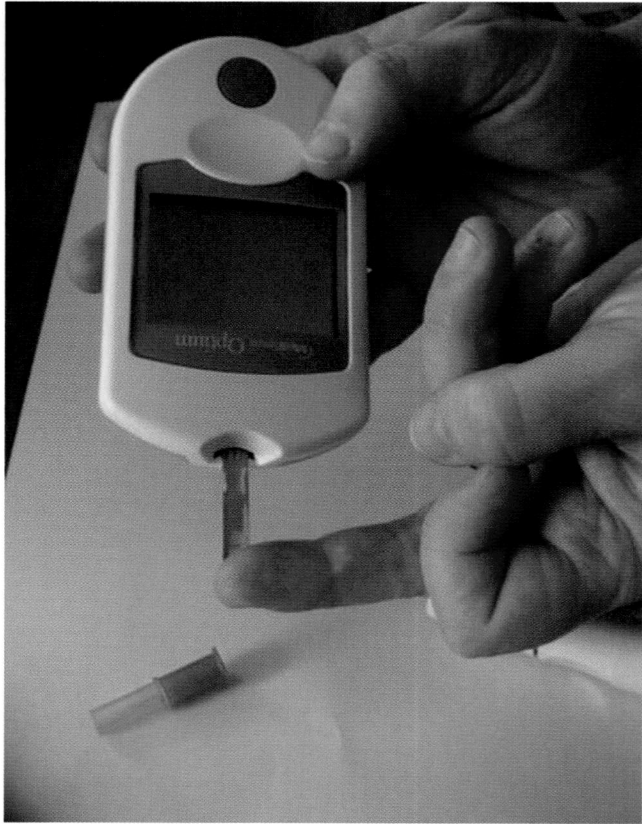

Figure 25.2 Correct technique for self-monitoring of blood glucose improves accuracy of testing.

Self-monitoring of blood glucose (SMBG) is a standard of care for patients with T1DM and necessary for insulin-treated patients with T2DM, although optimal use in this group is not established. SMBG may also be helpful for some non-insulin-treated patients with T2DM, although it is unlikely to offer benefit to well-controlled patients. SMBG requires a high level of motivation and if people using SMBG are not aware of how to interpret the results and what actions they should take, it is unlikely to be a clinically effective or cost-effective procedure. People with diabetes need to be taught how to perform the test accurately and how to use the data to adjust therapy in relation to food intake and physical activity. Correct technique involves obtaining the blood sample from the side of the finger pulp, wiping and using the second drop of hanging blood, using the meter correctly and disposing of the lancet (Figure 25.2). Alternative sites for sampling include the base of the thumb, forearm and thigh. Pre-meal readings will be the same between sites, but at times of rapid glucose change (in the post-prandial period or during hypoglycemia) forearm and thigh results will be different from the fingertip results.

Type 1 diabetes

For patients with T1DM, blood glucose control should be measured with HbA_{1c} every 2–6 months depending on the level and stability of blood glucose control and change in therapy. HbA_{1c} measurement should be provided either at site of care or carried out by the laboratory before clinical consultation. Patients should be encouraged to use SMBG using capillary blood glucose meters. With treatment regimens intended to produce intensive glycemic control, testing should be frequent (e.g. four or more times a day).

When using a typical basal bolus regimen including three injections of short-acting insulin and one or more injection of long-acting insulin, at least four time-points during the day need to be monitored, pre-breakfast, pre-lunch, pre-dinner and before bedtime. There is some evidence that tests 1 hour post meals may allow more accurate adjustment of pre-meal short-acting insulin although this needs to be offset against the greater inconvenience. Frequent glucose testing allows identification of periods during the day when plasma glucose levels are higher or lower than ideal and appropriate adjustment of the short-acting or bedtime injections. If the individual has regular routines and varies little in food intake and physical activity from day to day, then monitoring can take place at a frequency of less than four tests a day; for example, a daily fasting blood glucose with either 1 or 2 days a week with four-point sampling, or each day testing at one or more additional time-points to build a picture over the week. Until the dose of long-acting insulin has been established, a series of paired bedtime and fasting readings are needed.

Tight control brings with it the risk of hypoglycemia [4]. For some people (limited duration of life, inability to make the adjustments required for tight control) intensive control is inappropriate. Accepting less tight control allows use of less complicated regimens and less frequent monitoring.

For individuals using conventional rather than analog long-acting insulin, and with biphasic regimens more frequent monitoring may be required because of the less stable time course of the long-acting components of the insulin.

Glycated hemoglobin measurement complements blood glucose measurement by providing a check on the extent to which the glucose results are providing an accurate picture of overall blood glucose control. A schedule of blood glucose measurements indicating good control may need to be examined if an HbA_{1c} measure indicates that control is not so good. For example, timing of measurements and user technique may need reassessing.

SMBG should be carried out three or more times daily for patients using multiple insulin injections or insulin pump therapy. For patients using less frequent insulin injections, SMBG may be useful as an additional guide to the success of therapy and to support adjustment of insulin dose. In addition to measurement at defined time-points, additional checks on blood glucose levels can be made in relation to the risk of hypoglycemia, for example, before exercise or driving and in the presence of symptoms that may indicate hypoglycemia.

Glycemic targets for adults are for an HbA_{1c} of 48–59 mmol/mol (6.5–7.5%). Targets for children (aged 0–12 years) are higher because of the high risk of and vulnerability to hypoglycemia.

Adolescents and young adults are at particular risk with developmental and psychologic issues, but should nevertheless aim for control <59 mmol/mol (<7.5%).

Type 2 diabetes

For patients with T2DM, blood glucose control should be monitored using high precision methods for measurement of HbA_{1c} every 2–6 months depending on the level and stability of blood glucose control and change in therapy. HbA_{1c} measurements should be provided either at site of care or from the laboratory before clinical consultation.

Insulin-treated patients with T2DM need to make use of SMBG, particularly in the period of titration of insulin dose. For those patients using a long-acting insulin, fasting glucose readings can be used to guide incremental increases in insulin dose, with readings averaged over longer periods as the fasting glucose falls towards the target range. While fasting plasma glucose levels remain elevated, insulin dosage can be increased by up to 10%.

Although some patients report that they are able to gain motivation from regular blood glucose testing, others note their frustration when they are unable to make sense of what appears to be a random pattern of test results [19]. They report that health professionals do not appear interested in their carefully recorded results, and that this also leads them to question the value of the procedure. Many recent recommendations about the use of self-monitoring have stressed the need for self-monitoring to be accompanied by education about use of the results to promote optimal health behaviors. The extent to which understanding of test results might be improved by further support or training from health professionals is uncertain [19]. Other forms of evidence are therefore needed.

Evidence from large population-based clinical studies provides a mixed picture for the benefits of SMBG. Records from thousands of patients receiving care in the USA and Germany were examined to look at the outcomes of patients who were using SMBG compared with those who were not. Their results suggest that more frequent monitoring leads to improvements in glycemic control [20] and overall mortality [21]. Large studies of this type, however, have a high likelihood of bias. Although some statistical adjustments can be made for differences between users and non-users, there is likely to be a strong association between regular use of a blood glucose meter and take-up of other health promoting behaviors. In contrast, other studies using similar methods have identified no association between use of a blood glucose meter and improved outcomes [22]. Other research designs have therefore been used to identify an effect of SMBG.

Randomized trials provide an alternative approach to looking at the potential effectiveness of SMBG in improving outcomes for people with diabetes. Although they avoid potential bias through randomly allocating people to using or not using a meter, those people who agree to enter such a trial may not be completely typical of the wider group of people who might benefit from the intervention. Since the year 2000, there have been six randomized trials of at least 6 months' duration that compared the use of self-monitoring with no self-monitoring. These trials were summarized in a recent review. The overall identified benefit from use of self-monitoring in terms of improvement in glycemia was a decrease in HbA_{1c} of 0.2% [23]. Those trials that directly compared self-monitoring, and included state-of-the art patient education for both the SMBG user group and the non-user group, did not show a benefit [24]. These trials were also limited by including a substantial proportion of reasonably well-controlled patients. Other reviews have raised the possibility that, when used with patients who have less well-controlled diabetes, SMBG might be helpful [25]. Although most studies have focused their attention on potential benefits of SMBG, there is also the possibility of adverse outcomes. For example, two recent trials [26,27] have raised the possibility that, as the result of self-monitoring, some patients might become depressed or anxious compared to others not self-monitoring.

Most trials of self-monitoring have focused on the potential for SMBG to contribute to improved motivation and lifestyle adjustment. One recent trial has focused directly on adjustment of oral glucose-lowering medication. The study compared use of SMBG to titrate oral medication in comparison with usual care, and identified a small but significant improvement in glycemic control among patients allocated to self-testing compared with those assigned to usual care [28]. Further studies are needed to explore the extent to which there are long-term advantages of including SMBG compared to, for example, the more frequent use of HbA_{1c} measurement, as part of the management pathway for titration of glucose-lowering medication.

Some studies have also examined the costs that are associated with SMBG for non-insulin-treated patients. These studies vary in their assessment of the extent to which SMBG might be considered a cost-effective intervention. Some studies have used estimates of cost–benefit derived from selected cohort studies [29]. Other estimates of costs using more conservative estimates of SMBG efficacy and based on detailed cost data collected from clinical practice, suggest that any benefit in outcomes obtained from improved glucose control might be balanced out by the impact of a lower quality of life. Even when modeled over a long-term time horizon, use of SMBG failed to reach a conventional threshold of cost-effectiveness [27].

There are many unresolved questions about SMBG, including frequency and timing of testing, its value in new users and ongoing users, and if and how users act on the results. It is clear, however, that SMBG should only be used as part of a structured self-management program and when it serves an identified purpose in self-management.

Gestational diabetes mellitus

Women with diabetes should be advised to test fasting blood glucose levels and blood glucose levels 1 hour after every meal during pregnancy. Women should be able to adjust their insulin dose to maintain target blood glucose levels. Many oral glucose-lowering medicines are not recommended for use during pregnancy, particularly during the first trimester, so early training in the use of SMBG and insulin therapy is often necessary.

Monitoring diabetes in a hospital setting

Within a hospital setting, laboratory and point-of-care testing should be supported by certified quality assurance schemes. Some meters used in hospitals support quality assurance procedures by restricting access to trained personnel and transferring the results directly to the electronic patient record.

Blood glucose measurements should be available from meters situated on hospital wards. Measurement of glucose on admission to hospital is needed to identify hypoglycemia or hyperglycemia and to provide appropriate patient care. Confirmation from laboratory measurement is necessary for a proportion of these samples. Continuous monitoring may be appropriate for some patients while in hospital.

Critically ill surgical patients should have blood glucose levels maintained as close to 6.1 mmol/L as possible, and generally <7.8 mmol/L using an intravenous insulin protocol. Targets for non-surgical critically ill patients are less well defined, but some studies provide evidence for maintaining levels <7.8 mmol/L. For non-critically ill patients there is no evidence about optimum glycemic goals. Concerns about hypoglycemia mean that some institutions have concern about the safety of these goals as initial targets.

Self-management of diabetes in the hospital setting may be appropriate where adult patients are alert, able to self-manage their diabetes at home and have stable requirements for insulin. This may also provide an opportunity for providing support in learning techniques of insulin adjustment in line with carbohydrate intake.

Monitoring diabetes in a community setting

Glycated hemoglobin and SMBG testing are the two primary techniques for monitoring success in achieving glycemic goals, adjusting therapy and providing information to support lifestyle change.

Glycated hemoglobin testing

Glycated hemoglobin testing is usually carried out on a non-fasting venous sample obtained in EDTA tubes and sent to a locally accredited laboratory measured using one of the available techniques for measurement. In addition, capillary blood can be sent to the laboratory in capillary tubes or preserved as dry blood on a filter paper and sent to the laboratory, although chromatographic methods are less suitable for HbA_{1c} measurement in dry blood. Point-of-care testing systems are also available, either using an analyzer or small meters with test-strips.

HbA_{1c} provides a measure of glycemia that can be used to adjust treatment for patients with T1DM or T2DM. For patients with poorly controlled non-insulin-treated diabetes, advice about weight loss may bring about an improvement in glycemia, in the presence of some endogenous insulin secretion. Continuing poor control usually leads to initiation or increases in oral glucose-lowering medication as an appropriate further response. If these measures fail to improve glycemia, or there is concern about possible hypoglycemia, then characterizing the daily course of blood glucose in relation to food and physical activity may be appropriate.

To facilitate clinical decisions, patients are often asked to provide blood for HbA_{1c} testing before a clinic visit so that the results are available at a face-to-face consultation. Differences of 0.5% in HbA_{1c} in measurements made at the same laboratory using the same assays will indicate clinically relevant changes and provide a guide to the necessity of changes in treatment or facilitating lifestyle change.

Blood glucose testing

Blood glucose testing carried out by the patient with diabetes may enhance understanding of the impact of diabetes and treatment and adjust medication. For patients with T1DM and insulin-treated T2DM, the need to adjust insulin requires measurement, interpretation and appropriate adjustment to be carried out on a regular basis at home. Detailed records of blood glucose measurements and actions are needed to allow review by both the patient and their clinician. Blood glucose measurements are particularly helpful in situations where frequent adjustment of therapy is needed.

A single measurement of post-meal glucose used as a screening tool is likely to identify most inadequately controlled patients [10]. Blood glucose levels are usually high following meals, and thus contribute to overall blood glucose control. Some studies have been interpreted to suggest that post-prandial glucose levels correlate with development of complications better than fasting blood glucose levels (or that glycemic variability may be related to poor outcomes). Attempts to titrate oral hypoglycemic medication by taking account of post-meal measures, however, have not been successful [30].

Fasting blood glucose measurements can be used to inform management for patients with both T1DM and T2DM. Preprandial blood glucose levels are often equated with, but are not equivalent to, fasting blood glucose levels, which require an 8-hour fast. Preprandial measurements, however, may be useful for evaluating the impact of a complex insulin schedule, particularly with fast-acting analog insulin. For insulin treated patients, pre-breakfast levels, compared with the previous evening's readings, indicate the effectiveness of any long-acting insulin being taken.

For patients with non-insulin-treated T2DM, the within-person coefficient of variation of pre-fasting (pre-breakfast) blood glucose levels is low and measurements vary little from day to day. They are therefore a means of assessing day-to-day control and making adjustments to therapy or assessing the impact of lifestyle changes, although the cost-effectiveness in relation to HbA_{1c} testing has not been established. The frequency of fasting blood glucose measurement for non-insulin-treated T2DM has been suggested from once a week to once a day. The evidence for a particular frequency of testing, however, is lacking, and individual variations (familiarity with ensuring measurement techniques, variation in lifestyle, availability of professional help in supporting patients in interpretation of measurements) will require that a judgment is made on the precise purpose of monitoring.

SMBG may provide some patients with T2DM, not requiring glucose lowering therapy, with insight about the impact of day-to-day activities on blood glucose. Evidence to support the use of SMBG in this way derives from qualitative and observational studies. Measurement of fasting glucose, if HbA_{1c} is unavailable, may be used as an alternative indicator of overall glycemic control. It is also possible that, in patients unable to achieve target HbA_{1c}, characterizing the extent of hyperglycemia 1–2 hours after a meal, aiming to reduce post-meal levels below 10 mmol/L may be a recommendation worth further evaluation.

A target capillary plasma glucose of 3.9–7.2 mmol/L is recommended on the basis of outcome studies such as UKPDS and DCCT in which HbA_{1c} was shown to predict complications. Most patients with T2DM treated with long-acting insulin also continue oral glucose-lowering medication. The recommended schedules for monitoring are derived from trials that have sought to achieve reductions in HbA_{1c} to within recommended levels [20]. The intensity of these schedules has not yet been evaluated in wider populations and those more representative of primary care populations. Fasting blood glucose levels carried out twice a week will allow the weekly or 2-weekly titration of the long-acting insulin to achieve tight control. Additional 4 or 7-point profiles may be helpful every 3–4 weeks to identify patterns of blood glucose control that require further attention, for example, to address the possibility of hypoglycemia or to identify high levels of post-prandial glucose that may require the use of pre-meal short-acting insulin.

Continuous blood glucose measurement

The need to provide more frequent SMBG measurements to document glucose excursions and guide insulin therapy has led to the development of innovative technologies that can provide nearly 300 measurements a day. Detailed data on the magnitude and duration of glucose fluctuations can be used to guide lifestyle and drug therapy in an attempt to produce a near-physiologic control of glucose levels.

There are a number of different systems currently available. All require calibration using capillary blood glucose measurement and utilize a subcutaneously implanted sensor that can remain *in situ* for up to 7 days. All the continuous glucose monitoring systems (CGMS) are intended for intermittent use in order to identify periods of hyperglycemia that can be corrected by changing therapy (e.g. increasing the dose of insulin or changing timing of injections), or detecting periods of biochemical hypoglycemia that may be too brief to cause symptoms but may nevertheless cause some impairment in cognitive function.

Evidence for effectiveness of CGMS in selected patients aged over 25 years with T1DM using intensive insulin therapy comes from a randomized trial with 322 people with T1DM in which those allocated to the CGMS arm experienced a 0.5% (6 mmol/mol) reduction in HbA_{1c} from 7.6 to 7.1% (60 to 54 mmol/mol) compared to conventional therapy [31]. Evidence for HbA_{1c} lowering is less strong in children, teens and younger adults, although there may be specific clinical circumstances in which CGMS might be helpful. Success correlates with adherence to the ongoing use of the device.

Use of CGMS has also been evaluated for pregnant women with diabetes treated with insulin. In a randomized trial those women randomized to continuous glucose monitoring had lower mean HbA_{1c} levels from 32 to 36 weeks' gestation compared with women randomized to standard antenatal care. The authors concluded that continuous glucose monitoring during pregnancy is associated with improved glycemic control in the third trimester, lower birth weight and reduced risk of macrosomia [32].

CGMS is now being used as a research tool among patients with T2DM, but the extent to which the procedure is useful to the patient or to the clinician remains unclear and its use cannot be recommended in routine clinical practice. Advocates of the procedure suggest that it might be useful as a means of helping patients to recognize aspects of their lifestyle that lead to hyperglycemia [33].

Resource-poor settings

Costs of SMBG using test meters remain high in relative terms, and testing with this equipment may not be appropriate in a resource-poor setting. Particularly for patients with T1DM, there is an urgent need for lower cost test strips, although a requirement for rigorous quality control procedures to maintain accuracy limits the potential for lower cost equipment.

Urine glucose testing remains a viable alternative to blood testing or HbA_{1c} measurement for patients in a country where health care resources are limited, or in a health care setting where costs of testing equipment are borne directly by the patient. There are few data on self-monitoring using urine glucose testing. A meta-analysis from 2005 [34] included two studies that compared SMBG and self-monitoring of urine glucose and reported a non-significant reduction in HbA_{1c} of 2 mmol/mol (0.17%) in favor of SMBG. Many patients, however, do not find the procedure acceptable or helpful [35]. Measurement of urine glucose should therefore not be seen as a substitute for SMBG, but can be used as an alternative where SMBG is not accessible, affordable or desired. Interpretation of information needs to be focused on the period between last voiding and the production of the current urine specimen. Most people have a renal threshold for glucose of around 8 mmol/L, so information about glucose levels is limited below this threshold. The renal threshold can drop during pregnancy, and so glycosuria is more likely in this situation.

The future

Current research is focusing on a number of non-invasive methods to enable continuous monitoring. Methods being considered include using infrared, electric currents and ultrasound. Currently available continuous monitoring systems require calibration, but are then able to record blood glucose levels at 5-minute intervals for up to 72 hours. Efforts are currently being made to develop integrated systems with glucose meters and insulin pumps. Computerized algorithms for controlling insulin pumps on the basis of blood glucose levels have been developed and have already been evaluated in the setting of intensive care. Mobile phones have also been linked to blood glucose meters to allow easy review of charted data, real-time feedback of support and integration of data with medical records [36].

Conclusions

Glycemic control should be monitored regularly for all patients with diabetes. The optimal method of determining risk of long-term complications is through HbA_{1c} measurement, although if this is not available, then examination of a series of blood glucose measurements, including fasting tests, may provide some guidance. Management of therapy depends on the clinical setting and the type and stage of the patient's diabetes. Patients with non-insulin-treated diabetes have little scope for adjusting therapy on the basis of routine SMBG measurements, although some individuals may benefit from exploring the extent of glycemic variability, self-titration of glucose-lowering medication or checking whether symptoms are related to low-blood glucose readings. For adult patients with T1DM and pregnant women treated with insulin, the evidence for active and regular blood glucose testing (including use of continuous glucose monitoring) to achieve intensive blood glucose control through adjustment of insulin dose in relation to lifestyle is strong. There is also good evidence for the routine use of SMBG for insulin-treated patients with T2DM. Rigorous trials of SMBG in well-controlled non-insulin-treated patients do not demonstrate a clinically important effect. Until further studies suggest settings or groups of patients where SMBG is likely to contribute to the impact of an educational intervention, it should be used only in circumstances where the information obtained through testing can be used to adjust treatment actively, enhance understanding of diabetes and assess the effectiveness of the management plan on glycemic control.

References

1 Home P, Chacra A, Chan J, Emslie-Smith A, Sorensen L, Van Crombrugge P. Considerations on blood glucose management in type 2 diabetes mellitus. *Diabetes Metab Res Rev* 2002; **18**:273–285.

2 International Diabetes Federation. *Diabetes Facts and Figures.* Available from: www.diabetesatlas.org/content/diabetes-and-impaired-glucose-tolerance. Accessed on 18 December, 2009.

3 Stratton IM, Adler AI, Neil HAW, Matthews DR, Manley SE, Cull CA, *et al.* Association of glycaemia with macrovascular and microvascular complications of type 2 diabetes (UKPDS 35): prospective observational study. *Br Med J* 2000; **321**:405–412.

4 Diabetes Control and Complications Trial/Epidemiology of Diabetes Interventions and Complications (DCCT/EDIC) Study Research Group. Intensive diabetes treatment and cardiovascular disease in patients with type 1 diabetes. *N Engl J Med* 2005; **353**:2643–2653.

5 American Diabetes Association. Clinical practice recommendations 2009. *Diabetes Care* 2009; **32**(Suppl 1).

6 Holman RR, Paul SK, Bethel MA, Matthews DR, Neil HA. 10-year follow-up of intensive glucose control in type 2 diabetes. *N Engl J Med* 2008; **359**:1577–1589.

7 National Collaborating Centre for Chronic Conditions. *Type 2 Diabetes: National Clinical Guideline for Management in Primary and Secondary Care (Update).* London: Royal College of Physicians, 2008.

8 Sacks DB, Bruns DE, Goldstein DE, Maclaren NK, McDonald JM, Parrott M. Guidelines and recommendations for laboratory analysis in the diagnosis and management of diabetes mellitus. *Clin Chem* 2002; **48**:436–472.

9 Kilpatrick ES. Consensus meeting on reporting glycated haemoglobin and estimated average glucose in the UK: time for 'Kilpatrick's Kludge'? *Ann Clin Biochem* 2009; **46**:84–85.

10 Schwartz K, Monsur J, Bartoces M, West P, Neale A. Correlation of same-visit HbA1c test with laboratory-based measurements: a MetroNet study. *BMC Fam Pract* 2005; **6**:28.

11 Nathan DM, Kuenen J, Borg R, Zheng H, Schoenfeld D, Heine RJ, *et al.* Translating the A1C assay into estimated average glucose values. *Diabetes Care* 2008; **31**:1473–1478.

12 Manley SE, Sikaris KA, Lu ZX, Nightingale PG, Stratton IM, Round RA, *et al.* Validation of an algorithm combining haemoglobin A(1c) and fasting plasma glucose for diagnosis of diabetes mellitus in UK and Australian populations. *Diabet Med* 2009; **26**:115–121.

13 Khunti K, Stone MA, Burden AC, Turner D, Raymond NT, Burden M, *et al.* Randomised controlled trial of near-patient testing for glycated haemoglobin in people with type 2 diabetes mellitus. *Br J Gen Pract* 2006; **56**:511–517.

14 Stone MA, Burden AC, Burden M, Baker R, Khunti K. Near patient testing for glycated haemoglobin in people with type 2 diabetes mellitus managed in primary care: acceptability and satisfaction. *Diabet Med* 2007; **24**:792–795.

15 Smellie WS, Forth J, Bareford D, Twomey P, Galloway MJ, Logan EC, *et al.* Best practice in primary care pathology: review 3. *J Clin Pathol* 2006; **59**:781–789.

16 American Diabetes Association. Bedside blood glucose monitoring in hospitals. *Diabetes Care* 2003; **26**(Suppl 1):S119.

17 Brunner GA, Ellmerer M, Sendlhofer G, Wutte A, Trajanoski Z, Schaupp L, *et al.* Validation of home blood glucose meters with respect to clinical and analytical approaches. *Diabetes Care* 1998; **21**:585–590.

18 Tahara Y, Shima K. The response of GHb to stepwise plasma glucose change over time in diabetic patients. *Diabetes Care* 1993; **16**:1313–1314.

19 Peel E, Douglas M, Lawton J. Self monitoring of blood glucose in type 2 diabetes: longitudinal qualitative study of patients' perspectives. *Br Med J* 2007; **335**:493.

20 Karter AJ, Parker MM, Moffet HH, Spence MM, Chan J, Ettner SL, *et al.* Longitudinal study of new and prevalent use of self-monitoring of blood glucose. *Diabetes Care* 2006; **29**:1757–1763.

21 Martin S, Schneider B, Heinemann L, Lodwig V, Kurth J, Kolb H, *et al.* Self-monitoring of blood glucose in type 2 diabetes and long-term outcome: an epidemiological cohort study. *Diabetologia* 2006; **49**:271–278.

22 Davis WA, Bruce DG, Davis ME. Does self-monitoring of blood glucose improve outcome in type 2 diabetes? The Fremantle Diabetes Study. *Diabetologia* 2007; **50**:510–515.

23 Towfigh A, Romanova M, Weinreb JE, Munjas B, Suttorp MJ, Zhou A, *et al.* Self-monitoring of blood glucose levels in patients with type 2 diabetes mellitus not taking insulin: a meta-analysis. *Am J Manag Care* 2008; **14**:468–475.

24 Farmer A, Wade A, Goyder E, Yudkin P, French D, Craven A, *et al.* Impact of self monitoring of blood glucose in the management of patients with non-insulin treated diabetes: open parallel group randomised trial. *Br Med J* 2007; **335**:132.

25 Sarol JN Jr, Nicodemus NA Jr, Tan KM, Grava MB. Self-monitoring of blood glucose as part of a multi-component therapy among non-insulin requiring type 2 diabetes patients: a meta-analysis (1966–2004). *Curr Med Res Opin* 2005; **21**:173–184.

26 O'Kane MJ, Bunting B, Copeland M, Coates VE, on behalf of the ESMON study group. Efficacy of self monitoring of blood glucose in patients with newly diagnosed type 2 diabetes (ESMON study): randomised controlled trial. *Br Med J* 2008; **336**:1174–1177.

27 Simon J, Gray A, Clarke P, Wade A, Neil A, Farmer A, *et al.* Cost effectiveness of self monitoring of blood glucose in patients with non-insulin treated type 2 diabetes: economic evaluation of data from the DiGEM trial. *Br Med J* 2008; **336**:1177–1180.

28 Barnett AH, Krentz AJ, Strojek K, Sieradzki J, Azizi F, Embong M, *et al.* The efficacy of self-monitoring of blood glucose in the management of patients with type 2 diabetes treated with a gliclazide modified release-based regimen: a multicentre, randomized, parallel-group, 6-month evaluation (DINAMIC 1 study). *Diabetes Obes Metab* 2008; **10**:1239–1247.

29 Palmer AJ, Dinneen S, Gavin JR III, Gray A, Herman WH, Karter AJ. Cost–utility analysis in a UK setting of self-monitoring of blood glucose in patients with type 2 diabetes. *Curr Med Res Opin* 2006; **22**:861–872.

30 Gerstein HC, Garon J, Joyce C, Rolfe A, Walter CM. Pre-prandial vs. post-prandial capillary glucose measurements as targets for repaglinide dose titration in people with diet-treated or metformin-treated type 2 diabetes: a randomized controlled clinical trial. *Diabet Med* 2004; **21**:1200–1203.

31 Juvenile Diabetes Research Foundation Continuous Glucose Monitoring Study Group. Continuous glucose monitoring and i ntensive treatment of type 1 diabetes. *N Engl J Med* 2008; **359**:1464–1476.

32 Murphy HR, Rayman G, Lewis K, Kelly S, Johal B, Duffield K, *et al.* Effectiveness of continuous glucose monitoring in pregnant women with diabetes: randomised clinical trial. *Br Med J* 2008; **337**:a1680.

33 Harman-Boehm I. Continuous glucose monitoring in type 2 diabetes. *Diabetes Res Clin Pract* 2008; **82**(Suppl 2):S118–S121.

34 Welschen LMC, Bloemendal E, Nijpels G, Dekker JM, Heine RJ, Stalman WAB, *et al.* Self-monitoring of blood glucose in patients with type 2 diabetes who are not using insulin: a systematic review. *Diabetes Care* 2005; **28**:1510–1517.

35 Lawton J, Peel E, Douglas M, Parry O. Urine testing is a waste of time: newly diagnosed type 2 diabetes patients' perceptions of self-monitoring. *Diabet Med* 2004; **21**:1045–1048.

36 Farmer A, Gibson O, Hayton P, Bryden K, Dudley C, Neil A, *et al.* A real-time, mobile phone-based telemedicine system to support young adults with type 1 diabetes. *Inform Prim Care* 2005; **13**: 171–178.

26 Drug Therapy: Special Considerations in Diabetes

Bernard M.Y. Cheung[1] & Robin E. Ferner[1,2]

[1] College of Medical and Dental Sciences, University of Birmingham, Birmingham, UK

[2] West Midlands Centre for Adverse Drug Reactions, City Hospital, Birmingham, UK

Keypoints

- Many drugs interfere with glucose homeostasis or interact with antidiabetic agents and thus can disturb glycemic control in people with diabetes. Specific diabetic complications, such as nephropathy and neuropathy, may require particular drugs to be used with care.
- Hyperglycemia can be caused or worsened by numerous drugs. Those that induce insulin resistance include glucocorticoids, certain oral contraceptives, antipsychotic drugs, HIV protease inhibitors, the fluoroquinolone gatifloxacin and β-adrenoceptor antagonists. Diabetogenic drugs that damage the β-cell include pentamidine and cyclosporine (ciclosporin).
- Sulfonylureas and related agents commonly cause hypoglycemia by interacting with other drugs that block their metabolism in the liver, e.g. ciprofloxacin inhibits CYP2C9, which degrades glyburide (glibenclamide), or that impair renal function and decrease their elimination (e.g. non-steroidal anti-inflammatory agents).
- Hypoglycemia can be induced by drugs that stimulate insulin secretion (e.g. quinine, especially in children with cerebral malaria); and sulfamethoxazole, which binds to the sulfonylurea receptor. Pentamidine can induce transient hypoglycemia, by causing passive loss of insulin from the β-cell, as a prelude to permanent diabetes.
- Hypoglycemia can complicate overdosage with acetaminophen (paracetamol), following hepatic necrosis; or aspirin, which blocks hepatic glucose output and stimulates peripheral glucose uptake. Alcohol inhibits hepatic gluconeogenesis and can provoke, prolong or exacerbate hypoglycemia.
- Non-selective β-adrenoceptor antagonists inhibit insulin secretion and can impair glucose tolerance. They also decrease certain catecholamine-mediated symptomatic and metabolic responses to hypoglycemia; awareness of hypoglycemia may therefore be reduced, and recovery of normoglycemia delayed. These adverse effects are much less pronounced with cardioselective β_1-adrenoceptor antagonists.
- Thiazide diuretics used at low dosages (e.g. 2.5 mg/day bendroflumethiazide) lower blood pressure effectively and are suitable for use in patients with diabetes.
- Certain drugs require special consideration in patients with diabetic complications. Metformin and several sulfonylureas are cleared through the kidney; they are therefore contraindicated in advanced nephropathy and should not be co-administered with nephrotoxic drugs. Vasodilators and ganglion-blocking agents exacerbate postural hypotension.

This chapter discusses the problems posed by drug therapy in the management of people with diabetes. Numerous drugs can affect diabetic control, causing hyperglycemia or hypoglycemia, by interfering with insulin secretion or action or both, or by interacting with antidiabetic agents. Some important examples are illustrated in Figure 26.1. The special considerations that apply when using other drugs in patients with diabetes and in the presence of specific diabetic complications are also discussed.

Textbook of Diabetes, 4th edition. Edited by R. Holt, C. Cockram, A. Flyvbjerg and B. Goldstein.

Drugs that raise blood glucose concentrations

Drug-induced diabetes is now recognized as a distinct etiologic category, and diabetogenic drugs are discussed in detail in Chapter 16. The main culprits are shown in Table 26.1. Most of these drugs – notably glucocorticoids (a common and important cause of iatrogenic diabetes), contraceptive steroids and β-adrenoceptor antagonists – act by inhibiting insulin action. By contrast, insulin secretion is inhibited by diazoxide, while pentamidine can cause permanent β-cell damage. In recent years, antipsychotic drugs, HIV protease inhibitors and the fluoroqui-

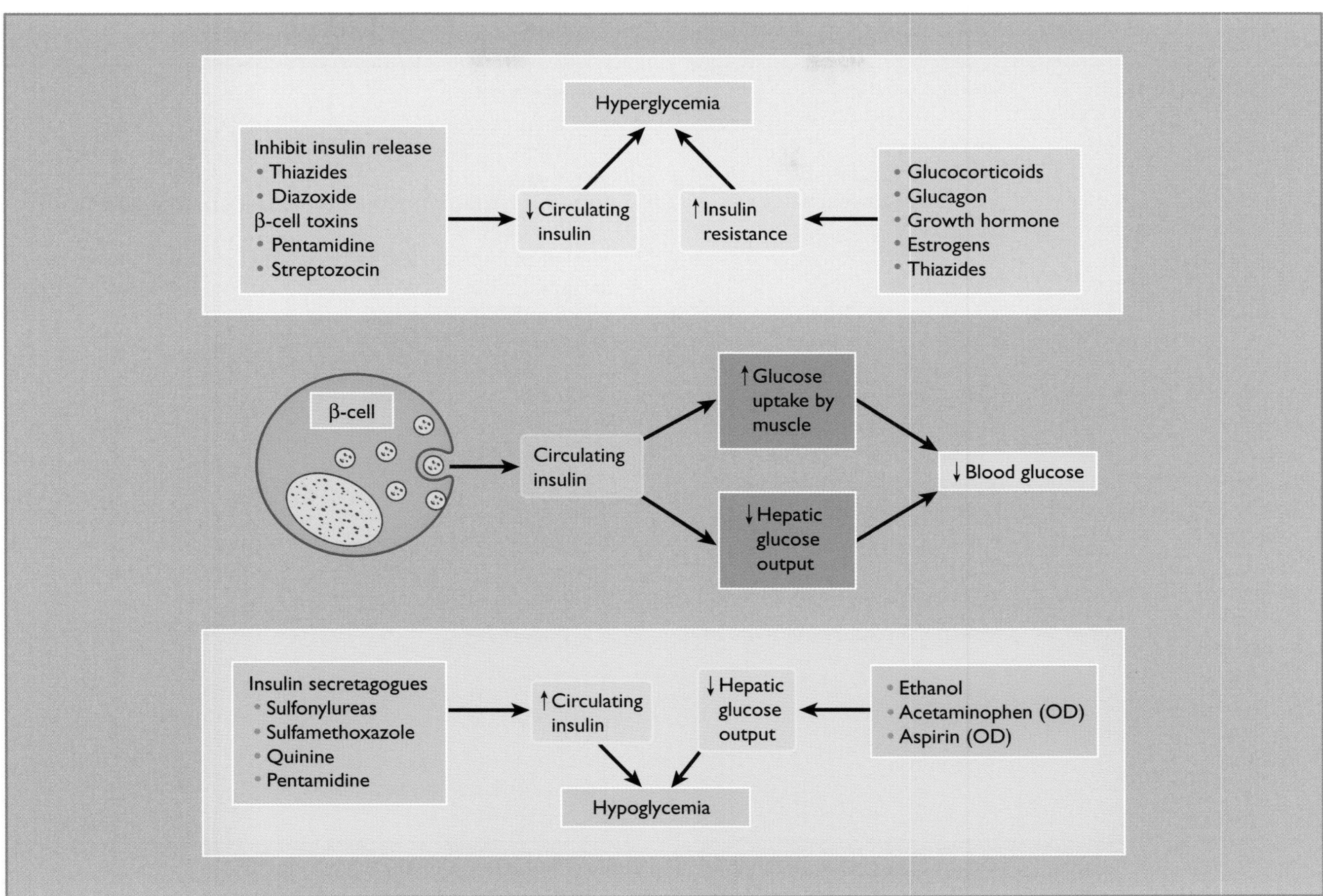

Figure 26.1 General mechanisms of drug-induced hyperglycemia and hypoglycemia. OD, overdose.

nolone antibiotic gatifloxacin have emerged as important causes of hyperglycemia.

Drugs that lower blood glucose concentration

Many drugs can cause hypoglycemia (Table 26.2) [1–10]. These include some that interact with and enhance the action of glucose-lowering drugs. Others act in their own right as insulin secretagogues, or to enhance or mimic the effect of insulin in suppressing glucose production by the liver and stimulating glucose uptake into peripheral tissues. Some drugs (e.g. non-selective β-adrenoceptor antagonists) specifically block the warning symptoms or the neuroendocrine counter-regulatory responses that are normally triggered by hypoglycemia, and so can prolong and intensify hypoglycemic episodes.

Drugs should always be suspected whenever patients with previously well-controlled diabetes experience unexplained hypoglycemic episodes, or if dosages of insulin or oral hypoglycemic agents decline. As well as prescription drugs, patients should be asked about herbal, traditional and other alternative medicines. These are now widely used by people with diabetes – up to one-third of patients in one study [11] – and some products may contain naturally occurring or synthetic glucose-lowering agents (Table 26.3).

Sulfonylureas

Sulfonylureas are an important and sometimes unrecognized cause of symptomatic hypoglycemia (see Chapter 33). They are also affected by numerous interactions with other drugs (Figure 26.2).

The long-acting sulfonylureas glibenclamide and chlorpropamide are especially troublesome. In one outpatient survey, 20% of patients treated with glibenclamide reported symptoms of hypoglycemia within the previous six months [12], while other surveys suggest that tolbutamide is much less likely to cause severe hypoglycemia (i.e. requiring hospital admission) than either glibenclamide or chlorpropamide [13,14]. A Swiss study [15] defined the risk of severe hypoglycemia as two episodes per 1000 persons per year in those given glibenclamide, over twice as high as in those taking shorter-acting sulfonylureas such as tolbutamide, gliclazide or glipizide. The novel sulfonylurea, glimepir-

Table 26.1 Drugs that may cause or exacerbate hyperglycemia.

Potentially potent effects	Minor or no effects
Glucocorticoids	Oral contraceptives
Oral contraceptives	Progestogen-only pills
High-dose oestrogen	Levonorgestrel in combination pills
Thiazide diuretics (especially high dosages)*	Loop diuretics
Non-selective β-adrenoceptor antagonists	Calcium-channel blockers
β_2-Adrenoceptor agonists	α_1-Adrenoceptor antagonists
Salbutamol	Growth hormone (physiologic doses)
Ritodrine	Somatostatin analogs†
Antipsychotics	Androgen deprivation therapy for prostate cancer
HIV protease inhibitors	Selective serotonin reuptake inhibitors
Indinavir, nelfinavir, ritonavir and others	Nicotinic acid
Others	Lamivudine
Pentamidine	Isoniazid
Gatifloxacin	
Streptozotocin	
Diazoxide	
Cyclosporine (ciclosporin)	
Tacrolimus	
Temsirolimus	
Interferon-α	
L-Asparaginase	

* "High" dosages of thiazides correspond to ≥5 mg/day bendroflumethazide.
† Somatostatin analogs may induce hyperglycemia in type 2 but not type 1 diabetes.

ide, is said to carry a relatively low risk of hypoglycemia because it binds to a different site on the sulfonylurea receptor from classic sulfonylureas and also has distinct pharmacokinetic properties. None the less, the rate of hypoglycemia is still substantial, with 10–20% of patients experiencing at least one mild episode each year [16].

Several factors other than the individual drug per se can increase the risk of hypoglycemia from sulfonylureas, notably increasing age and renal impairment [13,14,16–18]. Reduced food intake during intercurrent illness can also contribute [17,18]. Drug interactions that enhance the action of sulfonylureas are considered below.

Not all those who have sulfonylurea-induced hypoglycemia are patients with type 2 diabetes (T2DM): "bystanders" have included toddlers who ate a grandparent's tablet [19], nursing-home residents given the treatment of other patients [20] and people whose prescriptions for other drugs have been misread [21].

Sulfonylurea-induced hypoglycemia can be profound and prolonged, and difficult to manage. Patients with sulfonylurea-induced hypoglycemia may require admission and treatment with glucose until the effect of the sulfonylurea has worn off although caution is needed as indicated in the case report below.

Table 26.2 Drugs that may cause or exacerbate hypoglycemia.

Antidiabetic drugs
Insulins
Sulfonylureas, e.g. glimepiride
Repaglinide
Drugs that interact to enhance the actions of sulfonylureas (Table 26.4)
Quinolone antibacterials: Levofloxacin, gatifloxacin [4]
Corticosteroids, including inhaled corticosteroids (when withdrawn may lead to adrenal insufficiency) [5,6]
Other drugs
Aspirin (in overdosage)
Cibenzoline
Disopyramide
Doxycycline [7,8]
Etanercept
Ethanol
Hydroxychloroquine
Imatinib
Mefloquine
Non-selective β-adrenoceptor antagonists
Paracetamol (in overdosage)
Pentamidine
Quinidine
Quinine
Sulfamethoxazole (in co-trimoxazole)
Valproate (in neonates exposed *in utero*) [9]
Venlafaxine (in overdosage) [10]

Insulin hypersecretion induced by sulfonylureas can be suppressed effectively with either diazoxide (which opens the β-cell K_{ATP} channel that is closed by sulfonylureas) [22,23] or by the somatostatin analog octreotide [24].

Case report: Severe relapsing sulfonylurea-induced hypoglycemia

A 62-year-old woman was admitted with acute confusion and became unresponsive 2 hours after admission. She had type 2 diabetes with impaired renal function (serum creatinine 176 μmol/L) and had been taking 40 mg gliclazide twice a day. Her blood glucose concentration was 1.8 mmol/L. The hypoglycemia was reversed with an intravenous bolus of 50 mL 50% glucose but subsequently she had repeated episodes of hypoglycemia and required continuous intravenous glucose infusion for 3 days. A blood sample taken when she was hypoglycemic showed raised serum insulin and C peptide concentrations, indicating increased insulin secretion. This patient had impaired renal function. It is likely that this caused gliclazide to accumulate, leading to hypoglycemia. Intravenous glucose restored consciousness, but also stimulated further insulin secretion, leading to further episodes of hypoglycemia.

Adapted from Langford *et al. Postgrad Med J* 2003; **79**:120.

Table 26.3 Some herbal medicinal products and food supplements that can potentially interact with antidiabetic drugs to affect blood glucose concentrations. Data from Ernst E. *The Desktop Guide to Complementary and Alternative Medicine. An Evidence-Based Approach.* Edinburgh: Mosby, 2001.

Name	Effect on blood glucose	Name	Effect on blood glucose
Alfalfa	↓	Ginseng, *Eleutherococcus*	↓
Aloe vera	↓	Ginseng, *Panax*	↓
Basil	↓	Gotu kola	↑
Bee pollen	↑	Guar gum	↓
Bitter melon	↓	Horehound	↓
Burdock	↓	Hydrocotyle	↑
Celandine	↓	Juniper	↓
Celery	↓	Licorice	↑
Coriander	↓	Marshmallow	↓
Cornsilk	↓	Melatonin	↓
Damiana	↓	Myrrh	↓
Dandelion	↓	Myrtle	↓
Devil's claw	↑	Nettle	↓
Elecampane	↑	Night-blooming cereus	↓
Eucalyptus	↓	Onion	↓
Fenugreek	↓	Sage	↓
Figwort	↑	St. John's wort	↑
Garlic	↓	Tansy	↓

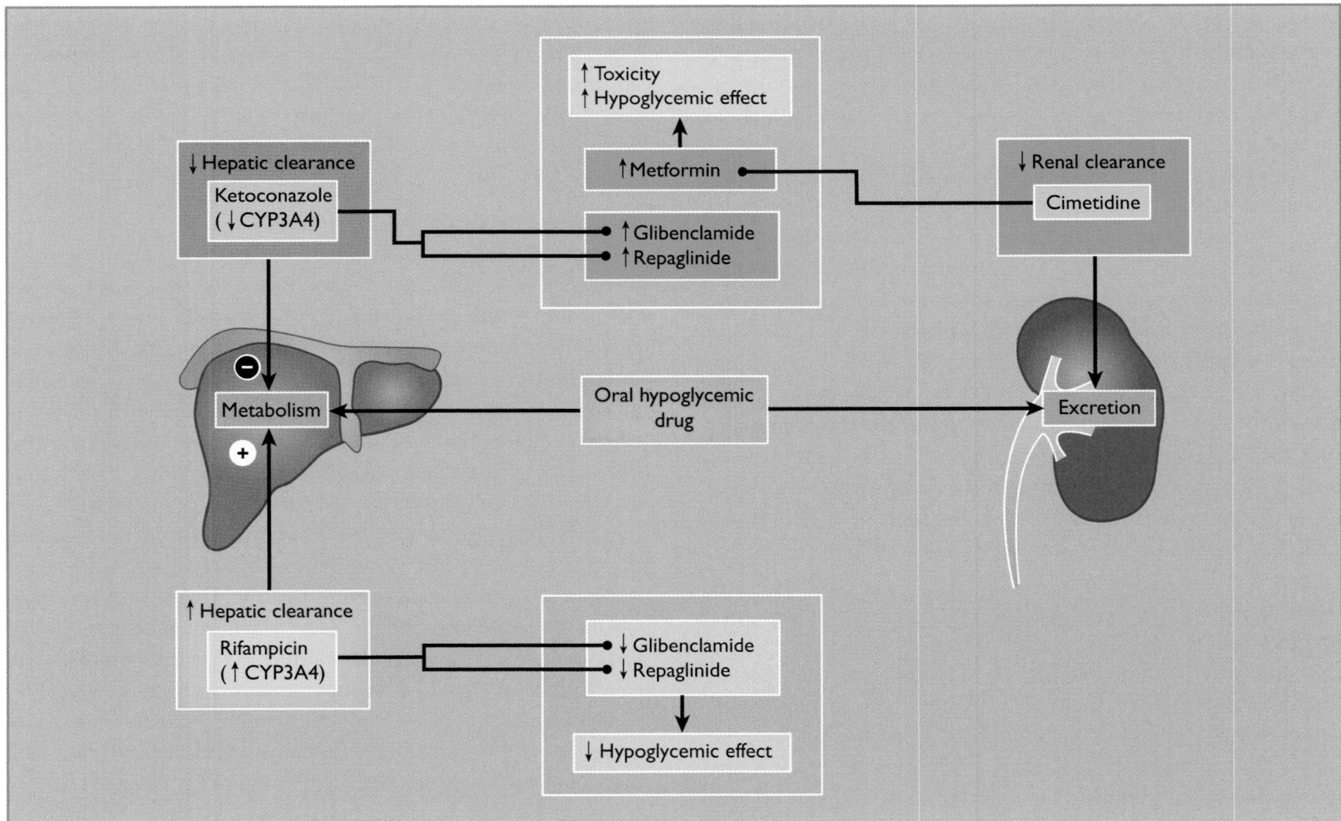

Figure 26.2 Interactions between oral hypoglycemic agents and other drugs.

Other antidiabetic agents

These are described in Chapter 29.

• *Metformin* used alone is not expected to cause hypoglycemia in therapeutic use; but instances of "hypoglycemia" were reported by the UK Prospective Diabetes Study (UKPDS) during metformin treatment [25]. They were not generally confirmed by blood glucose measurements.

• *Thiazolidinediones* (e.g. rosiglitazone and pioglitazone) potentiate the peripheral actions of insulin. They do not induce hypoglycemia in their own right, but can enhance hypoglycemia caused by sulfonylureas or insulin when used in combination with them.

• *Repaglinide* stimulates insulin release by a mechanism distinct from that of the sulfonylureas and so causes hyperinsulinemic hypoglycemia. A case of factitious hypoglycemia from repaglinide has been reported [26].

• *Acarbose* inhibits intestinal disaccharidase, and so reduces the hydrolysis of sucrose and thus glucose absorption. It does not cause hypoglycemia when used as monotherapy. Acarbose-treated patients who develop hypoglycemia from other glucose-lowering drugs should be warned that oral glucose, not sucrose, is needed to treat the episode.

• *Exenatide* and *liraglutide* are incretins, that is, peptide hormones that enhance the pancreatic insulin response to glucose in the gut. They are agonists of the glucagon-like peptide-1 (GLP-1) receptor. They slow down stomach emptying and stimulate insulin secretion. Unlike insulin, they do not tend to cause hypoglycemia. They also increase pancreatic β-cell mass and promote weight loss. The major disadvantages are nausea, the need for subcutaneous injections, and the high cost relative to sulfonylureas.

• *Gliptins* increase the circulating levels of incretins by inhibiting dipeptidyl peptidase 4 (DPP-4), the enzyme that breaks down incretins and other peptides. The oral route of administration is an advantage, but the long-term effects of DPP-4 inhibition remain unknown. Exenatide and gliptins are indicated for glycemic control as alternatives to thiazolidinediones or acarbose in patients with T2DM on metformin therapy in whom a sulfonylurea is not tolerated or inappropriate.

• *Inhaled insulin preparations* deliver insulin by the pulmonary route, and have a value in patients who have a phobia of needles. Because of poor sales and safety concerns, the first inhaled insulin marketed has been withdrawn. There could be a revival of interest in inhaled insulin if long-acting formulations become available.

Other drugs

Antimicrobials

• *Quinine and quinine derivatives.* Patients with falciparum malaria are often extremely ill, and may have hypoglycemia because of the effects of cytokines and malnutrition, both of which diminish hepatic gluconeogenesis. In this context, it is easy to overlook quinine-induced hypoglycemia, which can be profound, especially in children [27,28]. It is caused by insulin hypersecretion, as quinine has insulin secretagogue activity [29]. Octreotide (a long-acting somatostatin analogue) has been used successfully to inhibit insulin release and raise blood glucose concentrations under these conditions [30]. Quinidine and mefloquine may occasionally cause hypoglycemia, while chloroquine does not [28].

• *Sulfamethoxazole*, which is combined with trimethoprim in co-trimoxazole, has a sulfonylurea-like action and can stimulate insulin secretion; several cases of severe hypoglycemia have been described [31]. This tends to be long-lasting, perhaps because excessive amounts of glucose solution are infused; this may paradoxically worsen hypoglycemia by further stimulating insulin secretion. Elderly patients receiving high dosage, and patients in renal failure (which causes the drug to accumulate) are at particular risk [32], as are patients infected with HIV who receive high doses of co-trimoxazole to treat *Pneumocystis jirovecii* pneumonia (formerly known as *Pneumocystis carinii*) [33].

• *Pentamidine*, a drug used to treat and prevent *P. jirovecii* pneumonia, can also damage pancreatic β-cells. This initially leads to the passive leakage of insulin out of secretory vesicles, causing hypoglycemia, but diabetes may develop subsequently [34]. In two series of patients with HIV treated with pentamidine, 25% [35] and 14% [36] developed symptomatic hypoglycemia; they invariably developed renal damage from the drug as well. Even inhaled pentamidine can cause hypoglycemia [37].

• *Doxycycline* has been suggested to cause hypoglycemia, but the reaction is infrequent and no mechanism has been identified [38].

• *Quinolones*, particularly gatifloxacin, can cause hypoglycemia (and also hyperglycemia). A case–control study defined an adjusted odds ratio for hypoglycemia with gratifloxacin treatment of 4.3 (95% confidence interval [CI] 2.9–6.3) compared with macrolide treatment [4]. There was a small increase in risk with levofloxacin.

Miscellaneous drugs

• *Disopyramide* and *cibenzoline* (*cifenline*), class Ia antiarrhythmic agents, can rarely cause symptomatic hypoglycemia; this can occur either with or without hyperinsulinemia [39], suggesting that peripheral effects contribute. In normal subjects, disopyramide produces a small but statistically significant fall in fasting glucose concentration [40]. In a Japanese case–control study, cibenzoline treatment was associated with an eightfold increase in the risk of hypoglycemia; disopyramide did not significantly increase the overall risk, but the confidence intervals were wide [41]. The effect of disopyramide appears to be dose-dependent. In one case, a man developed severe hypoglycemia while taking disopyramide only after starting treatment with clarithromycin for an intercurrent infection [42]; clarithromycin inhibits the hepatic microsomal enzymes that metabolize disopyramide and so greatly increases serum disopyramide concentrations.

• *Antidepressants*, including monoamine oxidase inhibitors, selective serotonin reuptake inhibitors and nefazodone, have been reported to reduce blood glucose concentrations [43].

Drugs in overdose

• *Acetaminophen* (*paracetamol*), in overdose, can cause hypoglycemia as a complication of acute hepatic necrosis. Overdosage of *aspirin* and other salicylates inhibits hepatic glucose production and also increases peripheral glucose utilization, leading to hypoglycemia, especially in children. Paradoxically, and for unknown reasons, hyperglycemia can be encountered in adults.

• *Ethanol* inhibits gluconeogenesis; consequently, it can cause hypoglycemia in children or fasting adults and exacerbate hypoglycemia from another cause even when consumed in relatively modest amounts (see Chapter 24). Results of experimental studies are unclear: modest concentrations of ethanol impaired the growth hormone response to insulin-induced hypoglycemia in volunteers with type 1 diabetes (T1DM), but did not affect glucagon response [44]. The same dose of ethanol impaired glucagon, although not growth hormone (GH), response to the same degree of hypoglycemia in patients with diet-treated T2DM [45]. Rebound hypoglycemia can follow 2–3 hours after drinking alcohol with a glucose load in the form of sweet drinks or foods – so-called "gin-and-tonic hypoglycemia" [46]. Alcohol ingestion also increases the risk of severe brain damage or death in people who take an intentional overdose of insulin [47].

Non-pharmacopoeial drugs

Some "herbal," "traditional" and "folk" remedies contain compounds with glucose-lowering properties that are generally weak [48]. Some preparations, however, have caused severe hypoglycemia and have been found on analysis to contain an undeclared sulfonylurea [49].

Drug interactions that affect blood glucose concentrations

Several potential mechanisms underlying drug interaction cause hyperglycemia or hypoglycemia. Pharmacokinetic interactions can influence the effective concentrations of a glucose-modifying drug; examples are the increased concentrations of disopyramide following co-administration of clarithromycin, as described above, and the large number of drugs that increase or decrease circulating concentrations of sulfonylureas (see below).

Pharmacodynamic interactions occur when the observed action of one drug is modified by the action of another, without a change in the circulating concentration of either. The drugs can act at the same site (e.g. sulfamethoxazole is a ligand at the SUR-1 sulfonylurea receptor) or at different sites. Examples of the latter include β-adrenoceptor antagonists and other drugs that influence the physiologic response to hypoglycemia, and so alter the duration or severity of hypoglycemia from another cause.

Drugs that interact to enhance the actions of insulin secretagogues

Many drugs have pharmacokinetic or pharmacodynamic interactions with sulfonylureas that can cause clinically important disturbances in glycemic control. Some of the more important examples are shown in Table 26.4 and Figure 26.2. The most common outcome is hypoglycemia, brought about by reduced metabolic or renal clearance. Transient effects from displacement of protein-bound drug may occasionally also be important. Major dangers include the potentiation of the effects of tolbutamide, and possibly of chlorpropamide, glibenclamide and glipizide, by azapropazone (apazone), oral chloramphenicol and fluconazole. Miconazole interacts with glibenclamide and glipizide as well as tolbutamide. All these interactions are secondary to the inhibition of the metabolism of sulfonylurea in the liver. Similarly, ciprofloxacin increases the plasma concentrations and therefore enhances the hypoglycemic action of glibenclamide, apparently by inhibiting the hepatic CYP2C9 enzyme that metabolizes glibenclamide [50].

Table 26.4 Drugs that interact with sulfonylureas.

Drugs that may enhance the hypoglycemic effect of sulfonylureas
Azapropazone, phenylbutazone
Salicylates
Probenecid
Sulfonamides
Clarithromycin
Nicoumalone
Fluconazole, ketoconazole, miconazole, voriconazole
Drugs that may reduce the hypoglycemic effect of sulfonylureas
Rifampicin
Chlorpromazine

By contrast, rifampicin reduces the action of glibenclamide by inducing CYP2C9 and enhancing the hepatic clearance of sulfonylurea. Chlorpromazine also decreases the glucose-lowering effect of sulfonylurea, possibly by inhibiting insulin secretion.

Another important interaction with chlorpropamide (and, to a much lesser extent, with other sulfonylureas) is the cutaneous vasodilatation of the face and occasionally the trunk that is induced by ethanol, the chlorpropamide–alcohol flush (see Chapter 29).

Clarithromycin has been reported to interact with glibenclamide and glipizide, leading to hypoglycemia [51].

Some patients may be more susceptible to drug-induced hypoglycemia than others. For example, a Japanese case–control study suggested that patients taking levothyroxine and who also had liver disease were at substantially increased risk of mild hypoglycemia, with an odds ratio of 14.7 (range 1.6–137) [52].

Several oral hypoglycemic agents, including glimepiride, glipizide, glibenclamide, tolbutamide and nateglinide, are metabolized by CYP2C9, and a study suggests that among other factors, individuals with genetically determined low CYP2C9 activity are at an increased risk of sulfonylurea-associated severe hypoglycemia [53].

A meta-analysis confirms the impression that hypoglycemia is more likely with glibenclamide than other insulin secretagogues (relative risk 1.52 [95% CI 1.21–1.92]) [51].

Surreptitious ingestion of sulfonylureas such as glibenclamide in alternative medicines can cause hypoglycemia [54].

Interactions with metformin

Metformin has a high renal clearance. Cimetidine reduces the renal clearance of metformin, and causes it to accumulate (Figure 26.2). Drugs that impair renal function, such as non-steroidal anti-inflammatory agents and aminoglycosides, should be used with care, as they can also raise metformin concentrations, increasing the risk of lactic acidosis. Metformin should be stopped 24 hours before prolonged fasting (e.g. before surgery) and 48 hours before procedures requiring intravenous radiocontrast media. Patients on metformin are advised to avoid alcohol or to drink in moderation as hepatic damage poses a risk of hypoglycemia and lactic acidosis.

Interactions with other antidiabetic agents

- *Rosiglitazone* is metabolized by the hepatic microsomal enzyme CYP2C8, raising the theoretical possibility of interaction with other agents metabolized by the same enzyme. These include cerivastatin, now withdrawn in the USA and the UK, and paclitaxel [55], but no clinically significant interactions have yet been reported.
- *Repaglinide* is metabolized by CYP3A4, which also breaks down glibenclamide and several other important drugs, and is then excreted in the bile. Clarithromycin, an inhibitor of CYP3A4, has been reported to increase repaglinide concentration and the risk of hypoglycemia [56]. Rifampicin, which induces the same enzyme, reduces the effective concentrations of repaglinide by 25% in healthy volunteers, and could potentially worsen glycemic control in patients with T2DM [56]. Repaglinide is also metabolized by CYP2C8, and its plasma concentration is greatly increased by gemfibrozil, an inhibitor of CYP2C8. This interaction can result in hypoglycemia [56].
- *Glimepiride* is broken down by CYP2C9, and its metabolism is significantly inhibited by fluconazole, thus potentially enhancing its hypoglycemic action [57].

Hazards of general drugs when used in patients with diabetes

The presence of diabetes can influence the choice of agent for treating several important conditions. Drugs to treat cardiovascular diseases – hypertension, angina, arrhythmias and heart failure – and hyperlipidemia are of particular importance, because these conditions are common in people with diabetes.

Drugs with cardiovascular actions

β-Adrenoceptor antagonists

These are useful in the treatment of hypertension, angina, arrhythmias and in some cases of heart failure. There is also evidence that β-adrenoceptor antagonists (beta-blockers) are effective cardioprotective agents that reduce mortality following myocardial infarction in subjects both with and without diabetes [58,59]. β-Adrenoceptor antagonists are indicated in patients with chronic heart failure as they improve left ventricular function and reduce mortality [60]. The β-adrenoceptor antagonists should be started in stable patients, at a very low dose which should be escalated gradually.

β-Adrenoceptor antagonists can, theoretically at least, interfere with several aspects of glucose homeostasis (Figure 26.3). In the islets, insulin secretion is enhanced by β_2-adrenoceptor stimulation, while the β_2-adrenoceptor-mediated response to hypoglycemia in the liver promotes hepatic glycogenolysis and increases hepatic glucose output, a crucial part of the counter-regulatory response that restores blood glucose to normal.

Long-term treatment with β-adrenoceptor antagonists, especially in combination with high-dose thiazide diuretics, has been shown to be diabetogenic. This is discussed further in Chapter 16. β-Adrenoceptor antagonists were used in combination with thiazide diuretics in most of the early large clinical trials in patients with hypertension. In clinical trials testing a β-adrenoceptor antagonist on its own, its effect on stroke was less favorable than comparative drugs. This led to its relegation to fourth line treatment in the fourth British Hypertension Society guidelines [61]. In people with diabetes, their effect on insulin resistance may make them a less suitable choice than angiotensin-converting enzyme (ACE) inhibitors for example. People with diabetes, however, have a more stringent blood pressure target (130/85 mmHg), which necessitates the use of multiple classes to control blood pressure. In such instances, a beta-blocker could be added. People with diabetes frequently have ischemic heart disease, which is another indication for β-adrenoceptor antagonists.

β-Adrenoceptor stimulation is responsible for major hypoglycemic symptoms: the pounding heart and palpitation are secondary to β_1-adrenoceptor-mediated increases in heart rate and contractility, while tremor and sweating are both β_2-mediated (sweating also has a cholinergic component) (Figure 26.3). Non-selective β-adrenoceptor antagonists that antagonize both β_1- and β_2-receptors can therefore delay recovery from hypoglycemia and also reduce the patient's awareness of hypoglycemia.

Cardioselective β_1-adrenoceptor antagonists are less likely to interfere with awareness of or recovery from hypoglycemia, and so are preferable in patients treated with insulin or sulfonylureas. Even low doses of cardioselective β_1-adrenoceptor antagonists can modify some of the symptoms and signs of hypoglycemia (e.g. tachycardia), while other symptoms that are robust indicators of hypoglycemia (e.g. sweating) are unchanged or even more pronounced in the presence of β_1-blockade [62,63]. Overall, cardioselective β-adrenoceptor antagonists rarely impair recognition of hypoglycemia. The incidence of hypoglycemia is not increased during treatment with β_1-selective adrenoceptor antagonists, even in patients prone to the condition [64,65]. By contrast, the non-selective drugs can impair recovery from hypoglycemia [62,66,67].

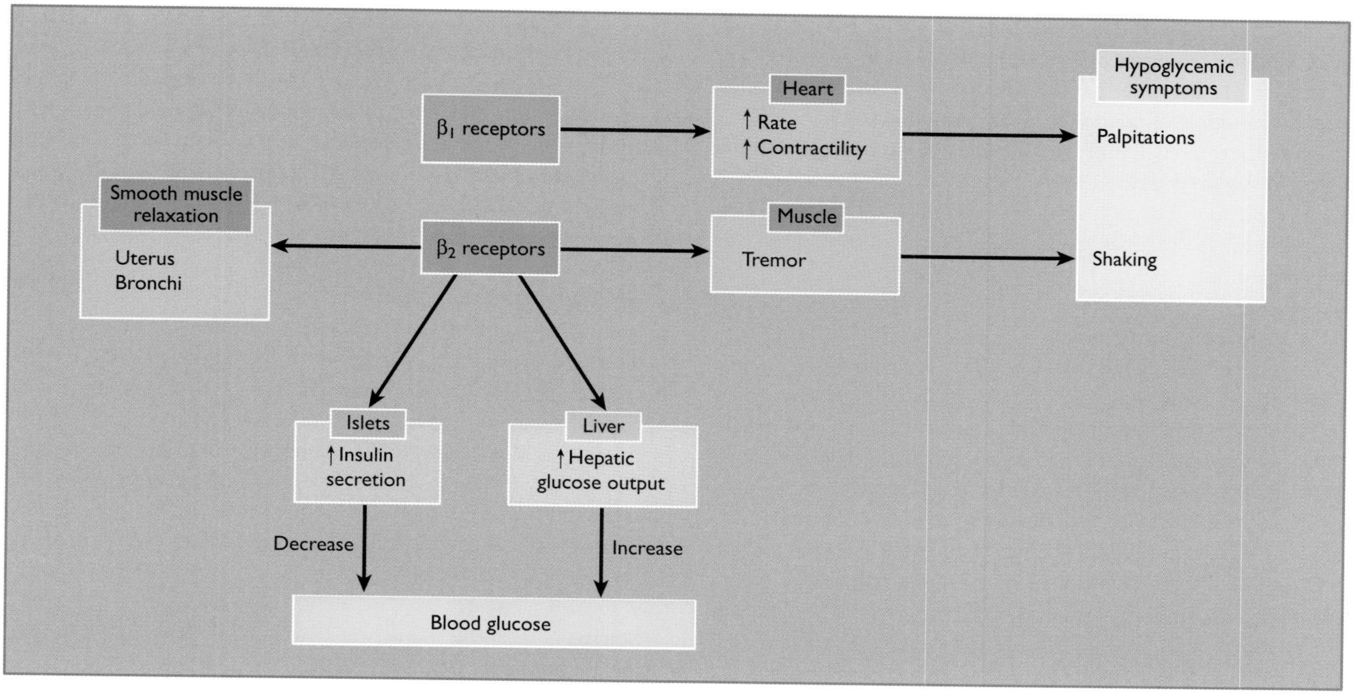

Figure 26.3 Effects mediated by β-adrenoceptors.

Concerns about the adverse metabolic effects of β_1-selective adrenoceptor antagonists have probably been exaggerated and the potential benefits of their cardioprotective effects underplayed [58]. Moreover, studies in heart failure have now provided extensive data showing that low-dose β-adrenoceptor antagonists are relatively safe in older, vulnerable patients [68].

Calcium-channel blockers

In vitro and *in vivo* studies have suggested that calcium-channel blockers may impair glucose metabolism, possibly because of impaired insulin secretion. Very few cases of clinically significant hyperglycemia, however, have been reported, and most of these were associated with excessive dosages of the drugs. When used appropriately, calcium-channel blockers are as safe in patients with diabetes as in people without diabetes (see Chapter 40). In people of Asian or African origin, calcium-channel blockers are relatively more efficacious in lowering blood pressure. This is especially relevant in populations that have a high incidence of stroke.

Angiotensin-converting enzyme inhibitors

ACE inhibitors are now widely used to treat hypertension and heart failure in both people with and without diabetes. The evidence of benefit of ACE inhibition after myocardial infarction, in systolic ventricular dysfunction and chronic heart failure is strong [69–71]. Similarly, ACE inhibitors reduce proteinuria and the endpoint of doubling of serum creatinine, or the need for dialysis or transplantation [72]. This protective effect on the kidney is encouraging their use in normotensive patients with early nephropathy (see Chapter 37). By contrast, the use of ACE inhibitors in patients with coronary heart disease without systolic ventricular dysfunction remains controversial. Two large randomized controlled trials showed reductions in cardiovascular events [73,74], but this was not confirmed in a third trial [75].

ACE inhibitors do not cause hyperglycemia, and neither do they adversely affect lipid metabolism [76,77]. Indeed, there is some evidence from the HOPE study that ACE inhibitors may reduce the likelihood of new-onset diabetes [78]. The DREAM study, which specifically addressed this issue, did not confirm this. In comparison with diuretics and beta-blockers, the effect is striking. ACE inhibitors can improve insulin sensitivity and lower blood glucose concentrations, occasionally causing severe hypoglycemia [79,80]. Case–control studies in the Netherlands and Scotland have demonstrated a threefold increase in the risk of severe hypoglycemia (requiring hospital admission) in patients with diabetes who were taking ACE inhibitors [81,82].

In people with and without diabetes, ACE inhibitors are contraindicated if the renal arteries are stenosed because of the high risk of renal impairment, which is usually reversible but sometimes permanent. There may be significant renal artery stenosis in up to 20% of patients with both hypertension and T2DM [83].

Angiotensin receptor blockers

Like ACE inhibitors, angiotensin receptor blockers (ARBs) are also indicated for hypertension, heart failure, post-myocardial infarction and diabetic nephropathy [84]. One study showed a marked reduction in stroke and mortality in patients with diabetes on an ARB-based regimen [85]. There is also evidence that ARBs reduce the risk of new-onset diabetes [86].

There are no trials demonstrating that ARBs are superior to ACE inhibitors in terms of outcome, and they are currently more expensive. On the other hand, ARBs do not cause the characteristic dry cough associated with ACE inhibitors.

Combining an ACE inhibitor and an ARB has no demonstrable value in coronary heart disease or diabetic nephropathy, other than reducing urinary albumin excretion further [87,88]. Furthermore, it may be associated with significant hyperkalemia.

α_1-Adrenoceptor antagonists

α_1-Adrenoceptor antagonists are effective hypotensive agents. They are generally thought to have beneficial metabolic effects, including improved insulin sensitivity, with falls in blood insulin, glucose and lipid concentrations [89–91], although one report [92] has suggested that the use of doxazosin may worsen glycemic control in patients with diabetes. Despite their potential advantages, these drugs are not currently in extensive use, perhaps because of the side effect of postural hypotension. In the Antihypertensive and Lipid-Lowering Treatment to Prevent Heart Attack Trial (ALLHAT), the α-blocker arm of the study was prematurely terminated because of an increased incidence of congestive heart failure compared to the diuretic arm [93]. This probably reflects the benefit of diuretics in treating the symptoms of heart failure rather than induction of heart failure by α-adrenoceptor antagonists.

Thiazides and other diuretics

Thiazides

It has become unfashionable to use thiazide diuretics in patients with diabetes, even though they are generally well tolerated, inexpensive and at least as effective as newer agents in preventing stroke and myocardial infarction. The concerns are the reversible impairment of glucose tolerance that can occur with thiazides, unfavorable changes in serum lipid profile and the worry that they may make men impotent [94–111]. Many of these concerns stem from old trials in which high doses of thiazide diuretics (e.g. 5 mg bendroflumethiazide) were used.

The diabetogenic potential of the thiazides is discussed in detail in Chapter 16. The consensus is that low dosages (e.g. 2.5 mg bendroflumethiazide), which are just as effective as higher dosages in lowering blood pressure, cause little if any deterioration in glycemic control [112]. The effects on lipids of low dosages are minor, and outweighed by the benefits of blood pressure reduction [109,110,113]. Finally, one large study (Treatment of Mild Hypertension Study) found no excess of impotence attributable to thiazide treatment among middle-aged hypertensive men, who had a high baseline incidence of this complaint [111]. Overall, the thiazides have a useful place in the treatment of hypertension in people with diabetes [114].

Loop diuretics

Loop diuretics, such as furosemide, ethacrynic acid and bumetanide, seem to have less impact on glucose homeostasis than thiazide diuretics, although several reports suggest that they can cause hyperglycemia [115,116]. Recent *in vitro* studies have shown that furosemide inhibits enzymes in the glycolytic pathway [117], so leading to poor glucose utilization and hyperglycemia. In practice, however, few problems are encountered in using loop diuretics in people with diabetes; it has been argued that any insulin resistance and hyperglycemia are not actually drug-induced, but instead are the consequence of the conditions that require potent diuretic therapy.

Antihyperlipidemic agents

The relationship between diabetes mellitus and dyslipidemia is discussed in detail in Chapter 40. Hypertriglyceridemia is often ameliorated by the effective treatment of hyperglycemia; conversely, some evidence indicates that lowering lipids (including free fatty acid concentrations) can improve blood glucose control. In practice, drugs are often prescribed independently for diet-resistant hyperglycemia and hyperlipidemia, so interactions between agents used to treat the conditions are potentially important.

Statins

Statins (hydroxymethyl-glutaryl coenzyme A inhibitors) seem to pose few problems in this respect. Meta-analysis has shown that people with diabetes treated by a statin enjoy the same relative risk reduction in major cardiovascular events as people without diabetes [118]. In general, people with diabetes have a higher absolute risk of myocardial infarction and stroke; their annual cardiovascular risk is comparable with that in non-diabetic patients with a history of myocardial infarction. Therefore, diabetes is regarded in many guidelines as an indication for lipid lowering therapy.

Fibrates

Early studies suggested that clofibrate could improve glycemic control in patients with poorly controlled T2DM taking sulfonylureas [119] or metformin [120]. More recently, similar benefits have been reported with bezafibrate [121], although these observations have not been widely pursued.

Nicotinic acid and its derivatives

Nicotinic acid (niacin) has recently been confirmed as an effective treatment for dyslipidemia in patients with diabetes; it does not appear to interact with antidiabetic therapy, and may be an alternative to fibrates or statins in those who are unable to tolerate them [122]. It can, however, cause hyperglycemia [123] and unpleasant flushing. A slow-release formulation that causes less flushing is now available. Acipimox is an analog of nicotinic acid that does not cause hyperglycemia (see Chapter 16) [124].

Anion-exchange resins

Anion-exchange resins such as cholestyramine could theoretically reduce the absorption of antidiabetic drugs from the gut, although clinically significant interference has not been reported. By contrast, ezetimibe does not have this effect.

Combined statin and fibrate therapy

This is sometimes indicated for dyslipidemia that is refractory to treatment with single agents. Myalgia and more serious muscle damage (with rhabdomyolysis and myoglobinuria) are rare but well-established complications of both statins and fibrates, and the risks are substantially increased by co-administration.

Other drugs

The UK Summaries of Product Characteristics of many products contain contraindications to using the product in patients with diabetes, or diabetic complications. Some of the less obvious examples are oxymetazoline hydrochloride nasal spray and verruca gels containing salicylic acid [125]. In addition, there is a wide range of warnings that medicines should be used with caution in diabetes; for example, oral rehydration solutions and ribavirin [125].

Special precautions in diabetic complications

Some drugs are relatively or absolutely contraindicated in the presence of certain diabetic complications. These include oral contraceptives or hormone replacement therapies in women with diabetes and severe vascular disease, the antiplatelet agents abciximab and cilostazol, and growth hormone in patients with proliferative retinopathy, and propranol by injection in patients prone to hypoglycemia [125]. Important examples are shown in Table 26.5.

Table 26.5 Drugs requiring caution in specific diabetic complications.

Complication and drug	Problem	Action to be taken
Nephropathy		
Sulfonylureas	Accumulate in renal failure; increased risk of hypoglycemia and toxicity	Use insulin or a sulfonylurea not cleared through the kidneys (e.g. gliquidone, gliclazide)
Metformin	Accumulates in renal failure; increased risk of lactic acidosis	Avoid
ACE inhibitors or ARBs	Initial rise in plasma creatinine; risk of hyperkalemia	Use with caution and appropriate monitoring of renal function
NSAIDs or COX-2 inhibitors	Further compromise renal function	Avoid if possible
Radiocontrast media	Reduce renal function	Adequate hydration before procedure
Cardiovascular disease		
β-Adrenoceptor antagonists	Accentuate hypoglycemia May cause modest VLDL elevation	Consider alternative antihypertensive, antianginal or antiarrhythmic drugs (e.g. ACE inhibitors, calcium-channel blockers)
Thiazide diuretics (high dose)	Worsen glycemic control in type 2 diabetes Exacerbate hyperlipidemia	Reduce dose, or use loop diuretic or alternative antihypertensive drugs
Retinopathy		
Mydriatics (eyedrops or systemic atropinic drugs)	In patients with rubeosis or previous eye surgery, glaucoma may be precipitated	Seek ophthalmologic advice before dilating pupils
Anticoagulants	May predispose to vitreous hemorrhage in patients with proliferative changes	Avoid if possible
Abciximab	May predispose to vitreous hemorrhage in patients with proliferative changes	Avoid if possible
Somatropin	Can worsen proliferative retinopathy	Avoid
Autonomic neuropathy		
Phosphodiesterase inhibitors (e.g. sildenafil)	Aggravates postural hypotension	Avoid, especially in the elderly and those taking nitrates
Ganglion-blocking agents and vasodilators	Aggravate postural hypotension	Use with caution
Impotence		
Ganglion-blocking agents β-Adrenergic blockers Clonidine α-Methyldopa	Aggravate erectile failure	Use alternative antihypertensive drugs (e.g. ACE inhibitor, calcium-channel blocker or α-adrenergic blocker)

ACE, angiotensin-converting enzyme; ARB, angiotensin receptor blocker; COX, cyclo-oxygenase; NSAID, non-steroidal anti-inflammatory drug; VLDL, very low density lipoprotein.

There has been controversy about the risks of inducing vitreous hemorrhage with thrombolytic treatment (e.g. streptokinase) for myocardial infarction in patients with proliferative retinopathy. Current advice is to give thrombolytic drugs according to the usual indications, as the likely benefits far outweigh the potential threat to vision.

Drug interference with monitoring of diabetic control

Urine testing for glucose, still favored by many elderly patients, is subject to interference by several drugs [126], including ascorbic acid, which can give false-negative urine glucose readings with glucose oxidase strips (see Chapter 25) [127].

Blood glucose measurements, using dry-reagent glucose oxidase test strips, can potentially be affected by drugs such as aspirin if present in very high concentrations [128]. Readings can also be misleading if fingers are contaminated with alcohol from swabs (which inactivates glucose oxidase) or with glucose (e.g. from sugary drinks) [129].

The complex sugar icodextrin, used as a peritoneal dialysate, can give spuriously high glucose concentrations; this can mask underlying hypoglycemia [130].

Conclusions

Rational prescribing is a difficult task whose success demands the integration of data about the drugs being used, the patient, and the conditions that affect the patient. There are three major areas of difficulty when prescribing for patients with diabetes. First, a large number of drugs affect glucose tolerance. They include important agents, such as oral corticosteroids, which can be life-saving but confound attempts to achieve euglycemia. Secondly, patients with diabetes are now commonly asked to take several medicines to control glycemia, and to treat the complications of diabetes. The number of potential interactions between pairs of drugs increases rapidly with the number of different drugs prescribed. As the number of prescribed medicines increases from 5 to 10, the number of possible pair-wise interactions increases from 10 to 45 (and the number of three-way interactions from 10 to 120). Thirdly, patients with diabetes are at high risk of other disorders whose management conventionally involves the prescribing of a range of medicines. For example, treatment of patients after myocardial infarction, five times more likely in the presence of diabetes, would commonly involve one or more antiplatelet agents, a statin, an ACE inhibitor, and a β-adrenoceptor antagonist.

Rational prescribers will consider, in consultation with the patient, therapeutic purpose, and the potential benefit and the possible harm of any additional treatment in the individual patient prior to prescribing. They will also review long-standing prescriptions from time to time to revisit previous decisions in the light of changes in the patient, the reason for prescribing, and the pharmacopoeia.

References

1 Seltzer HS. Drug-induced hypoglycemia: a review of 1418 cases. *Endocrinol Metab Clin North Am* 1989; **18**:163–183.
2 Marks V, Teale JD. Drug-induced hypoglycemia. *Endocrinol Metab Clin North Am* 1999; **28**:555–577.
3 Ben-Ami H, Nagachandran P, Mendelson A, Edoute Y. Drug-induced hypoglycemic coma in 102 diabetic patients. *Arch Intern Med* 1999; **59**:281–284.
4 Park-Wyllie LY, Juurlink DN, Kopp A, Shah BR, Stukel TA, Stumpo C, *et al.* Outpatient gatifloxacin therapy and dysglycemia in older adults. *N Engl J Med* 2006; **354**:1352–1361.
5 Todd GR, Acerini CL, Ross-Russell R, Zahra S, Warner JT, McCance D. Survey of adrenal crisis associated with inhaled corticosteroids in the United Kingdom. *Arch Dis Child* 2002; **87**:455–456.
6 Drake AJ, Howells RJ, Shield JPH, Prendiville A, Ward PS, Crowne EC. Lesson of the week: symptomatic adrenal insufficiency presenting with hypoglycemia in children with asthma receiving high dose inhaled fluticasone propionate. *Br Med J* 2002; **324**:1081–1083.
7 Odeh M, Oliven A. Doxycycline-induced hypoglycemia. *J Clin Pharmacol* 2000; **40**:1173–1174.
8 Basaria S, Braga M, Moore WT. Doxycycline-induced hypoglycemia in a nondiabetic young man. *South Med J* 2002; **95**:1353–1354.
9 Ebbesen F, Joergensen A, Hoseth E, Kaad PH, Moeller M, Holsteen V, *et al.* Neonatal hypoglycemia and withdrawal symptoms after exposure *in utero* to valproate. *Arch Dis Child Fetal Neonatal Ed* 2000; **83**:F124–129.
10 Meertens JH, Monteban-Kooistra WE, Ligtenberg JJ, Tulleken JE, Zijlstra JG. Severe hypoglycemia following venlafaxine intoxication: a case report. *J Clin Psychopharmacol* 2007; **27**:414–415.
11 Ryan EA, Pick ME, Marceau C. Use of alternative medicines in diabetes mellitus. *Diabet Med* 2001; **18**:242–245.
12 Jennings AM, Wilson RM, Ward JD. Symptomatic hypoglycemia in NIDDM patients treated with oral hypoglycemic agents. *Diabetes Care* 1989; **12**:203–208.
13 Ferner RE, Neil HA. Sulphonylureas and hypoglycemia. *Br Med J* 1988; **296**:949–950.
14 van Staa T, Abenhaim L, Leufkens H. Rates of hypoglycemia in users of sulfonylureas. *J Clin Epidemiol* 1997; **50**:735–741.
15 Stahl M, Berger W. Higher incidence of severe hypoglycemia leading to hospital admission in type 2 diabetic patients treated with long-acting versus short-acting sulphonylureas. *Diabet Med* 1999; **16**:586–590.
16 Langtry HD, Balfour JA. Glimepiride: a review of its use in the management of type 2 diabetes mellitus. *Drugs* 1998; **55**:563–584.
17 Shorr RI, Ray WA, Daugherty JR, Griffin MR. Incidence and risk factors for serious hypoglycemia in older persons using insulin or sulphonylureas. *Arch Intern Med* 1997; **157**:1681–1686.
18 Burge MR, Schmitz-Fiorentino K, Fischette C, Qualls CR, Schade DS. A prospective trial of risk factors for sulfonylurea-induced hypoglycemia in type 2 diabetes mellitus. *JAMA* 1988; **279**:137–143.
19 Szlatenyi CS, Capes KF, Wang RY. Delayed hypoglycemia in a child after ingestion of a single glipizide tablet. *Ann Emergency Med* 1998; **31**:773–776.

20 Kalimo H, Olsson Y. Effects of severe hypoglycemia on the human brain: neuropathological reports. *Acta Neurol Scand* 1980; **62**:345–356.

21 Ludman P, Mason P, Joplin GF. Dangerous misuse of sulphonylureas. *Br Med J* 1986; **293**:1287–1288.

22 Johnson SF, Schade DS, Peake GT. Chlorpropamide-induced hypoglycemia: successful treatment with diazoxide. *Am J Med* 1977; **63**:799–804.

23 Jeffery WH, Graham FM. Treatment of chlorpropamide over-dose with diazoxide. *Drug Intell Clin Pharm* 1983; **17**:372–374.

24 Boyle PJ, Justice K, Krentz AJ, Nagy RJ, Schade DS. Octreotide reverses hyperinsulinemia and prevents hypoglycemia induced by sulphonylurea overdoses. *J Clin Endocrinol Metab* 1993; **76**:752–756.

25 UK Prospective Diabetes Study (UKPDS) Group. Intensive blood-glucose control with sulphonylureas or insulin compared with conventional treatment and risk of complications in patients with type 2 diabetes (UKPDS 33). *Lancet* 1998; **352**:837–853.

26 Hirshberg B, Skarulis MC, Pucino F, Csako G, Brennan R, Gorden P. Repaglinide-induced factitious hypoglycemia. *J Clin Endocrinol Metab* 2001; **86**:475–477.

27 Okitolonda W, Delacollette C, Malengreau M, Henquin JC. High incidence of hypoglycemia in African patients treated with intravenous quinine for severe malaria. *Br Med J* 1987; **295**:716–718.

28 White NJ, Miller KD, Marsh K, Berry CD, Turner RC, Williamson DH, *et al.* Hypoglycemia in African children with severe malaria. *Lancet* 1987; **i**:708–711.

29 White NJ, Warrell DA, Chanthavanich P, Looareesuwan S, Warrell MJ, Krishna S, *et al.* Severe hypoglycemia and hyperinsulinemia in falciparum malaria. *N Engl J Med* 1983; **309**:61–66.

30 Phillips RE, Looareesuwan S, Molyneux ME, Hatz C, Warrell DA. Hypoglycemia and counterregulatory hormone responses in severe falciparum malaria: treatment with Sandostatin. *Q J Med* 1993; **86**:233–240.

31 Lee AJ, Maddix DS. Trimethoprim–sulfamethoxazole-induced hypoglycemia in a patient with acute renal failure. *Ann Pharmacother* 1997; **31**:727–732.

32 Johnson JA, Kappel JE, Sharif MN. Hypoglycemia secondary to trimethoprim–sulfamethoxazole administration in a renal transplant patient. *Ann Pharmacother* 1993; **27**:304–306.

33 Schattner A, Rimon E, Green L, Coslovsky R, Bentwich Z. Hypoglycemia induced by co-trimoxazole in AIDS. *Br Med J* 1988; **297**:742.

34 Assan R, Perronne C, Assan D, Chotard L, Mayaud C, Zucman D. Pentamidine-induced derangements of glucose homeostasis: determinant roles of renal failure and drug accumulation – a study of 128 patients. *Diabetes Care* 1995; **18**:47–55.

35 Stahl-Bayliss CM, Kalman CM, Laskin OL. Pentamidine-induced hypoglycemia in patients with the acquired immune deficiency syndrome. *Clin Pharmacol Ther* 1986; **39**:271–275.

36 Waskin H, Stehr-Green JK, Helmick CG, Sattler FR. Risk factors for hypoglycemia associated with pentamidine therapy for *Pneumocystis* pneumonia. *JAMA* 1988; **260**:345–347.

37 Karboski JA, Godley PJ. Inhaled pentamidine and hypoglycemia. *Ann Intern Med* 1988; **108**:490.

38 Odeh M, Oliven A. Doxycycline-induced hypoglycemia. *J Clin Pharmacol* 2000; **40**:1173–1174.

39 Goldberg IJ, Brown LK, Rayfield EJ. Disopyramide (Norpace) induced hypoglycemia. *Am J Med* 1980; **69**:463–466.

40 Strathman I, Schubert EN, Cohen A, Nitzberg DM. Hypoglycemia in patients receiving disopyramide phosphate. *Drug Intell Clin Pharm* 1983; **17**:635–638.

41 Takada M, Fujita S, Katayama Y, Harano Y, Shibakawa M. The relationship between risk of hypoglycemia and use of cibenzoline and disopyramide. *Eur J Clin Pharmacol* 1999; **56**:335–342.

42 Croxson MS, Shaw DW, Henley PG, Gabriel HD. Disopyramide-induced hypoglycemia and increased serum insulin. *N Z Med J* 1987; **100**:407–408.

43 Warnock JK, Biggs F. Nefazodone-induced hypoglycemia in a diabetic patient with major depression. *Am J Psychiatry* 1997; **154**:288–289.

44 Kerr D, Cheyne E, Thomas P, Sherwin R. Influence of acute alcohol ingestion on the hormonal responses to modest hypoglycemia in patients with type 1 diabetes. *Diabet Med* 2007; **24**:312–316.

45 Rasmussen BM, Orskov L, Schmitz O, Hermansen K. Alcohol and glucose counterregulation during acute insulin-induced hypoglycemia in type 2 diabetic subjects. *Metabolism* 2001; **50**:451–457.

46 O'Keefe SJ, Marks V. Lunchtime gin and tonic: a cause of reactive hypoglycemia. *Lancet* 1977; **i**:1286–1288.

47 Critchley JA, Proudfoot AT, Boyd SG, Campbell IW, Brown NS, Gordon A. Deaths and paradoxes after intentional insulin overdosage. *Br Med J* 1984; **289**:225.

48 Bailey CJ, Day C. Traditional plant medicines as treatment for diabetes. *Diabetes Care* 1989; **12**:553–564.

49 Baba T, Kataoka K, Itakura M. Hypoglycemia due to folk medicine. *Diabetes Care* 1999; **22**:1376.

50 Roberge RJ, Kaplan R, Frank R, Fore C. Glyburide–ciprofloxacin interaction with resistant hypoglycemia. *Ann Emerg Med* 2000; **36**:160–163.

51 Gangji AS, Cukierman T, Gerstein HC, Goldsmith CH, Clase CM. A systematic review and meta-analysis of hypoglycemia and cardiovascular events: a comparison of glyburide with other secretagogues and with insulin. *Diabetes Care* 2007; **30**:389–394.

52 Iihara N, Kurosaki Y, Takada M, Morita S. Risk of hypoglycemia associated with thyroid agents is increased in patients with liver impairment. *Int J Clin Pharmacol Ther* 2008; **46**:1–13.

53 Holstein A, Plaschke A, Ptak M, Egberts EH, El-Din J, Brockmöller J, *et al.* Association between CYP2C9 slow metabolizer genotypes and severe hypoglycemia on medication with sulphonylurea hypoglycemic agents. *Br J Clin Pharmacol* 2005; **60**:103–106.

54 Goudie AM, Kaye JM. Contaminated medication precipitating hypoglycemia. *Med J Aust* 2001; **175**:256–257.

55 Anon. Summary of product characteristics for "Avenida" brand of rosiglitazone. http://emc.vhn.net. Accessed August 7, 2001.

56 Anon. Summary of product characteristics for "Novonorm" brand of repaglinide. http://emc.vhn.net. Accessed August 7, 2001.

57 Niemi M, Backman JT, Neuvonen M, Laitila J, Neuvonen PJ, Kivisto KT. Effects of fluconazole and fluvoxamine on the pharmacokinetics and pharmacodynamics of glimepiride. *Clin Pharmacol Ther* 2001; **69**:194–200.

58 Tse WY, Kendall M. Is there a role for beta-blockers in hypertensive diabetic patients? *Diabet Med* 1994; **11**:137–144.

59 Kjekshus J, Gilpin E, Cali G, Blackey AR, Henning H, Ross J Jr. Diabetic patients and beta-blockers after acute myocardial infarction. *Eur Heart J* 1990; **11**:43–50.

60 Poole-Wilson PA, Swedberg K, Cleland JG, Di Lenarda A, Hanrath P, Komajda M, *et al.* Carvedilol Or Metoprolol European Trial Investigators. Comparison of carvedilol and metoprolol on clinical outcomes in patients with chronic heart failure in the Carvedilol Or

Metoprolol European Trial (COMET): randomised controlled trial. *Lancet* 2003; **362**:7–13.

61 Williams B, Poulter NR, Brown MJ, Davis M, McInnes GT, Potter JF, *et al.* BHS guidelines working party, for the British Hypertension Society. British Hypertension Society guidelines for hypertension management 2004 (BHS-IV): summary. *Br Med J* 2004; **328**:634–640.

62 Fagerberg B, Berglund A, Holme E, Wilhelmsen L, Elmfeldt D. Metabolic effects of controlled-release metoprolol in hypertensive men with impaired or diabetic glucose tolerance: a comparison with atenolol. *J Intern Med* 1990; **227**:37–43.

63 Clausen-Sjobom N, Lins P, Adamson U, Curstedt T, Hamberger B. Effects of metoprolol on the counter-regulation of prolonged hypoglycemia in insulin-dependent diabetics. *Acta Med Scand* 1987; **222**:57–63.

64 Barnett A, Leslie D, Watkins P. Can insulin-treated diabetics be given beta-adrenergic blocking drugs? *Br Med J* 1980; **2**:976–978.

65 Blohme G, Lager I, Lönnroth P, Smith U. Hypoglycemic symptoms in insulin-dependent diabetics: a prospective study on the influence of beta-blockade. *Diabète Métab* 1981; **7**:235–238.

66 Deacon S, Karunanayake A, Barnett D. Acebutolol, atenolol and propranolol and metabolic responses to acute hypoglycemia in diabetes. *Br Med J* 1977; **2**:1255–1257.

67 Lager I, Blohme G, Smith U. Effect of cardioselective beta-blockade on the hypoglycemic response in insulin-dependent diabetics. *Lancet* 1979; **i**:458–462.

68 Dargie HJ, Lechat P. The Cardiac Insufficiency Bisoprolol Study II (CIBIS-II): a randomised trial. *Lancet* 1999; **353**:9–13.

69 CONSENSUS Trial Study Group. Effects of enalapril on mortality in severe congestive heart failure: results of the Cooperative North Scandinavian Enalapril Survival Study (CONSENSUS). *N Engl J Med* 1987; **316**:1429–1435.

70 SOLVD investigators. Effect of enalapril on survival in patients with reduced left ventricular dysfunction after myocardial infarction. *N Engl J Med* 1991:**325**:293–302.

71 Pfeffer MA, Braunwald E, Moyet LA, Basta L, Brown EJ, Cuddy TE, *et al.* Effect of captopril on mortality and morbidity in patients with left ventricular dysfunction after myocardial infarction. *N Engl J Med* 1992; **327**:669–677.

72 Lewis EJ, Hunsicker LG, Bain RP, Rohde RD. The effect of angiotensin-converting enzyme inhibition on diabetic nephropathy. *N Engl J Med* 1993; **329**:1456.

73 Heart Outcomes Prevention Evaluation Study Investigators. Effects of an angiotensin-converting-enzyme inhibitor, ramipril, on cardiovascular events in high-risk patients. *N Engl J Med* 2000; **342**:145–153.

74 Fox KM; EURopean trial On reduction of cardiac events with Perindopril in stable coronary Artery disease Investigators. Efficacy of perindopril in reduction of cardiovascular events among patients with stable coronary artery disease: randomised, double-blind, placebo-controlled, multicentre trial (the EUROPA study). *Lancet* 2003; **362**:782–788.

75 Braunwald E, Domanski MJ, Fowler SE, Geller NL, Gersh BJ, Hsia J, *et al.* PEACE Trial Investigators. Angiotensin-converting-enzyme inhibition in stable coronary artery disease. *N Engl J Med* 2004; **351**:2058–2068.

76 Andronico G, Piazza G, Mangano MT, Mule G, Carone MB, Cerasola G. Nifedipine vs. enalapril in treatment of hypertensive patients with glucose intolerance. *J Cardiovasc Pharmacol* 1991; **18**(Suppl. 10):S52–S54.

77 Seefeldt T, Orskov L, Mengel A, Rasmussen O, Pedersen NM, Moller N, *et al.* Lack of effects of angiotensin-converting enzyme (ACE) inhibitors on glucose metabolism in type I diabetes. *Diabet Med* 1990; **7**:700–704.

78 Yusuf S, Gerstein H, Hoogwerf B, Pogue J, Bosch J, Wolffenbuttel BH, *et al.* HOPE Study Investigators. Ramipril and the development of diabetes. *JAMA* 2001; **286**:1882–1885.

79 Pollare T, Lithell H, Berne C. A comparison of the effects of hydrochlorothiazide and captopril in glucose and lipid metabolism in patients with hypertension. *N Engl J Med* 1989; **321**:868–873.

80 Torlone E, Britta M, Rambotti A. Improved insulin action and glycemic control after long-term angiotensin converting enzyme inhibition in subjects with arterial hypertension and type II diabetes. *Diabetes Care* 1993; **16**:1347–1355.

81 Herrings RMC, de Boer A, Stricker BHC, Leufkens HGM, Porsius A. Hypoglycemia associated with use of inhibitors of angiotensin converting enzyme. *Lancet* 1995; **345**:1195–1198.

82 Morris AD, Boyle DI, McMahon AD, Pearce H, Evans JM, Newton RW, *et al.* ACE inhibitor use is associated with hospitalization for severe hypoglycemia in patients with diabetes. DARTS/MEMO Collaboration. Diabetes Audit and Research in Tayside, Scotland: Medicines Monitoring Unit. *Diabetes Care* 1997; **20**:1363–1367.

83 Valabhji J, Robinson S, Poulter C, Robinson AC, Kong C, Henzen C, *et al.* Prevalence of renal artery stenosis in subjects with type 2 diabetes and coexistent hypertension. *Diabetes Care* 2000; **23**:539–545.

84 Barnett AH, Bain SC, Bouter P, Karlberg B, Madsbad S, Jervell J, *et al.* Diabetics Exposed to Telmisartan and Enalapril Study Group. Angiotensin-receptor blockade versus converting-enzyme inhibition in type 2 diabetes and nephropathy. *N Engl J Med* 2004; **351**:1952–1961.

85 Lindholm LH, Ibsen H, Dahlof B, Devereux RB, Beevers G, de Faire U, *et al.* LIFE Study Group. Cardiovascular morbidity and mortality in patients with diabetes in the Losartan Intervention For Endpoint reduction in hypertension study (LIFE): a randomised trial against atenolol. *Lancet* 2002; **359**:1004–1010.

86 Andraws R, Brown DL. Effect of inhibition of the renin-angiotensin system on development of type 2 diabetes mellitus (meta-analysis of randomized trials). *Am J Cardiol* 2007; **99**:1006–1012.

87 Yusuf S, Teo KK, Pogue J, Dyal L, Copland I, Schumacher H, *et al.* ONTARGET Investigators. Telmisartan, ramipril, or both in patients at high risk for vascular events. *N Engl J Med* 2008; **358**:1547–1559.

88 Mann JF, Schmieder RE, McQueen M, Dyal L, Schumacher H, Pogue J, *et al.* ONTARGET investigators. Renal outcomes with telmisartan, ramipril, or both, in people at high vascular risk (the ONTARGET study): a multicentre, randomised, double-blind, controlled trial. *Lancet* 2008; **372**:547–553.

89 Giorda C, Appendio M. Effects of doxazosin, a selective alpha 1-inhibitor, on plasma insulin and blood glucose response to a glucose tolerance test in essential hypertension. *Metabolism* 1993; **42**:1440–1442.

90 Pollare T, Lithell H, Selinus I, Berne C. Application of prazosin is associated with an increase of insulin sensitivity in obese patients with hypertension. *Diabetologia* 1988; **31**:415–420.

91 Swislocki A, Hoffman B, Sheu W, Chen YD, Reaven GM. Effect of prazosin treatment on carbohydrate and lipoprotein metabolism in patients with hypertension. *Am J Med* 1989; **86**:14–18.

92 McLaughlin B, Daly L, Devlin JG. Doxazosin in the management of hypertensive diabetes: a cautionary note? *Irish Med J* 1992; **161**:9–11.

93 ALLHAT Officers and Coordinators for the ALLHAT Collaborative Research Group. Major outcomes in high-risk hypertensive patients randomized to angiotensin-converting enzyme inhibitor or calcium channel blocker vs diuretic: The Antihypertensive and Lipid-Lowering Treatment to Prevent Heart Attack Trial (ALLHAT). *JAMA* 2002; **288**:2981–2997.

94 Duke M. Thiazide-induced hypokalemia: association with acute myocardial infarction and ventricular fibrillation. *JAMA* 1978; **239**: 43–49.

95 Goldner M, Zurkowitz H, Akgun S. Hyperglycemia and glycosuria due to thiazide derivatives administered in diabetes mellitus. *N Engl J Med* 1960; **262**:403–405.

96 Shapiro A, Benedek T, Small J. Effect of thiazides on carbohydrate metabolism in patients with hypertension. *N Engl J Med* 1961; **265**:1028–1033.

97 Lewis P, Petrie A, Kohner E. Deterioration of glucose tolerance in hypertensive patients on prolonged diuretic treatment. *Lancet* 1976; **i**:564–566.

98 Murphy M, Kohner E, Lewis P, Schumer B, Dollery CT. Glucose intolerance in hypertensive patients treated with diuretics: fourteen year follow up. *Lancet* 1982; **ii**:1293–1295.

99 Amery A, Wasir H, Bulpitt C, Conway J, Fagard R, Lijnen P, *et al.* Glucose intolerance during diuretic therapy: results of trial by the European Working Party on Hypertension in the Elderly. *Lancet* 1978; **i**:681–683.

100 Wilkins R. New drugs for the treatment of hypertension. *Ann Intern Med* 1959; **50**:1–10.

101 Nguyen K. Are thiazides diabetogenic? *Tidsskr Nor Legeforen* 1993; **113**:2587–2589.

102 Freis D. Adverse effects of diuretics. *Drug Saf* 1992; **7**:364–373.

103 Anderson O, Gudbrandsson T, Jamerson K. Metabolic adverse effects of thiazide diuretics: the importance of normokalemia. *J Intern Med* 1991; **735**(Suppl.):89–96.

104 Sagild U, Andersen V, Andreasen P. Glucose tolerance and insulin responsiveness in experimental potassium depletion. *Acta Med Scand* 1961; **169**:243–251.

105 Helderman JH, Elahi D, Andersen DK, Raizes GS, Tobin JD, Shocken D, *et al.* Prevention of the glucose intolerance of thiazide diuretics by maintenance of body potassium. *Diabetes* 1983; **32**:106–111.

106 Rapoport M, Hurd H. Thiazide-induced glucose tolerance treated with potassium. *Arch Intern Med* 1964; **113**:405–408.

107 Gorden P, Sherman B, Simopoulos A. Glucose intolerance with hypokalemia, an increased proportion of circulating proinsulin-like component. *J Clin Endocrinol Metabolism* 1972; **34**:235–240.

108 Schmitz O, Hermansen K, Hother Nielsen O. Insulin action in insulin-dependent diabetics after short term thiazide therapy. *Diabetes Care* 1986; **9**:630–637.

109 Hansson L, Lindholm LH, Ekbom T, Dahlöf B, Lanke J, Linjer E, *et al.* Comparison of old versus newer antihypertensive therapies in preventing cardiovascular mortality and morbidity in elderly hypertensives: principal results of the Swedish Trial in Old Patients with Hypertension-2 (STOP-Hypertension-2). *Lancet* 1999; **354**: 1751–1756.

110 Philipp T, Anlauf M, Distler A, Holzgreve H, Michaelis J, Wellek S. Randomised, double-blind, multicentre comparison of hydrochlorothiazide, atenolol, nitrendipine and enalapril in antihypertensive treatment: results of the HANE Study. *Br Med J* 1997; **315**:154–159.

111 Grimm RH, Grandits GA, Prineas RJ, McDonald RH, Lewis CE, Flack JM, *et al.* Long-term effects on sexual function of five antihypertensive drugs and nutritional hygienic treatment of hypertensive men and women: Treatment of Mild Hypertension Study (TOMHS). *Hypertension* 1997; **29**:8–14.

112 Harper R, Ennis CN, Sheridan B, Gormley M, Atkinson AB, Johnston GD, *et al.* Effects of low dose versus conventional dose thiazide diuretic in essential hypertension. *Br Med J* 1994; **309**:226–230.

113 Adler AI, Stratton IM, Neil HA, Yudkin JS, Matthews DR, Cull CA, *et al.* Association of systolic blood pressure with macrovascular and microvascular complications of type 2 diabetes (UKPDS 36): prospective observational study. *Br Med J* 2000; **321**:412–419.

114 Beevers DG, Ferner RE. Why are thiazide diuretics declining in popularity? *J Hum Hypertens* 2001; **15**:287–289.

115 Toivonen S, Mustala O. Diabetogenic actions of frusemide. *Br Med J* 1966; **1**:920–921.

116 Taylor R. Drugs and glucose tolerance. *Adverse Drug React Bull* 1986; **121**:452–455.

117 Dimitriodos G, Tegos C, Golfinopolou L, Roboti C, Raptis S. Furosemide-induced hyperglycemia: the implication of glycolytic kinases. *Horm Metab Res* 1993; **25**:557–559.

118 Kearney PM, Blackwell L, Collins R, Keech A, Simes J, Peto R, *et al.* Cholesterol Treatment Trialists' (CTT) Collaborators. Efficacy of cholesterol-lowering therapy in 18,686 people with diabetes in 14 randomised trials of statins: a meta-analysis. *Lancet* 2008; **371**:117–125.

119 Daubresse JC, Daigneux D, Bruwier M, Luyckx A, Lefebvre PJ. Clofibrate and diabetes control in patients treated with oral hypoglycemic agents. *Br J Clin Pharmacol* 1979; **7**:599–603.

120 De Silva SR, Betteridge DJ, Shawe JE, Cudworth AG, Alberti KGMM. Metformin and clofibrate in maturity onset diabetes mellitus: advantages of combined treatment. *Diabète Métab* 1979; **5**:223–229.

121 Jones IR, Swai A, Taylor R, Miller M, Laker MF, Alberti KG. Lowering of plasma glucose concentrations with bezafibrate in patients with moderately controlled NIDDM. *Diabetes Care* 1990; **13**:855–863.

122 Elam MB, Hunninghake DB, Davis KB, Garg R, Johnson C, Egan D, *et al.* Effect of niacin on lipid and lipoprotein levels and glycemic control in patients with diabetes and peripheral arterial disease: the Arterial Disease Multiple Intervention Trial (ADMIT) study: a randomized trial. *JAMA* 2000; **284**:1263–1270.

123 Schwartz M. Severe reversible hyperglycemia as a consequence of niacin therapy. *Arch Intern Med* 1993; **153**:2050–2052.

124 Dean JD, McCarthy S, Betteridge DJ, Whately-Smith C, Powell J, Owens DR. The effect of acipimox in patients with type 2 diabetes and persistent hyperlipidemia. *Diabet Med* 1992; **9**:611–615.

125 Association of British Pharmaceutical Industries. eMedicines Compendium. http://emc.medicines.org.uk/. Accessed on December 14, 2008.

126 Rotblatt MD, Koda-Kimble MA. Review of drug interference with urine glucose tests. *Diabetes Care* 1987; **10**:103–110.

127 Mayson JS, Schumaker O, Nakamura RM. False-negative tests for urine glucose. *Lancet* 1973; **1**:780–781.

128 Rice GK, Galt KA. *In vitro* drug interference with home blood-glucose-measurement systems. *Am J Hospital Pharm* 1985; **42**: 2202–2207.

129 Ferner RE. Superficial hyperglycemia. *Lancet* 1985; **ii**:618–619.

130 Kroll HR, Maher TR. Significant hypoglycemia secondary to icodextrin peritoneal dialysate in a diabetic patient. *Anesth Analg* 2007; **104**:1473–1474.

6 Treatment of Diabetes

27 Insulin and Insulin Treatment

Stephen Gough[1] & Parth Narendran[2]

[1]Oxford Centre for Diabetes, Endocrinology and Metabolism, University of Oxford and Churchill Hospital, Oxford, UK
[2]Institute of Biomedical Research, The Medical School, University of Birmingham, Birmingham, UK

Keypoints

- Insulin is a potent anabolic hormone essential for life. Insulin has a circulating concentration of 15–20 mU/L in the fasting state, and 60–80 mU/L post-prandially.
- Early insulins were extracted from the pancreata of pigs and cows but good glycemic control was difficult to achieve because of residual impurities after the purification process. The newer and purer animal insulins are better tolerated and can potentially achieve a level of glycemic control similar to synthetic human insulins. Clinically significant hypoglycemia rates between the human and animal insulins also appear to be similar.
- The challenge of insulin replacement therapy is to reproduce a normal physiologic insulin profile without incurring significant hypoglycemia. A range of insulin preparations with differing durations of actions are available to achieve this: rapid-acting insulin analogs (about 3 hours), soluble insulin (about 6–8 hours), neutral protamine Hagedorn (NPH) insulin (12–18 hours), lente insulins (about 12–24 hours), long-acting insulin analogs (about 24 hours).
- Current recommendations for the injection of insulin are that the skin is pinched to reduce the risk of injecting into muscle, and to inject at a right angle to the skin after which the fold should be held for 5–10 seconds before removing the needle. Injection needle lengths of 5–12 mm are available to ensure that the insulin is delivered deep enough into the subcutaneous tissue to prevent back-leakage, but not so deep that it is intramuscular. Alternative modes of insulin administration such as continuous subcutaneous insulin infusion can also be highly effective.
- Multiple-dose insulin therapy is an appropriate initial approach to reproducing the physiologic insulin profile in patients with absolute insulin deficiency such as those with type 1 diabetes. This consists of a long-acting insulin preparation administered once or twice a day to meet the basal insulin requirement, with the injection of a short-acting insulin preparation with each meal.
- A number of different insulin injection regimens are available for patients with type 2 diabetes who may already be treated with non-insulin-based therapies. These include a once daily injection of a long-acting insulin, a once daily injection of a long-acting insulin with an injection of a short-acting insulin with the main meal, twice a day injections of insulin mixtures, and multiple dose injections.

Life (and death) before insulin

Insulin is a potent anabolic hormone, and its absence induces a profound catabolic state that affects fat, carbohydrate and protein stores. Absolute insulin deficiency, such as that characterized by type 1 diabetes (T1DM), will result in death if left untreated (Figure 27.1). What the study of patients with diabetes in the pre-insulin era teaches us is the surprisingly long period that can be survived without insulin. Leonard Thompson was the first patient to have effective insulin treatment. He was 12 years old when he was diagnosed with diabetes in 1919 and had survived over 2 years when at 11 AM on January 22, 1922 he received his first injection of insulin. This said, it was a miserable existence without insulin. Other than the weight loss, constant tiredness, thirst, urination and frequent infections, there was the certain knowledge that a death sentence had been passed, and that death would be an agonizing and slow process. The most effective therapy available at that time appeared to be severe nutritional restriction, perhaps most popularly expounded by Allen [1] from the Rockefeller Institute in New York. However, this was a difficult regimen which did not appear to prolong life expectancy significantly, and when death came it was not clear whether it was the result of diabetes or starvation.

Textbook of Diabetes, 4th edition. Edited by R. Holt, C. Cockram, A. Flyvbjerg and B. Goldstein.

The discovery of insulin

Although there had been previous attempts to identify a pancreatic agent that could control blood sugar, most notably by the

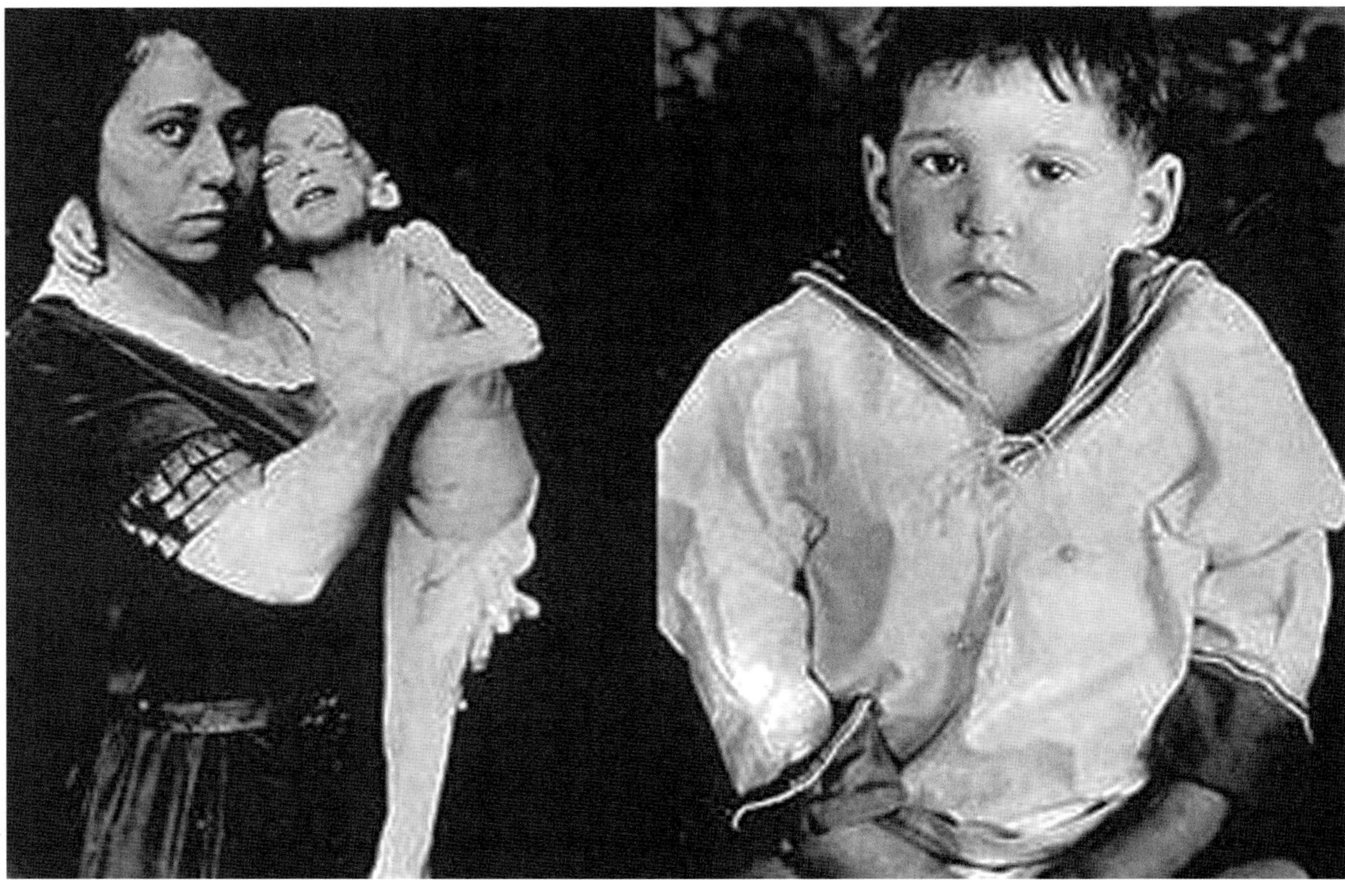

Figure 27.1 A patient with diabetes before and after insulin therapy.

Romanian physiologist Nicolas Paulesco, the story of insulin may be considered to start in the autumn of 1920 when Frederick Grant Banting who, while preparing a lecture on carbohydrate metabolism, considered a way to isolate the internal secretion of the pancreas. By the summer of the next year he had arranged with John Macleod, Professor of Physiology at the University of Toronto, for facilities and the support of a science student Charles Best to start experimentation (Figure 27.2). They showed that tying off the pancreatic ducts induced atrophy of the exocrine glands of the pancreas, thus allowing the "internal" secretions to be isolated. They tested the effect of this internal secretion on blood sugar by injecting it into dogs rendered diabetic through pancreatectomy. With the help of a biochemist, James Collip, they were able to purify this abstract sufficiently for the early experiments on patients. For this work, Banting and Macleod shared the Nobel Prize for Medicine in 1923.

By no means was this discovery a straightforward process, and according to one particularly harsh commentator, "the production of insulin … originated in wrongly conceived, wrongly conducted and wrongly interpreted series of experiments" [2]. The discovery of insulin nevertheless was a defining moment in the history of diabetes and the molecule has gone on to be well studied, with work contributing to three further Nobel Prizes: Frederick Sanger in 1958 for determining its primary amino acid sequence; Dorothy Hodgkin in 1964 for X-crystallographic studies; and Rosalyn Yalow *et al.* in 1977 for contributing to the development of radioimmunoassays.

The first insulins

Commercially available insulin was initially extracted from porcine and bovine pancreata. The organs would be freshly collected from abattoirs and frozen immediately to prevent the enzymatic degradation of the insulin protein. The tissue would undergo acid-ethanol treatment to solubilize insulin, which would then be salted out with sodium chloride, precipitated and then crystallized [3]. This procedure resulted in insulin with a purity of 80–90%, the contaminants largely being pancreatic polypeptides and glucagon. Although this insulin was effective, it was often complicated by immune-mediated side effects, in particular lipoatrophy and antibody-mediated insulin resistance [4], both of which that can profoundly influence the kinetics of insulin action. These impurities also contributed to an allergic

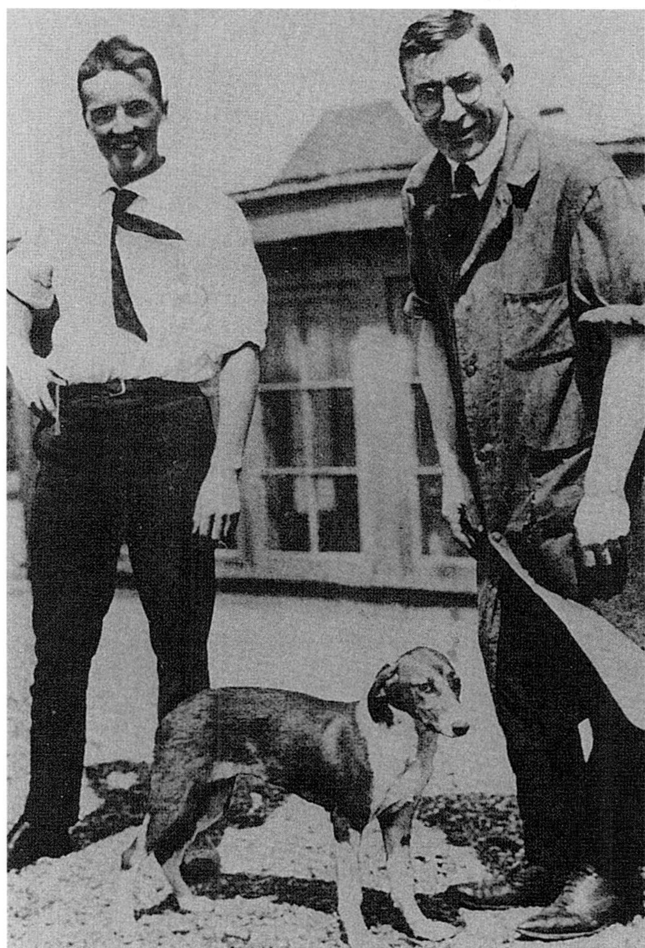

Figure 27.2 Charles Best and Frederick Banting on the roof of the medical building at the University of Toronto, summer 1921.

reaction which sometimes resulted in swelling and pain at the site of injection.

Animal and human insulins

Animal insulin continues to be porcine and bovine derived. The amino acid structure of bovine insulin differs from that of human by three amino acids (position 30 of the B chain, and 8 and 10 of the A chain) and that of porcine from human by just one amino acid (position 30 of the B chain) [5,6]. These differences aside, it was the purity of the insulin preparation that appeared to influence its immunogenicity.

In the 1970s, additional purification steps using gel filtration and ion exchange chromatography resulted in an insulin, called mono-component or single component insulin, with fewer side effects and which was better tolerated (Table 27.1). The incidence of lipoatrophy and allergy decreased as these purer insulins became more widely available. It was a logical step therefore to move on to treatment with human insulin in an effort to further reduce immune-mediated complications and improve glucose control.

Table 27.1 Insulin therapy milestones.

1922	Isolation of insulin and treatment of the first patient
1936	Protamine insulin
1946	NPH isophane insulin
1951	Zinc lente insulin
1959	Biphasic insulin
1977	Continuous subcutaneous insulin infusion
1980	rDNA human insulin in humans
1981	Insulin pens
1987	Monomeric short-acting insulins
1987	Soluble prolonged-action insulin
1996	Rapid-acting insulin analog
2001	Long-acting insulin analogs

Human insulin has been obtained using three techniques. The earliest attempts were to isolate and purify it directly from human cadaveric pancreata. The supply of human tissue, however, was never sufficient to enable this technique to provide sufficient quantities. The technique of "semi-synthesis" chemically converts porcine insulin to the human sequence through the substitution of the one amino acid difference in the primary sequence. It was only in 1980 with the introduction of recombinant DNA technology that human insulin therapy became widely available. The technique involves the insertion of the human DNA sequence into a host cell, usually bakers' yeast or the bacteria *Escherichia coli*, allowing it to synthesize the insulin molecule [7]. The protein would then be purified usually via chromatography columns to achieve a 99.5–99.9% insulin purity. The quality of the human insulin preparation achieved with this technique, as indeed with the purified porcine insulin, has virtually eliminated problems associated with immune-mediated side effects.

Counter to expectations, rigorous and well-designed studies comparing purified animal insulin with recombinant human insulin have yet to demonstrate a significant benefit in glycemic control. A recent meta-analysis of 45 randomized controlled trials involving a total of 2156 participants comparing animal and human insulin failed to show a significant difference between these two therapies [8]. Most (36 of the 45) studies used highly purified porcine insulin, which many believe to be less immunogenic than bovine insulin and this may explain the favorable results for animal insulins. Overall, there is a marked absence of good studies demonstrating a superiority of human over animal insulin with regard to glycemic control. Bovine insulin was associated with a higher titer of anti-insulin antibodies, but these titers did not appear to influence the dose of insulin required, or the level of glycemic control achieved.

The move from animal to human insulin was associated in some patients with reports of greater hypoglycemia, anecdotally brought about by changes in hypoglycemia warnings [9,10], but systematic reviews have failed to substantiate this finding in population studies [8,11].

There has been a large-scale uptake of recombinant human insulin such that less than 7% of global insulin sales are now animal insulin. This shift has probably resulted at least in part, because of the phasing out of animal insulins by the leading insulin manufacturers. Several companies continue to provide this alternate source, and both bovine and porcine-derived insulin remain available. Although cheaper to produce, the price of animal insulins in the UK is structured at a cost comparable to that of recombinant human insulin (£17–18 per 10 mL vial; BNF 2009). This pricing strategy is not the same worldwide; in the developing world for example, the cost of animal insulin is about half that of recombinant human insulin, a factor that may influence the choice of insulin preparation [12].

Soluble and long-acting insulin preparations

The biologic action of soluble insulin lasts about 5–6 hours and the early preparations were often also associated with pain and swelling at the site of injection. Attempts were therefore made in the 1920s and 1930s to provide the patient's daily insulin requirement in just one injection. To this end, modifying agents such as lecithin, oil and cholesterol were used [13]; however, their duration of action varied significantly from injection to injection which made their clinical use very difficult.

In 1936 a method for incorporating insulin into a poorly soluble complex, thus slowing its absorption, was reported [14]. This technique involved the addition of a highly basic protein, protamine, derived from the sperm of salmon or trout. The complex was further stabilized by the addition of a small amount of zinc such that it lasted about 24 hours, and this insulin was called protamine-zinc insulin. It was difficult to make consistent batches and absorption again tended to be erratic. In 1946, the technique was further refined such that protamine and zinc were added in stoichiometric proportions (so that there was no free protamine or zinc), which resulted in a preparation that was absorbed at a more consistent rate and lasted 12–24 hours. This insulin was called isophane or neutral protamine Hagedorn (NPH), and became available clinically in 1940.

In 1951, a development that prolonged the action of insulin without the need for protamine was reported; this required zinc to be added in excess and in acetate buffer, resulting in crystals of relatively insoluble zinc-insulin complexes, called the lente insulins [15]. The size of the crystals could be adjusted by changing the pH such that larger crystals, which were more slowly absorbed (ultralente), and smaller crystals (semilente) could be produced. A preparation containing a 70:30 ratio of the ultralente and semilente insulins (lente insulin) was the most popular form of the zinc insulins and was used widely in clinical practice.

Rapid and long-acting insulin analogs

Insulin circulates as single molecules in the blood at concentrations of approximately 10^{-9} mol/L. At higher concentrations, such as in commercial preparations, insulin molecules tend to associate non-covalently into dimers, tetramers and hexamers [16]. The presence of zinc further stabilizes the hexamer association. Following injection, fluid is drawn into the injected insulin depot through osmosis. This leads to dilution of the insulin and dissociation of the insulin molecules, a spontaneous but gradual process that must occur before insulin can cross the capillary walls as monomers into the blood circulation [17,18]. Patients are therefore advised to inject their soluble insulin 15–20 minutes before a meal so that circulating insulin levels are optimal at the time their meal is being absorbed (Figure 27.3). A significant

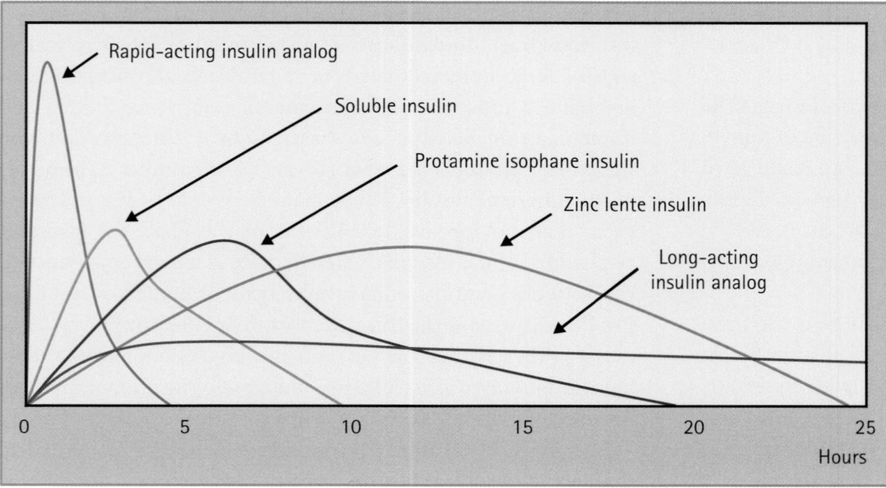

Figure 27.3 Time–action profiles of the different insulin formulations.

proportion of patients find it hard to follow this advice because of the planning required. Even when they do, the calculated doses may be inaccurate, particularly when the preparation of the meal is not under the patient's control.

The association between insulin molecules can be reduced by specific changes to the amino acid sequence of insulin [19]. These changes result in faster absorption of the insulin into the bloodstream, and allow it to be injected just before, or even immediately after eating a meal [20]. To date, three such rapid-acting analogs (RAIs) have become available: insulin lispro (Humalog®, Lilly), insulin aspart (Novorapid®, Novo Nordisk) and insulin glulisine (Apidra®, Sanofi-Aventis). These analogs act more quickly (within 10–20 minutes) and have a shorter duration of action (3–5 hours) than soluble insulin (30–60 minutes, and 6–8 hours, respectively) (Figure 27.3) [21]. A number of studies have now demonstrated the safety of RAIs in both T1DM and type 2 diabetes (T2DM), as part of a "basal bolus" insulin injection regimen combined with intermediate-acting insulins, and in continuous subcutaneous insulin infusion (CSII) [22]. The time–action profile of RAIs is well suited to mimicking the requirement at meal times, and therefore they probably control post-prandial hyperglycemia more effectively than soluble insulin. As a result, patients can achieve better glycemic control with fewer episodes of hypoglycemia with RAIs than with soluble insulin. The benefits of RAI over soluble insulin appears to be clearer in studies involving patients with T1DM than T2DM, and using CSII than for multiple dose injections [21].

Although delayed-action insulin such as insulin lente and isophane can cover the 12–24-hour period, their absorption from subcutaneous tissue can vary significantly [23]. Therefore, attempts at stringent glucose control can be associated with an increased risk of hypoglycemia. The modification of the primary amino acid sequence of the insulin molecule can result in a shift in the isoelectric point towards neutrality (the isoelectric point is that at which the molecule is least soluble). This shift in the isoelectric point therefore encourages insulin to precipitate following injection into the subcutaneous tissue (which is at neutral pH), and results in a slower and, more importantly, a more reproducible absorption [24]. Early studies of the long-acting analog insulins, designed to demonstrate equivalence rather than superiority over the isophane NPH insulins, have failed to show a clear benefit in glycemic control [25]. However, what the studies do appear to show is that achieving glycemic control with the long-acting insulin analogs is associated with less symptomatic and nocturnal hypoglycemia [26].

Reproducing physiologic insulin delivery – the size of the problem

In health, the background insulin secretion is low and stable between meals, with significant prandial surges (Figure 27.4). The stimulus and pattern of insulin secretion is reviewed in Chapter 6, but suffice it to say that the background as well as the prandial

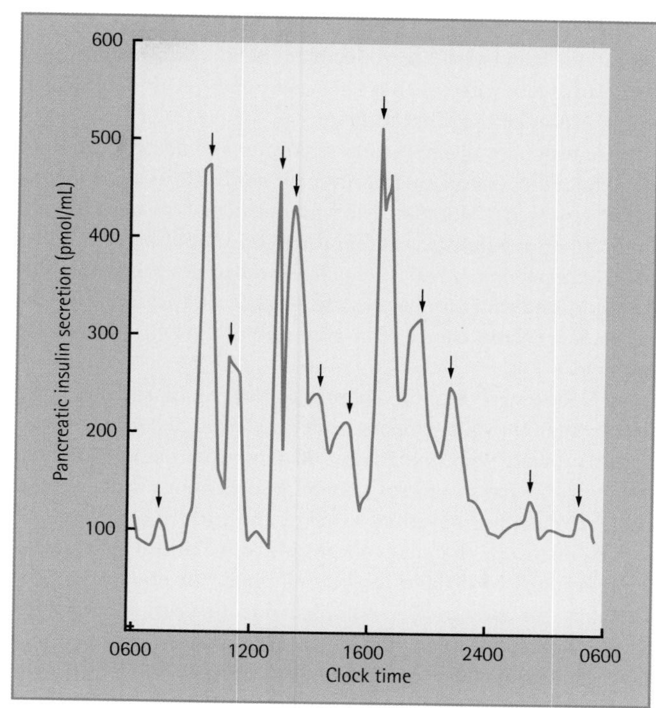

Figure 27.4 Pancreatic insulin secretion in a healthy non-obese individual. Meals were consumed at 0900, 1300 and 1800. Statistically significant pulses of secretion are shown by the arrows. Reproduced from Polonsky *et al.* [27], with permission from the American Society for Clinical Investigation.

insulin secretion can vary significantly within the same individual; the former according to the level of counter-regulatory hormones such as growth hormone and catecholamines, and the latter according to the carbohydrate and protein content of the meal [27].

Furthermore, the insulin is secreted into the portal circulation, with about 50% of the insulin removed in the first pass through the liver [28]. The continuous low levels (15–20 mU/L) of insulin secretion act to suppress hepatic glucose output. Peripheral tissues such as muscle also take up glucose but this is at higher insulin concentrations (60–80 mU/L) and tends to occur predominantly post-prandially.

The challenge of insulin replacement therapy is to reproduce the physiologic insulin profile without incurring significant risk of hypoglycemia.

Routes of insulin administration other than subcutaneous

The early experiments of Frederick Banting quickly revealed that the oral route of insulin administration was not an effective means of delivery, and subsequently that the insulin molecule was functionally degraded by gut peptides. Subcutaneous injection of insulin has become the most popular route of insulin delivery because of its relatively reproducible kinetics of absorption, and the relative ease with which it can be administered, but it is worth visiting some of the other routes.

Intramuscular injection is more painful and absorption more rapid than the subcutaneous route [29] but is useful, for example, in the emergency situation when intravenous access is difficult. Inadvertent intramuscular administration should be considered in the slim patient with diabetes who complains of pain on insulin injection, and who may have erratic glucose control and hypoglycemia. The correct choice of insulin needles can help address this problem.

Intraperitoneal insulin administration is absorbed more quickly than the subcutaneous route and has gained some interest recently for use with implantable insulin pump therapy [30]. An advantage is that the major part of absorbed insulin is into the portal circulation [31], thus reducing the risks of high levels of peripheral insulin that may conceivably contribute to the vascular complications of diabetes and development of obesity [32,33]. Certainly, the early studies of implantable intraperitoneal pumps appear to achieve better glucose control and less hypoglycemia than the subcutaneous route. A longer experience of intraperitoneal insulin delivery has been obtained in patients requiring renal replacement therapy using continuous ambulatory peritoneal dialysis where the insulin is administered along with the dialysis fluid. There are some reports that this route is associated with more consistent absorption and lower peripheral insulin levels; however, there are no robust trials to show that any one route is superior to another [34,35].

The oral administration of insulin is a route by which this drug can enter the portal circulation, thus avoiding high levels of peripheral insulin. There are emerging reports that such an approach may be possible. Techniques such as insulin modification to engender resistance to degradation [36,37] have been reported to increase circulating insulin concentrations effectively and decrease blood glucose in early phase clinical trials.

Subcutaneous route of insulin administration

Subcutaneous insulin administration is the most popular route of insulin therapy and suggested sites for injection are the abdomen, thigh and deltoid. Despite a scarcity of clinical trials on this subject, the current recommendations are that the skin is pinched to reduce the risk of injecting into muscle, and to inject at right angles to the skin, after which the fold should be held for 5–10 seconds before removing the needle (Figure 27.5) [38].

The increasing availability of insulin pens, which are easier to use than the traditional needle and syringe, has seen a shift towards this mode of delivery. A selection of the pen types available from the major insulin manufacturers is shown in Figure 27.6. Currently available needle lengths are 12.7, 8, 6 and 5 mm. There are few if any indications for prescribing the 12.7 mm

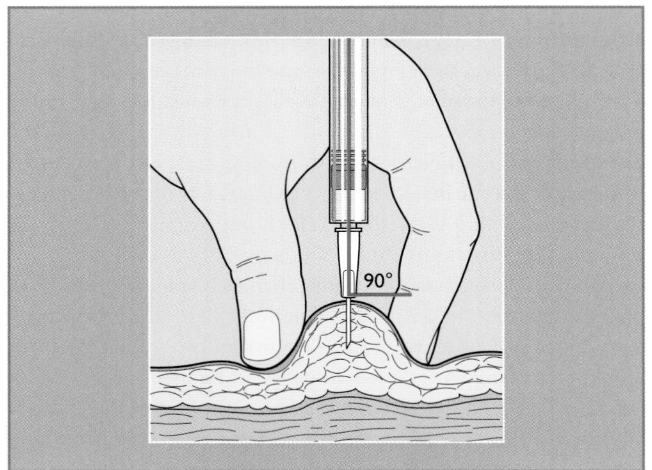

Figure 27.5 The recommended technique for the subcutaneous injection of insulin.

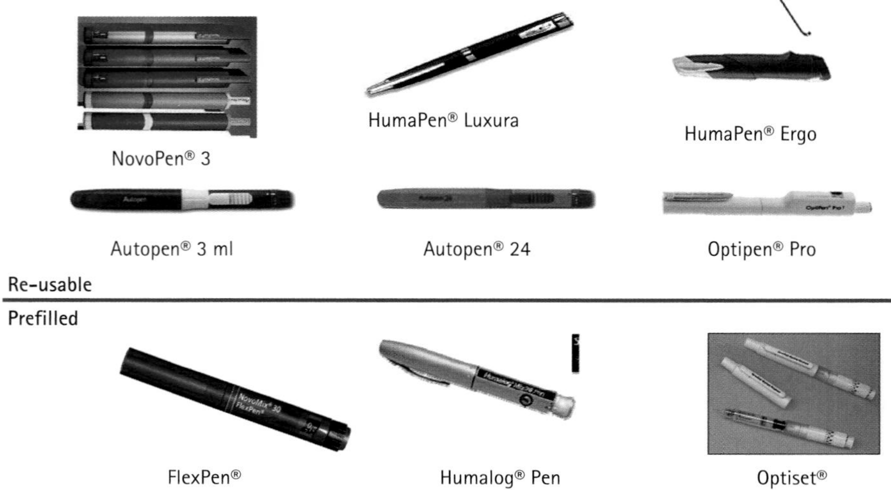

Figure 27.6 A selection of the available insulin injection devices. These are the most commonly used injection devices, although others are also available. Most are available on prescription.

needle, and shorter needles are associated with a lower risk of intramuscular injection and may well be perceived to be less traumatic. Nevertheless, there is some evidence that unless the injection technique is good, the shorter needles are associated with a greater risk of back-leakage of insulin. For a non-obese patient who uses the pinch technique on the abdomen, arm or legs, the 6–8 mm needle is usually the most appropriate.

Standard insulin preparations have a shelf life of 4–6 weeks when stored at under 25°C. Storage for longer periods will require that they be kept in a fridge (4°C), which then allows them to be stored till their expiry date. Exposure of insulin to high temperatures or to microwaves can render them inactive, a technique that may be employed by patients who wish to manipulate their treatment secretly.

Some preparations of delayed-action insulin exist in a two-phase solution which needs to be mixed adequately for complete suspension. It is important that patients are educated on the importance of this to ensure consistent amounts of insulin are drawn up on each occasion [39]. This mixing is not required for the long-acting insulin analogs.

Insulin preparations consist of insulin at or over 40 U/mL, which will exist largely as monomers, dimers or hexamers. Fluid drawn into the injected depot by osmosis following injection results in the dissociation of the oligomers into single molecules which are then able to traverse the capillary membrane and enter the circulation. Circulating insulin binds onto the insulin receptor on the target cell, is internalized and triggers a number of intracellular pathways. This internalization and degradation of insulin is the major route of insulin disposal, with less than 1% excreted by the kidney [40]. Overall, about 60–80% of insulin is degraded in the liver, 10–20% in the kidney and 10–20% in skeletal muscle and fat tissue [41]. Hence, failure of liver or renal function can and does result in the persistence of circulating insulin, with the risk of hypoglycemia.

Studies of absorption of subcutaneously administered insulin have used a variety of techniques including measuring the rate of loss of ^{125}I labeled insulin from the site of injection using a gamma counter [42]. Studies show that the rate can vary significantly between individuals, but also from one injection to another within the same individual [43]. Absorption rates in the obese patient are slower than in the non-obese patient, and there does not appear to be any clear differences in the rate of absorption between the different injection sites. In the non-obese patient, the absorption of soluble insulin from the abdomen appears to be faster than the arm or leg [44], and the upper abdomen faster than the lower abdomen [45]. These differences across injection sites appear to be less apparent with the insulin analogs than with soluble insulin [24,46].

Repeated injection of insulin at the same site results in local hypertrophy of adipose tissue, resulting in slower and more erratic insulin absorption. Patients should always be advised to rotate their insulin injection sites to avoid this complication, but the non-obese patient must also be warned that the rates may vary when they move from one part of the body to the other. Other local factors such as edema or local inflammation can influence rates of absorbtion. Exercise results in greater blood flow to the skin and can result in faster uptake of insulin, particularly when injected into an area close to the muscle groups being exercised; patients who are planning to run, for example, should be advised that injection into the leg may be less favorable than injecting into the arm or abdomen [47]. Similarly, temperature influences cutaneous blood flow and can influence insulin absorption [48]; hot climates or sitting in the sauna may result in a rapid surge in insulin levels whereas the converse, traveling to cooler climates, can result in a slower uptake. There are also reports that hypoglycemia and smoking can reduce the rate of insulin absorption [49,50].

Complications of subcutaneous insulin therapy

The most serious complication of insulin injection for most people is hypoglycemia. The causes, avoidance, consequences and management of hypoglycemia are discussed in Chapter 33. With respect to insulin treatment, the fear of hypoglycemia may be a major barrier to insulin initiation and achievement of tight glycemic control.

Insulin can not only restore fat and muscle mass in newly or suboptimally treated insulin-requiring patients, but can also lead to excessive weight gain [51,52]. This remains a major concern for many patients, particularly for the already overweight patient with T2DM who can no longer be controlled on oral hypoglycemic agents. Weight gain can be reduced by concomitant advice from the dietitian and an insulin regimen tailored to the individual needs of the patient, that wherever possible provides most insulin when needed (i.e. at meal times). Overaggressive insulin titration regimens leading to low blood glucose and stimulation in appetite can lead to excessive weight gain. Some patients, particularly but not exclusively young females, can pose a management challenge when they reduce their insulin dose to suboptimal levels to manipulate body weight (see Chapter 55).

Immune responses to the older animal insulins have been well reported but such responses to current human and analog insulins are extremely uncommon. Allergies may very rarely develop in response to both insulin and agents added to the insulin preparation. Most commonly, but again rarely, local acute urticarial reactions develop and are best treated by switching to an alternative insulin. Occasionally, the urticarial reaction may develop into a subcutaneous nodule. Antihistamines may be of benefit in such patients as too may be the use of high dose steroids in exceptional circumstances.

With the introduction of increasingly purified animal insulins, human insulin and analog insulin, antibodies to exogenous insulin are rare but, when detected, are usually induced by animal insulin products [53], polyclonal in nature, and directed against various parts of the insulin molecule. Clinically, they may lead to local allergic reactions described above and may have a retardant effect on short-acting insulins by reducing peak and raising trough levels. Such effects are likely to be unpredictable. While many clinicians speculate, in difficult to manage patients, over the potential effect of insulin antibodies on blood glucose levels and glycemic control, there is little evidence, outside anecdotal case reports, to substantiate any significant effect.

Lipoatrophy, in which subcutaneous tissue at the site of injection disappears or atrophies, is an allergic response seen predominantly with the older animal insulins; it is rarely seen today. In contrast, lipohypertrophy is not uncommon, is not an allergic response at all but develops as an increase in adipose tissue as a trophic response to insulin. It is most commonly seen in patients with a poor injection technique and usually in patients who do not rotate their insulin injection sites. The patient usually finds the appearance unsightly and further injections into sites of hypertrophy can lead to poor and delayed insulin absorption with consequent effects on blood glucose levels [54]. Lipohypertrophy tends to settle if injections are avoided in that particular area. Occasionally, mild ulceration, pitting and, more commonly, bruising can occur at injection sites. Moving to another area for injection is advisable and, particularly when bruising occurs, a shorter needle may be preferable.

Insulin regimens

As insulin preparations have evolved from the early animal insulins to both human and analog insulins we have also seen the development of more versatile and flexible treatment regimens that enable the doctor and nurse to provide the patient requiring insulin with a bespoke treatment that fits in better with their individual needs and lifestyle.

In people without diabetes it is well known that the β-cells of the pancreas have the ability to produce insulin both between meals and at meal times to maintain blood glucose values within a narrow physiologic range. In people with T1DM, who are no longer producing endogenous insulin, the administration of exogenous insulin is required to try, as far as is possible, to mimic physiologic insulin release using a combination of both fast or rapid-acting insulin to deal with the glucose challenge presented at meal times and more longer acting or basal insulin to provide a background control of glucose between meals. In people with T2DM, the principle is the same although as the β-cells may still be producing some insulin, the addition of exogenous insulin to existing oral hypoglycemic agents can be used to try to achieve control of blood glucose levels.

We discuss how each of the individual insulins discussed above can be used, alone or more often in combination, in conjunction with lifestyle and diet to control blood glucose.

Basal only regimen

In excess of 50% of people with T2DM will require insulin injections at some point in their lives [55]. Often, as T2DM progresses, the transition from oral hypoglycemic agents to insulin injections can be a time of great stress and anxiety to many people for a number of related reasons [56]. While health care professionals employ a variety of skills and techniques to minimize what people see as a life-changing event, we remain very aware of the many anxieties insulin injections can induce. These can include a sense of personal failure in not being able to control blood glucose levels with lifestyle, diet and oral therapy; a feeling that the diabetes is now much more serious than it was, as it now requires injections rather than tablets; apprehensions, fears and, very occasionally, real phobias over the need to self-inject a treatment [56]; worries of hypoglycemia leading to coma and death; concerns over weight gain; and also that the use of insulin may impact severely on a patient's occupation and lifestyle activities.

One way in which insulin injections can be introduced to people no longer able to manage their blood glucose on diet, lifestyle and oral therapy alone is to start with only one injection a day. This is usually added on to existing oral therapies rather than as a replacement therapy. An increasing number of studies have now been published demonstrating that a once a day basal insulin can be used as an add-on therapy to metformin, a sulfonylurea, the thiazolidinedione pioglitazone and as an add-on to these agents when used as a dual or triple oral therapy [57]. National and international guidelines in the UK, Europe and the USA also recommend the use of a basal insulin with oral therapy as a way of initiating insulin in patients with T2DM [58–60]. At the time of writing, some of the newer agents including the dipeptidyl peptidase 4 (DPP-4) inhibitors and the glucagon-like peptide 1 (GLP-1) receptor agonists do not have a license for use with insulin therapy in people with T2DM although trials are ongoing and this may change.

The initiation of insulin therapy, whether in the hospital or, more commonly, in the community, should only take place within a structured program employing active insulin dose titration. The program should include appropriate education, ongoing telephone, text and/or email support, the use of blood glucose self-monitoring to help with dose titration to an agreed target, an understanding of diet, avoidance and management of hypoglycemia and support from appropriately trained and experienced health care professionals.

A number of guidelines continue to recommend initiation with a human NPH insulin taken once or twice a day according to need [60]. However, many health care professionals opt for long-acting insulin analogs particularly in people who require assistance with injections from a carer or health care professional and where the use of an analog would reduce the number of injections from twice to once a day. Long-acting analog insulins may also be preferred in people whose lifestyle is restricted by recurrent symptomatic hypoglycemia, those who would otherwise need twice daily insulin injections in combination with oral therapy and those who have difficulties with the device required for injection of NPH insulin [57]. Similarly, indications for switching from NPH insulin to a long-acting basal analog include failure to reach an agreed HbA_{1c} target because of hypoglycemia regardless of HbA_{1c}.

Once started on a basal insulin it is important to adjust insulin doses appropriately to achieve an agreed target. A number of algorithms have been developed to assist with this with almost all based upon the fasting blood glucose measured in the patient's home and usually by patient themselves [57,61,62]. While self monitoring of blood glucose is important in the dose titration process, the ultimate measure that determines the success or otherwise of the basal insulin is the HbA_{1c} value. If this is proving difficult to control with satisfactory fasting plasma glucose values, the next step would be to add a prandial fast or rapid-acting insulin component.

Combinations of prandial and basal insulins

In patients with T2DM, a rising HbA_{1c} in the face of normal or near-normal fasting glucose values suggests significant post-prandial glucose excursions and the need for a meal time insulin. This can be achieved by the addition of a prandial insulin with the main meal followed as needed by the addition of a prandial insulin before every meal [57]. Alternatively, patients can be switched from a basal insulin to a premixed insulin which traditionally has been given twice daily, at breakfast and the evening meal, but which increasingly is also given initially once a day with the main meal and increased up to three times a day [59,63].

Clearly, for patients with T1DM, a basal insulin alone is inadequate and either a complete basal bolus regimen is required with prandial insulin before each meal alongside a basal insulin or alternatively a twice or thrice daily insulin premix can be used.

Basal plus

The addition of a fast-acting human insulin or rapid-acting analog insulin prior to the main meal of the day can be a useful next step in intensification after starting a basal insulin in patients with T2DM [59,64]. Increasingly, health care professionals are using rapid-acting insulin analogs over fast-acting human insulins for convenience, as they can be given immediately before, during and even immediately after a meal [65–67]. The dietary intake of the individual will determine which the main meal of the day is and therefore with which meal the single injection of fast- or rapid-acting insulin will be given. Once again it is important to titrate the prandial insulin to a glucose target. The ideal time to test the impact of the prandial insulin, and certainly a rapid-acting insulin analog, is 90 minutes to 2 hours after the meal. As with basal insulin adjustment it is advisable not to make too frequent a change in insulin dosage and ideally no less than every 3 days or no more than twice a week. The patient may vary the amount of insulin administered based upon the size of the meal, although as the insulin is given with the main meal of the day, the dose is usually fairly stable from one day to another. As glycemic control becomes more difficult to achieve a second prandial insulin injection may be necessary, taken before the second main meal of the day using a similar dose titration procedure as that for the single prandial injection [64].

Basal bolus

The use of the basal bolus regimen in patients with T1DM and T2DM attempts to mimick, as closely as possible, the normal physiologic secretion of insulin by providing a background 24-hour coverage of insulin along with a bolus injection at each meal time (Figure 27.7). In most patients, with the development of long-acting analog insulins, the basal injection is administered once a day. However, based on the results of pre-meal self-monitored blood glucose values some patients may require two basal injections approximately 12 hours apart to achieve satisfactory before meal glucose values without hypoglycemia.

Traditionally, with animal and then human insulins, basal injections are given in the evening, often before bed. This is less important with the basal analog insulins and indeed many patients benefit from having their once a day basal injection at the same time each morning. It is important that insulin doses are adequately titrated to achieve target glucose and HbA_{1c} values and for the basal bolus regimen the dose of the basal insulin is determined by measurement of fasting (pre-meal) glucose values and the most appropriate fast human or rapid-acting analog insulin dose is best determined by 2 hour post-prandial glucose values.

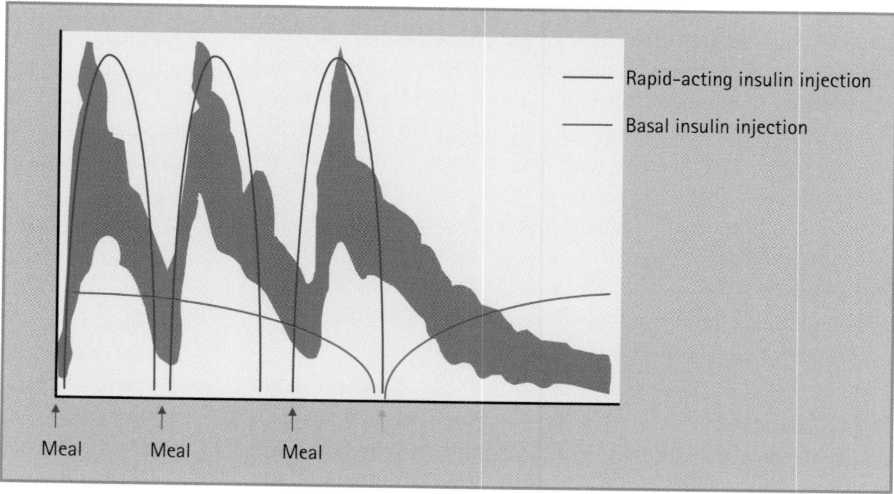

Figure 27.7 Schematic representation of the attempt to mimic physiologic insulin release following three main meals using a basal bolus regimen.

Insulin mixtures

While some patients still self-mix either animal or human fast-acting and long-acting insulins prior to injection, most people using insulin mixes inject premixed insulin preparations. In recent years, we have seen a whole spectrum of insulin premix insulins ranging from a 10:90 to 50:50 short:long-acting insulin ratios. In reality, many of these premixes were not required and consequently through lack of use the range of premixes has contracted down to 25:75, 30:70 and 50:50 mixes.

Most patients use premixed insulin twice a day, before breakfast and the evening meal. In people with T2DM, insulin initiation may start with a once a day premix insulin with the main meal, increasing up to two injections a day when needed based on self-monitored blood glucose values and the HbA_{1c} [59,64]. Some patients with T1DM, but more frequently patients with T2DM, move to three injections a day by also administering an injection before lunch. For patients moving up to three injections a day, the 50:50 mixture providing more rapid-acting insulin at meal times may be more appropriate than the more commonly used 25:75 or 30:70 mixture, usually given twice a day.

Selecting the most appropriate insulin regimen

Most people with T1DM and T2DM try a number of treatment regimens throughout their lives. There are many factors that influence the decision to opt for a specific regimen and ultimately the most important is patient choice rather than evidence from clinical trials.

Type 1 diabetes

All patients with T1DM, unless they have been fortunate enough to become insulin independent following a pancreas or islet cell transplant, will require exogenous insulin to provide 24-hour background and meal time coverage. For many patients this is provided by the basal bolus regimen. The advantages of such an approach are that it is generally better at providing a more physiologic insulin replacement with a greater degree of 24-hour flexibility than less frequent premixed insulin. While it has the disadvantage of more daily insulin injections and for many more frequent self blood glucose monitoring, which is not popular with some patients, particularly young and teenage children, it does provide a much greater degree of flexibility throughout the day. Importantly, it allows the patient to vary the meal time dose at up to three different time points during the day to accommodate different daily activities and meal sizes. For some, this "freedom" is less important and the administration of only two injections a day sways them towards an insulin premix.

Type 2 diabetes

While in some patients with T2DM insulin requirements are similar to those with T1DM, for many, insulin initiation and intensification is a more gradual process. Views differ on the insulin of choice for initiation, particularly as an add-on to oral hypoglycemic therapy. Prior to the introduction of the long-acting basal analogs, many patients requiring insulin were started on a twice a day premixed insulin often as an add-on to metformin. If patients were also on a sulfonylurea this was usually stopped. Supported by clinical trials, using long-acting basal analogs as an add-on to existing oral therapy and low rates of hypoglycemia compared to those seen with NPH insulin, once a day long-acting basal insulins are now recommended in T2DM treatment guidelines and have found significant popularity, particularly in the community as a means of introducing the patient to insulin [57,61]. Anecdotally, while this is a popular way of starting insulin, many health care professionals struggle to achieve satisfactory glycemic targets with this regimen and many patients will require a second insulin injection with a meal time component within 6–12 months.

Trials comparing twice daily premixed insulins with a long-acting basal analog when added to metformin in insulin-naïve patients appear to show a benefit in favor of twice daily premixed insulin with respect to the numbers of patients achieving target HbA_{1c} values [68,69]. The relative merits of basal only, prandial only and premixed insulin are unclear [70] and are currently being further evaluated [71]. Clearly, there are advantages and disadvantages associated with each approach. A pragmatic response is to consider each patient individually and their lifestyle, social circumstances and co-morbidities and taking into account what their insulin needs are likely to be in the longer term to make a clinical judgment. If it seems likely that if started on a basal insulin they are likely to remain on this as a single injection or as part of a basal bolus regimen in the future, the basal insulin may be the best option. However, if it seems likely that the patient will be switched to a premixed insulin if a long-acting bolus does not achieve target, then initiating with a premixed insulin would seem sensible. Starting the premixed insulin as a once a day injection increasing to two and sometimes three injections is also an option with some clinical evidence to support it.

Starting insulin for the first time

In the past, insulin initiation, particularly for people with T1DM, was conducted either as an inpatient or as a day case in a hospital diabetes center. As confidence grows with the development of purer animal insulins and most recently with human and analog insulins and also with the introduction of disposable syringes, pen injectors and needles, more insulin initiations are performed on an outpatient basis. Most recently, with an increased emphasis on community-based diabetes care, insulin initiation, particularly in patients with T2DM, is taking place in health centers and GP surgeries [72]. While older algorithms for helping to decide when and where insulin should be initiated have been published, national and local guidelines now seem more appropriate as varying levels of expertise, infrastructure and service delivery are present in different health settings.

Table 27.2 Outpatient/community pathway for people starting insulin for the first time.

Session 1
- The need for insulin has already been discussed with the patient by a doctor or diabetes nurse specialist and patient has been seen by a dietitian
- A regimen will have been agreed upon and the first prescription has been obtained by the patient
- A review of "what is diabetes" including what insulin does and the need for insulin injections usually takes place
- Nurse demonstrates the basics and use of insulin injection device and patient gives first injection
- Further discussions including:
  (i) sites for injection/site rotation
  (ii) timing of injections
  (iii) where and how to obtain equipment (insulin, pens, needles, self blood glucose monitoring equipment, sharps disposal equipment)
  (iv) recognition and management hypoglycemia and hyperglycemia
  (v) self blood glucose monitoring
  (vi) driving and legal issues surrounding insulin
- 24-hour contact details provided

Session 2 (around 2 weeks after insulin initiation)
- Prior to session 2 patient and nurse will usually have had telephone contact over insulin injections and blood glucose readings
- Review of information provided in session 1
- Review of insulin injection technique

Session 3 (around 4 weeks after insulin initiation)
- Review of session 1 and 2
- Further information provided about:
  (i) insulin on holiday and when traveling
  (ii) insulin injections when traveling through time zones (e.g. transatlantic travel)
  (iii) insulin management during periods of acute sickness
  (iv) foot care, other diabetes-related complications and in females of childbearing age, pregnancy

Session 4 (around 10 weeks after insulin initiation)
- Review of previous sessions
- Assessment of glycemic control and need for further doctor/nurse follow-up
- Book follow-up clinic/surgery appointment

Wherever insulin is initiated it is vital that for it to be successful a good insulin initiation program is in place, with a qualified and competent diabetes nurse specialist. A number of programs are available, most with appropriate training courses for health care professionals. Insulin initiation involves much more than teaching a patient how to use a needle and syringe and the process of starting and successfully stabilizing a patient on insulin will require a number of structured contacts with the nurse and also a 24-hour emergency contact number for any urgent problems that may arise (Table 27.2).

For those patients presenting acutely ill with nausea and vomiting, with or without ketosis, admission to hospital for insulin initiation and, where needed, intravenous fluids, is a necessity.

Use of animal, human and analog insulins

The evolution from animal to human and then analog insulins has been discussed at the start of this chapter. We have subsequently outlined above some of the advice included in national guidelines regarding the use of human and analog insulin. In clinical practice all three types of insulin are in regular use. At the present time, patients wishing to stay on animal insulin should, wherever possible, be allowed to do so. There are also advantages associated with the use of the analog insulins although generally they are more expensive to prescribe than human insulin and concerns have been raised over cost–benefit when prescribed routinely. While some of the individual benefits appear small, collectively these benefits are likely to have an impact on many patients [65]. While those responsible for health care budgets seek persuasive clinical trial data it is most unlikely that we will ever see direct head to head studies that provide incontrovertible data one way or another. Ultimately, it will come down to clinical judgment and a decision involving the patient.

Assessments of glycemic control

While national and international guidelines have made recommendations on glycemic targets based predominantly on the HbA_{1c} [58–60,73], self-monitoring of blood glucose not only helps patients achieve HbA_{1c} targets by adjustment of insulin doses, but also helps patients better understand their own diabetes and blood sugar levels better. The timing of glucose tests and their role in determining the most appropriate insulin dose is discussed above and is disscussed in greater detail in Chapter 25. Generally speaking, patients should be advised to test at different times on different days including pre-meal and 2 hours postprandial testing to obtain 24-hour glucose profiles over a number of days rather than performing a large number of tests every day. To achieve strict glycemic control, as seen in the T1DM DCCT [52], pre-meal blood sugar readings should fall between 4 and 7 mmol/L and post-meal levels from 4–10 mmol/L, with a value >7 mmol/L before bed. While individual specialists often follow their own dose adjustment algorithms, in general terms a change in dose of 2 units or 10% of a dose (whichever is the greater) is a sensible adjustment for most patients.

Similar targets may be sought for people with T2DM although recent trials based on achieving very tight HbA_{1c} values, with some aiming for <6%, serve to highlight the dangers of hypoglycemia [74]. The frequency of blood glucose testing is extremely variable, with patients being recommended to test anything from seven times a day to four or five tests a week. The most important aspect of regular self-monitoring by patients on insulin is that the test result should be used as part of a management plan to help decide prospectively on insulin dose. There are other points that should be considered when advising on the timing of self-testing, including intercurrent illness, symptoms and treatment of hypoglycemia, and foreign travel. While more frequent testing generally provides more information, it is also important to remember not to recommend unnecessary and costly testing as pricking the finger is painful and for most patients is worse that injecting insulin.

References

1 Allen FM. *Total Dietary Regulation in the Treatment of Diabetes*. 1919.
2 Roberts F. Letter. *Br Med J* 1922 [from *The Discovery of Insulin* by Michael Bliss].
3 Jorgensen KH, Brange J, Hallund O, Pingel M. A method for the preparation of essentially pure insulin. In: Rodriguez RR, Eblin FJG, Henderson I, Assan R, eds. *VII Congress of the International Diabetes Federation*. Amsterdam: Excerpta Medica, Int. Congress Series 1970; **209**:149 (Abstract 334).
4 Schlichtkrull J, Brange J, Christiansen AH, Hllund O, Heding LG, Jorgensen KH. Clinical aspects of insulin antigenicity. *Diabetes* 1972; **21**(Suppl. 2):649–656.
5 Brogden RN, Heel RC. Human insulin: a review of its biological activity, pharmacokinetics and therapeutic use. *Drugs* 1987; **34**:350–371.
6 Heinemann L, Richter B. Clinical pharmacology of human insulin. *Diabetes Care* 1993; **16**(Suppl. 3):90–100.
7 Chien YW. Human insulin: basic sciences to therapeutic uses. *Drug Dev Ind Pharm* 1996; **22**:753–789.
8 Richter B, Neises G. "Human" insulin versus animal insulin in people with diabetes mellitus. *Cochrane Database Syst Rev* 2005; **1**:CD003816.
9 Berger W, Keller U, Honegger B, Jaeggi E. Warning symptoms of hypoglycaemia during treatment with human and porcine insulin in diabetes mellitus. *Lancet* 1989; **1**:1041–1044.
10 Teuscher A, Berger WG. Hypoglycaemia unawareness in diabetics transferred from beef/porcine insulin to human insulin. *Lancet* 1987; **2**:382–385.
11 Airey CM, William DR, Martin PG, Bennett CM, Spoor PA. Hypoglycaemia induced by exogeneous insulin: "human" and animal insulin compared. *Diabet Med* 2000; **17**:416–432.
12 Yadav S, Parakh A. Insulin therapy. *Indian Pediatrics* 2006; **43**:863–872.
13 Bauman L. Clinical experience with globulin insulin. *Proc Soc Exp Biol Med* 1939; **40**:170–171.
14 Hagedorn HC, Jensen BN, Krarup NB, Woodstrup I. Protamin insulinate. *JAMA* 1936; **106**:177–180.
15 Hallas-Moller K, Peterson K, Schlichtkrull J. Crystalline and amorphous insulin-zinc compounds with prolonged action [in Danish]. *Ugeskr Laeger* 1951; **113**:1761–1767.
16 Søeborg T, Rasmussen CH, Mosekilde E, Colding-Jørgensen M. Absorption kinetics of insulin after subcutaneous administration. *Eur J Pharm Sci* 2009; **36**:78–90.
17 Brange J, Owens DR, Kang S, Volund A. Monomeric insulins and their experimental and clinical implications. *Diabetes Care* 1990; **13**:923–954.
18 Kang S, Brange J, Burch A, Volund A, Owens DR. Subcutaneous insulin absorption explained by insulin's physiochemical properties. *Diabetes Care* 1991; **14**:942–948.
19 Heinemann L, Heise T, Jorgensen LN, Starke AA. Action profile of the rapid acting insulin analogue: human insulin B28Asp. *Diabet Med* 1993; **10**:535–539.
20 Howey DC, Bowsher RR, Brunelle RL, Woodworth JR. [Lys(B28), Pro(B29)]-human insulin: a rapidly absorbed analogue of human insulin. *Diabetes* 1994; **43**:396–402.
21 Hirsch IB. Insulin analogues. *N Engl J Med* 2005; **352**:174–183.
22 Bode BW. Use of rapid-acting insulin analogues in the treatment of patients with type 1 and type 2 diabetes mellitus: insulin pump therapy versus multiple daily injections. *Clin Ther* 2007; **29**(Suppl D):S135–144.
23 Binder C, Lauritzen T, Faber O, Pramming S. Insulin pharmacokinetics. *Diabetes Care* 1984; **7**:188–199.
24 Owens DR, Coates PA, Luzio SD, Tinbergen JP, Kurzhals R. Pharmacokinetics of ^{125}I-labeled insulin glargine (HOE 901) in healthy men: comparison with NPH insulin and the influence of different subcutaneous injection sites. *Diabetes Care* 2000; **23**:813–819.
25 Horvath K, Jeitler K, Berghold A, Ebrahim SH, Gratzer TW, Plank J, *et al.* Long-acting insulin analogues versus NPH insulin (human isophane insulin) for type 2 diabetes mellitus. *Cochrane Database Syst Rev* 2007; **2**.
26 Monami M, Marchionni N, Mannucci E. Long-acting insulin analogues versus NPH human insulin in type 2 diabetes: a meta-analysis. *Diabetes Res Clin Pract* 2008; **81**:184–189.
27 Polonsky KS, Given BD, Van Cauter E. Twenty-four-hour profiles and pulsatile patterns of insulin secretion in normal and obese subjects. *J Clin Invest* 1988; **81**:442–448.
28 Duckworth WC, Bennett RG, Hamel FG. Insulin degradation: progress and potential. *Endocr Rev* 1998; **19**:608–612.
29 Vaag A, Handberg A, Lauritzen M, Henriksen JE, Pedersen KD, Beck-Nielsen H. Variation in absorption of NPH insulin due to intramuscular injection. *Diabetes Care* 1990; **13**:74.
30 Selam JL. External and implantable insulin pumps: current place in the treatment of diabetes. *Exp Clin Endocrinol Diabetes* 2001; **109**(Suppl 2):S333–340.
31 Duckworth WC, Saudek CD, Henry RR. Why intraperitoneal delivery of insulin with implantable pumps in NIDDM? *Diabetes* 1992; **41**:657–661.
32 Henry RR, Gumbiner B, Ditzler T, Wallace P, Lyon R, Glauber HS. Intensive conventional insulin therapy for type II diabetes: metabolic effects during a 6-mo outpatient trial. *Diabetes Care* 1993; **16**:21–31.
33 Feskens EJ, Kromhout D. Hyperinsulinemia, risk factors, and coronary heart disease. The Zutphen Elderly Study. *Arterioscler Thromb* 1994; **14**:1641–1647.
34 Chan E, Montgomery PA. Administration of insulin by continuous ambulatory peritoneal dialysis. *Pharmacotherapy* 1993; **13**:455–460.
35 Quellhorst E. Insulin therapy during peritoneal dialysis: pros and cons of various forms of administration. *J Am Soc Nephrol* 2002; **13**(Suppl 1):S92–96.
36 Kipnes M, Dandona P, Tripathy D, Still JG, Kosutic G. Control of postprandial plasma glucose by an oral insulin product (HIM2) in patients with type 2 diabetes. *Diabetes Care* 2003; **26**:421–426.
37 Silva CM, Ribeiro AJ, Ferreira D, Veiga F. Insulin encapsulation in reinforced alginate microspheres prepared by internal gelation. *Eur J Pharm Sci* 2006; **29**:148–159.
38 Strauss K. Insulin injection techniques. *Pract Diabetes Int* 1998; **15**:181–184.
39 Jehle PM, Micheler C, Jehle DR, Breitig D, Boehm BO. Inadequate suspension of neutral protamine Hagendorn (NPH) insulin in pens. *Lancet* 1999; **354**:1604–1607.
40 Rubenstein AH, Spitz I. Role of the kidney in insulin metabolism and excretion. *Diabetes* 1968; **17**:161–169.
41 Duckworth WC. Insulin degradation: mechanisms, products, and significance. *Endocr Rev* 1988; **9**:319–314.
42 Binder C. Absorption of injected insulin: a clinical pharmacological study. *Acta Pharmacol Toxicol (Copenh)* 1969; **27**(Suppl 2):1–84.

43 Binder C, Lauritzen T, Faber O, Pramming S. Insulin pharmacokinetics. *Diabetes Care* 1984; **7**:188–199.

44 Koivisto VA, Felig P. Alterations in insulin absorption and in blood glucose control associated with varying insulin injection sites in diabetic patients. *Ann Intern Med* 1980; **92**:59–61.

45 Frid A, Linde B. Intraregional differences in the absorption of unmodified insulin from the abdominal wall. *Diabet Med* 1992; **9**:236–239.

46 ter Braak EW, Woodworth JR, Bianchi R, Cerimele B, Erkelens DW, Thijssen JH, *et al.* Injection site effects on the pharmacokinetics and glucodynamics of insulin lispro and regular insulin. *Diabetes Care* 1996; **19**:1437–1440.

47 Koivisto VA, Felig P. Effects of leg exercise on insulin absorption in diabetic patients. *N Engl J Med* 1978; **298**:79–83.

48 Rönnemaa T, Koivisto VA. Combined effect of exercise and ambient temperature on insulin absorption and postprandial glycemia in type I patients. *Diabetes Care* 1988; **11**:769–773.

49 Fernqvist-Forbes E, Gunnarsson R, Linde B. Insulin-induced hypoglycaemia and absorption of injected insulin in diabetic patients. *Diabet Med* 1989; **6**:621–626.

50 Klemp P, Staberg B, Madsbad S, Kølendorf K. Smoking reduces insulin absorption from subcutaneous tissue. *Br Med J (Clin Res Ed)* 1982; **284**:237.

51 Wing RR, Klein R, Moss SE. Weight gain associated with improved glycemic control in population-based sample of subjects with type I diabetes. *Diabetes Care* 1990; **13**:1106–1109.

52 Diabetes Control and Complications Trial Research Group. The effect of intensive treatment of diabetes on the development and progression of long-term complications in insulin-dependent diabetes mellitus. *N Engl J Med* 1993; **329**:977–986.

53 Ratner RE, Phillips TM, Steiner M. Persistent cutaneous insulin allergy resulting from high-molecular-weight insulin aggregates. *Diabetes* 1990; **39**:728–733.

54 Young RJ, Hannan WJ, Frier BM, Steel JM, Duncan LJ. Diabetic lipohypertrophy delays insulin absorption. *Diabetes Care* 1984; **7**:479–480.

55 Mayfield JA, White RD. Insulin therapy for type 2 diabetes: rescue, augmentation, and replacement of beta-cell function. *Am Fam Physician* 2004; **70**:489–500.

56 Peyrot M, Rubin RR, Lauritzen T, Skovlund SE, Snoek FJ, Matthews DR, *et al.* The International DAWN Advisory Panel. Resistance to insulin therapy among patients and providers: results of the cross-national Diabetes Attitudes, Wishes, and Needs (DAWN) study. *Diabetes Care* 2005; **28**:2673–2679.

57 Raccah D, Bretzel RG, Owens D, Riddle M. When basal insulin therapy in type 2 diabetes mellitus is not enough: what next? *Diabetes Metab Res Rev* 2007; **23**:257–264.

58 Nathan DM, Buse JB, Davidson MB, Heine RJ, Holman RR, Sherwin R, *et al.* Management of hyperglycemia in type 2 diabetes. A consensus algorithm for the initiation and adjustment of therapy: a consensus statement from the American Diabetes Association and the European Association for the Study of Diabetes. *Diabetes Care* 2006; **29**:1963–1972.

59 Rodbard HW, Blonde L, Braithwaite SS, Brett EM, Cobin RH, Handelsman Y, *et al.* AACE Diabetes Mellitus Clinical Practice Guidelines Task Force. American Association of Clinical Endocrinologists medical guidelines for clinical practice for the management of diabetes mellitus. *Endocr Pract* 2007; **13**(Suppl 1):1–68.

60 National Collaborating Centre for Chronic Conditions. *Type 2 diabetes: national clinical guideline management in primary and secondary care (update)*. London: Royal College of Physicians, 2008.

61 Riddle MC, Rosenstock J, Gerich J; Insulin Glargine 4002 Study Investigators. The treat-to-target trial: randomized addition of glargine or human NPH insulin to oral therapy of type 2 diabetic patients. *Diabetes Care* 2003; **26**:3080–3086.

62 Davies M, Khunti K. Insulin management in overweight or obese type 2 diabetes patients: the role of insulin glargine. *Diabetes Obes Metab* 2008; **10**(Suppl 2):42–49.

63 Liebl A, Prager R, Binz K, Kaiser M, Bergenstal R, Gallwitz B; PREFER Study Group. Comparison of insulin analogue regimens in people with type 2 diabetes mellitus in the PREFER Study: a randomized controlled trial. *Diabetes Obes Metab* 2009; **11**:45–52.

64 Garber AJ, Wahlen J, Wahl T, Bressler P, Braceras R, Allen E, *et al.* Attainment of glycaemic goals in type 2 diabetes with once-, twice-, or thrice-daily dosing with biphasic insulin aspart 70/30 (The 1-2-3 study). *Diabetes Obes Metab* 2006; **8**:58–66.

65 Gough SC. A review of human and analogue insulin trials. *Diabetes Res Clin Pract* 2007; **77**:1–15.

66 Mannucci E, Monami M, Marchionni N. Short-acting insulin analogues vs. regular human insulin in type 2 diabetes: a meta-analysis. *Diabetes Obes Metab.* 2009; **11**:53–59.

67 Monami M, Marchionni N, Mannucci E. Long-acting insulin analogues vs. NPH human insulin in type 1 diabetes: meta-analysis. *Diabetes Obes Metab* 2009; **11**:372–378.

68 Raskin P, Allen E, Hollander P, Lewin A, Gabbay RA, Hu P, *et al.* INITIATE Study Group. Initiating insulin therapy in type 2 diabetes: a comparison of biphasic and basal insulin analogs. *Diabetes Care* 2005; **28**:260–265.

69 Malone JK, Kerr LF, Campaigne BN, Sachson RA, Holcombe JH; Lispro Mixture-Glargine Study Group. Combined therapy with insulin lispro mix 75/25 plus metformin or insulin glargine plus metformin: a 16-week, randomized, open-label, crossover study in patients with type 2 diabetes beginning insulin therapy. *Clin Ther* 2004; **26**:2034–2044. [Erratum in: *Clin Ther* 2005; 27:1112.]

70 Bretzel RG, Nuber U, Landgraf W, Owens DR, Bradley C, Linn T. Once-daily basal insulin glargine versus thrice-daily prandial insulin lispro in people with type 2 diabetes on oral hypoglycaemic agents (APOLLO): an open randomised controlled trial. *Lancet* 2008; **371**:1073–1084.

71 Holman RR, Thorne KI, Farmer AJ, Davies MJ, Keenan JF, Paul S, *et al.* 4-T Study Group. Addition of biphasic, prandial, or basal insulin to oral therapy in type 2 diabetes. *N Engl J Med* 2007; **357**:1716–1730.

72 Ligthelm R, Davidson J. Initiating insulin in primary care: the role of modern premixed formulations. *Prim Care Diabetes* 2008; **2**:9–16.

73 National Collaborating Centre for Chronic Conditions. *Type 1 diabetes in adults: national clinical guideline for diagnosis and management.* London: Royal College of Physicians, 2004.

74 Dluhy RG, McMahon GT. Intensive glycemic control in the ACCORD and ADVANCE trials. *N Engl J Med* 2008; **358**:2630–2633.

28 New Technologies for Insulin Administration and Glucose Monitoring

Howard Wolpert & Judy Shih
Joslin Diabetes Center, Boston, MA, USA

Keypoints

- Continuous subcutaneous insulin infusion pumps and continuous glucose monitors can be effective tools for improving metabolic control in patients with type 1 diabetes.
- Pump therapy provides increased lifestyle flexibility, and can reduce the risk for hypoglycemia.
- Real-time continuous glucose monitoring devices provide detailed information on glucose patterns and trends, and alarms that are triggered by both hyperglycemia and hypoglycemia.
- Randomized trials indicate that this technology can lead to a reduction in HbA_{1c} without an associated increase in hypoglycemia.

Introduction

The development of capillary blood glucose monitors set the stage for the era of intensive insulin therapy, and technologic advances continue to be an important driver for improvements in diabetes care. In this chapter we highlight the developments of the past decade focusing on those technologies that show the most promise in improving the lives of people with diabetes, in particular, insulin pump therapy and real-time continuous glucose monitoring. In recent years, inhaled insulin has been an area of intense investigation; however, interest in this mode of insulin delivery has been diminished by concerns about potential pulmonary toxicity.

Continuous subcutaneous insulin infusion pumps

Continuous subcutaneous insulin infusion (CSII) pumps were first introduced over 30 years ago [1,2]. They consist of an insulin reservoir and a delivery catheter that continuously infuses insulin into the subcutaneous tissue. In recent years, there has been growing adoption of this technology in diabetes care. Several factors have contributed to this increased use, including the focus on intensive therapy triggered by the Diabetes Control and Complications Trial (DCCT); improvements in the reliability and usability of pumps; patient preferences; and also the growing recognition by clinicians that CSII delivery is associated with reduced risk for hypoglycemia. Because a comprehensive review of insulin pump therapy is beyond the scope of this chapter, we focus on issues that have received most attention in the recent literature, including the potential advantages of pumps as a tool for insulin administration and newer developments in pump technology such as bolus calculator software. In addition, we provide some practical pointers about pump therapy for the clinician.

Glycemic control with insulin pumps compared with multiple daily insulin injections

Several published meta-analyses have examined the role of CSII pumps as a tool for intensifying glycemic control [3–5]. These meta-analyses of the randomized controlled trials in the published literature indicate that CSII use in patients with type 1 diabetes mellitus (T1DM) is associated with 0.4–0.5% (5–6 mmol/mol) lower HbA_{1c} than multiple daily injection (MDI) therapy. The improvements in HbA_{1c} with the change to pump therapy appear to be greater in individuals who have poorer glycemic control [6,7]. Most of the studies examined in these meta-analyses involved MDI regimens using NPH or ultralente insulins; however, more recent randomized controlled trials suggest that CSII is also superior to MDI regimens using the newer long-acting insulin analogs [8,9]. Data about potential complications of pump therapy (such as ketoacidosis, pump malfunction and insulin site problems) is not reported in many of the published randomized trials, and most evidence suggesting that CSII is associated with an increased risk for ketoacidosis date from the 1980s [10–12]; however, device malfunction and infusion site problems

Textbook of Diabetes, 4th edition. Edited by R. Holt, C. Cockram, A. Flyvbjerg and B. Goldstein.

do still occur with modern pump technology, which points to the importance of giving education on proper catheter site care and ketoacidosis prevention to all patients using pumps.

Because of the more controlled delivery of insulin, CSII can be an effective tool for reducing glycemic variability, and this can be of benefit for reducing the risk for hypoglycemia brought about by insulin replacement therapy [13]. Clinical guidelines from several national and international organizations recommend consideration of pump therapy for individuals with T1DM with suboptimal glycemic control and problematic hypoglycemia (Box 28.1) [14–16]. However, conclusions from the meta-analyses about whether the mode of insulin delivery has an impact on hypoglycemia have yielded conflicting results [5,17,18], in large part because of methodologic issues and differences in trial selection [19,20]. The meta-analysis of randomized controlled trials by Pickup & Sutton [17], which was restricted to studies published since 1995 (i.e. since the introduction of more reliable pump technology) with a baseline (pre-trial) rate of severe hypoglycemia of >10 episodes/100 patient years and ≥6 months of CSII use, showed that there was a 2.9-fold (95% confidence interval [CI] 1.45–5.76) reduction in severe hypoglycemia during CSII compared to MDI. The analysis also indicated that the benefit from pump therapy was greater in individuals with higher rates of severe hypoglycemia ($P < 0.001$) and those with longer duration of diabetes ($P = 0.025$) [17]. A meta-analysis commissioned by the Endocrine Society reached different findings, and concluded that in comparison with MDI, CSII was not associated with a significant reduction in severe or nocturnal hypoglycemia [18]. The validity of these conclusions is limited by the inclusion of studies of relatively short duration with low incidence rates of severe hypoglycemia that would bias against the detection of any potential benefit from pump therapy. In addition, the rates of minor and nocturnal hypoglycemia were determined using intermittent fingerstick glucose monitoring, which can be unreliable in detecting nocturnal hypoglycemic events [21] and would therefore be relatively insensitive to detecting treatment-related differences. Furthermore, it should also be noted that the studies examined in this analysis were almost entirely performed using older pump types that did not incorporate the bolus calculator software now available in updated pumps which can help to limit hypoglycemia related to doses stacking up from repeated boluses. These factors limit the generalizability of the conclusions from this analysis to clinical practice, and the weight of evidence from studies reported in the literature suggest that clinicians caring for motivated patients with T1DM who have recurrent hypoglycemia and especially a history of severe hypoglycemic reactions should recommend a trial of insulin pump therapy.

Evidence in insulin-requiring type 2 diabetes mellitus (T2DM) regarding the potential benefits of pump therapy in comparison with MDI is limited. The studies of Raskin *et al.* [22] and Herman *et al.* [23] showed similar HbA_{1c} changes with both modes of insulin delivery. A small-scale cross-over study in obese subjects with T2DM with insulin resistance has demonstrated a significant reduction in HbA_{1c} and postmeal glucose excursion with use of pump therapy [24]. Where patients are unable to achieve adequate glycemic control, several practical issues should be considered (Box 28.2).

Box 28.1 Pump therapy: indications and considerations

- Severe hypoglycemia and hypoglycemia unawareness
- HbA_{1c} above goal
  - *Caution:* Intentional insulin omission (to facilitate weight loss) is a not uncommon cause for poorly controlled diabetes, especially in young women [32]. Before initiating pump therapy, it is important to rule out this problem. Because these patients habitually underdose insulin and are frequently hyperglycemic, they do not routinely troubleshoot for insulin non-delivery by the pump and can therefore be at increased risk for developing ketoacidosis
- Diurnal variations in basal insulin requirements caused by the dawn phenomenon [33,34] and steroid therapy can be more readily managed using the multiple basal rates provided by the pump than by long-acting injected insulins [35]. Continuous subcutaneous insulin infusion can be of special benefit for the post-renal transplant diabetes patient on steroid therapy who is striving for intensive glycemic control
- Preconception and pregnancy
- Practical advantages of pumps for bolus insulin delivery include:
  - *Dosing precision:* The extra precision of insulin dosing with pumps can be an important advantage for young children (especially infants and neonates) [36] and adults who are on very low insulin doses. In addition, accurate dosing of insulin boluses in fractions of a unit allows the patient to correct hyperglycemia more precisely without overshooting and causing hypoglycemia. For those patients in whom fear of hypoglycemia is an impediment to tight glycemic control, this added assurance can be critical in overcoming reluctance to intensification. In practice, it can be helpful to reduce missed food boluses, facilitate interprandial "correction" bolusing, and help simplify eating at restaurants and social occasions (with the use of extended/square wave boluses and multiple bolusing)
  - *Optimizing post-prandial insulin coverage:* Facilitates dosing for higher fat, complex carbohydrate and/or larger meals. Dietary fat delays gastric emptying [37] and induces post-prandial insulin resistance [38], so high-fat meals cannot usually be adequately covered using a single injection of rapid-acting insulin [39]. Use of the extended/dual bolus and increased temporary basal can help optimize post-prandial glycemic control following these meals [40–42]. (For practical strategies see Wolpert [43].)
  - *Gastroparesis:* Use of the extended/dual wave bolus can allow for better matching of carbohydrate absorption and insulin action

Box 28.2 Practical issues to consider in the pump patient with erratic glucose control

- *Infusion site issues including scarring, lipohypertrophy and lipoatrophy:* Infusion sites should be routinely examined in pump users with unexplained glucose fluctuations
- *Infusion catheter kinking or dislodgement:* Plastic catheters that are perpendicular to the skin surface and have a small base for attachment (e.g. Medtronic MiniMed Sofset™, Disetronic Ultraflex™) are more prone to kink or become dislodged especially with activity or perspiration. Solutions include changing to metal needle infusion sets, plastic sets with a shorter cannula, or other types of plastic infusion sets that are less prone to kinking. These include the Medtronic MiniMed Quickset™ (which has a broad base of attachment to the skin), and sets that insert obliquely such as the Medtronic MiniMed Silouette™, Roche Disetronic Tender™ and Animas Comfort™
- *Failure to change the pump reservoir and infusion system on a regular basis:* This may manifest in a tendency for elevated and erratic glucose in the period preceding infusion set changes
- *Review of pump downloads can be helpful:*
  - Check priming history to assess how frequently the infusion system is being changed
  - Check bolus history to detect possible missed meal boluses
  - Check percentage of basal to bolus insulin. A high percentage of basal insulin in the patient with frequent hyperglycemia may indicate that bolus doses are frequently being missed. A high percentage of basal insulin in the patient with frequent hypoglycemia may indicate that high basal rates are contributing to hypoglycemia, and would point to a need to re-evaluate basal rate settings
  - Check for a history of pump suspension or basal rate reduction. Even temporary removal of the pump to bathe can lead to elevations in the glucose levels; patients need to be reminded to bolus to replace the missed basal when reconnecting the pump. Some patients using the pump will get in the practice of reducing the basal rate or suspending the pump when they are hypoglycemic; the end result will often be exaggerated rebound hyperglycemia
- *Insulin instability in the pump infusion system:* This can manifest as increases in the glucose levels in the period preceding infusion set changes or even precipitation in the infusion system [46]
- Pump malfunction
- Air bubbles in infusion system resulting from poor filling technique

Quality of life benefits and patient expectations

Many patients describe improvements in quality of life when they change to pump therapy; however, there have been few carefully designed studies that have examined patient perspectives of pump therapy, and differences in psychosocial functioning with CSII compared to MDI [4,25]. The published literature suggests that use of pumps is associated with improved quality of life compared to MDI [26–28]; however, this has not been confirmed in all studies [29]. Patients will vary in their perceptions about the potential quality of life benefits (including increased lifestyle flexibility, dietary freedom, reduced fear for hypoglycemia) relative to some of the potential drawbacks of CSII (including body image concerns and the need for frequent blood glucose monitoring) [30]. Wolpert and colleagues conducted a focus group investigation of 30 patients followed at the Joslin Diabetes Center to examine how psychosocial factors impacted the use of the pump [31]. Patients with better glycemic control viewed the pump as a tool for diabetes self-management rather than as a panacea. In contrast, the pump patients with poorer HbA_{1c} had more unrealistic expectations including the perception that use of technology was a substitute for attentiveness to self-care and that pump therapy allowed them to do whatever they wanted, particularly with regard to eating. Before initiating pump therapy, health care professionals need to assess patients' expectations of the pump, dispel unrealistic notions (often promoted by marketing materials) and ensure that patients recognize that while the pump allows life with diabetes to be more flexible and convenient, it is not a vehicle for total freedom from diabetes.

New developments in pump technology: bolus calculators

In recent years, new software programs that assist patients with bolus calculations have been incorporated into insulin pumps. The patient's insulin : carbohydrate ratio (the number of carbohydrate grams covered by 1 unit of insulin) and correction/sensitivity factor (a measure of the glucose-lowering effect of 1 unit of insulin) is programmed into the pump software. Based on planned carbohydrate intake of the patient and the blood glucose level, the bolus calculator will recommend a bolus dose. Although this dose calculation software can simplify the daily self-care routines of the pump users, patients should receive appropriate education to ensure that they can manually calculate bolus doses in the event they need to discontinue pump therapy. In addition, it is important that the programming of the bolus calculator software is adjusted to individual needs and not automatically left at the manufacturer's default settings. These bolus calculators have an important role in minimizing the risk for hypoglycemia from multiple boluses and dose stacking which are a common practical problem with some pump users [43]. When calculating an insulin dose, the pump software will consider the amount of active insulin-on-board (commonly referred to as IOB) and subtract this IOB from the recommended dose. This IOB calculation is based on insulin action plots which predict the amount of insulin remaining as a function of time; the assumed insulin duration of action used by the software in this calculation is individually programmed by the patient or health care professional, and can be varied from 2 to 8 hours depending on the pump type [44]. As outlined in Chapter 27 the absorption of insulin analogs can vary markedly even within individuals. In practice, the major consideration in setting the insulin duration of action in the bolus calculator software is usually a best guess based on a clinical assessment of the hypoglycemia risk of the patient and the imperative for achieving tight glycemic control (in particular, preconception and pregnancy) [45]. For individuals with frequent hypoglycemia, hypoglycemia unawareness or a history of severe hypoglycemic reactions, the duration of action should be set 5 hours or even longer, whereas for the woman who is pregnant or trying to conceive, the duration of action is often set at 2–3 hours. The glucose records of the patient can be assessed to determine if the duration of action settings are appropriate. If the duration of action time programmed into the software is less than the true duration of action, the pump will indicate that there is less IOB than is actually the case, and the patient will mistakenly take more insulin than required; the glucose records will show evidence of hypoglycemia from "stacking" of doses. Conversely, if the setting programmed into the pump is longer than the true duration of insulin action, this can lead to underdosing of insulin and hinder attempts to optimize glycemic control.

Real-time continuous glucose monitoring

In the last several years, several real-time continuous glucose monitoring (RT-CGM) devices (Abbott Freestyle Navigator®, DexCom Seven®, Medtronic Guardian®/Paradigm® system) have received the CE mark and approval from the US Food and Drug Administration (FDA) for long-term use in ambulatory patients with diabetes (Figure 28.1). These devices have transcutaneous glucose oxidase-based electrochemical sensors that measure the glucose concentration in the interstitial fluid every 1–5 minutes (Figure 28.2). Because of accuracy limitations [47,48], the current

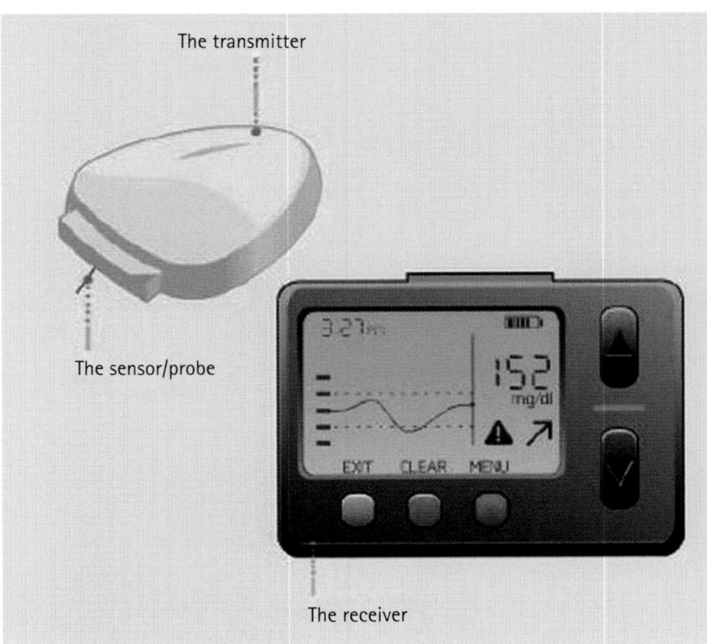

Figure 28.1 Three components of continuous glucose monitoring (CGM) device: sensor, transmitter and receiver unit.

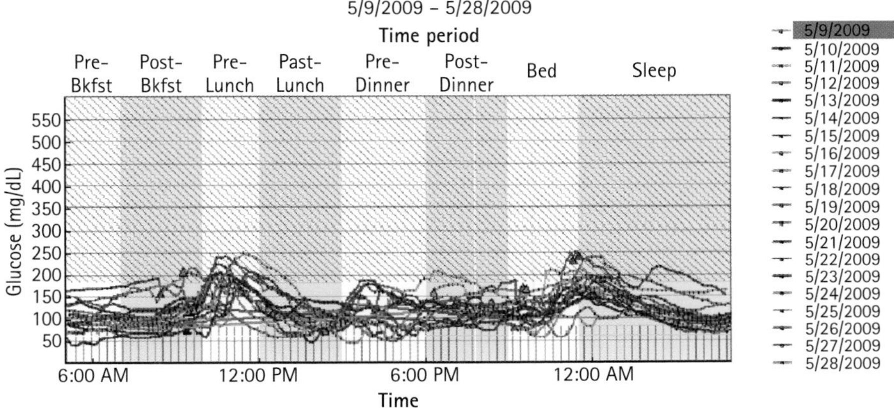

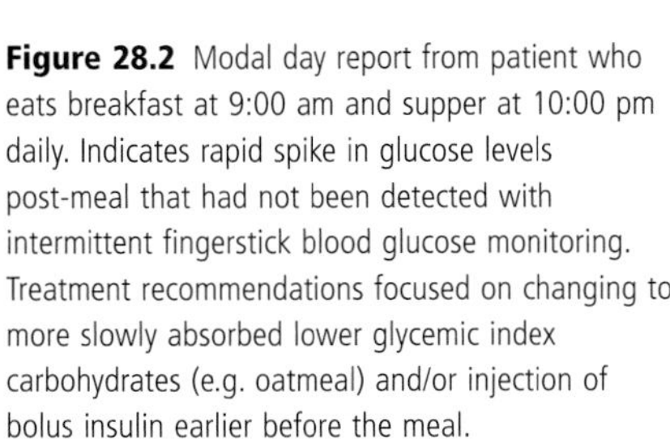

Figure 28.2 Modal day report from patient who eats breakfast at 9:00 am and supper at 10:00 pm daily. Indicates rapid spike in glucose levels post-meal that had not been detected with intermittent fingerstick blood glucose monitoring. Treatment recommendations focused on changing to more slowly absorbed lower glycemic index carbohydrates (e.g. oatmeal) and/or injection of bolus insulin earlier before the meal.

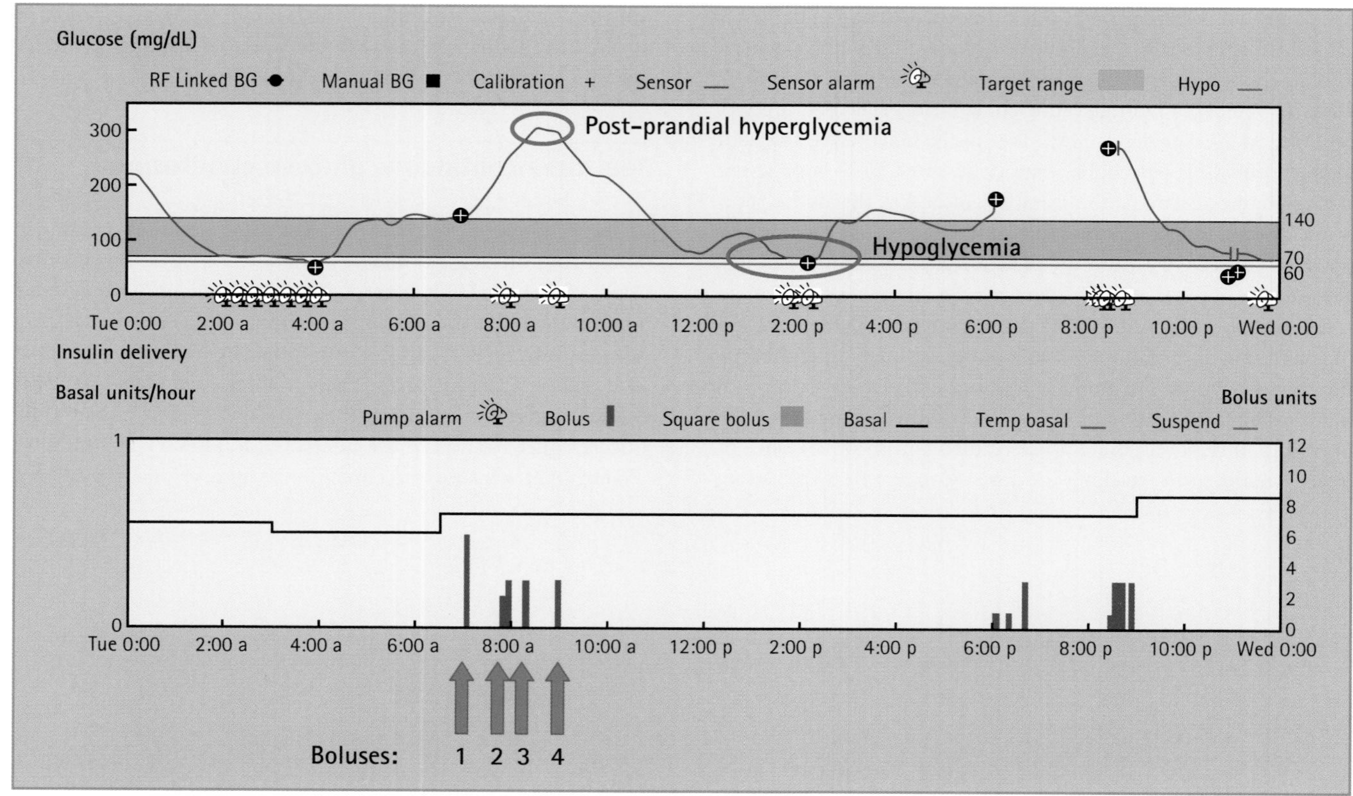

Figure 28.3 Device download: top panel shows continuous glucose tracing, and bottom panel shows insulin delivery (each blue bar represents an insulin bolus with units of insulin shown on the vertical axis on the right). Following breakfast the glucose level increased to 300 mg/dL (16.7 mmol/L) prompting the patient to take multiple boluses with resultant hypoglycemia.

generation of CGM devices do not have regulatory approval for use as stand-alone devices, and patients are required to perform adjunctive capillary blood glucose measurements; however, this limitation is compensated by the additional detailed information provided by the CGM about glucose patterns, the rate and direction of change in the glucose level and adjustable alarms that are triggered by both hyperglycemia and hypoglycemia (Figure 28.3) [49].

Clinical efficacy of RT-CGM

Because RT-CGM is a relatively new technology, to date only a few randomized controlled trials have been performed. The initial reported studies, which were only several days in duration, showed that use of RT-CGM leads to a reduction of both hyperglycemic and hypoglycemic excursions with more time in the target glucose range [50,51]. The GuardControl trial using the Medtronic Guardian was the first longer duration study of RT-CGM. This study enrolled 156 adults and children with T1DM using both pumps and MDI therapy [52]. At 3-month follow-up, the group randomized to RT-CGM use had 1.0 ± 1.1% (11 ± 12 mmol/mol) reduction in HbA_{1c} (down from 9.5 ± 1.1% [80 ± 12 mmol/mol] at baseline) compared to 0.4 ± 1.0% (5 ± 11 mmol/mol) reduction in the control group (P = 0.003). In addition, at 3 months, 50% of subjects in the CGM group had HbA_{1c} reductions of ≥1% compared to 15% of subjects in the control group, and 26% in the CGM group had HbA_{1c} reductions of ≥2% compared to 4% in the control arm. Reported results from this industry-supported study have not included any specific information on the treatment protocols used in the trial or data about the effect of CGM on hypoglycemia.

To date, the results of two large-scale multicenter randomized controlled trials of 6 months' duration have been published in the literature: the industry-supported Star 1 trial and the Juvenile Diabetes Research Foundation (JDRF) sponsored CGM trial. The Star 1 trial enrolled 146 subjects aged 12–72 years with T1DM treated with CSII pumps [53] who were randomized to pump therapy with RT-CGM using the Medtronic 722 pump system or pump therapy with fingerstick self-monitoring of blood glucose. The primary endpoint was not achieved; there was a similar reduction in HbA_{1c} (0.71 ± 0.71% in the sensor group vs 0.56 ± 0.072% in the control group; P = non-significant) over the 6-month trial. Importantly, in the subjects using RT-CGM, the improvement in glycemic control was accomplished without any change in biochemical hypoglycemia ($P < 0.0002$), whereas in the control subjects using fingerstick glucose monitoring there was an increase in biochemical hypoglycemia (documented with blinded CGM devices). More severe hypoglycemic events occurred in the group using RT-CGM than in the control group (11 vs 4; $P = 0.04$). During six of the 11 severe events in the RT-CGM group, subjects were not using a sensor. The Data Safety Monitoring Board determined that in the remaining five severe hypoglycemic events there was evidence of the following:

1 Failure of subjects to respond to alarm warnings of hypoglycemia;

2 Multiple insulin boluses without use of the pump bolus calculator, resulting in dose stacking; or

3 "Blind boluses" (i.e. treatment decision based on sensor readings showing hyperglycemia without confirmatory fingerstick capillary blood glucose measurements).

This clinical experience from the Star 1 trial was incorporated into the treatment protocols and patient education materials used in the JDRF CGM trial.

The JDRF CGM trial enrolled 451 patients with T1DM aged 8–74 years and HbA_{1c} <10% (86 mmol/mol) to a RT-CGM group or control group that continued with capillary blood glucose monitoring [54,55]. This study involved patients using both insulin pumps and injection therapy and used three different CGM devices (Abbott Navigator®, Dexcom Seven® and Medtronic Guardian/722® system), with assignment based on patient preference with investigator guidance. By design, the cohorts with HbA_{1c} at randomization of <7.0% (<53 mmol/mol; n = 129) and 7–10% (53–80 mmol/mol; n = 322) were analyzed separately.

For individuals with T1DM who have already managed to achieve HbA_{1c} levels in the optimal target range with intermittent capillary blood glucose monitoring, the main therapeutic challenge is minimizing the risk for hypoglycemia that accompanies intensive glucose control. Accordingly, for the cohort enrolled in this trial with baseline HbA_{1c} <7.0% (<53 mmol/mol), the pre-specified primary endpoints were focused on changes in hypoglycemia rather than HbA_{1c} per se. At 26 weeks, biochemical hypoglycemia ≤3.9 mmol/L (70 mg/dL) was less frequent in the CGM group than the control group using intermittent fingerstick monitoring (median 54 vs 91 minutes/day), but this was not statistically significant. Median time spent with glucose level ≤3.3 mmol/L (60 mg/dL) was 18 vs 15 minutes/day, respectively ($P = 0.05$). There were similar numbers of severe hypoglycemic events in the two groups; however, the trial was not adequately powered to detect a treatment group difference. More subjects in the CGM group than the control group had a decrease in HbA_{1c} of ≥0.3% without having a severe hypoglycemic event (28% vs 5%; $P < 0.01$) [56].

For the cohort with baseline HbA_{1c} 7–10% (53–86 mmol/mol), the pre-specified primary endpoint was HbA_{1c} reduction. A significant between-group difference in change in HbA_{1c} from baseline to 26 weeks was seen in patients ≥25 years old, favoring the continuous monitoring group (mean difference in change –0.53%; $P < 0.001$), but not in the younger subjects. Biochemical hypoglycemia evaluated by CGM was similar in the two treatment groups. Similarily, there were no significant differences in the incidence of severe hypoglycemic events between the study groups. In the adult cohort, the frequency of the combined outcome of 26-week HbA_{1c} <7.0% (<53 mmol/mol) and no severe hypoglycemic events was 30% in the CGM group and 7% in the control group ($P = 0.0006$) [55]. This finding, that RT-CGM leads to an improvement in glycemic control without an associated worsening in hypoglycemic events, is in direct contrast to other intervention studies such as the DCCT in which intermittent capillary glucose monitoring had been used to guide intensification of metabolic control, and points to the promise this new technology offers for people with T1DM.

Practical issues with use of RT-CGM

The randomized controlled trials that have demonstrated the benefits of RT-CGM have involved patients with a high level of engagement in their diabetes self-care (mean number of daily capillary blood glucose measurements performed by subjects enrolling in the JDRF trial was six). Furthermore, to use this technology successfully, patients need to have advanced diabetes self-management skills (Box 28.3). In the next sections we discuss several key issues that need to be addressed in the training of patients starting on CGM.

Physiologic lag between blood and interstitial glucose

The lag in the equilibration of glucose levels between the capillary blood (measured using home blood glucose monitoring device) and the interstitial fluid in the subcutaneous tissue (measured by the CGM device) [57,58] has important practical implications. In general, increases or decreases in the glucose concentration will first be apparent in the blood followed by the interstitial fluid. Currently available CGM devices are calibrated using fingerstick capillary blood glucose measurements, and to optimize sensor accuracy it is important that the device only be calibrated when the glucose level is relatively stable, and there is steady-state equilibration between glucose concentrations in the blood and interstitial fluid. In practice, calibrations should be performed

Box 28.3 Patient teaching points: Adjusting bolus doses based on rate of change of glucose [63]

- If glucose ↑ by 0.056–0.11 mmol/L/minute (1–2 mg/dL/minute): +10% to calculated food/correction bolus
- If glucose ↑ by >0.11 mmol/L/minute (>2 mg/dL/minute): +20% to calculated food/correction bolus
- If glucose ↓ by 0.056–0.11 mmol/L/minute (1–2 mg/dL/minute): –10% from calculated food/correction bolus
- If glucose ↓ by >0.11 mmol/L/minute (>2 mg/dL/minute): –20% from calculated food/correction bolus

Box 28.4 Patient teaching points: Calibration do's and don'ts

- Before calibrating the sensor, the patient should check to be sure that there are no arrows on the sensor display indicating that the glucose is changing rapidly
- Calibration should not be performed:
  - Within 3–4 hours of a meal or an insulin bolus
  - During exercise
  - After recovering from hypoglycemia

Box 28.5 Patient teaching points: Circumstances where fingerstick capillary glucose must be checked

- If the sensor indicates that the glucose is elevated, the reading must first be confirmed with a fingerstick capillary blood glucose measurement before the patient takes a corrective bolus
- Whenever subjective symptoms are not in keeping with the sensor reading, a fingerstick reading should be taken to confirm the glucose level
- Before or during driving, if the sensor reading is normal and the continuous glucose monitoring rate of change indicator or tracing indicates that the glucose level is falling, the patient must measure fingerstick blood glucose
- Following treatment of a low glucose, if the sensor still shows a low reading, the patient should check fingerstick blood glucose and use this measurement to decide whether to take in more carbohydrate. Reliance on the sensor reading to assess response can lead to overtreatment

preprandially or at least 3 hours after a bolus (Box 28.4). The first generation CGM devices need to be calibrated at least 4 times per day for optimal accuracy [59].

The physiologic lag has implications with regard to detection and treatment of hypoglycemia. Because of the lag of interstitial glucose behind blood glucose, when the glucose level is declining the interstitial (sensor) glucose can be in the normal range even though the actual blood glucose is low [60]. Patients should be instructed to perform a fingerstick blood glucose measurement before driving if the sensor glucose reading is normal and the trend graph or rate-of-change arrows on the sensor display indicate that the glucose level is declining (Box 28.5). As shown in the study by Wilson *et al.* [61], when the glucose is falling rapidly, the physiologic lag can also lead to underestimation by the rate-of-change indicator of the CGM device. The practical implication is that if the patient feels hypoglycemic or has reason to suspect that the glucose is declining, but this is not corroborated by the sensor, they should disregard the sensor data and carry out a fingerstick glucose measurement.

This lag phenomena also has practical implications for the treatment of hypoglycemia. During the recovery from hypoglycemia, the increase in the interstitial glucose will often lag behind the blood glucose [62], and at a time when blood glucose has already normalized the sensor/interstitial glucose may still be in the low range. Patients should be instructed of the need to perform fingerstick glucose measurements to assess the response to treatment of hypoglycemia accurately. Patients who rely on the RT-CGM to judge whether the glucose level is improving following ingestion of carbohydrates will mistakenly assume that they need to consume more.

Setting glucose alarms

The alarms for hypoglycemia and hyperglycemia are an important feature of RT-CGM devices. There are trade-offs in the adjustment of alarm thresholds, and settings need to be individualized based on specific clinical considerations [64]. If the alarm thresholds are set at target or ideal glucose levels (e.g. low = 5 mmol/L [90 mg/dL]; high = 10 mmol/L [180 mg/dL]), there will be increased sensitivity for detection of high and low glucoses; however, the frequent false alarms can be a source of irritation and disrupt sleep leading to "alarm fatigue" in some patients with a related tendency to ignore the alarms (Figure 28.4).

The adjustment of alarm thresholds is a stepwise process:

1 Deciding on initial thresholds when initiating use of the sensor; and

2 Optimizing alarm thresholds over time based on retrospective review of continuous glucose tracings.

For patients with hypoglycemia, unawareness or a history of severe hypoglycemic reactions, where the overriding imperative is on reducing hypoglycemia, the low glucose alarm threshold should be set at 4.5 mmol/L (80 mg/dL) or higher. Because of physiologic lag between blood and interstitial glucose, when the sensor alarm is triggered, the blood glucose level will often be lower than the sensor measurement.

For individuals without a history of problematic hypoglycemia, it is a common practice to set the initial glucose thresholds at 3–3.5 mmol/L (55–60 mg/dL) and ≥14 mmol/L (250 mg/dL). This ensures that during the initial period after starting use of CGM, while the patient is mastering use of the technology, there will be fewer intrusive and irritating alarms, and less risk for alarm burnout. Over time, as the patient uses the information from the sensor to reduce glucose excursions, the alarm settings can be brought closer to target glucose levels, and this can assist with further tightening of glycemic control.

During follow-up visits, the clinician should enquire whether the sensor alarm alerted the patient to low or markedly elevated glucose levels, and whether the patient was troubled by frequent false alarms. If there are frequent high glucoses (especially during the overnight period) and the patient is not being appropriately alerted by the sensor to take corrective action, the high alarm threshold should be reduced. Conversely, if the patient has experienced hypoglycemic reactions without being alerted by the

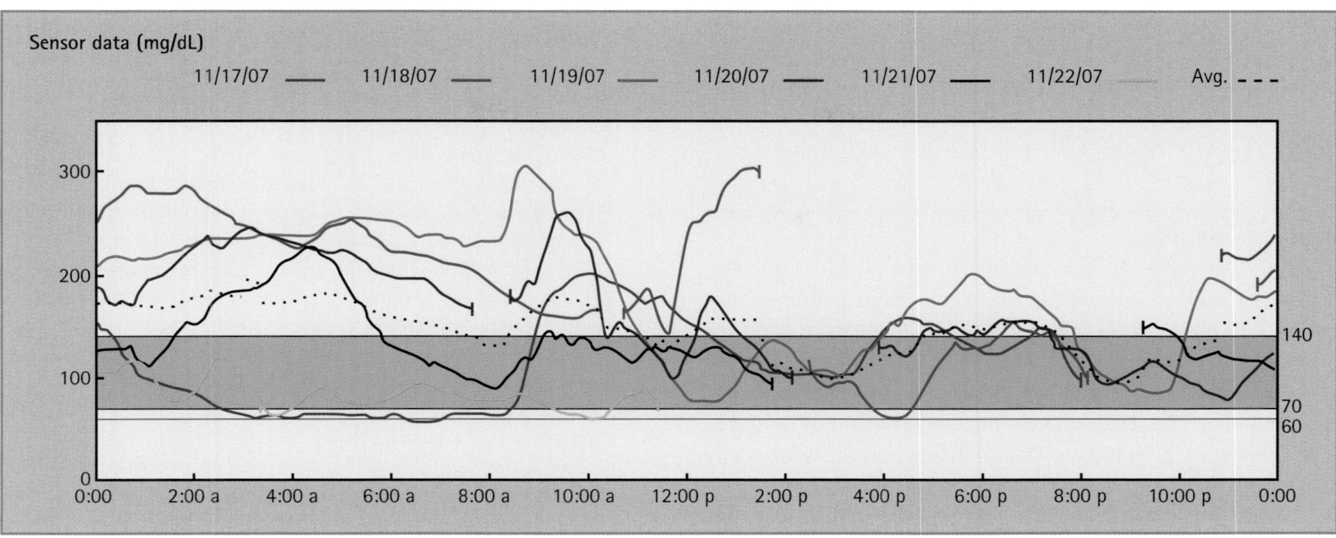

Figure 28.4 Sensor downloads indicated that this patient had marked variability in overnight glucose control because of snacking at bedtime. Sensor high alarm threshold was set at 300 mg/dL (16.7 mmol/L) and as a result the alarm was not sounding at night. Reduction in the alarm threshold to 220 mg/dL (12.2 mmol/L) resulted in improvement in overnight glucose control and HbA_{1c}.

CGM alarm, the low alarm threshold will need to be set at a higher level.

Risk for hypoglycemia from excessive post-prandial bolusing

While the glucose alarms and trend indicators on CGM devices can be helpful in minimizing hypoglycemia, some patients will overreact to the post-prandial glucose spikes revealed by the continuous sensor by taking excessive doses of insulin [65], leading to an increased risk for hypoglycemia. Minimizing this tendency for post-prandial overbolusing should be a major focus in the training of the patient using RT-CGM. Patients need to factor in the amount of residual IOB from the previous bolus before taking additional insulin to treat post-prandial hyperglycemia. The newer pumps with bolus calculator software can guide patients in making appropriate dose adjustments.

The glycemic index of the carbohydrates in the meal is another factor to consider in the decision about whether additional boluses may be required to treat post-prandial hyperglycemia. High glycemic index carbohydrates will often lead to an early spike in the glucose levels (because of the mismatch between the absorption of the carbohydrate and action of the insulin bolus), and correction boluses taken within 2–3 hours after the meal can result in hypoglycemia.

Closed-loop/artificial pancreas

Insulin pump therapy as it is currently used is considered to be an "open-loop system," in which the patient must make executive decisions about when to check the glucose level and what to do with the information. Clearly, there is inherent human error in this system and overdosing or underdosing of insulin based on a small miscalculation could result in subsequent hypoglycemic or hyperglycemic episodes, respectively. In a "closed-loop system" which integrates a continuous glucose monitor and insulin pump, together with an automated algorithm to control insulin delivery, the patient would be removed from the decision loop, and the system would essentially function as an artificial pancreas.

At present, one of the major challenges for the fully automated closed-loop system may be in the development of a fail-safe algorithm that is capable of "interpreting" a person's metabolic state based on data obtained from the continuous glucose monitor and then relaying this information to the pump for automatic insulin delivery of the appropriate dose of insulin. Several algorithms including model predictive control and proportional integral derivative control are already being evaluated in both *in vivo* and *in silico* settings [66]. There are also several technical obstacles to developing a closed-loop system including having glucose sensors that are both accurate and reliable (e.g. minimal calibration drift, limited potential mechanisms for sensor failure), and also physiologic lag which can be particularly problematic during times of rapid rates of change in blood glucose levels (e.g. during meals or exercise) [67]. Thus, development of a sensor with a short lag time would also be important. The first prototype closed-loop systems that can deliver glucagon to prevent hypoglycemia are currently being evaluated [68].

Development of the first generations of an artificial pancreas is underway and several studies have already demonstrated that glycemic control can be achieved with an automated closed loop system in investigational and controlled hospital settings [69–72]. Medtronic MiniMed has developed an external physiologic insulin delivery system that combines an external insulin pump and continuous glucose sensor with a variable insulin infusion rate algorithm designed to emulate the physiologic characteristics of the β-cell. Similar devices by other companies, including Abbott Laboratories, are also being developed and tested.

Inhaled insulin

Survey studies have indicated that fear of needles and discomfort and inconvenience from injecting insulin are barriers to the use of insulin by many patients with T2DM [73,74]. An effective alternative mode for insulin administration would therefore be of potential benefit. As insulin is a peptide hormone, it cannot be taken orally, as it would be quickly degraded by the digestive enzymes of the stomach. Alternative routes of administration that have been investigated include transdermal, transbuccal and transpulmonary (inhaled) delivery of insulin.

The lung is an attractive mode for administration of a systemic drug because of its large available area for drug absorption and accessibility. In January 2006, the FDA approved the use of Exubera® (Pfizer), the first inhalable insulin.

Clinical studies have shown that pre-meal inhaled insulin achieves comparable glycemic control to subcutaneous regular insulin administration [75–77]; however, smoking can significantly alter the pharmacokinetics of inhaled insulin [78,79], and even passive smoke exposure in non-smokers can affect bioavailability [80]. Follow-up of the patients who had used Exubera in clinical trials has raised concerns about the potential long-term toxicity of insulin delivered by the pulmonary route. As of April 2008, six of the 4740 patients who used Exubera in clinical trials had developed lung cancer, compared with only one of the 4292 patients in the placebo group. All six patients with lung cancer had a prior history of cigarette smoking (Exubera label, FDA approval September 29, 2008), and this association was not statistically significant because of the small numbers. However, because of these safety concerns, as well as failure of Exubera to gain acceptance by patients and physicians, Pfizer withdrew Exubera from the market, and Eli Lilly and Novo Nordisk also gave up their efforts to develop their own insulin inhalation systems.

At present, one company, MannKind Corporation, has continued to develop an inhaled insulin, Technosphere® insulin [81]. In March 2009, a new drug application to market this insulin was filed with the FDA. Technosphere insulin contains insulin particles that are optimized for inhalation (2.5 μm in diameter) and dissolve rapidly after inhalation (pH sensitive carrier particles). Pharmacokinetic studies have demonstrated that this formulation has very rapid systemic insulin uptake (insulin T_{max} approximately 12–14 minutes), a fast onset of action (maximum activity approximately 20–30 minutes) and a short duration of action (approximately 2–3 hours) [82] which could potentially provide better post-prandial control than subcutaneously injected insulin.

References

1 Pickup JC, Keen H, Parsons JA, Alberti KG. Continuous subcutaneous insulin infusion: an approach to achieving normoglycaemia. *Br Med J* 1978; **1**:204–207.

2 Tamborlane WV, Sherwin RS, Genel M, Felig P. Reduction to normal of plasma glucose in juvenile diabetes by subcutaneous administration of insulin with a portable infusion pump. *N Engl J Med* 1979; **300**:573–578.

3 Pickup J, Mattock M, Kerry S. Glycaemic control with continuous subcutaneous insulin infusion compared with intensive insulin injections in patients with type 1 diabetes: meta-analysis of randomised controlled trials. *Br Med J (Clin Res Edn)* 2002; **324**:705.

4 Weissberg-Benchell J, Antisdel-Lomaglio J, Seshadri R. Insulin pump therapy: a meta-analysis. *Diabetes Care* 2003; **26**:1079–1087.

5 Jeitler K, Horvath K, Berghold A, Gratzer TW, Neeser K, Pieber TR, *et al.* Continuous subcutaneous insulin infusion versus multiple daily insulin injections in patients with diabetes mellitus: systematic review and meta-analysis. *Diabetologia* 2008; **51**:941–951.

6 Retnakaran R, Hochman J, DeVries JH, Hanaire-Broutin H, Heine RJ, Melki V, *et al.* Continuous subcutaneous insulin infusion versus multiple daily injections: the impact of baseline A1c. *Diabetes Care* 2004; **27**:2590–2596.

7 Pickup JC, Kidd J, Burmiston S, Yemane N. Determinants of glycaemic control in type 1 diabetes during intensified therapy with multiple daily insulin injections or continuous subcutaneous insulin infusion: importance of blood glucose variability. *Diabetes Metab Res Rev* 2006; **22**:232–237.

8 Doyle EA, Weinzimer SA, Steffen AT, Ahern JA, Vincent M, Tamborlane WV. A randomized, prospective trial comparing the efficacy of continuous subcutaneous insulin infusion with multiple daily injections using insulin glargine. *Diabetes Care* 2004; **27**:1554–1558.

9 Hirsch IB, Bode BW, Garg S, Lane WS, Sussman A, Hu P, *et al.* Continuous subcutaneous insulin infusion (CSII) of insulin aspart versus multiple daily injection of insulin aspart/insulin glargine in type 1 diabetic patients previously treated with CSII. *Diabetes Care* 2005; **28**:533–538.

10 Levy-Marchal C, Czernichow P. Feasibility of continuous subcutaneous insulin infusion in young diabetic patients. *Diabete Metab* 1988; **14**:108–113.

11 Beck-Nielsen H, Richelsen B, Schwartz Sorensen N, Hother Nielsen O. Insulin pump treatment: effect on glucose homeostasis, metabolites, hormones, insulin antibodies and quality of life. *Diabetes Res* 1985; **2**:37–43.

12 Mecklenburg RS, Benson EA, Benson JW Jr, Fredlund PN, Guinn T, Metz RJ, *et al.* Acute complications associated with insulin infusion pump therapy: report of experience with 161 patients. *JAMA* 1984; **252**:3265–3269.

13 Pickup JC, Kidd J, Burmiston S, Yemane N. Effectiveness of continuous subcutaneous insulin infusion in hypoglycaemia-prone type 1 diabetes. *Pract Diabetes Int* 2005; **22**:10–14.

14 American Diabetes Association. Continuous subcutaneous insulin infusion. *Diabetes Care* 2004; **27**(Suppl 1):110.

15 Hammond P, Boardman S, Greenwood R. ABCD position paper on insulin pumps. *Pract Diabetes Int* **2006**; **23**:395–400.

16 Pickup JC, Hammond P. NICE guidance on continuous subcutaneous insulin infusion 2008: review of the technology appraisal guidance. *Diabet Med* 2009; **26**:1–4.

17 Pickup JC, Sutton AJ. Severe hypoglycemia and glycemic control in type 1 diabetes: meta-analysis of multiple daily insulin injections compared with continuous subcutaneous insulin infusion. *Diabet Med* 2008; **25**:765–774.

18 Fatourechi MM, Kudva YC, Murad MH, Elamin MB, Tabini CC, Montori VM. Hypoglycemia with intensive insulin therapy: a systematic review and meta-analyses of randomized trials of continuous subcutaneous insulin infusion versus multiple daily injections. *J Clin Endocrinol Metab* 2009; **94**:729–740.

19 Siebenhofer A, Jeitler K, Berghold A, Horvath K, Pieber TR. Severe hypoglycemia and glycemic control in type 1 diabetes: meta-analysis of multiple daily insulin injections compared with continuous subcutaneous insulin infusion. *Diabet Med* 2009; **26**:311–312.

20 Pickup JC. Author's response. *Diabet Med* 2009; **26**:312–313.

21 McGarraugh G, Bergenstal R. Detection of hypoglycemia with continuous interstitial and traditional blood glucose monitoring using the freestyle navigator continuous glucose monitoring system. *Diabetes Technol Ther* 2009; **11**:145–150.

22 Raskin P, Bode BW, Marks JB, Hirsch IB, Weinstein RL, McGill JB, *et al.* Continuous subcutaneous insulin infusion and multiple daily injection therapy are equally effective in type 2 diabetes: a randomized, parallel-group, 24-week study. *Diabetes Care* 2003; **26**:2598–2603.

23 Herman WH, Ilag LL, Johnson SL, Martin CL, Sinding J, Al Harthi A, *et al.* A clinical trial of continuous subcutaneous insulin infusion versus multiple daily injections in older adults with type 2 diabetes. *Diabetes Care* 2005; **28**:1568–1573.

24 Wainstein J, Metzger M, Boaz M, Minuchin O, Cohen Y, Yaffe A, *et al.* Insulin pump therapy vs. multiple daily injections in obese type 2 diabetic patients. *Diabet Med* 2005; **22**:1037–1046.

25 Barnard KD, Lloyd CE, Skinner TC. Systematic literature review: quality of life associated with insulin pump use in type 1 diabetes. *Diabet Med* 2007; **24**:607–617.

26 Barnard KD, Skinner TC. Cross-sectional study into quality of life issues surrounding insulin pump use in type 1 diabetes. *Pract Diabetes Int* 2008; **25**.

27 Linkeschova R, Raoul M, Bott U, Berger M, Spraul M. Less severe hypoglycemia, better metabolic control, and improved quality of life in type 1 diabetes mellitus with continuous subcutaneous insulin infusion (CSII) therapy; an observational study of 100 consecutive patients followed for a mean of 2 years. *Diabet Med* 2002; **19**:746–751.

28 Hoogma RPLM, Hammond PJ, Gomis R, Kerr D, Bruttomesso D, Bouter KP, *et al.* Comparison of the effects of continuous subcutaneous insulin infusion (CSII) and NPH-based multiple daily insulin injections (MDI) on glycemic control and quality of life: results of the 5-nations trial. *Diabet Med* 2006; **23**:141–147.

29 Tsui E, Barnie A, Ross S, Parkes R, Zinman B. Intensive insulin therapy with insulin lispro: a randomized trial of continuous subcutaneous insulin infusion versus multiple daily insulin injection. *Diabetes Care* 2001; **24**:1722–1727.

30 Speight J, Shaw JAM. Does one size really fit all? Only by considering individual preferences and priorities will the true impact of insulin pump therapy on quality of life be determined. *Diabet Med* 2007; **24**:693–695.

31 Ritholz MD, Smaldone A, Lee J, Castillo A, Wolpert H, Weinger K. Perceptions of psychosocial factors and the insulin pump. *Diabetes Care* 2007; **30**:549–554.

32 Polonsky WH, Anderson BJ, Lohrer PA, Aponte JE, Jacobson AM, Cole CF. Insulin omission in women with IDDM. *Diabetes Care* 1994; **17**:1178–1185.

33 Perriello G, De Feo P, Torlone E, Fanelli C, Santeusanio F, Brunetti P, *et al.* The dawn phenomenon in type 1 (insulin-dependent) diabetes mellitus: magnitude, frequency, variability, and dependency on glucose counterregulation and insulin sensitivity. *Diabetologia* 1991; **34**:21–28.

34 Koivisto VA, Yki-Jarvinen H, Helve E, Karonen SL, Pelkonen R. Pathogenesis and prevention of the dawn phenomenon in diabetic patients treated with CSII. *Diabetes* 1986; **35**:78–82.

35 Bevier W, Zisser H, Jovanovic L, Finan DA, Palerm C, Seborg D, *et al.* Use of continuous glucose monitoring to estimate insulin requirements in patients with type 1 diabetes mellitus during a short course of prednisone. *J Diabetes Sci Technol* 2008; **2**:578–583.

36 Phillip M, Battelino T, Rodriguez H, Danne T, Kaufman F. Use of insulin pump therapy in the pediatric age-group: consensus statement from the European Society for Pediatric Endocrinology, the Lawson Wilkins Pediatric Endocrine Society, and the International Society for Pediatric and Adolescent Diabetes, endorsed by the American Diabetes Association and the European Association for the Study of Diabetes. *Diabetes Care* 2007; **30**:1653–1662.

37 Marciani L, Wickham M, Singh G, Bush D, Pick B, Cox E, *et al.* Enhancement of intragastric acid stability of a fat emulsion meal delays gastric emptying and increases cholecystokinin release and gallbladder contraction. *Am J Physiol Gastrointest Liver Physiol* 2007; **292**:G1607–G1613.

38 Pedrini MT, Niederwanger A, Kranebitter M, Tautermann C, Ciardi C, Tatarczyk T, *et al.* Postprandial lipemia induces an acute decrease of insulin sensitivity in healthy men independently of plasma NEFA levels. *Diabetologia* 2006; **49**:1612–1618.

39 Ahern JA, Gatcomb PM, Held NA, Petit WA Jr, Tamborlane WV. Exaggerated hyperglycemia after a pizza meal in well-controlled diabetes. *Diabetes Care* 1993; **16**:578–580.

40 Jones SM, Quarry JL, Caldwell-McMillan M, Mauger DT, Gabbay RA. Optimal insulin pump dosing and postprandial glycemia following a pizza meal using the continuous glucose monitoring system. *Diabetes Technol Ther* 2005; **7**:233–240.

41 Lee SW, Cao M, Sajid S, Hayes M, Choi L, Rother C, *et al.* The dual-wave bolus feature in continuous subcutaneous insulin infusion pumps controls prolonged post-prandial hyperglycemia better than standard bolus in type 1 diabetes. *Diabetes Nutr Metab* 2004; **17**:211–216.

42 Chase HP, Saib SZ, MacKenzie T, Hansen MM, Garg SK. Post-prandial glucose excursions following four methods of bolus insulin administration in subjects with type 1 diabetes. *Diabet Med* 2002; **19**:317–321.

43 Wolpert H. *Smart Pumping: A Practical Approach to Mastering the Insulin Pump*, 2002.

44 Zisser H, Robinson L, Bevier W, Dassau E, Ellingsen C, Doyle FJ, *et al.* Bolus calculator: a review of four insulin pumps. *Diabetes Technol Ther* 2008; **10**:441–444.

45 Wolpert H, Schade DS. To pump or not to pump. *Diabetes Technol Ther* 2005; **7**:845–848.

46 Wolpert HA, Faradji RN, Bonner-Weir S, Lipes MA. Metabolic decompensation in pump users due to lispro insulin precipitation. *Br Med J (Clin Res edn)* 2002; **324**:1253.

47 Kovatchev B, Anderson S, Heinemann L, Clarke W. Comparison of the numerical and clinical accuracy of four continuous glucose monitors. *Diabetes Care* 2008; **31**:1160–1164.

48 Mastrototaro J, Shin J, Marcus A, Sulur G. The accuracy and efficacy of real-time continuous glucose monitoring sensor in patients with type 1 diabetes. *Diabetes Technol Ther* 2008; **10**:385–390.

49 Hirsch IB, Armstrong D, Bergenstal RM, Buckingham B, Childs BP, Clarke WL, *et al.* Clinical application of emerging sensor technologies in diabetes management: consensus guidelines for continuous glucose monitoring (CGM). *Diabetes Technol Ther* 2008; **10**:232–244; quiz 45–46.

50 Garg S, Zisser H, Schwartz S, Bailey T, Kaplan R, Ellis S, *et al.* Improvement in glycemic excursions with a transcutaneous, real-time continuous glucose sensor: a randomized controlled trial. *Diabetes Care* 2006; **29**:44–50.

51 Garg S, Jovanovic L. Relationship of fasting and hourly blood glucose levels to HbA1c values: safety, accuracy, and improvements in glucose profiles obtained using a 7-day continuous glucose sensor. *Diabetes Care* 2006; **29**:2644–2649.

52 Deiss D, Bolinder J, Riveline JP, Battelino T, Bosi E, Tubiana-Rufi N, *et al.* Improved glycemic control in poorly controlled patients with type 1 diabetes using real-time continuous glucose monitoring. *Diabetes Care* 2006; **29**:2730–2732.

53 Hirsch IB, Abelseth J, Bode BW, Fischer JS, Kaufman FR, Mastrototaro J, *et al.* Sensor-augmented insulin pump therapy: results of the first randomized treat-to-target study. *Diabetes Technol Ther* 2008; **10**: 377–383.

54 JDRF CGM. Study Group. JDRF randomized clinical trial to assess the efficacy of real-time continuous glucose monitoring in the management of type 1 diabetes: research design and methods. *Diabetes Technol Ther* 2008; **10**:310–321.

55 Tamborlane WV, Beck RW, Bode BW, Buckingham B, Chase HP, Clemons R, *et al.* Continuous glucose monitoring and intensive treatment of type 1 diabetes. *N Engl J Med* 2008; **359**:1464–1476.

56 Tamborlane WV, Beck RW, Bode BW, Buckingham B, Chase HP, Clemons R, *et al.* The effect of continuous glucose monitoring in well-controlled type 1 diabetes. *Diabetes Care* 2009; in print.

57 Monsod TP, Flanagan DE, Rife F, Saenz R, Caprio S, Sherwin RS, *et al.* Do sensor glucose levels accurately predict plasma glucose concentrations during hypoglycemia and hyperinsulinemia? *Diabetes Care* 2002; **25**:889–893.

58 Rebrin K, Steil GM, van Antwerp WP, Mastrototaro JJ. Subcutaneous glucose predicts plasma glucose independent of insulin: implications for continuous monitoring. *Am J Physiol* 1999; **277**:E561–E571.

59 Buckingham BA, Kollman C, Beck R, Kalajian A, Fiallo-Scharer R, Tansey MJ, *et al.* Evaluation of factors affecting CGMS calibration. *Diabetes Technol Ther* 2006; **8**:318–325.

60 Moberg E, Hagstrom-Toft E, Arner P, Bolinder J. Protracted glucose fall in subcutaneous adipose tissue and skeletal muscle compared with blood during insulin-induced hypoglycemia. *Diabetologia* 1997; **40**:1320–1326.

61 Wilson DM, Beck RW, Tamborlane WV, Dontchev MJ, Kollman C, Chase P, *et al.* The accuracy of the FreeStyle Navigator continuous glucose monitoring system in children with type 1 diabetes. *Diabetes Care* 2007; **30**:59–64.

62 Cheyne EH, Cavan DA, Kerr D. Performance of a continuous glucose monitoring system during controlled hypoglycemia in healthy volunteers. *Diabetes Technol Ther* 2002; **4**:607–613.

63 Buckingham B, Xing D, Weinzimer S, Fiallo-Scharer R, Kollman C, Mauras N, *et al.* Use of the DirecNet Applied Treatment Algorithm (DATA) for diabetes management with a real-time continuous glucose monitor (the FreeStyle Navigator). *Pediatr Diabetes* 2008; **9**:142–147.

64 Wolpert HA. Establishing a continuous glucose monitoring program. *J Diabetes Sci Technol* 2008; **2**:307.

65 Wolpert HA. The nuts and bolts of achieving end points with real-time continuous glucose monitoring. *Diabetes Care* 2008; **31**(Suppl 2):S146–S149.

66 Hovorka R. The future of continuous glucose monitoring: closed loop. *Curr Diabetes Rev* 2008; **4**:269–279.

67 Hovorka R. Continuous glucose monitoring and closed-loop systems. *Diabet Med* 2006; **23**:1–12.

68 Russell S. Continuous glucose monitoring awaits its "killer app". *J Diabetes Sci Technol* 2008; **2**:490–494.

69 Steil GM, Rebrin K, Darwin C, Hariri F, Saad MF. Feasibility of automating insulin delivery for the treatment of type 1 diabetes. *Diabetes* 2006; **55**:3344–3350.

70 Weinzimer SA, Steil GM, Swan KL, Dziura J, Kurtz N, Tamborlane WV. Fully automated closed-loop insulin delivery versus semi-automated hybrid control in pediatric patients with type 1 diabetes using an artificial pancreas. *Diabetes Care* 2008; **31**:934–939.

71 Plank J, Blaha J, Cordingley J, Wilinska ME, Chassin LJ, Morgan C, *et al.* Multicentric, randomized, controlled trial to evaluate blood glucose control by the model predictive control algorithm versus routine glucose management protocols in intensive care unit patients. *Diabetes Care* 2006; **29**:271–276.

72 Cordingley JJ, Vlasselaers D, Dormand NC, Wouters PJ, Squire SD, Chassin LJ, *et al.* Intensive insulin therapy: enhanced Model Predictive Control algorithm versus standard care. *Intensive Care Med* 2009; **35**:123–128.

73 Hunt LM, Valenzuela MA, Pugh JA. NIDDM patients' fears and hopes about insulin therapy. The basis of patient reluctance. *Diabetes Care* 1997; **20**:292–298.

74 Zambanini A, Newson RB, Maisey M, Feher MD. Injection related anxiety in insulin-treated diabetes. *Diabetes Res Clin Pract* 1999; **46**:239–246.

75 Ceglia L, Lau J, Pittas AG. Meta-analysis: efficacy and safety of inhaled insulin therapy in adults with diabetes mellitus. *Ann Intern Med* 2006; **145**:665–675.

76 Quattrin T, Belanger A, Bohannon NJ, Schwartz SL. Efficacy and safety of inhaled insulin (Exubera) compared with subcutaneous insulin therapy in patients with type 1 diabetes: results of a 6-month, randomized, comparative trial. *Diabetes Care* 2004; **27**:2622–2627.

77 Hollander PA, Blonde L, Rowe R, Mehta AE, Milburn JL, Hershon KS, *et al.* Efficacy and safety of inhaled insulin (exubera) compared with subcutaneous insulin therapy in patients with type 2 diabetes: results of a 6-month, randomized, comparative trial. *Diabetes Care* 2004; **27**:2356–2362.

78 Himmelmann A, Jendle J, Mellen A, Petersen AH, Dahl UL, Wollmer P. The impact of smoking on inhaled insulin. *Diabetes Care* 2003; **26**:677–682.

79 Becker RH, Sha S, Frick AD, Fountaine RJ. The effect of smoking cessation and subsequent resumption on absorption of inhaled insulin. *Diabetes Care* 2006; **29**:277–282.

80 Fountaine R, Milton A, Checchio T, Wei G, Stolar M, Teeter J, *et al.* Acute passive cigarette smoke exposure and inhaled human insulin (Exubera) pharmacokinetics. *Br J Clin Pharmacol* 2008; **65**:864–870.

81 Rosenstock J, Bergenstal R, Defronzo RA, Hirsch IB, Klonoff D, Boss AH, *et al.* Efficacy and safety of Technosphere inhaled insulin compared with Technosphere powder placebo in insulin-naive type 2 diabetes suboptimally controlled with oral agents. *Diabetes Care* 2008; **31**:2177–2182.

82 Pfutzner A, Mann AE, Steiner SS. Technosphere/Insulin: a new approach for effective delivery of human insulin via the pulmonary route. *Diabetes Technol Ther* 2002; **4**:589–594.

29 Oral Antidiabetic Agents

Clifford J. Bailey[1] & Andrew J. Krentz[2]

[1] School of Life and Health Sciences, Aston University, Birmingham, UK
[2] Formerly, Department of Diabetes and Endocrinology, Southampton University Hospitals NHS Trust, Southampton, UK

Keypoints

- Glycemic control is a fundamental part of the management of type 2 diabetes mellitus. Adequate glycemic control is necessary to address acute symptoms and to prevent, defer or reduce the severity of chronic microvascular and macrovascular complications.
- Treating type 2 diabetes is complicated by the multivariable and progressive natural history of the disease. Insulin resistance, a progressive decline in β-cell function, defects of other gluco-regulatory hormones and nutrient metabolism give rise to a continually changing presentation of the disease that requires therapy to be adjusted accordingly. Patients are often overweight or obese, exhibit substantial co-morbidity and elevated cardiovascular risk, and receive many other medications which further complicate treatment.
- Care plans and treatment programs should be tailored to fit the prevailing circumstances of the patient. Lifestyle management (diet and exercise) should be emphasized from the time of diagnosis and reinforced thereafter. Drug treatment should be undertaken promptly if lifestyle intervention does not achieve adequate glycemic control.
- Choice of drug therapy should ideally address underlying pathophysiology, but any safe means of restraining the escalating hyperglycemia may be appropriate. Combinations of differently acting agents are frequently required to provide additive efficacy, and single tablet, fixed dose combinations are available to facilitate combination therapy. Contraindications and precautions associated with each component must be respected.
- The biguanide metformin is often selected as initial oral antidiabetic drug therapy. It counters insulin resistance and lowers blood glucose through several insulin-dependent and independent mechanisms, notably reducing hepatic glucose production and also increasing glucose uptake by skeletal muscle. It does not stimulate insulin secretion, carries a low risk of frank hypoglycemia and does not cause weight gain. Metformin also exerts several potentially beneficial effects on cardiovascular risk factors independently of glycemic control, with evidence of improved long-term cardiovascular outcomes. Metformin may be conveniently combined with other classes of antidiabetic drugs. Gastrointestinal side effects including diarrhoea limit the use of metformin. The rare but serious adverse effect of lactic acidosis excludes the use of the drug in patients with significant renal insufficiency, significant liver disease or any condition predisposing to hypoxia or hypoperfusion including cardiac or respiratory failure.
- Sulfonylureas (e.g. gliclazide, glimepiride, glibenclamide/glyburide, glipizide) act on the pancreatic β-cells to stimulate insulin secretion. They bind to the transmembranal complex of sulfonylurea receptors SUR1 with ATP-sensitive Kir6.2 potassium efflux channels. This closes the channels, depolarizes the membrane, opens voltage-dependent calcium channels and raises intracellular free calcium concentrations. This in turn activates proteins regulating insulin secretion. The efficacy of sulfonylureas depends on adequate remaining function of the β-cells. Hypoglycemia is the most serious adverse effect, particularly with longer acting sulfonylureas and in the elderly. Caution with hepatic and/or renal insufficiency is warranted in accordance with the metabolism and elimination of individual preparations, and interactions with other protein-bound drugs can occur.
- Meglitinides (repaglinide and nateglinide), also known as prandial insulin releasers, are rapid and short-acting insulin secretagogues taken before meals to boost insulin levels during digestion, thereby reducing prandial hyperglycemia and decreasing risk of interprandial hypoglycemia. They act in a similar manner to sulfonylureas by binding to a "benzamido" site on the SUR1–Kir6.2 complex. They are conveniently used in combination with an agent that reduces insulin resistance.
- Thiazolidinediones (pioglitazone and rosiglitazone) produce a slow-onset glucose-lowering effect, attributed mainly to increased insulin sensitivity. They alter the expression of certain insulin-sensitive genes by stimulating the peroxisome proliferator-activated receptor γ, increasing adipogenesis, and rebalancing the glucose–fatty acid (Randle) cycle. Thiazolidinediones can be used as monotherapy or in combination with other classes of antidiabetic agents. They have low risk of hypoglycemia but often cause weight gain. The potential for fliud retention and an attendant risk of congestive heart failure should be borne in mind, especially in combination with insulin. Thiazolidinediones are not recommended for individuals at high risk of cardiac disease or women with reduced bone density.

Textbook of Diabetes, 4th edition. Edited by R. Holt, C. Cockram, A. Flyvbjerg and B. Goldstein. © 2010 Blackwell Publishing.

- Gliptins (sitagliptin, vildagliptin and saxagliptin) act predominantly as prandial insulin secretagogues by raising the circulating concentrations of endogenous incretin hormones, notably glucagon-like peptide 1 and glucose-dependent insulinotropic polypeptide. Incretin hormones are released from the intestine during a meal and potentiate nutrient-stimulated insulin secretion, but they are rapidly degraded by the enzyme dipeptidyl peptidase 4: gliptins inhibit this enzyme. Gliptins are weight neutral and, as monotherapy, they carry low risk of interprandial hypoglycemia. They are often used in combination with metformin or a thiazolidinedione.
- α-Glucosidase inhibitors (e.g. acarbose) slow the digestion of carbohydrates by competitive inhibition of intestinal α-glucosidase enzymes. This delays glucose absorption and reduces post-prandial glucose excursions without stimulating insulin secretion. These agents must be used in conjunction with meals rich in digestible complex carbohydrate. They do not cause weight gain or hypoglycemia as monotherapy and can be used alongside any other antidiabetic agents.
- In advanced stages of type 2 diabetes, β-cell function is often too severely compromised to support the continued use of oral agents alone. Insulin therapy should be initiated, continuing one or more oral agents where appropriate.

Table 29.1 Aims of appropriate glycemic control in type 2 diabetes. Adapted from Wallace & Matthews [1].

Purpose	Complications
Prevent acute symptoms of hyperglycemia	Dehydration, thirst, polyuria, blurred vision, increased infections
Prevent acute complications	Hyperosmolar non-ketotic state
Prevent, defer or reduce severity of chronic vascular complications	Microvascular: retinopathy, nephropathy, neuropathy Macrovascular: coronary, cerebrovascular, peripheral vascular

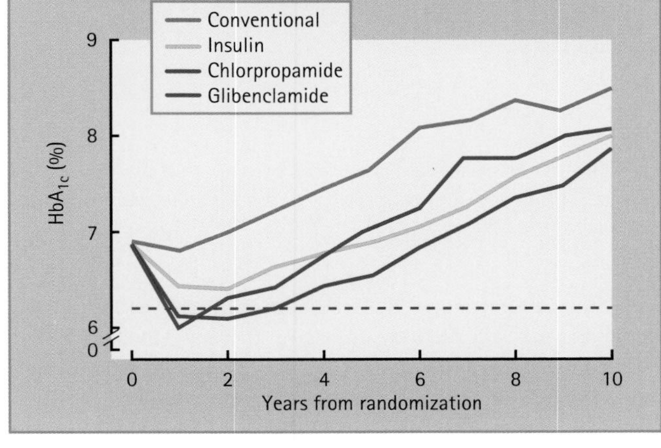

Figure 29.1 The UK Prospective Diabetes Study (UKPDS) shows the progressive rise in HbA_{1c} occurring with time in groups receiving "conventional" (diet) therapy and "intensive" therapy with various antidiabetic drugs (two sulfonylureas – chlorpropamide and glibenclamide – and insulin). Data from Wallace & Matthews [1] and UKPDS [12].

Introduction

Appropriate glycemic control is a fundamental pillar in the management of type 2 diabetes mellitus (T2DM). It is required to prevent and relieve acute symptoms and complications of hyperglycemia; prevent, defer and reduce the severity of microvascular complications; and afford some benefits against macrovascular complications (Table 29.1) (see Chapters 20) [1,2]. Treatment of the hyperglycemia is essential to an individualized care plan that takes account of coexistent diseases and personal circumstances, offers suitable advice on lifestyle and diet, includes other measures to address modifiable cardiovascular risk, selects realistic targets, and facilitates patient education and empowerment, as considered in detail in Part 5. This chapter focuses on the role of oral blood glucose-lowering agents (other antidiabetic therapies are addressed in Chapters 27 and 30) in the treatment of T2DM) [2–5].

Pathophysiologic considerations

The interdependent multiplicity of genetic and environmental factors underlying T2DM (see Chapters 12 and 14) give rise to a highly heterogeneous and progressive natural history [2,6,7]. The pathophysiology typically involves defects of insulin secretion *and* insulin action [8]. Obesity, especially visceral adiposity, and abnormalities of glucagon secretion commonly contribute to the disease process, while cellular disturbances of nutrient metabolism participate both as causes and consequences of glucotoxicity and lipotoxicity [9–11]. An ideal approach to therapy might therefore address the basic endocrine defects, but any other safe means of ameliorating the hyperglycemia and attendant biochemical disruptions should provide clinical benefits.

The progressive nature of T2DM was well-illustrated by the UK Prospective Diabetes Study (UKPDS), a randomized trial of 5102 patients with newly diagnosed T2DM followed for a median of 10 years while receiving either "conventional" (diet) therapy or "intensive" therapy with various oral antidiabetic agents or insulin (Figure 29.1). Note that insulin was introduced earlier than is usual in clinical practice, and insulin was also used as necessary when oral agents were deemed inadequate. Although glycemic control (illustrated by the HbA_{1c} level) deteriorated

Table 29.2 Trials comparing intensive with standard (conventional) glycemic control in type 2 diabetes.

Trial	Number	Duration of follow-up	Age	Duration of diabetes	Baseline HbA_{1c}%	Intensive HbA_{1c}%		Conventional HbA_{1c}%	Relative risk reduction			
									Microvascular		Macrovascular	
									%	*P*	%	*P*
UKPDS	3867[a]	10	53	New	7.1[b]	7.0	vs	7.9	↓ 25%	0.009	↓ 16%[c]	0.052[d]
UKPDS (post-trial follow-up)	2998	8.5	63	10	–		–		↓ 24%	0.001	↓ 15%[c]	0.014
ADVANCE	11,140	5	66	8	7.5	6.5	vs	7.3	↓ 14%	0.01	↓ 6%	0.32[b]
ACCORD[e]	10,251	3.5[e]	62	10	8.3	6.4[e]	vs	7.5	↓ 33%	0.005[f]	↓ 10%	0.16[b]
VADT	1791	5.6	60	11.5	9.4	6.9	vs	8.4	↓ 2.5[g]	0.05	↓ 12%	0.14[b]

ACCORD, Action to Control Cardiovascular Risk in Diabetes; ADVANCE, Action in Diabetes and Vascular Disease: Preterax and Diamicron-MR Controlled Evaluation; UKPDS, UK Prospective Diabetes Study; VADT, Veterans Affairs Diabetes Trial.

[a] Non-obese patients.

[b] After a 3-month dietary run-in.

[c] Myocardial infarction.

[d] Non-significant.

[e] Intensive therapy discontinued at median 3.5 years because of increased deaths in the intensive (257/5128; 5%) versus conventional (203/5123; 4%) group.

[f] Reduction in new or worsening nephropathy. No effect on incidence of progression of retinopathy.

[g] Any increase in albuminuria.

with time irrespective of the treatment, the improvement in glycemic control afforded by intensive therapy (median HbA_{1c} reduced by 0.9% [10 mmol/mol]) was associated with a 12% reduction in overall diabetes-related endpoints and a 25% reduction in microvascular endpoints [12]. An epidemiologic analysis showed that benefits of intensive therapy continued to accrue until glucose levels were returned to the normal range [13]. Moreover, the benefits of earlier "intensive" control were continued during an unrandomized post-trial follow-up (median 8.5 years) during which glycemic differences between the former groups were not maintained [14]. This illustrates the glycemic "legacy" effect in which early intensive glycemic control confers an extended reduction in complications, even when control deteriorates at later stages in the disease process.

Other large randomized trials [15–17] have confirmed fewer microvascular complications amongst those receiving more intensive glycemic management (Table 29.2). One such study, the Action to Control Cardiovascular Risk in Diabetes (ACCORD) study, noted increased mortality during highly intensified (5% mortality, 257/5128) versus standard (4% mortality, 205/5123) glycemic management. This may be ascribed to unique features of the trial design outside of normal practice in an aging population at high cardiovascular risk with a long previous duration of inadequately controlled diabetes given extensive medications and experiencing high rates of hypoglycemia. Indeed, an acceptable HbA_{1c} value does not preclude excessive daily fluctuations in glycemia with hyperglycemic excursions and hypoglycemic troughs, the latter often unrecognized nocturnally (see Chapter 33). Survival of a myocardial event appears to be reduced by hypoglycemia as well as hyperglycemia [18].

Guidelines and algorithms

Factors to consider when selecting a glycemic target for a particular patient are deliberated in detail in Chapter 20, but it is pertinent to reiterate here that the general principle is to safely return glycemia as close to normal as practicable, avoiding hypoglycemia, minimizing potential drug interactions, and observing other necessary cautions and contraindications. An individualized approach is recommended. Current treatment algorithms [19–25] provide a framework for initiating and intensifying therapy, but clinical judgment should be applied to harmonize this with patient circumstances. Thus, a younger, newly diagnosed individual without co-morbidity who is responsive to therapy might be expected to meet a more rigorous target, while an elderly infirm individual with co-morbidity and a long history of problems with diabetes control may require more flexiblity. Management of hyperglycemia should always be part of a comprehensive management program to address coexistent disease and modifiable cardiovascuar risk factors.

It is emphasized that diet, exercise and other lifestyle measures should be introduced at diagnosis and reinforced at every appropriate opportunity thereafter. These measures can provide valuable blood glucose lowering efficacy and may initially enable the desired glycemic target to be achieved (see Chapters 22 and 23); however, even when lifestyle advice is successfully implemented, the progressive natural history of the disease dictates that the majority of patients will later require pharmacologic therapy, and this should be introduced promply if the glycemic target is not met or not maintained.

The main classes of oral antidiabetic drugs and their principal modes of action are listed in Table 29.3. The main tissues through which they exert their glucose-lowering effects are illustrated in Figure 29.2, and the main cautions and contraindications associated with oral antidiabetic agents are listed in Table 29.4. Although there are several different classes from which to choose, many dilemmas continue to impinge on both strategy and individualization of treatment. For example, an increase in fasting glycemia usually accounts for the majority of the hyperglycemia in T2DM: ideally therefore, this should be adequately addressed during therapy [26]. It is also pertinent to note the link between postprandial hyperglycemic excursions and cardiovascular risk, which mandates the need to also address this component of the hyperglycemic day profile [27]. Additionally, consideration should be given to the improvements in glycemic control that can be achieved through the treatment of obesity (see Chapter 14) [28]. By the time of diagnosis, insulin resistance is usually well established and does not usually progress with extended duration of the disease [8]. Nevertheless, the association between insulin resistance and cardiovascular risk warrants the amelioration of insulin resistance as a valued therapeutic strategy. The ongoing deterioration in glycemic control after diagnosis is largely attributed to a further progressive decline in β-cell function [8]. Thus, preserving β-cell function and mass are important considerations in maintaining long-term glycemic control. If β-cell function deteriorates beyond the capacity of oral agents to provide adequate glycemic control, then the introduction of insulin should not be delayed. Incorporating some or all of the above into the treatment process is inevitably a challenge, and the need to explore suitable combinations of therapies to accommodate the changing status of the disease is now accepted practice.

The increasing prevalence of T2DM amongst younger adults and pre-adults adds an extra long-term dimension to risk–benefit

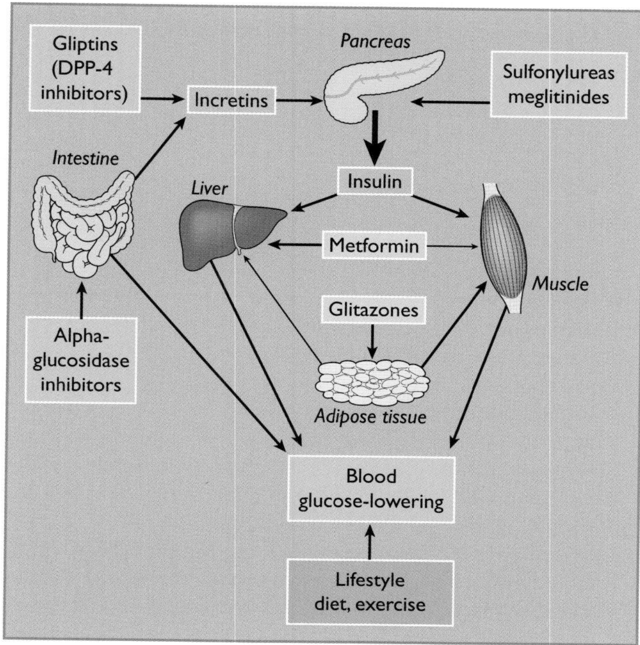

Figure 29.2 Main tissues through which oral antidiabetic agents exert their glucose-lowering effects.

Table 29.3 Classes of oral antidiabetic drugs and their main modes of action.

Class with examples	Main mode of glucose-lowering	Main cellular mechanism of action
Biguanide		
Metformin	Counter insulin resistance (especially decrease hepatic glucose output)	Enhance various insulin dependent and independent actions including AMPK
Sulfonylureas		
Glimepiride, gliclazide, glyburide/glibenclamide, glipizide	Stimulate insulin secretion (typically 6–24 hours)	Bind to SUR1 sulfonylurea receptors on pancreatic β-cells, which closes ATP-sensitive Kir6.2 potassium channels
Meglitinides		
Repaglinide, nateglinide	Stimulate insulin secretion (faster onset and shorter duration of action than sulfonylureas)	Bind to benzamido site on SUR1 receptors on pancreatic β-cells, which closes ATP-sensitive Kir6.2 potassium channels
Gliptins (DPP-4 inhibitors)		
Sitagliptin, vildagliptin, saxagliptin	Increase prandial insulin secretion	Inhibit DPP-4 enzyme, which increases plasma half-life of insulinotropic incretin hormones
Thiazolidinediones (PPAR-γ agonists)		
Pioglitazone, rosiglitazone	Increase insulin sensitivity (especially increase peripheral glucose utilization)	Activate nuclear receptor PPAR-γ mainly in adipose tissue, which affects insulin action and glucose–fatty acid cycle
α-Glucosidase inhibitors		
Acarbose, miglitol, voglibose	Slow rate of carbohydrate digestion	Competitive inhibition of intestinal α-glucosidase enzymes

AMPK, adenosine 5′-monophosphate-activated protein kinase; ATP, adenosine triphosphate; DPP-4, dipeptidyl peptidase 4; PPAR-γ, peroxisome proliferator-activated receptor γ.

Table 29.4 General features of oral antidiabetic treatments for type 2 diabetes including the main cautions and contraindications.

	Metformin	Sulfonylureas	Meglitinides	Thiazolidinediones	Gliptins	α-Glucosidase inhibitors
HbA_{1c}	↓ 1–2%	↓ 1–2%	↓ 0.5–1.5%[h]	↓ 1–1.5%	↓ 0.5–1.5%[h]	↓ 0.5–1%[h]
Body weight	–/↓	↑	↑/–	↑	–	–
Lipids	–/+	–	–	+/–/×	–	–/+
Blood pressure	–	–	–	↓/–	–	–
Tolerability	GI[a]	Hypo[f]	Hypo[i]	Fluid[d]	–	GI[a]
Safety	LA[b]	Hypo[f]	Hypo[i]	Edema Anemia Heart failure[e] Fractures	–	–
Cautions	Renal Liver Hypoxemia[c]	Liver Renal[g]	Liver Renal[g]	CV[e]	–[j]	–

CV, cardiovascular; GI, gastrointestinal; HbA_{1c}, glycated hemoglobin (1% = ~11 mmol/mol); Hypo, hypoglycemia; LA, lactic acidosis.
↑ Increased; ↓ decreased; – neutral; + benefit; × impair.
[a] Gastrointestinal side effects.
[b] Lactic acidosis (rare).
[c] Check for adequate renal and hepatic function, avoid in conditions with heightened risk of hypoxemia.
[d] Fluid retention, anemia, increased risk of heart failure in susceptible patients.
[e] Check for pre-existing cardiovascular disease or developing signs of heart disease: controversy regarding possible early increase in myocardial infarction with rosiglitazone not confirmed in long-term prospective studies.
[f] Risk of hypoglycemia, occasionally severe.
[g] Check liver and/or renal function relevant to mode of metabolism/elimination.
[h] Mostly act to lower post-prandial hyperglycemia – lesser impact on fasting glycemia and on HbA_{1c}.
[i] Lesser risk of severe hypoglycemia than sulfonylurea.
[j] Monitoring of liver function with vildagliptin.

considerations. While initial adequate intervention remains paramount, there is limited experience with oral antidiabetic agents in children and adolescents; metformin has been used safely in controlled pediatric practice from 10 years of age, and sulfonylureas have been used in pediatric presentations of certain forms of maturity-onset diabetes of the young (MODY). Treating T2DM in women who are of childbearing age carries the risk of unplanned pregnancy while receiving oral antidiabetic agents. Treatment with these agents at the time of conception and during the first trimester has not been shown to have any adverse effects on mother or fetus, and judicious use of metformin has been shown to reduce miscarriage and gestational diabetes. Insulin remains the preferred antidiabetic medication in pregnancy, however, having a substantial evidence base for safety and flexibility. A paucity of evidence contraindicates thiazolidinediones and gliptins during pregnancy and lactation.

Elderly patients are more vulnerable to most of the cautions and contraindications to glucose-lowering drugs, and deteriorations in their pathophysiologic status can occur rapidly, necessitating more frequent monitoring (see Chapter 54). Hypoglycemia is a particular concern in this age group. While safety must be judged on an individual drug–patient basis, it is noteworthy that several common medications can impair glycemic control (e.g. glucocorticoids, certain antipsychotics, diuretics and beta-blockers), while others may have their own minor glucose-lowering effect (e.g. aspirin, some angiotensin-converting enzyme [ACE] inhibitors and mineral supplements) (see Chapter 26). The most frequent interactions with glucose-lowering drugs are summarized in Table 29.5.

Terminology within the field of antidiabetic agents may simplify the usage of the different agents. Hypoglycemic agents have the capacity to lower blood glucose below normal to the extent of frank hypoglycemia (e.g. sulfonylureas and insulin). Antihyperglycemic agents can reduce hyperglycemia, but when acting alone they do not have the capability to lower blood glucose below normoglycemia to the extent of frank hypoglycema (e.g. metformin, thiazolidinediones, incretins, gliptins, α-glucosidase inhibitors).

Biguanides

Metformin (dimethylbiguanide) is the only biguanide currently used in most countries (Figure 29.3). The history of biguanides stems from a guanidine-rich herb *Galega officinalis* (goat's rue or French lilac) that was used as a traditional treatment for diabetes in Europe [29]. Guanidine has a glucose-lowering effect, and several guanidine derivatives were adopted for the treatment of

Table 29.5 Drug interactions with oral antidiabetic agents that may affect their glucose-lowering effects.

Antidiabetic agent	Increase glucose lowering	Decrease glucose lowering
Any	Combination with other antidiabetic drugs Minor insulin releasers (e.g. aspirin) Minor insulin sensitivity enhancers, e.g. ACE inhibitors, magnesium or chromium supplements	Agents that impair insulin action (e.g. glucocorticoids, some antipsychotics, minor effects of diuretics, beta-blockers, some β_2-agonists) Impair insulin secretion (e.g. octreotide, some calcium channel blockers)
Metformin	Renal cation secretion competition by cimetidine Minor PK interaction with furosemide and nifedipine	–
Sulfonylureas	Reduce hepatic metabolism (e.g. some antifungals and MAOIs) Displace plasma protein binding (e.g. coumarins, NSAIDs, sulfonamides) Decrease excretion (e.g. probenecid)	K^+–ATP channel openers (e.g. diazoxide) Metabolism secondary to enzyme induction (e.g. rifampicin)
Meglitinides	Reduce hepatic metabolism, gemfibrozil Potentially displace plasma protein binding	Metabolism secondary to enzyme induction (e.g rifampicin, barbiturates, carbamazepine)
Thiazolidinediones	Reduce hepatic metabolism, gemfibrozil Potentially displace plasma protein binding	Metabolism secondary to enzyme induction (e.g rifampicin)
Gliptins	Potential interactions with liver and renal metabolism and plasma protein binding	–
α-Glucosidase inhibitors	Slow gut motility (e.g. cholestyramine)	Potentially with agents that increase gut motility

ACE, angiotensin-converting enzyme; MAOI, mono oxidase inhibitor; NSAID, non-steroidal anti-inflammatory drug; PK, pharmacokinetic.

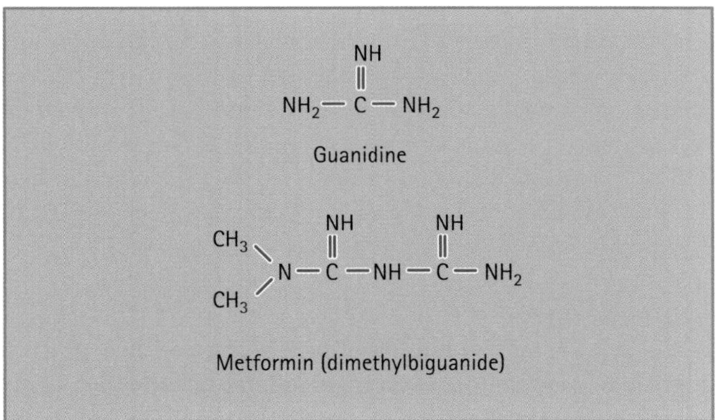

Figure 29.3 Chemical structures of guanidine and metformin.

diabetes in the 1920s [30]. These agents all but disappeared as insulin became available, but three biguanides – metformin, phenformin and buformin – were introduced in the late 1950s. Phenformin and buformin were withdrawn in many countries in the late 1970s because of a high incidence of lactic acidosis. Metformin remained and was introduced into the USA in 1995 [31], and this has since become the most prescribed antidiabetic agent worldwide [32].

Mode of action

Metformin exerts a range of actions that counter insulin resistance and lower blood glucose: the drug also offers some protection against vascular complications independently of its antihyperglycemic effect (Table 29.6) [33,34]. At the cellular

Table 29.6 Diverse metabolic and vascular effects of metformin.

Features associated with diabetes		Effects of metformin
Hyperglycemia	↓	↓ HGP, ↑ peripheral glucose uptake ↑ glucose turnover
Insulin resistance	↓	↑ Receptor–postreceptor insulin signals
Hyperinsulinemia	↓	↓ Fasting and often post-prandial insulin
Obesity	↓/–	↓ or stabilizes body weight
IGT	↓	↓ Progression to type 2 diabetes
Dyslipidemia	↓/–	Modest benefits if abnormal ↓ VLDL-TG, ↓ LDL, ↑ HDL May decrease FA oxidation
Blood pressure	–	No significant effect
Pro-coagulant state	↓	Antithrombotic (↓ fibrinogen, ↓PAI-1, ↓ platelet aggregation)
Endothelial function	↑	↓ Vascular adhesion molecules
Atherosclerosis	↓	↓ MI, ↓ stroke, ↑ vascular reactivity, ↓ cIMT, ↑ life expectancy, anti-atherogenic in animals

↑ Increase; ↓ decrease; – no significant effect; cIMT, carotid intima-media thickness; FA, fatty acid; HDL, high density lipoprotein cholesterol; HGP, hepatic glucose production; IGT, impaired glucose tolerance; LDL, low density lipoprotein cholesterol; MI, myocardial infarction; PAI-1, plasminogen-activator inhibitor-1; VLDL-TG, very low density lipoprotein cholesterol triglyceride.

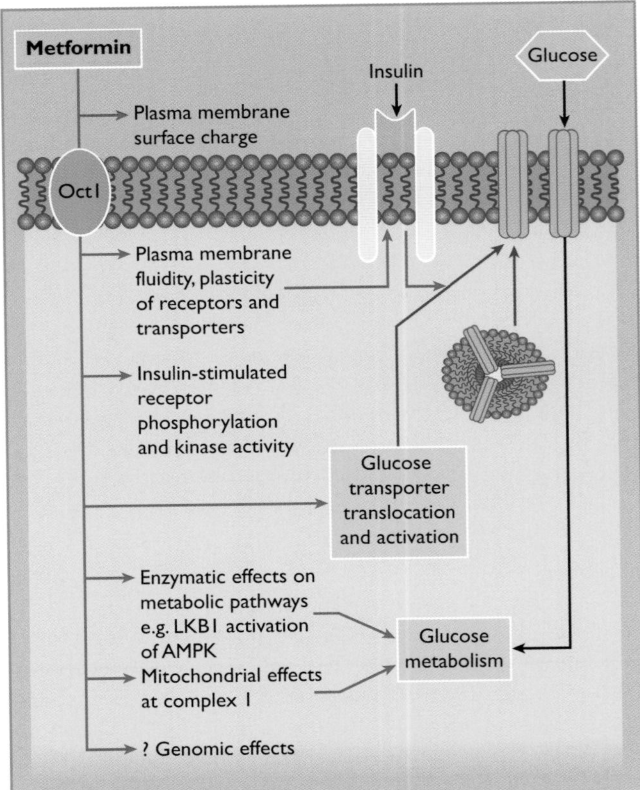

Figure 29.4 Multiple cellular action mechanisms of metformin involve insulin dependent and independent effects. For example, metformin can improve insulin sensitivity via effects on insulin receptor signaling and post-receptor signaling pathways of insulin action. Metformin also appears to influence cellular nutrient metabolism and energy production independently of insulin via activation of adenosine 5′-monophosphate (AMP) activated protein kinase (AMPK). Oct1, organic cation transporter 1; LKB1 protein kinase.

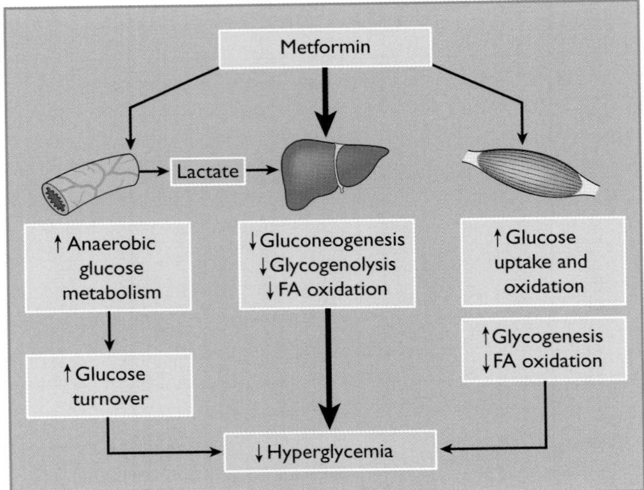

Figure 29.5 Main sites of action of metformin contributing to glucose-lowering effect.

level, metformin exerts insulin-dependent and independent effects on glucose metabolism (Figure 29.4). For example, metformin modestly improves insulin sensitivity probably via post-receptor signaling pathways for insulin, and it also appears to influence nutrient metabolism and energy production independently of insulin via activation of adenosine 5′-monophosphate-activated protein kinase (AMPK) [35].

The glucose-lowering efficacy of metformin requires a presence of at least some insulin because metformin does not mimic or activate the genomic effects of insulin. Also, metformin does not stimulate insulin release; its main glucose-lowering effect appears to be a reduction of hepatic glucose production, but not sufficiently to cause frank hypoglycemia when used as monotherapy. Metformin reduces gluconeogenesis by increasing hepatic insulin sensitivity and by decreasing hepatic extraction of some gluconeogenic substrates such as lactate (Figure 29.5). It also decreases hepatic glycogenolysis. Metformin can enhance insulin-stimulated glucose uptake in skeletal muscle by increasing translocation of insulin-sensitive glucose transporters (GLUT-4) into the cell membrane and increasing activity of glycogen synthase which promotes glycogen synthesis. Independently of insulin, metformin can suppress the oxidation of fatty acids and may reduce triglyceride levels in patients with hypertriglyceridemia. This restricts the supply of energy for hepatic gluconeogenesis and rebalances the glucose–fatty acid (Randle) cycle, allowing greater use of glucose relative to fatty acids as a cellular source of energy. Accumulation of a high cellular concentration of metformin (e.g. in the intestine) can suppress the mitochondrial respiratory chain at complex 1. This may contribute to the blood glucose-lowering effect of the drug, and help to prevent body weight gain by increasing glucose–lactate turnover.

Pharmacokinetics

Metformin is rapidly but incompletely absorbed, shows little binding to plasma proteins and is not metabolized, so it does not interfere with co-administered drugs. Metformin is widely distributed at concentrations similar to plasma (about 10^{-5} mol/L), but much higher concentrations are retained in the walls of the gastrointestinal tract. The plasma half-life ($t_{1/2}$) is about 6 hours with elimination of unchanged drug in the urine, mostly within 12 hours [36]. Although renal clearance is achieved more by tubular secretion than glomerular filtration, metformin is contraindicated for patients with significant impairment of glomerular filtration. Cimetidine is the only drug known to compete for clearance sufficiently to cause a clinically significant increase plasma metformin concentrations.

Indications and contraindications

Because metformin does not cause weight gain it is often preferred for overweight and obese people with T2DM, although it shows similar antihyperglycemic efficacy in normal weight patients [37]. To preclude drug accumulation, patient suitability should be considered very carefully if there is any evidence of impaired renal function (e.g. if serum creatinine >130 μmol/L or creatinine clearance <60 mL/min or estimated glomerular filtration rate [eGFR] <45 mL/min/1.73 m^2). Further contraindications include significant cardiac or respiratory insufficiency, or any other condition predisposing to hypoxia or reduced tissue perfusion (e.g. hypotension, septicemia), as well as significant liver disease, alcohol abuse or a history of metabolic acidosis. Because the potential for acute deterioration in renal, cardiopulmonary and hepatic function should be taken into account, it is not practicable to identify precise cutoffs for starting or stopping metformin therapy. With this in mind, metformin can be used in the elderly providing renal insufficiency and other exclusions are not present. Ovulation can resume in women with anovulatory polycystic ovarian syndrome (PCOS), which is an unlicensed application of the drug in the absence of diabetes [38].

A standard (so-called immediate release [IR]) tablet or liquid formulation of metformin should be taken with meals or immediately before meals to minimize possible gastrointestinal side effects. Start with 500 or 850 mg once daily, or 500 mg twice daily (divided between the morning and evening meals). The dosage is increased slowly – one tablet at a time – at intervals of about 1–2 weeks until the target level of blood glucose control is attained. If the target is not attained and an additional dose produces no further improvement, return to the previous dose. In the case of monotherapy, consider combination therapy by adding in another agent (e.g. an insulin secretagogue or thiazolidinedione). The maximal effective dosage of metformin is about 2000 mg/day, taken in divided doses with meals, and the maximum is 2550 or 3000 mg/day in different countries.

Slow-release formulations (XR/SR/ER) of metformin are available in most countries; they can be taken once daily in the morning, or if necessary morning and evening. Metformin can also be used in combination with any other class of antidiabetic agent including insulin, and several fixed dose combination tablets are available in which metformin is combined with either a sulfonylurea or thiazolidinedione or dipeptidyl peptidase 4 (DPP-4) inhibitor (see below). Recall that although metformin alone is unlikely to cause serious hypoglycemia, this can occur when metformin is used in combination with an insulin-releasing agent or insulin.

During long-term use of metformin it is advisable to check at least annually for emergence of contraindications, particularly renal (as a minimum, serum creatinine). Metformin can reduce gastrointestinal absorption of vitamin B_{12}, and although this is rarely a cause of frank anemia, an annual hemoglobin measurement is recommended especially for individuals with known or suspected nutritional deficiencies. Metformin should be temporarily stopped when using intravenous radiographic contrast media, or during surgery with general anesthesia or other intercurrent situations in which the exclusion criteria could be invoked. Substitution with insulin may be appropriate at such times.

Efficacy

As monotherapy in patients who are not adequately controlled by lifestyle management, optimally titrated metformin typically reduces fasting plasma glucose by 2–4 mmol/L, corresponding to a decrease in HbA_{1c} by approximately 1–2% (11–22 mmol/mol) [39]. This is largely independent of body weight, age and duration of diabetes provided that some β-cell function is still present. To accommodate the progressive nature of T2DM, it is likely that uptitration of dosage and addition of a second agent will be required to maintain glycemic control in the long term.

Metformin carries minimal risk of significant hypoglycemia or weight gain when used as monotherapy. It may lead to a reduction of basal insulin concentrations, notably in hyperinsulinemic patients, which should help to improve insulin sensitivity. Minor improvements in the blood lipid profile have been observed during metformin therapy, mostly in hyperlipidemic patients: plasma concentrations of triglycerides, fatty acids and low density lipoprotein (LDL) cholesterol tend to fall, whereas high density lipoprotein (HDL) cholesterol tends to rise [37]. These effects appear to be independent of the antihyperglycemic effect, although a lowering of triglyceride and free fatty acids is likely to help improve insulin sensitivity and benefit the glucose–fatty acid cycle.

In the UKPDS, overweight patients who started oral antidiabetic therapy with metformin showed a 39% reduced risk of myocardial infarction compared with conventional treatment ($P = 0.01$) [40]. There was no obvious relationship with metformin dosage, suggesting that patients who can only tolerate a low dosage of metformin may benefit from continuing the drug, even when other agents are required to achieve adequate glycemic control. The decrease in myocardial infarction was not related to the extent of the glucose-lowering effect of metformin, or effects on classic cardiovascular risk factors such as blood pressure or plasma lipids. Reported benefits of metformin on various atherothrombotic risk markers and factors have been reported, including reduced carotid intima-media thickness (cIMT) (Table 29.6), increased fibrinolysis and reduced concentrations of the antithrombolytic factor plasminogen activator inhibitor-1 (PAI-1) [34]. Detracting somewhat from the generally favorable cardiovascular risk reports there is evidence that combination of metformin with a sulfonylurea may initially increase cardiovascular mortality [40,41]. One potentially confounding factor might be greater cardiovascular risk caused by more severe metabolic disease in patients needing treatment with the combination [42]. Evidence from large databases with sulfonylurea plus metformin combination therapy have been reassuring [43,44]. Indeed, recent results from the post-trial follow-up of UKPDS (without continuation of randomized groups) showed that the cardiovascular benefits of metformin were maintained [14].

When metformin is added to the regimens of patients receiving insulin therapy, a reduction of insulin dosage is often required, consistent with the ability of metformin to improve insulin sensitivity. Similarly, addition of insulin in patients already receiving metformin usually requires lesser dosages of insulin and results in less weight gain. Lesser amounts of insulin are also associated with fewer and less severe episodes of hypoglycemia [44,45]. Although metformin is not indicated for the prevention of diabetes, it is noteworthy that the US Diabetes Prevention Program found metformin to reduce the incidence of new cases of diabetes in overweight and obese subjects with impaired glucose tolerance by 33%, compared with a reduced risk of 58% using an intensive regimen of diet and exercise [46]. The preventive effect of metformin was most evident amongst younger, more obese individuals.

Adverse effects

The main tolerability issue with metformin is abdominal discomfort and other gastrointestinal adverse effects, including diarrhea. These are often transient and can be ameliorated by taking the drug with meals and titrating the dose slowly. Symptoms may remit if the dose is reduced, but around 10% of patients cannot tolerate the drug at any dose. The most serious adverse event associated with metformin is lactic acidosis; it is rare (probably about 0.03 cases per 1000 patient-years), but about half of cases are fatal [31,47,48]. Because the background incidence of lactic acidosis amongst patients with T2DM has not been established, it is possible that some cases previously attributed to metformin were caused by other factors.

Most reported cases of lactic acidosis in patients receiving metformin have been caused by inappropriate prescription, particularly overlooking renal insufficiency. The resulting accumulation of metformin is likely to increase lactate production, and increasing lactate will be aggravated by any hypoxic condition or impaired liver function. Hyperlactatemia occurs in cardiogenic shock and other illnesses that decrease tissue perfusion, so metformin may only be an incidental factor in some cases. Nevertheless, metformin should be stopped immediately in all cases of suspected or proven lactic acidosis, regardless of cause.

Lactic acidosis is typically characterized by a raised blood lactate concentration (e.g. >5 mmol/L), decreased arterial pH and/or bicarbonate concentration with an increased anion gap ($[Na^+] - [Cl^- + HCO_3^-]$ >15 mmol/L). Presenting symptoms are generally non-specific, but often include hyperventilation, malaise and abdominal discomfort. Treatment should be commenced promptly without waiting to determine whether metformin is a cause; bicarbonate remains the usual therapy, but evidence of its efficacy is limited. Hemodialysis to remove excess metformin can be helpful, and may assist restoration of fluid and electrolyte balance during treatment with high-dose intravenous bicarbonate.

Sulfonylureas

Since their introduction in the 1950s, sulfonylureas have been used extensively as insulin secretagogues for the treatment of T2DM. Sulfonylureas were developed as structural variants of sulfonamides after the latter were reported to cause hypoglycemia [49]. Early sulfonylureas such as carbutamide, tolbutamide, acetohexamide, tolazamide and chlorpropamide are often referred to as "first generation." These have been largely superceded by more potent "second-generation" sulfonylureas, notably glibenclamide (glyburide), gliclazide, glipizide and most recently glimepiride (Figure 29.6).

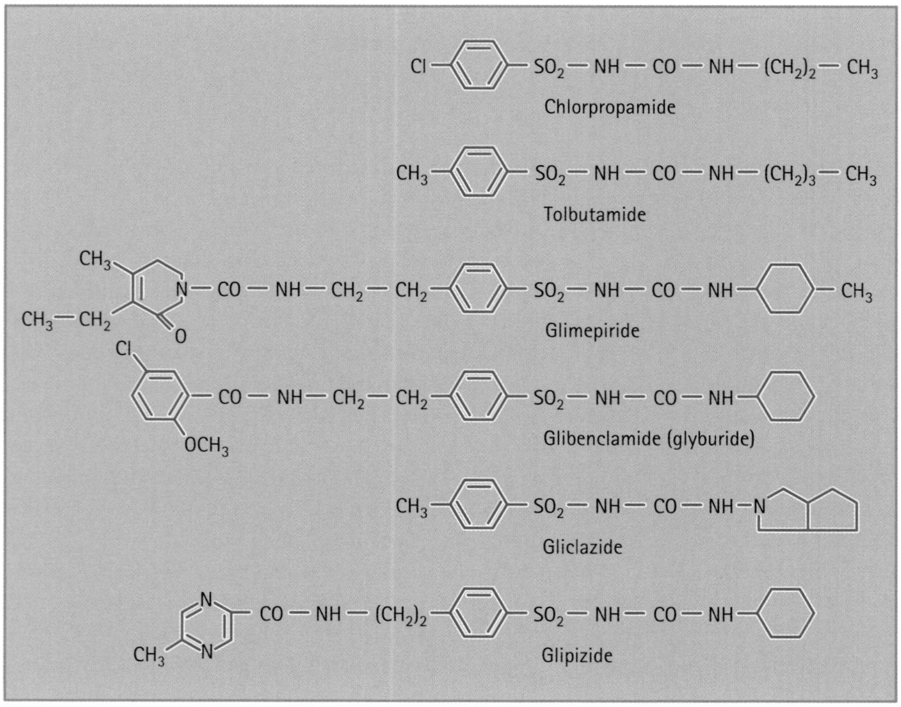

Figure 29.6 Chemical structures of sulfonylureas.

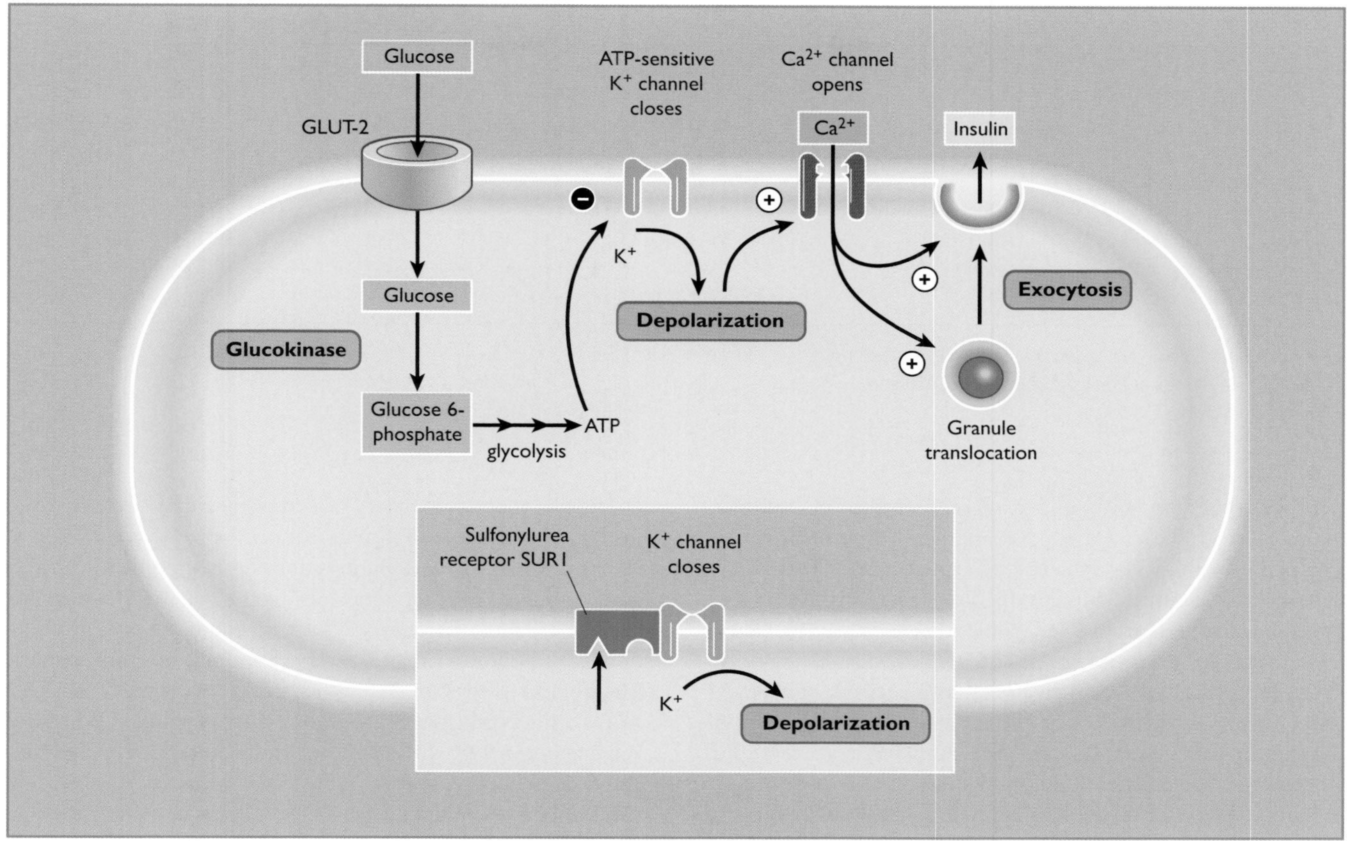

Figure 29.7 Sulfonylureas act on the pancreatic β-cell to stimulate insulin secretion. They bind to the cytosolic surface of the sulfonylurea receptor 1 (SUR1), causing closure of ATP-sensitive Kir6.2 potassium channels, depolarizing the plasma membrane, opening calcium channels, and activating calcium-dependent signaling proteins that control insulin exocytosis.

Mode of action

Sulfonylureas act directly on the β-cells of the islets of Langerhans to stimulate insulin secretion (Figure 29.7). They enter the β-cell and bind to the cytosolic surface of the sulfonylurea receptor 1 (SUR1), which forms part of a transmembrane complex with ATP-sensitive Kir6.2 potassium channels (K^+ATP channels) (Figure 29.8) [50,51]. Binding of a sulfonylurea closes the K^+ATP channel, reducing the efflux of potassium and enabling membrane depolarization. Localized membrane depolarization opens adjacent voltage-dependent L-type calcium channels, increasing calcium influx and raising the cytosolic free calcium concentration. This activates calcium-dependent signaling proteins that control the contractility of micotubules and mictrofilaments that mediate the exocytotic release of insulin granules. Preformed insulin granules adjacent to the plasma membrane are promptly released ("first phase" insulin release), followed by a protracted ("second phase") period of insulin release that begins about 10 minutes later [52]. The "second phase" of insulin release involves translocation of preformed and newly formed insulin granules to the plasma membrane for secretion. Sulfonylureas continue to stimulate insulin release while they are bound to the SUR1 provided that the β-cells are functionally competent. Some desensitization, however, occurs during repeated and protracted stimulation [53]. Because sulfonylureas can stimulate insulin release when glucose concentrations are below the normal threshold for glucose-stimulated insulin release (approximately 5 mmol/L), they are capable of causing hypoglycemia, mainly because of insulin-induced suppression of hepatic glucose production.

There is some evidence that sulfonylureas exert minor glucose-lowering effects independently of increased insulin secretion [54,55]. A small reduction in glucagon concentrations, increased peripheral glucose transport and increased hepatic glucose deposition have been reported, but these effects are not regarded to be of sufficient magnitude to be clinically relevant.

Pharmacokinetics

Sulfonylureas vary considerably in their pharmacokinetic properties (Table 29.7), which in turn affects their clinical suitability for different patients [54,55,56]. They are generally well absorbed, and reach peak plasma concentration in 2–4 hours. Sulfonylureas are highly bound to plasma proteins which can lead to interac-

Table 29.7 Sulfonylureas.

Agent	Dose range (mg/day)	Duration of action (h)	Metabolites	Elimination
Tolbutamide	500–2000	6–10	Inactive	Urine 100%
Glipizide	2.5–20	6–16	Inactive	Urine ~70%
Gliclazide	40–320	12–20	Inactive	Urine ~65%
Gliclazide MR	30–120	18–24	Inactive	Urine ~65%
Glimepiride	1.0–6.0	12–>24	Active	Urine ~60%
Glibenclamide	1.25–15	12–>24	Active	Bile >50%
Chlorpropamide	100–500	24–50	Active	Urine >90%

New patients are not usually started on first generation sulfonylureas (tolbutamide, chlorpropamide).
Glibenclamide is also known as glyburide in some countries.
MR, modified release.

tions with other protein-bound drugs such as salicylates, sulfonamides and warfarin. Also, displacement of protein-bound sulfonylurea can increase the risk of hypoglycemia (Table 29.5). Sulfonylureas are metabolized in the liver to varying extents to a range of active and inactive metabolites that are eliminated along with unchanged drug via the bile and urine. Longer acting sulfonylureas can be given once daily but carry greater risk of hypoglycemia, especially with active metabolites. Sites and rates of metabolism and elimination are also important considerations, especially in older patients and individuals with coexistent liver or kidney disease or taking several other medications.

The formulation of some sulfonylureas has been altered to modify the duration of action [3,4]. For example, a micronized formulation of glibenclamide (glyburide) in the USA increases the rate of gastrointestinal absorption for earlier onset of action. A longer acting ("extended release") formulation of glipizide and a "modified release" (MR) formulation of gliclazide have been introduced for once-daily dosing. Interestingly, the 30 mg preparation of gliclazide MR gives similar efficacy to 80 mg of unmodified gliclazide and reduces risk of severe hypoglycemia [57].

Indications and contraindications

Sulfonylureas are widely used as monotherapy and in combination with metformin or a thiazolidinedione. They can also be used with an α-glucosidase inhibitor, and there are individuals who can benefit from combination of a sulfonylurea with an incretin or DPP-4 inhibitor or insulin. Combination of a sulfonylurea with a different type of antidiabetic agent usually affords approximately additive glucose-lowering efficacy, at least initially, but there is increased risk of hypoglycemia. The additive efficacy of a sulfonylurea with another type of insulin secretagogue is dependent on different modes of action on the β-cell. (Meglinide prandial insulin secretagogues act via the SUR1 complex similarly to sulfonylureas, so they generally offer no extra benefit beyond uptitration of the sulfonylurea, except on rare occasions where the two types of agent are carefully timed to coincide with unusual or unpredictable meal patterns.)

The pharmacologic theory of adding a sulfonylurea (or other insulin secretagogue) to insulin therapy for patients with T2DM is that subcutaneous insulin injections do not mimic the normal endogenous delivery of more insulin to the liver than to the periphery. Thus, where there is residual endogenous β-cell function, a stimulus to increase delivery of endogenous insulin to the liver should assist in reducing hepatic glucose production particularly during digestion of a meal. Hence, daytime sulfonylurea is sometimes given with bedtime insulin, and this can substantially, if only temporarily, reduce the required insulin dose [45,56]. Present guidelines have tended to favor sulfonylureas as alternative first-line oral therapy where metformin is not appropriate or not tolerated. Because sulfonylurea therapy is associated with weight gain, these agents have customarily been preferred for patients who are not overweight.

Begin sulfonylurea therapy with a low dose, preferably with self-monitoring of blood glucose by the patient at least once daily during the first few weeks. This is especially recommended where there are strong concerns about the potential consequences of hypoglycemia (e.g. in elderly patients, those living alone, operating machinery or driving). In general, patients who have responded to some extent (but still inadequately) with lifestyle measures and have less marked fasting hyperglycemia are more likely to incur hypoglycemia with a sulfonylurea. Uptitrate the dosage at 2–4 week intervals as required. Hypoglycemia, or early hypoglycemic symptoms are the main limitation to dose escalation of sulfonylureas. If evidence of hypoglycemia occurs before the glycemic target is achieved, or if a dosage increment produces no further glycemic benefit, it is advisable to return to the previous dose. Adjustment of the administration regimen may assist or an alternative class of insulin secretagogue may be more suitable. Where the sulfonylurea is taken as monotherapy and the glycemic target is not achieved, then addition of an agent to reduce insulin resistance or an α-glucosidase inhibitor is the usual recourse. Note that the maximal blood glucose-lowering effect of a sulfonylurea is usually achieved at a dose that is well below the recommended maximum, indicating that maximum stimulation of insulin secretion has already been achieved.

Efficacy

As monotherapy in patients inadequately controlled by lifestyle measures, sulfonylureas can be expected to reduce fasting plasma glucose by about 2–4 mmol/L, equating to a decrease in HbA_{1c} of 1–2% (11–22 mmol/mol) [3,55,56]. The glucose-lowering effect of sulfonylureas is immediate, and sulfonylureas are particularly effective in the short-term. Efficacy is dependent, however, on sufficient reserve of β-cell function, and this is set against the inevitable decline in β-cell function as the natural history of T2DM proceeds. Thus, it is expected that the dose will need to be escalated to counter the progressive loss of β-cell function, which can reduce the durability of the glucose-lowering efficacy [3,55]. A rapid deterioration of glycemic control during sulfonylurea therapy (sometimes termed "secondary sulfonylurea failure") occurs in approximately 5–10% of patients per annum [55]. While this may possibly vary between compounds it largely reflects the progression of β-cell failure [3,54,56]. Early intervention in patients with a greater reserve of β-cell function usually produces a better and longer response to sulfonylureas, although not without risk of hypoglycemia, whereas late intervention in patients with severely compromised β-cell function is less effective.

Sulfonylureas generally have little effect on blood lipids. Occasionally, their use will cause a small decrease in plasma triglyceride or increase in HDL cholesterol.

Adverse effects

Weight gain, typically in the range of 1–4 kg, is common after initiation of sulfonylurea therapy; it stabilizes by about 6 months [1,3,12]. The weight gain probably reflects the anabolic effects of increased plasma insulin concentrations together with reduced loss of glucose in the urine.

Hypoglycemia is the most common and potentially most serious adverse effect of sulfonylurea therapy. Although it is only rarely life-threatening in patients with T2DM, even mild impairment of neural or motor function can endanger the patient and others, and may predispose to a poor prognosis after a myocardial infarction [3,18]. Patients treated with sulfonylureas should be given instruction on the prevention and recognition of hypoglycemia and the prompt actions required. In the UKPDS, about 20% of sulfonylurea-treated patients reported one or more episodes of hypoglycemic symptoms annually. Other studies have suggested similar rates [12,58]. Severe hypoglycemia (requiring third party assistance) during sulfonylurea therapy occurred in about 1% of patients annually in the UKPDS, and lower rates (approximately 0.2–2.5 episodes per 1000 patient-years) have been reported elsewhere. The mortality risk from sulfonylurea-induced hypoglycemia is reported to be 0.014–0.033 per 1000 patient-years [58]. Longer acting sulfonylureas, irregular meals, other antidiabetic drugs especially insulin, excessive alcohol consumption, already near-normal fasting glycemia, old age and interacting drugs can predispose to increased risk of hypoglycemia (see Chapter 33).

Sulfonylurea-induced hypoglycemia requires prompt admission to hospital. Treat with glucose by continuous intravenous infusion, probably for more than 1 day to guard against the tendency for a recurrence of hypoglycemia where long-acting sulfonylureas are concerned. If accumulation of chlorpropamide is suspected, renal elimination may be enhanced by forced alkaline diuresis. The vasodilator diazoxide and the somatostatin analog octreotide have been used successfully (but with extreme caution) to inhibit insulin secretion in severe sulfonylurea-induced hypoglycemia. Use of glucagon in patients with T2DM should be avoided as this is itself an insulin secretagogue.

Very occasionally, sulfonylureas produce sensitivity reactions, usually transient cutaneous rashes. Erythema multiforme is rare. Fever, jaundice, acute porphyria, photosensitivity and blood dyscrasias are also rare. Chlorpropamide (no longer in common use) was known for its propensilty to cause facial flushing with alcohol and increasing renal sensitivity to antidiuretic hormone, occasionally causing water retention and hyponatremia. Glibenclamide is claimed to have a mild diuretic action.

Although the efficacy of sulfonylureas depends on the stimulation of insulin secretion, this seldom raises plasma insulin concentrations beyond the range of normal (non-diabetic) and subjects with impaired glucose tolerance (IGT). The suggestion emanating from the University Group Diabetes Program study in the 1960s that tolbutamide-induced hyperinsulinemia might have a detrimental effect on the cardiovascular system remains unsubstantiated.

Further studies on the cardiovascular safety of sulfonylureas were prompted by the finding that two isoforms of the sulfonylurea receptor, SUR2A and SUR2B, are expressed in cardiac muscle and vascular smooth muscle, respectively. These isoforms lack the sulfonylurea binding site but they retain the benzamido binding site (Figure 29.8). Therefore, SUR2A/B can only bind those sulfonylureas that contain a benzamido group (glibenclamide, glipizide, glimepiride) [51]. Sulfonylureas without a benzamido group (e.g. tolbutamide, chlorpropamide and gliclazide) show very little interaction with the cardiac and vascular SUR receptors. The effects of the K^{+}ATP channel opener nicorandil (an anti-anginal drug with cardioprotective properties) are blocked by sulfonylureas that have a benzamido group. Although compounds with a benzamido group could theoretically interfere with ischemic preconditioning and increase vascular contractility at a time when this might be undesirable (e.g. severe myocardial ischemia), there is no clear evidence that therapeutic concentrations of sulfonylureas exert such an effect. Indeed, hyperglycemic states appear to obviate ischemic preconditioning; however, some authorities continue to advocate that use of sulfonylureas is kept to a minimum in patients with overt coronary artery disease [59].

Meglitinides (short-acting prandial insulin releasers)

Meglinide analogs were evaluated as potential antidiabetic agents after an observation in the 1980s that meglitinide – the non-

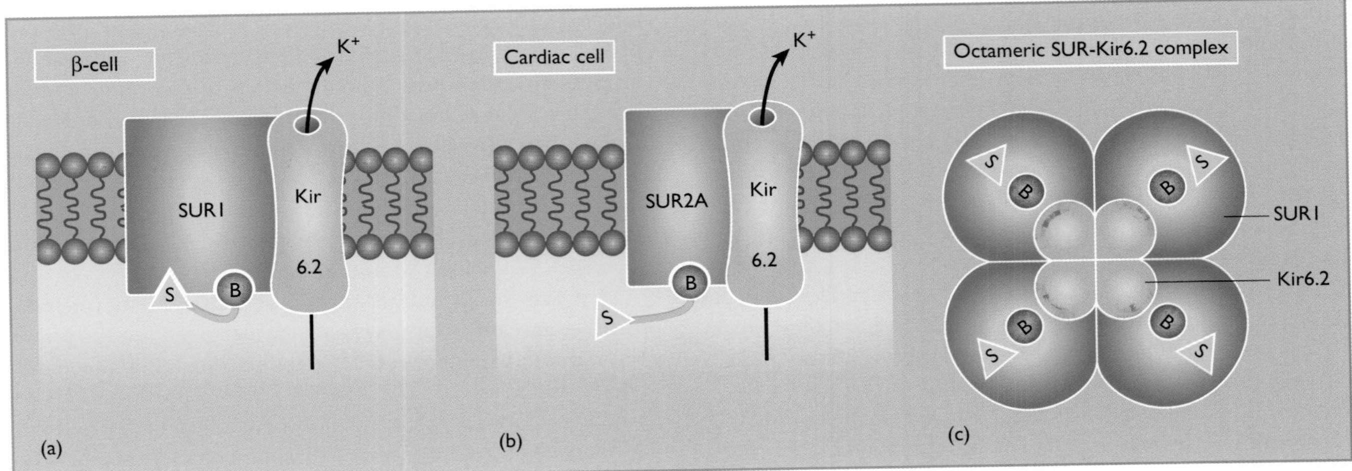

Figure 29.8 This illustrates the transmembrane complex of the SUR1 sulfonylurea receptor and the ATP-sensitive Kir6.2 potassium efflux channel on the pancreatic β-cells (a). Each SUR1 has a cytosolic sulfonylurea (S) binding site and a benzamido (B) binding site. SUR2A on cardiac muscle cells (and SUR2B on vascular smooth muscle cells) does not have a sulfonylurea binding site (b). The SUR1–Kir6.2 complex is a non-covalently bonded octamer comprising 4 × SUR1 and 4 × Kir6.2, illustrated from the cytosolic surface to show the sulfonylurea and benzamido binding sites (c). The Kir6.2 molecules are located at the centre and form the K^+ efflux pore. The Kir6.2 channel has a cytosolic binding region for ADP/ATP.

sulfonylurea moiety of glibenclamide which contains the benzamido group – could stimulate insulin secretion similarly to a sulfonylurea [60]. The pharmacokinetic properties of these compounds favored a rapid but short-lived insulin secretory effect that suited administration with meals to promote prandial insulin release. By generating a prompt increase of insulin to coincide with meal digestion these agents help to restore partially the first phase glucose-induced insulin response that is lost in T2DM. Specifically targeting post-prandial hyperglycemia might also address the vascular risk attributed to prandial glucose excursions, and reduce the risk of interprandial hypoglycemia [61–63]. Two agents, the meglitinide derivative repaglinide and the structurally related phenylalanine derivative nateglinide, were introduced in 1998 and 2001, respectively, as "prandial insulin releasers" (Figure 29.9). Although acting mainly during the prandial and early post-prandial period, their effects extend sufficiently to produce some reduction of fasting hyperglycemia, particularly with repaglinide.

Mode of action

Prandial insulin releasers bind to the benzamido site on the sulfonylurea receptor SUR1 in the plasma membrane of the islet β-cells (Figure 29.8). This site is distinct from the sulfonylurea site, but the response to binding is the same as for sulfonylureas, causing closure of the K^+ATP channel. Thus, there is no therapeutically additive advantage of the two types of agonists, but variations in their binding affinities and duration of action provide opportunities for the specialist to combine a meglitinide and a sulfonylurea to fit with an unusual meal pattern.

Pharmacokinetics

Repaglinide is almost completely and rapidly absorbed with peak plasma concentrations after about 1 hour. It is quickly metabolized in the liver to inactive metabolites, which are mostly excreted in the bile (Table 29.8). Taken about 15 minutes before a meal, repaglinide produces a prompt insulin response which lasts about 3 hours, coinciding with the duration of meal digestion. Nateglinide has a slightly faster onset and shorter duration of action [61–63].

Indications and contraindications

Prandial insulin releasers can be used as monotherapy in patients inadequately controlled by non-pharmacologic measures. They are perhaps most suited for individuals who exhibit post-prandial glycemic excursions while retaining near-normal fasting glycemia. As rapid-acting insulin releasers they can be helpful to individuals with irregular lifestyles with unpredictable or missed meals. The lower risk of hypoglycemia also provides a useful option for some elderly patients, particularly if other agents are contraindicated, although the need for multiple daily dosages may be a disincentive.

Repaglinide is ideally taken 15–30 minutes before a meal. Introduce therapy with a low dose (e.g. 0.5 mg) and monitor glycemic control during titration every 2 weeks up to a maximum of 4 mg before each main meal. When a meal is not consumed, the corresponding dose of repaglinide should be omitted. With appropriate caution and monitoring, repaglinide can be given to patients with moderate renal impairment where some sulfonylureas and metformin are contraindicated.

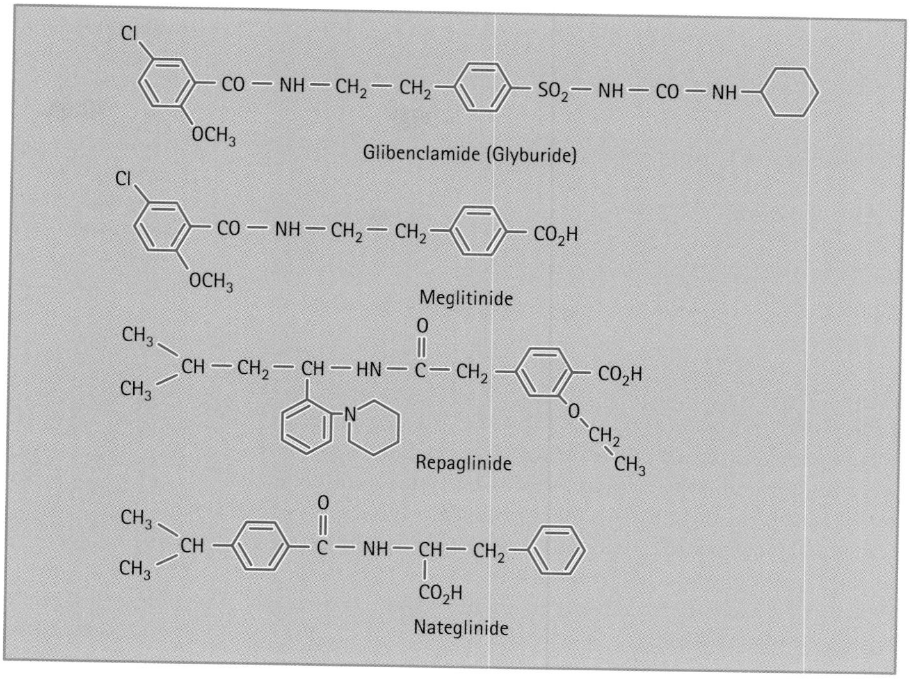

Figure 29.9 Chemical structures of meglitinide, and the prandial insulin releasers repaglinide and nateglinide compared with glibenclamide (glyburide).

Table 29.8 The meglitinides: repaglinide and nateglinide.

Agent	Dose range (mg/meal)	Max daily dose (mg)	Duration of action (h)	Metabolites	Elimination
Repaglinide	0.5–4.0	16	4–6	Inactive	Bile ~90%
Nateglinide	60–180	540	3–5	One slightly active	Urine ~80%

Nateglinide can be used as monotherapy in much the same way as repaglinide, although nateglinide tends to be faster and shorter acting and requires caution in patients with hepatic disease. Note that in some countries, such as the UK, nateglinide is not licensed for use as monotherapy, only for combination therapy.

If the desired glycemic target is not met with a prandial insulin releaser, consider early introduction of combination therapy (e.g. with an agent to reduce insulin resistance). Prandial insulin releasers can also be useful add-ons to monotherapy with metformin or a thiazolidinedione.

Efficacy

Consistent with their use to boost prandial insulin secretion, repaglinide (0.5–4 mg) or nateglinide (60–180 mg) taken before meals produce dose-dependent increases in insulin concentrations and reduce post-prandial hyperglycemia. There is usually a small reduction in fasting hyperglycemia. Reductions in HbA_{1c} are similar to or smaller than with sulfonylureas, as predicted by their shorter duration of action. As add-on to metformin, they can reduce HbA_{1c} by an additional 0.5–1.5% (6–17 mmol/mol).

Adverse effects

Hypoglycemic episodes are fewer and less severe with prandial insulin releasers than with sulfonylureas. Sensitivity reactions, usually transient, are uncommon. Plasma levels of repaglinide may be increased during co-administration with gemfibrozil. Prandial insulin releasers may cause a small increase in body weight when started as initial monotherapy, but body weight is little affected among patients switched from a sulfonylurea or when a prandial insulin releaser is combined with metformin.

Thiazolidinediones

The antidiabetic activity of a thiazolidinedione (ciglitazone) was reported in the early 1980s. In the early 1990s the peroxisome proliferator-activated receptor (PPAR) family was identified as part of the nuclear receptor superfamily 1, and it became evident that thiazolidinediones were potent agonists of PPAR-γ [64]. The PPAR-γ-mediated transcriptional effects of thiazolidinediones were shown to improve whole-body insulin sensitivity, and troglitazone became the first thiazolidinedione to enter routine

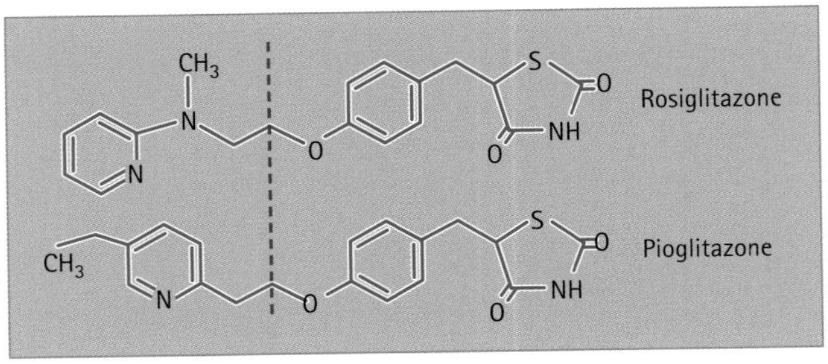

Figure 29.10 Chemical structures of thiazolidinediones rosiglitazone and pioglitazone.

clinical use, introduced in the USA in 1997. The drug, however, was associated with fatal cases of idiosyncratic hepatotoxicity and was withdrawn in 2000. Troglitazone was available for only a few weeks in 1997 in the UK. Two other thiazolidinediones, rosiglitazone and pioglitazone (Figure 29.10), which did not show hepatotoxicity, were introduced in the USA in 1999 and in Europe in 2000 [65]. Fixed-dose combinations of each agent with metformin are also available.

Mode of action

Most of the antidiabetic efficacy of thiazolidinediones appears to be achieved through stimulation of PPAR-γ leading to increased insulin sensitivity [66,67]. PPAR-γ is highly expressed in adipose tissue, and to a lesser extent in muscle and liver. When activated it forms a heterodimeric complex with the retinoid X receptor and binds to a nucleotide sequence (AGGTCAXAGGTCA) termed the peroxisome proliferator response element (PPRE) located in the promoter regions of PPAR-responsive genes. In conjunction with co-activators such as PGC-1, this alters the transcriptional activity of a range of insulin-sensitive and other genes (Table 29.9). Many of these genes participate in lipid and carbohydrate metabolism (Figure 29.11). Stimulation of PPAR-γ by a thiazolidinedione promotes differentiation of pre-adipocytes into mature adipocytes: these new small adipocytes are particularly sensitive to insulin, and show increased uptake of fatty acids with increased lipogenesis. This in turn reduces circulating free fatty acids which rebalances the glucose–fatty acid (Randle) cycle, facilitating glucose utilization and restricting fatty acid availability as an energy source for hepatic gluconeogenesis. By reducing circulating fatty acids, ectopic lipid deposition in muscle and liver is reduced which further contributes to improvements of glucose metabolism.

Thiazolidinediones also increase glucose uptake into adipose tissue and skeletal muscle via increased availability of GLUT 4 glucose transporters. Improvements in insulin sensitivity are likely to be assisted by reduced production of several adipocyte-derived pro-inflammatory cytokines, notably tumor necrosis factor α (TNF-α), which has been implicated in muscle insulin resistance. Thiazolidinediones also increase production of adiponectin, which enhances insulin action and exerts potentially beneficial effects on vascular reactivity [68]. Because PPAR-γ is

Table 29.9 Examples of key genes activated by thiazolidinediones via stimulation of the peroxisome propliferator-activated receptor γ (PPAR-γ). Not all genes appear to be activated in all tissues. The main effects are in adipose tissue.

↑ Lipoprotein lipase
↑ Fatty acid transporter protein (FATP/CD36)
↑ Adipocyte fatty acid binding protein (aP2)
↑ Acyl-CoA synthetase
↑ Malic enzyme
↑ Glycerol kinase (in adipocytes ?)
↑ PEPCK (adipocytes), ↑ perilipin
↑ GLUT-4 (by derepression), ↑ GLUT-2 (islet β-cells)
↓ 11β-hydroxysteroid dehydrogenase-1
↓ Resistin, ↓ RBP 4
↑ Adiponectin (↑ leptin ?)
↓ TNF-α, ↓ IL-6
↓ CRP and some proinflammatory cytokines, ↓ NFκB
↓ PAI-1, ↓ MMP-9
↑ UCP-1 (?)

↑ increase expression; ↓ decrease expression; ? unconfirmed.
CRP, C-reactive protein; GLUT, glucose transporter; IL-6, interleukin 6; NFκB, nuclear factor κB; PAI-1, plasminogen activator inhibitor 1; MMP-9, matrix metalloproteinase 9; PEPCK, phosphoenolpyruvate carboxy kinase; RBP, retinol binding protein; TNF-α, tumor necrosis factor α; UCP-1, uncoupling protein 1.

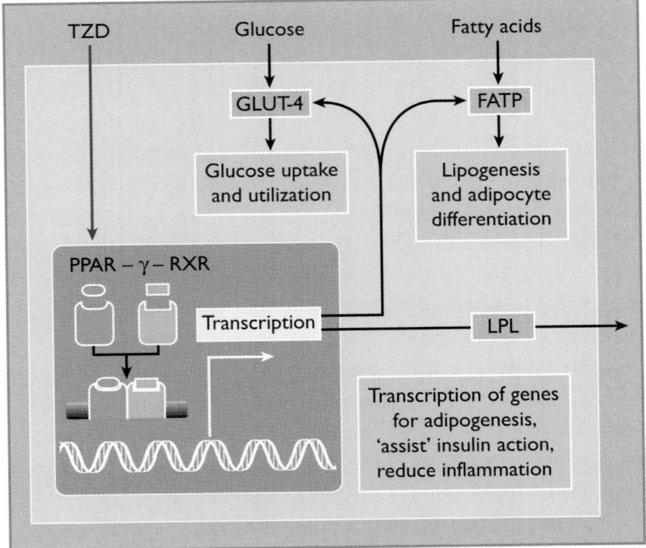

Figure 29.11 Mechanism of action of thiazolidinediones. Most actions of a thiazolidinedione (TZD) are mediated via stimulation of the nuclear peroxisome proliferator-activated receptor γ (PPAR-γ), which is highly expressed in adipose tissue. When stimulated, PPAR-γ forms a heterodimeric complex with the retinoid X receptor (RXR). The complex binds to the peroxisome proliferator response element (PPRE) nucleotide sequence (AGGTCAXAGGTCA) in the promoter regions of certain genes, recruits co-activators, and alters the transcriptional activity of these genes. This modifies nutrient uptake and metabolism, as well as the other functions of the cell.

expressed to a small extent in many tissues, thiazolidinediones can therefore affect responsive genes at these locations, and this has given rise to the tag "pleotropic effects."

Thiazolidinediones, like metformin, are antihyperglycemic agents and require the presence of sufficient insulin to generate their blood glucose-lowering effect. Plasma insulin concentrations are typically lowered by thiazolidinediones, and there is evidence that long-term viability of islet β-cells might be improved [69].

Pharmacokinetics

Absorption of rosiglitazone and pioglitazone is rapid and almost complete, with peak concentrations at 1–2 hours, but slightly delayed when taken with food. Both drugs are metabolized extensively by the liver. Rosiglitazone is metabolized mainly by cytochrome P450 isoform CYP2C8 to inactive or only very weakly active metabolites with a plasma $t_{1/2}$ of 100–160 hours; these are mostly eliminated in the urine. Pioglitazone is metabolized predominantly by CYP2C8 and CYP3A4 to active metabolites that are eliminated in the bile (Table 29.10). Rosiglitazone can interact with gemfibrozil. Pioglitazone does not appear to cause any clinically significant reductions in plasma concentrations of other drugs metabolized by CYP3A4 such as oral contraceptives. Both thiazolidinediones are almost completely bound to plasma proteins, but their concentrations are not sufficient to interfere with other protein-bound drugs.

Indications and contraindications

Thiazolidinediones can be used as monotherapy in non-obese and obese patients with T2DM in whom lifestyle does not afford adequate glycemic control. Various treatment algorithms ascribe different positions for thiazolidinediones, but in general they are used as monotherapy if metformin is inappropriate or not tolerated, and for patients in whom an insulin secretagogue is less favored. They are often used to gain additive efficacy in combination with other antidiabetic drugs, particularly metformin [70]. Because of their slow onset of action it is not straightforward to substitute a thiazolidinedione for either a sulfonylurea or metformin without a temporary deterioration in glycemic control. Combination of a thiazolidinedione with insulin can improve glycemic control while reducing insulin dosages, especially in obese patients, but requires extra caution as peripheral edema is more common [71].

A particular issue with thiazolidinediones is their propensity for fluid retention with increased plasma volume of up to 500 mL, a reduced hematocrit and a decrease in hemoglobin concentration of up to 1 g/dL. Thus, the use of thiazolidinediones is contraindicated in patients with evidence of heart failure. The exclusion criteria, based on cardiac status, vary between countries; for example, New York Heart Association classes I–IV are exclusions in Europe, while III and IV are exclusions in the USA [71]. Appropriate clinical monitoring is important, especially for patients considered at higher risk of cardiac failure and those showing marked initial weight gain. Current controversey has focused on a meta-analysis noting that rosiglitazone increased the risk of myocardial infarction during the first 6–12 months of therapy [72]. While this analysis has received much criticism, the labeling has been tightened to increase awareness of the issue. Despite an increased fluid volume, thiazolidinediones do not increase, and usually slightly decrease, blood pressure.

Although hepatotoxicity has not been a concern with either rosiglitazone or pioglitazone, the troglitazone experience prompted vigilance concerning liver function by measuring serum alanine aminotransferase (ALT) before starting therapy and periodically thereafter. Pre-existing liver disease, development of clinical hepatic dysfunction or elevated ALT levels >2.5 times the upper limit of normal are contraindications to thiazolidinediones. Interestingly, because of the effects of thiazolidinediones on hepatic fat metabolism, recent studies have suggested that this class of drug might even be useful for the treatment of non-alcoholic steatohepatitis.

If there are no contraindications, rosiglitazone and pioglitazone can be used in the elderly. They can also be considered for patients with mild renal impairment, but appreciating the potential for edema. Use of a thiazolidinedione in women with anovulatory PCOS can cause ovulation to resume, but thiazolidinediones should not be continued in pregnancy.

Efficacy

Thiazolidinediones produce a slowly generated antihyperglycemic effect which usually requires 2–3 months to reach maximum effect [65]. This tends to prolong the dose titration process, and because the therapeutic response can vary considerably between individuals, it is appropriate to consider the patient as a non-responder and to switch to another treatment if there is no clinically meaningful effect after 3 months. The two thiazolidinediones have similar blood glucose-lowering effects, reducing HbA_{1c} by around 0.5–1.5% (6–17 mmol/mol). In a long-term monotherapy comparison with metformin or a sulfonylurea (the ADOPT study), rosiglitazone showed a slower onset but a more durable

Table 29.10 The thiazolidinediones: pioglitazone and rosiglitazone.

Agent	Dose range (mg/day)	Duration of action (h)	Metabolites	Elimination
Pioglitazone	15–45	~24	Active	Bile > 60%
Rosiglitazone	4–8	~24	Inactive	Urine ~ 64%

glucose-lowering effect over more than 3 years [69]. Data from clinical trials suggest that the effect of thiazolidinediones may be better in patients with greater β-cell reserve and more overweight individuals, but a clear indicator of the best responders has not been established. Thiazolidinediones do not cause hypoglycemia as monotherapy.

Both thiazolidinediones substantially reduce circulating non-esterified (free) fatty acids, but effects on other components of the plasma lipid profile have been the subject of debate. Rosiglitazone tends to cause a small rise in the total cholesterol concentration, which stabilizes by about 3 months, although this may be mitigated by adequate statin therapy. The effect appears to reflect a rise in both LDL and HDL cholesterol, leaving the LDL : HDL cholesterol ratio and the total : HDL cholesterol ratio little changed or slightly improved. Pioglitazone generally appears to have little effect on total cholesterol, and has frequently reduced triglyceride concentrations in clinical trials. Both thiazolidinediones reduce the proportion of the smaller, more dense (more atherogenic) LDL particles [73].

Weight gain, similar in magnitude to sulfonylurea therapy (typically 1–4 kg) and stabilizing over 6–12 months, is usually observed after initiation of thiazolidinedione therapy. Several studies indicate that the distribution of body fat is altered. The visceral adipose depot is little changed or reduced, while the subcutaneous depot is increased as new small, insulin-sensitive adipocytes are formed [74].

Thiazolidinediones have been reported to exert beneficial effects on a selection of atherothrombotic risk markers, indices of vascular reactivity and components of the "metabolic syndrome" [69,75,76]. For example, thiazolidinediones downregulate PAI-1 expression, decrease urinary albumin excretion to a greater extent than expected for the improvement in glycemic control, reduce cIMT and coronary restenosis, and reduce circulating markers of chronic low-grade inflammation. Thiazolidinediones also reduce the occurrence of new onset diabetes in individuals with IGT or those with a history of gestational diabetes [77,78].

Adverse effects

Despite improvements in several atherothrombotic risk factors, the main concerns over thiazolidinediones focus on the cardiovascular impact of edema, reduced hemoglobin levels and congestive heart disease. Additionally, a meta-analysis has suggested increased risk of myocardial infarction during the initial period of treatment with rosiglitazone, although this has not been confirmed by scrutiny of large treatment databases or by long-term prospective studies [75]. Nevertheless, in a large prospective study, pioglitazone reduced long-term vascular events [76,79,80].

Hypoglycemia may occur several weeks after adding a thiazolidinedione to a sulfonylurea; self-monitoring of blood glucose can be helpful to identify when the dosage of the sulfonylurea should be reduced. It has been suggested that rosiglitazone is initiated at half maximal dosage with a sulfonylurea. Recent studies have also noted an approximate doubling of the risk of a bone fracture – notably at distal sites – amongst postmeopausal women receiving a thiazolidinedione, and possibly a slightly increased risk amongst men [81]. A check on bone density should exclude those at particular risk. Stimulation of PPAR-γ in colonic cells has been reported to both increase and decrease the risk of tumors in animals and cell models; thus, familial polyposis coli is a contraindication to thiazolidinediones on theoretical grounds.

Gliptins

Gliptins are DPP-4 inhibitors that enhance incretin levels. They act as selective inhibitors of the enzyme DPP-4 to enhance endogenous incretin activity by preventing the rapid degradation of the incretin hormones glucose-dependent insulinotropic polypeptide (GIP) and glucagon-like peptide 1 (GLP-1). The history, structure and function of incretin hormones, and the therapeutic role of subcutaneously injected incretin mimetics such as exenatide and liraglutide are covered in Chapter 30. Briefly, incretin hormones are secreted from the intestine in response to meal digestion: one of their key actions is to increase glucose-induced insulin secretion by the pancreatic islet β-cells, thereby reducing prandial glucose excursions [82,83]. GLP-1 also suppresses glucagon secretion from the islet α-cells.

It was noted in the 1980s that the incretin effect is reduced in T2DM, and this was attributed, at least in part, to reduced secretion of GLP-1 [84,85]. By contrast, the biologic actions of GLP-1 remained essentially intact in T2DM, suggesting that administration of extra GLP-1 might be useful therapeutically. This was not a straightforward option because the peptide is rapidly degraded ($t_{1/2} < 2$ minutes). Studies dating from the early 1990s had shown that degradation was mainly by the enzyme DPP-4. Thus, DPP-4-resistant constructs and analogs of GLP-1 have been developed.

An alternative therapeutic approach is to inhibit the action of DPP-4. The first DPP-4 inhibitors were tested in the late 1990s but were not specific enough for clinical use [85]. Several specific inhibitors have subsequently been developed [86], and sitagliptin (2007) and vildagliptin (2008) were introduced in several countries (Figure 29.12). Another DPP-4 inhibitor, saxagliptin, has recently been introduced (2009) and other DPP-4 inhibitors are currently being developed.

Mode of action

DPP-4 inhibitors act to prevent the aminopeptidase activity of DPP-4, an enzyme found free in the circulation and tethered to endothelia and other epithelial cells in most tissues, especially in the intestinal mucosa [87]. DPP-4 cleaves the N-terminal dipeptide from peptides that have either an alanine or a proline residue penultimate to the N-terminus. The incretins GLP-1 and GIP are prime targets for DPP-4, and DPP-4 inhibitors more than double their circulating concentrations, but this is not as high as the concentrations of subcutaneously administered incretin mimetic [88]. Raised endogenous incretin concentrations enhance nutrient-induced insulin secretion, and animal studies have demonstrated increased insulin biosynthesis and increased β-cell mass

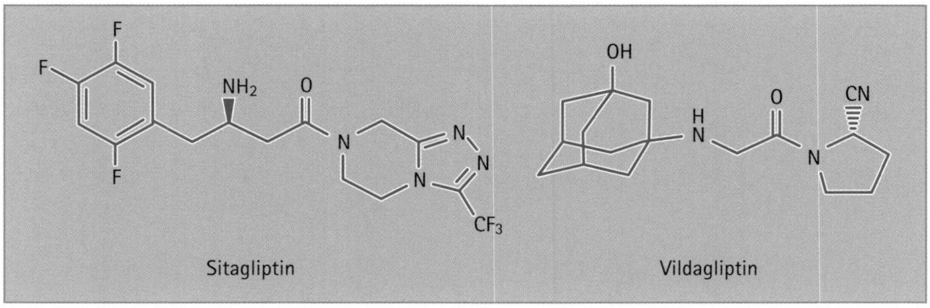

Figure 29.12 Chemical structures of the gliptins (DPP-4 inhibitors) sitagliptin and vildagliptin.

Table 29.11 Effects of the incretin hormones glucagon-like peptide 1 (GLP-1) and glucose-dependent insulinotropic polypeptide (GIP) on glucose homeostasis.

	GLP-1	GIP
Effects on pancreatic islets		
Increase nutrient-induced insulin secretion	✓	✓
Increase insulin biosynthesis*	✓	✓
Increase β-cell mass*	✓	✓
Suppress glucagon secretion	✓	–
Increase somatostatin secretion	✓	–
Extrapancreatic effects		
Slow gastric emptying	✓	–
Decrease gastric acid secretion	–	✓
Promote satiety and weight reduction	✓	–
Promote lipogenesis	–	✓

✓ yes, – no effect.
* Effect observed in animal studies but not confirmed by clinical studies in type 2 diabetes.

(Table 29.11). Increased GLP-1 concentrations also enhance suppression of glucagon secretion. Because these effects are glucose dependent, there is low risk of inducing significant hypoglycemia. The elevation of GLP-1 levels produced by DPP-4 inhibitors is not generally sufficient to create a measurable satiety effect or sufficient slowing of gastric emptying to cause any nausea, and body weight is usually little changed (Figure 29.13).

Because the incretin-mediated effect of DPP-4 inhibitors potentiates glucose-dependent insulin secretion, the activity period of these agents is mostly prandial. Although they are particularly effective in lowering post-prandial hyperglycemia, there is a substantial carry-over effect to benefit the control of interprandial glycemia [89]. By contrast, DPP-4 inhibitors do not initiate insulin secretion and so they do not increase basal insulin secretion. Also, they only suppress glucagon secretion in the hyperglycemic state, so there is low risk of interprandial "overshoot" into hypoglycemia.

Pharmacokinetics

Sitagliptin and vildagliptin are selective, competitive and reversible inhibitors of DPP-4 (IC50 approximately 18 and 3.5 nmol, respectively). Sitagliptin (piperazine derivative) and vildagliptin (cyanopyrrolidine derivative) are each highly bioavailable (approximately 87% and 85%, respectively), rapidly absorbed (t_{max} 1–4 and <2 hours, respectively), and show relatively low (approximately 38% and 9%, respectively) plasma protein binding. Sitagliptin has a plasma $t_{1/2}$ of 8–14 hours, and a small proportion is metabolized in the liver by CYP3A4 and CYP2C6. Most of a sitagliptin dose (approximately 79%) is eliminated unchanged in the urine through renal tubular secretion via the organic anion transporter OAT3. A single dose of 100 mg sitagliptin achieves near-complete inhibition of DPP-4 activity for about 12 hours and about 80% inhibition up to 24 hours. Vildagliptin has a shorter plasma $t_{1/2}$ of 1.5–4.5 hours: the majority (approximately 69%) undergoes mainly renal metabolism to inactive metabolites with negligible involvement of CYP450 isoforms, and most (approximately 85%) is eliminated in the urine. A dose of 50–100 mg vildagliptin gives almost complete inhibition of DPP-4 for about 12 hours and about 40% inhibition by 24 hours (Table 29.12).

Indications and contraindications

In principle, gliptins can be used as monotherapy in patients with T2DM who have responded inadequately to lifestyle measures, although this is not a licensed indication in all countries where available. Currently, as newly available agents, gliptins tend to be preferred as "add-on" therapy in patients inadequately controlled by metformin or a thiazolidinedione. Theoretically, they could be used with any other class of oral agent or insulin, as their mode of action on the β-cell is different from sulfonylureas and meglitinides, and their ability to reduce glucagon levels could be useful as add-on therapy to insulin even without β-cell function. In practice, however, full efficacy in T2DM requires adequate β-cell reserve. Lack of weight gain makes gliptins suitable for overweight and obese patients, and low risk of hypoglycemia when used as monotherapy (and when used with non-insulin releasing agents) favors their use in patients who have only slightly raised basal glycemia, are close to glycemic target or have unpredictable meal times [89,90].

Sitagliptin is taken once daily (100 mg) in the morning, and vildagliptin is usually twice daily (50 mg). The glucose-dependent mode of action reduces the risk of any significant glucose lowering effect unless there is hyperglycemia, lowering concern over

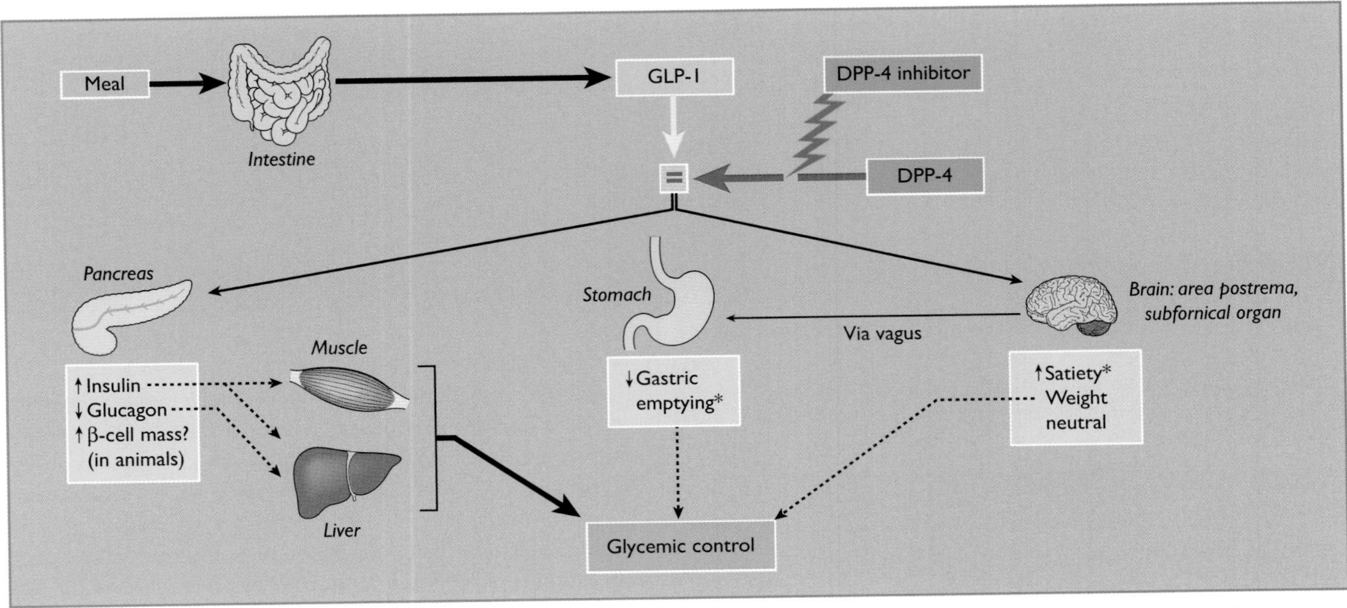

Figure 29.13 Sites of action of gliptins (DPP-4 inhibitors). Incretin hormones such as GLP-1 are released in reponse to a meal. These hormones are normally degraded rapidly by the enzyme DPP-4. Gliptins act as inhibitors of DPP-4, allowing the normal effects of the incretin hormones to be enhanced. The main site of the enhanced incretin effect is on the pancreas to increase nutrient-induced insulin secretion. GLP-1 also reduces glucagon secretion. * Potential effects to slow gastric emptying and increase satiety probably contribute little to the therapeutic efficacy of gliptins.

Table 29.12 Gliptins: sitagliptin and vildagliptin.

Agent	Dose (mg/day)	Duration of action (h)	Metabolites	Elimination
Sitagliptin	100	18–24	Nominal metabolism	Urine ~ 79%*
Vildagliptin	2 × 50	12–24	Inactive	Urine ~ 85%

* Unchanged drug.

missed meals. Thus, there is no dose titration, but it is recommended that fasting and post-prandial glycemia are reviewed after about 2 weeks of therapy, especially when added as a second agent.

Because sitagliptin is mostly eliminated unchanged in the urine, a reduced dose (50 mg once daily) is recommended for patients with moderate renal insufficiency (creatinine clearance ≥30 to <50 mL/min); for patients with severe renal insufficiency (creatinine clearance <30 mL/min) or with end-stage renal disease requiring hemodialysis or peritoneal dialysis, consider a dose of 25 mg once daily. Sitagliptin causes no apparent induction or inhibition of P450 isoforms, which allows its use in patients with mild or moderate impairment of liver function provided renal function is adequate.

In view of the renal metabolism and elimination of vildagliptin, this agent is not recommended in patients with moderate or severe renal impairment (e.g. creatinine clearance <50 mL/min). Some cases of reversibly raised ALT or aspartate aminotransferase (AST) have been observed in patients receiving vildagliptin, therefore a liver function check should be made before starting treatment and periodically thereafter. A marked rise in liver enzymes (e.g. ALT or AST >3× upper limits of normal) or other signs of hepatic impairment contraindicate treatment.

No significant drug interactions have been noted with either gliptin. As clinical experience is limited it is advisable to use these drugs cautiously in patients with heart disease and to stop gliptin therapy in pregnancy.

Efficacy

Sitagliptin

Administration of 100 mg/day sitagliptin as monotherapy or add-on therapy to other antidiabetic agents typically reduced HbA_{1c} (from a baseline of approximately 8% [64 mmol/mol]) by about 0.7–0.8% (8–9 mmol/mol) after 24–52 weeks [89–92]. Individuals with a high baseline HbA_{1c} usually showed reductions in HbA_{1c} of >1% (11 mmol/mol). Fasting plasma glucose concentrations were reduced by about 1.0–1.5 mmol/L, and post-prandial glucose levels measured 2 hours after a standard mixed meal were usually reduced by about 3 mmol/L. Sitagliptin therapy did not cause a clinically significant increase in the incidence of hypoglycemia, and a sitagliptin + metformin combination was associated with fewer hypoglycemic episodes than a combination of glipizide + metformin despite similar levels of HbA_{1c} [93]. Sitagliptin did not increase body weight compared with placebo in any of the trials.

Vildagliptin

In clinical trials a single daily dose of 50–100 mg/day vildagliptin showed similar efficacy and tolerability to sitagliptin when used as monotherapy or add-on to metformin or a thiazolidinedione [89–91,94]. Although several trials with vildagliptin produced slightly greater reductions in HbA_{1c}, this was mostly associated with a slightly higher average baseline (starting) HbA_{1c} (>8.5% [>69 mmol/mol]). Again there was no effect on hypoglycemia or body weight.

Adverse effects

Clinical experience to date with gliptins has not identified any serious adverse effects. In clinical trials (typically 6–12 months), measures of tolerability and adverse events were generally similar to placebo or comparator. There were some increases in liver enzymes with a 100 mg dose of vildagliptin, but not with the 50 mg dose that is marketed. Nominal increases in reported signs or symptoms of abdominal discomfort suggest that the potential to slow gastric emptying is unlikely to have a clinically significant impact.

Because there are many natural substrates for DPP-4 including bradykinin, enkephalins, neuropeptide Y, peptide YY1–36, gastrin releasing polypeptide, substance P, insulin-like growth factor I, vasostatin 1, the α chains of thyrotropin, luteinizing hormone and chorionic gonadotropin and several chemokines such as monocyte chemotactic protein 1 (MCP-1), gliptins have the potential to influence the hunger–satiety system, gastrointestinal motility, growth, vascular reactivity and immune mechanisms [88]. DPP-4 is also the CD26 T-cell activation antigen, but neither CD26 knockout mice nor the DPP-4-specific inhibitors used in animals or humans have yet shown any significant untoward immune-related effects. The importance of selective DPP-4 inhibition is also noted because inhibition of related enzymes such as DPP-8 and DPP-9 has produced blood dyscrasias and skin lesions in some species, but not in clinical use. Nevertheless, it is advisable to check for any evidence of skin lesions.

α-Glucosidase inhibitors

Studies conducted in the late 1970s noted that inhibitors of intestinal α-glucosidase enzymes could retard the final steps of carbohydrate digestion with consequent delay to the absorption of sugars. By the early 1980s it was demonstrated that this approach could reduce post-prandial hyperglycemia in diabetes [95]. Acarbose, the first α-glucosidase inhibitor, was introduced in the early 1990s. Subsequently, two further agents, miglitol and voglibose, were introduced in some countries (Figure 29.14). In patients

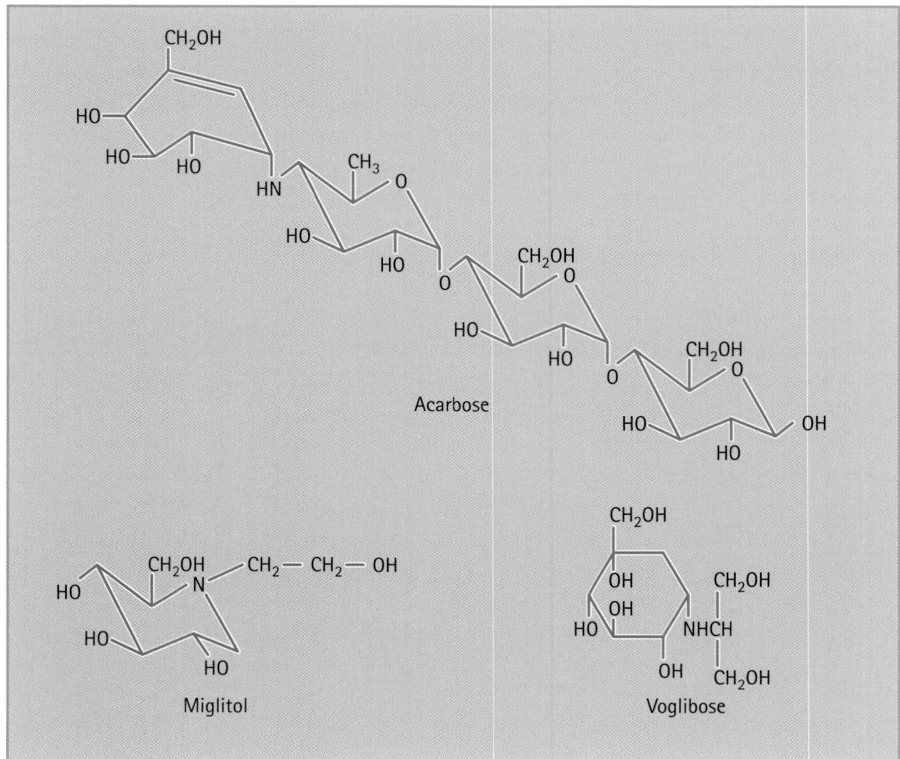

Figure 29.14 Chemical structures of the α-glucosidase inhibitors acarbose, miglitol and volglibose.

who consume meals containing complex carbohydrate, α-glucosidase inhibitors can effectively reduce post-prandial glucose excursions. These agents also have a good safety record but their application has been limited by gastrointestinal side effects.

Mode of action

α-Glucosidase inhibitors competitively inhibit the activity of α-glucosidase enzymes in the brush border of enterocytes lining the intestinal villi (Figure 29.15). They bind to the enzymes with high affinity, preventing the enzymes from cleaving disaccharides and oligosaccharides into monosaccharides. This delays completion of carbohydrate digestion and can defer the process distally along the intestinal tract, leading to a delay in glucose absorption [95]. Different α-glucosidase inhibitors have different affinities for the various α-glucosidase enzymes. This gives slightly different activity profiles (e.g. acarbose has greatest affinity for glycoamylase > sucrase > maltase > dextrinases, whereas miglitol is a stronger inhibitor of sucrase). It is emphasized that α-glucosidase inhibitors can only be effective if the patient is consuming complex digestible carbohydrate. These agents do not significantly affect the absorption of glucose per se. By moving glucose absorption more distally along the intestinal tract, α-glucosidase inhibitors may alter the release of glucose-dependent intestinal hormones such as GIP and GLP-1 which enhance nutrient-induced insulin secretion. Thus, release of GIP, which occurs mainly from the jejunal mucosa, may be reduced by α-glucosidase inhibitors, whereas secretion of GLP-1 (mostly from the ileal mucosa) is increased. α-Glucosidase inhibitors probably reduce post-prandial insulin concentrations through the attenuated rise in post-prandial glucose levels [95].

Pharmacokinetics

Acarbose is degraded by amylases in the small intestine and by intestinal bacteria; less than 2% of the unchanged drug is absorbed along with some of the intestinal degradation products. Absorbed material is mostly eliminated in the urine within 24 hours [95]. Miglitol is almost completely absorbed and eliminated unchanged in the urine.

Indications and contraindications

α-Glucosidase inhibitors can be used as monotherapy, usually for patients with T2DM with post-prandial hyperglycemia but only slightly raised fasting glycemia; however, they are more commonly used as add-on to other therapies, again to target post-prandial hyperglycemia [95]. α-Glucosidase inhibitors can also be used to extend the post-prandial period to reduce interprandial glycemic troughs or hypoglycemia in individuals receiving a sulfonylurea and/or insulin. Acarbose has also been shown to prevent progression of IGT to T2DM [96], although this is not a licensed use.

When starting an α-glucosidase inhibitor the patient should be advised that a diet containing complex digestible carbohydrate is important. α-Glucosidase inhibitors should be taken with meals, starting with a low dose (e.g. 50 mg/day acarbose) and slowly uptitrated over several weeks. Monitoring of post-prandial glycemia is often helpful. Hypoglycemia is unlikely when used as monotherapy, but gastrointestinal symptoms commonly limiting initial tolerability and dose titration. Symptoms tend to be reduced by slow titration and usually subside with time, possibly reflecting some adaptation of the intestinal tract, but tolerability is poor.

α-Glucosidase inhibitors are contraindicated for patients with a history of chronic intestinal disease, and high dosages of acarbose can occasionally increase liver enzyme concentrations; so it is recommended to measure transaminase concentrations periodically in patients receiving a maximum dosage (200 mg acarbose three times daily). Raised liver enzymes should remit as the dosage is reduced, otherwise alternative causes of hepatic dysfunction should be considered.

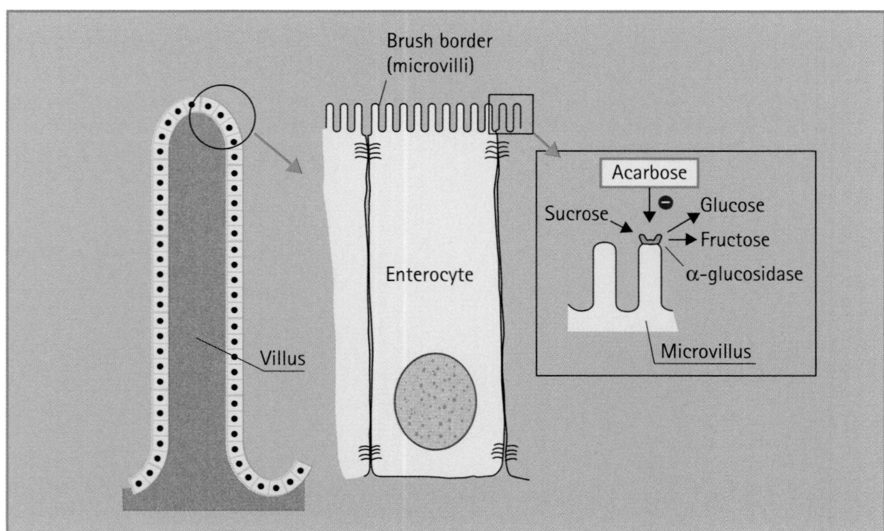

Figure 29.15 Mode of action of α-glucosidase inhibitors. α-Glucosidase inhibitors competitively inhibit the activity of α-glucosidase enzymes in the brush border of enterocytes lining the intestinal villi, preventing these enzymes from cleaving disaccharides and oligosaccharides into monosaccharides. This delays carbohydrate digestion.

Efficacy

Because α-glucosidase inhibitors target post-prandial glucose excursions during meals that contain complex carbohydrate, their effectiveness is entirely dependent on dietary compliance. As monotherapy, these agents can reduce peak post-prandial glucose concentrations by 1–4 mmol/L. The incremental area under the post-prandial plasma glucose curve can be more than halved in some individuals, and there is usually some extended duration of effect to modestly lower basal glycemia up to about 1 mmol/L. The decrease in HbA_{1c} is usually about 0.5–1.0% (6–11 mmol/mol), provided that a high dose of the drug is tolerated and dietary compliance is maintained [97].

Although overall reductions in HbA_{1c} are modest, α-glucosidase inhibitors offer several useful features: they do not cause weight gain or frank hypoglycemia and may reduce inter-prandial episodes of hypoglycemia. When combined with other antidiabetic agents, α-glucosidase inhibitors can reduce post-prandial hyperinsulinemia, and they often lower plasma triglyceride concentrations. Use of an α-glucosidase inhibitor can produce minor alterations to the intestinal absorption of other oral antidiabetic agents when used in combination therapy, but α-glucosidase inhibitors usually provide additive efficacy gains when used in combination with any other class of antidiabetic agent [95]. There is preliminary evidence that acarbose might reduce major cardiac events, including myocardial infarction, but this requires confirmation, and it is unclear if this could be caused by the targeting of post-prandial hyperglycemia or an independent effect of the drug [98].

Adverse effects

Gastrointestinal side effects represent the main problem with α-glucosidase inhibitors. For example, in the STOP-NIDDM trial, 31% of acarbose-treated patients compared with 19% on placebo discontinued treatment early [96]. If the dosage is too high (relative to the amount of complex carbohydrate in the meal), undigested oligosaccharides pass into the large bowel. These are fermented, causing flatulence, abdominal discomfort and sometimes diarrhea, but usually ameliorating with slower titration and time. Hypoglycemia is uncommon and there are no clinically significant drug interations, although use in conjunction with agents affecting gut motility or cholestyramine is not recommended.

Antiobesity therapies

Obesity, especially excess visceral adiposity, predisposes to diabetes, complicates glycemic control and substantially increases the risk of vascular disease (see Chapter 14). The blood glucose-lowering efficacy of lifestyle measures to reduce adiposity in obese T2DM is well appreciated, although it is often very difficult to achieve and maintain significant weight loss in these patients. Interestingly, several studies have suggested that additional glucose-lowering can be attained with pharmacologic antiobesity therapies. Whether this is entirely explained by greater weight loss and improved dietary compliance is unclear because it has been mooted that some antiobesity therapies could have some modest independent glucose-lowering effects.

In conjunction with a mildly hypocaloric and reduced fat diet, the intestinal lipase inhibitor orlistat (120 mg three times daily with meals) can reduce dietary fat absorption by up to 30%. In overweight and obese patients with T2DM this typically increases weight reduction by an extra 2–3 kg, and additional reductions in HbA_{1c} of 0.28–1.1% (3–12 mmol/mol) have been reported [28]. Potential improvements in the glucose–fatty acid cyle might be envisaged. The satiety-inducing serotonin–norepinephrine reuptake inhibitor sibutramine often enables slightly greater reductions of body weight in overweight and obese patients with T2DM, with extra reductions in HbA_{1c} of around 0.6% (7 mmol/mol)*. Sibutramine metabolites might have useful metabolic effects. Antiobesity therapies carry their own contraindications, cautions and side effects, and orlistat could interfere with the absorption and activity of some oral antidiabetic agents, particularly α-glucosidase inhibitors.

Fixed-dose combinations

As the target-driven early and intensified approach to management of hyperglycemia in T2DM gathers momentum, the use of combinations of two or more oral agents with *different* mechanisms of action has become commonplace [99]. To facilitate combination therapy, several fixed dose, single tablet combinations have been made available (Table 29.13). These are designed to provide bioequivalence and thereby similar efficacy, although minor adjustments to formulation may also enable some extra blood glucose-lowering efficacy. Fixed dose combinations can offer convenience, reduce the "pill burden," simplify administration regimens and they may increase patient adherence compared with equivalent combinations of separate tablets. Lower doses of two different types of agents rather than a high dose of one agent may also provide a way to achieve efficacy while circumventing dose-related side effects. Current fixed dose combinations of antidiabetic agents include metformin combined with a sulfonylurea, thiazolidinedione, gliptin or meglitinide, as well as thiazolidinedione–sulfonylurea combinations. Although single tablets could reduce titration flexibility, most of the commonly used dosage combinations have been accommodated. It is reiterated that any form of combination therapy necessitates the same

*The marketing authorization for sibutramine has recently been withdrawn in Europe following the publication of the SCOUT trial. In this trial which included 9,800 overweight or obese individuals at high risk of CVD events, treatment with sibutramine was associated with a 16% increased risk of non-fatal MI, non-fatal stroke, resuscitated cardiac arrest or CVD death. This result was driven by an increased incidence of non-fatal MI and stroke.

Table 29.13 Fixed-dose single-tablet combinations of antidiabetic agents. Adapted from Bailey and Day [99].

Tablet	Components	Strengths (mg)
Glucovance	Metformin +glibenclamide	250:1.25, 500:2.5, 500:5.0
Metaglip	Metformin + glipizide	250:2.5, 500:2.5, 500:5.0
Avandamet	Metformin + rosiglitazone	500:1.0, 500:4.0, 500:2.0, 1000:2.0, 1000:4.0
Competact (Actoplusmet)	Metformin + pioglitazone	500:15, 850:15
Eucreas	Metformin + vildagliptin	850:50, 1000:50
Janumet	Metformin + sitagliptin	500:50, 1000:50
Prandimet	Metformin + repaglinide	500:1, 500:2
Avaglim (Avandaryl)	Rosiglitazone + glimepiride	4:1, 4:2, 4:4, 8:2, 8:4
Tandemact (Duetact)	Pioglitazone + glimepiride	30:, 45:4

Availability of tablets and component strengths differ between countries. Names vary between Europe and USA. Alternative names are given in parentheses.
Glibenclamide = glyburide

cautions and contraindications that apply to each active component.

Conclusions

A minimalistic archetypal algorithm to treat hyperglycemia in T2DM is shown in Figure 29.16. This illustrates a typical stepped approach similar to that advocated in most current guidelines. Guidelines should be interpreted with flexibility, however, to ensure that the care plan, treatment targets and selection of therapies are individualized to suit the circumstances of the patient. The value of lifestyle intervention as initial and ongoing therapy in conjunction with pharmacologic agents should not be underestimated. In view of the progressive natural history of T2DM, the introduction of drug therapy, the need for periodic uptitration of dosage and the use of combination therapy can be expected for most patients (covered in further detail in Chapter 31).

A range of differently acting oral agents is available: metformin and thiazolidinediones counter insulin resistance; sulfonylureas, meglitinides and gliptins increase insulin secretion; and α-glucosidase inhibitors slow carbohydrate digestion. Additionally, injected incretin analogs increase insulin secretion. All of these blood glucose-lowering agents can only provide glycemic control if there is sufficient β-cell reserve. When adequate control is not achieved or not maintained, it is important to proceed to the next stage without delay to avoid periods of hyperglycemia. Insulin should be considered when other therapies do not provide adequate glycemic control or are unsuitable. Integrated management to address cardiovascular risk and co-morbid conditions is essential. Monitoring, therapeutic adjustments for efficacy, safety, avoidance of hypoglycemia and contraindications require constant vigilance, but early, effective and sustained glycemic control is essential to minimize vulnerability to vascular complications later in life.

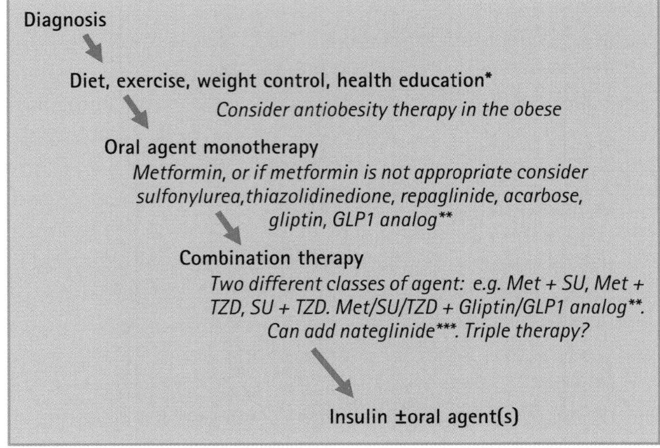

Figure 29.16 Archetypal algorithm used in the treatment of hyperglycemia in type 2 diabetes (except patients presenting with severe hyperglycemia who may require immediate insulin therapy). Start with lifestyle measures (diet and exercise). If the individualized glycemic target for the patient is not achieved quickly using lifestyle measures, then add pharmacologic therapy without delay. The selected monotherapy is uptitrated to achieve the desired glycemic effect. If an uptitration step does not add benefit or is not tolerated revert back a step. When the desired glycemic effect is not achieved or adequate titration is not tolerated, move promptly to the addition of a second agent and uptitrate. If the desired glycemic control is not achieved or maintained consider triple therapy or introduce insulin while maintaining one or two of the existing therapies where appropriate. Respect drug cautions and contraindications at all times, monitor as required, and try to select glycemic targets that are realistic, safely achievable and avoid hypoglycemia. * Lifestyle advice reinforced throughout. ** GLP1 analog given as subcutaneous injection. *** Nateglinide usually only as second agent.

References

1 Wallace TM, Matthews DR. The drug treatment of type 2 diabetes. In: Pickup JC, Williams G, eds. *Textbook of Diabetes*, 3rd edn. Oxford: Blackwell, 2003: 45.1–45.18.

2 Krentz AJ, Bailey CJ. *Type 2 Diabetes in Practice*, 2nd edn. London: Royal Society of Medicine Press, 2005.

3 Krentz AJ, Bailey CJ. Oral antidiabetic agents: current role in type 2 diabetes mellitus. *Drugs* 2005; **65**:385–411.

4 Krentz AJ, Patel MB, Bailey CJ. New drugs for type 2 diabetes: what is their place in therapy? *Drugs* 2008; **68**:2131–2162.

5 Bailey CJ. Antidiabetic drugs other than insulin. In: Offermans S, Rosenthal W, eds. *Encyclopedia of Molecular Pharmacology*, 2nd edn. Berlin: Springer, 2009: 116–125.

6 Sladek R, Rocheleau G, Rung J, Dina C, Shen L, Serre D, *et al.* A genome-wide association study identifies novel risk loci for type 2 diabetes. *Nature* 2007; **445**:881–885.

7 DeFronzo RA. Pathogenesis of type 2 diabetes mellitus: metabolic and molecular implications for identifying diabetes genes. *Diabetes Rev* 1997; **5**:177–269.

8 Kahn SE. The relative contributions of insulin resistance and beta-cell dysfunction to the pathophysiology of type 2 diabetes. *Diabetologia* 2003; **46**:3–19.

9 Kahn SE, Hull RL, Utzschneider KM. Mechanisms linking obesity to insulin resistance and type 2 diabetes. *Nature* 2006; **444**:840–846.

10 Brownlee M. Biochemistry and molecular cell biology of diabetic complications. *Nature* 2001; **414**:813–820.

11 McGarry JD. Dysregulation of fatty acid metabolism in the etiology of type 2 diabetes. *Diabetes* 2002; **51**:7–17.

12 UK Prospective Study (UKPDS) Group. Intensive blood-glucose control with sulphonylureas or insulin compared with conventional treatment and risk of complications in patients with type 2 diabetes (UKPDS 33). *Lancet* 1998; **352**:837–853.

13 Stratton IM, Adler AI, Neil HA, Matthews DR, Manley SE, Cull CA, *et al.* Association of glycaemia with macrovascular and microvascular complications of type 2 diabetes (UKPDS 35): prospective observational study. *Br Med J* 2000; **321**:405–412.

14 Holman RR, Paul SK, Bethel MA, Matthews DR, Neil HA. 10-year follow-up of intensive glucose control in type 2 diabetes. *N Engl J Med* 2008; **359**:1577–1589.

15 Action to Control Cardiovascular Risk in Diabetes Study Group. Effects of intensive glucose lowering in type 2 diabetes. *N Engl J Med* 2008; **358**:2545–2559.

16 ADVANCE Collaboratrive Group. Intensive blood glucose and vascular outcomes in patients with type 2 diabetes. *N Engl J Med* 2008; **358**:2560–2572.

17 Duckworth W, Abraira C, Moritz T, Reda D, Emanuele N, Reaven PD, *et al.* Glucose control and vascular complications in veterans with type 2 diabetes. *N Engl J Med* 2009; **360**;129–139.

18 Kosiborod M, Inzucchi SE, Krumholz HM, Xiao L, Jones PG, Fiske S, *et al.* Glucometrics in patients hospitalized with acute myocardial infarction. *Circulation* 2008; **117**:1018–1027.

19 American Diabetes Association. Standards of medical care in diabetes – 2009. *Diabetes Care* 2009; **32**(Suppl 1):13–61.

20 Nathan DM, Buse JB, Davidson MB, Ferrannini E, Holman RR, Sherwin R, *et al.* Management of hyperglycaemia in type 2 diabetes mellitus: a consensus algorithm for the initiation and adjustment of therapy – a consensus statement from the American Diabetes Association and the European Association for the Study of Diabetes. *Diabetologia* 2009; **52**:17–30.

21 International Diabetes Federation Clinical Guidelines Task Force. *Global Guideline for Type 2 Diabetes*. Brussels: International Diabetes Federation, 2005.

22 National Collaborating Centre for Chronic Conditions. *Type 2 diabetes: national clinical guideline for management of primary and secondary care (update)*. London: Royal College of Physicians, 2008.

23 Bailey CJ, Blonde L, Del Prato S, Leiter LA, Nesto R, *et al.* What are the practical implications for treating diabetes in light of recent evidence? Updated recommendations from the Global Partnership for Effective Diabetes Management. *Diabetes Vascular Dis Res* 2009; **6**:283–287.

24 Canadian Diabetes Association Clinical Practice Guidelines Expert Committee. Phamacologic management of type 2 diabetes. *Can J Diabetes* 2003; **27**(Suppl 2):37–42. www.diabetes.ca/cpg2003/downloads/pharmacologic.pdf

25 Matthaei S, Bierwirth R, Fritsche A, Gallwitz B, Haring HU, Joost HG, *et al.* Medical antihyperglycaemic treatment of type 2 diabetes mellitus. Update of the evidence-based guidelines of the German Diabetes Association. *Exp Clin Endocrinol Diabetes* 2009; **117**:522–557.

26 Bonora E, Calcaterra F, Lombardi S, Bonfante N, Formentini G, Bonandonna RC, *et al.* Plasma glucose levels throughout the day and HbA_{1c} interrelationships in type 2 diabetes. *Diabetes Care* 2001; **24**:2023–2029.

27 DECODE study group. Is the current definition for diabetes relevant to mortality risk from all causes and cardiovascular and noncardiovascular diseases. *Diabetes Care* 2003; **26**:688–696.

28 Lloret-Linares C, Greenfield JR, Czernichow S. Effects of weight-reducing agents on glycaemic parameters and progression to type 2 diabetes: a review. *Diabet Med* 2008; **25**:1142–1150.

29 Bailey CJ, Day C. Metformin: its botanical background. *Pract Diabet Int* 2004; **21**:115–117.

30 Bailey CJ. Biguandes and NIDDM. *Diabetes Care* 1992; **15**:755–772.

31 Bailey CJ, Turner RC. Metformin. *N Engl J Med* 1996; **334**:574–579.

32 Bailey CJ, Campbell IW, Chan JCN, Davidson JA, Howlett HCS, Ritz P. *Metformin: The Gold Standard*. Chichester: Wiley, 2007.

33 Bailey CJ. Metformin: effects on micro and macrovascular complications in type 2 diabetes. *Cardiovasc Drugs Ther* 2008; **22**:215–224.

34 Grant PJ. Beneficial effects of metformin on haemostasis and vascular function in man. *Diabetes Metab* 2003; **29**:6S44–52.

35 Zhou G, Myers R, Li Y, Chen Y, Shen X, Fenyk-Melody J, *et al.* Role of AMP-activated protein kinase in the mechanism of action of metformin. *J Clin Invest* 2001; **108**:1167–1174.

36 Scheen AJ. Clinical pharmacokinetics of metformin. *Clin Pharmacokinet* 1996; **30**:359–371.

37 Cusi K, DeFronzo RA. Metformin: a review of its metabolic effects. *Diabetes Rev* 1998; **6**:89–131.

38 Palumbo S, Falbo A, Zullo F, Orio F. Evidence-based and potential benefits of metformin in the polycystic ovary syndrome: a comprehensive review. *Endocr Rev* 2009; **30**:1–50.

39 Natali A, Ferrannini E. Effects of metformin and thiazolidinediones on suppression of hepatic glucose production and stimulation of glucose uptake in type 2 diabetes: a systematic review. *Diabetologia* 2006; **49**:434–441.

40 UK Prospective Diabetes Study Group. Effect of intensive blood-glucose control with metformin on complications in overweight patients with type 2 diabetes (UKPDS 34). *Lancet* 1998; **352**:854–865.

41 Rao AD, Reynolds K, Kuhadha N, Fonseca VA. Is the combination of sulphonylureas and metformin associated with an increased risk of cardiovascular disease or all-cause mortality? *Diabetes Care* 2008; **31**:1672–1678.

42 Hermann LS, Lindberg G, Lindblad U, Melander A. Efficacy, effectiveness and safety of sulphonylurea-metformin combination therapy in patients with type 2 diabetes. *Diabetes Obes Metab* 2002; **4**:296–304.

43 Johnson JA, Majumdar SR, Simpson SH, Toth EL. Decreased mortality associated with sulfonylurea monotherapy in type 2 diabetes. *Diabetes Care* 2002; **25**:2244–2248.

44 Douek IF, Allen SE, Ewings P, Gale EA, Bingley PJ; Metformin Trial Group. Continuing metformin when starting insulinin patients with type 2 diabetes: a double-blind randomized placebo-controlled trial. *Diabet Med* 2005; **22**:634–640.

45 Yki-Jarvinen H, RyysyL, Nikkila K, Tulokas T, Vanamo R, Heikkilä M. Comparison of bedtime insulin regimens in patients with type 2 diabetes mellitus: a randomized, controlled trial. *Ann Intern Med* 1999; **130**:389–396.

46 Diabetes Prevention Program Research Group. Reduction of the incidence of type 2 diabetes with lifestyle intervention or metformin. *N Engl J Med* 2002; **346**:393–403.

47 Salpeter SR, Greyber E, Pasternak GA, Salpeter EE. Risk of fatal and non-fatal lactic acidosis with metformin use in type 2 diabetes. *Arch Intern Med* 2003; **163**:2594–2602.

48 Lalau J-D, Race J-M. Metformin and lactic acidosis in diabetic humans. *Diabetes Obes Metab* 2000; **2**:131–137.

49 Henquin JC. The fiftieth anniversary of hypoglycaemic suphonamides: how did the mother compound work? *Diabetologia* 1992; **35**:907–912.

50 Ashcroft FM, Gribble FM. ATP-sensitive K^+ channels and insulin secretion: their role in health and disease. *Diabetologia* 1999; **42**:903–919.

51 Gribble FM, Reimann F. Pharmacological modulation of K-ATP channels. *Biochem Soc Trans* 2002; **30**:333–339.

52 Rorsman P, Renstrom E. Insulin granule dynamics in pancreatic beta cells. *Diabetologia* 2003; **46**:1029–1045.

53 Ball AJ, Flatt PR, McClenaghan NH. Desensitization of sulphonylurea- and nutrient-induced insulin secretion following prolonged treatment with glibenclamide. *Eur J Pharmacol* 2000; **408**:327–333.

54 Lebovitz HE. Insulin secretagogues: old and new. *Diabetes Rev* 1999; **7**:139–151.

55 Groop LC. Sulfonylureas in NIDDM. *Diabetes Care* 1992; **15**:1737–1754.

56 Rendell M. The role of sulfonylureas in the management of type 2 diabetes. *Drugs* 2004; **64**:1339–1358.

57 Schernthaner G, Grimaldi A, Di Mario U, Drzewoski J, Kempler P, Kvapil M, *et al.* GUIDE study: double-blind comparison of once-daily gliclazide MR and glimepiride in type 2 diabetic patients. *Eur J Clin Invest* 2004; **34**:535–542.

58 Krentz AJ, Ferner RE, Bailey CJ. Comparative tolerability profiles of oral antidiabetic agents. *Drug Saf* 1994; **11**:223–241.

59 Wilson SH, Kennedy FP, Garratt KN. Optimization of the management of patients with coronary heart disease and type 2 diabetes mellitus. *Drugs Aging* 2001; **18**:325–333.

60 Garrino MG, Schmeer W, Nenquin M, Meissner HP, Henquin JC. Mechanism of the stimulation of insulin release *in vitro* by HB 699, a benzoic acid derivative similar to the non-sulfonylurea moiety of glibenclamide. *Diabetologia* 1985; **28**:697–703.

61 Dornhorst A. Insulotropic meglitinide analogues. *Lancet* 2001; **358**:1709–1715.

62 Davies M. Nateglinide: better post-prandial glucose control. *Prescriber* 2002; **13**:17–27.

63 Blickle JF. Meglitinide analogues: a review of clinical data focused on recent trials. *Diabetes Metab* 2006; **32**:113–120.

64 Day C. Thiazolidinediones: a new class of antidiabetic drugs. *Diabet Med* 1999; **16**:1–14.

65 Yki-Jarvinen H. Thiazolidinediones. *N Engl J Med* 2004; **351**:1106–1118.

66 Staels B, Fruchart J. Therapeutic roles of peroxisome proliferator-activated receptor genes. *Diabetes* 2005; **54**:2460–2470.

67 Semple RK, Chatterjee VK, O'Rahilly S. PPAR gamma and human metabolic disease. *J Clin Invest* 2006; **116**:581–589.

68 Blaschke F, Spanheimer R, Khan M, Law RE. Vascular effects of TZDs: new implications. *Vasc Pharmacol* 2006; **45**:3–18.

69 Kahn SE, Haffner SM, Heise MA, Holman RR, Kravitz BG, Yu D, *et al.* Glycemic durability of rosiglitazone, metformin or glyburide monotherapy. *N Engl J Med* 2006; **355**:2427–2443.

70 Bailey CJ. Treating insulin resistance in type 2 diabetes with metformin and thiazolidinedione. *Diabetes Obes Metab* 2005; **7**:675–691.

71 Nesto RW, Bell D, Bonow RO, Fonseca V, Grundy SM, Horton ES, *et al.* Thiazolidinedione use, fluid retention, and congestive heart failure: a consensus statement from the American Heart Association and the American Diabetes Association. *Circulation* 2003; **108**:2941–2948.

72 Nissen SE, Wolski K. Effect of rosiglitazone on the risk of myocardial infarction and death from cardiovascular casuses. *N Engl J Med* 2007; **356**:2457–2471.

73 Goldberg RB, Kendall DM, Deeg MA, Buse JB, Zagar AJ, Pinaire JA, *et al.* A comparison of lipid and glycemic effects of pioglitazone and rosiglitazone in patients with type 2 diabetes and dyslipidemia. *Diabetes Care* 2005; **28**:1547–1554.

74 Hermansen K, Mortensen LS. Body weight changes associated with antihyperglycaemic agents in type 2 diabetes mellitus. *Drug Saf* 2007; **30**:1127–1142.

75 McGuire DK, Inzucchi SE. New drugs for the treatment of diabetes mellitus. Part 1. thiazolidinedione and their evolving cardiovascular impolications. *Circulation* 2008; **117**:440–449.

76 Dormandy JA, Charbonnel B, Eckland DJ, Erdmann E, Massi-Benedetti M, Moules IK, *et al.* Secondary prevention of macrovascular events in patients with type 2 diabetes in the PROactive study (PROspective pioglitAzone Clinical Trial In macroVascular Events): a randomised controlled trial. *Lancet* 2005; **366**:1279–1289.

77 DREAM Trial Investigators, Gerstein HC, Yusuf S, Bosch J, Pogue J, Sheridan P, Dinccaq N, *et al.* Effect of rosiglitazone on the frequency of diabetes in patients with impaired glucose tolerance or impaired fasting glucose: a randomized controlled trial. *Lancet* 2006; **368**:1096–1105.

78 Buchanan TA, Xiang AH, Peters RK, Kjos SL, Marroquin A, Goico J, *et al.* Preservation of pancreatic beta-cell function and prevention of type 2 diabetes by pharmacological treatment of insulin resistance in high-risk hispanic women. *Diabetes* 2002; **51**: 2796–2803.

79 Erdmann E, Dormandy JA, Charbonnel B, Massi-Benedetti M, Moules IK, Skene AM; PROactive Investigators. The effect of pioglitazone on recurrent myocardial infarction in 2,445 patients with type 2 diabetes and previous myocardial infarction. Results from the PROactive (PROactive 05) study. *J Am Coll Cardiol* 2007; **49**:1772–1780.

80 Wilcox R, Bousser MG, Betteridge DJ, Schernthaner G, Piraqs V, Kupfer S, *et al.* Effects of pioglitazone in patients with type 2 diabetes with or without previous stroke. Results from PROactive (PROspective pioglitAzone Clinical Trial In macroVascular Events 04). *Stroke* 2007; **38**:865–873.

81 Loke Y, Singh S, Furberg CD. Long-term use of thiazolidinediones and fractures in type 2 diabetes: a meta-analysis. *Can Med Assoc J* 2009; **180**:5–15.

82 Holst JJ. Glucagon-like peptide-1: from extract to agent. The Claude Bernard Lecture, 2005. *Diabetologia* 2006; **49**:253–260.

83 Drucker DJ. The role of gut hormones in glucose homeostasis. *J Clin Invest* 2007; **117**:24–32.

84 Nauck M, Stockmann F, Ebert R, Creutzfeldt W. Reduced incretin effect in type 2 (non-insulin-dependent diabetes. *Diabetologia* 1986; **29**:46–52.

85 Deacon CF. Therapeutic strategies based on glucagon-like peptide 1. *Diabetes* 2004; **53**:2181–2189.

86 Weber AE. Dipeptidyl peptidase IV inhibitors for the treatment of diabetes. *J Med Chem* 2004; **47**:4135–4141.

87 Gorrell MD. Dipeptidyl peptidase IV (DPP-IV) and related enzymes in cell biology and liver disorders. *Clin Sci* 2005; **108**:277–292.

88 Flatt PR, Bailey CJ, Green BD. Dipeptidyl peptidase IV (DPP IV) and related molecules in type 2 diabetes. *Frontiers Biosci* 2008; **13**:3648–3660.

89 Flatt PR, Bailey CJ, Green BD. Recent advances in antidiabetic drug therapies targeting the enteroinsular axis. *Curr Drug Metab* 2009; **10**:125–137.

90 Amori RE, Lau J, Pittas AG. Efficacy and safety of incretin therapy in type 2 diabetes: systematic review and meta-analysis. *JAMA* 2007; **298**:194–206.

91 Green BD, Flatt PR, Bailey CJ. Gliptins: dipeptidyl peptidase-4 (DPP-4) inhibitors to treat type 2 diabetes. *Future Prescriber* 2007; **8**: 7–13.

92 Campbell IW, Day C. Sitagliptin: enhancing incretin action. *Br J Diabetes Vasc Dis* 2007; **7**:134–139.

93 Nauck MA, Meininger G, Sheng D, Terranella L, Stein PP; Sitagliptin Study 024 Group. Efficacy and safety of the dipeptidly peptidase-4 inhibitor, sitagliptin, compared with the sulfonylurea, glipizide, in patients with type 2 diabetes inadequately controlled on metformin alone: a randomized, double-blind, non-inferiority trial. *Diabetes Obes Metab* 2007; **9**:194–205.

94 Croxtall JD, Keam SJ. Vildagliptin: a review of its use in the management of type 2 diabetes mellitus. *Drugs* 2008; **68**:2387–2409.

95 Lebovitz HE. Alpha-glucosidase inhibitors as agents in the treatment of diabetes. *Diabetes Rev* 1998; **6**:132–145.

96 Chiasson JL, Josse RG, Gomis R, Hanefeld M, Karasik A, Laakso M; STOP-NIDDM Trial Research Group. Acarbose for the prevention of diabetes mellitus: the STOP-NIDDM randomised trial. *Lancet* 2002; **359**: 2072–2077.

97 Holman RR, Cull CA, Turner RC. A randomised double-blind trial of acarbose in type 2 diabetes shows improved glycemic control over 3 years (UK Prospective Diabetes Study 44). *Diabetes Care* 1999; **22**:960–964.

98 Chiasson J-L, Josse RG, Gomis R, Hanefeld M, Karasik A, Laakso M; STOP-NIDDM Trial Research Group. Acarbose treatment and the risk of cardiovascular disease and hypertension in patients with impaired glucose tolerance: the STOP-NIDDM trial. *JAMA* 2003; **290**:486–494.

99 Bailey CJ, Day C. Fixed-dose single tablet antidiabetic combinations. *Diabetes Obes Metab* 2009; **11**:527–533.

30 Non-Insulin Parenteral Therapies

Jens Juul Holst,[1] Sten Madsbad[2] & Ole Schmitz[3]

[1] Department of Biomedical Sciences, The Panum Institute, University of Copenhagen, Copenhagen, Denmark
[2] Department of Endocrinology, Hvidovre Hospital, University of Copenhagen, Denmark
[3] Department of Clinical Pharmacology, Aarhus University Hospital, Denmark

Keypoints

- Incretins are gut hormones that enhance glucose-stimulated insulin secretion and have an important role in the regulation of post-prandial glucose levels.
- The major incretin hormones are glucagon-like peptide 1 (GLP-1) and glucose-dependent insulinotropic polypeptide (GIP).
- The physiologic actions of GLP-1 include potentiation of meal-induced insulin secretion, inhibition of glucagon secretion, delay in gastric emptying and suppression of food intake and appetite.
- Beneficial effects of parenteral administration of a synthetic GLP-1 receptor agonist (exenatide or liraglutide) in patients with type 2 diabetes include improved glycemic control and mild weight loss; nausea and vomiting are the most common adverse events.
- Amylin is a naturally occurring peptide that is co-secreted with insulin from the β-cells of the pancreatic islets.
- Physiologic actions of amylin include delayed gastric emptying, suppression of post-prandial glucagon secretion and increased satiety.
- Beneficial effects of parenteral administration of pramlintide, a synthetic amylin mimetic approved for use in insulin-treated subjects with either type 1 or type 2 diabetes, include improved glycemic control and mild weight loss; transient nausea and hypoglycemia are the most common adverse events.
- The non-insulin parenteral therapies include activators of the GLP-1 receptor, also called "incretin mimetics," as well as amylin mimetics.

GLP-1 receptor activators

The actions of glucagon-like peptide 1 (GLP-1) include the potentiation of meal-induced insulin secretion and, in preclinical models, proliferation and/or neogenesis of the β-cell and prevention of β-cell apoptosis has been observed. GLP-1 also inhibits glucagon secretion, delays gastric emptying and suppresses food intake and appetite. Cardiovascular effects include protection of the ischemic heart, improved left ventricular ejection fraction, endothelial function and blood pressure lowering. In animal models, GLP-1 may also possess neurotropic effects. GLP-1 receptor agonists improve glycemic control to a degree that is similar to or greater than oral antidiabetic drugs. Furthermore, they induce weight loss of 2–3 kg, on average. It is unknown whether GLP-1 receptor agonists can delay the progression of type 2 diabetes mellitus (T2DM). The GLP-1 receptor mimetics are well tolerated and the most common adverse events are gastrointestinal, including nausea and vomiting. The available GLP-1 receptor agonists require injection once or twice daily, but once-weekly GLP-1 receptor activators are in development.

The incretin effect

"The incretin effect" designates the amplification of insulin secretion elicited by hormones secreted from the gastrointestinal tract. It is quantified by comparing insulin responses to oral and intravenous glucose administration, where the intravenous infusion is adjusted so as to result in the same (isoglycemic) peripheral plasma glucose concentrations [1,2]. In healthy subjects, the oral administration of gluocose causes a two- to threefold larger insulin response than the intravenous route as a result of the actions of the "incretin hormones." Because of this, the incretin hormones are thought to have a particularly important role in the regulation of post-prandial glucose levels.

The two most important incretins are glucose-dependent insulinotropic polypeptide (GIP), previously designated gastric inhibitory polypeptide, and GLP-1. Both have been established as important incretin hormones in mimicry experiments in humans, where the hormones were infused together with intravenous glucose to concentrations approximately corresponding to those observed during oral glucose tolerance tests. Both hormones powerfully enhanced insulin secretion, to an extent that

Textbook of Diabetes, 4th edition. Edited by R. Holt, C. Cockram, A. Flyvbjerg and B. Goldstein.

could fully explain the insulin response [3,4], and recent experiments have documented that both are active with respect to enhancing insulin secretion from the beginning of a meal (even at fasting glucose levels), and that they contribute almost equally, but with the effect of GLP-1 predominating at higher glucose levels [5]. The effects of the two hormones with respect to insulin secretion have been shown to be additive in humans [6].

The incretin effect in T2DM

Original studies by Nauck *et al.* [7] and several subsequent studies have indicated that the incretin effect is severely reduced or lost in patients with T2DM [8,9]. Thus, there is little doubt that a defective incretin effect contributes to the glucose intolerance of these patients.

Given that GLP-1 and GIP are the most important incretin hormones, it is possible to analyze their contribution to the defective incretin action in patients with diabetes. Such contributions could consist of defects with respect to secretion, action or metabolism. Detailed studies of the secretion of GIP and GLP-1 in response to mixed meals in patients with T2DM revealed a slightly impaired secretion of GIP, but a more pronounced impairment with respect to the secretion of GLP-1. The reduction was particularly prominent during the second and third hour of the meal test, while the initial response was unimpaired. The decreased response was related to both body mass index (BMI; the higher the BMI, the lower the incretin response) and to the actual diabetic state [10]. A decreased GLP-1 secretion in obese subjects has been observed repeatedly [11] and is related to an impaired incretin effect [12,13]. Insulin resistance is also independently related to a decreased GLP-1 meal response [13,14]. A decreased secretion of GLP-1 may not be seen in all obese or insulin-resistant subjects. Experience from the authors' laboratory suggests that in addition to insulin resistance and obesity, longer duration of diabetes and, in particular, influence of therapy is important. For instance, it is now clear that metformin enhances GLP-1 secretion [15]. When present, impaired secretion of GLP-1 is likely to contribute to the failing incretin effect.

The metabolism of GLP-1 and GIP was compared by Vilsbøll *et al.* [16,17] in patients with diabetes and controls; both hormones were metabolized at similar rates, suggesting that differences in their elimination do not explain the reduced plasma concentrations in diabetes.

With respect to the actions of the incretin hormones, it was discovered in 1993 that infusion of large amounts of GLP-1 resulted in near-normal insulin responses in patients with T2DM, whereas GIP had no significant effect [18]. However, infusions of GIP and GLP-1 at rates resulting in physiologic elevations of the incretin levels (as observed after mixed meal ingestion) while glucose was clamped at 15 mmol/L, failed to affect insulin secretion at all, despite these infusion rates greatly (and equally) increasing insulin secretion in healthy subjects [19]. These findings illustrate the dramatic loss of potency of both GIP and GLP-1 in T2DM. By contrast, when infused to supraphysiologic levels, GLP-1, but not GIP, was capable of restoring the β-cell sensitivity to glucose to completely normal values [20]. The mechanisms whereby GLP-1, but not GIP, stimulates insulin secretion in T2DM remain unknown, but the observation suggested that GLP-1 in pharmacologic doses could be used clinically to enhance insulin secretion in T2DM.

Finally, one may ask whether the incretin defect is a primary event, perhaps a major etiologic contributor to the β-cell failure that characterizes T2DM. Several observations suggest that this is not the case [9], but may be related to insulin resistance and/or hyperglycemia [21], as reviewed recently [9]. Interestingly, there are now data to suggest that intensified treatment resulting in near-normal glucose levels may lead to a partial restoration of incretin action of GLP-1 and GIP [19,22] and induction of insulin resistance in healthy subjects is associated with a loss of the incretin effect [23].

Actions of GLP-1

The acute insulinotropic effects of GLP-1 raised interest in the use of this peptide for the treatment of diabetes. In addition, the peptide possesses a number of other effects, which in the context of diabetes treatment must be considered favorable (Figure 30.1).

Effects on the islets

The insulinotropic activity of GLP-1, which represents a potentiation of glucose-induced insulin secretion and therefore is strictly glucose-dependent, is, at least partly (see below), exerted via interaction with the GLP-1 receptor located on the cell membrane of the β-cells [24]. Binding of GLP-1 to the receptor causes activation of adenylate cyclase resulting in the formation of cyclic AMP (cAMP), via a stimulatory G-protein. Most of the actions of GLP-1 are secondary to the formation of cAMP and results in a plethora of events including altered ion channel activity, intracellular calcium handling and enhanced exocytosis of insulin-containing granules [25]. The effects of glucose and GLP-1 may converge at the level of the K_{ATP} channels of the β-cells. These channels are sensitive to the intracellular ATP levels and, thereby, to glucose metabolism of the β-cells, but may also be closed by protein kinase A activated by GLP-1, resulting in subsequent depolarization of the plasma membrane and opening of voltage-sensitive calcium channels [26–28]. This has clinical importance because sulfonylurea drugs, which bind to and close the K_{ATP} channels and thereby cause membrane depolarization and calcium influx, may uncouple the glucose dependency of GLP-1 [29]. Indeed, 30–40% of patients treated with both sulfonylurea compounds and a GLP-1 agonist (see below) experience, usually mild, hypoglycemia.

The transcription factor PDX-1, a key regulator of islet growth and insulin gene transcription, appears to be essential for most of the glucoregulatory, proliferative and cytoprotective actions of GLP-1 [30]. In addition, GLP-1 upregulates the genes for the cellular machinery involved in insulin secretion, such as the glucokinase and GLUT-2 genes [31]. For further discussion of the insulinotropic effects of GLP-1, see Holst [32].

Importantly, GLP-1 also has trophic effects on β-cells [33]. Not only does it stimulate β-cell proliferation [34,35], but it also

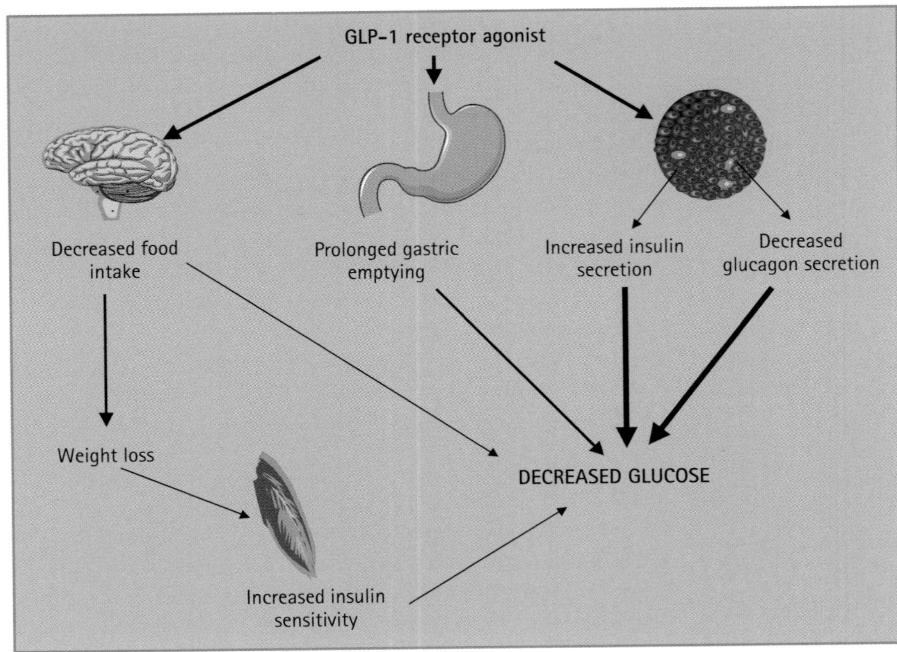

Figure 30.1 Effects of glucagon-like peptide 1 (GLP-1) receptor agonists on glucose metabolism.

enhances the differentiation of new β-cells from progenitor cells in the pancreatic duct epithelium [30,36] and inhibits apoptosis of β-cells including human β-cells [37,38]. Because the normal number of β-cells is maintained in a balance between apoptosis and proliferation [39], this observation is of considerable interest, and also raises the possibility that GLP-1 could be useful in conditions with increased β-cell apoptosis.

The complicated mechanisms whereby GLP-1 may exert trophic effects on the β-cells were reviewed recently by Drucker [40].

Reflex activation of the β-cell

GLP-1 is extensively degraded by the enzyme dipeptidyl peptidase 4 (DPP-4) and it has been demonstrated that only about one-quarter of the amount of GLP-1 leaving the gut (the endocrine organ) is still in the intact active form, and only about 8% of what is secreted actually reaches the pancreas as the intact peptide [41–43]. This has given rise to speculation that the actions of GLP-1 on the β-cells might be exerted indirectly via activation of long vagovagal reflexes [42]. Indeed, the GLP-1 receptor is expressed in cell bodies in the nodose ganglion from which the sensory afferents from the gastrointestinal tract emanate [44], and it has been demonstrated that blockade of the autonomic ganglia also blocked the effects of intraportally injected GLP-1 on insulin secretion [45]. Thus, it may be that under physiologic conditions the majority of the effects of GLP-1 on insulin secretion are transmitted via autonomic nerves.

Effects on glucagon secretion

GLP-1 also strongly inhibits glucagon secretion. Because in patients with T2DM there is fasting hyperglucagonemia as well as exaggerated glucagon responses to meal ingestion [46], and because it has been demonstrated that the hyperglucagonemia contributes to the hyperglycemia of patients [47], this effect may be as important as the insulinotropic effects. The mechanism whereby GLP-1 inhibits glucagon secretion remains unsettled but there is evidence that the somatostatin-producing D-cells of the islets transmit the effects of GLP-1 by paracrine inhibition of the α-cells [48].

Effects on the gastrointestinal tract

Further important effects of GLP-1 include inhibition of gastrointestinal secretion and motility, notably gastric emptying [49,50]. By this mechanism, GLP-1 may curtail post-prandial glucose excursions [51], and thereby reduce the number of episodes with high post-prandial glucose levels. There has been concern that the powerful inhibitory effect could represent a problem in patients with gastroparesis, but so far there have been no reported cases.

Effects on appetite and food intake

GLP-1 inhibits appetite and food intake in normal subjects [52] as well as in obese subjects with T2DM [53,54], and it is thought that GLP-1 is one of the gastrointestinal hormones that normally regulate food intake [32]. Clinical studies have shown that the effects on food intake are maintained for several years and lead to a sustained or progressive weight loss.

Cardiovascular effects

It has been known for some time that there are GLP-1 receptors in the heart [55]. A physiologic function for these receptors was indicated in recent studies in mice lacking the GLP-1 receptor,

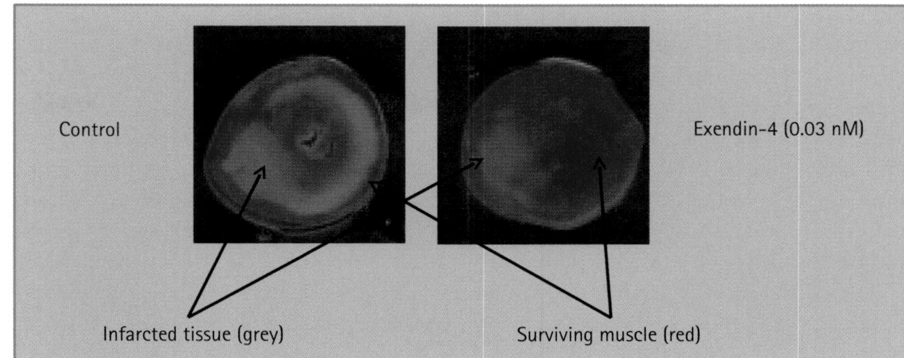

Figure 30.2 Cardioprotective effect of the GLP-1 receptor agonist, exendin-4. Post-conditioning with the GLP-1 receptor agonist, exendin-4 (i.e. addition of the agonist to the perfusate *after* the ischemia period) reduces infarct size in an isolated rat heart model of ischemia-reperfusion injury. Adapted from Sonne *et al.* [60]

which exhibit impaired left ventricular contractility and diastolic functions as well as impaired responses to exogenous epinephrine [56]. GLP-1 also increases left ventricular pressure and coronary blood flow in isolated mouse hearts [57], although in normal rat hearts, it reduces contractility [58]. However, further studies in rats showed that GLP-1 protects the ischemic and reperfused myocardium in rats by mechanisms independent of insulin [58,59]. Protective effects may be demonstrated by administration of GLP-1or GLP-1 receptor agonists both before and after ischemia (Figure 30.2) [57,60], and may involve the p70s6 kinase [61]. Surprisingly, some of the cardiac effects may also be elicited by the metabolite GLP-1 9-36 amide, which is formed rapidly in the circulation, but which has a strongly reduced activity on the classic GLP-1 receptor of the β-cells [57,60,62]. It has therefore been suggested that a different receptor mediates at least some of the cardiovascular effects, although not all studies support this [61]. Whatever the mechanism, these findings may have important clinical implications. Nikolaidis *et al.* [63] studied patients treated with angioplasty after acute myocardial infarction, but with postoperative left ventricular ejection fractions as low as 29%. In these patients, GLP-1 administration significantly improved the ejection fraction to 39% and improved both global and regional wall motion indices [63]. In studies of dogs with induced dilated cardiomyopathy, GLP-1 was reported to improve left ventricular and systemic hemodynamics dramatically, and it was suggested that GLP-1 may be a useful metabolic adjuvant in decompensated heart failure [64]. Indeed, addition of GLP-1 to standard therapy in patients with heart failure significantly improved left ventricular ejection fraction, myocardial oxygen uptake, 6-minute walking distance and quality of life [65]. In another study in which patients undergoing coronary artery bypass grafting were randomized to receive GLP-1 or conventional treatment, there was less use of inotropic and vasoactive drugs and fewer arrhythmias, as well as better glycemic control, in the GLP-1 group [66]. The cardioprotective actions of GLP-1 were recently reviewed by Fields *et al.* [67].

Furthermore, GLP-1 has been found to improve endothelial dysfunction in patients with T2DM and coronary heart disease, again a finding with interesting therapeutic perspectives [68]. An effect on endothelial dependent vasodilation was confirmed in healthy subjects [69], and functional receptors for GLP-1 have been identified on endothelial cells [57]. Chronic administration of GLP-1 agonists for clinical use is generally associated with small but significant decreases in blood pressure [70,71]. This may reflect the vasodilatory actions of GLP-1 as observed in various animal experimental models [57,72].

Neurotropic effects

Intracerebroventricular GLP-1 administration was associated with improved learning in rats and also displayed neuroprotective effects [73,74]. GLP-1 has also been proposed as a new therapeutic agent for neurodegenerative diseases, including Alzheimer disease [75], supported by observations that GLP-1 can modify processing of amyloid precursor protein and protect against oxidative injury [76]. Very recently, it was reported that the GLP-1 receptor agonist, exendin 4, promoted adult neurogenesis, normalized dopamine imbalance and increased the number of dopaminergic neurons in the substantia nigra in animal models of Parkinson disease [77].

Actions of GLP-1 in T2DM

In agreement with the findings of preserved insulinotropic actions of GLP-1 in T2DM [18], intravenous infusion of GLP-1 at 1.2 pmol/kg/minute was demonstrated to be capable of completely normalizing plasma glucose in patients with long-standing severe disease admitted to hospital for insulin treatment [78]. Subsequent studies in patients with moderate disease showed that plasma glucose concentrations could be near-normalized by an intravenous GLP-1 infusion covering the night-time and the next day, including two meals [79]. Continuous intravenous infusion of GLP-1 is not clinically practical and the effect of subcutaneous injections of GLP-1, given to both patients and healthy subjects [80], on plasma glucose and insulin concentrations turned out to be very short-lasting, because of an extremely rapid and extensive metabolism of GLP-1 in the body [81,82]. The intact peptide has an apparent intravenous half-life of 1–2 minutes and a plasma clearance amounting to 2–3 times the cardiac plasma output [16]. GLP-1 degradation is brought about by the actions of the ubiquitous enzyme, DPP-4, which catalyzes the removal of the two N-terminal amino acids of the molecule, thereby rendering it inactive [81] with respect to insulin secretion (but it may have cardiovascular effects, see above). The metabolic instability of

GLP-1 clearly restricts its clinical usefulness, but Zander *et al.* [83] carried out a clinical study in which GLP-1 or saline was administered as a continuous subcutaneous infusion (using insulin pumps) for 6 weeks to a group of patients with T2DM. The patients were evaluated before, after 1 week and after 6 weeks of treatment. No changes were observed in the saline-treated control group, whereas in the GLP-1 group, fasting and average plasma glucose concentrations were lowered by approximately 4–6 mmol/L, HbA_{1c} decreased by 1.2% (13 mmol/mol), free fatty acids were significantly lowered and the patients had a gradual weight loss of approximately 2 kg. In addition, insulin sensitivity, determined by a hyperinsulinemic euglycemic clamp, almost doubled, and insulin secretion capacity (measured using a 30 mmol/L glucose clamp + arginine) greatly improved. There was no significant difference between results obtained after treatment for 1 or 6 weeks, but there was a tendency towards further improvement of plasma glucose as well as insulin secretion. There were very few side effects and no differences between saline and GLP-1 treated patients in this respect. This study therefore provided "proof of concept" for the principle of GLP-based therapy of T2DM, and further attempts to utilize the therapeutic potential of GLP-1 have included, on one hand, the development of stable, DPP-4 resistant analogs [84] and, on the other hand, inhibitors of DPP-4 demonstrated to be capable of protecting the peptide from degradation and thereby augmenting its insulinotropic activity (see Chapter 29) [85].

GLP-1 receptor agonists

None of the per oral antidiabetics or insulin have been shown to stop the progressive decline of β-cell function, and none address the elevated glucagon secretion [86]. Some oral antidiabetics are associated with weight gain (sulfonylureas, glinides and glitazones), hypoglycemia (sulfonylureas and glinides), lactate acidosis (metformin), intestinal side effects (metformin and α-glucosidase inhibitors) or peripheral edema and fractures (glitazones) [86].

In contrast, GLP-1 receptor agonists regulate glucose metabolism and promote weight loss with a low risk of hypoglycemia. At present two GLP-1 receptor agonists are approved. Exenatide (Byetta®) was approved by the US Food and Drug Administration (FDA) in April 2005 and released in Europe in 2007 for the treatment of T2DM. Liraglutide (Victoza®), a once-daily human GLP-1 analog, was approved in Europe in May 2009 and by the FDA in January 2010.

Exenatide (Byetta)

Exendin-4, originally isolated from the saliva of the Gila monster, has 53% sequence homology with human GLP-1 in its first 30 amino acids [87]. Synthetic exendin-4, referred to as exenatide (1-39), is resistant to DPP-4 cleavage, and has a subcutaneous half-life in humans of approximately 2.5 hours after injection and a peak action 2–3 hours after injection [88], as reviewed in [89]. Exenatide is not recommended for patients with severe kidney failure (creatinine clearance <30 mL/minute), because it is predominantly eliminated by glomerular filtration with subsequent proteolytic degradation. Exenatide, administered twice daily within 60 minutes of morning and evening meals, lowers glucose for 5–7 hours and predominately affects post-prandial glycemic excursion, with only modest effects on lunch hyperglycemia and on fasting blood glucose [89–90]. The main side effect, nausea, is dose-dependent after subcutaneous injection, but may show some tachyphylaxis [88]. Therefore, it is recommended to start therapy with 5 μg twice daily for 1 month and subsequently to increase to 10 μg twice daily.

In clinical studies, exenatide exhibited actions that are similar to those of GLP-1, but the *in vivo* glucoregulatory potency of exenatide is significantly greater than that of native GLP-1 [91]. Increased insulin secretion, inhibition of glucagon secretion and delayed gastric emptying are the main mechanisms by which exenatide improves glucose metabolism (Figure 30.1) [88,89,92].

Clinical efficacy of exenatide

In the three so-called AMIGO (Diabetes Management for Improving Glucose Outcome) trials, the efficacy of exenatide in combination with metformin, sulfonylurea or a combination of the two was studied for 30 weeks [93–95]. Basal mean HbA_{1c} in the three studies was 8.3–8.6% (67–70 mmol/mol). The placebo-corrected reduction in HbA_{1c} with 10 μg b.i.d. was 0.9–1.0% (10–11 mmol/mol), and the weight loss was 1.6–2.6 kg after 30 weeks [94–95]. Body weight reductions were directly proportional to baseline BMI, with about 80% of subjects losing weight [93–95]. Improvements were observed in some cardiovascular risk factors and hepatic biomarkers [71]. Thus, increases in high density lipoprotein (HDL) cholesterol (+0.12 mmol/L), decreases in triglycerides (−0.43 mmol/L) and diastolic blood pressure (−2.7 mmHg) were achieved [71]. Two weeks' treatment with exenatide was associated with significantly decreased post-prandial triglycerides excursions [96].

In patients with T2DM treated with a glitazone and metformin, exenatide reduced HbA_{1c} (baseline mean HbA_{1c} 7.9%, 63 mmol/mol) by 1.0% (11 mmol/mol) and weight by 1.6 kg compared with placebo [97]. No clinically significant episodes of hypoglycemia were reported [97]. As in most of the other studies, the drop-out rate in the exenatide group was twice that in the placebo group (29% vs 14%) [97].

In an open-label trial, insulin glargine once daily or exenatide twice daily were added for patients inadequately controlled by metformin and sulfonylurea [98]. HbA_{1c} fell by 1.1% (12 mmol/mol) points in both groups (baseline mean HbA_{1c} 8.2%, 66 mmol/mol) [98]. Body weight increased by 1.8 kg with insulin glargine while a 2.3-kg weight loss was obtained with exenatide. Frequencies of hypoglycemia did not differ between treatments, but nocturnal hypoglycemia was less frequent with exenatide. Approximately 19% and 10% of the patients withdrew from the study in the exenatide and glargine groups, respectively [98]. In a 52-week trial, exenatide was compared with twice daily biphasic insulin aspart (baseline mean HbA_{1c} 8.6%, 70 mmol/mol) [99]. A greater proportion of exenatide-treated patients reached HbA_{1c} <7.0% (<53 mmol/mol, 32% vs 24%) [99]. Body weight changes (−2.5 kg vs +2.9 kg) also favored exenatide over insulin. Systolic (−5 mmHg) and diastolic (−2 mm Hg) blood pressures were significantly reduced with exenatide, but remained unchanged with insulin. No difference with respect to hypoglycemia was found between the two groups [99].

In obese subjects with T2DM treated with insulin plus oral antidiabetic drugs, addition of exenatide induced a 6.5-kg weight loss and lowered HbA_{1c} by 0.6% (7 mmol/mol) points over a 26-week follow-up period [100]. Rapid acting and premix insulin doses were reduced by 28% and 60%, respectively, while the dose of basal insulin was unchanged. In contrast, substitution of exenatide for insulin in insulin-treated patients with T2DM appears to be less successful, because such a switch resulted in a slight increase in HbA_{1c} (+0.3%, 3 mmol/mol) [101].

Other studies have shown that exenatide improved first-phase insulin responses to intravenous glucose and decreased the proinsulin : insulin ratio, indicating a beneficial effect of exenatide treatment on β-cell function [94,102]. Nevertheless, no human data indicate that exenatide can protect or restore the β-cell mass. Thus, the β-cell function did not change from before start of treatment when tested after 1 year treatment with exenatide followed by 1 month wash-out of exenatide [103].

Adverse effects with exenatide

Exenatide has generally been well tolerated and rarely causes treatment discontinuation because of side effects, but in the phase 3 studies drop-out rates in the exenatide groups were twice those in the placebo-treated groups [93–95]. Hypoglycemia is not a problem when exenatide is used in monotherapy or in combination with metformin [94], but mild hypoglycemia was observed in 15–36% of subjects receiving sulfonylurea in combination with exenatide [93,95]. Appropriate glucagon responses have been demonstrated during treatment with GLP-1 or exenatide, which may protect against severe hypoglycemia [104,105]. Mild to moderate nausea has been reported in up to 57% of patients treated with exenatide compared to about 7–23% on placebo in combination with oral antidiabetic drugs [93–95]. Nausea generally occurs during the first days of treatment and, in most patients, decreases with time. Vomiting and headache have also been observed in some patients. Other adverse effects reported include diarrhoea, dizziness and constipation [106]. About 40–50% of treated subjects develop antibodies to exenatide [93–95]; the importance of these is unknown, but they do not seem to influence efficacy on glucose control, except in some subjects with very high titers. Exenatide treatment has been associated with acute pancreatitis, and clinicians should be alert to this potential adverse effect [107]; however, it is not evident that the incidence of acute pancreatitis is higher in those receiving exenatide than in the background diabetic population. It has been recommended that exenatide should not be used in subjects at risk of pancreatitis (e.g. with alcoholism, cholecystolithiasis or hypertriglyceridemia), and if pancreatitis is suspected the drug should be discontinued.

Liraglutide

Liraglutide is a once daily human GLP-1 analog, with a half-life of about 13 hours following subcutaneous injection. Liraglutide is based on the structure of native GLP-1 with an amino acid substitution (lysine with arginine at position 34) and attachment of a C16 acyl chain via a glutamoyl spacer to lysine at position 26 [108]. Liraglutide is relatively stable towards DPP-4 degradation both intrinsically (because it may form heptameric aggregates) and as a consequence of binding to albumin [108]. After initiation of treatment, steady-state concentrations are obtained after 3–4 days [108].

Studies with liraglutide

In the clinical Liraglutide Effect and Action in Diabetes (LEAD) development program the initial dose of liraglutide was escalated weekly in a stepwise fashion from 0.6 mg/day to 1.2 mg/day, and in some patients to 1.8 mg/day. In monotherapy (basal mean HbA_{1c} 8.3%, 67 mmol/mol) liraglutide 1.2 and 1.8 mg reduced HbA_{1c} more than glimepiride (LEAD-3) over 52 weeks (0.84%, 1.14% [12 mmol/mol] and 0.5% [5 mmol/mol], respectively) [109]. The decrease in HbA_{1c} with 1.8 mg liraglutide was significantly greater than with 1.2 mg liraglutide, and the decrease was most pronounced in the group previously treated with only lifestyle changes (1.2 mg liraglutide, 1.2% [13 mmol/mol]; 1.8 mg liraglutide, 1.6% [17 mmol/mol]; and glimepiride, 0.9% [10 mmol/mol]) [109]. A weight decrease occurred in the liraglutide groups, compared to weight gain in the glimepiride group, resulting in a weight difference of 3.2–3.6 kg [109]. Nausea, mostly transient, occurred in 29% of the participants in the liraglutide groups compared with 9% in the glimepiride group. The rates of minor hypoglycemic episodes were significantly lower for the liraglutide groups versus glimepiride (12, 8 and 24 events/subjects/year) [109]. Two-year data showed that liraglutide had a long-lasting beneficial effect on glycemic control with a reduction in HbA_{1c} of −0.9% (10 mmol/mol), −1.1% (12 mmol/mol) and −0.6% (7 mmol/mol) in the 1.2 mg liraglutide, 1.8 mg liraglutide and glimepiride groups, respectively [110]. The weight loss was −2.1 kg, −2.7 kg and +1.1 kg in the three groups [110].

Liraglutide, when added to glimepiride (LEAD-1) reduced HbA_{1c} more than rosiglitazone over 26 weeks (1.1% vs 0.4%, 12 vs 4 mmol/mol) [111]. The changes in weight were superior for liraglutide compared with rosiglitazone [111].

Liraglutide was compared with 4 mg glimepiride when added to metformin (baseline mean HbA_{1c} 8.4%, 68 mmol/mol) in LEAD-2 [112]. The reduction in HbA_{1c} did not differ between glimepiride and liraglutide over 26 weeks (1.0% vs 1.0%, 11 mmol/mol). The reduction in weight in the two groups treated with 1.2 or 1.8 mg/day liraglutide was 2.6 and 2.8 kg, compared with an increase in weight of 1.0 kg in group the treated with glimepiride [112]. Mild hypoglycemic events were reported in up to 2.5% of the patients treated with metformin and liraglutide compared with 17% in the glimepiride group [112]. In LEAD-4, liraglutide, when added to metformin and rosiglitazone, reduced HbA_{1c} (−1.5% vs +0.5%, −16 vs +5 mmol/mol) and weight (−2.0 vs +0.6 kg) more than placebo [113].

In LEAD-5, patients treated with metformin plus a sulfonylurea were randomized to treatment with liraglutide (1.8 mg) or insulin glargine [114]. Mean reduction in HbA_{1c} was significantly greater with liraglutide than in insulin glargine treated groups (1.1% vs 0.9%, 12 vs 10 mmol/mol), and more than half of the patients treated with liraglutide reached the American Diabetes Association (ADA) target of HbA_{1c} <7.0% (<53 mmol/mol), and 36% reached HbA_{1c} <6.5% (<48 mmol/mol) [114]. With respect to body weight, liraglutide resulted in a weight difference of 3.5 kg compared to the insulin glargine treated group [114]. Five patients (2.2%) experienced major hypoglycemic episodes in the liraglutide treated group; there were no major episodes in the insulin glargine treatment group. It is well described that the combination of a sulfonylurea with a GLP-1 receptor agonist increases the risk of hypoglycemia. The mechanism behind this reflects an uncoupling of the glucose-dependent insulin secretion of GLP-1 when combined with a sulfonylurea [29]. Incidence of minor hypoglycemic events did not differ between the groups [114].

In LEAD-6, a head-to-head comparison of 1.8 mg liraglutide once daily with exenatide 10 μg twice daily, the reduction in HbA_{1c} was 1.1% (12 mmol/mol), compared to 0.8% (9 mmol/mol), respectively [115]. Both groups lost around 3 kg in weight. The most frequent reported adverse events for both liraglutide and exenatide treated groups were nausea at a level of around 25% when initiating therapy [115]. After week 8–10 the percentage of patients reporting nausea with liraglutide was well below 10%, while in the exenatide group the level remained at about 10%. The rate of minor hypoglycemia was significantly lower in the liraglutide group. After 30 weeks the patients treatment with exenatide were shifted to liraglutide, which resulted in a further 0.3% (3 mmol/mol) reduction in HbA_{1c}.

Treatment with liraglutide has been associated with improvement of several cardiovascular risk factors: C-reactive protein (CRP), tumor necrosis factor α (TNF-α) induced plasminogen activator inhibitor 1 (PAI-1), vascular cell adhesion molecule 1 (VCAM-1), intercellular adhesion molecule 1 (ICAM-1) and B-type natriuretic peptide (BNP) [116]. The weight reduction in the clinical studies depend on basal BMI, and was in subjects with BMI <25 kg/m^2 from 0–2 kg increasing to 1–4.5 kg in subjects with a BMI >35 kg/m^2 [117]. The greatest weight loss was observed with the combination of liraglutide and metformin, which may reflect that metformin is weight neutral while sulfonylureas such as glimepiride and rosiglitazone are associated with weight gain [117]. The highest dose of liraglutide (1.8 mg/day) reduces systolic blood pressure by 2.7–4.5 mmHg versus comparator treatment, but in patients with a systolic blood pressure greater than 140 mmHg the reduction was about 11 mmHg [118]. Lastly, liraglutide improved β-cell function evaluated by homeostasis model assessment (HOMA) and the proinsulin : insulin ratio [119]. The thyroid C-cell neoplastic changes, which have been observed in rodents and mice, have not been observed in humans [120]. Five cases of pancreatitis were described during the phase 3 program with liraglutide.

Comparison of GLP-1 receptor agonists with DPP-4 inhibitors

The GLP-1 receptor agonist and DPP-4 inhibitors differ in route of administration and may have differing side effect and tolerability profiles (Figure 30.3). Two head-to-head studies have

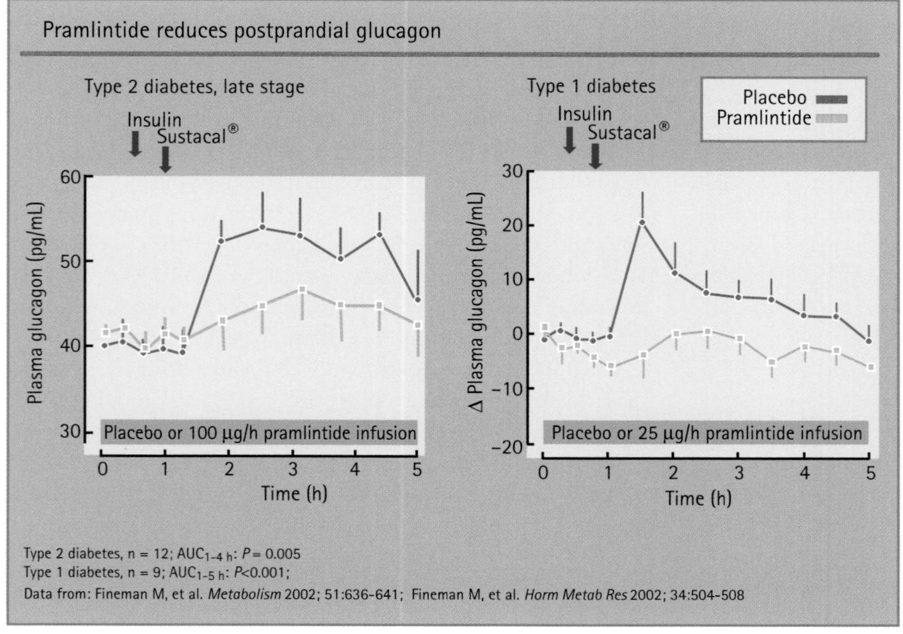

Figure 30.3 Dose-response relationships for the effects of GLP-1. The figure illustrates the relationship between the plasma concentrations of GLP-1 or GLP-1 mimetics and their clinical effects and side effects as observed during treatment with GLP-1 mimetics or incretin enhancers (DPP-4 inhibitors, see Chapter 29). With modestly elevated GLP-1 levels, as obtained with both mimetics and enhancers, there are significant effects on the pancreatic islets. Higher concentrations (which may not be reached during therapy with enhancers) are needed to slow down gastric emptying and to reduce appetite and food intake. At even higher concentrations, which may be reached with GLP-1 mimetics, side effects such as nausea, diarrhea and vomiting might result . Adapted from Holst JJ, Deacon CF, Vilsbøll T, Krarup T, Madsbad S: Glucagon-like peptide-1, glucose homeostasis and diabetes. *Trends Mol Med* 2008; 14: 161–168.

compared the efficacy of a GLP-1 receptor agonist and the DPP-4 inhibitor sitagliptin. Liraglutide reduced HbA_{1c} by 1.4% vs 0.9% (14 vs 10 mmol/mol) and weight by −3.5 vs −0.9 kg compared with sitagliptin. In another study, exenatide once weekly reduced HbA_{1c} by 1.7% vs 1.0% (19 vs 11 mmol/mol), and the weight by 2.8 vs 0.9 kg compared with sitagliptin [121].

Future GLP-1 receptor agonists

Exenatide once weekly

Exenatide once weekly, a preparation containing a polylactide-glycolide microsphere suspension, leads to a sustained release for up to 28 days after single subcutaneous injection and is currently in phase 3 clinical development [122]. Exenatide 10 μg twice daily and 2 mg once weekly reduced HbA_{1c} after 30 weeks' treatment by 1.9% vs 1.5% (21 vs 16 mmol/mol) from a baseline of 8.3% (67 mmol/mol) 77% vs 61% of patients reached an HbA_{1c} of 7.0% or less (<53 mmol/mol) without any reports of severe hypoglycemia [122]. Notably, 29% of once weekly treated patients taking exenatide with a baseline HbA_{1c} >9.0% (>75 mmol/mol) achieved levels <6.5% (<48 mmol/mol). About 26% vs 35% of the patients reported nausea with once weekly exenatide. Both groups lost about 4 kg in weight [123]. After 30 weeks the patients treated with exenatide twice daily were changed to treatment with exenatide once weekly [122]. After 1 year, the reduction in HbA_{1c} was about 2% (22 mmol/mol) in both groups and the mean HbA_{1c} was 6.6% (49 mmol/mol). Of the participants, 77% obtained a HbA_{1c} <7.0% (<53 mmol/mol). Weight loss was 4.5 kg, and one-third of the patients lost more than 5% in weight. In a group of participants with a HbA_{1c} >9.0% (>75 mmol/mol), the reduction in HbA_{1c} was 2.8% (31 mmol/mol). Systolic blood pressure was reduced by 6 mmHg in the whole group, and 11 mmHg in subjects with hypertension at baseline. About 74% developed antibodies to exenatide, and a small group of participants with high-titer antibodies showed attenuated glycemic response [122].

Albiglutide

Albiglutide is a long-acting GLP-1 receptor agonist, developed by fusion of two recombinant human GLP-1 molecules (with an ALA8→GLY amino acid substitution) to recombinant human albumin [124]. Despite the large size of the molecule, albiglutide inhibits gastric emptying and appetite, although it is unclear whether the anorectic effect is weaker than that of native GLP-1 because of an impaired blood–brain barrier permeability [125]. The circulating half-life is 6–7 days, and in phase 2 studies it has been administered weekly, biweekly or monthly [126]. The optimal dose seems to be 30 mg weekly in relation to reduction in HbA_{1c} and side effects, and this dose has been shown to be more potent than exenatide twice daily in reducing HbA_{1c} with less nausea [126]. Albiglutide is currently in phase 3 clinical development.

Taspoglutide

This a modified human GLP-1 receptor agonist resistant to DPP-4 degradation with a release profile extending up to 26 days, which make it suitable for once weekly administration [127]. The reduction in HbA_{1c} was 1.4–1.5% (15–16 mmol/mol) after 8 weeks' treatment with 10 and 20 mg once weekly. About 80% reached the goal of 7.0% (53 mmol/mol) from mean baseline of 7.9% (63 mmol/mol) [127]. The reduction in body weight after 8 weeks was about 2.1–2.8 kg. Taspoglutide is in phase 3 clinical development.

Other GLP-1 receptor agonists

Lixisenatide is a modified exendin 4 molecule which in phase 2 studies has been administered once or twice daily, and now is in phase 3 clinical development [128].

Other GLP-1 receptor agonists in development are CJC1134, which is a exendin 4 molecule linked covalently to serum albumin. Its half-life is similar to circulating albumin, approximately 10–15 days [129]. NN9535 from Novo Nordisk Pharmaceutical is a once weekly GLP-1 receptor agonist. Orally administered GLP-1 receptor agonists are in development, and also intranasal and pulmonary administration of GLP-1 is under investigation.

Comments on GLP-1 receptor agonists

The GLP-1 analog are attractive for treatment of people with T2DM because their effects on both insulin and glucagon secretion are glucose dependent, which reduces the risk of hypoglycemia. When GLP-1 analogs are combined with metformin or a glitazone the risk of hypoglycemia is minimal. GLP-1 receptor agonists induce weight loss, which is important because many people with T2DM are obese. The need for self-monitoring of blood glucose is minimal, especially when compared with insulin treatment. Whether the GLP-1 analogs can prevent the progression of the disease by preventing β-cell failure is yet unknown. The durability and magnitude of the weight loss induced by the GLP-1 analogs need to be established.

The observation that GLP-1 improves myocardial function in human patients after myocardial infarction, improves endothelial function and reduces blood pressure highlights the need for studies with cardiovascular endpoints [130]. GLP-1 analogs may be attractive to use in subjects with T2DM and heart failure because GLP-1 promotes renal sodium and water excretion and lowers blood pressure [70,131,132]. Long-term studies are also needed to obtain more data on the safety of the GLP-1 analogs. Lastly, studies in patients with newly diagnosed type 1 diabetes mellitus (T1DM) and in patients with T1DM of long duration and no residual β-cell function are needed to evaluate the ability of GLP-1 to prolong the remission, to reduce the insulin requirements and possibly the risk of hypoglycemia.

Amylin and amylin analogs

Amylin is a 37 amino acid peptide co-secreted with insulin. It delays gastric emptying, suppresses post-prandial glucagon secretion and increases satiety. Human amylin has an inherent

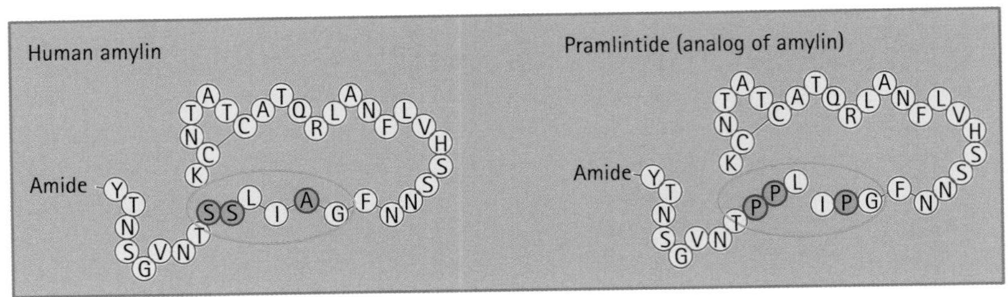

Figure 30.4 Human amylin, naturally occurring in β-cells. On the right-hand side is depicted the structure of the pramlintide molecule specifically engineered by three proline substitutions at amino acids 25, 28 and 29.

tendency to self-aggregate, forming fibrils and adhering to surfaces. Amylin Pharmaceuticals Inc. has developed an analog named pramlintide where the amino acid residues at positions 25, 28 and 29 are replaced with proline (Figure 30.4). Pramlintide was approved by the FDA in 2005 for use in insulin-treated subjects with either T1DM or T2DM. The results have been quite promising in that, when measured over a period of 6–12 months, treatment resulted in a decrease in HbA_{1c} of 0.4–0.6% (4–7 mmol/mol) compared with placebo. A small, but clinically significant, weight loss was observed (0.8–1.4 kg compared with placebo). Main side effects are nausea (often transient) and hypoglycemia but, when titrated, especially with a reduction in insulin dose, both have been reduced significantly.

Although amyloid deposits in the pancreas were first described more than a century ago as a major constituent in the islet of Langerhans of patients with T2DM, the primary component of these deposits was not identified until two decades ago by Cooper *et al.* [133] and Westermark *et al.* [134]. It is a 37 amino acid peptide, denoted islet amyloid polypeptide (IAPP) or amylin. Amylin has approximately 50% sequence identity to calcitonin gene-related peptide (CGRP) and is also structurally related to calcitonin, and belongs to the family of peptides, which also includes adrenomedullin. The amylin precursor, proamylin, is primarily co-localized in the secretory granules together with insulin and is processed by the same processing enzyme before being released from the pancreatic β-cells, co-secreted with insulin (Figure 30.5). Interestingly, similar to insulin and many other hormones, amylin is released in a high frequency pulsatile manner [135]. The peptide circulates in both a non-glycosylated form (approximately 50%) and a glycosylated form [136]. In contrast to insulin, amylin is mainly eliminated through renal metabolism. In healthy people its plasma concentrations are within the range of 4–25 pmol/L, and amylin is distributed, like insulin, in plasma and interstitial fluids. Smaller amounts of amylin are also present in the central nervous system, especially the caudal trigeminal nucleus and the amygdala area, and also in the gastric antrum and fundus, as well as being expressed in the entire gastrointestinal tract. The gene encoding the 89 amino acid prepolamylin precursor protein is located to chromosome 12 and consists of three exons and two introns. Functional amylin receptors can be generated by co-expression of the G-protein coupled calcitonin receptor gene and receptor activity modifying proteins.

Amylin effects

In vitro and animal studies

Most studies have been performed in rodents, and have demonstrated effects of amylin on glucose metabolism. In the rat skeletal muscle, amylin leads to insulin resistance in pharmacologic doses by inhibiting glycogen synthase activity and enhancing glycogen breakdown and subsequently lactate release. The influence of amylin *per se* on insulin secretion is controversial.

Amylin inhibits glucagon secretion in rats following an arginine infusion in a dose-dependent manner [137], but it does not suppress glucagon release in the isolated perfused pancreas, implying that its ability to inhibit glucagon secretion depends on extrapancreatic pathways. Amylin also delays gastric emptying. Dose–response studies have demonstrated that amylin is more potent in this respect than other gastrointestinal hormones. The ability of amylin to slowing down the gastric emptying process has, however, been shown to be overridden by hypoglycemia [138]. Finally, amylin reduces food intake and body weight in rodents. The inhibitory effect on food intake is present after both intracerebral and peripheral administration of amylin. These effects appear to be mediated mainly via central pathways that include high affinity binding sites in the area postrema in the hindbrain.

Amylin in human studies

Two studies, both from Bloom's group [139,140], have examined the possible impact of acute administration of native amylin on *in vivo* glucose metabolism in healthy humans. Despite using high pharmacologic doses of the hormone, resulting in circulating amylin levels 50–100 times above normal post-prandial concentrations, no effect of native amylin could be demonstrated on glucose uptake, neither as assessed by a hyperinsulinemic euglycemic clamp nor during an intravenous glucose tolerance test.

Effects of the amylin analog pramlintide in human studies

Acute and short-term studies

Human amylin has inappropriate physicochemical properties. It has an inherent tendency to self-aggregate, to form fibrils and to adhere to surfaces. Particularly, the amino residues in positions 20–29 are responsible for self-aggregation. Amylin Pharmaceuticals Inc. tested a number of different analogs of the human amylin

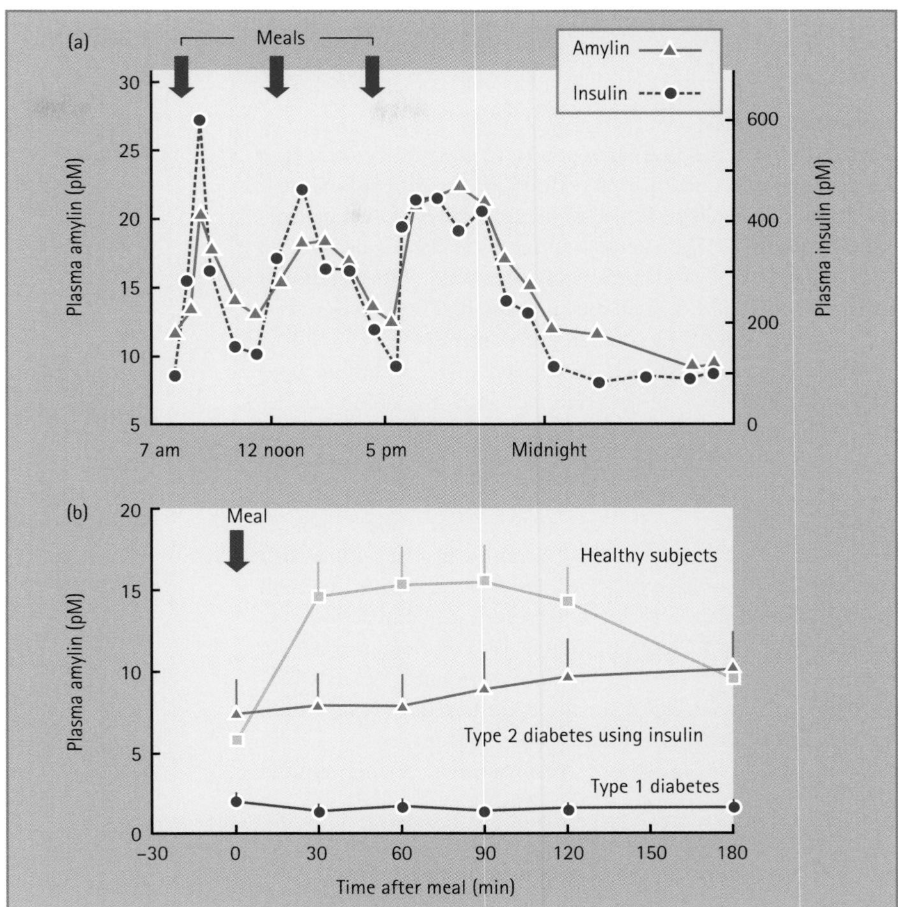

Figure 30.5 Plasma amylin concentrations in healthy subjects and patients with diabetes. (a) Mean 24-hour plasma profiles of insulin and amylin in six healthy males without diabetes. (b) Mean (±SE) amylin plasma concentrations following ingestion of a liquid Sustacal® meal. Similar to insulin secretion, amylin secretion is impaired in patients with type 2 diabetes (n = 12) and absent in patients with type 1 diabetes (n = 190) compared with healthy subjects (n = 27).

molecule including the originally designated peptide AC137 (pramlintide) in which the amino acid residues at positions 25, 28 and 29 were replaced with proline (Figure 30.2). Pramlintide was approved by the FDA in March 2005 for use in insulin-treated patients with T1DM and T2DM. At the time of writing, pramlintide has only been approved in the USA, where it has the tradename Symlin®. The plasma half-life of pramlintide is approximately 48 minutes [141] when given subcutaneously into the abdominal area or the thigh. The peptide is primarily eliminated by the kidneys. Normal dosing in patients with T1DM during gradual titration is often 60–90 μg three to four times per day prior to meals. In those with T2DM, doses may be somewhat higher and often administered subcutaneously twice per day. In order to optimize efficacy and also to minimize the often transient nausea, it is also important to titrate pramlintide dosing.

In the mid 1990s, Kolterman [142] performed a series of acute and short time studies with pramlintide given prior to a Sustacal meal (350 kcal, 24% protein, 21% fat and 55% carbohydrate). A considerable reduction in the glycemic levels after oral intake before the meal was observed in both patients with T1DM and T2DM in the acute studies as well as during the studies lasting 14–28 days. The efficacy of the acute and short-term pramlintide administration is probably because of the decreased gastric emptying and reduced glucagon response. The effect on gastric emptying in diabetes is well-documented [143]. The suppression of glucagon in subjects with diabetes and the ensuing decrease in endogenous glucose production as reported by Shah *et al.* [144] is considered important in view of the post-prandial glucagon excess characterizing T2DM. Fineman *et al.* [141] have convincingly described a significant, and probably clinical relevant, reduction in post-prandial circulation glucagon in patients with either T1DM or T2DM after pramlintide exposure together with a liquid Sustacal meal (Figure 30.4). It has been estimated that the influence of pramlintide on post-prandial glucagon is responsible for an approximately 25% reduction in plasma glucose which has also been confirmed by others. In a cross-over study during a stepwise hypoglycemic clamp in subjects with T1DM it was demonstrated that insulin sensitivity during euglycemia was normal (as shown in many other studies). During the hypoglycemic clamp with nadir of plasma glucose at 2.8 m/mol, plasma adrenalin and noradrenalin did not differ between pramlintide and placebo. Plasma glucagon tended to be higher during pramlintide administration ($P = 0.10$) as did cortisol. Growth hormone was significantly increased during hypoglycemia after pramlintide exposure. Recovery time after hypoglycemia did not differ [145].

Long-term studies

Several studies in the phase 3 program and many other interesting studies have subsequently been performed. The conclusion is that pramlintide, in double-blinded studies in insulin-treated patients with T1DM or T2DM, after 6–12 months leads to a decrease in HbA_{1c} of 0.4–0.6% (4–7 mmol/mol) compared with placebo. In patients with T2DM, a small but clinically significant weight loss was observed (0.8–1.4 kg compared to controls).

Other interesting findings have been made regarding lipid profile, combination of pramlintide with thiazolidinediones regarding weight, and the lowering of post-prandial glycemia during pramlintide administration. Previous exposure to pramlintide in humans significantly reduces the enthusiasm to eat a second meal [146]. In a recent study in very obese subjects without diabetes treated over a 12-month period with a high pramlintide dose as an adjunct to lifestyle intervention, a weight loss of approximately 8 kg was observed compared with the placebo group [147]. Recently, Roth *et al.* [148] demonstrated, in a proof of concept study, that pramlintide in humans acts synergistically with recombinant human leptin to reduce body weight in non-leptin deficient subjects and suggested that amylin agonism may restoring leptin responsiveness in diet-induced obesity.

Side effects and drawbacks of pramlintide treatment

The most common side effects are gastrointestinal, but these are generally transient and can be minimized by starting with a low dose of the compound. Another side effect is hypoglycemia, which is rare in T2DM. It should be noted that in the primary studies pramlintide and insulin doses were fixed, increasing the risk of hypoglycemia. Current recommendations suggest that titration is performed both with respect to both pramlintide dosing and reduction of insulin dose.

In spite of the availability of advanced injection devices, some patients feel it a burden to take these additional injections 2–4 times a day. For reasons of biochemical compatibility, it is unfortunately not possible to mix insulin and pramlintide in the same pen. It was demonstrated recently, however, that adjunctive pramlintide administration to individuals with T1DM, intensively treated with either multiple daily injection or pump therapy, in a double-blind non-inferiority trial, resulted in greater treatment satisfaction compared with placebo treatment, despite similar reductions in HbA_{1c} [149].

Conclusions and perspectives

Overall, pramlintide has proven effective in terms of reducing glycemia and weight, but must now prove efficacy against new drugs such as incretin mimetics. Conversely, pramlintide appears to be a safe antidiabetic drug, which can be used in combination with classic antidiabetic agents.

References

1 McIntyre N, Holdsworth CD, Turner DS. New interpretation of oral glucose tolerance. *Lancet* 1964; **2**:20–21.

2 Perley MJ, Kipnis DM. Plasma insulin responses to oral and intravenous glucose: studies in normal and diabetic subjects. *J Clin Invest* 1967; **46**:1954–1962.

3 Nauck M, Schmidt WE, Ebert R, Strietzel J, Cantor P, Hoffmann G, *et al.* Insulinotropic properties of synthetic human gastric inhibitory polypeptide in man: interactions with glucose, phenylalanine, and cholecystokinin-8. *J Clin Endocrinol Metab* 1989; **69**:654–662.

4 Kreymann B, Williams G, Ghatei MA, Bloom SR. Glucagon-like peptide-1 7-36: a physiological incretin in man. *Lancet* 1987; **2**:1300–1304.

5 Vilsboll T, Krarup T, Madsbad S, Holst JJ. Both GLP-1 and GIP are insulinotropic at basal and postprandial glucose levels and contribute nearly equally to the incretin effect of a meal in healthy subjects. *Regul Pept* 2003; **114**:115–121.

6 Nauck MA, Bartels E, Orskov C, Ebert R, Creutzfeldt W. Additive insulinotropic effects of exogenous synthetic human gastric inhibitory polypeptide and glucagon-like peptide-1-(7-36) amide infused at near-physiological insulinotropic hormone and glucose concentrations. *J Clin Endocrinol Metab* 1993; **76**:912–917.

7 Nauck M, Stockmann F, Ebert R, Creutzfeldt W. Reduced incretin effect in type 2 (non-insulin-dependent) diabetes. *Diabetologia* 1986; **29**:46–52.

8 Knop FK, Aaboe K, Vilsboll T, Madsbad S, Krarup T, Holst JJ. Reduced incretin effect in obese subjects with normal glucose tolerance as compared to lean control subjects. *Diabetologia* 2008; **51**:S258.

9 Holst JJ, Vilsboll T, Deacon CF. The incretin system and its role in type 2 diabetes mellitus. *Mol Cell Endocrinol* 2009; **297**:127–136.

10 Toft-Nielsen MB, Damholt MB, Madsbad S, Hilsted LM, Hughes TE, Michelsen BK, *et al.* Determinants of the impaired secretion of glucagon-like peptide-1 in type 2 diabetic patients. *J Clin Endocrinol Metab* 2001; **86**:3717–3723.

11 Naslund E, Backman L, Holst JJ, Theodorsson E, Hellstrom PM. Importance of small bowel peptides for the improved glucose metabolism 20 years after jejunoileal bypass for obesity. *Obes Surg* 1998; **8**:253–260.

12 Knop FK, Aaboe K, Vilsboll T, Madsbad S, Krarup T, Holst JJ. Reduced incretin effect in obese subjects with normal glucose tolerance as compared to lean control subjects. *Diabetologia* 2008; **51**:S258.

13 Muscelli E, Mari A, Casolaro A, Camastra S, Seghieri G, Gastaldelli A, *et al.* Separate impact of obesity and glucose tolerance on the incretin effect in normal subjects and type 2 diabetic patients. *Diabetes* 2008; **57**:1340–1348.

14 Rask E, Olsson T, Soderberg S, Johnson O, Seckl J, Holst JJ, *et al.* Impaired incretin response after a mixed meal is associated with insulin resistance in nondiabetic men. *Diabetes Care* 2001; **24**:1640–1645.

15 Migoya EM, Miller JL, Larson PJ, Tanen MR, Hilliard D, Deacon CF, *et al.* Sitagliptin, a selective DPP-4 inhibitor, and metformin have complementary effects to increase active GLP-1 concentrations. *Diabetologia* 2007; **50**:S52.

16 Vilsboll T, Agerso H, Krarup T, Holst JJ. Similar elimination rates of glucagon-like peptide-1 in obese type 2 diabetic patients and healthy subjects. *J Clin Endocrinol Metab* 2003; **88**:220–224.

17 Vilsboll T, Agerso H, Lauritsen T, Deacon CF, Aaboe K, Madsbad S, *et al.* The elimination rates of intact GIP as well as its primary metabolite, GIP 3-42, are similar in type 2 diabetic patients and healthy subjects. *Regul Pept* 2006; **137**:168–172.

18 Nauck MA, Heimesaat MM, Orskov C, Holst JJ, Ebert R, Creutzfeldt W. Preserved incretin activity of glucagon-like peptide 1 [7-36 amide] but not of synthetic human gastric inhibitory polypeptide in patients with type 2 diabetes mellitus. *J Clin Invest* 1993; **91**:301–307.

19 Hojberg PV, Vilsboll T, Rabol R, Knop FK, Bache M, Krarup T, *et al.* Four weeks of near-normalisation of blood glucose improves the insulin response to glucagon-like peptide-1 and glucose-dependent insulinotropic polypeptide in patients with type 2 diabetes. *Diabetologia* 2009; **52**:199–207.

20 Vilsboll T, Knop FK, Krarup T, Johansen A, Madsbad S, Larsen S, *et al.* The pathophysiology of diabetes involves a defective amplification of the late-phase insulin response to glucose by glucose-dependent insulinotropic polypeptide – regardless of etiology and phenotype. *J Clin Endocrinol Metab* 2003; **88**:4897–4903.

21 Jensen DH, Aaboe K, Henriksen JE, Madsbad S, Krarup T. Reduced incretin effect in dexamethasone-induced insulin resistance and glucose intolerance in diabetic offspring. *Diabetologia* 2009; **52**:S227–S228.

22 Hojberg PV, Zander M, Vilsboll T, Knop FK, Krarup T, Volund A, *et al.* Near normalisation of blood glucose improves the potentiating effect of GLP-1 on glucose-induced insulin secretion in patients with type 2 diabetes. *Diabetologia* 2008; **51**:632–640.

23 Jensen DH, Aaboe K, Henriksen JE, Madsbad S, Krarup T. Reduced incretin effect in dexamethasone-induced insulin resistance and glucose intolerance in diabetic offspring. *Diabetologia* 2009; **52**:S227–S228.

24 Holst JJ, Gromada J. Role of incretin hormones in the regulation of insulin secretion in diabetic and nondiabetic humans. *Am J Physiol Endocrinol Metab* 2004; **287**:E199–E206.

25 Holz GG. Epac: A new cAMP-binding protein in support of glucagon-like peptide-1 receptor-mediated signal transduction in the pancreatic beta-cell. *Diabetes* 2004; **53**:5–13.

26 Holz GG, Kuhtreiber WM, Habener JF. Pancreatic beta-cells are rendered glucose-competent by the insulinotropic hormone glucagon-like peptide-1(7-37). *Nature* 1993; **361**:362–365.

27 Gromada J, Bokvist K, Ding WG, Holst JJ, Nielsen JH, Rorsman P. Glucagon-like peptide 1 (7-36) amide stimulates exocytosis in human pancreatic beta-cells by both proximal and distal regulatory steps in stimulus-secretion coupling. *Diabetes* 1998; **47**: 57–65.

28 Light PE, Manning Fox JE, Riedel MJ, Wheeler MB. Glucagon-like peptide-1 inhibits pancreatic ATP-sensitive potassium channels via a protein kinase A- and ADP-dependent mechanism. *Mol Endocrinol* 2002; **16**:2135–2144.

29 de HJ, Holst JJ. Sulfonylurea compounds uncouple the glucose dependence of the insulinotropic effect of glucagon-like peptide 1. *Diabetes* 2007; **56**:438–443.

30 Li Y, Cao X, Li LX, Brubaker PL, Edlund H, Drucker DJ. Beta-cell Pdx1 expression is essential for the glucoregulatory, proliferative, and cytoprotective actions of glucagon-like peptide-1. *Diabetes* 2005; **54**:482–491.

31 Buteau J, Roduit R, Susini S, Prentki M. Glucagon-like peptide-1 promotes DNA synthesis, activates phosphatidylinositol 3-kinase and increases transcription factor pancreatic and duodenal homeobox gene 1 (PDX-1) DNA binding activity in beta (INS-1)-cells. *Diabetologia* 1999; **42**:856–864.

32 Holst JJ. The physiology of glucagon-like peptide 1. *Physiol Rev* 2007; **87**:1409–1439.

33 Egan JM, Bulotta A, Hui H, Perfetti R. GLP-1 receptor agonists are growth and differentiation factors for pancreatic islet beta cells. *Diabetes Metab Res Rev* 2003; **19**:115–123.

34 Xu G, Stoffers DA, Habener JF, Bonner-Weir S. Exendin-4 stimulates both beta-cell replication and neogenesis, resulting in increased beta-cell mass and improved glucose tolerance in diabetic rats. *Diabetes* 1999; **48**:2270–2276.

35 Stoffers DA, Kieffer TJ, Hussain MA, Drucker DJ, Bonner-Weir S, Habener JF, *et al.* Insulinotropic glucagon-like peptide 1 agonists stimulate expression of homeodomain protein IDX-1 and increase islet size in mouse pancreas. *Diabetes* 2000; **49**:741–748.

36 Zhou J, Wang X, Pineyro MA, Egan JM. Glucagon-like peptide 1 and exendin-4 convert pancreatic AR42J cells into glucagon- and insulin-producing cells. *Diabetes* 1999; **48**:2358–2366.

37 Farilla L, Bulotta A, Hirshberg B, Li CS, Khoury N, Noushmehr H, *et al.* Glucagon-like peptide 1 inhibits cell apoptosis and improves glucose responsiveness of freshly isolated human islets. *Endocrinology* 2003; **144**:5149–5158.

38 Buteau J, El-Assaad W, Rhodes CJ, Rosenberg L, Joly E, Prentki M. Glucagon-like peptide-1 prevents beta cell glucolipotoxicity. *Diabetologia* 2004; **47**:806–815.

39 Bonner-Weir S. Beta-cell turnover: its assessment and implications. *Diabetes* 2001; **50**(Suppl 1):S20–S24.

40 Drucker DJ. The biology of incretin hormones. *Cell Metab* 2006; **3**:153–165.

41 Hansen L, Deacon CF, Orskov C, Holst JJ. Glucagon-like peptide-1-(7-36)amide is transformed to glucagon-like peptide-1-(9-36) amide by dipeptidyl peptidase IV in the capillaries supplying the L cells of the porcine intestine. *Endocrinology* 1999; **140**:5356–5363.

42 Holst JJ, Deacon CF. Glucagon-like peptide-1 mediates the therapeutic actions of DPP-IV inhibitors. *Diabetologia* 2005; **48**:612–615.

43 Hjollund KR, Hughes TE, Deacon CF, Holst JJ. The dipeptidyl peptidase-4 inhibitor vildagliptin increases portal concentrations of active GLP-1 to a greater extent than the peripheral concentrations. *Diabetes* 2008; **57**:A411.

44 Nakagawa A, Satake H, Nakabayashi H, Nishizawa M, Furuya K, Nakano S, *et al.* Receptor gene expression of glucagon-like peptide-1, but not glucose-dependent insulinotropic polypeptide, in rat nodose ganglion cells. *Auton Neurosci* 2004; **110**:36–43.

45 Balkan B, Li X. Portal GLP-1 administration in rats augments the insulin response to glucose via neuronal mechanisms. *Am J Physiol Regul Integr Comp Physiol* 2000; **279**:R1449–R1454.

46 Toft-Nielsen MB, Damholt MB, Madsbad S, Hilsted LM, Hughes TE, Michelsen BK, *et al.* Determinants of the impaired secretion of glucagon-like peptide-1 in type 2 diabetic patients. *J Clin Endocrinol Metab* 2001; **86**:3717–3723.

47 Shah P, Vella A, Basu A, Basu R, Schwenk WF, Rizza RA. Lack of suppression of glucagon contributes to postprandial hyperglycemia in subjects with type 2 diabetes mellitus. *J Clin Endocrinol Metab* 2000; **85**:4053–4059.

48 de HJ, Rasmussen C, Coy DH, Holst JJ. Glucagon-like peptide-1, but not glucose-dependent insulinotropic peptide, inhibits glucagon secretion via somatostatin (receptor subtype 2) in the perfused rat pancreas. *Diabetologia* 2008; **51**:2263–2270.

49 Wettergren A, Schjoldager B, Mortensen PE, Myhre J, Christiansen J, Holst JJ. Truncated GLP-1 (proglucagon 78-107-amide) inhibits gastric and pancreatic functions in man. *Dig Dis Sci* 1993; **38**:665–673.

50 Nauck MA, Niedereichholz U, Ettler R, Holst JJ, Orskov C, Ritzel R, *et al.* Glucagon-like peptide 1 inhibition of gastric emptying outweighs its insulinotropic effects in healthy humans. *Am J Physiol* 1997; **273**:E981–E988.

51 Willms B, Werner J, Holst JJ, Orskov C, Creutzfeldt W, Nauck MA. Gastric emptying, glucose responses, and insulin secretion after a liquid test meal: effects of exogenous glucagon-like peptide-1 (GLP-1)-(7-36) amide in type 2 (noninsulin-dependent) diabetic patients. *J Clin Endocrinol Metab* 1996; **81**:327–332.

52 Naslund E, Barkeling B, King N, Gutniak M, Blundell JE, Holst JJ, *et al.* Energy intake and appetite are suppressed by glucagon-like peptide-1 (GLP-1) in obese men. *Int J Obes Relat Metab Disord* 1999; **23**:304–311.

53 Gutzwiller JP, Drewe J, Goke B, Schmidt H, Rohrer B, Lareida J, *et al.* Glucagon-like peptide-1 promotes satiety and reduces food intake in patients with diabetes mellitus type 2. *Am J Physiol* 1999; **276**:R1541–R1544.

54 Verdich C, Flint A, Gutzwiller JP, Naslund E, Beglinger C, Hellstrom PM, *et al.* A meta-analysis of the effect of glucagon-like peptide-1 (7-36) amide on ad libitum energy intake in humans. *J Clin Endocrinol Metab* 2001; **86**:4382–4389.

55 Bullock BP, Heller RS, Habener JF. Tissue distribution of messenger ribonucleic acid encoding the rat glucagon-like peptide-1 receptor. *Endocrinology* 1996; **137**:2968–2978.

56 Gros R, You X, Baggio LL, Kabir MG, Sadi AM, Mungrue IN, *et al.* Cardiac function in mice lacking the glucagon-like peptide-1 receptor. *Endocrinology* 2003; **144**:2242–2252.

57 Ban K, Noyan-Ashraf MH, Hoefer J, Bolz SS, Drucker DJ, Husain M. Cardioprotective and vasodilatory actions of glucagon-like peptide 1 receptor are mediated through both glucagon-like peptide 1 receptor-dependent and -independent pathways. *Circulation* 2008; **117**:2340–2350.

58 Zhao T, Parikh P, Bhashyam S, Bolukoglu H, Poornima I, Shen YT, *et al.* Direct effects of glucagon-like peptide-1 on myocardial contractility and glucose uptake in normal and postischemic isolated rat hearts. *J Pharmacol Exp Ther* 2006; **317**:1106–1113.

59 Bose AK, Mocanu MM, Carr RD, Brand CL, Yellon DM. Glucagon-like peptide 1 can directly protect the heart against ischemia/reperfusion injury. *Diabetes* 2005; **54**:146–151.

60 Sonne DP, Engstrom T, Treiman M. Protective effects of GLP-1 analogues exendin-4 and GLP-1 (9-36) amide against ischemia-reperfusion injury in rat heart. *Regul Pept* 2008; **146**:243–249.

61 Bose AK, Mocanu MM, Carr RD, Yellon DM. Myocardial ischaemia-reperfusion injury is attenuated by intact glucagon like peptide-1 (GLP-1) in the *in vitro* rat heart and may involve the p70s6K pathway. *Cardiovasc Drugs Ther* 2007; **21**:253–256.

62 Nikolaidis LA, Elahi D, Shen YT, Shannon RP. Active metabolite of GLP-1 mediates myocardial glucose uptake and improves left ventricular performance in conscious dogs with dilated cardiomyopathy. *Am J Physiol Heart Circ Physiol* 2005; **289**:H2401–H2408.

63 Nikolaidis LA, Mankad S, Sokos GG, Miske G, Shah A, Elahi D, *et al.* Effects of glucagon-like peptide-1 in patients with acute myocardial infarction and left ventricular dysfunction after successful reperfusion. *Circulation* 2004; **109**:962–965.

64 Nikolaidis LA, Elahi D, Hentosz T, Doverspike A, Huerbin R, Zourelias L, *et al.* Recombinant glucagon-like peptide-1 increases myocardial glucose uptake and improves left ventricular performance in conscious dogs with pacing-induced dilated cardiomyopathy. *Circulation* 2004; **110**:955–961.

65 Sokos GG, Nikolaidis LA, Mankad S, Elahi D, Shannon RP. Glucagon-like peptide-1 infusion improves left ventricular ejection fraction and functional status in patients with chronic heart failure. *J Card Fail* 2006; **12**:694–699.

66 Sokos GG, Bolukoglu H, German J, Hentosz T, Magovern GJ Jr, Maher TD, *et al.* Effect of glucagon-like peptide-1 (GLP-1) on glycemic control and left ventricular function in patients undergoing coronary artery bypass grafting. *Am J Cardiol* 2007; **100**:824–829.

67 Fields AV, Patterson B, Karnik AA, Shannon RP. Glucagon-like peptide-1 and myocardial protection: more than glycemic control. *Clin Cardiol* 2009; **32**:236–243.

68 Nystrom T, Gutniak MK, Zhang Q, Zhang F, Holst JJ, Ahren B, *et al.* Effects of glucagon-like peptide-1 on endothelial function in type 2 diabetes patients with stable coronary artery disease. *Am J Physiol Endocrinol Metab* 2004; **287**:E1209–E1215.

69 Basu A, Charkoudian N, Schrage W, Rizza RA, Basu R, Joyner MJ. Beneficial effects of GLP-1 on endothelial function in humans: dampening by glyburide but not by glimepiride. *Am J Physiol Endocrinol Metab* 2007; **293**:E1289–E1295.

70 Vilsboll T, Zdravkovic M, Le-Thi T, Krarup T, Schmitz O, Courreges JP, *et al.* Liraglutide, a long-acting human glucagon-like peptide-1 analog, given as monotherapy significantly improves glycemic control and lowers body weight without risk of hypoglycemia in patients with type 2 diabetes. *Diabetes Care* 2007; **30**:1608–1610.

71 Klonoff DC, Buse JB, Nielsen LL, Guan X, Bowlus CL, Holcombe JH, *et al.* Exenatide effects on diabetes, obesity, cardiovascular risk factors and hepatic biomarkers in patients with type 2 diabetes treated for at least 3 years. *Curr Med Res Opin* 2008; **24**:275–286.

72 Hansen L, Hartmann B, Mineo H, Holst JJ. Glucagon-like peptide-1 secretion is influenced by perfusate glucose concentration and by a feedback mechanism involving somatostatin in isolated perfused porcine ileum. *Regul Pept* 2004; **118**:11–18.

73 Perry T, Haughey NJ, Mattson MP, Egan JM, Greig NH. Protection and reversal of excitotoxic neuronal damage by glucagon-like peptide-1 and exendin-4. *J Pharmacol Exp Ther* 2002; **302**:881–888.

74 During MJ, Cao L, Zuzga DS, Francis JS, Fitzsimons HL, Jiao X, *et al.* Glucagon-like peptide-1 receptor is involved in learning and neuroprotection. *Nat Med* 2003; **9**:1173–1179.

75 Perry TA, Greig NH. A new Alzheimer's disease interventive strategy: GLP-1. *Curr Drug Targets* 2004; **5**:565–571.

76 Perry T, Lahiri DK, Sambamurti K, Chen D, Mattson MP, Egan JM, *et al.* Glucagon-like peptide-1 decreases endogenous amyloid-beta peptide (Abeta) levels and protects hippocampal neurons from death induced by Abeta and iron. *J Neurosci Res* 2003; **72**:603–612.

77 Bertilsson G, Patrone C, Zachrisson O, Andersson A, Dannaeus K, Heidrich J, *et al.* Peptide hormone exendin-4 stimulates subven-

tricular zone neurogenesis in the adult rodent brain and induces recovery in an animal model of Parkinson's disease. *J Neurosci Res* 2008; **86**:326–338.

78 Nauck MA, Kleine N, Orskov C, Holst JJ, Willms B, Creutzfeldt W. Normalization of fasting hyperglycaemia by exogenous glucagon-like peptide 1 (7-36 amide) in type 2 (non-insulin-dependent) diabetic patients. *Diabetologia* 1993; **36**:741–744.

79 Rachman J, Barrow BA, Levy JC, Turner RC. Near-normalisation of diurnal glucose concentrations by continuous administration of glucagon-like peptide-1 (GLP-1) in subjects with NIDDM. *Diabetologia* 1997; **40**:205–211.

80 Nauck MA, Wollschlager D, Werner J, Holst JJ, Orskov C, Creutzfeldt W, *et al.* Effects of subcutaneous glucagon-like peptide 1 (GLP-1 [7-36 amide]) in patients with NIDDM. *Diabetologia* 1996; **39**:1546–1553.

81 Deacon CF, Johnsen AH, Holst JJ. Degradation of glucagon-like peptide-1 by human plasma *in vitro* yields an N-terminally truncated peptide that is a major endogenous metabolite *in vivo*. *J Clin Endocrinol Metab* 1995; **80**:952–957.

82 Deacon CF, Nauck MA, Toft-Nielsen M, Pridal L, Willms B, Holst JJ. Both subcutaneously and intravenously administered glucagon-like peptide I are rapidly degraded from the NH2-terminus in type II diabetic patients and in healthy subjects. *Diabetes* 1995; **44**:1126–1131.

83 Zander M, Madsbad S, Madsen JL, Holst JJ. Effect of 6-week course of glucagon-like peptide 1 on glycaemic control, insulin sensitivity, and beta-cell function in type 2 diabetes: a parallel-group study. *Lancet* 2002; **359**:824–830.

84 Deacon CF, Knudsen LB, Madsen K, Wiberg FC, Jacobsen O, Holst JJ. Dipeptidyl peptidase IV resistant analogues of glucagon-like peptide-1 which have extended metabolic stability and improved biological activity. *Diabetologia* 1998; **41**:271–278.

85 Deacon CF, Hughes TE, Holst JJ. Dipeptidyl peptidase IV inhibition potentiates the insulinotropic effect of glucagon-like peptide 1 in the anesthetized pig. *Diabetes* 1998; **47**:764–769.

86 Nathan DM, Buse JB, Davidson MB, Ferrannini E, Holman RR, Sherwin R, *et al.* Medical management of hyperglycemia in type 2 diabetes: a consensus algorithm for the initiation and adjustment of therapy: a consensus statement of the American Diabetes Association and the European Association for the Study of Diabetes. *Diabetes Care* 2009; **32**:193–203.

87 Eng J, Kleinman WA, Singh L, Singh G, Raufman JP. Isolation and characterization of exendin-4, an exendin-3 analogue, from *Heloderma suspectum* venom: further evidence for an exendin receptor on dispersed acini from guinea pig pancreas. *J Biol Chem* 1992; **267**:7402–7405.

88 Kolterman OG, Kim DD, Shen L, Ruggles JA, Nielsen LL, Fineman MS, *et al.* Pharmacokinetics, pharmacodynamics, and safety of exenatide in patients with type 2 diabetes mellitus. *Am J Health Syst Pharm* 2005; **62**:173–181.

89 Cvetkovic RS, Plosker GL. Exenatide: a review of its use in patients with type 2 diabetes mellitus (as an adjunct to metformin and/or a sulfonylurea). *Drugs* 2007; **67**:935–954.

90 Fineman MS, Bicsak TA, Shen LZ, Taylor K, Gaines E, Varns A, *et al.* Effect on glycemic control of exenatide (synthetic exendin-4) additive to existing metformin and/or sulfonylurea treatment in patients with type 2 diabetes. *Diabetes Care* 2003; **26**:2370–2377.

91 Joy SV, Rodgers PT, Scates AC. Incretin mimetics as emerging treatments for type 2 diabetes. *Ann Pharmacother* 2005; **39**:110–118.

92 Cervera A, Wajcberg E, Sriwijitkamol A, Fernandez M, Zuo P, Triplitt C, *et al.* Mechanism of action of exenatide to reduce post-prandial hyperglycemia in type 2 diabetes. *Am J Physiol Endocrinol Metab* 2008; **294**:E846–E852.

93 Buse JB, Henry RR, Han J, Kim DD, Fineman MS, Baron AD. Effects of exenatide (exendin-4) on glycemic control over 30 weeks in sulfonylurea-treated patients with type 2 diabetes. *Diabetes Care* 2004; **27**:2628–2635.

94 DeFronzo RA, Ratner RE, Han J, Kim DD, Fineman MS, Baron AD. Effects of exenatide (exendin-4) on glycemic control and weight over 30 weeks in metformin-treated patients with type 2 diabetes. *Diabetes Care* 2005; **28**:1092–1100.

95 Kendall DM, Riddle MC, Rosenstock J, Zhuang D, Kim DD, Fineman MS, *et al.* Effects of exenatide (exendin-4) on glycemic control over 30 weeks in patients with type 2 diabetes treated with metformin and a sulfonylurea. *Diabetes Care* 2005; **28**:1083–1091.

96 Schwartz SL, Ratner RE, Kim DD, Qu Y, Fechner LL, Lenox SM, *et al.* Effect of exenatide on 24-hour blood glucose profile compared with placebo in patients with type 2 diabetes: a randomized, double-blind, two-arm, parallel-group, placebo-controlled, 2-week study. *Clin Ther* 2008; **30**:858–867.

97 Zinman B, Hoogwerf BJ, Duran GS, Milton DR, Giaconia JM, Kim DD, *et al.* The effect of adding exenatide to a thiazolidinedione in suboptimally controlled type 2 diabetes: a randomized trial. *Ann Intern Med* 2007; **146**:477–485.

98 Heine RJ, Van Gaal LF, Johns D, Mihm MJ, Widel MH, Brodows RG. Exenatide versus insulin glargine in patients with suboptimally controlled type 2 diabetes: a randomized trial. *Ann Intern Med* 2005; **143**:559–569.

99 Nauck MA, Duran S, Kim D, Johns D, Northrup J, Festa A, *et al.* A comparison of twice-daily exenatide and biphasic insulin aspart in patients with type 2 diabetes who were suboptimally controlled with sulfonylurea and metformin: a non-inferiority study. *Diabetologia* 2007; **50**:259–267.

100 Viswanathan P, Chaudhuri A, Bhatia R, Al-Atrash F, Mohanty P, Dandona P. Exenatide therapy in obese patients with type 2 diabetes mellitus treated with insulin. *Endocr Pract* 2007; **13**:444–450.

101 Davis SN, Johns D, Maggs D, Xu H, Northrup JH, Brodows RG. Exploring the substitution of exenatide for insulin in patients with type 2 diabetes treated with insulin in combination with oral antidiabetes agents. *Diabetes Care* 2007; **30**:2767–2772.

102 Fehse F, Trautmann M, Holst JJ, Halseth AE, Nanayakkara N, Nielsen LL, *et al.* Exenatide augments first- and second-phase insulin secretion in response to intravenous glucose in subjects with type 2 diabetes. *J Clin Endocrinol Metab* 2005; **90**:5991–5997.

103 Bunck MC, Diamant M, Corner A, Eliasson B, Malloy JL, Shaginian RM, *et al.* Beta-cell function and glycemic control following one year exenatide therapy, and after 12 week wash out, in patients with type 2 diabetes. *Diabetes* 2008; **57**:A32.

104 Degn KB, Brock B, Juhl CB, Djurhuus CB, Grubert J, Kim D, *et al.* Effect of intravenous infusion of exenatide (synthetic exendin-4) on glucose-dependent insulin secretion and counterregulation during hypoglycemia. *Diabetes* 2004; **53**:2397–2403.

105 Nauck MA, Heimesaat MM, Behle K, Holst JJ, Nauck MS, Ritzel R, *et al.* Effects of glucagon-like peptide 1 on counterregulatory

hormone responses, cognitive functions, and insulin secretion during hyperinsulinemic, stepped hypoglycemic clamp experiments in healthy volunteers. *J Clin Endocrinol Metab* 2002; **87**:1239–1246.

106 Amori RE, Lau J, Pittas AG. Efficacy and safety of incretin therapy in type 2 diabetes: systematic review and meta-analysis. *JAMA* 2007; **298**:194–206.

107 Denker PS, Dimarco PE. Exenatide (exendin-4)-induced pancreatitis: a case report. *Diabetes Care* 2006; **29**(2):471.

108 Agerso H, Vicini P. Pharmacodynamics of NN2211, a novel long acting GLP-1 derivative. *Eur J Pharm Sci* 2003; **19**:141–150.

109 Garber A, Henry R, Ratner R, Garcia-Hernandez PA, Rodriguez-Pattzi H, Olvera-Alvarez I, *et al.* Liraglutide versus glimepiride monotherapy for type 2 diabetes (LEAD-3 Mono): a randomised, 52-week, phase III, double-blind, parallel-treatment trial. *Lancet* 2009; **373**:473–481.

110 Garber AJ, Henry R, Ratner R, Hale P, Chang CT, Bode B. Liraglutide, a human GLP-1 analogue, maintains greater reductions in HbA(1c), FPG and weight than glimepiride over 2 years in patients with type 2 diabetes: LEAD-3 extension study. *Diabetologia* 2009; **52**:S287–S288.

111 Marre M, Shaw J, Brandle M, Bebakar WM, Kamaruddin NA, Strand J, *et al.* Liraglutide, a once-daily human GLP-1 analogue, added to a sulphonylurea over 26 weeks produces greater improvements in glycaemic and weight control compared with adding rosiglitazone or placebo in subjects with type 2 diabetes (LEAD-1 SU). *Diabet Med* 2009; **26**:268–278.

112 Nauck M, Frid A, Hermansen K, Shah NS, Tankova T, Mitha IH, *et al.* Efficacy and safety comparison of liraglutide, glimepiride, and placebo, all in combination with metformin, in type 2 diabetes: the LEAD (Liraglutide Effect and Action in Diabetes)-2 study. *Diabetes Care* 2009; **32**:84–90.

113 Zinman B, Gerich J, Buse JB, Lewin A, Schwartz S, Raskin P, *et al.* Efficacy and safety of the human glucagon-like peptide-1 analog liraglutide in combination with metformin and thiazolidinedione in patients with type 2 diabetes (LEAD-4 Met+TZD). *Diabetes Care* 2009; **32**:1224–1230.

114 Russell-Jones D, Vaag A, Schmitz O, Sethi BK, Lalic N, Antic S, *et al.* Liraglutide vs insulin glargine and placebo in combination with metformin and sulfonylurea therapy in type 2 diabetes mellitus (LEAD-5 met+SU): a randomised controlled trial. *Diabetologia* 2009; **52**:2046–2055.

115 Buse JB, Rosenstock J, Sesti G, Schmidt WE, Montanya E, Brett JH, *et al.* Liraglutide once a day versus exenatide twice a day for type 2 diabetes: a 26-week randomised, parallel-group, multinational, open-label trial (LEAD-6). *Lancet* 2009; **374**:39–47.

116 Courreges JP, Vilsboll T, Zdravkovic M, Le-Thi T, Krarup T, Schmitz O, *et al.* Beneficial effects of once-daily liraglutide, a human glucagon-like peptide-1 analogue, on cardiovascular risk biomarkers in patients with type 2 diabetes. *Diabet Med* 2008; **25**:1129–1131.

117 Russell-Jones D, Shaw JE, Brandle M, Matthews D, Frid A, Zdravkovic M, *et al.* The once-daily human GLP-1 analog liraglutide reduces body weight in subjects with type 2 diabetes, irrespective of body mass index at baseline. *Diabetes* 2008; **57**:A593–A594.

118 Colagiuri S, Frid A, Zdravkovic M, Le-Thi TD, Vaag A. The once-daily human GLP-1 analog-liraglutide reduces systolic blood pressure in patients with type 2 diabetes. *Diabetes* 2008; **57**:A164–A165.

119 Matthews D, Marre M, Le-Thl TUD, Zdravkovic M, Simo R. Liraglutide, a once-daily human GLP-1 analog, significantly improves beta-cell function in subjects with type 2 diabetes. *Diabetes* 2008; **57**:A150–A151.

120 Vilsboll T, Zdravkovic M, Le-Thi T, Krarup T, Schmitz O, Courreges JP, *et al.* Liraglutide, a long-acting human glucagon-like peptide-1 analog, given as monotherapy significantly improves glycemic control and lowers body weight without risk of hypoglycemia in patients with type 2 diabetes. *Diabetes Care* 2007; **30**:1608–1610.

121 Wysham C, Bergenstal R, Yan P, MacConell L, Malloy J, Porter L. DURATION-2: exenatide once weekly demonstrated superior glycaemic control and weight reduction compared to sitagliptin or pioglitazone after 26 weeks of treatment. *Diabetologia* 2009; **52**:S290.

122 Drucker DJ, Buse JB, Taylor K, Kendall DM, Trautmann M, Zhuang D, *et al.* Exenatide once weekly versus twice daily for the treatment of type 2 diabetes: a randomised, open-label, non-inferiority study. *Lancet* 2008; **372**:1240–1250.

123 Drucker DJ, Buse JB, Taylor K, *et al.* Exenatide once weekly results in significantly greater improvements in glycemic control compared to exenatide twice daily in patients with type 2 diabetes. *Diabetes* 2008; **57**(Suppl 1):A33.

124 Bush MA, Matthews JE, De Boever EH, Dobbins RL, Hodge RJ, Walker SE, *et al.* Safety, tolerability, pharmacodynamics and pharmacokinetics of albiglutide, a long-acting glucagon-like peptide-1 mimetic, in healthy subjects. *Diabetes Obes Metab* 2009; **11**:498–505.

125 Baggio LL, Huang Q, Brown TJ, Drucker DJ. A recombinant human glucagon-like peptide (GLP)-1-albumin protein (albugon) mimics peptidergic activation of GLP-1 receptor-dependent pathways coupled with satiety, gastrointestinal motility, and glucose homeostasis. *Diabetes* 2004; **53**:2492–2500.

126 Rosenstock J, Reusch J, Bush M, Yang F, Stewart M. Potential of albiglutide, a long-acting GLP-1 receptor agonist, in type 2 diabetes: a randomized controlled trial exploring weekly, biweekly, and monthly dosing. *Diabetes Care* 2009; **32**:1880–1886.

127 Nauck MA, Ratner RE, Kapitza C, Berria R, Boldrin M, Balena R. Treatment with the human once-weekly glucagon-like peptide-1 analog taspoglutide in combination with metformin improves glycemic control and lowers body weight in patients with type 2 diabetes inadequately controlled with metformin alone: a double-blind placebo-controlled study. *Diabetes Care* 2009; **32**:1237–1243.

128 Christensen M, Knop FK, Holst JJ, Vilsboll T. Lixisenatide, a novel GLP-1 receptor agonist for the treatment of type 2 diabetes mellitus. *IDrugs* 2009; **12**:503–513.

129 Sinclair EM, Drucker DJ. Proglucagon-derived peptides: mechanisms of action and therapeutic potential. *Physiology (Bethesda)* 2005; **20**:357–365.

130 Mannucci E, Rotella CM. Future perspectives on glucagon-like peptide-1, diabetes and cardiovascular risk. *Nutr Metab Cardiovasc Dis* 2008; **18**:639–645.

131 Moreno C, Mistry M, Roman RJ. Renal effects of glucagon-like peptide in rats. *Eur J Pharmacol* 2002; **434**:163–167.

132 Colagiuri S, Frid A, Zdravkovic M, Le-Thi TD, Vaag A. The once-daily human GLP-1 analog-liraglutide reduces systolic blood pressure in patients with type 2 diabetes. *Diabetes* 2008; **57**:A164–A165.

133 Cooper GJ, Willis AC, Clark A, Turner RC, Sim RB, Reid KB. Purification and characterization of a peptide from amyloid-rich pancreases of type 2 diabetic patients. *Proc Natl Acad Sci U S A* 1987; **84**:8628–8632.

134 Westermark P, Wernstedt C, O'Brien TD, Hayden DW, Johnson KH. Islet amyloid in type 2 human diabetes mellitus and adult diabetic cats contains a novel putative polypeptide hormone. *Am J Pathol* 1987; **127**:414–417.

135 Juhl CB, Porksen N, Sturis J, Hansen AP, Veldhuis JD, Pincus S, *et al.* High-frequency oscillations in circulating amylin concentrations in healthy humans. *Am J Physiol Endocrinol Metab* 2000; **278**:E484–E490.

136 Nyholm B, Fineman MS, Koda JE, Schmitz O. Plasma amylin immunoreactivity and insulin resistance in insulin resistant relatives of patients with non-insulin-dependent diabetes mellitus. *Horm Metab Res* 1998; **30**:206–212.

137 Gedulin BR, Rink TJ, Young AA. Dose–response for glucagonostatic effect of amylin in rats. *Metabolism* 1997; **46**:67–70.

138 Gedulin BR, Young AA. Hypoglycemia overrides amylin-mediated regulation of gastric emptying in rats. *Diabetes* 1998; **47**:93–97.

139 Bretherton-Watt D, Gilbey SG, Ghatei MA, Beacham J, Macrae AD, Bloom SR. Very high concentrations of islet amyloid polypeptide are necessary to alter the insulin response to intravenous glucose in man. *J Clin Endocrinol Metab* 1992; **74**:1032–1035.

140 Wilding JP, Khandan-Nia N, Bennet WM, Gilbey SG, Beacham J, Ghatei MA, *et al.* Lack of acute effect of amylin (islet associated polypeptide) on insulin sensitivity during hyperinsulinaemic euglycaemic clamp in humans. *Diabetologia* 1994; **37**:166–169.

141 Fineman MS, Koda JE, Shen LZ, Strobel SA, Maggs DG, Weyer C, *et al.* The human amylin analog, pramlintide, corrects postprandial hyperglucagonemia in patients with type 1 diabetes. *Metabolism* 2002; **51**:636–641.

142 Kolterman OG. Amylin and glycaemic regulation: a possible role for the human amylin analogue pramlintide. *Diabet Med* 1997; **14**(Suppl 2):S35–S38.

143 Macdonald IA. Amylin and the gastrointestinal tract. *Diabet Med* 1997; **14**(Suppl 2):S24–S28.

144 Shah P, Vella A, Basu A, Basu R, Schwenk WF, Rizza RA. Lack of suppression of glucagon contributes to postprandial hyperglycemia in subjects with type 2 diabetes mellitus. *J Clin Endocrinol Metab* 2000; **85**:4053–4059.

145 Nyholm B, Moller N, Gravholt CH, Orskov L, Mengel A, Bryan G, *et al.* Acute effects of the human amylin analog AC137 on basal and insulin-stimulated euglycemic and hypoglycemic fuel metabolism in patients with insulin-dependent diabetes mellitus. *J Clin Endocrinol Metab* 1996; **81**:1083–1089.

146 Chapman I, Parker B, Doran S, Feinle-Bisset C, Wishart J, Strobel S, *et al.* Effect of pramlintide on satiety and food intake in obese subjects and subjects with type 2 diabetes. *Diabetologia* 2005; **48**:838–848.

147 Smith SR, Aronne LJ, Burns CM, Kesty NC, Halseth AE, Weyer C. Sustained weight loss following 12-month pramlintide treatment as an adjunct to lifestyle intervention in obesity. *Diabetes Care* 2008; **31**:1816–1823.

148 Roth JD, Roland BL, Cole RL, Trevaskis JL, Weyer C, Koda JE, *et al.* Leptin responsiveness restored by amylin agonism in diet-induced obesity: evidence from nonclinical and clinical studies. *Proc Natl Acad Sci U S A* 2008; **105**:7257–7262.

149 Marrero DG, Crean J, Zhang B, Kellmeyer T, Gloster M, Herrmann K, *et al.* Effect of adjunctive pramlintide treatment on treatment satisfaction in patients with type 1 diabetes. *Diabetes Care* 2007; **30**:210–216.

31 How to Use Type 2 Diabetes Treatments in Clinical Practice: Combination Therapies

Joseph A. Aloi & Anthony L. McCall

Division of Endocrinology, University of Virginia Health System, Charlottesville, VA, USA

Keypoints

- Managing type 2 diabetes has become more complex as pharmacotherapy has expanded. Clinicians have more pharmaceutical agents targeted to hyperglycemia and obesity than before, but a relentlessly progressive disorder to overcome.
- Clinical trials continue to show that glycemic control is critical to reduce microvascular complications and in the long-term also cardiovascular events. Nonetheless, poor glycemic control, hypoglycemia and obesity remain stubborn barriers for clinicians.
- Few comparative data direct us in the best use of multiple drug therapies for the management of type 2 diabetes and its co-morbidities. One is guided by good clinical studies, the potential of therapeutic agents to reverse pathophysiology and ultimately the proper use of insulin which is eventually needed in most patients to replace the loss of β-cell function.

Introduction

The epidemic of type 2 diabetes mellitus (T2DM) presents the clinician as well as society with complex challenges in designing both prevention and treatment strategies for T2DM. T2DM is a worldwide epidemic with a global prevalence in 2009 of 285 million people, expected to increase to 435 million by 2030 [1]. The Centers for Disease Control and Prevention (CDC) estimates that in 2007 nearly 24 million people in the USA have diabetes [2], mostly T2DM. At least 57 million people have pre-diabetes (impaired fasting glucose or impaired glucose tolerance), providing an expanding pool of new patients with T2DM. Current prevalence represents a 90% increase in the new diagnosis of diabetes over the last decade [3] and more rapid increases in many parts of the world. This increasing prevalence of diabetes relates both to environmental and genetic factors, each of which may influence insulin sensitivity (e.g. insulin resistance) and insulin secretion capacity. Insulin resistance begins in early life and is fueled by obesity and a sedentary lifestyle which contribute to alterations in glucose homeostasis and to abnormal lipid and protein metabolism.

Relative insulin deficiency is the defining metabolic difference between obesity and the development of hyperglycemia with progression to T2DM. An inexorable progression of diabetes appears related to worsening insulin deficiency [4,5]. Most people therefore have gradually increasing needs for additional therapy. Combinations of therapy such as adopting a therapeutic lifestyle change, as well as oral and injectable medicines, are required to keep the glycemia under control. The failure to advance therapy at an early sign of therapeutic failure and, in particular, a reluctance to advance to insulin underlies the less than optimum control for many patients with diabetes.

Algorithms for management

Several approaches to the best management of T2DM have been proposed. All algorithms begin with therapeutic lifestyle change and are generally focused primarily upon controlling hyperglycemia. Consensus statements from the American Diabetes Association (ADA) have been recently revised in conjunction with the European Association for the Study of Diabetes (EASD) [6]. The most recent algorithm (Figure 31.1) moves away from the focus on glucose as the sole goal of therapy and tries to develop evidence-directed therapy to treating diabetes by normalizing hyperglycemia and minimizing cardiometabolic risk. The US Food and Drug Administration (FDA) has recently advised that new medicines for glycemic control in diabetes be routinely evaluated early for their effects upon cardiovascular disease. By doing so, they recognize atherosclerosis as the primary cause of cost and mortality in diabetes.

Textbook of Diabetes, 4th edition. Edited by R. Holt, C. Cockram, A. Flyvbjerg and B. Goldstein.

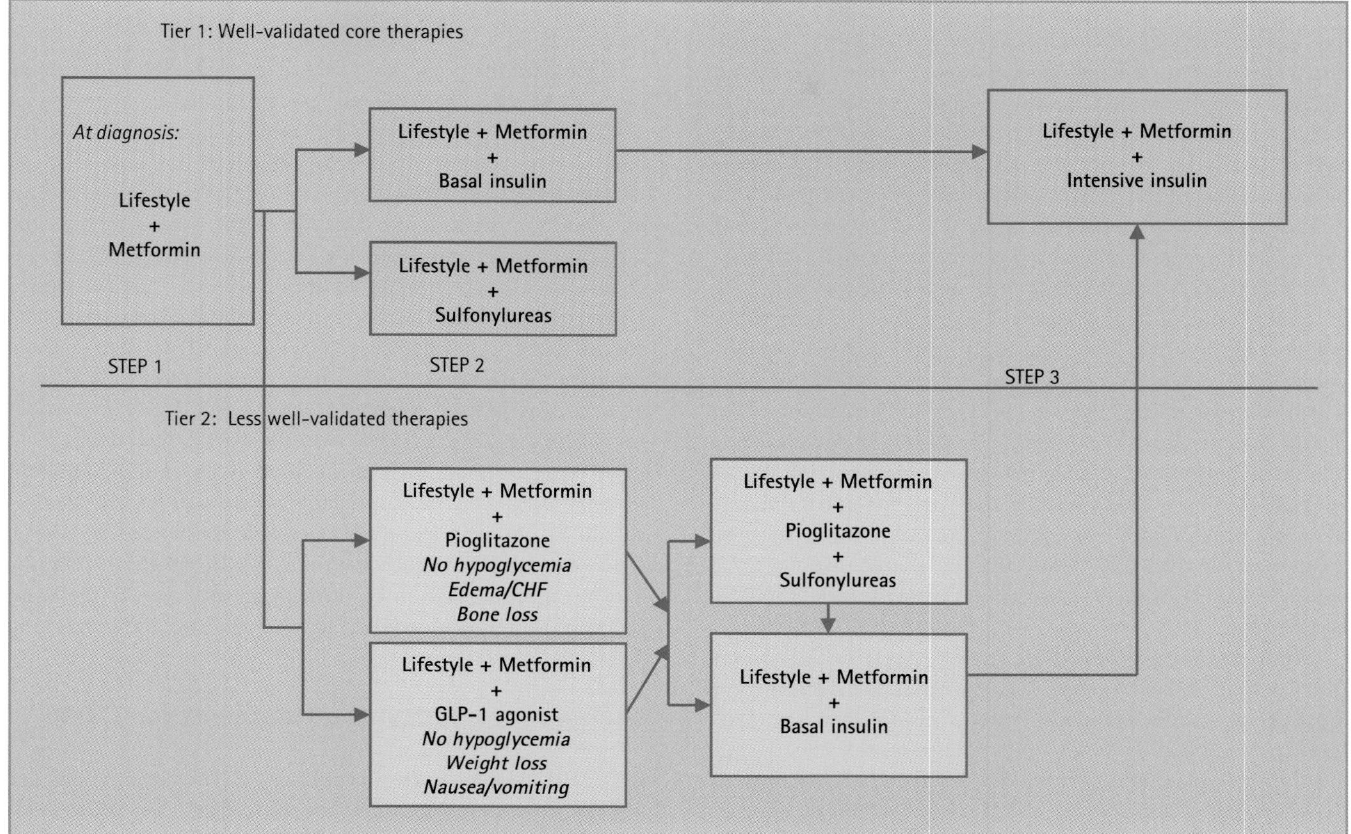

Figure 31.1 The ADA/EASD consensus statement on the recommended strategy to advance therapies to control hyperglycemia in diabetes. The top portion focuses on traditional well-validated therapies buttressed by large studies and long experience (metformin, sulfonylureas, insulin). The lower portion focuses on more recent emerging therapies that have less follow-up and validation in clinical trials (thiazolidinediones or glitazones as they are often called; e.g. pioglitazone, GLP-1 agonists such as exenatide). According to the authors, the amylin agonists, α-glucosidase inhibitors, glinides and DPP-4 inhibitors were not included in the two tiers of preferred agents in this algorithm, owing to their lower or equivalent overall glucose-lowering effectiveness compared with the first- and second-tier agents and/or to their limited clinical data or relative expense. However, they may be appropriate choices in selected patients. Similarly, colesevelam is not mentioned in this algorithm but may be appropriate for selected patients. Rosiglitazone is omitted from the algorithm because of unsettled concerns raised about cardiovascular side effects. Reproduced from the updated American Diabetes Association/European Association for the Study of Diabetes consensus statement [6].

The current consensus algorithm (Figure 31.1) moves quickly from metformin treatment failure to the addition of sulfonylurea or insulin. Newer classes of drugs (e.g. incretin mimetics, pioglitazone) are recommended later or as a secondary consideration because of the lack of compelling data to suggest their superiority compared to existing treatments and associated concerns for unintentional ill effects such as long bone fractures or increase in congestive heart failure (glitazones) or pancreatitis (exenatide). Ultimately, the treatment pathway must incorporate patient individualization, clinical acumen, and the broad experience gained from clinical trials.

Goals of treatment

Treatment goals for patients with diabetes have changed considerably over the past two decades. The Diabetes Control and Complications Trial (DCCT) [7] confirmed the concept of the relationship of glycemic control to microvascular complications in type 1 diabetes. Similar results were found for T2DM in the landmark UK Prospective Diabetes Study (UKPDS) [8,9]. Long-term analysis of subjects participating in these trials at 10 years following a period of improved glycemic control found cardiovascular risk reduction with insulin, metformin and sulfonylureas [10,11] and for T2DM also a mortality advantage.

In assigning patients to a treatment plan, consideration must be given to treatment goals. The ADA continues to recommend HbA_{1c} of <7% (<53 mmol/mol) as a general glycemic goal and individualization is recommended. For properly selected patients, either less tight control or alternatively more rigorous normalization of glycemia down to 6% (42 mmol/mol) HbA_{1c} can be recommended, if the latter can be achieved without hypoglycemia problems. Using similar data sources, the International Diabetes Federation (IDF) and American Association of Clinical Endocrinologists (AACE) suggest ≤6.5% (48 mmol/mol) as a general goal. All authorities recommend the need for individualization of goals based on co-morbidities and vulnerability to hypoglycemia among other criteria. The ACCORD trial hypothesized that close to normal glucose control (HbA_{1c} 6% or less [<42 mmol/mol]) would improve cardiovascular endpoints. Recent analysis of the ACCORD trial [12] cautions the provider against attempting to normalize glycemia in those with characteristics similar to this patient cohort (e.g. older and those with existing cardiovascular disease), as the intensively treated group had a 22% increase in mortality primarily from fatal cardiovascular events; very possibly, although unproven, this may have been as a result of hypoglycemia. This poses a dilemma to the practitioner: how best to normalize glycemia but avoid hypoglycemia. This practical consideration suggests newer therapies with a relatively low hypoglycemia risk should be considered for certain patient groups. Additionally, strategies to recognize and prevent hypoglycemia risk in patients at high risk should be adopted routinely. These include the need for self-monitored blood glucose (SMBG) tests, good communication and education about how to treat and adjust therapy should hypoglycemia become frequent or severe, especially if hypoglycemia unawareness occurs.

Ultimately, patients with T2DM require progression of therapy from combination oral therapy to combination injectable therapy (basal bolus insulin regimens, incretin insulin combinations). Initiating combination therapy early minimizes side effects while maximizing clinical effectiveness, decreasing pill counts and cost while facilitating compliance. New ACCE guidelines use all drugs and tailor their number and starting insulin to the baseline HbA_{1c} [13].

Lifestyle advice for diabetes and pre-diabetes

Lifestyle management is one of the most challenging barriers to successful diabetes control. Deriving recommendations for eating, physical activity and minimizing psychologic stressors is frequently frustrating for both the provider and patient [14]. The assumption that complex patterns of lifestyle behavior can be altered by dispensing general advice in the course of a busy medical visit is flawed, but unfortunately a reality for many providers. It should be replaced by an agreement that the patient is responsible for assisting in their disease management and is the only source of key information needed to manage their illness [15]. One strategy is to make patients more aware of their own lifestyle patterns. Developing a baseline for eating and exercise (type, frequency, duration, barriers) is as integral as obtaining initial laboratory testing in patients with T2DM to compile a treatment plan based on physiology as well as the psychology of the patient. Obtaining a narrow focus on a few behavioral objectives can increase success. Approaches we often use for patients are:

- Keep an eating behavior diary over the next week; and
- Wear a pedometer and keep track of your baseline steps for the next week.

The information almost always contains some surprises for patients but it helps them to identify personal behaviors and to focus and motivate them to take the lead in setting meaningful objectives.

The role of the physician is critical in emphasizing the importance of lifestyle change to the patient, initiating a process of working on lifestyle change, and reinforcing, and refining the education to achieve incremental obtainable objectives. Use of motivational interviewing and assessment of readiness to change are important aspects of evaluation of the patient by both the medical provider and diabetes educator. It is our practice to recommend strongly diabetes education for every patient who is willing to do so and to reinforce the recommendation for lifestyle change at any point when additional therapy needs occur. A useful acronym that we have used to help trainees remember how to assist patients in making lifestyle change is FIRM [15]. This stands for negotiating Few changes, typically 1–3 at any clinical visit; those changes should be Individualized by the patient's selection of what aspects of behavior change to embark on; the changes should be Realistic and therefore likely to succeed by setting moderate, achievable goals within a specific timeframe; and be Measureable and monitored through patient record-keeping to be shared with the provider or diabetes educator at the next visit.

Therapy for obesity as a treatment for T2DM

Because the vast majority of people with T2DM are overweight or obese, a serious consideration is the use of weight loss and increasing physical activity strategies as a useful treatment to gain control of glycemia and favorably influence multiple cardiovascular risk factors as well [16,17]. Prevention and/or treatment plans for T2DM could also legitimately consider use of pharmacotherapy for obesity. Successful weight loss of 10% or less has repeatedly been shown to improve glycemic control (HbA_{1c} reductions 0.3–0.5% [3–6 mmol/mol] and sometimes much more) as well as favorable improvements in lipids, hypertension as well as other cardiac risk factors. Currently, three drugs (phentermine, orlistat and sibutramine) are approved for management of obesity in the USA. Rimonabant was approved for use in several countries outside the USA, but recent withdrawal of support by the European Medicines Agency has ended its possibility of wider use. Other drugs of the endocannabinoid receptor blocker class have also been discontinued from clinical development. Phentermine is only approved for short-term use and is the least well-studied and is less commonly used and not generally recommended.

Orlistat is currently approved for use in the management of obesity. Orlistat functions as a gastric and pancreatic lipase inhibitor. When given at a dosage of 120 mg three times daily with meals, approximately 20–30% of ingested fat is passed into the feces. Large amounts of fat in the gastrointestinal tract result in the most difficult side effect to manage, namely anal leakage of oil to post-prandial diarrhea which may be abrupt. Attention to this expected effect as well as dietary counseling or use of daily or twice daily dosing can minimize patient's gastrointestinal accidents and may enhance patient adherence to low fat dietary regimens. No long-term malabsorption of fat-soluble vitamins has been seen but replacement with a multivitamin including vitamin D is recommended during therapy. A lower dosage (60 mg) over-the-counter form is now available.

Orlistat has been critically studied both in the prevention [18] and in the treatment of T2DM in patients receiving metformin or insulin [19,20]. In the XENDOS trial, 3305 obese subjects at risk for T2DM were randomized to therapeutic lifestyle change or therapeutic lifestyle change plus orlistat 120 mg three times daily over a study period of 4 years. The subset of subjects with impaired glucose tolerance at entry receiving orlistat enjoyed a 37% relative risk reduction in development of T2DM at study end. Favorable lipid effects were also seen.

In obese subjects with T2DM failing metformin monotherapy [19], the addition of orlistat to the treatment plan lowered HbA_{1c} by 0.35% (4 mmol/mol) and improved lipid as well as blood pressure control. Similarly, benefits were also seen in insulin-treated patients given orlistat for 1 year [20] with improved glycemia (HbA_{1c} −0.62 ± 0.08 for orlistat-treated vs −0.27 ± 0.08% given placebo; $P < 0.002$, 7 vs 3 mmol/mol) and improved lipids despite lowered diabetes medicine doses.

Sibutramine enhances satiety and diminishes appetite primarily through central pathways, involving the inhibition of synaptic reuptake of norepinephrine, serotonin and to a lesser extent dopamine.* Doses approved for use in the management of obesity range 5–15 mg, with greatest efficacy at the cost of highest frequency of side effects seen at the 15 mg dosage. Doses up to 20 mg have been used in the clinical trial setting with a similar observation. A recent meta-analysis studied eight of 30 available clinical trials using sibutramine in the management of diabetes [21]. The authors included studies using sibutramine in combinations with sulfonylureas, metformin or a hypo-caloric diet. In general, treatment effects were associated with a 5.5-kg loss in body weight versus an approximate 1-kg weight gain in comparator groups. On average, HbA_{1c} improved 0.28% (3 mmol/mol) with variability among the different studies included. Additional positive effects were noted in reducing triglycerides and raising high density lipoprotein (HDL) without any adverse effects on blood pressure. Small increases in heart rate were noted. The presence of hypertension, especially if not ideally controlled, should be considered a contraindication to use of sibutramine, especially given how sensitive patients with diabetes are to the adverse impact of modest blood pressure changes and the effects of blood pressure upon diabetes complications.

Rimonabant, an endocannabinoid CB1 receptor blocker, has recently been removed from the European market because of concerns over exacerbating mood disorders (depression). Ongoing clinical trials using rimonabant have also been halted, raising questions over both the utility and availability of drugs acting on the endocannabinoid system. Despite its removal from studies and failure to stay widely marketed, there are studies finding a substantial antihyperglycemia effect similar to that of some approved diabetes pills. Such work validates the notion that treatment directed toward obesity have glycemic effects that are similar to some of the already approved pharmacotherapy choices for diabetes. Safety concerns regarding depression appear unlikely to allow this type of medication to be marketed in the future.

Bariatric surgery for appropriate patients (typically BMI >40 kg/m^2 or >35 kg/m^2 with co-morbidities) who have failed successful lifestyle interventions and/or pharmacotherapy for obesity is an increasingly utilized option. Improved safety and standardization combined with expanding data for the surgical management of obesity with favorable effects including long-standing remissions of T2DM in most patients make this an increasingly employed procedure [22,23]. The physiology behind such benefits remains poorly understood. Paradigms for identifying patients best suited for surgical treatment of cardiometabolic risk are evolving. Typically, many patients who are candidates for bariatric surgery are already on a combination of therapies. Following surgery, most patients who have been on insulin will be able to stop unless there is a very long history of diabetes. During the hypocaloric diet employed in preparation for such surgery, significant decreases in the need for insulin and sometimes other diabetes medications occur. For those who undergo Roux-en-Y procedures it is common to have a rapid reduction of insulin requirements within days to weeks. Decreasing insulin dosage by half or more is frequently necessary to avoid hypoglycemia.

Combination pharmacotherapy for T2DM

Therapies for T2DM can be divided into drugs facilitating supply of endogenous insulin (secretagogues, incretins) or those enhancing insulin actions (biguanides, thiazolidinediones, incretins, α-glucosidase inhibitors, amylin analogs, colesevelam). Successful treatment of T2DM combines approaches to lifestyle modification frequently in conjunction with use of pharmacologic therapy.

We conclude from data found in the UKPDS that insulin secretory loss starts on average 10 years before the formal diagnosis of T2DM, followed by insulin deficiency on average 10–12 years after diagnosis [8]. The dual aspects of T2DM, insulin resistance and insulin deficiency, are important factors in therapy selection and the subsequent response to therapy. This chapter provides an update on combinations of therapies for T2DM, presents evidence and opinions on sequences of medications, reviews new insights into diabetes and obesity treatments, and briefly describes some new medications emerging for the treatment of T2DM.

Need for combination therapy

The management of T2DM, as with any chronic illness, requires individual assessment and involvement of patient with their care

*The marketing authorization for sibutramine has recently been withdrawn in Europe following the publication of the SCOUT trial. In this trial which included 9,800 overweight or obese individuals at high risk of CVD events, treatment with sibutramine was associated with a 16% increased risk of non-fatal MI, non-fatal stroke, resuscitated cardiac arrest or CVD death. This result was driven by an increased incidence of non-fatal MI and stroke.

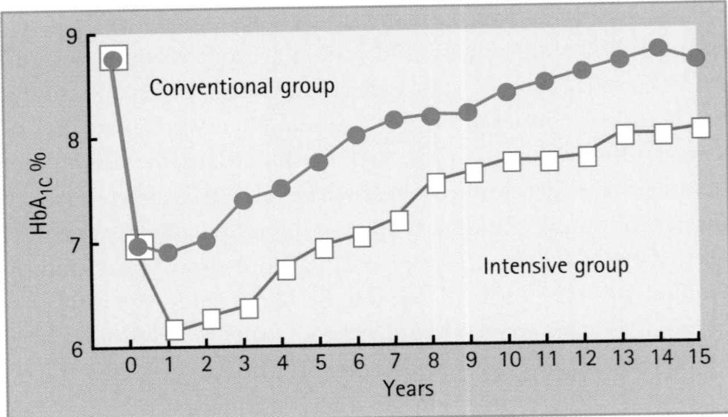

Figure 31.2 This figure, which is adapted from the UK Prospective Diabetes Study comparing conventional policy to intensive policy with sulfonylureas or insulin, shows the progressive rise of median HbA_{1c} that presumably is related to the progressive insulin secretory defect present in type 2 diabetes mellitus. A noteworthy aspect of this figure is the decline in HbA_{1c} from nearly 9% (75 mmol/mol) to around 7% (53 mmol/mol) in the first 3 months after initial evaluation. During this period, subjects in this study had visits with educators and dietitians helping them to improve lifestyle.

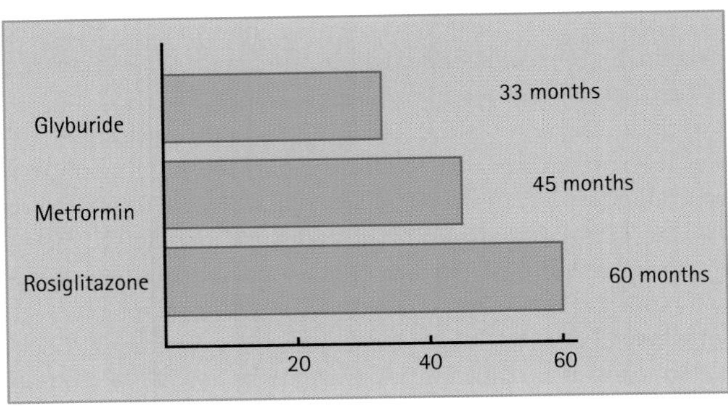

Figure 31.3 The ADOPT study examined the duration of maintenance of fasting glycemia in patients with diabetes on three monotherapies: glyburide (glibenclamide), metformin and rosiglitazone. As shown in this figure, rosiglitazone was superior to metformin which was in turn superior to glyburide in efficacy of maintenance of HbA_{1c}. Nonetheless, at 4 years most patients in each of the three groups did not maintain their HbA_{1c} goals and needed to progress to combination therapy. The analysis shown reflects time until mean HbA_{1c} within treatment group exceeds 7% (>53 mmol/mol) based on a repeated measures mixed model. Reproduced from Kahn *et al. N Engl J Med* 2006; **355**:2427–2443.

plans. Perhaps the original "combination therapy" for T2DM remains advice on flexible approaches to healthy eating styles coupled with encouragement and support to improve physical activity with consideration of the use of early pharmacologic treatment interventions in most patients. Most patients with T2DM eventually require combination pharmacologic therapy; some at the time of initial diagnosis, especially if they have a markedly elevated HbA_{1c}. Data from the UKPDS [5] showed that about 50% of patients required combination therapy within 3 years of diagnosis, and approximately 75% at 9 years after diagnosis (Figure 31.2).

Choice of initial therapy

No therapy has rigorously been proven to alter the natural history of progressive β-cell decline and the ultimate need for combination treatment. Nonetheless, randomization to rosiglitazone in the ADOPT trial [24] was associated with longer monotherapy success for a new diagnosis of T2DM (60 months) versus metformin (45 months) or glyburide (glibenclamide) (33 months). The data from this study (Figure 31.3) found that at the 4-year evaluation, 40% of the 1456 patients in the rosiglitazone group had a glycated hemoglobin level of less than 7% (<53 mmol/mol), compared with 36% of the 1454 patients in the metformin group ($P = 0.03$) and 26% of the 1441 patients in the glyburide group ($P < 0.001$). Thus, even with some superior durability of treatment-related glycemic response, it is clear that most patients with T2DM will require combination therapy within the first 3–6 years after medication is begun.

Rationale for combination therapy

In the context of at least two major physiologic defects in T2DM, insulin resistance and progressive insulin secretory failure, combining treatments with complementary actions can be a logical approach. Several distinct advantages of combining agents can be distinguished.

Efficacy

The first rationale for combination therapy (either with oral agents alone, with oral agents and insulin or oral agents with other injectable medicine such as incretin mimetics) is its superior efficacy. One principle that emerges from randomized controlled trials of antidiabetic therapies is that switching from one medication to another does not work as well as adding on or combining therapies. Figure 31.4 shows a classic study of combination oral agent therapy that illustrates this point [25]. Patients with inadequate glycemic control on maximal doses of glyburide were randomized to continuation of that monotherapy, to metformin monotherapy gradually titrated to maximal doses (850 mg orally three times a day), or to a combination of glyburide and metformin. Neither monotherapy resulted in any significant improvement in fasting plasma glucose (FPG), but combination therapy with an insulin secretagogue and metformin showed a dramatic improvement. Similarly, studies with other combination therapies showed no benefit of switching to a new agent class, but greater glucose-lowering efficacy through combining it with an agent with a different mechanism. A final benefit of combination treatment may add efficacy by using some agents that treat preprandial hyperglycemia and others that treat post-prandial hyperglycemia. As with basal and bolus insulin, it may be important to use both approaches in balance.

Tolerability and convenience

Most side effects of glycemic medications are dose-related. For example, hypoglycemia is a side effect of insulin or insulin secretagogues, gastrointestinal side effects are common with met-

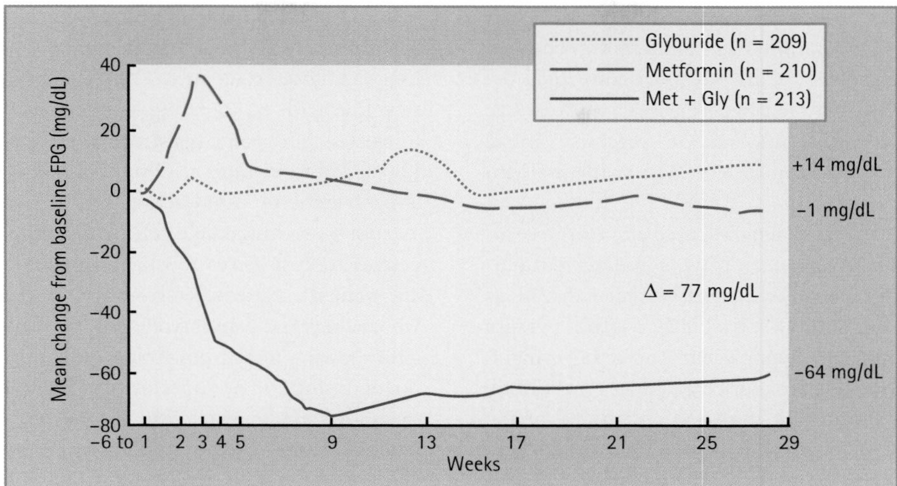

Figure 31.4 As shown by DeFronzo *et al.* [25] in subjects failing maximal dose glyburide (dotted line), continuation of the "failing" secretagogue led to gradually worse hyperglycemia. Likewise, a switch from glyburide to metformin (dashed line) showed little glycemic improvement. A worsening of hyperglycemia with increased fasting plasma glucose (FPG) was seen in the metformin group after glyburide had been stopped and before full dose titration of metformin had occurred. This study exemplifies the general principle that switching makes little sense as the combination of therapy (solid line) substantially improves FPG which is not observed with either monotherapy.

formin, incretin mimetics and α-glucosidase inhibitors, and fluid retention or weight gain may occur with the thiazolidinediones. In contrast to some of the adverse effects of diabetes agents noted above, the efficacy of oral agents in glucose lowering is often not linear with increasing dose. Thus, with dose escalation one may increase undesirable side effects while gaining little in efficacy. One option is to utilize lower doses of two complementary medications, which can minimize side effects while achieving equal or better glycemic control. This principle has been tested directly for the combination of glyburide and metformin [25].

Using combinations of oral agents may seem more complex than monotherapy, but in some cases their convenience can be enhanced. Combining a single dose of a long-acting sulfonylurea, such as glimepiride, with one or two tablets of metformin, may have greater benefit than three or four tablets of metformin alone. Metformin–secretagogue (metformin–glyburide, metformin–glipizide, metformin–repaglinide) combination pills, have been introduced. Similarly, metformin–thiazolidinedione (metformin–rosiglitazone, metformin–pioglitazone) combination pills are also available. Recently, thiazolidinediones–secretagogue (rosiglitazone–glimepiride, pioglitazone–glimepiride) combination pills have become available. Some newer agents such as sitagliptin have been approved for use when combined with metformin and are also available as a combination pill.

The trend to use combination pills will likely increase in the future. Formulations of two agents in a single pill with dual actions may appeal to many patients and practitioners. While separate titration of agents may be desirable for many patients, for others a case can be made for combination preparations. Side effects are often characteristic of a particular agent (e.g. sulfonylureas with hypoglycemia, metformin with gastrointestinal side effects, glitazones with fluid retention) and thus can be commonly attributed correctly to the specific agent in a combination pill. Occasionally, rarer or idiosyncratic side effects could be less readily attributed to the specific agent. This tactic may prove especially attractive for patients who must take not only two or more agents for glycemic control, but also other medications for manage blood pressure, lipid abnormalities, heart disease and other problems.

Secretagogues

Whether rapid or longer-acting, secretagogues work well with both metformin [25] and thiazolidinediones [26]. Their use with basal insulin therapy, such as evening NPH or glargine [27] is also evidence-based. Use of secretagogues with a mixture of evening basal plus mealtime insulin reduces insulin requirements and prevents interim hyperglycemia during insulin dose titration [28], however, their use with two or more mealtime insulin doses is considered superfluous, and might increase the risk of hypoglycemia. Insulin secretagogues work by binding to sulfonylurea receptors (SUR), which in the pancreas are of the SUR1A subtype. SUR are linked to potassium inward rectifier (Kir 6.2) channels. When Kir channels are closed by secretagogue binding to SUR, calcium channels are opened and insulin is released. The Diabetes mellitus, Insulin Glucose infusion in Acute Myocardial Infarction 1 (DIGAMI-1) study [29] showed that, compared with usual care, insulin treatment reduced mortality from acute myocardial infarction in diabetes mellitus; thus, it seems reasonable to avoid secretagogues, particularly glyburide, in patients with active ischemic heart disease (acute coronary syndromes or the presence of stable angina). DIGAMI-2 [30] did not confirm the mortality differential found in DIGAMI-1. The DIGAMI-2 study was limited by the inability to achieve targeted glycemic goals (5–7 mmol/L) and a small separation of glycemic control between treatment groups. Nevertheless, the investigators confirmed the epidemiologic relationship between hyperglycemia and cardiac mortality. Taken together, this information suggests cardiac ischemia with hyperglycemia may still be best managed with insulin.

The primary side effect of secretagogues, used alone or in combination, is hypoglycemia. Avoidance of hypoglycemia, particularly in older patients or patients with cardiovascular disease as recently highlighted by the ACCORD trial [12], restricts overuse of this class. For a few patients hypoglycemia occurs overnight. Chlorpropamide and glyburide are the secretagogues most likely to cause hypoglycemia although it may occur with any of the sulfonylureas. Nonetheless, daytime hypoglycemia, most commonly in the mid afternoon, with once daily morning dosing is a more common timing of hypoglycemia. It should lead to advice not to skip or delay lunch and may occasionally require a snack when patients are physically active in the middle of the day.

Loss of early prandial insulin release is thought to be an early event in the development of T2DM [31]. Epidemiologic studies suggest that post-prandial hyperglycemia or impaired glucose tolerance independently predicts risk for cardiovascular disease in patients with diabetes mellitus and normal fasting glycemia [32,33]. Several antidiabetes agents specifically target post-prandial hyperglycemia. These agents include the rapid-acting insulin analogs aspart, lispro and glulisine; α-glucosidase inhibitors; rapid-acting insulin secretagogues and incretins. Table 31.1 lists commonly used medication, their efficacy and their preprandial and post-prandial effects and side effects of different agents.

Rapid-acting secretagogues (glinides)

The meglitinide repaglinide and the phenylalanine derivative nateglinide have theoretical advantages, with rapid prandial insulin release potentially mimicking normal physiology. Some facilitation of prandial insulin release, however, does occur with long-acting secretagogues. The differential effect on early insulin secretion with rapid-acting secretagogues compared to sulfonylureas has not been consistently seen in all studies. Carroll *et al.* [34] failed to identify a substantial and consistent prandial glycemic benefit of rapid-acting secretagogues in comparison to extended- or immediate-release glipizide. Rapid-acting secretagogues are considered most appropriate for sulfonylurea-intolerant patients, patients with erratic food intake and patients in whom there is a demonstrated individual benefit. The absence of data showing improved clinical outcome, greater cost, more frequent dosing and no superiority in HbA_{1c} reduction limits enthusiasm for their wider use. Moreover, the rapid kinetics of nateglinide may explain its somewhat reduced overall antihyperglycemic efficacy. Secretagogues will retain their role in restoring insulin secretory deficits, especially in leaner patients, alone and in combination.

Biguanides

The antihyperglycemic effect of metformin is largely brought about by suppression of hepatic glucose release, thus reducing insulin resistance in the liver. Metformin may accomplish this by activation of the enzyme adenosine 5′-monophosphate-activated protein kinase (AMPK), which acts as a "fuel sensor." Although not approved by the FDA for the treatment of the metabolic syndrome or intermediate hyperglycemia, some clinicians have taken advantage of the insights from the Diabetes Prevention Program (DPP) [35]; in patients with impaired glucose tolerance, there was a delay in the onset of T2DM through the use of intensive lifestyle modification (58% reduction), metformin (31% reduction) and troglitazone (early DPP data suggest a benefit, but this study arm was discontinued because of the

Table 31.1 Diabetes drugs with efficacy, preprandial and post-prandial effects and side effects.

Drug type	HbA_{1c} lowering	Pre-prandial effect	Post-prandial effect	Actions	Side effects
Sulfonylureas and non-SU rapid secretagogues	1.0–2.0%	++	+	Direct/indirect secretagogue	Hypoglycemia, wt gain
Biguanides	1.0–2.0%	+++	–	↓ Hepatic glucose output	GI, lactic acidosis, wt neutral
Thiazolidinediones	0.5–1.6%	+++	–	↑ Muscle insulin sensitivity	Edema, CHF
Incretin agonists	0.9–1.1%	+	++	Strong GLP-1 effects ↑ insulin ↓ glucagon	Nausea, vomiting, wt loss
DPP-4 inhibitors	0.6–0.8%	+	++	Moderate GLP-1 effects ↑ Insulin ↓ glucagon	Nausea, wt neutral
Insulin Basal (NPH, glargine and detemir)	1.5–2.5%	+++	– Depends upon type	↓ Hepatic glucose output, ↑ muscle glucose disposal	Hypoglycemia, wt gain
Insulin Meal (analog and regular)	1.0–2.0%	–/+	++ Depends upon type	↓ Hepatic glucose output, ↑ muscle glucose disposal	Hypoglycemia, wt gain
Pramlintide	0.5–0.7%	–/+	++	↑ Insulin ↓ glucagon	Nausea, vomiting

CHF, congestive heart failure; DPP-4, dipeptidyl peptidase 4; GI, gastrointestinal; GLP-1, glucagon-like receptor 1; SU, sulfonylurea; wt, weight. HbA_{1c} 1%=11 mmol/mol.

hepatotoxicity observed). Thus, in patients with pre-diabetes or the metabolic syndrome, metformin is sometimes used in combination with intensive lifestyle modification for prevention of T2DM.

Metformin is usually the preferred initial treatment selection in most T2DM. Data, again from the UKPDS, demonstrate that metformin as monotherapy in overweight patients reduced mortality, myocardial infarction and weight gain [9]. Long-term follow-up from the UKPDS suggests this cardiovascular and mortality benefit persists [11]. The use of metformin in combination with secretagogues in T2DM is very common and two combination pills are available. One formulation combines metformin with glyburide, and the other combines metformin with glipizide. Combination medications are also available for metformin with thiazolidinediones, repaglinide and sitagliptin. The combination medications do not include the extended-release versions of metformin, and this may limit gastrointestinal tolerance for a few patients.

Thiazolidinediones

Thiazolidinediones (TZDs) are insulin-sensitizing agents that act as ligands of the nuclear transcription factor peroxisome proliferator-activated receptor γ (PPAR-γ) [36]. In so doing, they improve not only glycemia but may ameliorate dyslipidemia, inflammation and hypercoagulability associated with insulin resistance [37]. As a result, there is particular interest in their potential cardiovascular benefits in T2DM. The pleiotropic effects of TZDs beyond glycemic control lie in the role of their ligand, PPAR-γ, on lipid metabolism and inflammatory pathways. PPARs are members of a nuclear receptor superfamily that regulates gene expression in response to ligand binding. There are three known PPARs: α, δ (sometimes called β) and γ. PPAR-α is found in the liver, the heart, muscle and vascular walls, and binds fibrates, with subsequent free fatty acid oxidation, reduced triglycerides, improved high-density lipoprotein (HDL) cholesterol and a decrease in inflammation [37]. PPAR-γ is most abundant in adipose tissue, but also is in β-cells of pancreatic islets, vascular endothelium and macrophages. It regulates gene expression, influencing adipocyte differentiation, fatty acid uptake and storage, and glucose uptake [36,37].

Rosiglitazone and pioglitazone are both FDA approved for monotherapy and in combination with metformin and sulfonylureas [38–41]. Because of concerns about cardiovascular risk, rosiglitazone is no longer recommended with insulin or nitrate therapy. Pioglitazone is approved for use with insulin. A TZD predecessor, troglitazone, was FDA approved in 1997 but withdrawn in 2000 because of reports of fatal hepatotoxicity, which is not seen with current TZDs. In a meta-analysis of 13 randomized clinical trials, less than 0.3% of patients on pioglitazone or rosiglitazone had alanine aminotransferase (ALT) levels greater than three times the upper limit of normal, compared to nearly 2% of patients on troglitazone [42]. Nonetheless, it is recommended that liver function tests be performed prior to initiation of therapy and periodically thereafter. Of interest, recent reports suggest that TZD therapy may improve elevated transaminase values and even liver histology in patients with T2DM and non-alcoholic fatty liver disease or non-alcoholic steatohepatitis [43].

Both pioglitazone and rosiglitazone effectively lower HbA_{1c}, up to about 1–1.5% (11–16 mmol/mol), with maximum doses in monotherapy [44] but less on average. Glycemic control is improved on average more than with nateglinide or α-glucosidase inhibitors, but less than with sulfonylureas or metformin in unselected patients, partly because of a heterogeneous response; some patients have a small response, but others have a robust response. When TZDs are added to sulfonylureas, metformin or insulin, an additional 0.8–1.5% (9–16 mmol/mol) HbA_{1c} decline can generally be achieved [45]. A combination form of metformin and rosiglitazone is currently available. A combination pill of pioglitazone and metformin is now marketed. As with the sulfonylurea combination pills, the immediate-release form of metformin is used in these formulations. For very insulin-resistant patients (usually with high BMI, marked central obesity and hypertriglyceridemia) with preserved insulin secretion (shorter duration of diabetes), use of metformin with a TZD can be very effective. These same characteristics probably identify good TZD monotherapy responders. Combination pills of metformin and rosiglitazone or pioglitazone may be preferable for some patients because there are fewer pills to take or there is lower co-payment from insurance in some countries. TZD–secretagogue combinations are effective in insulin-resistant patients with moderate insulin secretory reserve. Combination pills are available, both for pioglitazone (with glimepiride) and rosiglitazone (with glimepiride).

As described above, the ADOPT (A Diabetes Outcome Progression Trial) trial (Figure 31.3) [24] assessed the durability of glycemic efficacy of glyburide, metformin and rosiglitazone as a monotherapy. It used as a primary endpoint the ability to maintain fasting plasma glucose less than 180 mg/dL. Secondary outcomes included time from randomization to FPG >140 mg/dL. Other prespecified outcomes included levels of FPG and glycated hemoglobin, weight and measures of insulin sensitivity and β-cell function as determined by homeostasis model assessment using the HOMA 2 method (Figure 31.5). The primary study endpoint, the proportion of those who failed to keep the FPG less than 180 mg/dL was achieved by 143 patients on rosiglitazone (2.9 per 100 patient-years), 207 on metformin (4.3 per 100 patient-years) and 311 on glyburide (7.5 per 100 patient-years). The percentages of patients HbA_{1c} achieving <7.0% (<53 mmol/mol) while on assigned therapy at study end were 26% for glyburide, 36% for metformin and 40% for rosiglitazone. Weight gain was greater with rosiglitazone than glyburide (2.5 kg) and greater still than metformin (6.9 kg) while hypoglycemia was more common with glyburide and gastrointestinal side effects with metformin as would be expected. Cardiovascular events were reduced with glyburide but not with the other two therapies.

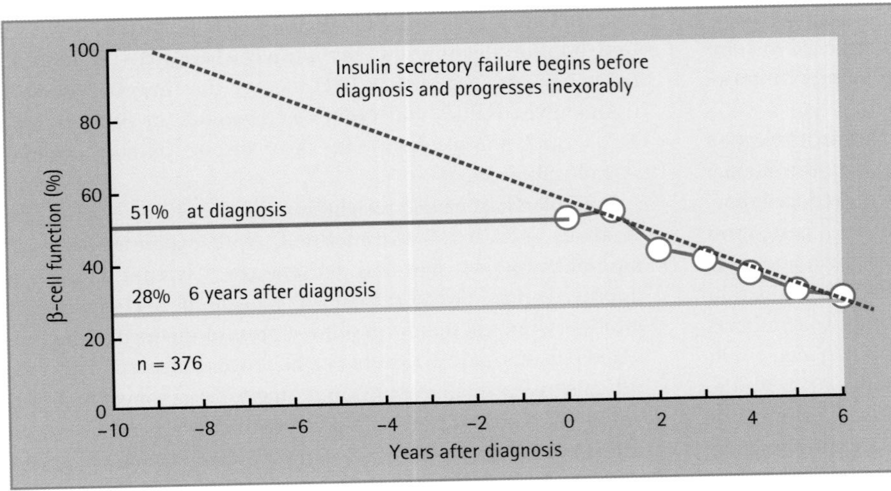

Figure 31.5 Based upon a homeostasis (HOMA) model, residual maximal insulin secretory reserve is depicted at the time of diagnosis and yearly for 6 years in subjects receiving diet only in the UK Prospective Diabetes Study. This figure illustrates that nearly half of insulin secretion is lost at diagnosis. It also shows the progressive loss of insulin secretory reserve, which predicts essentially complete insulin deficiency in about a dozen years if further loss were linear.

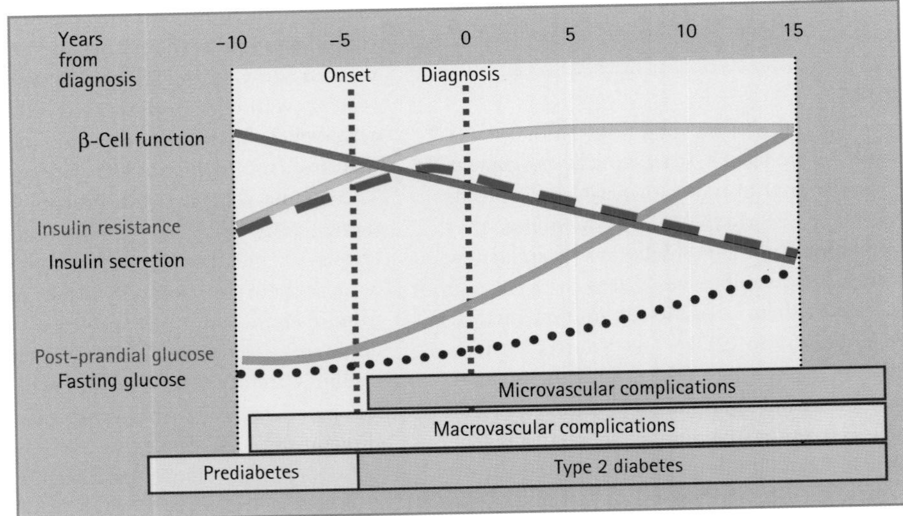

Figure 31.6 The natural history of type 2 diabetes mellitus. Long before diagnosis β-cell function begins a gradual and inexorable decline (solid red line at top of figure). Insulin resistance (solid orange line) begins to increase during early adulthood in conjunction with cardiovascular risks. The dashed green line depicts the initial compensatory increase in insulin secretion in response to increasing insulin resistance, which initially maintains euglycemia but which eventually fails and causes progression from euglycemia to prediabetes to diabetes. At the bottom of the figure post-prandial glucose levels rise (solid pink line) initially as insulin secretion fails to keep pace with insulin resistance. Later (dotted purple line) fasting glucose will also begin to rise progressively as insulin secretion wanes further. Progressive insulin deficiency requires progressive therapy combinations. After about 10 years of diagnosed diabetes frank insulin deficiency leads to the need for basal and then basal and meal insulin treatment in most people with type 2 diabetes. Microvascular complications occur only after several years of hyperglycemia. Macrovascular complications may precede or arrive simultaneously with diagnosis of diabetes because of the long prodrome of insulin resistance-related cardiovascular risks. Adapted from Holman RR. *Diabetes Res Clin Pract* 1998; **40**(suppl):S21–S25; Ramlo-Halsted BA, Edelman SV. *Prim Care* 1999; **26**:771–789; Nathan DM. *N Engl J Med* 2002; **347**:1342–1349; UKPDS Group. *Diabetes* 1995; **44**:1249–1258.

Overall, most editorialists have concluded that glitazones remain in the balance less attractive as initial therapy than metformin [46].

TZDs also stimulate the production and circulation of adiponectin [47], a fat-cell-derived hormone (or adipokine) that increases AMPK activity in the liver, adipose tissue and skeletal muscle. Low adiponectin levels are seen in patients with T2DM and are thought to contribute to insulin resistance and subsequent hyperglycemia [48]. The stimulation of adiponectin production, in addition to direct activation of AMPK, may explain some of the beneficial lipid effects of TZDs as well as their ability to increase insulin sensitivity [48]. Low adiponectin levels may predict a therapeutic response to TZDs, and polymorphisms in the PPAR-γ gene could potentially help to explain the variability of therapeutic response to TZDs and progression of diabetes (see Chapter 12) [48].

A recent meta-analysis raised the question of cardiac safety with rosiglitazone with findings of a 43% relative increased risk in ischemic heart disease events [49]. Some studies using the same data have confirmed this increase in risk while others have failed to do so. Further analysis, including interim safety analysis of the RECORD trial, failed to show increased rates of major adverse cardiac events (see below) [50]. Results from recently published prospective randomized controlled clinical trails (VADT, ADVANCE, ACCORD) [12,51,52] which had high rates of TZD usage failed to show reduction in major adverse cardiovascular events (MACE) with tighter glycemic control and did not suggest increases in MACE associated with TZD use. Nevertheless, the ADA/EASD algorithm has taken a conservative stance and has not included rosiglitazone in its standard alternative recommendations.

What does become clear in review of the available safety data for this class is their propensity for promoting fluid retention in some patients, who may be difficult to predict in advance. Close tracking of patient weight and reviewing medication dose or diuretic use may need to be performed when patients gain more than 5–7 lb (3 kg). This has lead to a re-emphasis on their potential for exacerbation of congestive heart failure particularly in patients with class III or IV heart failure [53].

Subsequent analysis of clinical trial data, both old and new, with an emphasis on analysis of those patients at risk for MACE lead to significant changes in the labeling for use of TZDs. In particular, concomitant usage of insulin or nitrates was associated with increased risk for congestive heart failure and other cardiovascular events, and combination therapy of insulin and/or nitrates with rosiglitazone is no longer indicated. Currently, neither pioglitazone nor rosiglitazone are indicated in patients with class III or IV heart failure.

The link between TZD usage and possible adverse cardiovascular events or potential cardiovascular risk reduction remains unanswered. Rosiglitazone was used in large numbers of patients in both the ACCORD [12] and VADT trial [52] without a clear MACE signal, suggesting the drug does not promote cardiovascular events. Pioglitazone was studied in the Prospective Pioglitazone Clinical Trial in Macrovascular Events (PROactive) to examine its effects on morbidity and cardiovascular mortality and the secondary cardiovascular endpoints of myocardial infarction, death and stroke were favorably affected [54]. This study of 2600 actively treated patients showed no increase in mortality or MACE. Future studies may assist the practitioner to reach a clearer answer to this important but unresolved question.

Two recent studies tend to affirm the cardiovascular safety of rosiglitazone. They are the RECORD trial [55] and the BARI 2D trial [56]. These studies compared the cardiovascular benefits of rosiglitazone to other monotherapy (RECORD) in a non-inferiority analysis, while an insulin sensitizing approach was compared with an insulin providing approach in the BARI 2D trial. In the BARI 2D trial [56], 2368 patients with both T2DM and heart disease were randomly assigned to either prompt revascularization with intensive medical therapy or intensive medical therapy alone. They were also assigned to either insulin-sensitization or insulin-provision therapy, with either insulin or secretagogues. The primary endpoints were the rate of death and a composite of death, myocardial infarction or stroke (major cardiovascular events). At 5 years, survival rates were similar with revascularization (88.3%) and medical therapy (87.8%; $P = 0.97$) or with insulin-sensitization (88.2%) and insulin-provision (87.9%; $P = 0.89$). Similarly, freedom from major cardiovascular events did not differ significantly among the groups: 77.2% with revascularization and 75.9% with medical treatment ($P = 0.70$) and 77.7% with insulin-sensitization and 75.4% with insulin-provision group ($P = 0.13$). Severe hypoglycemia was more common with insulin provision (9.2%) than with an insulin-sensitization strategy (5.9%; $P = 0.003$).

In the RECORD study [55], 4447 patients with T2DM on metformin or sulfonylurea monotherapy with mean HbA_{1c} of 7.9% (63 mmol/mol) were randomly assigned to added rosiglitazone (n = 2220) or to metformin and sulfonylurea (n = 2227). The primary endpoint was cardiovascular hospitalization or cardiovascular death, with a hazard ratio (HR) non-inferiority margin of 1:20; 321 people offered added rosiglitazone and 323 in the control group experienced the primary outcome during 5.5-year follow-up, meeting the criterion of non-inferiority (HR 0.99; 95% CI 0.85–1.16). HR was 0.84 (0.59–1.18) for cardiovascular death, 1.14 (0.80–1.63) for myocardial infarction, and 0.72 (0.49–1.06) for stroke. Although these cardiovascular endpoints did not differ significantly, heart failure leading to hospitalization or death occurred in 61 people with rosiglitazone and 29 in the control group (HR 2.10, 1.35–3.27). Limb fracture rates were increased (about double), mainly in women randomly assigned to rosiglitazone. Mean HbA_{1c} was lower (approximately 0.25% [3 mmol/mol]) in the rosiglitazone group than in the control group at 5 years. Although the preponderance of this evidence now appears to exculpate rosiglitazone from the concern regarding ischemic heart disease, it does not indicate a clear benefit in this regard either.

Lastly, an unanticipated complication seen with both TZDs is an increase in observed long bone fractures in woman participating in PROactive [54] and rosiglitazone trials (ADOPT) [24]. In both cases, the fracture rates were approximately double (5.1% vs 2.5%: PROactive) that of comparator groups, were seen early and were unrelated to diabetic control. A potential mechanism may relate to PPAR involvement in osteoblast cell differentiation [57], but this remains incompletely understood. Consideration should be given to screening for fracture risk including at the wrist to assess cortical bone in patients on TZD therapy at initiation and periodically thereafter until further information regarding the mechanism of the increased fracture rate associated with TZD usage is provided.

Taken together, the adverse event profile for the rosiglitazone without compelling evidence for specific cardiovascular benefit suggests use of this agent be reserved for patients unable to tolerate alternative drug regimens. This is in concordance with the current ADA/EASD recommendations. It should be acknowledged that this recommendation is controversial and we may see revision of this in due course.

Incretin therapy combinations

The recent availability of incretin mimetics, either glucagon-like peptide 1 (GLP-1) receptor agonists, such as exenatide and liraglutide, or dipeptidyl peptidase 4 (DPP-4) inhibitors, such as sitagliptin, saxagliptin, alogliptin and vildagliptin, has opened up new possibilities in combination therapy [58]. Exenatide is an injectable synthetic analog of the Gila monster (*Heloderma suspectum*) salivary protein exendin 4. This compound has substantial homology with GLP-1 and tightly binds to GLP-1 receptors and thereby mimics the actions of native GLP-1 when given in doses of 5 or 10 µg twice daily. Three registration trials of similar design show the use of exenatide in 30-week long studies in patients with oral agent failure with sulfonylureas [59], metformin [60] or both [61]. After a 4-week placebo run in, subjects were randomized to blinded placebo versus exenatide 5 µg twice daily for 1 month and then continued this dose or increased to 10 µg twice daily. All subjects continued their prior oral agents.

When exenatide versus placebo was added to metformin, 272 patients completed the study [60]. They were middle-aged (53 ± 10 years), obese (34.2 ± 5.9 kg/m^2 BMI) and with inadequate glycemic control (HbA_{1c} 8.2 ± 1.1% [66 mmol/mol]). At 30 weeks, the HbA_{1c} change from baseline was −0.78 ± 0.1% (10 µg), −0.4 ± 0.11% (5 µg) and 0.08 ± 0.1% for placebo; $P < 0.002$, (8, 4 and 1 mmol/mol, respectively). Exenatide was associated with weight loss: −2.8 ± 0.5 kg (10 µg), −1.6 ± 0.4 kg (5 µg); $P < 0.001$ versus placebo. Gastrointestinal side effects including nausea, vomiting and diarrhea were more common with exenatide but lessened toward the end of the trial. In the 5 and 10 µg groups, exenatide resulted in a placebo subtracted percentage for nausea of 11% and 22%, for vomiting 7% and 8%, and for diarrhea 4% and 8% overall during the study.

In the sulfonylurea failure study [59], the study population was similar with obese middle-aged subjects with slightly higher baseline glycemia (HbA_{1c} 8.6 ± 1.2% [70 mmol/mol]). The change from baseline HbA_{1c} at 30 weeks was −0.86 ± 0.11 (10 µg), −0.46 ± 0.12 (5 µg) and 0.12 ± 0.09% (placebo); $P < 0.001$, (9, 5 and 1 mmol/mol, respectively). Weight loss was somewhat less with 10 µg than in the metformin alone study (−1.6 kg). The third trial was for patients inadequately controlled on the combination of effective doses of sulfonylurea and metformin. Similar subjects were studied with middle-aged, obese, poorly controlled subjects (baseline HbA_{1c} 8.5 ± 1.0% [69 mmol/mol]). The change from baseline HbA_{1c} occurred at 30 weeks was −0.8 ± 0.1% (10 µg), −0.6 ± 0.1% (5 µg) and 0.2 ± 0.1% (placebo); $P < 0.0001$, (9, 7 and 2 mmol/mol, respectively). Weight loss in this study averaged 1.6 kg for the 10 µg dose group and was similar to the sulfonylurea alone study.

A similar study has been conducted showing comparable glycemic benefit in patients in a thiazolidinedione alone or with metformin to which 5 and then 10 µg doses of exenatide were added for 16 weeks [62]. Again, approximately 1% (11 mmol/mol) reduction in HbA_{1c} occurred from a baseline of 7.9% (63 mmol/mol) in comparison to placebo controls and approximately a 30 mg/dL (1.7 mmol/L) decline in fasting glucose occurred with a greater weight loss in the exenatide group (~1.5 kg). Nausea was more common with exenatide (40 vs 15% for placebo) and the drop-out rate was also higher.

Is it reasonable to choose exenatide as an alternative to basal insulin therapy? Perhaps if patients are not very far from glycemic goal the answer may be yes. Heine *et al.* [63] reported a study of 551 subjects with T2DM who were inadequately controlled. They were randomized to either insulin glargine once a day at bedtime or 5 µg for 1 month then 10 µg exenatide for the duration of this 26-week long trial. Baseline HbA_{1c} was 8.2% (66 mmol/mol) for patients receiving exenatide and 8.3% for those on insulin glargine. By study end, exenatide and insulin glargine therapies resulted in equal reduction of HbA_{1c} levels by 1.11% (12 mmol/mol). Exenatide reduced post-prandial plasma glucose levels more than insulin glargine, while insulin glargine reduced FPG levels more than exenatide. This is well illustrated in the seven-point self-monitored glucose levels before and after meals and at 3 AM performed at study beginning and end. Body weight decreased 2.3 kg with exenatide and increased 1.8 kg with insulin glargine. Rates of symptomatic hypoglycemia were similar, but nocturnal hypoglycemia occurred less frequently with exenatide (0.9 vs 2.4 events/patient-year). Gastrointestinal symptoms were more common in the exenatide group than in the insulin glargine group, including nausea (57.1% vs 8.6%), vomiting (17.4% vs 3.7%) and diarrhea (8.5% vs 3.0%). Despite similar lowering of HbA_{1c}, there were marked differences in prandial versus preprandial control, suggesting these interventions had different patterns of benefit.

In all of the studies of exenatide in which sulfonylureas were used, an increased risk of hypoglycemia occurred that sometimes required a reduction in sulfonylurea dose to reduce the risk of hypoglycemia symptoms. In patients on sulfonylureas treated with exenatide (and likely also with DPP-4 inhibitors), it may be appropriate to pre-emptively reduce sulfonylurea doses by half if patients' lowest blood sugars are less than 100 mg/dL because the glucose-dependent insulin secretion with this combination is lost as a result of the sulfonylurea. Taken together, these studies suggest that exenatide may represent a desirable alternative for overweight patients for whom lifestyle intervention alone is insufficient in improving weight and who also need improved glycemia control but are reluctant to use insulin.

One study by Nauck *et al.* [64] studied exenatide twice daily (n = 253) vs biphasic insulin aspart (70/30, n = 248) in patients poorly controlled on metformin and sulfonylureas in a non-inferiority analysis. Exenatide was found to be non-inferior with a mean ± SEM decrease in HbA_{1c} from baseline of −1.04 ± 0.07% (11 mmol/mol), and for biphasic insulin aspart it was −0.89 ± 0.06% (10 mmol/mol); the difference was −0.15% ((5% CI −0.32 to 0.01%). Exenatide-treated patients lost weight and had nausea in 35%, while patients treated with biphasic insulin aspart gained weight (between-group difference −5.4 kg; 95% CI −5.9 to 5.0 kg). Both treatments reduced fasting glucose (exenatide −1.8 ± 0.2 mmol/L, $P < 0.001$; biphasic insulin aspart −1.7 ± 0.2 mmol/L, $P < 0.001$). Greater reductions in post-prandial glucose excursions at all meals were observed with exenatide. The withdrawal rate was 21.3% (54/253) for exenatide and 10.1% (25/248) for biphasic insulin aspart.

In a second study which compared 70/30 insulin aspart analog mixture, as alternatives for patients failing oral agent therapy, Bergenstal *et al.* [65] found that more patients responded to the biphasic insulin than to exenatide. The higher baseline HbA_{1c} (10.2% [88 mmol/mol]) was thought to reflect more advanced disease and thus would be associated with less β-cell function, which is a requirement for full clinical response to exenatide.

Although not approved for use together, exenatide with insulin therapy is reportedly used in patients with T2DM. The rationale is based upon the potential insulin sparing effects of exenatide presumably through its multiple effects to augment insulin and reduce glucagon at meals as well as its effects upon gastric emptying, appetite and weight loss. Sheffield *et al.* [66] described a series of 134 patients initiating exenatide in combination with insulin in private endocrine practice with a 1-year follow-up. Exenatide use resulted in a 0.87% (9 mmol/mol) reduction of HbA_{1c}, despite a 45% discontinuation of premeal insulin, reduction in insulin injection number and discontinuation of sulfonylureas. Its use resulted in reduced weight slightly over 5 kg, although some weight loss was observed in 72% of patients. Slightly over one-third of patients (36%) discontinued the exenatide primarily because of gastrointestinal side effects, while 10% of patients had hypoglycemia. The authors have some experience with the use of exenatide with a basal insulin as an alternative for selected patients who have difficulty with accurate dosing of meal insulin in combination with basal insulin, which mirrors the experience reported in this case series.

Liraglutide is a GLP-1 analog with 97% homology to human GLP-1 which has now had several clinical trials, and has now been approved by the US FDA and European Medicines Agency. Phase 3 trials have included monotherapy and trials in combination with either metformin, with sulfonylureas or the combination of the two oral agents. In a 52-week study [67], doses of 1.2 and 1.8 mg were given once daily to 746 patients with early T2DM. The subjects in this study were randomly assigned to once daily liraglutide (1.2 mg [n = 251] or 1.8 mg [n = 247]) or glimepiride 8 mg (n = 248). The primary outcome was change in HbA_{1c} from baseline. The analysis was by intention-to-treat. At 52 weeks, the HbA_{1c} was decreased by 0.51% (SD 1.20%) with glimepiride, compared with 0.84% (1.23%) with liraglutide 1.2 mg (difference −0.33%; 95% CI −0.53 to −0.13; $P = 0.0014$) and 1.14% (1.24%) with liraglutide 1.8 mg (−0.62; −0.83 to −0.42; $P < 0.0001$). Five patients in the 1.2 mg liraglutide, and one in 1.8 mg groups discontinued the treatment because of vomiting, but none in the glimepiride group did so. The frequently self-monitored blood glucose profiles appear to show very good fasting glucose control, although interestingly a bit less marked blunting of post meal glucose than in some of the exenatide studies. There is no direct comparison with exenatide in this study.

In a multiple-arm study [68] of 1041 adults with T2DM with an average age of 56 ± 10 years (mean ± SD) over 26 weeks, liraglutide (0.6, 1.2 or 1.8 mg/day) or rosiglitazone (4 mg/day) or placebo was added to glimepiride monotherapy. Liraglutide (1.2 or 1.8 mg) reduced HbA_{1c} from baseline more (−1.1% [12 mmol/mol]; baseline 8.5% [69 mmol/mol]) when compared with placebo (+0.2% [2 mmol/mol]; $P < 0.0001$; baseline 8.4% [68 mmol/mol]) or rosiglitazone (−0.4% [4 mmol/mol]; $P < 0.0001$; baseline 8.4% [68 mmol/mol]). A lower dose of liraglutide was less effective and only reduced HbA_{1c} by 0.6% (7 mmol/mol). Fasting plasma glucose decreased by week 2, with a 1.6 mmol/L decrease from baseline at 26 weeks with liraglutide 1.2 mg (baseline 9.8 mmol/L) or 1.8 mg (baseline 9.7 mmol/L) compared with a 0.9 mmol/L increase with placebo ($P < 0.0001$; baseline 9.5 mmol/L) or 1.0 mmol/L decrease with rosiglitazone ($P < 0.006$; baseline 9.9 mmol/L). Post-prandial plasma glucose decreased more from baseline with liraglutide 1.2 or 1.8 mg (−2.5 to −2.7 mmol/L [baseline 12.9 mmol/L for both]) compared with placebo (−0.4 mmol/L; $P < 0.0001$; baseline 12.7 mmol/L) or rosiglitazone (−1.8 mmol/L; $P < 0.05$; baseline 13.0 mmol/L). Changes in body weight with liraglutide 1.8 mg (−0.2 kg; baseline 83.0 kg), 1.2 mg (+0.3 kg; baseline 80.0 kg) or placebo (−0.1 kg; baseline 81.9 kg) were less than with rosiglitazone (+2.1 kg; $P < 0.0001$; baseline 80.6 kg). The adverse events for all treatments were minor hypoglycemia (<10%), nausea (<11%), vomiting (<5%) and diarrhea (<8%).

A recently published article studied the addition of liraglutide [69] in 533 patients with diabetes failing on oral agents, randomizing them in a 1 : 1 : 1 ratio to liraglutide 1.2 or 1.8 mg daily or placebo in addition to rosiglitazone 4 mg twice daily and metformin 1 g twice daily for 26 weeks. HbA_{1c} values decreased significantly more in the liraglutide groups vs placebo (1.5 ± 0.1% for both liraglutide 1.2 and 1.8 mg and −0.5 ± 0.1% for placebo [mean ± SE]). FPG decreased by 40, 44 and 8 mg/dL for liraglutide 1.2, 1.8 and placebo, respectively, and 90 minutes post meal post-prandial plasma glucose (PPG) decreased by 47, 49 and 14 mg/dL, respectively ($P < 0.001$ for all liraglutide groups vs placebo). Dose-dependent weight loss occurred with liraglutide 1.2 and 1.8 mg (1.0 ± 0.3 and 2.0 ± 0.3 kg, respectively; $P < 0.0001$) as compared to weight gain with placebo (0.6 ± 0.3 kg). Interestingly systolic blood pressure decreased by 6.7, 5.6 and 1.1 mmHg with liraglutide 1.2, 1.8 mg, and placebo, respectively. These data, dissimilar to some with exenatide, suggest a greater effect on fasting glucose control and a more commensurate change in fasting with post-prandial control. A 26-week head-to-head comparison of exenatide 10 μg twice daily with liraglutide 1.8 mg daily showed a 0.3% (3 mmol/mol) greater reduction in HbA_{1c} with liraglutide in a population of adults with inadequately controlled T2DM on maximally tolerated doses of metformin, sulphonylurea, or both [70]. Furthermore, more patients receiving liraglutide achieved an HbA_{1c} of less than 7% (54%vs 43%). Liraglutide also reduced mean fasting plasma glucose more than did exenatide. Both drugs promoted similar weight losses but nausea was less persistent and minor hypoglycaemia was less frequent with liraglutide.

Drucker *et al.* [71] have compared exenatide with a longer acting preparation given once weekly of the same agent. This randomized non-inferiority study compared long-acting release exenatide 2 mg once weekly with 10 µg exenatide administered twice daily, in 295 patients with T2DM (HbA_{1c} 8.3% ± 1.0 SD [67 mmol/mol]), mean fasting glucose 9 ± 2 mmol/L, weight 102 ± 20 kg and diabetes duration of 6.7 ± 5.0 years. The patients were either naive to drug therapy or on one or more oral antidiabetic agents. The primary endpoint was change in HbA_{1c} at 30 weeks. At study endpoint the patients given exenatide once a week had lower HbA_{1c} than those on exenatide twice daily (−1.9 ± 0.1%; SE vs −1.5 ± 0.1%; (95% CI −0.54% to −0.12%; $P = 0.0023$). More patients receiving treatment once weekly vs twice daily achieved HbA_{1c} levels of 7.0% (53 mmol/mol) or less (77% vs 61%; $P = 0.0039$). Again, in this trial as in the liraglutide studies there appears to be more effect upon fasting glycemic control than with twice daily exenatide. It is a little difficult to know if in this study differences were to be attributed mostly to kinetics differences or changes in the achieved levels of the incretin mimetic in the blood at the end of the study. However, the ability to lower fasting control to a greater degree than currently available with exenatide seems an important observation and may relate to overall antihyperglycemic efficacy.

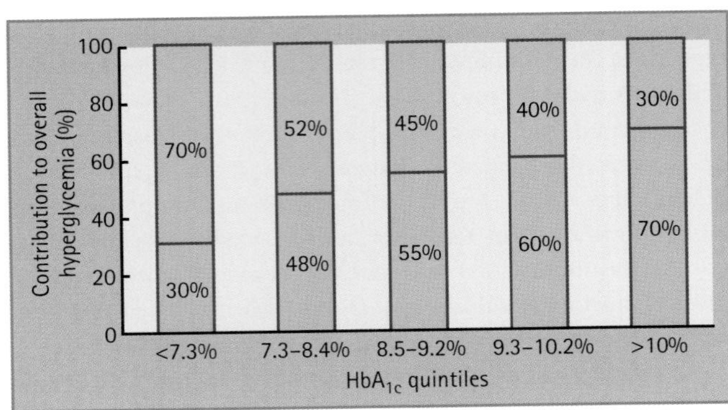

Figure 31.7 The relative contribution of fasting plasma glucose (FPG; shown in the open bars) and the post-prandial plasma glucose (PPG; shown in the shaded bars) to overall hyperglycemia. An area-under-the-curve analysis suggests that as HbA_{1c} approaches the ADA goal for minimum desirable glycemic control (<7.0% [53 mmol/mol]), the PPG makes a greater contribution to overall hyperglycemia. Conversely, as the HbA_{1c} rises far from goal, the contribution of FPG to overall hyperglycemia is greater. For patients with poor hyperglycemia a focus on the fasting glucose thus becomes an important priority. As patient approach targeted glycemic goals a greater attention should be directed to post-prandial hyperglycemia. The equivalent IFCC units for the quintiles are: <56 mmol/mol, 56–58 mmol/mol, 69–77 mmol/mol, 78–88 mmol/mol, >88 mmol/mol,

DPP-4 inhibitors

Incretin action can also be provided by inhibiting the rapid degradation of GLP-1 and glucose-dependent insulinotropic peptide (GIP). Although with DPP-4 inhibition the level of circulating GLP-1 agonist activity probably does not rise to a degree similar to that seen with receptor agonists such as exenatide and liraglutide, the glycemic lowering efficacy of sitagliptin and vildagliptin is close to that seen with injectable receptor agonists. Vildagliptin 50 mg once daily added to patients inadequately controlled on metformin (baseline HbA_{1c} 7.7% [61 mmol/mol]) resulted in a placebo subtracted difference in HbA_{1c} at 52 weeks of −1.0 ± 0.2% (11 mmol/mol, $P < 0.001$) [72].

Vildagliptin combined with a sulfonylurea or a thiazolidinedione also improved glycemia in patients with T2DM in trials of 24–52 weeks. In patients inadequately controlled with metformin, added vildagliptin 100 mg/day was non-inferior to add on therapy with pioglitazone; each treatment reducing HbA_{1c} an additional 1% (11 mmol/mol) [73]. Vildagliptin is also available as a fixed-dose formulation with metformin. Vildagliptin has also been studied by Fonseca *et al.* [74] added to insulin treatment and has a small additional effect (approximately 0.3% [3 mmol/mol] HbA_{1c} lowering) when compared with placebo. In an interested recent physiologic study, Ahren *et al.* [75] have found that glucagon responsiveness is not only suppressed with a glucose challenge with vildagliptin, but there is also a slight improvement in glucagon increment to insulin hypoglycemia.

DPP-4 inhibitors do not cause nausea and vomiting and are weight neutral, lacking the weight-reduction effects of the GLP-1 agonists observed at 1 year. This is likely because of lower levels of GLP-1 activity. Sitagliptin has been studied as monotherapy [76,77] and as additional treatment for those not meeting glycemic goals on either metformin [78] or a thiazolidinedione [79]. In doses of 100 mg for patients with normal renal function in two monotherapy studies of 18 and 24 weeks' duration, sitagliptin reduced HbA_{1c} by 0.6% (7 mmol/mol) and 0.8% (9 mmol/mol), respectively. Added to either metformin or pioglitazone, it further reduced HbA_{1c} by 0.7% (8 mmol/mol) in 24-week duration studies. DPP-4 inhibitors are weight neutral, probably because of an appetite effect of raising endogenous GLP-1 levels. Their glycemic effects on peak prandial control appear superior to effects on preprandial control. This should complement the primarily preprandial effects of metformin or thiazolidinediones. Incretin drugs appear especially favorable for prandial glycemic control and may be favored also because of positive effects of weight loss or minimal weight gain. Prandial control has been observed by Monnier *et al.* [80,81] to be important particularly as HbA_{1c} nears goal (Figure 31.7). Also, if prandial euglycemia contributes to decreased cardiovascular risk through reducing oxidative stress then incretins could have an additional favorable action.

Colesevelam

After a pilot trial of 12 weeks' duration, 65 subjects with T2DM showed that the addition of the bile acid sequestrant colesevelam reduced HbA_{1c} by 0.5% (5 mmol/mol, $P < 0.007$) as well as the expected lipid benefit [82]. Further studies have examined combination therapy in several different groups. Bays *et al.* [83] looked at its effects in doses of 3.75 g/day (n = 159) compared with matched placebo (n = 157) in subjects with T2DM on metformin and other diabetes oral agents, confirming the early pilot with a reduction of HbA_{1c} of 0.54% (6 mmol/mol, $P < 0.001$). Those on metformin alone were reduced by 0.47% compared with placebo; those on combined therapy (mostly sulfonylureas, or glitazones and a few other agents) were reduced by 0.62% (7 mmol/mol). Goldberg *et al.* [84] found that patients who were on insulin therapy but not adequately controlled also show the similar level of glycemic benefit after 16 weeks when compared with placebo (−0.41% HbA_{1c} for colesevelam vs +0.09% for the placebo group; $P < 0.001$). Fonseca *et al.* [85] found that patients on sulfonylureas given colesevelam 3.75 g/day for 26 weeks showed a placebo corrected difference of −0.54% (6 mmol/mol) HbA_{1c}. Overall, these data suggest a modest consistent benefit of colesevelam, on average of 0.5% (6 mmol/mol) reduction in HbA_{1c}, in people with T2DM on a variety of combination regimens. The drug is well known and may certainly cause hypertriglyceridemia in those who have pre-existing high levels of triglycerides (usually >250 mg/dL would be high risk). In addition, like other bile acid sequestrants it may cause constipation. With absent high triglycerides at baseline, it is both safe and likely in patients on statins to reduce low density lipoprotein (LDL) cholesterol significantly and contribute to achieving cardiovascular risk reduction.

Transition to insulin

Current consensus guidelines endorse early adoption of insulin therapy. In general, insulin is an underutilized therapy as a result of both patient and provider hesitance to adopt an injectable therapy associated with weight gain and potential severe life-threatening hypoglycemia. Attention to patient reluctance and provider barriers can maximize successful initiation of insulin therapy. Providing simple patient titration schemes enhance practitioner and patient acceptance [86]. Combination insulin (parenteral) and sulfonylurea (oral) therapy has been widely studied and provides a basis for many later basal insulin studies. Twice daily (bedtime insulin, daytime sulfonylurea) therapy [87–90] was shown to be an effective therapy prior to the widespread use of metformin in the USA. The use of bedtime insulin suppressed hepatic glucose output and facilitated the use of sulfonylurea for prandial insulin support.

Initiation of insulin therapy can be performed safely and efficiently with the addition of a basal insulin (NPH, glargine, detemir) with titration of dosage to desired target blood glucose. Several studies and reviews support the safety and effectiveness of this approach [6,91–95].

An alternative to a single dose of basal insulin, which has similar overall efficacy but a different pattern of control, is prandial dosing. The APOLLO trial (Figure 31.8) [93] examined basal once daily insulin glargine in comparison to three times a day insulin lispro at meals in 418 subjects with inadequate glycemic control while on oral diabetes agents. In this study, which was 44 weeks in duration, the HbA_{1c} drop was similar (−1.7% [19 mmol/mol] for glargine −8.7% [72 mmol/mol] to 7% [53 mmol/mol], −1.9% [21 mmol/mol] for lispro – from 8.7% [72 mmol/mol] to 6.8% [51 mmol/mol]), and as might be expected from the kinetics and timing of the insulin preparations showed superior fasting glycemic control with insulin glargine (−4.3 vs −1.8 mmol/L; 77 vs 32 mg/dL) and better nocturnal control but less effective daytime control (each by about 0.5 or 10 mg/dL). Not surprisingly in this open label study, patients found it preferable to use once daily injection. Subjects taking glargine had fewer hypoglycemia episodes than those on lispro. This study suggests that either meal insulin or basal can be used to achieve improved control although patient preference suggests a basal insulin strategy.

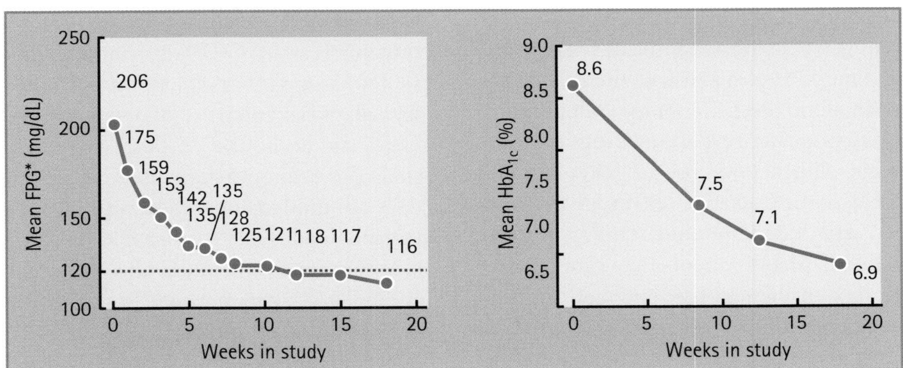

Figure 31.8 From the APOLLO study, nine-point self-monitored blood glucose profiles in the APOLLO trial. This open labeled study compared the effects of once daily insulin glargine in comparison to lispro three times daily at meals. Average glycemia and HbA_{1c} were similar, although hypoglycemia was increased with lispro while weight gain was similar in the two groups. The pattern of glycemia reveals that fasting glucose control improved to a greater degree with glargine and that as one would expect prandial control is better with lispro. These two strategies are complementary in the glycemic patterns suggesting that using basal insulin and some meal analog insulin may be a useful strategy for many patients. The highest increase in prandial glycemia occurred at breakfast and dinner [94].

Combining insulin and oral agent therapy

Insulin therapy is eventually needed for most patients with T2DM. An evening insulin strategy is a simple way to begin insulin therapy that will achieve glycemic goals and is easily understood by patients. The rationale for evening insulin has previously been reviewed [86,91,92]. In brief, an evening injection of intermediate- or long-acting insulin addresses a fundamental need in management of T2DM by suppressing overnight endogenous glucose production and thereby preventing hyperglycemia prior to the first meal of the day. This approach is useful for most patients with T2DM, with the notable exception of patients taking morning glucocorticoid therapy.

There are several versions of this strategy, including the use of intermediate-acting insulin at bedtime, intermediate and quick-acting insulin mixed in a single injection at dinnertime, and insulin glargine or insulin detemir at bedtime. For some patients, an alternate timing of glargine may be used earlier in the day; for those using large doses (0.8 units/kg) of detemir use early in the day may also be possible. Most of the evidence for these regimens comes from trials of insulin combined with oral agents, such as a sulfonylurea alone or with metformin, with the oral agents continued while the insulin dosage is gradually increased until control is re-established.

NPH at bedtime

Addition of an injection of NPH insulin within an hour of bedtime is usually able to restore adequate fasting glycemic control for patients who are no longer well-controlled with one or more oral agents alone. This tactic may be best employed in patients who do not eat a very large meal toward the end of the day and thus do not need short-acting insulin at suppertime. A multicenter trial has shown bedtime NPH insulin plus daytime oral agents achieves glycemic control as effectively as insulin taken in the morning with oral agents, or mixed intermediate and regular insulin twice daily without oral agents; however, there is less weight gain with evening NPH [89]. Other trials show better glycemic control with bedtime NPH plus a sulfonylurea than with a single injection of insulin alone [87,88]. Evening NPH insulin also reduces free fatty acids to a greater degree than use of daytime insulin. Patients can begin with a low dose of NPH insulin, usually about 10 units. They are instructed to self-titrate the dose up by 2–4 units every 3–7 days based upon the stability of their fasting glycemic response [86]. Stable patients may titrate more quickly, based upon the pattern of response, but there is little reason to hurry because glucose control will steadily improve at any rate of titration so long as the oral agents are continued. The insulin dosage required is frequently in the range of 30–50 units daily [91], or about 0.4–0.5 units/kg body weight. The target for fasting glucose should be individualized and adjusted when hypoglycemia occurs, but often can be ADA recommended 90–130 mg/dL (5–7.2 mmol/L) value in plasma-referenced home glucose-monitoring systems. Patients need to wake at a reasonably consistent time and eat breakfast consistently. Oral agents are continued, although sulfonylureas are usually given only with the first meal of the day. A randomized trial has examined the choice of daytime therapy accompanying bedtime NPH insulin [89]. This study compared four different regimens in a prospective 1-year randomized controlled trial. The four regimens included bedtime insulin combined with morning insulin, glyburide alone, metformin alone or glyburide combined with metformin. The least weight gain occurred when metformin was the only oral agent, and hypoglycemia was a limiting factor when glyburide was used.

Pre-mixed insulin with the evening meal

A second form of evening insulin that appears to work better for more obese patients (BMI >30 kg/m^2) is the combination of morning sulfonylureas and suppertime mixed insulin, the latter commonly offered as 70/30 (70% NPH with 30% Regular) insulin. In a multicenter study using the long-acting sulfonylurea glimepiride [90], patients achieved a more rapid restoration of glycemic control with self-titration of 70/30 insulin while continuing the oral agent, rather than with insulin alone. Insulin was started at 10 units and titrated weekly, seeking FPG equivalent to 140 mg/dL (7.8 mmol/L, plasma-referenced). Nearly all subjects using the combination regimen reached the titration target rapidly, but 15% of the subjects in the placebo plus insulin group dropped out, mainly because of hyperglycemia during the transition to insulin. The mean HbA_{1c} declined from almost 10% (86 mmol/mol) to 7.6% (60 mmol/mol) for subjects completing the trial in both groups. The mean dose in the insulin alone group was 78 units and for the glimepiride plus insulin combination was 49 units. More subjects in this study who were on insulin alone needed doses higher than 100 units daily, and so had to take more than one injection. A smaller study with a more aggressive titration scheme found better glycemic control using 70/30 insulin with the evening meal plus glyburide once daily than with evening insulin alone [83]. Premixed rapid analog mixes [e.g. lispro–neutral protamine lispro (25/75%) and aspart–neutral protamine aspart (30/70%)] similarly may achieve control with somewhat more convenient meal timing of insulin. It is critical for safety that patients understand the appropriate timing of meals and do not skip meals. Garber *et al.* [96] have reported a small observational study using either once, twice or three times daily administration at meal time of the 70/30 aspart mixture in patients inadequately controlled or oral agents with or without basal insulin treatment. In this study, once daily administration at dinner of 70/30 reduced HbA_{1c} by 1.4% (15 mmol/mol), twice daily at breakfast and supper by 1.9% (21 mmol/mol) and thrice daily with an added lunch dose by 1.8% (20 mmol/mol). Use of insulin pens at meal times is often desirable especially for those who eat outside the home frequently. Pre-mixed insulins are commonly given twice a day, sometimes more or less frequently. When given more frequently they may become somewhat non-intuitive as to which dose to adjust and this may confuse some patients.

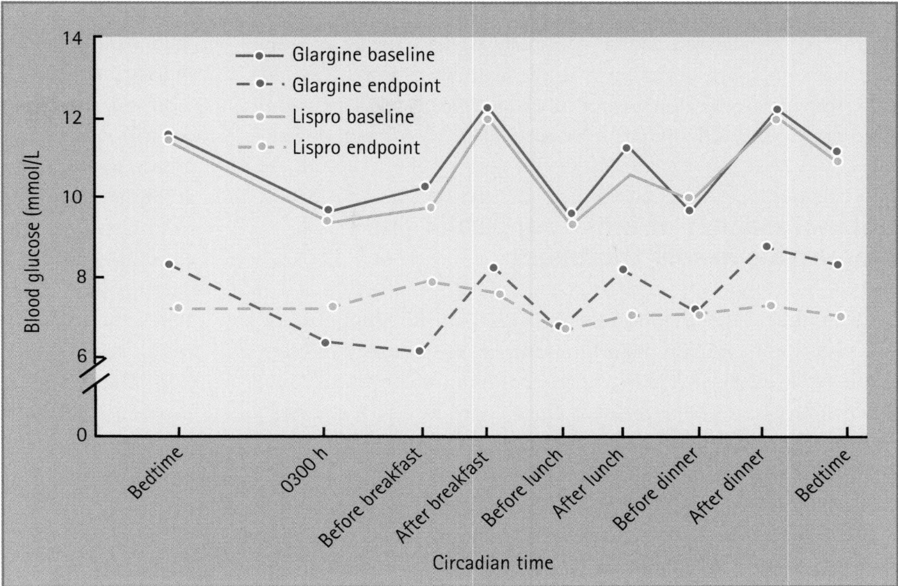

Figure 31.9 Improved metabolic control with patient titration of insulin. Metabolic control (FPG and HbA_{1c}) improved in all insulin-treated patients in the treat to target study. Based upon a forced titration strategy of increases between 2 and 8 units each week based upon average fasting plasma glucose (FPG; an average of 2 days) after starting with 10 units, the course of FPG (solid line) and HbA_{1c} (dotted line) are depicted on the left and right of the above figure. By week 18, FPG decreased from 206 mg/dL to 116 mg/dL ($P = 0.0001$) and HbA_{1c} decreased from 8.6% to 6.9%. To convert to mmol/L divide FPG values by 18. DCCT result (%) = (0.0915 × IFCC result in mmol/mol) + 2.15.

Insulin glargine at bedtime

A study using insulin glargine [97] suggested this agent offers another option for starting insulin with an evening injection. In this 1-year European study, 426 subjects were randomly assigned to either insulin glargine or NPH insulin at bedtime, while continuing previous oral therapy. The therapeutic target was a fasting blood glucose <120 mg/dL (6.7 mmol/L), using a method that was probably not plasma-referenced. The insulin dosages used (23 units for glargine and 21 for NPH) and HbA_{1c} values achieved (8.3% and 8.2%, 67 mmol/mol and 66 mmol/mol) were similar with the two insulins, but the rates of hypoglycemia were significantly less for the group using glargine (33% vs 51% for all symptomatic hypoglycemia), despite similar average insulin doses. Nocturnal hypoglycemia occurred in less than half as many subjects using glargine (13% vs 28%). Moreover, glucose control was better in the afternoon and evening with glargine, presumably because of its longer duration of action than NPH.

The Treat to Target Trial (Figure 31.9) [91], also compared insulin glargine with NPH insulin at bedtime. Subjects in this study averaged a baseline HbA_{1c} of 8.6% (70 mmol/mol). Both NPH and glargine study groups were instructed to initiate doses of 10 units of insulin at bedtime and each week the dose was raised between 0 and 8 units based upon how close the subjects were to the glycemic goal (<5.5 mmol/L; 100 mg/dL). This forced weekly titration of dose based upon fasting glucose concentration with patient self-adjustment according to the pattern of therapy response was a key concept in reaching the targeted goal of HbA_{1c} <7% (<53 mmol/mol) in about 60% of patients in this study on both NPH and glargine insulin. Subjects in this study did not need to achieve the targeted FPG because hypoglycemia would have been too frequent. Hypoglycemia overnight was more common with NPH insulin as might be expected based upon the differences in kinetics of NPH versus glargine with the former having a greater peak effect usually within the first 4–8 hours after subcutaneous administration.

Insulin detemir

Insulin detemir is a newer formulation of intermediate- to long-acting insulin with a duration of effect in type 1 diabetes single-dose studies that is dose-dependent. Based upon a common dosage of 0.4 units/kg, an average duration of action of about 20 hours is predicted. With higher doses a longer duration approaching 24 hours is achieved [98]. In one study [99], twice daily insulin therapy with NPH versus detemir was compared in subjects with T2DM inadequately controlled (HbA_{1c} 8.5% [69 mmol/mol] and 8.6% [70 mmol/mol] for NPH and detemir, respectively) on therapy (mostly metformin plus secretagogues with some use of α-glucosidase inhibitors and about 30% of subjects not on oral agents when insulin was used). A total of 475 subjects were randomized to participate in a 24-week study comparing twice daily administration of these two insulins at breakfast and bedtime. Starting with 10 units per injection subjects were instructed to titrate doses every 3 days based upon pre-dinner and pre-breakfast self-monitored glucose averages from 2 up to 10 units per injection. At 24 weeks, subjects with insulin detemir decreased HbA_{1c} by 1.8% (20 mmol/mol) to an average value of 6.8% (51 mmol/mol), while subjects on NPH decreased the HbA_{1c} by 1.9% (21 mmol/mol) to an average value of 6.6% (49 mmol/mol). Most subjects (about 70%) achieved HbA_{1c} less than 7% (<53 mmol/mol) but more subjects on detemir achieved the goal without hypoglycemia. Overall hypoglycemia was significantly less on detemir, which by non-inferiority analysis was comparable in overall glycemic lowering efficacy to NPH. Doses of insulin were a bit higher than might have been expected (36.1 units in the morning and 29.5 units in the afternoon for detemir; and 25.3 units in the morning and 19.7 units in the afternoon for

NPH) given that the average BMI of these patients was a little over 29 kg/m^2. Detemir can be administered once in the evening or twice daily. Its desirable features include a lower rate of hypoglycemia, somewhat greater consistency in glycemic response from day to day, and possibly a reduced tendency for weight gain.

Optimal manner of initiating insulin and progressive insulin treatment

Recent studies have tried to readdress the issue of whether there is a best way to initiate insulin treatment. The strategy of basal insulin only vs the alternative of basal and prandial insulin combined continues to be addressed. The 4-T Study, which is a multicenter multiyear trial of insulin therapy carried out in an open-label manner is one such study [100]. In this study, 708 patients with HbA_{1c} of 7–10% (53–86 mmol/mol) while on maximally tolerated doses of metformin and sulfonylureas were randomized to receive biphasic insulin aspart (70/30) twice daily at breakfast and supper, prandial insulin aspart three times daily, or basal insulin detemir once daily or twice if required. The outcomes of this study included mean glycated hemoglobin level, the proportion of patients with a glycated hemoglobin level of 6.5% or less (<48 mmol/mol), the rate of hypoglycemia, and weight gain. At 1 year, mean HbA_{1c} levels were similar in the biphasic group (7.3%, 56 mmol/mol) and the prandial group (7.2% [55 mmol/mol]; $P = 0.08$) but higher in the basal group (7.6% [60 mmol/mol]; $P < 0.001$) for both comparisons. The proportions of patients with HbA_{1c} level of 6.5% or less were 17.0%, 23.9% and 8.1% in mixed insulin, prandial insulin and basal insulin, respectively. The average of hypoglycemic events per patient-year was 5.7, 12.0 and 2.3, respectively. The mean weight gains were 4.7, 5.7 and 1.9 kg, respectively. Rates of adverse events were similar among the three groups. After 3-years of treatment, the median HbA_{1c} ranged from 6.8–7.1% (51–54 mmol/mol) and did not differ between groups [101]; however, there were important differences between the regimens. Fewer participants receiving biphasic insulin reached a target of either of 6.5% (48 mmol/mol) or 7.0% (53 mmol/mol) than the other groups. Hypoglycemia rates were lowest in those who began with basal insulin while weight gain was highest in those who began with prandial insulin. The authors concluded that this study provides evidence to support the addition of basal insulin to oral therapy with subsequent intensification to a basal-bolus regimen as the preferred method of insulin initiation in people with type 2 diabetes. A subsequent editorial, however, felt that while it was clear that insulin initiation with basal insulin is preferred to prandial insulin, biphasic insulin may still provide an effective means of obtaining glycemia control for patients and clinicians wanting a less intensive insulin regimen [102].

In general, the authors' practice is to begin patients on either a weight-based dose (e.g. 0.2 unit/kg) or an arbitrary starting dose and titrate basal insulin weekly or every 3 days if quite stable with the dose, increase by 2–4 units if on low doses or by 10–20% of basal dose if higher insulin doses are needed or if the patient is poorly controlled. Patient self-titration is clearly more effective than waiting until the next physician visit and involves the patient in their own care.

When patients no longer can continue adequate glycemic control despite fasting glycemia in a desirable range or if erratic fasting control exists, the authors often add meal insulin at dinner or at the largest meal of the day based on weight (0.1 units/kg) or an arbitrary low dose and titrate upward by assessing 2-hour post-prandial glucose levels [93]. The overuse of basal insulin alone can lead to serious hypoglycemia overnight. When there is a history of overnight or early morning hypoglycemia, testing of post-prandial control is very important. Commonly, one needs to make at least a unit for unit trade-off between meal insulin and basal insulin; as the former increases, an equal decrease in basal insulin helps to minimize nocturnal hypoglycemia.

References

1 International Diabetes Federation. *Diabetes Facts and Figures*. Available from: http://www.diabetesatlas.org/content/diabetes-and-impaired-glucose-tolerance. Accessed on 18 December, 2009.

2 http://www.cdc.gov/diabetes/pubs/pdf/ndfs_2007.pdf

3 Centers for Disease Control and Prevention (CDC). State-specific incidence of diabetes among adults: participating states, 1995–1997 and 2005–2007. *MMWR Morb Mortal Wkly Rep* 2008; **57**: 1169–1173.

4 UKPDS Study Group. Overview of 6 years' therapy of type II diabetes: a progressive disease (UKPDS 16). *Diabetes* 1995; **44**:1249–1258.

5 Turner RC, Cull CA, Frighi V, Holman RR. Glycemic control with diet, sulfonylurea, metformin, or insulin in patients with type 2 diabetes mellitus: progressive requirement for multiple therapies (UKPDS 49). *JAMA* 1999; **281**:2005–2012.

6 Nathan DM, Buse JB, Davidson MB, Ferrannini E, Holman RR, Sherwin R, *et al*. Medical management of hyperglycemia in type 2 diabetes: a consensus algorithm for the initiation and adjustment of therapy. A consensus statement of the American Diabetes Association and the European Association for the Study of Diabetes. *Diabetes Care* 2009; **32**:193–203.

7 Diabetes Control and Complications Trial Research Group. The effect of intensive treatment of diabetes on the development and progression of long-term complications in insulin-dependent diabetes mellitus. *N Engl J Med* 1993; **329**:977–986.

8 UK Prospective Diabetes Study Group (UKPDS). Intensive blood-glucose control with sulphonylureas or insulin compared with conventional treatment and risk of complications in patients with type 2 diabetes. *Lancet* 1998; **352**:837–853.

9 UK Prospective Diabetes Study Group (UKPDS). Effect of intensive blood-glucose control with metformin on complications in overweight patients with type 2 diabetes (UKPDS 34). *Lancet* 1998; **352**:854–865.

10 Nathan DM, Cleary PA, Backlund JY, Genuth SM, Lachin JM, Orchard TJ, *et al*; Diabetes Control and Complications Trial/Epidemiology of Diabetes Interventions and Complications (DCCT/EDIC) Study Research Group. Intensive diabetes treatment and cardiovascular disease in patients with type 1 diabetes. *N Engl J Med* 2005; **353**:2643–2653.

11 Holman RR, Paul SK, Bethel MA, Matthews DR, Neil HA. 10-year follow-up of intensive glucose control in type 2 diabetes. *N Engl J Med* 2008; **359**:1577–1589.

12 Action to Control Cardiovascular Risk in Diabetes Study Group. Effects of intensive glucose lowering in type 2 diabetes. *N Engl J Med* 2008; **358**:2545–2559.

13 Rodbard HW, Jellinger PS, Davidson JA, Einhorn D, Garber AJ, Grundberger G, *et al.* Statement by an American Association of Clinical Endocrinologists/American College of Endocrinology consensus panel on type 2 diabetes mellitus: an algorithm for glycemic control. *Endocr Pract* 2009; **15**(6):540–559.

14 Whittemore R, Melkus G, Wagner J, Dziura J, Northup V, Grey M. Translating the Diabetes Prevention Program to primary care: a pilot study. *Nurs Res* 2009; **58**:2–12.

15 Saunders JT, Pastors JG. Practical tips on lifestyle management of type 2 diabetes for the busy clinician. *Curr Diab Rep* 2008; **8**:353–360.

16 Yates T, Khunti K, Troughton J, Davies M. The role of physical activity in the management of type 2 diabetes mellitus. *Postgrad Med J* 2009; **85**:129–133.

17 Choussein S, Makri AA, Frangos CC, Petridou ET, Daskalopoulou SS. Effect of antiobesity medications in patients with type 2 diabetes mellitus. *Diabetes Obes Metab* 2009; **11**:641–664.

18 Torgerson JS, Hauptman J, Boldrin MN, Sjostrom L. XENical in the Prevention of Diabetes in Obese Subjects (XENDOS) Study: a randomized study of orlistat as an adjunct to lifestyle changes for the prevention of type 2 diabetes in obese patients. *Diabetes Care* 2004; **27**:155–161.

19 Miles JM, Leiter L, Hollander P, Wadden T, Anderson JW, Doyle M, *et al.* Effect of orlistat in overweight and obese patients with type 2 diabetes treated with metformin. *Diabetes Care* 2002; **25**:1123–1128.

20 Kelley DE, Bray GA, Pi-Sunyer FX, Klein S, Hill J, Miles J, *et al.* Clinical efficacy of orlistat therapy in overweight and obese patients with insulin-treated type 2 diabetes: a 1-year randomized controlled trial. *Diabetes Care* 2002; **25**:1033–1041.

21 Vettor R, Serra R, Fabris R, Pagano C, Federspil G. Effect of sibutramine on weight management and metabolic control in type 2 diabetes: a meta-analysis of clinical studies. *Diabetes Care* 2005; **28**:942–949.

22 Pories WJ. Bariatric surgery: risks and rewards. *J Clin Endocrinol Metab* 2008; **93**(Suppl 1):89–96.

23 Vetter ML, Cardillo S, Rickels MR, Iqbal N. Narrative review: effect of bariatric surgery on type 2 diabetes mellitus. *Ann Intern Med* 2009; **150**:94–103.

24 Kahn SE, Haffner SM, Heise MA, Herman WH, Holman RB, Jones NP, *et al*; ADOPT Study Group. Glycemic durability of rosiglitazone, metformin, or glyburide monotherapy. *N Engl J Med* 2006; **355**:2427–2443.

25 DeFronzo RA, Goodman AM; Multicenter Metformin Study Group. Efficacy of metformin in patients with non-insulin-dependent diabetes mellitus. *N Engl J Med* 1995; **333**:541–549.

26 Horton ES, Whitehouse F, Ghazzi MN, Venable TC, Whitcombe RW; Troglitazone Study Group. Troglitazone in combination with sulfonylurea restores glycemic control in patients with type 2 diabetes. *Diabetes Care* 1998; **21**:1462–1469.

27 Riddle MC. Combined therapy with a sulfonylurea plus evening insulin: safe, reliable, and becoming routine. *Horm Metabol Res* 1996; **28**:430–433.

28 Riddle MC, Schneider J; Glimepiride Combination Group. Beginning insulin treatment of obese patients with evening 70/30 insulin plus glimepiride versus insulin alone. *Diabetes Care* 1998; **217**:1052–1057.

29 Malmberg K; DIGAMI (Diabetes Mellitus, Insulin Glucose Infusion in Acute Myocardial Infarction) Study Group. Prospective randomised study of intensive insulin treatment on long term survival after acute myocardial infarction in patients with diabetes mellitus. *Br Med J* 1997; **314**:1512–1515.

30 Malmberg K, Ryden L, Wedel H, Birkeland K, Bootsma A, Dickstein K, *et al.* DIGAMI 2 Investigators. Intense metabolic control by means of insulin in patients with diabetes mellitus and acute myocardial infarction (DIGAMI 2): effects on mortality and morbidity. *Eur Heart J* 2005; **26**:650–661.

31 Gerich JE. Metabolic abnormalities in impaired glucose tolerance. *Metabolism* 1997; **46**(Suppl 1):40–43.

32 DECODE Study Group, the European Diabetes Epidemiology Group. Glucose tolerance and cardiovascular mortality: comparison of fasting and 2-hour diagnostic criteria. *Arch Intern Med* 2001; **161**:397–405.

33 Bonora E, Muggeo M. Postprandial blood glucose as a risk factor for cardiovascular disease in type II diabetes: the epidemiological evidence. *Diabetologia* 2001; **44**:2107–2114.

34 Carroll MF, Gutierrez A, Castro M, Tsewang D, Schade DS. Targeting postprandial hyperglycemia: a comparative study of insulinotropic agents in type 2 diabetes. *J Clin Endocrinol Metab* 2003; **88**:5248–5254.

35 Knowler WC, Barrett-Connor E, Fowler SE, Hamman RF, Lachin JM, Walker EA, *et al.* Reduction in the incidence of type 2 diabetes with lifestyle intervention or metformin. *N Engl J Med* 2002; **346**:393–403.

36 Berger J, Moller DE. The mechanisms of action of PPARs. *Annu Rev Med* 2002; **53**:409–435.

37 Barbier O, Torra IP, Duguay Y, Blanguart C, Fruchart JC, Glineur C, *et al.* Pleiotropic actions of peroxisome proliferator activated receptors in lipid metabolism and atherosclerosis. *Arterioscler Thromb Vasc Biol* 2002; **22**:712–726.

38 Wolffenbuttel BH, Gomis R, Squatrito S, Jones NP, Patwardhan RN. Addition of low dose rosiglitazone to sulphonylurea therapy improves glycaemic control in type 2 diabetic patients. *Diabet Med* 2000; **17**:40–47.

39 Kipnes MS, Krosnick A, Rendell MS, Egan JW, Mathisen AL, Schneider RL. Pioglitazone hydrochloride in combination with sulfonylurea therapy improves glycemic control in patients with type 2 diabetes mellitus: a randomized, placebo-controlled study. *Am J Med* 2001; **111**:10–17.

40 Einhorn D, Rendell M, Rosenzweig J, Egan JW, Mathisen AL, Schneider RL; Pioglitazone 027 Study Group. Pioglitazone hydrochloride in combination with metformin in the treatment of type 2 diabetes mellitus: a randomized, placebo-controlled study. *Clin Ther* 2000; **22**:1395–1409.

41 Fonseca V, Rosenstock J, Patwardhan R, Salzman A. Effect of metformin and rosiglitazone combination therapy in patients with type 2 diabetes mellitus: a randomized controlled trial. *JAMA* 2000; **2835**:1695–1702.

42 Lebovitz HE, Krieder M, Freed MI. Evaluation of liver function in type 2 diabetic patients during clinical trials: evidence that rosiglitazone does not cause hepatic dysfunction. *Diabetes Care* 2002; **25**:815–882.

43 Belfort R, Harrison SA, Brown K, Darland C, Finch J, Hardies J, *et al.* A placebo-controlled trial of pioglitazone in subjects with nonalcoholic steatohepatitis. *N Engl J Med* 2006; **355**:2297–2307.

44 DeFronzo RA. Pharmacologic therapy for type 2 diabetes mellitus. *Ann Intern Med* 1999; **131**:281–303 [Review].

45 Yki-Jarvinen H. Combination therapies with insulin in type 2 diabetes. *Diabetes Care* 2001; **24**:758–767.

46 Nathan DM. Thiazolidinediones for initial treatment of type 2 diabetes? *N Engl J Med* 2006; **355**:2477–2480.

47 Lihn AS, Pedersen SB, Richelsen B. Adiponectin: action, regulation and association to insulin sensitivity. *Obes Rev* 2005; **6**:13–21.

48 Kang ES, Park SY, Kim HJ, Ahn CW, Nam M, Cha BS, *et al.* The influence of adiponectin gene polymorphism on the rosiglitazone response in patients with type 2 diabetes. *Diabetes Care* 2005; **28**:1139–1144.

49 Nissen SE, Wolski K. Effect of rosiglitazone on the risk of myocardial infarction and death from cardiovascular causes. *N Engl J Med* 2007; **356**:2457–2471.

50 Home PD, Pocock SJ, Beck-Nielsen H, Gomis R, Hanefield M, Jones NP, *et al.*, for the RECORD study group. Rosiglitazone evaluated for cardiovascular outcomes: an interim analysis. *N Engl J Med* 2007; **357**:28–38.

51 ADVANCE Collaborative Group. Intensive blood glucose control and vascular outcomes in patients with type 2 diabetes. *N Engl J Med* 2008; **358**:2560–2572.

52 Duckworth W, Abraira C, Moritz T, Reda D, Emanuele N, Reaven PD, *et al.* for the VADT investigators. Glucose control and vascular complications in veterans with type 2 diabetes. *N Engl J Med* 2009; **360**:129–139.

53 Dormandy JA, Charbonnel B, Eckland DJ, Erdmann E, Massi-Benedetti M, Moules IK, *et al.* Secondary prevention of macrovascular events in patients with type 2 diabetes in the PROactive Study (PROspective pioglitAzone Clinical Trial In macroVascular Events): a randomised controlled trial. *Lancet* 2005; **366**:1279–1289.

54 Nesto RW, Bell D, Bonow RO, Fonseca V, Grundy SM, Horton ES, *et al.* Thiazolidinedione use, fluid retention, and congestive heart failure: a consensus statement from the American Heart Association and American Diabetes Association. *Diabetes Care* 2004; **27**:256–263.

55 Home PD, Popcock SJ, Beck-Nielsen H, Curtis PS, Gomis R, Hanefeld M, *et al.* for the RECORD Study Team. Rosiglitazone evaluated for cardiovascular outcomes in oral agent combination therapy for type 2 diabetes (RECORD): a multicenter, randomized, open-label trial. *Lancet* 2009; **373**:2125–2135.

56 BARI 2D Study Group. A randomized trial of therapies for type 2 diabetes and coronary artery disease. *N Engl J Med* 2009; **360**:2503–2515.

57 McDonough AK, Rosenthal RS, Cao X, Saag KG. The effect of thiazolidinediones on BMD and osteoporosis. *Nat Clin Pract Endocrinol Metab* 2008; **4**:507–513.

58 Pratley RE, Gilbert M. Targeting incretins in type 2 diabetes: role of GLP-1 receptor agonists and DPP-4 inhibitors. *Rev Diabet Stud* 2008; **5**:94.

59 Buse JB, Henry RR, Han J, Kim DD, Fineman MS, Baron AD. Effects of exenatide (exendin-4) on glycemic control over 30 weeks in sulfonylurea-treated patients with type 2 diabetes. *Diabetes Care* 2004; **27**:2628–2635.

60 DeFronzo RA, Ratner RE, Han J, Kim DD, Fineman MS, Baron AD. Effects of exenatide (exendin-4) on glycemic control and weight over 30 weeks in metformin-treated patients with type 2 diabetes. *Diabetes Care* 2005; **28**:1092–1100.

61 Kendall DM, Riddle MC, Rosenstock J, Zhuang D, Kim DD, Fineman MS, *et al.* Effects of exenatide (exendin-4) on glycemic control over 30 weeks in patients with type 2 diabetes treated with metformin and a sulfonylurea. *Diabetes Care* 2005; **28**:1083–1091.

62 Zinman B, Hoogwerf BJ, Durán GS, Milton DR, Giaconia JM, Kim DD, *et al.* The effect of adding exenatide to a thiazolidinedione in suboptimally controlled type 2 diabetes: a randomized trial. *Ann Intern Med* 2007; **146**:477–485.

63 Heine RJ, Van Gaal LF, Johns D, Mihm MJ, Widel MH, Brodows RG, for the GWAA Study Group. Exenatide versus insulin glargine in patients with suboptimally controlled type 2 diabetes: a randomized trial. *Ann Intern Med* 2005; **143**:559–569.

64 Nauck M, Duran S, Kim D, Johns D, Northrup D, Festa A, *et al.* A comparison of twice-daily exenatide and biphasic insulin aspart in patients with type 2 diabetes who were suboptimally controlled with sulfonylurea and metformin: a non-inferiority study. *Diabetologia* 2007; **50**:259–267.

65 Bergenstal R, Lewin A, Bailey T, Chang D, Gylvin T, Roberts V. NovoLog Mix-vs.-Exenatide Study Group. Efficacy and safety of biphasic insulin aspart 70/30 versus exenatide in type 2 diabetes failing to achieve glycemic control with metformin and a sulfonylurea. *Curr Med Res Opin* 2009; **25**:65–75.

66 Sheffield CA, Kane MP, Busch RS, Basket G, Abelseth JM, Hamilton RA. Safety and efficacy of exenatide in combination with insulin in patients with type 2 diabetes mellitus. *Endocr Pract* 2008; **14**:285–292.

67 Garber A, Henry R, Ratner R, Garcia-Hernandez PA, Rodriguez-Pattzi H, Olvera-Alvarez I, *et al.* Liraglutide versus glimepiride monotherapy for type 2 diabetes (LEAD-3 Mono): a randomised, 52-week, phase III, double-blind, parallel-treatment trial. *Lancet* 2009; **373**:473–481.

68 Marre M, Shaw J, Brändle M, Bebakar WMW, Kamaruddin NA, Strand J, *et al.* on behalf of the LEAD-1 SU study group. Liraglutide, a once-daily human GLP-1 analogue, added to a sulphonylurea over 26 weeks produces greater improvements in glycaemic and weight control compared with adding rosiglitazone or placebo in subjects with type 2 diabetes (LEAD-1 SU). *Diabet Med* 2009; **26**:268–278.

69 Zinman B, Gerich J, Buse JB, Lewin A, Schwartz S, Raskin P, *et al.* Efficacy and safety of the human GLP-1 analog liraglutide in combination with metformin and TZD in patients with type 2 diabetes mellitus (LEAD-4 Met+TZD). *Diabetes Care* 2009; **32**:1224–1230.

70 Buse JB, Rosenstock J, Sesti G, Schmidt WE, Montanya E, Brett JH, Zychma M, Blonde L; LEAD-6 Study Group. Liraglutide once a day versus exenatide twice a day for type 2 diabetes: a 26-week randomised, parallel-group, multinational, open-label trial (LEAD-6). *Lancet*. 2009;**374**(9683):39–47. Epub 2009 Jun 8.

71 Drucker DJ, Buse JB, Taylor K, Kendall DM, Trautmann M, Zhuang D, *et al.* for the DURATION-1 Study Group. Exenatide once weekly versus twice daily for the treatment of type 2 diabetes: a randomised, open-label, non-inferiority study. *Lancet* 2008; **372**:1240–1250.

72 Ahren B, Pacini G, Foley JE, Schweizer A. Improved meal-related beta-cell function and insulin sensitivity by the dipeptidyl peptidase-IV inhibitor vildagliptin in metformin-treated patients with type 2 diabetes over 1 year. *Diabetes Care* 2005; **28**:1936–1940.

73 Bolli G, Dotta F, Rochotte E, Cohen SE. Efficacy and tolerability of vildagliptin vs. pioglitazone when added to metformin: a 24-week,

randomized, double-blind study. *Diabetes Obes Metab* 2008; **10**:82–90.

74 Fonseca V, Baron M, Shao Q, Dejager S. Sustained efficacy and reduced hypoglycemia during one year of treatment with vildagliptin added to insulin in patients with type 2 diabetes mellitus. *Horm Metab Res* 2008; **40**:427–430.

75 Ahren B, Schweizer A, Dejager S, Dunner BE, Nilsson PM, Persson M, *et al.* Vildagliptin enhances islet responsiveness to both hyper- and hypoglycemia in patients with type 2 diabetes. *J Clin Endocrinol Metab* 2009; **94**:1236–1243.

76 Raz I, Hanefeld M, Xu L, Caria C, Williams-Herman D, Khatami H; Sitagliptin Study 023 Group. Efficacy and safety of the dipeptidyl peptidase-4 inhibitor sitagliptin as monotherapy in patients with type 2 diabetes mellitus. *Diabetologia* 2006; **49**:2564–2571.

77 Aschner P, Kipnes MS, Lunceford JK, Sanchez M, Mickel C, Williams-Herman DE. Effect of the dipeptidyl peptidase-4 inhibitor sitagliptin as monotherapy on glycemic control in patients with type 2 diabetes. *Diabetes Care* 2006; **29**:2632–2637.

78 Charbonnel B, Karasik A, Liu J, Wu M, Meininger G. Efficacy and safety of the dipeptidyl peptidase-4 inhibitor sitagliptin added to ongoing metformin therapy in patients with type 2 diabetes inadequately controlled with metformin alone. *Diabetes Care* 2006; **29**:2638–2643.

79 Rosenstock J, Brazg R, Andryuk PJ, Lu K, Stein P. Efficacy and safety of the dipeptidyl peptidase-4 inhibitor sitagliptin added to ongoing pioglitazone therapy in patients with type 2 diabetes: a 24-week, multicenter, randomized, double-blind, placebo-controlled, parallel-group study. *Clin Ther* 2006; **28**:1556–1568.

80 Monnier L, Mas E, Ginet C, Michel F, Villon L, Cristol JP, *et al.* Activation of oxidative stress by acute glucose fluctuations compared with sustained chronic hyperglycemia in patients with type 2 diabetes. *JAMA* 2006; **295**:1681–1687.

81 Monnier L, Lapinski H, Colette C. Contributions of fasting and postprandial plasma glucose increments to the overall diurnal hyperglycemia of type 2 diabetic patients: variations with increasing levels of HbA(1c). *Diabetes Care* 2003; **26**:881–885.

82 Zieve FJ, Kalin MF, Schwartz, SL, Jones MR, Bailey, WL. Results of the glucose-lowering effect of WelChol study (GLOWS): a randomized, double-blind, placebo-controlled pilot study evaluatinig the effect of colesevelam hydrochloride on glycemic control in subjects with type 2 diabetes. *Clin Ther* 2007; **29**:74–83.

83 Bays HE, Goldberg RB, Truitt KE, Jones MR. Colesevelam hydrochloride therapy in patients with type 2 diabetes mellitus treated with metformin: glucose and lipoid effects. *Arch Intern Med* 2008; **168**:1975–1983.

84 Goldberg RB, Fonseca VA, Truitt KE, Jones MR. Efficacy and safety of colesevelam in patients with type 2 diabetes mellitus and inadequate glycemic control receiving insulin-based therapy. *Nat Clin Pract Endocrinol Metab* 2009; **5**:16–17.

85 Fonseca VA, Rosenstock J, Wang AC, Truitt KE, Jones MR. Colesevelam HCl improves glycemic control and reduces LDL cholesterol in patients with inadequately controlled type 2 diabetes on sulfonylurea-based therapy. *Diabetes Care* 2008; **31**:1479–1484.

86 Hirsch IB, Bergenstal RM, Parkin CG, *et al.* A real-world approach to insulin therapy in primary care practice. *Clin Diabetes* 2005; **23**:78–86.

87 Riddle M, Hart J, Bingham P, Garrison C, McDaniel P. Combined therapy for obese type 2 diabetes: suppertime mixed insulin with daytime sulfonylurea. *Am J Med Sci* 1992; **303**:151–156.

88 Shank ML, Del Prato S, DeFronzo RA. Bedtime insulin/daytime glipizide: effective therapy for sulfonylurea failures in NIDDM. *Diabetes* 1995; **44**:165–172.

89 Yki-Jarvinen H, Ryysy L, Nikkila K, Tulokas T, Vanamo R, Heikkila M. Comparison of bedtime insulin regimens in patients with type 2 diabetes mellitus: a randomized, controlled trial. *Ann Intern Med* 1999; **130**:389–396.

90 Riddle MC, Schneider J; Glimepiride Combination Group. Beginning insulin treatment of obese patients with evening 70/30 insulin plus glimepiride versus insulin alone. *Diabetes Care* 1998; **217**:1052–1057.

91 Riddle MC, Rosenstock J, Gerich J. The treat-to-target trial: randomized addition of glargine or human NPH insulin to oral therapy of type 2 diabetic patients. *Diabetes Care* 2003; **26**:3080–3086.

92 Meneghini LF, Rosenberg KH, Koenen C, Merilainen MJ, Lüddeke HJ. Insulin detemir improves glycaemic control with less hypoglycaemia and no weight gain in patients with type 2 diabetes who were insulin naive or treated with NPH or insulin glargine. *Diabetes Obes Metab* 2007; **9**:418–427.

93 Bretzel RG, Nuber U, Landgraf W, Owens DR, Bradley C, Linn T. Once-daily basal insulin glargine versus thrice-daily prandial insulin lispro in people with type 2 diabetes on oral hypoglycemic agents (APOLLO): an open randomized controlled trial. *Lancet* 2008; **371**:1073–1084.

94 Karl DM. The use of bolus insulin and advancing insulin therapy in type 2 diabetes. *Curr Diabetes Rep* 2004; **4**:352–357.

95 Mooradian AD, Bernbaum M, Albert SG. Narrative review: a rational approach to starting insulin therapy. *Ann Intern Med* 2006; **145**:125–134.

96 Garber AJ, Wahlen J, Wahl T, Bressler P, Braceras R, Allen E, *et al.* Attainment of glycaemic goals in type 2 diabetes with once-, twice-, or thrice-daily dosing with biphasic insulin aspart 70/30 (The 1-2-3 study). *Diabetes Obes Metab* 2006; **8**:58–66.

97 Yki-Jarvinen H, Dressler A, Ziemen M; HOE 901/300s Study Group. Less nocturnal hypoglycemia and better post-dinner glucose control with bedtime insulin glargine compared with bedtime NPH insulin during insulin combination therapy in type 2 diabetes. *Diabetes Care* 2000; **23**:1130–1136.

98 Plank J, Bodenlenz M, Sinner F, Magnes C, Gorzer E, Regittnig W, *et al.* A double-blind, randomized, dose–response study investigating the pharmacodynamic and pharmacokinetic properties of the long-acting insulin analog detemir. *Diabetes Care* 2005; **28**:1107–1112.

99 Hermansen K, Davies M, Derezinski T, Martinez Ravn G, Clausen P, Home P; on behalf of the Levemir Treat-to-Target Study Group. A 26-week, randomized, parallel, treat-to-target trial comparing insulin detemir with NPH insulin as add-on therapy to oral glucose-lowering drugs in insulin-naive people with type 2 diabetes. *Diabetes Care* 2006; **29**:1269–1274.

100 Holman RR, Thorne KI, Farmer AJ, Davies MJ, Keenan JF, Paul S; for the 4-T Study Group. Addition of biphasic, prandial, or basal insulin to oral therapy in type 2 diabetes. *N Engl J Med* 2007; **357**:1716–1730.

101 Holman RR, Farmer AJ, Davies MJ, Levy JC, Darbyshire JL, Keenan JF, Paul SK; 4-T Study Group. Three-year efficacy of complex insulin regimens in type 2 diabetes. *N Engl J Med* 2009; **361**(18): 1736–1747.

102 Holt RIG. Insulin initiation in type 2 diabetes: the implications of the 4-T study. *Diabetic Medicine* 2010; **27**(1):1–3.

32 In-Hospital Treatment and Surgery in Patients with Diabetes

Maggie Sinclair Hammersley[1] & June James[2]

[1] Nuffield Department of Medicine, University of Oxford, Oxford, UK
[2] University Hospitals of Leicester, Leicester, UK

Keypoints

- The diabetes epidemic is not sparing hospital practice. Approximately 12–24% of all hospital inpatients have diabetes.
- A significant proportion of hospital inpatients with hyperglycemia have undiagnosed diabetes and stress hyperglycemia.
- Hospitalization frequently presents a missed opportunity to diagnose diabetes and to identify those at risk for diabetes.
- In-hospital hyperglycemia and hypoglycemia are associated with poor outcomes in a broad range of specialties.
- There are few randomized controlled trials demonstrating benefit from interventions in the inpatient care setting.
- Hospital inpatients with diabetes frequently have multiple co-morbidities and complex medical and nursing requirements.
- Ward-based staff are frequently poorly trained and therefore ill-equipped to manage diabetes care safely and effectively.
- Care of the critically ill patient with diabetes and hyperglycemia requires highly skilled and appropriately trained staff.
- Insulin and diabetes management errors continue to compromise patient safety.
- Structured diabetes care delivered by appropriately trained staff and supported by a dedicated specialist inpatient team in partnership with the patient improves the patient experience, reduces diabetes prescribing and management errors and length of stay in many clinical settings in hospital.
- Patients with diabetes are more likely to undergo in-hospital procedures and should be individually managed by agreed and audited protocols.
- Patients undergoing surgery should have a preoperative assessment, a robust risk assessment and an individualized care plan including a safe and effective discharge plan.
- Standards of care for hospital inpatients have been defined by professional organizations but are not globally implemented.
- Audit of inpatient care reveals poor standards of care and patient experience and demonstrates the inadequacy of present systems and processes.

Introduction

Known diabetes in hospital

The global burden of diagnosed diabetes has reached epidemic proportions. The International Diabetes Federation predicts that by the year 2030 prevalence rates of type 2 diabetes will have increased by approximately 20% in Europe and by 65–98% in less economically developed countries [1]. Disproportionate numbers of people admitted to hospital have diabetes. The prevalence of diabetes in the inpatient population is almost certainly underestimated because of poor coding of diabetes as a co-morbidity. This applies equally to both planned and emergency care. Conservative estimates of diagnosed diabetes are between 12% and 24% of all inpatients in the USA [2]. Every year people with diabetes spend approximately 1.34 million days in hospital and it is estimated that in the UK there are 80 000 excess bed days per year. The cost of caring for inpatients with diabetes is around £485 million per year [3].

Undiagnosed diabetes and stress hyperglycemia in hospital

The number of hospital inpatients with diabetes has increased and is rising inexorably. This only represents the tip of the iceberg, however, as it takes no account of those patients with a raised plasma glucose level without a diagnosis of diabetes. In addition to those with diagnosed diabetes, there are two other groups of patients with hyperglycemia in hospital. First, there are those with unrecognized diabetes occurring during hospitalization and subsequently confirmed after discharge and, secondly, those with so-called "hospital-related" hyperglycemia (fasting plasma glucose >126 mg/dL (7 mmol/L) or random >198 mg/dL (11 mmol/L), occurring during hospitalization, which reverts to normal after discharge (also known as "stress hyperglycemia"). Recent studies suggest that these two groups may add a further 30% to the total numbers with raised plasma glucose levels [4].

Textbook of Diabetes, 4th edition. Edited by R. Holt, C. Cockram, A. Flyvbjerg and B. Goldstein.

So when the burden of "in-hospital hyperglycemia" is considered to include all three groups, then the prevalence is approximately 40% of all hospital inpatients.

Evidence of harm from in-hospital hyperglycemia and benefit of glucose lowering

There is compelling evidence that poorly controlled blood glucose levels are associated with a higher in-hospital morbidity and mortality, prolonged length of stay, unfavorable post-discharge outcomes and significant excess health care costs [5–9]. Umpierrez *et al.* [4] showed that patients with new hyperglycemia had an 18-fold increased in-hospital mortality and patients with known diabetes had a 2.7-fold increased in-hospital mortality when compared with normoglycemic patients [4]. In 2004, a joint position statement from the American College of Endocrinology (ACE) and the American Association of Clinical Endocrinologists (AACE) on inpatient diabetes and metabolic control concluded that hyperglycemia in hospitalized patients is a common, serious and costly health care problem [10]. There was a strong recommendation for early detection of hyperglycemia and an aggressive management approach to improve outcomes.

Randomized trials have demonstrated improved outcomes resulting from more aggressive management of hyperglycemia in the following areas.

Acute coronary syndromes

It is not clear whether high glucose is a marker or mediator of poor outcomes in acute coronary syndromes (ACS). In the management of myocardial infarction a meta-analysis of 15 studies showed that blood glucose (BG) >120 mg/dL (6.1 mmol/L), with or without a prior diagnosis of diabetes, was associated with an increased in-hospital mortality and subsequent heart failure [11]. Current evidence supports the use of intravenous insulin in the first 24 hours and intensified subcutaneous insulin for 3 months in the setting of ST-segment elevation myocardial infarction (STEMI) where the DIGAMI 1 study showed a 29% reduction in mortality at 1 year [12]. Other randomized controlled trials such as DIGAMI-2 and CREATE-ECLAT have failed to reproduce these findings [13,14].

Observational data from the UK Myocardial Infarction National Audit Programme (MINAP) of patients with troponin-positive ACS demonstrated poorer outcomes in those with an elevated BG on admission, with 30-day mortality of 20.2% in those with BG >170 mg/dL (9.4 mmol/L) compared with 3.3% in those with BG <170 mg/dL (9.4 mmol/L). Of 38 864 patients recorded on the MINAP database, around 10% (of those with no prior diagnosis of diabetes) had an admission BG >250 mg/dL (14 mmol/L). Patients who did not receive treatment with intravenous insulin had a relative increased risk of death of 56% at 7 days and 51% at 30 days [15].

Cardiac surgery

Most of the outcome data for patients undergoing cardiac surgery relates to the Portland Diabetic Project, which was a non-randomized observational study of 5510 patients undergoing cardiac surgery during 1987–2005. This has shown that patients with hyperglycemia managed with an intravenous infusion titrated to normoglycemia for 3 days postoperatively had improved mortality, reduction in deep sternal wound infections and reduction in length of stay [16].

Critical care setting

The landmark study by Van den Berge *et al.* [17] showed that postoperative intensive insulin therapy (IIT) reduced mortality and morbidity in patients in the surgical intensive treatment unit (ITU). In a later study by the same group in medical ITU patients, IIT reduced morbidity but not mortality [18]. Randomized trials of IIT have shown inconsistent effects on mortality and increased rates of severe hypoglycemia. A recent meta-analysis of 26 trials involving 13 567 patients including the recent NICE-SUGAR trial, the pooled relative risk of death with IIT compared with conventional therapy was 0.93 (95% CI 0.83–1.04). Fourteen trials reported hypoglycemic events and showed a significant increase in severe hypoglycemia with a relative rate (RR) of 6.0 (95% CI 4.5–8.0). The different targets of IIT did not influence either mortality or risk of hypoglycemia [19].

Pathophysiology of hyperglycemia in acute illness

A key goal of inpatient diabetes management is minimizing the metabolic decompensation from the stress of illness and surgery. Stress-induced hyperglycemia is caused by the combined effects of integrated endogenous hormonal, cytokines and counter-regulatory nervous system signals on glucose metabolic pathways [20]. Inflammatory and counter-regulatory responses to critical illness alter the effect of insulin on hepatic glucose production and skeletal muscle. Stress leads to the increased secretion of counter-regulatory hormones (glucagon, epinephrine, norepinephrine, cortisol and growth hormone), which stimulates hepatic glycogenolysis and gluconeogenesis. Peripheral uptake of glucose is inhibited. A major consequence of severe hyperglycemia is osmotic diuresis accompanied by dehydration and electrolyte disturbances (sodium, potassium, magnesium and phosphate). This increased osmotic state is procoagulant.

The stress hormones also accelerate fat and protein breakdown leading to a generalized catabolic state. In the surgical setting, starvation preoperatively and postoperatively can be a large contributor to this process. In people without diabetes, a compensatory increase in insulin secretion helps to mediate against these catabolic effects. Patients with an absolute insulin deficiency are prone to unopposed lipolysis and ketone body formation that can ultimately result in diabetic ketoacidosis.

Stress increases the release of inflammatory mediators, leading to insulin resistance and hyperglycemia [21]. Inflammatory cytokines interleukin-1, interleukin-6 and tumor necrosis factor α (TNF-α) may directly or indirectly enhance both hepatic gluconeogenesis and glycogenolysis. TNF-α alters the signaling properties of insulin receptor substrate, leading to enhanced target organ insulin resistance.

Wound healing and the susceptibility to infection are also affected by hyperglycemia and insulin deficiency, as demonstrated by *in vitro* studies looking at white blood cell functioning [22]. Hyperglycemia-induced abnormalities in the phagocytic and bactericidal actions of neutrophils are reversed with improved glucose control.

There are other causes of hyperglycemia, which may be more specifically related to the hospital admission [23]. These include co-administered medications such as corticosteroids and immunosuppressants (e.g. cyclosporine, tacrolimus). Immobility secondary to surgery, trauma or acute illness can accelerate both hyperglycemic and procoagulant states.

Effects of glucose lowering and intravenous insulin therapy

The mechanisms behind the improved outcomes from intravenous insulin are numerous. The vasodilatory, anti-inflammatory and anti-atherogenic effects of insulin have been studied. *In vitro*, insulin induces a dose-dependent increase in nitrous oxide synthase production in the endothelium. Ultimately, insulin treatment may improve endothelial function in patients with diabetes [24].

Current recommended standards of care for hospital inpatients with diabetes

Several professional organizations from different countries have published suggested standards of care for hospital inpatients. The International Diabetes Federation (IDF) is an umbrella organization of over 200 national diabetes associations in over 160 countries which has also published a standards document about inpatient care in type 2 diabetes. The content of the major publications are reviewed below. There are a number of recurring themes which include equitable access to specialist services, empowerment of patients, delivery of care by agreed guidelines, setting of glycemic targets and embedding effective and audited hyperglycemic management protocols.

International Diabetes Federation 2005

Within the guideline produced by the IDF on the care of patients with type 2 diabetes, a number of recommendations were made concerning inpatient care [25]. The standard recommendation of the IDF group fell broadly into four categories:

1 *Inpatient care organization.* This should be undertaken by a trained diabetes care health care professional with focus on individual plans including discharge and follow-up, access to the multidisciplinary team and appropriate laboratory and investigative procedures, increasing staff awareness of the needs of people with diabetes and implementing strategies to prevent patient disempowerment by promotion of self-management of diabetes.

2 *General ward care.* Patients should be empowered to self-manage where appropriate with regard to glucose monitoring, food choices and insulin administration.

3 *Care of patients undergoing inpatient procedures.* There should be provision for assessment of glycemic control and of metabolic and vascular risk for those undergoing planned procedures and agreed protocols should be in place. Staff should be made aware of the special risks associated with diabetes such as development of new ulceration, cardiac risk and renal failure.

4 *Care of the critically ill.* Patients should be managed according to a strict glycemic protocol with glucose levels kept <110 mg/dL (6.1 mmol/L) and an active avoidance of hypoglycemia.

American Diabetes Association and American Association of Clinical Endocrinologists 2006

The American Diabetes Association (ADA) *Technical Review on the Management of Diabetes and Hyperglycemia in Hospital* was published as an in-depth review of the literature on this topic and outlined practical management strategies [26]. The implementation of these policies and recommendations had remained an elusive goal in everyday clinical practice. Therefore, in 2006, the ADA and the American Association of Clinical Endocrinologists (AACE) produced a further consensus statement entitled *Inpatient Diabetes and Glycemic Control: A call to action* in an attempt to identify and overcome barriers to change in practice to facilitate improvement in inpatient diabetes care [27]. This was updated in 2009 with new glycemic targets based on recent publications that have demonstrated concern about the harmful effect of in-hospital hypoglycemia in some clinical settings [28].

Canadian Diabetes Association

The Canadian guidelines include separate sections on peri-operative and peri-acute coronary syndrome glycemic control, recommending glucose levels of 6.1 mmol/L in post surgical ITU patients and 128–180 mg/dL (7.1–10 mmol/L) in peri-myocardial infarction patients [29].

UK Diabetes Services

National Service Framework for Diabetes 2004

The Diabetes National Service Framework set out the first set of national standards for the treatment of diabetes [30]. Two standards were set for hospital care.

1 *Standard 7.* The NHS will develop, implement and monitor agreed protocols for rapid and effective treatment of diabetic emergencies by appropriately trained health care professionals. Protocols will include the management of acute complications and procedures to minimize the risk of recurrence.

2 *Standard 8.* All children, young people and adults with diabetes admitted to hospital, for whatever reason, will receive effective care of their diabetes. Wherever possible, they will continue to be involved in decisions concerning the management of their diabetes.

National Diabetes Support Group (NHS Diabetes) 2008

In 2008, the National Diabetes Support Group produced a document focusing on improvement of diabetes inpatient services and the commissioning of these services [31]. NHS Diabetes has now updated the commissioning toolkit to include the commissioning of emergency and inpatient care [31].

Diabetes UK 2009

Diabetes UK has produced a document for patients entitled "What care to expect in hospital", available from Diabetes UK [32]. It is hoped that this empowerment of patients will help to drive up in-hospital standards of care. Diabetes UK in partnership with NHS Diabetes and a number of other professional bodies through the "Putting Feet First' campaign have recently promoted the dissemination of a national guideline for the management of patients with acute diabetic foot problems in hospital.

National Health Institute of Innovation and Implementation 2009

The National Health Institute of Innovation and Implementation recently launched a package of recommendations to improve standards of care in hospital inpatients. This was branded the "Think Glucose" campaign and has been cascaded to all UK hospitals. Each acute hospital in the UK has been provided with a set of recommendations and a toolkit to drive improvement in standards [33].

Aims of diabetes inpatient care

Diabetes care in hospital inpatients poses a real challenge as most patients are admitted to a hospital bed with a condition unrelated to their diabetes, be that electively or as an emergency. Non-diabetes specialists are often in charge of their care, and they may often have little understanding of diabetes management and its importance on patient outcomes. As a result, there can be an increased risk of harm from issues such as lack of insulin dose adjustment or prescribing errors.

Achieving a good outcome

Patients should come to no harm because of their diabetes management. Hypoglycemia and excessive hyperglycemia are both are associated with poorer clinical outcomes and should be managed according to local protocols. Clinical guidelines supported by the use of integrated care pathways should be in place to drive up standards of care. Management by a specialist team with agreed protocols against agreed standards improves care for those admitted to hospital [34].

Supporting a rapid recovery

Patients with diabetes are twice as likely to be admitted to hospital and stay twice as long in a hospital bed [35]. Minimizing excess length of stay should be one of the principal aims of good inpatient care. Prolonged length of stay occurs for a multiplicity of reasons but is often because of diabetes mismanagement secondary to poor staff knowledge and lack of education. There is evidence that involvement of the specialist diabetes team, and in particular diabetes inpatient specialist nurses (DISNs), significantly reduces length of stay and insulin errors and improves the patient experience [36–38]. This requires a culture that invests in excellent communication between the person with diabetes, diabetes specialists and non-specialist teams to activate timely intervention by avoiding glycemic deterioration during hospital stay.

Facilitating a good patient experience and patients expressed concerns about inpatient care

Patients are accustomed to managing their own diabetes. Traditionally, patients are disempowered in the management of their diabetes as soon as they are admitted to a hospital bed. For those people with diabetes accustomed to self-management by insulin adjustment this is a negative experience [35]. The ADA [28] and Diabetes UK [32], while acknowledging the importance of diabetes self-management, highlighted the need to educate people with diabetes to deliver safe self-care in the hospital setting. Individuals suitable for self-management in hospital must be competent adults with a stable level of consciousness who successfully manage their diabetes at home. In addition, while in hospital it is advised that these patients have the physical skills appropriate to self-administer insulin; be accustomed to performing self-monitoring of blood glucose; and have adequate oral intake. In the event that self-care is deemed unsafe or impossible (e.g. critically ill, post surgery or unwilling), then there must be a governance arrangement to assess patient competency and if necessary supersede patients' right to self-care.

Encouraging and supporting patients to have as much responsibility for their diabetes management as they wish for, and their clinical status allows, is likely to enhance the patient experience during a hospital stay. The Diabetes UK position statement on what care adults with diabetes should expect in hospital clearly focuses on the importance of patient self-management, while reminding health care professionals of the importance of policies and strategies being in place to support this concept in the ward setting (Table 32.1).

Barriers to safe and effective diabetes care delivery in hospital

Systems failures

It is essential that the patient with diabetes is identified and flagged at an early stage of the admission process. The ADA recommends that all patients admitted to hospital should be identified in the medical record as having diabetes. The UK NHS

Table 32.1 Patients' experiences of in-hospital diabetes care [60].

1	Experiences of disempowerment and distress. Patients felt that they were not engaged as partners in their care during their admissions, and in some cases patronized by staff members
2	Food/food timings and their coordination with medication. This often reflected a lack of understanding amongst staff of the relationship between food and good diabetes management
3	Medicines mismanagement in hospital. People were given the wrong medication or dose
4	Lack of communication between different multidisciplinary team members and with the person with diabetes. This led to basic failures in communication such as notification of both changes in timings of procedures and dosages of medications to the patient
5	Lack of hospital staff knowledge of diabetes management both in terms of basic care and respecting patient autonomy
6	Importance of people with diabetes being allowed to self-manage and thereby respecting the role of the person with diabetes in usually self-managing their condition on a daily basis
7	Positive experiences of good diabetes management and proactively allowing patients to self-manage

Institute for Innovation and Improvement also recommends a diabetes identifier as a prerequisite for ensuring quality of care [33]. Yet this has not been achievable in the UK in secondary care because of systems failure as a result of poor coding and inadequate information systems technology. In addition, if we are to identify those patients with undiagnosed diabetes and stress hyperglycemia and make an impact on their poor outcomes there needs to be a policy of routine blood glucose screening for all hospital inpatients. This is not standard practice in the UK.

Ward environment factors

Basic diabetes care is often not well delivered in hospital. An analysis of 44 US hospitals revealed persistent shortcomings in diabetes management, including persistent excessive hyperglycemia [39]. The hospital environment is one that is characterized by instability and unpredictability for the patient. It is a major contributor to the difficulty of managing inpatient diabetes well. Intercurrent illness, in-hospital changes to a patient's usual outpatient regimen, and the scheduling and unpredictability of tests and procedures contribute to glycemic instability [40]. A patient's dietary intake may also be erratic, because of poor appetite, palatability of food or timeliness of delivery.

Staff training challenges

In the UK, qualified staff numbers have been reduced to a minimum and ward staff have little or no protected time for education and training other than mandatory training (fire, manual handling, back care, infection control) defined by the employing organization. Despite the large numbers of patients with diabetes in hospital, the only mandatory training in diabetes is in blood glucose monitoring. People with diabetes, who generally have a high level of knowledge about their condition, are therefore often being managed by nursing and medical staff with only a rudimentary training in diabetes care [41].

Box 32.1 Defining adverse events and medical errors

Adverse events are described as: An unintentional injury caused by medical management rather than the underlying disease or condition of the patient. This can include physical or emotional harm [61]

Medical errors are described as: The failure to complete a planned action as intended or the use of a wrong plan to achieve an aim [61]

Insulin prescribing and delivery errors

Insulin treatment in hospital can be life-saving. It also has the potential to be life-threatening given its narrow therapeutic index. The prescribing of insulin is a minefield of ignorance and error. Insulin has been identified as one of the top five high-risk medications in the inpatient environment [42,43]. There is a wealth of material, predominantly from the USA and the UK, describing both medical errors and adverse events in the general inpatient population (Box 32.1). Medical errors, including those related to insulin treatment, are described as common in hospitals worldwide [44,45]. Insulin medication errors can occur at any stage in the process of prescribing, preparing and delivering the medication to the patient [46]. The potential consequences of error can be catastrophic. One-third of all inpatient medical errors that cause death within 48 hours of the error involve insulin administration [47].

Medical prescribing

A common recommendation emerging in both diabetes management and prescribing errors has been the need for appropriate medical staff education in diabetes and insulin treatment. Hellman [47] suggests that endocrinologists take on this role and maintain that junior doctors should be taught the principles of drug dosage and prescription writing before starting their ward placements. A report from the National Patient Safety Agency 2007 [49] devotes one entire page to insulin errors and advocates changes to pre-registration training to incorporate the principles and therapeutics of safe prescribing. The curriculum for junior doctors has been revised in recent years and new models of education have been implemented yet this has not reduced insulin prescribing errors in junior hospital doctors and therefore the process merits review.

Non-medical prescribing

In the UK, legislation for nurse prescribing, now known as non-medical prescribing, was implemented in 2003. The editorial by Aronson *et al.* [50] compared medical student training (approximately 61 hours) to that of nurse prescribers (162 hours of theory and 90 hours in practice). The authors called for the adoption of the British Pharmacological Society's prescribing and assessment processes to be applied for doctors in training in the teaching of diabetes and insulin treatment. Aronson also called for the formation of an independent systematic review of medical prescribing and teaching by a multi-organizational body in order to inform practice. This process has yet to be implemented but if introduced could form the basis for training in diabetes medicines management.

Delivering effective diabetes care: the role of diabetes inpatient team

Diabetes inpatient teams are multidisciplinary; the health care professionals involved individually contribute specialist skills and together provide a holistic approach to patient care. As well as operating as a discreet unit, the team works closely with other medical specialities including the specialist diabetic foot team. The defined roles forming the diabetes specialist inpatient team include the following.

The Patient

Central to the diabetes team is the patient. The majority of people living with diabetes have developed highly competent and individualized management skills, therefore it is essential, where possible, that the patient is encouraged to participate in the formulation and conduct of their own care plan while in the ward setting.

Consultant physician

The primary role of the consultant physician is as leader of the multidisciplinary team. The consultant physician has ultimate responsibility for the clinical care of diabetes inpatients. They work closely to provide clinical support to diabetes specialist nurses (DSNs) and certified diabetes educators (CDEs), while being heavily involved in the training and education of other diabetes and non-diabetes health care professionals. With the need to maintain standards of care and update clinical guidelines, physicians are also frequently involved in audit and research work in order to ensure the highest quality of diabetes care for inpatients with diabetes.

Certified Diabetes Educator

In 2009, the Association of Diabetes Educators published a position statement, which emphasized the key role of CDEs in patient and staff education, the promotion and implementation of glycemic control strategies and appropriate nutritional therapies. In close partnership with social work, case managers and home care coordinators, they are able to facilitate a smooth patient pathway from hospital to home at discharge.

Diabetes specialist nurse

The work of DSNs is exclusively in diabetes care. In 2009, there were 1361 DSNs in the UK working in primary and/or secondary care settings. DSNs deliver patient-centered care wherever required and influence care delivery at every stage of the patient journey, including inpatient care. The role of the DISN has evolved in recent times and specifically focuses on supporting inpatients and the ward staff caring for them. Aside from clinical care, DISNs are frequently involved in medical and nursing education and also in guideline production and update. Not only can DISNs significantly reduce inpatient length of stay [36,37], but if they also obtain non-medical prescribing skills, have also been seen to reduce insulin and diabetes management errors significantly [38].

Diabetes specialist dietitian

Diabetes specialist dietitians have a pivotal role in the care of diabetic inpatients with complex nutritional needs, in particular those patients who are unable to swallow or those required to adhere to a complex dietary regimen as in renal failure, cystic fibrosis and the elderly.

Other team members may include ward-based diabetes link nurses and diabetes specialist pharmacists.

Which type of patient needs to be seen by the diabetes specialist team?

The correct answer to this question is that all patients with diabetes should have access to specialist diabetes services; however, given that up to 20% of all inpatients now have diabetes then in real world it is going to be almost impossible for specialist team members to see every patient. Specialist teams therefore, driven by need, have drawn up a priority list for which patients should be referred for assessment. An example of one of these referral criteria documents from Leicester, UK, is seen in Table 32.2.

Management of in-hospital hyperglycemia

All hospitals should have a policy for glycemic management and or blood glucose monitoring in place according to the ADA [28] or the National Institute for Health, Innovation and Improvement (NHSIII) standards of care. The newly introduced UK "Think Glucose" campaign from the NHSIII has as its mantra, "It is as unacceptable for hospitals not to have a glycemic management policy as it is for them not to have an infection control policy" [33].

Hyperglycemia in hospital is a common problem and occurs in around 25% of all hospital inpatients. The majority of patients with diabetes are not admitted to hospital to address and treat complications associated with the disease. Control of blood glucose often becomes secondary to the care of the primary diagnosis requiring admission. In patients without diabetes who develop hyperglycemia during an acute illness, high glucose levels are often ignored or treated inappropriately. Poor glycemic control is common among inpatients with diabetes, particularly

Table 32.2 Indications for referral to diabetes inpatient specialist nurses (DISN). Adapted from University of Leicester Hospitals, UK.

Always refer	Hyperglycemic emergencies (e.g. DKA, HHS) Acute coronary syndromes Severe or repeated hypoglycemia New diagnosis of diabetes Problems with intravenous insulin infusion or duration >48 hours Active foot ulceration Reduced consciousness Enteral or parenteral nutrition Vomiting and sepsis Patient request Persisitent hyperglycemia Pregnancy
Consider refer	Educational needs Stress hyperglycemia NBM >24 hours Poor wound healing
Rarely refer	Minor hypoglycemia Routine dietetic advice Simple educational needs Well-controlled and managed diabetes

DKA, diabetic ketoacidosis; HSS, hyperosmolar hyperglycemic syndrome; NBM, nil by mouth.

in those treated with insulin, for many reasons. Poorly defined management plans, poor coordination of care, overly high or absent glycemic targets, lack of therapeutic adjustment, over utilization of "sliding scales" which are often not adjusted to optimize control and under-utilization of insulin infusions represent some of the reasons for poor control of blood glucose. A further important contributing factor has been the fear of provoking hypoglycemia.

Intravenous insulin to treat in-hospital hyperglycemia

Insulin provides the greatest flexibility in the hospital setting to achieve optimal blood glucose control. As protocols for tight glucose control are introduced in a variety of hospital settings it will be essential to implement safeguards to minimize the risk of hypoglycemia and ensure patient safety. The systemic problems that create obstacles to appropriate and safe care of patients receiving insulin in hospital are well recognized [45]. Insulin administration errors could be minimized and clinical outcomes improved by thorough analysis of the setting, additional training for ward staff, setting of goals focused on patient safety, double checking of insulin prescription and administration and regular audit of adverse incidents.

Indications for an intravenous insulin infusion

Whether the patient has previously recognized diabetes or not, insulin provides the greatest flexibility to meet rapidly changing

Box 32.2 Indications for an intravenous insulin infusion

- To treat critical care illness
- Acute coronary syndromes
- Postoperative periods following heart surgery
- Patients on "nil by mouth" status
- Type 1 diabetes
- General preoperative, intra-operative and postoperative care
- Organ transplantation
- Stroke
- Hyperglycemia during high-dose corticosteroid therapy
- Labor and delivery
- Other acute illness for which prompt glycemic control is judged important to recovery such as prevention or treatment of infection
- Diabetes emergencies such as diabetic ketoacidosis or hyperosmolar hyperglycemic syndrome

requirements in different hospital settings to achieve optimal blood glucose control. Intravenous infusion of insulin is the only insulin treatment strategy specifically developed for use in the hospital setting. The American College of Endocrinologists advised that intravenous insulin infusion should be used to control glycemia in certain indications (Box 32.2).

Insulin infusion protocols

The ideal insulin protocol should be safe, understandable, easily ordered and implemented. It should be effective in correcting hyperglycemia quickly and in maintaining glucose levels within a defined target range. The provision of an algorithm for making incremental changes to the infusion rate, which can be executed by nursing staff, is likely to improve the efficacy of the protocol. Hypoglycemia is a potential complication of intensified insulin therapy and is associated with poor outcomes. It is for this reason that intravenous insulin infusions should be supported by caloric input. In most patients this is in the form of a simultaneous infusion of dextrose but calories can be provided by other routes (e.g. enteral, parenteral or in a diasylate). If hypoglycemia develops despite adequate provision of calories then the patient should be treated promptly for hypoglycemia according to local protocol and the insulin infusion adjusted accordingly.

Successful implementation of an insulin infusion protocol is best achieved with the appointment of a champion to lead the multidisciplinary team. The protocol should be submitted to a medicines advisory or therapeutics committee and implemented with a widespread educational program to include medical, nursing and pharmacy staff. Adherence to a standard protocol is likely to reduce adverse events for patients and limit medical errors in insulin prescribing.

Table 32.3 Insulin infusion table adapted from Oxford Radcliffe NHS Trust, UK.

Blood glucose (mmol/L)	Insulin infusion rate (unit/hour)				
	Rate A	Rate B	Rate C	Rate D	Tailored rate
0–4.0	0 and treat hypo	0 and treat hypo	0 and treat hypo	0 and treat hypo	0 and treat hypo
4.1–6.0	1	1	2	3	
6.1–8.0	2	3	4	5	
8.1–10.0	3	4	6	8	
>10.1	4	6	8	10	

>10 mmol/L

If blood glucose remains >10.1 for 4 hours move to the next infusion rate (e.g. A to B)

Prescriptions should include the signature, bleep and date as well as the time and date infusion started

Box 32.3 AACE/ADA recommendations for in-hospital glycemic control

A target of 140–180 mg/dL (7.8–10.0 mmol/L) is preferable in *most* patients

A target of 110–140 mg/dL (6.1–7.8 mmol/L) may be appropriate in *selected* patients

A target of >180 mg/dL (10 mmol/L) or <110 mg/dL (6.1 mmol/L) is *not* recommended

Preparation and delivery of an insulin infusion

The insulin infusion is prepared by adding 50 units of soluble insulin to 49.5 mL normal saline, which will provide 1 unit of insulin in 1 mL saline, which is delivered via an infusion pump. This insulin infusion can be piggy-backed into the infusion of dextrose using a three-way connector and a non-return valve. All patients should commence on algorithm A and uptitrate to achieve target glucose range (Table 32.3).

Targets for glycemic control

The AACE/ADA has recently set new targets for the management of hyperglycemia in hospital (Box 32.3) [62]. The recommendation is that once intravenous insulin has been commenced the blood glucose level should be maintained at 140–180 mg/dL (7.8–10 mmol/L) with greater benefit possibly realized at the lower end of the target. There is recognition that lower targets may be beneficial in specified groups but there is insufficient evidence to make firm recommendations. It is recommended that target glucose should not fall below a level of 110 mg/dL (6.1 mmol/L). Where lower targets are being used, patients should be treated in sites with extensive experience and appropriate support such as areas caring for coronary artery bypass graft patients, sites with low rates of hypoglycemia, patients on total parenteral nutrition and those in ITUs.

Transition from intravenous to subcutaneous insulin

Conversion to subcutaneous insulin should be delayed until patients are able to eat and drink normally without nausea or emesis. The most appropriate time to switch from IV to subcutaneous insulin is at the usual time of the patient's insulin administration, before a meal. Patients with known type 1 diabetes will become insulin deficient within minutes of the IV infusion being stopped because of the short half-life of IV insulin. It is therefore good practice to continue the infusion of insulin for 1 hour after the subcutaneous insulin has been administered to allow time for the insulin to be absorbed.

If the patient has been on an established insulin regimen, then this regimen should be restarted, but doses may have to be adjusted depending on the patient's clinical condition. If the patient is new to insulin therapy, then a rough estimation of the total daily dose (TDD) of insulin can be made from a simple calculation using the hourly rates delivered in the IV insulin infusion (Box 32.4a). Estimation of insulin doses can also be made

Box 32.4 Converting patients to subcutaneous insulin

(a) *Estimation of insulin dose for a patient being converted from an intravenous insulin infusion*
- Calculate average hourly insulin dose by totaling the last 6 hours' doses on the chart and dividing by 6 (e.g. 15 units divide by 6 = 2.5 units/hour. Multiply by factor of 20 to get the total daily dose (TDD) insulin (e.g. 50 units)
- For a basal : bolus insulin regimen, divide 50 : 50 basal : bolus (e.g. 25 units as basal; 25 units as bolus. Give 25 units as a basal insulin (e.g. Lantus). Divide total bolus dose by three to get bolus for each meal (e.g. 8 units short-acting insulin, e.g. Novorapid)
- For a twice daily fixed mixture regime divide 60 : 40 morning : evening (e.g. Humalog Mix 25, Novomix 30). Give 36 units am; 14 units pm

(b) *Estimation of insulin dose when no insulin infusion has been used*

Calculate the total daily insulin dose insulin according to diabetes type
- Known type 2 diabetes 0.5–0.7 unit/kg
- Known type 1 diabetes 0.3–0.5 unit/kg
- Unsure 0.3–0.5 unit/kg
- Divide insulin 50 : 50 for basal bolus regime (see above)
- Divide 60 : 40 for twice daily mixed insulin (see above)

Table 32.4 Causes of in-hospital hypoglycemia.

Cause of in-hospital hypoglycemia	Example
Primary reason for hospital stay	Medical causes: hepatic failure, cardiogenic shock, severe sepsis Surgical causes: nil by mouth for operation or procedure
Inappropriate food administration	Change of meal times, missed meals, poor access to snacks
Errors of insulin prescription or administration	Poorly written medication charts (e.g. writing of "U" instead of units) so that 4 U becomes 40 units, poor injection technique
Inappropriate use of "stat" insulin doses	Corrective dosing of insulin prescribed by untrained staff
Inappropriate use of sulfonylureas or interactions with other prescribed medication	Long-acting hypoglycemic agents should be avoided in hospital
Inappropriately timed diabetes medication for meal/enteral feed	Food and insulin or oral hypoglycemic agents mismatch
Use of unopposed intravenous insulin therapy	Dextrose infusion should be prescribed concurrently
Mobilization after acute illness	Insulin requirements may decrease with exercise

according to body weight, which is useful in calculating TDD in patients who are new to insulin but have not required an insulin infusion (Box 32.4b).

Avoiding and treating in-hospital hypoglycemia

There is an increasing body of evidence supporting the widespread occurrence of hypoglycemia in hospitals and poor knowledge of how to detect and manage it. Acute hypoglycemia is associated with significant morbidity and more rarely mortality as it causes an intense hemodynamic response that can lead to potentially fatal cardiac arrhythmias, myocardial ischemia, cerebrovascular accidents, coma and death. In-hospital hypoglycemia is defined as a blood glucose level equal or below 72 mg/dL (4.0 mmol/L).

Causes of in-hospital hypoglycemia

There are many reasons why hypoglycemia is more likely to be to occur during hospitalization but most of these relate to insulin administration and prescribing errors and inappropriate food administration (Table 32.4).

Management of in-hospital hypoglycemia

In 2005, Tomky *et al.* [51] gave a clear overview of the topic in their article. 2006 saw the introduction of Hypoboxes™ for the management of hypoglycemia in the UK [52]. These boxes are often in a prominent place (e.g. on resuscitation trolleys) and are brightly colored for instant recognition. They contain all the equipment required to treat hypoglycemia, from cartons of fruit juice to intravenous 20% glucose. There are general guidelines for the treatment of in-hospital hypoglycemia and these should be available in each ward and outpatient setting; however, each patient developing in-hospital hypoglycemia should be assessed as an individual and diabetes teams should agree local guidance for self-management. Certain conditions such as renal impairment or heart failure may require tailored treatment to avoid fluid overload. Many people with diabetes carry their own treatment supplies for hypoglycemic events and should be supported to self-manage when capable and appropriate. This information regarding capacity to self-manage should be recorded in the patient notes at the time of the admission assessment.

If the patient is not capable and/or uncooperative but is able to swallow, give either 1.5–2 tubes GlucoGel™ squeezed into the mouth between the teeth and gums or, if this is ineffective, give 1 mg glucagon intramuscularly (Figure 32.1). Monitor the blood glucose levels after 15 minutes. If the blood glucose levels are still less than 4 mmol/L, GlucoGel treatment can be repeated up to three times. If the hypoglycemia does not resolve at this stage, IV 10% glucose infusion at 100 mL/hour should be considered. Once the blood glucose is above 4 mmol/L and patient has recovered, a long-acting carbohydrate snack should be offered.

In adults who are unconscious with or without seizure activity and/or very aggressive, the patient's airway, breathing and circulation should be assessed, any insulin infusion *in situ* should be discontinued and a medical practitioner summoned. At this stage any of the following treatments can be considered for use.

Treatments such as 15–20 g quick-acting carbohydrate (e.g. 50–60 mL of Ensure Plus juice or Fortijuice 25 mL original or 3–4 heaped teaspoons sugar dissolved in water) can be administered via a feed tube. The capillary blood glucose measurement should be repeated 5–10 minutes later. If blood glucose is still less than 4 mmol/L, repeat this step up to three times. If the hypoglycemia is still not resolved after 15 minutes or three cycles, IV 10% glucose infusion at 100 mL/hour can be considered as a treatment option. Once the blood glucose is above 4 mmol/L and patient has recovered, a long-acting carbohydrate such as 200 mL milk (not soya) can be given and the feed. Insulin should not be omitted and regular continued capillary blood glucose level monitoring should be recorded for 24–48 hours.

Prevention of recurrent in-hospital hypoglycemia

When hypoglycemia has been successfully treated it is important that the reason for hypoglycemia is ascertained and the treatment documented in the patient notes. If the hypoglycemic episode was severe or a recurrent event, or if patient has concerns regarding treatment of further recurrence of hypoglycemia and its treatment, then referral should be made to the CDE, DISN or specialist medical team. Measures such as medication adjustment or timing of meals should be introduced to prevent further episodes of hypoglycemia.

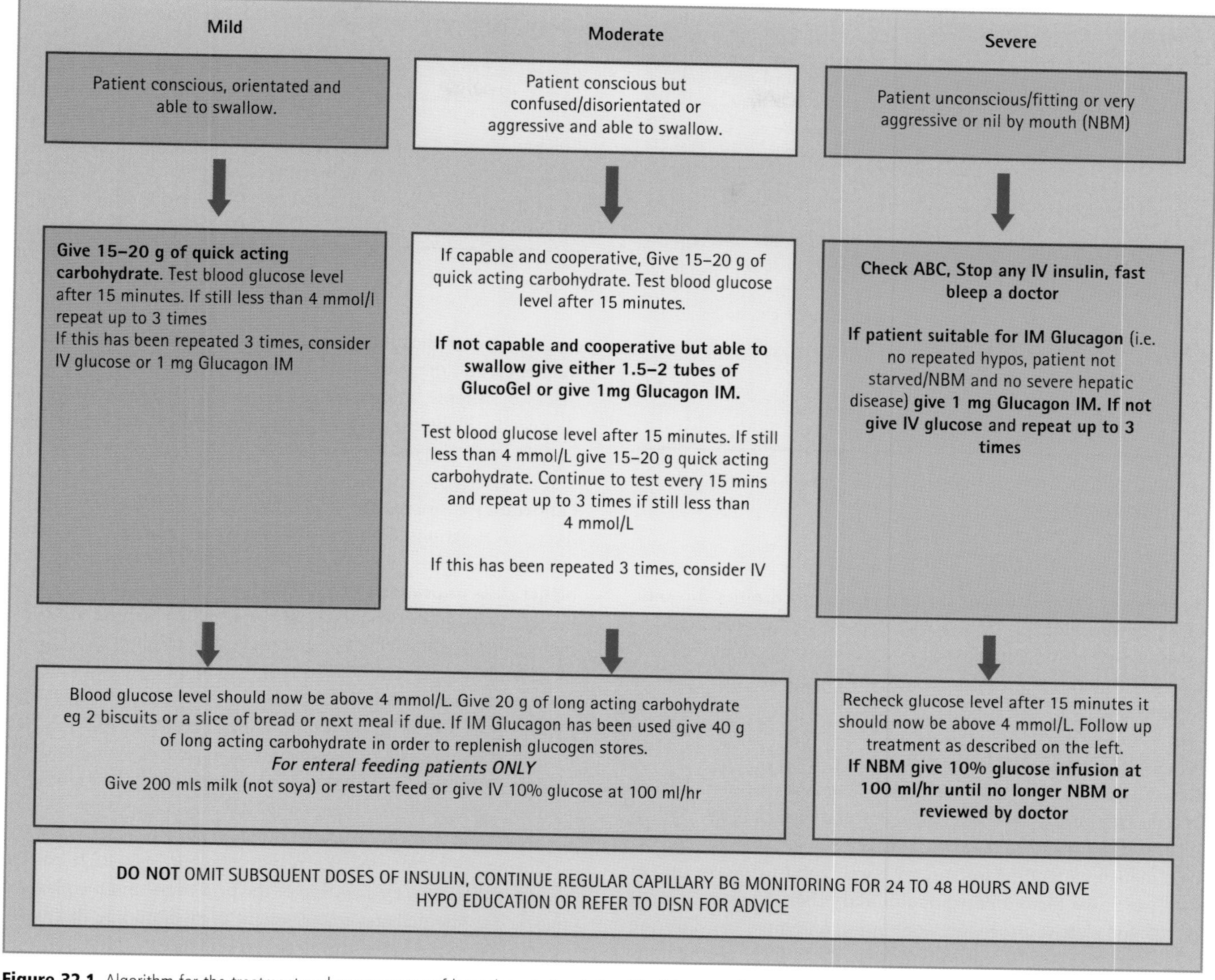

Figure 32.1 Algorithm for the treatment and management of hypoglycemia in adults with diabetes mellitus in hospital. Hypoglycemia is defined as blood glucose of <4 mmol/L (if not <4 mmol/L but symptomatic, give a small carbohydrate snack for symptom relief). ABC, Airway, Breathing and Circulation; DISN, diabetes inpatient specialist nurse; IM, intramuscularly; IV, intravenously; NBM, nil by mouth.

Surgery in patients with diabetes

Patients with diabetes have poorer health than those without diabetes so this means they are more likely to undergo surgery. It is estimated that 50% of those with diabetes will require surgery in their lifetime. Diabetes is associated with increased risk of perioperative infection and postoperative cardiovascular morbidity and mortality. The complex interplay of the operative procedure, anesthesia, fasting and additional postoperative factors such as artificial feeding and emesis all contribute to labile glycemic control in the perioperative period.

Metabolic response to surgery

Surgery and anesthesia causes a state of relative insulin hyposecretion and insulin resistance. It induces a complex series of hormonal and metabolic changes [53,54]. The secretion of the counter-regulatory or "stress" hormones, particularly cortisol and catecholamines, is greatly increased, and this can lead to an acute decrease in insulin sensitivity [54,55]. Enhanced sympathetic activity, together with raised circulating catecholamine concentrations, tends to inhibit insulin secretion. The net result of these changes is to push metabolism towards catabolism, leading to increased hepatic glucose production and hyperglycemia and enhanced breakdown of protein and fat. The magnitude of the counter-regulatory response varies in each individual and is greater with prolonged surgery and other factors such as postoperative sepsis.

Preoperative evaluation

Nowadays, most patients are admitted on the same day as scheduled surgery. Pre-assessment planning in diabetes can prevent

Table 32.5 Goldmann risk index [56].

Risk	Patient characteristics	Preoperative investigation
Low	<60 years old No history of cardiopulmonary disease Non-specific ECG changes	No further investigation necessary
Medium	All patients >60 years old Stable angina or previous MI Compensated heart failure	Determine functional capacity using ECG, exercise stress test (has a predictive value of 81% detection of multivessel disease)
High	Acute coronary syndromes Decompensated heart failure Supraventricular arrhythmias Known COPD	Consider preoperative coronary angiography

COPD, chronic obstructive pulmonary disease; ECG, electrocardiogram; MI, myocardial infarction.

unnecessary cancellation of surgery, give opportunities for joint care planning with the person with diabetes and enables optimization of glycemic control prior to surgery which can reduce length of stay, medication errors and improve the patient experience.

Assessing cardiac risk

Careful assessment of patients with diabetes is required because of their complexity and high risk of coronary heart disease, which is sometimes asymptomatic. It is therefore vital that all patients with diabetes attending for surgery have a robust risk assessment with particular focus on cardiopulmonary risk. In the assessment of risk for elective procedures one must one must consider the risk associated with the procedure itself in addition to the individual patient risk associated with pre-existing co-morbidities. Those at highest risk are those in whom there is significant cardiorespiratory pathology. There are several cardiac risk stratification indexes in the literature but essentially all use clinical variables that allow patients to be classified as low, intermediate or high risk of a major cardiac event during or after surgery. The Goldmann cardiac risk index [56] is widely used in clinical practice (Table 32.5).

Assessing surgical risk

The American College of Cardiology/American Heart Association guidelines introduce the concept of "surgery-specific risk." Risk stratification is based on the degree of hemodynamic stress associated with specific procedures [57]. Table 32.6 summarizes the risk associated with various types of surgery.

Physical assessment

All patients require a careful history and physical examination. Key aspects of this should include assessment of glycemic control, long-term complications, occurrence of hypoglycemia and its frequency, and the patient's awareness and knowledge of all drug therapy. Patients should be given written information about changes in diabetes-specific and other medication in the days leading up to surgery.

Table 32.6 Surgery-specific risk.

	Procedure
Low	Peripheral and laparoscopic procedures
Medium	Orthopedic and prostatic operations
High	Major abdominal and thoracic operations, particularly major vascular surgery and ones where there are anticipated major fluid or blood loss

Laboratory assessment

Basic investigations should include HbA_{1c} as there is a suggestion that elevated levels over 7% (>53 mmol/mol) are associated with higher risks of postoperative infections [58].

There is good evidence that effective pre-assessment of people with diabetes will enable a safe and effective discharge from hospital. In Bolton, UK, a DSN has implemented a patient pathway from pre-assessment to discharge. This pathway includes assessment, optimization of glycemic control, the writing up of an insulin infusion scale preoperatively and the implementation of planning for routine diabetes care postoperatively. This work has resulted in significant improvement in reduced length of stay, medication errors and positive patient experience [59].

During the course of the pre-assessment visit each patient should undergo an explanation of the procedure and the planned anesthesia. The diabetes management plan should be discussed, thus enabling the patient to make an informed decision around the diabetes care to be offered. Further appointments should be offered if optimization of glycemic control is required. All information should be supported with appropriate literature. All recommendations for treatment should be written in the patient's notes and in a handheld record kept by the patient.

Same-day admissions and specific preparations

High-risk patients are not suitable for same-day admission and should be admitted the day before surgery for assessment and optimization of glycemic control. There is evidence that elevated preoperative glucose levels >200 mg/dL (11 mmol/L) were associated with deep wound infections in a case–control study.

On the day of admission the patient's notes including the diabetes management plan should be available to all staff caring for that individual. All guidelines pertaining to the plan of care should be in place and accessible for staff. If the blood glucose is unacceptably high on the day of admission, plans should be in place for rapid optimization of glycemic control including the use of an intravenous infusion of insulin.

Table 32.7 Instructions for diabetes management on day of minor or intermediate surgery. Adapted from Nottingham University Trust, UK.

Morning list	Day before: normal food and medication. NBM from 02.00 Day of surgery: fast from 02.00 On tablets: omit diabetes tablets On insulin: omit any short-acting insulin, withhold insulin mixtures Give stat dose of isophane insulin, give 75% total daily dose if on once day insulin and 50% TDD if on twice daily insulin Continue long-acting analogs (Lantus, Levemir) at full dose Postoperative: lunch and normal insulin or tablets
Afternoon list	Day of surgery: light breakfast, fast from 08.00 On tablets: take diabetes tablets On insulin: take 50% normal insulin dose Continue long-acting analogs (Lantus, Levemir) at full dose Postoperative: late lunch and normal insulin or tablets

NBM, nil by mouth; TDD, total daily dose.

Individual intra-operative diabetes care treatment plan

Management of the individual patient is determined by the following:

- Severity and nature of surgery (major or minor surgery)
- Duration of perioperative fast
- Timing of surgery
- Pre-existing diabetes treatment

Major surgery (prolonged fast >6 hours)

All patients with diabetes undergoing major surgery should have a dextrose and insulin infusion.

Minor surgery (short fast <6 hours)

Table 32.7 shows an example of the various treatment options for patients being admitted for minor surgery.

Goals of glycemic management

The goals of perioperative diabetes care are avoidance of marked hyperglycemia and of hypoglycemia. Patients with type 1 diabetes have no endogenous insulin and will therefore require exogenous insulin to prevent the development of severe hyperglycemia and subsequent life-threatening complications such as diabetic ketoacidosis. Such patients will also need a continuous supply of glucose of 5–10 g/hour to prevent hypoglycemia.

It is not clear how "tight" glucose control needs to be during surgery. There are a paucity of clinical trials to inform clinical practice in the surgical arena with the exception of cardiac surgery where there is evidence that good control, defined as BG 80–110 mg/dL (4.4–6.1 mmol/L), may reduce mortality.

The lack of clear evidence on glycemic specific targets is reflected in the varying glucose targets recommended by national guidelines [24,27,28]. It would seem reasonable therefore to advise treatment regimens to aim for as near normal glycemia with avoidance of hypoglycemia (80 mg/dL, 4 mmol/L). This range seems to be a safe and practicable target during the perioperative period.

Intra-operative management of glycemia

Use of an IV insulin infusion to control glycemia has the advantage of easy titration to the glucose level because of the short half-life of IV insulin. Its safety has been demonstrated in many studies and is therefore the treatment of choice during surgery. The infusion requires close monitoring of blood glucose and potassium as well as appropriate interpretation by well-trained staff.

Types of intravenous insulin infusion

No type of insulin infusion used during surgery has been shown to be superior in either safety or effectiveness in achieving glucose control. The fixed rate insulin infusion and the intermittent bolus regimens have failed to gain popularity and are little used in clinical practice and are therefore not discussed further.

Variable rate separate insulin and glucose intravenous infusions

In this commonly used regimen, intravenous dextrose is infused at a rate of 5–10 g/hour and a separate insulin infusion is given. The rate varies depending on the procedure and the level of insulin resistance. Following coronary artery bypass graft operations, insulin requirements may increase 10-fold [38]. Glucose should be measured hourly and electrolytes every 4 hours.

Glucose insulin potassium infusion

The glucose, insulin and potassium infusion is a single solution infusion comprising 500 mL 5% dextrose, 10 mmol/L potassium chloride and 15 units of soluble insulin. This is infused at a rate of 100 mL/hour. Glucose is usually measured 2-hourly and the insulin content of the infusion can be changed if necessary. This method has the disadvantage of inflexibility and wastefulness as the entire infusion has to be discarded and replaced if insulin requirements change.

Postoperative care and discharge

For those undergoing minor surgery characterized by a short fast, generally the preoperative diabetes treatment can be reinstated at an early stage once the patient is eating well. For those undergoing major surgery, particularly abdominal surgery where there may be several days of fasting, then it is better to keep these patients on IV insulin infusion with appropriate fluid replacement. The IV fluid regimen should consist of replacement crystalloid, a minimum of 2 L/day (normal saline, Hartmann solution, Ringer lactate) and a supply of substrate (e.g. 100 mL/hour 5% dextrose) to prevent onset of catabolism. Conversion to normal therapy, whether insulin or oral hypoglycemic therapy, should occur when the patient is eating and drinking and free from nausea and emesis.

For patients with prolonged periods of nil by mouth or who are severely unwell or malnourished, hyperalimentation may be introduced. In these circumstances, insulin requirements may increase considerably and so these patients are better managed on high dose IV insulin with the support of the specialist diabetes team. Hospitals should have protocols in place to support this practice.

Conclusions

Patients with diabetes are twice as likely to be admitted to hospital and stay twice as long as those without diabetes. They have worse outcomes and a poorer patient experience than those without diabetes. Diabetes inpatient care and training has become the Cinderella area of diabetes care delivery despite the setting of clinical standards by several professional bodies. Although there is now a wealth of evidence that specialist inpatient diabetes teams reduce length of stay, reduce errors in prescribing, improve the patient experience and clinical outcomes, many hospitals across the world still lack inpatient specialist teams.

Patients voices are being raised in anger against this imbalance in care delivery. Providers of care need to listen to patients and professionals and ensure the delivery of a high quality inpatient service to include appropriate medical and nursing staff training, an equitable access to specialist services across the board, and an active partnership with patients to deliver a comprehensive range of services. Systems need to be in place to enable patients to self-manage where it is clinically appropriate. If standards are to be improved there needs to be agreed national targets and key performance indicators for diabetes inpatient care for which health care providers should be held accountable.

Acknowledgment

The authors thank Dr. Rif Malik for his contribution to this chapter.

References

1 International Diabetes Federation. *Diabetes Facts and Figures*. Available from: http//www.diabetesatlas.org/content/diabetes-and-impaired-glucose-tolerance. Accessed on 8 January, 2010.

2 Cowie CC, Rust KF, Byrd-Holt DD, Eberhardt MS, Flegal KM, Engelgau MM, *et al.* Prevalence of diabetes and impaired fasting glucose in adults in the US population: National Health and Nutrition Examination Survey 1999–2002. *Diabetes Care* 2006; **29**:1263–1268.

3 National Diabetes Support team. *Improving emergency and inpatient care for diabetes 2008*. Available from: http://www.diabetes.nhs.uk/document.php?o=324. Accessed on 18 January, 2010.

4 Umpierrez GE, Isaacs SD, Bazargan N, You X, Thaler LM, Kitabchi AE. Hyperglycemia: an independent marker of in-hospital mortality in patients with undiagnosed diabetes. *J Clin Endocrinol Metab* 2002; **87**:978–982.

5 Yendamuri S, Fulda GJ, Tinkoff GH. Admission hyperglycemia as a prognostic indicator in trauma. *J Trauma* 2003; **55**:33–38.

6 Capes SE, Hunt D, Malmberg K, Pathak P, Gerstein HC. Stress hyperglycemia and prognosis of stroke in nondiabetic and diabetic patients: a systematic overview. *Stroke* 2001; **32**:2426–2432.

7 Golden S, Peart-Vigilance C, Kao WH, Brancati FL. Perioperative glycemic control and risk of infectious complications in a cohort of adult with diabetes. *Diabetes Care* 1999; **22**:1408–1414.

8 Pomposelli JJ, Baxter JK, Babineau TJ, Pomfret EA, Driscoll DF, Forse RA, *et al.* Early postoperative glucose control predicts nosocomial infection rate in diabetic patients. *J Parenter Enteral Nutr* 1998; **22**:77–81.

9 McAlister FA, Majumdar SR, Blitz S, Rowe BH, Romney J, Marrie TJ. The relation between hyperglycemia and outcomes in 2,471 patients admitted to the hospital with community-acquired pneumonia. *Diabetes Care* 2005; **28**:810–815.

10 Moghissi ES, Korytkowski MT, DiNardo M, Einhorn D, Hellman R, Hirsch IB, *et al.* ACCE/ADA Consensus Statement on inpatient glycaemia control. *Diabetes Care* 2009; **32**:1119–1131.

11 Capes SE, Hunt D, Malmberg K, Gerstein HC. Stress hyperglycemia and increased risk of death after myocardial infarction in patients with and without diabetes: a systematic overview. *Lancet* 2000; **355**:773–778.

12 Malmberg K, for the DIGAMI Study Group. Prospective randomised study of intensive insulin treatment on long term survival after acute myocardial infarction in patients with diabetes mellitus. *Br Med J* 1997; **314**:1512–1515.

13 Malmberg K, Ryden L, Wedel H, and the DIGAMI 2 Investigators. Intense metabolic control by means of insulin in patients with diabetes mellitus and acute myocardial infarction (DIGAMI 2): effects on mortality and morbidity. *Eur Heart J* 2005; **26**:650–661.

14 Mehta SR, Yusuf S. Effect of glucose-insulin-potassium infusion on mortality in patients with acute ST-segment elevation myocardial infarction: the CREATE-ECLA randomized controlled trial. *JAMA* 2005; **293**:437–446.

15 Weston C, Walker L, Birkhead J. Early impact of insulin treatment on mortality for hyperglycaemic patients without known diabetes who present with an acute coronary syndrome. *Heart* 2007; **93**:1542–1546.

16 Funary AP, Wu Y. Clinical effects of hyperglycaemia in the cardiac surgery population: the Portland Diabetic Project. *Endocr Pract* 2006; **12**(Suppl 3):22–26.

17 Van den Berge G, Wooters P, Weekers F, Verwaest C, Bruyninckx F, Schetz M, *et al.* Intensive insulin therapy in critically ill patients. *N Engl J Med* 2001; **345**:1359–1367.

18 Van den Berge G, Wilmer, Hermans G. Intensive insulin therapy in the medical ICU. *N Engl J Med* 2006; **354**:449–461.

19 Griesdale DE, de Souza RJ, van Dam RM, Heyland DK, Cook DJ, Malhotra A, *et al.* Intensive insulin therapy and mortality among critically ill patients: a meta-analysis including NICE-SUGAR study data. *CMAJ* 2009; **180**:821–882.

20 Mesotten D, Van den Berghe G. Clinical potential of insulin therapy in critically ill patients. *Drugs* 2003; **63**:625–636.

21 Lewis KS, Kane-Gill SL, Bobek MB, Dasta JF. Intensive insulin therapy for critically ill patients. *Ann Pharmacother* 2004; **38**:1243–1251.

22 McMahon MM, Bistrian BR. Host defenses and susceptibility to infection in patients with diabetes mellitus. *Infect Dis Clin North Am* 1995; **9**:1–9.

23 Montori VM, Bistrian BR, McMahon MM. Hyperglycemia in acutely ill patients. *JAMA* 2002; **288**:2167–2169.

24 Aljada A, Dandona P. Effect of insulin on human aortic endothelial nitric oxide synthase. *Metabolism* 2000; **49**:147–150.

25 International Diabetes Federation 2005. Clinical Guidelines Taskforce. Global Guideline for type 2 Diabetes. Chapter 19: Inpatient care.

Available from: http://www.idf.org/Global_guideline. Accessed on 17 January, 2010.

26 Clement S, Braithwaite SS, Magee MF, Ahmann A, Smith EP, Schafer RG, *et al.* American Diabetes Association Diabetes in Hospitals Writing Committee. Management of diabetes and hyperglycemia in hospitals. *Diabetes Care* 2004; **27**:553–591.

27 Garber A, Moghissi E, *et al.* ACE/ADA Inpatient Diabetes and Glycemic Control Consensus Statement. American College of Endocrinology and American Diabetes Association Consensus statement on inpatient diabetes and glycemic control: a call to action. *Diabetes Care* 2006; **29**:1955–1962.

28 American Diabetes Association. Standards of medical care in diabetes. *Diabetes Care* 2009; **32**(Suppl 1):S13–61.

29 Canadian Diabetes Association Clinical Practice Guidelines Expert Committee. Canadian Diabetes Association 2003 clinical practice guidelines for the prevention and management of diabetes in Canada. *Can J Diabetes* 2003; **27**(Suppl 2):S113–S116.

30 Department of Health. *Department of Health Five years on: delivering the diabetes National Service Framework 2008*. Available from: http://www.dh.gov.uk/prod_consum_dh/groups/dh_digitalassets/@dh/@en/documents/digitalasset/dh_087122.pdf. Accessed on 18 January, 2010.

31 National Diabetes Support Team. Improving emergency and inpatient care for people with diabetes. 2008. Available from: www.diabetes.nhs.uk/news-1/Inpatient care.pdf. Accessed on 18 January, 2010; and www.diabetes.nhs.uk/commissioning-resource. Accessed on 19 March, 2010.

32 What care to expect in hospital. www.diabetes.org.uk.

33 National Institute of Innovation and Improvement. Delivering quality and value and focus on: inpatient care for people with diabetes. 2008. Available from: http://www.diabetes.nhs.uk/news-1/focus-on-inpatient-care-for-people-with-diabetes-published-by-the-nhs-institute-for-innovation-and-improvement/?searchterm=inpatient. Accessed on 17 January, 2010.

34 Levetan CS, Salas JR, Wilets IF, Zumoff B. Impact of endocrine and diabetes team consultation on hospital length of stay for patients with diabetes. *Am J Med* 1995; **99**:22–28.

35 Audit Commission. *Audit Commission Testing times: a review of diabetes services in England and Wales 2000*. Available from: http://www.audit-commission.gov.uk/nationalstudies/health/primarycare/Pages/testingtimes.aspx. Accessed on 18 January, 2010.

36 Cavan DA, Hamilton P, Everett J, Kerr D. Reducing hospital inpatient length of stay for patients with diabetes. *Diabet Med* 2001; **18**:162–164.

37 Davies M, Dixon S, Currie CJ, Davis RE, Peters JR. Evaluation of a hospital diabetes specialist nursing service: a randomized controlled trial. *Diabet Med* 2001; **18**:301–307.

38 Courtenay M, Carey N, James J, Hills M, Roland J. An evaluation of a diabetes specialist nurse prescriber on the system of delivering medicines to patients with diabetes. *J Clin Nurs* 2008; **17**:1635–1644.

39 Wexler DJ, Meigs JB, Cagliero E, Nathan D, Grant RW. Prevalence of hyper- and hypoglycemia among inpatients with diabetes. *Diabetes Care* 2007; **30**:367–369.

40 Inzucchi SE. Management of hyperglycaemia in the hospital setting. *N Engl J Med* 2006: **355**:1903–1911.

41 Lansang MC, Harrell H. Knowledge on inpatient diabetes among fourth year medical students. *Diabetes Care* 2007; **30**:1088–1091.

42 "High-alert" medications and patient safety. *Int J Qual Health Care* 2001; **13**:339–340.

43 Department of Health. *Department of Health Building a Safer NHS. Improving medication safety 2004*. Available from: http://www.dh.gov.uk/prod_consum_dh/groups/dh_digitalassets/@dh/@en/documents/digitalasset/dh_4077110.pdf. Accessed on 18 January, 2010.

44 Kowiatek J, Skledar S, Potoski B. Insulin medication error reduction: a quality improvement initiative. *Hosp Pharm* 2001; **36**:639–644.

45 Clinical Resource Efficiency Support Team (CREST). Safe and effective use of insulin in secondary care: recommendations for treating hyperglycaemia in adults. 2006. Available from: www.crestni.org.uk/publications/insulin.pdf. Accessed on 17 January, 2010.

46 Metchick LN, Petit WA Jr, Inzucchi SE. Inpatient management of diabetes management. *Am J Med* 2002; **113**:317–323.

47 Hellman R. A systems approach to reducing errors in insulin therapy in the inpatient setting. *Endocr Pract* 2004; **10**:100–108.

48 Winterstein AG, Hatton RC, Gonzalez-Rothi R, Johns TE, Segal R. Identifying clinically significant preventable adverse drug events through a hospital's database of adverse drug reaction reports. *Am J Health Syst Pharm* 2002; **59**:1742–1749.

49 National Patient Safety Agency. Available from: http://www.patientsafetyfirst.nhs.uk/Content.aspx?path=/interventions/High-riskmedication. Accessed on 17 January, 2010.

50 Aronson JK, Henerson G, Webb DJ, Rawlins MD. A prescription for better prescribing. *Br Med J* 2006; **333**:459–460.

51 Tomky D. Detection, prevention, and treatment of hypoglycemia in the hospital. *Diabetes Spectrum* 2005; **18**:39–45.

52 Baker H, Horton A, Low P, *et al.* "HYPOBOX": a practical aid in the management of hypoglycaemia in hospital. *Diabet Med* 2006; **23**:P186.

53 Elliott MJ, Alberti KGMM. Carbohydrate metabolism: effects of preoperative starvation and trauma. *Clin Anaesthesiol* 1983; **1**:527–550.

54 Frayn KN. Hormonal control of metabolism in trauma and sepsis. *Clin Endocrinol* 1986; **24**:577–599.

55 Nygren JO, Thorell A, Soop M, Efendic S, Brismar K, Karpe F, *et al.* Perioperative insulin and glucose infusion maintains normal insulin sensitivity after surgery. *Am J Physiol* 1998; **275**:E140–E148.

56 Goldman L, Caldera DL, Nussbaum SR. Multifactorial index of cardiac risk in noncardiac surgical procedures. *N Engl J Med* 1977; **297**:845–50.

57 Eagle KA, Brundage BH, Chaitman BR, Ewy GA, Fleisher LA, Hertzer NR, *et al.* Guidelines for perioperative cardiovascular evaluation for noncardiac surgery. Report of the American College of Cardiology/American Heart Association Task Force on Practice Guidelines. Committee on Perioperative Cardiovascular Evaluation for Noncardiac Surgery. *Circulation* 1996; **93**:1278–1317.

58 Pomposelli JJ, Baxter JK 3rd, Babineau TJ, Pomfret EA, Driscoll DF, Forse RA, *et al.* Early postoperative glucose control predicts nosocomial infection rate in diabetic patients. *J Parenter Enteral Nutr* 1998; **22**:77–81.

59 Hilton L, Digner M. Developing a pathway of preoperative assessment and care planning for people with diabetes. *J Diabetes Nurs* 2006; **10**:89–94.

60 Diabetes UK. *Collation of inpatient experiences 2007*. Available from: http://diabetes.org.uk/Professionals/Publications-reports-and-resources/Reports-statistics-and-case-studies/reports/Collation-of-inpatient-Experiences. Accessed on 19 January, 2010.

61 DeLisa JA. Physiatry:medical errors, patient safety, patient injury, and quality of care. *Am J Physical Med Rehab* 2004: **83**(8); 575–83.

62 AACE/ADA. *American Association of Clinical Endocrinologists and American Diabetes Association Consensus statement on inpatient diabetes glycemic control 2009*. Available from: http://www.aace.com/pub/pdf/guidelines/InpatientGlycemicControlConsensusStatement.pdf. Accessed on 18 January, 2010.

33 Hypoglycemia in Diabetes

Philip E. Cryer
Division of Endocrinology, Metabolism and Lipid Research, Washington University School of Medicine, St. Louis, MO, USA

Keypoints

- Iatrogenic hypoglycemia is the limiting factor in the glycemic management of diabetes. It occurs during treatment with an insulin secretagogue or with insulin.
- The key physiologic defenses against falling plasma glucose concentrations are decrements in insulin and increments in glucagon and epinephrine. The behavioral defense is carbohydrate ingestion prompted by symptoms that are largely the result of sympathetic neural activation.
- Hypoglycemia in diabetes is the result of therapeutic hyperinsulinemia. As glucose levels fall, decrements in insulin and increments in glucagon are lost, because of β-cell failure, in type 1 diabetes mellitus (T1DM) and advanced type 2 diabetes mellitus (T2DM). In that setting, attenuated increments in epinephrine cause the syndrome of defective glucose counter-regulation. Attenuated increments in sympathetic neural activity largely bring about the syndrome of hypoglycemia unawareness.
- The concept of hypoglycemia-associated autonomic failure (HAAF) in diabetes posits that recent antecedent hypoglycemia, as well as prior exercise or sleep, causes both defective glucose counter-regulation and hypoglycemia unawareness by attenuating the sympathoadrenal response to subsequent hypoglycemia.
- Hypoglycemia unawareness and, in part, the reduced epinephrine component of defective glucose counter-regulation are reversible in 2–3 weeks with scrupulous avoidance of hypoglycemia in most affected patients.
- The risk factors for hypoglycemia, based on this pathophysiology, include relative as well as absolute therapeutic insulin excess, and factors indicative of HAAF which include absolute endogenous insulin deficiency, a history of severe hypoglycemia, hypoglycemia unawareness, or both as well as prior exercise or sleep, and aggressive glycemic therapy per se.
- This pathophysiology explains why the incidence of iatrogenic hypoglycemia increases over time in T2DM, approaching that in T1DM. Most episodes of hypoglycemia occur in people with T2DM.
- Minimizing the risk of iatrogenic hypoglycemia requires acknowledging the problem, applying the principles of aggressive glycemic therapy and considering the risk factors for relative as well as absolute therapeutic insulin excess and for HAAF.
- Maintenance of the greatest degree of glycemic control that can be accomplished safely in a given patient at a given stage of that individual's diabetes is in the patient's best interest. Concerns about hypoglycemia should not be an excuse for poor glycemic control.

Overview of the clinical problem

Iatrogenic hypoglycemia is the most important limiting factor in the glycemic management of diabetes [1,2]. It causes recurrent morbidity in most people with type 1 diabetes mellitus (T1DM) and many with advanced type 2 diabetes mellitus (T2DM), and is sometimes fatal. It compromises physiologic and behavioral defenses against subsequent falling plasma glucose concentrations and thus causes a vicious cycle of recurrent hypoglycemia. It precludes maintenance of euglycemia over a lifetime of diabetes and thus full realization of the vascular benefits of glycemic control.

Hypoglycemia in diabetes is fundamentally iatrogenic, the result of pharmacokinetically imperfect treatments with an insulin secretagogue (e.g. a sulfonylurea or a glinide) or with exogenous insulin that results in episodes of hyperinsulinemia. Nonetheless, hypoglycemia is typically the result of the interplay of relative or absolute therapeutic insulin excess and comprised physiologic and behavioral defenses against falling plasma glucose concentrations [1,2].

The problem of hypoglycemia in diabetes has been summarized [1] and reviewed in detail [2]. My premise is that understanding of the pathophysiology of glucose counter-regulation, the mechanisms that normally prevent or rapidly correct hypoglycemia, leads to insight into the frequency of, risk factors for and prevention of iatrogenic hypoglycemia. Therefore, the physiology of glucose counter-regulation and its pathophysiology in diabetes are addressed first, followed by a summary of the magnitude of the clinical problem. With that background, a clinical approach to the prevention of iatrogenic hypoglycemia, and if necessary its treatment, is discussed.

Textbook of Diabetes, 4th edition. Edited by R. Holt, C. Cockram, A. Flyvbjerg and B. Goldstein.

Physiology of glucose counter-regulation

Hypoglycemia and the brain

Glucose is an obligate oxidative fuel for the brain under physiologic conditions [1–4]. The brain accounts for more than 50% of whole body glucose utilization. Because it cannot synthesize glucose, utilize physiologic concentrations of circulating non-glucose fuels effectively or store more than a few minutes supply as glycogen [1,2], the brain requires a virtually continuous supply of glucose from the circulation. Because facilitated blood–brain glucose transport is a direct function of the arterial plasma glucose concentration, that requires maintenance of the physiologic plasma glucose concentration. Hypoglycemia causes functional brain failure, which is typically reversed after the plasma glucose concentration is raised [4]. Rarely, profound prolonged hypoglycemic causes brain death [4].

Responses to hypoglycemia

Falling plasma glucose concentrations cause a sequence of responses in individuals without diabetes (Table 33.1) [1,5–8]. The first physiologic response, which occurs as plasma glucose concentrations decline within the postabsorptive plasma glucose concentration range, is a decrease in insulin secretion. The secretion of glucose counter-regulatory (plasma glucose raising) hormones, including glucagon and epinephrine, increases as plasma glucose concentrations fall just below the physiologic range. Lower plasma glucose levels cause a more intense sympathoadrenal – sympathetic neural as well as adrenomedullary – response and symptoms. Even lower plasma glucose concentrations cause functional brain failure [4].

Clinical manifestations of hypoglycemia

The symptoms and signs of hypoglycemia are not specific [8,9]. Thus, clinical hypoglycemia is most convincingly documented by Whipple's triad: symptoms, signs, or both, consistent with hypoglycemia; a low measured plasma glucose concentration; and resolution of those symptoms and signs after the plasma glucose concentration is raised.

Neuroglycopenic symptoms, which are the result of brain glucose deprivation per se, include cognitive impairments, behavioral changes and psychomotor abnormalities and, at lower plasma glucose concentrations, seizure and coma [1,2,4,8,9]. Neurogenic (or autonomic) symptoms, which are largely the result of the perception of physiologic changes caused by the sympathoadrenal – particularly the sympathetic neural [9] – discharge triggered by hypoglycemia, include both adrenergic (e.g. palpitations, tremulousness and anxiety/arousal) and cholinergic (e.g. sweating, hunger and paresthesias) symptoms [8]. Central mechanisms may also be involved in some of the latter symptoms such as hunger [10]. Awareness of hypoglycemia is largely the result of the perception of neurogenic symptoms [8].

Signs of hypoglycemia include pallor and diaphoresis, the result of adrenergic cutaneous vasoconstriction and cholinergic activation of sweat glands, respectively [1,2]. Neuroglycopenic manifestations are often observable.

Table 33.1 Physiologic responses to decreasing plasma glucose concentrations.

Response	Glycemic threshold* (mg/dL [mmol/L])	Physiologic effects	Role in prevention or correction of hypoglycemia (glucose counter-regulation)
↓ Insulin	80–85 [4.4–4.7]	↑R_a (↓R_d)	Primary glucose regulatory factor, first defense against hypoglycemia
↑ Glucagon	65–70 [3.6–3.9]	↑R_a	Primary glucose counter-regulatory factor, second defense against hypoglycemia
↑ Epinephrine	65–70 [3.6–3.9]	↑R_a, ↓R_d	Involved, critical when glucagon is deficient, third defense against hypoglycemia
↑ Cortisol and growth hormone	65–70 [3.6–3.9]	↑R_a, ↓R_d	Involved but not critical
Symptoms	50–55 [2.8–3.1]	↑ Exogenous glucose	Prompt behavioral defense (food ingestion)
↓ Cognition	<50 [<2.8]	–	Compromises behavioral defense

R_a, rate of glucose appearance, glucose production by the liver and kidneys; R_d, rate of glucose disappearance, glucose utilization by insulin-sensitive tissues such as skeletal muscle (no direct effect on central nervous system glucose utilization).
*Arterialized venous, not venous, plasma glucose concentrations.
Reproduced from Cryer PE. Glucose homeostasis and hypoglycemia. In: Kronenberg HM, Melmed S, Polonsky KS, Larsen PR, eds. *Williams Textbook of Endocrinology*, 11th edn. Philadelphia: Saunders, 2008: 1503–1533, with permission.

Maintenance of systemic glucose balance

Because obligatory glucose utilization, largely by the brain, is fixed and exogenous glucose delivery from ingested carbohydrates is intermittent, systemic glucose balance is maintained, and hypoglycemia (as well as hyperglycemia) is prevented, by dynamic regulation of endogenous glucose production from the liver (and the kidneys) and of glucose utilization by non-neural tissues such as muscle [1,11]. Although an array of hormones, neurotransmitters and metabolic substrates are involved, endogenous glucose production and glucose utilization by non-neural tissues are regulated primarily by insulin (Figure 33.1; Table 33.1) [11].

The first physiologic defense against hypoglycemia is a decrease in pancreatic islet β-cell insulin secretion. That occurs as plasma glucose concentrations decline within the physiologic range (Table 33.1) and favors increased hepatic (and renal) glucose production with virtual cessation of glucose utilization by insu-

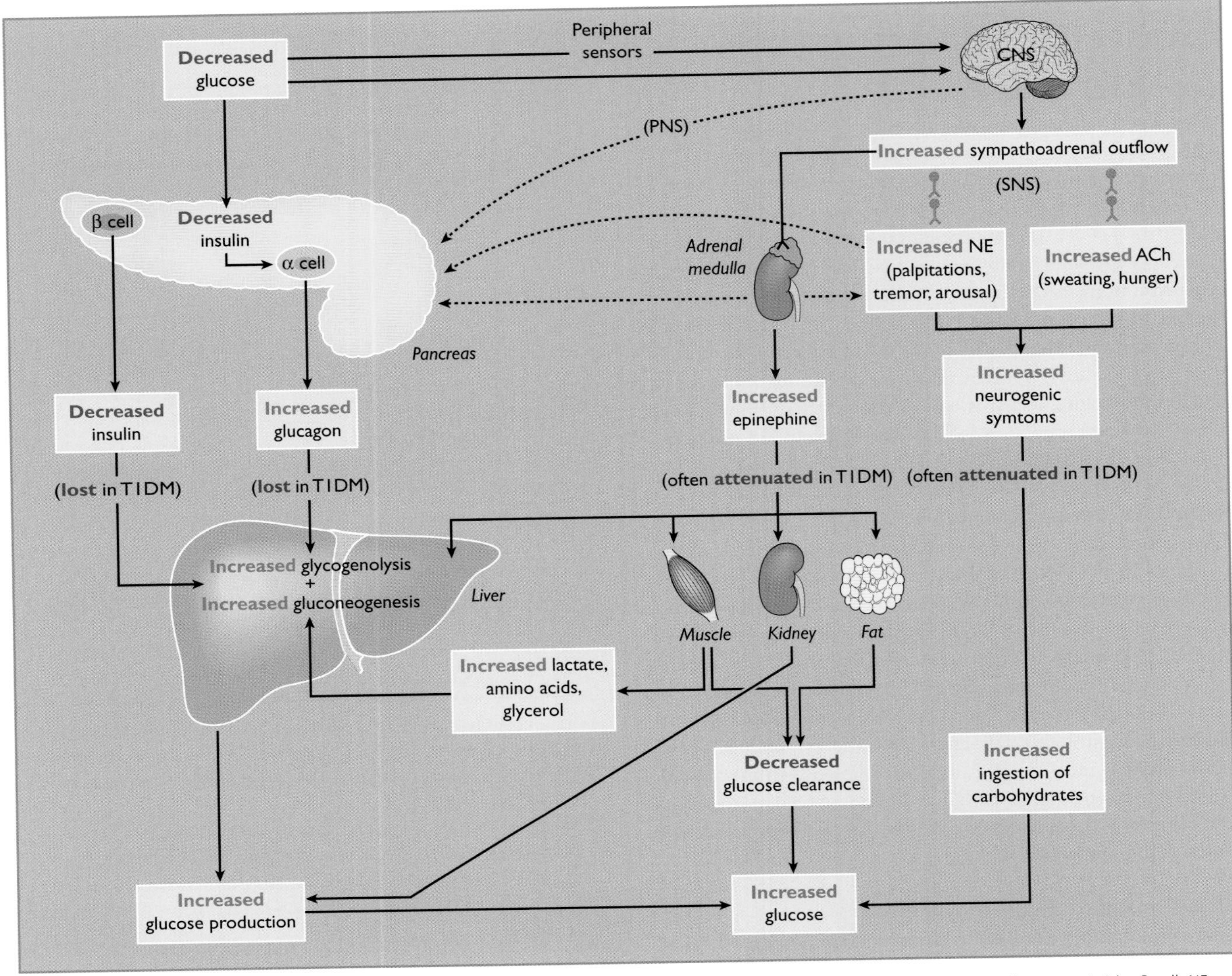

Figure 33.1 Physiologic and behavioral defenses against hypoglycemia in humans. ACh, acetylcholine; α-cell, pancreatic islet α-cell; β-cell, pancreatic islet β-cell; NE, norepinephrine; PNS, parasympathetic nervous system; SNS, sympathetic nervous system; T1DM, type 1 diabetes mellitus. Reproduced from Cryer PE. Mechanisms of sympathoadrenal failure and hypoglycemia in diabetes. *J Clin Invest* 2006; **116**:1470–1473, with permission from the American Society for Clinical Investigation.

lin-sensitive tissues such as muscle (Figure 33.1). The second physiologic defense is an increase in pancreatic islet α-cell glucagon secretion. That occurs as plasma glucose concentrations fall just below the physiologic range (Table 33.1) and stimulates hepatic glucose production (largely by stimulating glycogenolysis) (Figure 33.1). Increased glucagon secretion is signaled primarily by a decrease in intra-islet insulin, perhaps among other β-cell secretory products, in the setting of low glucose concentrations [1,2,12] and secondarily by increased autonomic nervous system – sympathetic, parasympathetic and adrenomedullary – inputs [1,2,13]. The third physiologic defense, which becomes critical when glucagon is deficient, is an increase in adrenomedullary epinephrine secretion [1,2,11]. That, too, occurs as plasma glucose concentrations fall just below the physiologic range (Table 33.1). It raises plasma glucose concentrations largely by β_2-adrenergic stimulation of hepatic (and renal) glucose production (Figure 33.1), but the glucose-raising actions of epinephrine also involve limitation of glucose clearance by insulin sensitive tissues, mobilization of gluconeogenic substrates such as lactate and amino acids from muscle and glycerol from fat and α_2-adrenergic limitation of insulin secretion [1,2,14]. Sympathoadrenal activity, including epinephrine secretion, is regulated in the brain [1,2,11]. Circulating epinephrine is almost exclusively derived from the adrenal medulle [9]; while circulating norepinephrine is largely derived from sympathetic nerves under resting and many stimulated (e.g. exercise) conditions, the plasma norepinephrine response to hypoglycemia is also largely adrenomedullary in origin [9].

Table 33.2 Responses to falling plasma glucose concentrations in humans.

Plasma glucose	Individuals	Plasma		
		Insulin	Glucagon	Epinephrine
↓	Non-diabetic	↓	↑	↑
↓	T1DM*	No ↓	No ↑	Attenuated ↑
↓	Early T2DM	↓	↑	↑
↓	Late T2DM*	No ↓	No ↑	Attenuated ↑

*These alterations account for the appearance of defective glucose counter-regulation and hypoglycemia unawareness in T1DM and late T2DM.

If these physiologic defenses fail to abort an episode of developing hypoglycemia, lower plasma glucose concentrations cause a more intense sympathoadrenal response that causes neurogenic symptoms (Figure 33.1) [1,2,11]. Those symptoms cause awareness of hypoglycemia that prompts the behavioral defense of ingestion of carbohydrates [1,2,11].

All of these defenses against hypoglycemia, not just insulin secretion, are typically compromised in people with T1DM and those with advanced (i.e. absolutely endogenous insulin deficient) T2DM (Figure 33.1) [1,2].

Pathophysiology of glucose counter-regulation in diabetes

Insulin excess

While substantial insulin excess alone can cause hypoglycemia, the integrity of the defenses against falling plasma glucose concentrations determines whether a typical episode of therapeutic hyperinsulinemia results in clinical hypoglycemia [1,2]. Thus, iatrogenic hypoglycemia is typically the result of the interplay of relative or absolute therapeutic hyperinsulinemia and compromised physiologic and behavioral defenses against falling plasma glucose concentrations (Figure 33.1; Table 33.2) [1,2,15,16].

Defective glucose counter-regulation and hypoglycemia unawareness

In fully developed (i.e. C peptide negative) T1DM circulating insulin concentrations cannot decrease as plasma glucose concentrations fall in response to therapeutic (exogenous) hyperinsulinemia (Table 33.2) [1,2,15]. That is the result of β-cell failure which also causes loss of the increase in circulating glucagon concentrations (Figure 33.2; Table 33.2) [1,2,12,15]. The latter conclusion is based on the finding that indirect reciprocal β-cell-mediated signaling normally predominates over direct α-cell signaling in the regulation of glucagon secretion in humans [1,2,12]. Thus, the absence of a decrease in intra-islet insulin, perhaps among other β-cell secretory products, in concert with low glucose levels, plausibly explains loss of the glucagon response [1,2,12]. Therefore, both the first and second physiologic defenses against hypoglycemia are lost. Furthermore, the increase in circulating epinephrine, the third physiologic defense, is typically attenuated (Figure 33.2; Table 33.2) [1,15]. In the setting of absent insulin and glucagon responses, the attenuated epinephrine response causes the clinical syndrome of defective glucose counter-regulation (Table 33.2) [1,2,15,17,18] which is associated with a 25-fold [17] or greater [18] increased risk of severe iatrogenic hypoglycemia in T1DM. In addition, the attenuated epinephrine response is a marker for an attenuated sympathoadrenal, including sympathetic neural, response (Table 33.2) which is largely responsible for reduced neurogenic symptom responses and therefore the clinical syndrome of hypoglycemia unawareness [1,2,9] which is associated with a sixfold increased risk of severe iatrogenic hypoglycemia in T1DM [19]. Attenuated sympathoadrenal responses to falling plasma glucose concentrations can be caused by recent antecedent hypoglycemia (Figures 33.3 and 33.4) [1,2,15,16,20], prior exercise [1,2,21–23] or sleep [1,2,24–26].

While hypoglycemia unawareness is largely the result of reduced release of the neurotransmitters norepinephrine and acetylcholine [1,9], there is evidence of decreased β-adrenergic sensitivity, specifically reduced cardiac chronotropic sensitivity to isoproterenol, in affected patients [27,28]. However, vascular sensitivity to β_2-adrenergic agonism was not found to be reduced in patients with unawareness [29], reduced sensitivity to β-adrenergic signaling of neurogenic symptoms remains to be demonstrated in patients with unawareness and it would be necessary to postulate decreased cholinergic sensitivity as well to explain reduced cholinergic symptoms such as sweating.

The pathophysiology of glucose counterregulation is the same in T1DM and advanced (i.e. absolutely endogenous insulin deficient) T2DM, albeit with different time courses (Table 33.2) [1,2,15,16]. The pathogenesis of an episode of iatrogenic hypoglycemia involves therapeutic hyperinsulinemia resulting in falling plasma glucose concentrations and loss of the appropriate decrements in insulin and increments in glucagon. The hypoglycemia, in turn, reduces the sympathoadrenal responses to subsequent hypoglycemia. Because β-cell failure, which causes loss of both the insulin and the glucagon responses [1,2,15,16], occurs rapidly in T1DM but slowly in T2DM, the syndromes of defective glucose counterregulation and hypoglycemia unawareness develop early in T1DM but later in T2DM. This temporal pattern of compromised glycemic defenses explains why iatrogenic hypoglycemia becomes progressively more frequent as patients approach the insulin deficient end of the spectrum of T2DM as discussed later in this chapter.

Hypoglycemia-associated autonomic failure

The concept of hypoglycemia-associated autonomic failure (HAAF) in diabetes posits that recent antecedent hypoglycemia (Figures 33.3 and 33.4) [1,2,15,16,20] – as well as prior exercise [1,2,21–23] or sleep [1,2,24–26] – causes both defective glucose counter-regulation (by attenuating the epinephrine responses to subsequent hypoglycemia in the setting of absent decrements in

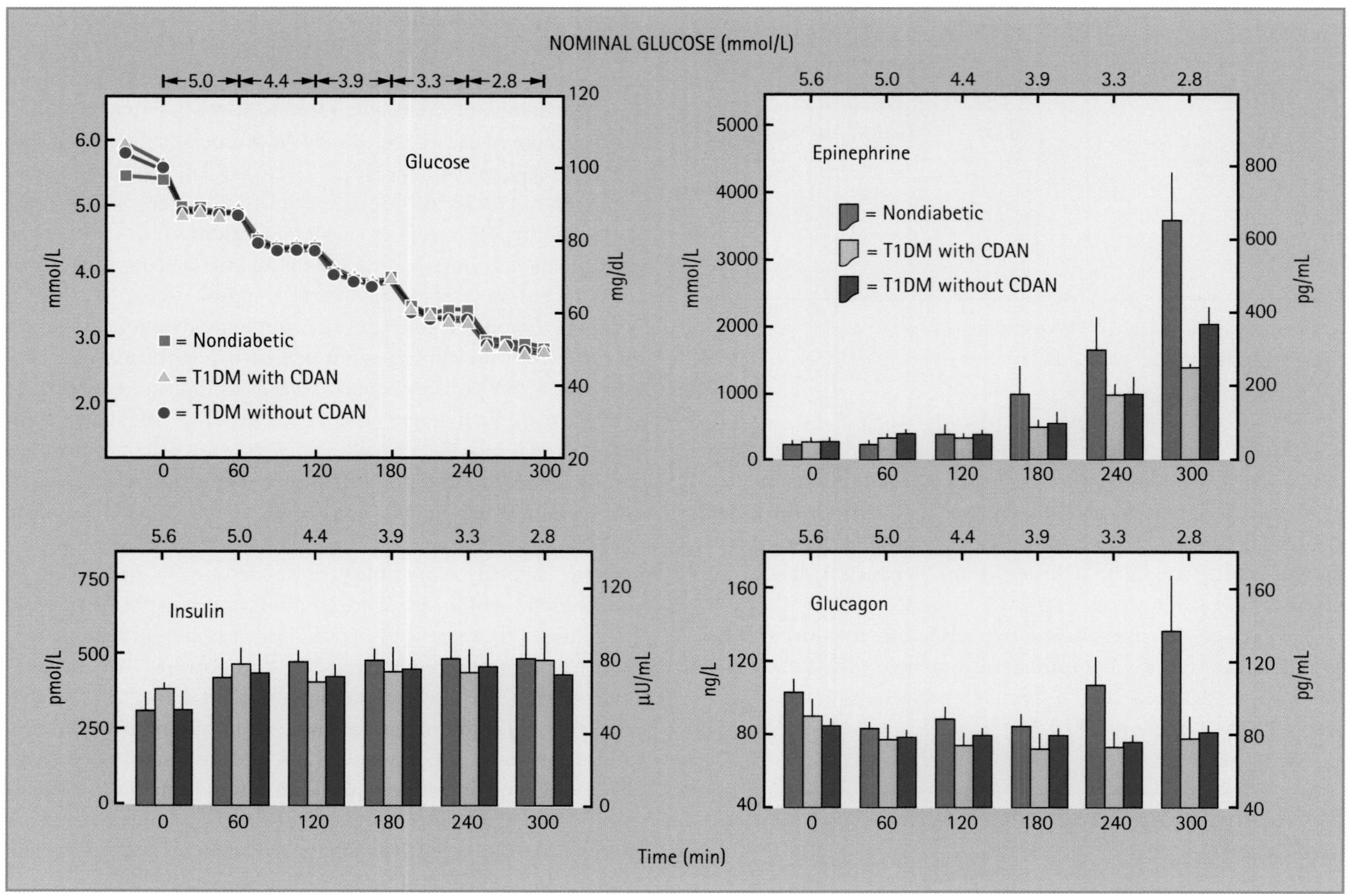

Figure 33.2 Mean (± SE) plasma glucose, insulin, epinephrine and glucagon concentrations during hyperinsulinemic stepped hypoglycemic glucose clamps in individuals without diabetes (red squares and columns), people with type 1 diabetes (T1DM, insulin-dependent diabetes mellitus) with classic diabetic autonomic neuropathy (CDAN) (yellow triangles and columns) and people with type 1 diabetes without CDAN (blue circles and columns). Reproduced from Dagogo-Jack *et al.* [15] with permission from the American Society for Clinical Investigation.

insulin and absent increments in glucagon) and hypoglycemia unawareness (by attenuating the sympathoadrenal, including the sympathetic neural, and resulting neurogenic symptom responses to subsequent hypoglycemia). It therefore leads to a vicious cycle of recurrent iatrogenic hypoglycemia (Figure 33.5). Thus, HAAF is, at least in large part, a dynamic functional disorder that is distinct from classic diabetic autonomic neuropathy [1,2]. Nonetheless, the key feature of HAAF, an attenuated sympathoadrenal response to a given level of hypoglycemia, is more prominent in patients with diabetic autonomic neuropathy (Figure 33.2) [30,31].

The clinical impact of HAAF is well established in T1DM [1,2,15,32–37]. Recent antecedent hypoglycemia, even asymptomatic nocturnal hypoglycemia, reduces epinephrine, symptomatic and cognitive dysfunction responses to a given level of subsequent hypoglycemia [32], reduces detection of hypoglycemia in the clinical setting [33] and reduces defense against hyperinsulinemia [15] in T1DM. Perhaps the most compelling support for the concept of HAAF is the finding, initially by three independent research teams [34–37], that as little as 2–3 weeks of scrupulous avoidance of hypoglycemia reverses hypoglycemia unawareness (Figure 33.6) and improves the attenuated epinephrine component of defective glucose counter-regulation in most affected patients.

People with advanced T2DM are also at risk for HAAF [1,2,16]. Glucagon responses to hypoglycemia are lost [16], as they are in T1DM. Furthermore, the glycemic thresholds for sympathoadrenal and symptomatic (among other) responses to hypoglycemia are shifted to lower plasma glucose concentrations by recent antecedent hypoglycemia [16], as they are in T1DM.

The three recognized causes of HAAF each cause attenuated sympathoadrenal and symptomatic (among other) responses to a given level of hypoglycemia [1,2]. Antecedent hypoglycemia-related HAAF [1,2,15,16,20] led to the concept. Exercise-related HAAF [1,2,21–23] is exemplified by late post-exercise hypoglycemia which typically occurs 6–15 hours after strenuous exercise and is often nocturnal [38,39]. Sleep-related HAAF [1,2,24–26] is the result of further attenuation of the sympathoadrenal response to hypoglycemia during sleep. Sleeping patients are

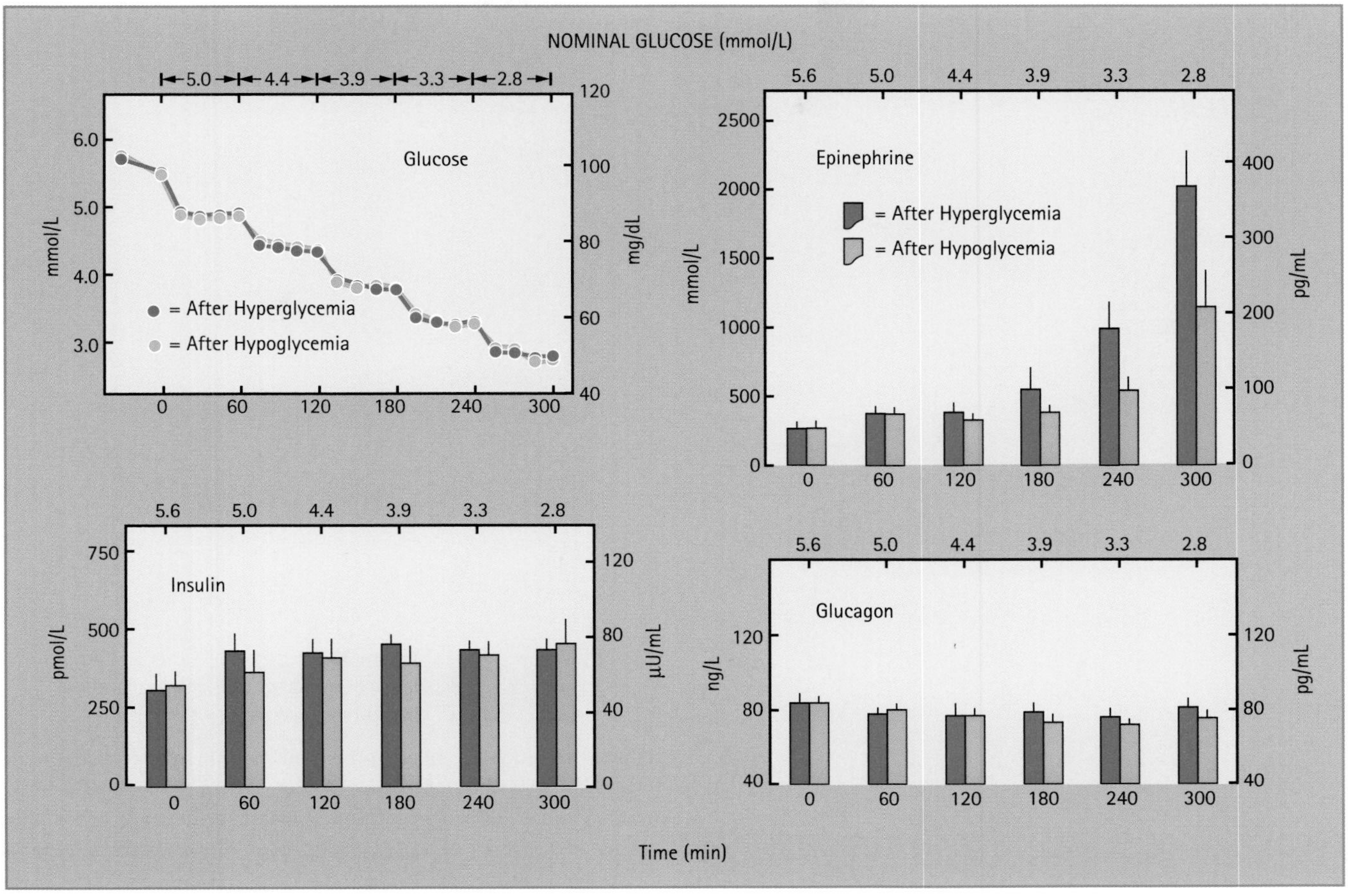

Figure 33.3 Mean (± SE) plasma glucose, insulin, epinephrine and glucagon concentrations during hyperinsulinemic stepped hypoglycemic glucose clamps in patients with type 1 diabetes without classic diabetic autonomic neuropathy on mornings following afternoon hyperglycemia (red circles and columns) and on mornings following afternoon hypoglycemia (yellow circles and columns). From Dagogo-Jack *et al.* [15] with permission from the American Society for Clinical Investigation.

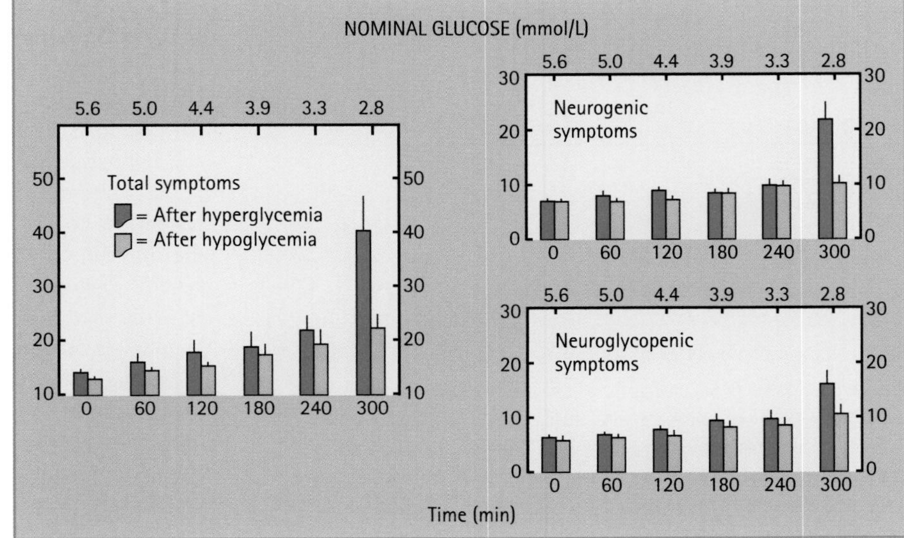

Figure 33.4 Mean (± SE) total, neurogenic and neuroglycopenic symptom scores during hyperinsulinemic stepped hypoglycemic clamps in patients with type 1 diabetes without classic diabetic autonomic neuropathy on mornings following afternoon hyperglycemia (red columns) and on mornings following afternoon hypoglycemia (yellow columns). Reproduced from Dagogo-Jack *et al.* [15] with permission from the American Society for Clinical Investigation.

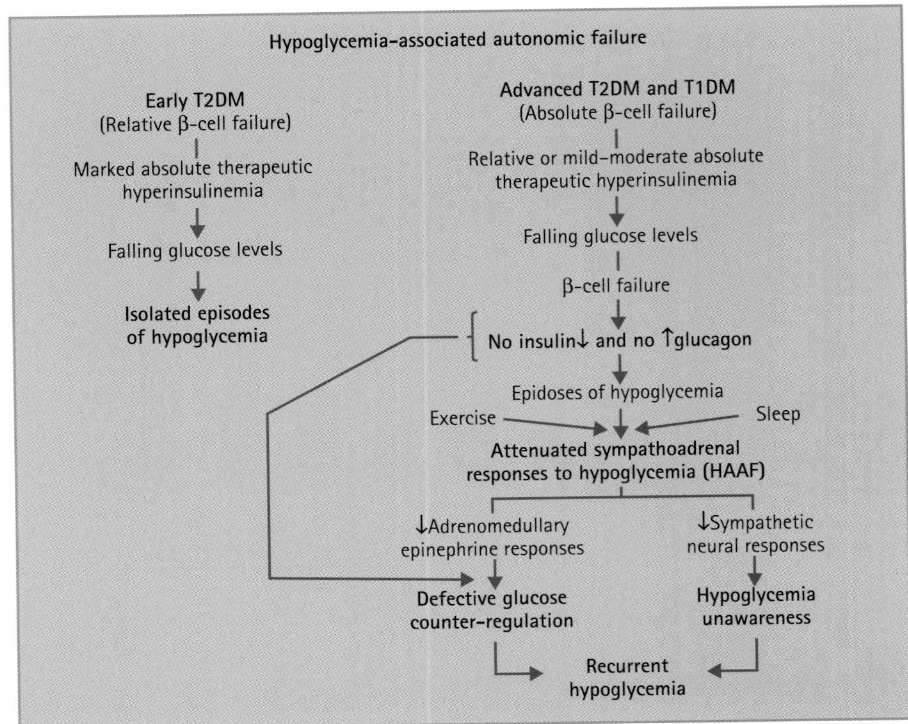

Figure 33.5 Hypoglycemia-associated autonomic failure (HAAF) in the pathogenesis of iatrogenic hypoglycemia in diabetes.

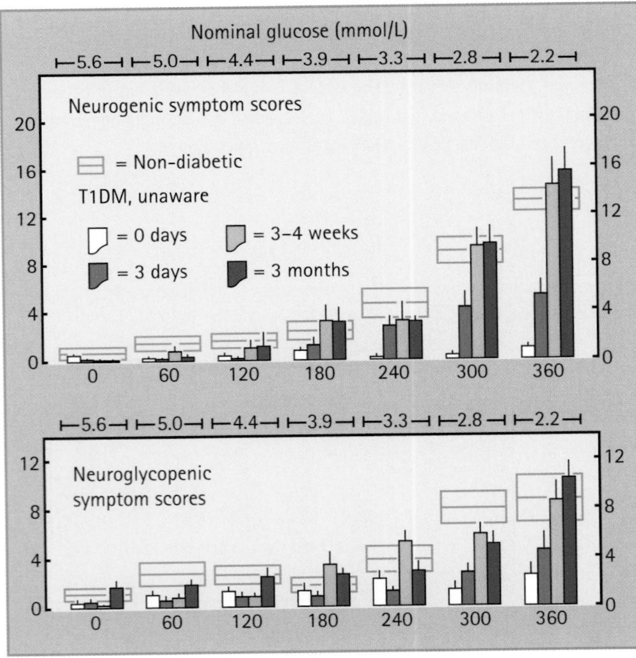

Figure 33.6 Mean (± SE) neurogenic and neuroglycopenic symptom scores during hyperinsulinemic stepped hypoglycemic clamps in individuals without diabetes (open rectangles) and in patients with T1DM (columns) at baseline (0 days), after 3 days of inpatient strict avoidance of hypoglycemia and after 3–4 weeks and 3 months of outpatient scrupulous avoidance of hypoglycemia. From Dagogo-Jack *et al.* [37] with permission from the American Diabetes Association.

therefore much less likely to be awakened by hypoglycemia than individuals without diabetes [25,26]. There may well be additional, as yet unrecognized, functional, and therefore potentially reversible, causes of HAAF [1,2]. In addition, there may be a structural component [1,2].

The mechanisms of HAAF are summarized in Figure 33.7 [1,2]. Loss of the insulin and glucagon responses to falling plasma glucose concentrations caused by therapeutic hyperinsulinemia is the result of β-cell failure in T1DM and advanced T2DM. Because normal insulin and glucagon responses to low glucose concentrations occur in patients with a transplanted (i.e. denervated) pancreas [40] and in dogs with a denervated pancreas [41] – as well as from the perfused pancreas and perifused pancreatic islets – innervation is not required.

In the setting of absent insulin and glucagon responses to falling plasma glucose concentrations, attenuated sympathoadrenal responses cause both defective glucose counter-regulation and hypoglycemia unawareness, the two components of HAAF [1,2]. The mechanism of the attenuated sympathoadrenal response is not known, but it must be at the level of the brain (or the afferent or efferent components of the sympathoadrenal system) (Figure 33.7). The proposed mechanisms include the systemic mediator, brain fuel transport and brain metabolism hypotheses, all of which have been reviewed [1,2,42,43].

Much of the research into the pathogenesis of HAAF has focused on the hypothalamus, the central integrator of the sympathoadrenal responses to hypoglycemia [43]. While the primary alteration could reside in the hypothalamus, the changes in hypothalamic function could be secondary to those in other brain regions. For example, measurements of regional cerebral blood

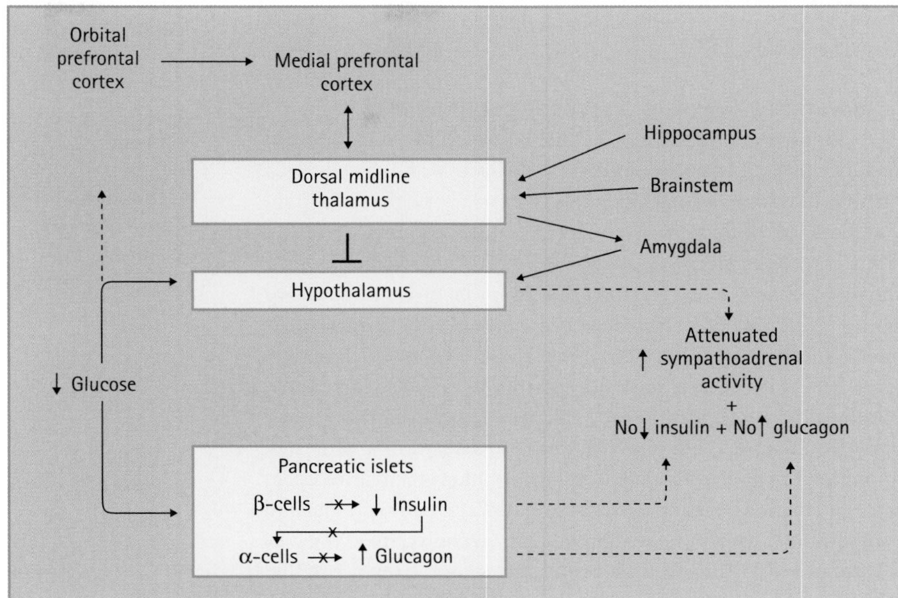

Figure 33.7 Pancreatic islet, hypothalamic and cerebral network mechanisms of hypoglycemia-associated autonomic failure (HAAF) in diabetes. Reproduced from Cryer [1] with permission from the American Diabetes Association.

flow with [^{15}O] water and positron emission tomography (PET) [44] indicate that hypoglycemia activates widespread but interconnected brain regions, including the medial prefrontal cortex, the lateral orbitofrontal cortex, the thalamus, the globus pallidus and the periaqueductal gray. These studies also show that recent antecedent hypoglycemia both reduces the sympathoadrenal and symptomatic responses (a model of HAAF) and causes a greater increase in synaptic activity in the dorsal midline thalamus during subsequent hypoglycemia [45]. Thus, it has been suggested that there may be a cerebral network that results in thalamic inhibition of hypothalamic activity in HAAF (Figure 33.7) [45]. That suggestion is generically consistent with the findings of various patterns of [^{18}F] deoxyglucose uptake in T1DM patients with and without hypoglycemia unawareness [46].

Table 33.3 Risk factors for hypoglycemia in diabetes.

Relative or absolute insulin excess
1. Insulin or insulin secretagogue doses are excessive, ill-timed or of the wrong type
2. Exogenous glucose delivery is decreased (e.g. following missed meals and during the overnight fast)
3. Glucose utilization is increased (e.g. during and shortly after exercise)
4. Endogenous glucose production is decreased (e.g. following alcohol ingestion)
5. Sensitivity to insulin is increased (e.g. in the middle of the night and following weight loss or improved glycemic control)
6. Insulin clearance is decreased (e.g. with renal failure)

Hypoglycemia-associated autonomic failure
1. Absolute endogenous insulin deficiency
2. A history of severe hypoglycemia, hypoglycemia unawareness, or both as well as recent antecedent hypoglycemia, prior exercise and sleep
3. Aggressive glycemic therapy per se (lower HbA_{1c} levels, lower glycemic goals)

Risk factors for hypoglycemia in diabetes

The risk factors for hypoglycemia in diabetes follow directly from the pathophysiology of glucose counter-regulation and are based on the principle that iatrogenic hypoglycemia is typically the result of the interplay of relative or absolute therapeutic insulin excess and compromised physiologic and behavioral defenses against falling plasma glucose concentrations (i.e. HAAF) in T1DM and advanced T2DM [1,2,47].

Absolute or relative insulin excess

The conventional risk factors for hypoglycemia in diabetes are based on the premise that absolute or relative therapeutic insulin excess is the sole determinant of risk (Table 33.3) [1,2,47]. Absolute therapeutic insulin excess occurs when insulin secretagogue or insulin doses are excessive, ill-timed or of the wrong type, or when insulin clearance is reduced as in renal failure. Relative therapeutic insulin excess occurs under a variety of conditions. It occurs when exogenous glucose delivery is decreased (as following missed or low carbohydrate meals and during the overnight fast), when glucose utilization is increased (as during and shortly after exercise), when endogenous glucose production is decreased (as following alcohol ingestion) and when sensitivity to insulin is increased (as following weight loss or improved glycemic control and in the middle of the night). People with diabetes and their caregivers must consider each of these risk factors when the problem of iatrogenic hypoglycemia is recognized. Overall, however, they explain only a minority of episodes of hypoglycemia [48].

Compromised defenses against hypoglycemia

The risk factors indicative of HAAF (Table 33.3) [1,2,47,49–55] include absolute endogenous insulin deficiency [1,2,47,49–53], a history of severe iatrogenic hypoglycemia, hypoglycemia unawareness, or both as well as recent antecedent hypoglycemia, prior exercise or sleep [1,2,47,50–52,54] and aggressive glycemic therapy per se (i.e. lower HbA_{1c} levels, lower glycemic goals, or both) [1,2,47,50–55]. The degree of endogenous insulin deficiency (i.e. β-cell failure) determines the extent to which insulin levels will not decrease and glucagon levels will not increase as plasma glucose concentrations fall in response to therapeutic hyperinsulinemia. A history of severe hypoglycemia indicates, and that of hypoglycemia unawareness implies, recent antecedent hypoglycemia. The latter causes attenuated sympathoadrenal and symptomatic responses to subsequent hypoglycemia, the key feature of HAAF. In addition, prior exercise and sleep cause that feature of HAAF. Studies of intensive glycemic therapy with a control group treated to a higher HbA_{1c} level consistently report higher rates of hypoglycemia in the group treated to lower HbA_{1c} levels in T1DM [56–58] and T2DM [54,59,60]. That does not mean that one cannot both improve glycemic control and minimize the risk of hypoglycemia [1,2,47] as discussed below.

Magnitude of the clinical problem of hypoglycemia in diabetes

Diabetes is an increasingly common disease. It has been estimated that its prevalence will rise from 285 million people in the year 2009 to 435 million people by the year 2030 [61]. Iatrogenic hypoglycemia affects most of the minority with T1DM and many of the majority with T2DM [1,2]. Indeed, because it precludes maintenance of euglycemia over a lifetime of diabetes, the barrier of hypoglycemia ultimately affects all people with diabetes [1,2].

Frequency of hypoglycemia

Hypoglycemia is a fact of life for people with T1DM (Table 33.4) [1,2,55,62,63]. The average patient has untold numbers of episodes of asymptomatic hypoglycemia and experiences two episodes of symptomatic hypoglycemia per week – thousands of such episodes over a lifetime of diabetes – and one or more episodes of severe, temporarily disabling hypoglycemia, often with seizure or coma, per year. There is no evidence that this problem has abated since it was highlighted by the report of the Diabetes Control and Complications Trial (DCCT) in 1993 [56]. For example, in 2007 the UK Hypoglycemia Study Group [63] reported an incidence of severe hypoglycemia that was twice that in the DCCT in patients with T1DM for <5 years and an incidence fivefold higher than that in the DCCT in those with T1DM for >15 years (Table 33.4). An incidence comparable to the latter was also found in a large observational study [55].

Table 33.4 Event rates for severe hypoglycemia (that requiring the assistance of another person), expressed as episodes per 100 patient-years, in insulin-treated diabetes [2].

Citation	n	Event rate	Comment
Type 1 diabetes			
UK Hypoglycemia Study Group [63]	57*	320	Prospective multicenter study
	50†	110	
MacLeod *et al.* [64]	544	170	Retrospective clinic survey, randomly selected sample
Donnelly *et al.* [65]	94	115	Prospective study, population-based random sample
Reichard & Pihl [66]	48	110	Clinical trial, intensive insulin group
DCCT Research Group [67]	711	62	Clinical trial, intensive insulin group
Type 2 diabetes			
MacLeod *et al.* [64]	56	73	Retrospective clinic survey, randomly selected sample
UK Hypoglycemia Study Group [63]	77‡	70	Prospective multicenter study
	89§	10	
Akram *et al.* [69]	401	44	Retrospective clinic survey
Donnelly *et al.* [65]	173	35	Prospective study, population-based random sample
Henderson *et al.* [70]	215	28	Retrospective clinic survey, randomly selected sample
Murata *et al.* [71]	344	21	Prospective study, random Veterans Affairs sample
Saudek *et al.* [72]	62	18¶	Clinical trial, multiple insulin injection group
Gürlek *et al.* [73]	114	15	Retrospective clinic survey
Abraira *et al.* [74]	75	3	Clinical trial, intensive insulin group
Yki-Järvinen *et al.* [75]	88	0	Clinical trial, initial insulin therapy
Ohkubo *et al.* [76]	52	0	Clinical trial, initial insulin therapy

* Insulin treatment for >15 years.
† Insulin treatment for <5 years.
‡ Insulin treatment for >5 years.
§ Insulin treatment for <2 years.
¶ Definite (8 per 100 patient-years) plus suspected (10 per 100 patient-years).
Reproduced from Cryer PE, Axelrod L, Grossman AB, Heller SR, Montori VM, Seaquist ER, Service FJ. Evaluation and management of adult hypoglycemic disorders: an Endocrine Society clinical practice guideline. *J Clin Endocrinol Metab* 2009, with permission from the Endocrine Society.

Overall, hypoglycemia is less frequent in T2DM (Table 33.4) [1,2,55,63–80], but for the pathophysiologic reasons discussed, hypoglycemia becomes progressively more frequent as patients approach the insulin deficient end of the spectrum of T2DM [1,2,63,78]. Indeed, its frequency has been reported to be similar in those with T2DM and T1DM matched for duration of insulin therapy [78]. When the UK Hypoglycemia Study Group [63] contrasted patients with T2DM treated with insulin for <2 years with those treated with insulin for >5 years they found severe hypoglycemia prevalences of 7% and 25% and incidences of 10 and 70 episodes per 100 patient-years, respectively. The pattern for self-treated hypoglycemia was similar [63]. Thus, while the incidence of iatrogenic hypoglycemia is relatively low (with current less than euglycemic goals) in the first few years of insulin treatment of T2DM, the risk increases substantially, approaching that in T1DM, in advanced of T2DM.

Because asymptomatic episodes will almost invariably be missed, symptomatic episodes may not be recognized as the result of hypoglycemia [81] and, even if they are, they are not long remembered [82,83], estimates of the frequency of iatrogenic hypoglycemia are underestimates. Although they represent only a small fraction of the total hypoglycemic experience, because they are dramatic events that are more likely to be reported (by the patient or an associate) [82,83], estimates of the frequency of severe hypoglycemia, requiring the assistance of another person, are more reliable, particularly if they are determined in population-based prospective studies that include a focus on hypoglycemia [1,2].

The prospective population-based data of Donnelly *et al.* [65] indicate that the overall incidence of hypoglycemia in insulin treated T2DM is approximately one-third of that in T1DM (Table 33.4). The incidence of any and of severe hypoglycemia was approximately 4300 and 115 episodes per 100 patient-years, respectively, in T1DM and approximately 1600 and 35 episodes per 100 patient-years, respectively, in insulin-treated T2DM. In addition, in population-based studies the incidence of severe hypoglycemia requiring emergency treatment in insulin-treated T2DM was approximately 40% [79] and approximately 100% [80] of that in T1DM. Because the prevalence of T2DM is approximately 20-fold greater than that of T1DM, and most people with T2DM ultimately require treatment with insulin, these data suggest that most episodes of iatrogenic hypoglycemia, including severe hypoglycemia, occur in people with T2DM.

Impact of hypoglycemia

Iatrogenic hypoglycemia causes recurrent physical and psychologic morbidity, and some mortality, impairs defenses against subsequent hypoglycemia and precludes maintenance of euglycemia over a lifetime of diabetes [1,2]. In the short-term it causes brain fuel deprivation that, if unchecked, results in functional brain failure that is typically corrected after the plasma glucose concentration is raised [4]. Rarely, it causes sudden, presumably cardiac arrhythmic [84,85], death or, if it is profound and prolonged, brain death [4].

The physical morbidity of an episode of hypoglycemia ranges from unpleasant symptoms to seizure and coma [1,2,4]. It can impair judgment, behavior and performance of physical tasks. Permanent neurologic damage is rare. While there is concern that recurrent hypoglycemia might cause chronic cognitive impairment, long-term follow-up of the DCCT patients is reassuring in that regard [86]. Nonetheless, the possibility that it does so in young children remains [87,88], and there are no corresponding data in the elderly [86]. The psychologic morbidity includes fear of hypoglycemia [89], which can be a barrier to glycemic control.

Three early reports indicated that 2–4% of people with diabetes die from hypoglycemia [90–92]. More recent reports indicated that 6% [86], 7% [93] and 10% [94] of deaths of people with T1DM were the result of hypoglycemia. Similar data are not available for T2DM but mortality rates of up to 10% during episodes of severe sulfonylurea induced hypoglycemia have been reported [95,96].

The cause of excess mortality during intensive glycemic therapy of patients with T2DM in the large Action to Control Cardiovascular Risk in Diabetes (ACCORD) study [60] is not known, and likely will not be known with certainty [1,2]. It could have been chance; excessive mortality during intensive glycemic therapy was not observed in the ADVANCE trial [59] although there was less glycemic separation between the groups. It could have been the result of a non-glycemic effect of the intensive therapy regimen (e.g. an adverse effect of a drug, weight gain or something else). Nonetheless, the most plausible cause of excess mortality during intensive glycemic therapy in ACCORD is hypoglycemia [1,2]:

1 Median glycemia (HbA_{1c}) was lower in the intensive glycemic therapy group.
2 Lower median glycemia is associated with a higher frequency of hypoglycemia in T2DM [59,60,68].
3 Hypoglycemia can be fatal in T2DM [4,84,85,95,96].
4 More patients died in the intensive glycemic therapy group.

Clinical definition and classification of hypoglycemia

The American Diabetes Association (ADA) Workgroup on Hypoglycemia [97] defined hypoglycemia in diabetes as "all episodes of abnormally low plasma glucose concentration that expose the individual to potential harm." It is not possible to state a specific plasma glucose concentration that defines clinical hypoglycemia. Although symptoms typically develop at a plasma glucose concentration of approximately 50–55 mg/dL (2.8–3.1 mmol/L) (Table 33.1) [11] in individuals without diabetes, the glycemic threshold for symptoms (as well as those for glucose counter-regulatory and cognitive dysfunction responses) shift to lower plasma glucose concentrations in people with tightly controlled diabetes and recurrent hypoglycemia [98,99] and to higher plasma glucose concentrations in those with poorly controlled diabetes [98,100].

The ADA Workgroup recommended that people with drug-treated diabetes (implicitly those treated with an insulin secretagogue or insulin) become concerned about the possibility of developing hypoglycemia at a plasma glucose concentration of ≤70 mg/dL (3.9 mmol/L) [97]. Within the error of self-monitoring of blood glucose (or continuous glucose sensing), that conservative alert value approximates the lower limit of the non-diabetic post-absorptive plasma glucose concentration range [11] and the normal glycemic thresholds for activation of physiologic glucose counter-regulatory systems [11], and is low enough to reduce glycemic defenses against subsequent hypoglycemia

Table 33.5 American Diabetes Association Workgroup on Hypoglycemia classification of hypoglycemia in people with diabetes [97].

Severe hypoglycemia
An event requiring assistance of another person to administer actively carbohydrate, glucagon or other resuscitative actions. Plasma glucose measurements may not be available during such an event, but neurologic recovery attributable to the restoration of plasma glucose to normal is considered sufficient evidence that the event was induced by a low plasma glucose concentration

Documented symptomatic hypoglycemia
An event during which typical symptoms of hypoglycemia are accompanied by a measured plasma glucose concentrations ≤70 mg/dL (3.9 mmol/L)

Asymptomatic hypoglycemia
An event not accompanied by typical symptoms of hypoglycemia but with a measured plasma glucose concentration ≤70 mg/dL (3.9 mmol/L)

Probable symptomatic hypoglycemia
An event during which symptoms typical of hypoglycemia are not accompanied by a plasma glucose determination but that was presumably caused by a plasma glucose concentration ≤70 mg/dL (3.9 mmol/L)

Relative hypoglycemia
An event during which the person with diabetes reports any of the typical symptoms of hypoglycemia, and interprets those as indicative of hypoglycemia, with a measured plasma glucose concentration >70 mg/dL (3.9 mmol/L) but approaching that level

[101], in individuals without diabetes. It also generally provides some margin for the relative inaccuracy of glucose monitors at low plasma glucose concentrations [102]. The use of this plasma glucose cutoff value, compared with lower values, will result in higher frequencies of hypoglycemia, and a greater proportion of episodes that are asymptomatic.

The recommended generic alert value does not mean that people with diabetes should always treat for hypoglycemia at an estimated plasma glucose concentration of ≤70 mg/dL (3.9 mmol/L). Rather, it indicates that they should consider actions ranging from repeating the measurement in the near-term through behavioral changes such as avoiding exercise or driving without treatment to carbohydrate ingestion and subsequent regimen adjustments.

The ADA Workgroup also recommended a clinical classification of hypoglycemia (Table 33.5) [97].

Prevention and treatment of hypoglycemia in diabetes

Prevention of hypoglycemia: hypoglycemia risk factor reduction

Iatrogenic hypoglycemia is a barrier to glycemic control in people with diabetes [1,2], but that barrier can be lowered in individual patients with diabetes by the practice of hypoglycemia risk factor reduction (Table 33.6) [1,2,47]. That involves four steps:

Table 33.6 Hypoglycemic risk factor reduction.

1 Acknowledge the problem
2 Apply the principles of aggressive glycemic therapy
- Diabetes self-management (patient education and empowerment)
- Frequent self-monitoring of blood glucose (and in some instances continuous glucose sensing)
- Flexible and appropriate insulin (and other drug) regimens
- Individualized glycemic goals
- Ongoing professional guidance and support

3 Consider the conventional risk factors for hypoglycemia (Table 33.3)
4 Consider the risk factors indicative of hypoglycemia-associated autonomic failure (Table 33.3)

1 Acknowledge the problem;
2 Apply the principles of aggressive glycemic therapy [1,2,47,103–107];
3 Consider the conventional risk factors for hypoglycemia (Table 33.3); and
4 Consider the risk factors for hypoglycemia-associated autonomic failure (HAAF) in diabetes (Table 33.3).

The issue of hypoglycemia should be addressed in every contact with people with diabetes, at least those treated with an insulin secretagogue or with insulin [1,2,47]. Acknowledging the problem allows the caregiver either to move on if hypoglycemia is not an issue or to address it, and keep it in perspective, if hypoglycemia is an issue. Patient concerns about the reality, or even the possibility, of hypoglycemia can be a barrier to glycemic control [108,109]. It is often also helpful to question close associates of the patient because they may have observed clues to episodes of hypoglycemia not recognized by the patient. Even if no concerns are expressed, examination of the self-monitoring of blood glucose records (or continuous glucose sensing data) will often disclose that hypoglycemia is a problem.

If hypoglycemia is an issue, the principles of aggressive glycemic therapy in diabetes [1,2,47,103–107] should be reviewed and applied. Those include diabetes self-management based on patient education and empowerment, frequent self-monitoring of blood glucose (and in some instances continuous glucose sensing), flexible and appropriate insulin (and other drug) regimens, individualized glycemic goals, and ongoing professional guidance and support (Table 33.6).

Patient education and empowerment are fundamentally important. As the therapeutic regimen becomes progressively more complex – early in T1DM and later in T2DM – the success of glycemic management becomes progressively more dependent on the many management decisions and skills of the well-informed person with diabetes. In addition to basic training about diabetes, people with insulin secretagogue or insulin-treated diabetes need to be taught about hypoglycemia [110]. They need to know the common symptoms of hypoglycemia, and their individual most meaningful symptoms, and how to treat (and not overtreat) an episode. Close associates also need to be taught the symptoms and signs of hypoglycemia, and when and how to administer glucagon. Patients need to understand the relevant conventional risk factors for hypoglycemia (Table 33.3) including the effects of the dose and timing of their individual secretagogue or insulin preparation(s) as well as the effects of missed meals and the overnight fast, exercise and alcohol ingestion. They also need to know that episodes of hypoglycemia signal an increased likelihood of future, often more severe, hypoglycemia [50–52,54,110–113]. Finally, patients using an online glucose sensor need to apply those data critically to their attempts to minimize hypoglycemia as well as hyperglycemia.

In patients treated with an insulin secretagogue, and particularly those treated with insulin, frequent self-monitoring of blood glucose becomes progressively more key to diabetes self-management as the therapeutic regimen becomes more complex, early in T1DM and later in T2DM. Ideally, patients should estimate their glucose levels whenever they suspect hypoglycemia. That would not only confirm or deny an episode of hypoglycemia, it would also help the individual learn the key symptoms of their hypoglycemic episodes and might lead to regimen adjustments. It is particularly important for people with hypoglycemia unawareness to monitor their glucose level before performing a critical task such as driving. Self-monitoring of blood glucose provides a glucose estimate only at one point in time; it does not indicate whether glucose levels are falling, stable or rising. That limitation is addressed by evolving technologies for continuous glucose sensing [114–118]. While the utility of such data seems self-evident, critical clinical data on that point are needed.

Flexible and appropriate drug regimens are key components of hypoglycemia risk factor reduction [1,2,47]. Hypoglycemia is typically the result of relative or absolute therapeutic (endogenous or exogenous) insulin excess and compromised defenses against falling plasma glucose concentrations. The relevant treatments include insulin or an insulin secretagogue such as a sulfonylurea (e.g. glibenclamide [glyburide], glipizide, glimepiride and gliclazide) or a glinide (e.g. repaglinide or nateglinide). Early in the course of T2DM, patients may respond to drugs that do not raise insulin levels at low or normal plasma glucose concentrations and therefore should not, and probably do not, cause hypoglycemia [119]. Those include the biguanide metformin, which nonetheless has been reported to cause self-reported hypoglycemia [68,120], thiazolidinediones (e.g. pioglitazone, rosiglitazone), α-glucosidase inhibitors (e.g. acarbose, miglitol), glucagon-like peptide 1 (GLP-1) receptor agonists (e.g. exenatide, liraglutide) and dipeptidyl peptidase 4 (DPP-4) inhibitors (e.g. sitagliptin, vildagliptin). All of these drugs require endogenous insulin secretion to lower plasma glucose concentrations, and insulin secretion declines appropriately as glucose levels fall into the normal range. That is true even for the GLP-1 receptor agonists and the DPP-4 inhibitors which enhance glucose stimulated insulin secretion (among other actions). They do not stimulate insulin secretion at normal or low plasma glucose concentrations (i.e. they increase insulin secretion in a glucose-dependent fashion); however, the latter feature may be lost, and hypoglycemia can occur, when they are used with an insulin secretagogue [121]. Indeed, all five categories of drugs increase the risk of hypoglycemia if used with an insulin secretagogue or insulin.

Among the commonly used sulfonylureas, the longer acting glibenclamide (glyburide) is more often associated with hypoglycemia than the shorter acting glimepiride [122,123]. The use of long-acting insulin analogs (e.g. glargine or detemir), rather than neutral protamine Hagedorn (NPH) insulin, as the basal insulin in a multiple daily injection (MDI) insulin regimen reduces at least the incidence of nocturnal hypoglycemia, and perhaps that of total, symptomatic and nocturnal hypoglycemia as well, in T1DM and T2DM [124–126]. The use of a rapid-acting analog (e.g. lispro, aspart or glulisine) as the prandial insulin in a MDI regimen reduces the incidence of nocturnal hypoglycemia, at least in T1DM [124,126]. Albeit conceptually attractive, the superiority of continuous subcutaneous insulin infusion (CSII) over MDI with insulin analogs with respect to the frequency and severity of hypoglycemia at comparable levels of glycemic control remains to be established convincingly [127,128]. In addition to the use of insulin analogs [124–126], approaches to the prevention of nocturnal hypoglycemia include attempts to produce sustained delivery of exogenous carbohydrate or sustained endogenous glucose production throughout the night [129].

Partial glycemic control reduces, but does not eliminate, the development of microvascular complications of diabetes, namely retinopathy, nephropathy and neuropathy, in T1DM [56,57] and in T2DM [67,130]. Extrapolation of the DCCT retinopathy data suggests that long-term maintenance of euglycemia might eliminate those complications [131]. Follow-up of the DCCT patients seemingly indicates that a period of earlier partial glycemic control also reduces macrovascular complications in T1DM [132]. Aside from the metformin subset of the UK Prospective Diabetes Study (UKPDS) [130], randomized controlled trials have not documented a cardiovascular mortality benefit of partial glycemic control in T2DM [59,60,67]; however, those trials do not exclude a macrovascular benefit of glycemic control, or even partial glycemic control, if that could be maintained over a longer period of time. Indeed, follow-up of the UKPDS patients also seemingly indicates a macrovascular benefit of a period of earlier partial glycemic control [133]. In any event, given its documented microvascular benefit, maintenance of euglycemia over a lifetime of diabetes would be in the best interests of people with diabetes if that could be accomplished safely [1,2]. Unfortunately, it cannot be accomplished safely in the vast majority of patients with currently available treatment methods because of the barrier of hypoglycemia [1,2]. Thus, the generic glycemic goal is a HbA_{1c} level as close to the non-diabetic range as can be accomplished safely in a given patient [134,135] at a given point in the evolution of his or her diabetes. Nonetheless, there is substantial long-term benefit from reducing HbA_{1c} levels from higher to lower, although still above recommended levels [56,57,67,130,136]. Clearly, glycemic goals should be individualized and may need to be reconsidered over time because of progression of endogenous insulin deficiency, the development of co-morbid illness and functional impairment that negates the benefit of glycemic control, or both [137].

Because the glycemic management of diabetes is empirical, caregivers should work with each individual patient over time to find the most effective and safest method of glycemic control at a given point in the course of that patient's diabetes. Care is best accomplished by a team that includes, in addition to a physician, professionals trained in, and dedicated to, translating the standards of care into the care of individual patients and making full use of modern communication and computing technologies.

Having recognized the problem and reviewed and applied the principles of aggressive glycemic therapy, the next step is to consider the conventional risk factors for hypoglycemia, those that result in relative as well as absolute therapeutic insulin excess. In addition to insulin secretagogue or insulin doses, timing and type, those include conditions in which exogenous glucose delivery or endogenous glucose production is decreased, glucose utilization or sensitivity to insulin is increased, or insulin clearance is reduced (Table 33.3).

Finally, the risk factors for HAAF need to be considered. Those include the degree of endogenous insulin deficiency, a history of severe hypoglycemia, hypoglycemia unawareness, or both, as well as any relationship between hypoglycemic episodes and recent antecedent hypoglycemia, prior exercise or sleep, and lower HbA_{1c} levels (Table 33.3). Unless the cause is easily remediable, a history of severe hypoglycemia should prompt consideration of a fundamental regimen adjustment. Without that, the risk of a subsequent episode of severe hypoglycemia is high [50–52,54,110–113]. Given a history of hypoglycemia unawareness, a 2–3 week period of scrupulous avoidance of hypoglycemia, which may require acceptance of somewhat higher glycemic goals in the short term, is advisable because that can be expected to restore awareness [34–37]. A history of late post-exercise hypoglycemia, nocturnal hypoglycemia, or both, should prompt appropriately timed regimen adjustments (generically, less insulin action, more carbohydrate ingestion, or both).

When prevention fails, treatment of hypoglycemia becomes necessary. Most episodes of asymptomatic hypoglycemia (detected by self-monitoring of blood glucose or continuous glucose sensing) and of mild–moderate symptomatic hypoglycemia are effectively self-treated by ingestion of glucose tablets or carbohydrate containing juice, soft drinks, candy, other snacks or a meal [138,139]. A reasonable dose is 20 g glucose [139]. Clinical improvement should occur in 15–20 minutes, however, in the setting of ongoing hyperinsulinemia, the glycemic response to oral glucose is transient, typically less than 2 hours [139]. Thus, ingestion of a more substantial snack or meal shortly after the plasma glucose concentration is raised is generally advisable.

Parenteral treatment is required when a hypoglycemic patient is unwilling (because of neuroglycopenia) or unable to take carbohydrate orally. Glucagon, injected subcutaneously or intramuscularly (in a usual dose of 1.0 mg in adults) by an associate of the patient, is often used. That can be life-saving, but it often causes substantial, albeit transient, hyperglycemia and it can cause nausea or even vomiting. Smaller doses of glucagon (e.g. 150 μg), repeated if necessary, have been found to be effective without side effects [140]. Because it acts by stimulating hepatic glycogenolysis, glucagon is ineffective in glycogen depleted individuals (e.g. following a binge of alcohol ingestion).

Although glucagon can be administered intravenously by medical personnel, intravenous glucose is the standard parenteral therapy. A common initial dose is 25 g [138]. The glycemic response to intravenous glucose is, of course, transient in the setting of ongoing hyperinsulinemia.

The duration of an episode of iatrogenic hypoglycemia is a function of its cause. An episode caused by a rapid-acting insulin secretagogue or insulin analog will be relatively brief, that caused by a long-acting sulfonylurea or insulin analog substantially longer. The latter can result in prolonged hypoglycemia requiring hospitalization.

Perspective on hypoglycemia in diabetes

Glycemic control, a focus of this chapter, is but one aspect of the management of diabetes. It is now possible to drive plasma low density lipoprotein (LDL) cholesterol concentrations to subphysiologic levels and to normalize blood pressure pharmacologically, usually without major side effects, in most people with diabetes. Weight loss and smoking cessation are more challenging. While it is not possible to maintain euglycemia over a lifetime of diabetes, because of the barrier of hypoglycemia, maintenance of the lowest mean glycemia that can be accomplished safely is in the best interest of people with diabetes.

Despite the difficulty, people with diabetes and their caregivers should keep the problem of iatrogenic hypoglycemia in perspective. Early in the course of T2DM, by far the most common type of diabetes, hyperglycemia may respond to lifestyle changes, specifically weight loss, or to glucose lowering drugs that do not raise insulin levels and therefore do not cause hypoglycemia. In theory, when such drugs are effective in the absence of side effects there is no reason not to accelerate their dosing until euglycemia is achieved. Over time, however, as people with T2DM become progressively more insulin deficient, those drugs, even in combination, fail to maintain glycemic control. Insulin secretagogues are also effective early in the course of T2DM, but they cause hyperinsulinemia and therefore introduce the risk of hypoglycemia. Euglycemia is not an appropriate goal during therapy with an insulin secretagogue or with insulin. Nonetheless, as discussed earlier, the frequency of hypoglycemia is relatively low (with current less than euglycemic goals) during treatment with an insulin secretagogue or even with insulin early in the course of T2DM when glycemic defenses against falling plasma glucose concentrations are still intact. Thus, over much of the course of the most common type of diabetes it is possible to maintain a meaningful degree of glycemic control with no risk or relatively low risk of hypoglycemia.

The challenge is greater in people with advanced T2DM and T1DM caused by compromised defenses against falling plasma glucose concentrations and the resulting higher barrier of iatrogenic hypoglycemia. In such patients therapy with insulin is demonstrably effective, but it is not demonstrably safe. Nonetheless, concerns about hypoglycemia should not be used as a excuse for poor glycemic control. It should be recalled that the DCCT data [56,136] document that the relationship between microvascular complications and mean glycemia is curvilinear; some degree of glycemic control puts the patient at substantially lower risk than little or no glycemic control.

Diabetes will someday be cured and prevented. Pending that, elimination of hypoglycemia from the lives of people with diabetes will likely be accomplished by new treatment methods that provide plasma glucose regulated insulin replacement or secretion. In the meantime, innovative research is needed if we are to improve the lives of all people affected by diabetes by lowering the barrier of iatrogenic hypoglycemia.

Acknowledgments

The author's original work cited has been supported, in part, by US Public Health Service, National Institutes of Health grants R37 DK27085, MO1 RR00036 (now UL1 RR24992), P60 DK20579 and T32 DK07120 and by a fellowship award from the American Diabetes Association. The author is grateful for the contributions of the postdoctoral fellows who did the bulk of the work and made the work better by their conceptual input, and the skilled nursing, technical, dietary and data management/statistical assistance of the staff of the Washington University General Clinical Research Center. Ms. Janet Dedeke prepared this manuscript.

This chapter was written shortly after completion of the author's Perspective in Diabetes [1] and his book *Hypoglycemia in Diabetes: Pathophysiology, Prevalence and Prevention* [2]. Therefore, much of the factual and interpretive content here is the same, as is no small part of the phraseology.

Disclosures

The author has served as a consultant to several pharmaceutical and device firms, including Amgen Inc., Johnson & Johnson, MannKind Corp., Marcadia Biotech, Medtronic MiniMed Inc., Merck and Co., Novo Nordisk A/S, Takeda Pharmaceuticals North America and TolerRx Inc., in recent years. He does not receive research funding from, hold stock in or speak for any of these firms.

References

1 Cryer PE. The barrier of hypoglycemia in diabetes. *Diabetes* 2008; **57**:3169–3176.

2 Cryer PE. *Hypoglycemia in Diabetes: Pathophysiology, Prevalence and Prevention*. Alexandria, VA: American Diabetes Association, 2009.

3 Clarke DD, Sokoloff L. Circulation and energy metabolism of the brain. In: Siegel G, Agranoff B, Albers RW, Molinoff P, eds. *Basic Neurochemistry: Molecular, Cellular and Medical Aspects*, 5th edn. New York: Raven Press, 1994: 645–680.

4 Cryer PE. Hypoglycemia, functional brain failure, and brain death. *J Clin Invest* 2007; **117**:868–870.

5 Schwartz NS, Clutter WE, Shah SD, Cryer PE. Glycemic thresholds for activation of glucose counterregulatory systems are higher than the threshold for symptoms. *J Clin Invest* 1987; **79**:777–781.

6 Mitrakou A, Ryan C, Veneman T, Mokan M, Jenssen T, Kiss I, *et al.* Hierarchy of glycemic thresholds for counterregulatory hormone secretion, symptoms and cerebral dysfunction. *Am J Physiol Endocrinol Metab* 1991; **260**:E67–74.

7 Fanelli C, Pampanelli S, Epifano L, Rambotti AM, Ciofetta M, Modarelli F, *et al.* Relative roles of insulin and hypoglycemia on induction of neuroendocrine responses to, symptoms of, and deterioration of cognitive function in hypoglycemia in male and female humans. *Diabetologia* 1994; **37**:797–807.

8 Towler DA, Havlin CE, Craft S, Cryer PE. Mechanism of awareness of hypoglycemia: perception of neurogenic (predominantly cholinergic) rather than neuroglycopenic symptoms. *Diabetes* 1993; **42**:1791–1798.

9 DeRosa MA, Cryer PE. Hypoglycemia and the sympathoadrenal system: neurogenic symptoms are largely the result of sympathetic neural, rather than adrenomedullary, activation. *Am J Physiol Endocrinol Metab* 2004; **287**:E32–41.

10 Schultes B, Oltmanns KM, Kern W, Fehm HL, Born J, Peters A. Modulation of hunger by plasma glucose and metformin. *J Clin Endocrinol Metab* 2003; **88**:1133–1141.

11 Cryer PE. The prevention and correction of hypoglycemia. In: Jefferson LS, Cherrington AD, eds. *Handbook of Physiology. Section 7, The Endocrine System.* Vol. II, *The Endocrine Pancreas and Regulation of Metabolism*. New York: Oxford University Press, 2001: 1057–1092.

12 Raju B, Cryer PE. Loss of the decrement in intraislet insulin plausibly explains loss of the glucagon response to hypoglycemia in insulin-deficient diabetes. *Diabetes* 2005; **54**:757–764.

13 Taborsky GJ Jr, Ahrén B, Havel PJ. Autonomic mediation of glucagon secretion during hypoglycemia. *Diabetes* 1998; **47**:995–1005.

14 Berk MA, Clutter WE, Skor D, Shah SD, Gingerich RP, Parvin CA, *et al.* Enhanced glycemic responsiveness to epinephrine in insulin-dependent diabetes mellitus is the result of the inability to secrete insulin. *J Clin Invest* 1985; **75**:1842–1851.

15 Dagogo-Jack SE, Craft S, Cryer PE. Hypoglycemia-associated autonomic failure in insulin-dependent diabetes mellitus. *J Clin Invest* 1993; **91**:819–828.

16 Segel SA, Paramore DS, Cryer PE. Hypoglycemia-associated autonomic failure in advanced type 2 diabetes. *Diabetes* 2002; **51**:724–733.

17 White NH, Skor DA, Cryer PE, Levandoski LA, Bier DM, Santiago JV. Identification of type 1 diabetic patients at increased risk for hypoglycemia during intensive therapy. *N Engl J Med* 1983; **308**:485–491.

18 Bolli GB, De Feo P, De Cosmo S, Perriello G, Ventura MM, Benedetti MM, *et al.* A reliable and reproducible test for adequate glucose counter-regulation in type 1 diabetes mellitus. *Diabetes* 1984; **33**:732–737.

19 Geddes J, Schopman JE, Zammitt NN, Frier BM. Prevalence of impaired awareness of hypoglycemia in adults with type 1 diabetes. *Diabet Med* 2008; **25**:501–504.

20 Heller SR, Cryer PE. Reduced neuroendocrine and symptomatic responses to subsequent hypoglycemia after 1 episode of hypoglycemia in nondiabetic humans. *Diabetes* 1991; **40**:223–226.

21 Galassetti P, Mann S, Tate D, Neill RA, Costa F, Wasserman DH, *et al.* Effects of antecedent prolonged exercise on subsequent counterregulatory responses to hypoglycemia. *Am J Physiol Endocrinol Metab* 2001; **280**:E908–917.

22 Sandoval DA, Aftab Guy DL, Richardson MA, Ertl AC, Davis SN. Effects of low and moderate antecedent exercise on counterregulatory responses to subsequent hypoglycemia in type 1 diabetes. *Diabetes* 2004; **53**:1798–1806.

23 Ertl AC, Davis SN. Evidence for a vicious cycle of exercise and hypoglycemia in type 1 diabetes mellitus. *Diabetes Metab Res Rev* 2004; **20**:124–130.

24 Jones TW, Porter P, Sherwin RS, Davis EA, O'Leary P, Frazer F, *et al.* Decreased epinephrine responses to hypoglycemia during sleep. *N Engl J Med* 1998; **338**:1657–1662.

25 Banarer S, Cryer PE. Sleep-related hypoglycemia-associated autonomic failure in type 1 diabetes: reduced awakening from sleep during hypoglycemia. *Diabetes* 2003; **52**:1195–1203.

26 Schultes B, Jauch-Chara K, Gais S, Hallschmid M, Reiprich E, Kern W, *et al.* Defective awakening response to nocturnal hypoglycemia in patients with type 1 diabetes mellitus. *PLoS Medicine* 2007; **4**:e69.

27 Berlin I, Grimaldi A, Payan C, Sachon C, Bosquet F, Thervet F, *et al.* Hypoglycemic symptoms and decreased β-adrenergic sensitivity in insulin dependent diabetic patients. *Diabetes Care* 1987; **10**:742–747.

28 Fritsche A, Stefan N, Häring H, Gerich J, Stumvoll M. Avoidance of hypoglycemia restores hypoglycemia awareness by increasing β-adrenergic sensitivity in type 1 diabetes. *Ann Intern Med* 2001; **134**:729–736.

29 de Galan BE, De Mol P, Wennekes L, Schouwenberg BJJ, Smits P. Preserved sensitivity to β_2-adrenergic receptor agonists in patients with type 1 diabetes mellitus and hypoglycemia unawareness. *J Clin Endocrinol Metab* 2006; **91**:2878–2881.

30 Bottini P, Boschetti E, Pampanelli S, Ciofetta M, Del Sindaco P, Scionti L, *et al.* Contribution of autonomic neuropathy to reduced plasma adrenaline responses to hypoglycemia in IDDM: evidence for a nonselective defect. *Diabetes* 1997; **46**:814–823.

31 Meyer C, Grossman R, Mitrakou A, Mahler R, Veneman T, Gerich J, *et al.* Effects of autonomic neuropathy on counterregulation and awareness of hypoglycemia in type 1 diabetic patients. *Diabetes Care* 1998; **21**:1960–1966.

32 Fanelli CG, Paramore DS, Hershey T, Terkamp C, Ovalle F, Craft S, *et al.* Impact of nocturnal hypoglycemia on hypoglycemic cognitive dysfunction in type 1 diabetes. *Diabetes* 1998; **47**:1920–1927.

33 Ovalle F, Fanelli CG, Paramore DS, Hershey T, Craft S, Cryer PE. Brief twice-weekly episodes of hypoglycemia reduce detection of clinical hypoglycemia in type 1 diabetes mellitus. *Diabetes* 1998; **47**:1472–1479.

34 Fanelli CG, Epifano L, Rambotti AM, Pampanelli S, Di Vincenzo A, Modarelli F, *et al.* Meticulous prevention of hypoglycemia normalizes the glycemic thresholds and magnitude of most of neuroendocrine responses to, symptoms of, and cognitive function during hypoglycemia in intensively treated patients with short-term IDDM. *Diabetes* 1993; **42**:1683–1689.

35 Cranston I, Lomas J, Maran A, Macdonald I, Amiel SA. Restoration of hypoglycemia awareness in patients with long-duration insulin-dependent diabetes. *Lancet* 1994; **344**:283–287.

36 Fanelli C, Pampanelli S, Epifano L, Rambotti AM, Di Vincenzo A, Modarelli F, *et al.* Long-term recovery from unawareness, deficient counterregulation and lack of cognitive dysfunction during hypoglycemia, following institution of rational, intensive therapy in IDDM. *Diabetologia* 1994; **37**:1265–1276.

37 Dagogo-Jack S, Rattarasarn C, Cryer PE. Reversal of hypoglycemia unawareness, but not defective glucose counterregulation, in IDDM. *Diabetes* 1994; **43**:1426–1434.

38 MacDonald MJ. Post exercise late onset hypoglycemia in insulin-dependent diabetic patients. *Diabetes Care* 1987; **10**:584–588.

39 Tansey MJ, Tsalikian E, Beck RW, Mauras N, Buckingham BA, Weinzimer SA, *et al.* for the Diabetes Research in Children Network (DirecNet) Study Group. The effects of erobic exercise on glucose and counterregulatory hormone concentrations in children with type 1 diabetes. *Diabetes Care* 2006; **29**:20–25.

40 Diem P, Redmon JB, Abid M, Moran A, Sutherland DE, Halter JB, *et al.* Glucagon, catecholamine and pancreatic polypeptide secretion in type 1 diabetic recipients of pancreatic allografts. *J Clin Invest* 1990; **86**:2008–2013.

41 Sherck SM, Shiota M, Saccomando J, Cardin S, Allen EJ, Hastings JR, *et al.* Pancreatic response to mild non-insulin induced hypoglycemia does not involve extrinsic neural input. *Diabetes* 2001; **50**:2487–2496.

42 Cryer PE. Mechanisms of hypoglycemia-associated autonomic failure and its component syndromes in diabetes. *Diabetes* 2005; **54**:3592–3601.

43 Sherwin RS. Bringing light to the dark side of insulin: a journey across the blood–brain barrier. *Diabetes* 2008; **57**:2259–2268.

44 Teves D, Videen TO, Cryer PE, Powers WJ. Activation of human medial prefrontal cortex during autonomic responses to hypoglycemia. *Proc Natl Acad Sci U S A* 2004; **101**:6217–6221.

45 Arbelez AM, Powers WJ, Videen TO, Price JL, Cryer PE. Attenuation of counterregulatory responses to recurrent hypoglycemia by active thalamic inhibition: a mechanism for hypoglycemia-associated autonomic failure. *Diabetes* 2008; **57**:470–475.

46 Dunn JT, Cranston I, Marsden PK, Amiel SA, Reed LJ. Attenuation of amygdala and frontal cortical responses to low blood glucose concentration in asymptomatic hypoglycemia in type 1 diabetes. *Diabetes* 2007; **56**:2766–2773.

47 Cryer PE, Davis SN, Shamoon H. Hypoglycemia in diabetes. *Diabetes Care* 2003; **26**:1902–1912.

48 Diabetes Control and Complications Trial Research Group. Epidemiology of severe hypoglycemia in the Diabetes Control and Complications Trial. *Am J Med* 1991; **90**:450–459.

49 Fukuda M, Tanaka A, Tahara Y, Ikegami H, Yamamoto Y, Kumahara Y, *et al.* Correlation between minimal secretory capacity of pancreatic β-cells and stability of diabetic control. *Diabetes* 1988; **37**:81–88.

50 Diabetes Control and Complications Trial Research Group. Hypoglycemia in the Diabetes Control and Complications Trial. *Diabetes* 1997; **46**:271–286.

51 Mühlhauser I, Overmann H, Bender R, Bott U, Berger M. Risk factors for severe hypoglycemia in adult patients with type 1 diabetes: a prospective population based study. *Diabetologia* 1997; **41**:1274–1282.

52 Allen C, LeCaire T, Palta M, Daniels K, Meredith M, D'Alessio DJ; Wisconsin Diabetes Registry Project. Risk factors for frequent and severe hypoglycemia in type 1 diabetes. *Diabetes Care* 2001; **24**:1878–1881.

53 Steffes MW, Sibley S, Jackson M, Thomas W. β-Cell function and the development of diabetes related complications in the Diabetes Control and Complications Trial. *Diabetes Care* 2003; **26**:832–836.

54 Wright AD, Cull CA, MacLeod KM, Holman RR; for the UKPDS Group. Hypoglycemia in type 2 diabetic patients randomized to and maintained on monotherapy with diet, sulfonylurea, metformin or insulin for 6 years from diagnosis: UKPDS 73. *J Diabetes Complications* 2006; **20**:395–401.

55 Lüddeke H-J, Sreenan S, Aczel S, Maxeiner S, Yenigun M, Kozlovski P, *et al.* on behalf of the PREDICTIVE Study Group. PREDICTIVE – a global, prospective observational study to evaluate insulin detemir treatment in types 1 and 2 diabetes: baseline characteristics and predictors of hypoglycemia from the European cohort. *Diabetes Obes Metab* 2007; **9**:428–434.

56 Diabetes Control and Complications Trial Research Group. The effect of intensive treatment of diabetes on the development and progression of long-term complications in insulin dependent diabetes mellitus. *N Engl J Med* 1993; **329**:977–986.

57 Reichard P, Pihl M. Mortality and treatment side-effects during long-term intensified conventional insulin treatment in the Stockholm Diabetes Intervention Study. *Diabetes* 1994; **43**:313–317.

58 Egger M, Davey Smith G, Stettler C, Diem P. Risk of adverse effects of intensified treatment in insulin-dependent diabetes mellitus: a meta-analysis. *Diabet Med* 1997; **14**:919–928.

59 ADVANCE Collaborative Group. Intensive blood glucose control and vascular outcomes in patients with type 2 diabetes. *N Engl J Med* 2008; **358**:2560–2572.

60 Action to Control Cardiovascular Risk in Diabetes Study Group. Effects of intensive glucose lowering in type 2 diabetes. *N Engl J Med* 2008; **358**:2545–2559.

61 International Diabetes Federation. *Diabetes Facts and Figures*. Available from: http://www.diabetesatlas.org/content/diabetes-and-impaired-glucose-tolerance. Accessed on 8 January, 2010.

62 Diabetes Control and Complications Trial Research Group. Hypoglycemia in the Diabetes Control and Complications Trial. *Diabetes* 1997; **46**:271–286.

63 UK Hypoglycemia Study Group. Risk of hypoglycemia in type 1 and 2 diabetes: effects of treatment modalities and their duration. *Diabetologia* 2007; **50**:1140–1147.

64 MacLeod KM, Hepburn DA, Frier BM. Frequency and morbidity of severe hypoglycemia in insulin-treated diabetic patients. *Diabet Med* 1993; **10**:238–245.

65 Donnelly LA, Morris AD, Frier BM, Ellis JD, Donnan PT, Durrant R, *et al.* Frequency and predictors of hypoglycemia in type 1 and insulin-treated type 2 diabetes: a population-based study. *Diabet Med* 2005; **22**:749–755.

66 Reichard P, Pihl M. Mortality and treatment side-effects during long-term intensified conventional insulin treatment in the Stockholm Diabetes Intervention Study. *Diabetes* 1994; **43**:313–317.

67 UK Prospective Diabetes Study (UKPDS) Group. Intensive blood-glucose control with sulphonylureas or insulin compared with conventional treatment and risk of complications in patients with type 2 diabetes (UKPDS 33). *Lancet* 1998; **352**:837–853.

68 Wright AD, Cull CA, MacLeod KM, Holman RR; for the UKPDS Group. Hypoglycemia in type 2 diabetic patients randomized to and maintained on monotherapy with diet, sulfonylurea, metformin, or insulin for 6 years from diagnosis: UKPDS73. *J Diabetes Complications* 2006; **20**:395–401.

69 Akram K, Pedersen-Bjergaard U, Carstensen B, Borch-Johnsen K, Thorsteinsson B. Frequency and risk factors for severe hypoglycemia in insulin-treated type 2 diabetes: a cross-sectional survey. *Diabet Med* 2006; **23**:750–756.

70 Henderson JN, Allen KV, Deary IJ, Frier BM. Hypoglycemia in insulin-treated type 2 diabetes: frequency, symptoms and impaired awareness. *Diabet Med* 2003; **20**:1016–1021.

71 Murata GH, Duckworth WC, Shah JH, Wendel CS, Mohler MJ, Hoffman RM. Hypoglycemia in stable, insulin-treated veterans with type 2 diabetes: a prospective study of 1662 episodes. *J Diabetes Complications* 2005; **19**:10–17.

72 Saudek CD, Duckworth WC, Giobbie-Hurder A, Henderson WG, Henry RR, Kelley DE, *et al.* Implantable insulin pump vs. multiple dose insulin for non-insulin dependent diabetes mellitus: a randomized clinical trial. *JAMA* 1996; **276**:1322–1327.

73 Gürlek A, Erbas T, Gedik O. Frequency of severe hypoglycemia in type 1 and type 2 diabetes during conventional insulin therapy. *Exp Clin Endocrinol Diabetes* 1999; **107**:220–224.

74 Abraira C, Colwell JA, Nuttall FQ, Sawin CT, Nagel NJ, Comstock JP, *et al.* Veterans Affairs cooperative study on glycemic control and complications in type II diabetes (VA CSCM). *Diabetes Care* 1995; **18**:1113–1123.

75 Yki-Järvinen H, Ryysy L, Nikkilä K, Tulokas T, Vanamo R, Heikkilä M. Comparison of bedtime insulin regimens in patients with type 2 diabetes mellitus. *Ann Intern Med* 1999; **130**:389–396.

76 Ohkubo Y, Kishikawa H, Araki E, Miyata T, Isami S, Motoyoshi S, *et al.* Intensive insulin therapy prevents the progression of diabetic microvascular complications in Japanese patients with non-insulin dependent diabetes mellitus: a randomized prospective 6-year study. *Diabetes Res Clin Pract* 1995; **28**:103–117.

77 UK Prospective Diabetes Study Group. UK Prospective Diabetes Study 24: a six year, randomized, controlled trial comparing sulfonylurea, insulin and metformin therapy in patients with newly diagnosed type 2 diabetes that could not be controlled with diet therapy. *Ann Intern Med* 1998; **128**:165–175.

78 Hepburn DA, MacLeod KM, Pell AC, Scougal IJ, Frier BM. Frequency and symptoms of hypoglycemia experienced by patients with type 2 diabetes treated with insulin. *Diabet Med* 1993; **10**:231–237.

79 Holstein A, Plaschke A, Egberts E-H. Clinical characterization of severe hypoglycemia – a prospective population-based study. *Exp Clin Endocrinol Diabetes* 2003; **111**:364–369.

80 Leese GP, Wang J, Broomhall J, Kelly P, Marsden A, Morrison W, *et al.*; DARTS/MEMO Collaboration. Frequency of severe hypoglycemia requiring emergency treatment in type 1 and type 2 diabetes: a population based study of health service resource use. *Diabetes Care* 2003; **26**:1176–1180.

81 Clarke WL, Cox DJ, Gonder-Frederick LA, Julian D, Schlundt D, Polonsky W. Reduced awareness of hypoglycemia in IDDM adults: a prospective study of hypoglycemia frequency and associated symptoms. *Diabetes Care* 1995; **18**:517–522.

82 Pramming S, Thorsteinsson B, Bendtson I, Binder C. Symptomatic hypoglycemia in 411 type 1 diabetic patients. *Diabet Med* 1991; **8**:217–222.

83 Pedersen-Bjergaard U, Pramming S, Thorsteinsson B. Recall of severe hypoglycemia and self-estimated state of awareness in type 1 diabetes. *Diabetes Metab Res Rev* 2003; **19**:232–240.

84 Lee SP, Yeoh L, Harris ND, Davies CM, Robinson RT, Leathard A, *et al.* Influence of autonomic neuropathy on QTc interval lengthening during hypoglycemia in type 1 diabetes. *Diabetes* 2004; **53**:1535–1542.

85 Adler GK, Bonyhay I, Failing H, Waring E, Dotson S, Freeman R. Antecedent hypoglycemia impairs autonomic cardiovascular function: implications for rigorous glycemic control. *Diabetes* 2009; **58**:360–366.

86 Diabetes Control and Complications Trial/Epidemiology of Diabetes Interventions and Complications Study Research Group. Long-term effect of diabetes and its treatment on cognitive function. *N Engl J Med* 2007; **356**:1842–1852.

87 Hershey T, Perantie DC, Warren SL, Zimmerman EC, Sadler M, White NH. Frequency and timing of severe hypoglycemia affects spatial memory in children with type 1 diabetes. *Diabetes Care* 2005; **28**:2372–2377.

88 Perantie DC, Wu J, Koller JM, Lim A, Warren SL, Black KJ, *et al.* Regional brain volume differences associated with hyperglycemia and severe hypoglycemia in youth with type 1 diabetes. *Diabetes Care* 2007; **30**:2331–2337.

89 Jacobsen AM. The psychological care of patients with insulin-dependent diabetes mellitus. *N Engl J Med* 1996; **344**:1249–1253.

90 Deckert T, Poulsen JE, Larsen M. Prognosis of diabetics with diabetes before the age of 31. I. Survival, cause of deaths and complications. *Diabetologia* 1978; **14**:363–370.

91 Tunbridge WMG. Factors contributing to deaths of diabetics under 50 years of age. *Lancet* 1981; **2**:569–572.

92 Laing SP, Swerdlow AJ, Slater SD, Botha JL, Burden AC, Waugh NR, *et al.* The British Diabetic Association Cohort Study. I. All-cause mortality in patients with insulin-treated diabetes mellitus. *Diabetic Med* 1999; **16**:459–465.

93 Feltbower RG, Bodansky HJ, Patterson CC, Parslow RC, Stephenson CR, Reynolds C, *et al.* Acute complications and drug misuse are important causes of death for children and young adults with type 1 diabetes. *Diabetes Care* 2008; **31**:922–926.

94 Skrivarhaug T, Bangstad H-J, Stene LC, Sandvik L, Hanssen KF, Joner G. Long-term mortality in a nationwide cohort of childhood-onset type 1 diabetic patients in Norway. *Diabetologia* 2006; **49**:298–305.

95 Gerich JE. Oral hypoglycemic agents. *N Engl J Med* 1989; **34**:1231–1245.

96 Holstein A, Egberts EH. Risk of hypoglycemia with oral antidiabetic agents in patients with type 2 diabetes. *Exp Clin Endocrinol Metab* 2003; **111**:405–414.

97 American Diabetes Association Workgroup on Hypoglycemia. Defining and reporting hypoglycemia in diabetes. *Diabetes Care* 2005; **28**:1245–1249.

98 Amiel SA, Sherwin RS, Simonson DC, Tamborlane WV. Effect of intensive insulin therapy on glycemic thresholds for counterregulatory hormone release. *Diabetes* 1988; **37**:901–907.

99 Mitrakou A, Fanelli C, Veneman T, Perriello G, Calderone S, Platanisiotis D, *et al.* Reversibility of hypoglycemia unawareness in patients with an insulinoma. *N Engl J Med* 1993; **329**:834–839.

100 Boyle PJ, Schwartz NS, Shah SD, Clutter WE, Cryer PE. Plasma glucose concentrations at the onset of hypoglycemic symptoms in patients with poorly controlled diabetes and in nondiabetics. *N Engl J Med* 1988; **318**:1487–1492.

101 Davis SN, Shavers C, Mosqueda-Garcia R, Costa F. Effects of differing antecedent hypoglycemia on subsequent counterregulation in normal humans. *Diabetes* 1997; **46**:1328–1335.

102 Diabetes Research in Children Network (DirecNet) Study Group. A multicenter study of the accuracy of the One Touch Ultra home glucose meter in children with type 1 diabetes. *Diabetes Technol Ther* 2003; **5**:933–941.

103 Davis S, Alonso MD. Hypoglycemia as a barrier to glycemic control. *J Diabetes Complications* 2004; **18**: 60–68.

104 de Galan BE, Schouwenberg BJJW, Tack CJ, Smits P. Pathophysiology and management of recurrent hypoglycemia and hypoglycemia unawareness in diabetes. *Neth J Med* 2006; **64**:269–279.

105 Boyle PJ, Zrebiec J. Management of diabetes-related hypoglycemia. *Southern Med J* 2007; **100**:183–194.

106 Rossetti P, Porcellati F, Bolli GB, Fanelli CG. Prevention of hypoglycemia while achieving good glycemic control in type 1 diabetes. *Diabetes Care* 2008; **31**(Suppl 2):S113–120.

107 Heller SR. Minimizing hypoglycemia while maintaining glycemic control in diabetes. *Diabetes* 2008; **57**:3177–3183.

108 Gonder-Frederick LA, Fisher CD, Ritterband LM, Cox DJ, Hou L, DasGupta AA, *et al.* Predictors of fear of hypoglycemia in adolescents with type 1 diabetes and their parents. *Pediatr Diabetes* 2006; **7**:215–222.

109 Nordfeldt S, Ludvigsson J. Fear and other disturbances of severe hypoglycemia in children and adolescents with type 1 diabetes mellitus. *J Pediatr Endocrinol Metab* 2005; **18**:83–91.

110 Cox DJ, Kovatchev B, Koev D, Koeva L, Dachev S, Tcharakchiev D, *et al.* Hypoglycemia anticipation, awareness and treatment training (HAATT) reduces occurrence of severe hypoglycemia among adults with type with type 1 diabetes mellitus. *Int J Behav Med* 2004; **11**:212–218.

111 Kovatchev BP, Cox DJ, Gonder-Frederick LA, Young-Hyman D, Schlundt D, Clarke WL. Assessment of risk for severe hypoglycemia among adults with 1DDM: validation of the Low Blood Glucose Index. *Diabetes Care* 1998; **21**:1870–1875.

112 Kovatchev BP, Cox DJ, Kumar A, Gonder-Frederick LA, Clarke WL. Algorithmic evaluation of metabolic control and risk of severe hypoglycemia in type 1 and type 2 diabetes using self-monitoring blood glucose (SMBG) data. *Diabetes Technol Ther* 2003; **5**:817–828.

113 Cox DJ, Gonder-Frederick L, Ritterband L, Clarke W, Kovatchev BP. Prediction of severe hypoglycemia. *Diabetes Care* 2007; **30**:1370–1373.

114 Hovorka R. Continuous glucose monitoring and closed-loop systems. *Diabet Med* 2005; **23**:1–12.

115 Ellis SL, Bookout T, Garg SK, Izuora KE. Use of continuous glucose monitoring to improve diabetes mellitus management. *Endocrinol Metab Clinics NA* 2007; **36**(Suppl 2):46–68.

116 Deiss D, Hartmann R, Schmidt J, Kordonouri O. Results of a randomized controlled cross-over trial on the effect of continuous subcutaneous glucose monitoring (CSGM) on glycemic control in children and adolescents with type 1 diabetes. *Exp Clin Endocrinol Diabetes* 2006; **114**:63–67.

117 Wilson DM, Beck RW, Tamborlane WV, Dontchev MJ, Kollman C, Chase P, *et al.* and The DirecNet Study Group. The accuracy of the FreeStyle Navigator continuous glucose monitoring system in children with type 1 diabetes. *Diabetes Care* 2007; **30**:59–64.

118 Buckingham B, Caswell K, Wilson DM. Real-time continuous glucose monitoring. *Curr Opin Endocrinol Diabetes Obes* 2007; **14**:288–295.

119 Bolen S, Feldman L, Vassy J, Wilson L, Yeh HC, Marinopoulos S, *et al.* Systematic review: comparative effectiveness and safety of oral medications for type 2 diabetes mellitus. *Ann Intern Med* 2007; **147**:386–399.

120 UK Prospective Diabetes Study Group. Overview of 6 years of therapy of type II diabetes: a progressive disease. *Diabetes* 1995; **44**:1249–1258.

121 de Heer J, Holst JJ. Sulfonylurea compounds uncouple the glucose dependence of the insulinotropic effect of glucagon-like peptide 1. *Diabetes* 2007; **56**:438–443.

122 Holstein A, Egberts EH. Risk of hypoglycemia with oral antidiabetic agents in patients with type 2 diabetes. *Exp Clin Endocrinol Metab* 2003; **111**: 405–414.

123 Gangji AS, Cukierman T, Gerstein HC, Goldsmith GH, Clase CM. A systematic review and meta-analysis of hypoglycemia and cardiovascular events. *Diabetes Care* 2007; **30**:389–394.

124 Hirsch IB. Insulin analogues. *N Engl J Med* 2005; **352**:174–183.

125 Horvath K, Jeitler K, Berghold A, Ebrahim SH, Gratzer TW, Plank J, *et al.* Long-acting insulin analogues versus NPH insulin (human isophane insulin) for type 2 diabetes. *Cochrane Database Syst Rev* 2007; **2**:CD005613.

126 Gough SCL. A review of human and analogue insulin trials. *Diabetes Res Clin Pract* 2007; **77**:1–15.

127 Fatourechi MM, Kudva YC, Murad MH, Elamin MB, Tabini CC, Montori VM. Hypoglycemia with intensive insulin therapy: a systematic review and meta-analysis of randomized trials of continuous subcutaneous insulin infusion versus multiple daily injections. *J Clin Endocrinol Metab* 2009; **94**:729–740.

128 Mukhopadhyay A, Farrell T, Fraser RB, Ola B. Continuous subcutaneous insulin infusion vs intensive conventional insulin therapy in pregnant diabetic women: a systematic review and metaanalysis of randomized, controlled trials. *Am J Obstet Gynecol* 2007; **197**:447–456.

129 Raju B, Arbelez AM, Breckenridge SM, Cryer PE. Nocturnal hypoglycemia in type 1 diabetes: an assessment of preventive bedtime treatments. *J Clin Endocrinol Metab* 2006; **91**:2087–2092.

130 UK Prospective Diabetes Study (UKPDS) Group. Effect of intensive blood-glucose control with metformin on complications in overweight patients with type 2 diabetes (UKPDS 34). *Lancet* 1998; **352**:854–865.

131 Diabetes Control and Complications Trial Research Group. The relationship of glycemic exposure (HbA_{1c}) to the risk of development and progression of retinopathy in the Diabetes Control and Complications Trial. *Diabetes* 1995; **44**:968–983.

132 Diabetes Control and Complications Trial/Epidemiology of Diabetes Interventions and Complications Study Research Group. Intensive diabetes treatment and cardiovascular disease in patients with type 1 diabetes. *N Engl J Med* 2005; **353**:2643–2653.

133 Holman RR, Paul SK, Bethel MA, Matthews DR, Neil HA. 10-year follow-up of intensive glucose control in type 2 diabetes. *N Engl J Med* 2008; **359**:1577–1589.

134 American Diabetes Association. Standards of medical care in diabetes, 2008. *Diabetes Care* 2008; **31**(Suppl 1):S12–54.

135 Qaseem A, Vijan S, Snow V, Cross JT, Weiss KB, Owens DK; for the Clinical Efficacy Assessment Subcommittee of the American College of Physicians. Glycemic control and type 2 diabetes mellitus: the optimal hemoglobin A_{1C} targets: a guidance statement from the American College of Physicians. *Ann Intern Med* 2007; **147**:417–422.

136 Lachin JM, Genuth S, Nathan DM, Zinman B, Rutledge BN for the DCCT/EDIC Research Group. Effect of glycemic exposure on the risk of microvascular complications in the Diabetes Control and Complications Trial – revisited. *Diabetes* 2008; **57**:995–1001.

137 Huang ES, Zhang Q, Gandra N, Chin MH, Meltzer DO. The effect of comorbid illness and functional status on the expected benefits of intensive glucose control in older patients with type 2 diabetes: a decision analysis. *Ann Intern Med* 2008; **149**:11–19.

138 MacCuish AC. Treatment of hypoglycemia. In: Frier BM, Fisher BM, eds. *Diabetes and Hypoglycemia*. London: Edward Arnold, 1993: 212–221.

139 Wiethop BV, Cryer PE. Alanine and terbutaline in the treatment of hypoglycemia in IDDM. *Diabetes Care* 1993; **16**:1131–1136.

140 Haymond MW, Schreiner B. Mini-dose glucagon rescue to children with type 1 diabetes. *Diabetes Care* 2001; **24**:643–645.

34 Acute Metabolic Complications of Diabetes: Diabetic Ketoacidosis and Hyperosmolar Hyperglycemia

Troels Krarup Hansen & Niels Møller
Medical Department M (Endocrinology and Diabetes), Aarhus University Hospital, Arhus, Denmark

Keypoints

Diabetic ketoacidosis

- Lack of insulin is the culprit in diabetic ketoacidosis.
- The most common precipitating cause is infection.
- The classic signs include polyuria and polydipsia, rapid weight loss, weakness, Kussmaul respiration, drowsiness and, rarely, coma.
- The cornerstones of treatment are rehydration, IV insulin and potassium supplementation.
- Intravenous insulin administration should continue until the acidosis is normalized (i.e. not merely until euglycemia is achieved).

Hyperosmolar non-ketotic hyperglycemia

- This is characterized by hyperosmolality with progressive hyperglycemia of >35–40 mmol/L and an effective serum osmolality of >320 mOsm/kg.
- It typically affects elderly patients with type 2 diabetes.
- The most common precipitating causes are infection and cardiovascular disease.
- Treatment involves aggressive rehydration and IV insulin.

Introduction

Both diabetic ketoacidosis (DKA) and hyperosmolar non-ketotic hyperglycemia (HH) are caused by a lack of insulin leading to unrestricted flux of stored lipid, carbohydrate and amino acid nutrients into the blood. These conditions are both acute and life-threatening, and represent the ultimate metabolic consequences of deranged type 1 (T1DM) and type 2 diabetes mellitus (T2DM), respectively [1–3]. The hallmark of DKA is a high-anion-gap metabolic acidosis caused by a rapidly progressive excess of ketoacids (3-hydroxybutyrate and acetoacetate – "ketone bodies") while severe hyperosmolarity caused by hyperglycemia is the most notable feature of HH. The distinction is not always obvious on clinical grounds; patients with DKA may be very hyperosmolar and ketone body levels are in general somewhat elevated in HH. Although the clinical picture may vary considerably depending on co-morbidities, differential diagnosis seldom poses any major problem and in the rare cases in which distinction remains difficult, treatment generally follows the same principles, regardless of whether ketosis or hyperglycemia is the most urgent clinical challenge.

Mortality rates have been steadily declining over the past few years [4], but remain close to 5% for DKA and 10–15% for HH [2,5]. The decline in mortality may be a consequence of lower incidence of DKA and HH, earlier diagnosis, improved treatment or, more plausibly, all of these effects combined. Improved education schedules and self-monitoring (e.g. blood ketone testing), organization of specialized diabetes clinics and the use of standardized low-dose insulin regimens have also contributed to this favorable trend [2,6].

Diabetic ketoacidosis

Definitions

Diabetic ketoacidosis is the most common, serious and demanding medical emergency within the fields of diabetology and endocrinology. There is no generally accepted definition of DKA and, in particular, very mild cases may be difficult to diagnose. At a minimum, it is reasonable to require that pH is below the normal range and that the levels of ketoacids (ketone bodies) in the blood or urine are markedly elevated. As outlined in Table 34.1, there is a continuous deterioration from clinically insignificant "stress" ketosis to full-blown severe ketoacidosis. In the US population,

Textbook of Diabetes, 4th edition. Edited by R. Holt, C. Cockram, A. Flyvbjerg and B. Goldstein.

Table 34.1 Classification of clinical pictures and diagnostic criteria. Adapted from Standards of Medical Care in Diabetes – 2004/2006 position statement. *Diabetes Care* 2004; **27**:S94–S101, with permission from the American Diabetes Association.

	Stress ketosis	Compensated DKA	Diabetic ketoacidosis			Hyperosmolar hyperglycemia
			Mild	Moderate	Severe	
Plasma glucose	Variable	Generally increased	Generally increased	Generally increased	Generally increased	>35–40 mmol/L
Arterial pH	Normal	Normal	Decreased >7.25	7.0–7.25	<7.0	Generally normal
Serum bicarbonate	Normal	Marginally decreased	15–18 mmol/L	10–15 mmol/L	<10 mmol/L	>15 mmol/L
Urine ketones	Increased	Increased	Increased	Increased	Increased	Normal/marginally increased
Blood ketones	Increased	Increased	Increased	Increased	Increased	Normal/marginally increased
Anion gap*	Normal/marginally increased	Marginally increased	>10	>12	>12	Variable
Mental status	Normal	Normal	Normal	Normal/drowsy	Drowsy–coma	Drowsy–coma

DKA, diabetic ketoacidosis.
* Anion gap can be calculated as: $[Na^+]-([Cl^-]+[HCO^{-3}])$.

it has been estimated that 2–8% of hospital admissions in children with diabetes are a result of DKA and that the annual incidence rate of DKA in children is around 5 per 1000 patients [1].

Pathogenesis and pathophysiology

Insulin deficiency

DKA is caused by insulin deficiency. Insulin deficiency may be relative (e.g. in the setting of severe infection) where normal amounts of insulin are insufficient, or absolute when insulin therapy is neglected. Lack of insulin leads to uncontrolled lipolysis and ketogenesis and increases plasma glucose. Although often disregarded it should also be borne in mind that insulin deficiency, most particularly when longstanding, causes increased breakdown of body protein, as evidenced by the extreme sarcopenia and cachexia of patients with T1DM prior to the insulin era. Excessive protein breakdown and ensuing release of ketogenic and gluconeogenic amino acids may contribute to ketosis and hyperglycemia.

Stress hormones and cytokines

At some stage insulin deficiency becomes coupled with excess of "counter-regulatory" or "stress" hormones and cytokines [7,8]. Release of stress hormones may in part be triggered by cytokines and in part by general stress, such as dehydration, hypotension and hypoperfusion. It has been shown that both endotoxin and tumor necrosis factor (TNF) mimics all metabolic responses to infection including hyperthermia and stress hormone release [9,10]. The traditional stress hormones include glucagon, epinephrine, growth hormone (GH) and cortisol, all of which have well-described metabolic actions. Glucagon and epinephrine have a rapid onset of action, whereas GH and cortisol act with a latency of hours.

Cytokine levels are elevated in DKA, even in the absence of infection. The metabolic actions of cytokines are in general not so well understood and it is possible that many of these actions are mediated by hypothalamo-pituitary activation and subsequent stress hormone release. Certain cytokines, such as TNF-α, may impair insulin sensitivity in peripheral tissues [11,12] and a vicious circle may thus be initiated with self-perpetual increments in blood glucose and cytokine levels. Insulin has anti-inflammatory properties in critically ill patients [13], and administration of exogenous insulin may in itself increase insulin sensitivity [14], conceivably to some extent by breaking this vicious circle but also because glucotoxicity and lipotoxicity wane.

Lipid metabolism

Contrary to popular belief, deranged lipid – not carbohydrate – metabolism is the main cause of DKA. In essence, DKA is brought about by uncontrolled lipolysis in adipose tissue and uncontrolled ketogenesis in liver.

Adipose tissue is present in regional depots such as subcutaneous upper and lower body and visceral fat [15]. Apart from these classic depots, fat is present in most other tissues (e.g. connective tissue, bone marrow, liver and muscle). The picture is further complicated by the fact that within each tissue fat is distributed in compartments. In muscle, for instance, fat is present intramyocellularly, intermyocellularly and intermuscularly. Under physiologic conditions, lipolysis is tightly controlled by lipases. Hormone-sensitive lipase and probably also adipose triglyceride lipase stimulate release of free fatty acids and glycerol into the circulation. This process is inhibited by insulin and low insulin levels increase lipolysis swiftly. The stress hormones, such as epinephrine, growth hormone and cortisol, stimulate lipolysis. It is plausible that dehydration per se also participates in the stimulation of lipolysis [16]. These events take place in the course of hours and may rapidly triple or quadruple blood concentrations of free fatty acids.

Ketogenesis occurs in the liver by oxidation of free fatty acids to ketoacids or ketone bodies (Figure 34.1). Ketone bodies, in

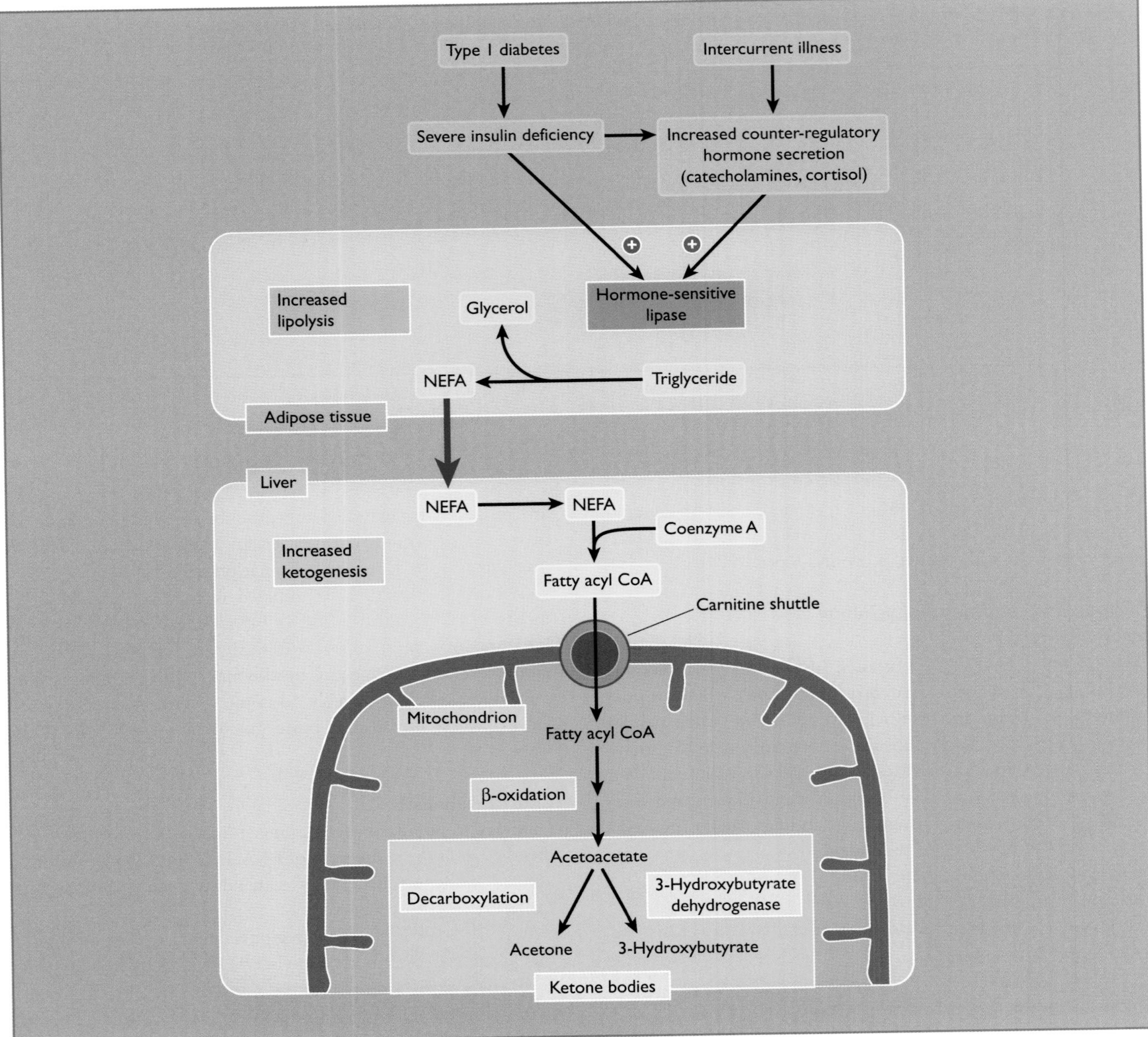

Figure 34.1 Mechanisms of ketogenesis. NEFA, non-esterified fatty acids.

particular 3-OH-butyrate, are phylogenetically ancient fuel compounds, which are present and prominent in very primitive species [17], suggesting that they have had an important role throughout evolution for the past 2–3 billion years. Physiologically, ketone bodies provide important fuel energy for the brain and other tissues under fasting, prolonged exercise and other conditions of fuel shortage. In DKA, ketogenesis becomes uncontrolled and circulating levels of ketone bodies rise rapidly and excessively. This occurs because of both increased supply of fatty acids to the liver and because low levels of insulin and high levels of glucagon in the liver promotes ketogenesis [18]. In normal individuals this unrestrained process is prevented by compensatory rises in insulin secretion, but this does not occur in those with T1DM.

Glucose metabolism

Hyperglycemia is usually present in DKA, but it is important to stress that DKA not infrequently presents with normal or modestly elevated glucose concentrations [19]. This may particularly be the case during caloric deprivation caused by gastrointestinal disease, for example. Hyperglycemia is caused by a combination of lack of insulin and an excess of stress hormones, leading to insulin resistance. In the liver this increases gluconeogenesis and hepatic glucose production. The kidney is unlikely to have any significant role in the initial stages of DKA [20]. The ensuing high glucose levels generate a high flux state with increased peripheral glucose disposal, but the increased mass action of glucose is generally insufficient to compensate fully. Muscle glucose metabolism is characterized by insulin resistance because of high levels of stress hormones, high levels of free fatty acids and varying degrees of dehydration.

Precipitating factors

In patients with known diabetes, DKA is usually precipitated by a coexisting illness or by omission of insulin therapy. The most common factor is infection, ranging from trivial viral infections to full-blown septicemia. Other precipitating factors include cardiovascular events (myocardial infarction, stroke), gastrointestinal disease, inflammatory diseases, pancreatitis, trauma and major surgery, alcohol abuse and drugs, especially glucocorticoids. All of these factors induce insulin resistance because of the stress hormone responses. Furthermore, poor appetite and food deprivation will often lead the patient to take less insulin. In this context, gastrointestinal disease with nausea and vomiting pose a specific problem and it may be necessary to admit such patients to the hospital for intravenous glucose and insulin therapy. Diabetes ketoacidosis may be a presenting feature of new onset T1DM (see Chapter 19).

Psychologic factors also play an important part. Poor compliance is commonly seen in younger patients, patients with psychiatric illnesses and in minority groups who unfortunately may have a poor understanding of diabetes care principles for linguistic or cultural reasons.

Diagnosis and clinical presentation

DKA usually develops over a short period of time, generally in less than 24 hours. There may have been some antecedent days with general malaise and poor metabolic control. Depending on the degree of hyperglycemia, the history will include symptoms of polydipsia and polyuria (Table 34.2). Specific symptoms depend on the precipitating factors and other co-morbidities that might be present. Physical examination may reveal poor skin turgor, hyperventilation (Kussmaul respirations), hypotension, tachycardia and impairment of mental state. Many patients have infections but with normothermia or even hypothermia, caused by peripheral vasodilatation brought about by the acidemia.

Table 34.2 Common clinical features of diabetic ketoacidosis.

Polyuria, polydipsia
Rapid weight loss
Muscular weakness
Visual disturbance
Air hunger with Kussmaul respiration, dry lips
Abdominal pain, leg cramps
Nausea, vomiting
Confusion, drowsiness, coma

Prompt diagnosis and initial treatment rests on:

1 Careful clinical examination;
2 Determination of plasma glucose;
3 Measurement of ketones in blood or urine;
4 Measurement of plasma potassium and other electrolytes; and
5 Assessment of acidemia.

If glucose is high and blood or urine ketones are markedly elevated, DKA is likely and fluid and insulin therapy can usually be intiated, unless the patient is severely hypokalemic (<3.5 mmol/L). If potassium is very low, supplementation must be given prior to insulin therapy; however, rehydration should not be delayed while waiting for a potassium measurement.

The next diagnostic steps usually include arterial blood gas analysis, blood electrolytes (including anion gap), serum lactate (if there is doubt about the cause of the acidemia), complete blood cell count, biochemical assessment of liver and renal function, blood and urine cultures, myocardial biomarkers (if there is suspicion of a myocardial infarction), electrocardiogram (ECG) and chest X-ray. In this context it is advantageous that most modern gas analyzers also readily provide potassium concentrations. Another recent advantage is the advent of bedside ketone body monitors. Thus, it is now possible to have a quick and reliable measure of 3-hydroxybutyrate concentrations in blood, as opposed to unreliable measurements of acetoacetate in urine or the time-consuming conventional laboratory methods used in the past. The diagnostic criteria are shown in Table 34.1.

Despite potassium depletion, serum potassium is typically either normal or elevated because of water deficiency and an intracellular to extracellular shift caused by insulin deficiency and acidemia. Patients with potassium in the low range have a severe total body potassium deficiency and should receive vigorous replacement therapy guided by cardiac monitoring. Sodium concentrations can be normal or low, as a result of osmotic shifts. It can be calculated that for every 3 mmol/L rise in plasma glucose the plasma sodium falls by 1 mmol/L. Thus, there is often a real hypernatremia with sodium levels rising as the glucose is brought under control. A majority of patients will have a leukocytosis, which correlates with ketone body levels rather than with the presence of infection. There is also a water deficit of around 10% of body weight. Non-specific elevations of amylase and liver enzymes are also common.

Differential diagnoses include all other causes of acidosis. Note that many acute medical conditions induce a stress ketosis and may be associated with acidosis. DKA is a metabolic acidosis characterized by a high anion gap and varying degrees of respiratory compensation. Thus, it is crucial to obtain measures of ketone body concentrations and perform an arterial gas analysis. If there is a major discrepancy between the extent of the ketonemia and the acidemia then lactate measurements are warranted. Starvation ketosis and alcoholic ketoacidosis can usually be identified by clinical history. Other conditions causing metabolic acidosis include lactic acidosis and intoxication with salicylate, methanol, ethylene glycol (antifreeze) and paraldehyde. The clinical picture may be blurred whenever the acidosis is aggravated by renal failure or respiratory failure. In addition, DKA may imitate other diseases. High levels of potassium may also cause ECG changes suggestive of myocardial infarction and elevation of myocardial enzymes and biomarkers may occur in the absence of a clinical myocardial infarction [21]. DKA may also mimic an acute abdomen, particularly in younger patients.

Management

Management and treatment of DKA rests on four pillars:

1 Fluid and electrolyte therapy;
2 IV insulin therapy;
3 Treatment of co-morbidities; and
4 Careful monitoring of the clinical course.

It is particularly important that treatment is initiated without delay and that the patient is monitored frequently and carefully, preferably in a highly specialized unit. Severe cases should be treated and monitored in an intensive care unit where possible. Useful algorithms for treatment are available from many sources including the American Diabetes Association. In general, the overall goal is a controlled, gradual correction of metabolic abnormalities and fluid and electrolyte deficiencies in the course of around 24 hours.

Treatment of DKA in children and young adolescents follows slightly different guidelines than those presented below (see Chapter 51) [22]. It is recommended that in children insulin is given continuously intravenously (0.1 IU/kg body weight/hour) after initiation of fluid and electrolyte therapy in order to minimize the risk of cerebral edema. Otherwise children are in general treated with weight reduced doses as indicated below.

Fluid/saline therapy

The first priority is to start to replace fluids. Water and sodium deficits typically are around 10% of body weight and 10 mmol/kg and isotonic saline (0.154 mmol/L; 0.9% NaCl) is given at a rate of approximately 15–20 mL/kg/hour or 1 L/hour initially, followed by 250 mL/hour after the first 2–3 hours depending on the state of dehydration. Depending on prevailing sodium concentrations and hydration, hypotonic saline may also be used, but this is rarely necessary. Urine production as well as cardiovascular, renal and mental performance should be monitored frequently.

Insulin

Lack of insulin is the culprit in DKA and insulin treatment is mandatory. Insulin therapy in adults is given by infusion of 0.1 IU/kg body weight/hour or more simply as 6 units/hour. An IV bolus of 0.15 IU/kg body weight (or 10 IU) of regular insulin can be given initially but is not really required, as most of the initial improvement in metabolic status is brought about by rehydration. Alternatively, a bolus of 0.15 IU/kg body weight (or 10 IU) may be given every hour or a 20 unit bolus IM followed by 6 units every hour. If the patient is very insulin resistant as assessed by daily insulin requirements, dosage can be increased and vice versa if the patient is insulin sensitive. Considering the short half-life of IV administered insulin, it is imperative that insulin is given at least every hour, regardless of the prevailing blood glucose.

Insulin therapy is adjusted based on hourly measurements of blood glucose and – if possible – blood ketones, with the overall aim being a gradual decline in both. The initial decline is to a large extent caused by rehydration and expansion of the extracellular volume. Repeated analysis of arterial blood gases may be indicated but only in those patients with very low pH values and/or poor clinical condition. Measurements of ketone levels in urine is in general unreliable in this phase; these methods measure acetoacetate, which is quantitatively of minor importance compared to 3-OH-butyrate and acetoacetate in urine may exhibit an paradoxical initial increase because of increasing blood concentrations (and low urine production), despite successful treatment. In particular, acetone is also measured by standard urine dipstick methods and may continue to be excreted for up to 48 hours after the onset of treatment as it is fat soluble and leaches out slowly during treatment.

When glucose concentrations are 10–15 mmol/L, glucose is given IV and/or orally to avoid hypoglycemia. It is usually possible to taper IV insulin treatment when 3-hydroxybutyrate concentrations are well below 3 mmol/L. Ten percent glucose should be used for IV replacement as this provides some extra anabolic substrate. If the patient is still dehydrated then the saline infusion should be continued.

Potassium, bicarbonate and phosphate

Potassium

Even though the body is potassium depleted, with a typical deficit of around 5 mmol/kg, initial potassium values are usually normal or elevated. Insulin therapy, rehydration and correction of acidosis all cause a decrease in serum potassium and 20–30 mmol potassium/hour may be administered once potassium levels are below 5.0 mmol/L, provided renal function is intact. Subsequent potassium administration is guided by frequent concentration measurements; adjuvant oral administration may be used in very mild cases of DKA. It is a frequent practical problem that there may be some delay before values are available from the laboratory; gas analyzers that provide instant bedside potassium concentrations greatly facilitate this process.

Bicarbonate

Bicarbonate use in DKA is a matter of controversy [23], but it is empirically recommended that 25–50 mmol sodium bicarbonate is given hourly for 1–2 hours if the pH is below 7.0.

Phosphate

Phosphate deficiency of around 1 mmol/kg is typically present in DKA, but there is no evidence that phosphate supplementation should be given routinely. In patients with severe hypophosphatemia and/or cardiac and skeletal or respiratory muscle weakness, 20–30 mmol potassium phosphate can be given hourly for 1–2 hours.

Co-morbidity

Coexisting diseases precipitate DKA and DKA precipitates coexisting disease. Most often, patients with DKA have infectious disease and signs of infection should be vigorously sought for and treatment should be instituted as appropriate. Other prominent co-morbidities include cardiovascular events (myocardial infarction, stroke, thrombophlebitis, pulmonary embolism), acute gastrointestinal disorders and a variety of intoxications.

Complications

Iatrogenic hypoglycemia and hypokalemia are common and preventable, provided there is access to rapid analysis of glucose and potassium and – not less important – a competent and experienced medical team. Another frequent complication is recurrence of DKA or unnecessary protraction of the course, typically caused by insufficient insulin therapy. Thrombotic events are also not uncommon although more often in HH than DKA.

Cerebral edema is a rare, but often fatal, complication preponderant in children and adolescents. The pathophysiology is poorly understood, but may relate to overly aggressive therapy, the use of hypotonic replacement fluids, local cerebral overhydration and abnormalities of vasogenic function [22]. Symptoms frequently develop 4–12 hours after initiation of therapy and include headache, altered mental status, specific neurologic deficits and signs of increased intracranial pressure. Treatment with mannitol or hypertonic saline may be beneficial in this condition.

In some patients, the high anion-gap ketoacidosis may be further complicated by the appearance of a non-anion-gap hyperchloremic acidosis during treatment with insulin and saline infusions [24]. This is because of loss of alkali in the form of ketoanions with sodium or potassium in the urine. This component often results in protracted acidosis, which can confuse clinical assessment. Some of these patients may benefit from bicarbonate therapy.

Prevention

Implementation of self-care and shared-care principles is crucial. Patients should learn about symptoms of DKA and be able to measure ketones in blood or urine when they feel ill or if their blood glucose is high. A common lapse is the omission or reduction of insulin during episodes with impaired well-being and poor appetite. Persistent ketosis should be treated with extra insulin, fluid and carbohydrate, when necessary. Furthermore, it is very important that the individual patient has ready, 24 hours/day access to diabetologic expertise, preferably in a specialized diabetes center.

Hyperosmolar hyperglycemia

Hyperosmolar hyperglycemia (HH) is generally the fulminant result of poorly treated T2DM or delayed diagnosis of previously unknown T2DM. HH is less frequent than DKA, but mortality is higher and remains close to 15% in many centers [2,25]. As implied, hyperosmolality is the primary clinical problem accompanied by hyperglycemia of >35–40 mmol/L and an effective serum osmolality of >320 mOsm/kg (Table 34.1). HH most often occurs in frail patients in combination with other potentially fatal conditions. Strict differentiation between DKA and HH can be difficult, because some degree of ketosis may be present in HH and because lactic acidosis, respiratory and renal failure may also be present. In practice this dilemma is mainly ornamental, because diagnostic and therapeutic efforts follow the same principles.

In line with DKA, HH is most often precipitated by infectious diseases or cardiovascular events and symptoms of hyperglycemia usually have been present for some days. Hyperglycemia is caused by a vicious cycle, in which relative insulin deficiency and high levels of stress hormones lead to increased endogenous glucose production and decreased peripheral glucose utilization; hyperglycemia in turn induces hyperosmolality and dehydration, which amplifies the stress hormone response and further impairs insulin secretion and vice versa.

At presentation, the patient's clinical condition is poor, with severe dehydration, poor skin turgor and often an altered level of consciousness (ranging from drowsiness to coma) and signs of hypovolemic shock. In general, the diagnostic procedures are similar to DKA. Typically, there will be a water deficit of 10–20% of body weight together with sodium, chloride and potassium deficits of 5–10 mmol/kg body weight.

Treatment of HH in general follows the same guidelines as for DKA, the main aim being a controlled correction of hyperglycemia, hyperosmolality and water and electrolyte deficits over 24 hours. Patients are generally more sensitive to insulin and an infusion of 0.1 IU/kg body weight/hour is more than adequate in most cases. Repeated hourly boluses of 0.15 IU/kg body weight (or 10 IU) may also be used. As with DKA, the dosage should be adjusted according to normal daily insulin needs and depending on the therapeutic response. Usually 1 L isotonic saline is infused in the first hour but after that slower rehydration is advisable. Hemodynamic performance should be monitored carefully and it should be borne in mind that many of the patients have pre- or coexisting cardiac disease. The use of a central venous pressure line is helpful. It should be noted that a significant proportion of HH patients are hypernatremic. In this case hypotonic saline can be used but more slowly. Potassium is administered along the same lines as with DKA and it is often prudent to monitor the patient in the intensive care unit.

References

1 Eledrisi MS, Alshanti MS, Shah MF, Brolosy B, Jaha N. Overview of the diagnosis and management of diabetic ketoacidosis. *Am J Med Sci* 2006; **331**:243–251.

2 Kitabchi AE, Umpierrez GE, Murphy MB, Kreisberg RA. Hyperglycemic crises in adult patients with diabetes: a consensus statement from the American Diabetes Association. *Diabetes Care* 2006; **29**:2739–2748.

3 Kitabchi AE, Umpierrez GE, Fisher JN, Murphy MB, Stentz FB. Thirty years of personal experience in hyperglycemic crises: diabetic ketoacidosis and hyperglycemic hyperosmolar state. *J Clin Endocrinol Metab* 2008; **93**:1541–1552.

4 Wang J, Williams DE, Narayan KM, Geiss LS. Declining death rates from hyperglycemic crisis among adults with diabetes, US, 1985–2002. *Diabetes Care* 2006; **29**:2018–2222.

5 Freire AX, Umpierrez GE, Afessa B, Latif KA, Bridges L, Kitabchi AE. Predictors of intensive care unit and hospital length of stay in diabetic ketoacidosis. *J Crit Care* 2002; **17**:207–211.

6 Alberti KG. Low-dose insulin in the treatment of diabetic ketoacidosis. *Arch Intern Med* 1977; **137**:1367–1376.

7 Barnes AJ, Kohner EM, Bloom SR, Johnston DG, Alberti KG, Smythe F. Importance of pituitary hormones in aetiology of diabetic ketoacidosis. *Lancet* 1978; **1**:1171–1174.

8 Stentz FB, Umpierrez GE, Cuervo R, Kitabchi AE. Proinflammatory cytokines, markers of cardiovascular risks, oxidative stress, and lipid peroxidation in patients with hyperglycemic crises. *Diabetes* 2004; **53**:2079–2086.

9 Fong YM, Marano MA, Moldawer LL, Wei H, Calvano SE, Kenney JS, *et al.* The acute splanchnic and peripheral tissue metabolic response to endotoxin in humans. *J Clin Invest* 1990; **85**:1896–1904.

10 Van der Poll T, Romijn JA, Endert E, Borm JJ, Büller HR, Sauerwein HP. Tumor necrosis factor mimics the metabolic response to acute infection in healthy humans. *Am J Physiol* 1991; **261**:E457–E465.

11 Hansen TK, Thiel S, Wouters PJ, Christiansen JS, Van den Berghe G. Intensive insulin therapy exerts antiinflammatory effects in critically ill patients and counteracts the adverse effect of low mannose-binding lectin levels. *J Clin Endocrinol Metab* 2003; **88**:1082–1088.

12 Lang CH, Dobrescu C, Bagby GJ. Tumor necrosis factor impairs insulin action on peripheral glucose disposal and hepatic glucose output. *Endocrinology* 1992; **130**:43–52.

13 Langouche L, Vanhorebeek I, Vlasselaers D, Vander Perre S, Wouters PJ, Skogstrand K, *et al.* Intensive insulin therapy protects the endothelium of critically ill patients. *J Clin Invest* 2005; **115**:2277–2286.

14 Langouche L, Vander Perre S, Wouters PJ, D'Hoore A, Hansen TK, Van den Berghe G. Effect of intensive insulin therapy on insulin sensitivity in the critically ill. *J Clin Endocrinol Metab* 2007; **92**:3890–3897.

15 Koutsari C, Jensen MD. Thematic review series: patient-oriented research. Free fatty acid metabolism in human obesity. *J Lipid Res* 2006; **47**:1643–1650.

16 Keller U, Szinnai G, Bilz S, Berneis K. Effects of changes in hydration on protein, glucose and lipid metabolism in man: impact on health. *Eur J Clin Nutr* 2003; **57**(Suppl 2):S69–S74.

17 Cahill GF Jr. Fuel metabolism in starvation. *Annu Rev Nutr* 2006; **26**:1–22.

18 Foster DW, McGarry JD. The metabolic derangements and treatment of diabetic ketoacidosis. *N Engl J Med* 1983; **309**:159–169.

19 Burge MR, Hardy KJ, Schade DS. Short-term fasting is a mechanism for the development of euglycemic ketoacidosis during periods of insulin deficiency. *J Clin Endocrinol Metab* 1993; **76**:1192–1198.

20 Moller N, Jensen MD, Rizza RA, Andrews JC, Nair KS. Renal amino acid, fat and glucose metabolism in type 1 diabetic and non-diabetic humans: effects of acute insulin withdrawal. *Diabetologia* 2006; **49**:1901–1908.

21 Moller N, Foss AC, Gravholt CH, Mortensen UM, Poulsen SH, Mogensen CE. Myocardial injury with biomarker elevation in diabetic ketoacidosis. *J Diabetes Complications* 2005; **19**:361–363.

22 Wolfsdorf J, Glaser N, Sperling MA. Diabetic ketoacidosis in infants, children, and adolescents: a consensus statement from the American Diabetes Association. *Diabetes Care* 2006; **29**:1150–1159.

23 Latif KA, Freire AX, Kitabchi AE, Umpierrez GE, Qureshi N. The use of alkali therapy in severe diabetic ketoacidosis. *Diabetes Care* 2002; **25**:2113–2114.

24 Oh MS, Carroll HJ, Goldstein DA, Fein IA. Hyperchloremic acidosis during the recovery phase of diabetic ketoacidosis. *Ann Intern Med* 1978; **59**:925–927.

25 Gaglia JL, Wyckoff J, Abrahamson MJ. Acute hyperglycemic crisis in the elderly. *Med Clin North Am* 2004; **88**:1063–1084, xii.

7 Microvascular Complications in Diabetes

35 Pathogenesis of Microvascular Complications

Ferdinando Giacco & Michael Brownlee
Diabetes Research Center, Departments of Medicine and Endocrinology, Albert Einstein College of Medicine, NY, USA

Keypoints

- Microvascular complications are caused by prolonged exposure to hyperglycemia.
- Hyperglycemia damages cell types that cannot downregulate glucose uptake, causing intracellular hyperglycemia.
- Intracellular hyperglycemia damages tissues by five major mechanisms: increased flux of glucose and other sugars through the polyol pathway; increased intracellular formation of advanced glycation end-products (AGEs); increased expression of the receptor for AGEs and its activating ligands; activation of protein kinase C isoforms; and overactivity of the hexosamine pathway.
- A single process – increased mitochondrial production of oxygen free radicals – activates each of these mechanisms.
- Persistent consequences of hyperglycemia-induced mitochondrial superoxide production may also explain the continuing progression of tissue damage after improvement of glycemic levels ("hyperglycemic memory").
- Different individual susceptibility to microvascular complications have been linked to polymorphisms in the superoxide dismutase 1 gene.
- Hyperglycemia-induced mitochondrial reactive oxygen species production impairs the neovascular response to ischemia by blunting hypoxia-inducible factor 1 transactivation.
- Hypertension accelerates microvascular damage by increasing intracellular hyperglycemia through upregulation of the glucose transporter 1.
- Potential mechanism-based therapeutic agents for diabetic microvascular complications include transketolase activators, poly(ADP-ribose) polymerase inhibitors and catalytic antioxidants.

Overview of diabetic complications

All forms of diabetes are characterized by hyperglycemia, a relative or absolute lack of insulin action, and the development of diabetes-specific pathology in the retina, renal glomerulus and peripheral nerve. Diabetes is also associated with accelerated atherosclerotic disease affecting arteries that supply the heart, brain and lower extremities. As a consequence of its disease-specific pathology, diabetes mellitus is now the leading cause of new blindness in people 20–74 years of age and the leading cause of end-stage renal disease (ESRD) in the developed world. Survival of patients with diabetic ESRD on dialysis is half that of those without diabetes. More than 60% of patients with diabetes are affected by neuropathy, which includes distal symmetrical polyneuropathy, mononeuropathies and a variety of autonomic neuropathies causing erectile dysfunction, urinary incontinence, gastroparesis and nocturnal diarrhoea. Diabetic accelerated lower extremity arterial disease in conjunction with neuropathy accounts for 50% of all non-traumatic amputations in the USA. Diabetes and impaired glucose tolerance increase cardiovascular disease (CVD) risk three- to eightfold. Thus, over 40% of patients hospitalized with acute myocardial infarction (MI) have diabetes and 35% have impaired glucose tolerance. Finally, new blood vessel growth in response to ischemia is impaired in diabetes, resulting in decreased collateral vessel formation in ischemic hearts, and in non-healing foot ulcers. The focus of this chapter is on the microvascular complications comprising retinopathy, nephropathy and peripheral neuropathy.

Much of the impact of chronic diabetes falls on the microcirculation [1,2]. With long-standing disease, there is progressive narrowing and eventual occlusion of vascular lumina, resulting in impaired perfusion, ischemia and dysfunction of the affected tissues. Several processes contribute to microvascular occlusion. One of the earliest is increased vascular permeability, allowing extravasation of plasma proteins that accumulate as periodic acid–Schiff-positive deposits in the vessel walls. In addition, the extracellular matrix elaborated by perivascular cells such as pericytes (retina) and mesangial cells (glomerulus) is increased, brought about by changes in synthesis and turnover of its component proteins and glycosaminoglycans. As a result, the basement membrane is thickened in many tissues, including retinal capillaries and the vasa nervorum, while mesangial matrix is

Textbook of Diabetes, 4th edition. Edited by R. Holt, C. Cockram, A. Flyvbjerg and B. Goldstein. © 2010 Blackwell Publishing.

expanded in the renal glomerulus. Hypertrophy and hyperplasia of endothelial, mesangial and arteriolar smooth muscle cells also contribute to vessel wall thickening. Finally, increased coagulability of the blood and adhesion of platelets and leukocytes to the endothelial surface lead to microthrombus formation and luminal occlusion.

The progressive narrowing and blockage of diabetic microvascular lumina are accompanied by loss of microvascular cells. In the retina, diabetes induces apoptosis of Müller cells and ganglion cells [3], pericytes and endothelial cells [4]. In the glomerulus, widespread capillary occlusion and declining renal function are associated with podocyte loss. In the vasa nervorum of diabetic nerves, endothelial cell and pericyte degeneration occur [5] and appear to precede functional abnormalities of peripheral nerves [6]. Increased apoptosis of cells in the retina, renal glomerulus and peripheral neurons is a prominent feature of diabetic microvascular tissue damage [7–11] and may also cause damage to adjacent cells.

Role of hyperglycemia in microvascular complications

Overall, diabetic microvascular complications are caused by prolonged exposure to high glucose levels. This has been established by large-scale prospective studies for both type 1 diabetes (T1DM) by the Diabetes Control and Complications Trial/Epidemiology of Diabetes Interventions and Complications Study [DCCT/EDIC] [12] and for type 2 diabetes (T2DM) by the UK Prospective Diabetes Study [UKPDS] [13]). Similar data have been reported by the Steno-2 study [14].

Because every cell in the body of people with diabetes is exposed to abnormally high glucose concentrations, why does hyperglycemia selectively damage some cell types and not others? The targeting of specific cell types by generalized hyperglycemia reflects the failure of those cells to downregulate their uptake of glucose when extracellular glucose concentrations are elevated. Cells that are not directly susceptible to direct hyperglycemic damage such as vascular smooth muscle show an inverse relationship between extracellular glucose concentrations and glucose transport. In contrast, vascular endothelial cells, a major target of hyperglycemic damage, show no significant change in glucose transport rate when glucose concentration is elevated, resulting in intracellular hyperglycemia (Figure 35.1). These differences are caused in part by tissue-specific differences in expression and function of different glucose transporter (GLUT) proteins [15].

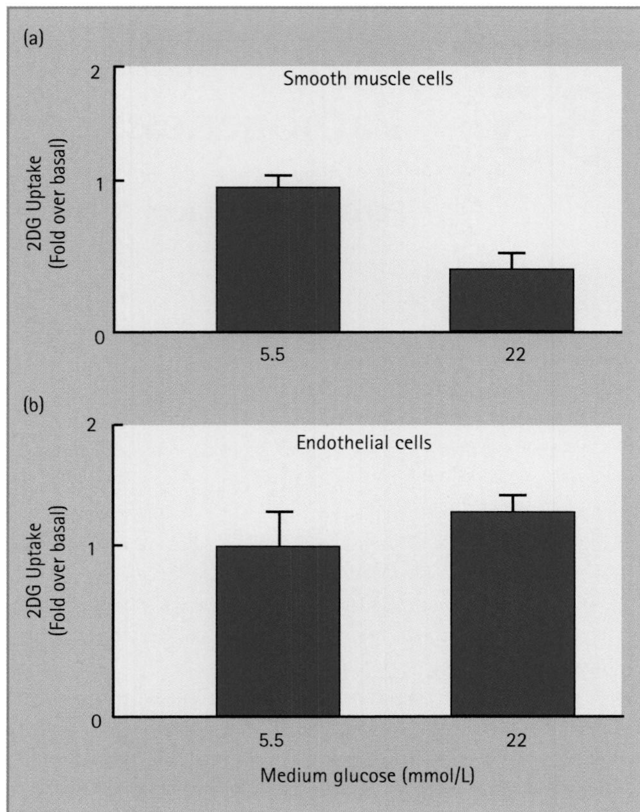

Figure 35.1 Lack of downregulation of glucose transport by hyperglycemia in cells affected by diabetic complications. (a) 2-Deoxyglucose uptake in vascular smooth muscle cells pre-exposed to 5.5 or 22 mmol/L glucose. (b) 2-Deoxyglucose uptake in aortic endothelial cells pre-exposed to 5.5 or 22 mmol/L glucose. Data from Kaiser N, Sasson S, Feener EP, Boukobza-Vardi N, Higashi S, Moller DE, *et al.* Differential regulation of glucose transport and transporters by glucose in vascular endothelial and smooth muscle cells. *Diabetes* 1993; **42**:80–89.

Mechanisms of hyperglycemia-induced damage

There are nearly 2000 publications supporting five major mechanisms by which hyperglycemia causes diabetic complications:

1 Increased flux of glucose and other sugars through the polyol pathway;

2 Increased intracellular formation of advanced glycation end-products (AGEs);

3 Increased expression of the receptor for AGEs (RAGE) and its activating ligands;

4 Activation of protein kinase C (PKC) isoforms; and

5 Overactivity of the hexosamine pathway.

Despite this, the results of clinical studies in which one of these pathways is blocked have been disappointing. This led to the hypothesis in 2000 that all five mechanisms are activated by a single upstream event: mitochondrial overproduction of the reactive oxygen species (ROS) superoxide as a result of intracellular hyperglycemia. This provides a unifying hypothesis for the pathogenesis of diabetic complications.

Increased polyol pathway flux

The polyol pathway is based on a family of aldoketo reductase enzymes which can utilize as substrates a wide variety of sugar-derived carbonyl compounds and reduce these by nicotinic acid

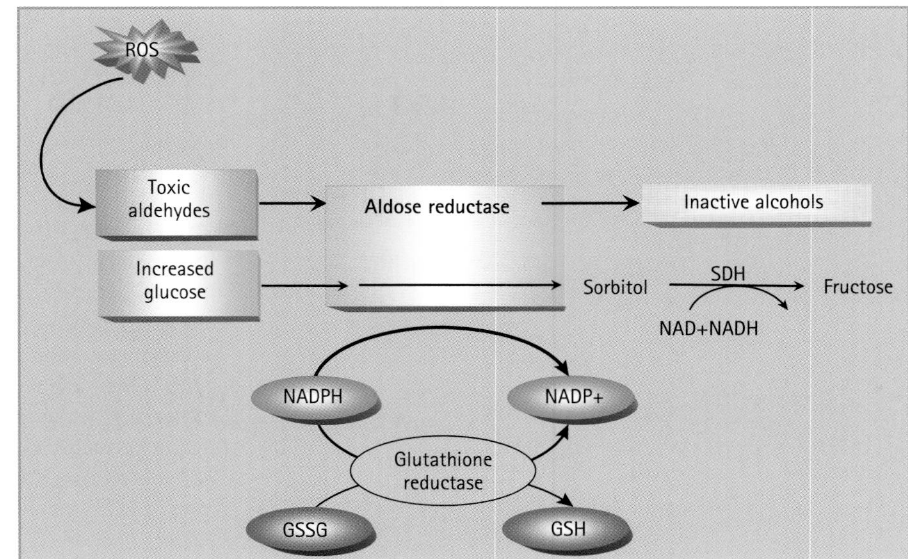

Figure 35.2 The polyol pathway. When glucose concentration is normal, aldose reductase reduces toxic aldehydes generated by reactive oxygen species (ROS) to inactive alcohols. With intracellular hyperglycemia, it can also reduce glucose to sorbitol. Both reactions use nicotinic acid adenine dinucleotide phosphate (NADPH) as a co-factor. When aldose reductase activity is sufficient to deplete reduced glutathione (GSH), oxidative stress is augmented. Sorbitol-dehydrogenase (SDH) oxidizes sorbitol to fructose using NAD^+ as a co-factor. GSSG, glutathione disulfide (oxidized glutathione).

adenine dinucleotide phosphate (NADPH) to their respective sugar alcohols (polyols). The classic representation holds that glucose is converted to sorbitol, and galactose to galactitol. Sorbitol is then oxidized to fructose by the enzyme sorbitol dehydrogenase (SDH), with NAD^+ being reduced to NADH (Figure 35.2).

The first and rate-limiting step of the polyol pathway is governed by aldose reductase, which is found in tissues such as nerve, retina, lens, glomerulus and blood vessel wall. In these tissues, glucose uptake is mediated by GLUT proteins other than GLUT-4 and so does not require insulin; intracellular glucose concentrations therefore rise in parallel with hyperglycemia.

Several mechanisms have been proposed to explain how hyperglycemia-induced increases in polyol pathway flux could damage the tissues involved. These include sorbitol-induced osmotic stress, decreased cytosolic Na/K^+-ATPase activity, increased cytosolic $NADH/NAD^+$, and decreased cytosolic NADPH. It was originally suggested that intracellular accumulation of sorbitol, which does not diffuse easily across cell membranes, could result in osmotic damage, but it is now clear that sorbitol levels in diabetic vessels and nerves are far too low to do this. Another early suggestion was that increased flux through the polyol pathway led to decreased phosphatidylinositol synthesis, and that this inhibited Na/K^+-ATPase activity. The latter abnormality does occur in diabetes, but has recently been shown to result from hyperglycemia-induced activation of PKC which increases the production of two inhibitors of Na/K^+-ATPase, arachidonate and prostaglandin E_2 [16].

It has also been suggested that the reduction of glucose to sorbitol by NADPH (Figure 35.2) consumes the latter. NADPH is a co-factor required to regenerate reduced glutathione (GSH); as GSH is an important scavenger of ROS, this could induce or exacerbate intracellular oxidative stress. Indeed, overexpression of human aldose reductase increased atherosclerosis in diabetic mice and reduced the expression of genes that regulate regeneration of GSH [17]. Reduced GSH is depleted in the lens of transgenic mice that overexpress aldose reductase and in diabetic rat lens compared with non-diabetic lens [18,19]. It has also been recently demonstrated that decreased glutathiolation of cellular proteins is related to decreased nitric oxide (NO) availability in diabetic rats which would decrease S-nitrosoglutathione (GSNO). Restoring the NO levels in diabetic animals increases glutathiolation of cellular proteins, inhibits aldose reductase activity and prevents sorbitol accumulation.

Moreover, hyperglycemia can also inhibit glucose-6-phosphate dehydrogenase, the major source of NADPH regeneration, which may further reduce NADPH concentration in some vascular cells and neurons [20].

In diabetic vascular cells, however, glucose does not appear to be the substrate for aldose reductase, because the Michaelis constant (Km) of aldose reductase for glucose is 100 mmol/L, while the intracellular concentration of glucose in diabetic retina is 0.15 mmol/L [21,22]. Glycolytic metabolites of glucose such as glyceraldehyde-3-phosphate, for which aldose reductase has much higher affinity, may be the physiologically relevant substrate.

Increased intracellular AGE formation

AGEs are formed by the reaction of glucose and other glycating compounds (e.g. dicarbonyls such as 3-deoxyglucosone, methylglyoxal and glyoxal) with proteins and, to a lesser extent, nucleic acids. The reactions proceed through a series of stages that are initially reversible and yield early glycation products, but eventually undergo irreversible changes that markedly impair the structural, enzymatic or signaling functions of the glycated proteins (Figure 35.3). A familiar example of this process yields glycated hemoglobin (HbA_{1c}). AGEs are found in increased amounts in

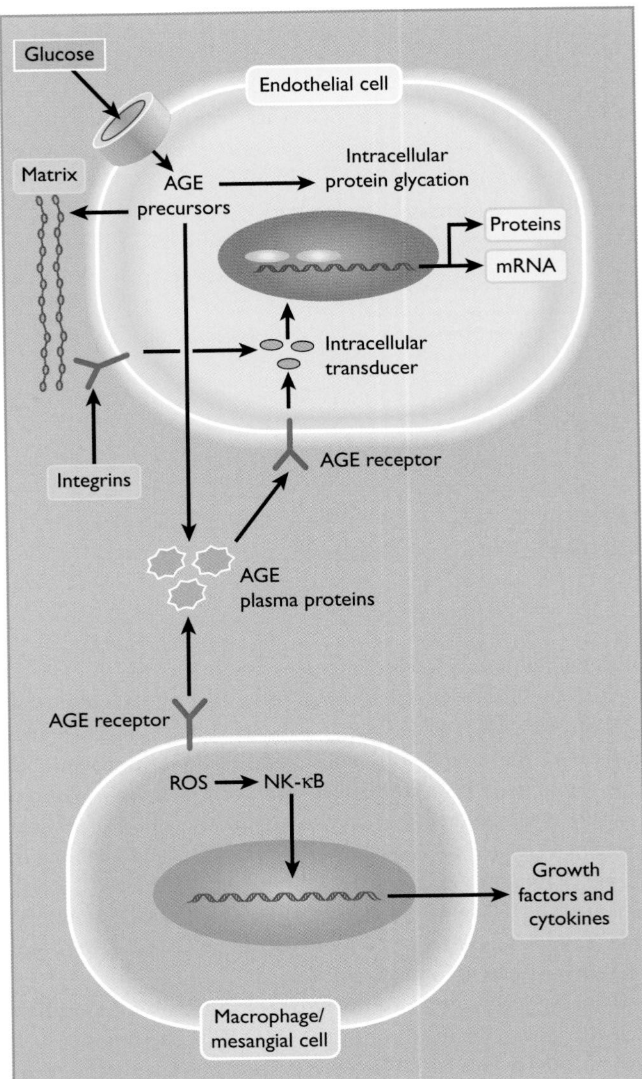

Figure 35.3 Increased production of intracellular advanced glycation end-products (AGE) precursors damages cells by three mechanisms: modification of intracellular proteins; modification of the extracellular matrix (upper panel); and interactions with AGE receptors such as RAGE in endothelial cells and macrophages. NFκB, nuclear factor κB; ROS, reactive oxygen species.

extracellular structures of diabetic retinal vessels [23–25] and renal glomeruli [26–28], where they can cause damage through the mechanisms described below.

These AGEs were originally thought to arise from non-enzymatic reactions between extracellular proteins and glucose; however, the rate of AGE formation from glucose is orders of magnitude slower than that induced by glucose-derived dicarbonyl precursors generated intracellularly, and it now seems likely that raised intracellular glucose is the primary initiating event in the formation of both intracellular and extracellular AGEs [29]. AGEs can arise intracellularly from the autooxidation of glucose to glyoxal [30], the decomposition of an Amadori product to the 3-deoxyglucosone, or the fragmentation of glyceraldehyde-3-phosphate to yield methylglyoxal [31]. All these reactive intracellular dicarbonyls react readily with uncharged amino groups of intracellular and extracellular proteins to form AGEs. Methylglyoxsal is the major intracellular AGE precursor [32,33].

Intracellular effects of AGEs

Intracellular production of AGE precursors can damage cells by three general mechanisms. First, intracellular proteins modified by AGEs have altered function. Secondly, extracellular matrix components modified by AGE precursors interact abnormally with other matrix components and with matrix receptors (integrins) which are expressed on the surface of cells. Finally, plasma proteins modified by AGE precursors bind to AGE receptors on cells such as macrophages; binding induces the production of ROS, which in turn activates the pleiotropic transcription factor, nuclear factor κB (NFκB), causing multiple pathologic changes in gene expression [34].

It has been recently demonstrated that AGE modification of intracellular protein can be involved in diabetic retinopathy. In diabetes, retinal capillary formation is regulated by complex context-dependent interactions among pro- and anti-angiogenic factors [35,36], including angiopoietin-2 (Ang-2). When vascular endothelial growth factor (VEGF) levels are insufficient, Ang-2 causes endothelial cell death and vessel regression. Diabetes induces a significant increase in retinal expression of Ang-2 in rat [37], and diabetic Ang-2 +/– mice have both decreased pericyte loss and reduced acellular capillary formation [38].

Moreover, in mouse kidney endothelial cells, high glucose causes increased methylglyoxal modification of the corepressor mSin3A. Methylglyoxal modification of mSin3A results in increased recruitment of O-GlcNAc-transferase, with consequent increased modification of Sp3 by *O*-linked *N*-acetylglucosamine. This modification of Sp3 causes decreased binding to a glucose-responsive GC-box in the Ang-2 promoter, resulting in increased Ang-2 expression. Increased Ang-2 expression induced by high glucose in renal endothelial cells increased expression of intracellular adhesion molecule 1 (ICAM-1) and vascular cell adhesion molecule 1 (VCAM-1) in cells and in kidneys from diabetic mice and sensitized microvascular endothelial cells to the pro-inflammatory effects of tumor necrosis factor α (TNF-α) [39].

Effects of AGEs on extracellular matrix

AGE formation alters the functional properties of several important matrix molecules. Collagen was the first matrix protein in which glucose-derived AGEs were shown to form covalent intermolecular bonds. This process is partly mediated by H_2O_2 production [40,41]. With type I collagen, this cross-linking causes expansion of molecular packing [42], while AGE formation on type IV collagen from basement membrane inhibits the normal lateral association of these molecules into a network-like structure by interfering with binding of the non-collagenous NC1 domain to the helix-rich domain [43]. AGE formation on laminin prevents the molecules from self-assembling into a polymer and also decreases binding with type IV collagen and heparan sulfate proteoglycan [44].

These AGE-induced cross-links alter tissue function, notably in blood vessels. AGEs decrease elasticity in arteries from diabetic rats, even after vascular tone is abolished, and increase fluid filtration across the carotid artery [45]. *In vitro*, AGE formation on intact glomerular basement membrane increases its permeability to albumin in a manner that resembles the abnormal permeability of diabetic nephropathy [46,47].

AGE formation on extracellular matrix also interferes with the ways in which cells interact with the matrix. For example, methylglyoxal modification of type IV collagen's cell-binding domains decreases endothelial cell adhesion and inhibits angiogenesis [48].

AGE formation on a 6-amino acid, growth-promoting sequence in the A chain of the laminin molecule markedly reduces neurite outgrowth [49], while AGE modification of vitronectin reduces its ability to promote cell attachment [50]. In addition, matrix glycation impairs agonist-induced Ca^{2+} increases which might adversely affect the regulatory functions of endothelium [51].

Receptor-mediated biologic effects of AGEs

AGE-modified proteins in the circulation can affect a range of cells and tissues. Specific receptors for AGEs were first identified on monocytes and macrophages. Two AGE-binding proteins isolated from rat liver, identified as OTS-48 (60 kDa) and 80K-H (90 kDa) [52], are both present on monocytes and macrophages; antisera against either protein block AGE binding [53]. AGE protein binding to this receptor stimulates macrophages to produce cytokines, including interleukin-1, TNF-α, transforming growth factor β (TGF-β), macrophage colony-stimulating factor and granulocyte–macrophage colony-stimulating factor, as well as insulin-like growth factor I (IGF-I). These factors appear to be produced at concentrations that can increase glomerular synthesis of type IV collagen and induce chemotaxis and proliferation of both arterial smooth muscle cells and macrophages [54–62]. The macrophage scavenger receptor type II (class A), galectin-3 and CD36 (a member of the class B macrophage scavenger receptor family) have also been shown to recognize AGEs [63–67].

AGE receptors have also been identified on glomerular mesangial cells. *In vitro*, AGE protein binding to its receptor on mesangial cells stimulates secretion of platelet-derived growth factor which in turn mediates mesangial cells to produce type IV collagen, laminin and heparan sulfate proteoglycan [68,69].

Vascular endothelial cells and other cell types also express specific AGE receptors (RAGEs), notably 35-kDa and 46-kDa AGE-binding proteins that have been purified to homogeneity [70–72]. The N-terminal sequence of the 35-kDa protein is identical to lactoferrin, whereas the 46-kDa AGE-binding protein is a novel member of the immunoglobulin superfamily, containing three disulfide-bonded immunoglobulin homology units. RAGE have been shown to mediate signal transduction via generation of ROS, activation of NFκB, and p21 *ras* [73–75]. AGE signaling can be blocked in cells by expression of RAGE antisense cDNA [76] or anti-RAGE ribozyme [77]. It has been also recently demonstrated that a RAGE–NFκB axis operates in diabetic neuropathy by mediating functional sensory deficits [78].

In endothelial cells, AGE binding to its receptor alters the expression of several genes, including thrombomodulin, tissue factor and VCAM-1 [79–81]. These effects induce procoagulatory changes on the endothelial cell surface and increase the adhesion of inflammatory cells to the endothelium. In addition, endothelial AGE receptor binding appears to mediate in part the increased vascular permeability induced by diabetes, probably through the induction of VEGF [82–85]. RAGE deficiency attenuates the development of atherosclerosis in the diabetic apoE(−/−) model of accelerated atherosclerosis. Diabetic RAGE(−/−)/apoE(−/−) mice had significantly reduced atherosclerotic plaque area. These beneficial effects on the vasculature were associated with attenuation of leukocyte recruitment, decreased expression of pro-inflammatory mediators, including the NFκB subunit p65, VCAM-1, and monocyte chemotactic protein 1 (MCP-1) and reduced oxidative stress [86].

It is important to note that more recent studies indicate that AGEs at the concentrations found in diabetic sera are not the major ligand for RAGE. Rather, several pro-inflammatory protein ligands have been identified, which activate RAGE at low concentrations. These include several members of the S100 calgranulin family and high mobility group box 1 (HMGB1), all of which are increased by diabetic hyperglycemia. Binding of these ligands with RAGE causes cooperative interaction with the innate immune system signaling molecule toll-like receptor 4 (TLR-4) [87,88].

Increased protein kinase C activation

The group of PKCs consist of at least 11 isoforms that are widely distributed in mammalian tissues. The activity of the classic isoforms is dependent on both Ca^{2+} ions and phosphatidylserine and is greatly enhanced by diacylglycerol (DAG). Persistent and excessive activation of several PKC isoforms might also operate as a third common pathway mediating tissue injury induced by hyperglycemia and associated biochemical and metabolic abnormalities. This results primarily from enhanced *de novo* synthesis of DAG from glucose via triose phosphates, whose availability is increased because raised intracellular glucose levels enhance glucose flux through the glycolytic pathway [89–92]. Finally, recent evidence suggests that the enhanced activity of PKC isoforms could also result from the interaction between AGEs and their cell-surface receptors [93]. Hyperglycemia primarily activates the β and δ isoforms of PKC, both in cultured vascular cells [94–96] and in the retina and glomeruli of diabetic animals [91,92,93], but increases in other isoforms have also been found, such as PKC-α and PKC-ε isoforms in the retina [89] and PKC-α and PKC-δ in the glomerulus of diabetic rats [97,98] (Figure 35.4).

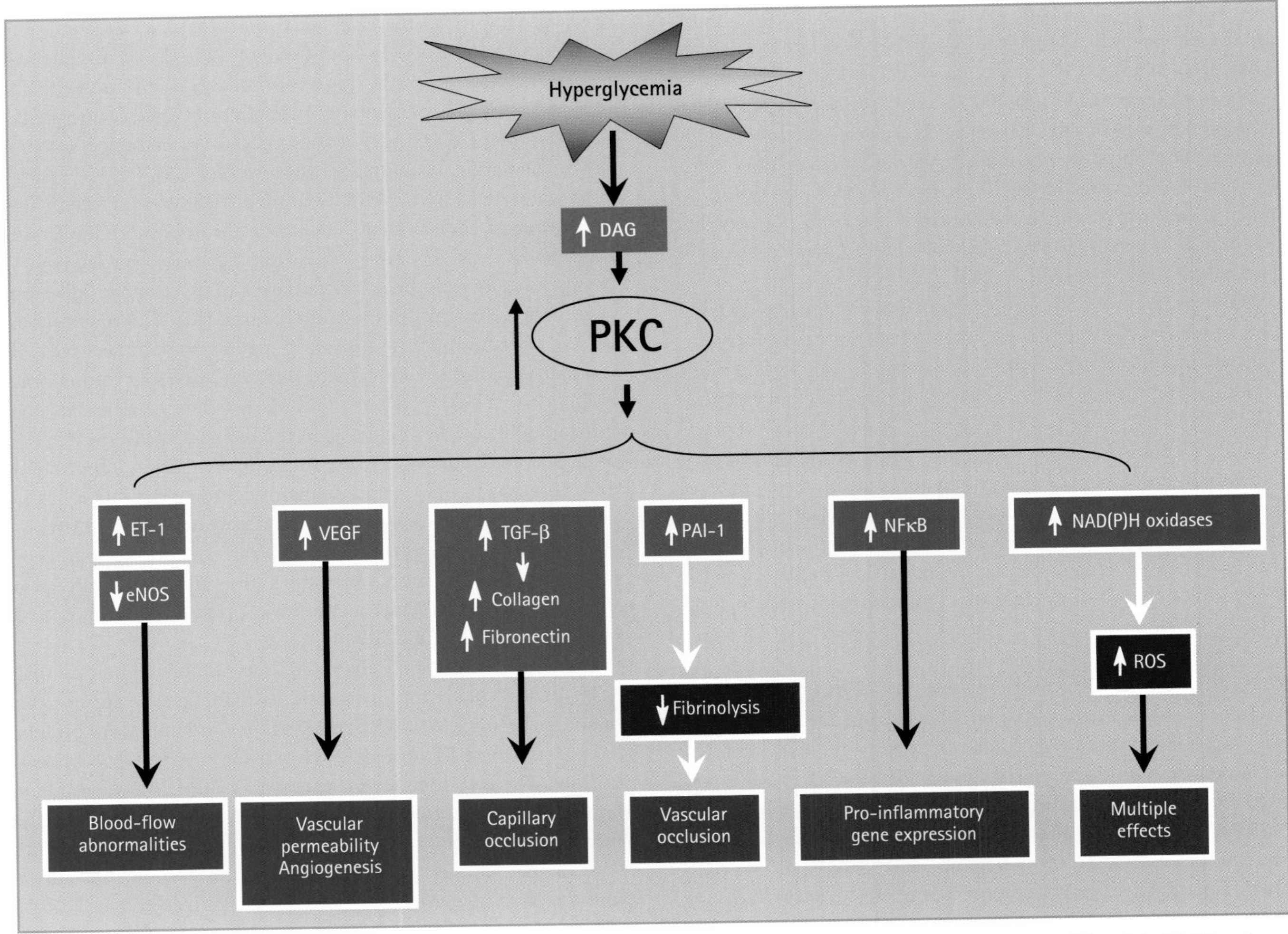

Figure 35.4 Activation of protein kinase C (PKC) by *de novo* synthesis of diacylglycerol (DAG) and some of its pathologic consequences. eNOS, endothelial NO synthase; ET-1, endothelin-1; NADPH, nicotinic acid adenine dinucleotide phosphate; NFκB, nuclear factor κB; PAI-1, plasminogen activator inhibitor 1; ROS, reactive oxygen species; TGF-β, transforming growth factor β; VEGF, vascular endothelial growth factor.

In early experimental diabetes, activation of PKC-β isoforms has been shown to mediate the diabetes-related decreases in retinal and renal blood flow [99], perhaps by depressing the production of the vasodilator NO and/or increasing endothelin-1, a potent vasoconstrictor. Overactivity of PKC has been implicated in the decreased NO production by the glomerulus in experimental diabetes [100] and by smooth muscle cells in the presence of high glucose levels [101], and has been shown to inhibit insulin-stimulated expression of endothelial NO synthase (eNOS) in cultured endothelial cells [102]. Hyperglycemia increases the ability of endothelin-1 to stimulate mitogen activated protein kinase (MAPK) activity in glomerular mesangial cells, and this occurs by activating PKC isoforms [103]. The increased endothelial cell permeability induced by high glucose in cultured cells is mediated by activation of PKC-α [104]; activation of PKC by high glucose also induces expression of the permeability-enhancing factor VEGF in smooth muscle cells [105].

In addition to mediating hyperglycemia-induced abnormalities of blood flow and permeability, activation of PKC may contribute to the accumulation of microvascular matrix protein by inducing expression of TGF-β1, fibronectin and type IV collagen in both cultured mesangial cells [106,107] and in glomeruli of diabetic rats [97]. This effect also appears to be mediated through the inhibition of NO production by PKC [108]. Hyperglycemia-induced activation of PKC has also been implicated in the overexpression of the fibrinolytic inhibitor, plasminogen activator inhibitor 1 (PAI-1) [109], and in the activation of NFκB in cultured endothelial cells and vascular smooth muscle cells [110,111].

Increased hexosamine pathway flux

Several data suggest that hyperglycemia could cause diabetic complications by shunting glucose into the hexosamine pathway [112–115]. Here, fructose-6-phosphate is diverted from glycolysis to provide substrates for reactions that utilize UDP-*N*-

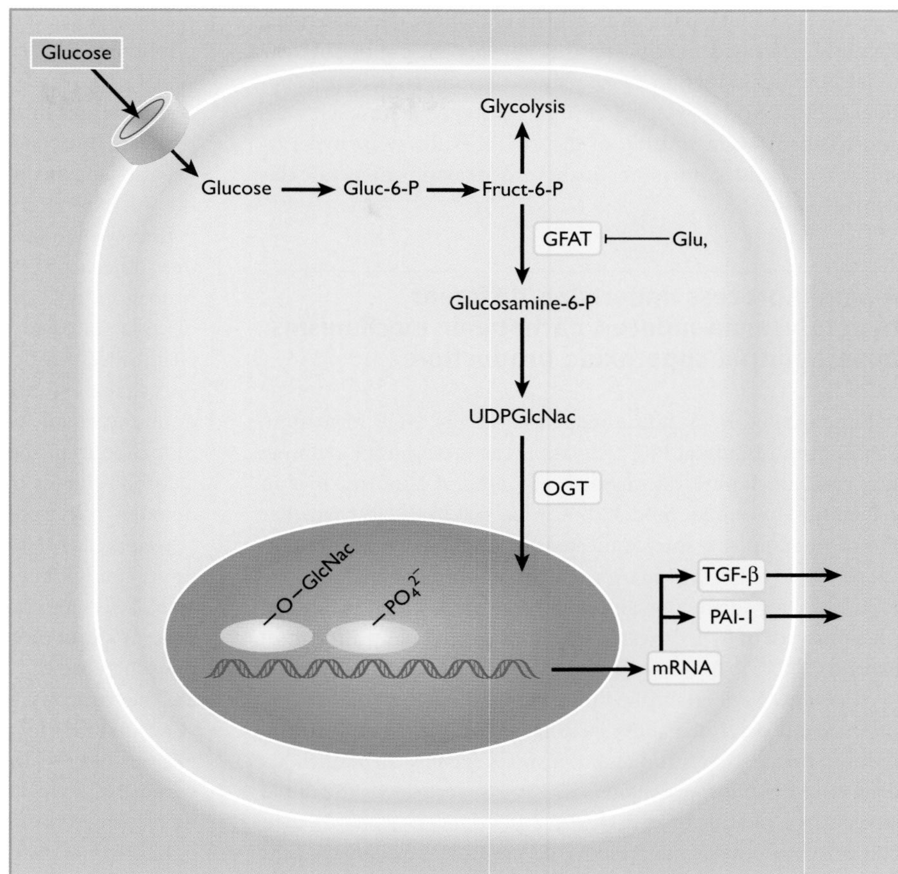

Figure 35.5 The glucosamine pathway. Glucosamine-6-phosphate is generated from fructose-6-phosphate and glutamine, by glutamine: fructose-6-phosphate amidotransferase (GFAT), the rate-limiting enzyme of this pathway. Glucosamine-6-phosphate is converted to UDP-*N*-acetylglucosamine (UDP-GlcNac), which can glycosylate transcription factors and thus enhance transcription of genes including plasminogen activator inhibitor 1 (PAI-1) and transforming growth factor β1 (TGF-β1). OGT, O-linked N-acetylglucosamine (GLcNac) transferase.

acetylglucosamine, particularly the formation of *O*-linked *N*-acetylglucosamine. This pathway has been shown to have an important role in hyperglycemia-induced and fat-induced insulin resistance [116–118]. The rate-limiting step in the conversion of glucose to glucosamine is regulated by glutamine:fructose-6-phosphate amidotransferase (GFAT), and inhibition of this enzyme blocks hyperglycemia-induced increases in the transcription of both TGF-α [112] and TGF-β1 [113].

It is not entirely clear how increased glucose flux through the hexosamine pathway mediates hyperglycemia-induced increases in the gene transcription of key genes such as TGF-α, TGF-β1 and PAI-1, however, it has been shown that the transcription factor Sp1 regulates hyperglycemia-induced activation of the PAI-1 promoter in vascular smooth muscle cells [119], raising the possibility that covalent glycation of Sp1 by *N*-acetylglucosamine to form its *O*-GlcNacylated derivative could explain how hexosamine pathway activation might operate. Virtually every RNA polymerase II transcription factor examined is *O*-GlcNacylated [120], and this glycosylated form of Sp1 appears to be more transcriptionally active than its non-glycosylated counterpart [121]. A fourfold increase in Sp1 *O*-GlcNacylation (caused by inhibition of the enzyme *O*-GlcNac-β-*N*-acetylglucosaminidase) resulted in a reciprocal 30% decrease in the level of serine/threonine phosphorylation of Sp1; thus, *O*-GlcNacylation and phosphorylation may compete to modify the same sites on Sp1 (Figure 35.5) [122].

GlcNac modification of Sp1 may regulate other glucose-responsive genes in addition to TGF-β1 and PAI-1. Glucose-responsive transcription of the acetylcoenzyme A carboxylase gene (the rate-limiting enzyme for fatty acid synthesis) is regulated by Sp1 sites, and post-transcriptional modification of Sp1 may similarly be responsible [123,124]. Because so many RNA polymerase II transcription factors are *O*-GlcNacylated [120], others in addition to Sp1 may be regulated by reciprocal modification (glycosylation vs phosphorylation) at key serine and threonine residues and so cause gene transcription to be glucose-responsive. In addition to transcription factors, many other nuclear and cytoplasmic proteins can be modified by *O*-GlcNac moities perturbing their normal function and regulation. One example relevant to diabetes is the inhibition of eNOS activity by *O*-GlcNacylation at the Akt site of eNOS protein [125–127]. Hyperglycemia also increases GFAT activity in aortic smooth muscle cells which increases *O*-GlcNac modification of several proteins in these cells [128]. Overall, activation of the hexosamine pathway by hyperglycemia may result in many changes in both gene expression and in protein function that together contribute to the pathogenesis of diabetic complications. Recently, increased modification of key signaling molecules by *O*-GlcNAc was shown to cause reduced insulin signal transduction [129]. Pathway selective insulin resistance in vascular cells and resultant overactivation of the MAPK pathway by hyperinsulinemia could contribute further to diabetic microvascular damage [130].

A single process underlying different hyperglycemia-induced pathogenic mechanisms: mitochondrial superoxide production

Specific inhibitors of aldose-reductase activity, AGE formation, RAGE ligand binding, PKC activation and hexosamine pathway flux each ameliorate various diabetes-induced abnormalities in cell culture or animal models, but it has not been clear whether these processes are interconnected or might have a common cause [99,131–134]. Moreover, all the above abnormalities are rapidly corrected when euglycemia is restored, which makes the phenomenon of hyperglycemic memory conceptually difficult to explain.

It has now been established that all of the different pathogenic mechanisms described above stem from a single hyperglycemia-induced process, overproduction of superoxide by the mitochondrial electron-transport chain [135,136]. Superoxide is the initial oxygen free radical formed by the mitochondria which is then converted to other, more reactive species that can damage cells in numerous ways. [137]. To understand how this occurs, mitochondrial glucose metabolism is briefly reviewed (Figure 35.6).

Intracellular glucose oxidation begins with glycolysis in the cytoplasm, which generates NADH and pyruvate. Cytoplasmic NADH can donate reducing equivalents to the mitochondrial electron-transport chain via two shuttle systems, or it can reduce pyruvate to lactate, which leaves the cell to act as a substrate for hepatic gluconeogenesis. Pyruvate can also be transported into the mitochondria where it is oxidized by the tricarboxylic acid (TCA) cycle to produce CO_2, H_2O, four molecules of NADH and one molecule of reduced flavine adenine dinucleotide ($FADH_2$). Mitochondrial NADH and $FADH_2$ provide energy for ATP production via oxidative phosphorylation by the electron transport chain. Electron flow through the mitochondrial electron transport chain is effected by four enzyme complexes, plus cytochrome *c* and the mobile carrier ubiquinone, all of which lie in the inner mitochondrial membrane [137]. NADH derived from both cytosolic glucose oxidation and mitochondrial TCA cycle activity donates electrons to NADH:ubiquinone oxidoreductase (Complex I) which ultimately transfers its electrons to ubiquinone. Ubiquinone can also be reduced by electrons donated from several $FADH_2$-containing dehydrogenases, including succinate:ubiquinone oxidoreductase (Complex II) and glycerol-3-phosphate dehydrogenase. Electrons from reduced ubiquinone are then transferred to ubiquinol:cytochrome *c* oxidoreductase (Complex III) by the Q cycle which generates ubisemiquinone radicals [138]. Electron transport then proceeds through cytochrome *c*, cytochrome *c* oxidase (Complex IV) and, finally, molecular oxygen.

Electron transfer through Complexes I, III and IV extrudes protons outwards into the intermembrane space, generating a proton gradient that drives ATP synthase (Complex V) as protons

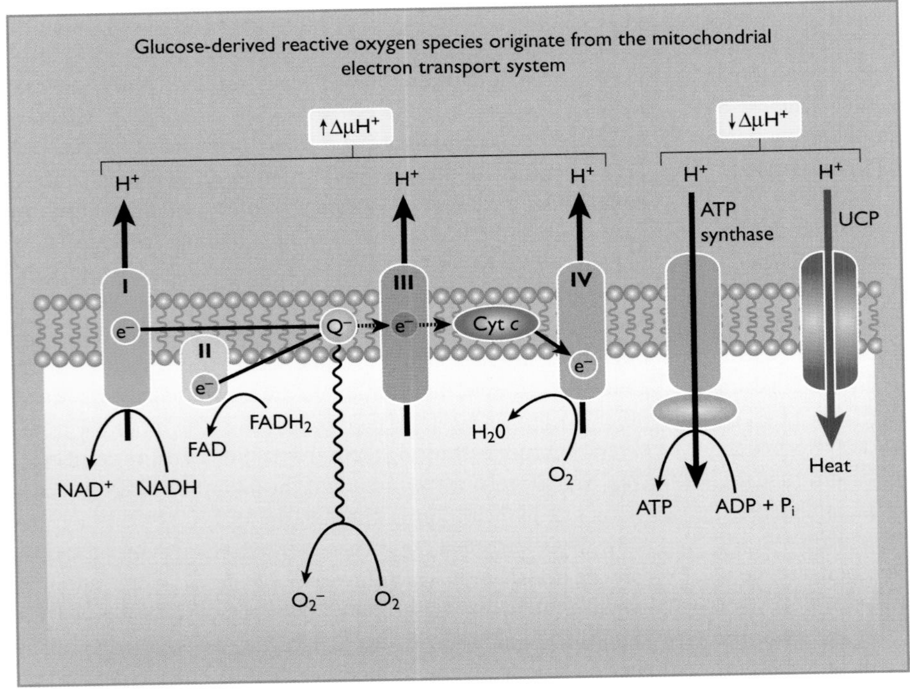

Figure 35.6 Mitochondrial metabolism. Flow of electrons (e^-) through the electron transport chain in the inner mitochondrial membrane pumps H^+ ions into the intermembrane space; superoxide is generated as a consequence of one electron leak. H^+ ions can pass back across the inner membrane along their concentration gradient, either via ATP synthase (to produce ATP) or via uncoupling proteins (UCP). When intracellular hyperglycemia increases electron flux by generating more NADH and $FADH_2$, more superoxide is produced. Cyt c, cytochrome *c*; Q, ubiquinone.

pass back through the inner membrane into the matrix. That is what happens in normal cells. In contrast, in diabetic cells with high glucose inside, there is more glucose being oxidized in the TCA cycle which in effect pushes more electron donors (NADH and $FADH_2$) into the electron transport chain. As a result of this, the voltage gradient across the mitochondrial membrane increases until a critical threshold is reached. At this point, electron transfer inside Complex III is blocked [139], causing the electrons to back up to co-enzyme Q which donates the electrons one at a time to molecular oxygen and thereby generating superoxide. The mitochondrial isoform of the enzyme superoxide dismutase degrades this oxygen free radical to hydrogen peroxide which is then converted to H_2O and O_2 by other enzymes. Intracellular hyperglycemia did, indeed, increase the voltage across the mitochondrial membrane above the critical threshold necessary to increase superoxide formation [140] and, subsequently, increase in production of ROS.

It has been also recently demonstrated that dynamic changes in mitochondrial morphology are associated with high glucose-induced overproduction of ROS and inhibition of mitochondrial fission prevented periodic fluctuation of ROS production during high glucose exposure [141]. Hyperglycemia does not increase ROS and does not activate any of the pathways when either the voltage gradient across the mitochondrial membrane is collapsed by uncoupling protein 1 (UCP-1), or when the superoxide produced is degraded by manganese superoxide dismutase (MnSOD) [142]. Overexpression of either MnSOD and UCP-1 also prevents inhibition of eNOS activity by hyperglycemia [125]. Importantly, inhibition of hyperglycemia-induced superoxide overproduction using a transgenic approach (superoxide dismutase [SOD]) also prevents long-term experimental diabetic nephropathy and retinopathy [143]. In humans, skin fibroblast gene expression profiles from two groups of patients with T1DM – 20 with very fast (fast track) versus 20 with very slow (slow track) rate of development of diabetic nephropathy lesions – showed that the fast-track group has increased expression of oxidative phosporylation genes, electron transport system Complex II and TCA cycle genes compared to that of the slow track group. This association is consistent with a central role for mitochondrial ROS production in the pathogenesis of diabetic complications [144].

Hyperglycemia-induced mitochondrial superoxide production activates the five damaging pathways by inhibiting GAPDH

Diabetes in animals and humans and hyperglycemia in cells decrease the activity of the key glycolytic enzyme glyceraldehyde-3 phosphate dehydrogenase (GAPDH) in cell types that develop intracellular hyperglycemia. Inhibition of GAPDH activity by hyperglycemia does not occur when mitochondrial overproduction of superoxide is prevented by either UCP-1 or MnSOD [145]. When GAPDH activity is inhibited, the level of all the glycolytic intermediates that are upstream of GAPDH increase. An increased level of the upstream glycolytic metabolite glyceraldehyde-3-phosphate activates two major pathways. It activates the AGE pathway because the major intracellular AGE precursor methylglyoxal is formed non-enzymatically from glyceraldehyde-3 phosphate. Hyperglycemia-induced methylglyoxal formation has recently been shown to cause both increased expression of RAGE and its activating ligands S100 calgranulins and HMGB1 (M. Brownlee, unpublished).

Increased glyceraldehyde-3-phosphate also activates the classic PKC pathway, because the activator of PKC, DAG, is also formed from glyceraldehyde-3 phosphate. Further upstream, levels of the glycolytic metabolite fructose-6 phosphate increase, which increases flux through the hexosamine pathway, where fructose-6 phosphate is converted by the enzyme GFAT to UDP–*N*-acetylglucosamine (UDP-GlcNAc). Finally, inhibition of GAPDH increases intracellular levels of the first glycolytic metabolite, glucose. This increases flux through the polyol pathway where the enzyme aldose reductase reduces it (or glyceraldehyde-3-phosphate), consuming NADPH in the process (Figure 35.7). Inhibition of GAPDH in 5 mmol/L activity using antisense DNA elevates the activity of each of the major pathways of hyperglycemic damage to the same extent as that induced by hyperglycemia [146].

Hyperglycemia-induced mitochondrial superoxide production inhibits GAPDH by activating poly(ADP-ribose) polymerase

Hyperglycemia-induced superoxide inhibits GAPDH activity *in vivo* by modifying the enzyme with polymers of ADP-ribose [146]. By inhibiting mitochondrial superoxide production with either UCP-1 or MnSOD, both modification of GAPDH by ADP-ribose and reduction of its activity by hyperglycemia are prevented. Most importantly, both modification of GAPDH by ADP-ribose and reduction of its activity by hyperglycemia are also prevented by a specific inhibitor of poly(ADP-ribose) polymerase (PARP), the enzyme that makes these polymers of ADP ribose. Normally, PARP resides in the nucleus in an inactive form, waiting for DNA damage to activate it. When increased intracellular glucose generates increased ROS in the mitochondria, free radicals induce DNA strand breaks, thereby activating PARP. Both hyperglycemia-induced processes are prevented by either UCP-1 or MnSOD [146]. Once activated, PARP splits the NAD^+ molecule into its two component parts: nicotinic acid and ADP ribose. PARP then proceeds to make polymers of ADP ribose, which accumulate on GAPDH and other nuclear proteins. GAPDH is commonly thought to reside exclusively in the cytosol. In fact, it normally shuttles in and out of the nucleus, where it has a critical role in DNA repair (a summary of the integrated mechanism is shown in Figure 35.8) [147,148].

Glycemic memory

In 1993, the results of the landmark DCCT study showed that, in people with short-duration T1DM, intensive glycemic

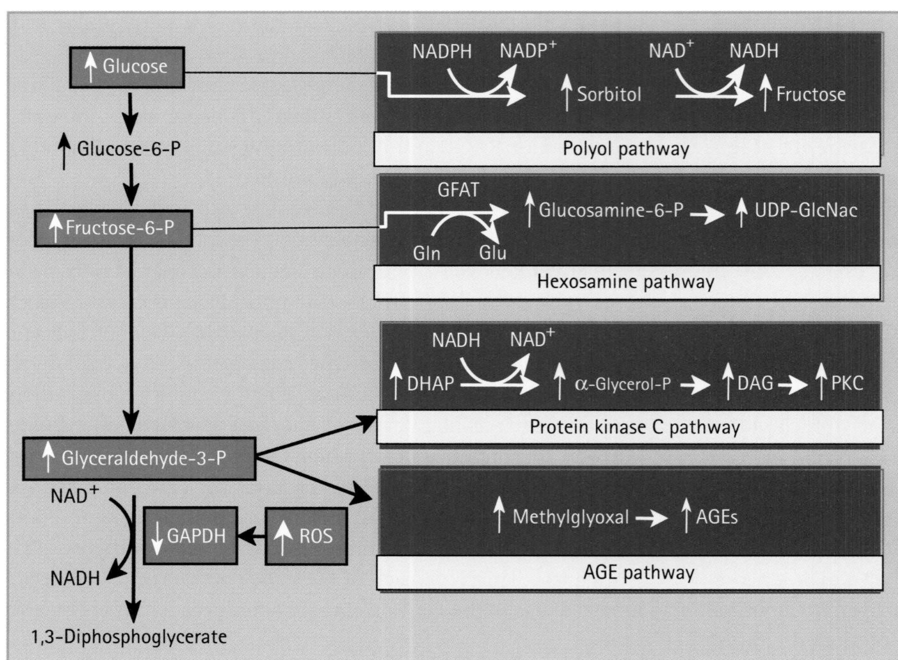

Figure 35.7 Mitochondrial overproduction of superoxide activates the major pathways of hyperglycemic damage by inhibiting glyceraldehyde-3 phosphate dehydrogenase (GAPDH).

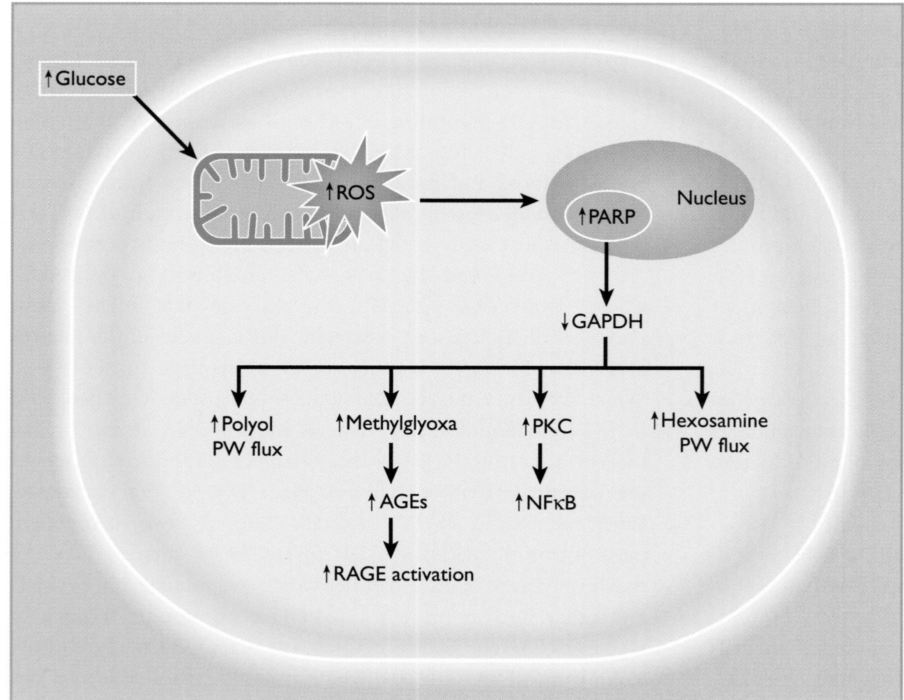

Figure 35.8 The unifying mechanism of hyperglycemia-induced cellular damage.

control dramatically reduced the occurrence and severity of diabetic microvascular complications. After the announcement of the DCCT results, many patients who had been in the standard therapy group adopted more intensive therapeutic regimens, and their level of glycemic control improved, as measured by HbA_{1c}. At the same time, the mean level of HbA_{1c} worsened for patients who had been in the intensive therapy group. The post-DCCT HbA_{1c} values for both groups became statistically identical during the approximate 14 years of follow-up in the ongoing EDIC Study.

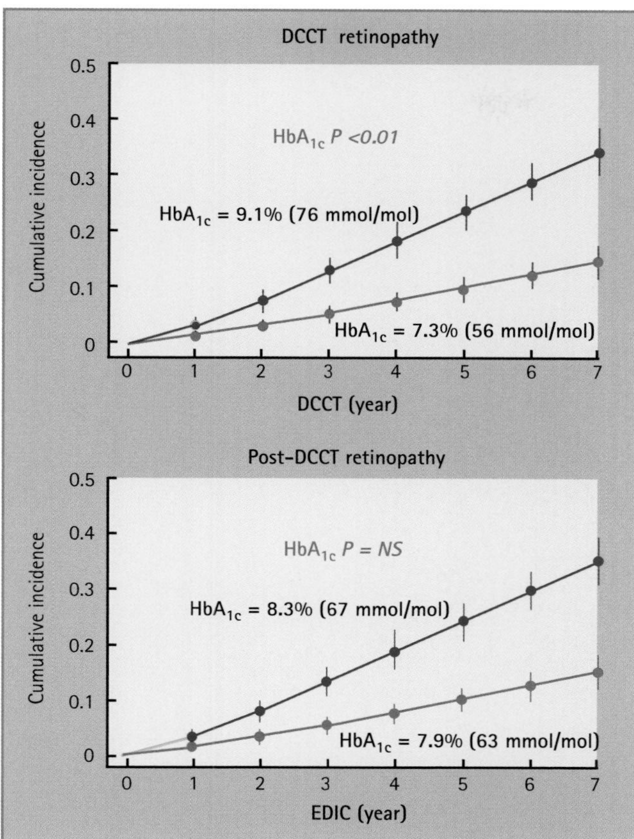

Figure 35.9 "Hyperglycemic memory": previous higher blood glucose levels make people with diabetes more susceptible to damage from subsequent lower blood glucose exposure. After the end of the Diabetes Control and Complications Trial (DCCT) study, the group that had been poorly controlled on conventional insulin therapy continued to have a higher incidence of diabetic retinopathy than the tightly controlled group given intensive therapy, even though post-trial HbA_{1c} levels were comparable in the two groups. EDIC, Epidemiology of Diabetes Interventions and Complications Study.

Surprisingly and provocatively, however, the effects of a 6.5-year difference in HbA_{1c} during the DCCT on the incidence of retinopathy and nephropathy have persisted and have even become greater over the subsequent 14 years of follow-up. People in the standard therapy group continue to have a higher incidence of complications, even with an improvement in glycemic control during the 14 years of EDIC, while people in the intensive therapy group continue to have a lower incidence of complications, even with a deterioration in glycemic control during the EDIC years. This phenomenon has been given the name "glycemic memory" (Figure 35.9). More recent data indicate that glycemic memory also occurs in patients with T2DM. Indeed, the tight glucose control group from the UKPDS demonstrated a continued reduction in microvascular risk and emergent risk reductions for myocardial infarction and death from any cause, despite an early loss of glycemic differences (also termed "the legacy effect"). A continued benefit was evident during the 10-year post-trial follow-up among overweight patients [149–151]. Glycemic memory has several important clinical implications:

1 Early tight control is very important;
2 Cure of diabetes may not prevent subsequent development of complications; and
3 Novel therapies that reverse hyperglycemic memory may be needed.

Hyperglycemia-induced mitochondrial superoxide production may provide an explanation for the continuing progression of tissue damage after the correction of hyperglycemia ("hyperglycemic memory"). Post-translational modifications of histones cause chromatin remodeling and changes in levels of gene expression [152–154]. Because these modifications do not involve differences in DNA sequence, they are called "epigenetic" (Figure 35.10a). Transient hyperglycemia was recently shown to induce long-lasting activating epigenetic changes in the promoter of the NFκB-subunit p65 in human aortic endothelial cells (16 hours exposure) and in aortic cells *in vivo* in non-diabetic mice (6 hours exposure) which cause sustained increases in p65 gene expression (Figure 35.10b) and in the expression of p65-dependent pro-inflammatory genes. Both the epigenetic changes and the gene expression changes persist for at least 6 days of subsequent normal glycemia. Hyperglycemia-induced epigenetic changes and increased p65 expression are prevented by normalizing mitochondrial superoxide production or superoxide-induced methylglyoxal (Figure 35.10b,c) [155]. These results highlight the dramatic and long-lasting effects that short-term hyperglycemic spikes can have on vascular cells and suggest that transient spikes of hyperglycemia may be an HbA_{1c}-independent risk factor for diabetic complications.

Demethylation of another histone lysine residue, H3K9, is also induced by hyperglycemia-induced overproduction of ROS. This reduces inhibition of p65 gene expression, and thus acts synergistically with the activating methylation of histone 3 lysine 4 [156]. Consistent with these observations, others have shown similar epigenetic changes in lymphocytes from patients with T1DM [157] and in vascular smooth muscle cells derived from *db/db* mice [158,159].

Determinants of individual susceptibility to hyperglycemia-induced damage

As with all complex diseases, the occurrence and progression of diabetic complications vary markedly among patients. Some patients have T1DM for over 50 years with minimal complications, while others manifest severe disease or death within 15 years after diagnosis. The control of blood glucose, as well as blood pressure and blood lipid profiles, are important factors in predicting the risk of complications, but they only partially explain the risk of complications for an individual patient. Therefore, genetic factors have been investigated for their influence on the risk of developing complications. An understanding of the genes involved in the susceptibility to or protection from

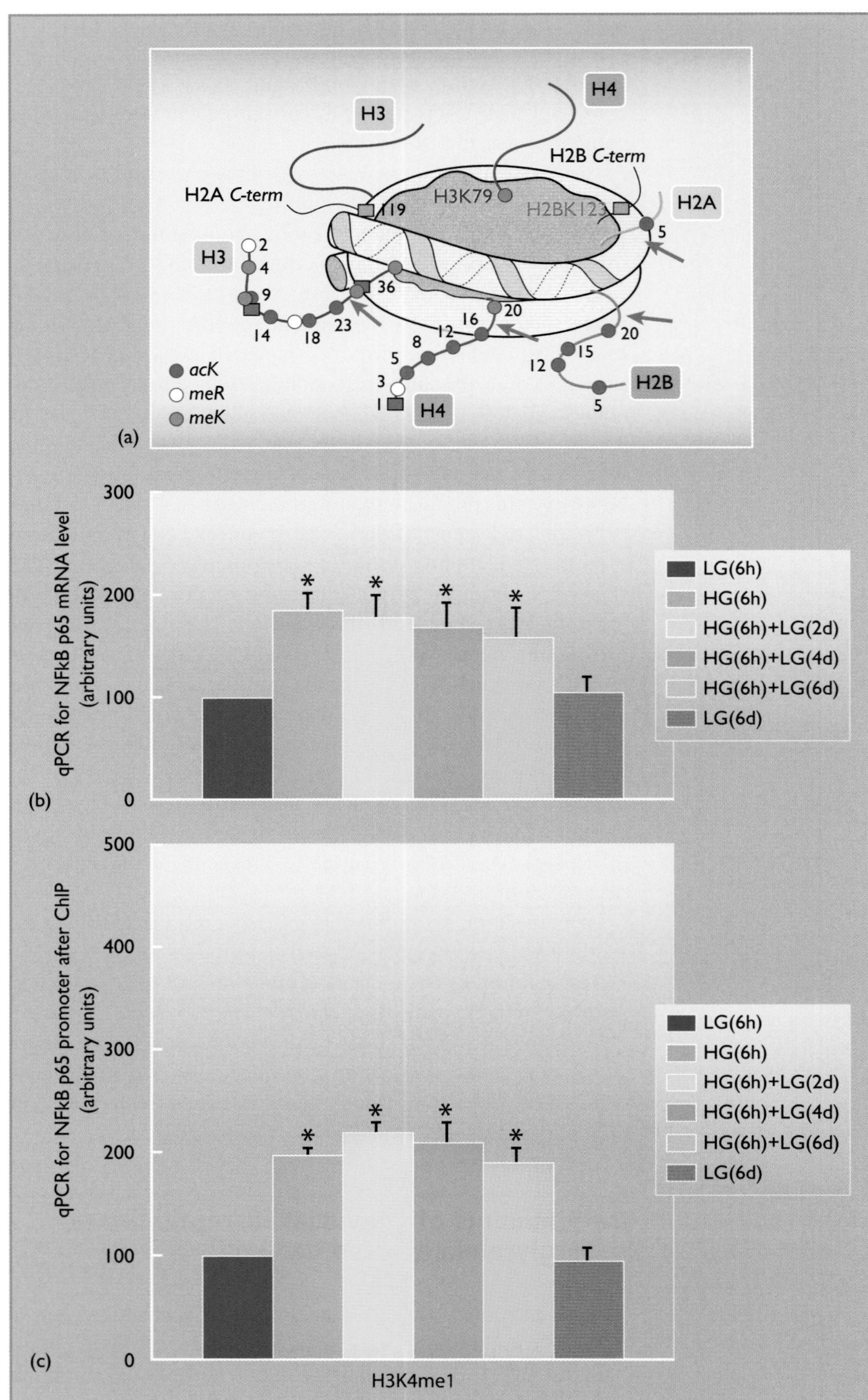

Figure 35.10 Transient hyperglycemia causes persistent epigenetic changes and altered gene expression during subsequent normoglycemia. (a) Schematic representation of several histone modifications (acK: acetylated lysine; meK, methylated lysine; meR: metylated arginine). (b and c) Transient hyperglycemia induces persistent increased expression of the NFκB-p65 subunit, caused by persistent epigenetic changes, including histone 3 lysine 4 monomethylationn (H3K4me1) in the proximal promoter of the NFκB-subunit p65. HG, high glucose; LG, low glucose. Data from El-Osta A, Brasacchio D, Yao D, Pocai A, Jones PL, Roeder RG, *et al.* Transient high glucose causes persistent epigenetic changes and altered gene expression during subsequent normoglycemia. *J Exp Med* 2008; **205**:2409–2417.

diabetic complications can lead to both a better understanding of the pathophysiologic mechanisms, as well as new biomarkers and molecular targets for drug development. Familial clustering studies strongly support a role for genetic determinants of susceptibility to hyperglycemic damage.

In two studies of families that have two or more siblings with T1DM, if one sibling had advanced diabetic nephropathy, the other sibling with diabetes had a nephropathy risk of 83% and 72%, respectively. By contrast, the risk was only 17% or 22% if the index patient did not have diabetic nephropathy [160,161] or retinopathy. Numerous associations have been made between various genetic polymorphisms and the risk of various diabetic complications. Those include the HLA-DQB10201/0302 alleles [162], polymorphisms of the aldose reductase gene [163], of the sorbitol dehydrogenase gene [164] and of the promoter of erythropoietin gene [165]. Study in European descent families of patients with T1DM showed a positive linkage and association with diabetic nephropathy of simple tandem repeat polymorphisms and single nucleotide polymorphisms in 20 genes. Five genes code for transcription factors and signaling molecules (*HNF1B1/TCF2, NRP1, PRKCB1, SMAD3* and *USF1*). Three genes code for components of the extracellular matrix (*COL4A1, LAMA4* and *LAMC1*), and two are involved in its degradation (*MMP9* and *TIMP3*). Three genes code for growth factors or growth factors receptors (*IGF-IR, TGFBR-2* and *TGFBR-3*). The others are genes likely to be important in kidney function (*AGRT1, AQP1, BCL2, CAT, GPX1, LPL* and *p22phox*) [166].

The DCCT/EDIC trial also reported familial clustering and association with gene polymorphisms. The odds ratio for risk of severe retinopathy in diabetic relatives of positive versus negative subjects from the conventional treatment group is 5.4; coronary artery calcification also showed familial clustering [167]. In the same cohort, an association of multiple superoxide dismutase 1 variants is associated with the development and progression of diabetic nephropathy [168].

In the future, the challenge will be to identify specific genes involved in the varying clinical severity of diabetic complications. Recent emphasis in human disease genetics has been on so-called modifying genes, i.e. genetic variants that are distinct from disease susceptibility genes and that modify the phenotypic and clinical expression of the disease genes. Studies show that genetic modifiers can be "tipping point" genes. This means that one gene changes the whole phenotype in an all-or-nothing fashion, in contrast with the incremental effects seen with changes in a large number of non-modifier genes. Many examples of modifier genes are known in model organisms, and several have been identified in humans [169,170].

Impaired neovascular response to ischemia

Tissue ischemia promotes vasculogenesis through chemokine-induced recruitment of bone marrow-derived endothelial progenitor cells (EPCs). Diabetes significantly impairs this process in tissues whose cells develop intracellular hyperglycemia. Many of the defects responsible for impaired vasculogenesis involve hypoxia-inducible factor 1 (HIF-1) regulated genes. Recently, HIF-1 function was shown to be impaired in diabetes because of ROS-induced modification of HIF-1α and its coactivator p300 by the glyoxalase 1 (GLO1) substrate methylglyoxal (Brownlee, unpublished data) [171]. Decreasing superoxide in diabetic mice by either transgenic expression of MnSOD or by administration of a small molecular weight SOD mimetic corrected post-ischemic defects in neovascularization, oxygen delivery and chemokine expression, and normalized tissue survival. In hypoxic fibroblasts cultured in high glucose, overexpression of GLO1 prevented reduced expression of both the EPC mobilizing chemokine stromal cell-derived factor 1 (SDF-1) and of VEGF which modulates growth and differentiation of recruited EPCs. In hypoxic EPCs cultured in high glucose, overexpression of GLO1 prevented reduced expression of both the SDF-1 receptor CXCR4, and endothelial nitric-oxide synthase, an enzyme essential for EPC mobilization. HIF-1α modification by methylglyoxal reduced heterodimer formation, and HIF-1α binding to all relevant promoters [171]. These results provide a basis for the rational design of new therapeutics to normalize impaired ischemia-induced vasculogenesis in patients with diabetes such as occurs in non-healing foot ulcers.

Hemodynamic factors

Hypertension is one of the most significant secondary risk factors for the development of microvascular vascular diabetic complications. In both retina and glomerulus, reduction of vascular surface area appears to occur first in microvessels with high perfusion pressure, and in patients with unilateral ophthalmic or renal artery stenosis there is a pronounced decrease in the severity of retinopathy or nephropathy on the affected side.

Tight control of blood pressure delays the progression of retinopathy and nephropathy, while elevated blood pressure accelerates the onset of nephropathy and its progression [172–174]. In the kidney, glomerular hypertension occurs with diabetes as a result of altered afferent and efferent arteriolar tone, increasing renal damage. This is one of the major targets of blockers of the angiotensin system (ARBs). How might hypertension connect to intracellular ROS generation, and activation of the five mechanisms of hyperglycemic damage? In hypertensive rats with glomerular hypertension, there is an 80% increase in glomerular GLUT-1 expression, associated with glomerulosclerosis and proteinuria. When mesangial cells, an important target for mechanically induced glomerular injury, were subjected to mechanical stretch, GLUT-1 protein expression was also upregulated, causing an increase in basal glucose transport. It has also been demonstrated that overexpression of GLUT-1 in mesangial cells grown in normal glucose concentration induces a diabetic cellular phenotype, with diabetic changes in gene expression [175,176]. Together, these data suggest that hypertension contributes to diabetic microvascular complications by further increasing intracellular hyperglycemia.

Potential mechanism-based therapeutic agents for diabetic complications

Transketolase activators

The first new class of potential therapeutic agents is transketolase activators. This concept originated from a feature of the unifying mechanism. When increased superoxide inhibits GAPDH activity, the glycolytic intermediates above the enzyme accumulate and are then shunted into the four pathways of hyperglycemic damage. Two of these glycolytic intermediates, fructose-6-phosphate and glyceraldehyde-3-phosphate, are also the final products of the transketolase reaction, which is the rate-limiting enzyme in another metabolic pathway, the pentose phosphate pathway [177]. Because in diabetes the concentration of these two glycolytic intermediates is high, activating transketolase could reduce their concentration by converting them to pentose phosphates. This would divert their flux away from three of the damaging pathways normally activated by hyperglycemia. This enzyme requires the vitamin thiamine as a co-factor. Although thiamine itself only activated transketolase by 25% in arterial endothelial cells, the thiamine derivative benfotiamine activated transketolase 250% in arterial endothelial cells.

Based on those findings, several groups have demonstrated the effectiveness of benfotiamine to counteract glucose-mediated toxicity in cultured endothelial cells, endothelial progenitor and endothelial cells and mouse models of diabetes [177–179]. Most importantly, it has been recently demonstrated that beneficial effects of benfotiamine on complication-causing pathways in rodent models of diabetic complications and in humans with T1DM [180]. Benfotiamine treatment prevented experimental diabetic retinopathy and nephropathy in mice, and treatment with high-dose thiamine reduced albuminuria in patients with T2DM. Diabetes has recently been implicated as a cause of intracellular thiamine depletion, which would impair normal transketolase conversion of hyperglycemia-induced elevation of glycolytic intermediates, further exacerbating activation of the five damaging pathways [181–183].

PARP inhibitors

The second new class of potential therapeutic agents based on the unified mechanism is PARP inhibitors. In cultured endothelial cells, a specific PARP inhibitor prevents hyperglycemia-induced activation of PKC, NFκB, intracellular AGE formation, and the hexosamine pathway [146]. In animal models of diabetes, PARP inhibition prevents podocyte apoptosis, ameliorates nephropathy and alleviates sensory neuropathy [184,185].

Catalytic antioxidants

Although increased superoxide activates the five damaging pathways implicated in the pathogenesis of microvascular complications, it is important to recognize that excess superoxide itself can also directly inhibit critical endothelial enzymes without any involvement of these four mechanisms. Two of these enzymes that are particularly important for vascular biology are eNOS and prostacyclin synthase. Both are dramatically inhibited in diabetic patients with diabetes and diabetic animals. To prevent direct oxidative inactivation of these key enzymes, it is necessary to directly reduce the amount of superoxide directly; however, conventional antioxidants are unlikely to do this effectively because conventional antioxidants neutralize reactive oxygen molecules on a one-for-one basis, while hyperglycemia-induced overproduction of superoxide is a continuous process. What is needed then is a new type of antioxidant, a catalytic antioxidant, such as an SOD/catalase mimetic [186], that works continuously. Hyperglycemia-induced reactive oxygen overproduction directly reduces eNOS activity in diabetic aortas by 65%; however, when these diabetic animals are treated with an SOD/catalase mimetic, there is no reduction in activity of this anti-atherogenic enzyme. Similarly, but more dramatically, hyperglycemia-induced reactive oxygen overproduction directly reduces prostacyclin synthase activity in diabetic aortas by 95%. Treatment of these diabetic animals with an SOD/catalase mimetic completely prevents diabetes-induced oxidative inactivation of aortic prostacyclin synthase, and also normalizes all five of the pathways implicated in hyperglycemic damage. Inhibition of hyperglycemia-induced ROS production in diabetic mice using either transgenic antioxidant enzyme expression or combinations of antioxidant compounds prevents the development of experimental diabetic retinopathy, nephropathy, neuropathy and cardiomyopathy [143,187–192]. Together, these data strongly suggest that therapeutic correction of diabetes-induced superoxide overproduction may be a powerful approach for preventing diabetic microvascular complications.

References

1 Nathan D. Relationship between metabolic control and long term complications of diabetes. In: Kahn CR, Weir G, eds. *Joslin's Diabetes*. Philadelphia: Lea & Febiger, 1994: 620–30.
2 Skyler J. Diabetic complications: the importance of glucose control. *Endocrinol Metab Clin North Am* 1996; **25**:243–254.
3 Hammes HP, Federoff HJ, Brownlee M. Nerve growth factor prevents both neuroretinal programmed cell death and capillary pathology in experimental diabetes. *Mol Med* 1995; **1**:527–534.
4 Mizutani M, Kern TS, Lorenzi M. Accelerated death of retinal microvascular cells in human and experimental diabetic retinopathy. *J Clin Invest* 1996; **97**:2883–2890.
5 Giannini C, Dyck PJ. Ultrastructural morphometric features of human sural nerve endoneurial microvessels. *J Neuropathol Exp Neurol* 1993; **52**:361–369.
6 Giannini C, Dyck PJ. Basement membrane reduplication and pericyte degeneration precede development of diabetic polyneuropathy and are associated with its severity. *Ann Neurol* 1995; **37**:498–504.
7 Mizutani M, Kern TS, Lorenzi M. Accelerated death of retinal microvascular cells in human and experimental diabetic retinopathy. *J Clin Invest* 1996; **97**:2883–2890.
8 Hammes HP. Pericytes and the pathogenesis of diabetic retinopathy. *Horm Metab Res* 2005; **37**(Suppl 1):39–43.
9 Susztak K, Raff AC, Schiffer M, Böttinger EP. Glucose-induced reactive oxygen species cause apoptosis of podocytes and podocytedepletion at the onset of diabetic nephropathy. *Diabetes* 2006; **55**: 225–233.
10 Isermann B, Vinnikov IA, Madhusudhan T, Herzog S, Kashif M, Blautzik J, *et al.* Activated protein C protects against diabetic nephropathy by inhibiting endothelial and podocyte apoptosis. *Nat Med* 2007; **13**:1349–1358.

11 Russell JW, Sullivan KA, Windebank AJ, Herrmann DN, Feldman EL. Neurons undergo apoptosis in animal and cell culture models of diabetes. *Neurobiol Dis* 1999; **6**:347–363.

12 Diabetes Control and Complications Trial Research Group. The effect of intensive treatment of diabetes on the development and progression of long-term complications in insulin-dependent diabetes mellitus. *N Engl J Med* 1993; **329**:977–986.

13 UK Prospective Diabetes Study (UKPDS) Group. Intensive blood-glucose control with sulphonylureas or insulin compared with conventional treatment and risk of complications in patients with type 2 diabetes (UKPDS 33). *Lancet* 1998; **352**:837–853.

14 Gaede P, Lund-Andersen H, Parving HH, Pedersen O. Effect of a multifactorial intervention on mortality in type 2 diabetes. *N Engl J Med* 2008; **358**:580–591.

15 Giardino I, Edelstein D, Brownlee M. BCL-2 expression or antioxidants prevent hyperglycemia-induced formation of intracellular advanced glycation endproducts in bovine endothelial cells. *J Clin Invest* 1996; **97**:1422–1428.

16 Xia P, Kramer RM, King GL. Identification of the mechanism for the inhibition of Na/K-adenosine triphosphatase by hyperglycaemia involving activation of protein kinase C and cytosolic phospholipase A_2. *J Clin Invest* 1995; **96**:733.

17 Vikramadithyan RK, Hu Y, Noh HL, Liang CP, Hallam K, Tall AR, *et al.* Human aldose reductase expression accelerates diabetic atherosclerosis in transgenic mice. *J Clin Invest* 2005; **115**: 2434–2443.

18 Lee AY, Chung SS. Contributions of polyol pathway to oxidative stress in diabetic cataract. *FASEB J* 1999; **13**:23–30.

19 Chung SS, Ho EC, Lam KS, Chung SK. Contribution of polyol pathway to diabetes-induced oxidative stress. *J Am Soc Nephrol* 2003; **14**(Suppl 3):S233–236. [Review]

20 Zhang Z, Apse K, Pang J, Stanton RC. High glucose inhibits glucose-6-phosphate dehydrogenase via cAMP in aortic endothelial cells. *J Biol Chem* 2000; **275**:40042–40047.

21 Bohren KM, Grimshaw CE, Gabbay KH. Catalytic effectiveness of human aldose reductase. Critical role of C-terminal domain. *J Biol Chem* 1992; **267**:20965–20970.

22 Zhang JZ, Gao L, Widness M, Xi X, Kern TS. Captopril inhibits glucose accumulation in retinal cells in diabetes. *Invest Ophthalmol Vis Sci* 2003; **44**:4001–4005.

23 Hammes HP, Martin S, Federlin K, Geisen K, Brownlee M. Aminoguanidine treatment inhibits the development of experimental diabetic retinopathy. *Proc Natl Acad Sci USA* 1991; **88**:11555–11558.

24 Stitt AW, Moore JE, Sharkey JA, Murphy G, Simpson DA, Bucala R, *et al.* Advanced glycation end products in vitreous: structural and functional implications for diabetic vitreopathy. *Invest Ophthalmol Vis Sci* 1998; **39**:2517–2523.

25 Stitt AW, Li YM, Gardiner TA, Bucala R, Archer DB, Vlassara H. Advanced glycation end products (AGEs) co-localize with AGE receptors in the retinal vasculature of diabetic and of AGE-infused rats. *Am J Pathol* 1997; **150**:523–531.

26 Nishio T, Horii Y, Shiiki H, Yamamoto H, Makita Z, Bucala R, *et al.* Immunohistochemical detection of advanced glycosylation end products within the vascular lesions and glomeruli in diabetic nephropathy. *Hum Pathol* 1995; **26**:308–313.

27 Horie K, Miyata T, Maeda K, Miyata S, Sugiyama S, Sakai H, *et al.* Immunohistochemical colocalization of glycoxidation products and lipid peroxidation products in diabetic renal glomerular lesions: implication for glycoxidative stress in the pathogenesis of diabetic nephropathy. *J Clin Invest* 1997; **100**:2995–3004.

28 Niwa T, Katsuzaki T, Miyazaki S, Miyazaki T, Ishizaki Y, Hayase F, *et al.* Immunohistochemical detection of imidazolone, a novel advanced glycation end product, in kidneys and aortas of diabetic patients. *J Clin Invest* 1997; **99**:1272–1280.

29 Degenhardt TP, Thorpe SR, Baynes JW. Chemical modification of proteins by methylglyoxal. *Cell Mol Biol* 1998; **44**:1139–1145.

30 Wells-Knecht KJ, Zyzak DV, Litchfield JE, Thorpe SR, Baynes JW. Mechanism of autoxidative glycosylation: identification of glyoxal and arabinose as intermediates in the autoxidative modification of proteins by glucose. *Biochemistry* 1995; **34**:3702–3709.

31 Thornalley PJ. The glyoxalase system: new developments towards functional characterization of a metabolic pathway fundamental to biological life. *Biochem J* 1990; **269**:1–11.

32 Ahmed N, Battah S, Karachalias N, Babaei-Jadidi R, Horanyi M, Baroti K, *et al.* Increased formation of methylglyoxal and protein glycation, oxidation and nitrosation in triosephosphate isomerase deficiency. *Biochim Biophys Acta* 2003; **1639**:121–132.

33 Takahashi M, Fujii J, Teshima T, Suzuki K, Shiba T, Taniguchi N. Identity of a major 3-deoxyglucosone-reducing enzyme with aldehyde reductase in rat liver established by amino acid sequencing and cDNA expression. *Gene* 1993; **127**:249–253.

34 Chang EY, Szallasi Z, Acs P, Raizada V, Wolfe PC, Fewtrell C, *et al.* Functional effects of overexpression of protein kinase C-alpha-beta-delta-epsilon, and -eta in the mast cell line RBL-2H3. *J Immunol* 1997; **159**:2624–2632.

35 Carmeliet P. Angiogenesis in health and disease. *Nat Med* 2003; **9**:653–660.

36 Hanahan D. Signaling vascular morphogenesis and maintenance. *Science* 1997; **277**:48–50.

37 Hammes HP, Lin J, Wagner P, Feng Y, Vom Hagen F, Krzizok T, *et al.* Angiopoietin-2 causes pericyte dropout in the normal retina: evidence for involvement in diabetic retinopathy. *Diabetes* 2004; **53**:1104–1110.

38 Hammes HP, Lin J, Renner O, Shani M, Lundqvist A, Betsholtz C, *et al.* Pericytes and the pathogenesis of diabetic retinopathy. *Diabetes* 2002; **51**:3107–3112.

39 Yao D, Taguchi T, Matsumura T, Pestell R, Edelstein D, Giardino I, *et al.* High glucose increases angiopoietin-2 transcription in microvascular endothelial cells through methylglyoxal modification of mSin3A. *J Biol Chem* 2007; **282**:31038–31045.

40 Elgawish A, Glomb M, Friedlander M, Monnier VM. Involvement of hydrogen peroxide in collagen cross-linking by high glucose *in vitro* and *in vivo*. *J Biol Chem* 1996; **271**:12964–12971.

41 Brownlee M, Vlassara H, Kooney A, Ulrich P, Cerami A. Aminoguanidine prevents diabetes-induced arterial wall protein cross-linking. *Science* 1986; **232**:1629–1632.

42 Tanaka S, Avigad G, Brodsky B, Eikenberry EF. Glycation induces expansion of the molecular packing of collagen. *J Mol Biol* 1988; **203**:495–505.

43 Tsilibary EC, Charonis AS, Reger LA, Wohlhueter RM, Furcht LT. The effect of non-enzymatic glycosylation on the binding of the main noncollagenous NC1 domain to type IV collagen. *J Biol Chem* 1988; **263**:4302–4308.

44 Charonis AS, Reger LA, Dege JE, Kouzi-Koliakos K, Furcht LT, Wohlhueter RM, *et al.* Laminin alterations after *in vitro* nonenzymatic glycosylation. *Diabetes* 1990; **39**:807–814.

45 Huijberts MS, Wolffenbuttel BH, Boudier HA, Crijns FR, Kruseman AC, Poitevin P, *et al.* Aminoguanidine treatment increases elasticity and decreases fluid filtration of large arteries from diabetic rats. *J Clin Invest* 1993; **92**:1407–1411.

46 Cochrane SM, Robinson GB. *In vitro* glycation of glomerular basement membrane alters its permeability: a possible mechanism in diabetic complications. *FEBS Lett* 1995; **375**:41–44.

47 Boyd-White J, Williams JC Jr. Effect of cross-linking on matrix permeability: a model for AGE-modified basement membranes. *Diabetes* 1996; **45**:348–353.

48 Dobler D, Ahmed N, Song L, Eboigbodin KE, Thornalley PJ. Increased dicarbonyl metabolism in endothelial cells in hyperglycemia induces anoikis and impairs angiogenesis by RGD and GFOGER motif modification. *Diabetes* 2006; **55**:1961–1969.

49 Federoff HJ, Lawrence D, Brownlee M. Nonenzymatic glycosylation of laminin and the laminin peptide CIKVAVS inhibits neurite outgrowth. *Diabetes* 1993; **42**:509–513.

50 Hammes HP, Weiss A, Hess S, Araki N, Horiuchi S, Brownlee M, *et al.* Modification of vitronectin by advanced glycation alters functional properties *in vitro* and in the diabetic retina. *Lab Invest* 1996; **75**:325–338.

51 Bishara NB, Dunlop ME, Murphy TV, Darby IA, Sharmini Rajanayagam MA, Hill MA. Matrix protein glycation impairs agonist-induced intracellular Ca^{2+} signaling in endothelial cells. *J Cell Physiol* 2002; **193**:80–92.

52 Li YM, Mitsuhashi T, Wojciechowicz D, Shimizu N, Li J, Stitt A, *et al.* Molecular identity and cellular distribution of advanced glycation endproduct receptors: relationship of p60 to OST-48 and p90–80K-H membrane proteins. *Proc Natl Acad Sci U S A* 1996; **93**:11047–11052.

53 Yang Z, Makita Z, Horii Y, Brunelle S, Cerami A, Sehajpal P, *et al.* Two novel rat liver membrane proteins that bind advanced glycosylation endproducts: relationship to macrophage receptor for glucose-modified proteins. *J Exp Med* 1991; **74**:515–524.

54 Vlassara H, Brownlee M, Manogue KR, Dinarello CA, Pasagian A. Cachectin/TNF and IL-1 induced by glucose-modified proteins: role in normal tissue remodeling. *Science* 1988; **240**:1546–1548.

55 Kirstein M, Aston C, Hintz R, Vlassara H. Receptor-specific induction of insulin-like growth factor I in human monocytes by advanced glycosylation end product-modified proteins. *J Clin Invest* 1992; **90**:439–446.

56 Yui S, Sasaki T, Horiuchi S, Yamazaki M. Induction of macrophage growth by advanced glycation end products of the Maillard reaction. *J Immunol* 1994; **152**:1943–1949.

57 Higashi T, Sano H, Saishoji T, Ikeda K, Jinnouchi Y, Kanzaki T, *et al.* The receptor for advanced glycation end products mediates the chemotaxis of rabbit smooth muscle cells. *Diabetes* 1997; **46**:463–472.

58 Westwood ME, Thornalley PJ. Induction of synthesis and secretion of interleukin 1 beta in the human monocytic THP-1 cells by human serum albumins modified with methylglyoxal and advanced glycation endproducts. *Immunol Lett* 1996; **50**:17–21.

59 Abordo EA, Westwood ME, Thornalley PJ. Synthesis and secretion of macrophage colony stimulating factor by mature human monocytes and human monocytic THP-1 cells induced by human serum albumin derivatives modified with methylglyoxal and glucose-derived advanced glycation endproducts. *Immunol Lett* 1996; **53**:7–13.

60 Abordo EA, Thornalley PJ. Synthesis and secretion of tumor necrosis factor-alpha by human monocytic THP-1 cells and chemotaxis induced by human serum albumin derivatives modified with methylglyoxal and glucose-derived advanced glycation endproducts. *Immunol Lett* 1997; **58**:139–147.

61 Webster L, Abordo EA, Thornalley PJ, Limb GA. Induction of TNF alpha and IL-1 beta mRNA in monocytes by methylglyoxal- and advanced glycated endproduct-modified human serum albumin. *Biochem Soc Trans* 1997; **25**:250S.

62 Pugliese G, Pricci F, Romeo G, Pugliese F, Mené P, Gianni S, *et al.* Upregulation of mesangial growth factor and extracellular matrix synthesis by advanced glycation end products via a receptor-mediated mechanism. *Diabetes* 1997; **46**:1881–1887.

63 Smedsrod B, Melkko J, Araki N, Sano H, Horiuchi S. Advanced glycation end products are eliminated by scavenger-receptor-mediated endocytosis in hepatic sinusoidal Kupffer and endothelial cells. *Biochem J* 1997; **322**:567–573.

64 Horiuchi S, Higashi T, Ikeda K, Saishoji T, Jinnouchi Y, Sano H, *et al.* Advanced glycation end products and their recognition by macrophage and macrophage-derived cells. *Diabetes* 1996; **45**:S73–76.

65 Sano H, Higashi T, Matsumoto K, Melkko J, Jinnouchi Y, Ikeda K, *et al.* Insulin enhances macrophage scavenger receptor-mediated endocytic uptake of advanced glycation end products. *J Biol Chem* 1998; **273**: 8630–8637.

66 Vlassara H, Li YM, Imani F, Wojciechowicz D, Yang Z, Liu FT, *et al.* Identification of galectin-3 as a high-affinity binding protein for advanced glycation end products (AGE): a new member of the AGE-receptor complex. *Mol Med* 1995; **1**:634–646.

67 Ohgami N, Nagai R, Ikemoto M, Arai H, Kuniyasu A, Horiuchi S, *et al.* Cd36, a member of the class b scavenger receptor family, as a receptor for advanced glycation end products. *J Biol Chem* 2001; **276**:3195–3202.

68 Skolnik EY, Yang Z, Makita Z, Radoff S, Kirstein M, Vlassara H. Human and rat mesangial cell receptors for glucose-modified proteins: potential role in kidney tissue remodelling and diabetic nephropathy. *J Exp Med* 1991; **174**:931–939.

69 Doi T, Vlassara H, Kirstein M, Yamada Y, Striker GE, Striker LJ. Receptor-specific increase in extracellular matrix production in mouse mesangial cells by advanced glycosylation end products is mediated via platelet-derived growth factor. *Proc Natl Acad Sci U S A* 1992; **89**:2873–2877.

70 Schmidt AM, Vianna M, Gerlach M, Brett J, Ryan J, Kao J, *et al.* Isolation and characterization of two binding proteins for advanced glycosylation end products from bovine lung which are present on the endothelial cell surface. *J Biol Chem* 1992; **267**:14987–14997.

71 Neeper M, Schmidt AM, Brett J, Yan SD, Wang F, Pan YC, *et al.* Cloning and expression of a cell surface receptor for advanced glycosylation end products of proteins. *J Biol Chem* 1992; **267**:14998–5004.

72 Schmidt AM, Mora R, Cao R, Yan SD, Brett J, Ramakrishnan R, *et al.* The endothelial cell binding site for advanced glycation end products consists of a complex: an integral membrane protein and a lactoferrin-like polypeptide. *J Biol Chem* 1994; **269**:9882–9888.

73 Yan SD, Schmidt AM, Anderson GM, Zhang J, Brett J, Zou YS, *et al.* Enhanced cellular oxidant stress by the interaction of advanced glycation end products with their receptors/binding proteins. *J Biol Chem* 1994; **269**:9889–9897.

74 Lander HM, Tauras JM, Ogiste JS, Hori O, Moss RA, Schmidt AM. Activation of the receptor foe advanced glycation end products trig-

gers a p21(ras)-dependent mitogen-activated protein kinase pathway regulated by oxidant stress. *J Biol Chem* 1997; **272**:17810–17814.
75 Li J, Schmidt AM. Characterization and functional analysis of the promoter of RAGE, the receptor for advanced glycation end products. *J Biol Chem* 1997; **272**:16498–16506.
76 Yamagishi S, Fujimori H, Yonekura H, Yamamoto Y, Yamamoto H. Advanced glycation endproducts inhibit prostacyclin production and induce plasminogen activator inhibitor-1 in human microvascular endothelial cells. *Diabetologia* 1998; **41**:1435–1441.
77 Tsuji H, Iehara N, Masegi T, Imura M, Ohkawa J, Arai H, *et al.* Ribozyme targeting of receptor for advanced glycation end products in mouse mesangial cells. *Biochem Biophys Res Commun* 1998; **245**:583–588.
78 Bierhaus A, Haslbeck KM, Humpert PM, Liliensiek B, Dehmer T, Morcos M, *et al.* Loss of pain perception in diabetes is dependent on a receptor of the immunoglobulin superfamily. *J Clin Invest* 2004; **114**:1741–1751.
79 Vlassara H, Fuh H, Donnelly T, Cybulsky M. Advanced glycation endproducts promote adhesion molecule (VCAM-1, ICAM-1) expression and atheroma formation in normal rabbits. *Mol Med* 1995; **1**:447–456.
80 Schmidt AM, Hori O, Chen JX, Li JF, Crandall J, Zhang J, *et al.* Advanced glycation endproducts interacting with their endothelial receptor induce expression of vascular cell adhesion molecule-1 (VCAM-1) in cultured human endothelial cells and in mice: a potential mechanism for the accelerated vasculopathy of diabetes. *J Clin Invest* 1995; **96**:1395–1403.
81 Schmidt AM, Crandall J, Hori O, Cao R, Lakatta E. Elevated plasma levels of vascular cell adhesion molecule-1 (VCAM-1) in diabetic patients with microalbuminuria: a marker of vascular dysfunction and progressive vascular disease. *Br J Haematol* 1996; **92**:747–750.
82 Sengoelge G, Födinger M, Skoupy S, Ferrara I, Zangerle C, Rogy M, *et al.* Endothelial cell adhesion molecule and PMNL response to inflammatory stimuli and AGE-modified fibronectin. *Kidney Int* 1998; **54**:1637–1651.
83 Wautier JL, Zoukourian C, Chappey O, Wautier MP, Guillausseau PJ, Cao R, *et al.* Receptor-mediated endothelial cell dysfunction in diabetic vasculopathy: soluble receptor for advanced glycation end products blocks hyperpermeability in diabetic rats. *J Clin Invest* 1996; **97**:238–243.
84 Lu M, Kuroki M, Amano S, Tolentino M, Keough K, Kim I, *et al.* Advanced glycation end products increase retinal vascular endothelial growth factor expression. *J Clin Invest* 1998; **101**:1219–1224.
85 Hirata C, Nakano K, Nakamura N, Kitagawa Y, Shigeta H, Hasegawa G, *et al.* Advanced glycation end products induce expression of vascular endothelial growth factor by retinal Muller cells. *Biochem Biophys Res Commun* 1997; **236**:712–715.
86 Soro-Paavonen A, Watson AM, Li J, Paavonen K, Koitka A, Calkin AC, *et al.* Receptor for advanced glycation end products (RAGE) deficiency attenuates the development of atherosclerosis in diabetes. *Diabetes* 2008; **57**:2461–2469.
87 Bierhaus A, Humpert PM, Morcos M, Wendt T, Chavakis T, Arnold B, *et al.* Understanding RAGE, the receptor for advanced glycation end products. *J Mol Med* 2005; **83**:876–886.
88 Rong LL, Gooch C, Szabolcs M, Herold KC, Lalla E, Hays AP, *et al.* RAGE: a journey from the complications of diabetes to disorders of the nervous system – striking a fine balance between injury and repair. *Restor Neurol Neurosci* 2005; **23**:355–365.
89 Koya D, King GL. Protein kinase C activation and the development of diabetic complications. *Diabetes* 1998; **47**:859–866.
90 Inoguchi T, Battan R, Handler E, Sportsman JR, Heath W, King GL. Preferential elevation of protein kinase C isoform beta II and diacylglycerol levels in the aorta and heart of diabetic rats: differential reversibility to glycemic control by islet cell transplantation. *Proc Natl Acad Sci U S A* 1992; **89**:11059–11063.
91 Craven PA, Davidson CM, DeRubertis FR. Increase in diacylglycerol mass in isolated glomeruli by glucose from de novo synthesis of glycerolipids. *Diabetes* 1990; **39**:667–674.
92 Shiba T, Inoguchi T, Sportsman JR, Heath WF, Bursell S, King GL. Correlation of diacylglycerol level and protein kinase C activity in rat retina to retinal circulation. *Am J Physiol* 1993; **265**:E783–793.
93 Scivittaro V, Ganz MB, Weiss MF. AGEs induce oxidative stress and activate protein kinase C-beta (II) in neonatal mesangial cells. *Am J Physiol* 2000; **278**:F676–683.
94 Derubertis FR, Craven PA. Activation of protein kinase C in glomerular cells in diabetes: mechanism and potential links to the pathogenesis of diabetic glomerulopathy. *Diabetes* 1994; **43**:1–8.
95 Xia P, Inoguchi T, Kern TS, Engerman Rl, Oates PJ, King GL. Characterization of the mechanism for the chronic activation of diacylglycerol-protein kinase C pathway in diabetes and hypergalactosemia. *Diabetes* 1994; **43**:1122–1129.
96 Ayo SH, Radnik R, Garoni JA, Troyer DA, Kreisberg JI. High glucose increases diacylglycerol mass and activates protein kinase C in mesangial cell cultures. *Am J Physiol* 1991; **261**:F571–577.
97 Koya D, Jirousek MR, Lin YW, Ishii H, Kuboki K, King GL. Characterization of protein kinase C beta isoform activation on the gene expression of transforming growth factor-beta, extracellular matrix components, and prostanoids in the glomeruli of diabetic rats. *J Clin Invest* 1997; **100**:115–126.
98 Kikkawa R, Haneda M, Uzu T, Koya D, Sugimoto T, Shigeta Y. Translocation of protein kinase C alpha and zeta in rat glomerular mesangial cells cultured under high glucose conditions. *Diabetologia* 1994; **37**:838–841.
99 Ishii H, Jirousek MR, Koya D, Takagi C, Xia P, Clermont A, *et al.* Amelioration of vascular dysfunctions in diabetic rats by an oral PKC beta inhibitor. *Science* 1996; **272**:728–731.
100 Craven PA, Studer RK, DeRubertis FR. Impaired nitric oxide-dependent cyclic guanosine monophosphate generation in glomeruli from diabetic rats: evidence for protein kinase C-mediated suppression of the cholinergic response. *J Clin Invest* 1994; **93**:311–320.
101 Ganz MB, Seftel A. Glucose-induced changes in protein kinase C and nitric oxide are prevented by vitamin E. *Am J Physiol* 2000; **278**:E146–152.
102 Kuboki K, Jiang ZY, Takahara N, Ha SW, Igarashi M, Yamauchi T, *et al.* Regulation of endothelial constitutive nitric oxide synthase gene expression in endothelial cells and *in vivo*: a specific vascular action of insulin. *Circulation* 2000; **101**:676–681.
103 Glogowski EA, Tsiani E, Zhou X, Fantus IG, Whiteside C. High glucose alters the response of mesangial cell protein kinase C isoforms to endothelin-1. *Kidney Int* 1999; **55**:486–499.
104 Hempel A, Maasch C, Heintze U, Lindschau C, Dietz R, Luft FC, *et al.* High glucose concentrations increase endothelial cell permeability via activation of protein kinase C alpha. *Circ Res* 1997; **81**:363–371.
105 Williams B, Gallacher B, Patel H, Orme C. Glucose-induced protein kinase C activation regulates vascular permeability factor mRNA

expression and peptide production by human vascular smooth muscle cells *in vitro*. *Diabetes* 1997; **46**:1497–1503.

106 Studer RK, Craven PA, DeRubertis FR. Role for protein kinase C in the mediation of increased fibronectin accumulation by mesangial cells grown in high-glucose medium. *Diabetes* 1993; **42**:118–126.

107 Pugliese G, Pricci F, Pugliese F, Mene P, Lenti L, Andreani D, *et al.* Mechanisms of glucose-enhanced extracellular matrix accumulation in rat glomerular mesangial cells. *Diabetes* 1994; **43**:478–490.

108 Craven PA, Studer RK, Felder J, Phillips S, DeRubertis FR. Nitric oxide inhibition of transforming growth factor-beta and collagen synthesis in mesangial cells. *Diabetes* 1997; **46**:671–681.

109 Feener EP, Xia P, Inoguchi T, Shiba T, Kunisaki M, King GL. Role of protein kinase C in glucose- and angiotensin II-induced plasminogen activator inhibitor expression. *Contrib Nephrol* 1996; **118**:180–187.

110 Pieper GM, Riaz-ul-Haq. Activation of nuclear factor-kappaB in cultured endothelial cells by increased glucose concentration: prevention by calphostin C. *J Cardiovasc Pharmacol* 1997; **30**:528–532.

111 Yerneni KK, Bai W, Khan BV, Medford RM, Natarajan R. Hyperglycemia-induced activation of nuclear transcription factor kappaB in vascular smooth muscle cells. *Diabetes* 1999; **48**:855–864.

112 Sayeski PP, Kudlow JE. Glucose metabolism to glucosamine is necessary for glucose stimulation of transforming growth factor-alpha gene transcription. *J Biol Chem* 1996; **271**:15237–15243.

113 Kolm-Litty V, Sauer U, Nerlich A, Lehmann R, Schleicher ED. High glucose-induced transforming growth factor beta1 production is mediated by hexosamine pathway in porcine glomerular mesangial cells. *J Clin Invest* 1998; **101**:160–169.

114 Daniels MC, Kansal P, Smith TM, Paterson AJ, Kudlow JE, McClain DA. Glucose regulation of transforming growth factor-alpha expression is mediated by products of the hexosamine biosynthesis pathway. *Mol Endocrinol* 1993; **7**:1041–1048.

115 McClain DA, Paterson AJ, Roos MD, Wei X, Kudlow JE. Glucose and glucosamine regulate growth factor gene expression in vascular smooth muscle cells. *Proc Natl Acad Sci U S A* 1992; **89**:8150–8154.

116 Marshall S, Bacote V, Traxinger RR. Discovery of a metabolic pathway mediating glucose-induced desensitization of the glucose transport system: role of hexosamine biosynthesis in the induction of insulin resistance. *J Biol Chem* 1991; **266**:4706–4712.

117 Rossetti L, Hawkins M, Chen W, Gindi J, Barzilai N. *In vivo* glucosamine infusion induces insulin resistance in normoglycemic but not in hyperglycemic conscious rats. *J Clin Invest* 1995; **96**:132–140.

118 Hawkins M, Barzilai N, Liu R, Hu M, Chen W, Rossetti L. Role of the glucosamine pathway in fat-induced insulin resistance. *J Clin Invest* 1997; **99**:2173–2182.

119 Chen YQ, Su M, Walia RR, Hao Q, Covington JW, Vaughan DE. Sp1 sites mediate activation of the plasminogen activator inhibitor-1 promoter by glucose in vascular smooth muscle cells. *J Biol Chem* 1998; **273**:8225–8231.

120 Hart GW. Dynamic O-linked glycosylation of nuclear and cytoskeletal proteins. *Annu Rev Biochem* 1997; **66**:315–335.

121 Kadonaga JT, Courey AJ, Ladika J, Tjian R. Distinct regions of Sp1 modulate DNA binding and transcriptional activation. *Science* 1988; **242**:1566–1570.

122 Haltiwanger RS, Grove K, Philipsberg GA. Modulation of O-linked N-acetylglucosamine levels on nuclear and cytoplasmic proteins in vivo using the peptide O-GlcNAc-beta-N-acetylglucosaminidase inhibitor O-(2-acetamido-2-deoxy-D-glucopyranosylidene) amino-N-phenylcarbamate. *J Biol Chem* 1998; **273**:3611–3617.

123 Daniel S, Zhang S, DePaoli-Roach AA, Kim KH. Dephosphorylation of Sp1 by protein phosphatase 1 is involved in the glucose-mediated activation of the acetyl-CoA carboxylase gene. *J Biol Chem* 1996; **271**:14692–14697.

124 Daniel S, Kim KH. Sp1 mediates glucose activation of the acetyl-CoA carboxylase promoter. *J Biol Chem* 1996; **271**:1385–1392.

125 Yamagishi SI, Edelstein D, Du XL, Brownlee M. Hyperglycemia potentiates collagen-induced platelet activation through mitochondrial superoxide overproduction. *Diabetes* 2001; **50**:1491–1494.

126 Hart GW. Dynamic O-linked glycosylation of nuclear and cytoskeletal proteins. *Annu Rev Biochem* 1997; **66**:315–335.

127 Musicki B, Kramer MF, Becker RE, Burnett AL. Inactivation of phosphorylated endothelial nitric oxide synthase (Ser-1177) by O-GlcNAc in diabetes-associated erectile dysfunction. *Proc Natl Acad Sci U S A* 2005; **102**:11870–11875.

128 Akimoto Y, Kreppel LK, Hirano H, Hart GW. Hyperglycemia and the O-GlcNAc transferase in rat aortic smooth muscle cells: elevated expression and alteredpatterns of O-GlcNAcylation. *Arch Biochem Biophys* 2001; **389**:166–175.

129 Yang X, Ongusaha PP, Miles PD, Havstad JC, Zhang F, So WV, *et al.* Phosphoinositide signalling links O-GlcNAc transferase to insulin resistance *Nature* 2008; **451**:964–969.

130 Jiang ZY, He Z, King B, Kuroki T, Opland DM, Suzuma I, *et al.* Characterization of multiple signaling pathways of insulin in the regulation of vascular endothelial growth factor expression in vascular cells and angiogenesis. *J Biol Chem* 2003; **278**:31964–31971.

131 Engerman RL, Kern TS, Larson ME. Nerve conduction and aldose reductase inhibition during 5 years of diabetes or galactosaemia in dogs. *Diabetologia* 1994; **37**:141–144.

132 Sima AA, Prashar A, Zhang WX, Chakrabarti S, Greene DA. Preventive effect of long-term aldose reductase inhibition (ponalrestat) on nerve conduction and sural nerve structure in the spontaneously diabetic Bio-Breeding rat. *J Clin Invest* 1990; **85**:1410–1420.

133 Lee AY, Chung SK, Chung SS. Demonstration that polyol accumulation is responsible for diabetic cataract by the use of transgenic mice expressing the aldose reductase gene in the lens. *Proc Natl Acad Sci U S A* 1995; **92**:2780–2784.

134 Brownlee M. Advanced protein glycosylation in diabetes and aging. *Annu Rev Med* 1995; **46**:223–234.

135 Nishikawa T, Du Edelstein DXL, Yamagishi S, *et al.* Normalizing mitochondrial superoxide production blocks three pathways of hyperglycaemic damage. *Nature* 2000; **404**:787–790.

136 Du XL, Edelstein D, Rossetti L, Fantus IG, Goldberg H, Ziyadeh F, *et al.* Hyperglycemia-induced mitochondrial superoxide overproduction activates the hexosamine pathway and induces plasminogen activator inhibitor-1 expression by increasing Sp1 glycosylation. *Proc Natl Acad Sci U S A* 2000; **97**:12222–12226.

137 Wallace DC. Disease of the mitochondrial DNA. *Annu Rev Biochem* 1992; **61**:1175–212.

138 Trumpower BL. The protonmotive Q cycle: energy transduction by coupling of proton translocation to electron transfer by the cytochrome bc1 complex. *J Biol Chem* 1990; **265**:11409–11412.

139 Korshunov SS, Skulachev VP, Starkov AA. High protonic potential actuates a mechanism of production of reactive oxygen species in mitochondria. *FEBS Lett* 1997; **416**:15–18.

140 Du XL, Edelstein D, Dimmeler S, Ju Q, Sui C, Brownlee M. Hyperglycemia inhibits endothelial nitric oxide synthase activity by posttranslational modification at the Akt site. *J Clin Invest* 2001; **108**:1341–1348.

141 Yu T, Robotham JL, Yoon Y. Increased production of reactive oxygen species in hyperglycemic conditions requires dynamic change of mitochondrial morphology. *Proc Natl Acad Sci U S A* 2006; **103**:2653–2658.

142 Nishikawa T, Edelstein D, Du XL, Yamagishi S, Matsumura T, Kaneda Y, *et al.* Normalizing mitochondrial superoxide production blocks three pathways of hyperglycaemic damage. *Nature* 2000; **404**:787–790.

143 DeRubertis FR, Craven PA, Melhem MF, Salah EM. Attenuation of renal injury in *db/db* mice overexpressing superoxide dismutase: evidence for reduced superoxide–nitric oxide interaction. *Diabetes* 2004; **53**:762–768.

144 Huang C, Kim Y, Caramori ML, Moore JH, Rich SS, Mychaleckyj JC, *et al.* Diabetic nephropathy is associated with gene expression levels of oxidative phosphorylation and related pathways. *Diabetes* 2006; **55**:1826–1831.

145 Du XL, Edelstein D, Rossetti L, Fantus IG, Goldberg H, Ziyadeh F, *et al.* Hyperglycemia-induced mitochondrial superoxide overproduction activates the hexosamine pathway and induces plasminogen activator inhibitor-1 expression by increasing Sp1 glycosylation. *Proc Natl Acad Sci U S A* 2000; **97**:12222–12226.

146 Du X, Matsumura T, Edelstein D, Rossetti L, Zsengellér Z, Szabó C, *et al.* Inhibition of GAPDH activity by poly(ADP-ribose) polymerase activates three major pathways of hyperglycemic damage in endothelial cells. *J Clin Invest* 2003; **112**:1049–1057.

147 Sawa A, Khan AA, Hester LD, Snyder SH. Glyceraldehyde-3-phosphate dehydrogenase: nuclear translocation participates in neuronal and nonneuronal cell death. *Proc Natl Acad Sci U S A* 1997; **94**:11669–11674.

148 Schmidtz HD: Reversible nuclear translocation of glyceraldehyde-3-phosphate dehydrogenase upon serum depletion. *Eur J Cell Biol* 2001; **80**:419–427.

149 Diabetes Control and Complications Trial (DCCT) Research Group. Effect of intensive therapy on the development and progression of diabetic nephropathy in the Diabetes Control and Complications Trial. *Kidney Int* 1995; **47**:1703–1720.

150 Diabetes Control and Complications Trial Research Group. The effect of intensive diabetes therapy on the development and progression of neuropathy. *Ann Intern Med* 1995; **122**:561–568.

151 Diabetes Control and Complications Trial/Epidemiology of Diabetes Interventions and Complications Research Group. Retinopathy and nephropathy in patients with type 1 diabetes four years after a trial of intensive therapy. *N Engl J Med* 2000; **342**:381–389.

152 Vaissière T, Sawan C, Herceg Z. Epigenetic interplay between histone modifications and DNA methylation in gene silencing. *Mutat Res* 2008; **659**:40–48.

153 Probst AV, Dunleavy E, Almousni G. Epigenetic inheritance during the cell cycle. *Nat Rev Mol Cell Biol* 2009; **10**:192–206.

154 Göndör A, Ohlsson R. Replication timing and epigenetic reprogramming of gene expression: a two-way relationship? *Nat Rev Genet* 2009; **10**:269–276.

155 El-Osta A, Brasacchio D, Yao D, Pocai A, Jones PL, Roeder RG, *et al.* Transient high glucose causes persistent epigenetic changes and altered gene expression during subsequent normoglycemia. *J Exp Med* 2008; **205**:2409–2417.

156 Brasacchio D, Okabe J, Tikellis C, Balcerczyk A, George P, Baker EK, *et al.* Hyperglycemia induces a dynamic cooperativity of histone methylase and demethylase enzymes associated with gene-activating epigenetic marks that co-exist on the lysine tail. *Diabetes* 2009; **58**:1229–1236.

157 Miao F, Smith DD, Zhang L, Min A, Feng W, Natarajan R. Lymphocytes from patients with type 1 diabetes display a distinct profile of chromatin histone H3 lysine 9 dimethylation: an epigenetic study in diabetes. *Diabetes* 2008; **57**:3189–3198.

158 Reddy MA, Villeneuve LM, Wang M, Lanting L, Natarajan R. Role of the lysine-specific demethylase 1 in the proinflammatory phenotype of vascular smooth muscle cells of diabetic mice. *Circ Res* 2008; **103**:615–623.

159 Villeneuve LM, Reddy MA, Lanting LL, Wang M, Meng L, Natarajan R. Epigenetic histone H3 lysine 9 methylation in metabolic memory and inflammatory phenotype of vascular smooth muscle cells in diabetes. *Proc Natl Acad Sci U S A* 2008; **105**:9047–9052.

160 Seaquist ER, Goetz FC, Rich S, Barbosa J. Familial clustering of diabetic kidney disease. Evidence for genetic susceptibility to diabetic nephropathy. *N Engl J Med* 1989; **320**:1161–1165.

161 Quinn M, Angelico MC, Warram JH, Krolewski AS. Familial factors determine the development of diabetic nephropathy in patients with IDDM. *Diabetologia* 1996; **39**:940–945.

162 Agardh D, Gaur LK, Agardh E, Landin-Olsson M, Agardh CD, Lernmark A. HLA-DQB1*0201/0302 is associated with severe retinopathy in patients with IDDM. *Diabetologia* 1996; **39**:1313–1317.

163 Oates PJ, Mylari BL. Aldose reductase inhibitors: therapeutic implications for diabetic complications. *Expert Opin Investig Drugs* 1999; **8**:2095–2119.

164 Szaflik JP, Majsterek I, Kowalski M, Rusin P, Sobczuk A, Borucka AI, *et al.* Association between sorbitol dehydrogenase gene polymorphisms and type 2 diabetic retinopathy. *Exp Eye Res* 2008; **86**:647–652.

165 Tong Z, Yang Z, Patel S, Chen H, Gibbs D, Yang X, *et al.* Promoter polymorphism of the erythropoietin gene in severe diabetic eye and kidney complications. *Proc Natl Acad Sci U S A* 2008; **105**:6998–7003.

166 Ewens KG, George RA, Sharma K, Ziyadeh FN, Spielman RS. Assessment of 115 candidate genes for diabetic nephropathy by transmission/disequilibrium test. *Diabetes* 2005; **54**:3305–3318.

167 Diabetes Control and Complications Trial Research Group. Clustering of long-term complications in families with diabetes in the diabetes control and complications trial. *Diabetes* 1997; **46**:1829–1839.

168 Al-Kateb H, Boright AP, Mirea L, Xie X, Sutradhar R, Mowjoodi A, *et al.* Diabetes Control and Complications Trial/Epidemiology of Diabetes Interventions and Complications Research Group. Multiple superoxide dismutase 1/splicing factor serine alanine 15 variants are associated with the development and progression of diabetic nephropathy: the Diabetes Control and Complications Trial/Epidemiology of Diabetes Interventions and Complications Genetics study. *Diabetes* 2008; **57**:218–228.

169 Drumm ML, Konstan MW, Schluchter MD, Handler A, pace R, Zou F, *et al.* Genetic modifiers of lung disease in cystic fibrosis. *N Engl J Med* 2005; **353**:1443–1453.

170 Bremer LA, Blackman SM, Vanscoy LL, *et al.* Interaction between a novel TGFB1 haplotype and CFTR genotype is associated with improved lung function in cystic fibrosis. *Hum Mol Genet* 2008; **17**:2228–2237.

171 Ceradini DJ, Yao D, Grogan RH, Callaghan MJ, Edelstein D, Brownlee M, *et al.* Decreasing intracellular superoxide corrects defective ischemia-induced new vessel formation in diabetic mice. *J Biol Chem* 2008; **283**:10930–10938.

172 McGill JB. Improving microvascular outcomes in patients with diabetes through management of hypertension. *Postgrad Med* 2009; **121**:89–101.

173 Zannad F. Implications of the ADVANCE study for clinical practice. *J Hypertens* 2008; **26**(Suppl 3):S31–34.

174 Earle KA, Morocutti A, Viberti G. Permissive role of hypertension in the development of proteinuria and progression of renal disease in insulin-dependent diabetic patients. *J Hypertens* 1997; **1**:191–196.

175 Gnudi L, Thomas SM, Viberti G. Mechanical forces in diabetic kidney disease: a trigger for impaired glucose metabolism. *J Am Soc Nephrol* 2007; **18**:2226–2232.

176 Gnudi L, Viberti G, Raij L, Rodriguez V, Burt D, Cortes P, *et al.* GLUT-1 overexpression: Link between hemodynamic and metabolic factors in glomerular injury? *Hypertension* 2003; **42**:19–24.

177 Hammes HP, Du X, Edelstein D, Taguchi T, Matsumura T, Ju Q, *et al.* Benfotiamine blocks three major pathways of hyperglycemic damage and prevents experimental diabetic retinopathy. *Nat Med* 2003; **9**:294–299.

178 Berrone E, Beltramo E, Solimine C, Ape AU, Porta M. Regulation of intracellular glucose and polyol pathway by thiamine and benfotiamine in vascular cells cultured in high glucose. *J Biol Chem* 2006; **281**:9307–9313.

179 Marchetti V, Menghini R, Rizza S, Vivanti A, Feccia T, Lauro D, *et al.* Benfotiamine counteracts glucose toxicity effects on endothelial progenitor cell differentiation via Akt/FoxO signaling. *Diabetes* 2006; **55**:2231–2237.

180 Du X, Edelstein D, Brownlee M. Oral benfotiamine plus alpha-lipoic acid normalises complication-causing pathways in type 1 diabetes. *Diabetologia* 2008; **51**:1930–1932.

181 Rabbani N, Alam SS, Riaz S, Larkin JR, Akhtar MW, Shafi T, *et al.* High-dose thiamine therapy for patients with type 2 diabetes and-microalbuminuria: a randomised, double-blind placebo-controlled pilot study. *Diabetologia* 2009; **52**:208–212.

182 Thornalley PJ. The potential role of thiamine (vitamin B1) in diabetic complications. *Curr Diabetes Rev* 2005; **1**:287–298.

183 Thornalley PJ, Babaei-Jadidi R, Al Ali H, Rabbani N, Antonysunil A, Larkin J, *et al.* High prevalence of low plasma thiamine concentration in diabetes linked to a marker of vascular disease. *Diabetologia* 2007; **50**:2164–2170.

184 Szabó C, Biser A, Benko R, Böttinger E, Suszták K. Poly(ADP-ribose) polymerase inhibitors ameliorate nephropathy of type 2 diabetic Leprdb/db mice. *Diabetes* 2006; **55**:3004–3012.

185 Ilnytska O, Lyzogubov VV, Stevens MJ, Drel VR, Mashtalir N, Pacher P, *et al.* Poly(ADP-ribose) polymerase inhibition alleviates experimental diabetic sensory neuropathy. *Diabetes* 2006; **55**:1686–1694.

186 Salvemini D, Wang ZQ, Zweier JL, Samouilov A, Macarthur H, Misko TP, *et al.* A nonpeptidyl mimic of superoxide dismutase with therapeutic activity in rats. *Science* 1999; **286**:304–306.

187 Vincent AM, Russell JW, Sullivan KA, Backus C, Hayes JM, McLean LL, *et al.* SOD2 protects neurons from injury in cell culture and animal models of diabetic neuropathy. *Exp Neurol* 2007; **208**: 216–227.

188 Otero P, Bonet B, Herrera E, Rabano A. Development of atherosclerosis in the diabetic BALB/c mice. Prevention with Vitamin E administration. *Atherosclerosis* 2005; **182**:259–265.

189 Shen X, Zheng S, Metreveli NS, Epstein PN. Protection of cardiac mitochondria by overexpression of MnSOD reduces diabetic cardiomyopathy. *Diabetes* 2006; **55**:798–805.

190 Zhang Y, Wada J, Hashimoto I, Eguchi J, Yasuhara A, Kanwar YS, *et al.* Therapeutic approach for diabetic nephropathy using gene delivery of translocase of inner mitochondrial membrane 44 by reducing mitochondrial superoxide production. *J Am Soc Nephrol* 2006; **17**:1090–1101.

191 Kowluru RA, Kowluru V, Xiong Y, Ho YS. Overexpression of mitochondrial superoxide dismutase in mice protects the retina from diabetes-induced oxidative stress. *Free Radic Biol Med* 2006; **41**:1191–1196.

192 DeRubertis FR, Craven PA, Melhem MF. Acceleration of diabetic renal injury in the superoxide dismutase knockout mouse: effects of tempol. *Metabolism* 2007; **56**:1256–1264.

36 Diabetic Retinopathy

Peter H. Scanlon
Gloucestershire and Oxford Eye Units, University of Oxford, Oxford, UK

Keypoints

- In the Wisconsin study [1], proliferative diabetic retinopathy (PDR) occurred in 67% of persons with type 1 diabetes mellitus (T1DM) for 35 or more years. One would therefore expect that two-thirds of people with T1DM would need laser treatment for PDR during their lifetime.
- In the same study, the 4-year incidence of panretinal photocoagulation was 2.5 times higher than the rate of macular laser.
- In patients with type 2 diabetes mellitus (T2DM), the rate of PDR is not as high but it is estimated that 1 in 3 patients with T2DM will develop sight-threatening diabetic retinopathy requiring laser during their lifetime.
- The prevalence of blindness is influenced by duration of diabetes, blood glucose and blood pressure control, and by the presence or absence of screening and preventive laser treatment.
- Achieving a high compliance as achieved in Iceland [2] can lower the risk of blindness to very low levels.

Introduction – a historical perspective

In 1877, Mackenzie and Nettleship [3], in one of the first pathologic reports on diabetic retinopathy (DR), observed capillary aneurysms. In 1900, the average life expectancy for men was 48.5 years and for women was 52.4 years and this rose over the next century to 76.0 years for men and 80.6 years for women. In 1921, Banting and Best discovered insulin in the laboratory of Dr. J. MacLeod. In 1923, Banting and MacLeod were awarded the Nobel Prize for Medicine. In 1943, Ballantyne and Loewenstein [4] examining flat unstained retinas, noted many capillary aneurysms and they first coined the phrase "diabetic retinopathy." In 1953, Ashton [5] described changes in the arterioles in DR, studied in retinas removed postmortem. Examples of the Indian ink preparations published in his article [5] written in 1953 are shown in Figure 36.1.

The normal eye

The eye is an approximate globe with the innermost surface of the eye, the retina, containing specialized photoreceptor cells (Figure 36.2).

The central foveal region is thinner and is devoid of retinal blood supply; essential supply is provided through diffusion from the capillaries of the innermost vascular layer of underlying choroid through contact with the retinal pigment epithelium. The majority of the retina is provided with oxygen by means of the retinal vascular circulation (Figure 36.3).

The blood vessels in the retina exhibit tight junctions between adjacent cells maintaining the blood–retinal barrier. The normal structure of retinal vessels is shown in Figure 36.4.

The cells of the choroidal circulation have small gaps (fenestrations) between the cells in the walls of smaller choroidal vessels allowing transport of essential nutrients and other small molecules and hence support the nutrition and oxygenation of the foveal region through the retinal pigment epithelium.

Risk factors for diabetic retinopathy

Major international epidemiologic trials have established that the development of DR is related to the following modifiable and non-modifiable risk factors.

Modifiable risk factors

Blood glucose

Evidence for the link between poor glucose control and greater progression of DR was provided by numerous early studies.

The study that confirmed that intensive blood glucose control reduces the risk of new onset DR and slows the progression of existing DR for patients with type 1 diabetes mellitus (T1DM) was the Diabetes Control and Complications Trial (DCCT) [6]. In the DCCT [7], early worsening of DR was reported at the 6- and/or 12-month visit in 13.1% of patients assigned to intensive

Textbook of Diabetes, 4th edition. Edited by R. Holt, C. Cockram, A. Flyvbjerg and B. Goldstein.

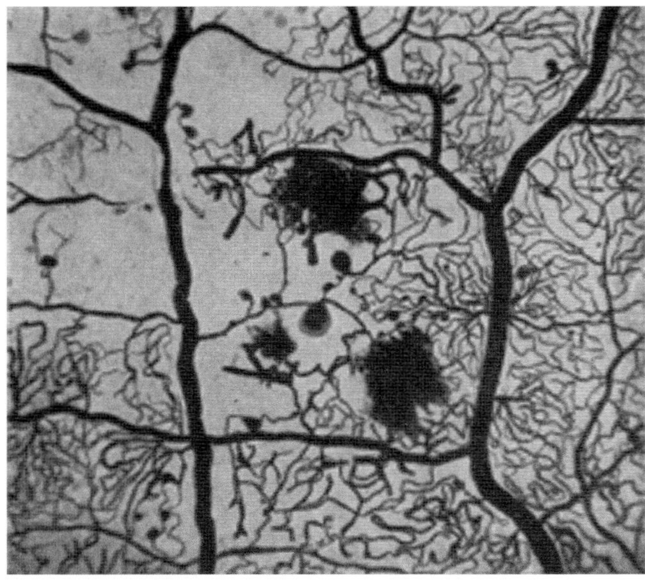

Figure 36.1 Diabetic retinopathy showing an artery on the left and vein on the right. Hemorrhages and microaneurysms are present; in the center of the picture they are seen on an arteriole. The arteriolar side of the circulation is extensively atrophied. Injected Indian ink. Periodic acid–Schiff stain ×44. Reproduced from Ashton N. Arteriolar involvement in diabetic retinopathy. *Br J Ophthalmol* 1953; **37**:282–292.

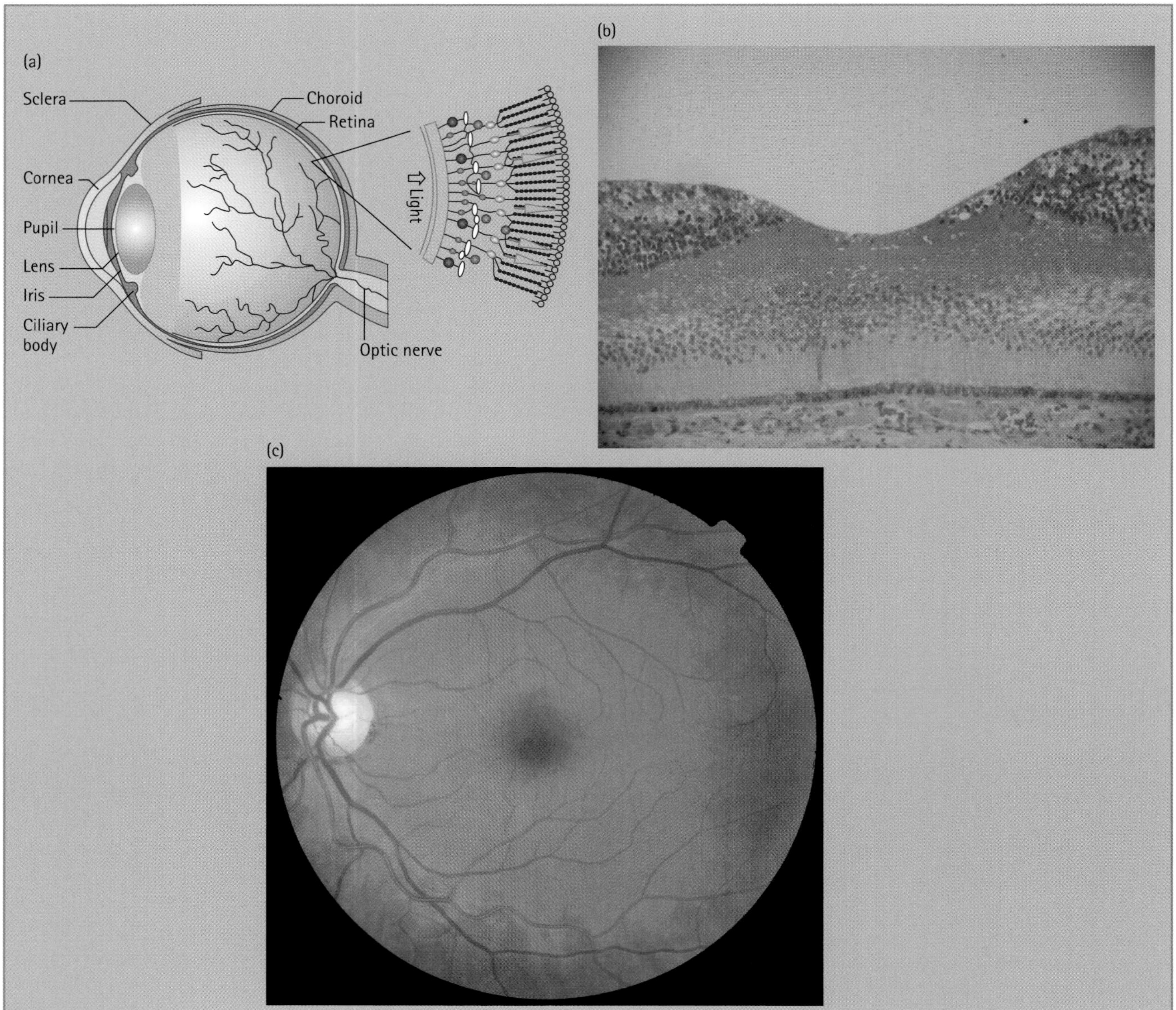

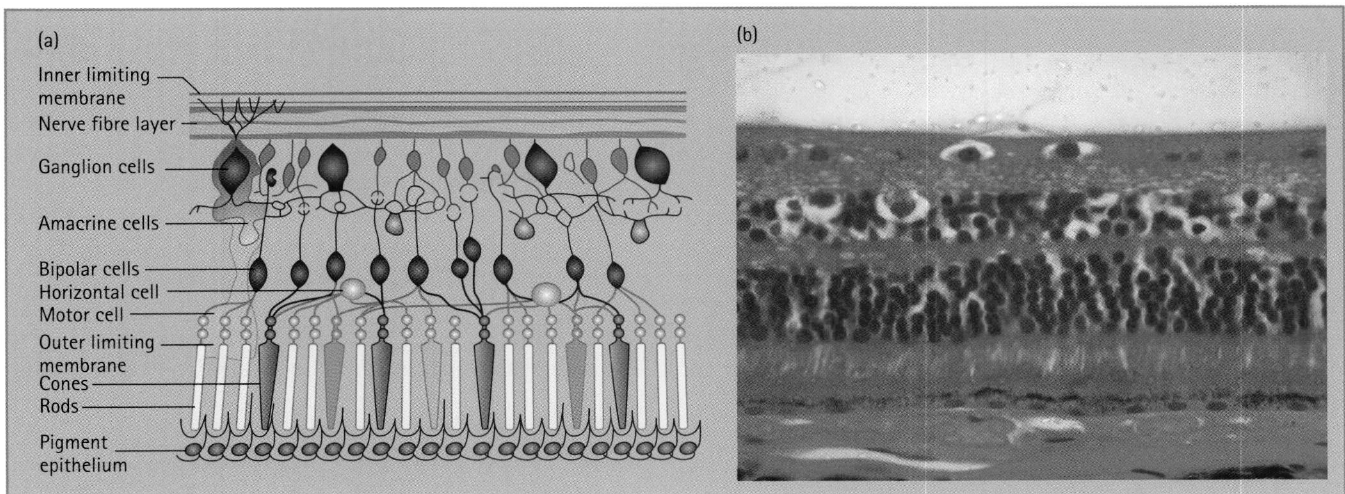

Figure 36.3 (a) This figure shows a retinal structure cross-section diagram. Reproduced from Scanlon PH, Wilkinson CP, Aldington SJ, Matthews DR. *A Practical Manual of Diabetic Retinopathy Management*. Published 2009 by Blackwell Publishing. (b) A histologic section showing the ganglion cell layer, the bipolar layer, the nuclei of the cones and rods, the pigment epithelium, Bruchs membrane and choroids vessels. Reproduced from Scanlon PH, Wilkinson CP, Aldington SJ, Matthews DR. *A Practical Manual of Diabetic Retinopathy Management*. Published 2009 by Blackwell Publishing.

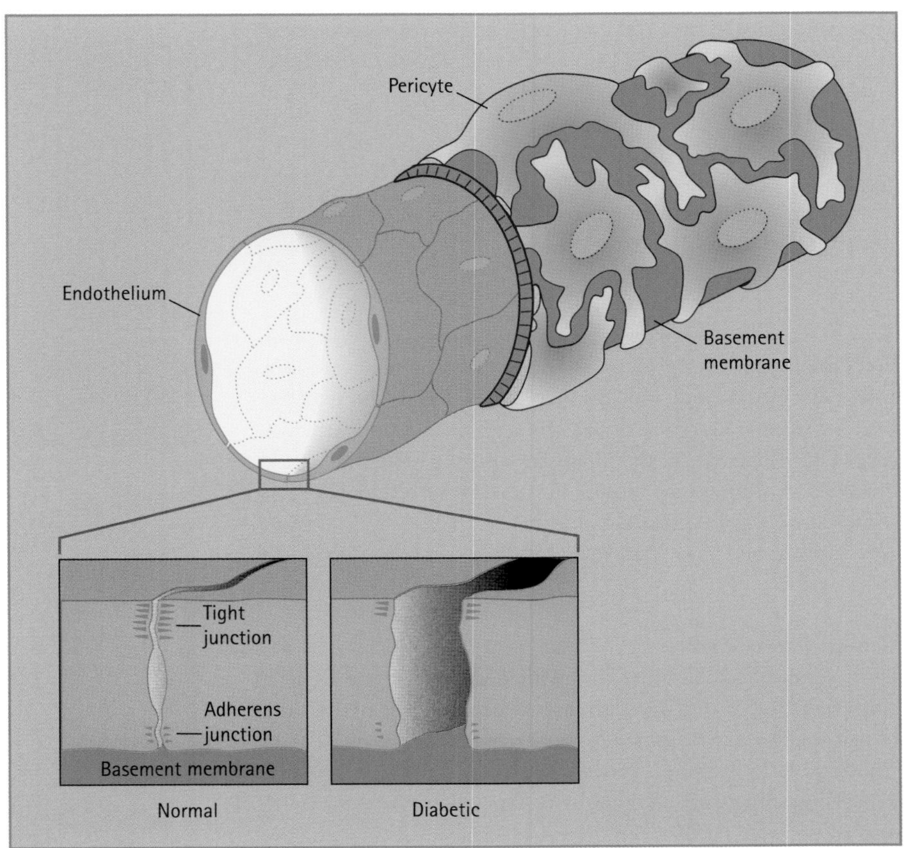

Figure 36.4 An inner layer of endothelial cells is enclosed by a tube of basement membrane, which in turn is surrounded by pericytes.

Figure 36.2 (a) Cross-section diagram of the eye and major structures. Reproduced from Scanlon PH, Wilkinson CP, Aldington SJ, Matthews DR. *A Practical Manual of Diabetic Retinopathy Management*. Published 2009 by Blackwell Publishing. (b) Normal human fovea. This shows the inner and outer nuclear cell layers at the edge of the fovea and the concentration of cones centrally. Reproduced from Scanlon PH, Wilkinson CP, Aldington SJ, Matthews DR. *A Practical Manual of Diabetic Retinopathy Management*. Published 2009 by Blackwell Publishing. (c) Color photograph of the left central retina, including the macula and disc. Reproduced from Scanlon PH, Wilkinson CP, Aldington SJ, Matthews DR. *A Practical Manual of Diabetic Retinopathy Management*. Published 2009 by Blackwell Publishing.

treatment; however, the long-term benefits of intensive insulin treatment greatly outweighed the risks of early worsening.

Similarly, for type 2 diabetes (T2DM) the UK Prospective Diabetes Study (UKPDS) [8] demonstrated that intensive blood glucose control reduces the risk of new onset DR and slows the progression of existing DR for patients with T2DM.

Blood pressure

Control of systemic hypertension has been shown to reduce the risk of new onset DR and slow the progression of existing DR [9,10].

Lipid levels

There is evidence that elevated serum lipids are associated with macular exudates and moderate visual loss; partial regression of hard exudates may be possible by reducing elevated lipid levels [11,12].

Smoking

There is some evidence that smoking may be a risk factor in the progression of DR in T1DM as described by Muhlhauser *et al.* [13] and Karamanos *et al.* [14]; however, in T2DM the evidence is controversial.

Non-modifiable risk factors

Duration

The major non-modifiable determinant of progression of DR is duration of diabetes [15,16].

Age

There is a rather complex link with age, with the Wisconsin Epidemiological Study [1,17,18] demonstrating that in those whose age of diagnosis was less than 30 years and who had diabetes of 10 years' duration or less, the severity of retinopathy was related to older age at examination, whereas when the age at diagnosis was 30 years or more, the severity of retinopathy was related to younger age at diagnosis. In the UKPDS [19], in those who already had retinopathy, progression was associated with older age.

Genetic predisposition

Early studies of identical twins with diabetes suggest familial clustering of DR. An association between severity of DR and human leukocyte antigens has been suggested in a number of studies [20,21], although this has not been uniformly accepted [22]. The majority of candidate genes studied exhibit weak or no association with retinopathy status, and where associations have been detected these results have not been replicated in multiple populations.

Ethnicity

Emanuele *et al.* [23] reported a higher prevalence of DR scores >40 in Latin Americans (36%) and African-Americans (29%) than for whites of Northern European ancestry (22%). Simmons *et al.* [24] compared ethnic differences in the prevalence of DR in European, Maori and Pacific peoples with diabetes in Auckland, New Zealand. They demonstrated that moderate or more severe DR is more common in Polynesians than Europeans. In neither of these two studies could the differences be accounted for by an imbalance in traditional risk factors such as age, duration of diagnosed diabetes, HbA_{1c} and blood pressure.

Pathophysiologic events in diabetic retinopathy

Basement membrane thickening

An early histopathologic sign of DR is thickening of the basement membrane (Figure 36.5) [25].

Pericyte loss

Fallout of pericytes, which are sensitive to high glucose concentrations and undergo apoptosis [26], is an early and crucial event

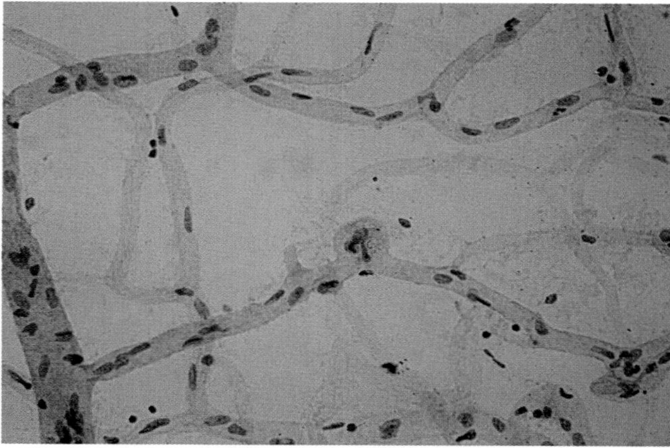

Figure 36.5 (a) Basement membrane thickening (arrow) in a retinal arteriole. Periodic acid–Schiff stain, original magnification ×250. (b) Pericyte loss, in a flat-mounted tryptic digest of retina. Pericytes (small, dark nuclei) normally occur in a 1 : 1 ratio with the endothelial cells (pale, elongated nuclei). Original magnification ×400.

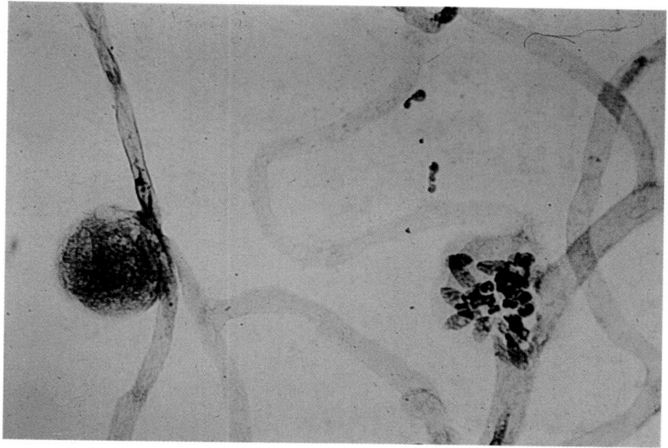

Figure 36.6 Tryptic digest of diabetic retina, showing two large microaneurysms in an area of acellular capillaries. One aneurysm (left) appears to be filled with clotted blood, while the second is hypercellular. Hematoxylin and eosin stain, original magnification ×400.

in DR (Figure 36.5b). Loss of retinal capillary endothelial cells follows soon after pericyte loss with the formation of acellular capillaries.

Increased capillary permeability

Endothelial cells form a continuous sheet with each cell being fused to neighbors by tight junctions that maintain the inner blood–retinal barrier, which may break down in DR leading to leakage of plasma proteins. Focal leakage is also observed around microaneurysms but this is likely to be caused by local endothelial cell damage caused by inflammatory mediators released from adherent leukocytes [27].

Microaneurysms

The microaneurysm is the hallmark of retinal microvascular disease in patients with diabetes (Figure 36.6). It has been suggested that microaneurysms may be asymmetric dilatations of the capillary wall where it is weakened or damaged, following the loss of the supporting pericytes (Figure 36.5b) and localized increases in hydrostatic pressure [28]. Early stage microaneurysms may be extensively infiltrated with large numbers of monocyte and polymorphonuclear cells (Figure 36.6) [28].

Smooth muscle death

Progressive death of vascular smooth muscle cells in the retinal arteries and arterioles has been established in the diabetic human retina [29].

Capillary weakening

Increasing closure of capillaries may be linked with the occurrence of intraretinal microvascular abnormalities (IRMA). These structures contain large numbers of endothelial-like cells and occur in association with acellular capillaries close to the arterial side of the circulation [29].

Retinal blood flow

Most clinical hemodynamic studies in diabetes conclude that increased blood flow and impaired autoregulation are features of DR [30]. Persistent dilatation of retinal arterioles is a well-known phenomenon in diabetes [31]. As DR progresses, increasingly large and widespread areas of retinal ischemia develop, caused by capillary occlusion and intravascular coagulation, which is considered to be enhanced by increased platelet stickiness in some studies [32], but not others [33].

The consultation

A carefully taken history and high quality clinical examination is a vital component of the care of any patient with DR.

Practical assessment

- History, which includes past ocular, diabetes, medical, family, drug and psychosocial history.
- Eye examination, which includes assessment of visual acuity and, where appropriate, color vision, inspection of external structures, visual fields to confrontation, ocular movement, pupillary reactions to light and accommodation, red reflex with an ophthalmoscope and slit-lamp biomicroscopy of the anterior eye.
- Both pupils are dilated with 1% tropicamide and in many patients 2.5% phenylephrine as well.
- Direct ophthalmoscopy has a limited two-dimensional field of view and has been shown to have a limited sensitivity and specificity for the detection of sight-threatening DR but is useful for ad hoc detection of DR.
- Slit-lamp biomicroscopy of the retina is the most common method employed by ophthalmologists to diagnose and monitor retinal disease using condensing lenses or fundus contact lenses (contact lens biomicroscopy).
- Binocular indirect ophthalmoscopy is useful for evaluating the posterior segment and retinal periphery. A larger area can be viewed than with slit-lamp biomicroscopy but this view is less magnified.

Multidisciplinary management

It is very important for an ophthalmologist to be aware of the control of risk factors in the individual patient and to have good communication with the diabetic physician or general practitioner who is looking after this aspect of the patient's management.

Investigative techniques to assess diabetic retinopathy

Retinal photography

Digital color retinal photography is increasingly being used as a record of retinal lesions.

Fundus fluorescein angiography

This is a diagnostic procedure, when sodium fluorescein injection is given rapidly into the arm and the fluorescence of the dye in

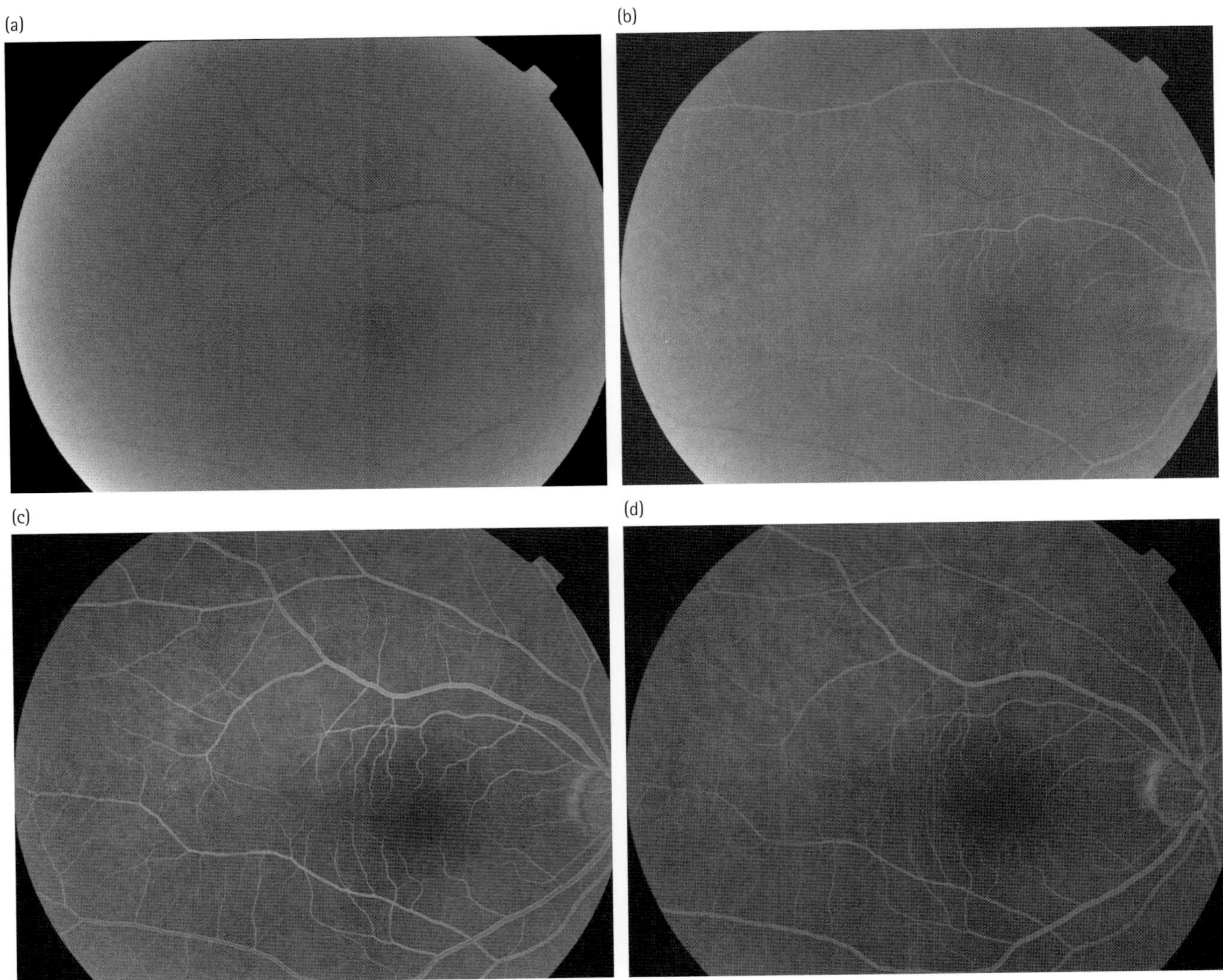

Figure 36.7 Fundus fluorescein angiography. (a) Choroidal flush. (b) Retinal arterial stage with very early signs of fluorescein in veins. (c) Arteriovenous phase. (d) Venous phase.

blue light enables photographs to be taken as it appears in the retina (Figure 36.7). The fluorescein dye causes a few side effects such as nausea, vomiting, occasional syncope, skin rashes and itching. More serious side effects of bronchospasm, anaphylactic shock and cardiac arrest are extremely rare.

Optical coherence tomography

Optical coherence tomography (OCT) is an imaging technique that interprets reflected optical waves using interferometry. OCT images can be presented as either cross-sectional images or as topographic maps (Figure 36.8).

Ultrasound B scan examination

Ultrasound B scan examination uses high frequency ultrasound to examine the density and extent of a vitreous hemorrhage and the presence or absence of a retinal detachment where the retinal view is obscured.

Perimetry

Perimetry is the systematic measurement of differential light sensitivity in the visual field by the detection of the presence of test targets on a defined background in order to map and quantify the visual field, normally testing each eye independently but binocularly for driving field assessment.

Screening for diabetic retinopathy

The definition of screening that was adapted by the World Health Organization (WHO) [34] in 1968 was "the presumptive identification of unrecognized disease or defect by the application of tests, examinations or other procedures which can be applied rapidly. Screening tests sort out apparently well persons who probably have a disease from those who probably do not. A screening test is not intended to be diagnostic. Persons with posi-

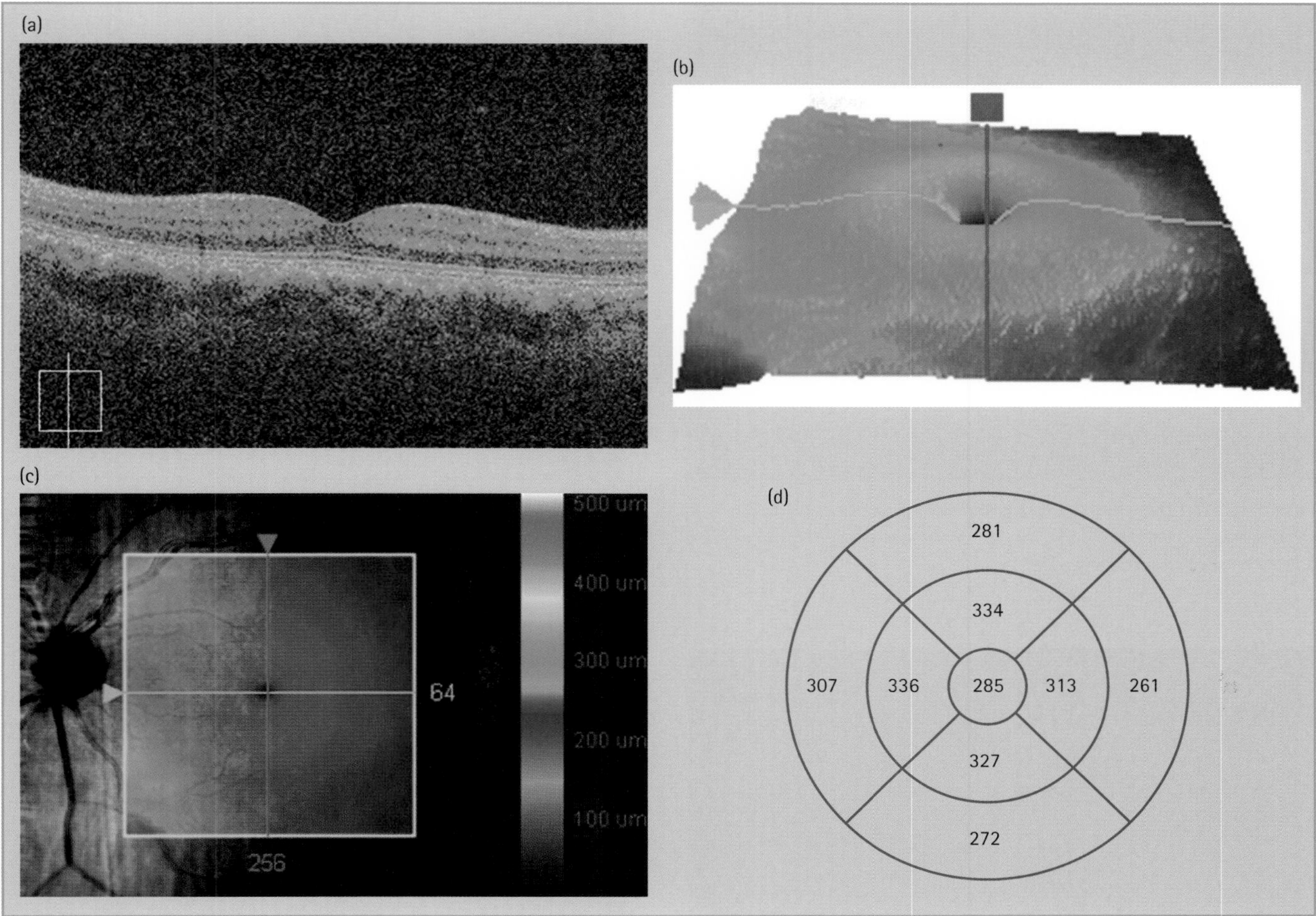

Figure 36.8 (a) Normal cross-sectional optical coherence tomography (OCT) image. (b) Topographic map of macular area. (c) Topographic map superimposed on red free image of macular area. (d) Measurements of thickness in macular area.

tive or suspicious findings must be referred to their physicians for diagnosis and necessary treatment."

Applying this definition to DR demonstrates that it is a very suitable condition for screening:

- Sight-threatening DR is an important public health problem [35,36].
- The incidence of sight-threatening DR is going to become an even greater public health problem; the International Diabetes Federation (IDF) has predicted a worldwide increase in diabetes and DR.
- Sight-threatening DR has a recognizable latent stage [19,37].
- Laser treatment for sight-threatening DR is effective [38,39] and agreed universally. Favorable long-term visual results have been reported [40–42] and there is also evidence that intensive control of blood glucose control [6,19] and systemic hypertension [10] reduces the risk of new onset DR and slows the progression of existing DR.
- A suitable and reliable screening test is available (digital photography) for sight-threatening DR [43–46], and is acceptable to both health care professionals and to the public.
- The costs of screening and effective treatment of sight-threatening DR balance economically in relation to total expenditure on health care [47–50], including the consequences of leaving the disease untreated.

Lesions and classifications of diabetic retinopathy

Microaneurysms and retinal hemorrhages

The lesions that the Early Treatment Diabetic Retinopathy Study (ETDRS) (Table 36.1) [51] described as critical to the stages of progression of DR were:

- *Microaneurysms* – a microaneurysm is defined as a red spot <125 μm (approximate width of vein at disc margin) and sharp margins.
- *Small retinal hemorrhages* – a hemorrhage is defined as a red spot, which has irregular margins and/or uneven density, particularly when surrounding a smaller central lesion considered to be a microaneurysm.

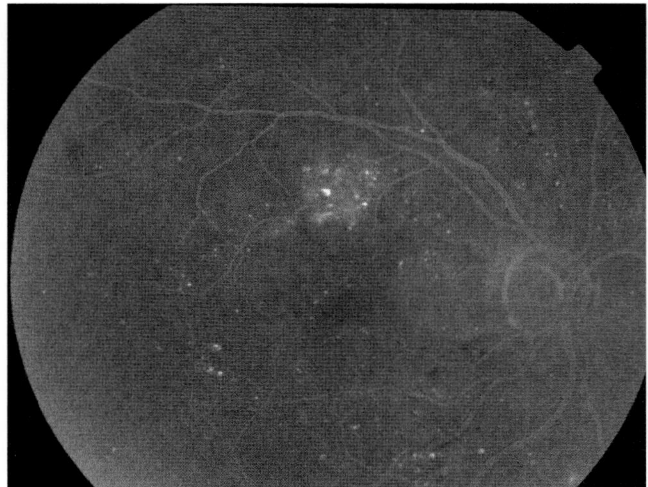

Figure 36.9 An example of the venous phase of a fluorescein angiogram showing small hemorrhages (dark), microaneurysms fluorescing, some of which are leaking shown by the fluffy edge.

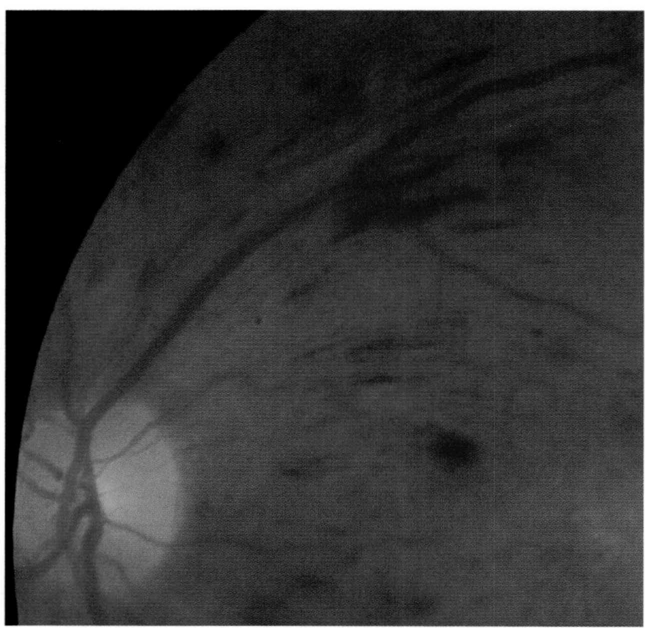

Figure 36.10 An example of more elongated lighter red flame hemorrhages and more oval and darker red blot hemorrhages.

- *Hemorrhage/microaneurysm* (HMa) – because the ETDRS recognized that it was very difficult to differentiate between microaneurysms and small hemorrhages, the concept of HMa was introduced, which is a small hemorrhage or microaneurysm (Figure 36.9).

Other larger retinal hemorrhages

- *Flame hemorrhages* – superficial hemorrhages just under the nerve fiber layer (Figure 36.10).

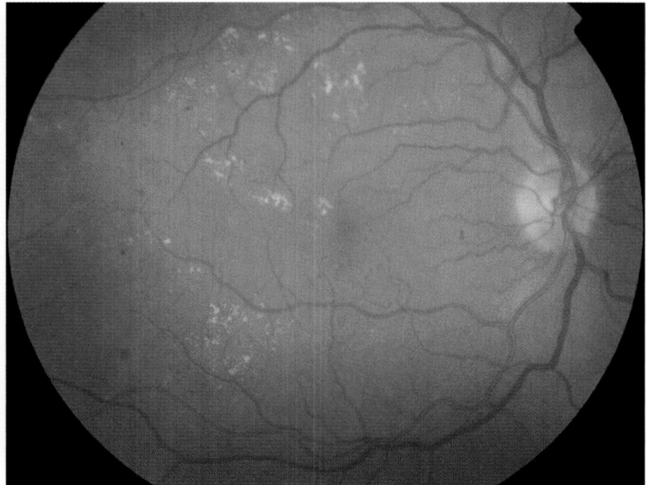

Figure 36.11 An example of exudates in the right macular area.

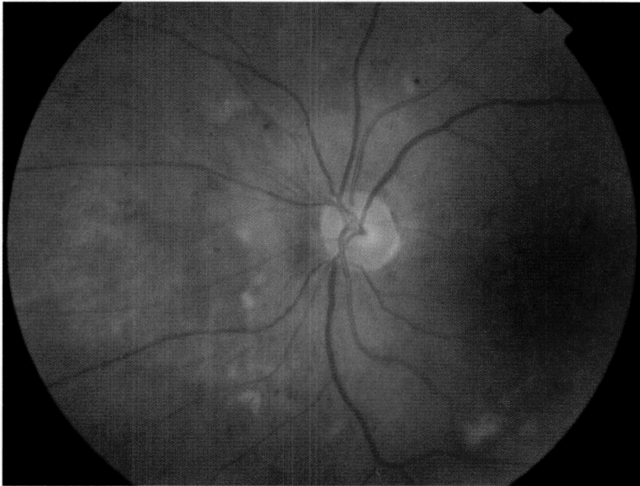

Figure 36.12 An example of cotton wool spots. Reproduced from Scanlon PH, Wilkinson CP, Aldington SJ, Matthews DR. *A Practical Manual of Diabetic Retinopathy Management.* Published 2009 by Blackwell Publishing.

- *Blot hemorrhages* – deeper hemorrhages, which are a sign of retinal ischemia in the area of the retina in which they occur.

Hard exudates

Hard exudates (sometimes now just referred to as exudates) are defined as small white or yellowish-white deposits with sharp margins, located typically in the outer layers of the retina, but they may be more superficial, particularly when retinal edema is present (Figure 36.11).

Cotton wool spots

Cotton wool spots (referred to as soft exudates in the ETDRS, but this term is now rarely used) are fluffy white opaque areas caused by an accumulation of axoplasm in the nerve fiber layer of the retina, which is caused by an arteriolar occlusion in that area of retina that is apparent on a fluorescein angiogram (Figure 36.12).

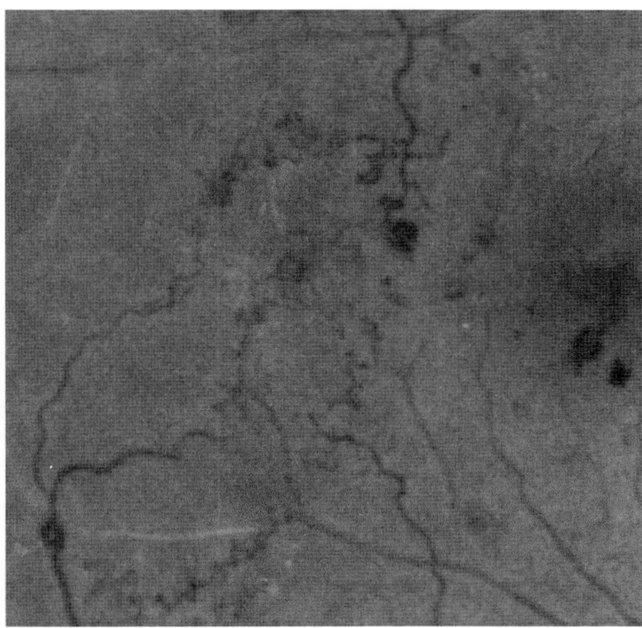

Figure 36.13 An example of intraretinal microvascular abnormality (IRMA) in the temporal retina of the right eye (the right macula is seen in the right side of this red free photograph).

Intraretinal microvascular abnormalities

IRMA are defined as tortuous intraretinal vascular segments, varying in caliber, derived from remodeling of the retinal capillaries and small collateral vessels in areas of microvascular occlusion and are therefore a sign of retinal ischemia (Figure 36.13).

Venous abnormalities

- *Venous loops* – abrupt curving deviations of a vein from its normal path (Figure 36.14).
- *Venous beading* – in the ETDRS, venous beading is described as a localized increase in caliber of the vein and the severity is dependent on the increase in caliber and the length of vein involved. It is associated with retinal ischemia (Figure 36.15).

Other venous changes that occur in DR are as follow:

- Venous dilatation;
- Venous narrowing;
- Opacification of the venous wall; and
- Perivenous exudate.

Arteriolar abnormalities

Other arteriolar changes that occur in DR are as follow:

- Arteriolar narrowing;
- Opacification of arteriolar walls; and
- Arteriovenous nipping.

Fibrous proliferation at the disc

Fibrous proliferation at the disc (FPD) usually occurs when new vessels at the disc start to regress and fibrosis occurs.

Fibrous proliferation elsewhere

Fibrous proliferation elsewhere (FPE) usually occurs when new vessels elsewhere start to regress and fibrosis occurs.

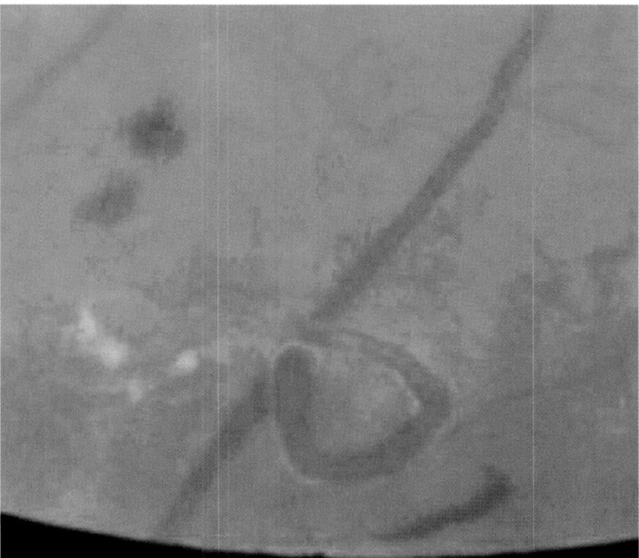

Figure 36.14 An example of a venous loop.

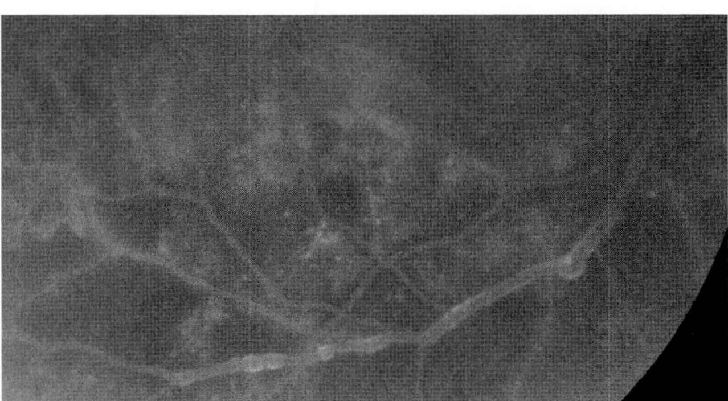

Figure 36.15 A fluorescein angiogram showing venous beading adjacent to an ischemic area of retina. Reproduced from Scanlon PH, Wilkinson CP, Aldington SJ, Matthews DR. *A Practical Manual of Diabetic Retinopathy Management.* Published 2009 by Blackwell Publishing.

New vessels on and/or within 1 disc diameter of the disc

For new vessels on and/or within 1 disc diameter (DD) of the disc (NVD), see Figure 36.16.

New vessels elsewhere

For new vessels elsewhere (NVE), see Figure 36.17.

Vitreous hemorrhage

Vitreous hemorrhage (VH) is a hemorrhage that is in the vitreous gel.

Preretinal hemorrhage

Preretinal hemorrhages (PRH) are boat-shaped hemorrhages and roughly round, confluent or linear patches of hemorrhage just anterior to the retina or under the internal limiting membrane (Figure 36.18).

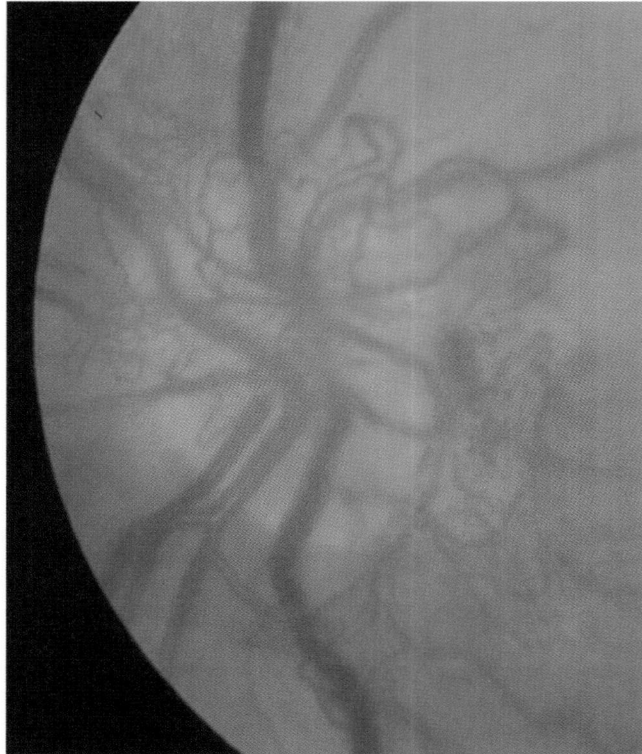

Figure 36.16 An example of new vessels on disc (NVD).

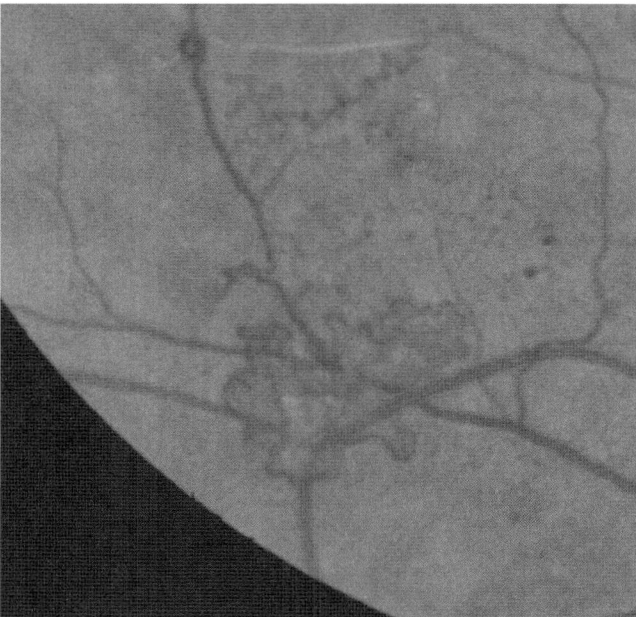

Figure 36.17 An example of new vessels elsewhere (NVE).

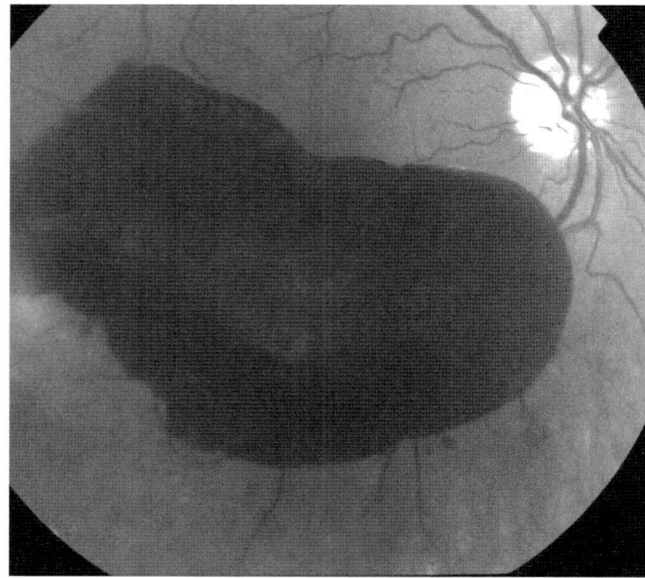

Figure 36.18 An example of preretinal hemorrhage.

Post laser treatment

Photocoagulation laser scars may be seen both after macular or panretinal laser treatment (Figure 36.19; Tables 36.1–36.4).

Maculopathy

Clinical classification of diabetic maculopathy

Diabetic maculopathy may be classified into focal (subdivided into focal exudates and focal/multifocal edema), diffuse and ischemic diabetic maculopathy (Tables 36.2 and 36.4).

Pathophysiology of macular edema

In focal macular edema, focal leakage tends to occur from microaneurysms, often with extravascular lipoprotein in a circinate pattern around the focal leakage [57].

In diffuse macular edema, there is a generalized breakdown of the blood–retina barrier and profuse early leakage from the entire capillary bed of the posterior pole [58] causing extracellular fluid accumulation, often accompanied by cystoid macular edema [57], which is caused by cellular swelling. In ischemic maculopathy, enlargement of the foveal avascular zone as a result of capillary closure is found.

The fluorescein angiographic appearance

In diabetic maculopathy, most leakage occurs in the venous phase of the angiogram and hence examples of venous phase angiograms are shown in Figure 36.20.

Optical coherence tomography

An example of diabetic maculopathy is shown in Figure 36.21. Macular traction can occur from contracture of fibrotic proliferations, particularly as new vessels regress after panretinal photocoagulation, and also from a taut posterior hyaloid. If macular traction is severe, surgical intervention is required (Figure 36.22).

Laser treatment for diabetic maculopathy

In 1985, the ETDRS [59] demonstrated that focal (direct/grid) laser photocoagulation reduces moderate vision loss caused by

Table 36.1 Early Treatment Diabetic Retinopathy Study (ETDRS) Research Group diabetic retinopathy classification of progression to proliferative diabetic retinopathy based on 7 × 30° field stereo photographs of each eye.

ETDRS final Retinopathy Severity Scale [37]	ETDRS (final) grade	Lesions	Risk of progression to PDR in 1 year (ETDRS Interim)	Practical clinic follow-up intervals (not ETDRS)
No apparent retinopathy	10	DR absent		1 year
	14, 15	DR questionable		
Mild NPDR	20	Microaneurysms only		1 year
	35	One or more of the following:	Level 30 = 6.2%	6–12 months
	a	Venous loops ≥ definite in 1 field		
	b	SE, IRMA, or VB questionable		
	c	Retinal hemorrhages present		
	d	HE ≥ definite in 1 field		
	e	SE ≥ definite in 1 field		
Moderate NPDR	43a	H/Ma moderate in 4-5 fields or severe in 1 field *or*	Level 41 = 11.3%	6 months
	b	IRMA definite in 1–3 fields		
Moderately severe NPDR	47	Both level 43 characteristics – H/Ma moderate in 4–5 fields or severe in 1 field and IRMA definite in 1–3 fields	Level 45 = 20.7%	4 months
	a			
	b	*or* any one of the following:		
	c	IRMA in 4–5 fields		
	d	HMa severe in 2–3 fields		
		VB definite in 1 field		
Severe NPDR	53	One or more of the following:	Level 51 = 44.2%	3 months
	a	≥2 of the 3 level 47 characteristics		
	b	H/Ma severe in 4–5 fields		
	c	IRMA ≥ moderate in 1 field	Level 55 = 54.8%	
	d	VB ≥ definite in 2–3 fields		
Mild PDR	61a	FPD or FPE present with NVD absent *or*	1976. Diabetic Retinopathy Study [52] protocol changed to treat untreated eyes with high risk characteristics	
	b	NVE = definite		
Moderate PDR	65a	**1** NVE ≥ moderate in 1 field or definite NVD with VH and PRH absent or questionable *or*		
	b	**2** VH or PRH definite and NVE < moderate in 1 field and NVD absent	1981. Diabetic Retinopathy Study [53] recommendation to treat – eyes with new vessels on or within 1 DD of the optic disc (NVD) ≥0.25 –0.33 disc area, even in the absence of preretinal or vitreous hemorrhage. Photocoagulation, as used in the study, reduced the risk of severe visual loss by 50% or more	
High risk PDR	71	Any of the following:		
	a	**1** VH or PRH ≥ moderate in 1 field		
	b	**2** NVE ≥ moderate in 1 field and VH or PRH definite in 1 field		
	c	**3** NVD = 2 and VH or PRH definite in 1 field		
	d	**4** NVD ≥ moderate		
High risk PDR	75	NVD ≥ moderate and definite VH or PRH		
Advanced PDR	81	Retina obscured due to VH or PRH		

DD, disc diameter; DR, diabetic retinopathy; HE, hard exudate; HMa, small hemorrhage or microaneurysm; IRMA, intraretinal microvascular abnormality; NPDR, non-proliferative DR; NVD, new vessels on disc; NVE, new vessels elsewhere; PDR, proliferative diabetic retinopathy; PRH, preretinal hemorrhage; SE, soft exudate, a term that has now been replaced by cotton wool spot; VB, venous beading; VH, vitreous hemorrhage.

Table 36.2 Early Treatment Diabetic Retinopathy Study (ETDRS) maculopathy classification.

ETDRS	Outcome
Clinically significant macular edema [54] as defined by:	
• A zone or zones of retinal thickening one disc area or larger, any part of which is within one disc diameter of the center of the macula	Consider laser
• Retinal thickening at or within 500 μm of the center of the macula	Consider laser
• Hard exudates at or within 500 μm of the center of the macula, if associated with thickening of the adjacent retina (not residual hard exudates remaining after disappearance of retinal thickening)	Consider laser

Because of the difficulty in correlating 7 field stereo-photography to the clinical setting, two further simplified classifications have been developed (International Classification and the English Screening Classification).

Table 36.3 International and English retinopathy classifications.

International clinical classification of diabetic retinopathy severity or diabetic macular edema [55]	Recommended International outcome	English Screening program levels [56] and recommended outcome
Microaneurysms only	Optimize medical therapy, screen at least annually	**R0**: no DR Outcome: currently screen annually
More than just microaneurysms but less severe than severe NPDR	Refer to ophthalmologist	**R1**: background DR Microaneurysm(s) Retinal hemorrhage(s) ± any exudate Outcome: currently screen annually
Severe NPDR Any of the following: (a) Extensive intraretinal hemorrhage (>20) in 4 quadrants (b) Definite venous beading in 2+ quadrants (c) Prominent IRMA in 1+ quadrant *and* no signs of PDR	Consider scatter photocoagulation for T2DM	**R2**: preproliferative DR venous beading venous loop or reduplication IRMA, multiple deep, round or blot hemorrhages Outcome: refer to ophthalmologist
Neovascularization Vitreous/preretinal hemorrhage	Scatter Photocoagulation without delay for patients with vitreous hemorrhage or neovascularization within 1 DD of the optic nerve head	**R3:** proliferative NVD NVE Preretinal or vitreous hemorrhage Preretinal fibrosis ± tractional retinal detachment Outcome: urgent referral to ophthalmologist

DD, disc diameter; DR, diabetic retinopathy; IRMA, intraretinal microvascular abnormality; NPDR, non-proliferative DR; NVD, new vessels on disc; NVE, new vessels elsewhere; PDR, proliferative diabetic retinopathy.

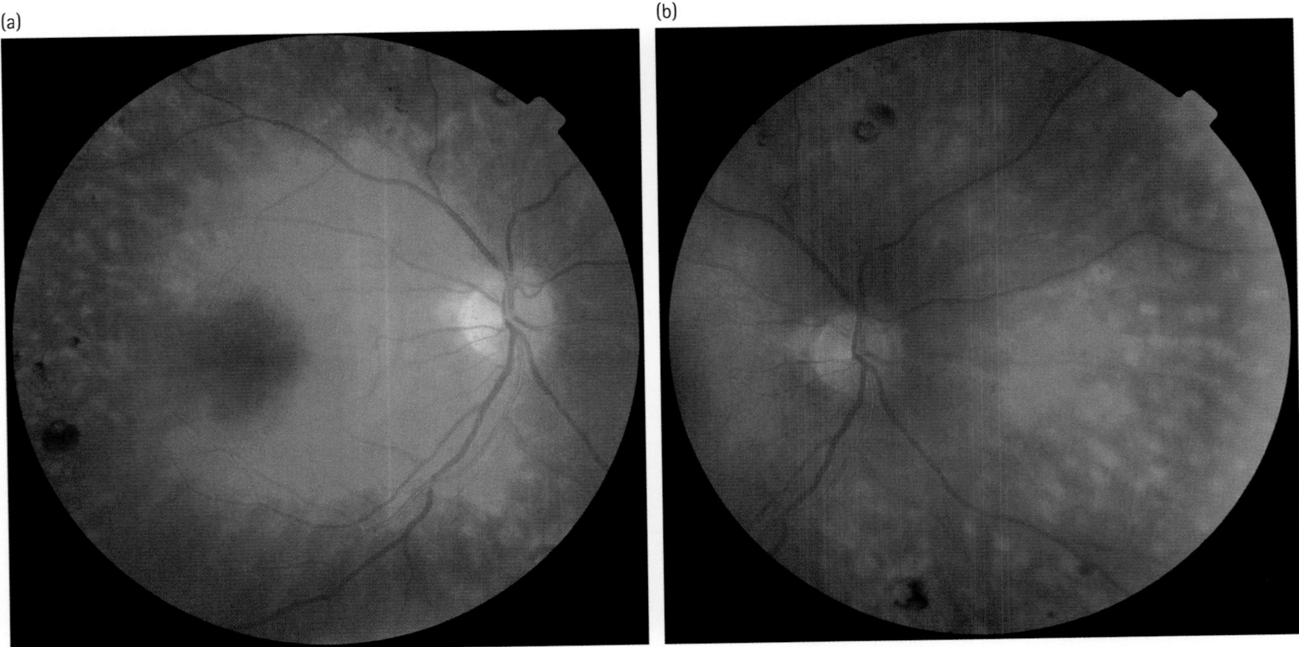

Figure 36.19 (a,b) Right macular and nasal views following panretinal photocoagulation to show laser treatment scars in the superior, inferior, temporal and nasal retina.

Table 36.4 International and English maculopathy classification.

International classification [55]	Outcome	English classification [56]	Outcome
Diabetic macular edema present as defined by some retinal thickening or hard exudates in the posterior pole and subclassified into: Mild diabetic macular edema: Some retinal thickening or hard exudates in the posterior pole but distant from the macula	Referral	Circinate or group of exudates within the macula (The macula is defined as that part of the retina that lies within a circle centered on the fovea whose radius is the distance between the center of the fovea and the temporal margin of the disc) Any microaneurysm or hemorrhage within 1 DD of the center of the fovea only if associated with a best VA of ≤6/12 (if no stereo)	Referral Referral
Moderate diabetic macular edema: Retinal thickening or hard exudates approaching the center of the macula but not involving the center	Referral	Exudate within 1 DD of the center of the fovea	Referral
Severe diabetic macular edema: Retinal thickening or hard exudates involving the center of the macula	Referral	Retinal thickening within 1 DD of the center of the fovea (if stereo available)	Referral

DD, disc diameter; VA, visual acuity.

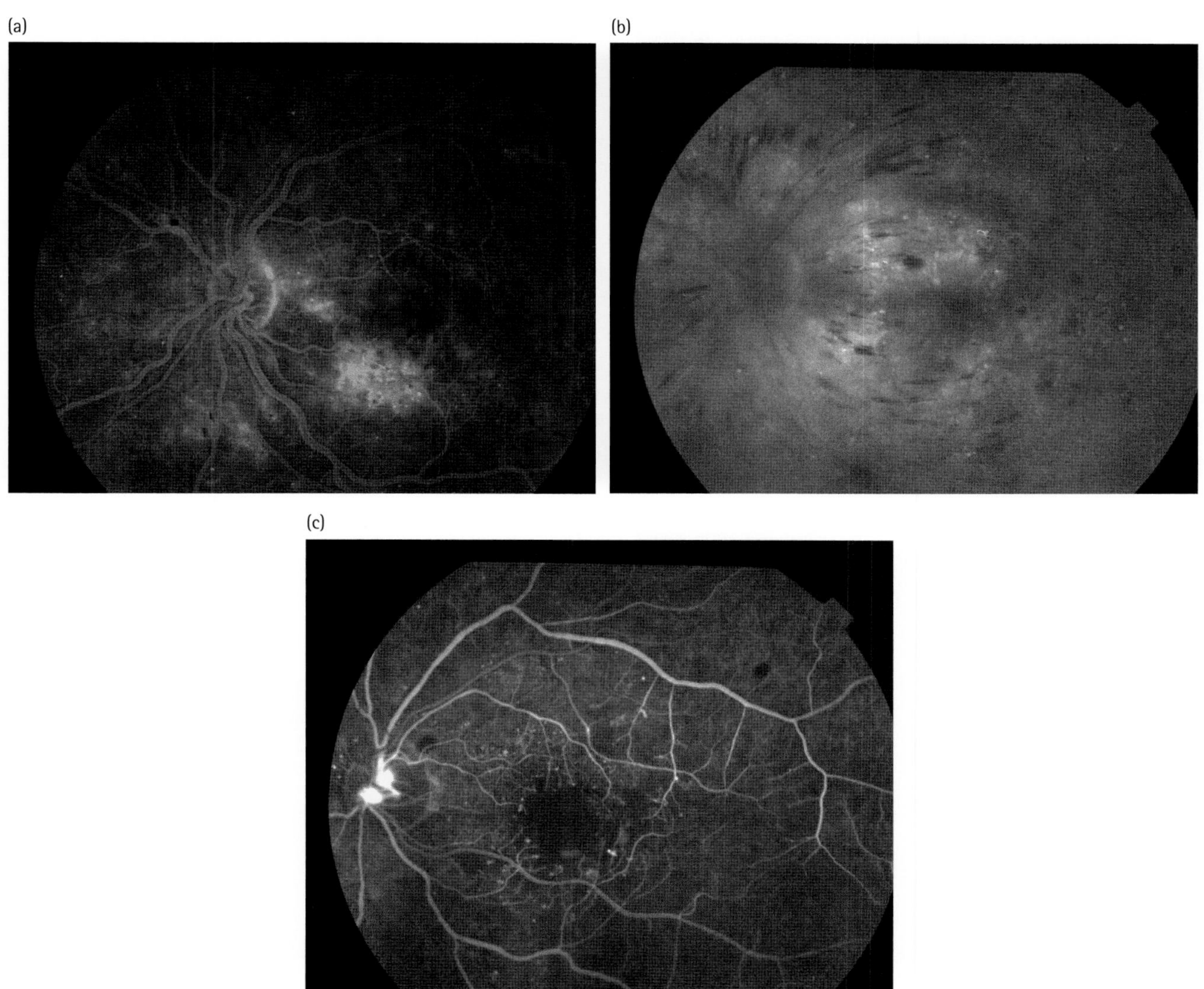

Figure 36.20 (a) Focal maculopathy. Reproduced from Scanlon PH, Wilkinson CP, Aldington SJ, Matthews DR. *A Practical Manual of Diabetic Retinopathy Management*. Published 2009 by Blackwell Publishing. (b) Diffuse maculopathy. Reproduced from Scanlon PH, Wilkinson CP, Aldington SJ, Matthews DR. *A Practical Manual of Diabetic Retinopathy Management*. Published 2009 by Blackwell Publishing. (c) Ischemic maculopathy. Reproduced from Scanlon PH, Wilkinson CP, Aldington SJ, Matthews DR. *A Practical Manual of Diabetic Retinopathy Management*. Published 2009 by Blackwell Publishing.

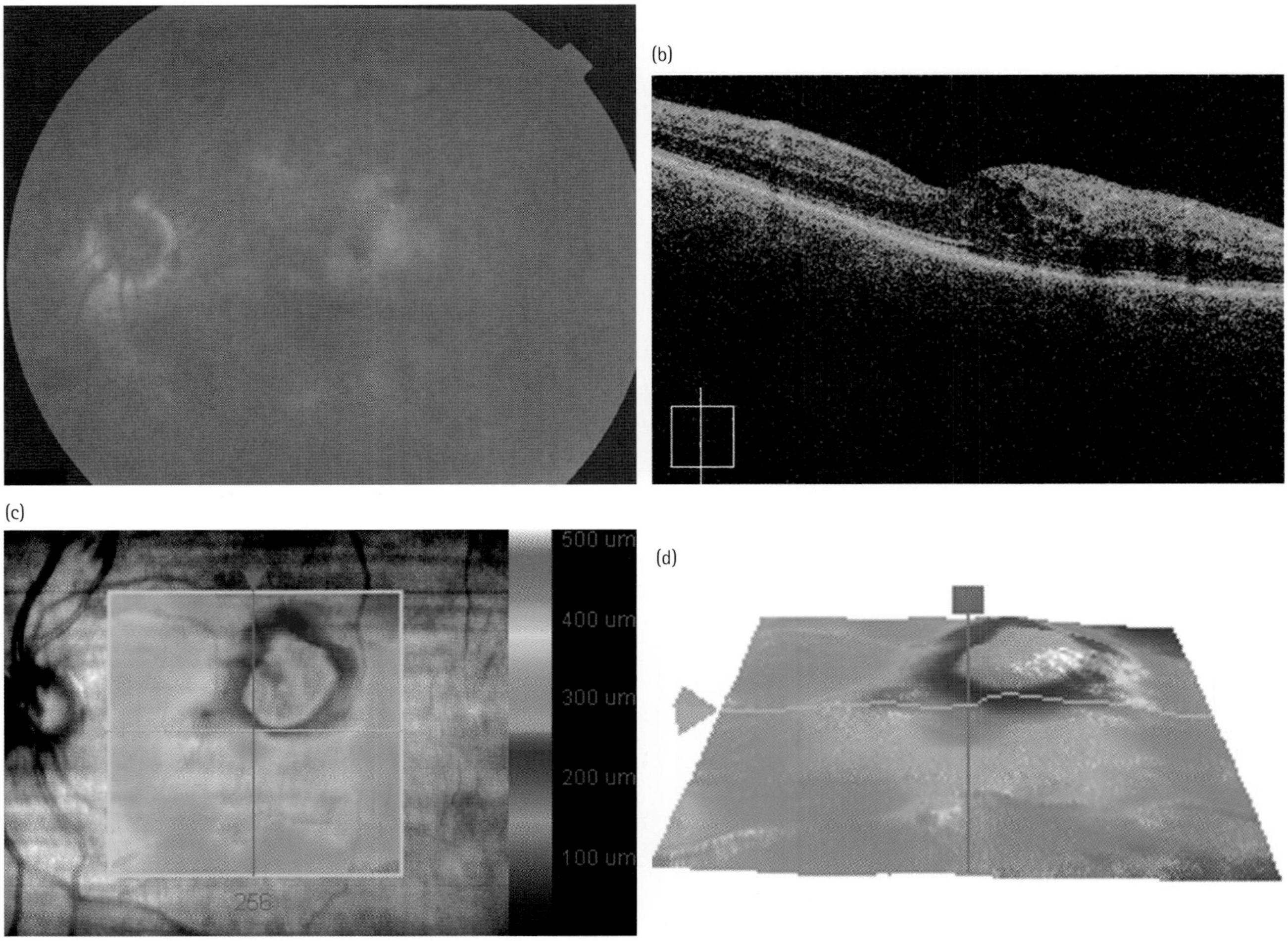

Figure 36.21 (a) Venous phase fluorescein angiogram showing leakage superotemporal to the macula. (b) Cross-sectional optical coherence tomography (OCT) image showing clinically significant macular edema. (c) Topographic map superimposed on red free photograph. (d) Topographic map of clinically significant macular edema.

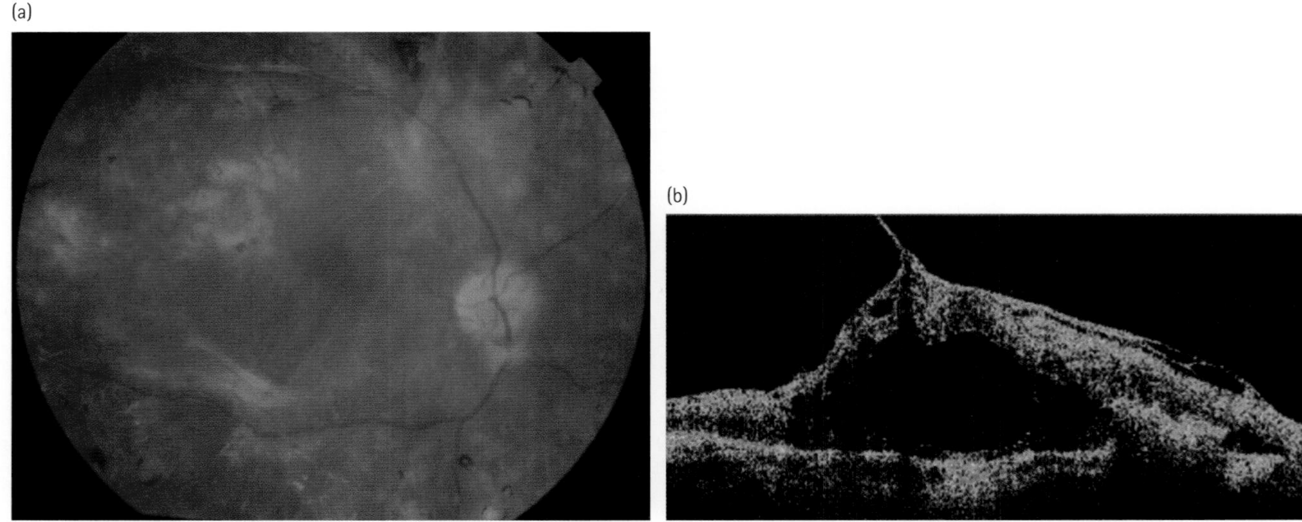

Figure 36.22 (a) Fibrotic proliferations causing macular traction following panretinal photocoagulation. Reproduced from Scanlon PH, Wilkinson CP, Aldington SJ, Matthews DR. *A Practical Manual of Diabetic Retinopathy Management.* Published 2009 by Blackwell Publishing. (b) A cross-sectional optical coherence tomography (OCT) image showing macular traction. Reproduced from Scanlon PH, Wilkinson CP, Aldington SJ, Matthews DR. *A Practical Manual of Diabetic Retinopathy Management.* Published 2009 by Blackwell Publishing.

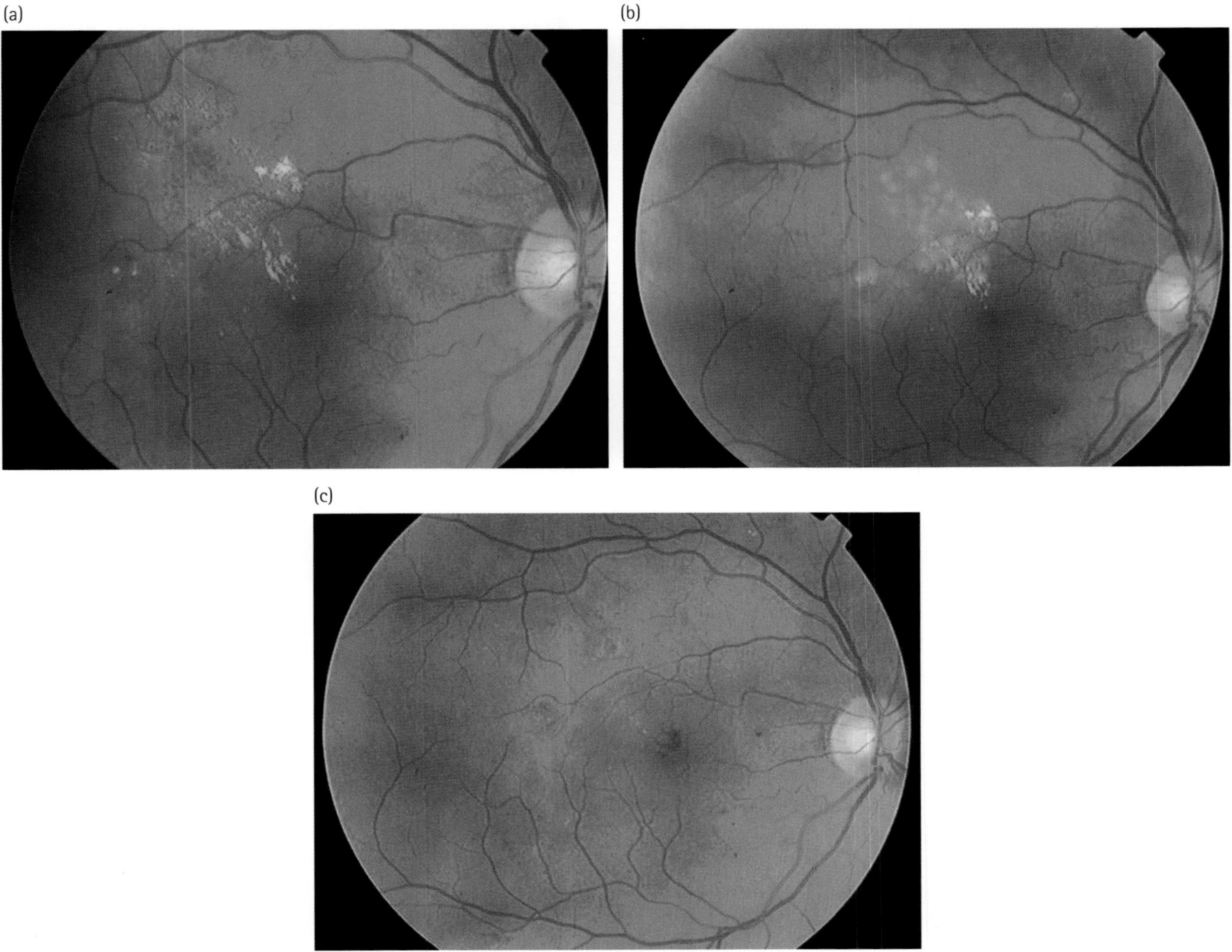

Figure 36.23 (a) Focal maculopathy pretreatment. (b) Focal maculopathy immediately after treatment showing blanching from laser treatment. (c) Focal maculopathy 6 months after treatment showing clearing of the exudate.

diabetic maculopathy edema by 50% or more. It also described "clinically significant macular edema," which defined the parameters for treatment as [54]:

- Thickening of the retina at or within 500 μm of the center of the macula;
- Hard exudates at or within 500 μm of the center of the fovea, if associated with thickening of the adjacent retina (not residual hard exudates remaining after disappearance of retinal thickening);
- A zone or zones of retinal thickening 1 disc area or larger, any part of which is within 1 DD of the center of the macula (Figure 36.23).

Mechanisms of action of laser for macular edema

The effectiveness of focal laser treatment may be caused, in part, by the closure of leaky microaneurysms. Other methods suggested have been histopathologic changes [60], biochemical changes [61] and the application of Starling's law and improved oxygenation [62].

Adverse effects of macular laser treatment

Potential side effects specific to macular laser are:

- Laser close to the central fovea, resulting in a drop in visual acuity. Laser burns may be associated with paracentral scotomas and may become larger than the original spot size [63] and encroach on fixation.
- Choroidal neovascular membrane developing in an area that has received laser treatment – this complication is extremely rare.

Intravitreal triamcinolone

Promising results in the short term for improving the vision in eyes with chronic diabetic macular edema unresponsive to conventional laser treatment, reducing macular thickness and inducing reabsorption of hard exudates, have been described in numerous studies [64–67]. The effects are reported to last for 3–8 months, which may be partially dependent on the dose given, varying between 1 and 25 mg.

Serious side effects, however, have been reported such as early rapid increases in intraocular pressure requiring surgical intervention [68] and infectious endophthalmitis [69]. Randomized controlled trials utilizing varying doses of steroid are now required to assess the long-term efficacy, safety and to define optimum treatment regimens.

Vascular endothelial growth factor treatments

For anti-vascular endothelial growth factor (anti-VEGF) treatments, see the section on the use of intravitreal vascular endothelial growth factor inhibitors later in this chapter.

Mild non-proliferative diabetic retinopathy (ETDRS & International) and background diabetic retinopathy (English Screening)

The earliest sign of mild non-proliferative DR (mild NPDR) or background DR is microaneurysms.

Microaneurysms

Patients with no DR and microaneurysms only were not included in the ETDRS study. In the Wisconsin Epidemiological Study of Diabetic Retinopathy, the rate of progression to proliferative retinopathy 4 years after the initial evaluation showed "no DR" was 0.4% for young patients <30 years with T1DM, 0% for older patients ≥30 years with diabetes taking insulin and 0.6% for those not using insulin. For those with microaneurysms or one hemorrhage in one eye only, the rate of progression to proliferative retinopathy 4 years after the initial evaluation was 3.0% for young patients <30 years with T1DM, 0% for older patients ≥30 years with T1DM and 1.5% for those not using insulin.

The other signs of mild NPDR are one or more of the following:

- *Retinal hemorrhages.* In mild NPDR, retinal hemorrhages are usually small dot hemorrhages or flame-shaped hemorrhages (Figures 36.9 and 36.10). Because small retinal hemorrhages can be difficult to differentiate from microaneurysms they are commonly referred to as HMa.
- *Exudates* (or hard exudates) are a feature of mild NPDR (Figure 36.11).
- *Cotton wool spots* may be present in mild NPDR or background DR but are caused by an arteriolar occlusion in that area of retina, but despite this being the underlying cause, they are not a good sign of increasing retinal ischemia. They are often associated with hypertension (Figure 36.12).
- *A single venous loop.* The ETDRS included a single venous loop in their classification of mild NPDR; however, this rarely occurs in isolation without other significant signs of retinal ischemia and a venous loop is therefore not a feature of the English Screening definition of background DR (Figure 36.14).

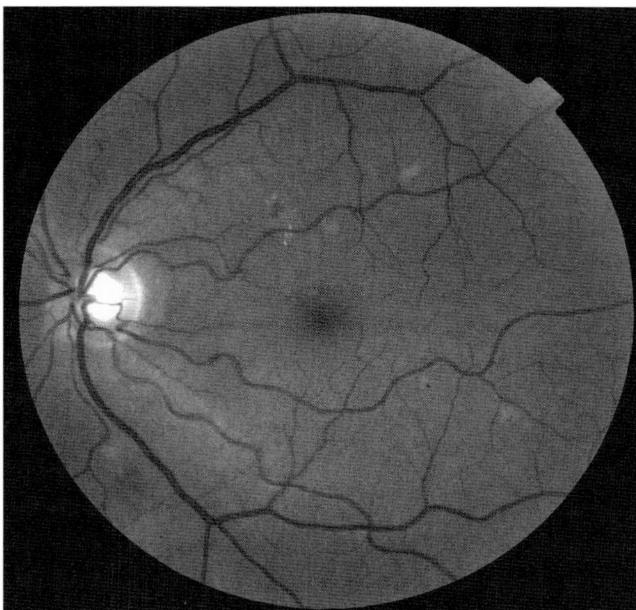

Figure 36.24 Red free photograph showing microaneurysms, hemorrhages, hard exudates and cotton wool spots.

For mild NPDR, there is a 6.2% risk of progression to proliferative retinopathy within 1 year.

The International classification of DR recommends that anyone who has a more severe disorder than microaneurysms is referred to an ophthalmologist [55]. In the UK, patients who are screened and who show signs of background DR are only rescreened annually. For the purposes of the English National Screening Programme, background DR is defined by the following lesions [56]:

- Microaneurysm(s); and
- Retinal hemorrhage(s) with or without any exudate (Figure 36.24).

Moderate and severe non-proliferative diabetic retinopathy (ETDRS & International) and pre-proliferative diabetic retinopathy (English Screening)

The main features that warrant classifying a DR level in the higher levels of moderate and severe NPDR [55] (or pre-proliferative DR [56]) are increasing signs of retinal ischemia.

Lesions associated with increasing retinal ischemia:

- Retinal hemorrhages especially blot hemorrhages (Figure 36.25).
- Intraretinal microvascular abnormality (Figure 36.25). Intraretinal microvascular abnormalities are derived from remodeling of the retinal capillaries and small collateral vessels in

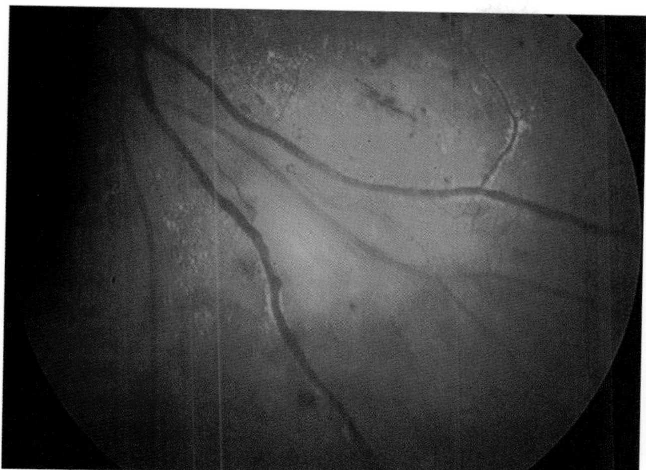

Figure 36.25 Photograph showing venous beading, intraretinal microvascular abnormality, perivenous exudate and a small number of blot hemorrhages. Reproduced from Scanlon PH, Wilkinson CP, Aldington SJ, Matthews DR. *A Practical Manual of Diabetic Retinopathy Management.* Published 2009 by Blackwell Publishing.

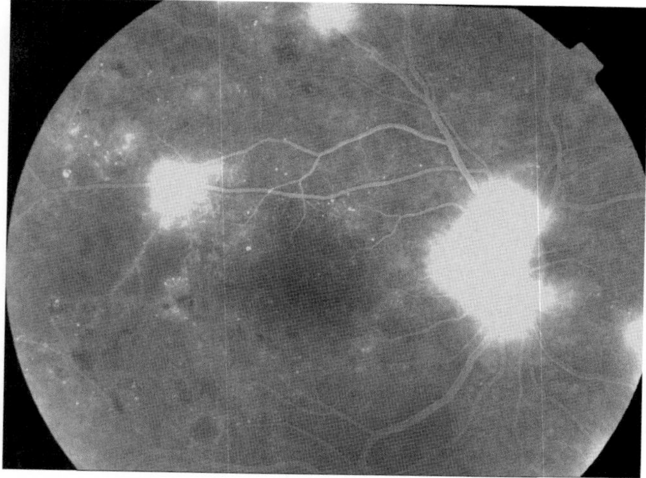

Figure 36.26 Profuse leakage of fluorescein from new vessels on disc (NVD) and new vessels elsewhere (NVE) in the arteriovenous phase of this angiogram.

areas of microvascular occlusion. They are usually found on the borders of areas of non-perfused retina.

- Venous beading (VB; Figure 36.25) is found to be associated with retinal ischemia and is used for assessment of severity of DR.

With increasing ischemia, there is an increasing risk of progression to proliferative in 1 year. The risk increases from approximately 11.3% in the lower levels of moderate NPDR to 54.8% progression to proliferative in 1 year in the most severe NPDR level.

ETDRS definitions have been simplified to make them easier for everyday clinical use both in the International classification and in the English classification for screening.

The ETDRS "4:2:1 rule" indicates that the presence of severe hemorrhages in four quadrants (≥20), VB in two quadrants or IRMA in a single quadrant represents this severity of retinopathy, severe NPDR.

In the International classification, severe NPDR is defined by any of the following:

- Extensive intraretinal hemorrhages (>20) in four quadrants;
- Definite VB in two or more quadrants;
- Prominent IRMA in one or more quadrant, and no signs of PDR.

Moderate NPDR is classified in the International classification as more than "microaneurysms only" and less severe than the 4:2:1 rule.

In the English Screening classification, pre-proliferative DR is defined by any of the following:

- VB;
- Venous loop or reduplication;
- IRMA; or
- Multiple deep, round or blot hemorrhages.

Proliferative diabetic retinopathy and advanced diabetic retinopathy

Pathogenesis of retinal angiogenesis (new vessel formation)

New vessels arise from the post capillary venule in areas of ischemic retina. New vessel growth originates either within 1 DD of the optic disc (new vessels at the disc [NVD]) or developing from retinal vessels more than 1 DD away from the edge of the optic disc (new vessels elsewhere [NVE]).

The central role of growth factors in retinal neovascularization was suggested as early as 1948 by Michaelson [70], who proposed that a diffusible factor released from the ischemic retina was responsible for angiogenesis. The growth factors that have been extensively studied are fibroblast-derived growth factor (FDGF) [71], insulin-like growth factor I (IGF-I) [72], platelet-derived growth factor (PDGF) [73], hepatocyte growth factor (HGF) [74] and VEGF [75]. Another consequence of generalized retinal ischemia can be neovascularization in the anterior chamber on the iris (rubeosis iridis).

Fluorescein angiographic appearance

The characteristic appearance of new vessels on the fluorescein angiogram, once they have penetrated the internal limiting membrane, is leakage appearing in the arteriovenous phase of the angiogram and increasing through the angiogram (Figure 36.26).

Presentation

Some patients present asymptomatically from screening, others with visual loss arising from hemorrhage from new vessels.

Laser treatment for proliferative diabetic retinopathy

For laser treatment for proliferative diabetic retinopathy (PDR), see Figure 36.27.

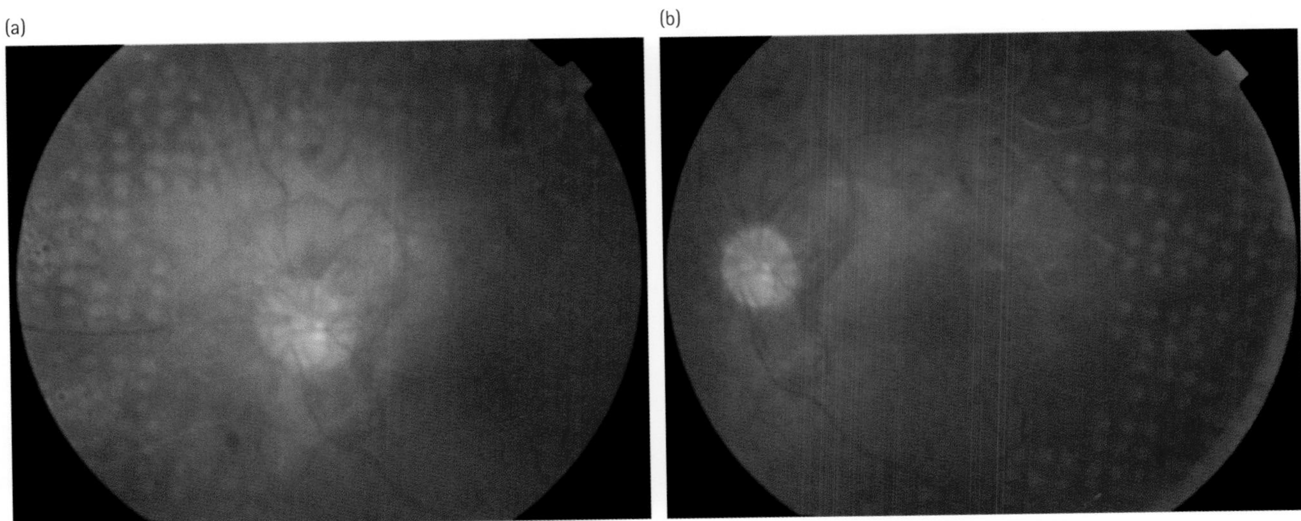

Figure 36.27 Disc and macular photographs taken immediately after panretinal laser treatment on a patient with proliferative diabetic retinopathy. Reproduced from Scanlon PH, Wilkinson CP, Aldington SJ, Matthews DR. *A Practical Manual of Diabetic Retinopathy Management*. Published 2009 by Blackwell Publishing.

Diabetic Retinopathy Study

The Diabetic Retinopathy Study (DRS) [53] recommended prompt treatment in the presence of DRS high-risk characteristics, which reduced the 2-year risk of severe visual loss by 50% or more and were defined by:

- Presence of preretinal or vitreous hemorrhage;
- Eyes with NVD equalling or exceeding one-quarter to one-third disc area in extent with no hemorrhage;
- NVE equalling more than half disc area with hemorrhage.

Untreated, eyes with high risk characteristics had a 25.6–36.9% chance of severe visual loss within 2 years, depending on the size and location of the new vessels and whether or not hemorrhage was present.

"Low risk" proliferative patients

In eyes with PDR without high risk characteristics, there were still the following risks of severe visual loss:

- Untreated: 2 year 7.0%, 4 years 20.9%;
- Treated: 2 year 3.2%, 4 years 7.4%.

These risks need to be balanced against the potential adverse effects of laser treatment.

Adverse effects of laser treatment

Adverse effects of laser treatment described in the DRS [76] and other studies are as follow:

- Loss of peripheral areas of visual field was attributed to argon laser in approximately 10% of eyes and field loss was nearly three times more common in the xenon arc treated group.
- Visual acuity loss at the 6-week follow-up visit was assumed to be brought about by treatment. Among eyes with NPDR, 14.3% more argon-treated and 29.7% of xenon-treated eyes than control subjects had an early persistent loss of one or more lines.

Other possible adverse effects of panretinal laser treatment are as follow:

- Unintended laser absorption (e.g. to the lens) or uptake of laser from a flame-shaped hemorrhage, which may result in a burn and destruction of the nerve fiber layer that lies on its surface.
- Inadvertent coagulation (e.g. to the fovea).
- Choroidal detachment is usually as a result of a large dose of laser treatment being applied in a single session, which usually resolves spontaneously within 10 days.

Risks to the ophthalmologist

There has been some concern in the past that the ophthalmologist is exposed to excessive amounts of reflected light, particularly blue light; however, modern technology with appropriate filters has significantly reduced this risk.

Risks to an observer

The risk to an observer is extremely small but, as a precaution, it is advised that any observer wears the appropriate spectacle protection.

Factors other than high risk characteristics influencing the decision to laser

Anterior segment neovascularization

Extensive neovascularization in the anterior chamber angle is an urgent indication for scatter laser photocoagulation, if it is feasible (Figure 36.28).

Signs of ischemia

Large IRMA, VB in more than one quadrant, extensive retinal hemorrhages and opaque small arteriolar branches are signs suggesting severe retinal ischemia.

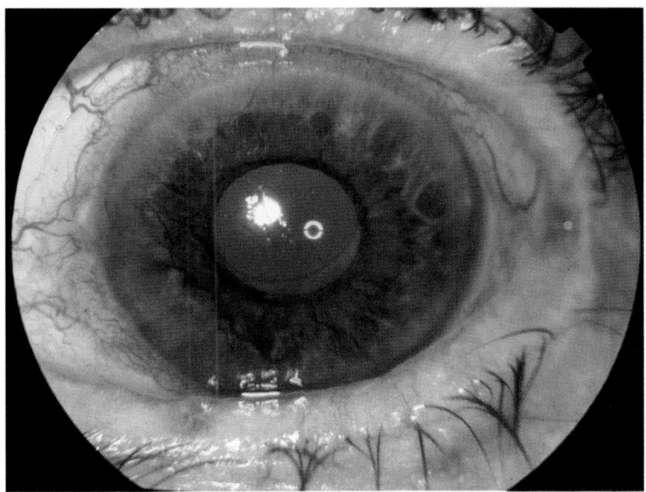

Figure 36.28 Iris neovascularization.

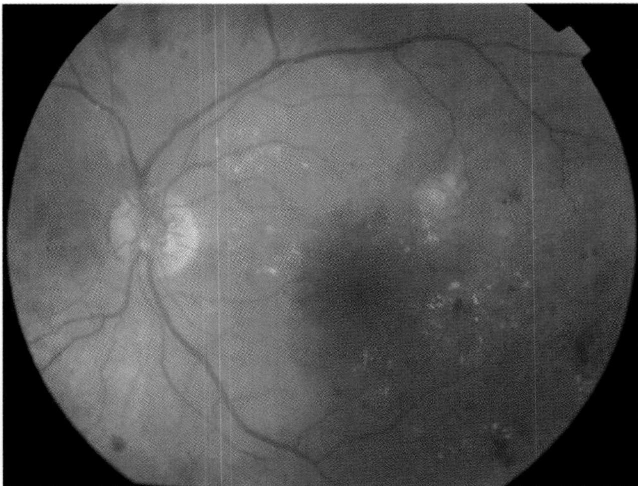

Figure 36.29 Proliferative diabetic retinopathy and concurrent maculopathy.

Macular edema

See the section on laser for PDR and concurrent diabetic maculopathy.

Pregnancy

See the section on pregnancy and DR (below).

Renal failure

Treatment needs to coincide with renal dialysis or transplantation. It is also important to control hypertension.

Past history

The past history of retinopathy, both in the eye for which scatter laser photocoagulation and in the fellow eye, needs to be considered.

Duration of the laser burn

There has been an increasing tendency in the last year for operators to reduce the duration of the burn and increase the power to produce an apparently similar mild bleaching because of the clinical impression that this is more comfortable for the patient.

Pattern scan laser

With conventional methods of retinal laser photocoagulation, the ophthalmologist uses a mechanical joystick and foot pedal to deliver single 100-ms laser pulses to the peripheral retina. With the pattern scan laser, the laser pulse time is reduced from 100 ms to just 10–20 ms, and automated multiple spots are produced with each depression of the foot pedal. Higher power is required for shorter burns. Predetermined pattern types can administer up to 25 spots at a time for scatter laser treatment.

Stage R3 with M1: proliferative diabetic retinopathy with maculopathy

The ETDRS [77] compared giving immediate panretinal photocoagulation with either simultaneous or delayed focal treatment. The conclusion was that, where possible, clinically significant macular edema should be treated by applying focal/grid photocoagulation for macular edema before beginning scatter laser treatment. When the risk of vitreous hemorrhage or neovascular glaucoma seems high, combine treatment of clinically significant macular edema by applying focal/grid photocoagulation for macular edema with panretinal photocoagulation to the inferior half of the peripheral retina, followed 2 weeks later by panretinal photocoagulation to the superior half.

Hamilton *et al.* [78] recommended an exception to this approach for young patients with T1DM who have rapidly accelerating peripheral ischemia associated with macular edema that may resolve following panretinal photocoagulation (Figure 36.29).

Use of intravitreal vascular endothelial growth factor inhibitors

Ocular neovascularization (angiogenesis) and increased vascular permeability have been associated with VEGF, which does also has a neuroprotective effect. There are three potential VEGF inhibitors:

1 Pegaptanib (Macugen);
2 Ranibizumab (Lucentis);
3 Bevacizumab (Avastin).

Ranibizumab (Lucentis) is an antibody fragment derived from bevacizumab (Avastin), which is a full-length humanized monoclonal antibody against human VEGF.

There are reports of reduction in macular thickness using intravitreal injections of these agents [79]; however, the effect does not last and repeated injections would be required to sustain any beneficial effects.

Favorable results have been reported with some regression of neovascularization and reduction in fluorescein leakage in some studies using bevacizumab [80,81] and using pegaptanib [82] but the effect is only transient (2–11 weeks [81]).

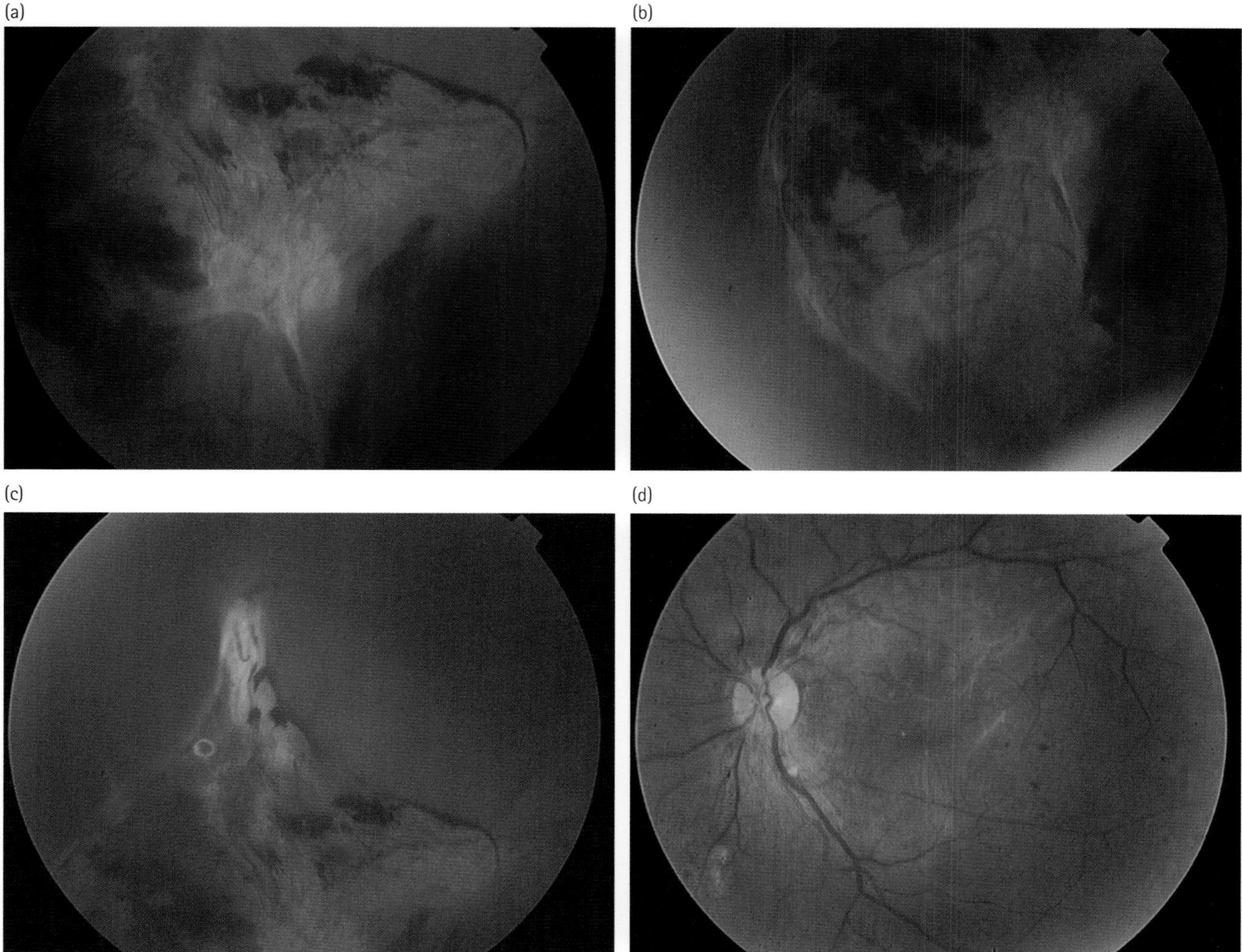

Figure 36.30 Vitrectomy for tractional detachment shown in (a–c) with postoperative photograph in (d). Reproduced from Scanlon PH, Wilkinson CP, Aldington SJ, Matthews DR. *A Practical Manual of Diabetic Retinopathy Management*. Published 2009 by Blackwell Publishing.

Intravitreal injection is an effective means of delivering anti-VEGF drugs to the retina but has the potential complications of endophthalmitis and retinal detachment. Randomized controlled trials utilizing varying doses of the VEGF inhibitors are required to assess the long-term efficacy, safety and to define optimum treatment regimens.

Vitrectomy

Smiddy and Flynn [83] wrote an excellent review where they noted that, according to the ETDRS, at least 5% of eyes receiving optimal medical treatment will still have progressive retinopathy that requires laser treatment and pars plana vitrectomy.

Two recent reports of vitrectomy case series have demonstrated that the most common reason for vitrectomy for DR is vitreous hemorrhage [84,85]. In the latter study, the indications for vitrectomy were:

- Vitreous hemorrhage in 80 patients (86.1%);
- Tractional retinal detachment in three patients (3.2%); and
- Vitreous hemorrhage associated with tractional retinal detachment in 10 patients (10.7%).

Lewis [86] suggested that for clinically significant macular edema, OCT should be performed to test for posterior hyaloid thickening and vitrectomy should be considered when a shallow macular detachment is found. Studies by Okamoto *et al.* [87] and Emi *et al.* [88] have shown that vitrectomy is effective in increasing the quality of life of patients with DR (Figure 36.30).

Pregnancy and the diabetic eye

Risk factors for progression of diabetic retinopathy in pregnancy

The known risk factors for progression of DR in pregnancy are:

- Pregnancy itself is independently associated with progression of DR [89,90];
- Baseline severity of DR [91–93];
- Poor metabolic control at conception [91];
- Rapid improvement of glycemic control [90–93];
- Poor metabolic control during pregnancy or the early postpartum period [89,90,93,94];
- Duration of diabetes [93,95,96]; and
- Chronic hypertension and pregnancy-induced hypertension [93].

Recommendations for patients

- Plan pregnancies early in life – women with T1DM should be encouraged to plan pregnancies early in life [94].
- Improving metabolic control before conception is recommended both for the mother and infant [91].
- Improving metabolic control during pregnancy is recommended both for the mother and infant [89,90,93,94].
- Control of hypertension both before conception and during pregnancy is recommended both for the mother and infant [93].
- Photocoagulation before conception and during pregnancy [95]. It is recommended that, if a patient is found to have significant retinopathy before conception, pregnancy is delayed where possible until appropriate laser treatment has been applied and good metabolic control has been achieved for a 9-month period to overcome any effects of the early worsening phenomenon [7]. Photocoagulation before pregnancy may protect against rapidly progressive PDR. Aggressive treatment of PDR developing in pregnancy may prevent further progression of the disease.

Low vision and blindness from diabetic retinopathy

In 2001, Cunningham [97] reported that 45 million people worldwide fulfil the WHO criteria for blindness. Twenty-four percent of all blindness, affecting people in both developed and developing nations, is caused by a combination of DR and macular degeneration with a small contribution from other eye diseases. In 2002, Kocur and Resnikoff [36] reported that in people of working age in Europe, DR is the most frequently reported cause of serious visual loss, confirmed in the UK by two studies [98,99].

In 2004, Fong *et al.* [100] reported that DR is a leading cause of adult blindness in the USA, resulting in blindness for more than 10 000 people per year.

The most progress in reduction of blindness has been made in Iceland [2] where the prevalence of legal blindness from DR dropped from 4.0% to 0.5% over 15 years, beginning in 1980.

References

1 Klein R, Klein BE, Moss SE, Davis MD, DeMets DL. The Wisconsin epidemiologic study of diabetic retinopathy. II. Prevalence and risk of diabetic retinopathy when age at diagnosis is less than 30 years. *Arch Ophthalmol* 1984; **102**:520–526.

2 Stefansson E. Prevention of diabetic blindness. *Br J Ophthalmol* 2006; **90**:2–3.

3 Mackenzie S, Nettleship E. *Royal Ophthalmic London Hospital Report 9 (part 2)*. 1877: 134.

4 Ballantyne A, Loewenstein A. Diseases of the retina: the pathology of diabetic retinopathy. *Trans Ophthalmol Soc UK* 1943; **63**:95–115.

5 Ashton N. Arteriolar involvement in diabetic retinopathy. *Br J Ophthalmol* 1953; **37**:282–292.

6 Diabetes Control and Complications Trial Research Group. The effect of intensive treatment of diabetes on the development and progression of long-term complications in insulin-dependent diabetes mellitus. *N Engl J Med* 1993; **329**:977–986.

7 Early worsening of diabetic retinopathy in the Diabetes Control and Complications Trial. *Arch Ophthalmol* 1998; **116**:874–886.

8 UK Prospective Diabetes Study (UKPDS) Group. Intensive blood-glucose control with sulphonylureas or insulin compared with conventional treatment and risk of complications in patients with type 2 diabetes (UKPDS 33). *Lancet* 1998; **352**:837–853.

9 Chase HP, Garg SK, Jackson WE, Thomas MA, Harris S, Marshall G, *et al.* Blood pressure and retinopathy in type 1 diabetes. *Ophthalmology* 1990; **97**:155–159.

10 Matthews DR, Stratton IM, Aldington SJ, Holman RR, Kohner EM. Risks of progression of retinopathy and vision loss related to tight blood pressure control in type 2 diabetes mellitus: UKPDS 69. *Arch Ophthalmol* 2004; **122**:1631–1640.

11 Chew EY, Klein ML, Ferris FL 3rd, Remaley NA, Murphy RP, Chantry K, *et al.* Association of elevated serum lipid levels with retinal hard exudate in diabetic retinopathy. Early Treatment Diabetic Retinopathy Study (ETDRS) Report 22. *Arch Ophthalmol* 1996; **114**:1079–1084.

12 Cusick M, Chew EY, Chan CC, Kruth HS, Murphy RP, Ferris FL 3rd. Histopathology and regression of retinal hard exudates in diabetic retinopathy after reduction of elevated serum lipid levels. *Ophthalmology* 2003; **110**:2126–2133.

13 Muhlhauser I, Bender R, Bott U, Jörgens V, Grüsser M, Wagener W, *et al.* Cigarette smoking and progression of retinopathy and nephropathy in type 1 diabetes. *Diabet Med* 1996; **13**:536–543.

14 Karamanos B, Porta M, Songini M, Metelko Z, Kerenyi Z, Tamas G, *et al.* Different risk factors of microangiopathy in patients with type I diabetes mellitus of short versus long duration. The EURODIAB IDDM Complications Study. *Diabetologia* 2000; **43**:348–355.

15 Klein R, Klein BE, Moss SE, Davis MD, DeMets DL. The Wisconsin Epidemiologic Study of Diabetic Retinopathy. IX. Four-year incidence and progression of diabetic retinopathy when age at diagnosis is less than 30 years. *Arch Ophthalmol* 1989; **107**:237–243.

16 Klein R, Klein BE, Moss SE, Davis MD, DeMets DL. The Wisconsin Epidemiologic Study of Diabetic Retinopathy. X. Four-year incidence and progression of diabetic retinopathy when age at diagnosis is 30 years or more. *Arch Ophthalmol* 1989; **107**:244–249.

17 Klein R, Klein BE, Moss SE, Davis MD, DeMets DL. The Wisconsin epidemiologic study of diabetic retinopathy. III. Prevalence and risk of diabetic retinopathy when age at diagnosis is 30 or more years. *Arch Ophthalmol* 1984; **102**:527–532.

18 Klein R, Klein BE, Moss SE, Cruickshanks KJ. The Wisconsin Epidemiologic Study of diabetic retinopathy. XIV. Ten-year inci-

dence and progression of diabetic retinopathy. *Arch Ophthalmol* 1994; **112**:1217–1228.
19 Stratton IM, Kohner EM, Aldington SJ, Turner RC, Holman RR, Manley SE, *et al.* UKPDS 50: risk factors for incidence and progression of retinopathy in type II diabetes over 6 years from diagnosis. *Diabetologia* 2001; **44**:156–163.
20 Birinci A, Birinci H, Abidinoglu R, Durupinar B, Oge I. Diabetic retinopathy and HLA antigens in type 2 diabetes mellitus. *Eur J Ophthalmol* 2002; **12**:89–93.
21 Mimura T, Funatsu H, Uchigata Y, Kitano S, Shimizu E, Amano S, *et al.* Glutamic acid decarboxylase autoantibody prevalence and association with HLA genotype in patients with younger-onset type 1 diabetes and proliferative diabetic retinopathy. *Ophthalmology* 2005; **112**:1904–1909.
22 Wong TY, Cruickshank KJ, Klein R, Moss SE, Palta M, Riley WJ, *et al.* HLA-DR3 and DR4 and their relation to the incidence and progression of diabetic retinopathy. *Ophthalmology* 2002; **109**:275–281.
23 Emanuele N, Sacks J, Klein R, Reda D, Anderson R, Duckworth W, *et al.* Ethnicity, race, and baseline retinopathy correlates in the Veterans Affairs Diabetes Trial. *Diabetes Care* 2005; **28**:1954–1958.
24 Simmons D, Clover G, Hope C. Ethnic differences in diabetic retinopathy. *Diabet Med* 2007; **24**:1093–1098.
25 Ljubimov AV, Burgeson RE, Butkowski RJ, Couchman JR, Zardi L, Ninomiya Y, *et al.* Basement membrane abnormalities in human eyes with diabetic retinopathy. *J Histochem Cytochem* 1996; **44**: 1469–1479.
26 Podesta F, Romeo G, Liu WH, Krajewski S, Reed JC, Gerhardinger C, *et al.* Bax is increased in the retina of diabetic subjects and is associated with pericyte apoptosis *in vivo* and *in vitro*. *Am J Pathol* 2000; **156**:1025–1032.
27 Joris I, Majno G, Corey EJ, Lewis RA. The mechanism of vascular leakage induced by leukotriene E4: endothelial contraction. *Am J Pathol* 1987; **126**:19–24.
28 Stitt AW, Gardiner TA, Archer DB. Histological and ultrastructural investigation of retinal microaneurysm development in diabetic patients. *Br J Ophthalmol* 1995; **79**:362–367.
29 Gardiner TA, Archer DB, Curtis TM, Stitt AW. Arteriolar involvement in the microvascular lesions of diabetic retinopathy: implications for pathogenesis. *Microcirculation* 2007; **14**:25–38.
30 Schmetterer L, Wolzt M. Ocular blood flow and associated functional deviations in diabetic retinopathy. *Diabetologia* 1999; **42**:387–405.
31 Kristinsson JK, Gottfredsdottir MS, Stefansson E. Retinal vessel dilatation and elongation precedes diabetic macular oedema. *Br J Ophthalmol* 1997; **81**:274–278.
32 Collier A, Tymkewycz P, Armstrong R, Young RJ, Jones RL, Clarke BF. Increased platelet thromboxane receptor sensitivity in diabetic patients with proliferative retinopathy. *Diabetologia* 1986; **29**:471–474.
33 Alessandrini P, McRae J, Feman S, FitzGerald GA. Thromboxane biosynthesis and platelet function in type 1 diabetes mellitus. *N Engl J Med* 1988; **319**:208–212.
34 Wilson J, Jungner G. *The Principles and Practice of Screening for Disease.* Public Health Papers 34. Geneva: World Health Organization, 1968.
35 Kempen JH, O'Colmain BJ, Leske MC, Haffner SM, Klein R, Moss SE, *et al.* The prevalence of diabetic retinopathy among adults in the United States. *Arch Ophthalmol* 2004; **122**:552–563.
36 Kocur I, Resnikoff S. Visual impairment and blindness in Europe and their prevention. *Br J Ophthalmol* 2002; **86**:716–722.
37 Early Treatment Diabetic Retinopathy Study Research Group. Fundus photographic risk factors for progression of diabetic retinopathy. ETDRS Report no. 12. *Ophthalmology* 1991; **98**(Suppl):823–833.
38 Diabetic Retinopathy Study Research Group. Four risk factors for severe visual loss in diabetic retinopathy: the third report from the Diabetic Retinopathy Study. *Arch Ophthalmol* 1979; **97**:654–655.
39 Early Treatment Diabetic Retinopathy Study Research Group. Photocoagulation for diabetic macular edema: Early Treatment Diabetic Retinopathy Study Report no. 4. *Int Ophthalmol Clin* 1987; **27**:265–272.
40 Davies EG, Petty RG, Kohner EM. Long-term effectiveness of photocoagulation for diabetic maculopathy. *Eye* 1989; **3**:764–767.
41 Sullivan P, Caldwell G, Alexander N, Kohner E. Long-term outcome after photocoagulation for proliferative diabetic retinopathy. *Diabet Med* 1990; **7**:788–794.
42 Chew EY, Ferris FL 3rd, Csaky KG, Murphy RP, Agrón E, Thompson DJ, *et al.* The long-term effects of laser photocoagulation treatment in patients with diabetic retinopathy: the early treatment diabetic retinopathy follow-up study. *Ophthalmology* 2003; **110**:1683–1689.
43 Olson JA, Strachan FM, Hipwell JH, Groatman KA, McHardy KC, Forrester JV, *et al.* A comparative evaluation of digital imaging, retinal photography and optometrist examination in screening for diabetic retinopathy. *Diabet Med* 2003; **20**:528–534.
44 Scanlon PH, Malhotra R, Thomas G, Foy C, Kirkpatrick JN, Lewis-Barned N, *et al.* The effectiveness of screening for diabetic retinopathy by digital imaging photography and technician ophthalmoscopy. *Diabet Med* 2003; **20**:467–474.
45 Scanlon PH, Malhotra R, Greenwood RH, Aldington SJ, Foy C, Flatman M, *et al.* Comparison of two reference standards in validating two field mydriatic digital photography as a method of screening for diabetic retinopathy. *Br J Ophthalmol* 2003; **87**:1258–1263.
46 Williams GA, Scott IU, Haller JA, Maguire AM, Marcus D, McDonald HR. Single-field fundus photography for diabetic retinopathy screening: a report by the American Academy of Ophthalmology. *Ophthalmology* 2004; **111**:1055–1062.
47 Javitt JC, Aiello LP. Cost-effectiveness of detecting and treating diabetic retinopathy. *Ann Intern Med* 1996; **124**:164–169.
48 Dasbach EJ, Fryback DG, Newcomb PA, Klein R, Klein BE. Cost-effectiveness of strategies for detecting diabetic retinopathy. *Med Care* 1991; **29**:20–39.
49 Fendrick AM, Javitt JC, Chiang YP. Cost-effectiveness of the screening and treatment of diabetic retinopathy: what are the costs of underutilization? *Int J Technol Assess Health Care* 1992; **8**:694–707.
50 James M, Turner DA, Broadbent DM, Vora J, Harding SP. Cost effectiveness analysis of screening for sight threatening diabetic eye disease. *Br Med J* 2000; **320**:1627–1631.
51 Early Treatment Diabetic Retinopathy Study Research Group. Grading diabetic retinopathy from stereoscopic color fundus photographs: an extension of the modified Airlie House classification. ETDRS Report no. 10. *Ophthalmology* 1991; **98**(Suppl):786–806.
52 Spalter HF. Photocoagulation of circinate maculopathy in diabetic retinopathy. *Am J Ophthalmol* 1971; **1**:242–250.
53 Diabetic Retinopathy Study Research Group. Photocoagulation treatment of proliferative diabetic retinopathy. Clinical application of Diabetic Retinopathy Study (DRS) findings. DRS Report no. 8. *Ophthalmology* 1981; **88**:583–600.

54 Early Treatment Diabetic Retinopathy Study Research Group. Treatment techniques and clinical guidelines for photocoagulation of diabetic macular edema. Early Treatment Diabetic Retinopathy Study Report no. 2. *Ophthalmology* 1987; **94**:761–774.

55 Wilkinson CP, Ferris FL 3rd, Klein RE, Lee PP, Agardh CD, Davis M, *et al.* Proposed international clinical diabetic retinopathy and diabetic macular edema disease severity scales. *Ophthalmology* 2003; **110**:1677–1682.

56 Harding S, Greenwood R, Aldington S, Gibson J, Owens D, Taylor R, *et al.* Grading and disease management in national screening for diabetic retinopathy in England and Wales. *Diabet Med* 2003; **20**:965–971.

57 Bresnick GH. Diabetic macular edema: a review. *Ophthalmology* 1986; **93**:989–997.

58 Kearns M, Hamilton AM, Kohner EM. Excessive permeability in diabetic maculopathy. *Br J Ophthalmol* 1979; **63**:489–497.

59 Early Treatment Diabetic Retinopathy Study Research Group. Photocoagulation for diabetic macular edema: Early Treatment Diabetic Retinopathy Study Report no. 1. *Arch Ophthalmol* 1985; **103**:1796–1806.

60 Apple DJ, Goldberg MF, Wyhinny G. Histopathology and ultrastructure of the argon laser lesion in human retinal and choroidal vasculatures. *Am J Ophthalmol* 1973; **75**:595–609.

61 Ogata N, Tombran-Tink J, Jo N, Mrazek D, Matsumura M. Upregulation of pigment epithelium-derived factor after laser photocoagulation. *Am J Ophthalmol* 2001; **132**:427–429.

62 Arnarsson A, Stefansson E. Laser treatment and the mechanism of edema reduction in branch retinal vein occlusion. *Invest Ophthalmol Vis Sci* 2000; **41**:877–879.

63 Schatz H, Madeira D, McDonald HR, Johnson RN. Progressive enlargement of laser scars following grid laser photocoagulation for diffuse diabetic macular edema. *Arch Ophthalmol* 1991; **109**: 1549–1551.

64 Ciardella AP, Klancnik J, Schiff W, Barile G, Langton K, Chang S. Intravitreal triamcinolone for the treatment of refractory diabetic macular oedema with hard exudates: an optical coherence tomography study. *Br J Ophthalmol* 2004; **88**:1131–1136.

65 Ozkiris A, Evereklioglu C, Erkilic K, Tamcelik N, Mirza E. Intravitreal triamcinolone acetonide injection as primary treatment for diabetic macular edema. *Eur J Ophthalmol* 2004; **14**:543–549.

66 Spandau UH, Derse M, Schmitz-Valckenberg P, Papoulis C, Jonas JB. Dosage dependency of intravitreal triamcinolone acetonide as treatment for diabetic macular oedema. *Br J Ophthalmol* 2005; **89**:999–1003.

67 Jonas JB, Martus P, Degenring RF, Kreissig I, Akkoyun I. Predictive factors for visual acuity after intravitreal triamcinolone treatment for diabetic macular edema. *Arch Ophthalmol* 2005; **123**:1338–1343.

68 Singh IP, Ahmad SI, Yeh D, Challa P, Herndon LW, Allingham RR, *et al.* Early rapid rise in intraocular pressure after intravitreal triamcinolone acetonide injection. *Am J Ophthalmol* 2004; **138**: 286–287.

69 Sutter FK, Simpson JM, Gillies MC. Intravitreal triamcinolone for diabetic macular edema that persists after laser treatment: three-month efficacy and safety results of a prospective, randomized, double-masked, placebo-controlled clinical trial. *Ophthalmology* 2004; **111**:2044–2049.

70 Michaelson IC. The mode of development of retinal vessels. *Trans Ophthalmol Soc UK* 1948; **68**:137–138.

71 Beranek M, Kolar P, Tschoplova S, Kankova K, Vasku A. Genetic variation and plasma level of the basic fibroblast growth factor in proliferative diabetic retinopathy. *Diabetes Res Clin Pract* 2008; **79**:362–367.

72 Simo R, Lecube A, Segura RM, Garcia Arumi J, Hernandez C. Free insulin growth factor-I and vascular endothelial growth factor in the vitreous fluid of patients with proliferative diabetic retinopathy. *Am J Ophthalmol* 2002; **134**:376–382.

73 Lindblom P, Gerhardt H, Liebner S, Abramsson A, Enge M, Hellstrom M, *et al.* Endothelial PDGF-B retention is required for proper investment of pericytes in the microvessel wall. *Genes Dev* 2003; **17**:1835–1840.

74 Simo R, Vidal MT, García-Arumí J, Carrasco E, García-Ramírez M, Segura RM, *et al.* Intravitreous hepatocyte growth factor in patients with proliferative diabetic retinopathy: a case–control study. *Diabetes Res Clin Pract* 2006; **71**:36–44.

75 Takagi H. Molecular mechanisms of retinal neovascularisation in diabetic retinopathy. *Intern Med* 2003; **42**:299–301.

76 Diabetic Retinopathy Study Research Group. Indications for photocoagulation treatment of diabetic retinopathy: Diabetic Retinopathy Study Report no. 14. *Int Ophthalmol Clin* 1987; **27**:239–253.

77 Early Treatment Diabetic Retinopathy Study Research Group. Early photocoagulation for diabetic retinopathy. ETDRS Report no. 9. *Ophthalmology* 1991; **98**(Suppl):766–785.

78 Hamilton A, Ulbig M, Polkinghorne P. *Management of Diabetic Retinopathy*. London: BMJ Publishing Group, 1996.

79 Arevalo JF, Fromow-Guerra J, Quiroz-Mercado H, Sanchez JG, Wu L, Maia M, Berrocal MH, *et al.* Primary intravitreal bevacizumab (Avastin) for diabetic macular edema: results from the Pan-American Collaborative Retina Study Group at 6-month follow-up. *Ophthalmology* 2007; **114**:743–750.

80 Jorge R, Costa RA, Calucci D, Cintra LP, Scott IU. Intravitreal bevacizumab (Avastin) for persistent new vessels in diabetic retinopathy (IBEPE study). *Retina* 2006; **26**:1006–1013.

81 Avery RL, Pearlman J, Pieramici DJ, Rabena MD, Castellarin AA, Nasir MA, *et al.* Intravitreal bevacizumab (Avastin) in the treatment of proliferative diabetic retinopathy. *Ophthalmology* 2006; **113**:1695. e1–15.

82 Adamis AP, Altaweel M, Bressler NM, Cunningham ET Jr, Davis MD, Goldbaum M, *et al.* Changes in retinal neovascularisation after pegaptanib (Macugen) therapy in diabetic individuals. *Ophthalmology* 2006; **113**:23–28.

83 Smiddy WE, Flynn HW Jr. Vitrectomy in the management of diabetic retinopathy. *Surv Ophthalmol* 1999; **43**:491–507.

84 Lahey JM, Francis RR, Kearney JJ. Combining phacoemulsification with pars plana vitrectomy in patients with proliferative diabetic retinopathy: a series of 223 cases. *Ophthalmology* 2003; **110**:1335–1339.

85 Schrey S, Krepler K, Wedrich A. Incidence of rhegmatogenous retinal detachment after vitrectomy in eyes of diabetic patients. *Retina* 2006; **26**:149–152.

86 Lewis H. The role of vitrectomy in the treatment of diabetic macular edema (Editorial). *Am J Ophthalmol* 2001; **131**:123–125.

87 Okamoto F, Okamoto Y, Fukuda S, Hiraoka T, Oshika T. Vision-related quality of life and visual function following vitrectomy for proliferative diabetic retinopathy. *Am J Ophthalmol* 2008; **146**: 318–322.

88 Emi K, Oyagi T, Ikeda T, Bando H, Okita T, Kashimoto D, *et al.* Influence of vitrectomy for diabetic retinopathy on health-related

quality of life. [In Japanese] *Nippon Ganka Gakkai Zasshi* 2008; **112**:141–147.

89 Klein BE, Moss SE, Klein R. Effect of pregnancy on progression of diabetic retinopathy. *Diabetes Care* 1990; **13**:34–40.

90 Diabetes Control and Complications Trial Research Group. Effect of pregnancy on microvascular complications in the diabetes control and complications trial. *Diabetes Care* 2000; **23**:1084–1091.

91 Chew EY, Mills JL, Metzger BE, Remaley NA, Jovanovic-Peterson L, Knopp RH, *et al.* Metabolic control and progression of retinopathy. The Diabetes in Early Pregnancy Study. National Institute of Child Health and Human Development Diabetes in Early Pregnancy Study. *Diabetes Care* 1995; **18**:631–637.

92 Phelps RL, Sakol P, Metzger BE, Jampol LM, Freinkel N. Changes in diabetic retinopathy during pregnancy: correlations with regulation of hyperglycemia. *Arch Ophthalmol* 1986; **104**:1806–1810.

93 Rosenn B, Miodovnik M, Kranias G, Khoury J, Combs CA, Mimouni F, *et al.* Progression of diabetic retinopathy in pregnancy: association with hypertension in pregnancy. *Am J Obstet Gynecol* 1992; **166**:1214–1218.

94 Lauszus F, Klebe JG, Bek T. Diabetic retinopathy in pregnancy during tight metabolic control. *Acta Obstet Gynecol Scand* 2000; **79**:367–370.

95 Dibble CM, Kochenour NK, Worley RJ, Tyler FH, Swartz M. Effect of pregnancy on diabetic retinopathy. *Obstet Gynecol* 1982; **59**:699–704.

96 Temple RC, Aldridge VA, Sampson MJ, Greenwood RH, Heyburn PJ, Glenn A. Impact of pregnancy on the progression of diabetic retinopathy in type 1 diabetes. *Diabet Med* 2001; **18**:573–577.

97 Cunningham ET Jr. World blindness: no end in sight. *Br J Ophthalmol* 2001; **85**:253.

98 Evans J. *Causes of Blindness and Partial Sight in England and Wales 1990–1991*. London: OPCS, 1995: 1–29.

99 Bunce C, Wormald R. Leading causes of certification for blindness and partial sight in England & Wales. *BMC Public Health* 2006; **6**:58.

100 Fong DS, Aiello LP, Ferris FL 3rd, Klein R. Diabetic retinopathy. *Diabetes Care* 2004; **27**:2540–2553.

37 Diabetic Nephropathy

Sally M. Marshall[1] & Allan Flyvbjerg[2]

[1] Diabetes Research Group, Institute of Cellular Medicine, Newcastle University, Newcastle upon Tyne, UK
[2] Department of Endocrinology and Internal Medicine, Aarhus University Hospital – Aarhus University, Aarhus, Denmark

Keypoints

- Diabetic nephropathy is characterized by gradually increasing urine albumin excretion (UAE) over many years, accompanied by slowly rising blood pressure (BP); the decline in glomerular filtration rate (GFR) occurs late.
- Individuals with nephropathy are at greatly increased risk of other microvascular and macrovascular complications of diabetes.
- The risk of cardiovascular disease increases as UAE increases and as GFR decreases.
- Approximately 30–50% of Caucasian people with diabetes will develop microalbuminuria; the prevalence is higher in non-Caucasians.
- One-third of people with diabetes will progress to proteinuria and be at high risk of end-stage renal disease (ESRD).
- Factors most closely associated with progression of nephropathy are poor glucose and BP control, and baseline UAE.
- Screening for diabetic nephropathy should be performed annually, by measuring urine albumin : creatinine ratio and estimated GFR (eGFR).
- Good blood glucose and BP control are key to prevention of nephropathy.
- If UAE is raised, an inhibitor of the renin angiotensin system should be commenced and titrated up to the maximum tolerated dose.
- Maintaining BP <125/75 mmHg will reduce the rate of decline of GFR from 10–12 to 3–5 mL/min/1.73 m^2.
- Reducing dietary protein intake to 0.7–1.0 g/kg body weight per day may slow the deterioration in renal function.
- Aggressive management of other cardiovascular risk factors and prescription of aspirin reduces the incidence of cardiovascular events and of progression to nephropathy by around 60%.
- Renal failure from diabetes is the most common single cause of entry to renal replacement programs worldwide; the majority of patients have type 2 diabetes plus major co-morbidities.
- Patients with ESRD and significant co-morbidities should be offered dialysis. Fitter patients benefit from kidney or kidney–pancreas transplantation, but need full cardiovascular assessment and treatment before transplantation if necessary.

Introduction

Diabetic nephropathy remains an important common complication of diabetes. End-stage renal disease (ESRD) is devastating to the individual and of enormous financial and social consequences to society. In 2006, the proportion of individuals with diabetes beginning renal replacement therapy (RRT) was 20–44% in most countries reporting to the US Renal Disease Registry [1]. The number of people with diabetes requiring RRT in the USA increased 50% between 1996 and 2006. The increasing numbers are accounted for primarily by individuals with type 2 diabetes mellitus (T2DM), often with severe co-morbidities [2]. A European report covering 1998–2002 demonstrated a 9.9% per year increase in the numbers of Europid patients with T2DM beginning RRT, with no change in non-Europid populations [3]. ESRD caused by T2DM currently is uncommon before age 45 years, although the annual increase in patients with diabetes beginning RRT may be greatest in this age group [4]. The numbers of patients with type 1 diabetes mellitus (T1DM) entering RRT has not changed dramatically over the same time [2,3].

Textbook of Diabetes, 4th edition. Edited by R. Holt, C. Cockram, A. Flyvbjerg and B. Goldstein.

Definitions

Classic diabetic nephropathy is a chronic condition developing over many years, characterized by gradually increasing urinary albumin excretion (UAE) and blood pressure (BP). Declining glomerular filtration rate (GFR) is a relatively late event. As nephropathy progresses, the risk of other chronic complications of diabetes increases, so that if other complications of diabetes are absent, an alternative cause of the renal disease should be considered. In particular, the risk of cardiovascular disease (CVD) increases dramatically as renal disease progresses.

Kidney disease is staged on the basis of both the level of UAE and GFR. In diabetic nephropathy, UAE increases gradually from

Table 37.1 Definitions of normal urinary albumin excretion (UAE), microalbuminuria and proteinuria.

	Normal UAE	Microalbuminuria	Proteinuria
Albumin : creatinine ratio (mg/mmol)	<3.5 (female) <2.5 (male)	3.5–30.0 (female) 2.5–30.0 (male)	>30
Timed overnight urine albumin excretion rate (μg/min)	<20	20–200	>200
24-hour urine collection (mg/24 h)	<30	30–300	>300

Table 37.2 Staging of chronic kidney disease on the basis of estimated glomerular filtration rate (eGFR) and urine albumin excretion (UAE).

Stage	eGFR description	UAE
Normal	GFR >90 mL/min/1.73 m²	Normal
1	GFR >90 mL/min/1.73 m² with other evidence of kidney disease*	Normal / micro / proteinuria
2	Mild impairment; GFR 60–90 mL/min/1.73 m² with other evidence of kidney disease*	Normal / micro / proteinuria
3a	Moderate impairment; GFR 45–59 mL/min/1.73 m²	Normal / micro / proteinuria
3b	Moderate impairment; GFR 30–44 mL/min/1.73 m²	Normal / micro / proteinuria
4	Severe impairment; GFR 15–29 mL/min/1.73 m²	Normal / micro / proteinuria
5	Established renal failure; GFR <15 mL/min/1.73 m² or on dialysis	Normal / micro / proteinuria

*Other evidence of kidney disease may be: microalbuminuria, persistent proteinuria, persistent hematuria after exclusion of all other causes, structural abnormalities of the kidney demonstrated on ultrasound, or biopsy-proven glomerular nephritis.

normal, through microalbuminuria to proteinuria. Consensus definitions of normal UAE, microalbuminuria and proteinuria are given in Table 37.1.

Serum creatinine is a relatively poor reflection of GFR, but more precise direct measures of GFR are inappropriate in routine clinical practice. Calculation of an "estimated" GFR (eGFR) is now recommended, using the four variable Modification of Diet in Renal Disease study equations [5]. The agreed staging of chronic kidney disease (CKD) on the basis of the eGFR and UAE is shown in Table 37.2.

Natural history

The development of diabetic nephropathy generally takes at least 20 years. Gradually increasing UAE is the hallmark (Figure 37.1).

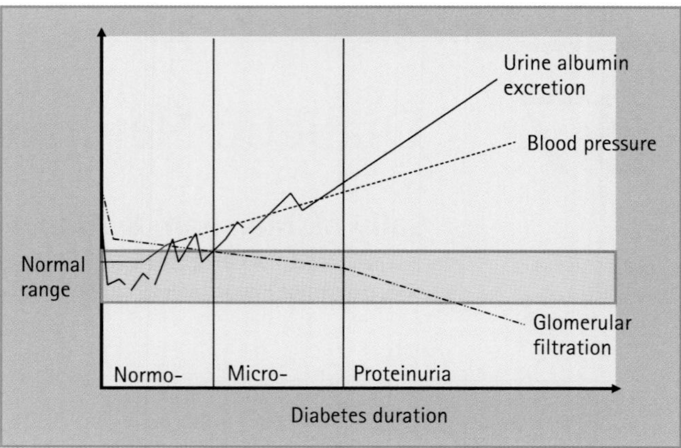

Figure 37.1 Development of diabetic nephropathy. Micro-, microalbuminuria; Normo-, normal urine albumin excretion.

Type 1 diabetes

During the acute presentation of T1DM, UAE and GFR may both be increased above normal. With insulin therapy, UAE returns to normal in most if not all individuals. GFR also returns to normal in the majority, but remains above normal in 25–40%. The implications of this have long been debated. A recent meta-analysis of 10 cohort studies concluded that individuals with persistently elevated GFR were at increased risk of progression to diabetic nephropathy [6].

In those patients who will never develop nephropathy, UAE remains normal, except during periods of particularly poor glucose control, or during acute intercurrent illness, when a transient increase in UAE may occur. In those who will develop diabetic nephropathy, UAE increases gradually, with microalbuminuria usually appearing within 5–15 years of diabetes. Untreated, the mean increase in UAE is 20% per year. Patients may go through a phase of "transient microalbuminuria" as they approach the cut-off, when sequential samples may vary from normal to microalbuminuria, but eventually they become persistently microalbuminuric. In patients with normal UAE, approximately 1.5–2.5% per year develop microalbuminuria [7,8], and 50% develop persistent microalbuminuria at some point in their life [9–11]. One recent study reported an estimated cumulative incidence of microalbuminuria of 25.4% after 40 years of diabetes, suggesting that the incidence of microalbuminuria may be falling [12]. Approximately one-third of patients with T1DM microalbuminuria will progress gradually over a further 5–15 years to proteinuria, one-third will remain microalbuminuric and one-third will revert to normal UAE (Figure 37.2) [13–15]. In the short term, reversion from microalbuminuria to normal UAE may be even more common, one study reporting regression in 58% of patients over 6 years [16]. Short-duration microalbuminuria, and lower HbA_{1c}, systolic BP, total cholesterol and triglycerides were all independently associated with regression. The eventual outcome in those who regress, or who do not initially progress, remains unclear; however, they probably remain

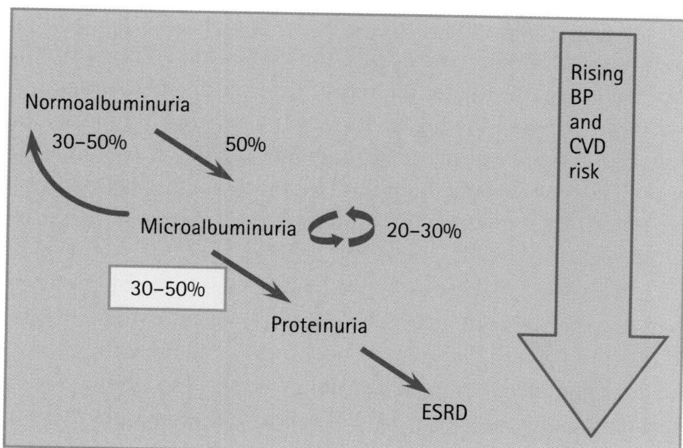

Figure 37.2 Progression of albuminuria in type 1 diabetes mellitus (T1DM). Approximately 50% of individuals with T1DM will develop microalbuminuria at some time. Of these, around one-third will regress to normal urinary albumin excretion (UAE), at least temporarily, one-third will remain microalbuminuric and one-third will progress to proteinuria. Once proteinuria is present, progression to end-stage renal disease (ESRD) is usually inevitable. BP, blood pressure; CVD, cardiovascular disease. Reproduced from Marshall SM, Flyvbjerg A. Prevention and early detection of vascular complications of diabetes. *Br Med J* 2006; **333**:475–480, with permission.

at increased risk of nephropathy compared to individuals who have never had microalbuminuria.

Older data suggest that the cumulative incidence of proteinuria is around 40%, but in several Scandinavian studies, the cumulative incidence has fallen in individuals diagnosed after 1970 to around 10–14% after 20–25 years' duration [17,18]. In the Pittsburgh cohort, the incidence has remained relatively steady at 32% after 25 years [19]. Almost all patients with T1DM with proteinuria eventually progress to ESRD, if untreated in a mean time of 9 years. GFR is generally relatively stable in microalbuminuria but begins to fall when proteinuria develops, with a mean annual rate of decline in GFR of 10–12 mL/min/1.73 m^2 in a patient without good BP control. Low eGFR occurs very rarely without preceding microalbuminuria in patients with T1DM [20].

Several countries report a declining incidence of ESRD in T1DM. In Sweden, at a maximum duration of diabetes of 27 years (mean 21 years), only 33 of 12 032 cases with childhood-onset diabetes had developed ESRD, all with diabetes duration >15 years [21]. With diabetes duration >15 years, the cumulative incidence of ESRD was 0.7%. Data from the Pittsburgh Epidemiology of Diabetes Complications Study also suggests a declining incidence, but after 30 years' duration, the cumulative incidence remained higher at 18% in those diagnosed 1965–1969 [19]. Analyses of data combined from several individual registries confirms that between 1991 and 2000, the numbers of people with T1DM entering RRT has either remained static [2] or even decreased slightly [3], at a time when the incidence of T1DM is rising. Survival once ESRD has developed may also have improved [22,23].

Thus, the incidence of all stages of diabetic nephropathy may be declining, at least in some centers. Whether this represents true prevention, or perhaps more likely delay in progression, remains to be seen.

Type 2 diabetes

Classic diabetic nephropathy

The natural history of nephropathy in T2DM is not unlike that of T1DM, with some notable exceptions. At diagnosis, UAE may be raised but with good glycemic control generally returns to normal; however, in 10–48% microalbuminuria persists [24,25]. Those with persistently raised UAE probably have had diabetes for some time before diagnosis, and have established kidney changes. The reported prevalence of hyperfiltration at diagnosis of T2DM varies between studies, reflecting diabetes undiagnosed for some time and the presence of co-morbidities including pre-existing hypertension.

Longitudinal studies in the Pima Indians show that GFR is generally increased in subjects with impaired glucose tolerance (IGT) who later progress to frank diabetes [26]. In one study, 16% of newly diagnosed patients had hyperfiltration [27]. After 6 months' treatment, GFR fell significantly only in those with GFR initially >120 mL/min [28]. GFR remains stable with the onset of microalbuminuria, only beginning to decline when proteinuria develops [26,29]. No relationship of hyperfiltration at diagnosis to subsequent nephropathy has been found.

In cross-sectional studies in established diabetes, the prevalence of microalbuminuria is 10–42%, depending on population selection [30–36]. Higher prevalences are reported in UK Asians [31], Pima Indians [35], African-Americans [37] and in Maori and Pacific Islanders [33] than Europid patients. The relationship of microalbuminuria to duration of T2DM is not as strong as in T1DM. Many longitudinal studies suggest that the rate of progression from normal UAE to microalbuminuria is 3–4% per annum which is at least as high as, if not higher than, in T1DM [35,38–41].

In Caucasian populations, approximately 7% of microalbuminuric patients with T2DM develop proteinuria per year [42–44]. In an older study, after 20 years' duration of T2DM, the cumulative incidence of proteinuria was 27%, similar to that in T1DM [45]. In the Pima Indians, more than 50% develop proteinuria within 20 years [26]. In contrast to the decline in the cumulative incidence of proteinuria in T1DM, the incidence has doubled in Pima Indians in the last 40 years [46], despite improvements in glucose and BP control and probably as a consequence of increasing survival and therefore duration of diabetes [47].

Once proteinuria develops, the untreated rate of decline of GFR is similar to that in T1DM at 10–12 mL/min/1.73 m^2 [45,48], although it may be greater in non-Europid subjects [49]. Rates for acceptance on to RRT are higher in African-Caribbean and Indo-Asian than Europid people with diabetes [50–52]. In the Pima Indians, the age- and sex-adjusted incidence of ESRD has declined since 1990, suggesting slowing of progression [47].

Overall, the course of nephropathy in Europid T2DM is similar to that in T1DM, the differences probably relating to delayed diagnosis, older age and more CVD of the subjects with T2DM. In the ethnic minorities, the prevalence of nephropathy is higher, and progression to ESRD may be faster.

Non-classic diabetic nephropathy

One-third of Europid patients with T2DM with raised UAE do not have classic histologic changes of diabetic glomerulosclerosis; arterial hyalinization is the most common abnormality. Conversely, some patients with T2DM with a progressive decline in GFR have normal albumin excretion or only low levels of microalbuminuria which do not progress. In the UK Prospective Diabetes Study (UKPDS), 51% of those who developed renal impairment did not have preceding albuminuria [53]. Identification of patients with non-diabetic changes on the basis of clinical features, including the absence of diabetic retinopathy [54,55], is difficult. The underlying disease process probably reflects a combination of diabetes, hypertension and atherosclerotic vascular disease, or a specific obesity-related glomerulopathy [56].

Risk factors for diabetic nephropathy

Diabetes duration is one of the strongest risk factors for nephropathy, along with glycemic control, BP and blood lipid levels (Figure 37.3) [12]. "White coat" hypertension, reflecting higher 24-hour BP, doubles the risk of proteinuria [57] and, in young people, microalbuminuria is associated with higher nocturnal diastolic BP and loss of diastolic dipping [58]. Although blood lipids contribute to the development and progression of nephropathy, the lipid phenotype alters as nephropathy progresses [59,60]. Current smoking also predicts the development of albuminuria [61].

Both patients with T1DM and T2DM with nephropathy are more likely to have the metabolic syndrome [62–65].

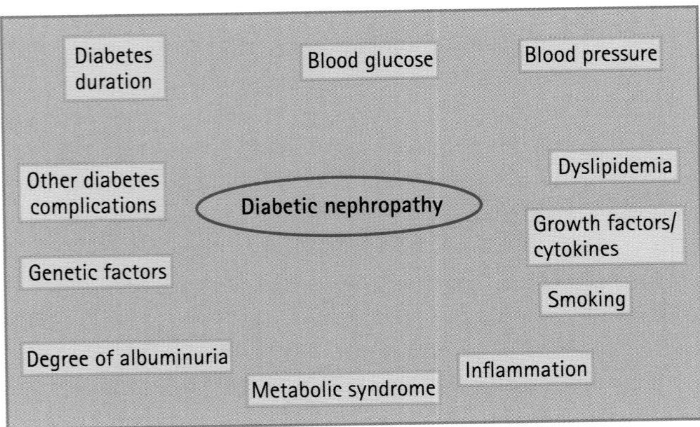

Figure 37.3 Factors associated with the development and/or progression of diabetic nephropathy.

The degree of albuminuria is also an independent predictor at each stage of nephropathy; thus, the higher the UAE within the normal range, the higher the risk of developing microalbuminuria [66]. Likewise, the higher the level of microalbuminuria, the higher the risk of developing proteinuria. Baseline albuminuria was the strongest predictor of ESRD in the Reduction of Endpoints in NIDDM with the Angiotensin II Antagonist Losartan (RENAAL) study [67].

Several lines of evidence suggest a genetic susceptibility to diabetic nephropathy in T1DM, as only 40% of patients are at risk. If one sibling with diabetes has nephropathy, the risk to a second sibling is increased four- to eightfold compared to siblings where neither has nephropathy [68]. The clustering of conventional cardiovascular risk factors and CVD in patients with diabetes and nephropathy also occurs in their parents [69]. This suggests that the genetic susceptibility to nephropathy also influences the development of CVD. Multiple genes are likely to be involved and different loci may influence UAE and GFR separately [70]. Many candidate genes suggested in small studies have not been confirmed in adequately powered cohorts.

Other possible risk factors for nephropathy include pre-eclampsia, but not pregnancy-induced hypertension [71], inflammatory markers [72], cytokines and growth factors [73] and periodontitis [74]. High levels of mannose-binding lectin (MBL) predict progression from normoalbuminuria to micro- and/or macro-albuminuria in T1DM and T2DM [75,76]. In patients with T1DM, higher baseline levels of the bone-related peptide osteoprotegerin (OPG) [77] predicted higher risk of progression to ESRD. Patients with T2DM and non-alcoholic fatty liver disease are more likely to have CKD [78].

Association of diabetic nephropathy with other complications of diabetes

The prognosis for diabetic patients with any degree of diabetic nephropathy is much poorer than for individuals without nephropathy. The risk of CVD and of other microvascular complications is greatly increased. Indeed, diabetic nephropathy may be a vascular disease [79].

Cardiovascular disease

In T1DM, the relative risk of CVD is 1.2-fold in microalbuminuric [80,81] and 10-fold higher in proteinuric than normoalbuminuric patients (Figure 37.4) [82,83]. The cumulative incidence of CVD by the age of 40 years is 43% in patients with T1DM with diabetic nephropathy, compared to 7% in patients without diabetic nephropathy, with a 10-fold increased risk of coronary heart disease and stroke. In ESRD the risk is even higher.

In T2DM, with microalbuminuria, the risk is increased two- to fourfold [84] and with proteinuria ninefold [85]. Once serum creatinine is outwith the normal range, cardiovascular risk increases exponentially [86,87]. Survival with ESRD is very limited: 20–25% of individuals with T2DM die in the first year of dialysis, and almost all are dead within 4–5 years.

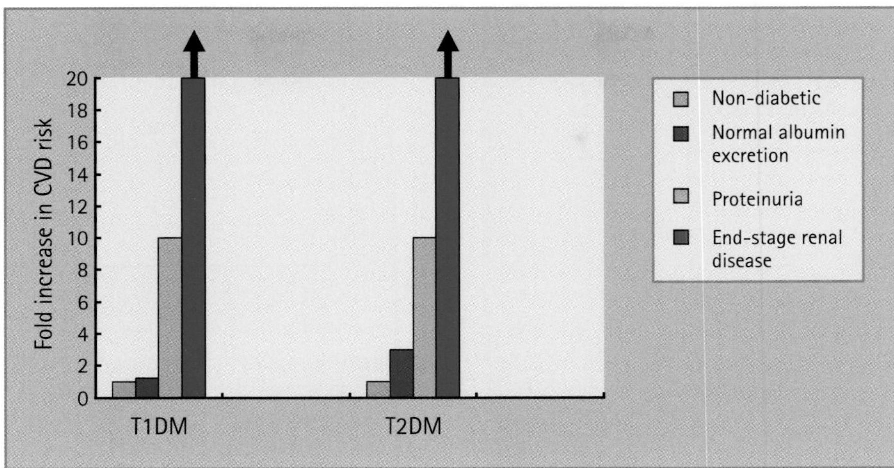

Figure 37.4 Increasing cardiovascular risk with the development of nephropathy in type 1 diabetes mellitus (T1DM) and type 2 diabetes mellitus (T2DM). Compared with normoalbuminuric individuals with T1DM, cardiovascular disease (CVD) risk is increased 1.2-fold in microalbuminuria, 10-fold in proteinuria and at least 20-fold in patients with T1DM with declining glomerular filtration rate (GFR). In T2DM, the risk is increased 2-4 fold in microalbuminuria, 10-fold in proteinuria and at least 20-fold in those with declining GFR.

In both T1DM and T2DM, all-cause and cardiovascular mortality increases as eGFR decreases [88]. UAE and declining GFR may have independent effects [89–91].

Hypertension

Hypertension is an invariable accompaniment of persistent proteinuria and ESRD. The excess prevalence of hypertension in T1DM is confined to patients with nephropathy, individuals with normal UAE having a prevalence of hypertension similar to the non-diabetic population [92]. This suggests that hypertension is an integral part of diabetic nephropathy, perhaps arising from the same underlying mechanisms. In support of this, BP rises very early in the development of nephropathy. Accordingly, patients with UAE in the high normal range, who are at increased risk of progression to microalbuminuria, have a higher BP than those with lower UAE [7,93]. Changes in BP are very subtle at this stage and may only be documented on 24-hour BP monitoring, perhaps as reduced dipping in nocturnal diastolic BP [94].

In most cross-sectional studies, patients with T1DM with microalbuminuria have higher BP than those with normal UAE, although the levels may not meet a formal definition of hypertension. Once proteinuria is present, untreated BP is >140/90 mmHg in over 80% of patients, and in ESRD hypertension is almost universal.

In T2DM, because hypertension is common, the link between hypertension and renal disease is less striking; however, almost all patients with microalbuminuria or more severe renal disease have hypertension, and the more severe the renal disease, the higher the BP.

Other microvascular complications

Patients with nephropathy are also much more likely to have other microvascular complications. Indeed, the absence of other microvascular disease should make one question the diagnosis of diabetic nephropathy as the cause for the renal disease. Significant retinopathy is almost invariably present in patients with T1DM with microalbuminuria or more severe renal disease. In patients with T2DM, the relationship is less clear-cut. Those with classic nephropathy and progressively increasing UAE usually have significant retinopathy. In those with non-classic disease, with non-progressive low levels of microalbuminuria, retinopathy may be absent.

Peripheral neuropathy is also more common in patients with diabetes and renal disease, associating with both albuminuria and declining GFR [95]. Autonomic neuropathy, perhaps relating to loss of nocturnal BP dipping, occurs frequently [96,97].

Testing for kidney disease in diabetes

Screening

Early identification of CKD in people with diabetes allows intensification of therapy to slow the progression of the kidney disease and to manage the increased risk of other complications, particularly CVD. All guidelines suggest systematic screening, generally as part of the "annual review." Both UAE and GFR should be measured, as the combination improves prediction of ESRD [98]. Screening should be undertaken when the person is free of acute illness and in stable glucose control, because many acute illnesses and acute hyperglycemia increase UAE temporarily.

As UAE may increase in the upright posture and with exercise, measurements are best made in an early morning urine sample; however, a spot urine sample can be used if there is no alternative. Timed overnight or 24-hour urine collections are only required for research purposes. A plan for screening is shown in Figure 37.5. Urine albumin is stable at room temperature; the patient

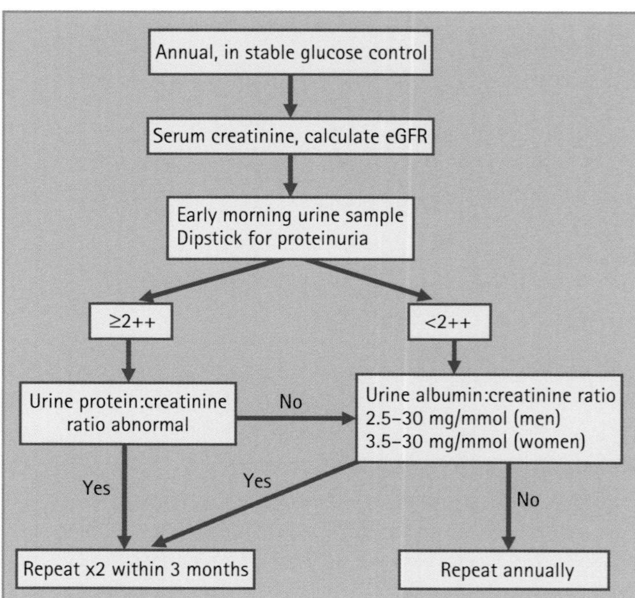

Figure 37.5 A suggested plan for annual screening for kidney disease in diabetes. eGFR, estimated glomerular filtration rate. Adapted from Marshall SM, Flyvbjerg A. Prevention and early detection of vascular complications of diabetes. *Br Med J* 2006; **333**:475–480.

can collect two or three early morning urine samples on consecutive days and return them all at the same time. Because of the high day-to-day variation in UAE, at least two out of three measurements should be abnormal before a diagnosis of microalbuminuria or proteinuria is made.

Serum creatinine should also be measured annually, using an accredited assay standardized to the recommended isotope dilution mass spectroscopy reference method. Using the four variable Modification of Diet in Renal Disease equations, which adjust for age, sex and ethnicity, eGFR is calculated from the serum creatinine [99]. Although the validity of this equation in diabetes has been debated, there is general agreement that it provides information that is more reliable than serum creatinine and is sufficiently accurate for clinical use when eGFR is $<60\,\mathrm{mL/min/1.73\,m^2}$ [100–103]; however, the equation underestimates the rate of change of GFR at higher levels and is not a good indicator of hyperfiltration [104,105].

The final screening stage should indicate both the GFR and UAE status, as in Table 37.2. For example, stage 3 CKD with proteinuria or stage 2 CKD with microalbuminuria.

Serum cystatin C has been suggested as an alternative to creatinine. Cystatin C is a naturally circulating protein that is freely filtered by the glomerulus and almost completely reabsorbed and catabolized by tubular cells. Although levels reflect trends in GFR $<40\,\mathrm{mL/min/1.73\,m^2}$, there is doubt about its ability to detect changes in GFR before the serum creatinine has risen [105–108]. Thus, it seems premature to use cystatin C as a marker of GFR.

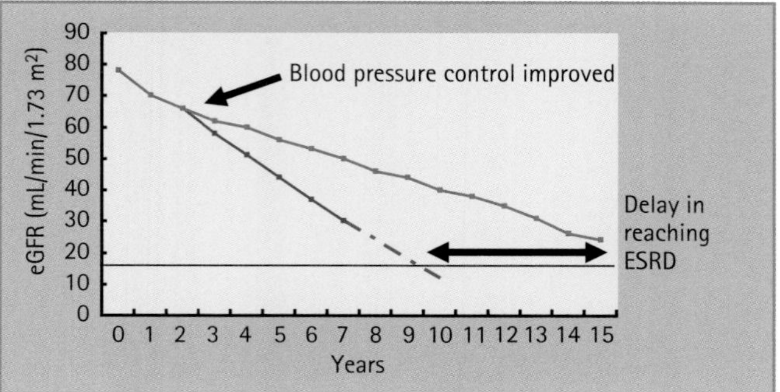

Figure 37.6 Monitoring changes in estimated glomerular filtration rate (eGFR). Solid black line: end-stage renal disease (ESRD). Blue line: actual linear decline in eGFR of $5–6\,\mathrm{mL/min/1.73\,m^2}$ in an individual with modest blood pressure (BP) control. Green dotted line: estimated further fall in eGFR in the same individual in the blue line, showing that they will reach ESRD in 9–10 years. Red line: fall in eGFR in an individual whose BP control was tightened between years 2 and 3. The rate of decline of eGFR is reduced, delaying ESRD by at least 5 years (illustrated by thick, black, double-ended arrow).

Excluding other treatable causes of kidney disease

It is uncommon to find a specific treatable cause of CKD if the natural history is classic, with slowly progressive rise in albuminuria and BP in the presence of retinopathy; however, if there is doubt, ultrasound of the renal tract and measurement of autoantibodies and immunoglobulins may help. If the diagnosis remains unclear, referral to a nephrologist is appropriate.

Monitoring kidney disease

Once abnormal UAE has been detected, the albumin : creatinine ratio should be measured every 3 months, preferably on the three consecutive mornings before the clinic visit. This provides sufficient information to identify true changes in UAE with time, as opposed to day-to-day variation. Serum creatinine and eGFR should also be measured 3–6 monthly. Once renal function begins to decline, there is a linear relationship between eGFR, or the inverse of the serum creatinine, which is useful in assessing changes in rate of decline of GFR in response to therapy and to estimate when an individual will reach ESRD (Figure 37.6).

Prevention of kidney disease

Prevention of kidney disease is crucial (Table 37.3). Although much can be done to slow progression when UAE is raised or GFR has begun to decline, it may not be possible to avoid ESRD. The risk of developing diabetic nephropathy is greatly reduced by good blood glucose control. In T2DM, BP control is also crucial. Studies have generally used the development of microalbuminuria as their primary endpoint, with data on preservation of GFR being limited.

Table 37.3 Factors important in prevention of nephropathy in T1DM and T2DM.

	T1DM	T2DM
Blood glucose control	Yes	Yes
Hypertension	Probably	Yes
RAS inhibition in "normotension"	No	Yes
Dyslipidemia treatment	Possibly	Possibly
Smoking cessation	Possibly	Possibly

RAS, renin angiotensin system.

Prevention in type 1 diabetes

Glucose control

In initially normoalbuminuric patients in the Diabetes Control and Complications Trial (DCCT), the relative risk reduction for development of microalbuminuria was 39% and for proteinuria 54% in those allocated to the intensively treated group compared to those in the conventionally managed group over the 6.5-year study [109]. Mean achieved HbA_{1c} was approximately 7.0% (53 mmol/mol) and 9.1% (76 mmol/mol), respectively. There is no HbA_{1c} threshold below which risk is not reduced, implying that the lower the HbA_{1c}, the lower the risk of nephropathy [110]. Thus, any reduction in HbA_{1c} is beneficial.

In the open follow-up of the DCCT cohort, the Epidemiology of Diabetes Interventions and Complications (EDIC) study, the difference in HbA_{1c} between the previously intensively and conventionally managed groups narrowed over 4 years of follow-up to a mean of 7.9% (63 mmol/mol) and 8.2% (66 mmol/mol), respectively [111]. Despite this, after 8 years, 6.8% in the intensively treated group and 15.8% in the conventionally treated group had developed new microalbuminuria, a 59% reduction in odds [112]. The 84% reduction in new proteinuria was even more impressive: 1.4 vs 9.4%. In addition, fewer participants in the intensive group developed hypertension (29.9 vs 40.3%) and serum creatinine >176 µmol/L (5 vs 19 patients; $P = 0.004$). Thus, the beneficial renal effects of intensive glucose therapy extend far beyond the actual period of good control, a phenomenon termed "metabolic memory."

Blood pressure control

No trials have specifically addressed the question of whether improved control of hypertension in patients with T1DM reduces the risk of renal disease, but given the weight of evidence in the general population, this would seem likely. Two trials have explored the effects of renin angiotensin system (RAS) inhibitors in patients with T1DM with normal UAE and BP [113,114]. In the Eurodiab Controlled Trial of Lisinopril in Insulin-Dependent Diabetes Mellitus (EUCLID) study, patients with T1DM receiving lisinopril for 2 years had significantly lower UAE than those receiving placebo [113]; however, the clinical relevance of the small difference (1 µg/min) is questionable. In the The DIabetic REtinopathy Candesartan Trials (DIRECT) study, candesartan 32 mg/day for 4.7 years did not prevent microalbuminuria [114]. Thus, there is no evidence that in normotensive patients with T1DM, prescription of agents that block the RAS prevents the onset of microalbuminuria.

Prevention in type 2 diabetes

Glucose control

In the UKPDS, although the mean achieved HbA_{1c} in the intensively managed group was 7.0% (53 mmol/mol), compared to 7.9% (63 mmol/mol) in the less strictly managed group, there was a reduction in the relative risk of developing microalbuminuria and proteinuria of approximately 30% after 9–12 years [115]. Different glucose lowering therapies had similar effects, although the UKPDS was not powered to detect small differences between therapies. As in the DCCT, no threshold of HbA_{1c} and risk was observed, again suggesting that the lower the HbA_{1c}, the lower the risk of nephropathy. For a 1% (11 mmol/mol) reduction in HbA_{1c}, there was a 37% reduction in the risk of microvascular complications [116]. In the open follow-up of the UKPDS cohort, HbA_{1c} was similar in the previously intensively and conventionally managed groups after 1 year [117]. Despite this, microvascular risk remained lower, confirming the "metabolic memory" seen in the DCCT/EDIC study.

In the Action in Diabetes and Vascular Disease: Preterax and Diamicron MR Controlled Evaluation (ADVANCE) study, intensive therapy was based on modified release gliclazide, with other agents added if the target HbA_{1c} of 6.5% (48 mmol/mol) was not reached [118]. The lower HbA_{1c} in the intensive group (6.5% [48 mmol/mol] compared to 7.3% [56 mmol/mol] in the standard group) was associated with a 9% relative risk reduction in new onset microalbuminuria over 5 years.

Blood pressure control

Control of hypertension reduces the risk of developing microalbuminuria. In the UKPDS [119], tight BP control (achieved mean 144/82 mmHg) compared to less tight control (achieved mean 154/87 mmHg) resulted in a 29% reduction in risk of microalbuminuria over 6 years. There is no BP level below which risk rises again (i.e. no "J" shape) [120]. Treatment with captopril and atenolol was equally effective, although the study was not powered to detect differences between treatment modalities [121]. In the subset of normoalbuminuric patients with diabetes in the Heart Outcomes Prevention Evaluation (HOPE) study [122], addition of ramipril to background antihypertensive therapy reduced the risk of developing proteinuria, compared to the addition of placebo. In the Bergamo Nephrologic Diabetes Complications Trial (BENEDICT) study, hypertensive (BP > 130/85 mmHg), but normoalbuminuric patients with T2DM receiving trandolapril alone or in combination with verapamil were approximately 50% less likely to develop microalbuminuria than subjects taking verapamil alone or placebo [41]. In the ADVANCE trial, there was a significant 17% reduction in the incidence of microalbuminuria in those receiving perindopril indapamide [123]. Thus, there may be a particular benefit of RAS inhibition in prevention of nephropathy, as seen in a meta-analysis [124].

Overall, there is no doubt that tight BP control (achieved BP of approximately 140/80 mmHg) reduces the risk of microalbuminuria in T2DM. First-line therapy with RAS inhibitors may be most effective, but lowering BP sufficiently is more important than the type of first line agent used. Many guidelines now suggest a BP target of 130/80 mmHg for people with T2DM, based on the evidence around prevention of CVD events and not on renal outcomes; of note, achieved BP in the specific renal studies has been around 140/80 mmHg.

In contrast to the "metabolic memory" demonstrated with glucose control, the benefits of BP reduction are lost when BP control deteriorates [125]. Tight BP control must be continued long-term if the benefits are to be maintained.

Management of diabetic kidney disease

Rigorous intervention, particularly to control BP tightly, can alter the gloomy prognosis in diabetic nephropathy (Table 37.4). Conservative estimates suggest that good management can double the time taken from first appearance of proteinuria to need for RRT, from a mean of 9 years to a mean of 18 years. More optimistically, improved management of microalbuminuria may prevent progression to proteinuria.

Type 1 diabetes

Glucose control

Once UAE is abnormal, there is little evidence that tight blood glucose control influences progression. The studies that have been performed were all small, of short duration or did not achieve sufficiently tight glucose control [13,14,126–128]. In a highly selected group of patients undergoing serial renal biopsies after pancreas transplantation, renal structural changes regressed [129], but only after 10 years. Thus, very prolonged periods of extremely good control may be necessary to reverse renal structural changes, indicated by microalbuminuria or proteinuria.

Table 37.4 Factors important in delaying progression of nephropathy in T1DM and T2DM.

Factor	Target
Glucose control	HbA_{1c} as low as possible without undue hypoglycemia
RAS inhibition	For all, unless absolutely contraindicated
Blood pressure	As low as possible; <125/75 mmHg if proteinuric or eGFR <60 mL/min/1.73 m^2; others <130/80 mmHg
Lipids	Statin for all; additional therapy if total cholesterol >4.0 mmol/L or LDL cholesterol >2.0 mmol/L or triglycerides >2.1 mmol/L
Aspirin	75 mg/day for all
Smoking	Stop
Weight	BMI <25.0 kg/m^2
Dietary protein intake	If proteinuria: 6-month trial of reduction to 0.9 g/kg body weight per day

BMI, body mass index; eGFR, estimated glomerular filtration rate; LDL, low density lipoprotein; RAS, renin angiotensin system.

Inhibition of the RAS in microalbuminuria and proteinuria

A meta-analysis of 12 studies (698 individuals) summarized the effects of treatment with angiotensin-converting enzyme (ACE) inhibitors in microalbuminuric patients with T1DM [130]. The odds ratio of progression to persistent proteinuria was reduced by ACE inhibition to 0.35, and the odds ratio for regression to normal UAE increased to 3.07, compared to placebo treatment. After 2 years' treatment, the mean reduction in UAE was 50.5% with ACE inhibition. The reduction in UAE was greatest in those with highest baseline UAE, but the response to treatment plateaued with time, suggesting that treatment delays, rather than prevents, progression.

Addition of an ACE inhibitor to non-ACE inhibitor antihypertensive therapy reduced the risk of a doubling of the serum creatinine by 48% and the composite endpoint of death, need for dialysis or renal transplantation by 50%, in patients with T1DM with proteinuria and hypertension [131]. Both benefits were independent of BP. In short-term studies, the effects of angiotensin II receptor blockers (ARBs) on BP and UAE are similar to those of ACE inhibitors in proteinuric patients with T1DM [132].

For a similar reduction in BP, there is a greater reduction in protein excretion using ACE inhibitors compared with other classes of antihypertensive agents [133]. This may be especially beneficial, as the passage of protein across the glomerular filtration barrier may accelerate the progression of nephropathy [134].

On the basis of the above, and of animal data showing preferential reduction in intraglomerular pressure with ACE inhibitors [135], ACE inhibitors should be offered to all patients with T1DM with abnormal UAE, even if BP is normal. The dose should be titrated up to the maximum recommended or tolerated doses, to obtain maximal antiproteinuric effect.

Blood pressure control

Tight BP control is crucial in slowing the progression of diabetic kidney disease. GFR and renal structural variables remain relatively stable in proteinuric patients with T1DM who do not have hypertension [136,137]. Reduction of BP to <140/80 mmHg reduces the rate of decline of GFR from 10–12 mL/min/year untreated to <5 mL/min/year [138]. Regression from persistent proteinuria to microalbuminuria has been reported, with the fall in GFR reduced to <1 mL/min/year for a substantial time in a significant number of patients [139].

If BP remains >125/75 mmHg on maximum dose of ACE inhibitor or ARB, antihypertensive therapy should be intensified. The choice of agent should be made on an individual basis, as there is no evidence in T1DM that any one add-on agent is better than any other. In the short term, addition of an ARB to therapy with an ACE inhibitor gives further reduction in BP and UAE [140,141], in line with a systematic review of data in proteinuric patients generally [142]; however, there is no evidence of long-term benefit, and some concern about hyperkalemia [142]. Addition of spironolactone to other antihypertensive therapy, including RAS blockade, reduces UAE in the short term [143]. There are no good data on direct renin inhibition in T1DM.

Type 2 diabetes

Glucose control

There is some evidence that improved glucose control delays progression of microalbuminuria. In the ADVANCE study, a difference in HbA_{1c} of 6.5% (48 mmol/mol) vs 7.3% (56 mmol/mol) over 5 years was associated with a relative risk reduction in the development of proteinuria of 21% [118]. In a small study of Japanese patients with T2DM, with normal UAE or microalbuminuria at baseline, the proportion of patients with worsening of nephropathy (an increase of one or more steps in the three stages of normoalbuminuria, microalbuminuria and proteinuria), was significantly lower after 6–8 years of intensive glucose management [144,145].

Inhibition of RAS

As with T1DM, there is now good evidence in T2DM that inhibition of the RAS should be the backbone of therapy. In microalbuminuric patients with T2DM with BP > 135/85 mmHg, a large randomized controlled study compared the ARB irbesartan, 150 or 300 mg/day, with placebo [44]. Over 2 years, the proportion of patients developing persistent proteinuria was as follows: high dose irbesartan 5.2% (hazard ratio 0.30); low dose irbesartan 9.7% (hazard ratio 0.61) and placebo 14.9%. The proportion of patients becoming normoalbuminuric was 34%, 24% and 21%, respectively. A much smaller study in similar patients demonstrated that ACE inhibition reduces the rise in UAE and stabilized serum creatinine over 4 or 5 years [146,147]. Thirty-two percent of the patients with T2DM in the HOPE study had microalbuminuria [122]. There was a significant reduction in the risk of developing proteinuria in those receiving ramipril, independent of BP.

Two large studies of patients with T2DM with advanced nephropathy have been conducted [148,149]. In the RENAAL study [148], the effects of the ARB losartan were compared with placebo, in addition to conventional antihypertensive therapy. In the group taking losartan, 43.5% reached the primary outcome (doubling of serum creatinine, ESRD or death), compared to 47.1% in the control group, a 16% risk reduction. In the second study, another ARB, irbesartan, was compared with the calcium-channel blocking agent amlodipine and placebo, in addition to conventional antihypertensive therapy [149]. Treatment with irbesartan was associated with a 20% reduction in the primary endpoint (doubling of serum creatinine, ESRD or death) compared to placebo and 23% compared to amlodipine.

Direct comparisons of ACE inhibitors and ARBs in microalbuminuric patients with T2DM suggest no clinically important differences in renal outcomes [150–152]; however, even the largest of these was not powered to detect small differences [150]. Thus, as in T1DM, patients with T2DM with high UAE should be prescribed an RAS inhibitor, which should be titrated up to the maximum tolerated dose.

Blood pressure control

Most patients with T2DM with elevated UAE will require additional antihypertensive therapy. The guideline target BP in proteinuric patients of <125/75 mmHg is extremely difficult to reach. The choice of additional agents should be made on an individual basis, with diuretics and calcium-channel blockers often being appropriate. A direct renin inhibitor, aliskiren, added to 100 mg/day losartan in hypertensive patients with T2DM with nephropathy, reduced UAE by 20% compared to placebo, with no increase in adverse events [153]. Spironolactone, with or without background ACE inhibitor or ARB, reduces UAE and BP but may cause glycemic control to deteriorate [154,155].

Short-term studies have suggested greater reduction in BP and UAE when ACE inhibitors and ARBs are used in combination than when they are used separately [152]; however, in a study designed to assess CVD outcomes, and which included individuals with diabetes, combination therapy with an ACE inhibitor and ARB did not improve CVD outcomes, and was associated with more adverse events [156]. In particular, the incidences of renal dysfunction and renal failure were higher in those on combination therapy than those taking ACE inhibitor or ARB monotherapy. Thus, combination therapy is not advisable.

Low protein diet

A Cochrane meta-analysis concluded that reducing dietary protein intake non-significantly reduces progression to ESRD [157]. Questions about the level of protein intake required and compliance with diet were raised. Large variability between patients was seen, so that a 6-month trial of dietary restriction might be appropriate, with only those patients who respond continuing thereafter. Dietary protein intake should not be restricted to <0.7 g/kg body weight/day.

Cardiovascular risk: smoking, lipids, aspirin

The above measures, particularly RAS blockade and controlling BP, reduce both CVD and renal risk. There are no good trials of smoking cessation, lipid control and use of aspirin individually in diabetic kidney disease, but the Steno-2 study in patients with T2DM and microalbuminuria addressed all modifiable CVD risk factors aggressively [158,159]. Although the proportion of patients reaching these strict targets was disappointing low, there was a large reduction in the proportion of the intensively managed group having a CVD event. The risk of developing proteinuria was also reduced (relative risk 0.39 [0.17–0.87];

Table 37.5 The Steno-2 study. Aggressive multifactorial management in patients with T2DM and microalbuminuria. Outcomes after 7.8 years of intensive or conventional management, plus 5.5 years observational follow-up.

Event	Intensive group	Conventional group
Proteinuria	20	37
Dialysis	1	6
Laser therapy	14	27
All deaths	24	40
CVD deaths	9	19
CVD events	42	139

CVD, cardiovascular disease. Figures are number of patients.

P = 0.003), as was the risk of retinopathy and autonomic neuropathy.

After the 8-year randomized trial, participants were followed observationally for a further 5.5 years [160]. Twenty four patients in the initially intensively managed group died, compared to 40 in the conventional therapy group (hazard ratio 0.54 [0.32–0.89]; P = 0.02). The risk of cardiovascular death and of cardiovascular events was significantly lower in the intensively treated group. One patient in the intensive group compared to six in the conventional group developed ESRD. Thus, intensive intervention with lifestyle modification and multiple drug combinations had sustained beneficial effects on both cardiovascular and renal outcomes (Table 37.5).

Management of chronic kidney disease stage 3 or poorer

Monitoring renal function

Serum creatinine, eGFR and UAE should be measured every 3 months, and more often if clinically indicated. In progressive CKD from stage 3 onwards, bone chemistry, full blood count and iron stores should be assessed 3–6 monthly.

Monitoring glucose control

Red blood cell turnover is abnormal in CKD, so that HbA_{1c} results may be misleading. One uncontrolled study suggested HbA_{1c} values fell by approximately 1% (11 mmol/mol) when hemoglobin rose from 10.6 to 11.8 g/dL with treatment with erythropoietin [161]. Thus, more reliance should be placed on self-monitoring of blood glucose and continuous glucose monitoring. As albumin turnover is also abnormal, interpretation of fructosamine is difficult.

Glucose control

Metformin is excreted mainly by the kidney (Table 37.6). In renal failure, metformin accumulates and inhibits oxidation of lactate. Lactic acidosis arises and may be fatal. Metformin should therefore be used cautiously in patients with eGFR <40 mL/min/1.73 m^2, and stopped completely when eGFR <35 ml/min/1.73 m^2.

Table 37.6 Managing glucose control in chronic kidney disease.

Drug	Comment
Metformin	Risk of accumulation and lactic acidosis; Caution when eGFR <40 mL/min/1.73 m^2; Stop when eGFR <35 mL/min/1.73 m^2
Sulfonylureas	Glibenclamide, gliclazide and tolbutamide predominantly renally excreted; may need to reduce dose
Meglitinides	~10% excreted via kidney; usually safe
Thiazolidenediones	Predominantly hepatic metabolism; use may be limited by fluid retention
DPP-4 inhibitors	Sitagliptin: 80% renally excreted, may need to reduce dose Vildagliptin: hepatic metabolism; probably safe
GLP-1 analogs	Exenatide: renal excretion; contraindicated in ESRD Liraglutide: no renal excretion; probably safe
Insulin	Excreted by kidney; may need to reduce dose and/or switch to shorter-acting preparations

DPP-4, dipeptidyl peptidase 4; eGFR, estimated glomerular filtration rate; ESRD, end-stage renal disease; GLP-1, glucagon-like peptide 1.

The sulfonylureas glibenclamide, gliclazide and tolbutamide are predominantly renally excreted and so accumulate in renal failure. Their dosage, and indeed the dosage of any sulfonylurea, may need to be reduced as CKD progresses. Only approximately 10% of the meglitinides, repaglinide and nateglinide, is renally excreted and so they may be suitable alternative agents. The thiazolidenediones, roziglitazone and pioglitazone are predominantly metabolized in the liver, but their use in ESRD may be limited by fluid retention. Insulin is also excreted by the kidney and so a reduced dosage, and perhaps a switch to shorter-acting preparations may be required.

The DPP-4 inhibitor, sitagliptin, is predominantly renally excreted and so a reduction in dose may be needed; vildagliptin is probably safe as this compound is not renally excreted. The GLP-1 analog, exenatide, is renally excreted and contraindicated in ESRD, while liraglutide probably is safe, as it is not excreted through the kidney.

Anemia

Anemia is common in people with diabetes and CKD stage 3 or poorer [162]. Investigation may be needed to exclude a non-renal cause. Anemic patients have a higher mortality, higher rates of hospital admission with heart failure and poorer quality of life. Oral iron should be given to replete iron stores, but parenteral iron may be necessary. The level of hemoglobin at which to commence erythropoietin replacement, and the target treatment level, is unclear.

When to refer to nephrology

Patients who begin dialysis as an emergency do less well than those in whom treatment is planned. Referral to nephrology

Table 37.7 When to refer to nephrology.

eGFR <45 mL/min/1.73 m^2 or serum creatinine 150–200 μmol/L
Diagnosis unclear
Blood pressure uncontrolled
eGFR falls by >5 mL/min/1.73 m^2
Nephrotic syndrome
Hb <10.0 g/dL and other causes of anemia have been excluded
Abnormalities in bone chemistry

should be made when serum creatinine is in the range 150–200 μmol/L or eGFR <45 mL/min/1.73 m^2. This allows structured physical and psychologic preparation for RRT. Earlier referral may be necessary in particular circumstances (Table 37.7). Early referral also allows specialist management of renal bone disease and anemia. The need for RRT should be discussed with all patients, and those who wish it should have access. Patients without significant co-morbidities will usually be offered transplantation. In the work-up for transplantation, full cardiovascular assessment is essential, with exercise testing, (stress)-echocardiography and angiography as indicated. Coronary angioplasty or bypass surgery may be required before transplantation.

Organization of care

A retrospective audit of a joint diabetes–renal clinic showed improved systolic BP, diastolic BP and cholesterol compared to at presentation to the joint clinic [163]. Analysis of a subset of patients showed that the rate of decline of GFR fell from 1.09 mL/min/month in the first year to 0.39 mL/min/month in the third year. Thus, joint diabetes–renal clinics may be useful.

Pregnancy in women with diabetes and chronic kidney disease

Recent studies have confirmed the poor pregnancy outcomes in women with diabetic nephropathy (see Chapter 53). Women with T1DM and vascular disease (retinopathy and/or nephropathy and/or pre-existing hypertension) are at increased risk of pre-eclampsia and abnormal fetal growth [164,165]. Women with any evidence of CKD therefore should be counseled about their increased risks. Inhibitors of the RAS should be stopped before trying to conceive. The incidence of congenital malformations is increased in babies exposed to ACE inhibitors in the first trimester, and there is an increased risk of fetopathy with exposure in the second and third trimesters [166]. Alternative therapies known to be safe in pregnancy, such as methyldopa, labetolol and nifedipine, should be substituted. Strict glucose and BP control may improve pregnancy outcome for mother and baby [167]. In an uncontrolled prospective study of 117 pregnant women with T1DM, methyldopa was given to maintain BP <135/85 mmHg and proteinuria <300 mg/24 hours. Gestational age was longer and birth weight higher than in previous studies.

References

1 US Renal Data System, USRDS. Annual Data Report: *Atlas of Chronic Kidney Disease and End-Stage Renal Disease in the United States*. Bethesda, MD: National Institutes of Health, National Institute of Diabetes and Digestive and Kidney Diseases, 2008.

2 Van Dijk PC, Jager KJ, Stengel B, Gronhagen-Riska C, Feest TG, Briggs JD. Renal replacement therapy for diabetic end-stage renal disease: data from 10 registries in Europe (1991–2000). *Kidney Int* 2005; **67**:1489–1499.

3 Stewart JH, McCredie MR, Williams SM, Jager KJ, Trpeski L, McDonald SP; ESRD Incidence Study Group. Trends in incidence of treated end-stage renal disease, overall and by primary renal disease, in persons aged 20–64 years in Europe, Canada and the Asia-Pacific region, 1998–2002. *Nephrology* 2007; **12**:520–527.

4 Stewart JH, McCredie MR, Williams SM; ESRD Incidence Study Group. Divergent trends in the incidence of end-stage renal disease due to type 1 and type 2 diabetes in Europe, Canada and Australia during 1998–2002. *Diabet Med* 2006; **23**:1364–1369.

5 Levey AS, Coresh J, Balk E, Kausz AT, Levin A, Steffes MW, *et al.* National Kidney Foundation practice guidelines for chronic kidney disease: evaluation, classification, and stratification. *Ann Intern Med* 2003; **139**:137–147.

6 Magee GM, Bilous RW, Cardwell CR, Hunter SJ, Kee F, Fogarty DG. Is hyperfiltration associated with the future risk of developing diabetic nephropathy? A meta-analysis. *Diabetologia* 2009; **52**:691–697.

7 Microalbuminuria Collaborative Study Group. Predictors of the development of microalbuminuria in patients with type 1 diabetes mellitus: a seven year prospective study. *Diabet Med* 1999; **16**:918–925.

8 Chaturvedi N, Bandinelli S, Mangili R, Penno G, Rottiers RE, Fuller JH. Microalbuminuria in type 1 diabetes: rates, risk factors and glycemic threshold. *Kidney Int* 2001; **60**:219–227.

9 Mackin P, MacLeod JM, New J, Marshall SM. Renal function in long-duration type diabetes. *Diabetes Care* 1996; **19**:249–251.

10 Orchard TJ, Dorman JS, Maser RE, Becker DJ, Drash AL, Ellis D, *et al.* Prevalence of complications in IDDM by sex and duration. *Diabetes* 1990; **39**:1116–1124.

11 Warram JH, Gearin G, Laffel L, Krolewski AS. Effect of duration of type 1 diabetes on the prevalence of stages of diabetic nephropathy defined by urinary albumin/creatinine ratio. *J Am Soc Nephrol* 1996; **7**:930–937.

12 Raile K, Galler A, Hofer S, Herbst A, Dunstheimer D, Busch P, *et al.* Diabetic nephropathy in 27805 children, adolescents and adults with type 1 diabetes: effect of diabetes duration, A1C, hypertension, dyslipidemia, diabetes onset and sex. *Diabetes Care* 2007; **30**:2523–2528.

13 Diabetes Control and Complications Trial (DCCT) Research Group. Effect of intensive therapy on the development and progression of diabetic nephropathy in the Diabetes Control and Complications Trial. *Kidney Int* 1995; **47**:1703–1720.

14 Microalbuminuria Collaborative Study Group UK. Intensive therapy and progression to clinical albuminuria in patients with insulin dependent diabetes mellitus and microalbuminuria. *Br Med J* 1995; **311**:973–977.

15 Giorgino F, Laviola L, Cavallo Perin P, Solnica B, Fuller J, Chaturvedi N. Factors associated with progression to macroalbuminuria in microalbuminuric type 1 diabetic patients: the EURODIAB prospective Complications Study. *Diabetologia* 2004; **47**:1020–1028.

16 Perkins BA, Ficociello LH, Silva KH, Finkelstein DM, Warram JH, Krolewski AS. Regression of microalbuminuria in type 1 diabetes. *N Engl J Med* 2003; **348**:2285–2293.

17 Nordwall M, Bojestig M, Arnqvist HJ, Ludvigsson J. Declining incidence of severe retinopathy and persisting decrease of nephropathy in an unselected population of type 1 diabetes: the Linkoping Diabetes Complications Study. *Diabetologia* 2004; **46**:1266–1272.

18 Hovind P, Tarnow L, Rossing K, Rossing P, Eising S, Larsen N, *et al.* Decreasing incidence of severe diabetic microangiopathy in type 1 diabetes. *Diabetes Care* 2003; **26**:1258–1264.

19 Pambianco G, Costacou T, Ellis D, Becker DJ Klein R, Orchard TJ. The 30-year natural history of type 1 diabetes complications: the Pittsburgh Epidemiology of Diabetes Complications Study experience. *Diabetes* 2006; **55**:1463–1469.

20 Costacou T, Ellis D, Fried L, Orchard TJ. Sequence of progression of albuminuria and decreased GFR in persons with type 1 diabetes: a cohort study. *Am J Kidney Dis* 2007; **50**:721–732.

21 Svensson M, Nyström L, Schon S, Dahlquist G. Age at onset of childhood-onset type 1 diabetes and the development of end-stage renal disease: a nationwide population-based study. *Diabetes Care* 2006; **29**:538–542.

22 Sørensen VR, Mathiesen ER, Watt T, Bjorner JB, Andersen MV, Feldt-Rasmussen B. Diabetic patients treated with dialysis: complications and quality of life. *Diabetologia* 2007; **50**:2254–2262.

23 Astrup AS, Tarnow L, Rossing P, Pietraszek L, Riis Hansen P, Parving HH. Improved prognosis in type 1 diabetic patients with nephropathy: a prospective follow-up study. *Kidney Int* 2005; **68**:1250–1257.

24 Schmitz A, Hvid Hansen H, Christensen T. Kidney function in newly diagnosed type 2 (non-insulin-dependent) diabetes before and during treatment. *Diabetologia* 1989; **32**:434–439.

25 Patrick AW, Leslie PJ, Clarke BF, Frier BM. The natural history and associations of microalbuminuria in type 2 diabetes during the first year after diagnosis. *Diabet Med* 1990; **7**:902–908.

26 Nelson RG, Meyer TN, Myers BD, Bennett PH. Course of renal disease in Pima Indians with NIDDM. *Kidney Int* 1997; **52**(Suppl. 63):45–48.

27 Vora JP, Dolben J, Deane JD, Thomas D, Williams JD, Owens DR, *et al.* Renal haemodynamics in newly presenting non-insulin dependent diabetes mellitus. *Kidney Int* 1992; **41**:829–835.

28 Vora JP, Dolben J, Williams JD, Peters JR, Owens DR. Impact of initial treatment on renal function in newly-diagnosed type 2 (non-insulin-dependent) diabetes mellitus. *Diabetologia* 1993; **36**:734–740.

29 Vedel P, Obel J, Nielsen FS, Bang LE, Svendsen TL, Pedersen OB, *et al.* Glomerular hyperfiltration in microalbuminuric NIDDM patients. *Diabetologia* 1996; **39**:1584–1589.

30 Marshall SM, Alberti KGMM. Comparison of the prevalence and associated features of abnormal albumin excretion in insulin dependent and non-insulin-dependent diabetes. *Q J Med* 1989; **70**:61–71.

31 Allawi J, Rao PV, Gilbert P, Scott G, Jarrett RJ, Keen H, *et al.* Microalbuminuria in non-insulin-dependent diabetes: its prevalence in Indian compared with Europid patients. *Br Med J* 1988; **296**:462–464.

32 Gall MA, Rossing P, Skøtt P, Damsbo P, Vaag A, Bech K, *et al.* Prevalence of micro- and macroalbuminuria, arterial hypertension, retinopathy and large vessel disease in European type II (non-insulin-dependent) diabetic patients. *Diabetologia* 1991; **34**:655–661.

33 Collins VR, Dowse GK, Finch CF, Zimmet PZ, Linnane AW. Prevalence and risk factors for micro and macroalbuminuria in diabetic subjects and entire population of Nauru. *Diabetes* 1989; **38**:1602–1610.

34 Damsgaard EM, Mogensen CE. Microalbuminuria in elderly hyperglycaemic patients and controls. *Diabet Med* 1986; **3**:430–435.

35 Nelson RG, Knowler WC, Pettitt DJ, Hanson RL, Bennett PH. Incidence and determinants of elevated urinary albumin excretion in Pima Indians with NIDDM. *Diabetes Care* 1995; **18**:182–187.

36 Unnikrashnan RI, Rema M, Pradeepa R, Deepa M, Shanthirani CS, Deepa R, *et al.* Prevalence and risk factors of diabetic nephropathy in an urban South Indian population: the Chennai Urban Rural Epidemiology Study (CURES 45). *Diabetes Care* 2007; **30**:2019–2024.

37 Dasmahapatra A, Bale A, Raghuwanshi MP, Reddi A, Byrne W, Suarez S, *et al.* Incipient and overt nephropathy in African Americans with NIDDM. *Diabetes Care* 1994; **17**:297–304.

38 Gall MA, Hougaard P, Borch-Johnsen K, Parving H-H. Risk factors for development of incipient and overt diabetic nephropathy in patients with non-insulin dependent diabetes mellitus. *Br Med J* 1997; **314**:783–788.

39 Ravid M, Brosh D, Ravid-Safran D, Levy Z, Rachmani R. Main risk factors for nephropathy in type 2 diabetes mellitus are plasma cholesterol levels, mean blood pressure and hyperglycemia. *Arch Intern Med* 1998; **158**:998–1004.

40 Forsblom CM, Groop PH, Ekstrand A, Totterman KJ, Sane T, Saloranta C, *et al.* Predictors of progression from normoalbuminuria to microalbuminuria in NIDDM. *Diabetes Care* 1998; **21**:1932–1938.

41 Ruggenenti P, Fassi A, Ilieva AP, Bruno S, Iliev IP, Brusegan V, *et al*: Bergamo Nephrologic Diabetes Complications Trial (BENEDICT) Investigators. Preventing microalbuminuria in type 2 diabetes. *N Engl J Med* 2004; **351**:1941–1951.

42 Schmitz A, Væth M, Mogensen CE. Systolic blood pressure relates to the rate of progression of albuminuria in NIDDM. *Diabetologia* 1994; **37**:1251–1258.

43 Ravid M, Lang R, Rachmani R, Lishner M. Long-term renoprotective effect of angiotensin-converting enzyme inhibition in non-insulin-dependent diabetes mellitus: a 7-year follow-up study. *Arch Intern Med* 1996; **156**:286–289.

44 Parving HH, Lehnert H, Brøchner-Mortensen J, Gomis R, Andersen S, Arner P. The effect of irbesartan on the development of diabetic nephropathy in patients with type 2 diabetes. *N Engl J Med* 2001; **345**:870–878.

45 Hasslacher C, Ritz E, Wahl P, Michael C. Similar risks of nephropathy in patients with type I or type II diabetes mellitus. *Nephrol Dial Transplant* 1989; **4**:859–863.

46 Nelson RG, Morgenstern H, Bennett PH. An epidemic of proteinuria in Pima Indians with type 2 diabetes. *Kidney Int* 1998; **54**:2081–2088.

47 Pavkov ME, Knowler WC, Bennett PH, Looker HC, Krakoff J, Nelson RG. Increasing incidence of proteinuria and declining incidence of end-stage renal disease in diabetic Pima Indians. *Kidney Int* 2006; **70**:1840–1846.

48 Myers BD, Nelson RG, Tan M, Beck GJ, Bennett PH, Knowler WC, *et al.* Progression of overt nephropathy in non-insulin-dependent diabetes. *Kidney Int* 1995; **47**:1781–1789.

49 Earle KA, Porter KK, Ostberg J, Yudkin JS. Variation in the progression of diabetic nephropathy according to racial origin. *Nephrol Dial Transplant* 2001; **16**:286–290.

50 Roderick PJ, Jones J, Raleigh VS, McGeown M, Mallick N. Population need for renal replacement therapy in Thames regions: ethnic dimension. *Br Med J* 1994; **309**:1111–1114.

51 Cowie CC, Port FK, Wolfe RA, Savage PJ, Moll PP, Hawthorne VM. Disparities in incidence of diabetic end-stage renal disease according to race and type of diabetes. *N Engl J Med* 1989; **321**:1074–1079.

52 Hebet LA, Kusek JW, Greene T, Agodoa LY, Jones CA, Levey AS, *et al.* Effects of blood pressure control on progression of renal disease in Blacks and Whites: Modification of Diet in Renal Disease Study Group. *Hypertension* 1997; **30**:428–435.

53 Retnakaran R, Cull CA, Thorne KI, Adler AI, Holman RR; UK Prospective Diabetes Study Group. Risk factors for renal dysfunction in type 2 diabetes: UKPDS 74. *Diabetes* 2006; **55**:1832–1839.

54 Fioretto P, Mauer M, Brocco E, Velussi M, Frigato F, Muollo B, *et al.* Patterns of renal injury in NIDDM patients with microalbuminuria. *Diabetologia* 1996; **39**:1569–1576.

55 Christensen PK, Larsen S, Horn T, Olsen S, Parving HH. Causes of albuminuria in patients with type 2 diabetes without diabetic retinopathy. *Kidney Int* 2000; **58**:1719–1731.

56 Ross WR, MaGill JB. Epidemiology of obesity and chronic kidney disease. *Adv Chronic Kidney Dis* 2006; **13**:325–335.

57 Kramer CK, Leitao CB, Canani LH, Gross JL. Impact of white coat hypertension on microvascular complications in type 2 diabetes. *Diabetes Care* 2008; **31**:2233–2237.

58 Dost A, Klinkert C, Kapellen T, Lemmer A, Naeke A, Grabert M, *et al.* Arterial hypertension determined by ambulatory blood pressure profiles: contribution to microalbuminuria risk in a multicenter investigation in 2105 children and adolescents with type 1 diabetes. *Diabetes Care* 2008; **31**:720–725.

59 Thomas MC, Rosengard-Barlund M, Mills V, Ronnback M, Thomas S, Forsblom C, *et al.* Serum lipids and the progression of nephropathy in type 1 diabetes. *Diabetes Care* 2006; **29**:317–322.

60 Tolonen N, Forsblom C, Thorn L, Waden J, Rosengard-Barlund M, Saraheimo M, *et al.* Relationship between lipid profiles and kidney function in patients with type 1 diabetes. *Diabetologia* 2008; **51**:12–20.

61 Xu J, Lee ET, Devereux RB, Umans JG, Bella JN, Shara NM, *et al.* A longitudinal study of risk factors for incident albuminuria in diabetic American Indians: the Strong Heart Study. *Am J Kidney Dis* 2008; **51**:415–424.

62 Thorn LM, Forsblom C, Fagerudd J, Thomas MC, Pettersson-Fernholm K, Saraheimo M, *et al.* Metabolic syndrome in type 1 diabetes: association with diabetic nephropathy and glycemic control (the FinnDiane study). *Diabetes Care* 2005; **28**:2019–2024.

63 Kilpatrick ES, Rigby AS, Atkin SL. Insulin resistance, the metabolic syndrome, and complication risk in type 1 diabetes: "double diabetes" in the Diabetes Control and Complications Diabetes. *Diabetes Care* 2007; **30**:707–712.

64 Costa LA, Canani LH, Lisboa HR, Tres GS, Gross JL. Aggregation of features of the metabolic syndrome is associated with increased prevalence of chronic complications in type 2 diabetes. *Diabet Med* 2004; **21**:252–253.

65 Bonadonna RC, Cucinotta D, Fedele D, Riccardi G, Tiengo A; Metascreen Writing Committee. The metabolic syndrome is a risk indicator of microvascular and macrovascular complications in diabetes: results from Metascreen, a multicenter diabetes clinic-based survey. *Diabetes Care* 2006; **29**:2701–2710.

66 Murussi M, Campagnolo N, Beck MO, Gross JL, Silveiro SP. High-normal levels of albuminuria predict the development of micro- and macroalbuminuria and increased mortality in Brazilian type 2 diabetic patients: an 8-year follow-up study. *Diabet Med* 2007; **24**:1136–1142.

67 De Zeeuw D, Ramjit D, Zhang Z, Ribeiro AB, Kurokawa K, Lash JP, *et al.* Renal risk and renoprotection among ethnic groups with type 2 diabetic nephropathy: a post hoc analysis of RENAAL. *Kidney Int* 2006; **69**:1675–1682.

68 Seaquist ER, Goetz FC, Rich S, Barbosa J. Familial clustering of diabetic kidney disease. *N Engl J Med* 1989; **320**:1161–1165.

69 Thorn LM, Forsblom C, Fagerudd J, Pettersson-Fernholm K, Kilpikari R, Groop PH; FinnDiane Study Group. Clustering of risk factors in parents of patients with type 1 diabetes and nephropathy. *Diabetes Care* 2007; **30**:1162–1167.

70 Schelling JR, Abboud HE, Nicholas SB, Pahl MV, Sedor JR, Adler SG, *et al.* Genome-wide scan for estimated glomerular filtration rate in multi-ethnic diabetic populations: the Family Investigation of Nephropathy and Diabetes (FIND). *Diabetes* 2008; **57**:235–243.

71 Gordin D, Hiilesmaa V, Fagerudd J, Ronnback M, Forsblom C, Kaaja R, *et al*; FinnDiane Study Group. Pre-eclampsia but not pregnancy-induced hypertension is a risk factor for diabetic nephropathy in type 1 diabetic women. *Diabetologia* 2007; **50**:516–522.

72 Lopes-Virella MF, Carter RE, Gilbert GE, Klein RL, Jaffa M, Jenkins AJ, *et al*; Diabetes Control and Complications Trial/Epidemiology of Diabetes Intervention and Complications Cohort Study Group. Risk factors related to inflammation and endothelial dysfunction in the DCCT/EDIC cohort and their relationship with nephropathy and macrovascular complications. *Diabetes Care* 2008; **31**: 2006–2012.

73 Schrijvers BF, de Vriese AS, Flyvbjerg A. From hyperglycemia to diabetic kidney disease: the role of metabolic, hemodynamic and intracellular factors and growth factors/cytokines. *Endocrine Rev* 2004; **25**:971–1010.

74 Shultis WA, Weil EJ, Looker HC, Curtis JM, Shlossman M, Genco RJ, *et al.* Effect of periodontitis on overt nephropathy and end-stage renal disease in type 2 diabetes. *Diabetes Care* 2007; **30**:306–311.

75 Hovind P, Hansen TK, Tarnow L, Steffensen R, Flyvbjerg A, Parving HH. Mannose-binding lectin as a predictor of microalbuminuria in type 1 diabetes: an inception cohort study. *Diabetes* 2005; **54**:1523–1527.

76 Hansen TK, Gall MA, Tarnow L, Thiel S, Stehouwer CD, Schalkwijk CG, *et al.* Mannose-binding lectin and mortality in type 2 diabetes. *Ann Intern Med* 2006; **166**:2007–2013.

77 Jorsal A, Tarnow L, Flyvbjerg A, Parving HH, Rossing P, Rasmussen LM. Plasma osteoprotegerin levels predict cardiovascular and all-cause mortality and deterioration of kidney function in type 1 diabetic patients with nephropathy. *Diabetologia* 2008; **51**:2100–2107.

78 Targher G, Bertolini L, Rodella S, Zoppini G, Lippi G, Day C, *et al.* Non-alcoholic fatty liver disease is independently associated with an

increased prevalence of chronic kidney disease and proliferative/laser-treated retinopathy in type 2 diabetic patients. *Diabetologia* 2008; **51**:444–450.

79 Aso Y. Cardiovascular disease in patients with diabetic nephropathy. *Curr Mol Med* 2008; **8**:533–543.

80 Deckert T, Yokoyama H, Mathiesen E, Rønn B, Jensen T, Feldt-Rasmussen B, *et al.* Cohort study of predictive value of urinary albumin excretion for atherosclerotic vascular disease in patients with insulin dependent diabetes. *Br Med J* 1996; **312**:871–874.

81 Rossing P, Hougaard P, Borch-Johnsen K, Parving HH. Predictors of mortality in IDDM: 10 year observational follow-up study. *Br Med J* 1996; **313**:779–784.

82 Borch-Johnsen K, Kreiner S. Proteinuria: value as predictor of cardiovascular mortality in insulin-dependent diabetes mellitus. *Br Med J* 1989; **294**:1651–1654.

83 Tuomilehto J, Borch-Johnsen K, Molarius A, Forsen T, Rastenyte D, Sarti C, *et al.* Incidence of cardiovascular disease in type 1 (insulin-dependent) diabetic patients with and without diabetic nephropathy in Finland. *Diabetologia* 1998; **41**:784–790.

84 Dinneen SF, Gerstein HC. The association of microalbuminuria and mortality in non-insulin-dependent diabetes mellitus: a systematic overview of the literature. *Arch Intern Med* 1997; **157**:1413–1418.

85 Fuller JH, Stevens LK, Wang SL, WHO Multinational Study Group. Risk factors for cardiovascular mortality and morbidity: the WHO Multinational Study of Vascular Disease in Diabetes. *Diabetologia* 2001; **44**(Suppl. 2):54–64.

86 Mann JF, Gerstein HC, Pogue J, Bosch J, Yusef S. Renal insufficiency as a predictor of cardiovascular outcomes and the impact of ramipril: the HOPE randomised trial. *Ann Intern Med* 2001; **134**:629–636.

87 Adler AI, Stevens RJ, Manley SE, Bilous RW, Cull CA, Holman RR; UKPDS Group. Development and progression of nephropathy in type 2 diabetes: the United Kingdom Prospective Diabetes Study (UKPDS 64). *Kidney Int* 2003; **63**:225–232.

88 Nag S, Bilous R, Kelly W, Jones S, Roper N, Connolly V. All-cause and cardiovascular mortality in diabetic subjects increases significantly with reduced estimated glomerular filtration rate (eGFR): 10 years' data from the South Tees Diabetes Mortality study. *Diabet Med* 2007; **24**:10–17.

89 McCullough PA, Jurkovitz CT, Pergola PE, McGill JB, Brown WW, Collins AJ, *et al.* Independent components of chronic kidney disease as a cardiovascular risk state: results from the Kidney Early Evaluation Program (KEEP). *Arch Intern Med* 2007; **167**:1122–1129.

90 So WY, Kong AP, Ma RC, Ozaki R, Szeto CC, Chan NN, *et al.* Glomerular filtration rate, cardiorenal end points, and all-cause mortality in type 2 diabetic patients. *Diabetes Care* 2006; **29**:2046–2052.

91 Bruno G, Merietti F, Bargero G, Novelli G, Melis D, Soddu A, *et al.* Estimated glomerular filtration rate, albuminuria and mortality in type 2 diabetes: the Casale Monferrato study. *Diabetologia* 2007; **50**:941–948.

92 Norgaard K, Feldt-Rasmussen B, Borch-Johnsen K, Saelan H, Deckert T. Prevalence of hypertension in type 1 (insulin-dependent) diabetes mellitus. *Diabetologia* 1990; **33**:407–410.

93 Chase HP, Garg SK, Harris S, Hoops SL, Marshall G. High normal blood pressure and early diabetic nephropathy. *Arch Intern Med* 1990; **150**:639–641.

94 Poulsen PL, Hansen KW, Mogensen CE. Ambulatory blood pressure in the transition from normo- to microalbuminuria: a longitudinal study in IDDM patients. *Diabetes* 1994; **43**:1248–1253.

95 Margolis DJ, Hofstad O, Feldman HI. Association between renal failure and foot ulcer or lower-extremity amputation in patients with diabetes. *Diabetes Care* 2008; **31**:1331–1336.

96 Ko SH, Park SA, Cho JH, Song KH, Yoon KH, Cha BY, *et al.* Progression of cardiovascular autonomic dysfunction in patients with type 2 diabetes: a 7-year follow-up study. *Diabetes Care* 2008; **31**:1832–1836.

97 Moran A, Palmas W, Field L, Bhattarai J, Schwartz JE, Weinstock RS, *et al.* Cardiovascular autonomic neuropathy is associated with microalbuminuria in older patients with type 2 diabetes. *Diabetes Care* 2004; **27**:972–977.

98 Hallan SI, Ritz E, Lydersen S, Romundstad S, Kvenild K, Orth SR. Combining GFR and albuminuria to classify CKD improves prediction of ESRD. *J Am Soc Nephrol* 2009; **20**:1069–1077.

99 Levey AS, Coresh J, Greene T; for the Chronic Kidney Disease Epidemiology Collaboration. Using standardized serum creatinine values in the modification of diet in renal disease study equation for estimating glomeurlar filtration rate. *Ann Intern Med* 2006; **145**:247–254.

100 Stevens LA, Coresh J, Feldman HI, Greene T, Lash JP, Nelson RG, *et al.* Evaluation of the modification of diet in renal disease study equation in a large diverse population. *J Am Soc Nephrol* 2007; **18**:2749–2757.

101 Basker V, Venugopal H, Holland MR, Singh BM. Clinical utility of estimated glomerular filtration rates in predicting renal risk in a district diabetes population. *Diabet Med* 2006; **23**:1057–1060.

102 Fontsere N, Bonal J, Salinas I, de Arellano MR, Rios J, Torres F, *et al.* Is the new Mayo Clinic quadratic equation useful of the estimation of glomerular filtration rate in type 2 diabetic patients? *Diabetes Care* 2008; **31**:2265–2267.

103 Chudleigh RA, Dunseath G, Evans W, Harvey JN, Evans P, Ollerton R, *et al.* How reliable is estimation of glomerular filtration rate at diagnosis of type 2 diabetes? *Diabetes Care* 2007; **30**:300–305.

104 Rossing P, Rossing K, Gæde P, Pedersen O, Parving HH. Monitoring kidney function in type 2 diabetic patients with incipient and overt nephropathy. *Diabetes Care* 2006; **29**:1024–1030.

105 Beauvieux MC, Le Moigne F, Lasseur C, Raffaitin C, Perlemoine C, Berthe N, *et al.* New predictive equations improve monitoring of kidney function in patients with diabetes. *Diabetes Care* 2007; **30**:1988–1994.

106 Tan GD, Lewis AV, James TJ, Altmann P, Taylor RP, Levy JC. Clinical usefulness of cystatin C for the estimation of glomerular filtration rate in type 1 diabetes: reproducibility and accuracy compared with standard measures and iohexol clearance. *Diabetes Care* 2002; **25**:2000–2004.

107 Perkins BA, Nelson RG, Ostrander BE, Blouch KL, Krolewski AS, Myers BD, *et al.* Detection of renal function decline in patients with diabetes and normal or elevated GFR by serial measurements of serum cystatin C concentration: results of a 4-year follow-up study. *J Am Soc Nephrol* 2005; **16**:1404–1412.

108 MacIsaac RJ, Tsalamandris C, Thomas MC, Premaratne E, Panagiotopoulos S, Smith TJ, *et al.* Estimating glomerular filtration rate in diabetes: a comparison of cystatin C and creatinine-based methods. *Diabetologia* 2006; **49**:1686–1689.

109 Diabetes Control and Complications Trial Research Group. The effect of intensive treatment of diabetes on the development and

progression of long-term complications in insulin-dependent diabetes mellitus. *N Engl J Med* 1993; **329**:977–986.

110 Diabetes Control and Complications Trial Research Group. The absence of a glycaemic threshold for the development of long-term complications: the prospective of the Diabetes Control and Complications Trial. *Diabetes* 1996; **45**:1289–1298.

111 Diabetes Control and Complications Trial/Epidemiology of Diabetes Interventions and Complications Research Group. Retinopathy and nephropathy in patients with type 1 diabetes four years after a trial of intensive therapy. *N Engl J Med* 2000; **342**:381–389.

112 Writing Team for the Diabetes Control and Complications Trial/Epidemiology of Diabetes Interventions and Complications Research Group. Sustained effect of intensive treatment of type 1 diabetes mellitus on development and progression of diabetic nephropathy. Epidemiology of Diabetes Interventions and Complications (EDIC) Study. *JAMA* 2003; **290**:2159–2167.

113 EUCLID Study Group. Randomised placebo-controlled trial of lisinopril in normotensive patients with insulin-dependent diabetes and normoalbuminuria or microalbuminuria. *Lancet* 1997; **349**:1787–1792.

114 Bilous RW, Chaturvedi N, Sjølie AK, Fuller J, Klein R, Orchard T, *et al.* Effect of candesartan on microalbuminuria and albumin excretion rate in diabetes: three randomised trials. *Ann Intern Med* 2009; **151**:11–20.

115 UK Prospective Diabetes Study. Intensive blood-glucose control with sulphonylureas or insulin compared with conventional treatment and risk of complications in patients with type 2 diabetes. *Lancet* 1998; **352**:837–853.

116 Stratton IM, Adler AI, Neil HA, Matthews DR, Manley SE, Cull CA, *et al.* Association of glycaemia with macrovascular and microvascular complications of type 2 diabetes (UKPDS 35): prospective observational study. *Br Med J* 2000; **321**:405–412.

117 Holman RR, Paul SK, Bethel MA, Matthews DR, Neil HA. 10-year follow-up of intensive glucose control in type 2 diabetes. *N Engl J Med* 2008; **359**:1577–1589.

118 ADVANCE Collaborative Group. Intensive blood glucose control and vascular outcomes in patients with type 2 diabetes. *N Engl J Med* 2008; **358**:2560–2572.

119 UK Prospective Diabetes Study Group. Tight blood pressure control and risk of macrovascular and microvascular complications in type 2 diabetes (UKPDS 38). *Br Med J* 1998; **317**:703–713.

120 Adler AI, Stratton IM, Neil HA, Yudkin JS, Matthews DR, Cull CA, *et al.* Association of systolic blood pressure with macrovascular and microvascular complications of type 2 diabetes: prospective observational study (UKPDS 36). *Br Med J* 2000; **321**:412–419.

121 UK Prospective Diabetes Study Group. Efficacy of atenolol and captopril in reducing risk of macrovascular and microvascular complications in type 2 diabetes (UKPDS 39). *Br Med J* 1998; **317**:713–720.

122 Heart Outcomes Prevention Evaluation (HOPE) Study Investigators. Effects of ramipril on cardiovascular and microvascular outcomes in people with diabetes mellitus: results of the HOPE study and MICRO-HOPE substudy. *Lancet* 2000; **355**:253–259.

123 Patel A; ADVANCE Collaborative Group. Effects of a fixed combination of perindopril and indapamide on macrovascular and microvascular outcomes in patients with type 2 diabetes mellitus (the ADVANCE trial): a randomised controlled trial. *Lancet* 2007; **370**:829–840.

124 Strippoli GF, Craig M, Schena FP, Craig JC. Antihypertensive agents for primary prevention of diabetic nephropathy. *J Am Soc Nephrol* 2005; **16**:3081–3091.

125 Holman RR, Paul SK, Bethel MA, Neil HA, Matthews DR. Long-term follow-up after tight control of blood pressure in type 2 diabetes. *N Engl J Med* 2008; **359**:1565–1576.

126 Bending JJ, Viberti GC, Watkins PJ, Keen H. Intermittent clinical proteinuria and renal function in diabetes: evolution and the effect of glycaemic control. *Br Med J* 1986; **292**:83–86.

127 Feldt-Rasmussen B, Mathiesen ER, Deckert T. Effect of two years of strict metabolic control on progression of incipient nephropathy in insulin-dependent diabetes. *Lancet* 1986; **ii**:1300–1304.

128 Feldt-Rasmussen B, Mathiesen ER, Hegedus L, Deckert T. Kidney function during 12 months of strict metabolic control in insulin-dependent diabetic patients with incipient nephropathy. *N Engl J Med* 1986; **314**:665–670.

129 Fioretto P, Steffes MW, Sutherland DE, Goetz FC, Mauer M. Reversal of lesions of diabetic nephropathy after pancreas transplantation. *N Engl J Med* 1998; **339**:115–117.

130 ACE Inhibitors in Diabetic Nephropathy Trialist Group. Should all patients with type 1 diabetes mellitus and microalbuminuria receive angiotensin-converting enzyme inhibitors? A meta-analysis of individual patient data. *Ann Intern Med* 2001; **134**:370–379.

131 Lewis EJ, Hunsicker LG, Bain RP, Rohde RD. The effect of angiotensin-converting enzyme inhibition on diabetic nephropathy. *N Engl J Med* 1993; **329**:1456–1462.

132 Andersen S, Tarnow L, Rossing P, Hansen BV, Parving HH. Renoprotective effects of angiotensin II receptor blockade in type 1 diabetic patients with diabetic nephropathy. *Kidney Int* 2000; **57**:601–606.

133 Kasiske BL, Kalil RSN, Ma JZ, Liao M, Keane WF. Effect of antihypertensive therapy on the kidney in patients with diabetes: a meta-regression analysis. *Ann Intern Med* 1993; **118**:129–138.

134 Remuzzi G. A unifying hypothesis for renal scarring linking protein trafficking to the different mediators of injury. *Nephrol Dial Transplant* 2000; **15**(Suppl. 6):58–60.

135 Zatz R, Dunn BR, Meyer TW, Brenner B. Prevention of diabetic glomerulopathy by pharmacological amelioration of glomerular capillary hypertension. *J Clin Lab Invest* 1986; **77**:1925–1930.

136 European Study for the Prevention of Renal Disease in Type 1 Diabetic Patients (ESPRIT) Research Group. Effect of 3 years antihypertensive therapy on renal structure in type 1 diabetic patients with albuminuria. *Diabetes* 2001; **50**:843–580.

137 Hovind P, Rossing P, Tarnow L, Smidt UM, Parving HH. Progression of diabetic nephropathy. *Kidney Int* 2001; **59**:702–709.

138 Parving HH, Hommel E, Jensen BR, Hansen HP. Long-term beneficial effect of ACE inhibition on diabetic nephropathy in normotensive type 1 diabetic patients. *Kidney Int* 2001; **60**:228–324.

139 Hovind P, Rossing P, Tarnow L, Smidt UM, Parving HH. Remission and regression in the nephropathy of type 1 diabetes when blood pressure is controlled aggressively. *Kidney Int* 2001; **60**:277–283.

140 Jacobsen P, Andersen S, Rossing K, Jensen BR, Parving HH. Dual blockade of the renin-angiotensin system versus maximal recommended dose of ACE inhibition in diabetic nephropathy. *Kidney Int* 2003; **63**:1874–1880.

141 Jacobsen P, Andersen S, Jensen BR, Parving HH. Additive effect of ACE inhibition and angiotensin II receptor blockade in type 1 diabetic patients with diabetic nephropathy. *Kidney Int* 2003; **63**:1874–1880.

142 MacKinnon M, Shurraw S, Akbari A, Knoll GA, Jaffey J, Clark HD. Combination therapy with an angiotensin receptor blocker and an ACE inhibitor in proteinuric renal disease: a systematic review of the efficacy and safety data. *Am J Kidney Dis* 2006; **48**:8–20.

143 Schødt KJ, Rossing K, Juhl TR, Boomsma F, Rossing P, Tarnow L, *et al.* Beneficial impact of spironolactone in diabetic nephropathy. *Kidney Int* 2005; **68**:2829–2836.

144 Ohkubo Y, Kishikawa H, Araki E, Miyata T, Isami S, Motoyoshi S, *et al.* Intensive insulin therapy prevents the progression of diabetic microvascular complications in Japanese patients with non-insulin-dependent diabetes: a randomised prospective 6-year study. *Diabetes Res Clin Pract* 1995; **28**:103–117.

145 Shichiri M, Kishikawa H, Ohkubo Y, Wake N. Long-term results of the Kumamoto Study on optimal diabetes control in type 2 diabetic patients. *Diabetes Care* 2000; **23**(Suppl 2):B21–29.

146 Sano T, Hotta N, Kawamura T, Matsumae H, Chaya S, Sasaki H, *et al.* Effects of long-term enalapril treatment on persistent microalbuminuria in normotensive type 2 diabetic patients: results of a 4-year, prospective, randomised study. *Diabet Med* 1996; **13**:120–124.

147 Ravid M, Savin H, Jutrin I, Bental T, Katz B, Lishner M. Long-term stabilizing effect of angiotensin-converting enzyme inhibition on plasma creatinine and on proteinuria in normotensive type II diabetic patients. *Ann Intern Med* 1993; **118**:577–581.

148 Brenner BM, Cooper ME, de Zeeuw D, Keane WF, Mitch WE, Parving HH, *et al.* Effects of losartan on renal and cardiovascular outcomes in patients with type 2 diabetes and nephropathy. *N Engl J Med* 2001; **345**:861–869.

149 Lewis EJ, Hunsicker LG, Clarke WR, Berl T, Pohl MA, Lewis JB, *et al.* Renoprotective effect of the angiotensin-receptor antagonist irbesartan in patients with nephropathy due to type 2 diabetes. *N Engl J Med* 2001; **345**:851–860.

150 Barnett AH, Bain SC, Bouter P, Karlberg B, Madsbad S, Jervell J, *et al.* Angiotensin-receptor blockade versus converting enzyme inhibition in type 2 diabetes and nephropathy. *N Engl J Med* 2004; **351**:1952–1961.

151 Lacourciere Y, Belanger A, Godin C, Halle JP, Ross S, Wright N, *et al.* Long-term comparison of losartan and enalapril on kidney function in hypertensive type 2 diabetics with early nephropathy. *Kidney Int* 2000; **58**:762–769.

152 Mogensen CE, Neldam S, Tikkanen I, Oren S, Viskoper R, Watts RW, *et al.* Randomised controlled trial of dual blockade of renin–angiotensin system in patients with hypertension, microalbuminuria, and non-insulin dependent diabetes: the candesartan and lisinopril microalbuminuria (CALM) study. *Br Med J* 2000; **321**:1440–1444.

153 Parving HH, Persson F, Lewis JB, Lewis EJ, Hollenberg NK; AVOID Study Investigators. Aliskiren combined with losartan in type 2 diabetes and nephropathy. *N Engl J Med* 2008; **358**:2433–2446.

154 Ustundag A, Tugrul A, Ustundag S, Sut N, Demirkan B. The effects of spironolactone on nephrin function in patients with diabetic nephropathy. *Ren Fail* 2008; **30**:982–991.

155 Swaminathan K, Davies J, George J, Rajendra NS, Morris AD, Struthers AD. Spironolactone for poorly controlled hypertension in type 2 diabetes: conflicting effects on blood pressure, endothelial function, glycemic control and hormonal profiles. *Diabetologia* 2008; **51**:762–768.

156 Mann JF, Schmieder RE, McQueen M, Dyal L, Schumacher H, Poque J, *et al.* Renal outcomes with telmisartan, ramipril, or both, in people at high risk (the ONTARGET study): a multi-centre, randomized, double-blind, controlled trial. *Lancet* 2008; **372**:547–553.

157 Robertson L, Waugh N, Robertson A. Protein restriction for diabetic renal disease. *Cochrane Database Syst Rev* 2007; **17**:CD002181.

158 Gæde P, Vedel P, Parving HH, Pedersen O. Intensive multifactorial intervention in patients with type 2 diabetes and microalbuminuria (the Steno 2 Study). *Lancet* 1999; **353**:617–622.

159 Gæde P, Vedel P, Larsen N, Jensen GV, Parving HH, Pedersen O. Multifactorial intervention and cardiovascular disease in patients with type 2 diabetes. *N Engl J Med* 2003; **348**:383–393.

160 Gæde P, Lund-Andersen H, Parving HH, Pedersen O. Effect of a multifactorial intervention on mortality in type 2 diabetes. *N Engl J Med* 2008; **358**:580–591.

161 Ng JM, Jennings PE, Laboi P, Jayagopal V. Erythropoietin treatment significantly alters measured glycated haemoglobin (HbA1c). *Diabet Med* 2008; **25**:239–242.

162 New JP, Aung T, Baker PG, Yongsheng G, Pylypczuk R, Houghton J, *et al.* The high prevalence of unrecognized anaemia in patients with diabetes and chronic kidney disease: a population-based study. *Diabet Med* 2008; **25**:564–567.

163 Jayapaul MK, Messersmith R, Bennett-Jones DN, Mead PA, Large DM. The joint diabetes–renal clinic in clinical practice: 10 years of data from a district general hospital. *Q J Med* 2006; **99**:153–160.

164 Howarth C, Gazis A, James D. Association of type 1 diabetes mellitus, maternal vascular disease and complications of pregnancy. *Diabet Med* 2007; **24**:1229–1234.

165 Haeri S, Khoury J, Kovilam O, Miodovnik M. The association of intrauterine growth abnormalities in women with type 1 diabetes mellitus complicated by vasculopathy. *Am J Obstet Gynecol* 2008; **199**:278e1–5.

166 Cooper WO, Hernandez-Diaz S, Arboqast PG, Dudley JA, Dyer S, Gideon PS, *et al.* Major congenital malformations after first trimester exposure to ACE inhibitors. *N Engl J Med* 2006; **354**:2443–2451.

167 Nielsen LR, Damm P, Mathiesen ER. Improved pregnancy outcome in type 1 diabetic women with microalbuminuria or diabetic nephropathy: effect of intensified antihypertensive therapy? *Diabetes Care* 2009; **32**:38–44.

38 Diabetic Peripheral Neuropathy

Dan Ziegler

Institute for Clinical Diabetology, German Diabetes Center at the Heinrich Heine University, Leibniz Center for Diabetes Research; Department of Metabolic Diseases, University Hospital, Düsseldorf, Germany

Keypoints

- Approximately one in three people with diabetes is affected by distal symmetric polyneuropathy (DPN), which represents a major health problem as it may present with excruciating neuropathic pain and is responsible for substantial morbidity, increased mortality and impaired quality of life.
- Neuropathic pain exerts a substantial impact on quality of life, particularly by causing considerable interference with sleep, daily activities and enjoyment of life.
- Treatment is based on four cornerstones: (1) intensive diabetes therapy and multifactorial risk intervention; (2) treatment based on pathogenetic mechanisms; (3) symptomatic treatment; and (4) avoidance of risk factors and complications.
- Recent experimental studies suggest a multifactorial pathogenesis of diabetic neuropathy. From the clinical point of view, it is important to note that, based on these pathogenetic mechanisms, therapeutic approaches could be derived, some of which are currently being evaluated in clinical trials.
- Management of chronic painful DPN remains a challenge for the physician and should consider the following practical rules: the appropriate and effective drug has to be tried and identified in each patient by carefully titrating the dosage based on efficacy and side effects; lack of efficacy should be judged only after 2–4 weeks of treatment using an adequate dosage. Analgesic combination therapy may be useful, and potential drug interactions have to be considered given the frequent polypharmacy in people with diabetes.
- Epidemiologic data indicate that not only increased alcohol consumption but also the traditional cardiovascular risk factors such as visceral obesity, hypertension, hyperlipidemia and smoking have a role in the development and progression of diabetic neuropathy and hence need to be prevented or treated.

Classification and epidemiology

Diabetic neuropathy has been defined as a demonstrable disorder, either clinically evident or subclinical, that occurs in the setting of diabetes without other causes for peripheral neuropathy. It includes manifestations in the somatic and/or autonomic parts of the peripheral nervous system [1] which are being classified along clinical criteria; however, because of the variety of the clinical syndromes with possible overlaps there is no universally accepted classification. The most widely used classification of diabetic neuropathy proposed by Thomas [2] has subsequently been modified [3]. This proposal differentiates between rapidly reversible, persistent symmetric polyneuropathies and focal or multifocal neuropathies (Table 38.1). Diabetic distal symmetrical sensory or sensorimotor polyneuropathy (DPN) represents the most relevant clinical manifestation affecting approximately 30% of community-based people with diabetes [4]. There is emerging evidence to suggest that intermediate hyperglycemia is associated with an increased risk of DPN. In the general population living in the region of Augsburg, Southern Germany, the prevalence of DPN was 28.0% in subjects with diabetes, 13.0% in those with impaired glucose tolerance (IGT), 11.3% in those with impaired fasting glucose (IFG) and 7.4% in those with normal glucose tolerance (NGT) [5]. The incidence of DPN is approximately 2% per year.

The most important etiologic factors that have been associated with DPN are poor glycemic control, visceral obesity, diabetes duration, height, hypertension, age, smoking, hypoinsulinemia and dyslipidemia [4]. The clinical impact of DPN is illustrated in Figure 38.1. DPN is related to both lower extremity impairments such as diminished position sense and functional limitations such as walking ability [6]. There is accumulating evidence suggesting that not only surrogate markers of microangiopathy such as albuminuria, but also those used for DPN such as nerve conduction velocity and vibration perception threshold (VPT) may predict mortality in people with diabetes [7,8]. Elevated VPT also predicts the development of neuropathic foot ulceration, one of the most common causes for hospital admission and lower limb amputations among patients with diabetes [9].

Pain is a subjective symptom of major clinical importance as it is often this complaint that motivates patients to seek health

Textbook of Diabetes, 4th edition. Edited by R. Holt, C. Cockram, A. Flyvbjerg and B. Goldstein. © 2010 Blackwell Publishing.

Table 38.1 Classification of diabetic neuropathies. Adapted from Sima *et al.* [3].

1 Rapidly reversible
Hyperglycemic neuropathy
2 Persistent symmetric polyneuropathies
Distal somatic sensory/motor polyneuropathies involving predominantly large fibers
Autonomic neuropathies
Small-fiber neuropathies
3 Focal/multifocal neuropathies
Cranial neuropathies
Thoracoabdominal radiculopathies
Focal limb neuropathies
Proximal neuropathies
Compression and entrapment neuropathies

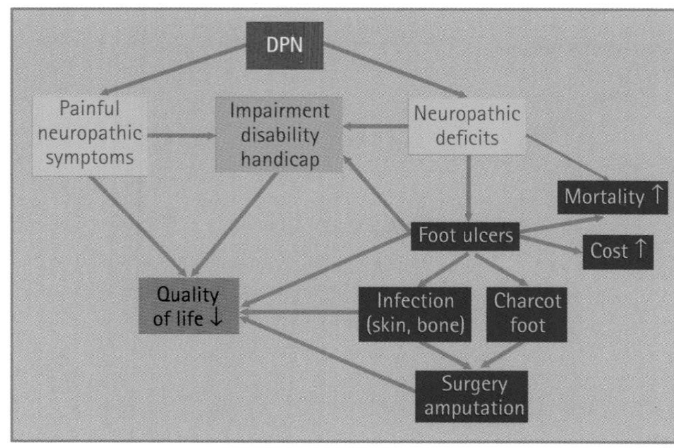

Figure 38.1 Clinical impact of diabetic distal symmetric polyneuropathy (DPN).

care. Pain associated with diabetic neuropathy exerts a substantial impact on quality of life, particularly by causing considerable interference in sleep and enjoyment of life [10]; however, in one UK survey, only 65% of patients with diabetes received treatment for their neuropathic pain, although 96% had reported the pain to their physician [11]. Pain treatment consisted of antidepressants in 43.5% of cases, anticonvulsants in 17.4%, opiates in 39% and alternative treatments in 30%. While 77% of the patients reported persistent pain over 5 years, 23% were pain-free over at least 1 year [11]. Thus, neuropathic pain persists in the majority of patients with diabetes over periods of several years.

Chronic painful DPN is present in up to 26% of patients with diabetes [11–14]. As well as the high prevalence of painful neuropathy among people with diabetes and intermediate hyperglycemia described previously, subjects with macrovascular disease appear to be particularly prone to neuropathic pain [14]. Among survivors of myocardial infarction (MI) from the Augsburg MI Registry, the prevalence of neuropathic pain was 21.0% in the people with diabetes, 14.8% in those with IGT, 5.7% in those with IFG and 3.7% in those with NGT [15]. The most important risk factors of DPN and neuropathic pain in these surveys were age, obesity and low physical activity, while the predominant comorbidity was peripheral arterial disease, highlighting the paramount role of cardiovascular risk factors and diseases in DPN.

Clinical manifestations

Distal symmetric polyneuropathy

The term "hyperglycemic neuropathy" has been used to describe sensory symptoms in people with poorly controlled diabetes that are rapidly reversible following institution of near-normoglycemia [2]; however, the most frequent form is DPN, commonly associated with autonomic involvement. Its onset is insidious and, in the absence of intervention, the course is chronic and progressive. It seems that the longer axons to the lower limbs are more vulnerable to the nerve lesions induced by diabetes (length-related distribution). This notion is supported by the correlation found between the presence of DPN and height. DPN typically develops as a "dying-back" neuropathy, affecting the most distal extremities (toes) first. The neuropathic process then extends proximally up the limbs and later it may also affect the anterior abdominal wall and then spread laterally around the trunk. Occasionally, the upper limbs are involved with the fingertips being affected first ("glove and stocking" distribution; Figure 38.2).

Variants including painful small-fiber or pseudosyringomyelic syndromes and an atactic syndrome (diabetic pseudotabes) have been described. Small-fiber unmyelinated (C) and thinly myelinated (Aδ) fibers as well as large-fiber myelinated (Aα, Aβ) neurons are typically involved. It is as yet uncertain whether the various fiber type damage develops following a regular sequence, with small fibers being affected first, followed by larger fibers, or whether the small-fiber or large-fiber involvement reflects either side of a continuous spectrum of fiber damage. Nevertheless, there is evidence suggesting that small-fiber neuropathy may occur early, often presenting with pain and hyperalgesia before sensory deficits or nerve conduction slowing can be detected [2]. The reduction or loss of small fiber-mediated sensation results in loss of pain sensation (heat pain, pinprick) and temperature perception to cold (Aδ) and warm (C) stimuli. Large-fiber involvement leads to nerve conduction slowing and reduction or loss of touch, pressure, two-point discrimination and vibration sensation which may lead to sensory ataxia (atactic gait) in severe cases. A typical example for the distribution of sensory deficits is shown in Figure 38.3. Sensory fiber involvement causes "positive" sensory symptoms such as paresthesia, dysesthesia and pain, as well as "negative" symptoms such as reduced sensation.

Persistent or episodic pain that typically worsens at night and improves during walking is localized predominantly in the feet. The pain is often described as a deep-seated aching but there may

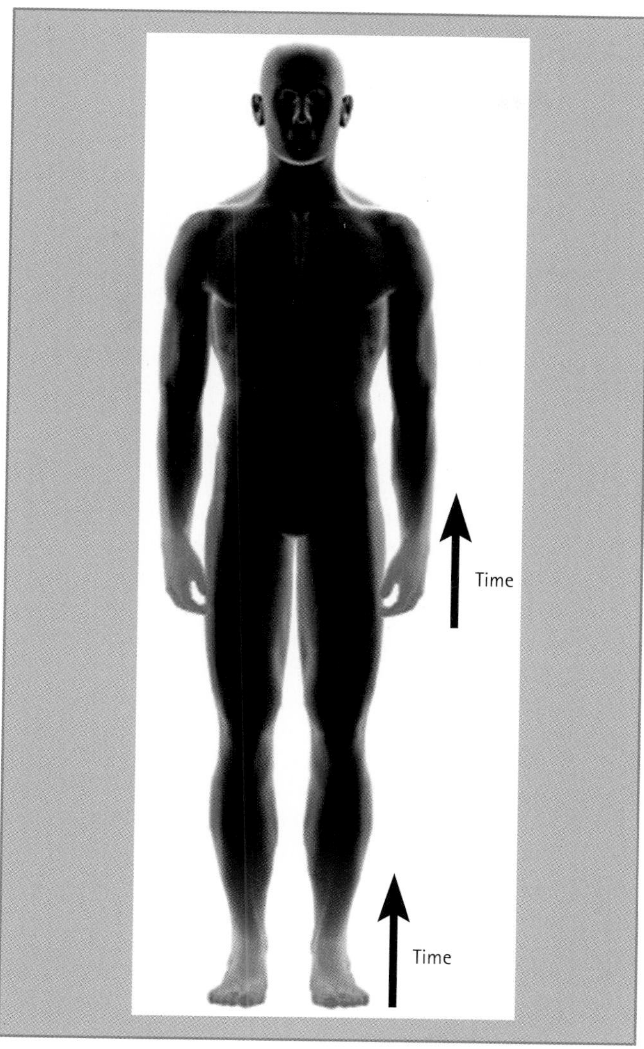

Figure 38.2 The typical "glove and stocking" distribution of diabetic distal symmetric sensory or sensorimotor polyneuropathy (DPN).

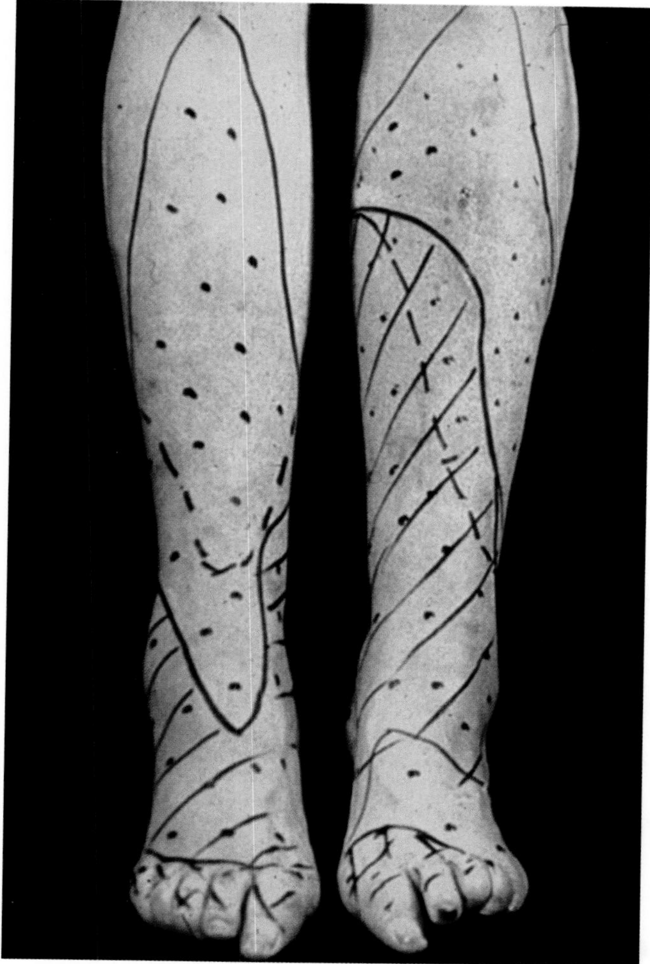

Figure 38.3 A typical example for the distribution of sensory deficits (dots: reduced thermal sensation; lines: reduced pain sensation; crossed lines: reduced touch sensation) in a patient with distal symmetric sensory or sensorimotor polyneuropathy (DPN).

be superimposed lancinating stabs or it may have a burning thermal quality. In a clinical survey including 105 patients with painful DPN, the following locations of pain were most frequent: 96% feet, 69% balls of feet, 67% toes, 54% dorsum of foot, 39% hands, 37% plantum of foot, 37% calves and 32% heels. The pain was most often described by the patients as "burning/hot," "electric," "sharp," "achy" and "tingling" and was worse at night time and when tired or stressed [10]. The average pain intensity was moderate, approximately 5.75/10 on a 0–10 scale, with the "least" and "most" pain 3.6 and 6.9/10, respectively. Allodynia (pain from a stimulus that does not normally cause pain; e.g. stroking) may occur. The symptoms may be accompanied by sensory loss, but patients with severe pain may have few clinical signs. Pain may persist over several years [16] causing considerable disability and impaired quality of life in some patients [10], whereas it remits partially or completely in others [17,18], despite further deterioration in small-fiber function [18]. Pain remission tends to be associated with sudden metabolic change, short duration of pain or diabetes, preceding weight loss and less severe sensory loss [17,18].

Compared with the sensory deficits, motor involvement is usually less prominent and restricted to the distal lower limbs resulting in muscle atrophy and weakness at the toes and foot. Ankle reflexes are frequently reduced or absent. At the foot level, the loss of the protective sensation (painless feet), motor dysfunction and reduced sweat production, resulting in dry and chapped skin and which is caused by autonomic involvement, increase the risk of callus and foot ulcers. Thus, the neuropathic patient has a high-risk of developing severe and potentially life-threatening foot complications such as ulceration, osteoarthropathy (Charcot foot) and osteomyelitis as well as medial arterial calcification and neuropathic edema. Because DPN is the major contributory factor for diabetic foot ulcers, and the lower limb amputation rates in subjects with diabetes are 15 times higher than in the non-diabetic population, early detection of DPN by screening is of paramount importance [9]. This is even more imperative because many patients with DPN are asymptomatic or have only mild symptoms. In view of these causation pathways, the majority of amputations should be potentially preventable if appropriate screening and preventative measures were adopted.

Acute painful neuropathy

Acute painful neuropathy has been described as a separate clinical entity [19]. It is encountered infrequently in patients with type 1 (T1DM) and type 2 diabetes mellitus (T2DM) and presents with continuous burning pain particularly in the soles ("like walking on burning sand") with nocturnal exacerbation. A characteristic feature is a cutaneous contact discomfort to clothes and sheets which can be objectified as hypersensitivity to tactile (allodynia) and painful stimuli (hyperalgesia). Motor function is preserved, and sensory loss may be only slight, being greater for thermal than for vibration sensation. The onset is associated with and preceded by precipitous and severe weight loss. Depression and impotence are constant features. The weight loss has been shown to respond to adequate glycemic control and the severe manifestations subsided within 10 months in all cases. No recurrences were observed after follow-up periods of up to 6 years [19]. The syndrome of acute painful neuropathy seems to be equivalent to diabetic cachexia as described by Ellenberg [20]. It has also been described in girls with anorexia nervosa and diabetes in association with weight loss [21].

The term "insulin neuritis" was used by Caravati [22] to describe a case with precipitation of acute painful neuropathy several weeks following the institution of insulin treatment. In a recent series, painful symptoms gradually improved in all patients, allowing discontinuation of analgesic therapy within 3–8 months. Thus, careful correction of glucose levels should be considered in patients with long-standing uncontrolled diabetes [23]. Sural nerve biopsy shows signs of chronic neuropathy with prominent regenerative activity [24] as well as epineurial arteriovenous shunting and a fine network of vessels, resembling the new vessels of the retina which may lead to a steal effect rendering the endoneurium ischemic [25]. This may happen in analogy to the transient deterioration of a pre-existing retinopathy following rapid improvement in glycemic control.

Focal and multifocal neuropathies

Most of the focal and multifocal neuropathies tend to occur in long-term patients with diabetes of middle age or older. The outlook for most of them is for recovery, either partial or complete, and for eventual resolution of the pain that frequently accompanies them [26]. With this in mind, physicians should always maintain an optimistic outlook in dealing with patients with these afflictions.

Cranial neuropathy

Palsies of the third cranial nerve (diabetic ophthalmoplegia) are painful in about 50% of cases. The onset is usually abrupt. The pain is felt behind and above the eye and at times precedes the ptosis and diplopia (with pupillary dysfunction in 14–18% of the cases) by several days. Oculomotor findings reach their nadir within a day or at most a few days, persist for several weeks and then begin gradually to improve. Full resolution is the rule and generally takes place within 3–5 months. The fourth, sixth and seventh cranial nerves are next in frequency [26].

Mononeuropathy of the limbs

Focal lesions affecting the limb nerves, most commonly the ulnar, median, radial and peroneal may be painful, particularly if of acute onset, as may entrapment neuropathies, such as the carpal tunnel syndrome which is associated with painful paresthesia [26].

Diabetic truncal neuropathy

Mononeuropathy of the trunk (thoracoabdominal neuropathy or radiculopathy) presents with an abrupt onset with pain or dysesthesia being the heralding feature, sometimes accompanied by cutaneous sensory impairment or hyperesthesia. Pain has been described as deep, aching or boring, but also the descriptors of jabbing, burning, sensitive skin or tearing have been used. The neuropathy is almost always unilateral or predominantly so. As a result, the pain felt in the chest or the abdomen may be confused with pain of pulmonary, cardiac or gastrointestinal origin. Sometimes, it may have a radicular or girdling quality, half encircling the trunk in a root-like distribution. Pain may be felt in one or several dermatomal distributions and, almost universally, it is worst at night. Rarely, abdominal muscle herniation may occur, predominantly in middle-aged men, involving 3–5 adjacent nerve roots between T6 and T12 (Figure 38.4). The time from first symptom to the peak of the pain syndrome is often just a few days, although occasionally spread of the pain to adjacent dermatomes may continue for weeks or even months. Weight loss of 15–40 pounds (7–18 kg) occurs in >50% of the cases. The course of truncal neuropathy is favorable, and pain subsides within months to a maximum of 1.5–2 years [26].

Diabetic amyotrophy

Asymmetric or symmetric proximal muscle weakness and muscle wasting (iliopsoas, obturator and adductor muscles) are easily recognized clinically in the syndrome of lower limb proximal motor neuropathy (synonyms: Bruns–Garland syndrome, diabetic amyotrophy, proximal diabetic neuropathy, diabetic lumbosacral plexopathy, ischemic mononeuropathy multiplex, femoral–sciatic neuropathy, femoral neuropathy). Pronounced bilateral atrophy and paresis of the quadriceps muscle is shown in Figure 38.5. Pain is nearly universal in this syndrome. Characteristically, it is deep, aching, constant and severe, invariably worse at night and may have a burning raw quality. It is usually not frankly dysesthetic or cutaneous. Frequently, pain is first experienced in the lower back or buttock on the affected side or may be felt as extending from hip to knee. Although severe and tenacious, the pain of proximal motor neuropathy has a good

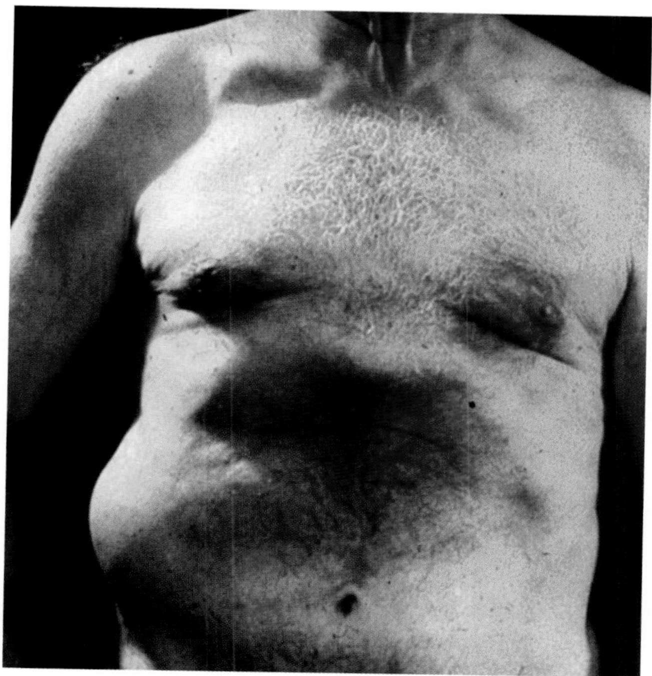

Figure 38.4 Diabetic truncal neuropathy (thoracoabdominal neuropathy or radiculopathy) leading to herniation of the oblique abdominal muscle.

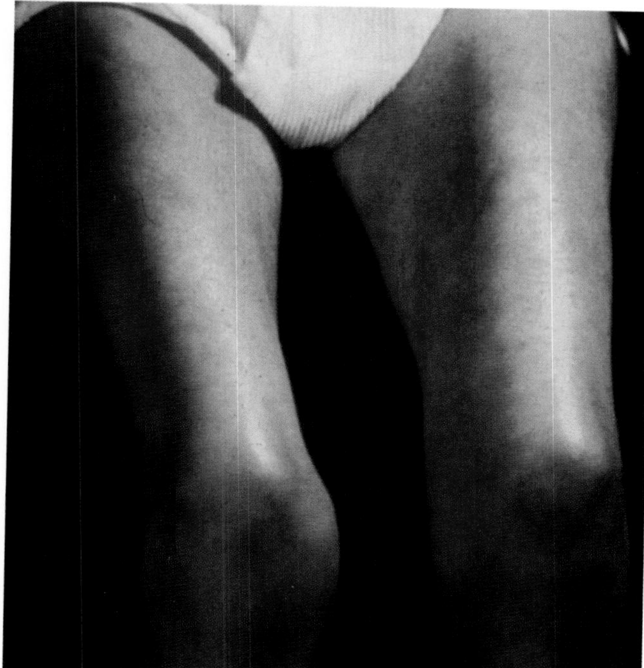

Figure 38.5 Diabetic amyotrophy (proximal neuropathy): pronounced bilateral atrophy and paresis of the quadriceps muscle.

prognosis. Concurrent distal sensory polyneuropathy is frequently present. Weight loss is also a frequently associated feature and may be as much as 35–40 pounds (16–18 kg). The weight is generally regained during the recovery phase [27,28].

Central nervous system dysfunction

Relatively little attention has been directed toward impairment of the central nervous system (CNS) in patients with DPN. Previous autopsy studies in people with diabetes have demonstrated diffuse degenerative lesions in the CNS, including demyelination and loss of axon cylinders in the posterior columns [29,30], degeneration of cortical neurons [31] and abnormalities in the midbrain and cerebellum [31,32] which have been described as diabetic myelopathy [30] and diabetic encephalopathy [32].

Studies that evaluated CNS function in people with diabetes using evoked potentials in response to stimulation of peripheral nerves, event-related potentials and neuropsychologic tests have yielded variable results as to the existence of spinal or supraspinal (central) conduction deficits or cognitive dysfunction; however, the author has shown that the degree of dysfunction along the somatosensory afferent pathways in patients with T1DM depends on the stage of peripheral neuropathy, is not related to the duration of diabetes or glycemic control and can be characterized by an alteration of the cortical sensory complex and peripheral rather than spinal or supraspinal conduction deficits [33]. Magnetic resonance imaging (MRI) showed an increased frequency of subcortical and brainstem lesions in patients with T1DM with DPN [34]. Moreover, patients with DPN showed a smaller cross-sectional chord area at C4/5 and T3/4 [35]. Using positron emission tomography (PET) and [^{18}F]-2-deoxy-2-fluoro-D-glucose (FDG), we have demonstrated reduced cerebral glucose metabolism in patients with T1DM with DPN as compared with newly diagnosed people with diabetes and healthy subjects (Figure 38.6) [36]. Spectroscopic measurement of brain metabolites such as N-acetyl aspartate (NAA) in the thalamus revealed a lower NAA : creatine ratio, suggesting thalamic neuro-

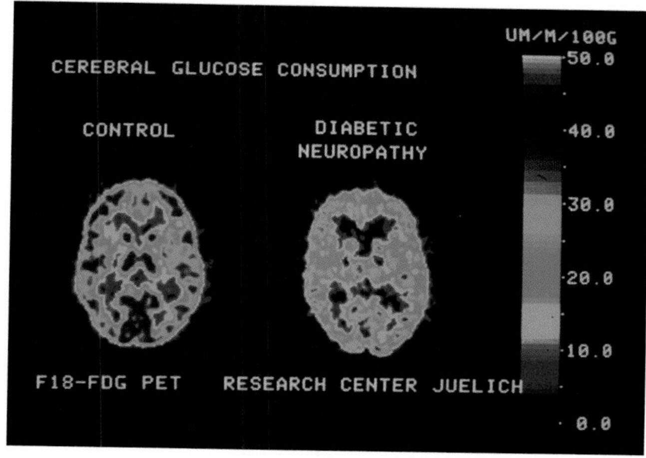

Figure 38.6 Positron emission tomography (PET) and [^{18}F]-2-deoxy-2-fluoro-D-glucose (FDG) showing reduced cerebral glucose metabolism in a patient with T1DM with polyneuropathy compared to a healthy subject.

nal dysfunction in DPN [37]. Thus, there is accumulating evidence suggesting that neuropathic involvement at central and spinal levels is a feature of DPN, but it is not clear whether these are primary or secondary events.

Pathogenetic mechanisms

Recent experimental studies suggest a multifactorial pathogenesis of diabetic neuropathy [38–40]. Most data have been generated in the diabetic rat model on the basis of which two approaches have been chosen to contribute to the clarification of the pathogenesis of diabetic neuropathy. First, it has been attempted to characterize the pathophysiologic, pathobiochemical and structural abnormalities that result in experimental diabetic neuropathy. Secondly, specific therapeutic interventions have been employed to prevent the development of these alterations, to halt their progression or to induce their regression despite concomitant hyperglycemia. At present, the following six pathogenetic mechanisms are being discussed which, in contrast to previous years, are no longer regarded as separate hypotheses, but as a complex interplay with multiple interactions between metabolic and vascular factors (see Chapter 35):

- Increased flux through the polyol pathway that leads to accumulation of sorbitol and fructose, *myo*-inositol depletion and reduction in Na^+-K^+-ATPase activity.
- Disturbances in n-6 essential fatty acid and prostaglandin metabolism which result in alterations of nerve membrane structure and microvascular and hemorrheologic abnormalities.
- Endoneural microvascular deficits with subsequent ischemia and hypoxia, generation of reactive oxygen species (oxidative stress), activation of the redox-sensitive transcription factor nuclear factor κB (NFκB), and increased activity of protein kinase C (PKC).
- Deficits in neurotrophism leading to reduced expression and depletion of neurotrophic factors such as nerve growth factor (NGF), neurotrophin-3, and insulin-like growth factor I (IGF-I) and alterations in axonal transport.
- Accumulation of non-enzymatic advanced glycation endproducts on nerve and/or vessel proteins.
- Immunologic processes with autoantibodies to vagal nerve, sympathetic ganglia and adrenal medulla as well as inflammatory changes.

From the clinical point of view it is important to note that, based on these pathogenetic mechanisms, therapeutic approaches could be derived, some of which have been evaluated in randomized clinical trials.

Diagnostic assessment

As a result of the increasing recognition of diabetic neuropathy as a major contributor to morbidity and the recent burst of clinical trials in this field, several consensus conferences have been convened to overcome the current problems that arise from the lack of agreement about the definition and diagnostic assessment of neuropathy. The Consensus Development Conference on Standardized Measures in Diabetic Neuropathy [41] recommended the following five measures to be employed in the diagnosis of diabetic neuropathy:

1 Clinical measures;
2 Morphologic and biochemical analyses;
3 Electrodiagnostic assessment;
4 Quantitative sensory testing; and
5 Autonomic nervous system testing.

Clinical measures

Clinical measures include:

1 General medical history and neurologic history;
2 Neurologic examination consisting of:
- Sensory (pain, light touch, vibration, position);
- Motor (graded as normal = 0, weak = 1–4 [25–100%]);
- Reflexes (present or absent); and
- Autonomic (bedside tests including heart rate variation during deep breathing and postural blood pressure response) examination.

The basic neurologic assessment comprises the general medical and neurologic history, inspection of the feet and neurologic examination of sensation using simple semi-quantitative bedside instruments such as the 10 g Semmes–Weinstein monofilament (Figure 38.7a), e.g. the Neuropen (touch) [42], NeuroQuick (Figure 38.7b) [43] or Tiptherm (temperature) [44], calibrated Rydel–Seiffer tuning fork (vibration) (Figure 38.7a), pinprick (pain) and tendon reflexes (knee and ankle). In addition, assessment of joint-position and motor power may be indicated. The normal range for the tuning fork on the dorsal distal joint of the great toe is ≥5/8 scale units in persons ≤20–40 years of age, ≥4.5/8 in those aged 41–60 years, ≥4/8 in individuals aged 61–71 years and ≥3/8 scale units in those aged 72–82 years [45]. An indicator test for the detection of sudomotor dysfunction is the Neuropad which assesses plantar sweat production by means of a color change from blue to pink. The patch contains the complex salt anhydrous cobalt-II-chloride. In the presence of water, this salt absorbs water molecules, normally changing its color from blue to pink. If the patch remains completely or partially blue within 10 minutes, the result is considered abnormal (Figure 38.7b) [46].

Clinical assessment should be standardized using validated scores for both the severity of symptoms and the degree of neuropathic deficits such as the Michigan Neuropathy Screening Instrument [47], Neuropathy Symptom Score for neuropathic symptoms and Neuropathy Disability Score for neuropathic deficits (impairments) [48] which appear to be sufficiently reproducible. The neurologic history and examination should be performed once a year. Minimum criteria for the clinical diagnosis of neuropathy according to the Neuropathy Symptom Score and Neuropathy Disability Score are:

- Moderate signs with or without symptoms; or
- Mild signs with moderate symptoms.

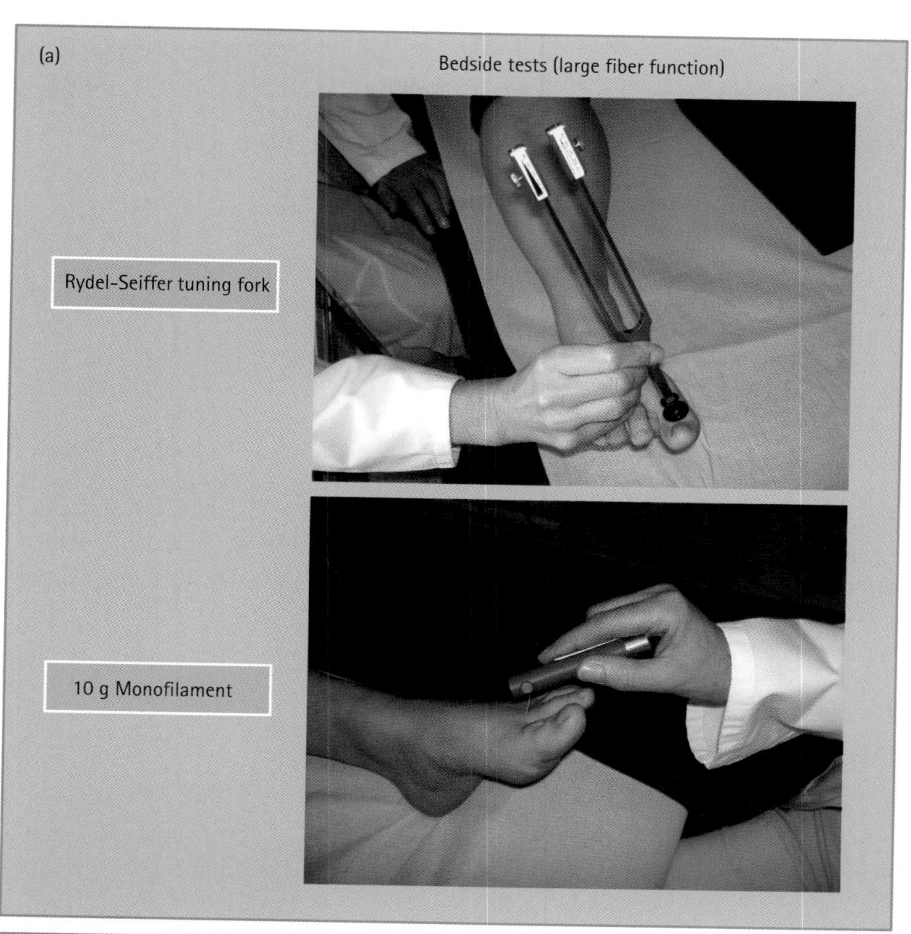

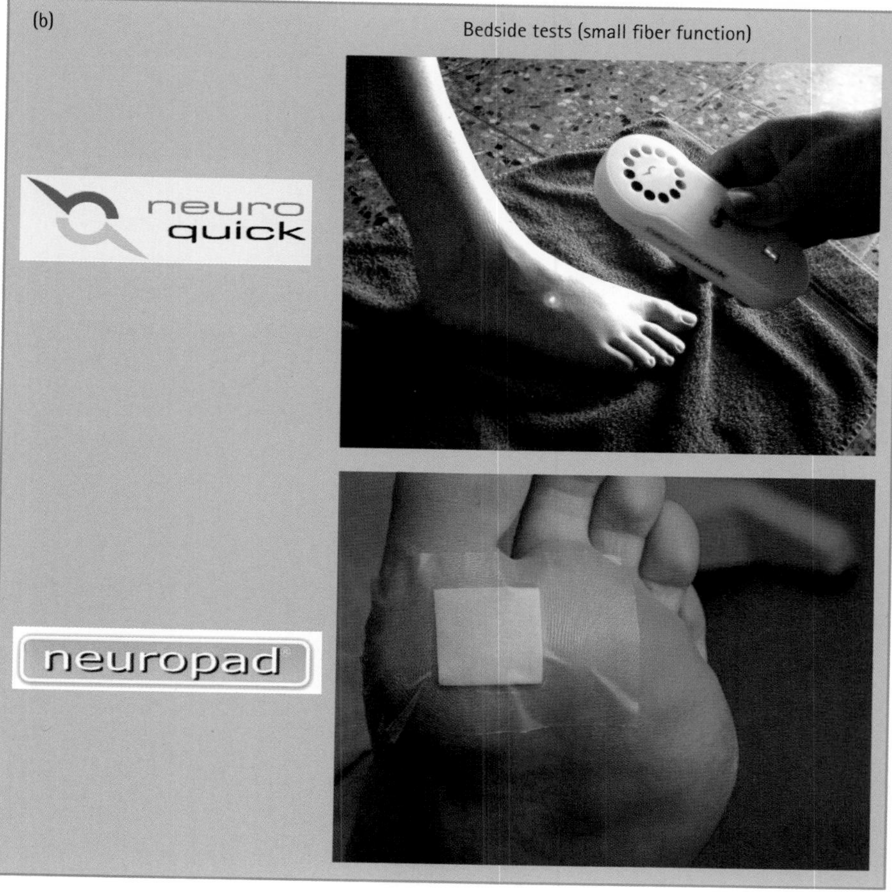

Figure 38.7 (a) Bedside tests for assessment of large fiber function. (b) Bedside tests for assessment of small fiber function.

This means that the exclusive presence of neuropathic symptoms without deficits is not sufficient to diagnose DPN. Therefore, early stages of DPN or a painful small-fiber neuropathy without or with minimal deficits can only be verified using more sophisticated tests such as thermal thresholds or skin biopsy.

The intensity (severity) of neuropathic pain and its course should be assessed using an 11-point numerical rating scale (Likert scale) or a visual analog scale. Various screening tools (with or without limited bedside testing) have been developed to identify neuropathic pain such as the PainDetect, LANSS, NPQ, DN-4, ID-Pain). These questionnaires use verbal descriptors and pain qualities as a basis for distinguishing neuropathic pain from other types of chronic pain such as nociceptive pain [49].

The following findings should alert the physician to consider causes for DPN other than diabetes and referral for a detailed neurologic work-up:

- Pronounced asymmetry of the neurologic deficits;
- Predominant motor deficits, mononeuropathy, cranial nerve involvement;
- Rapid development or progression of the neuropathic impairments;
- Progression of the neuropathy despite optimal glycemic control;
- Symptoms predominantly in the upper limbs;
- Family history of non-diabetic neuropathy; or
- Diagnosis of DPN cannot be ascertained by clinical examination.

The most important differential diagnoses from the general medicine perspective include neuropathies caused by alcohol abuse, uremia, hypothyroidism, vitamin B_{12} deficiency, peripheral arterial disease, paraneoplastic syndromes, inflammatory and infectious diseases and neurotoxic drugs.

Clinical measures are used to:

- Establish the presence or absence of neurologic dysfunction in diabetes;

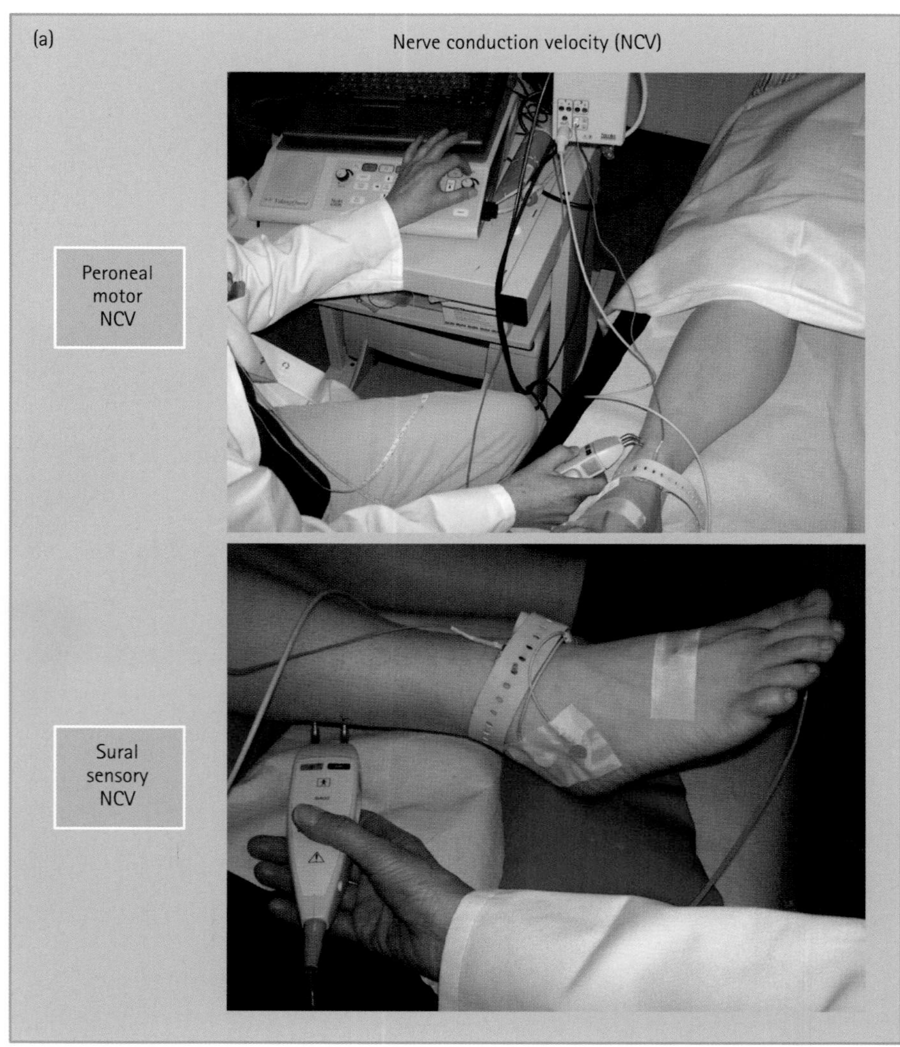

Figure 38.8 (a) Measurement of motor and sensory nerve conduction velocity.

- Exclude non-neuropathic causes of neurologic dysfunction;
- Eliminate non-diabetic causes of neuropathy;
- Distinguish and classify the different forms of diabetic neuropathy; and
- Monitor progression and provide a clinical correlate of outcome in trials.

The limitations to clinical measures include:

- Lack of sensitivity to change once they become abnormal; and
- Limited reliability and reproducibility.

Positive symptoms may reflect different pathophysiology than deficits (i.e. pain or paresthesia may be related to the degree of compensatory regeneration rather than to the degree of nerve fiber damage). Hence, it has been suggested that symptom or pain scores should not be used to evaluate overall presence or progression of diabetic neuropathy but only to assess pain severity [41].

Electrodiagnostic measures

Electrophysiologic techniques have the advantage of being the most objective, sensitive, specific and reproducible methods that are available in many neurophysiologic laboratories worldwide (Figure 38.8).

Electrodiagnostic measures have also limitations in as much as they:

- Measure only function in the largest fastest conducting myelinated fibers;
- Have relatively low specificity in detecting diabetic neuropathy;
- Show relatively high intra-individual variability for certain variables (amplitudes);
- Are vulnerable to external factors such as electrode locations or limb temperature; and
- Provide only indirect information about symptoms and deficits [41].

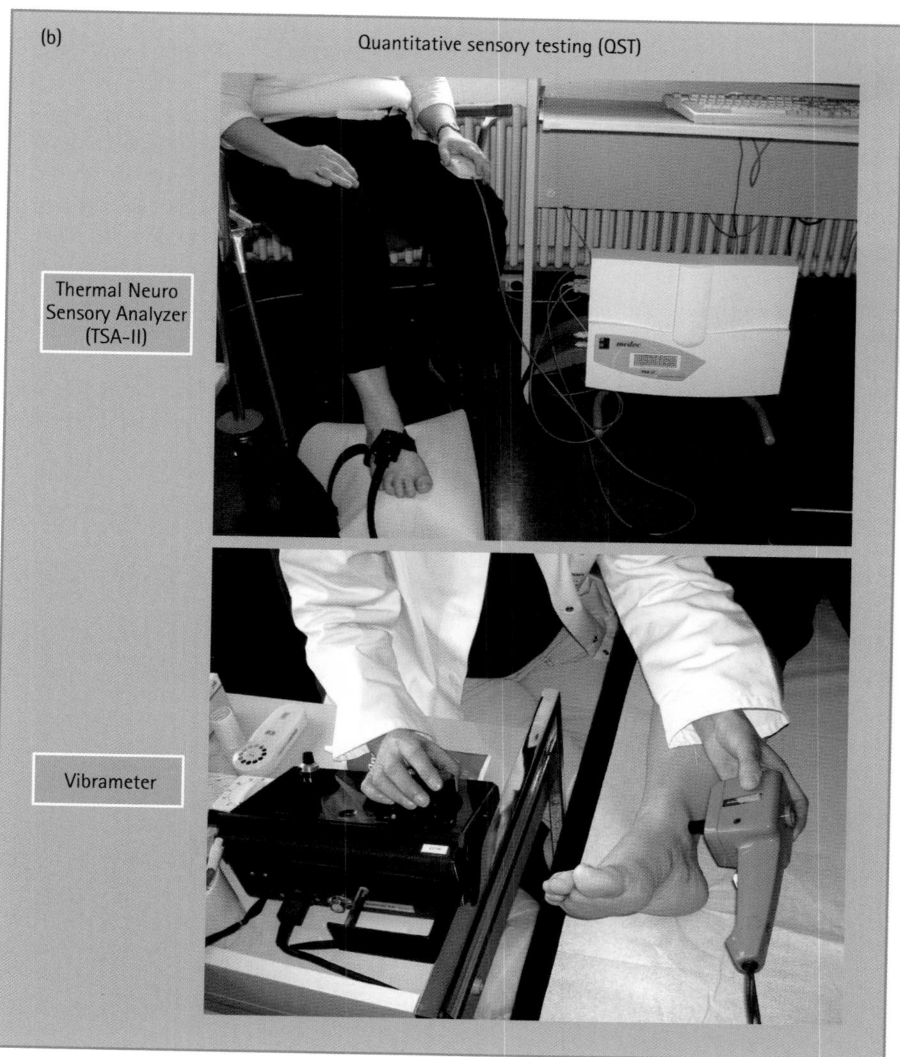

Figure 38.8 (b) Quantitative sensory testing.

Quantitative sensory testing

Quantitative sensory testing (QST) is the "determination of the absolute sensory threshold, defined as the minimal energy reliably detected for a particular modality." The Peripheral Nerve Society has recommended that detection thresholds of touch-pressure, vibration (Figure 38.8b), coolness, warmth (Figure 38.8b), heat pain, cold pain and mechanical pain be used to characterize cutaneous sensation [50].

The procedures that are being used for QST include:

- The method of limits (continuous increase or decrease in intensity to appearance or disappearance threshold);
- Threshold tracking (combination of appearance or disappearance threshold);
- Titration method (graded steps to appearance and disappearance threshold); and
- Two-alternative forced-choice method (pairs of stimulus and null-stimulus phases) [50].

The advantages of QST techniques are that they:

- Are highly sensitive, relatively simple, non-invasive and non-aversive;
- Afford precise control over stimulus intensity and testing algorithms;
- Contribute to differentiation of the relative deficit in small vs large fibers; and
- Are particularly valuable in screening large populations or in longitudinal trials.

The limitations to QST procedures include that they:

- Constitute psychophysical methods vulnerable to the effects of alertness, mood, concentration, ambient noise, etc.;
- Show a relatively high intra-individual variability;
- Have not been adequately standardized; and
- May be time-consuming (forced-choice methods), which may lead to a decline in concentration or boredom in the person tested and thereby result in diagnostic errors [41].

The method of limits has been criticized, because it may be associated with a response delay caused by reaction time which may vary between subjects, but it has been demonstrated that this approach yields a degree of sensitivity and reliability that is similar to the forced-choice techniques. The reproducibility of the QST indices is less favorable than that of nerve conduction but still in an acceptable range.

Morphologic assessment

Sural nerve biopsy

Sural nerve biopsy does not represent a routine method in the diagnosis of diabetic neuropathy. It may be used to establish the diagnosis when the etiology of the neuropathy is in doubt (Figure 38.9). The limitations to this technique are that the information from the biopsy is of no direct benefit to the patient and that the procedure is associated with a certain morbidity and may result in complications [41].

Skin biopsy

Skin biopsy has become a widely used tool to investigate small caliber sensory nerves including somatic unmyelinated intra-epidermal nerve fibers (IENF), dermal myelinated nerve fibers and autonomic nerve fibers in peripheral neuropathies and other conditions (Figure 38.10). Different techniques for tissue processing and nerve fiber evaluation have been used. A task force of the European Federation of Neurological Societies recently developed guidelines on the use of skin biopsy in the diagnosis of peripheral neuropathies [51]. For diagnostic purposes in peripheral neuropathies, the guideline recommends performing a 3-mm punch skin biopsy at the distal leg and quantifying the linear density of IENF in at least three 50-mum thick sections per biopsy, fixed in 2% periodate-lysine-paraformaldehyde (PLP) or Zamboni solution, by bright-field immunohistochemistry or immunofluorescence with antiprotein gene product 9.5 anti-

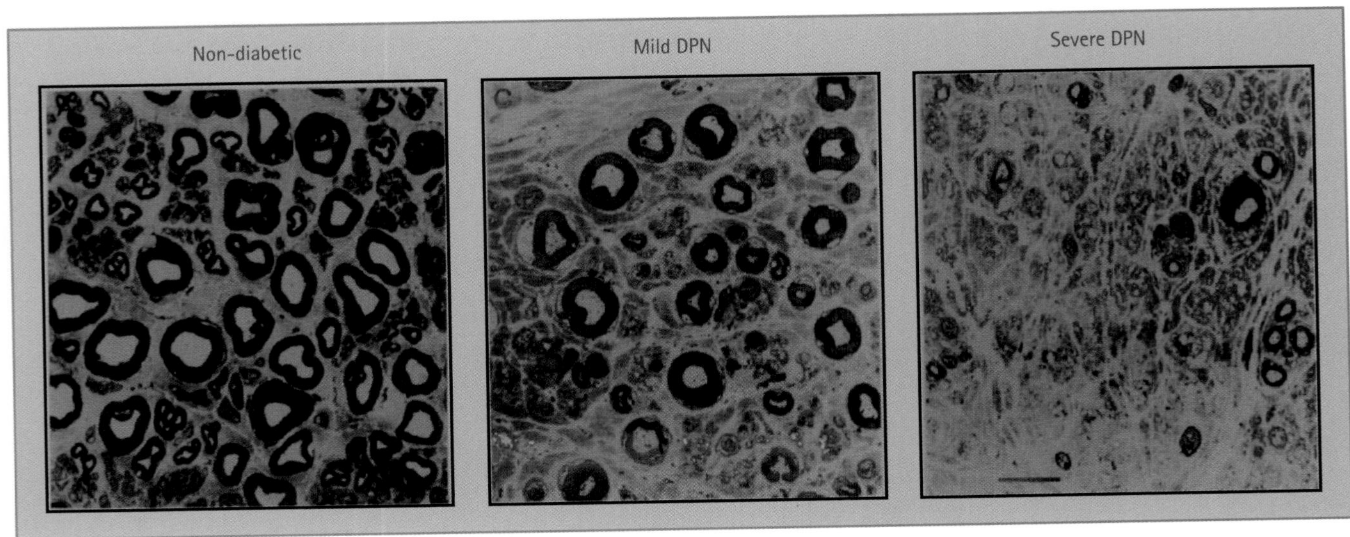

Figure 38.9 Normal sural nerve pathology (left panel) compared to mild (mid panel) and severe (right panel) axonal loss in mild and severe diabetic polyneuropathy (DPN). Copyright 1990 American Diabetes Association. Reproduced from *Diabetes* 1990; **39**:898–908, with permission from the American Diabetes Association.

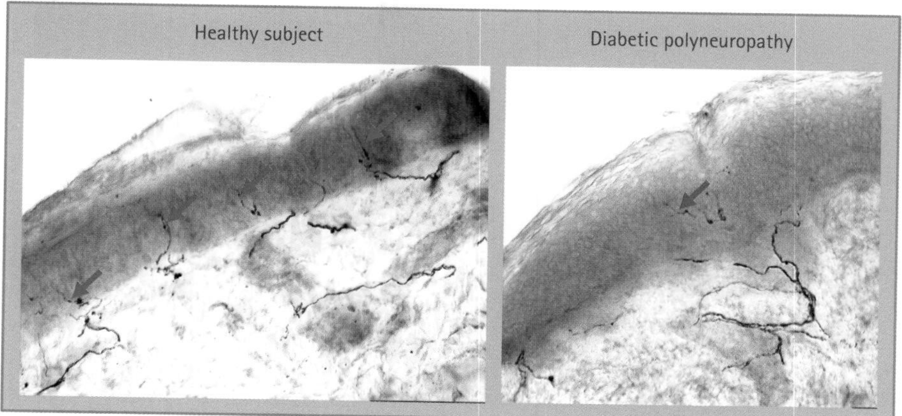

Figure 38.10 Loss of intra-epidermal nerve fibers (IENF) in skin biopsy from the lateral lower leg in a patient with diabetic polyneuropathy compared to a healthy subject (red arrows indicate IENF). Bright-field immunohistochemistry with antiprotein gene product 9.5 antibody (PGP 9.5).

bodies (level A recommendation). Quantification of IENF density closely correlated with warm and heat pain threshold, and appeared more sensitive than sensory nerve conduction study and sural nerve biopsy in diagnosing small-fiber sensory neuropathy. Diagnostic efficiency and predictive values of this technique were very high (level A recommendation). Longitudinal studies of IENF density and regeneration rate are warranted to correlate neuropathologic changes with progression of neuropathy and to assess the potential usefulness of skin biopsy as an outcome measure in peripheral neuropathy trials (level B recommendation). In conclusion, punch skin biopsy is a safe and reliable technique (level A recommendation).

Treatment

Role of intensive diabetes therapy in treatment and prevention of diabetic neuropathy

Several long-term prospective studies that assessed the effects intensive diabetes therapy on the prevention and progression of chronic diabetic complications have been published. The large randomized trials such as the Diabetes Control and Complications Trial (DCCT) and UK Prospective Diabetes Study (UKPDS) were not designed to evaluate the effects of intensive diabetes therapy on DPN, but rather to study the influence of such treatment on the development and progression of the chronic diabetic complications [52,53]. Thus, only a minority of the patients enrolled in these studies had symptomatic DPN at entry.

Studies in patients with T1DM show that intensive diabetes therapy retards but does not completely prevent the development of DPN. In the Epidemiology of Diabetes Interventions and Complications (EDIC) study, the benefits of 6.5 years of intensive therapy on neuropathy status extended for at least 8 years beyond the end of the DCCT despite equal HbA_{1c} levels (hyperglycemic memory), similar to the findings described for diabetic retinopathy and nephropathy [54]. In patients with T1DM with most advanced stages of peripheral neuropathy, the progression of nerve conduction deficits is halted after 3–4 years of normoglycemia following pancreatic transplantation, but no effect is seen in autonomic neuropathy. Although observational studies suggested a glycemic threshold for the development and progression of the long-term complications in T1DM, the DCCT data do not support such an assumption. Thus, attempts to achieve optimal glycemic control should not aim at a certain HbA_{1c} threshold within the diabetic range but follow the goal of achieving normal glycemia as early as possible in as many patients with T1DM as is safely possible. In general, intensive diabetes therapy is associated with a moderately increased risk of weight gain and hypoglycemia.

In contrast, in patients with T2DM, who represent the vast majority of people with diabetes, the results were largely negative. The UKPDS showed a lower rate of impaired VPT (VPT > 25 V) after 15 years for intensive vs conventional therapy (31 vs 52%), but the only additional time point at which VPT reached a significant difference between intensive and conventional therapy was the 9-year follow-up, whereas the rates after 3, 6 and 12 years did not differ between the groups. Likewise, the rates of absent knee and ankle reflexes as well as the heart rate responses to deep breathing did not differ between the groups [53]. In the ADVANCE study, which included 11 140 patients with T2DM randomly assigned to either standard glucose control or intensive glucose control, the relative risk reduction (95% confidence interval [CI]) for new or worsening neuropathy for intensive vs. standard glucose control after a median of 5 years of follow-up was 4% (−10% to 2%), without a significant difference between the groups [55]. Likewise, in the Veterans Affairs Diabetes Trial (VADT) [56] study including 1791 military veterans (mean age 60.4 years) who had a suboptimal response to therapy for T2DM, after a median follow-up of 5.6 years, no differences between the two groups on intensive or standard glucose control were observed for DPN or microvascular complications.

In the Steno 2 study, intensified multifactorial risk intervention including intensive diabetes treatment, angiotensin-converting enzyme (ACE) inhibitors, antioxidants, statins, aspirin and smoking cessation in patients with microalbuminuria did not have an effect on the progression of DPN after 3.8 years but on other microvascular complications such as diabetic nephropathy and retinopathy were beneficially affected. A positive effect of this approach was seen on autonomic neuropathy (increase in heart rate variability) only. After 7.8 (range 6.9–8.8) years, the same results were reported with a relative risk of 1.09 (95% CI 0.54–2.22) for the development or progression of DPN ($P = 0.66$) and 0.37 (95% CI 0.18–0.79) for autonomic neuropathy ($P = 0.002$) and again at 13.3 years, after the patients were subsequently followed observationally for a mean of 5.5 years. Autonomic neuropathy progressed in 39 patients in the intensive therapy group and in 52 patients in the conventional therapy group (relative risk 0.53; 95% CI 0.34–0.81; $P = 0.004$), and peripheral neuropathy progressed in 44 and 46 patients in the two groups, respectively (relative risk 0.97; 95% CI 0.62–1.51; $P = 0.89$) [57]. Thus, there is no evidence that intensive diabetes therapy or a target-driven intensified intervention aimed at multiple risk factors favorably influence the development or progression of DPN in patients with T2DM.

Treatment based on pathogenetic concepts

Recent experimental studies suggest a multifactorial pathogenesis of diabetic neuropathy. From the clinical point of view it is important to note that, based on the various pathogenetic mechanisms, several therapeutic approaches could be developed, some of which have been evaluated in randomized clinical trials including the aldose reductase inhibitors (alrestatin, sorbinil, ponalrestat, tolrestat, epalrestat, zopolrestat, zenarestat, fidarestat, ranirestat), the antioxidant α-lipoic acid (thioctic acid), essential fatty acid (γ-linolenic acid), ACE inhibitors (trandolapril), prostacyclin (PGI_2) analogs (iloprost, beraprost), prostaglandin derivatives (PGE_1 αCD), NGF, PKCβ inhibitor (ruboxistaurin), C-peptide, vascular endothelial growth factor and benfotiamine (vitamin B_1 derivative) [58]. These drugs have been designed to influence the underlying neuropathic process in a favorable manner, rather than for symptomatic pain treatment. Because, in the foreseeable future, normoglycemia will not be achievable in the majority of people with diabetes, the advantage of the aforementioned treatment approaches is that they may exert their effects despite prevailing hyperglycemia. Experimental studies of low-dose combined drug treatment suggest enhanced drug efficacy mediated by facilitatory interactions between drugs. Although considerable improvement in the quality of controlled trials has recently been achieved, no major breakthrough in slowing the progression of diabetic neuropathy in the long run has been achieved with drugs used on the basis of present pathogenetic concepts. Some of the newer drugs have shown promising results in phase II trials which require confirmation from large phase III trials. It is conceivable that drugs interfering with the pathogenesis of diabetic neuropathy may be most effective in terms of prevention, rather than intervention.

Only α-lipoic acid and benfotiamine are licensed for clinical use to treat symptomatic DPN in several countries, while epalrestat is marketed in Japan and India. The available evidence to support the use of benfotiamine in DPN is weak [59,60]. In contrast, according to a meta-analysis comprising 1258 patients, infusions of α-lipoic acid (600 mg/day IV) ameliorated neuropathic symptoms and deficits after 3 weeks [61]. Moreover, the SYDNEY 2 trial suggests that treatment for 5 weeks using 600 mg α-lipoic acid orally four times daily reduces the chief symptoms of DPN including pain, paresthesias and numbness to a clinically meaningful degree [62]. In a multicenter randomized double-masked parallel-group clinical trial (NATHAN 1), 460 patients with stage 1 or stage 2a DPN were randomly assigned to oral treatment with 600 mg α-lipoic acid four times daily (n = 233) or placebo (n = 227) for 4 years. After 4 years, some neuropathic deficits and symptoms, but not nerve conduction velocity, were improved, and the drug was well tolerated throughout the trial [63]. Clinical and post-marketing surveillance studies have revealed a highly favorable safety profile [64].

Pharmacologic treatment of painful neuropathy

Painful symptoms in DPN constitute a considerable management problem. The efficacy of a single therapeutic agent is not the rule, and simple analgesics are usually inadequate to control the pain. There is agreement that patients should be offered the available therapies in a stepwise fashion [65–68]. Effective pain treatment considers a favorable balance between pain relief and side effects without implying a maximum effect. The following general considerations in the pharmacotherapy of neuropathic pain require attention:

- The appropriate and effective drug has to be tried and identified in each patient by carefully titrating the dosage based on efficacy and side effects.
- Lack of efficacy should be judged only after 2–4 weeks of treatment using an adequate dose.
- Because the evidence from clinical trials suggests only a maximum response of ≈50% for any monotherapy, analgesic combinations may be useful.
- Potential drug interactions have to be considered given the frequent use of polypharmacy in people with diabetes.

A rational treatment algorithm including the various causal and symptomatic options is summarized in Table 38.2. Certain antidepressants (tricyclic drugs, duloxetine) and anticonvulsants (pregabalin, gabapentin) are considered as first-line treatments, while opioids are recommended as second-line options [66]. The advantages and disadvantages of the various drugs and drug classes used for treatment of painful diabetic neuropathy under consideration of the various co-morbidities and complications associated with diabetes are summarized in Table 38.3. Prior to any decision regarding appropriate treatment, the diagnosis of the underlying neuropathic manifestation allowing the estimatation of its natural history should be established. In contrast to the agents that have been derived from the pathogenetic mechanisms of diabetic neuropathy, those used for symptomatic therapy were designed to modulate the pain, without favorably influencing the underlying neuropathy.

The relative benefit of an active treatment over placebo treatment in clinical trials is usually expressed as the relative risk, the relative risk reduction or the odds ratio; however, to estimate the extent of a therapeutic effect (i.e. pain relief) that can be translated into clinical practice, it is useful to apply a simple measure that serves the physician to select the appropriate treatment for

Table 38.2 Treatment options for painful diabetic neuropathy.

Approach	Compound/measure	Dose per day	Remarks	NNT
Optimal diabetes control	Lifestyle modification, OAD, insulin	Individual adaptation	Aim: HbA_{1c} ≤6.5% (48 mmol/mol)	–
Pathogenetically oriented treatment	α-Lipoic acid (thioctic acid)‡	600 mg IV infusion	Duration: 3 weeks	6.3*
		1200–1800 mg orally	Favorable safety profile	2.8–4.2*
Symptomatic treatment	First line TCA			
	Amitriptyline	(10–)25–150 mg	NNMH: 15	2.1
	Desipramine	(10–)25–150 mg	NNMH: 24	2.2/3.2
	Imipramine	(10–)25–150 mg	CRR	1.3/2.4/3.0
	Clomipramine	(10–)25–150 mg	NNMH: 8.7	2.1
	Nortriptyline	(10–)25–150 mg	plus fluphenazine	1.2†
	SNRI			
	Duloxetine§	60–120 mg	NNT with 120 mg, 60 mg	5.3, 4.9
	Anticonvulsants-calcium channel modulators (α2-δ ligands)			
	Gabapentin	900–3600 mg	High dose	3.8/4.0
	Pregabalin§	300–600 mg	NNT with 600 mg, 300 mg	5.9, 4.2
	Second line weak opioids			
	Tramadol	50–400 mg	NNMH: 7.8	3.1/4.3
	Local treatment			
	Capsaicin (0.025%) cream	q.i.d. topically	Max. duration: 6–8 weeks	5.7
Pain resistant to standard pharmacotherapy	Strong opioids			
	Oxycodone		Add-on treatment	2.6
	ESCS		Invasive, specialist required	

CRR, concentration–response relationship; ESCS, electrical spinal cord stimulation; NNMH, number needed for major harm; NNT, number needed to treat; ns: not significant; OAD, oral antidiabetic drugs; TCA, tricyclic antidepressants; TENS, transcutaneous electrical nerve stimulation; SNRI, selective serotonin norepinephrine reuptake inhibitors.

*≥50% symptom relief after 3 and 5 weeks.

†Combined with fluphenazine.

‡Available only in some countries.

§Licensed in USA and EU.

Table 38.3 Differential treatment of painful neuropathy considering frequent co-morbidities and side-effects.

	Duloxetine	Pregabalin	Tricyclics	Opioids	α-Lipoic acid
Depression	+	n	+	n	n
Obesity	n	–	–	n	n
Generalized anxiety disorder	+	+	na	na	na
Sleep disturbances	+	+	+	+	na
Coronary heart disease	n	n	–	n	n
Autonomic neuropathy	na	na	–	–	+
Fasting glucose	(–)	n	–	n	n*
Hepatic failure	–	n	†	†	n
Renal failure	–	Adapt dose	†	†	n
Drug interactions	–	n	–	n	n

Effect: +, favorable; –, unfavorable; n, neutral; na, not available.

*Slight decrease possible.

†Dependent on individual agent.

the individual patient. Such a practical measure is the number needed to treat (NNT; i.e. the number of patients that need to be treated with a particular therapy to observe a clinically relevant effect or adverse event in one patient). This measure is expressed as the reciprocal of the absolute risk reduction (i.e. the difference between the proportion of events in the control group [Pc] and the proportion of events in the intervention group [Pi]: NNT = 1/[*Pc–Pi*]). The 95% CI of NNT can be obtained from the reciprocal value of the 95% CI for the absolute risk reduction. The NNT and number needed to harm (NNH) for the individual agents used in the treatment of painful diabetic neuropathy are given in Table 38.2. Some authors have cautioned that summary NNT estimates may have limited clinical relevance, because of problems of heterogeneity. The most that can be extracted from systematic reviews published to date is the identity of drugs that have demonstrated efficacy for specific types of neuropathic pain, and the strength of such evidence [69].

Tricyclic antidepressants

Psychotropic agents, among which tricyclic antidepressants (TCAs) have been evaluated most extensively, constitute an important component in the treatment of chronic pain syndromes for more than 30 years. Putative mechanisms of pain relief by antidepressants include the inhibition of norepinephrine and/or serotonin reuptake at synapses of central descending pain control systems and the antagonism of the *N*-methyl-D-aspartate receptor that mediates hyperalgesia and allodynia. Imipramine, amitriptyline and clomipramine induce a balanced reuptake inhibition of both norepinephrine and serotonin, while desipramine is a relatively selective norepinephrine inhibitor. The NNT (CI) for a ≥50% pain relief by TCAs is 2.4 (2.0–3.0) [65]. The NNH is 2.8 for minor adverse events and 19 for major adverse events (Table 38.2). Thus, among 100 patients with diabetes and neuropathic pain who are treated with antidepressants, 30 will experience pain relief by >50%, 30 will have mild adverse events and five will discontinue treatment because of severe adverse events. The mean NNT for drugs with balanced reuptake inhibition is 2.2, while it is 3.6 for the noradrenergic agents [65].

The most frequent adverse events of TCAs include tiredness and dry mouth. The starting dose should be 25 mg (10 mg in frail patients) and taken as a single night time dose 1 hour before sleep. It should be increased by 25 mg at weekly intervals until pain relief is achieved or adverse events occur. The maximum dose is usually 150 mg/day.

The notion that the character of the neuropathic pain is predictive of response, so that burning pain should be treated with antidepressants and shooting pain with anticonvulsants, is obviously unfounded because both pain qualities respond to TCAs. Most evidence of efficacy of antidepressants comes from studies that have been conducted over only several weeks, but many patients continue to achieve pain relief for months to years, although this is not true for everybody. TCAs should be used with caution in patients with orthostatic hypotension and are contraindicated in patients with unstable angina, recent (<6 months) MI, heart failure, history of ventricular arrhythmias, significant conduction system disease and long QT syndrome. Several authors consider TCAs to be the drug treatment of choice for neuropathic pain [65,70], but their use is limited by relative high rates of adverse events and several contraindications. Thus, there is a need for agents that exert efficacy equal to or better than that achieved with TCAs but with a more favorable side effect profile.

Selective serotonin reuptake inhibitors (SSRI)

Because of the relative high rates of adverse effects and several contraindications of TCA, it has been reasoned that patients who do not tolerate them because of adverse events could alternatively be treated with selective serotonin reuptake inhibitors (SSRI). SSRIs specifically inhibit presynaptic reuptake of serotonin, but not norepinephrine, and unlike the tricyclics they lack the postsynaptic receptor blocking effects and quinidine-like membrane stabilization. Only weak or no effects on neuropathic pain were observed after treatment with fluoxetine, paroxetine, citalopram and escitalopram [65,71]. Because of these limited efficacy data, SSRIs have not been licensed for the treatment of neuropathic pain.

Serotonin noradrenaline reuptake inhibitors (SNRI)

Because SSRI have been found to be less effective than TCAs, recent interest has focused on antidepressants with dual selective inhibition of serotonin and noradrenaline such as duloxetine and venlafaxine. The efficacy and safety of duloxetine was evaluated in three controlled studies using a dose of 60 and 120 mg/day over 12 weeks [72]. In all three studies, the average 24-hour pain intensity was significantly reduced with both doses compared with placebo treatment, the difference between active and placebo being achieving statistical significance after 1 week. The response rates defined as ≥50% pain reduction were 48.2% (120 mg/day), 47.2% (60 mg/day) and 27.9% (placebo), giving a NNT of 4.9 (95% CI 3.6–7.6) for 120 mg/day and 5.3 (3.8–8.3) for 60 mg/day. Pain severity, but not variables related to diabetes or neuropathy, predicts the effects of duloxetine in diabetic peripheral neuropathic pain. Patients with higher pain intensity tend to respond better than those with lower pain levels [73]. The most frequent side effects of duloxetine (60/120 mg/day) include nausea (16.7/27.4%), somnolence (20.2/28.3%), dizziness (9.6/23%), constipation 14.9/10.6%), dry mouth (7.1/15%) and reduced appetite (2.6/12.4%). These adverse events are usually mild to moderate and transient. To minimize them, the starting dose should be 30 mg/day for 4–5 days. In contrast to TCAs and some anticonvulsants, duloxetine does not cause weight gain, but a small increase in fasting blood glucose may occur [74].

In a 6-week trial comprising 244 patients, the analgesic response rates were 56%, 39% and 34% in patients given 150–225 mg venlafaxine, 75 mg venlafaxine and placebo, respectively. Because patients with depression were excluded, the effect of venlafaxin (150–225 mg) was attributed to an analgesic, rather than antidepressant, effect. The most common adverse events were tiredness and nausea [75]. Duloxetine, but not venlafaxine, has been licensed for the treatment of painful diabetic neuropathy.

Anticonvulsants

Calcium channel modulators (α2-δ ligands)

Gabapentin is an anticonvulsant structurally related to γ-aminobutyric acid (GABA), a neurotransmitter that has a role in pain transmission and modulation. The exact mechanisms of action of this drug in neuropathic pain are not fully elucidated. Among others, they involve an interaction with the system L-amino acid transporter and high affinity binding to the α2-δ subunit of voltage-activated calcium channels. In an 8-week multicenter dose-escalation trial including 165 patients with painful diabetic neuropathy, 60% of the patients on gabapentin (3600 mg/day achieved in 67%) had at least moderate pain relief compared to 33% on placebo. Dizziness and somnolence were the most frequent adverse events in about 23% of the patients each [76]. Pregabalin is a more specific α2-δ ligand with a sixfold higher binding affinity than gabapentin. The efficacy and safety of pregabalin was reported in a pooled analysis of 6 studies over 5–11 weeks in 1346 patients with painful diabetic neuropathy. The response rates defined as ≥50% pain reduction were 46% (600 mg/day), 39% (300 mg/day), 27% (150 mg/day) and 22% (placebo), giving a NNT of 4.2, 5.9 and 20.0 [33]. The most frequent side effects for 150–600 mg/day are dizziness (22.0%), somnolence (12.1%), peripheral edema (10.0%), headache (7.2%) and weight gain (5.4%) [77]. The evidence supporting a favorable effect in painful diabetic neuropathy is more solid and dose titration is considerably easier for pregabalin than gabapentin.

Sodium channel blockers

Although carbamazepine has been widely used for treating neuropathic pain, it cannot be recommended in painful diabetic neuropathy as there are very limited data. Its successor drug, oxcarbazepine [78,79] as well as other sodium channel blockers such as valproate, mexiletine, topiramate [80] and lamotrigine [81] showed only marginal efficacy and have not been licensed for the treatment of painful diabetic neuropathy.

A single IV infusion of lidocaine (5 mg/kg body weight over 30 minutes during continuous ECG monitoring) resulted in a significant pain relief after 1 and 8 days in a controlled study including 15 patients with chronic painful diabetic neuropathy [82]. Potential adverse systemic effects associated with IV lidocaine have led to the development of a newer and potentially safer agent, the topical lidocaine patch 5% (Lidoderm), a targeted peripheral analgesic. In patients with post-herpetic neuralgia, the lidocaine patch 5% has demonstrated relief of pain and tactile allodynia with a minimal risk of systemic adverse effects or drug–drug interactions [83]. Studies in patients with DPN are underway.

Lacosamide

Lacosamide is a novel anticonvulsant that selectively enhances the slow inactivation of voltage dependent sodium channels but, in contrast to the sodium channel blockers, does not influence the fast sodium channel inactivation. Its second putative mechanism is an interaction with a neuronal cytosolic protein, the collapsin response mediator protein 2 which has an important role in nerve sprouting and excitotoxicity. Lacosamide has been evaluated in several studies in painful diabetic neuropathy [84], but the drug has not been approved by the Food and Drug Administration (FDA) and the European Medicines Agency (EMEA) for painful diabetic neuropathy; further clinical trials may follow.

Topical capsaicin

Capsaicin (trans-8-methyl-*N*-vanillyl-6-nonenamide) is an alkaloid and the most pungent ingredient in the red pepper. It depletes tissues of substance P and reduces neurogenic plasma extravasation, the flare response and chemically induced pain. Substance P is present in afferent neurones innervating skin, mainly in polymodal nociceptors, and is considered the primary neurotransmitter of painful stimuli from the periphery to the central nervous system. Several studies have demonstrated significant pain reduction and improvement in quality of life in patients with painful diabetic neuropathy after 8 weeks of treatment with capsaicin cream (0.075%) [85]. It has been criticized that a double-blind design is not feasible for topical capsaicin because of the transient local hyperalgesia (usually mild burning sensation >50% of the cases), it may produce as a typical adverse event. Treatment should be restricted to a maximum of 8 weeks, as during this period no adverse effects on sensory function (brought about by the mechanism of action) were noted in patients with diabetes.

Opioids

Tramadol acts directly via opioid receptors and indirectly via monoaminergic receptor systems. Because the development of tolerance and dependence during long-term tramadol treatment is uncommon and its abuse liability appears to be low, it is an alternative to strong opioids in neuropathic pain. In painful diabetic neuropathy, tramadol (up to 400 mg/day orally, mean dose: 210 mg/day orally) has been studied in a 6-week multicenter trial including 131 patients [86]. Pain relief was 44% on tramadol vs 12% on placebo. The most frequent adverse events were nausea and constipation. The NNH of 7.8 for drop-outs because of adverse events was relatively low, indicating significant toxicity. In a 4-week study including patients with painful neuropathy of different origins, one-third of which being diabetes, tramadol significantly relieved pain (NNT 4.3 [2.4–20]) and mechanical allodynia. One conceivable mechanism for the favorable effect of tramadol could be a hyperpolarization of post-synaptic neurons via post-synaptic opioid receptors. Alternatively, the reduction in central hyperexcitability by tramadol could be from a monoaminergic or a combined opioid and monoaminergic effect.

Most severe pain requires administration of strong opioids such as oxycodone. Although there are few data available on combination treatment, combinations of different substance classes have to be used in patients with pain resistant to monotherapy. Several add-on trials have demonstrated significant pain relief and improvement in quality of life following treatment with controlled-release oxycodone, a pure μ-agonist in patients with painful DPN whose pain was not adequately controlled on standard treatment with antidepressants and anticonvulsants [87–89]. As expected, adverse events were frequent and typical of opioid-related side effects. A cross-over study examined the maximum tolerable dose of a combination treatment of gabapentin and morphine compared to monotherapy of each drug. The maximum tolerable dose was significantly lower and efficacy was better during combination therapy than with monotherapy, suggesting an additive interaction between the two drugs [90]. The results of these studies suggest that opioids should be included among the therapeutic options for painful DPN, provided that careful selection of patients unresponsive to standard treatments, regular monitoring, appropriate dose titration and management of possible opioid-specific problems (analgesic misuse or addiction, tolerance, opioid-induced hyperalgesia) are ensured. Recent recommendations have emphasized the need for clinical skills in risk assessment and management as a prerequisite to safe and effective opioid prescribing [66]. Treatment of painful DPN with opioid agonists should generally be reserved for patients who have failed to respond to or cannot tolerate the first-line medications.

Although several novel analgesic drugs have recently been introduced into clinical practice, the pharmacologic treatment of chronic painful diabetic neuropathy remains a challenge for the physician. Individual tolerability remains a major aspect in any treatment decision. Little information is available from controlled trials on long-term analgesic efficacy, head-to-head comparisons of individual analgesics, and only a few studies have used drug combinations. Combination drug use or the addition of a new drug to a therapeutic regimen may lead to increased efficacy. In future, drug combinations may include those drugs aimed at symptomatic pain relief and quality of life with those aimed at improvement or slowing of the progression of the underlying neuropathic process.

Non-pharmacologic treatment of painful neuropathy

Because there is no entirely satisfactory pharmacotherapy of painful diabetic neuropathy, non-pharmacologic treatment options should always be considered. As for the pharmacologic treatment, considerable efforts must also be made to develop effective non-pharmacologic approaches. A recent systematic review assessed the evidence from rigorous clinical trials and meta-analyses of complementary and alternative therapies for treating neuropathic and neuralgic pain. Data on the following complementary and alternative medicine treatments were identified: acupuncture, electrostimulation, herbal medicine, magnets, dietary supplements, imagery and spiritual healing. The conclusion was that the evidence is not fully convincing for most complementary and alternative medicine modalities in relieving neuropathic or neuralgic pain. The evidence can be classified as encouraging and warrants further study for cannabis extract, magnets, carnitine and electrostimulation [91].

Psychologic support

A psychologic component to pain should not be underestimated. Hence, an explanation to the patient that even severe pain may remit, particularly in poorly controlled patients with acute painful neuropathy or in those painful symptoms precipitated by intensive insulin treatment. Thus, the emphatic approach addressing the concerns and anxieties of patients with neuropathic pain is essential for their successful management [92].

Physical measures

The temperature of the painful neuropathic foot may be increased by arteriovenous shunting. Cold water immersion may reduce shunt flow and relieve pain. Allodynia may be relieved by wearing silk pyjamas or the use of a bed cradle. Patients who describe painful symptoms on walking likened to walking on pebbles may benefit from the use of comfortable footwear [92].

Acupuncture

In a 10-week uncontrolled study in patients with diabetes on standard pain therapy, 77% showed significant pain relief after up to six courses of traditional Chinese acupuncture without any side effects. During a follow-up period of 18–52 weeks, 67% were able to stop or significantly reduce their medications and only 24% required further acupuncture treatment [93]. Controlled studies using placebo needles should be performed to confirm these findings.

Electrical stimulation

Transcutaneous electrical nerve stimulation

Transcutaneous electrical nerve stimulation (TENS) influences neuronal afferent transmission and conduction velocity, increases the nociceptive flexion reflex threshold and changes the somatosensory evoked potentials. In a 4-week study of TENS applied to the lower limbs, each for 30 minutes daily, pain relief was noted in 83% of patients compared to 38% of a sham-treated group. In patients who only marginally responded to amitriptyline, pain reduction was significantly greater following TENS given for 12 weeks than with sham treatment. Thus, TENS may be used as an adjunctive modality combined with pharmacotherapy to augment pain relief [94].

Mid-frequency external muscle stimulation

One randomized controlled study showed a better effect of mid-frequency external muscle stimulation than TENS on neuropathic symptoms after 1 week [95], but longer-term controlled studies are not available.

Frequency-modulated electromagnetic nerve stimulation

Frequency-modulated electromagnetic nerve stimulation applied during 10 sessions over 3 weeks resulted in a significant pain reduction compared to placebo stimulation [96]. A larger-scale multicenter study is currently ongoing.

Electrical spinal cord stimulation

It is generally agreed that electrical spinal cord stimulation (ESCS) is effective in neurogenic forms of pain. Experiments indicate that electrical stimulation is followed by a decrease in the excitatory amino acids glutamate and aspartate in the dorsal horn. This effect is mediated by a GABAergic mechanism. In diabetic painful neuropathy that was unresponsive to drug treatment, ESCS with electrodes implanted between T9 and T11 resulted in a pain relief >50% in 8 out of 10 patients. In addition, exercise tolerance was significantly improved. Complications of ESCS included superficial wound infection in two patients, lead migration requiring reinsertion in two patients, and "late failure" after 4 months in a patient who had initial pain relief [97]. This invasive treatment option should be reserved for patients who do not respond to drug treatment.

Monochromatic infrared energy

Monochromatic infrared energy has been shown to reduce neuropathic symptoms and signs in patients with diabetes in uncontrolled studies. By contrast, two controlled studies showed that monochromatic infrared energy was no more effective than placebo in increasing sensation in patients with DPN [98,99], emphasizing the need for controlled studies in this area to allow an evidence-based treatment decision.

Surgical decompression

Surgical decompression at the site of anatomic narrowing has been promoted as an alternative treatment for patients with symptomatic DPN. A systematic review of the literature revealed only Class IV studies concerning the utility of this therapeutic approach. Given the current evidence available, this treatment alternative should be considered unproven (Level U). Prospective randomized controlled trials with standard definitions and outcome measures are necessary to determine the value of this therapeutic intervention [100,101].

References

1 Consensus statement. Report and recommendations of the San Antonio conference on diabetic neuropathy. *Diabetes Care* 1988; **11**:592–597.

2 Thomas PK. Metabolic neuropathy. *J R Coll Phys Lond* 1973; **7**:154–160.

3 Sima AAF, Thomas PK, Ishii D, Vinik A. Diabetic neuropathies. *Diabetologia* 1997; **40**:B74–B77.

4 Shaw JE, Zimmet PZ, Gries FA, Ziegler D. Epidemiology of diabetic neuropathy. In: Gries FA, Cameron NE, Low PA, Ziegler D, eds. *Textbook of Diabetic Neuropathy*. Stuttgart/New York: Thieme, 2003; 64–82.

5 Ziegler D, Rathmann W, Dickhaus T, Meisinger C, Mielck A; KORA Study Group. Prevalence of polyneuropathy in pre-diabetes and diabetes is associated with abdominal obesity and macroangiopathy: the MONICA/KORA Augsburg Surveys S2 and S3. *Diabetes Care* 2008; **31**:464–469.

6 Resnick HE, Vinik AI, Schwartz AV, Leveille SG, Brancati FL, Balfour J, *et al.* Independent effects of peripheral nerve dysfunction on lower-extremity physical function in old age. The Women's Health and Aging Study. *Diabetes Care* 2000; **23**:1642–1647.

7 Forsblom CM, Sane T, Groop PH, Totterman KJ, Kallio M, Saloranta C, *et al.* Risk factors for mortality in type II (non-insulin-dependent) diabetes: evidence of a role for neuropathy and a protective effect of HLA-DR4. *Diabetologia* 1998; **4**:1253–1262.

8 Coppini DV, Bowtell PA, Weng C, Young PJ, Sönksen PH. Showing neuropathy is related to increased mortality in diabetic patients: a survival analysis using an accelerated failure time model. *J Clin Epidemiol* 2000; **53**:519–523.

9 Abbott CA, Vileikyte L, Williamson S, Carrington AL, Boulton AJM. Multicenter study of the incidence of and predictive risk factors for diabetic neuropathic foot ulceration. *Diabetes Care* 1998; **21**:1071–1075.

10 Galer BS, Gianas A, Jensen MP. Painful diabetic neuropathy: epidemiology, pain description, and quality of life. *Diabetes Res Clin Pract* 2000; **47**:123–128.

11 Daousi C, Benbow SJ, Woodward A, MacFarlane IA. The natural history of chronic painful peripheral neuropathy in a community diabetes population. *Diabet Med* 2006; **23**:1021–1024.

12 Davies M, Brophy S, Williams R, Taylor A. The prevalence, severity, and impact of painful diabetic peripheral neuropathy in type 2 diabetes. *Diabetes Care* 2006; **29**:1518–1522.

13 Wu EQ, Borton J, Said G, Le TK, Monz B, Rosilio M, *et al.* Estimated prevalence of peripheral neuropathy and associated pain in adults with diabetes in France. *Curr Med Res Opin* 2007; **23**:2035–2042.

14 Ziegler D, Rathmann W, Dickhaus T, Meisinger C, Mielck A; KORA Study Group. Neuropathic pain in diabetes, pre-diabetes and normal glucose tolerance. The MONICA/KORA Augsburg Surveys S2 and S3. *Pain Med* 2009; **10**:393–400.

15 Ziegler D, Rathmann W, Meisinger C, Dickhaus T, Mielck A; KORA Study Group. Prevalence and risk factors of neuropathic pain in survivors of myocardial infarction with pre-diabetes and diabetes. The KORA Myocardial Infarction Registry. *Eur J Pain* 2008; **31**:464–469.

16 Boulton AJM, Scarpello JHB, Armstrong WD, Ward JD. The natural history of painful diabetic neuropathy: a 4-year study. *Postgrad Med J* 1983; **59**:556–559.

17 Young RJ, Ewing DJ, Clarke BF. Chronic and remitting painful diabetic neuropathy. *Diabetes Care* 1988; **11**:34–40.

18 Benbow SJ, Chan AW, Bowsher D, MacFarlane IA, Williams G. A prospective study of painful symptoms, small-fibre function and peripheral vascular disease in chronic painful diabetic neuropathy. *Diabet Med* 1993; **11**:17–21.

19 Archer AG, Watkins PJ, Thomas PK, Sharma AK, Payan J. The natural history of acute painful neuropathy in diabetes mellitus. *J Neurol Neurosurg Psychiat* 1983; **46**:491–499.

20 Ellenberg M. Diabetic neuropathic cachexia. *Diabetes* 1974; **23**:418–423.

21 Steele JM, Young RJ, Lloyd GG, Clarke BF. Clinically apparent eating disorders in young diabetic women: associations with painful neuropathy and other complications. *Br Med J* 1987; **294**:859–866.

22 Caravati CM. Insulin neuritis: a case report. *Va Med Mon* 1933; **59**:745–746.

23 Dabby R, Sadeh M, Lampl Y, Gilad R, Watemberg N. Acute painful neuropathy induced by rapid correction of serum glucose levels in diabetic patients. *Biomed Pharmacother* 2009; **63**:707–709.

24 Llewelyn JG, Thomas PK, Fonseca V, King RHM, Dandona P. Acute painful diabetic neuropathy precipitated by strict glycemic control. *Acta Neuropathol* 1986; **72**:157–163.

25 Tesfaye S, Malik R, Harris N, Jakubowski JJ, Mody C, Rennie IG, *et al.* Arterio-venous shunting and proliferating new vessels in acute painful neuropathy of rapid glycaemic control (insulin neuritis). *Diabetologia* 1996; **39**:329–335.

26 Asbury AK. Focal and multifocal neuropathies of diabetes. In: Dyck PJ, Thomas PK, Asbury AK, Winegrad AI, Porte D, eds. *Diabetic Neuropathy*. Philadelphia: Saunders, 1987; 45–55.

27 Said G, Goulon-Goeau C, Lacroix C, Moulonguet A. Nerve biopsy findings in different patterns of proximal diabetic neuropathy. *Ann Neurol* 1994; **35**:559–569.

28 Said G, Elgrably F, Lacroix C, Planté V, Talamon C, Adams D, *et al.* Painful proximal diabetic neuropathy: inflammatory nerve lesions and spontaneous favorable outcome. *Ann Neurol* 1997; **41**:762–770.

29 Reske-Nielsen E, Lundbaek K. Pathological changes in the central and peripheral nervous system of young long-term diabetics. II. The spinal cord and peripheral nerves. *Diabetologia* 1968; **4**:34–43.

30 Slager U. Diabetic myelopathy. *Arch Pathol Lab Med* 1978; **102**:467–469.

31 Olsson Y, Säve-Söderbergh J, Sourander P, Angervall L. A patho-anatomical study of the central and peripheral nervous system in diabetics of early onset and long duration. *Path Europ* 1968; **3**:62–79.

32 Reske-Nielsen E, Lundbaek K, Rafaelsen OJ. Pathological changes in the central and peripheral nervous system of young long-term diabetics. I. Diabetic encephalopathy. *Diabetologia* 1965; **1**:233–241.

33 Ziegler D, Mühlen H, Dannehl K, Gries FA. Tibial nerve somatosensory evoked potentials at various stages of peripheral neuropathy in type 1 diabetic patients. *J Neurol Neurosurg Psychiatry* 1993; **56**:58–64.

34 Dejgaard A, Gade A, Larsson H, Balle V, Parving A, Parving HH. Evidence for diabetic encephalopathy. *Diabet Med* 1991; **8**:162–167.

35 Eaton SE, Harris ND, Rajbhandari SM, Greenwood P, Wilkinson ID, Ward JD, *et al.* Spinal-chord involvement in diabetic peripheral neuropathy. *Lancet* 2001; **358**:35–36.

36 Ziegler D, Langen K-J, Herzog H, Kuwert T, Mühlen H, Feinendegen LE, *et al.* Cerebral glucose metabolism in type 1 diabetic patients. *Diabet Med* 1994; **11**:205–209.

37 Selvarajah D, Wilkinson ID, Emery CJ, Shaw PJ, Griffiths PD, Gandhi R, *et al.* Thalamic neuronal dysfunction and chronic sensorimotor distal symmetrical polyneuropathy in patients with type 1 diabetes mellitus. *Diabetologia* 2008; **51**:2088–2092.

38 Tomlinson DR, Gardiner NJ. Glucose neurotoxicity. *Nat Rev Neurosci* 2008; **9**:36–45.

39 Figueroa-Romero C, Sadidi M, Feldman EL. Mechanisms of disease: the oxidative stress theory of diabetic neuropathy. *Rev Endocr Metab Disord* 2008; **9**:301–314.

40 Cameron NE, Cotter MA. Pro-inflammatory mechanisms in diabetic neuropathy: focus on the nuclear factor kappa B pathway. *Curr Drug Targets* 2008; **9**:60–67.

41 Consensus Development Conference on Standardized Measures in Diabetic Neuropathy. Proceedings of a consensus development conference on standardized measures in diabetic neuropathy. *Diabetes Care* 1992; **15**(Suppl 3):1080–1107.

42 Paisley AN, Abbott CA, van Schie CH, Boulton AJ. A comparison of the Neuropen against standard quantitative sensory-threshold measures for assessing peripheral nerve function. *Diabet Med* 2002; **19**:400–405.

43 Ziegler D, Siekierka-Kleiser E, Meyer B, Schweers M. Validation of a novel screening device (NeuroQuick) for quantitative assessment of small nerve fiber dysfunction as an early feature of diabetic polyneuropathy. *Diabetes Care* 2005; **28**:1169–1174.

44 Viswanathan V, Snehalatha C, Seena R, Ramachandran A. Early recognition of diabetic neuropathy: evaluation of a simple outpatient procedure using thermal perception. *Postgrad Med J* 2002; **78**:541–542.

45 Martina IS, van Koningsveld R, Schmitz PI, van der Meché FG, van Doorn PA. Measuring vibration threshold with a graduated tuning fork in normal aging and in patients with polyneuropathy. *J Neurol Neurosurg Psychiatry* 1998; **65**:743–747.

46 Papanas N, Papatheodorou K, Christakidis D, Papazoglou D, Giassakis G, Piperidou H, *et al.* Evaluation of a new indicator test for sudomotor function (Neuropad) in the diagnosis of peripheral neuropathy in type 2 diabetic patients. *Exp Clin Endocrinol Diabetes* 2005; **113**:195–198.

47 Feldman EL, Stevens MJ, Thomas PK, Brown MB, Canal N, Greene DA. A practical two-step quantitative clinical and electrophysiological assessment for the diagnosis and staging of diabetic neuropathy. *Diabetes Care* 1994; **17**:1281–1289.

48 Young MJ, Boulton AJM, Macleod AF, Williams DRR, Sonksen PH. A multicentre study of the prevalence of diabetic peripheral neuropathy in the United Kingdom hospital clinic population. *Diabetologia* 1993; **36**:150–154.

49 Bennett MI, Attal N, Backonja MM, Baron R, Bouhassira D, Freynhagen R, *et al.* Using screening tools to identify neuropathic pain. *Pain* 2007; **127**:199–203.

50 Quantitative sensory testing: a consensus report from the Peripheral Neuropathy Association. *Neurology* 1993; **43**:1050–1052.

51 Lauria G, Cornblath DR, Johansson O, McArthur JC, Mellgren SI, Nolano M, *et al.*; European Federation of Neurological Societies. EFNS guidelines on the use of skin biopsy in the diagnosis of peripheral neuropathy. *Eur J Neurol* 2005; **12**:747–758.

52 Diabetes Control and Complications Trial Research Group. The effect of intensive treatment of diabetes on the development and progression of long-term complications in insulin-dependent diabetes mellitus. *N Engl J Med* 1993; **329**:977–986.

53 UK Prospective Diabetes Study (UKPDS) Group. Intensive blood-glucose control with sulphonylureas or insulin compared with conventional treatment and risk of complications in patients with type 2 diabetes (UKPDS 33). *Lancet* 1998; **352**:837–853.

54 Martin CL, Albers J, Herman WH, Cleary P, Waberski B, Greene DA, *et al.*; DCCT/EDIC Research Group. Neuropathy among the diabetes control and complications trial cohort 8 years after trial completion. *Diabetes Care* 2006; **29**:340–344.

55 ADVANCE Collaborative Group. Intensive blood glucose control and vascular outcomes in patients with type 2 diabetes. *N Engl J Med* 2008; **358**:2560–2572.

56 Duckworth W, Abraira C, Moritz T, Reda D, Emanuele N, Reaven PD, *et al.*; VADT Investigators. Glucose control and vascular com-

plications in veterans with type 2 diabetes. *N Engl J Med* 2009; **360**:129–139.

57 Gaede P, Lund-Andersen H, Parving HH, Pedersen O. Effect of a multifactorial intervention on mortality in type 2 diabetes. *N Engl J Med* 2008; **358**:580–591.

58 Boulton AJ, Vinik AI, Arezzo JC, Bril V, Feldman R, Freeman R, *et al.* Diabetic neuropathies: a statement by the American Diabetes Association. *Diabetes Care* 2005; **28**:956–962.

59 Ang CD, Alviar MJ, Dans AL, Bautista-Velez GG, Villaruz-Sulit MV, Tan JJ, *et al.* Vitamin B for treating peripheral neuropathy. *Cochrane Database Syst Rev* 2008; **3**:CD004573.

60 Stracke H, Gaus W, Achenbach U, Federlin K, Bretzel RG. Benfotiamine in diabetic polyneuropathy (BENDIP): results of a randomised, double blind, placebo-controlled clinical study. *Exp Clin Endocrinol Diabetes* 2008; **116**:600–605.

61 Ziegler D, Nowak H, Kempler P, Vargha P, Low PA. Treatment of symptomatic diabetic polyneuropathy with the antioxidant α-lipoic acid: a meta-analysis. *Diabetic Med* 2004; **21**:114–121.

62 Ziegler D, Ametov A, Barinov A, Dyck PJ, Gurieve I, Low PA, *et al.* Oral treatment with alpha-lipoic acid improves symptomatic diabetic polyneuropathy: the SYDNEY 2 trial. *Diabetes Care* 2006; **29**:2365–2370.

63 Ziegler D, Low PA, Boulton AJM, *et al.* Antioxidant treatment with α-lipoic acid in diabetic polyneuropathy: a 4-year randomised double-blind trial (NATHAN 1 Study). *Diabetologia* 2007; **50**(Suppl 1):63.

64 Ziegler D. Thioctic acid for patients with symptomatic diabetic neuropathy: a critical review. *Treat Endocrinol* 2004; **3**:1–17.

65 Finnerup NB, Otto M, McQuay HJ, Jensen TS, Sindrup SH. Algorithm for neuropathic pain treatment: an evidence based proposal. *Pain* 2005; **118**:289–305.

66 Dworkin RH, O'Connor AB, Backonja M, Farrar JT, Finnerup NB, Jensen TS, *et al.* Pharmacologic management of neuropathic pain: evidence-based recommendations. *Pain* 2007; **132**:237–251.

67 Ziegler D. Painful diabetic neuropathy. Advantage of novel drugs over old drugs? *Diabetes Care* 2009; **32**(Suppl 2):S414–S419.

68 Ziegler D. Painful diabetic neuropathy: treatment and future aspects. *Diabetes Metab Res Rev* 2008; **24**(Suppl 1):S52–S57.

69 Edelsberg J, Oster G. Summary measures of number needed to treat: how much clinical guidance do they provide in neuropathic pain? *Eur J Pain* 2009; **13**:11–16.

70 Wong MC, Chung JW, Wong TK. Effects of treatments for symptoms of painful diabetic neuropathy: systematic review. *Br Med J* 2007; **335**:87.

71 Otto M, Bach FW, Jensen TS, Brøsen K, Sindrup SH. Escitalopram in painful polyneuropathy: a randomized, placebo-controlled, cross-over trial. *Pain* 2008; **139**:275–283.

72 Kajdasz DK, Iyengar S, Desaiah D, Backonja MM, Farrar JT, Fishbain DA, *et al.* Duloxetine for the management of diabetic peripheral neuropathic pain: evidence-based findings from post hoc analysis of three multicenter, randomized, double-blind, placebo-controlled, parallel-group studies. *Clin Ther* 2007; **29**:2536–2546.

73 Ziegler D, Pritchett YL, Wang F, Desaiah D, Robinson MJ, Hall JA, *et al.* Impact of disease characteristics on the efficacy of duloxetine in diabetic peripheral neuropathic pain. *Diabetes Care* 2007; **30**:664–669.

74 Hardy T, Sachson R, Shen S, Armbruster M, Boulton AJ. Does treatment with duloxetine for neuropathic pain impact glycemic control? *Diabetes Care* 2007; **30**:21–26.

75 Rowbotham MC, Goli V, Kunz NR, Lei D. Venlafaxine extended release in the treatment of painful diabetic neuropathy: a double-blind, placebo-controlled study. *Pain* 2004; **110**:697–706.

76 Backonja M, Beydoun A, Edwards KR, Schwartz SL, Fonseca V, Hes M, *et al.* Gabapentin for the symptomatic treatment of painful neuropathy in patients with diabetes mellitus. *JAMA* 1998; **280**:1831–1836.

77 Freeman R, Durso-Decruz E, Emir B. Efficacy, safety, and tolerability of pregabalin treatment for painful diabetic peripheral neuropathy: findings from seven randomized, controlled trials across a range of doses. *Diabetes Care* 2008; **31**:1448–1454.

78 Grosskopf J, Mazzola J, Wan Y, Hopwood M. A randomized, placebo-controlled study of oxcarbazepine in painful diabetic neuropathy. *Acta Neurol Scand* 2006; **114**:177–180.

79 Beydoun A, Shaibani A, Hopwood M, Wan Y. Oxcarbazepine in painful diabetic neuropathy: results of a dose-ranging study. *Acta Neurol Scand* 2006; **113**:395–404.

80 Thienel U, Neto W, Schwabe SK, Vijapurkar U; Topiramate Diabetic Neuropathic Pain Study Group. Topiramate in painful diabetic polyneuropathy: findings from three double-blind placebo-controlled trials. *Acta Neurol Scand* 2004; **110**:221–231.

81 Vinik AI, Tuchman M, Safirstein B, Corder C, Kirby L, Wilks K, *et al.* Lamotrigine for treatment of pain associated with diabetic neuropathy: results of two randomized, double-blind, placebo-controlled studies. *Pain* 2007; **128**:169–179.

82 Mo J, Chen LL. Systemic lidocaine for neuropathic pain relief. *Pain* 2000; **87**:7–17.

83 Davies PS, Galer BS. Review of lidocaine patch 5% studies in the treatment of postherpetic neuralgia. *Drugs* 2004; **64**:937–947.

84 Ziegler D, Hidvégi T, Gurieva I, Bongardt S, Freynhagen R, Sen D, Sommerville K. Efficacy and safety of lacosamide in painful diabetic neuropathy. *Diabetes Care* 2010; Jan 12 [Epub ahead of print].

85 Mason L, Moore RA, Derry S, Edwards JE, McQuay HJ. Systematic review of topical capsaicin for the treatment of chronic pain. *Br Med J* 2004; **328**:991–995.

86 Harati Y, Gooch C, Swenson M, Edelman S, Greene D, Raskin P, *et al.* Double-blind randomized trial of tramadol for the treatment of the pain of diabetic neuropathy. *Neurology* 1998; **50**:1842–1846.

87 Watson CP, Moulin D, Watt-Watson J, Gordon A, Eisenhoffer J. Controlled-release oxycodone relieves neuropathic pain: a randomized controlled trial in painful diabetic neuropathy. *Pain* 2003; **105**:71–78.

88 Gimbel JS, Richards P, Portenoy RK. Controlled-release oxycodone for pain in diabetic neuropathy: a randomized controlled trial. *Neurology* 2003; **60**:927–934.

89 Gilron I, Bailey JM, Tu D, Holden RR, Weaver DF, Houlden RL. Morphine, gabapentin, or their combination for neuropathic pain. *N Engl J Med* 2005; **31**:1324–1334.

90 Hanna M, O'Brien C, Wilson MC. Prolonged-release oxycodone enhances the effects of existing gabapentin therapy in painful diabetic neuropathy patients. *Eur J Pain* 2008; **12**:804–813.

91 Pittler MH, Ernst E. Complementary therapies for neuropathic and neuralgic pain: systematic review. *Clin J Pain* 2008; **24**:731–733.

92 Tesfaye S. Painful diabetic neuropathy: aetiology and nonpharmacological treatment. In: Veves A, ed. *Clinical Management of Diabetic Neuropathy*. Totowa, NJ: Humana Press, 1998; 369–386.

93 Abuaisha BB, Costanzi, Boulton AJM. Acupuncture for the treatment of chronic painful peripheral diabetic neuropathy: a long-term study. *Diabetes Res Clin Pract* 1998; **39**:115–121.

94 Kumar D, Alvaro MS, Julka IS, Marshall HJ. Diabetic peripheral neuropathy. Effectiveness of electrotherapy and amitriptyline for symptomatic relief. *Diabetes Care* 1998; **21**:1322–1325.

95 Reichstein L, Labrenz S, Ziegler D, Martin S. Effective treatment of symptomatic diabetic polyneuropathy by high-frequency external muscle stimulation. *Diabetologia* 2005; **48**:824–828.

96 Bosi E, Conti M, Vermigli C, Cazzetta G, peretti E, Cordoni MC, *et al.* Effectiveness of frequency-modulated electromagnetic neural stimulation in the treatment of painful diabetic neuropathy. *Diabetologia* 2005; **48**:817–823.

97 Tesfaye S, Watt J, Benbow SJ, Pang KA, Miles J, MacFarlane IA. Electrical spinal-cord stimulation for painful diabetic peripheral neuropathy. *Lancet* 1996; **348**:1696–1701.

98 Clifft JK, Kasser RJ, Newton TS, Bush AJ. The effect of monochromatic infrared energy on sensation in patients with diabetic peripheral neuropathy: a double-blind, placebo-controlled study. *Diabetes Care* 2005; **28**:2896–2900.

99 Lavery LA, Murdoch DP, Williams J, Lavery DC. Does anodyne light therapy improve peripheral neuropathy in diabetes? A double-blind, sham-controlled, randomized trial to evaluate monochromatic infrared photoenergy. *Diabetes Care* 2008; **31**:316–321.

100 Chaudhry V, Stevens JC, Kincaid J, So YT; Therapeutics and Technology Assessment Subcommittee of the American Academy of Neurology. Practice Advisory: utility of surgical decompression for treatment of diabetic neuropathy: report of the Therapeutics and Technology Assessment Subcommittee of the American Academy of Neurology. *Neurology* 2006; **66**:1805–1808.

101 Chaudhry V, Russell J, Belzberg A. Decompressive surgery of lower limbs for symmetrical diabetic peripheral neuropathy. *Cochrane Database Syst Rev* 2008; **16**(3):CD006152.

8 Macrovascular Complications in Diabetes

39 The Pathogenesis of Macrovascular Complications Including Atherosclerosis in Diabetes

Riccardo Candido[1,2], Mark E. Cooper[1] & Karin A.M. Jandeleit-Dahm[1]

[1]Baker IDI Heart and Diabetes Institute, Danielle Alberti JDRF Center for Diabetes Complications, Melbourne, Australia
[2]Diabetic Center, A.S.S. 1 Triestina, Trieste, Italy

Keypoints

- Diabetes accounts for 75–90% of excess coronary artery disease risk seen in people with diabetes and enhances the effects of other cardiovascular risk factors.
- A range of hemodynamic and metabolic factors contribute to macrovascular disease in diabetes.
- The link between glucose control and cardiovascular disease (CVD) is not as strong as that seen with microvascular complications of diabetes.
- There is clear *in vitro* and *in vivo* evidence that glucose exerts direct and indirect toxic effects on the vasculature.
- Glycemic memory describes the deferred long-term injurious effects of prior glycemic status; early glycemic control appears to be important to reduce vascular complications in subsequent decades.
- Specific insulin resistance pathways appear to contribute to atherogenesis in diabetes.
- The accumulation of advanced glycation end-products (AGEs) exerts pro-inflammatory and pro-fibrotic effects on the vasculature via receptor independent and receptor dependent effects. The AGE receptor (RAGE) is pivotally involved in the pathogenesis of diabetes accelerated atherosclerosis.
- The components of the classic renin angiotensin system (RAS) and in particular more recently discovered components such as angiotensin converting enzyme 2 appear to contribute to macrovascular disease in diabetes. Inhibitors of the RAS have consistently demonstrated reduced endothelial dysfunction and atherosclerosis in animal models via suppression of inflammation, fibrosis and oxidative stress. There is also strong clinical evidence for vasculoprotection by RAS blockade.
- Other vasoactive components such as endothelin and urotensin II are also likely to contribute to macrovascular complications in diabetes and interact with the RAS. Furthermore, the role of novel tumor necrosis factor (TNF) related ligands, such as TNF-related apoptosis inducing ligand and osteoprotegerin, and the complement system in atherosclerosis are currently under evaluation.
- Treatments that reduce oxidative stress and inhibit inflammation such as peroxisome proliferator activated receptor agonists have been shown to be anti-atherosclerotic in experimental studies with some evidence, albeit not uniform, also having been obtained in clinical studies.
- A multifactorial approach treating conventional cardiovascular risk factors as well as diabetes specific risk factors is currently viewed as the optimal strategy to reduce the burden of CVD in diabetes.

Epidemiology of diabetic macrovascular complications

Macrovascular complications develop in patients with type 1 (T1DM) [1–3] and type 2 diabetes mellitus (T2DM) [4–6]. This is of a particular concern as the increasing prevalence of diabetes now also affects adolescents and younger adults, thus promoting the earlier development of long-term cardiovascular complications. Even after adjusting for concomitant risk factors such as hypertension and hyperlipidemia there remains an excess risk for cardiovascular disease (CVD) in people with diabetes [7,8]. Indeed, diabetes itself accounts for 75–90% of the excess coronary artery disease (CAD) risk and enhances the effects of other cardiovascular risk factors. Death from stroke and myocardial infarction (MI) are the leading causes of mortality in T1DM and T2DM [2,9].

A range of hemodynamic and metabolic factors have been considered responsible for the development and progression of macrovascular disease in diabetes (Figure 39.1) [10]. In terms of hemodynamic factors, in particular the hormonal cascade known as the renin angiotensin system (RAS) has been shown to have a pivotal role in diabetes-associated atherosclerosis; however, other vasoactive hormone systems such as the endothelin (ET)

Textbook of Diabetes, 4th edition. Edited by R. Holt, C. Cockram, A. Flyvbjerg and B. Goldstein.

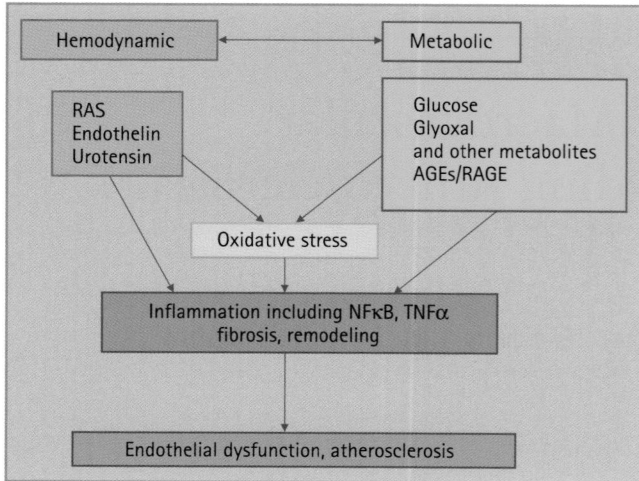

Figure 39.1 Hemodynamic and metabolic mediators contribute to the pathogenesis of diabetic vascular complications. Hemodynamic factors include the renin angiotensin system (RAS), and other vasoactive factors. Metabolic factors include glucose and glucose metabolites such as the formation of advanced glycation end-products (AGEs). Both pathways interact with each other and lead to oxidative stress and inflammation, thus promoting endothelial dysfunction and atherosclerosis. NFκB, nuclear transcription factor κB; TNF-α, tumor necrosis factor α.

[11] and urotensin systems [12,13] have also been implicated in diabetic macrovascular disease. More recently, a role for novel factors such as tumor necrosis factor (TNF) related apoptosis inducing ligand (TRAIL) [14] and the complement system has also been suggested [15].

Pathogenesis of diabetic macrovascular disease

Atherosclerosis is initiated by the adhesion of monocytes to the vascular wall, particularly to endothelial cells, followed by transmigration of monocytes into the subendothelial space [16]. Monocytes differentiate into macrophages which, via uptake of lipids, transform into foam cells and accumulate in the vascular wall. The early atherosclerotic process results in the formation of fatty streak lesions which over time develop into more advanced lesions, characterized by infiltration with vascular smooth muscle cells (VSMC), formation of a necrotic core and further lipid accumulation [16]. In humans, these lesions can demonstrate features of instability and plaque rupture including intraplaque hemorrhages as well as heightened thrombogenicity.

Role of hyperglycemia

A pivotal role for glycemic control and duration of diabetes exposure has been well established for microvascular complications in the UK Prospective Diabetes Study (UKPDS) study [4,17], although the data are not as convincing for macrovascular disease. The importance of glycemic control for macrovascular injury has only recently been extensively investigated in a series of studies that were reported over the last 12 months. It has been suggested that HbA_{1c} acts as an independent and continuous risk factor for macrovascular disease [18–21]; however, this link is not as strong as has been identified with respect to microvascular complications. For an increase in HbA_{1c} from 5.5% (37 mmol/mol) to 9.5% (80 mmol/mol) there is a 10-fold increase in microvascular disease endpoints, whereas the risk for macrovascular disease endpoints increases only twofold.

Clinical trials and hyperglycemia

Recently, clinical trials such as the Action to Control Cardiovascular Risk in Diabetes trial (ACCORD) [22], Action in Diabetes and Vascular disease: PreterAx and DiamicroN-MR Controlled Evaluation (ADVANCE) trial [23] and the Veterans Affairs Diabetes Trial (VADT) [24], which explored tight glycemic control in patients with T2DM with established CVD, have investigated the association between tight glycemic control and cardiovascular endpoints. As observed in the initial reports of the Diabetes Control and Complications Trial (DCCT) in patients with T1DM and in the UKPDS trial in patients with T2DM, tight blood glucose control had little effect on macrovascular outcomes. This was further emphasized by the recent studies including the ADVANCE study [23] and ACCORD trial [22]. Both studies failed to demonstrate significant cardiovascular benefits, with the ACCORD study suggesting possibly deleterious cardiovascular outcomes in association with tight glucose control.

One possible explanation for the lack of a positive effect of tight glycemic control on cardiovascular outcomes may be the short duration of these trials (less than 5 years). Indeed, as best seen with respect to the longer follow-up of the Steno-2 study [25] and a recent long-term follow-up of the UKPDS [26], the benefits of prior intensified cardiovascular risk management including aggressive glucose control may not appear for up to 10 years after initiation of the studies. Thus, in view of the relative lack of an impact on CVD with intensive glucose control, other risk factor modification strategies need to be emphasized.

Direct and indirect glycotoxicity

Hyperglycemia is thought to have direct and indirect toxic effect on vascular cells. It has been suggested that increased glucose levels enter the polyol pathway at an increased flux rate leading to heightened formation of diacylglycerol. In addition, increased flux of glucose into the hexosamine pathway may contribute to glucose mediated vascular injury in diabetes. To investigate specifically hyperglycemia mediated atherosclerosis, aldose reductase, transgenic mice have been investigated [27]. These mice demonstrated increased glucose delivery via the polyol pathway and also showed early atherosclerosis, but did not develop advanced vascular lesions.

In vitro studies

Studies in cell culture experiments have obtained clear evidence that hyperglycemia induces a range of pro-atherogenic effects.

Glucose directly activates monocytes–macrophages *in vitro* initiating increased expression of cytokines such as interleukin 1β (IL-1β) and IL-6 [28]. Furthermore, this leads to protein kinase C (PKC) and nuclear factor κB (NFκB) activation resulting in increased production of reactive oxygen species (ROS). Autooxidation of glucose can also lead to the formation of ROS and can mediate low density lipoprotein (LDL) oxidation. Scavenger receptors on activated macrophages can mediate the uptake of modified lipids such as the pro-atherogenic oxidized LDL. The formation of advanced glycation end-products (AGEs) in the hyperglycemic milieu can lead to the formation of modified albumin which inhibits scavenger receptor class B type 1 mediated efflux of cholesterol to high density lipoprotein (HDL). Therefore, prolonged hyperglycemia can indirectly lead to a range of secondary changes including changes in lipid profile, cellular lipid accumulation and foam cell formation as well as AGE mediated modification of proteins leading to altered cellular structure and function.

Animal models

The study of atherosclerosis in diabetes has long been hampered by the lack of an appropriate animal model. Our group and others have developed a murine model of diabetes associated macrovascular disease, the apoE knockout (KO) mouse rendered diabetic by multiple low doses of streptozotocin injections. This model is currently considered by the National Institutes of Health/Juvenile Diabetes Research Foundation (NIH/JDRF) co-sponsored Animal Models for Diabetes Complications Consortium (AMDCC) to be an appropriate model to study macrovascular disease in diabetes [29].

To address the separate roles of hyperglycemia and dyslipidemia in diabetes-associated atherosclerosis, mice deficient in the LDL receptor were bred with transgenic mice expressing a viral protein under control of the insulin promoter [30]. When infected with the virus, T cells mediate destruction of pancreatic β-cells that express the viral protein, thus closely mimicking the autoimmune response in human T1DM. In these animals, atherosclerosis development was accelerated even on a normal diet suggesting that hyperglycemia was driving atherosclerosis in these mice [30,31]. When animals were placed on a high fat diet, a further acceleration of atherosclerosis occurred suggesting that glucose and lipids may act through synergistic mechanisms to accelerate atherosclerosis. Furthermore, plaque disruption and intraplaque hemorrhages, features of plaque instability and potential plaque rupture were observed in this model [30].

Metabolic memory

The concept of "glycemic memory" describes the deferred effects of prior glycemic status on the subsequent development of diabetic complications. Episodes of poor glycemic control during the earlier stages of diabetes can precipitate or accelerate the development of complications later in the course of diabetes even when glycemic control is subsequently improved. Two studies have provided evidence for such a metabolic imprint, the DCCT/EDIC trial in T1DM [2] and the UKPDS in T2DM [26]. Both studies have shown that poor glycemic control was associated with an increased subsequent burden of complications. Another study in patients with T2DM, the VADT study, compared intensive with standard glucose control (6.9 vs. 8.4%, 52 vs 68 mmol/mol), but did not demonstrate significant cardiovascular protection after patients had been exposed to hyperglycemia for long periods of time (12–15 years) [24]. Therefore, it appears that early glycemic control is crucial for a long-term beneficial outcome on diabetic complications.

The concept of "metabolic memory" raises two important issues. First, hyperglycemia may expose patients to the harmful effects of hyperglycemia years before T2DM is diagnosed. Indeed, 25% of patients show complications at the time of diagnosis of T2DM. Therefore, it has been postulated that early diagnosis and strict glycemic control may be pivotal to reduce the induction of this metabolic memory with subsequent development of long-term diabetic vascular complications. Secondly, glycemic oscillations including peaks and troughs are not reflected in the HbA_{1c} levels [32,33] but may have a key role in mediating growth factor and cytokine expression as well as inducing chromatin remodeling [34].

There are many cellular and molecular processes that may contribute to the mechanisms underlying metabolic memory with most of those relating to glycotoxicity. These pathways include the formation of AGEs, glycation of DNA, increased flux of glucose metabolism, leading to increased oxidative damage, overproduction of PKC-β as well as mitochondrial stress. Recently, it has been shown that transient hyperglycemia induces long-lasting activation of epigenetic changes in the promoter region of the NFκB subunit p65 in aortic endothelial cells both *in vitro* and *in vivo*. These hyperglycemia induced epigenetic changes and increased p65 expression were prevented by reducing mitochondrial superoxide production or superoxide induced generation of α-oxoaldehydes such as methylglyoxal (Figure 39.2) [34]. These studies suggest that transient hyperglycemia

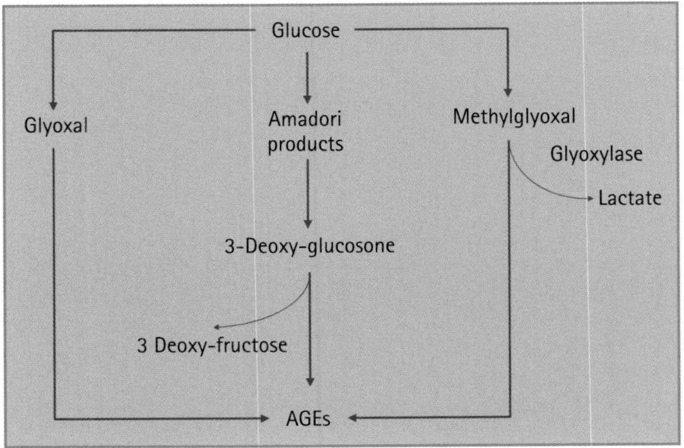

Figure 39.2 The formation of advanced glycation end-products (AGEs) can involve early glucose metabolites such as glyoxal and methylglyoxal, highly reactive dicarbonyls and key precursors of AGEs.

causes persistent atherogenic effects during subsequent normoglycemia by inducing long-lasting changes in chromatin remodeling. Specifically, hyperglycemia results in recruitment of the histone methyl transferase Set7 with increased H3K4 monomethylation of the proximal promoter region of the NFκB subunit p65 gene leading to increased expression of pro-atherogenic pathways including monocyte chemotactic protein 1 (MCP-1) and vascular cell adhesion molecule 1 (VCAM-1) [34]. Subsequent studies in mice, which were initially diabetic but returned spontaneously to normoglycemia, have also demonstrated persistent upregulation of pro-inflammatory genes such as p65 and MCP-1 as a result of prior hyperglycemia. Furthermore, more detailed epigenetic studies revealed that changes in histone modifications as a result of prior hyperglycemia also included changes in H3K9 methylation of the p65 promoter as well as effects on various histone methyl transferases and interestingly also demethylases such as LSD-1 [35].

Insulin resistance

Insulin resistance occurs in T2DM and in patients with impaired glucose tolerance, and has been associated with increased cardiovascular risk [36–38]. There is now increasing evidence that insulin resistance promotes atherogenesis as an independent risk factor [39–41]. Furthermore, insulin resistance is often associated with a pro-atherogenic lipid profile that includes a high very low-density lipoprotein (VLDL) component, a low HDL and small dense LDL.

In vitro studies have shown that insulin exerts both pro-atherogenic and anti-atherogenic effects [42,43]. This has led to the hypothesis of pathway specific insulin resistance (Figure 39.3). It has been suggested that insulin resistance towards glucose transport also affects resistance to the antiproliferative effects of insulin, whereas the signaling pathways leading to cellular proliferation remain intact (Figure 39.3). Insulin signaling via phosphatidylinositol 3 kinase (PI3K) has been associated with antiproliferative and antithrombogenic effects with decreased adhesion molecule expression such as MCP-1, VCAM-1 and intercellular adhesion molecule 1 (ICAM-1). Furthermore, nitric oxide (NO) production is mediated via the PI3K signal transduction pathway and therefore is impaired in insulin resistance. NO has been shown to reduce LDL oxidation and proliferation of VSMC. In contrast, effects on VSMC proliferation and migration are mediated via the Ras/Raf/MEKK/MAPK signal transduction pathway which is further stimulated in the context of hyperinsulinemia, thus suggesting that pathway specific insulin resistance contributes to the pro-atherogenic effects of insulin. More recently, it has been shown that IL-6 decreases insulin stimulated NO production from endothelial cells via decreased activity of insulin signaling mediated by enhanced TNF-α production [44]. Paradoxically, IL-6 increases insulin stimulated glucose uptake into skeletal muscle and adipose tissue via enhanced insulin signaling, yet IL-6 and insulin have not been linked to increased TNF-α expression in skeletal muscle [44].

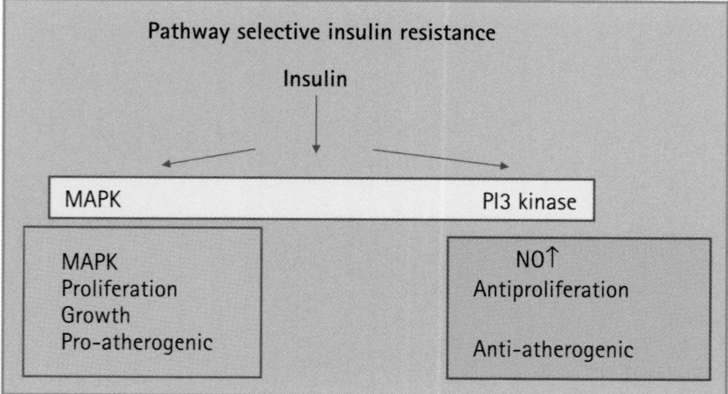

Figure 39.3 Pathway selective insulin resistance leading to endothelial dysfunction and atherosclerosis. MAPK, mitogen activated protein kinase; NO, nitric oxide; PI3 kinase, phosphatidylinositol 3 kinase.

Formation of AGE

AGE formation originates from early glycation products, the Schiff bases, which form the more stable Amadori products such as 1-amino-1-deoxyfructose derivatives. The Amadori products undergo further enzymatic modifications resulting in a number of reactive intermediates such as 3-deoxyglucosone and methylglyoxal (Figure 39.2). Methylglyoxal reacts with amino, sulfudryl and guanidine functional groups in proteins causing the browning, denaturation and redox active di-amine cross-linking between lysine residues of the target amino acids. Methylglyoxal also generates hydroimidazolones, N-E-(carboxyethyl) lysine, a homolog of carboxymethyl lysine (CML) and methylglyoxal lysine dimer [45,46]. The AGE-based cross-links are resistant to enzymatic degradation and therefore very stable [47]. The rate of AGE formation is dependent on multiple factors including the ambient concentrations of various sugars including glucose, the extent of oxidative stress and the duration of exposure to these various stimuli [48,49].

Direct effects of vascular AGE accumulation

There is evidence from experimental studies that AGEs directly influence endothelial function [50] as well as enhancing the evolution of macrovascular disease [51,52]. AGEs mediate their effects both directly and via receptor-mediated mechanisms. AGE accumulation in the vascular wall is associated with changes in the structural integrity of proteins, disturbance of their cellular function and degradation of these proteins [28]. AGEs accumulate on many proteins including collagen, albumin and apolipoproteins. Furthermore, the cross-linking of AGEs with matrix molecules can disrupt matrix–matrix and matrix–cell interactions. It has been shown that AGE cross-linking to collagens decreases vascular elasticity and reduces vascular compliance resulting in increased vascular stiffness [53,54]. In addition, AGEs are also able to quench NO [50,55] and generate ROS by stimulating nicotinic acid adenine dinucleotide phosphate (NADPH) oxidase activity [56].

AGE binding proteins

The receptor-mediated effects of AGEs occur via binding to proteins such as RAGE [57], AGE-R1 (p60), AGE-R2 (p90) and AGE-R3 (galectin-3), the ezrin-radixin-moesin (ERM) family of proteins [58] macrophage scavenger receptor ScR-11 and CD-36 [59]. The exact roles of AGE-R1, AGE-R2 and AGE-R3 have not been fully elucidated. Finally, the interaction between AGEs and several macrophage scavenger receptors, such as CD36 [59], has been postulated to also promote atherosclerosis with studies using CD36-knockout mice supporting the view that CD36 promotes atherosclerosis [60].

Receptor for AGEs, RAGE

RAGE is a multiligand signal transduction receptor of the immunoglobulin superfamily of cell surface molecules that acts as a pattern recognition receptor [57]. In addition to binding ligands actively participating in inflammation and immune responses, RAGE serves as an endothelial adhesion receptor for leukocyte integrins and promotes leukocyte recruitment and extravasation of infiltrating cells. Of direct relevance to diabetic macrovascular complications, RAGE is found on endothelial cells and monocytes–macrophages [52,61,62], with RAGE having been implicated in inflammatory lesions in many disorders [63].

Downstream effects of RAGE activation

Engagement of RAGE leads to activation of the pro-inflammatory transcription factor NFκB (Figure 39.4) [64]. AGE binding to RAGE activates various signaling pathways, including NADPH oxidase [56], MAPKs, $p21^{ras}$ [65], extracellular signal-regulated kinases (ERKs) [66] and PKC causing activation and translocation of NFκB [64]. Furthermore, expression of RAGE itself can be induced by NFκB [67]. RAGE expression within tissues is markedly enhanced in response to metabolic disturbances such as diabetes, dyslipidemia, uremia and aging, possibly because of accumulation of AGEs in these conditions [61,63]. In plaques from diabetic apoE KO mice, upregulation of connective tissue growth factor (CTGF) has been demonstrated that appears to be AGE dependent [51] and may be mediated via RAGE. Intracellular accumulation of AGEs may also promote phenotypic conversion of VSMCs into foam cells within atherosclerotic plaques [68].

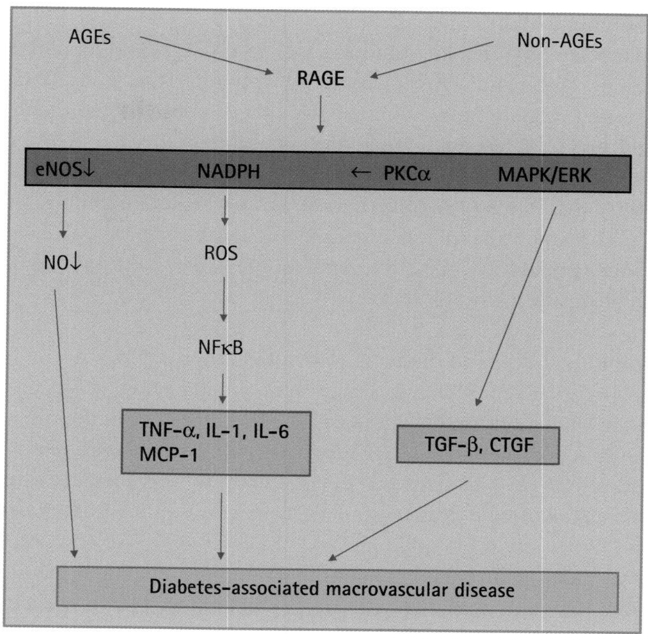

Figure 39.4 Activation of AGE receptor (RAGE) contributes to diabetes associated macrovascular disease via increased production of reactive oxygen species (ROS), decrease in nitric oxide (NO) availability, activation of the nuclear transcription factor κB (NFκB) and tumor necrosis factor α (TNF-α) as well as activation of profibrotic growth factors such as transforming growth factor β (TGF-β) and connective tissue growth factor (CTGF) associated with vascular remodeling. eNOS, endothelial nitric oxide synthase; ERK, extracellular signal-regulated kinase; MAPK, mitogen activated protein kinase; MCP, monocyte chemotactic protein; NADPH, nicotinic acid adenine dinucleotide phosphate; PKC, protein kinase C.

Studies reducing vascular AGE accumulation

A variety of pharmacologic interventions have been used to reduce the accumulation of AGEs via decreasing the total AGE load or via chemical modification of existing AGEs into inactive forms [69,70]. Aminoguanidine is a potent inhibitor of the formation of AGEs, scavenges reactive dicarbonyl AGE precursors [69,70] and decreases oxidative damage to mitochondrial proteins [71]. In experimental and clinical diabetes, aminoguanidine treatment has been shown to reduce microvascular [72] and more recently macrovascular complications in a model of accelerated atherosclerosis, the diabetic apoE KO mouse [51].

Another potential agent which inhibits AGE accumulation is ALT-711 or alagebrium [73]. Based initially on a range of *in vitro* studies, this thiazolium compound and its original prototype, phenylthiazolium bromide [74], have been shown to cleave preformed AGEs and thus one of the postulated mechanisms of ALT-711 is as an AGE cross-link breaker [73].

The removal of established cross-links in diabetic rats with ALT-711 has been shown to be associated with reversal of the diabetes-induced increase in large artery stiffness, increased collagen solubility and reduced vascular and cardiac AGE accumulation [54,75–77]. In addition, alagebrium prevents the progression of nephropathy [78,79] possibly via direct inhibition of PKC-α phosphorylation [80], thus reducing renal expression of vascular endothelial growth factor (VEGF). Treatment with ALT 711 in diabetic apoE KO mice was associated with a significant reduction in atherosclerosis [51]. This anti-atherosclerotic effect was associated with reduced vascular AGE accumulation and RAGE expression. Alagebrium treatment was also associated with less inflammation and reduced expression of pro-fibrotic growth factors, in particular CTGF [81,82]. In the clinical setting, ALT 711 has been shown to reduce pulse pressure and improve vascular compliance in patients with systolic hypertension [54].

Soluble RAGE

There are three major splice variants of RAGE [83]. First, there is the full-length RAGE receptor; secondly, the N-terminal variant, that does not contain the AGE-binding domain; and, thirdly, a C-terminal splice variant, soluble RAGE (sRAGE), which does not contain the *trans*-membrane and effector domains. It remains controversial as to whether the effects of sRAGE are primarily as a decoy to ligands such as AGEs or whether sRAGE acts as a competitive antagonist to the full-length biologically active RAGE [83,84].

Soluble RAGE and diabetes associated atherosclerosis

Soluble RAGE (sRAGE) has been identified as having therapeutic value in a model of diabetes associated atherosclerosis, the streptozotocin diabetic Apo E KO mouse [85,86]. In the original study, Park *et al.* [85] reported that diabetic apoE KO mice treated with sRAGE showed a dose-dependent suppression of atherosclerosis and reduced plaque complexity. These beneficial effects were independent of effects on glucose or lipid levels. Furthermore, AGE levels in these diabetic mice were suppressed in a dose-dependent manner by sRAGE to levels similar to those seen in non-diabetic animals. Furthermore, the effect of RAGE blockade with sRAGE was investigated in established atherosclerosis [86]. Administration of sRAGE decreased the expression of RAGE, as well as reducing the number of infiltrating inflammatory cells and gene expression for transforming growth factor β (TGF-β), fibronectin and type IV collagen in both the aorta and the kidney in association with reduced plaque area. Therefore, it was concluded by these investigators that RAGE activation not only contributes to lesion formation, but also to the progression of atherosclerosis.

Soluble RAGE treatment has also been reported to be effective in reducing vascular complications in other models of atherosclerosis and diabetes. Atherosclerosis in the LDL receptor –/– mouse made diabetic by streptozotocin injection [87] was significantly attenuated by sRAGE treatment. ApoE KO mice bred onto a *db/db* background, a model of T2DM and deficient leptin receptor signaling, showed increased atherosclerosis which was significantly attenuated by daily sRAGE treatment [88].

To understand better the specific role of RAGE in the genesis of vascular lesions, animals selectively deficient in RAGE/apoE (RAGE –/–) have been created [89,90]. These mice completely lack not only tissue bound full-length RAGE, but also soluble RAGE. As had been predicted by the pharmacologic intervention studies directed towards the RAGE ligands and AGEs, RAGE-knockout mice bred onto an apoE –/– background showed a marked reduction in plaque area in the presence and absence of diabetes [89,90]. More recently, the effect of RAGE deletion on atherosclerosis development has been investigated in streptozotocin diabetic RAGE/apoE KO mice and showed a significant reduction in atherosclerotic plaque area when compared with diabetic apoE KO mice expressing RAGE. These vascular changes seen in the streptozotocin diabetic double RAGE/apoE KO mice were associated with reduced inflammation, less accumulation of RAGE ligands such as S100/CML, decreased infiltration by macrophages and T lymphocytes and a reduction in expression of pro-fibrotic and pro-inflammatory growth factors and cytokines [90].

These promising results with RAGE antagonism have encouraged the development of RAGE neutralizing compounds for clinical use. The RAGE modulating agent TTP488 is currently being considered in phase II clinical trials in patients with Alzheimer disease and in patients with diabetic nephropathy. Another compound, TP4000, will soon enter phase I clinical trials (www.Clinicaltrials.gov and www.ttpharma.com); however, currently, the major focus of antagonizing RAGE does not appear to involve studies addressing CVD in the absence or presence of diabetes.

Interaction with the renin angiotensin system

Because diabetic complications appear to be multifactorial in origin and involve interactions between hemodynamic pathways such as the RAS and metabolic pathways such as hyperglycemia and the formation of AGEs, there has been increasing investigation of the potential links between these various pathways (Figure 39.1) [91]. There is increasing evidence that AGE accumulation can induce an upregulation of certain components of the RAS, although these studies have been performed predominantly in the renal context [92]. Furthermore, angiotensin-converting enzyme (ACE) inhibition has been reported to confer its end-organ protective effect, partly via a reduction in AGEs and an increase in sRAGE [93]. Therefore, the status of the RAS could represent a key modulator in AGE-induced diseases. More recently, other therapeutic interventions shown to be anti-atherosclerotic have been reported to exert part of their vasculoprotective effect via inhibition of the AGE/RAGE pathway. These include angiotensin II receptor blockers (ARBs), peroxisome proliferator-activated receptor α (PPAR-α) and PPAR-γ agonists and statins [94–96].

Role of vasoactive hormones in diabetes-related atherosclerosis

Classic RAS

Renin was described more than 100 years ago by Tigerstedt & Bergman [97]. Nevertheless, our understanding of the RAS is still not complete and has grown increasingly complex over the last decade. The classic pathway is now very well characterized (Figure 39.5). The generation of angiotensin (AT) I and II is not restricted to the systemic circulation but this production also takes place in vascular and other tissues (Figure 39.5) [98].

Novel aspects of the RAS: ACE2

In 2000, a further enzyme associated with the generation of AT peptides was identified – ACE2, a carboxypeptidase with sequence similarity to ACE [99]. ACE2 does not generate AT II but increases the formation of AT 1-7 (Figure 39.6). This heptapeptide causes vasodilatation and has growth inhibitory effects [100]. Further

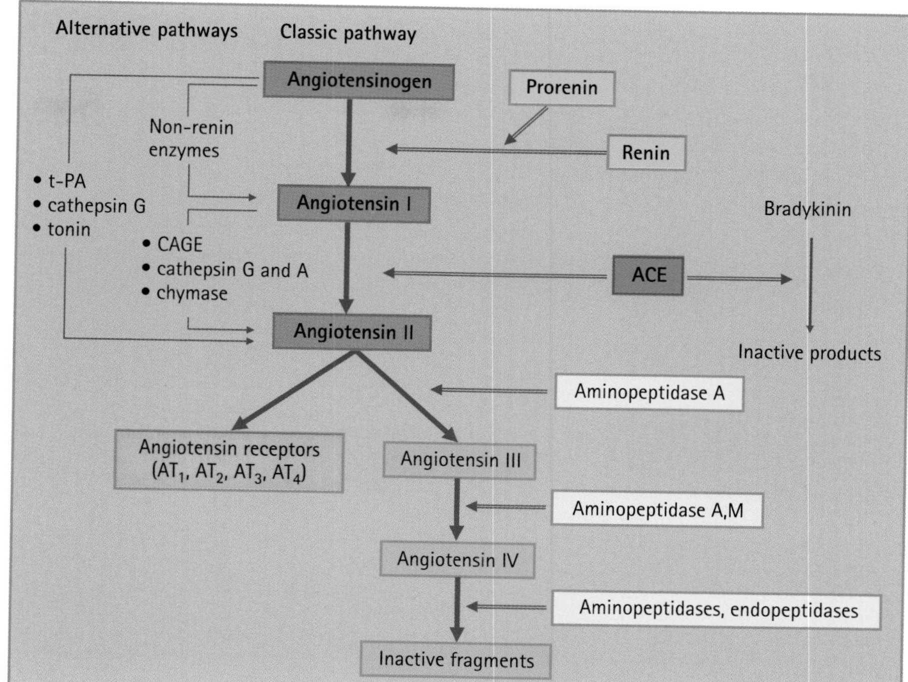

Figure 39.5 Overview of the enzymatic cascade of the renin angiotensin system (RAS): classic and alternative pathways. In the classic pathway, renin cleaves the decapeptide angiotensin I from angiotensinogen. Angiotensin I is then converted to angiotensin II which acts through several receptor subtypes, being AT_1 and AT_2 receptors the more relevant in the vasculature. CAGE, chymostatin-sensitive angiotensin II-generated enzyme; t-PA, tissue plasminogen activator.

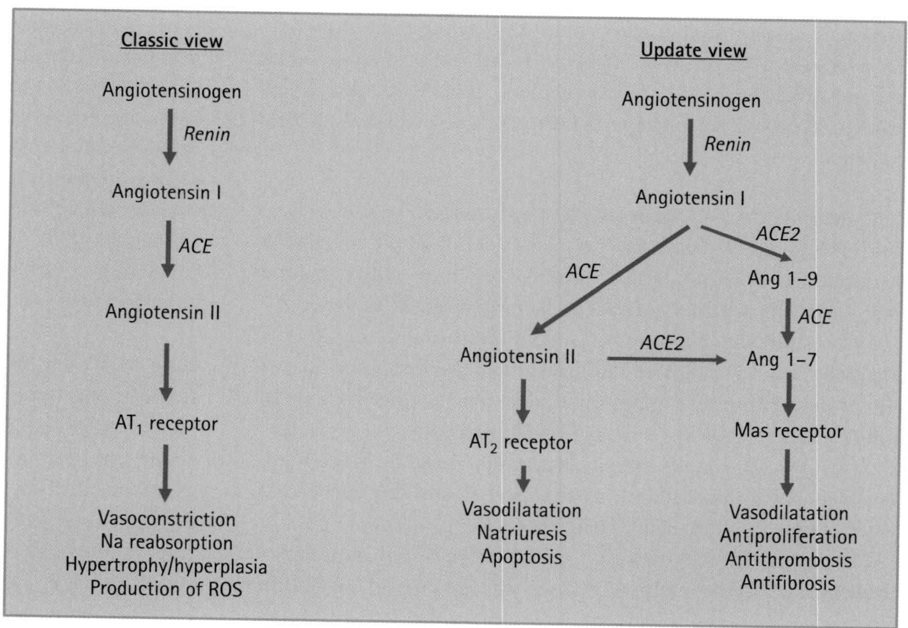

Figure 39.6 New aspects of the renin angiotensin system (RAS) components and its interactions. The classic RAS illustrates the main pathway for angiotensin II (AT II) generation from angiotensin I (AT I) via ACE, with effects being mediated via AT_1 receptor. The updated view illustrates the new components of the RAS in which ACE2 has a role to degrade AT I to AT 1-9, and AT II to the vasodilatator AT 1-7 which acts through the Mas receptor.

research, including into specific inhibitors, is needed to understand the many functions of ACE2 inside and outside the RAS.

AT receptors

The effects of all AT peptides are mediated through specific cell surface receptors (Figures 39.5 and 39.6). The AT_1 receptor mediates most of the effects usually associated with AT II. The role of the AT_2 receptor subtype remains controversial, but it appears to antagonise certain effects of AT II mediated via the AT_1 receptor [101].

Role of the RAS in macrovascular disease

It is now recognized that local RAS activation has an important role in the pathogenesis of diabetes-induced endothelial

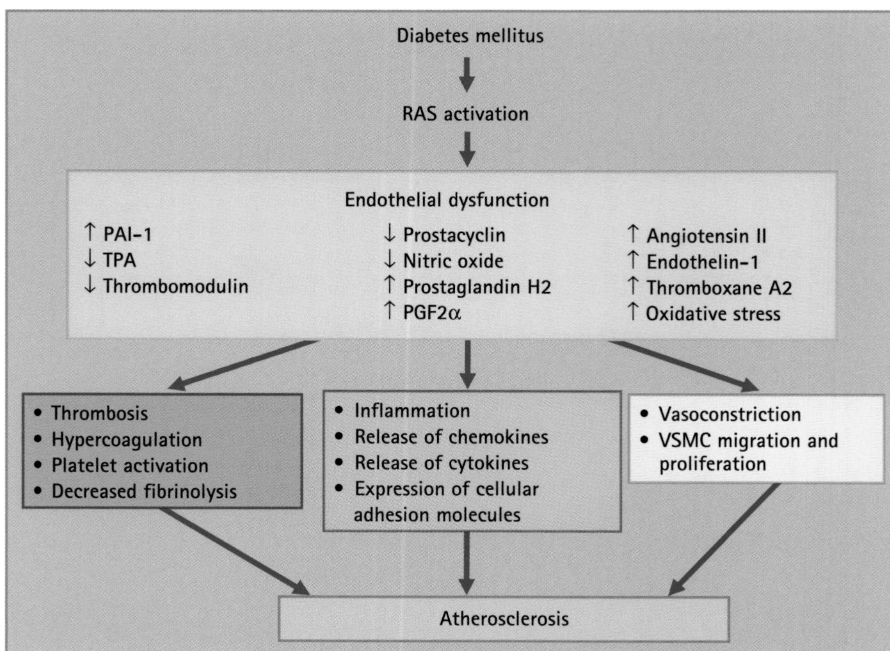

Figure 39.7 Effects of diabetes-induced renin angiotensin system (RAS) activation on mechanisms associated with endothelial dysfunction and atherosclerosis. In diabetes, activation of RAS induces endothelial dysfunction which is characterized by vasoconstriction, inflammation, cellular growth and thrombosis. By losing its protective properties, dysfunctional endothelium is a major promoter of atherogenesis and, consequently, cardiovascular events. PAI-1, plasminogen activator inhibitor-1; TPA, tissue plasminogen activator; VSMC, vascular smooth muscle cells.

dysfunction and atherosclerosis [102–104]. As a result, there is a strong rationale for blockade of the RAS to prevent cardiovascular events in patients with diabetes. In addition, several recent clinical trials [105–110] have suggested that blockade of the RAS may protect against the development of T2DM in at-risk patients.

RAS activation and endothelial dysfunction

Endothelial dysfunction has been considered as an imbalance between vasoconstrictors and vasodilatators in the vascular tone [111] associated with a decrease in NO activity and increased AT II and endothelin (ET) activity [112]. Endothelial dysfunction is characterized by defective endothelium-dependent vasorelaxation in association with inflammatory cytokine-induced increased interactions with blood leukocytes, in which adhesion molecules such as VCAM-1 and chemo-attractants such as MCP-1 are essential [113]. Endothelial dysfunction is strongly associated with atherosclerosis (Figure 39.7) [114,115].

Crucial to the pathogenesis of diabetes-induced endothelial dysfunction in the early stages, in the absence of structural changes of the vessel wall, is the activation of the RAS. Although measurements of components of the RAS in plasma have, in general, suggested suppression of this system in diabetes, there is increasing evidence for activation of the local cardiovascular RAS in the diabetic context [116,117]. It has been demonstrated that there is an increase in ACE expression and activity, in AT II expression, and in AT_1 receptor expression in the aortic wall of diabetic apoE KO mice suggesting a key role for RAS activation in the pathogenesis of diabetes associated endothelial dysfunction [102,118].

RAS and regenerative endothelial cell repair

A role for the RAS has also been demonstrated in affecting the number of regenerative endothelial progenitor cells in patients with diabetes. An increased concentration of circulating endothelial progenitor cells, which are believed to maintain the integrity of the vascular endothelium, has been associated with a favorable cardiovascular outcome in patients with CAD [119]. A study in patients with T2DM [120] suggested that treatment with an ARB (olmesartan) increases the number of regenerative endothelial progenitor cells, which could contribute to the beneficial cardiovascular effects seen with AT_1 receptor blockade.

Role of AT 1-7 and ACE2 in endothelial dysfunction

It has been hypothesized that disruption of the ACE–ACE2 balance may result in abnormal blood pressure, with increased ACE2 expression protecting against hypertension, and ACE2 deficiency causing hypertension (Figure 39.6) [121]. As reported above, it is well established that AT II produces endothelial dysfunction through different pathways, such as increasing oxidative stress and exerting proliferative and pro-thrombotic activities [122]. Recently, it has been observed that AT 1-7, which is generated by the enzyme ACE2, promotes the release of NO and prostaglandins [123,124] and potentiates bradykinin effects in different experimental models [124,125]. In addition, AT 1-7 inhibits growth of VSMC [126], platelet aggregation and thrombosis [127], inflammation, fibrosis [128] and oxidative stress [129] which in turn might lead to restoration of endothelial function. It appears that AT 1-7 can antagonize AT II effects, not only by the stimulation of other vasodilatators but also through AT_1 receptor inhibition. In this regard, Kostenis *et al.* [130] reported that the Mas receptor, which is increasingly considered to be the major receptor conferring the biologic effects of AT 1-7, seems to act as a physiologic antagonist of AT_1 receptor and thus counteracting many of the actions of AT II at the endothelial level.

RAS activation and atherosclerosis

Clinical and experimental evidence clearly indicates that activation of the RAS is central to almost all these pro-atherosclerotic pathways (Figure 39.7) [103,131]. Diet *et al.* [104] observed increased ACE protein accumulation within the atherosclerotic plaque in human coronary arteries suggesting that ACE may contribute to an increased production of local AT II which may participate in the pathophysiology of artery disease. In addition, there is evidence that AT II and the AT_1 receptor are overexpressed in atherosclerotic plaques [102,132,133]. Indeed, blockade of the RAS with an ACE inhibitor or an AT_1 receptor antagonist prevents atherosclerosis by mechanisms involving inhibition of pro-inflammatory molecules such as VCAM-1 and MCP-1 and pro-sclerotic and pro-proliferative cytokines such as CTGF and platelet derived growth factor. These observations confirm a key role for RAS activation in the development and progression of atherosclerosis.

Production of pro-inflammatory cytokines, such as IL-1β, TNF-α and IL-6, have a major role in the pathogenesis of atherosclerosis [134]. IL-6, ACE and AT_1 receptors have been detected in stable and unstable atherosclerotic plaques [132,135]. AT II stimulates the redox sensitive nuclear transcription factor, NFκB, which could serve as a unifying signaling system for inflammatory stimuli in atherogenesis through enhanced expression of adhesion molecules ICAM-1 and VCAM-1, E-selectin, MCP-1 and IL-8. Several clinical and experimental studies have demonstrated that both ACE inhibitors and AT_1 receptor blockers decrease the expression of several adhesion molecules, thus confirming that the chronic inflammatory response associated with atherosclerosis appears to be modulated by AT II at every level and can be targeted therapeutically by RAS inhibition [103,116,136].

Moreover, the sustained pro-inflammatory state seems to play an important part in the transformation of a stable atherosclerotic plaque into a vulnerable plaque prone to rupture. Plaque rupture has been connected with activation of matrix metalloproteinases in the fibrous cap of the atherosclerotic lesion [137], and there is evidence that AT II is implicated in matrix metalloproteinase activation, both through a direct action and through induction of pro-inflammatory cytokines such as IL-6.

ACE2 and diabetes accelerated atherosclerosis

Although studies on the expression and activity of ACE2 in atherosclerosis are limited, there is increasing evidence that such more recently identified components of the RAS may be involved in the development and progression of atherosclerosis. Recently, Zulli *et al.* [138] have shown very high expression of ACE2 in endothelial cells, macrophages and α-smooth muscle cells within atherosclerotic plaques in a rabbit model of atherosclerosis. It is not clear whether this increase in ACE2 is in response to injury in an attempt to protect the vessel by increasing levels of AT 1-7.

In the human context, there is evidence for a significant activation of the cardiac RAS after coronary artery occlusion, and it is well known that RAS blockade reduces remodeling and improves survival in humans after an MI. In recent studies [139], cardiac ACE2 expression and activity are also increased with experimental MI. All these observations suggest that an imbalance in the RAS activity has a central role in the pathogenesis of atherosclerosis. Nevertheless, as yet, it is unknown if deficiency of ACE2 contributes to the accelerated atherosclerotic disease process seen in diabetes.

RAS and oxidative stress

There is increasing evidence that the local production of ROS has a pivotal role in atherosclerosis, specifically in the diabetic milieu. Increased vascular superoxide production in aortas from diabetic atherosclerotic apoE KO mice has been demonstrated [94]. These changes were mediated by increased NAD(P)H oxidase (Nox) activity in the aorta with increased expression of various Nox subunits including p47phox, gp91phox and rac-1 [94]. Evidence of increased local vascular ROS generation in diabetes is further supported by the demonstration of increased nitrotyrosine staining in these diabetic plaques. Indeed, interventions that reduce vascular superoxide production such as PPAR-α and PPAR-γ agonists have been associated with reduced plaque formation, further emphasizing the link between vascular oxidative stress and atherosclerosis [94,140]. Furthermore, the deletion of antioxidant enzymes such as glutathione peroxidase, specifically the Gpx1 isoform in the vascular wall, results in an increase in plaque area particularly in the diabetic context via increases in inflammatory mediators including adhesion molecules and chemokines [141]. More recently, it has been shown that treatment of GPx1 deficient mice with the Gpx1 analog, ebselen, reduced oxidative stress variables and atherosclerosis in diabetic GPx1/apoE KO mice [142]. Furthermore, in the Gpx1/apo E double KO mice, there was associated upregulation of RAGE further linking vascular RAGE expression to increased oxidative stress and accelerated atherosclerosis in settings such as diabetes [141].

Therapeutic implications

RAS blockade and endothelial dysfunction

As a result of previous observations, RAS blockade has emerged as an obvious and attractive therapeutic target. Early evidence for a clinical beneficial effect of inhibition of this system on impaired endothelial function was derived from the Trial on Reversing Endothelial Dysfunction (TREND) [143] which showed that ACE inhibition improves endothelial function in subjects with coronary artery disease. Moreover, O'Driscoll *et al.* [144] observed that ACE inhibition with enalapril improved both basal and stimulated NO-dependent endothelial function in normotensive patients with T2DM.

Data are also available for the role of ARBs in improving endothelial function such as the AT_1 receptor antagonist, losartan

[145,146]. Furthermore, in patients with T1DM treated with the ACE inhibitor ramipril or the ARB losartan for 3 weeks [147] improved endothelial dysfunction potentially mediated by increased bradykinin levels with ACE inhibition or increased levels of AT 1-7 levels.

RAS inhibition and cardiovascular protection

There is accumulative evidence that pharmacologic therapy that interrupts the RAS may afford special benefits in reducing CVD in people with diabetes [109,148,149]. In a *post hoc* subgroup analysis of the Captopril Prevention Project (CAPP) study, the patients with diabetes treated with captopril fared significantly better compared with those treated with conventional therapy (beta-blockers and diuretics) in terms of primary endpoint as well as for MI, all cardiac events and total mortality [148]. These relative beneficial effects of ACE inhibitor therapy were particularly striking in those at highest risk, specifically those with the highest median fasting glucose or those with more elevated blood pressure (BP). This is in contrast to the UKPDS [150], in which there was comparable CVD benefits for patients with T2DM who were randomized to captopril or atenolol, perhaps reflecting a lower CVD risk in the newly diagnosed patients with diabetes studied in the UKPDS.

In a sub-study of the Hypertensive Old People in Edinburgh (HOPE) study, the MICRO-HOPE [151], of the relative risk reduction in the 3577 patients who had diabetes and one other CVD risk factor, there was a risk reduction of 25% for combined CVD events, 37% for CVD mortality, 22% for MI and 33% for stroke. In the Fosinopril versus Amlodipine Cardiovascular Events Trial (FACET) study, the incidence of CVD events was less in hypertensive patients with T2DM treated with fosinopril than the amlodipine-treated group [152]. The European Trial on Reduction of Cardiac Events with Perindopril in Stable Coronary Artery Disease (EUROPA) [153] has shown that ACE inhibition reduced cardiovascular mortality and morbidity in patients with established CAD without left ventricular dysfunction. The data from these trials were pooled with those of the Quinapril Ischemic Event Trial (QUIET) [154] study in a meta-analysis that included a total of 31 555 patients [155]. This analysis showed that, compared with placebo, ACE inhibitor therapy produced a significant 14% reduction in all-cause mortality and MI, a 23% reduction in stroke and a 7% statistically significant reduction in revascularization procedures. Recently, the ADVANCE study [23] has shown that the administration of the ACE inhibitor perindopril and the diuretic indapamide in high-risk patients with T2DM induced a reduction in macrovascular outcome when compared with placebo.

Recent reports of trials with ARBs indicate that these agents have CVD protection effects in patients with T2DM similar to those observed with ACE inhibitors. In the Losartan Intervention For Endpoint reduction in hypertension (LIFE) study [109], treatment with losartan in patients with T2DM and left ventricular hypertrophy (LVH) resulted in a significant reduction in death from CVD and in particular all cause mortality. An analysis from the large Reduction of Endpoints in NIDDM with Angiotensin II Antagonist Losartan (RENAAL) study has shown that treatment with losartan in patients with T2DM, nephropathy and LVH reduced the cardiovascular risk to levels similar to those observed in patients without LVH [156]. Recently, the Ongoing Telmisartan Alone and in combination with Ramipril Global Endpoint Trial (ONTARGET) has shown that the ARB telmisartan provides a benefit similar to that of a proven ACE inhibitor such as ramipril in high risk patients with CVD or subjects with diabetes who have end-organ damage. This is a population similar to that examined previously in the HOPE study [157]. Furthermore, in the ONTARGET study the combination of ramipril with telmisartan, despite the further lowering of BP, did not reduce the risk of cardiovascular events, compared with an ACE inhibitor alone, but was associated with additional adverse effects including hypotension and renal dysfunction. Thus, an ACE inhibitor, or possibly an ARB, is an initial antihypertensive agent of choice in patients with diabetes because these agents have been shown to have the capacity to prevent or retard the development of diabetic macrovascular complications, thus significantly reducing cardiovascular mortality and morbidity.

The endothelin system

Endothelin (ET) was first discovered in 1988 by Yanagisawa *et al.* [158] and is one of the most potent vasoconstrictors known. There are three distinct ET genes that encode different mature ET sequences, designated ET-1, ET-2 and ET-3. Big ET-1 is converted into mature 21 amino acid ET-1 by ET-converting enzyme. ET-1 is predominantly present in endothelial cells. In 1990, the ET_A and ET_B receptor subtypes [159], were cloned. ET_A receptors are found in VSMCs and mediate vasoconstriction and cell proliferation (Figure 39.8). ET_B receptors are found in endothelial cells (ET_{B1}) where they mediate vasodilation via the release of NO and on smooth muscle cells, where they may elicit vessel contraction and cell proliferation (Figure 39.8).

Role of ET in diabetic macrovascular complications

Plasma concentrations of ET-1 are increased in patients with T2DM complicated with atherosclerosis, compared with patients without diabetes with atherosclerosis and healthy subjects [160]. Kalogeropoulou *et al.* [161] demonstrated increased ET-1 levels in subjects with diabetes and carotid atherosclerosis. ET stimulates the production and release of inflammatory cytokines from monocytes [162] and enhances the uptake of LDL cholesterol by these cells, promoting a phenotypic change into foam cells [163]. Cytokines released from monocytes–macrophages, in turn, stimulate ET-1 production, providing positive feedback for further cytokine production [164].

In several animal models, both ET_A receptor-selective and non-selective ET_A/ET_B receptor blockade have been shown to inhibit the development of atherosclerotic lesions suggesting that elevated vascular ET-1 tissue levels promote endothelial dysfunction

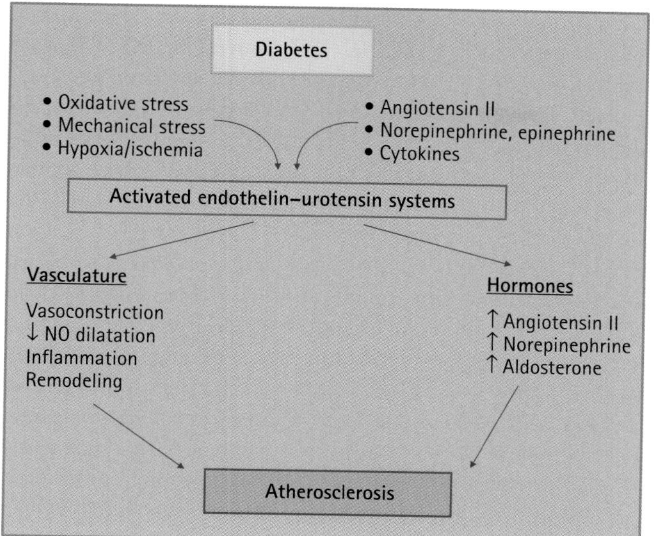

Figure 39.8 Proposed mechanisms of the endothelin and urotensin systems on atherosclerosis in diabetes. In diabetes, activation of the endothelin system induces vasoconstriction, vascular smooth muscle cells proliferation, wall thickening, inflammation and tissue remodeling thus leading to the development and progression of atherosclerosis.

and vascular structural alterations *via* the activation of ET_A receptors [163,165]. Treatment with an ET_A receptor antagonist decreased atherosclerotic lesion area in the aorta in apoE KO mice [11]. Similar results have been reported with a non-selective ET_A/ET_B receptor blocker in rabbits. The role of the ET_B receptor in atherosclerosis remains controversial at this stage although it has been shown to have anti-atherosclerotic effects via stimulation of NO production [166].

Finally, some of the beneficial effects of ACE-inhibitors in term of cardiovascular protection may be at least in part mediated by ET inhibition. Captopril inhibits the release of ET from cultured human endothelial cells and decreases 24-h urinary ET-1 excretion [167,168]. Furthermore, ET_A receptor antagonism appears to be beneficial in the treatment of diabetic nephropathy, but there are currently no data to support a protective effect on macrovascular disease in people with diabetes.

Urotensin II

Several recent reports have revealed the powerful vasocontractile effect of urotensin II (UT II) consistent with a potential importance of this peptide in cardiovascular physiology and diseases (Figure 39.8) [169]. A specific UT II receptor was identified in 1999 [170]. Elevated circulating concentrations of UT II have been detected in patients with various CVD states including heart failure, hypertension [171], carotid atherosclerosis, pre-eclampsia and eclampsia, renal dysfunction and diabetes mellitus [172]. In addition, upregulation of the UT receptor system has been found in patients with congestive heart failure and pulmonary hypertension [173].

Role of urotensin II in atherosclerosis

Expression of UT II is upregulated in endothelial, myointimal and medial smooth muscle cells of atherosclerotic human coronary arteries. Bousette *et al.* [12] have demonstrated that UT II expression is increased in both atherosclerotic carotid arteries and aortas. It has been shown that the plasma UT II level is correlated positively with carotid atherosclerosis in patients with essential hypertension [174]. In apoE KO mice, UT expression was significantly higher than in wild-type control mice [175]. Chronic infusion of UT II enhances atherosclerotic lesion in the aorta of apoE KO mice by increasing ROS production and acyl-CoA-cholesterol acyl-transferase 1 expression. UT II expression in endothelial cells and VSMCs is increased following balloon injury in rat carotid arteries [176]. Furthermore, treatment with a UT II receptor blocker was associated with a 60% reduction in intima lesion development.

UT II is linked to the activation of the redox-sensitive enzyme NADPH oxidase in the vascular wall and increased expression of inflammatory cytokines (Figure 39.8). In human peripheral blood mononuclear cells, inflammatory stimuli including IL-1β and TNF-α strongly enhance UT receptor mRNA and protein expression [177]. Of direct relevance to atherosclerosis, UT II has been shown, predominantly in *in vitro* studies to enhance LDL cholesterot and ROS production via NADPH oxidase and to promote monocyte recruitment.

TNF-related apoptosis inducing ligand and osteoprotegerin

Tumor necrosis factor (TNF) related apoptosis inducing ligand (TRAIL) is a member of the TNF ligand family [178]. Both the membrane-bound and soluble forms of TRAIL rapidly induce apoptosis in multiple transformed cell lines and tumor cells, but not in normal cells [178,179].

Osteoprotegerin (OPG) is a member of TNF-receptor superfamily [180], which is produced by a variety of tissues including the cardiovascular system. OPG has two known TNF family ligands: receptor activator of NFκB ligand (RANKL) [181] and TRAIL [182]. Increasing experimental evidence suggests that both TRAIL and OPG are involved in vascular pathophysiology.

Recently, the potential role of soluble recombinant (sr) TRAIL in the pathogenesis and/or treatment of diabetes-induced atherosclerosis has been investigated *in vivo*, in streptozotocin-diabetic apoE KO mice [183]. Repeated intraperitoneal injections of srTRAIL significantly attenuated plaque development and contributed to stabilize atherosclerotic lesions by selectively decreasing the number of infiltrating macrophages and increasing the VSMCs within the atherosclerotic plaques [183]. The potential clinical relevance of these results is corroborated by two studies in patients with acute coronary syndrome, revealing significantly lower sTRAIL serum levels in these subjects when compared to patients with stable angina or normal coronary arteries [184,185].

OPG-deficient mice demonstrated calcifications of the aorta and renal arteries [186], suggesting that OPG might have a role in protecting from vascular calcification. Interestingly, a study in elderly women found a significant correlation between elevated OPG serum levels and cardiovascular mortality [187]. The potential links between OPG and vascular disease in humans have been further supported by the detection of a single nucleotide polymorphism in the promoter region of the human gene for OPG related to vascular morphology and function [188]. Several independent studies have reported elevated serum and/or plasma OPG levels in people with diabetes, and in particular in people with diabetes and vascular complications [189]. Although some authors have proposed that the increase in OPG levels may represent a defence mechanism against other factors that promote vascular pathologies, other studies support a pro-atherosclerotic role for OPG in the vasculature [190].

Complement activation

The complement system consists of approximately 30 proteins that provide an important component of the innate immune system. The complement system is activated through three different pathways: the classic, the alternative and the mannose-binding lectin (MBL) complement pathway, respectively. These three pathways merge and stimulate the formation of a C3 convertase (Figure 39.9).

Recently, an increasing amount of evidence indicates that the complement system activation may have a role in the development of diabetic macrovascular complications [15], in particular the MBL pathway as the initiating pathway of complement activation in patients with diabetes [15]. Patients with T1DM with nephropathy and CVD have significantly higher circulating levels of MBL than normoalbuminuric patients [191]. Furthermore, there is evidence that MBL levels may have prognostic relevance in people with diabetes. Several observations have suggested that MBL may be involved in the pathogenesis of microvascular and macrovascular complications in T1DM and that determination of MBL status might be useful to identify patients at increased risk of developing these complications [191,192]. High levels of MBL early in the course of T1DM are significantly associated with later development of persistent microalbuminuria and macroalbuminuria [193]. In addition, in patients with T2DM, measurement of MBL has been shown to provide prognostic information on mortality and development of microalbuminuria [194]. The mechanism responsible for this potential activation of the complement system in patients with diabetes is still unknown. It has been hypothesized that hyperglycemia in people with diabetes may activate the complement system via mitochondrial ROS production or enhanced RAGE activation.

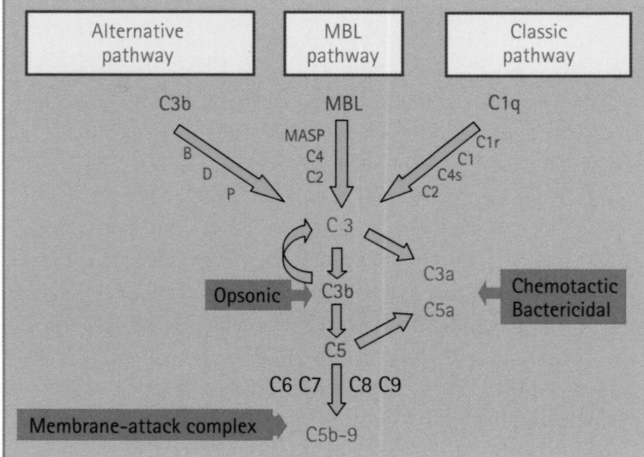

Figure 39.9 Schematic presentation of the complement system. The complement cascade is activated by either of the three pathways: the classic, the mannose-binding lectin (MBL) pathway, or the alternative pathway. Activation leads to formation of the membrane-attack complex as well as formation of opsonic, chemotactic and bactericidal factors.

Clinical studies using pexelizumab, an inhibitor of C5, have recently demonstrated a significant reduction in mortality following acute MI as well as reducing the incidence of death or MI in patients after coronary artery bypass graft surgery [195]. Further studies are needed to determine in particular if manipulation of the complement system may represent a promising target in the treatment and prevention of diabetes associated macrovascular disease.

Interventions to reduce diabetes associated macrovascular complications

A range of interventions has been proposed to reduce the macrovascular complications of diabetes including lifestyle modification, weight reduction, dietary changes and regular exercise.

Glucose control

Optimal glucose control is pivotal for the prevention and treatment of microvascular complications of diabetes; however, based on the recent clinical trials [22,23], the evidence for beneficial effects on macrovascular outcomes is less clear. Nevertheless, it has been suggested to aim for a HbA_{1c} <7% (53 mmol/mol), but to be more cautious in patients with underlying and pre-existing CVD.

Hypertension

Epidemiologic studies have shown that the risk for cardiovascular events and mortality starts at BP values as low as 115/75 mmHg for the general population and doubles for every increase in 20 mmHg systolic and 10 mmHg diastolic (see Chapter 40). The question of what systolic or diastolic BP level should be targeted has not been completely answered by currently available outcome trials. Based on studies such as the Hypertension Optimal Treatment (HOT) study [196], UKPDS [197] and the Appropriate Blood Pressure Control in type 2 Diabetes (ABCD) trial [198], a maximum systolic BP of 130–135 mmHg should be the goal for people with diabetes.

The more recently completed ADVANCE trial [23] evaluated the effect of a fixed dose of perindopril and indapamide on macrovascular and microvascular outcomes in subjects with T2DM. The treatment group showed a mean reduction in systolic and diastolic BP of 5.6 and 2.2 mmHg respectively, which was associated with a 18% reduction in cardiovascular deaths and a 14% reduction in coronary events in comparison to the control group. No lower limit for BP reduction appears to exist at which benefits related to cardiovascular outcomes are not observed with a similar pattern recently reported for renal disease [199]. The ACCORD trial is currently testing the effects of lowering BP below 140/90 mmHg on cardiovascular outcomes. Specifically, it will evaluate if a BP reduction to 120 mmHg systolic will further reduce the cardiovascular event rate.

Choice of antihypertensive treatment

Experimental studies have clearly demonstrated a reduction in atherosclerosis with RAS inhibitors with a possible superiority of ACE inhibitors compared to ARBs in T2DM; however, in the human setting, there are no conclusive studies as yet to show clear superiority of one class of antihypertensive drugs over another. The majority of the beneficial effects on cardiovascular events appear to be related to the antihypertensive actions of these agents. The ONTARGET study was the first study to evaluate the effect of combined RAS blockade in comparison to full-dose ramipril and telmisartan alone [200]. There was no superiority of the ACE inhibitor versus the ARB in terms of cardiovascular events, and dual blockade did not confer greater cardiovascular protection and indeed was associated with more adverse events; however, only 30% of all subjects enrolled in this study had diabetes, and no specific subgroup analysis has been reported so far. Therefore, this study cannot conclusively answer the question of superiority of different blockers of the RAS and combination RAS-blockade on microvascular and macrovascular outcomes in diabetes.

Dyslipidemia

The lipid profile is usually altered in the diabetic milieu and further altered in the context of liver or renal disease. Dyslipidemia further accelerates atherosclerosis development and progression (see Chapter 40). At any given level of cholesterol, a person with diabetes has a two- to threefold increased cardiovascular risk than a person without diabetes.

Current guidelines based on numerous studies particularly with statins (Heart Protective Study [HPS] [201], the Collaborative Atorvastatin Diabetes Study [CARDS] [202]) suggest to reduce LDL levels below 2.5 mmol/L with some more recent evidence suggesting enhanced benefits if LDL is lowered <2 mmol/L, triglycerides <1 mmol/L and HDL> 1 mmol/L according to pre-existing CVD and risk [203].

Hypercoagulability

Diabetes is associated with pro-thrombotic changes and enhanced coagulability, thus increasing cardiovascular risk [204,205]. Although not studied in detail, agents such as aspirin may be useful in people with diabetes, with increasing evidence that higher doses of these agents are often required in people with diabetes to confer cardiovascular benefits. Other drugs to consider in diabetes are clopidogrel as well as the use of drugs such as abciximab [206], which has been reported to be particularly effective in people with diabetes.

Novel therapies

Several approaches have been used to intervene in diabetes-associated complications including aldose reductase inhibitors, PKC isoform inhibitors, in particular PKC β, but most of the evidence for a potential role for these agents has been obtained in the context of microvascular complications. Furthermore, inhibitors of glucose induced ROS formation, such as benfotiamine, have been investigated in clinical trials with variable results. AGE inhibitors and RAGE antagonism have also been employed, mainly in the context of diabetic nephropathy. The cross-link breaker, alagebrium, has shown to reduce arterial stiffness in hypertensive patients and to improve left ventricular function. Direct antagonists of RAGE and human chimeric sRAGE are also currently being investigated in early clinical trials, however, not as yet with respect to macrovascular disease.

The role of PPAR-α and PPAR-γ agonists have also been investigated with modest or no effects on cardiovascular outcomes [207–209]. The dual PPAR-α/γ agonists such as muraglitazar do not appear to be likely to be introduced as a result of adverse side effects and the possibility of adverse cardiovascular events [210].

Multifactorial approaches

The Steno-2 study, using a multifactorial approach addressing lipids, BP and hyperglycemia, demonstrated significant improvements on cardiovascular outcomes [25]. Thus, a synergistic multifactorial approach addressing glycemic control in the context of additional strategies to reduce concomitant cardiovascular risk factors remains the best approach to be currently considered. Furthermore, strategies directed towards a reduction in activation of vasoactive systems such as the RAS, the ET and UT systems, the AGE/RAGE axis, novel proteins such as TRAIL and the complement system as well as oxidative stress and inflammation may additional promising approaches to prevent and minimize macrovascular disease in diabetes.

References

1 Nathan DM, Lachin J, Cleary P, Orchard T, Brillon DJ, Backlund JY, *et al.* Intensive diabetes therapy and carotid intima-media thickness in type 1 diabetes mellitus. *N Engl J Med* 2003; **348**: 2294–2303.

2 Nathan DM, Cleary PA, Backlund JY, Genuth SM, Lachin JM, Orchard TJ, *et al.* Intensive diabetes treatment and cardiovascular disease in patients with type 1 diabetes. *N Engl J Med* 2005; **353**:2643–2653.

3 Turner RC, Millns H, Neil HA, Stratton IM, Manley SE, Matthews DR, *et al.* Risk factors for coronary artery disease in non-insulin dependent diabetes mellitus: United Kingdom Prospective Diabetes Study (UKPDS 23). *Br Med J* 1998; **316**:823–828.

4 Turner R, Cull C, Holman R. UK Prospective Diabetes Study 17: a 9-year update of a randomized, controlled trial on the effect of improved metabolic control on complications in non-insulin-dependent diabetes mellitus. *Ann Intern Med* 1996; **124**:136–145.

5 Holman RR, Paul SK, Bethel MA, Neil HA, Matthews DR. Long-term follow-up after tight control of blood pressure in type 2 diabetes. *N Engl J Med* 2008; **359**:1565–1576.

6 Califf RM, Boolell M, Haffner SM, Bethel MA, McMurray J, Duggal A, *et al.* Prevention of diabetes and cardiovascular disease in patients with impaired glucose tolerance: rationale and design of the Nateglinide and Valsartan in Impaired Glucose Tolerance Outcomes Research (NAVIGATOR) Trial. *Am Heart J* 2008; **156**:623–632.

7 Stamler J, Vaccaro O, Neaton JD, Wentworth D. Diabetes, other risk factors, and 12-yr cardiovascular mortality for men screened in the Multiple Risk Factor Intervention Trial. *Diabetes Care* 1993; **16**:434–444.

8 Fitzgerald AP, Jarrett RJ. Are conventional risk factors for mortality relevant in type 2 diabetes? *Diabet Med* 1991; **8**:475–480.

9 Dale AC, Vatten LJ, Nilsen TI, Midthjell K, Wiseth R. Secular decline in mortality from coronary heart disease in adults with diabetes mellitus: cohort study. *Br Med J* 2008; **337**:a236.

10 Calcutt NA, Cooper ME, Kern TS, Schmidt AM. Therapies for hyperglycaemia-induced diabetic complications: from animal models to clinical trials. *Nat Rev Drug Discov* 2009; **8**:417–429.

11 Barton M, Haudenschild CC, d'Uscio LV, Shaw S, Munter K, Luscher TF. Endothelin ETA receptor blockade restores NO-mediated endothelial function and inhibits atherosclerosis in apolipoprotein E-deficient mice. *Proc Natl Acad Sci U S A* 1998; **95**:14367–14372.

12 Bousette N, Patel L, Douglas SA, Ohlstein EH, Giaid A. Increased expression of urotensin II and its cognate receptor GPR14 in atherosclerotic lesions of the human aorta. *Atherosclerosis* 2004; **176**:117–123.

13 Hassan GS, Douglas SA, Ohlstein EH, Giaid A. Expression of urotensin-II in human coronary atherosclerosis. *Peptides* 2005; **26**:2464–2472.

14 Secchiero P, Zerbinati C, Rimondi E, Corallini F, Milani D, Grill V, *et al.* TRAIL promotes the survival, migration and proliferation of vascular smooth muscle cells. *Cell Mol Life Sci* 2004; **61**: 1965–1974.

15 Østergaard J, Hansen TK, Thiel S, Flyvbjerg A. Complement activation and diabetic vascular complications. *Clin Chim Acta* 2005; **361**:10–19.

16 Libby P. Current concepts of the pathogenesis of the acute coronary syndromes. *Circulation* 2001; **104**:365–372.

17 UK Prospective Diabetes Study (UKPDS) Group. Intensive blood-glucose control with sulphonylureas or insulin compared with conventional treatment and risk of complications in patients with type 2 diabetes (UKPDS 33). *Lancet* 1998; **352**:837–853.

18 Gall MA, Borch-Johnsen K, Hougaard P, Nielsen FS, Parving H-H. Albuminuria and poor glycemic control predict mortality in NIDDM. *Diabetes* 1995; **44**:1303–1309.

19 Salomaa V, Miettinen H, Kuulasmaa K, Niemelä M, Ketonen M, Vuorenmaa T, *et al.* Decline of coronary heart disease mortality in Finland during 1983 to 1992: roles of incidence, recurrence, and case-fatality. The FINMONICA MI Register Study. *Circulation* 1996; **94**:3130–3137.

20 Kuusisto J, Mykkanen L, Pyorala K, Laakso M. Non-insulin-dependent diabetes and its metabolic control are important predictors of stroke in elderly subjects. *Stroke* 1994; **25**:1157–1164.

21 Gerstein HC. Is glucose a continuous risk factor for cardiovascular mortality? *Diabetes Care* 1999; **22**:659–660.

22 Gerstein HC, Miller ME, Byington RP, Goff DC Jr, Bigger JT, Buse JB, *et al.* Effects of intensive glucose lowering in type 2 diabetes. *N Engl J Med* 2008; **358**:2545–2559.

23 Patel A, MacMahon S, Chalmers J, Neal B, Billot L, Woodward M, Marre M, *et al.*; ADVANCE Collaborative Group. Intensive blood glucose control and vascular outcomes in patients with type 2 diabetes. *N Engl J Med* 2008; **358**:2560–2572.

24 Duckworth W, Abraira C, Moritz T, Reda D, Emanuele N, Reaven PD, *et al.* Glucose control and vascular complications in veterans with type 2 diabetes. *N Engl J Med* 2009; **360**:129–139.

25 Gæde P, Lund-Andersen H, Parving H-H, Pedersen O. Effect of a multifactorial intervention on mortality in type 2 diabetes. *N Engl J Med* 2008; **358**:580–591.

26 Holman RR, Paul SK, Bethel MA, Matthews DR, Neil HA. 10-year follow-up of intensive glucose control in type 2 diabetes. *N Engl J Med* 2008; **359**:1577–1589.

27 Vikramadithyan RK, Hu Y, Noh HL, Liang CP, Hallam K, Tall AR, *et al.* Human aldose reductase expression accelerates diabetic atherosclerosis in transgenic mice. *J Clin Invest* 2005; **115**: 2434–2443.

28 Brownlee M. Biochemistry and molecular cell biology of diabetic complications. *Nature* 2001; **414**:813–820.

29 Hsueh W, Abel ED, Breslow JL, Maeda N, Davis RC, Fisher EA, *et al.* Recipes for creating animal models of diabetic cardiovascular disease. *Circ Res* 2007; **100**:1415–1427.

30 Renard CB, Kramer F, Johansson F, Lamharzi N, Tannock LR, von Herrath MG, *et al.* Diabetes and diabetes-associated lipid abnormalities have distinct effects on initiation and progression of atherosclerotic lesions. *J Clin Invest* 2004; **114**:659–668.

31 Johansson F, Kramer F, Barnhart S, Kanter JE, Vaisar T, Merrill RD, *et al.* Type 1 diabetes promotes disruption of advanced atherosclerotic lesions in LDL receptor-deficient mice. *Proc Natl Acad Sci U S A* 2008; **105**:2082–2087.

32 Brownlee M, Hirsch IB. Glycemic variability: a hemoglobin A1c-independent risk factor for diabetic complications. *JAMA* 2006; **295**:1707–1708.

33 Monnier L, Mas E, Ginet C, Michel F, Villon L, Cristol JP, *et al.* Activation of oxidative stress by acute glucose fluctuations compared with sustained chronic hyperglycemia in patients with type 2 diabetes. *JAMA* 2006; **295**:1681–1687.

34 El-Osta A, Brasacchio D, Yao D, Pocai A, Jones PL, Roeder RG, *et al.* Transient high glucose causes persistent epigenetic changes and altered gene expression during subsequent normoglycemia. *J Exp Med* 2008; **205**:2409–2417.

35 Brasacchio D, Okabe J, Tikellis C, Balcerczyk A, George P, Baker EK, *et al.* Hyperglycemia induces a dynamic cooperativity of histone methylase and demethylase enzymes associated with gene-activating epigenetic marks that coexist on the lysine tail. *Diabetes* 2009; **58**:1229–1236.

36 Saydah SH, Loria CM, Eberhardt MS, Brancati FL. Subclinical states of glucose intolerance and risk of death in the US. *Diabetes Care* 2001; **24**:447–453.

37 Haffner S. Mortality from coronary heart disease in subjects with type 2 diabetes and in nondiabetic subjects with and without prior myocardial infarction. *N Engl J Med* 1998; **339**:229–234.
38 Hu G, Qiao Q, Tuomilehto J, Balkau B, Borch-Johnsen K, Pyorala K. Prevalence of the metabolic syndrome and its relation to all-cause and cardiovascular mortality in nondiabetic European men and women. *Arch Intern Med* 2004; **164**:1066–1076.
39 Yip J, Facchini FS, Reaven GM. Resistance to insulin-mediated glucose disposal as a predictor of cardiovascular disease. *J Clin Endocrinol Metab* 1998; **83**:2773–2776.
40 Hanley AJ, Williams K, Stern MP, Haffner SM. Homeostasis model assessment of insulin resistance in relation to the incidence of cardiovascular disease: the San Antonio Heart Study. *Diabetes Care* 2002; **25**:1177–1184.
41 Hanley AJ, McKeown-Eyssen G, Harris SB, Hegele RA, Wolever TM, Kwan J, *et al.* Association of parity with risk of type 2 diabetes and related metabolic disorders. *Diabetes Care* 2002; **25**:690–695.
42 Hsueh WA, Law RE. Cardiovascular risk continuum: implications of insulin resistance and diabetes. *Am J Med* 1998; **105**:4S–14S.
43 King GL, Brownlee M. The cellular and molecular mechanisms of diabetic complications. *Endocrinol Metab Clin North Am* 1996; **25**:255–270.
44 Yuen DY, Dwyer RM, Matthews VB, Zhang L, Drew BG, Neill B, *et al.* Interleukin-6 attenuates insulin-mediated increases in endothelial cell signaling but augments skeletal muscle insulin action via differential effects on tumor necrosis factor-alpha expression. *Diabetes* 2009; **58**:1086–1095.
45 Lo TW, Westwood ME, McLellan AC, Selwood T, Thornalley PJ. Binding and modification of proteins by methylglyoxal under physiological conditions: a kinetic and mechanistic study with N alpha-acetylarginine, N alpha-acetylcysteine, and N alpha-acetyllysine, and bovine serum albumin. *J Biol Chem* 1994; **269**:32299–32305.
46 Ahmed N, Thornalley PJ, Dawczynski J, Franke S, Strobel J, Stein G, *et al.* Methylglyoxal-derived hydroimidazolone advanced glycation end-products of human lens proteins. *Invest Ophthalmol Vis Sci* 2003; **44**:5287–5292.
47 Thornalley PJ, Langborg A, Minhas HS. Formation of glyoxal, methylglyoxal and 3-deoxyglucosone in the glycation of proteins by glucose. *Biochem J* 1999; **344**:109–116.
48 Brownlee M. Advanced protein glycosylation in diabetes and aging. *Annu Rev Med* 1995; **46**:223–234.
49 Vlassara H, Fuh H, Makita Z, Krungkrai S, Cerami A, Bucala R. Exogenous advanced glycosylation end products induce complex vascular dysfunction in normal animals: a model for diabetic and aging complications. *Proc Natl Acad Sci U S A* 1992; **89**:12043–12047.
50 Bucala R, Tracey KJ, Cerami A. Advanced glycosylation products quench nitric oxide and mediate defective endothelium-dependent vasodilatation in experimental diabetes. *J Clin Invest* 1991; **87**:432–438.
51 Forbes JM, Yee LT, Thallas V, Lassila M, Candido R, Jandeleir-Dahm KA, *et al.* Advanced glycation end product interventions reduce diabetes-accelerated atherosclerosis. *Diabetes* 2004; **53**:1813–1823.
52 Kislinger T, Tanji N, Wendt T, Qu W, Lu Y, Ferran LJ Jr, *et al.* Receptor for advanced glycation end products mediates inflammation and enhanced expression of tissue factor in vasculature of diabetic apolipoprotein E-null mice. *Arterioscler Thromb Vasc Biol* 2001; **21**:905–910.
53 Aronson D. Cross-linking of glycated collagen in the pathogenesis of arterial and myocardial stiffening of aging and diabetes. *J Hypertens* 2003; **21**:3–12.
54 Kass DA, Shapiro EP, Kawaguchi M, Capriotti AR, Scuteri A, deGroof RC, *et al.* Improved arterial compliance by a novel advanced glycation end-product crosslink breaker. *Circulation* 2001; **104**:1464–470.
55 Hogan M, Cerami A, Bucala R. Advanced glycosylation endproducts block the antiproliferative effect of nitric oxide: role in the vascular and renal complications of diabetes mellitus. *J Clin Invest* 1992; **90**:1110–1115.
56 Wautier MP, Chappey O, Corda S, Stern DM, Schmidt AM, Wautier JL. Activation of NADPH oxidase by AGE links oxidant stress to altered gene expression via RAGE. *Am J Physiol Endocrinol Metab* 2001; **280**:E685–694.
57 Neeper M, Schmidt AM, Brett J, Yan SD, Wang F, Pan YC, *et al.* Cloning and expression of a cell surface receptor for advanced glycosylation end products of proteins. *J Biol Chem* 1992; **267**:14998–15004.
58 McRobert EA, Gallicchio M, Jerums G, Cooper ME, Bach LA. The amino-terminal domains of the ezrin, radixin, and moesin (ERM) proteins bind advanced glycation end products, an interaction that may play a role in the development of diabetic complications. *J Biol Chem* 2003; **278**:25783–25789.
59 Ohgami N, Nagai R, Ikemoto M, Arai H, Kuniyasu A, Horiuchi S, *et al.* CD36, a member of the class b scavenger receptor family, as a receptor for advanced glycation end products. *J Biol Chem* 2001; **276**:3195–3202.
60 Febbraio M, Guy E, Silverstein RL. Stem cell transplantation reveals that absence of macrophage CD36 is protective against atherosclerosis. *Arterioscler Thromb Vasc Biol* 2004; **24**:2333–2338.
61 Soulis T, Thallas V, Youssef S, Gilbert RE, McWilliam BG, Murray-McIntosh RP, *et al.* Advanced glycation end products and their receptors co-localize in rat organs susceptible to diabetic microvascular injury. *Diabetologia* 1997; **40**:619–628.
62 Brett J, Schmidt AM, Yan SD, Zou YS, Weidman E, Pinsky D, *et al.* Survey of the distribution of a newly characterized receptor for advanced glycation end products in tissues. *Am J Pathol* 1993; **143**:1699–1712.
63 Bierhaus A, Stern DM, Nawroth PP. RAGE in inflammation: a new therapeutic target? *Curr Opin Investig Drugs* 2006; **7**:985–991.
64 Schmidt AM, Yan SD, Yan SF, Stern DM. The multiligand receptor RAGE as a progression factor amplifying immune and inflammatory responses. *J Clin Invest* 2001; **108**:949–955.
65 Lander HM, Tauras JM, Ogiste JS, Hori O, Moss RA, Schmidt AM. Activation of the receptor for advanced glycation end products triggers a p21(ras)-dependent mitogen-activated protein kinase pathway regulated by oxidant stress. *J Biol Chem* 1997; **272**:17810–17814.
66 Li JH, Wang W, Huang XR, Oldfield M, Schmidt AM, Cooper ME, *et al.* Advanced glycation end products induce tubular epithelial-myofibroblast transition through the RAGE-ERK1/2 MAP kinase signaling pathway. *Am J Pathol* 2004; **164**:1389–1397.
67 Li J, Schmidt AM. Characterization and functional analysis of the promoter of RAGE, the receptor for advanced glycation end products. *J Biol Chem* 1997; **272**:16498–16506.
68 Higashi T, Sano H, Saishoji T, Ikeda K, Jinnouchi Y, Kanzaki T, *et al.* The receptor for advanced glycation end products mediates the chemotaxis of rabbit smooth muscle cells. *Diabetes* 1997; **46**:463–472.

69 Miyata T, Ueda Y, Asahi K, Izuhara Y, Inagi R, Saito A, *et al.* Mechanism of the inhibitory effect of OPB-9195 ((+/−)-2-isopropylidenehydrazono-4-oxo-thiazolidin-5-yla cetanilide) on advanced glycation end product and advanced lipoxidation end product formation. *J Am Soc Nephrol* 2000; **11**:1719–1725.

70 Thornalley PJ, Yurek-George A, Argirov OK. Kinetics and mechanism of the reaction of aminoguanidine with the alpha-oxoaldehydes glyoxal, methylglyoxal, and 3-deoxyglucosone under physiological conditions. *Biochem Pharmacol* 2000; **60**:55–65.

71 Rosca MG, Mustata TG, Kinter MT, Ozdemir AM, Kern TS, Szweda LI, *et al.* Glycation of mitochondrial proteins from diabetic rat kidney is associated with excess superoxide formation. *Am J Physiol Renal Physiol* 2005; **289**:F420–430.

72 Soulis-Liparota T, Cooper M, Papazoglou D, Clarke B, Jerums G. Retardation by aminoguanidine of development of albuminuria, mesangial expansion, and tissue fluorescence in streptozocin-induced diabetic rat. *Diabetes* 1991; **40**:1328–1334.

73 Coughlan MT, Thallas-Bonke V, Pete J, Long DM, Gasser A, Tong DC, *et al.* Combination therapy with the advanced glycation end product cross-link breaker, alagebrium, and angiotensin converting enzyme inhibitors in diabetes: synergy or redundancy? *Endocrinology* 2007; **148**:886–895.

74 Vasan S, Zhang X, Kapurniotu A, Bernhagen J, Teichberg S, Basgen J, *et al.* An agent cleaving glucose-derived protein crosslinks *in vitro* and *in vivo*. *Nature* 1996; **382**:275–278.

75 Asif M, Egan J, Vasan S, Jyothirmayi GN, Masurekar MR, Lopez S, *et al.* An advanced glycation endproduct cross-link breaker can reverse age-related increases in myocardial stiffness. *Proc Natl Acad Sci U S A* 2000; **97**:2809–2813.

76 Wolffenbuttel BH, Boulanger CM, Crijns FR, Huijberts MS, Poitevin P, Swennen GN, *et al.* Breakers of advanced glycation end products restore large artery properties in experimental diabetes. *Proc Natl Acad Sci U S A* 1998; **95**:4630–4634.

77 Candido R, Forbes JM, Thomas MC, Thallas V, Dean RG, Burns WC, *et al.* A breaker of advanced glycation end products attenuates diabetes-induced myocardial structural changes. *Circ Res* 2003; **92**:785–792.

78 Lassila M, Seah KK, Allen TJ, Thallas V, Thomas MC, Candido R, *et al.* Accelerated nephropathy in diabetic apolipoprotein e-knockout mouse: role of advanced glycation end products. *J Am Soc Nephrol* 2004; **15**:2125–2138.

79 Forbes JM, Thallas V, Thomas MC, Founds HW, Burns WC, Jerums G, *et al.* The breakdown of preexisting advanced glycation end products is associated with reduced renal fibrosis in experimental diabetes. *Faseb J* 2003; **17**:1762–1764.

80 Thallas-Bonke V, Lindschau C, Rizkalla B, Bach LA, Boner G, Meier M, *et al.* Attenuation of extracellular matrix accumulation in diabetic nephropathy by the advanced glycation end product cross-link breaker ALT-711 via a protein kinase C-alpha-dependent pathway. *Diabetes* 2004; **53**:2921–2930.

81 Burns WC, Twigg SM, Forbes JM, Pete J, Tikellis C, Thallas-Bonke V, *et al.* Connective tissue growth factor plays an important role in advanced glycation end product-induced tubular epithelial-to-mesenchymal transition: implications for diabetic renal disease. *J Am Soc Nephrol* 2006; **17**:2484–2494.

82 Twigg SM, Cao Z, MCLennan SV, Burns WC, Brammar G, Forbes JM, *et al.* Renal connective tissue growth factor induction in experimental diabetes is prevented by aminoguanidine. *Endocrinology* 2002; **143**:4907–4915.

83 Yonekura H, Yamamoto Y, Sakurai S, Petrova RG, Abedin MJ, Li H, *et al.* Novel splice variants of the receptor for advanced glycation end-products expressed in human vascular endothelial cells and pericytes, and their putative roles in diabetes-induced vascular injury. *Biochem J* 2003; **370**:1097–1109.

84 Hanford LE, Enghild JJ, Valnickova Z, Petersen SV, Schaefer LM, Schaefer TM, *et al.* Purification and characterization of mouse soluble receptor for advanced glycation end products (sRAGE). *J Biol Chem* 2004; **279**:50019–50024.

85 Park L, Raman KG, Lee KJ, Ferran LJ Jr, Chow WS, Stern D, *et al.* Suppression of accelerated diabetic atherosclerosis by the soluble receptor for advanced glycation endproducts. *Nat Med* 1998; **4**:1025–1031.

86 Bucciarelli LG, Wendt T, Qu W, Lu Y, Lalla E, Rong LL, *et al.* RAGE blockade stabilizes established atherosclerosis in diabetic apolipoprotein E-null mice. *Circulation* 2002; **106**:2827–2835.

87 Naka Y, Bucciarelli LG, Wendt T, Lee LK, Rong LL, Ramasamy R, *et al.* RAGE axis: animal models and novel insights into the vascular complications of diabetes. *Arterioscler Thromb Vasc Biol* 2004; **24**:1342–1349.

88 Wendt T, Harja E, Bucciarelli L, Qu W, Lu Y, Rong LL, *et al.* RAGE modulates vascular inflammation and atherosclerosis in a murine model of type 2 diabetes. *Atherosclerosis* 2006; **185**:70–77.

89 Wendt TM, Tanji N, Guo J, Kislinger TR, Qu W, Lu Y, *et al.* RAGE drives the development of glomerulosclerosis and implicates podocyte activation in the pathogenesis of diabetic nephropathy. *Am J Pathol* 2003; **162**:1123–1137.

90 Soro-Paavonen A, Watson AM, Li J, paavonen K, Koitka A, Calkin AC, *et al.* Receptor for advanced glycation end products (RAGE) deficiency attenuates the development of atherosclerosis in diabetes. *Diabetes* 2008; **57**:2461–2469.

91 Cooper ME. Interaction of metabolic and hemodynamic factors in mediating experimental diabetic nephropathy. *Diabetologia* 2001; **44**:1957–1972.

92 Thomas MC, Tikellis C, Burns WM, Bialkowski K, Cao Z, Coughlan MT, *et al.* Interactions between renin angiotensin system and advanced glycation in the kidney. *J Am Soc Nephrol* 2005; **16**:2976–2984.

93 Forbes JM, Thorpe SR, Thallas-Bonke V, Pete J, Thomas MC, Deemer ER, *et al.* Modulation of soluble receptor for advanced glycation end products by angiotensin-converting enzyme-1 inhibition in diabetic nephropathy. *J Am Soc Nephrol* 2005; **16**:2363–2372.

94 Calkin AC, Cooper ME, Jandeleit-Dahm KA, Allen TJ. Gemfibrozil decreases atherosclerosis in experimental diabetes in association with a reduction in oxidative stress and inflammation. *Diabetologia* 2006; **49**:766–774.

95 Yoshida T, Yamagishi S, Nakamura K, Matsui T, Imaizumi T, Takeuchi M, *et al.* Telmisartan inhibits AGE-induced C-reactive protein production through downregulation of the receptor for AGE via peroxisome proliferator-activated receptor-gamma activation. *Diabetologia* 2006; **49**:3094–3099.

96 Cuccurullo C, Iezzi A, Fazia ML, De Cesare D, Di Francesco A, Muraro R, *et al.* Suppression of RAGE as a basis of simvastatin-dependent plaque stabilization in type 2 diabetes. *Arterioscler Thromb Vasc Biol* 2006; **26**:2716–2723.

97 Tigerstedt R, Bergman PG. Niere und Kreislauf. *Scand Arch Physiol* 1898; **8**:223–228.

98 Admiraal PJ, Derkx FH, Danser AH, Pieterman H, Schalekamp MA. Metabolism and production of angiotensin I in different vascular beds in subjects with hypertension. *Hypertension* 1990; **15**: 44–55.

99 Donoghue M, Hsieh F, Baronas E, Godbout K, Gosselin M, Stagliano N, *et al.* A novel angiotensin-converting enzyme-related carboxypeptidase (ACE2) converts angiotensin I to angiotensin 1-9. *Circ Res* 2000; **87**:E1–9.

100 Ferrario CM. Angiotensin-converting enzyme 2 and angiotensin-(1-7): an evolving story in cardiovascular regulation. *Hypertension* 2006; **47**:515–521.

101 Stoll M, Steckelings UM, Paul M, Bottari SP, Metzger R, Unger T. The angiotensin AT2-receptor mediates inhibition of cell proliferation in coronary endothelial cells. *J Clin Invest* 1995; **95**:651–657.

102 Candido R, Jandeleit-Dahm KA, Cao Z, Nesteroff SP, Burns WC, Twigg SM, *et al.* Prevention of accelerated atherosclerosis by angiotensin-converting enzyme inhibition in diabetic apolipoprotein E-deficient mice. *Circulation* 2002; **106**:246–253.

103 Schmieder RE, Hilgers KF, Schlaich MP, Schmidt BM. Renin-angiotensin system and cardiovascular risk. *Lancet* 2007; **369**:1208–1219.

104 Diet F, Pratt RE, Berry GJ, Momose N, Gibbons GH, Dzau VJ. Increased accumulation of tissue ACE in human atherosclerotic coronary artery disease. *Circulation* 1996; **94**:2756–2767.

105 Hansson L, Lindholm LH, Niskanen L, Lanke J, Hedner T, Niklason A, Luomanmäki K, *et al.* Effect of angiotensin-converting-enzyme inhibition compared with conventional therapy on cardiovascular morbidity and mortality in hypertension: the Captopril Prevention Project (CAPP) randomised trial. *Lancet* 1999; **353**:611–616.

106 Yusuf S, Ostergren JB, Gerstein HC, Pfeffer MA, Swedberg K, Granger CB, *et al.*; Candesartan in Heart Failure-Assessment of Reduction in Mortality and Morbidity Program Investigators. Effects of candesartan on the development of a new diagnosis of diabetes mellitus in patients with heart failure. *Circulation* 2005; **112**:48–53.

107 Lindholm LH, Ibsen H, Borch-Johnsen K, Olsen MH, Wachtell K, Dahlöf B, *et al.* Risk of new-onset diabetes in the Losartan Intervention For Endpoint reduction in hypertension study. *J Hypertens* 2002; **20**:1879–1886.

108 Lindholm LH, Persson M, Alaupovic P, Carlberg B, Svensson A, Samuelsson O. Metabolic outcome during 1 year in newly detected hypertensives: results of the Antihypertensive Treatment and Lipid Profile in a North of Sweden Efficacy Evaluation (ALPINE study). *J Hypertens* 2003; **21**:1563–1574.

109 Lindholm LH, Ibsen H, Dahlof B, Devereux RB, Beevers G, de Faire U, *et al.* Cardiovascular morbidity and mortality in patients with diabetes in the Losartan Intervention For Endpoint reduction in hypertension study (LIFE): a randomised trial against atenolol. *Lancet* 2002; **359**:1004–1010.

110 Yusuf S, Sleight P, Pogue J, Bosch J, Davies R, Dagenais G; Heart Outcomes Prevention Evaluation Study Investigators. Effects of an angiotensin-converting-enzyme inhibitor, ramipril, on cardiovascular events in high-risk patients. *N Engl J Med* 2000; **342**:145–153.

111 Jansson PA. Endothelial dysfunction in insulin resistance and type 2 diabetes. *J Intern Med* 2007; **262**:173–183.

112 Pechanova O, Simko F. The role of nitric oxide in the maintenance of vasoactive balance. *Physiol Res* 2007; **56**(Suppl 2):S7–S16.

113 De Caterina R. Endothelial dysfunctions: common denominators in vascular disease. *Curr Opin Lipidol* 2000; **11**:9–23.

114 Perticone F, Ceravolo R, Pujia A, Ventura G, Iacopino S, Scozzafava A, *et al.* Prognostic significance of endothelial dysfunction in hypertensive patients. *Circulation* 2001; **104**:191–196.

115 Halcox JP, Schenke WH, Zalos G, Mincemoyer R, Prasad A, Waclawiw MA, *et al.* Prognostic value of coronary vascular endothelial dysfunction. *Circulation* 2002; **106**:653–658.

116 Ribeiro-Oliveira A Jr, Nogueira AI, Pereira RM, Boas WW, Dos Santos RA, Simoes e Silva AC. The renin-angiotensin system and diabetes: an update. *Vasc Health Risk Manag* 2008; **4**:787–803.

117 Sechi LA, Griffin CA, Schambelan M. The cardiac renin-angiotensin system in STZ-induced diabetes. *Diabetes* 1994; **43**:1180–1184.

118 Candido R, Allen TJ, Lassila M, Cao Z, Thallas V, Cooper ME, *et al.* Irbesartan but not amlodipine suppresses diabetes-associated atherosclerosis. *Circulation* 2004; **109**:1536–1542.

119 Werner N, Kosiol S, Schiegl T, Ahlers P, Walenta K, Link A, *et al.* Circulating endothelial progenitor cells and cardiovascular outcomes. *N Engl J Med* 2005; **353**:999–1007.

120 Bahlmann FH, de Groot K, Mueller O, Hertel B, Haller H, Fliser D. Stimulation of endothelial progenitor cells: a new putative therapeutic effect of angiotensin II receptor antagonists. *Hypertension* 2005; **45**:526–529.

121 Yagil Y, Yagil C. Hypothesis: ACE2 modulates blood pressure in the mammalian organism. *Hypertension* 2003; **41**:871–873.

122 Watanabe T, Barker TA, Berk BC. Angiotensin II and the endothelium: diverse signals and effects. *Hypertension* 2005; **45**:163–169.

123 Porsti I, Bara AT, Busse R, Hecker M. Release of nitric oxide by angiotensin-(1-7) from porcine coronary endothelium: implications for a novel angiotensin receptor. *Br J Pharmacol* 1994; **111**:652–654.

124 Brosnihan KB, Li P, Ferrario CM. Angiotensin-(1-7) dilates canine coronary arteries through kinins and nitric oxide. *Hypertension* 1996; **27**(3 Pt 2):523–528.

125 Maia LG, Ramos MC, Fernandes L, de Carvalho MH, Campagnole-Santos MJ, Souza dos Santos RA. Angiotensin-(1-7) antagonist A-779 attenuates the potentiation of bradykinin by captopril in rats. *J Cardiovasc Pharmacol* 2004; **43**:685–691.

126 Freeman EJ, Chisolm GM, Ferrario CM, Tallant EA. Angiotensin-(1-7) inhibits vascular smooth muscle cell growth. *Hypertension* 1996; **28**:104–108.

127 Fraga-Silva RA, Pinheiro SV, Goncalves AC, Alenina N, Bader M, Santos RA. The antithrombotic effect of angiotensin-(1-7) involves mas-mediated NO release from platelets. *Mol Med* 2008; **14**:28–35.

128 Pereira RM, Dos Santos RA, Teixeira MM, Leite VH, Costa LP, da Costa Dias FL, *et al.* The renin-angiotensin system in a rat model of hepatic fibrosis: evidence for a protective role of angiotensin-(1-7). *J Hepatol* 2007; **46**:674–681.

129 Benter IF, Yousif MH, Dhaunsi GS, Kaur J, Chappell MC, Diz DI. Angiotensin-(1-7) prevents activation of NADPH oxidase and renal vascular dysfunction in diabetic hypertensive rats. *Am J Nephrol* 2008; **28**:25–33.

130 Kostenis E, Milligan G, Christopoulos A, Sanchez-Ferrer CF, Heringer-Walther S, Sexton PM, *et al.* G-protein-coupled receptor Mas is a physiological antagonist of the angiotensin II type 1 receptor. *Circulation* 2005; **111**:1806–1813.

131 Uusitupa MI, Niskanen LK, Siitonen O, Voutilainen E, Pyorala K. 5-Year incidence of atherosclerotic vascular disease in relation to general risk factors, insulin level, and abnormalities in lipoprotein composition in non-insulin-dependent diabetic and nondiabetic subjects. *Circulation* 1990; **82**:27–36.

132 Schieffer B, Schieffer E, Hilfiker-Kleiner D, Hilfiker A, Kovanen PT, Kaartinen M, *et al.* Expression of angiotensin II and interleukin 6 in human coronary atherosclerotic plaques: potential implications for inflammation and plaque instability. *Circulation* 2000; **101**: 1372–1378.
133 Gross CM, Gerbaulet S, Quensel C, Krämer J, Mittelmeier HO, Luft FC, *et al.* Angiotensin II type 1 receptor expression in human coronary arteries with variable degrees of atherosclerosis. *Basic Res Cardiol* 2002; **97**:327–333.
134 Boring L, Gosling J, Cleary M, Charo IF. Decreased lesion formation in CCR2–/– mice reveals a role for chemokines in the initiation of atherosclerosis. *Nature* 1998; **394**:894–897.
135 Wassmann S, Stumpf M, Strehlow K, Schmid A, Schieffer B, Böhm M, *et al.* Interleukin-6 induces oxidative stress and endothelial dysfunction by overexpression of the angiotensin II type 1 receptor. *Circ Res* 2004; **94**:534–541.
136 Jandeleit-Dahm K, Cooper ME. Hypertension and diabetes: role of the renin-angiotensin system. *Endocrinol Metab Clin North Am* 2006; **35**:469–490, vii.
137 Rabbani R, Topol EJ. Strategies to achieve coronary arterial plaque stabilization. *Cardiovasc Res* 1999; **41**:402–417.
138 Zulli A, Burrell LM, Widdop RE, Black MJ, Buxton BF, Hare DL. Immunolocalization of ACE2 and AT2 receptors in rabbit atherosclerotic plaques. *J Histochem Cytochem* 2006; **54**:147–150.
139 Burrell LM, Risvanis J, Kubota E, Dean RG, MacDonald PS, Lu S, *et al.* Myocardial infarction increases ACE2 expression in rat and humans. *Eur Heart J* 2005; **26**:369–375; discussion 22–24.
140 Calkin AC, Forbes JM, Smith CM, Lassila M, Cooper ME, Jandeleit-Dahm KA, *et al.* Rosiglitazone attenuates atherosclerosis in a model of insulin insufficiency independent of its metabolic effects. *Arterioscler Thromb Vasc Biol* 2005; **25**:1903–1909.
141 Lewis P, Stefanovic N, Pete J, Calkin AC, Giunti S, Thallas-Bonke V, *et al.* Lack of the antioxidant enzyme glutathione peroxidase-1 accelerates atherosclerosis in diabetic apolipoprotein E-deficient mice. *Circulation* 2007; **115**:2178–2187.
142 Chew P, Yuen DY, Koh P, Stefanovic N, Febbraio MA, Kola I, *et al.* Site-specific antiatherogenic effect of the antioxidant ebselen in the diabetic apolipoprotein E-deficient mouse. *Arterioscler Thromb Vasc Biol* 2009; **29**:823–830.
143 Mancini GB, Henry GC, Macaya C, O'Neill BJ, Pucillo AL, Carere RG, *et al.* Angiotensin-converting enzyme inhibition with quinapril improves endothelial vasomotor dysfunction in patients with coronary artery disease. The TREND (Trial on Reversing ENdothelial Dysfunction) Study. *Circulation* 1996; **94**:258–265.
144 O'Driscoll G, Green D, Maiorana A, Stanton K, Colreavy F, Taylor R. Improvement in endothelial function by angiotensin-converting enzyme inhibition in non-insulin-dependent diabetes mellitus. *J Am Coll Cardiol* 1999; **33**:1506–1511.
145 Cheetham C, Collis J, O'Driscoll G, Stanton K, Taylor R, Green D. Losartan, an angiotensin type 1 receptor antagonist, improves endothelial function in non-insulin-dependent diabetes. *J Am Coll Cardiol* 2000; **36**:1461–1466.
146 Hornig B, Landmesser U, Kohler C, Ahlersmann D, Spiekermann S, Christoph A, *et al.* Comparative effect of ace inhibition and angiotensin II type 1 receptor antagonism on bioavailability of nitric oxide in patients with coronary artery disease: role of superoxide dismutase. *Circulation* 2001; **103**:799–805.
147 Komers R, Simkova R, Kazdova L, Ruzickova J, Pelikanova T. Effects of ACE inhibition and AT1-receptor blockade on haemodynamic responses to L-arginine in Type 1 diabetes. *J Renin Angiotensin Aldosterone Syst* 2004; **5**:33–38.
148 Niskanen L, Hedner T, Hansson L, Lanke J, Niklason A. Reduced cardiovascular morbidity and mortality in hypertensive diabetic patients on first-line therapy with an ACE inhibitor compared with a diuretic/beta-blocker-based treatment regimen: a subanalysis of the Captopril Prevention Project. *Diabetes Care* 2001; **24**:2091–2096.
149 Brenner BM, Cooper ME, de Zeeuw D, Keane WF, Mitch WE, Parving HH, *et al.* Effects of losartan on renal and cardiovascular outcomes in patients with type 2 diabetes and nephropathy. *N Engl J Med* 2001; **345**:861–869.
150 UK Prospective Diabetes Study Group. Efficacy of atenolol and captopril in reducing risk of macrovascular and microvascular complications in type 2 diabetes: UKPDS 39. *Br Med J* 1998; **317**:713–720.
151 Heart Outcomes Prevention Evaluation Study Investigators. Effects of ramipril on cardiovascular and microvascular outcomes in people with diabetes mellitus: results of the HOPE study and MICRO-HOPE substudy. *Lancet* 2000; **355**:253–259.
152 Tatti P, Pahor M, Byington RP, Di Mauro P, Guarisco R, Strollo G, *et al.* Outcome results of the Fosinopril Versus Amlodipine Cardiovascular Events Randomized Trial (FACET) in patients with hypertension and NIDDM. *Diabetes Care* 1998; **21**:597–603.
153 Fox KM. Efficacy of perindopril in reduction of cardiovascular events among patients with stable coronary artery disease: randomised, double-blind, placebo-controlled, multicentre trial (the EUROPA study). *Lancet* 2003; **362**:782–788.
154 Pitt B, O'Neill B, Feldman R, Schwartz L, Mudra H, Bass T, *et al.* The QUinapril Ischemic Event Trial (QUIET): evaluation of chronic ACE inhibitor therapy in patients with ischemic heart disease and preserved left ventricular function. *Am J Cardiol* 2001; **87**:1058–1063.
155 Friedrich EB, Teo KK, Bohm M. ACE inhibition in secondary prevention: are the results controversial? *Clin Res Cardiol* 2006; **95**:61–67.
156 Boner G, Cooper ME, McCarroll K, Brenner BM, de Zeeuw D, Kowey PR, *et al.* Adverse effects of left ventricular hypertrophy in the reduction of endpoints in NIDDM with the angiotensin II antagonist losartan (RENAAL) study. *Diabetologia* 2005; **48**:1980–1987.
157 Yusuf S, Teo K, Anderson C, Pogue J, Dyal L, Copland I, *et al.* Telmisartan Randomised AssessmeNt Study in ACE iNtolerant subjects with cardiovascular Disease (TRANSCEND) Investigators. Effects of the angiotensin-receptor blocker telmisartan on cardiovascular events in high-risk patients intolerant to angiotensin-converting enzyme inhibitors: a randomised controlled trial. *Lancet* 2008; **372**:1174–1183.
158 Yanagisawa M, Kurihara H, Kimura S, Tomobe Y, Kobayashi M, Mitsui Y, *et al.* A novel potent vasoconstrictor peptide produced by vascular endothelial cells. *Nature* 1988; **332**:411–415.
159 Sakurai T, Yanagisawa M, Takuwa Y, Miyazaki H, Kimura S, Goto K, *et al.* Cloning of a cDNA encoding a non-isopeptide-selective subtype of the endothelin receptor. *Nature* 1990; **348**:732–735.
160 Perfetto F, Tarquini R, Tapparini L, Tarquini B. Influence of non-insulin-dependent diabetes mellitus on plasma endothelin-1 levels in patients with advanced atherosclerosis. *J Diabetes Complication* 1998; **12**:187–192.
161 Kalogeropoulou K, Mortzos G, Migdalis I, Velentzas C, Mikhailidis DP, Georgiadis E, *et al.* Carotid atherosclerosis in type 2 diabetes

mellitus: potential role of endothelin-1, lipoperoxides, and prostacyclin. *Angiology* 2002; **53**:279–285.

162 Cunningham ME, Huribal M, Bala RJ, McMillen MA. Endothelin-1 and endothelin-4 stimulate monocyte production of cytokines. *Crit Care Med* 1997; **25**:958–964.

163 Babaei S, Picard P, Ravandi A, Monge JC, Lee TC, Cernacek P, *et al.* Blockade of endothelin receptors markedly reduces atherosclerosis in LDL receptor deficient mice: role of endothelin in macrophage foam cell formation. *Cardiovasc Res* 2000; **48**:158–167.

164 Woods M, Wood EG, Bardswell SC, Bishop-Bailey D, Barker S, Wort SJ, *et al.* Role for nuclear factor-κB and signal transducer and activator of transcription 1/interferon regulatory factor-1 in cytokine-induced endothelin-1 release in human vascular smooth muscle cells. *Mol Pharmacol* 2003; **64**:923–931.

165 Schneider MP, Boesen EI, Pollock DM. Contrasting actions of endothelin ET(A) and ET(B) receptors in cardiovascular disease. *Annu Rev Pharmacol Toxicol* 2007; **47**:731–759.

166 King JM, Srivastava KD, Stefano GB, Bilfinger TV, Bahou WF, Magazine HI. Human monocyte adhesion is modulated by endothelin B receptor-coupled nitric oxide release. *J Immunol* 1997; **158**:880–886.

167 Lam HC. Role of endothelin in diabetic vascular complications. *Endocrine* 2001; **14**:277–284.

168 Ferri C, Laurenti O, Bellini C, Faldetta MR, Properzi G, Santucci A, *et al.* Circulating endothelin-1 levels in lean non-insulin-dependent diabetic patients: influence of ACE inhibition. *Am J Hypertens* 1995; **8**:40–47.

169 Douglas SA, Sulpizio AC, Piercy V, Sarau HM, Ames RS, Aiyar NV, *et al.* Differential vasoconstrictor activity of human urotensin-II in vascular tissue isolated from the rat, mouse, dog, pig, marmoset and cynomolgus monkey. *Br J Pharmacol* 2000; **131**:1262–1274.

170 Ames RS, Sarau HM, Chambers JK, Willette RN, Aiyar NV, Romanic AM, *et al.* Human urotensin-II is a potent vasoconstrictor and agonist for the orphan receptor GPR14. *Nature* 1999; **401**:282–286.

171 Cheung BM, Leung R, Man YB, Wong LY. Plasma concentration of urotensin II is raised in hypertension. *J Hypertens* 2004; **22**:1341–1344.

172 Totsune K, Takahashi K, Arihara Z, Sone M, Ito S, Murakami O. Increased plasma urotensin II levels in patients with diabetes mellitus. *Clin Sci (Lond)* 2003; **104**:1–5.

173 Pakala R. Role of urotensin II in atherosclerotic cardiovascular diseases. *Cardiovasc Revasc Med* 2008; **9**:166–178.

174 Suguro T, Watanabe T, Ban Y, Kodate S, Misaki A, Hirano T, *et al.* Increased human urotensin II levels are correlated with carotid atherosclerosis in essential hypertension. *Am J Hypertens* 2007; **20**:211–217.

175 Wang ZJ, Shi LB, Xiong ZW, Zhang LF, Meng L, Bu DF, *et al.* Alteration of vascular urotensin II receptor in mice with apolipoprotein E gene knockout. *Peptides* 2006; **27**:858–863.

176 Rakowski E, Hassan GS, Dhanak D, Ohlstein EH, Douglas SA, Giaid A. A role for urotensin II in restenosis following balloon angioplasty: use of a selective UT receptor blocker. *J Mol Cell Cardiol* 2005; **39**:785–791.

177 Segain JP, Rolli-Derkinderen M, Gervois N, Raingeard de la Bletiere D, Loirand G, Pacaud P. Urotensin II is a new chemotactic factor for UT receptor-expressing monocytes. *J Immunol* 2007; **179**:901–909.

178 Wiley SR, Schooley K, Smolak PJ, Din WS, Huang CP, Nicholl JK, *et al.* Identification and characterization of a new member of the TNF family that induces apoptosis. *Immunity* 1995; **3**:673–682.

179 Marsters SA, Pitti RM, Donahue CJ, Ruppert S, Bauer KD, Ashkenazi A. Activation of apoptosis by Apo-2 ligand is independent of FADD but blocked by CrmA. *Curr Biol* 1996; **6**:750–752.

180 Simonet WS, Lacey DL, Dunstan CR, Kelley M, Chang MS, Lüthy R, *et al.* Osteoprotegerin: a novel secreted protein involved in the regulation of bone density. *Cell* 1997; **89**:309–319.

181 Yasuda H, Shima N, Nakagawa N, Yamaguchi K, Kinosaki M, Mochizuki S, *et al.* Osteoclast differentiation factor is a ligand for osteoprotegerin/osteoclastogenesis-inhibitory factor and is identical to TRANCE/RANKL. *Proc Natl Acad Sci U S A* 1998; **95**:3597–3602.

182 Emery JG, McDonnell P, Burke MB, Deen KC, Lyn S, Silverman C, *et al.* Osteoprotegerin is a receptor for the cytotoxic ligand TRAIL. *J Biol Chem* 1998; **273**:14363–14367.

183 Secchiero P, Candido R, Corallini F, Zacchigna S, Toffoli B, Rimondi E, *et al.* Systemic tumor necrosis factor-related apoptosis-inducing ligand delivery shows antiatherosclerotic activity in apolipoprotein E-null diabetic mice. *Circulation* 2006; **114**:1522–1530.

184 Schoppet M, Sattler AM, Schaefer JR, Hofbauer LC. Osteoprotegerin (OPG) and tumor necrosis factor-related apoptosis-inducing ligand (TRAIL) levels in atherosclerosis. *Atherosclerosis* 2006; **184**:446–447.

185 Michowitz Y, Goldstein E, Roth A, Afek A, Abashidze A, Ben Gal Y, *et al.* The involvement of tumor necrosis factor-related apoptosis-inducing ligand (TRAIL) in atherosclerosis. *J Am Coll Cardiol* 2005; **45**:1018–1024.

186 Bennett BJ, Scatena M, Kirk EA, Rattazzi M, Varon RM, Averill M, *et al.* Osteoprotegerin inactivation accelerates advanced atherosclerotic lesion progression and calcification in older ApoE–/– mice. *Arterioscler Thromb Vasc Biol* 2006; **26**:2117–2124.

187 Yano K, Tsuda E, Washida N, Kobayashi F, Goto M, Harada A, *et al.* Immunological characterization of circulating osteoprotegerin/osteoclastogenesis inhibitory factor: increased serum concentrations in postmenopausal women with osteoporosis. *J Bone Miner Res* 1999; **14**:518–527.

188 Hofbauer LC, Schoppet M. Osteoprotegerin gene polymorphism and the risk of osteoporosis and vascular disease. *J Clin Endocrinol Metab* 2002; **87**:4078–4079.

189 Knudsen ST, Foss CH, Poulsen PL, Andersen NH, Mogensen CE, Rasmussen LM. Increased plasma concentrations of osteoprotegerin in type 2 diabetic patients with microvascular complications. *Eur J Endocrinol* 2003; **149**:39–42.

190 Hofbauer LC, Schoppet M. Osteoprotegerin: a link between osteoporosis and arterial calcification? *Lancet* 2001; **358**:257–259.

191 Hansen TK, Tarnow L, Thiel S, Steffensen R, Stehouwer CD, Schalkwijk CG, *et al.* Association between mannose-binding lectin and vascular complications in type 1 diabetes. *Diabetes* 2004; **53**:1570–1576.

192 Saraheimo M, Forsblom C, Hansen TK, Teppo AM, Fagerudd J, Pettersson-Fernholm K, *et al.* Increased levels of mannan-binding lectin in type 1 diabetic patients with incipient and overt nephropathy. *Diabetologia* 2005; **48**:198–202.

193 Hovind P, Hansen TK, Tarnow L, Thiel S, Steffensen R, Flybjerg A, *et al.* Mannose-binding lectin as a predictor of microalbuminuria in type 1 diabetes: an inception cohort study. *Diabetes* 2005; **54**:1523–1527.

194 Hansen TK, Gall MA, Tarnow L, Thiel S, Stehouwer CD, Schalkwijk CG, *et al.* Mannose-binding lectin and mortality in type 2 diabetes. *Arch Intern Med* 2006; **166**:2007–2013.

195 Verrier ED, Shernan SK, Taylor KM, Van de Werf F, Newman MF, Chen JC, *et al.* Terminal complement blockade with pexelizumab during coronary artery bypass graft surgery requiring cardiopulmonary bypass: a randomized trial. *JAMA* 2004; **291**:2319–2327.

196 Hansson L, Zanchetti A, Carruthers SG, Dahlöf B, Elmfeldt D, Julius S, *et al.*; HOT Study Group. Effects of intensive blood-pressure lowering and low-dose aspirin in patients with hypertension: principal results of the Hypertension Optimal Treatment (HOT) randomised trial. *Lancet* 1998; **351**:1755–1762.

197 UK Prospective Diabetes Study Group. Tight blood pressure control and risk of macrovascular and microvascular complications in type 2 diabetes: UKPDS 38. *Br Med J* 1998; **317**:703–713.

198 Estacio RO, Jeffers BW, Hiatt WR, Biggerstaff SL, Gifford N, Schrier RW. The effect of nisoldipine as compared with enalapril on cardiovascular outcomes in patients with non-insulin-dependent diabetes and hypertension. *N Engl J Med* 1998; **338**:645–652.

199 de Galan BE, Perkovic V, Ninomiya T, Pillai A, Patel A, Cass A, *et al.* Lowering blood pressure reduces renal events in type 2 diabetes. *J Am Soc Nephrol* 2009; **20**:883–892.

200 Yusuf S, Teo KK, Pogue J, Dyal L, Copland I, Schumacher H, *et al.*; ONTARGET Investigators. Telmisartan, ramipril, or both in patients at high risk for vascular events. *N Engl J Med* 2008; **358**:1547–1559.

201 Collins R, Armitage J, Parish S, Sleigh P, Peto R. MRC/BHF Heart Protection Study of cholesterol-lowering with simvastatin in 5963 people with diabetes: a randomised placebo-controlled trial. *Lancet* 2003; **361**:2005–2016.

202 Colhoun HM, Betteridge DJ, Durrington PN, Hitman GA, Neil HA, Livingstone SJ, *et al.* Primary prevention of cardiovascular disease with atorvastatin in type 2 diabetes in the Collaborative Atorvastatin Diabetes Study (CARDS): multicentre randomised placebo-controlled trial. *Lancet* 2004; **364**:685–696.

203 American Diabetes Association. Management of dyslipidemia in adults with diabetes. *Diabetes Care* 2000; **23**(Suppl 1):S57–60.

204 Bhatt DL. What makes platelets angry: diabetes, fibrinogen, obesity, and impaired response to antiplatelet therapy? *J Am Coll Cardiol* 2008; **52**:1060–1061.

205 Jackson SP, Calkin AC. The clot thickens: oxidized lipids and thrombosis. *Nat Med* 2007; **13**:1015–1016.

206 Berry C, Tardif JC, Bourassa MG. Coronary heart disease in patients with diabetes: II. Recent advances in coronary revascularization. *J Am Coll Cardiol* 2007; **49**:643–656.

207 Keech A, Simes RJ, Barter P, Best J, Scott R, Taskinen MR, *et al.* Effects of long-term fenofibrate therapy on cardiovascular events in 9795 people with type 2 diabetes mellitus (the FIELD study): randomised controlled trial. *Lancet* 2005; **366**:1849–1861.

208 Dormandy JA, Charbonnel B, Eckland DJ, Erdmann E, Massi-Benedetti M, Moules IK, *et al.* Secondary prevention of macrovascular events in patients with type 2 diabetes in the PROactive Study (Prospective Pioglitazone Clinical Trial in Macrovascular Events): a randomised controlled trial. *Lancet* 2005; **366**:1279–1289.

209 Home PD, Pocock SJ, Beck-Nielsen H, Curtis PS, Gomis R, Hanefeld M, *et al.* Rosiglitazone evaluated for cardiovascular outcomes in oral agent combination therapy for type 2 diabetes (RECORD): a multicentre, randomised, open-label trial. *Lancet* 2009; **373**:2125–2135.

210 Nissen SE, Wolski K, Topol EJ. Effect of muraglitazar on death and major adverse cardiovascular events in patients with type 2 diabetes mellitus. *JAMA* 2005; **294**:2581–2586.

40 Cardiovascular Risk Factors

Hypertension

Peter M. Nilsson
Department of Clinical Sciences, Lund University, University Hospital, Malmö, Sweden

Dyslipidemia: Diabetes Lipid Therapies

Adie Viljoen[1] & Anthony S. Wierzbicki[2]
[1] Department of Chemical Pathology, Lister Hospital, Stevenage, UK
[2] Guy's & St Thomas' Hospitals, London, UK

Hypertension

Peter M. Nilsson

Keypoints

- Hypertension is up to twice as common in people with diabetes as in the general population, affecting 10–30% of people with type 1 diabetes mellitus (T1DM) and 60–80% of those with type 2 diabetes (T2DM).
- Hypertension is associated with insulin resistance and other features of the metabolic syndrome. Insulin resistance could raise blood pressure (BP) by loss of insulin's normal vasodilator activity or through effects of the accompanying hyperinsulinemia.
- BP rises during the early microalbuminuric phase of diabetic nephropathy, especially in young patients with T1DM.
- Hypertension worsens both macrovascular and microvascular complications in diabetes. The effects of BP on the risk of fatal coronary heart disease are 2–5 times greater than in people without diabetes. The risks of nephropathy and end-stage renal failure are also increased 2–3 times by hypertension.
- All people with diabetes should be carefully screened for hypertension and evidence of hypertensive tissue damage at diagnosis and at least annually thereafter. Treatment is required for values that consistently exceed 130–140/80–85 mmHg – lower than the World Health Organization/International Society of Hypertension thresholds defined for hypertension in the general population. The blood lipid profile should also be checked.
- The treatment of hypertension begins with lifestyle management, including reduced dietary fat and salt intakes, weight loss for obese patients, smoking cessation and increased regular physical activity. These measures can lower BP by up to 11/8 mmHg.
- First-line antihypertensive drugs suitable for use in patients with diabetes are diuretics, such as low dose bendroflumethiazide (bendrofluazide); or cardioselective beta-blockers, calcium-channel antagonists (CCAs), angiotensin-converting enzyme (ACE) inhibitors and angiotensin II type 1 (AT1) receptor blockers (ARBs). Subjects of African decent tend to have low renin hypertension, and may not respond to beta-blockers or ACE inhibitors. Drugs can be selected for their beneficial effects on coexistent problems, e.g. angina or arrhythmia (beta-blockers, CCAs), heart failure (ACE inhibitors, certain beta-blockers), previous myocardial infarction (ACE inhibitors, beta-blockers) or nephropathy (ACE inhibitors, ARBs).
- Over two-thirds of people with diabetes need combinations of two or more antihypertensive drugs to control hypertension. Effective combinations include beta-blocker plus CCAs; ACE inhibitor/ARB plus diuretic (non-potassium-sparing); and CCA plus ACE inhibitor/ARB.

Textbook of Diabetes, 4th edition. Edited by R. Holt, C. Cockram, A. Flyvbjerg and B. Goldstein.

Introduction

Hypertension often accompanies diabetes mellitus, both type 1 (T1DM) and type 2 (T2DM). The association between the two conditions has long been recognized. In 1923, the Swedish physician Eskil Kylin described a syndrome of diabetes, hypertension and hyperuricemia [1], which are now regarded as aspects of the broader "metabolic syndrome" that has been linked to insulin resistance (IR) [2,3]. The relationship between diabetes and hypertension is complex. Both are common and so are likely to be associated by chance, but in some instances, they may have a common cause; moreover, hypertension can develop as a consequence of diabetic nephropathy, while some drugs used to treat hypertension can induce diabetes in susceptible subjects.

Hypertension is important because, like diabetes, it is a major cardiovascular risk factor and one that synergizes with the deleterious effects of diabetes. It is also a risk factor for microvascular complications: nephropathy and retinopathy. The management of hypertension in diabetes has been widely debated, and there is still a need to agree on treatment targets and strategies. During the last decade, several well-constructed trials have added considerably to the evidence base [4–8], demonstrating convincingly the benefits of lowering blood pressure (BP), but also highlighting how difficult this can be to achieve in practice.

Table 40.1 Criteria for hypertension and related tissue damage, defined by the World Health Organization (WHO) and the International Society for Hypertension, 1999 [33].

Category	Systolic (mmHg)	Diastolic (mmHg)
WHO criteria for the general population*		
Optimal	<120	<80
Normal	<130	<85
High normal	130–139	85–89
Grade 1 hypertension (mild)	140–159	90–99
Subgroup: borderline	140–149	90–94
Grade 2 hypertension (moderate)	160–179	100–109
Grade 3 hypertension (severe)	≥180	≥110
Isolated systolic hypertension	≥140	<90
Subgroup: borderline	140–149	<90
Hypertension-related tissue damage (WHO criteria)		
Grade I: none		
Grade II: subclinical damage (e.g. retinopathy, proteinuria)		
Grade III: clinical damage (e.g. heart failure, ischemia)		
Degree of proteinuria		
Microalbuminuria: 30–300 mg/24 hours (20–200 mg/min)		
Macroalbuminuria: >300 mg/24 hours (>300 mg/min)		

* Desirable blood pressure limits in the diabetic population are suggested in Figure 40.6.

Size of the problem

Hypertension is widely defined according to the World Health Organization/International Society of Hypertension (WHO/ISH) criteria (Table 40.1). People with diabetes are still at risk of macrovascular and microvascular complications at BP levels below these thresholds, and the treatment target range is therefore lower (130–140/80–85 mmHg).

Overall, hypertension (according to the WHO criteria) is up to twice as common in people with diabetes as in the general population [9]. In white Europeans, 10–30% of subjects with T1DM and 60–80% of those with newly diagnosed T2DM are hypertensive [10]. There are racial and ethnic differences in the prevalence of hypertension, which presumably are at least partly genetically determined: for example, hypertension (and macrovascular disease) is less frequent among the Pima Indians and Mexican-Americans [11]. Impaired glucose tolerance (IGT) is also associated with hypertension (20–40% of cases), perhaps reflecting the common origins of these aspects of the metabolic syndrome [12].

There is evidence that the true prevalence of hypertension is increasing in the diabetic population (especially T2DM) after allowing for the greater number of cases identified through improved screening and the lowering of thresholds for treatment of BP [13]. The causes probably include the rising prevalence of obesity and longer survival of older people with diabetes.

Causes of hypertension in diabetes

Associations between hypertension and diabetes are listed in Table 40.2. Essential hypertension and isolated systolic hypertension are both common in the non-diabetic population (especially in the elderly). It is estimated that essential hypertension accounts for about 10% of cases in people with diabetes. Other important causes are the hypertension that coexists with IR, obesity and IGT in the metabolic syndrome, and hypertension secondary to diabetic nephropathy, as discussed in detail below.

Hypertension in the metabolic syndrome

This syndrome consists of IR, IGT (including T2DM), a characteristic dyslipidemia – hypertriglyceridemia, low high-density lipoprotein (HDL) cholesterol, and raised low density lipoprotein (LDL), with an excess of small dense LDL particles – truncal obesity, procoagulant changes (raised plasminogen activator inhibitor 1 and fibrinogen levels) and hyperuricemia [2,14,15]. As these abnormalities are all risk factors for atherogenesis, the syndrome is completed by a marked tendency to vascular aging leading to macrovascular disease, especially coronary heart disease (CHD) and stroke (Figure 40.1). As discussed in Chapter 11, IR has been proposed by Reaven [2], DeFronzo and Ferrannini [14] and others [15] to be a fundamental cause of hypertension and cardiovascular disease (CVD) as well as T2DM. IR is partly genetically determined, and acquired factors such as obesity,

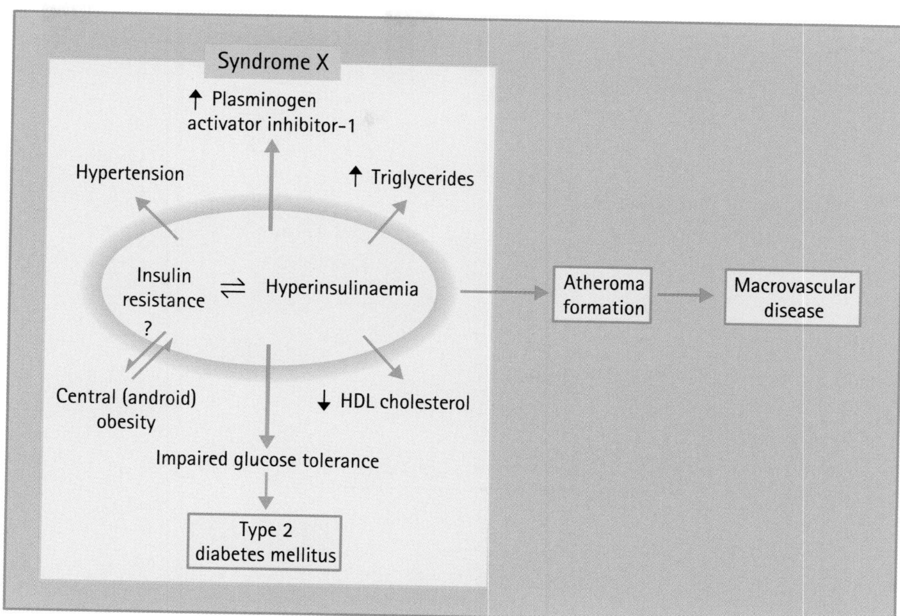

Figure 40.1 The metabolic syndrome. HDL, high density lipoprotein.

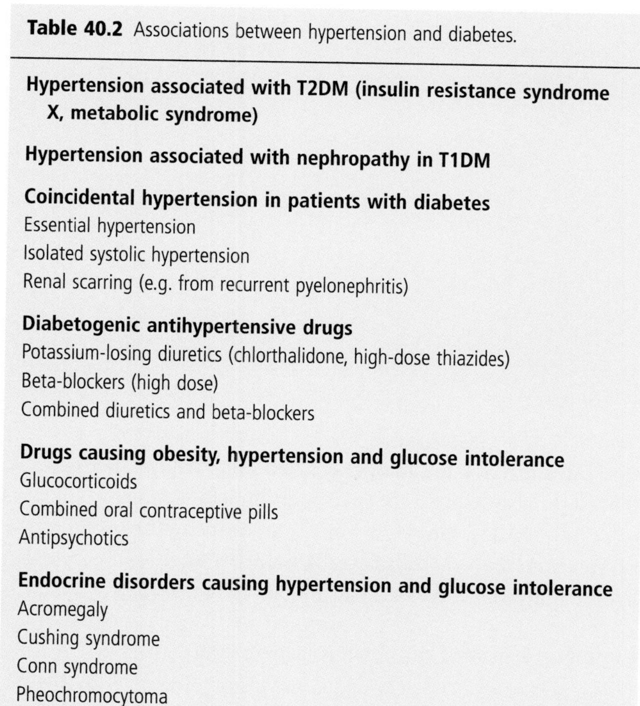

Table 40.2 Associations between hypertension and diabetes.

Hypertension associated with T2DM (insulin resistance syndrome X, metabolic syndrome)
Hypertension associated with nephropathy in T1DM
Coincidental hypertension in patients with diabetes
Essential hypertension
Isolated systolic hypertension
Renal scarring (e.g. from recurrent pyelonephritis)
Diabetogenic antihypertensive drugs
Potassium-losing diuretics (chlorthalidone, high-dose thiazides)
Beta-blockers (high dose)
Combined diuretics and beta-blockers
Drugs causing obesity, hypertension and glucose intolerance
Glucocorticoids
Combined oral contraceptive pills
Antipsychotics
Endocrine disorders causing hypertension and glucose intolerance
Acromegaly
Cushing syndrome
Conn syndrome
Pheochromocytoma

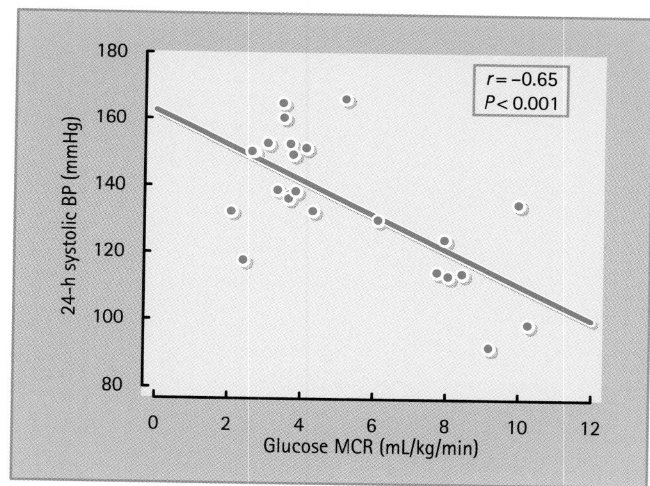

Figure 40.2 Hypertension is associated with insulin resistance. Insulin sensitivity, measured as the metabolic clearance rate (MCR) of glucose during an insulin clamp study, is inversely related to the mean 24-hour systolic and ambulatory blood pressure. Reproduced from Pinkney *et al.* [17], with permission from the Editor.

physical inactivity and perhaps malnutrition *in utero* and during early infancy may also contribute [16]. In support of the latter, family studies have revealed a correlation between the BP of the mother and her offspring that appears to be non-hereditary in origin; early growth retardation is suggested to program abnormal development of the vasculature as well as the tissues that regulate glucose homeostasis.

IR is closely associated with high BP in both humans and animals. Experimental induction of IR (e.g. feeding rats with fructose) is accompanied by a rise in BP. More persuasively, an inverse relationship has been demonstrated in humans between BP and insulin sensitivity [17] (Figure 40.2). Various mechanisms have been proposed to explain how IR and/or the hyperinsulinemia that accompanies it could increase BP (Figure 40.3). First, there is some evidence that insulin is an endothelium-dependent vasodilator, releasing nitric oxide (NO) from the endothelium, which relaxes vascular smooth muscle [18,19]; blunting of this

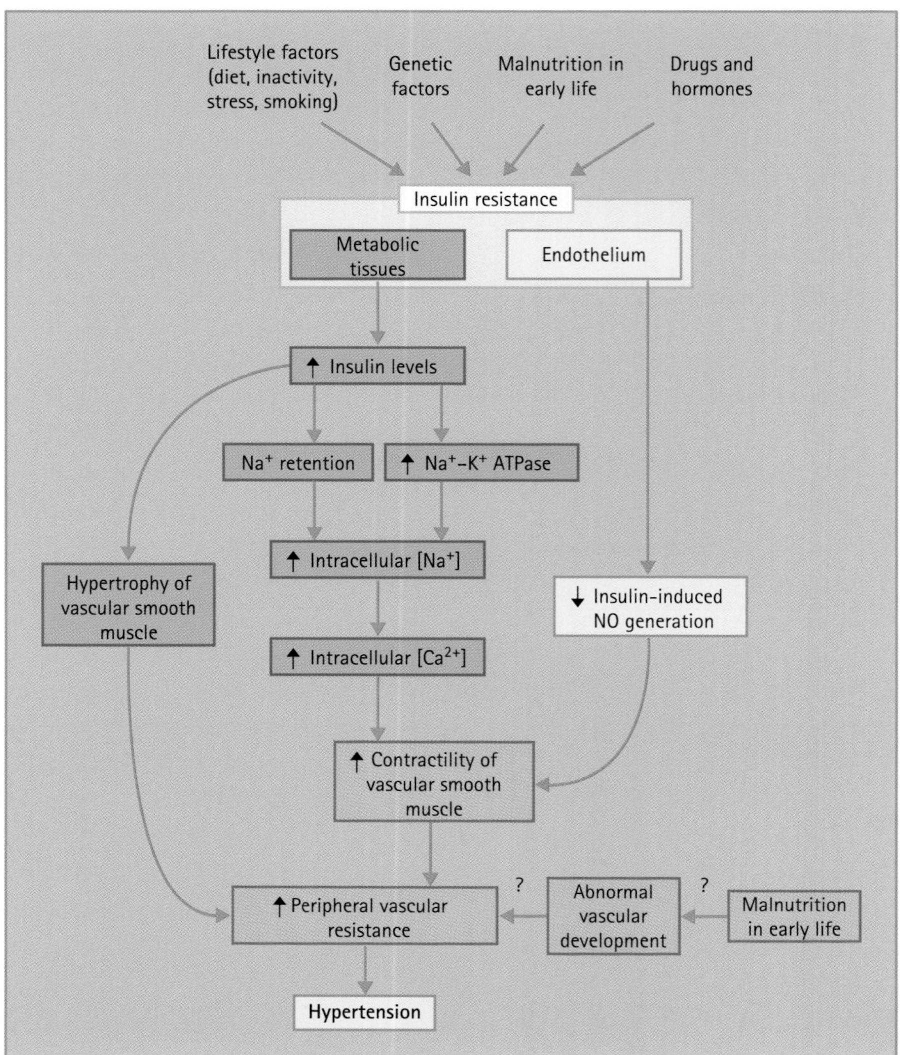

Figure 40.3 Possible mechanisms of hypertension in conditions of insulin resistance. NO, nitric oxide.

effect, caused by insensitivity to the action of insulin on the endothelium as well as on metabolically important tissues, could contribute to the increased peripheral resistance that is the hallmark of hypertension in obesity and T2DM. Impaired endothelium-mediated vasodilatation is associated with IR states and may have a key role in the initiation and progression of atherosclerosis [20].

By contrast, insulin also has several actions that tend to raise BP, and there is some evidence that these are accentuated in IR states, presumably because sensitivity is preserved to the effects of the raised insulin levels. Insulin acts on the distal renal tubule to retain Na^+ ions and water [20,21], an effect that still operates in IR subjects [22], and so could contribute to the rise in total body Na^+ content that occurs in obesity and T2DM [23]. Insulin also stimulates the cell membrane Na^+–K^+ ATPase, which would raise intracellular Na^+ concentrations in vascular smooth muscle and, by increasing systolic Ca^{2+} levels, would enhance contractility and increase peripheral resistance [22,23]. Through its effects on the CNS, insulin may stimulate the sympathetic outflow. Theoretically, this could also increase BP, although direct evidence in humans is lacking [22,24]. Finally, insulin may stimulate the proliferation of vascular smooth muscle cells, which could lead to medial hypertrophy and increased peripheral resistance [22,25].

Hypertension and diabetic nephropathy

This association is most obvious in young patients with T1DM, in whom the presence of hypertension is strikingly related to renal damage and even minor degrees of proteinuria. BP begins to rise when the urinary albumin excretion (UAE) enters the microalbuminuric range (>30 mg/24 hours) and is usually over the WHO threshold when UAE reaches the macroalbuminuric stage (>300 mg/24 hours) [26]. The association may be partly genetically determined: subjects with diabetes and microalbuminuria commonly have parents with hypertension and may also inherit overactivity of the cell-membrane Na^+–H^+ pump (indicated by increased Na^+–Li^+ counter-transport in red blood cells), which would tend to raise intracellular Na^+ concentrations and thus increase vascular smooth muscle tone [27].

The basic mechanisms of hypertension include decreased Na^+ excretion with Na^+ and water retention. Peripheral resistance is increased, to which raised intracellular Na^+ will contribute. The role of the renin angiotensin aldosterone system (RAS) is uncertain, as both increased and decreased activity has been reported [28,29]. These discrepancies may be explained by differences in diet, treatment, metabolic control and the type and duration of diabetes. Na^+ retention and hypertension would be predicted to suppress the RAS, while renin levels may be influenced by other complications of diabetes: renal tubular acidosis type 4 causes hyporeninemic hypoaldosteronism and neuropathy can also lower plasma renin, while renin may be raised in retinopathy and advanced nephropathy. Patients with microalbuminuria who are insulin-resistant appear to be particularly susceptible to hypertension [30].

Impact of hypertension in diabetes

A large proportion of hypertensive people with diabetes show signs of cardiovascular aging and target-organ damage [10]. Hypertension, as an independent risk factor for atherogenesis, synergizes with the effects of diabetes and significantly increases the development and progression of CHD, cerebrovascular and peripheral vascular disease. Overall, the effects of hypertension on deaths from CHD are increased by 2–5 times in people with diabetes, with the greatest increase occurring at the lowest BP levels (Figure 40.4).

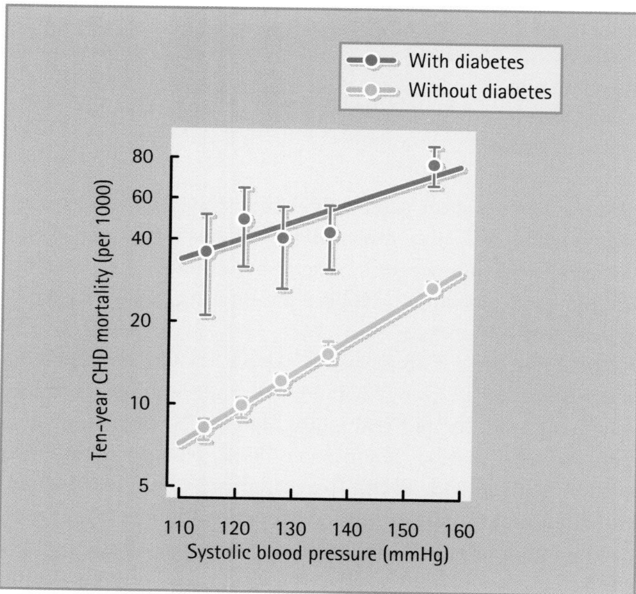

Figure 40.4 Synergistic effects of diabetes and hypertension on deaths from coronary heart disease (CHD). Data from 342 815 people without diabetes and 5163 people with diabetes aged 35–57 years, free from myocardial infarction at entry. Reproduced with permission from O. Vaccaro, paper presented at the 26th Annual Meeting of the European Diabetes Epidemiology Group, Lund, 1991.

The deleterious effects of hypertension on left ventricular function are also accentuated by the presence of diabetes. These include impaired left ventricular relaxation [31] and increased left ventricular mass [32], the latter being an independent predictor of premature death from CHD.

Hypertension also predisposes to the development of certain microvascular complications, particularly nephropathy and end-stage renal failure (ESRF), for which the risk is increased by 2–3 times (see Chapter 37). Hypertension is also a risk factor for retinopathy, as has been confirmed by the beneficial effects of improved BP control in patients with T2DM, reported by the UK Prospective Diabetes Study (UKPDS) [4].

Screening for hypertension in diabetes

As the two conditions are so commonly associated, people with diabetes must be regularly screened for hypertension and vice versa. Hypertensive patients, especially if obese or receiving treatment with potentially diabetogenic drugs, should be screened for diabetes at diagnosis and during follow-up. Should hyperglycemia be detected, potentially diabetogenic antihypertensive drugs should be reduced or changed to others or used in combinations that do not impair glucose tolerance, and normoglycemia can then often be restored.

All people with diabetes should have their BP checked at diagnosis and at least annually thereafter. This is especially important in those with other cardiovascular risk factors, such as nephropathy (which is associated with a substantial increase in the cardiovascular mortality rate), obesity, dyslipidemia, smoking or poor glycemic control.

Measurement of blood pressure

BP should be measured with the patient in the supine or sitting position, with an accurate sphygmomanometer and a cuff of appropriate size (i.e. wider for obese subjects with an arm circumference of >32 cm). Systolic and diastolic BP should be recorded, to the nearest 2 mmHg if using a manual sphygmomanometer, from phases I and V (i.e. appearance and final disappearance of the sounds of Korotkoff). Usual precautions should be taken to ensure reliability and avoid "white coat" stress effects which can acutely raise BP. Conditions should be quiet and relaxed, and at least two readings should be taken initially and then repeated at intervals over weeks or months to determine the subject's typical values and any trend to change. Office BP could be complemented by repeated home BP recordings.

BP should also be checked with the patient in the upright position (1 minute after standing), because there may be a significant postural fall (>20 mmHg systolic) in patients with diabetic autonomic neuropathy, the elderly or those treated with vasodilators or diuretics. Marked postural hypotension, which can coexist with supine hypertension, may indicate the need to change or reduce antihypertensive medication, especially if symptoms are provoked.

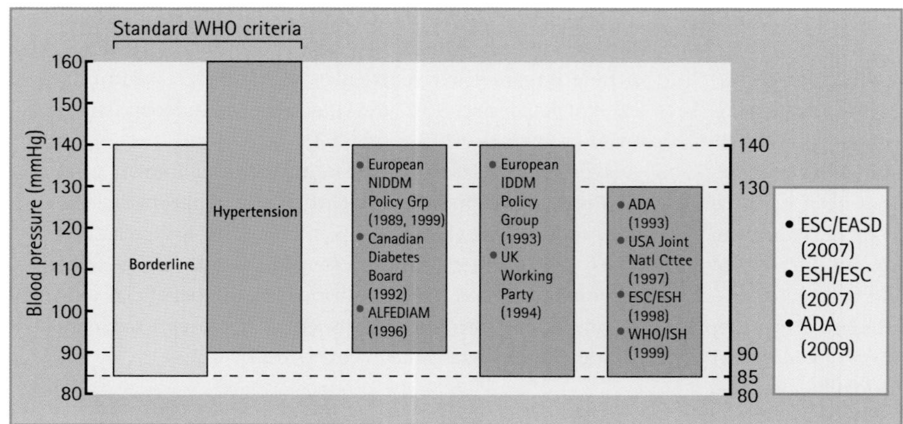

Figure 40.5 Blood pressure treatment targets suggested for subjects with diabetes, compared with the World Health Organization/International Society of Hypertension definition of hypertension and borderline hypertension [34]. ALFEDIAM, Association de langue française pour l'étude du diabète et des maladies métaboliques; ADA, American Diabetes Association; ESC, European Society of Cardiology; EASD, European Association for the Study of Diabetes; ESH, Europe Society of Hypertension.

Ambulatory BP monitoring over 24 hours may be useful in some cases to exclude "white coat" effects, and in patients with early nephropathy who have nearly normal BP during the day, but who may be at risk of hypertensive tissue damage because they fail to show the physiologic BP dip during sleep [33].

Diagnosis of hypertension in diabetes

The criteria issued in 1999 by WHO and ISH [34] define hypertension as an office BP exceeding 140/90 mmHg (Korotkoff I–V), and borderline hypertension as being below these limits but above 130 mmHg systolic and/or 85 mmHg diastolic (Figure 40.5) [34]. Established hypertension is diagnosed when readings consistently exceed 140/90 mmHg over several weeks, or when the BP is very high (diastolic BP >110 mmHg), or when there are clinical signs of tissue organ damage from long-standing hypertension.

It is clear from numerous epidemiologic studies that the WHO/ISH threshold is too high in people with diabetes because of their additional risk of both macrovascular and microvascular disease, and that there are definite benefits from treating microalbuminuric subjects whose diastolic BP is <90 mmHg [35]. Various other expert bodies have suggested alternative, generally lower target levels (Figure 40.5). A consensus would be to aim for a BP of less than 130–140 mmHg systolic and below 80–85 mmHg diastolic, and to treat any subject whose BP is consistently above one or both of these thresholds.

Investigation of hypertension in diabetes

Initial investigation of the hypertensive patient with diabetes aims to exclude rare causes of secondary hypertension (Table 40.2), to assess the extent of tissue organ damage caused by hypertension and diabetes (Table 40.1) and to identify other potentially treatable risk factors for vascular disease. The major points in the medical history and examination are shown in Table 40.3.

• *Cardiac function.* A standard 12-lead electrocardiogram may show obvious ischemia, arrhythmia or left ventricular hypertrophy; the latter is more accurately demonstrated by echocardiography, which will also reveal left ventricular dysfunction and decreased ejection fraction. Exercise testing (or stress-echo) testing and 24-hour Holter monitoring may also be appropriate.

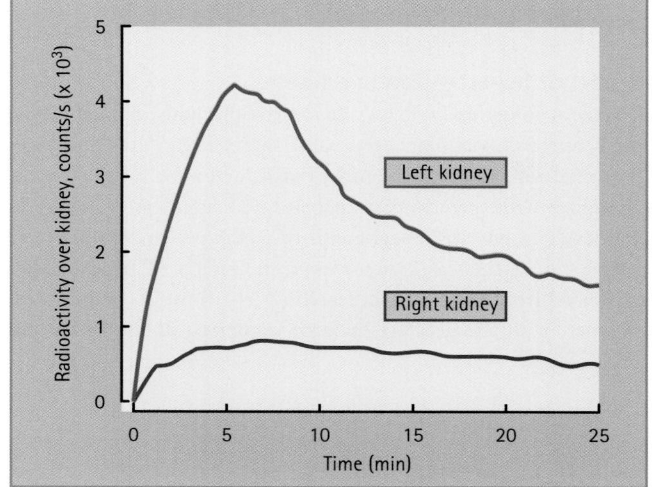

Figure 40.6 Renal artery stenosis affecting the right kidney, in a patient with diabetes and hypertension. Uptake of the isotope on this side is markedly reduced and delayed.

• *Renal function.* A fresh urine sample should be tested for microalbuminuria (see Chapter 37) and another examined microscopically for red and white blood cells, casts, and other signs of renal disease. Microscopic hematuria can occasionally occur in patients with T1DM (particularly children) in the apparent absence of significant renal dysfunction, but coexistent renal disease must always be excluded. Serum urea, creatinine and electrolytes should be checked. If the serum creatinine concentration is raised, measurement of the glomerular filtration rate (GFR) should be considered, ideally using a specific clearance method such as chromium ethylenediamine tetra-acetic acid (Cr-EDTA), iohexol or cystatin C. Further specialist investigations that may be needed include an isotope renogram and other tests for renal artery stenosis (Figure 40.6). This complication of renal

Table 40.3 Investigation of the patient with diabetes and hypertension.

Investigations	Questions to be answered
History Cardiovascular symptoms	Is hypertension significant? Does hypertension have an underlying cause?
Previous urinary disease Smoking and alcohol use Medication	• Renal • Endocrine • Drug-induced
Family history of hypertension or cardiovascular disease **Examination** Blood pressure erect and supine Left ventricular hypertrophy Cardiac failure Peripheral pulses (including renal bruits and radiofemoral delay) Ankle–brachial index	Has hypertension caused tissue damage? • Left ventricular hypertrophy • Ischemic heart disease • Cardiac failure • Peripheral vascular disease • Renal impairment • Fundal changes
Fundal changes of hypertension Evidence of underlying endocrine or renal disease **Electrocardiography** Left ventricular hypertrophy Ischemic changes Rhythm	Are other cardiovascular risk factors present? • Smoking • Hyperlipidemia • Poor glycemic control • Positive family history of cardiovascular disease
Chest radiography Cardiac shadow size Left ventricular failure **Echocardiography** Left ventricular hypertrophy Dyskinesia related to ischemia **Blood tests** Urea, creatinine, electrolytes Fasting lipids **Urinary tests** (Micro-)albuminuria	

arterial atherosclerosis may affect up to 20% of older patients with T2DM and, if bilateral, can lead to severe and sometimes permanent renal impairment if angiotensin-converting enzyme (ACE) inhibitors are given.

• *Lipid profile.* Fasting serum lipid concentrations should be checked. If total cholesterol or triglyceride levels are found to be elevated after repeated measurements, further investigation of lipoprotein subclasses – very low density lipoprotein (VLDL), LDL, HDL, as well as the apo-B : apo-A1 lipoprotein ratio – is recommended. Treatment for hyperlipidemia should be considered if the total cholesterol is >4.5 mmol/L, the LDL cholesterol level is >2.5 mmol/L or the LDL : HDL cholesterol ratio is >4 [36]. This is discussed in more detail in the second half of this chapter.

Other forms of secondary hypertension may be indicated by clinical findings of endocrine or renal disease, significant hypokalemia (plasma potassium <3.5 mmol/L without previous diuretic treatment), failure of hypertension to respond to standard treatment or a sudden decline in GFR after starting treatment with ACE inhibitors (suggestive of renal artery stenosis).

Management of hypertension in diabetes

Strict BP control is the primary goal of treatment. In recent years, target treatment levels have declined progressively to the current recommendation of a mean office BP less than 130–140/80–85 mmHg, for all patients who can tolerate this without side effects such as orthostatic reactions or compromising arterial circulation in critical vascular beds. Recent observations indicate that subgroups of susceptible patients might exist who will not tolerate a dramatic BP reduction below 130 mmHg systolic BP and so caution should be exercised.

Management begins with lifestyle modification, but few patients respond to this alone, and most will require more than one antihypertensive drug to control BP adequately [4,5].

Non-pharmacologic treatment

The treatment of hypertension in patients with diabetes must be based on structured lifestyle intervention. This means weight reduction or weight stabilization in the obese, sodium restriction, diet modification and regular physical exercise (moderate intensity, 40–60 minutes, 2–3 times weekly). Dietary intake of saturated fat has been associated with impaired in insulin sensitivity and should therefore be reduced [37]. Alcohol should be restricted to 2–3 units/day in men and 2 units/day in women, but omitted altogether if hypertension proves difficult to control.

Smoking causes an acute increase in blood pressure and greater variability overall [38]. Smoking cessation is especially important, as smoking not only accelerates the progression of atherosclerosis and vascular aging, but also impairs insulin sensitivity [39] and worsens albuminuria [40]. Treatment with nicotine supplementation for 4–6 weeks (chewing gum or patches), bupropion or varenicline may be useful.

When adopted in full by the patient, lifestyle modification can be extremely effective. The above measures can lower systolic and diastolic BP by 11 and 8 mmHg, respectively [41] – as much as many antihypertensive drugs – and sometimes enough to obviate the need for drug therapy. Weight reduction in obese patients can similarly reduce BP.

Antihypertensive drug therapy

Numerous drugs are available to lower BP, but some are better suited than others to the particular needs of subjects with diabetes because of their favorable or neutral effects on glucose metabolism and other factors. Most patients (at least two-thirds) will require combinations of antihypertensive drugs to control BP – an average of around three different drugs in two large studies [4,5]. Accordingly, the clinician must be able to use a wide variety of antihypertensive drugs and to choose combinations that exploit pharmacologic synergy. Combination therapy usually means that lower dosages of individual drugs can often be used, thus reducing the risk of their adverse effects.

Diuretics

Diuretics are often effective antihypertensive agents for people with diabetes, in whom the total body sodium load is increased and the extracellular fluid volume expanded [42]; however, diuretics that increase urinary potassium and magnesium losses can worsen hyperglycemia, as insulin secretion is impaired by potassium depletion, and insulin sensitivity in peripheral tissues may also be decreased [43]. The use of high-dose thiazide diuretics – equivalent to ≥5 mg/day bendroflumethiazide (bendrofluazide) – is reported to increase the risk of hypertensive patients developing diabetes by up to threefold; this does not seem to occur with low dosages (up to 2.5 mg/day bendroflumethiazide) [44]. Potassium depletion is particularly severe with high-dose chlortalidone (chlorthalidone), less with furosemide (frusemide) and bendroflumethiazide and apparently negligible with indapamide. This mechanism is irrelevant to C-peptide-negative subjects with T1DM who are totally dependent on exogenous insulin. Thiazides may also aggravate dyslipidemia [45], although low dosages probably carry a small risk. Thiazides have also been associated with gout and impotence and are generally avoided in middle-aged men with diabetes and hyperuricemia or erectile dysfunction; nevertheless some evidence suggests that the risk of erectile failure may have been overstated. Diuretics may precipitate hyperosmolar hyperglycemia syndrome and should be avoided or used at the lowest effective dose in patients with a history of this complication.

Diuretics have been shown to prevent CVD successfully in elderly subjects with T2DM and systolic hypertension [46], but one observational study suggested that the use of diuretics increased cardiovascular mortality in hypertensive patients with T2DM who were still hyperglycemic in spite of treatment [47]. Overall, these drugs are effective and safe when used appropriately in patients with diabetes.

Diuretics suitable for use in diabetic hypertension include furosemide, bendroflumethiazide (≤2.5 mg/day), hydrochlorothiazide, spironolactone and indapamide. Low dosages should be used, sometimes in combination with potassium supplements or potassium-sparing drugs, such as amiloride. If ineffective, diuretics should be combined with another first-line drug (e.g. an ACE inhibitor or an angiotensin II-receptor antagonist [ARB]), rather than given at increased dosage. Spironolactone is best not combined with an ACE inhibitor, as this increases the risk of hyperkalemia. Furosemide is useful in patients with renal impairment (serum creatinine >150 μmol/L) or edema.

Serum urea, creatinine and potassium should be checked when starting diuretic therapy and every 6–12 months thereafter, as dangerous disturbances in plasma potassium levels can develop, especially in patients with diabetes and renal impairment.

β-Adrenergic blocking agents

Beta-blockers may significantly lower BP levels in patients with diabetes and hypertension, even though renin release (a major target for these drugs) is commonly reduced in diabetes because of Na^+ and fluid retention. These drugs are often ineffective in Afro-Caribbean patients, who commonly have low renin hypertension. Other mechanisms of action that reduce BP include reductions in heart rate and cardiac output via interaction with β_1- and β_2-receptors in the myocardium and in the vessel wall.

Like diuretics, beta-receptor blockers may aggravate both hyperglycemia and dyslipidemia [48]. These effects depend on both the dosage and the degree of selectivity of the individual drug. The hyperglycemic effect is attributed to inhibition of β_2-adrenergic-mediated insulin release and decreased insulin action in peripheral tissues; the long-term risks of a person without diabetes developing the disease may be increased by sixfold [49] and even more if given together with thiazides. Some studies suggest that the hazards of both hyperglycemia and hyperlipidemia have been exaggerated and may be both dose-dependent and secondary to weight gain [50]. The metabolic side effects of beta-blockers can be reduced by using low dosages combined with other agents, particularly dihydropyridine calcium channel antagonists (CCAs), or by intensifying non-pharmacologic efforts to decrease weight and improve physical activity.

Beta-blockers have other side effects relevant to diabetes. They may interfere with the counter-regulatory effects of catecholamines released during hypoglycemia, thereby blunting manifestations such as tachycardia and tremor and delaying recovery from hypoglycemia [51]. In clinical practice, however, this rarely presents a serious problem, especially when cardioselective β_1-blockers are used. Beta-blockers may also aggravate impotence, and are generally contraindicated in second- or third-degree atrioventricular (AV) heart block, severe peripheral vascular disease, asthma and chronic airway obstruction. Recent studies have shown that certain beta-blockers such as metoprolol and carvedilol [52,53] can be used favorably in cardiac failure in patients with diabetes, as shown in the Metoprolol CR/XL Randomized Intervention Trial in congestive heart failure (MERIT-HF) study, in which 25% of the patients had diabetes [52].

Atenolol is a commonly used drug, as it is cardioselective and water soluble, which reduces CNS side effects and renders its metabolism and dosage more predictable. It is mostly effective as a single daily dose, which probably encourages compliance. In the UKPDS, its effect was comparable to that of the ACE inhibitor, captopril [54]; however, it should be kept in mind that the stroke preventive effect of atenolol is 16% less than other antihypertensive drugs, based on data from meta-analyses. Metoprolol is an alternative, in moderate dosages. Both non-selective and selective beta-blockers are effective in the secondary prevention of myocardial infarction (MI) after an initial event in patients with diabetes [55]. Metoprolol or carvedilol may be indicated in patients who also have heart failure [52,53], and beta-blockers in general are useful in patients who also have angina or tachyarrhythmias.

Calcium-channel antagonists

These useful vasodilator agents do not generally worsen metabolic control when used at conventional dosages, although sporadic cases of hyperglycemia have been reported after starting a calcium-channel antagonist (CCA) of the dihydropyridine class [56]. This may be caused by inhibition of insulin secretion (a calcium-dependent process) in susceptible patients, or a compensatory sympathetic nervous activation, which antagonizes both insulin secretion and action, following vasodilatation.

CCAs have a slight negative inotropic effect and are contraindicated in significant cardiac failure; they often cause mild ankle edema, but this is caused by relaxation of the peripheral precapillary sphincters and raised capillary pressure rather than to right ventricular failure. Because of their potent vasodilator properties, these drugs can cause postural hypotension and can aggravate that brought about by autonomic neuropathy. Non-dihydropyridine CCAs (e.g. verapamil) reduce proteinuria in diabetic nephropathy, but this effect is not seen with dihydropyridine derivatives such as nifedipine, amlodipine, felodipine and isradipine [57].

Because of their other cardiac actions, these drugs are particularly indicated in hypertensive patients who also have angina (e.g. sustained-release nifedipine and diltiazem) or supraventricular tachycardia (e.g. verapamil). Their vasodilator properties may also be beneficial in peripheral vascular disease. CCAs are ideally combined with selective β_1-blockers, but the specific combination of verapamil and beta-blockers (especially together with digoxin) must be avoided because of the risk of conduction block and asystole. Overall, CCAs appear less or similarly cardioprotective but better at preventing stroke than either beta-blockers or thiazide diuretics [58,59].

Amlodipine given once daily is an evidence-based and convenient preparation for general use, and felodipine, isradipine and sustained-release nifedipine are suitable alternatives.

Angiotensin-converting enzyme inhibitors

ACE inhibitors may be used in diabetic hypertension, even in cases where the general RAS is not activated as the drugs may interfere with local angiotensin action in specific target tissues. When used alone, however, these agents have a limited hypotensive action in many black patients, who tend to have suppressed RAS activity.

ACE inhibitors have no adverse metabolic effects and may even improve insulin sensitivity [60]; hypoglycemia has rarely been reported [61]. These drugs are particularly beneficial in diabetic nephropathy by reducing albuminuria and possibly delaying progression of renal damage [62]. Their antiproteinuric effect may be caused specifically by relaxation of the efferent arterioles in the glomerulus, which are highly sensitive to vasoconstriction by angiotensin II, thus reducing the intraglomerular hypertension that is postulated to favor albumin filtration; however, the importance of this mechanism remains controversial [63]. ACE inhibitors are also indicated in cardiac failure, in combination with relatively low dosages of diuretics.

A dry cough is reported by 10–15% of patients treated with ACE inhibitors, because these drugs also interfere with the breakdown of kinins in the bronchial epithelium. Changing to another ACE inhibitor or an ARB may avoid this problem. ACE inhibitors occasionally precipitate acute renal failure, particularly in the elderly and in subjects taking non-steroidal anti-inflammatory drugs (NSAIDs), or who have bilateral renal artery stenosis. Other side effects (rashes, neutropenia, taste disturbance) are unusual with the low dosages currently recommended, but become more prominent in renal failure. Because ACE inhibitors cause potassium retention, they should not generally be taken concurrently with potassium-sparing diuretics (spironolactone and amiloride) or potassium supplements. Serum creatinine and potassium levels should be monitored regularly, especially in patients with renal failure or type 4 renal tubular acidosis, in whom hyperkalemia can rapidly reach dangerous levels.

Ramipril, enalapril, captopril, lisinopril and perindopril are all established ACE inhibitors that are suitable for use in people with diabetes; enalapril, lisinopril, perindopril and ramipril are given once daily for hypertension. The first dose of an ACE inhibitor should be small and taken just before bedtime to minimize postural hypotension, which may be marked in subjects receiving diuretics or on a strict sodium-restricted diet. The same problem may arise in patients with autonomic neuropathy. ACE inhibitors are now recommended in patients with left ventricular dysfunction following MI (see Chapter 41). Ramipril has been shown to prevent cardiovascular morbidity and mortality in high-risk patients with diabetes, with or without pre-existing ischemic heart disease [64].

Angiotensin II type 1 receptor blockers

This promising new class includes losartan, irbesartan, valsartan, candesartan and telmisartan, which act on the AT1 receptor to decrease BP. They are metabolically neutral [65] and, unlike the ACE inhibitors, do not cause cough. They are effective antihypertensive drugs in people with diabetes [66] and have been shown to slow the progression of nephropathy in patients with diabetes and varying degrees of albuminuria (in the RENAAL, IDNT and PRIME-2 studies) [67–69]. Losartan has also been shown (in a subgroup of the LIFE study) to be better than atenolol in reducing both cardiovascular endpoints (by 25%) and total mortality (by 40%) in high-risk patients with T2DM with hypertension and left ventricular hypertrophy [70]. Interestingly, the combination of an ACE inhibitor (lisinopril) with an AT1-antagonist (candesartan) was more effective than either agent alone in lowering BP and UAE in patients with T2DM [71]; however, in the recent ONTARGET study, no extra benefits were recorded for the combination of telmisartan and ramipril on cardiovascular endpoints compared to monotherapy [72].

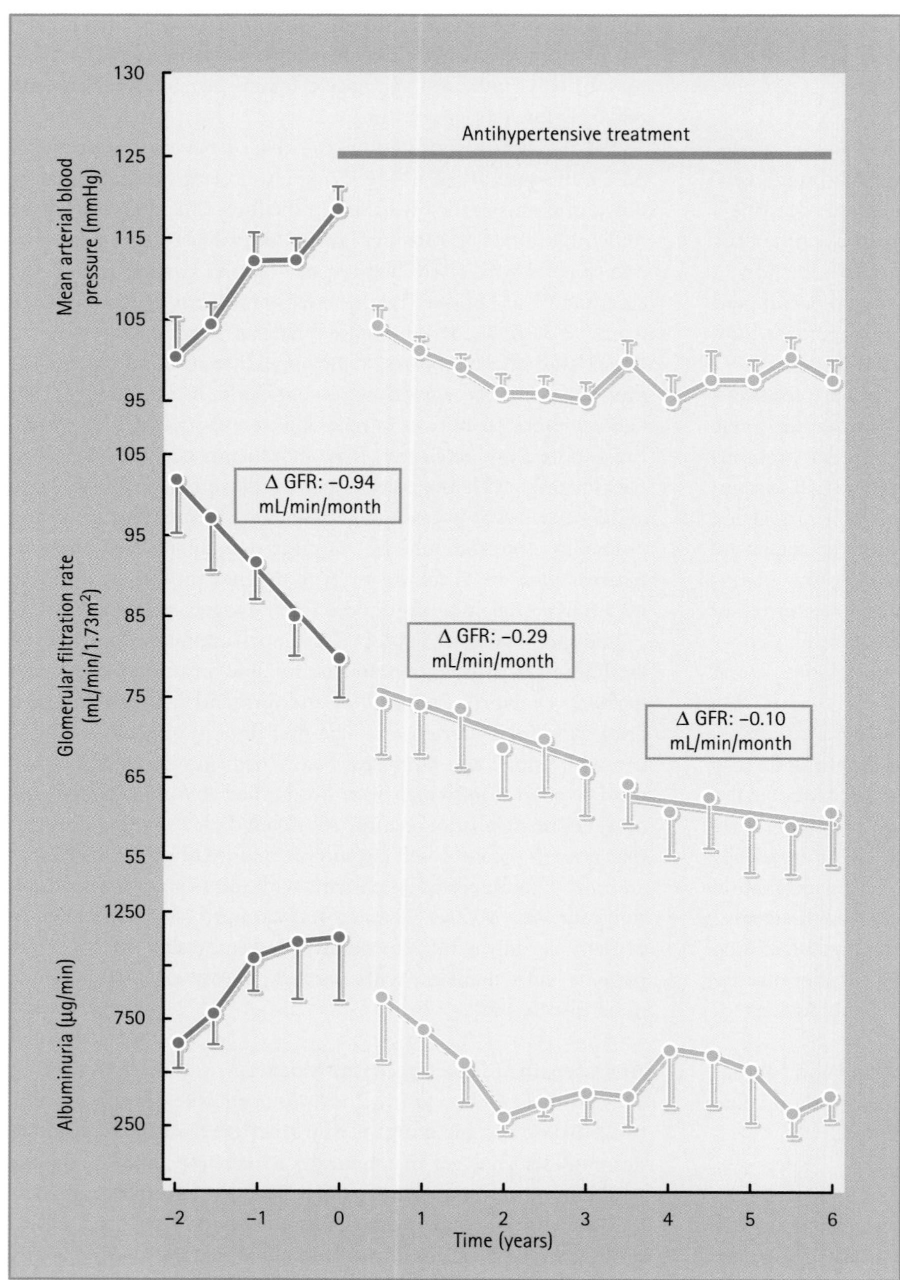

Figure 40.7 Treating hypertension slows the progression of diabetic nephropathy. Lowering blood pressure significantly decreased the rate of decline in the glomerular filtration rate (GFR) and urinary albumin excretion. Reproduced from Parving *et al.* [79], with permission.

α_1-Adrenoceptor antagonists

α_1-Blockers can lower BP effectively and also improve dyslipidemia and insulin sensitivity. Doxazosin is normally well tolerated, especially in combination therapy; side effects include nasal congestion and postural hypotension. Doxazosin has been reported to be inferior to the diuretic chlortalidone in the prevention of stroke and heart failure [73].

Treatment strategies

In general, lifestyle modification should be tried initially for 3 months or so. If moderate hypertension (diastolic BP >100 mmHg, or systolic BP >160 mmHg) or signs of hypertensive tissue damage are present, then drug therapy should be started at the outset. Initially, monotherapy with one of the first-line drugs suggested above should be used, the choice being influenced by other factors such as coexistence of angina, heart failure or nephropathy. All drug treatment should aim for being evidence-based and cost-effective in the individual patient.

Hypertension in T1DM

ACE inhibitors are especially suitable if the patient has albuminuria or more advanced stages of diabetic nephropathy. Diuretics, β_1-selective blockers and CCAs are equally valid alternatives with regard to BP reduction.

If renal function is moderately impaired (serum creatinine values >150 μmol/L), thiazide diuretics become less effective, and furosemide or other loop diuretics should be used instead; however, in established ESRF (serum creatinine >500 μmol/L) furosemide may be toxic, and dialysis must be started. In some patients, hypoglycemia attacks may be masked by use of beta-blockers.

Hypertension in T2DM

BP control is generally more important than the choice of individual drugs. First-line agents, according to evidence from clinical studies, are ACE inhibitors, ARBs, beta-blockers, low-dose thiazide diuretics (in the elderly), furosemide and CCAs [4–8].

Ramipril has evidence-based support for its use in patients with T2DM because of their high cardiovascular risk [64]. Beta-blockers (in combination with low-dose aspirin) are indicated as secondary prevention for patients who have had a MI, as long as no serious contraindications are present. Low doses of thiazide diuretics are useful in elderly patients with diabetes, as this class of drugs has proven efficacy in preventing stroke and all-cause mortality in elderly hypertensive patients [8].

α_1-Blockers may be used as part of combination therapy, especially in patients with dyslipidemia (high triglycerides and low HDL cholesterol levels) and prostatic hyperplasia. Indapamide is well tolerated and has no metabolic side effects. Spironolactone may also be of value [74], especially for elderly obese female patients with hypertension and hypervolemia with a low renin profile.

Combination therapy

Combination therapy is needed in most people with diabetes (especially those with T2DM) to achieve satisfactory BP control [4,5]. It is often better to use low dose combinations than to increase dosages of single agents, as side effects are commonly dose-dependent. As already mentioned, potassium-sparing agents (spironolactone and amiloride) should not be combined with an ACE inhibitor, because of the increased risk for hyperkalemia.

Certain combinations of antihypertensive drugs have proved very safe and effective in low to moderate doses, e.g. ACE inhibitor plus diuretic, for example in the ADVANCE study [75]; CCA plus ACE inhibitor, for example in the ACCOMPLISH study [76]; selective β_1-blocker plus CCA; or β_1-blocker plus α_1-blocker. In some high risk patients a combination treatment could also be considered as initial therapy.

Special considerations in ethnic groups

Hypertension in diabetes represents a serious medical problem in many ethnic groups, such as African-Americans [77]. In non-white European patients, beta-blockers and ACE inhibitors are often less effective at lowering BP because the RAS is already underactive. Diuretics and CCAs are often drugs to be preferred, particularly in African-Americans [78].

Outcome of treating hypertension in diabetes

It has long been recognized that effective treatment of hypertension can slow the progression of diabetic nephropathy, lowering UAE and decreasing the rate of fall of the GFR [79] (Figure 40.7).

The assumptions that improved BP control would improve cardiovascular and other prognoses in T2DM have been confirmed by the UKPDS [4]. In this study, tighter BP control (averaging 144/82 mmHg) for over 8 years led to significant improvements in several outcomes, compared with less strict control that averaged 154/87 mmHg (Table 40.4). Interestingly, the most powerful effects were related to microvascular complications (retinopathy and nephropathy), although significant reductions were seen in the risk of stroke (44%) and heart failure (56%). MI and peripheral vascular disease showed non-significant reductions (Table 40.4; Figures 40.8 and 40.9).

Overall, therefore, tight BP control has been proven to provide substantial benefits for hypertensive patients with diabetes. Moreover, this treatment strategy seems to be cost-effective, at least according to the health economics analyses in the UKPDS [80]; however, it must be kept in mind that these benefits will not last if a continuous BP reduction cannot be achieved long-term, as shown by the 10-year follow-up of the UKPDS [81].

Conclusions

The diagnosis and treatment of hypertension is of great importance for the person with diabetes [34,36,82–84]. The treatment targets are demanding and require considerable effort from both patient and physicians, but the benefits are now undisputed.

New antihypertensive drugs are constantly being introduced but have to prove themselves for both efficacy and tolerability. Even some antidiabetic drugs appear to lower BP as well as blood glucose [85], but safety concerns are important (see Chapter 29).

In the future, the application of cardiovascular genomics may substantially change the approach to treating hypertension in

Table 40.4 Impact of stricter control of hypertension on diabetic complications, macrovascular disease and diabetes-related deaths in T2DM. Data from the UKPDS [4].

Measure	Relative risk with tight control (mean, 95% confidence intervals)	*P* value
Diabetes-related deaths	0.76 (0.62–0.92)	0.19
All-cause mortality	0.82 (0.63–1.08)	0.17
Myocardial infarction	0.79 (0.59–1.07)	0.13
Stroke	0.56 (0.35–0.89)	0.013
Peripheral vascular disease	0.51 (0.19–1.37)	0.17
Microvascular disease	0.63 (0.44–0.89)	0.009

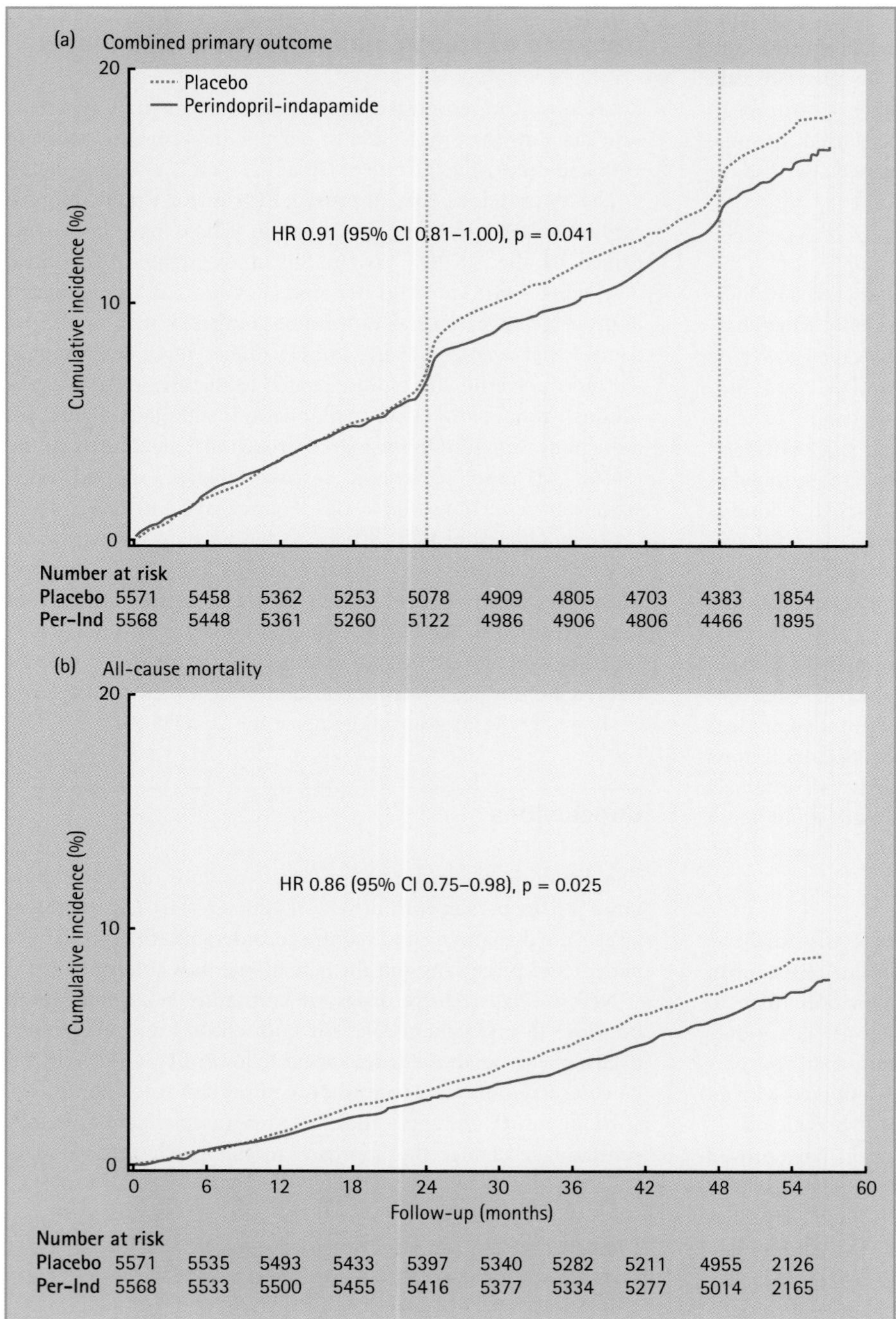

Figure 40.8 Kaplan–Meier curves for the primary outcome and all-cause mortality in the two study groups in the ADVANCE Trial [74]. The combined primary outcome were composites of major macrovascular and microvascular events. Major macrovascular events were cardiovascular death, non-fatal myocardial infarction, or non-fatal stroke. Major microvascular events were new or worsening nephropathy or retinopathy.

diabetes [86], aiming at tailoring treatment according to the genotype of the individual patient.

In addition, further large-scale studies with large numbers of hypertensive patients with T2DM are awaited [87]. In the recent ACCORD-Blood pressure study [88] there was no significant difference in the primary composite outcome of cardiovascular events between patients randomized to achieve a systolic blood pressure goal below 120 mmHg versus below 140 mmHg, even if a reduction in stroke was noticed (secondary end-point) in the intensive arm. This means that the optimal blood pressure goal for patients with hypertension and T2DM is still not established [89].

Finally, it takes a multifactorial approach to address and to treat all major cardiovascular risk factors, not only BP, to achieve lasting cardiovascular protection, as evidenced by the Steno-2 trial [90].

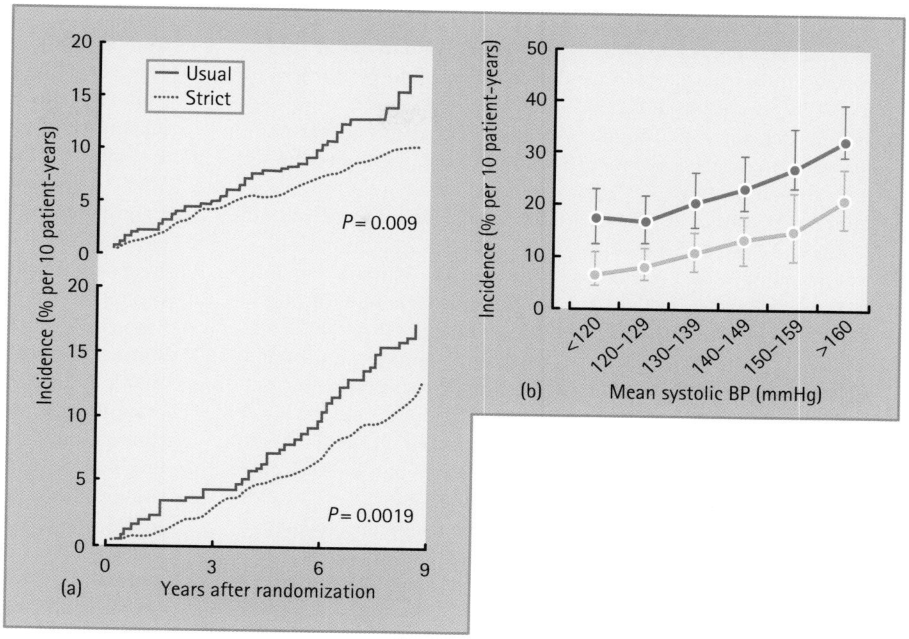

Figure 40.9 Treating hypertension improves the prognosis in T2DM. (a) Stricter BP control (mean pressure 144/82 mmHg) significantly reduced the risks of both microvascular complications (*top*) and diabetes-related death (*bottom*), compared with less strict control (mean 154/82 mmHg).
(b) The relationship between BP and rates of microvascular disease and MI. Lowering the BP progressively reduced the risk of microvascular complications, but there was no significant effect on MI. The red line represents MI and the yellow line represents microvascular complications. Reproduced from UKPDS [4,91], with permission.

References

1 Kylin E. Studien über das Hypertone-Hyperglykämie-Hyperurikämisyndrom. *Zeitschrift Inn Med* 1923; **7**:105–112.

2 Reaven GM. Role of insulin resistance in human disease. *Diabetes* 1988; **37**:1595–1607.

3 Meigs JB, D'Agostino RB Sr, Wilson P, Cupples LA, Nathan DM, Singer DE. Risk variable clustering in the insulin resistance syndrome: the Framingham Offspring Study. *Diabetes* 1997; **46**:1594–1600.

4 UK Prospective Diabetes Study Group. Tight blood pressure control and risk of macrovascular and microvascular complications in type 2 diabetes: UKPDS 38. *Br Med J* 1998; **317**:703–713.

5 Hansson L, Zanchetti A, Carruthers SG, Dahlöf B, Elmfeldt D, Julius S, *et al.* Effects of intensive blood-pressure lowering and low-dose aspirin in patients with hypertension: principal results of the Hypertension Optimal Treatment (HOT) randomised trial. *Lancet* 1998; **351**:1755–1762.

6 Estacio RO, Jeffers BW, Hiatt WR, Biggerstaff SL, Gifford N, Schrier RW. The effect of nisoldipine as compared with enalapril on cardiovascular outcomes in patients with non-insulin-dependent diabetes and hypertension. *N Engl J Med* 1998; **338**:645–652.

7 Tuomilehto J, Rastenyte D, Birkenhäger WH, Thijs L, Antikainen R, Bulpitt CJ, *et al.* Effects of calcium-channel blockade in older patients with diabetes and systolic hypertension. *N Engl J Med* 1999; **340**:677–684.

8 Lindholm LH, Hansson L, Ekbom T, Dahlöf B, Lanke J, Linjer E, *et al.* Comparison of antihypertensive treatments in preventing cardiovascular events in elderly diabetic patients: results from the Swedish Trial in Old Patients with Hypertension-2 Study Group. *J Hypertens* 2000; **18**:1671–1675.

9 Wiseman MJ, Viberti GC, Mackintosh D, Jarrett RJ, Keen H. Glycaemia, arterial pressure and microalbuminuria in type 1 (insulin-dependent) diabetes mellitus. *Diabetologia* 1984; **26**:401–405.

10 Hypertension in Diabetes Study Group. Hypertension in Diabetes Study (HDS). II. Increased risk of cardiovascular complications in hypertensive type 2 diabetic patients. *J Hypertens* 1993; **11**:319–325.

11 Haffner S, Mitchell B, Stern M, Hazuda HP, Patterson JK. Decreased prevalence of hypertension in Mexican-Americans. *Hypertension* 1990; **16**:225–232.

12 Salomaa VV, Strandberg TE, Vanhanen H, Naukkarinen V, Sarna S, Miettinen TA. Glucose tolerance and blood pressure: long-term follow up in middle aged men. *Br Med J* 1991; **302**:493–496.

13 Cooper R, Cutler J, Desvigne-Nickens P, Fortmann SP, Friedman L, Havlik R, *et al.* Trends and disparities in coronary heart disease, stroke, and other cardiovascular diseases in the United States: findings of the national conference on cardiovascular disease prevention. *Circulation* 2000; **102**:3137–3147.

14 DeFronzo R, Ferrannini E. Insulin resistance: a multifaceted syndrome responsible for NIDDM, obesity, hypertension, dyslipidemia, and atherosclerotic disease. *Diabetes Care* 1991; **14**:173–194.

15 Pyörälä M, Miettinen H, Halonen P, Laakso M, Pyörälä K. Insulin resistance syndrome predicts the risk of coronary heart disease and stroke in healthy middle-aged men: the 22-year follow-up results of the Helsinki Policemen Study. *Arterioscler Thromb Vasc Biol* 2000; **20**:538–544.

16 Barker DJP, ed. *Fetal and Infant Origins of Adult Disease.* London: British Medical Journal, 1992.

17 Pinkney JH, Mohamed-Ali V, Denver AE, Foster C, Sampson MJ, Yudkin JS. Insulin resistance, insulin, proinsulin, and ambulatory blood pressure in type II diabetes. *Hypertension* 1994; **24**:362–367.

18 Scherrer U, Randin D, Vollenweider P, Vollenweider L, Nicod P. Nitric oxide release accounts for insulin's vascular effects in humans. *J Clin Invest* 1994; **94**:2511–2515.

19 Rongen GA, Tack CJ. Triglycerides and endothelial function in type 2 diabetes. *Eur J Clin Invest* 2001; **31**:560–562.

20 DeFronzo RA, Goldberg M, Agus ZS. The effects of glucose and insulin on renal electrolyte transport. *J Clin Invest* 1976; **58**:83–90.

21 Natali A, Quiñones Galvan A, Santora D, Pecori N, Taddei S, Salvetti A, *et al.* Relationship between insulin release, antinatriuresis and hypokalaemia after glucose ingestion in normal and hypertensive man. *Clin Sci* 1993; **85**:327–335.

22 Hall JE, Summers RL, Brands MW, Keen H, Alonso-Galicia M. Resistance to metabolic actions of insulin and its role in hypertension. *Am J Hypertens* 1994; **7**:772–788.

23 Morris AD, Petrie JR, Connell JMC. Insulin and hypertension. *J Hypertens* 1994; **12**:633–642.

24 Anderson EA, Balon TW, Hoffman RP, Sinkey CA, Mark AL. Insulin increases sympathetic activity but not blood pressure in borderline hypertensive humans. *Hypertension* 1992; **19**:621–627.

25 Capron L, Jarnet J, Kazandjian S, Housset E. Growth-promoting effects of diabetes and insulin on arteries: an *in vivo* study of rat aorta. *Diabetes* 1986; **35**:973–978.

26 Mathiesen ER, Rønn B, Jensen T, Storm B, Deckert T. Relationship between blood pressure and urinary albumin excretion in development of microalbuminuria. *Diabetes* 1990; **39**:245–249.

27 Walker JD, Tariq T, Viberti GC. Sodium–lithium countertransport activity in red cells of patients with insulin-dependent diabetes and nephropathy and their parents. *Br Med J* 1990; **301**: 635–638.

28 Drury PL, Bodansky HJ, Oddie CJ, Edwards CRW. Factors in the control of plasma renin activity and concentration in type 1 diabetics. *Clin Endocrinol* 1984; **20**:607–618.

29 Zatz R, Brenner BM. Pathogenesis of diabetic microangiopathy: the hemodynamic view. *Am J Med* 1986; **80**:443–453.

30 Groop L, Ekstrand A, Forsblom C, Widen E, Groop PH. Insulin resistance, hypertension and microalbuminuria in patients with type II (non-insulin-dependent) diabetes mellitus. *Diabetologia* 1993; **36**: 642–647.

31 Liu JE, Palmieri V, Roman NJ, Bella JN, Fabsitz R, Hoard BV, *et al.* The impact of diabetes in left ventricular filling pattern in normotensive and hypertensive adults: the strong heart study. *J Am Coll Cardiol* 2001; **37**:1943–1949.

32 Kuperstein R, Hanly P, Niroamand M, Fasson Z. The importance of age and obesity on the relation between diabetes and left ventricular mass. *J Am Coll Cardiol* 2001; **37**:1957–1962.

33 Schernthaner G, Ritz E, Phillipp T, Bretzel R. The significance of 24-hour blood pressure monitoring in patients with diabetes mellitus. *Dtsch Med Wochenschrift* 1999; **124**:393–395.

34 World Health Organization–International Society of Hypertension Guidelines for the Management of Hypertension, 1999. Guidelines Subcommittee. *J Hypertens* 1999; **17**:151–183.

35 Stamler J, Vaccaro O, Neaton JD, Wentworth D. Diabetes, other risk factors, and 12-yr cardiovascular mortality for men screened in the Multiple Risk Factor Intervention Trial. *Diabetes Care* 1993; **16**:434–444.

36 Prevention of coronary heart disease in clinical practice. Recommendations of the Second Joint Task Force of European and other Societies on coronary prevention. Summary of recommendations. *Eur Heart J* 1998; **19**:1434–1503.

37 Vessby B, Tengblad S, Lithell H. Insulin sensitivity is related to the fatty acid composition of serum lipids and skeletal muscle phospholipids in 70-year old men. *Diabetologia* 1994; **37**: 1044–1050.

38 Stewart MJ, Jyothinagaram S, McGinley IM, Padfield PL. Cardiovascular effects of cigarette smoking: ambulatory blood pressure and BP variability. *J Hum Hypertens* 1994; **8**:19–22.

39 Facchini F, Hollenbeck C, Jeppesen J, Chen YD, Reaven GM. Insulin resistance and cigarette smoking. *Lancet* 1992; **339**:1128–1130.

40 Chase PH, Garg SK, Marshall G, Berg CL, Harris S, Jackson WE, *et al.* Cigarette smoking increases the risk of albuminuria among subjects with type 1 diabetes. *JAMA* 1991; **265**:614–617.

41 Treatment of Mild Hypertension Research Group. The Treatment of Mild Hypertension Study: a randomized, placebo-controlled trial of a nutritional-hygienic regimen along with various drug monotherapies. *Arch Intern Med* 1991; **151**:1413–1423.

42 Weidman P, Beretta-Piccoli C, Keusch G, Glück Z, Mujagic M, Grimm M, *et al.* Sodium-volume factor, cardiovascular reactivity and hypotensive mechanism of diuretic therapy in mild hypertension associated with diabetes mellitus. *Am J Med* 1979; **67**:779–784.

43 Pollare T, Lithell H, Berne C. A comparison of the effects of hydrochlorothiazide and captopril on glucose and lipid metabolism in patients with hypertension. *N Engl J Med* 1989; **321**:868–873.

44 Berglund G, Andersson O, Widgren B. Low-dose antihypertensive treatment with a thiazide diuretic is not diabetogenic: a 10-year controlled trial with bendroflumethiazide. *Acta Med Scand* 1986; **220**:419–424.

45 MacMahon SW, Macdonald GJ. Antihypertensive treatment and plasma lipoprotein levels: the associations in data from a population study. *Am J Med* 1987; **80**(Suppl. 2A):40–47.

46 Curb JD, Pressel SL, Cutler JA, Savage PJ, Applegate WB, Black H, *et al.*; Systolic Hypertension in the Elderly Program Cooperative Research Group. Effect of diuretic-based anti-hypertensive treatment on cardiovascular disease risk in older diabetic patients with isolated systolic hypertension. *JAMA* 1996; **276**:1886–1892.

47 Alderman MH, Cohen H, Madhavan S. Diabetes and cardiovascular events in diabetes patients. *Hypertension* 1999; **33**:1130–1134.

48 Pollare T, Lithell H, Selinus I, Berne C. Sensitivity to insulin during treatment with atenolol and metoprolol: a randomized, double blind study of effects on carbohydrate and lipoprotein metabolism in hypertensive patients. *Br Med J* 1989; **198**:1152–1157.

49 Gress TW, Nieto FJ, Shahar E, Wofford MR, Brancati FL. Hypertension and antihypertensive therapy as risk factors for type 2 diabetes mellitus. Atherosclerosis Risk in the Community Study. *N Engl J Med* 2000; **342**:905–912.

50 Sawicki PT, Siebenhofer A. Beta-blocker treatment in diabetes mellitus. *J Intern Med* 2001; **250**:11–17.

51 Lager I, Blohme G, Smith U. Effect of cardioselective and non selective beta-blockade on the hypoglycemic response in insulin-dependent diabetics. *Lancet* 1979; **i**:458–462.

52 Hjalmarson A, Goldstein S, Fagerberg B, Wedel H, Waagstein F, Kjekshus J, *et al.*; MERIT-HF Study Group. Effects of controlled-release metoprolol on total mortality, hospitalizations, and well-being in patients with heart failure: the Metoprolol CR/XL Randomized Intervention Trial in congestive heart failure (MERIT-HF). *JAMA* 2000; **283**:1295–1302.

53 Krum H, Ninio D, MacDonald P. Baseline predictors of tolerability to carvedilol in patients with chronic heart failure. *Heart* 2000; **84**:615–619.

54 UK Prospective Diabetes Study Group. Efficacy of atenolol and captopril in reducing risk of macrovascular and microvascular complications in type 2 diabetes: UKPDS 39. *Br Med J* 1998; **317**: 713–720.

55 Kjekshus J, Gilpin E, Cali G, Blackey AR, Henning H, Ross J Jr. Diabetic patients and beta-blockers after acute myocardial infarction. *Eur Heart J* 1990; **11**:43–50.

56 Chellingsworth MC, Kendall MJ, Wright AD, Singh BM, Pasi J. The effects of verapamil, diltiazem, nifedipine and propranolol on metabolic control in hypertensives with non-insulin-dependent diabetes mellitus. *J Hum Hypertens* 1989; **3**:35–39.

57 Bakris GL, Weir MR, DeQuattro V, McMahon FG. Effects of an ACE inhibitor/calcium antagonist combination on proteinuria in diabetic nephropathy. *Kidney Int* 1998; **54**:1283–1289.

58 Pahor M, Psaty BM, Alderman MH, Applegate WB, Williamson JD, Cavazzini C, *et al.* Health outcomes associated with calcium antagonists compared with other first-line antihypertensive therapies: a meta-analysis of randomised controlled trials. *Lancet* 2000; **356**:1949–1954.

59 Neal B, MacMahon S, Chapman N; Blood Pressure Lowering Treatment Trialists' Collaboration. Effects of ACE inhibitors, calcium antagonists, and other blood-pressure-lowering drugs: results of prospectively designed overviews of randomised trials. *Lancet* 2000; **356**:1955–1964.

60 Lithell HO. Effects of antihypertensive drugs on insulin, glucose and lipid metabolism. *Diabetes Care* 1991; **14**:203–209.

61 Herings RM, de Boer A, Stricker BH, Leufkens HG, Porsius A. Hypoglycaemia associated with use of inhibitor of angiotensin converting enzyme. *Lancet* 1995; **345**:1195–1198.

62 Lewis EJ, Hunsickler LG, Bain RP, Rohde RD. The effect of angiotensin-converting-enzyme inhibition on diabetic nephropathy. *N Engl J Med* 1993; **329**:1456–1462.

63 Bank N, Klose R, Aynedjan HS, Nguyen D, Sablay LB. Evidence against increased glomerular pressure initiating diabetic nephropathy. *Kidney Int* 1987; **31**:898–905.

64 Heart Outcomes Prevention Evaluation Study Investigators. Effects of ramipril on cardiovascular and microvascular outcomes in people with diabetes mellitus: results of the HOPE study and MICRO-HOPE substudy. *Lancet* 2000; **355**:253–259.

65 Goodfriend TL, Elliott ME, Catt KJ. Angiotensin receptors and their antagonists. *N Engl J Med* 1996; **334**:1649–1654.

66 Ruilope L. RAS blockade: new possibilities in the treatment of complications of diabetes. *Heart* 2000; **84**:32–34.

67 Brenner B, Cooper ME, de Zeeuw D, de Zeeuw D, Keane WF, Mitch WE, *et al.* Effects of losartan on renal and cardiovascular outcomes in patients with type 2 diabetes and nephropathy. *N Engl J Med* 2001; **345**:861–869.

68 Lewis EJ, Hunsicker LG, Clarke WR, Berl T, Pohl MA, Lewis JB, *et al.* Renoprotective effect of the angiotensin-receptor antagonist irbesartan in patients with nephropathy due to type 2 diabetes. *N Engl J Med* 2001; **345**:851–859.

69 Parving HH, Lehnert H, Bröckner-Mortensen J, Gomis R, Andersen S, Arner P; Irbesartan in Patients with Type 2 Diabetes and Microalbuminuria Study Group. The effect of irbesartan on the development of diabetic nephropathy in patients with type 2 diabetes. *N Engl J Med* 2001; **345**:870–878.

70 Lindholm LH, Ibsen H, Dahlöf B, Devereux RB, Beevers G, de Faire U, *et al.* Cardiovascular morbidity and mortality in patients with diabetes in the Losartan Intervention For Endpoint reduction in hypertension study (LIFE): a randomised trial against atenolol. *Lancet* 2002; **359**:1004–1008.

71 Mogensen CE, Neldam S, Tikkanen I, Oren S, Viskoper R, Watts RW, *et al.* Randomized controlled trial of dual blockage of renin-angiotensin and non-insulin dependent diabetes: the Candesartan and Lisinopril Microalbuminuria (CALM) Study. *Br Med J* 2000; **321**:1440–1444.

72 ONTARGET Investigators. Telmisartan, ramipril, or both in patients at high risk for vascular events. *N Engl J Med* 2008; **358**:1547–1559.

73 ALLHAT Collaborative Research Group. Major cardiovascular events in hypertensive patients randomized to doxazosin vs chlorthalidone: the antihypertensive and lipid-lowering treatment to prevent heart attack trial (ALLHAT). *JAMA* 2000; **283**:1967–1975.

74 Ramsay LE, Yeo WW, Jackson PR. Diabetes, impaired glucose tolerance and insulin resistance with diuretics. *Eur Heart J* 1992; **13**(Suppl. G):68–71.

75 Patel A; ADVANCE Collaborative Group. Effects of a fixed combination of perindopril and indapamide on macrovascular and microvascular outcomes in patients with type 2 diabetes mellitus (the ADVANCE trial): a randomised controlled trial. *Lancet* 2007; **370**:829–840.

76 Jamerson K, Weber MA, Bakris GL, Dahlöf B, Pitt B, Shi V, *et al.*; ACCOMPLISH Trial Investigators. Benazepril plus amlodipine or hydrochlorothiazide for hypertension in high-risk patients. *N Engl J Med* 2008; **359**:2417–2428.

77 Jamerson K, de Quattro V. The impact of ethnicity on response to antihypertensive therapy. *Am J Med* 1996; **101**:22S–32S.

78 Flack JM, Hamaty M. Difficult-to-treat hypertensive populations: focus on African-Americans and people with type 2 diabetes. *J Hypertens* 1999; **17**(Suppl.):S19–S24.

79 Parving HH, Andersen AR, Smidt UM, Hommel E, Mathiesen ER, Svendsen PA. Effect of antihypertensive treatment on kidney function in diabetic nephropathy. *Br Med J (Clin Res Ed)* 1987; **294**:1443–1447.

80 UK Prospective Diabetes Study Group. Cost effectiveness analysis of improved blood pressure control in hypertensive patients with type 2 diabetes: UKPDS 40. *Br Med J* 1998; **317**:720–726.

81 Holman RR, Paul SK, Bethel MA, Neil HA, Matthews DR. Long-term follow-up after tight control of blood pressure in type 2 diabetes. *N Engl J Med* 2008; **359**:1565–1576.

82 Chobanian AV, Bakris GL, Black HR, Cushman WC, Green LA, Izzo JL Jr, *et al.*; National Heart, Lung, and Blood Institute Joint National Committee on Prevention, Detection, Evaluation, and Treatment of High Blood Pressure; National High Blood Pressure Education Program Coordinating Committee. The Seventh Report of the Joint National Committee on Prevention, Detection, Evaluation, and Treatment of High Blood Pressure: the JNC 7 report. *JAMA* 2003; **289**:2560–2572.

83 Rydén L, Standl E, Bartnik M, Van den Berghe G, Betteridge J, de Boer MJ, *et al.*; Task Force on Diabetes and Cardiovascular Diseases of the European Society of Cardiology (ESC); European Association for the Study of Diabetes (EASD). Guidelines on diabetes, pre-diabetes, and cardiovascular diseases: executive summary. *Eur Heart J* 2007; **28**:88–136.

84 Mancia G, De Backer G, Dominiczak A, Cifkova R, Fagard R, Germano G, *et al.*; The Task Force for the Management of Arterial Hypertension of the European Society of Hypertension (ESH) and of the European Society of Cardiology (ESC). Management of arterial hypertension of the European Society of Hypertension; European Society of Cardiology: 2007 guidelines for the management of arterial hypertension: *J Hypertens* 2007; **25**:1105–1187.

85 Sarafidis P, Nilsson PM. The effects of thiazolidinedione compounds on blood pressure levels: a systematic review. *Blood Pressure* 2006; **15**:135–150.

86 Pratt RE, Dzau VJ. Genomics and hypertension: concepts, potentials, and opportunities. *Hypertension* 1999; **33**:238–247.

87 Lauritzen T, Griffin S, Borch-Johnsen K, Wareham NJ, Wolffenbuttel BH, Rutten G; Anglo-Danish-Dutch Study of Intensive Treatment in People with Screen Detected Diabetes in Primary Care. The ADDITION study: proposed trial of the cost-effectiveness of an intensive multifactorial intervention on morbidity and mortality among people with type 2 diabetes detected by screening. *Int J Obes Relat Metab Disord* 2000; **24**(Suppl 3):S6–11.
88 The ACCORD Study Group. Effects of Intensive Blood-Pressure Control in Type 2 Diabetes Mellitus. *N Engl J Med* 2010; Mar 14. [Epub ahead of print].
89 Mancia G, Laurent S, Agabiti-Rosei E, Ambrosioni E, Burnier M, Caulfield MJ, *et al.*; Reappraisal of European guidelines on hypertension management: a European Society of Hypertension Task Force document. *J Hypertens* 2009, Oct 15. [Epub ahead of print].
90 Gaede P, Lund-Andersen H, Parving H-H, Pedersen O. Effect of a multifactorial intervention on mortality in type 2 diabetes. *N Engl J Med* 2008; **358**:580–591.
91 Adler AI, Stratton IM, Neil HA, Yudkin JS, Matthews DR, Cull CA, *et al.* Association of systolic blood pressure with macrovascular and microvascular complications of type 2 diabetes (UKPDS 36): prospective observational study. *BMJ* 2000; **321**(7258):412–419.

Dyslipidemia: Diabetes Lipid Therapies

Adie Viljoen[1] and Anthony S. Wierzbicki[2]

Keypoints

- The greatest long-term risk in diabetes is cardiovascular disease (CVD), with macrovascular disease being the cause of 80% of mortality in people with diabetes.
- Epidemiologic studies have established that glycemic control, nephropathy and lipids are risk factors for CVD in type 1 diabetes.
- Low density lipoprotein (LDL) cholesterol, high density lipoprotein (HDL) cholesterol, smoking and hypertension are the principal risk factors in type 2 diabetes mellitus (T2DM).
- In T2DM, optimized glycemic control has modest effects in reducing CVD endpoints.
- Reduction of LDL cholesterol with statins has consistently shown cardiovascular event reductions >30%.
- The dyslipidemia of T2DM is associated with elevated triglycerides, reduced HDL cholesterol and small dense particles.
- Fibrates, when used as monotherapy, have shown a modest reduction in events in T2DM in the FIELD study.
- Post hoc analysis of the Coronary Drug Project with niacin suggests possible benefits on cardiovascular endpoints.
- Trials now underway will allow the efficacy of combination lipid-lowering therapies in diabetes to be determined.
- Optimal control of all risk factors can reduce cardiovascular events and mortality in diabetes by 50%.

Introduction

An association between diabetes and heart disease was described more than a century ago. Two decades later, in 1906, it was hypothesized that this association was caused by atherosclerosis. The importance of diabetes as a cardiovascular disease (CVD) risk factor became established following the Framingham Study and this was subsequently confirmed by other landmark studies [1,2]. The magnitude of diabetes as a CVD risk factor is substantial, with the increase in cardiovascular risk being two- to fourfold. Many guidelines regard diabetes as a coronary heart disease (CHD) risk equivalent [3–5]. This concept is based originally on a Finnish cohort [6], which showed comparable risk of CHD outcomes such as myocardial infarction (MI) and CHD death between subjects with type 2 diabetes mellitus (T2DM) for >10 years and subjects with established CHD (Figure 40.10). This was still apparent after adjusting for known risk factors such as age, sex, hypertension, total cholesterol and smoking. The Organization to Assess Strategies for Ischemic Syndromes (OASIS) study showed that patients with diabetes and no previous CVD have the same long-term morbidity and mortality as patients with established CVD but no diabetes after hospitalization for unstable coronary artery disease (CAD) [7]; however, there is a wide variation in the rate of CHD in diabetes which depends on the population studied, duration of diabetes, as well as existing risk factors [8,9]. This equivalence has not been confirmed by a subsequent study and it also seems less valid in older subjects where those with existing CHD have a greater risk than non-CHD patients with diabetes [9,10]. Most of the literature that reports on CVD risk and diabetes only considers T2DM. Even though people with type 1 diabetes mellitus (T1DM) are clearly at increased risk for CVD [11,12], no study has specifically examined whether subjects with T1DM have a CVD risk that is comparable or higher than those with T2DM. In T1DM there may even be a higher risk of premature CVD. In a cohort of 292 patients with T1DM followed for 20–40 years, the cumulative mortality rate from CAD was 35% by age 55 [11]. As T1DM mostly presents at an earlier age, it remains more difficult to assess and compare this but rates of CVD are increased at all ages [13].

Concomitant CVD risk factors also differ according to the type of diabetes. For example, those with T1DM have a two- to threefold increase in risk of developing CHD and stroke in later life. This risk is notably increased in those developing diabetic neph-

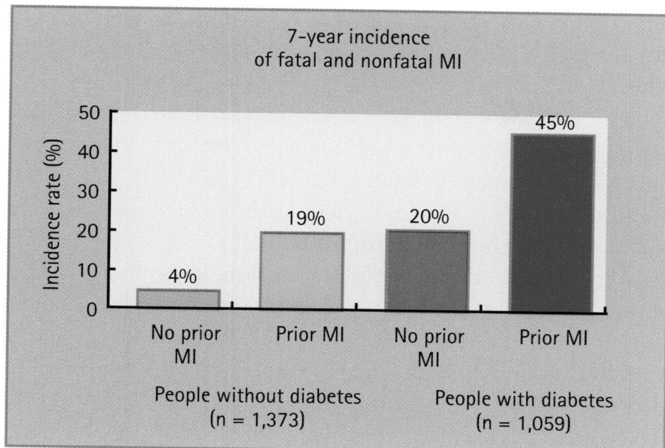

Figure 40.10 Equivalence of cardiovascular risk in patients with previous coronary heart disease (CHD) and those with diabetes. MI, myocardial infarction. Reproduced from Haffner *et al.* [6], with permission from Massachusetts Medical Society.

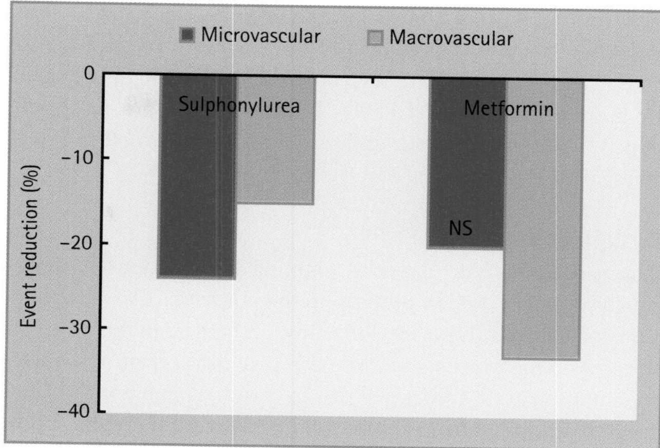

Figure 40.11 Results of the UK Prospective Diabetes Study (UKPDS) at 10 years follow-up. Reproduced from Holman *et al.* [24], with permission from Massachusetts Medical Society.

ropathy. Other markers of CVD risk in people with diabetes include diabetic retinopathy, autonomic neuropathy, erectile dysfunction, microalbuminuria and proteinuria [14].

In general, people with diabetes have a two- to fourfold CVD risk compared with the non-diabetic population [15]. Even though guidelines do not recommend formal CVD risk estimation in those with diabetes because of the significant risk these patients already have and the tendency of the Framingham algorithm to underestimate risk in this group, clinicians may still opt to estimate the risk by employing various risk calculators of which the UK Prospective Diabetes Study (UKPDS) is the most used [16]. It should be noted however, that these risk calculators predict risk with variable accuracy [17]. As all methods of CVD risk estimation suffer from distinct limitations, clinical judgment remains necessary to assess risk accurately and select and titrate appropriate treatment [18,19].

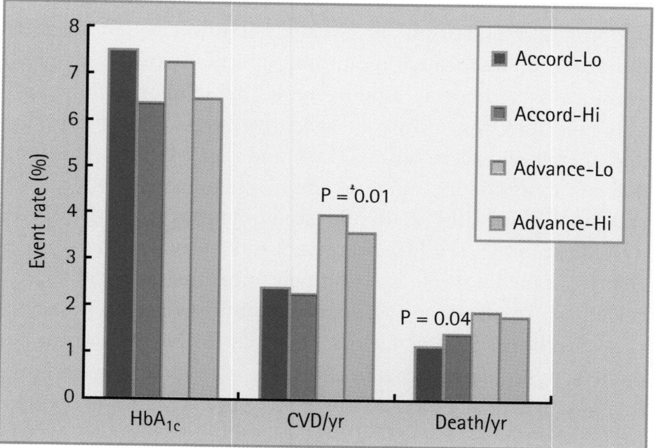

Figure 40.12 Effects of improved diabetes control to an HbA_{1c} <6.5% (48 mmol/mol) in the ACCORD and ADVANCE studies. CVD, cardiovascular disease; Lo, intensive glycemic control; Hi, conventional glycemic control. Data from ACCORD group *N Engl J Med* 2008; **358**:2545 and ADVANCE group *N Engl J Med* 2008; **358**:2560.

Cardiovascular disease risk factors in diabetes

Glucose

A risk continuum exists across a broad glucose concentration range which incorporates individuals without diabetes, with the risk of CVD being the lowest when the fasting blood glucose is 4–4.9 mmol/L [20–22]. Despite the well-established association between blood glucose and atherosclerosis, surprisingly few studies have been able to show an improvement in cardiovascular outcome by reduction in blood glucose. In T1DM, the Epidemiology of Diabetes Interventions and Complications (EDIC) study [23] which followed subjects after the completion the Diabetes Control and Complications Trial found that glucose lowering was associated with a long-term benefit with regard to cardiovascular complications that became apparent only years after recruitment. In T2DM, 10-year follow-up data from the UKPDS intensive glucose therapy showed long-term beneficial effects on macrovascular outcomes [24]; however, unlike the microvascular benefits, risk reductions for MI and death from any cause were observed only with extended post-trial follow-up (Figure 40.11). These results suggested that improved glucose control may result in a larger cardiovascular risk reduction in patients with T1DM than among those with T2DM, which is consistent with the results of one meta-analysis. Furthermore, neither the recent Action in Diabetes and Vascular Disease: Preterax and Diamicron Modified Release Controlled Evaluation (ADVANCE) [25] nor the Action to Control Cardiovascular Risk in Diabetes (ACCORD) [26] trials, each including in excess of 10 000 participants, could not show a significant beneficial effect on CVD outcome when targeting near-normal glucose levels in T2DM as determined by a HbA_{1c} <6.5% (48 mmol/mol) (Figure 40.12). More worrying was the finding in the ACCORD trial that near-normal glucose control was actually associated with a significantly increased risk of death from any cause and death from cardiovascular causes, the very outcomes the trial was designed to prevent [27]. Several other outcomes trials are underway, which should improve our understanding of the problem of glycemic control and CVD [28].

Dyslipidemia

Compared with hyperglycemia, targeting dyslipidemia has proven much more effective in preventing the macrovascular complications of diabetes; however, for many years the benefits of intervention on lipoproteins as cardiovascular risk factors in diabetes were uncertain. The principal reason was that people with diabetes were excluded from trials of lipid-lowering therapies. Thus, virtually no data exist from early studies with bile acid sequestrants, fibrates or nicotinic acid.

The reasons for the excess CVD risk in diabetes are numerous and varied and in part relate to the lipid abnormalities seen in diabetes. Enhanced glycation of lipoproteins has direct effects on lipoprotein metabolism as glycated lipoproteins are handled differently by lipoprotein receptors, particularly of the scavenger group, thus promoting atherogenesis [29]. Enhanced glycation also amplifies the effects of oxidative stress on lipoproteins and therefore affects both T1DM and T2DM [30]. The term diabetic dyslipidemia refers to the lipid abnormalities typically seen in persons with T2DM and is synonymous with atherogenic dyslipidemia [31,32]. It is characterized by elevated triglyceride-rich remnant lipoproteins (routinely measured as hypertriglyceridemia), small dense LDL particles and low HDL cholesterol concentrations. Several factors are likely to be responsible for diabetic dyslipidemia: insulin effects on liver apolipoprotein production, downregulation of lipoprotein lipase (LPL) as opposed to hepatic lipase, increased cholesteryl ester transfer protein (CETP) activity, and peripheral actions of insulin on adipose and muscle.

Low density lipoprotein cholesterol

LDL cholesterol is identified as the primary target of lipid-lowering therapy. Analysis of the UKPDS showed that LDL cholesterol was the strongest risk factor for CHD in this population and HDL cholesterol was the second strongest [33]. Even relatively modern studies discouraged recruitment or restricted entry to patients with hypercholesterolemia and reasonable glycemic control (HbA_{1c} <8% [64 mmol/mol]) as in the Scandinavian Simvastatin Survival Study (4S) [34]. Only recently have studies been performed recruiting large groups of people with T2DM. The 4S trial included only 202 people with diabetes out of 4444 participants. In this small group of subjects, simvastatin therapy was associated with a 55% reduction in major CHD (fatal and non-fatal CHD) ($P = 0.002$) compared with a 32% reduction in major CHD in subjects without diabetes [35]. It was concluded that the absolute benefit of cholesterol lowering in patients with diabetes may be greater than that in patients without diabetes because the patients with diabetes have a higher absolute risk of atherosclerotic events and CHD. This notion was later confirmed in several other studies that also recruited people with diabetes as a subgroup [36].

A number of studies have been specifically performed with statins in diabetes. Most notable of these were the Collaborative Atorvastatin Diabetes Study (CARDS) [37] and the Heart Protection Study (HPS) [38] where subjects were randomized in a double-blind placebo-controlled fashion to 10 mg/day atorvastatin in CARDS and to 40 mg/day simvastatin in the HPS. This produced, respectively, a 40% and 33% reduction in LDL cholesterol associated with a 37% and 31% reduction in combined cardiovascular endpoints. The HPS is the largest statin study to date and included a subgroup of 5963 patients with diabetes (29% of the total study group) [39]. The CARDS trial only included people with diabetes and more than one additional risk factor (e.g. uncontrolled hypertension and/or microalbuminuria) but without prior overt CVD. The study was terminated 2 years prematurely having shown unexpected early benefit. By contrast, the Atorvastatin Study for Prevention of Coronary Heart Disease Endpoints in Non-Insulin-Dependent Diabetes Mellitus (ASPEN) study of similar design to CARDS and also using atorvastatin showed a non-significant 15% reduction in events [40]. In end-stage diabetes with renal failure, aggressive LDL cholesterol reduction reduced events by a non-significant 8% despite a 41% reduction in LDL cholesterol [41]. Thus, the benefits of statin therapy seem to occur early in disease in diabetes.

Overall, the accumulated evidence therefore supports the efficacy of statin therapy in reducing cardiovascular risk in patients with diabetes. A meta-analysis, which evaluated the efficacy of cholesterol-lowering therapy in 18 686 people with diabetes in 14 randomized trials of statins, reported a 9% proportional reduction in all-cause mortality and a 21% proportional reduction in major vascular events per 1 mmol/L reduction in LDL cholesterol (Figure 40.13) [42].

There are few data on diabetes and other drugs that reduce LDL cholesterol as people with diabetes were excluded from trials of bile acid sequestrants. The cholesterol absorption inhibitor, ezetimibe, works by reducing the upper intestinal cholesterol

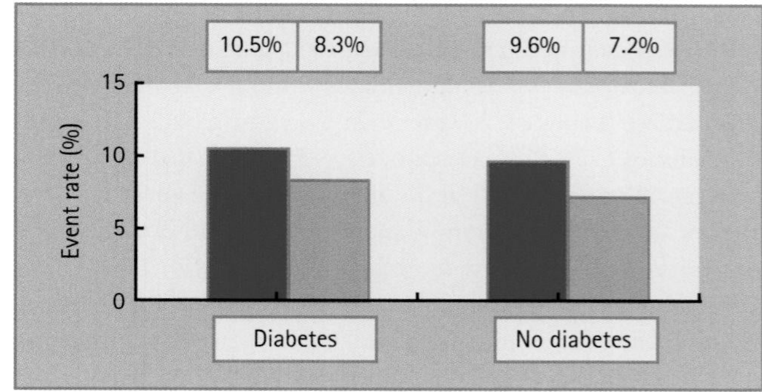

Figure 40.13 Comparison of the effects of reducing low density lipoprotein (LDL) cholesterol on cardiovascular events in patients with and without diabetes. Reproduced from Cholesterol Treatment Triallists Collaborators. *Lancet* 2005; **366**:1267–1278, with permission from Elsevier.

absorption to produce in monotherapy a 20–25% reduction in LDL cholesterol and, in contrast to bile acid sequestrants, it has remarkably little effect on other lipid fractions. People with diabetes were excluded from the Simvasatatin Ezetimibe Aortic Stenosis study [43]. More recently, it has received several potential setbacks with respect to surrogate marker measurements as well as pointers of potential detrimental effects [44]. Two ongoing trials, the Improved Reduction of Outcomes: Vytorian Efficacy International Trial (IMPROVE-IT), in which simvastatin plus ezetimibe is compared with simvastatin plus placebo, and the Study of Heart and Renal Protection (SHARP) trial, in which simvastatin plus ezetimibe is compared with placebo, will hopefully provide answers to these questions.

Low density lipoprotein subfractions

The LDL class comprises a heterogeneous population of particles [45]. LDL is heterogeneous with respect to lipid composition, charge, density, and particle size and shape. The sizes of LDL particles fall between the large triglyceride-enriched very low density lipoprotein (VLDL) particles and the dense and small protein-rich HDL. In addition, these small dense LDL particles may be more atherogenic than would be suspected by their concentration alone, because *in vitro* and cell culture studies suggest they may be more readily oxidized and glycated. Oxidized LDL delivers cholesterol to the atherosclerotic plaque in an unregulated way through uptake by the macrophage and is increased in diabetes [46].

Another aspect is the fatty acid composition of the LDL particle. Linoleic acid is the main polyunsaturated fatty acid in the LDL particle, and this is increased in diabetes. The reason for this may be because of the decreased activity of the insulin sensitive enzyme, 5α-desaturase. There is a strong correlation between linoleic acid in the LDL particle and propensity of the LDL particle to be oxidized. Uncontrolled diabetes results in increased free radical formation which leads to increased oxidation. The fact that the LDL particles are smaller and denser means that they carry relatively less cholesterol per particle. Estimation of the LDL cholesterol may therefore be misleading as there will be more LDL particles for any cholesterol concentration.

Large numbers of studies, including the Quebec Cardiovascular study [47], have confirmed the association of small dense LDL with CVD which reported that men with small dense LDL particles had an increased risk of CAD compared with men with normal-sized LDL particles, independent of LDL cholesterol, triglyceride and the total cholesterol : HDL cholesterol ratio; however, no prospective studies have specifically examined whether altering particle size profiles results in benefits on cardiovascular events although analysis of the Veterans Affairs High Density Lipoprotein Cholesterol Intervention Trial (VA-HIT) study does suggest some role for this mechanism [48].

Even with effective LDL cholesterol treatment, the residual risk of further cardiovascular events remains high, emphasizing the importance of improving other abnormalities and other CVD risk factors commonly observed in these patients.

Triglycerides

The reason for the elevated triglycerides in diabetes is complex, however, because of this derangement, it has been suggested that diabetes should not be called mellitus but rather lipidus [49]. Defects in insulin action and hyperglycemia can lead to changes in plasma lipoproteins in patients with diabetes. Alternatively, especially in the case of T2DM, the obesity and insulin-resistant metabolic disarray that are at the root of this form of diabetes could, themselves, lead to lipid abnormalities exclusive of hyperglycemia [32]. This molecular interplay between lipid and carbohydrate metabolism has led to what might be termed a "lipocentric" view of the pathogenesis of insulin resistance and T2DM [50]. As fatty acids have such a central role in insulin sensitivity, obesity and T2DM, it follows that the major disturbance in lipoprotein metabolism in diabetes is found in the triglyceride-rich lipoproteins, stemming from abnormalities in chylomicron synthesis and clearance [51].

Triglycerides (also referred to as triacylglycerol) are formed from a single molecule of glycerol combines with three fatty acids and represent a heterogeneous group of molecules which most frequently are measured collectively, as a "family" of analytes [52]. Elevated serum triglyceride levels are associated with increased risk for atherosclerotic events [53,54]. As high serum triglyceride levels are associated with abnormal lipoprotein metabolism, as well as with other cardiovascular risk factors including obesity, insulin resistance, diabetes and low levels of HDL cholesterol, it becomes more difficult to distinguish between cause and effect and to establish hypertriglyceridemia as an independent cardiovascular risk factor. Some causes of hypertriglyceridemia have no apparent effect on atherosclerotic vascular disease, making it difficult to prove that elevated triglycerides are a risk factor [55]. Nevertheless, several meta-analyses have found that triglycerides are an independent risk factor for CHD [54,56,57].

The two main sources of plasma triglycerides are exogenous (i.e. from dietary fat) carried in chylomicrons and endogenous (from the liver) and carried in VLDL particles. In capillaries within fat and muscle tissue, these lipoproteins and chylomicrons are hydrolyzed by LPL into free fatty acids. LPL is activated by apolipoprotein C-II, cleaving the triglyceride core and releasing free fatty acids, which can be oxidized by muscle for energy or kept in adipose tissue for future use, and inhibited by the action of apolipoprotein C-III [58]. In routine clinical practice, hypertriglyceridemia is the most frequent lipoprotein abnormality found in uncontrolled diabetes. The mechanisms for these include increased production or absorption, or reduced catabolism (mainly because of decreased activity of LPL). Liver apolipoprotein B production (the major protein component of VLDL and LDL) is increased in T2DM. This is indirectly brought about by increased lipolysis which occurs in adipose tissue, a consequence of insulin resistance and/or insulin deficiency. The increased lipolysis results in increased fatty acid release from fat cells with increase in fatty acid transport to the liver. Studies in tissue cultures, animal experiments [59] and humans [60] suggest that fatty acids modulate liver apolipoprotein B secretion.

Microsomal triglyceride transfer protein (MTP) assembles the chylomicron in the intestine and the VLDL particle in the liver. MTP has been shown to be increased in the intestine of subjects with diabetes [61]. Cholesterol absorption also seems to be adversely influenced in subjects with diabetes. The Niemann–Pick C1-like 1 protein, which has a critical role in the absorption of cholesterol, is increased in people with diabetes. The ATP-binding cassette transporters ABC-G5 and ABC-G8 dimerize to form a functional complex necessary for efflux of dietary cholesterol and non-cholesterol sterols from the intestine and liver. These proteins have been shown to be reduced in diabetes in both liver and intestine. LPL is an insulin-dependent enzyme being responsible for the conversion of lipoprotein triglyceride into free fatty acids. It has several other activities relating to lipid and carbohydrate metabolism [62]. Both patients with T1DM and T2DM have reduced LPL activity which is further suppressed by adipose-derived cytokines such as tumor necrosis factor α (TNF-α) and interleukin 6 (IL-6) [32].

Statins form the mainstay of lipid management based on their efficacy in lowering LDL cholesterol, but their effects on components of the atherogenic dyslipidemia associated with T2DM are more modest, reducing triglycerides at most by 15–30% and raising HDL cholesterol typically by less than 10%. There is no clear consensus on the benefits of directly targeting hypertriglyceridemia [63]. As the interventions usually affect both triglycerides and HDL cholesterol, it also becomes more difficult to distinguish between the individual benefits.

Fibrates

The "fibrate" class of lipid-lowering drugs is useful for lowering elevated triglyceride or non-HDL cholesterol levels as these agents, which act on peroxisomal proliferator-activated receptor α (PPARα), increase lipoprotein lipase activity, reduce apolipoprotein C-III and may increase HDL cholesterol or decrease fibrinogen [64]. Despite this, clinical trials of these drugs have reported mixed results in general, and most early trials recruited only a few patients with diabetes [65,66].

The VA-HIT study evaluated the potential benefits of gemfibrozil in 2531 men with an acute MI. Patients with relatively low LDL cholesterol (<3.6 mmol/L) and low HDL cholesterol (<1.0 mmol/L) were recruited. A significant reduction in the primary endpoint (fatal and non-fatal MI) of 22% was achieved [67]. One-third of participants had T2DM. These outcomes were achieved despite relatively small changes in HDL cholesterol (8%) and no change in LDL cholesterol (0%). An exploration of the effect of gemfibrozil showed that the principal effect of the fibrate treatment was a 31% reduction in triglycerides which reflects changes in particle sizes, but was not related to event reduction [68]. A subgroup analysis of the subjects with diabetes showed a relative risk reduction of 32% compared to 18% in the non-diabetic group [69], however, the enthusiasm for fibrate use has been considerably dampened by results of the Fenofibrate Intervention and Event Lowering in Diabetes (FIELD) study [70]. This trial randomized 9795 subjects with T2DM to fenofibrate (200 mg/day) or placebo who were not on statin treatment at the beginning of the study, and participants in the trial were treated for 5 years. The study reported a non-significant 11% reduction in the primary endpoint of CHD although a significant reduction in total cardiovascular events was achieved with fenofibrate therapy (P = 0.035) (Figure 40.14). The study was confounded by asymmetrical statin drop-in with many more patients on placebo arm being initiated on statin therapy during the trial (17%) than those on the fenofibrate arm (8%) [65]. It is therefore difficult to compare fibrate trials as they seem to give heterogenous results depending on the compound used, and no fibrate trials have shown to reduce all cause mortality. Nevertheless, meta-analayses suggest they may reduce non-fatal MI [71]. It is hoped that the ACCORD trial, which randomized fenofibrate in addition to baseline 20–40 mg simvastatin, can provide more definitive answers.

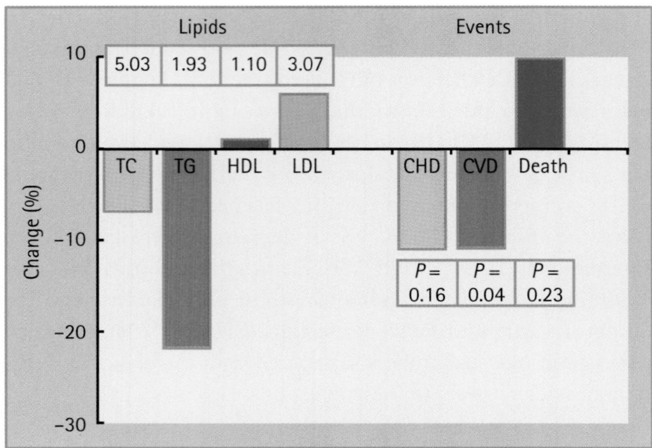

Figure 40.14 Reductions in mortality, coronary heart disease (CHD) and cardiovascular events with fenofibrate therapy in the FIELD study. HDL, high density lipoprotein; LDL, low density lipoprotein; TC, total cholesterol; TG, triglycerides. Reproduced from Keech *et al.* [70], with permission from Elsevier.

Niacin

Nicotinic acid (niacin) is another potential drug to address the combination of hypertriglyceridemia and low HDL cholesterol. Because of its favorable effects on LDL cholesterol, it has been referred to as the "broad-spectrum" lipid drug [72]. Nicotinic acid was the first lipid-lowering agent to show a significant reduction in cardiovascular events, but not in mortality. The Coronary Drug Project randomized 3908 men with previous MI to either nicotinic acid or placebo [73]. Major CHD events, non-fatal MI and cerebrovascular events were reduced, but there was no effect on mortality; however, in the 15-year post-trial follow-up, nearly 9 years after termination of the trial, mortality from all causes was 11% lower in the nicotinic acid group [74]. Several long-term clinical studies with niacin have since demonstrated a reduction in CHD events and mortality when used in combination with other lipid-modifying drugs which include: colestipol (a bile acid sequestrant) [75], fibrate [76] and statins [77]. Unfortunately,

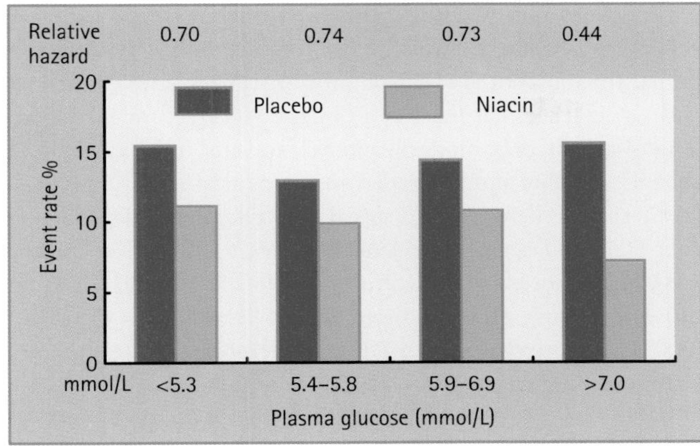

Figure 40.15 Reduction in coronary heart disease in patients with a fasting plasma glucose >7 mmol/L from a post hoc analysis of the Coronary Drug Project. Reproduced from Canner *et al.* [81], with permission from Excerpta Medica.

niacin has been hampered by its side effects, particularly flushing, although strategies exist to reduce this [78], and by hyperglycemia [79]. No long-term outcome trials with niacin in people with diabetes have been conducted. Furthermore, niacin adversely affects glycemic control. This effect is related to the dose of nicotinic acid. The study of the effect of extended release niacin on diabetic dyslipidemia found that, at week 16, whereas the HbA_{1c} did not change significantly in the 1 g group, in the 1.5 g group there was an increase from 7.2% (55 mmol/mol) to 7.5% (58 mmol/mol) [80]. Wider variations are seen in clinical practice [79]. Analysis of data from the Coronary Drug Project showed that regardless of how patients were grouped, niacin appeared as effective in lowering cardiovascular outcomes in patients with hyperglycemia as patients with normoglycemia (Figure 40.15) [81].

Guidelines are conflicting on the use of niacin in diabetes. The current position statement from the American Diabetes Association (ADA) suggests the use of nicotinic acid as an option in treating lipoprotein fractions other then LDL cholesterol [82]. It reports that only modest changes in glucose occur and that these are generally amenable to adjustment of diabetes therapy. A previous statement discouraged its routine use as do the recent National Institute for Health and Clinical Excellence (NICE) guidelines for management of diabetes in England and Wales [83]. Large outcome studies are currently underway. The Atherothrombosis Intervention in Metabolic syndrome with low HDL cholesterol/high triglyceride and Impact on Global Health outcomes (AIM-HIGH) hopes to report in 2011 [84]. The large Oxford-based outcome trial with extended release niacin/laropiprant (an inhibitor of prostaglandin receptor D1 which reduces the flushing), the Heart Protection Study 2-Treatment of HDL to Reduce the Incidence of Vascular Events (HPS2-THRIVE) [85], includes 28 000 patients with cardiovascular disease or at high risk of developing it, including a pre-specified subgroup of 6000 with diabetes, and is scheduled to report in 2013.

Other triglyceride-reducing agents

Hypoglycemic agents may also have an effect on triglyceride concentrations because of the peripheral actions of insulin on adipose and muscle or via their action on LPL. In poorly controlled T1DM and even ketoacidosis, hypertriglyceridemia and reduced HDL cholesterol is seen to occur, and this is most often corrected with insulin therapy. In T2DM, metformin [86], sulfonylureas [87] and acarbose [88] all show modest reductions in triglycerides which correlate with glycemic control [89,90]. In general, thiazolidinediones have better overall effects on lipids than sulfonylureas or insulin [91], but pioglitazone and rosiglitazone have distinctly different effects on the lipid profile [64,92]. Pioglitazone is associated with a reduction in triglycerides whereas rosiglitazone is associated with increased concentrations. Both medications raised LDL cholesterol, but the increase was significantly greater with rosiglitazone than pioglitazone. Pioglitazone did not significantly change apolipoprotein B levels but did reduce LDL particle concentration. Conversely, rosiglitazone increased both apolipoprotein B and LDL particle concentrations. Both medications increased HDL cholesterol, with pioglitazone having no effect on serum apolipoprotein AI levels while rosiglitazone was associated with a decrease in apolipoprotein AI levels. Differential effects on CVD outcomes in recent meta-analyses have recently been reported. Outcome data for rosiglitazone are awaited. In the Rosiglitazone Evaluated for Cardiac Outcomes and Regulation of Glycaemia in Diabetes (RECORD) trial, a prospective trial in patients with T2DM, no evidence for an increased cardiovascular event rate was found [93]. An outcome trial for pioglitazone, the PRO spective pioglitAzone Clinical Trial In macroVascular Events (PROACTIVE) study, which added pioglitazone to the current treatment in patients with T2DM, showed that treatment with pioglitazone was associated with reductions in major atherosclerotic events as defined in the main secondary endpoint [94]. The differential effects on lipid profiles may in part explain the differences these two drugs have on CVD outcomes as reported by recent meta-analyses (Figure 40.16) [95,96].

A number of other existing interventions reduce triglycerides secondary to their action in reducing weight [97]. Orlistat has been shown to prevent progression to diabetes in the XENical in the prevention of diabetes in obese subjects (XENDOS) study [98], and both sibutramine [99] and rimonabant [100,101] (prior to their suspension) showed benefits on lipids in patients with the metabolic syndrome and diabetes. Rimonabant had a non-significant benefit on coronary atherosclerosis as assessed by intravascular ultrasound in line with its lipid effects [102,103].

High density lipoprotein cholesterol

Analogous to LDL, the HDL class also comprises a heterogeneous population of particles. The inverse relationship between HDL cholesterol levels and atherosclerotic CVD provides the epidemiologic basis for the widely accepted hypothesis that HDL is atheroprotective [104,105]. Experimental studies, which include limited work on humans, have shown that HDL has several

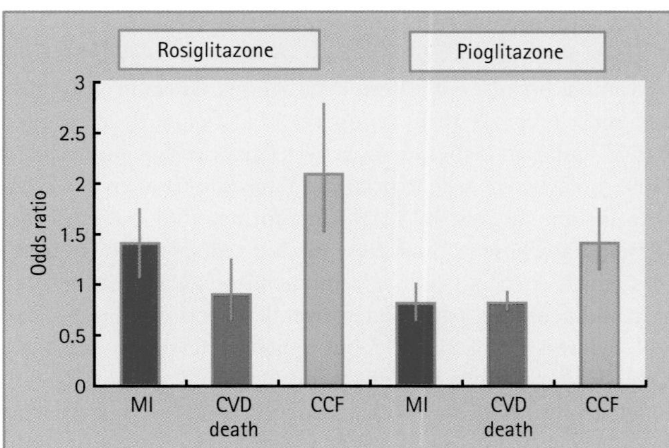

Figure 40.16 Effects of thiazolidinedione drugs on coronary heart disease (CHD) in trials using rosiglitazone and pioglitazone. CCF, congestive cardiac failure; CVD, cardiovascular disease; MI, myocardial infarction. Reproduced from Singh *et al. JAMA* 2007; **298**:1189, with permission from the American Medical Association.

distinct but potentially overlapping atheroprotective functions. These include the well-known reverse cholesterol transport [106] as well as reductions in oxidative stress and innate immune inflammation [107]. More HDL-associated proteins are involved in immune/inflammatory functions than in lipid transport and metabolism, suggesting the fundamental role for HDL in innate immunity [108]. There are several reasons that could account for the decrease in HDL cholesterol in diabetes [32]. CETP-mediated exchange of VLDL triglyceride for HDL cholesteryl esters is accelerated in the presence of hypertriglyceridemia [45]. The clinical laboratory measures the cholesterol component of HDL; substitution of triglyceride for cholesteryl ester in the core of the HDL particle therefore leads to a decrease in this measurement of HDL cholesterol. The triglyceride, but not cholesteryl ester, in HDL is a substrate for plasma lipases, especially hepatic lipase which converts HDL to a smaller particle being more rapidly cleared from the plasma. Precursors of advanced glycation end-products (AGEs) can also impair reverse cholesterol transport by HDL.

As opposed to LDL cholesterol lowering, therapies to intervene in order to raise HDL cholesterol have proven to be "not that simple." Some HDL therapies may reduce CVD without actually changing HDL cholesterol concentrations [109]. The Intravascular Ultrasound Study (IVUS) of the effects of 5 weekly infusions of a hyperfunctional apolipoprotein A-1 (apoA-1)$_{\text{Milano}}$ produced significant regression of coronary atherosclerosis after 3 months. In contrast, in the Investigation of Lipid Level Management to Understand Its Impact in Atherosclerotic Events (ILLUMINATE) trial, which investigated the CETP inhibitor, torcetrapib, in 15 000 patients, HDL cholesterol increased by 72% and LDL cholesterol decreased by 25%, although this trial was terminated early as the treatment arm had an increase of major cardiovascular events by 25% and death from cardiovascular causes by 40%, possibly related to the hypertensive properties of this particular molecule [110].

Guidelines vary when it comes to treatment targets for HDL cholesterol, mostly because there is no evidence base for intervention at the moment [111]. The Joint British Societies Guidelines and NICE argue that there is no treatment target for HDL cholesterol as it is only modestly altered, and not independently of changes in other lipid variables in the clinical trials [5,83,112]. Furthermore, there are no drugs available yet that independently alter HDL cholesterol. The American Heart Association and the ADA suggest lowering triglycerides to below 1.7 mmol/L (150 mg/dL) and raising HDL to more than 1.15 mmol/L (40 mg/dL) [3,82,113]. In women, an HDL cholesterol goal of 0.3 mmol/L (10 mg/dL) higher than this should be considered.

Future drug developments and drug targets

Drugs that target the exogenous and or the endogenous pathways of cholesterol metabolism may prove to be useful in the future [114,115]. These include Niemann–Pick C1-like 1 protein inhibitors, new PPAR agents and MTP inhibitors. Interventions that regulate fatty acid synthesis may also prove to be beneficial. Stearoyl-coenzyme A desaturase 1 catalyzes the synthesis of monounsaturated fatty acids and has emerged as a key regulator of metabolism [116]. Recent studies in human and animal models have highlighted that modulation of stearoyl-coenzyme A desaturase 1 activity by dietary intervention or genetic manipulation strongly influences several facets of energy metabolism to affect susceptibility to obesity, insulin resistance, diabetes and hyperlipidemia. HDL mimetic therapies may also prove to be beneficial. Other CETP inhibitors are also still under investigation [117]. Although numerous drug classes have been devised, many, such as torcetrapib, have recently failed in late phase III trials even after showing good initial results on lipids in human and in animal models. Other drugs, such as rimonabant, have shown unfavorable side effect profiles which led to the suspension of marketing in the European Union. Given the importance of atherosclerosis as a cause of morbidity and mortality in diabetes, numerous therapeutic approaches are in development, and all will require systematic evaluation through endpoint clinical trials to validate their effects in animal models or on surrogate markers [103].

Conclusions

CVD is a very common complication of diabetes. Up to 80% of all people with diabetes will die from macrovascular complications. Lifestyle intervention is both effective and paramount to prevent and treat diabetes and its dyslipidemia. Statins have revolutionized preventive cardiovascular medicine and this has formed the foundation of therapeutic lipid intervention (Figure 40.17). The abnormalities in lipids and lipoproteins represent only one factor among several that are responsible for the increased risk in persons with diabetes (Table 40.5) and therefore multifactorial intervention is required, and this reduces events and mortality by 50% (Figure 40.18) [118,119].

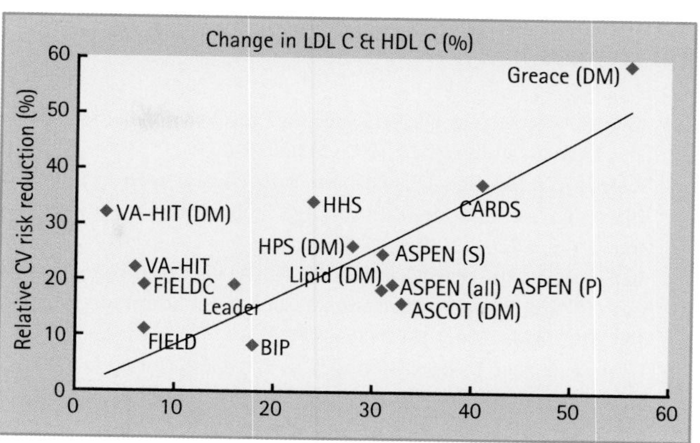

Figure 40.17 Comparative effects of different lipid lowering drugs on cardiovascular disease (CVD) in patients with diabetes. ASPEN, Atorvastatin Study for the Prevention of Coronary Heart Disease Endpoints in Non-Insulin-Dependent Diabetes Mellitus; BIP, Bezafibrate Infarct Prevention; CARDS, Collaborative Atorvastatin Diabetes Study; FIELD, Fenofibrate Intervention and Event Lowering in Diabetes; FIELDc, FIELD study (corrected data); GREACE; Greek Evaluation of Atorvastatin in Coronary Events; HHS, Helsinki Heart Study; HPS, Heart Protection Study; LEADER, Lower Extremity Arterial Disease Event Reduction; LIPID, Lipid Intervention with Pravastatin in Ischaemic Disease; VA-HIT, Veterans Affairs High Density Lipoprotein Cholesterol Intervention Trial; DM, diabetes sub-group; P, primary prevention subgroup; S, secondary prevention subgroup; HDL C, high density lipoprotein cholesterol; LDL C, low density lipoprotein cholesterol. Reproduced from Wierzbicki AS. *Diab Vasc Dis Res* 2006; **3**:166–171, with permission from Medinews.

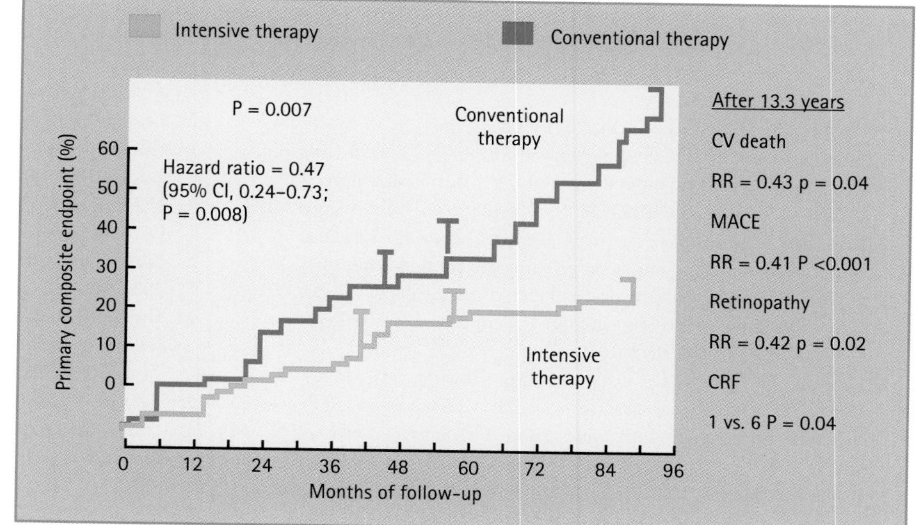

Figure 40.18 Effects of improved multiple risk factor intervention on mortality and cardiovascular events in diabetes. CABG, coronary artery bypass graft; CV, cardiovascular; MI, myocardial infarction; PAD, peripheral arterial disease; PC, percutaneous coronary intervention. Data from Gaede *et al. N Engl J Med* 2003; **348**:383–393 and Gaede *et al. N Engl J Med* 2008; **358**:580–591.

Table 40.5 Effects of different cardiovascular therapies on lipids and other cardiovascular risk factors and endpoint trial evidence of effects in prevention of diabetes and cardiovascular disease.

Drug/treatment group	Component of the cardiometabolic syndrome Change (%)					DM risk reduction (%)	CVD risk reduction (%)
	LDL decrease	HDL increase	TG decrease	SBP decrease	Glucose decrease		
Metformin	0–10	15	15	0–5	10	45–48	35
SU	0–5	0	0	3	0	?	20
TZD	–5 to 10	9	12	5	8	51–58	–10 to +43
Statin	20–55	0–15	15–25	0	0	0–14	20–55
Fibrate	0–10	2–16	15–24	0–8	0–6	0–23	10–34
Niacin	10–20	10–25	15–35	0	(+5)	?	22–31
Orlistat	0–5	+3	1	1	4	43	?
Sibutramine	0–5	+9	25	+4	4	?	?

CVD, cardiovascular disease; DM, diabetes mellitus; HDL, high density lipoprotein; LDL, low density lipoprotein; SBP, systolic blood pressure; SU, sulfonylurea; TG, triglycerides; TZD, thiazolidinedione.

References

1 Kannel WB, McGee DL. Diabetes and cardiovascular disease: the Framingham study. *JAMA* 1979; **241**:2035–2038.

2 Kannel WB, McGee DL. Diabetes and glucose tolerance as risk factors for cardiovascular disease: the Framingham study. *Diabetes Care* 1979; **2**:120–126.

3 Expert Panel on Detection EAToHBCIAATPI. Executive Summary of the Third Report of the National Cholesterol Education Program (NCEP). *JAMA* 2001; **285**:2486–2497.

4 Graham I, Atar D, Borch-Johnsen K, Boysen G, Burell G, Cifkova R, *et al.* Fourth Joint Task Force of the European Society of Cardiology and other societies on cardiovascular disease prevention in clinical practice (constituted by representatives of nine societies and by invited experts). *Eur J Cardiovasc Prev Rehabil* 2007; **14**(Suppl 2):S1–113.

5 British Cardiac Society, British Hypertension Society, Diabetes UK, *et al.* JBS 2: the Joint British Societies' guidelines for prevention of cardiovascular disease in clinical practice. *Heart* 2005; **91**(Suppl 5):1–52.

6 Haffner SM, Lehto S, Ronnemaa T, Pyörälä K, Laakso M. Mortality from coronary heart disease in subjects with type 2 diabetes and in nondiabetic subjects with and without prior myocardial infarction. *N Engl J Med* 1998; **339**:229–234.

7 Malmberg K, Yusuf S, Gerstein HC, Brown J, Zhao F, Hunt D, *et al.* Impact of diabetes on long-term prognosis in patients with unstable angina and non-Q-wave myocardial infarction: results of the OASIS (Organization to Assess Strategies for Ischemic Syndromes) Registry. *Circulation* 2000; **102**:1014–1019.

8 Howard BV, Best LG, Galloway JM, Howard WJ, Jones K, Lee ET, *et al.* Coronary heart disease risk equivalence in diabetes depends on concomitant risk factors. *Diabetes Care* 2006; **29**:391–397.

9 Evans JM, Wang J, Morris AD. Comparison of cardiovascular risk between patients with type 2 diabetes and those who had had a myocardial infarction: cross sectional and cohort studies. *Br Med J* 2002; **324**:939–942.

10 Simons LA, Simons J. Diabetes and coronary heart disease. *N Engl J Med* 1998; **339**:1714–1715.

11 Krolewski AS, Kosinski EJ, Warram JH, Leland OS, Busick EJ, Asmal AC, *et al.* Magnitude and determinants of coronary artery disease in juvenile-onset, insulin-dependent diabetes mellitus. *Am J Cardiol* 1987; **59**:750–755.

12 Jensen T, Borch-Johnsen K, Kofoed-Enevoldsen A, Deckert T. Coronary heart disease in young type 1 (insulin-dependent) diabetic patients with and without diabetic nephropathy: incidence and risk factors. *Diabetologia* 1987; **30**:144–148.

13 Soedamah-Muthu SS, Fuller JH, Mulnier HE, Raleigh VS, Lawrenson RA, Colhoun HM. All-cause mortality rates in patients with type 1 diabetes mellitus compared with a non-diabetic population from the UK general practice research database, 1992–1999. *Diabetologia* 2006; **49**:660–606.

14 Mogensen CE. Microalbuminuria predicts clinical proteinuria and early mortality in maturity-onset diabetes. *N Engl J Med* 1984; **310**:356–360.

15 Kannel WB. Lipids, diabetes, and coronary heart disease: insights from the Framingham Study. *Am Heart J* 1985; **110**:1100–1107.

16 Stevens RJ, Kothari V, Adler AI, Stratton IM. The UKPDS risk engine: a model for the risk of coronary heart disease in type II diabetes (UKPDS 56). *Clin Sci (Lond)* 2001; **101**:671–679.

17 Coleman RL, Stevens RJ, Retnakaran R, Holman RR. Framingham, SCORE, and DECODE risk equations do not provide reliable cardiovascular risk estimates in type 2 diabetes. *Diabetes Care* 2007; **30**:1292–1293.

18 Viljoen A. Cardiovascular risk estimation: making sense of the numbers. *Int J Clin Pract* 2008; **62**:1300–1303.

19 Reynolds TM, Twomey PJ, Wierzbicki AS. Concordance evaluation of coronary risk scores: implications for cardiovascular risk screening. *Curr Med Res Opin* 2004; **20**:811–818.

20 DECODE Study Group. Is fasting glucose sufficient to define diabetes? Epidemiological data from 20 European studies. European Diabetes Epidemiology Group. Diabetes epidemiology: collaborative analysis of diagnostic criteria in Europe. *Diabetologia* 1999; **42**:647–654.

21 Meigs JB, Nathan DM, Wilson PW, Cupples LA, Singer DE. Metabolic risk factors worsen continuously across the spectrum of nondiabetic glucose tolerance. The Framingham Offspring Study. *Ann Intern Med* 1998; **128**:524–533.

22 Levitan EB, Song Y, Ford ES, Liu S. Is nondiabetic hyperglycemia a risk factor for cardiovascular disease? A meta-analysis of prospective studies. *Arch Intern Med* 2004; **164**:2147–2155.

23 Nathan DM, Cleary PA, Backlund JY, Genuth SM, Lachin JM, Orchard TJ, *et al.* Intensive diabetes treatment and cardiovascular disease in patients with type 1 diabetes. *N Engl J Med* 2005; **353**:2643–2653.

24 Holman RR, Paul SK, Bethel MA, Matthews DR, Neil HA. 10-year follow-up of intensive glucose control in type 2 diabetes. *N Engl J Med* 2008; **359**:1577–1589.

25 Patel A, MacMahon S, Chalmers J, Neal B, Billot L, Woodward M, *et al.* Intensive blood glucose control and vascular outcomes in patients with type 2 diabetes. *N Engl J Med* 2008; **358**:2560–2572.

26 Gerstein HC, Miller ME, Byington RP, Goff DC Jr, Bigger JT, Buse JB, *et al.* Effects of intensive glucose lowering in type 2 diabetes. *N Engl J Med* 2008; **358**:2545–2559.

27 Dluhy RG, McMahon GT. Intensive glycemic control in the ACCORD and ADVANCE trials. *N Engl J Med* 2008; **358**:2630–2633.

28 Cefalu WT. Glycemic targets and cardiovascular disease. *N Engl J Med* 2008; **358**:2633–2635.

29 Beauchamp MC, Michaud SE, Li L, Sartippour MR, Renier G. Advanced glycation end products potentiate the stimulatory effect of glucose on macrophage lipoprotein lipase expression. *J Lipid Res* 2004; **45**:1749–1757.

30 Lyons TJ, Jenkins AJ. Lipoprotein glycation and its metabolic consequences. *Curr Opin Lipidol* 1997; **8**:174–180.

31 Durrington PN. Diabetic dyslipidaemia. *Baillieres Best Pract Res Clin Endocrinol Metab* 1999; **13**:265–278.

32 Goldberg IJ. Diabetic dyslipidemia: causes and consequences. Clinical review 124. *J Clin Endocrinol Metab* 2001; **86**:965–971.

33 Turner RC, Millns H, Neil HA, *et al.* Risk factors for coronary artery disease in non-insulin dependent diabetes mellitus: United Kingdom Prospective Diabetes Study (UKPDS: 23). *Br Med J* 1998; **316**:823–828.

34 Scandinavian Simvastatin Survival Study (4S) Investigators. Randomised trial of cholesterol lowering in 4444 patients with coro-

nary heart disease: the Scandinavian Simvastatin Survival Study (4S). *Lancet* 1994; **344**:1383–1389.

35 Pyorala K, Pedersen TR, Kjekshus J, Faergeman O, Olsson AG, Thorgeirsson G. Cholesterol lowering with simvastatin improves prognosis of diabetic patients with coronary heart disease: a subgroup analysis of the Scandinavian Simvastatin Survival Study (4S). *Diabetes Care* 1997; **20**:614–620.

36 Sacks FM, Tonkin AM, Shepherd J, Braunwald E, Cobbe S, Hawkins CM, *et al.* Effect of pravastatin on coronary disease events in subgroups defined by coronary risk factors: the Prospective Pravastatin Pooling Project. *Circulation* 2000; **102**:1893–1900.

37 Colhoun HM, Betteridge DJ, Durrington PN, Hitman GA, Neil HA, Livingstone SJ, *et al.* Primary prevention of cardiovascular disease with atorvastatin in type 2 diabetes in the Collaborative Atorvastatin Diabetes Study (CARDS): multicentre randomised placebo-controlled trial. *Lancet* 2004; **364**:685–696.

38 MRC/BHF Heart Protection Study Investigators. MRC/BHF Heart Protection Study of cholesterol lowering with simvastatin in 20,536 high-risk individuals: a randomised placebo-controlled trial. *Lancet* 2002; **360**:7–22.

39 Collins R, Armitage J, Parish S, Sleigh P, Peto R; Heart Protection Study Collaborative Group. MRC/BHF Heart Protection Study of cholesterol-lowering with simvastatin in 5963 people with diabetes: a randomised placebo-controlled trial. *Lancet* 2003; **361**:2005–2016.

40 Knopp RH, d'Emden M, Smilde JG, Pocock SJ. Efficacy and safety of atorvastatin in the prevention of cardiovascular end points in subjects with type 2 diabetes: the Atorvastatin Study for Prevention of Coronary Heart Disease Endpoints in Non-Insulin-Dependent Diabetes Mellitus (ASPEN). *Diabetes Care* 2006; **29**:1478–1485.

41 Wanner C, Krane V, Marz W, Olschewski M, Mann JF, Ruf G, *et al.* Atorvastatin in patients with type 2 diabetes mellitus undergoing hemodialysis. *N Engl J Med* 2005; **353**:238–248.

42 Kearney PM, Blackwell L, Collins R, Keech A, Simes J, Peto R, *et al.* Efficacy of cholesterol-lowering therapy in 18,686 people with diabetes in 14 randomised trials of statins: a meta-analysis. *Lancet* 2008; **371**:117–125.

43 Rossebo AB, Pedersen TR, Boman K, Brudi P, Chambers JB, Egstrup K, *et al.* Intensive lipid lowering with simvastatin and ezetimibe in aortic stenosis. *N Engl J Med* 2008; **359**:1343–1356.

44 Wierzbicki AS. Muddy waters: more stormy SEAS for ezetimibe. *Int J Clin Pract* 2008; **62**:1470–1473.

45 Austin MA. Triglyceride, small, dense low-density lipoprotein, and the atherogenic lipoprotein phenotype. *Curr Atheroscler Rep* 2000; **2**:200–207.

46 Scheffer PG, Teerlink T, Heine RJ. Clinical significance of the physicochemical properties of LDL in type 2 diabetes. *Diabetologia* 2005; **48**:808–816.

47 St-Pierre AC, Cantin B, Dagenais GR, St-Pierre AC, Cantin B, Dagenais GR, *et al.* Low-density lipoprotein subfractions and the long-term risk of ischemic heart disease in men: 13-year follow-up data from the Quebec Cardiovascular Study. *Arterioscler Thromb Vasc Biol* 2005; **25**:553–559.

48 Otvos JD, Collins D, Freedman DS, Shalauvova I, Schaefer EJ, McNamara JR, *et al.* Low-density lipoprotein and high-density lipoprotein particle subclasses predict coronary events and are favorably changed by gemfibrozil therapy in the Veterans Affairs High-Density Lipoprotein Intervention Trial. *Circulation* 2006; **113**:1556–1563.

49 Shafrir E, Raz I. Diabetes: mellitus or lipidus? *Diabetologia* 2003; **46**:433–440.

50 Savage DB, Petersen KF, Shulman GI. Disordered lipid metabolism and the pathogenesis of insulin resistance. *Physiol Rev* 2007; **87**:507–520.

51 Kahn SE, Hull RL, Utzschneider KM. Mechanisms linking obesity to insulin resistance and type 2 diabetes. *Nature* 2006; **444**:840–846.

52 Thienpont LM, Van UK, De Leenheer AP. Reference measurement systems in clinical chemistry. *Clin Chim Acta* 2002; **323**:73–87.

53 McBride P. Triglycerides and risk for coronary artery disease. *Curr Atheroscler Rep* 2008; **10**:386–390.

54 Sarwar N, Danesh J, Eiriksdottir G, Sigurdsson G, Wareham N, Bingham S, *et al.* Triglycerides and the risk of coronary heart disease: 10,158 incident cases among 262,525 participants in 29 Western prospective studies. *Circulation* 2007; **115**:450–458.

55 Austin MA, McKnight B, Edwards KL, Bradley CM, McNeely MJ, Psaty BM, *et al.* Cardiovascular disease mortality in familial forms of hypertriglyceridemia: a 20-year prospective study. *Circulation* 2000; **101**:2777–2782.

56 Austin MA, Hokanson JE, Edwards KL. Hypertriglyceridemia as a cardiovascular risk factor. *Am J Cardiol* 1998; **81**:7B–12B.

57 Assmann G, Schulte H, von EA. Hypertriglyceridemia and elevated lipoprotein(a) are risk factors for major coronary events in middle-aged men. *Am J Cardiol* 1996; **77**:1179–1184.

58 Grundy SM. Hypertriglyceridemia, atherogenic dyslipidemia, and the metabolic syndrome. *Am J Cardiol* 1998; **81**:18B–25B.

59 Taghibiglou C, Carpentier A, Van Iderstine SC, Chen B, Rudy D, Aiton A, *et al.* Mechanisms of hepatic very low density lipoprotein overproduction in insulin resistance: evidence for enhanced lipoprotein assembly, reduced intracellular ApoB degradation, and increased microsomal triglyceride transfer protein in a fructose-fed hamster model. *J Biol Chem* 2000; **275**:8416–8425.

60 Lewis GF, Uffelman KD, Szeto LW, Weller B, Steiner G. Interaction between free fatty acids and insulin in the acute control of very low density lipoprotein production in humans. *J Clin Invest* 1995; **95**:158–166.

61 Lally S, Tan CY, Owens D, Tomkin GH. Messenger RNA levels of genes involved in dysregulation of postprandial lipoproteins in type 2 diabetes: the role of Niemann–Pick C1-like 1, ATP-binding cassette, transporters G5 and G8, and of microsomal triglyceride transfer protein. *Diabetologia* 2006; **49**:1008–1016.

62 Mead JR, Irvine SA, Ramji DP. Lipoprotein lipase: structure, function, regulation, and role in disease. *J Mol Med* 2002; **80**:753–769.

63 Garg A, Simha V. Update on dyslipidemia. *J Clin Endocrinol Metab* 2007; **92**:1581–1589.

64 Rubenstrunk A, Hanf R, Hum DW, Fruchart JC, Staels B. Safety issues and prospects for future generations of PPAR modulators. *Biochim Biophys Acta* 2007; **1771**:1065–1081.

65 Wierzbicki AS. FIELDS of dreams, fields of tears: a perspective on the fibrate trials. *Int J Clin Pract* 2006; **60**:442–429.

66 Wierzbicki AS. Interpreting clinical trials of diabetic dyslipidaemia: new insights. *Diabetes Obes Metab* 2007; **11**:261–270.

67 Rubins HB, Robins SJ, Collins D, Fye CL, Anderson JW, Elam MB, *et al.* Gemfibrozil for the secondary prevention of coronary heart disease in men with low levels of high-density lipoprotein cholesterol. Veterans Affairs High-Density Lipoprotein Cholesterol Intervention Trial Study Group. *N Engl J Med* 1999; **341**:410–418.

68 Robins SJ, Collins D, Wittes JT, Papademetriou V, Deedwania PC, Schaefer EJ, *et al.* Relation of gemfibrozil treatment and lipid levels with major coronary events: VA-HIT: a randomized controlled trial. *JAMA* 2001; **285**:1585–1591.

69 Robins SJ, Rubins HB, Faas FH, Schaefer EJ, Elam MB, Anderson JW, *et al.* Insulin resistance and cardiovascular events with low HDL cholesterol: the Veterans Affairs HDL Intervention Trial (VA-HIT). *Diabetes Care* 2003; **26**:1513–1517.

70 Keech A, Simes RJ, Barter P, Best J, Scott R, Taskinen MR, *et al.* Effects of long-term fenofibrate therapy on cardiovascular events in 9795 people with type 2 diabetes mellitus (the FIELD study): randomised controlled trial. *Lancet* 2005; **366**:1849–1861.

71 Saha SA, Kizhakepunnur LG, Bahekar A, Arora RR. The role of fibrates in the prevention of cardiovascular disease: a pooled meta-analysis of long-term randomized placebo-controlled clinical trials. *Am Heart J* 2007; **154**:943–953.

72 Carlson LA. Nicotinic acid: the broad-spectrum lipid drug – a 50th anniversary review. *J Intern Med* 2005; **258**:94–114.

73 Coronary Drug Project Research Group. Clofibrate and niacin in coronary heart disease. *JAMA* 1975; **231**:360–381.

74 Canner PL, Berge KG, Wenger NK, Stamler J, Friedman L, Prineas RJ, *et al.* Fifteen year mortality in Coronary Drug Project patients: long-term benefit with niacin. *J Am Coll Cardiol* 1986; **8**:1245–1255.

75 Blankenhorn DH, Nessim SA, Johnson RL, Sanmarco ME, Azen SP, Cashin-Hemphill L. Beneficial effects of combined colestipol–niacin therapy on coronary atherosclerosis and coronary venous bypass grafts. *JAMA* 1987; **257**:3233–3240.

76 Carlson LA, Rosenhamer G. Reduction of mortality in the Stockholm Ischaemic Heart Disease Secondary Prevention Study by combined treatment with clofibrate and nicotinic acid. *Acta Med Scand* 1988; **223**:405–418.

77 Brown BG, Zhao XQ, Chait A, Fisher LD, Cheung MC, Morse JS, *et al.* Simvastatin and niacin, antioxidant vitamins, or the combination for the prevention of coronary disease. *N Engl J Med* 2001; **345**:1583–1592.

78 Oberwittler H, Baccara-Dinet M. Clinical evidence for use of acetyl salicylic acid in control of flushing related to nicotinic acid treatment. *Int J Clin Pract* 2006; **60**:707–715.

79 Vogt A, Kassner U, Hostalek U, Steinhagen-Thiessen E. Evaluation of the safety and tolerability of prolonged-release nicotinic acid in a usual care setting: the NAUTILUS study. *Curr Med Res Opin* 2006; **22**:417–425.

80 Grundy SM, Vega GL, McGovern ME, Tulloch BR, Kendall DM, Fitz-Patrick D, *et al.* Efficacy, safety, and tolerability of once-daily niacin for the treatment of dyslipidemia associated with type 2 diabetes: results of the assessment of diabetes control and evaluation of the efficacy of niaspan trial. *Arch Intern Med* 2002; **162**:1568–1576.

81 Canner PL, Furberg CD, Terrin ML, McGovern ME. Benefits of niacin by glycemic status in patients with healed myocardial infarction (from the Coronary Drug Project). *Am J Cardiol* 2005; **95**:254–257.

82 Standards of medical care in diabetes, 2008. *Diabetes Care* 2008; **31**(Suppl 1):S12–S54.

83 National Institute for Health and Clinical Excellence (NICE). *Type 2 Diabetes: The Management of Type 2 Diabetes (update).* London: National Institute for Health and Clinical Excellence; 2008 Dec 5. Report No.: CG66.

84 National Heart LaBIN. Niacin plus statin to prevent vascular events: AIM-HIGH. ClinicalTrials gov, 2006. Available at: http://www.clinicaltrials.gov/ct/show/NCT00120289. Accessed July 18, 2006.

85 A randomized trial of the long-term clinical effects of raising HDL cholesterol with extended release niacin/laropiprant. Clinical Trials Gov, 2007. Available at: http://clinicaltrials.gov/ct2/show/NCT00461630. Accessed January 26, 2009.

86 Saenz A, Fernandez-Esteban I, Mataix A, Ausejo Segura M, Roqué i Figuls M, Moher D. Metformin monotherapy for type 2 diabetes mellitus. *Cochrane Database Syst Rev* 2005; **3**:CD002966.

87 Howard BV, Xiaoren P, Harper I, Foley JE, Cheung MC, Taskinen MR. Effect of sulfonylurea therapy on plasma lipids and high-density lipoprotein composition in non-insulin-dependent diabetes mellitus. *Am J Med* 1985; **79**:78–85.

88 Van de Laar FA, Lucassen PL, Akkermans RP, van de Lisdonk EH, Rutten GE, van Weel C. Alpha-glucosidase inhibitors for patients with type 2 diabetes: results from a Cochrane systematic review and meta-analysis. *Diabetes Care* 2005; **28**:154–163.

89 Bolen S, Feldman L, Vassy J, Wilson L, Yeh HC, Marinopoulos S, *et al.* Systematic review: comparative effectiveness and safety of oral medications for type 2 diabetes mellitus. *Ann Intern Med* 2007; **147**:386–399.

90 Huupponen RK, Viikari JS, Saarimaa H. Correlation of serum lipids with diabetes control in sulfonylurea-treated diabetic patients. *Diabetes Care* 1984; **7**:575–578.

91 Yki-Jarvinen H. Thiazolidinediones. *N Engl J Med* 2004; **351**:1106–1118.

92 Deeg MA, Tan MH. Pioglitazone versus rosiglitazone: effects on lipids, lipoproteins, and apolipoproteins in head-to-head randomized clinical studies. *PPAR Res* 2008; **2008**:520465.

93 Home PD, Pocock SJ, Beck-Nielsen H, Curtis PS, Gomis R, Hanefeld M, Jones NP, Komajda M, McMurray JJ; RECORD Study Team. Rosiglitazone evaluated for cardiovascular outcomes in oral agent combination therapy for type 2 diabetes (RECORD): a multicentre, randomised, open-label trial. *Lancet* 2009; **373**:2125–2135.

94 Dormandy JA, Charbonnel B, Eckland DJ, Erdmann E, Massi-Benedetti M, Moules IK, *et al.* Secondary prevention of macrovascular events in patients with type 2 diabetes in the PROactive Study (PROspective pioglitAzone Clinical Trial In macroVascular Events): a randomised controlled trial. *Lancet* 2005; **366**:1279–1289.

95 Nissen SE, Wolski K. Effect of rosiglitazone on the risk of myocardial infarction and death from cardiovascular causes. *N Engl J Med* 2007; **356**:2457–2471.

96 Lincoff AM, Wolski K, Nicholls SJ, Nissen SE. Pioglitazone and risk of cardiovascular events in patients with type 2 diabetes mellitus: a meta-analysis of randomized trials. *JAMA* 2007; **298**:1180–1188.

97 Wierzbicki AS. Low HDL-cholesterol: common and under-treated, but which drug to use? *Int J Clin Pract* 2006; **60**:1149–1153.

98 Torgerson JS, Hauptman J, Boldrin MN, Sjostrom L. XENical in the prevention of diabetes in obese subjects (XENDOS) study: a randomized study of orlistat as an adjunct to lifestyle changes for the prevention of type 2 diabetes in obese patients. *Diabetes Care* 2004; **27**:155–161.

99 Fujioka K, Seaton TB, Rowe E, Jelinek CA, Raskin P, Lebovitz HE, *et al.* Weight loss with sibutramine improves glycaemic control and other metabolic parameters in obese patients with type 2 diabetes mellitus. *Diabetes Obes Metab* 2000; **2**:175–187.

100 Scheen AJ, Finer N, Hollander P, Jensen MD, Van Gaal LF, RIO-Diabetes Study Group. Efficacy and tolerability of rimonabant in

overweight or obese patients with type 2 diabetes: a randomised controlled study. *Lancet* 2006; **368**:1660–1672.

101 Rosenstock J, Hollander P, Chevalier S, Iranmanesh A. SERENADE: the Study Evaluating Rimonabant Efficacy in Drug-naive Diabetic Patients: effects of monotherapy with rimonabant, the first selective CB1 receptor antagonist, on glycemic control, body weight, and lipid profile in drug-naive type 2 diabetes. *Diabetes Care* 2008; **31**:2169–2176.

102 Nissen SE, Nicholls SJ, Wolski K, Rodés-Cabau J, Cannon CP, Deanfield JE, *et al.* Effect of rimonabant on progression of atherosclerosis in patients with abdominal obesity and coronary artery disease: the STRADIVARIUS randomized controlled trial. *JAMA* 2008; **299**:1547–1560.

103 Wierzbicki AS. Surrogate markers, atherosclerosis and cardiovascular disease prevention. *Int J Clin Pract* 2008; **62**:981–987.

104 Abbott RD, Wilson PW, Kannel WB, Castelli WP. High density lipoprotein cholesterol, total cholesterol screening, and myocardial infarction: the Framingham Study. *Arteriosclerosis* 1988; **8**: 207–211.

105 Boden WE. High-density lipoprotein cholesterol as an independent risk factor in cardiovascular disease: assessing the data from Framingham to the Veterans Affairs High-Density Lipoprotein Intervention Trial. *Am J Cardiol* 2000; **86**:19L–22L.

106 Cuchel M, Rader DJ. Macrophage reverse cholesterol transport: key to the regression of atherosclerosis? *Circulation* 2006; **113**:2548–2555.

107 Barter P. Effects of inflammation on high-density lipoproteins. *Arterioscler Thromb Vasc Biol* 2002; **22**:1062–1063.

108 Vaisar T, Pennathur S, Green PS, Gharib SA, Hoofnagle AN, Cheung MC, *et al.* Shotgun proteomics implicates protease inhibition and complement activation in the antiinflammatory properties of HDL. *J Clin Invest* 2007; **117**:746–756.

109 Nissen SE, Tsunoda T, Tuzcu EM, Schoenhagen P, Cooper CJ, Yasin M, *et al.* Effect of recombinant ApoA-I Milano on coronary atherosclerosis in patients with acute coronary syndromes: a randomized controlled trial. *JAMA* 2003; **290**:2292–2300.

110 Barter PJ, Caulfield M, Eriksson M, Grundy SM, Kastelein JJ, Komajda M, *et al.* Effects of torcetrapib in patients at high risk for coronary events. *N Engl J Med* 2007; **357**:2109–2122.

111 Sacks FM. The role of high-density lipoprotein (HDL) cholesterol in the prevention and treatment of coronary heart disease: expert group recommendations. *Am J Cardiol* 2002; **90**:139–143.

112 National Institute for Health and Clinical Excellence (NICE). *Lipid Modification.* London, UK: NICE, June 17, 2008. Report no. CG67.

113 Grundy SM, Cleeman JI, Merz CN, Brewer HB Jr, Clark LT, Hunninghake DB, *et al.* Implications of recent clinical trials for the National Cholesterol Education Program Adult Treatment Panel III guidelines. *Circulation* 2004; **110**:227–239.

114 Wierzbicki AS. Lipid-altering agents: the future. *Int J Clin Pract* 2004; **58**:1063–1072.

115 Viljoen A. New approaches in the diagnosis of atherosclerosis and treatment of cardiovascular disease. *Recent Pat Cardiovasc Drug Discov* 2008; **3**:84–91.

116 Flowers MT, Ntambi JM. Role of stearoyl-coenzyme A desaturase in regulating lipid metabolism. *Curr Opin Lipidol* 2008; **19**:248–256.

117 Krishna R, Anderson MS, Bergman AJ, Jin B, Fallon M, Cote J, *et al.* Effect of the cholesteryl ester transfer protein inhibitor, anacetrapib, on lipoproteins in patients with dyslipidaemia and on 24-h ambulatory blood pressure in healthy individuals: two double-blind, randomised placebo-controlled phase I studies. *Lancet* 2007; **370**:1907–1914.

118 Gaede P, Vedel P, Larsen N, Jensen GV, Parving HH, Pedersen O. Multifactorial intervention and cardiovascular disease in patients with type 2 diabetes. *N Engl J Med* 2003; **348**:383–393.

119 Gaede P, Lund-Andersen H, Parving HH, Pedersen O. Effect of a multifactorial intervention on mortality in type 2 diabetes. *N Engl J Med* 2008; **358**:580–591.

41 Congestive Heart Failure

Inga S. Thrainsdottir[1] & Lars Rydén[2]

[1] Department of Cardiology, Landspitali University Hospital, Reykjavik, Iceland
[2] Department of Cardiology, Karolinska University Hospital, Stockholm, Sweden

Keypoints

- There is a strong link between congestive heart failure (CHF), and diabetes and both conditions are becoming increasingly more common.
- The prevalence of the combination of CHF and diabetes was 0.5% in men and 0.4% in women increasing by age in a recent population-based study. Diabetes was found in 12% of those with CHF compared with only 3% of the controls without CHF.
- Diabetes is a serious prognostic factor for cardiovascular mortality in patients with left ventricular dysfunction caused by ischemic heart disease.
- A 1% (11 mmol/mol) reduction in glycated hemoglobin (HbA_{1c}) has been found to reduce CHF by 16%. In this study, the prognosis improved with a decrease in HbA_{1c} without any threshold or observed upper limit.
- Available data favor a proportionately similar efficacy of evidence-based CHF therapy in patients with and without diabetes. The impact expressed as number of patients needed to treat to avoid one event is lower among people with diabetes because of their higher absolute risk.
- Further studies have to be conducted before an aggressive glucose normalization can be recommended as a possibility to improve the prognosis in patients with diabetes and CHF.
- Thiazolidinediones can provoke or worsen CHF. These drugs should be used with great caution in patients with diabetes and heart failure.

Introduction

The concept that there may be a direct relation between diabetes and congestive heart failure (CHF) is not new. In 1954, Lundbaek [1,2] published an article on clinically important complications in patients with diabetes underlining that heart disease was common in patients with diabetes; indeed, it was present in two-thirds of elderly subjects. He was the first to suggest the presence of a diabetes-specific cardiomyopathy. Twenty years later, Rubler *et al.* [3] published supporting data, concluding that myocardial disease seemed to be a complication of the diabetic state and not merely caused by coronary artery disease (CAD). Shortly thereafter, the Framingham study presented epidemiologic evidence for a strong relation between CHF and diabetes. The latter study clearly indicated that the relation between diabetes and CHF was not only caused by traditional risk factors for coronary heart disease (CHD), but also involved other mechanisms [4].

The prevalence of CHF is increasing in Western societies because of an aging population and also because of increased survival following ischemic heart disease (IHD), and in particular myocardial infarction (MI) [5]. There are many known causes of CHF, including hypertension, CAD, valvular dysfunction, arrhythmias, anemia, renal failure and thyroid dysfunction [5–9]. Risk factors for the development of CHF include increasing age, valvular heart disease and IHD, particularly previous MI, electrocardiographic signs of left ventricular hypertrophy, cardiomegaly detected by chest X-ray, increased heart rate, hypertension and decreased pulmonary vital capacity; diabetes should be added to this list as a strong risk factor. The Framingham study used several of these risk factors to construct a multivariate risk formula to identify high-risk candidates for CHF [10].

Currently, IHD is the leading cause of CHF in industrialized societies with diabetes as a rapidly emerging risk factor for both CHF and IHD [8,11]. Considering the rapidly growing prevalence of diabetes [12], this means that the combination of diabetes and CHF will become increasingly more common in the future. Poor glucose control contributes to the development of CHF as reflected by the relation between an increase in glycated hemoglobin (HbA_{1c}) and the risk of developing CHF [13]. In an epidemiologic study of an elderly Italian cohort, 9.5% of the participants had CHF and 14.7% diabetes. Interestingly, the prevalence of diabetes among subjects with CHF was high, almost 30%. The association was strengthened

Textbook of Diabetes, 4th edition. Edited by R. Holt, C. Cockram, A. Flyvbjerg and B. Goldstein.

during follow-up, indicating that CHF predicted the appearance of diabetes [14].

In summary, there is a strong link between the existence of CHF and diabetes, and both conditions are becoming increasingly more common. The links between these disorders are complex and not yet fully explored.

Symptoms and diagnosis

Diagnosis and definition of congestive heart failure

The state of the art diagnosis of CHF is based on a combination of clinical symptoms combined with characteristic signs of myocardial dysfunction [5]. In clinical practice, CHF is commonly divided into systolic and diastolic myocardial dysfunction, the latter also being known as heart failure with preserved left ventricular function, with systolic dysfunction representing an impaired capacity to eject blood from the left ventricle and diastolic dysfunction an impaired ventricular filling caused by relaxation abnormalities. Echocardiography is the preferred method for documentation of such dysfunction, and left ventricular ejection fraction is the most commonly used expression for impaired systolic dysfunction. Evidence of abnormal left ventricular relaxation, reduced diastolic distensibility or diastolic stiffness are the echocardiographic signs of diastolic dysfunction. Echocardiography, including tissue Doppler imaging (TDI), is useful in detecting myocardial diastolic dysfunction in people with diabetes as well as in the non-diabetic population [15,16]. Plasma concentrations of natriuretic peptides or their precursors are also helpful for diagnosing CHF in patients, including those with diabetes [5,17]. The main clinical classification of the severity of CHF is that presented by the New York Heart Association (Table 41.1). This classification is used for all patients with CHF irrespective if seen in a hospital or outpatient setting and irrespective of etiology.

Diagnosis and definition of glucose abnormalities

Diabetes and other glucose abnormalities are a group of metabolic disorders characterized by hyperglycemia caused by defects in insulin secretion, insulin action or both. Diabetes is associated with damage, dysfunction and failure of various organs [18]. The metabolic syndrome is an entity that has been defined in various ways [19,20], combining different cardiovascular risk factors including abnormalities in glucose homeostasis. Further details on the classification and diagnosis of different glucose abnormalities are given elsewhere in this book.

Table 41.1 Classification of congestive heart failure (CHF) according to New York Heart Association (NYHA).

NYHA Class I	No limitation of physical activities Patients without symptoms during ordinary activities
NYHA Class II	Slight to mild limitation of physical activity Patients comfortable at rest and mild exertion
NYHA Class III	Marked limitation of activity Patients comfortable only at rest
NYHA Class IV	Confined to complete rest in a bed or a chair

Epidemiology

Risk factors for CHF and diabetes

The most important risk factors for cardiovascular disease (CVD) and MI are family history, smoking, abnormal blood lipids, hypertension, diabetes, obesity and socioeconomic factors [21]. Many of the risk factors for CHF are by necessity similar to those for CVD, with IHD and hypertension as leading causes. Other common factors influencing the occurrence of CHF are male gender, smoking, overweight, physical inactivity and valvular heart disease [5]. Type 2 diabetes mellitus (T2DM) as well as poor glucose control observed as high fasting plasma glucose and elevated HbA_{1c} are also of considerable importance [22–27].

Risk factors for T2DM are family history, age, overweight or increased waist : hip ratio and a sedentary lifestyle [28,29]. The morbidity is known to increase progressively with the number of existing risk factors [30]. Particular risk factors for CAD in T2DM are lipid perturbations, including small, dense, easily oxidized low density lipoprotein (LDL) particles, low high density lipoprotein (HDL) cholesterol and increased triglycerides. Moreover, poor glucometabolic control observed as high fasting plasma glucose and elevated HbA_{1c} contribute [31]. Hypertension is another important factor. The Reykjavík Study showed a strong relation between fasting and post load glucose levels and subsequent risk for hypertension, even after adjustment for age, body mass index (BMI) and weight gain, which is interesting because hypertension is one of the main risk factors for CHF [24,25]. Patients with diabetes and CHF have more IHD, increased systolic blood pressure (BP), lower diastolic BP and a higher HbA_{1c} than their counterparts without diabetes [26]. Accordingly, there are many mutual risk factors for CHF and glucose abnormalities.

Prevalence of CHF and glucose abnormalities

The prevalence of CHF varies somewhat in different studies, partly because of differences in the definition of this disease [5]. The demand that a heart failure diagnosis should be supported by evidence of systolic dysfunction on echocardiography may be difficult to fulfill in epidemiologic studies. Modern echocardiographic techniques did not exist when several of the studies, still serving as important sources of information, were conducted [4,32]. The prevalence of CHF has been estimated to be 0.6–6.2% in Swedish men with an increase by age [32]. This is similar to the overall prevalence of CHF among both genders in the Rotterdam population and in the Reykjavík Study [33,34]. The prevalence of CHF was 1–10% in a British outpatient population [35]. It increases considerably when looking at elderly populations as exemplified by the Italian Campania study, in which the prevalence was 9.5%, once more underlining the impact of age [14].

It has been estimated that at least 30% of patients with diabetes are undetected [20]. When screening a Belgian outpatient population with one known cardiovascular risk factor, diabetes was detected in 11% and an additional proportion of 3% had impaired glucose tolerance (IGT) [36]. The prevalence of diabetes was 7.8% in Swedish men and 5.1% in women aged 35–79 years with similar proportions reported from a Finnish middle-aged population [37,38]. The prevalence of diabetes may be considerably higher in selected high risk populations not the least those with CAD. In the Euro Heart Survey Diabetes and the Heart, patients admitted to hospital because of acute and stable CAD were investigated for the presence of diabetes and IGT. Only 29% of the 4961 patients had a normal glucose metabolism while 31% had known and 12% previously unknown diabetes. The remaining 28% of the patients had IGT [39]. Similar proportions were detected in patient populations with cerebral and peripheral vascular disease [40]. Thus, the combination of CVD and glucose perturbations is very common but underestimated in many previous studies because of lack of diagnostic accuracy in combination with a thorough investigation of the glucometabolic state.

Considerably less is known about the prevalence of the combination of diabetes and CHF. The most recent and extensive study of the prevalence of diabetes and CHF is that from the Reykjavík population [34], in which the prevalence of the combination of CHF and diabetes was 0.5% in men and 0.4% in women, increasing by age. Diabetes was found in 12% of those with CHF compared to only 3% of the controls without CHF. Thus, there was a strong association between diabetes and CHF (Figure 41.1).

Based on Framingham data, Rutter *et al.* [41] noted that the heart is prone to changes in the form of increased left ventricular mass and wall thickness with worsening glucose tolerance. Kannel *et al.* [4] and Gustafsson *et al.* [42] reported on the role of diabetes in CHF from a general and a hospitalized population, respectively. Their findings indicated a strong association between CHF and diabetes. Iribarren *et al.* [43], Bertoni *et al.* [44] and Nichols *et al.* [26], focusing on the role of CHF in patients with diabetes, noted that the prevalence of CHF varied between 1.9 and 22.3%. Finally, Amato *et al.* [14] found a strong association between diabetes and CHF in a population of elderly people. The outcomes of these studies have been summarized in Table 41.2.

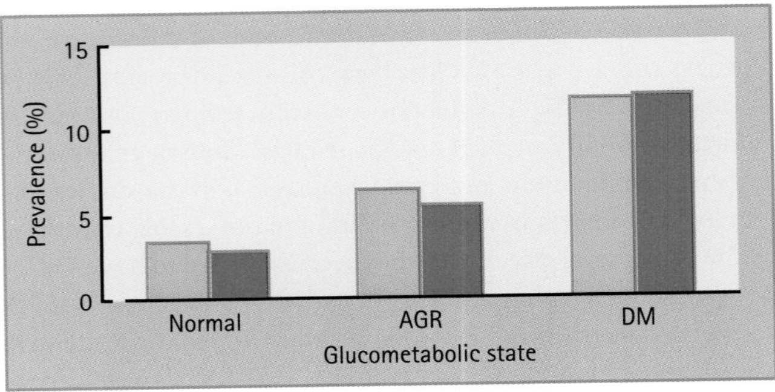

Figure 41.1 Prevalence of congestive heart failure (CHF) in relation to glucometabolic state. Yellow bars, males; red bars, females; AGR, abnormal glucose regulation; DM, diabetes. Reproduced from Thrainsdottir *et al.* [34], with permission from American Diabetes Association.

Incidence of CHF and glucose abnormalities

Recent results from the Framingham study indicate that the incidence of CHF has declined during the last five decades [45], but these data are not supported in other studies [46]. On the contrary, it seems that hospital admissions for CHF are increasing, resulting in higher health care expenditures for patients with this diagnosis [47]. Among British outpatients, the incidence of CHF has been reported to be 4.4/1000 person-years in men and 3.9/1000 in women, rising with age in both genders [48]. The incidence in Finland is similar among men, 4.0/1000 person-years, but lower in women 1.0/1000 person-years [49].

The age-standardized annual incidence of diabetes, reported to be 2.2 and 2.3/1000 person-years in Dutch men and women, respectively, is rather uniform in several European countries [50]. When turning to an elderly population, however, as in the Italian Campania study, the incidence was considerably higher at 6.1% per year. This is somewhat different from the observation in the Netherlands where the incidence decreased in the oldest age group [14,50].

Considerably less is known about the incidence of the combination of diabetes and CHF. Once more it seems as if the most recent and extensive study originates from the Reykjavík population. In this study, the age and gender standardized incidence of abnormal glucose regulation was 12.6/1000/year, diabetes 4.6/1000/year and CHF 5.3/1000/year (Figure 41.2). In addition, there was a strong association between the incidence of glucose abnormalities and CHF [51].

In the Framingham study, the incidence of CHF was twice that among males and five times higher in females with diabetes during 18 years of follow-up than patients free from diabetes. The excessive risk of CHF remained high even after the exclusion of patients with prior CAD [4]. In a general population of elderly Italians, the prevalence of diabetes was 9.6% per year in CHF patients [14].

Pathophysiology

Myocardial structural and biochemical alterations can be identified in the failing heart, and many of them seems to be independent of the etiology of myocardial dysfunction. They include changes in myocardial energy production, altered expression of contractile proteins, a desynchronized excitation–contraction coupling, β-adrenergic receptor stimulation, myocyte depletion and increased activity of a number of cytokines. Many of these aberrations are found in diabetic heart. Here, some general features of the pathophysiology are followed by a discussion of more diabetes-specific factors.

Table 41.2 Comparison of the prevalence, incidence and prediction of heart failure and diabetes in general populations and among patients.

Study name	Campania	Heart failure in patients with diabetes			Patients with diabetes and heart failure	
		Medicare sample	Kaiser Permanente	Kaiser Permanente	DIAMOND	Framingham
Authors [ref]	Amato *et al.* [14]	Bertoni *et al.* [44]	Iribarren *et al.* [43]	Nichols *et al.* [26]	Gustafsson *et al.* [42]	Kannel *et al.* [4]
Participants (no)	1339	151 738	48 858	9591	5491	5209
Follow-up (years)	3	5	2.2	2.5	5–8	18
Period	<1997	1994–1999	1995–1997	<1997	1993–2003	1949–
Age	74 (mean) (all >65)	73–76 (all >65)	58 (mean)		52–86, (mean 73)	30–62
CHF prevalence	9.5 %	22.3%	1.9%	11.8% in people with DM, 4.5% in controls	–	–
Diabetes prevalence	14.7	–	–	–	14.7% (T2DM)	–
Diabetes and CHF association	OR 2.0 CI (1.6–2.5)	–	–	–	–	RR men 2.4 women 5.1
Diabetes incidence	9.6%/year in CHF patients 6.1%/year in controls	–	–	–	–	
CHF incidence	–	12.6/100 PY	–	3.3/100 PY in people with DM, 1.5/100 PY in controls	–	17.5/1000 PY among men, 18.5/1000 PY among women In people with DM 9/1000 PY in men, 14/1000 PY in women
Diabetes predictive factors	CHF OR 1.4 (1.1–1.8)	–	–	–	–	–
CHF predictive factors	BMI, Waist : hip ratio	Men, Caucasians, IHD, hypertension, stroke, PVD, nephropathy, retinopathy, neuropathy	–	Age, female, diabetes duration, insulin, IHD, creatinine, glucose	–	Diabetes, males
Diabetes mortality	–	–		–	RR 1.5 in diabetes patients	–
Other endpoint	–	–	1% (11 mmol/mol) increase in HbA_{1c} => increased risk of CHF by 8%	–	–	–

BMI, body mass index; CHF, congestive heart failure; CI, confidence interval; DM, diabetes mellitus; IHD, ischemic heart disease; OR, odds ratio; PVD, peripheral vascular disease; PY, person-years; RR, relative rate.

Congestive heart failure

CHF is a clinical syndrome originally induced by myocardial damage but subsequently influenced by the induction of an untoward neurohormonal response. Thus, norepinephrine, angiotensin II, endothelin and aldosterone are all linked to the vicious cycle of myocardial remodeling (Figure 41.3) which unopposed will cause successive deterioration of myocardial performance [52].

Metabolic conditions have a significant role in cardiac adaptation and remodeling. This leads to an increase of myosin heavy chain beta, altered troponin T (TnT) molecules, diminished storage of creatinine phosphatases, and decreased sarcoplasmatic ATPase activity, which may result in myocyte hypertrophy associated with impaired contractile function and less effective energy supply [53,54].

The myocardium has a high energy turnover with ATP as an important source of energy. The two pathways for energy supply are via the breakdown of free fatty acids (FFA) and of carbohydrates (Figure 41.4). The lipolytic pathway transfers FFA via β-oxidation to acetyl co-enzyme A (ACA), which enters the citric acid or Krebs cycle. The carbohydrate pathway produces pyruvate via glycolysis, glycogenolysis and lactate oxidation. Pyruvate is

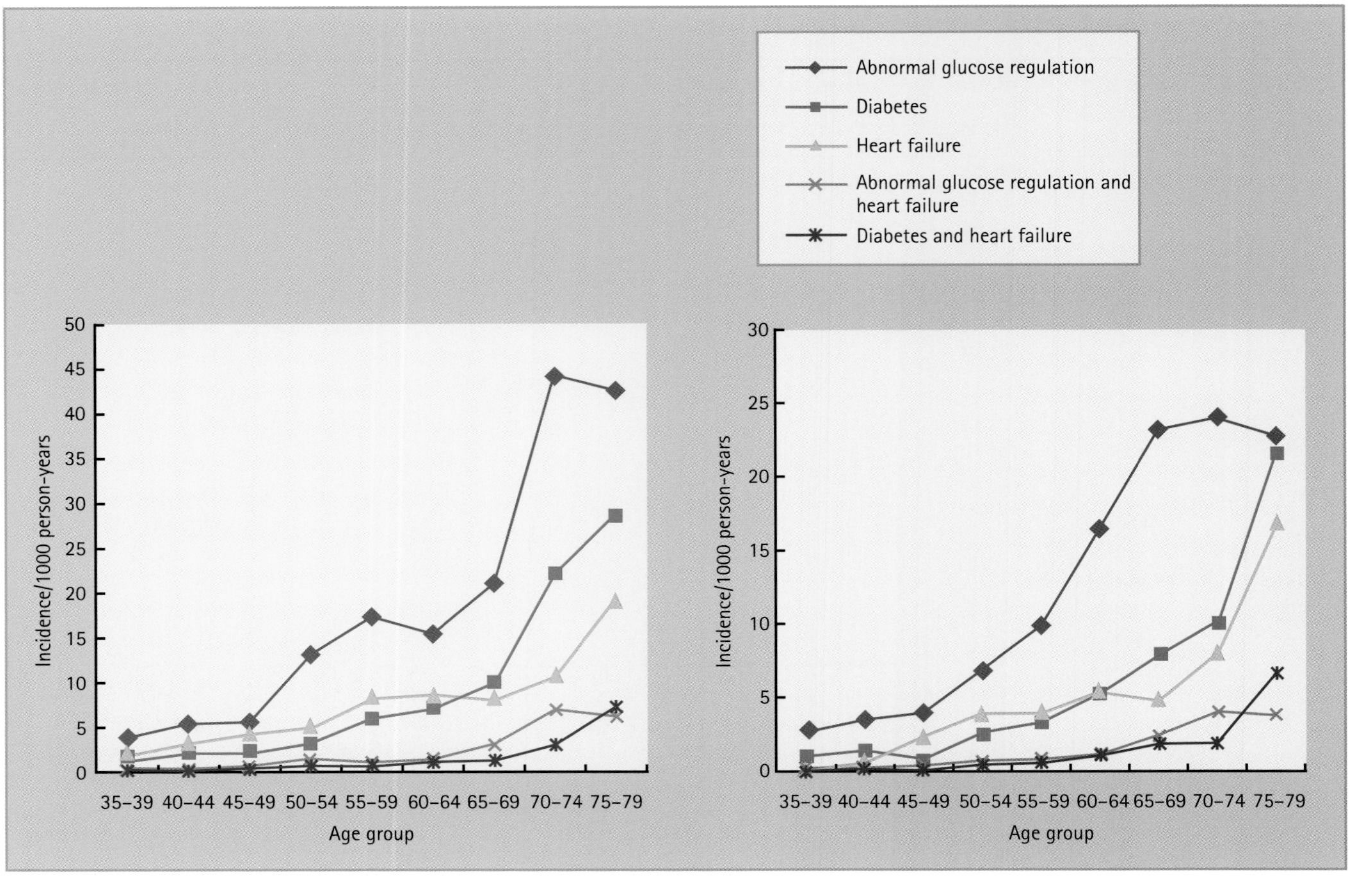

Figure 41.2 Incidence of abnormal glucose regulation, diabetes, congestive heart failure (CHF), abnormal glucose regulation and CHF, and diabetes and CHF expressed as number of incident cases/1000 person years among men (left) and women (right) by age. Reproduced from Thrainsdottir *et al.* [51], with permission from Oxford University Press.

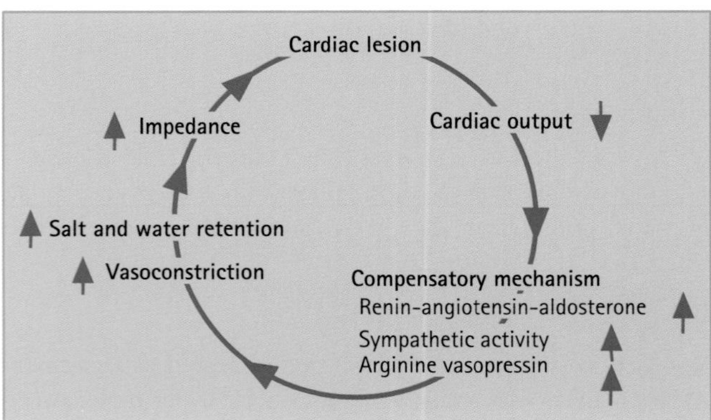

Figure 41.3 Neurohormonal activation caused by depressed myocardial function leads to a vicious circle further compromising the already compromised myocardial function.

decarboxylated via pyruvate dehydrogenase to ACA, which enters the Krebs cycle. The dominant pathway for myocardial energy production is β-oxidation of FFA, but the myocardium is also dependent on glucose oxidation [55].

When the heart is subjected to ischemic stress or exposed to sustained enhancement of intraventricular pressure, it tends to change towards a more dominant glucose oxidation [56]. This may be counteracted by a reduction of the glucose transporter 4 (GLUT-4), which becomes reduced in CHF, hampering glucose transport over the cell membrane. At the same time, the heart is subjected to increased FFA concentrations, released via stress influenced by an increased sympathetic tone [57]. It is assumed that prolonged intracellular accumulation of FFA and its metabolites may cause myocardial dysfunction [58].

Besides these mechanisms, alterations in gene expression and inflammatory activity have been suggested to cause metabolic and mechanical disturbances in CHF [59–62]. All nucleated cells, including the cardiomyocyte, can produce pro-inflammatory cytokines as a response to injury such as MI, myocarditis or when the heart fails. Both tumor necrosis factor α (TNF-α) and interleukin 6 (IL-6) levels increase in proportion to the severity and duration of CHF [59,60]. This cytokine release may trigger a cascade of events leading to myocardial structural alterations further deteriorating the clinical picture of CHF.

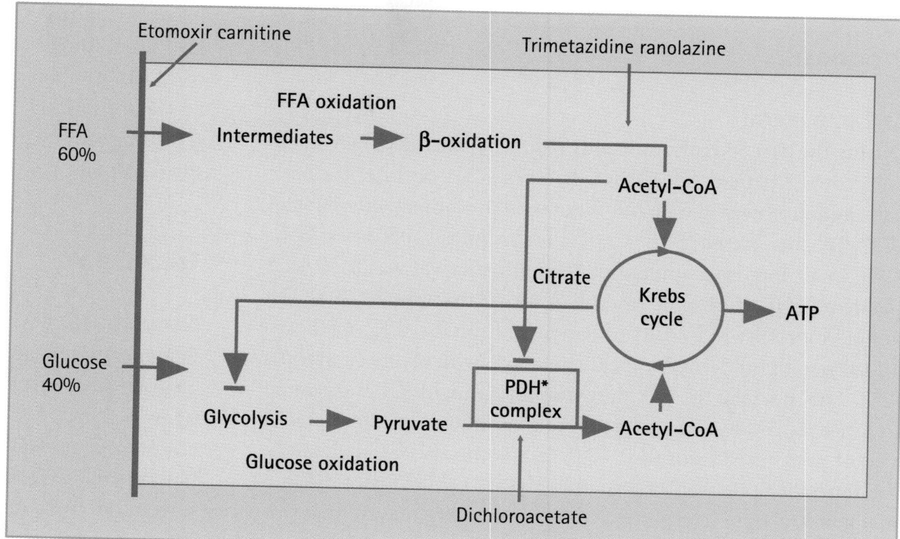

Figure 41.4 Schematic illustration of myocardial energy production of relevance for congestive heart failure (CHF) patients with and without diabetes. The site of action for metabolic modulators are indicated. See text for further information. CoA, co-enzyme A; FFA, free fatty acids; PDH, pyruvate dehydrogenase.

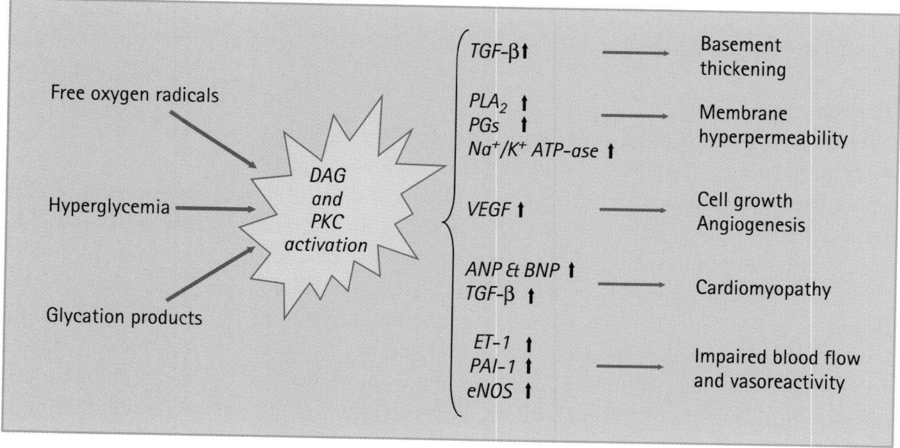

Figure 41.5 Metabolic effects of hyperglycemia induced activation of protein kinase C (PKC) and diacyloglycerol (DAG). See text for further explanation. ANP and BNP, atrial and brain natriuretic peptide; eNOS, endothelial nitrous oxide synthase; ET-1, endothelin 1; PAI-1, plasminogen activating inhibitor 1; PG, prostaglandin; PLA_2, phospholipase A_2; TGF-β, transforming growth factor β; VEGF, vascular endothelial growth factor.

CHF and diabetes

The main myocardial energy production is normally based on β-oxidation of FFA (70%) with a smaller contribution from glucose oxidation (30%) and lactate. FFA are produced by lipolysis of endogenous cardiac or exogenous stores of triglycerides. Oxidation of FFA is an effective supplier of energy in the form of ATP if the oxygen supply is sufficient. In conditions with limited oxygen availability, glucose oxidation will provide more energy per mole oxygen and support more work than FFA [63]. In the person with diabetes, glucose utilization for energy production is substantially lower, about 10% (Figure 41.4). The shift to an even more pronounced β-oxidation of FFA causes a higher oxygen utilization than under normal circumstances [64]. The major restriction to glucose utilization in the diabetic heart is the slow rate of glucose transport across the sarcolemmal membrane in the myocardium [65,66]. The impaired glucose oxidation in the diabetic heart can also result from a decreased rate of phosphorylation of glucose which subsequently limits the entry of glucose into the cell. The depressed phosphorylation is triggered by the increased metabolism of FFA [64]. Insulin deficiency enhances lipolysis thereby increasing circulating FFA [67]. People with diabetes are also known to have increased risk for other disturbances such as reduced myocardial blood flow and blunted hyperkinetic response to myocardial ischemia resulting in diminished myocardial function [68–71]. Indeed, CHF is an insulin-resistant state with an increased release of non-esterified fatty acids which are taken up in muscular tissue and downregulate glucose uptake and utilization [72].

Another consequence of hyperglycemia is oxidative stress and activation of processes triggered by an increased level of diacylglycerol and protein kinase C as depicted in Figure 41.5. Besides, many other unfavorable effects of the increased levels of inflammatory cytokines in heart failure patients may enhance insulin resistance [71,72].

Prognosis

CHF in general

During the past 30 years, mortality from CHD has declined markedly among patients free from diabetes. This decline has been substantially lower in men but is not seen in women with diabetes [73]. In the presence of CHF, the prognosis becomes poor [74]. In an English population, 1 month survival was 81% after incident CHF, declining to 57% after 18 months [8,75]. The annual mortality in a study of patients hospitalized for CHF was 10–20% with mild–moderate and 40–60% with severe symptoms [35]. The mortality in an elderly population with CHF recruited in Rotterdam was 47% during 6 years of follow-up. This is twice that of persons without CHF [74]. In a comparable Italian study, the mortality rate was 21.3% after 3 years [14]. Thus, CHF is a malignant disease irrespective of the underlying reason for myocardial dysfunction. Recent reports have been somewhat more encouraging. A 50-year follow-up of the Framingham data indicates that CHF survival has improved to some extent [45]. This observation is supported by a report based on the Swedish hospital discharge registry [76].

Diabetes and CHF

CVD is the most prevalent complication of diabetes and is of major importance. Cardiovascular mortality in men with diabetes lies between the mortality for men with angina and MI [77]. In the USA, it has been estimated that 77% of all hospitalizations for chronic complications of diabetes are attributable to CVD [78]. T2DM doubles the risk of death from CHD, and T2DM diagnosed at the age of 55 years reduces life expectancy by about 5 years [79]. This makes mortality from CVD in people with diabetes but without previous MI similar to the mortality in patients with a history of MI but without diabetes [80].

The prognosis of patients with diabetes becomes even worse in the presence of CHF [81–84]. In the first DIGAMI study, performed in patients with diabetes and acute MI, CHF was the most common reason for morbidity and mortality, accounting for 66% of the total mortality during the first year of follow-up [85]. Diabetes is a serious prognostic factor for cardiovascular mortality in patients with left ventricular dysfunction caused by IHD [86]. In a general population in Reykjavík, the survival decreased significantly with the concomitant presence of both CHF and glucose abnormality even after adjustment for cardiovascular risk factors and IHD [87], which may serve as an indicator of the serious implication of the presence of diabetes along with CHF.

Hyperglycemia and prognosis

The relationship between plasma glucose and mortality has been elucidated in several studies. According to the UK Prospective Diabetes Study (UKPDS), a 1% (11 mmol/mol) reduction in HbA_{1c} is associated with a reduction of MI by 14% and CHF by 16%. In this study, the prognosis improved with a decrease in HbA_{1c} without any threshold or observed upper limit [88]. In the DECODE study, a 2-hour post load glucose was a better predictor of mortality than fasting blood glucose [89]. This may perhaps be seen as an indicator of the importance of post-prandial hyperglycemia and the potentially serious implication of IGT for myocardial function.

Treatment

General aspects

Evidence-based treatment of CHF relies on a combination of angiotensin-converting enzyme (ACE) inhibitors and/or angiotensin receptor blockers (ARBs), beta-blockers, diuretics and aldosterone antagonists [5]. ACE inhibitors, ARBs and beta-blockers reduce mortality and improve symptoms in moderate to severe CHF with or without diabetes [90–93]. Diuretics are mandatory for symptomatic treatment of fluid overload, but should not be used in excess because they induce neurohormonal activation [94]. The addition of aldosterone antagonists is indicated in severe forms of CHF and may then improve longevity [95]; however, many patients are, although symptomatically improved, left with an unfavorable vital prognosis despite the best available pharmacologic treatment. A search for novel treatment modalities is therefore still ongoing. One of these is metabolic modulation with compounds that influence the disturbed metabolic pathways in CHF and which are thought to be of particular importance in patients with diabetes [55]. Attention has been paid to compounds that shift energy production from β-oxidation of FFA towards the energetically more efficient glucose oxidation under such conditions as in myocardial ischemia and CHF. Examples of such drugs are trimetazidine, ranolazine, etomoxir and dichloroacetate [96,97].

Various techniques have been used to study the efficacy of pharmacologic treatment in CHF. Among them are the general feeling of well-being as assessed by means of different questionnaires, and an estimation of physical capacity tested by exercise tolerance on a bicycle ergometer or treadmill. Two-dimensional echocardiography is the most commonly applied technique for investigating myocardial function [98–101]. A relatively newly developed technique, TDI assesses myocardial function in different myocardial segments. This technique is useful for diagnosing left ventricular dysfunction even before any symptoms or signs of CHF appear in subjects with diabetes [102–104].

Guidelines that specifically deal with diabetes and CVD including CHF have not been available until recently. Through a combined initiative by the European Society of Cardiology (ESC) and the European Association of the Study of Diabetes (EASD), guidelines on the management of diabetes, pre-diabetes and CVD were published in 2007 [105]. As outlined in this document, there are few trials that specificially address the treatment of patients with the combination of glucose abnormalities and CHF, causing a lack of specific evidence regarding the management of such patients. Current data are mostly based on analyses of subgroups

Table 41.3 The effect of inhibition of the renin angiotensin system in congestive heart failure (CHF) trials by diabetic state.

Study [ref]	Participants (no)	Diabetes (%)	Outcome
CONSENSUS [109]	253	18	31% reduction of 1-year mortality
SAVE [114]	2231	22	19% all cause mortality risk reduction 21% risk reduction of cardiovascular morbidity
ATLAS [112]	3164	19	14% mortality risk reduction with high dose ACE inhibitor treatment
GISSI 3 [115]	18 131	15	30% reduction in mortality after 6 weeks

ACE, angiotensin-converting enzyme.

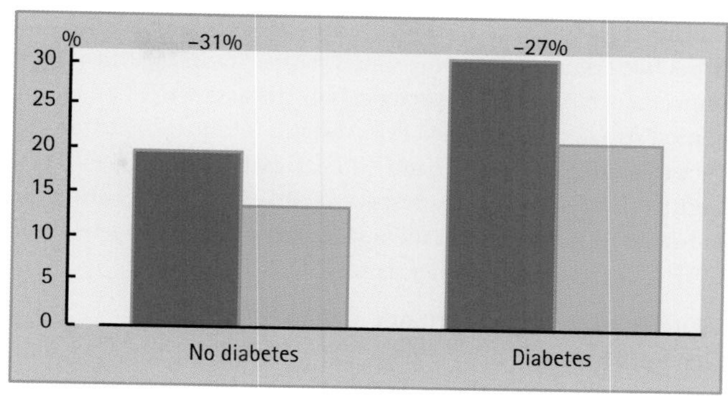

Figure 41.6 The impact of the beta-blocker metoprolol on the combined end-point mortality or hospitalization in congestive heart failure (CHF) patients with and without diabetes participating in the MERIT-HF trial [124,125]. Note that the relative risk reduction (given in % above bars) is independent of diabetic state but that the absolute mortality even with metoprolol treatment is considerably higher in the diabetic subgroup. Dark green bars, placebo; light green bars, metoprolol.

of patients with diabetes in large CHF trials. This results in potential shortcomings related to a poor definition of diabetes and hidden diabetes, actual glucose lowering therapy and also a risk for selection biases with an overrepresentation of less severe diabetes. With these limitations in mind, available data favor a proportionately similar efficacy in patients with and without diabetes. Because the absolute prognosis is considerably worse in patients with diabetes, the impact of therapy expressed as number of patients needed to treat to avoid an event (e.g. hospitalization for CHF or death) is considerably lower among these patients than their counterparts without diabetes.

Pharmacologic therapy of CHF

ACE inhibition

ACE inhibitors are recommended both in asymptomatic myocardial dysfunction and overt CHF. As shown in Table 41.3, they reduce mortality and improve symptoms in moderate to severe CHF with and without diabetes [106–110]. Patients with diabetes represent rather large subgroups in several trials. In SOLVD, the effect of enalapril on compromised left ventricular function was similar in patients with and without diabetes [111]. In ATLAS, comparing a high and a low dose lisinopril treatment strategy, mortality reduction was at least as good in patients with as in those without diabetes [112]. The GISSI 3 and the SAVE trials reported beneficial effects on morbidity and mortality of ACE inhibitor treatment in post-MI patients with diabetes [113–115].

Because hypoglycemic episodes may be provoked by ACE inhibitor therapy in patients on glucose lowering therapy, it is recommended that plasma glucose is monitored in the early phase of the institution of an ACE inhibitor in patients on glucose lowering treatment [116,117].

Angiotensin receptor blockers

The use of ARBs is an alternative to ACE inhibition and may even be used in combination with ACE inhibition in severe CHF. ARBs improve morbidity and mortality in CHF patients with and without diabetes [118,119].

Beta-blockers

Beta-blockade decreases myocardial FFA exposure and therefore such treatment has the capacity to influence the metabolic pathway favorably in patients with T2DM and CHF [120,121]. Subgroup analyses of patients with diabetes and moderate to severe CHF participating in large trials reveal that beta-blockers reduce mortality and improve symptoms. Therefore, beta-blockers are indicated as first-line treatment in patients with the combination of CHF and diabetes [122–126]. An example of the impact of beta-blockade (metoprolol) added to treatment with ACE inhibitors and diuretics in CHF patients with and without diabetes is given in Figure 41.6. It is worthy of note that the relative risk reduction following metoprolol is similar in the two groups. The remaining event rate is still substantially higher in the diabetic cohort than among those without diabetes.

Diuretics and aldosterone antagonists

Diuretics are mandatory for symptomatic relief of fluid overload. As already underlined, they should not be used in excess because they induce neurohormonal activation [94]. Loop diuretics are recommended rather than diuretics that may further impair glucose metabolism. The addition of aldosterone antagonists is indicated in severe forms of CHF and may improve longevity [127]; however, no information is available on the administration of aldosterone antagonists in patients with diabetes and CHF.

Statins

It has been debated for some time whether statin treatment may impact morbidity and longevity in patients with CHF. Two recent clinical trials, the Controlled Rosuvastatin Multinational Study in Heart Failure (CORONA) and GISSI Heart Failure (GISSI-HF), were both negative in this respect [128,129]. It is therefore not indicated to include statin therapy as part of the management of CHF if not needed for other reasons.

Glucose lowering treatment

General aspects

In accordance with the pathophysiologic aspects on CHF in patients with diabetes, it has been postulated that meticulous metabolic control may have beneficial effects on progress and prognosis. The European guidelines for the management of diabetes recommend that HbA_{1c} should be <6.5% (48 mmol/mol) and plasma glucose fasting <6 mmol/L (<108 mg/dL) and postprandial <7.5 mmol/L (<135 mg/dL) [105]. The scientific evidence, as derived from properly designed clinical trials, behind these recommendations seem sparse even if they are somewhat more solid for type 1 diabetes (T1DM) than T2DM [130]. The negative outcome of some recent trials on aggressive glucose lowering have further underlined the uncertainty in this respect [131,132]; however, these trials did not specifically look at patients with CHF. Further studies are yet to be conducted on this category of patient before aggressive glucose normalization can be recommended as a possibility to improve their situation. Currently, it seems as if such assumptions reflect information from epidemiologic studies showing increased risk with increasing levels of plasma glucose and HbA_{1c} starting well below what has currently been labeled as normal.

Glucose lowering agents

Regarding specific glucose lowering agents, there is some information available of importance for the choice of treatment in patients with or at risk for heart failure. The insulin sensitizers thiazolidinediones can provoke or worsen CHF because of their propensity to induce fluid retention. These drugs should be used with great caution in patients in New York Heart Association class I–II and are considered contraindicated in those in class III–IV [133–136]. Metformin is also contraindicated in CHF because of the risk of lactic acidosis.

Insulin treatment in patients with diabetes and CHF is under debate. The main effect of insulin is to decrease blood glucose, but it may also increase myocardial blood flow, decrease heart rate and cause a modest increase in cardiac output [137,138]. Beneficial effects on myocardial function have been reported, but also that insulin may be associated with increased morbidity [139] and mortality [140,141]. Further studies are needed to establish the specific role of insulin beyond the role as a glucose lowering agent in patients with diabetes and CHF.

In general, it may be summarized that there is very little information available of importance for the choice of agents for glycemic control in patients with diabetes and CHF. Thus, generally accepted management rules should apply [142].

Diastolic congestive heart failure

Impaired myocardial diastolic function and endothelial dysfunction are early expressions of diabetes-related cardiovascular involvement causing a decreased myocardial blood flow reserve. It has been suggested that hyperglycemia-related early myocardial and microcirculatory disturbances are dynamic and that they may be reversed by improved metabolic control [143]. An observational study by von Bibra *et al.* [144], on patients subjected to intensified glucose control in clinical routine, gave support to the assumption that particularly insulin-based glycemic control may be useful. Unfortunately, these observations were not verified in a recent prospective study, the Diabetes mellitus And Diastolic Dysfunction (DADD) trial, randomly distributing patients with T2DM and early signs of diastolic dysfunction to insulin or oral based glucose normalization. The patients were selected to be free from previous cardiovascular events and signs of CHF or CAD [145]. It should be underlined that it is still too early to abandon the hypothesis of a favorable relation between glycemic control and myocardial diastolic dysfunction. It may be that the DADD patients were too healthy to react to normalization of glucose control. Thus, it would be of value to study new agents, such as incretins, in future trials and to recruit patients at a more advanced disease stage than those selected for the DADD study. The problem is then the obvious risk for biases caused by hypertension and CAD and other complications to diabetes. Accordingly, such protocols must include detailed examinations of the patients with this in mind.

Metabolic modulators

Drugs, such as trimetazidine, etomoxir and dichloroacetate, whose mode of action is to shift myocardial metabolism from oxidation of FFA towards glycolysis have been tested in patients with myocardial dysfunction and diabetes. They act on different parts of the metabolic pathways as indicated in Figure 41.4. Their usefulness must be further explored in clinical trials of appropriate design until their therapeutic role can be considered established despite some recent promising results [146–148].

References

1 Lundbaek K. Diabetic angiopathy: a specific vascular disease. *Lancet* 1954; **263**:377–379.

2 Lundbaek K. Is there a diabetic cardiopathy? In: Schettler G, ed. *Pathogenetishe Faktoren des Myokardinfarkts*. Stuttgart: Schattauer, 1969: 63–71.

3 Rubler S, Dlugash J, Yuceoglu YZ, Kumral T, Branwood AW, Grishman A. New type of cardiomyopathy associated with diabetic glomerulosclerosis. *Am J Cardiol* 1972; **30**:595–602.

4 Kannel WB, Hjortland M, Castelli WP. Role of diabetes in congestive heart failure: the Framingham study. *Am J Cardiol* 1974; **34**:29–34.

5 Dickstein K, Cohen-Solal A, Filippatos G, McMurray JJ, Ponikowski P, Poole-Wilson PA, *et al.*; Task Force for Diagnosis and Treatment of Acute and Chronic Heart Failure 2008 of European Society of

Cardiology. ESC Guidelines for the diagnosis and treatment of acute and chronic heart failure 2008: the Task Force for the Diagnosis and Treatment of Acute and Chronic Heart Failure 2008 of the European Society of Cardiology. Developed in collaboration with the Heart Failure Association of the ESC (HFA) and endorsed by the European Society of Intensive Care Medicine (ESICM). *Eur Heart J* 2008; **29**:2388–2442.

6 Eriksson H, Svärdsudd K, Larsson B, Ohlson LO, Tibblin G, Welin L, *et al.* Risk factors for heart failure in the general population: the study of men born in 1913. *Eur Heart J* 1989; **10**:647–656.

7 Schocken DD, Arrieta MI, Leaverton PE, Ross EA. Prevalence and mortality rate of congestive heart failure in the United States. *J Am Coll Cardiol* 1992; **20**:301–306.

8 Massie BM, Shah NB. Evolving trends in the epidemiologic factors of heart failure: rationale for preventive strategies and comprehensive disease management. *Am Heart J* 1997; **133**:703–712.

9 Chae CU, Pfeffer MA, Glynn RJ, Mitchell GF, Taylor JO, Hennekens CH. Increased pulse pressure and risk of heart failure in the elderly. *JAMA* 1999; **281**:634–639.

10 Kannel WB, D'Agostino RB, Silbershatz H, Belanger AJ, Wilson PW, Levy D. Profile for estimating risk of heart failure. *Arch Intern Med* 1999; **159**:1197–1204.

11 Soläng L, Malmberg K, Rydén L. Diabetes mellitus and congestive heart failure. *Eur Heart J* 1999; **20**:789–795.

12 King H, Aubert RE, Herman WH. Global burden of diabetes, 1995–2025: prevalence, numerical estimates, and projections. *Diabetes Care* 1998; **21**:1414–1431.

13 Chae CU, Glynn RJ, Manson JE, Guralnik JM, Taylor JO, Pfeffer MA. Diabetes predicts congestive heart failure risk in the elderly. *Circulation* 1998; **98**(Suppl 1):721.

14 Amato L, Paolisso G, Cacciatore F, Ferrara N, Ferrara P, Canonico S, *et al.*; Osservatorio Geriatrico Regione Campania Group. Congestive heart failure predicts the development of non-insulin-dependent diabetes mellitus in the elderly. *Diabetes Metab* 1997; **23**:213–218.

15 Hatle L. How to diagnose diastolic heart failure a consensus statement. *Eur Heart J* 2007; **28**:2421–2423.

16 Paulus WJ, Tschöpe C, Sanderson JE, Rusconi C, Flachskampf FA, Rademakers FE, *et al.* How to diagnose diastolic heart failure: a consensus statement on the diagnosis of heart failure with normal left ventricular ejection fraction by the Heart Failure and Echocardiography Associations of the European Society of Cardiology. *Eur Heart J* 2007; **28**:2539–2550.

17 Epshteyn V, Morrison K, Krishnaswamy P, Kazanegra R, Clopton P, Mudaliar S, *et al.* Utility of B-type natriuretic peptide (BNP) as a screen for left ventricular dysfunction in patients with diabetes. *Diabetes Care* 2003; **26**:2081–2087.

18 Alberti KG, Zimmet PZ. Definition, diagnosis and classification of diabetes mellitus and its complications. Part 1: Diagnosis and classification of diabetes mellitus provisional report of a WHO consultation. *Diabet Med* 1998; **15**:539–553.

19 WHO. *Definition, diagnosis and classification of diabetes mellitus and its complications. Report of a WHO consultation. Part 1: Diagnosis and classification of diabetes mellitus.* Geneva: World Health Organization, Department of Noncommunicable Disease Surveillance, 1999.

20 American Diabetes Association. Clinical practice recommendations 2004. *Diabetes Care* 2004; **27**(Suppl 1):5–19.

21 Yusuf S, Hawken S, Ounpuu S, Dans T, Avezum A, Lanas F, *et al.*; INTERHEART Study Investigators. Effect of potentially modifiable risk factors associated with myocardial infarction in 52 countries (the INTERHEART study): case–control study. *Lancet* 2004; **364**:937–952.

22 He J, Ogden LG, Bazzano LA, Vupputuri S, Loria C, Whelton PK. Risk factors for congestive heart failure in US men and women. NHANES I. Epidemiologic follow-up study. *Arch Intern Med* 2001; **161**:996–1002.

23 Stratton IM, Adler AI, Neil HAW, Matthews DR, Manley SE, Cull CA, *et al.* Association of glycaemia with macrovascular and microvascular complications of type 2 diabetes (UKPDS 35): prospective observational study. *Br Med J* 2000; **321**:405–412.

24 Kristiansson K, Sigfusson N, Sigvaldason H, Thorgeirsson G. Glucose tolerance and blood pressure in a population-based cohort study of males and females: the Reykjavik Study. *J Hypertens* 1995; **13**:581–586.

25 McKee PA, Castelli WP, McNamara PM, Kannel WB. The natural history of congestive heart failure: the Framingham Study. *N Engl J Med* 1971; **285**:1441–1446.

26 Nichols GA, Gullion CM, Koro CE, Ephross SA, Brown JB. The incidence of congestive heart failure in type 2 diabetes: an update. *Diabetes Care* 2004; **27**:1879–1884.

27 Kenchaiah S, Evans JC, Levy D, Wilson PW, Benjamin EJ, Larson MG, *et al.* Obesity and the risk of heart failure. *N Engl J Med* 2002; **347**:305–313.

28 Tuomilehto J, Lindström J, Eriksson JG, Valle TT, Hämäläinen H, Ilanne-Parikka P, *et al.*; Finnish Diabetes Prevention Study Group. Prevention of type 2 diabetes mellitus by changes in lifestyle among subjects with impaired glucose tolerance. *N Engl J Med* 2001; **344**:1343–1350.

29 Simpson RW, Shaw JE, Zimmet PZ. The prevention of type 2 diabetes: lifestyle change or pharmacotherapy? A challenge for the 21st century. *Diabetes Res Clin Pract* 2003; **59**:165–180.

30 Stamler J, Vaccaro O, Neaton JD, Wentworth D. Diabetes, other risk factors, and 12-yr cardiovascular mortality for men screened in the Multiple Risk Factor Intervention Trial. *Diabetes Care* 1993; **16**:434–444.

31 Turner RC, Millns H, Neil HA, Stratton IM, Manley SE, Matthews DR, *et al.*; UK Prospective Diabetes Study Group. Risk factors for coronary artery disease in non-insulin dependent diabetes mellitus: UK Prospective Diabetes Study (UKPDS: 23). *Br Med J* 1998; **316**:823–828.

32 Wilhelmsen L, Rosengren A, Eriksson H, Lappas G. Heart failure in the general population of men: morbidity, risk factors and prognosis. *J Intern Med* 2001; **249**:253–261.

33 Mosterd A, Hoes AW, de Bruyne MC, Deckers JW, Linker DT, Hofman A, *et al.* Prevalence of heart failure and left ventricular dysfunction in the general population: the Rotterdam Study. *Eur Heart J* 1999; **20**:447–455.

34 Thrainsdottir IS, Aspelund T, Thorgeirsson G, Gudnason V, Hardarson T, Malmberg K, *et al.* The association between glucose abnormalities and heart failure in the population based Reykjavík study. *Diabetes Care* 2005; **28**:612–616.

35 Dargie HJ, McMurray JJ, McDonagh TA. Heart failure: implications of the true size of the problem. *J Intern Med* 1996; **239**:309–315.

36 Buysschaert M, Vandenbroucke C, Barsoum S. A type 2 diabetes screening program by general practitioners in a Belgian at risk population. *Diabetes Metab* 2001; **27**:109–114.

37 Andersson DK, Svardsudd K, Tibblin G. Prevalence and incidence of diabetes in a Swedish community 1972–1987. *Diabet Med* 1991; **8**:428–434.

38 Tuomilehto J, Korhonen HJ, Kartovaara L, Salomaa V, Stengård JH, Pitkänen M, *et al.* Prevalence of diabetes mellitus and impaired glucose tolerance in the middle-aged population of three areas in Finland. *Int J Epidemiol* 1991; **20**:1010–1017.

39 Bartnik M, Rydén L, Ferrari R, Malmberg K, Pyörälä K, Simoons M, *et al.*; Euro Heart Survey Investigators. The prevalence of abnormal glucose regulation in patients with coronary artery disease across Europe: the Euro Heart Survey on diabetes and the heart. *Eur Heart J* 2004; **25**:1880–1890.

40 Johansen OE, Birkeland KI, Brustad E, Aaser E, Lindahl AK, Midha R, *et al.* Undiagnosed dysglycaemia and inflammation in cardiovascular disease. *Eur J Clin Invest* 2006; **36**:544–551.

41 Rutter MK, Parise H, Benjamin EJ, Levy D, Larson MG, Meigs JB, *et al.* Impact of glucose intolerance and insulin resistance on cardiac structure and function: sex-related differences in the Framingham Heart Study. *Circulation* 2003; **107**:448–454.

42 Gustafsson I, Brendorp B, Seibaek M, Burchardt H, Hildebrandt P, Kober L, *et al.*; DIAMOND Study Group. Influence of diabetes and diabetes–gender interaction on the risk of death in patients hospitalized with congestive heart failure. *J Am Coll Cardiol* 2004; **43**:771–777.

43 Iribarren C, Karter AJ, Go AS, Ferrara A, Liu JY, Sidney S, *et al.* Glycemic control and heart failure among adult patients with diabetes. *Circulation* 2001; **103**:2668–2673.

44 Bertoni AG, Hundley WG, Massing MW, Bonds DE, Burke GL, Goff DC. Heart failure prevalence, incidence, and mortality in the elderly with diabetes. *Diabetes Care* 2004; **27**:699–703.

45 Levy D, Kenchaiah S, Larson MG, Benjamin EJ, Kupka MJ, Ho KK, *et al.* Long-term trends in the incidence of and survival with heart failure. *N Engl J Med* 2002; **347**:1397–1402.

46 Senni M, Tribouilloy CM, Rodeheffer RJ, Jacobsen SJ, Evans JM, Bailey KR, *et al.* Congestive heart failure in the community: trends in incidence and survival in a 10-year period. *Arch Intern Med* 1999; **159**:29–34.

47 Dominguez LJ, Parrinello G, Amato P, Licata G. Trends of congestive heart failure epidemiology: contrast with clinical trial results. *Cardiologia* 1999; **44**:801–808.

48 Johansson S, Wallander MA, Ruigómez A, Garcia Rodríguez LA. Incidence of newly diagnosed heart failure in UK general practice. *Eur J Heart Fail* 2001; **3**:225–231.

49 Remes J, Reunanen A, Aromaa A, Pyörala K. Incidence of heart failure in eastern Finland: a population-based surveillance study. *Eur Heart J* 1992; **13**:588–593.

50 Ubink-Veltmaat LJ, Bilo HJ, Groenier KH, Houweling ST, Rischen RO, Meyboom-de Jong B. Prevalence, incidence and mortality of type 2 diabetes mellitus revisited: a prospective population-based study in the Netherlands (ZODIAC-1). *Eur J Epidemiol* 2003; **18**:793–800.

51 Thrainsdottir I, Aspelund T, Gudnason V, Malmberg K, Sigurdsson G, Thorgeirsson G, *et al.* Increasing glucose levels and BMI predict future heart failure: experiences from the Reykjavik Study. *Eur J Heart Fail* 2007; **9**:1051–1057.

52 Mann DL. Mechanisms and models in heart failure: a combinatorial approach. *Circulation* 1999; **100**:999–1008.

53 Young ME, McNulty P, Taegtmeyer H. Adaptation and maladaptation of the heart in diabetes. Part II: potential mechanisms. *Circulation* 2002; **105**:1861–1870.

54 Guzik TJ, Mussa S, Gastaldi D, Sadowski J, Ratnatunga C, Pillai R, *et al.* Mechanisms of increased vascular superoxide production in human diabetes mellitus: role of NAD(P)H oxidase and endothelial nitric oxide synthase. *Circulation* 2002; **105**:1656–1662.

55 Stanley WC. Metabolic dysfunction in the diabetic heart. In: Stanley WC, Rydén L, eds. *The Diabetic Coronary Patient*. London: Science Press, 1999: 13–28.

56 Taegtmeyer H. Cardiac metabolism as a target for the treatment of heart failure. *Circulation* 2004; **110**:894–896.

57 Murray AJ, Anderson RE, Watson GC, Radda GK, Clarke K. Uncoupling proteins in human heart. *Lancet* 2004; **364**:1786–1788.

58 Pogatsa G: Metabolic energy metabolism in diabetes: therapeutic implications. *Coron Artery Dis* 2001; **12**(Suppl 1):S29–S33.

59 Torre-Amione G, Kapadia S, Benedict C, Oral H, Young JB, Mann DL. Proinflammatory cytokine levels in patients with depressed left ventricular ejection fraction: a report from the Studies of Left Ventricular Dysfunction (SOLVD). *J Am Coll Cardiol* 1996; **27**:1201–1206.

60 Dibbs Z, Thornby J, White BG, Mann DL. Natural variability of circulating levels of cytokines and cytokine receptors in patients with heart failure: implications for clinical trials. *J Am Coll Cardiol* 1999; **33**:1935–1942.

61 Sack MN, Rader TA, Park S, Bastin J, McCune S, Kelly DP. Fatty acid oxidation enzyme gene expression is downregulated in the failing heart. *Circulation* 1996; **94**:2837–2842.

62 Razeghi P, Young ME, Alcorn JL, Moravec CS, Frazier OH, Taegtmeyer H. Metabolic gene expression in fetal and failing human heart. *Circulation* 2001; **104**:2923–2931.

63 Wolff AA, Rotmensch HH, Stanley WC, Ferrari R. Metabolic approaches to the treatment of ischemic heart disease: the clinicians' perspective. *Heart Fail Rev* 2002; **7**:187–203.

64 Rodrigues B, Cam MC, McNeill JH, Metabolic disturbances in diabetic cardiomyopathy. *Mol Cell Biochem* 1998; **180**:53–57.

65 Randle PJ, Garland PB, Hales CN, Newsholme EA. The glucose fatty-acid cycle: its role in insulin sensitivity and the metabolic disturbances of diabetes mellitus. *Lancet* 1963; **1**:785–789.

66 Garvey WT, Hueckesteadt TP, Birnbaum MJ. Pretranslational suppression of an insulin-responsive glucose transporter in rats with diabetes mellitus. *Science* 1989; **245**:60–63.

67 Rodrigues B, McNeill JH. The diabetic heart: metabolic causes for the development of a cardiomyopathy. *Cardiovasc Res* 1992; **26**:913–922.

68 Williams SB, Goldfine AB, Timimi FK, Ting HH, Roddy MA, Simonson DC, *et al.* Acute hyperglycemia attenuates endothelium-dependent vasodilation in humans *in vivo*. *Circulation* 1998; **97**:1695–1701.

69 Yokoyama I, Momomura S, Ohtake T, Yonekura K, Nishikawa J, Sasaki Y, *et al.* Reduced myocardial flow reserve in non-insulin-dependent diabetes mellitus. *J Am Coll Cardiol* 1997; **30**:1472–1477.

70 Woodfield SL, Lundergan CF, Reiner JS, Greenhouse JS, Thompson MA, Rohrbeck SC, *et al.* Angiographic findings and outcome in diabetic patients treated with thrombolytic therapy for acute myocardial infarction: the GUSTO-I experience. *J Am Coll Cardiol* 1996; **28**:1661–1669.

71 Kannel WB, McGee DL. Diabetes and cardiovascular disease: the Framingham study. *JAMA* 1979; **241**:2035–2038.

72 Swan JW, Anker SD, Walton C, Godsland IF, Clark AL, Leyva F, *et al.* Insulin resistance in chronic heart failure: relation to severity and etiology of heart failure. *J Am Coll Cardiol* 1997; **30**:527–532.

73 Gu K, Cowie CC, Harris MI. Diabetes and decline in heart disease mortality in US adults. *JAMA* 1999; **281**:1291–1297.

74 Mosterd A, Cost B, Hoes AW, de Bruijne MC, Deckers JW, Hofman A, *et al.* The prognosis of heart failure in the general population: the Rotterdam Study. *Eur Heart J* 2001; **22**:1318–1327.

75 Cowie MR, Wood DA, Coats AJ, Thompson SG, Suresh V, Poole-Wilson PA, *et al.* Survival of patients with a new diagnosis of heart failure: a population based study. *Heart* 2000; **83**:505–510.

76 Schaufelberger M, Swedberg K, Koster M, Rosen M, Rosengren A. Decreasing one-year mortality and hospitalization rates for heart failure in Sweden: data from the Swedish Hospital Discharge Registry 1988 to 2000. *Eur Heart J* 2004; **25**:300–307.

77 Wannamethee SG, Shaper AG, Lennon L. Cardiovascular disease incidence and mortality in older men with diabetes and in men with coronary heart disease. *Heart* 2004; **90**:1398–1403.

78 Wingard DL, Barrett-Connor E. Heart disease and diabetes. In: Harris MI, Cowie CC, Stern MP, Boyko EJ, Reiber GE, Bennet PH, eds. *Diabetes in America*, 2nd edn. Washington DC: US Government Office, 1995: 429–448.

79 Vilbergsson S, Sigurdsson G, Sigvaldason H, Sigfusson N. Coronary heart disease mortality amongst non-insulin-dependent diabetic subjects in Iceland: the independent effect of diabetes. The Reykjavik Study 17-year follow up. *J Intern Med* 1998; **244**:309–316.

80 Haffner SM, Lehto S, Ronnemaa T, Pyörala K, Laakso M. Mortality from coronary heart disease in subjects with type 2 diabetes and in nondiabetic subjects with and without prior myocardial infarction. *N Engl J Med* 1998; **339**:229–234.

81 Stone PH, Muller JE, Hartwell T, York BJ, Rutherford JD, Parker CB, *et al.*; MILIS Study Group. The effect of diabetes mellitus on prognosis and serial left ventricular function after acute myocardial infarction: contribution of both coronary disease and diastolic left ventricular dysfunction to the adverse prognosis. *J Am Coll Cardiol* 1989; **14**:49–57.

82 Gwilt DJ, Petri M, Lewis PW, Nattrass M, Pentecost BL. Myocardial infarct size and mortality in diabetic patients. *Br Heart J* 1985; **54**:466–472.

83 Singer DE, Moulton AW, Nathan DM. Diabetic myocardial infarction: interaction of diabetes with other preinfarction risk factors. *Diabetes* 1989; **38**:350–357.

84 Melchior T, Gadsboll N, Hildebrandt P, Kober L, Torp-Pedersen C. Clinical characteristics, left and right ventricular ejection fraction, and long-term prognosis in patients with non-insulin-dependent diabetes surviving an acute myocardial infarction. *Diabet Med* 1996; **13**:450–456.

85 Malmberg K, Rydén L, Hamsten A, Herlitz J, Waldenström A, Wedel H; DIGAMI study group. Effects of insulin treatment on cause-specific one-year mortality and morbidity in diabetic patients with acute myocardial infarction. Diabetes Insulin-Glucose in Acute Myocardial Infarction. *Eur Heart J* 1996; **17**:1337–1344.

86 De Groote P, Lamblin N, Mouquet F, Plichon D, McFadden E, Van Belle E, *et al.* Impact of diabetes mellitus on long-term survival in patients with congestive heart failure. *Eur Heart J* 2004; **25**:656–662.

87 Thrainsdottir IS, Aspelund T, Hardarson T, Malmberg K, Sigurdsson G, Thorgeirsson G, *et al.* Glucose abnormalities and heart failure predict poor prognosis in the population-based Reykjavík Study. *Eur J Cardiovasc Prev Rehab* 2005; **12**:465–471.

88 Stratton IM, Adler AI, Neil HA, Matthews DR, Manley SE, Cull CA, *et al.*; UK Prospective Diabetes Study Group. Association of glycaemia with macrovascular and microvascular complications of type 2 diabetes (UKPDS 35): prospective observational study. *Br Med J* 2000; **321**:405–412.

89 DECODE Study Group, European Diabetes Epidemiology Group. Glucose tolerance and cardiovascular mortality: comparison of fasting and 2-hour diagnostic criteria. *Arch Intern Med* 2001; **161**:397–405.

90 CIBIS-II Investigators and Committees. The Cardiac Insufficiency Bisoprolol Study II (CIBIS-II): a randomised trial. *Lancet* 1999; **353**:9–13.

91 CONSENSUS Trial Study Group. Effects of enalapril on mortality in severe congestive heart failure: results of the Cooperative North Scandinavian Enalapril Survival Study (CONSENSUS). *N Engl J Med* 1987; **316**:1429–1435.

92 Haas SJ, Vos T, Gilberg RE, Krum H. Are β-blockers as efficacious in patients with diabetes mellitus as in patients without diabetes mellitus who have chronic heart failure? A meta-analysis of large-scale clinical trials. *Am Heart J* 2003; **146**:848–853.

93 Pitt B, Poole-Wilson PA, Segal R, Martinez FA, Dickstein K, Camm AJ, *et al.*; ELITE II investigators. Effect of losartan compared with captopril on mortality in patients with symptomatic heart failure: randomised trial – the Losartan Heart Failure Survival Study ELITE-II. *Lancet* 2000; **355**:1582–1587.

94 Vargo DL, Kramer WG, Black PK, Smith WB, Serpas T, Brater DC. Bioavailability, pharmacokinetics, and pharmacodynamics of torsemide and furosemide in patients with congestive heart failure. *Clin Pharmacol Ther* 1995; **57**:601–609.

95 Van Vliet AA, Donker AJ, Nauta JJ, Verheugt FW. Spironolactone in congestive heart failure refractory to high-dose loop diuretic and low-dose angiotensin-converting enzyme inhibitor. *Am J Cardiol* 1993; **71**:21A–28A.

96 Vitale C, Wajngaten M, Sposato B, Gebara O, Rossini P, Fini M, *et al.* Trimetazidine improves left ventricular function and quality of life in elderly patients with coronary artery disease. *Eur Heart J* 2004; **25**:1814–1821.

97 Bersin RM, Wolfe C, Kwasman M, Lau D, Klinski C, Tanaka K, *et al.* Improved hemodynamic function and mechanical efficiency in congestive heart failure with sodium dichloroacetate. *J Am Coll Cardiol* 1994; **23**:1617–1624.

98 Poirier P, Bogaty P, Garneau C, Marois L, Dumesnil JG. Diastolic dysfunction in normotensive men with well-controlled type 2 diabetes: importance of maneuvers in echocardiographic screening for preclinical diabetic cardiomyopathy. *Diabetes Care* 2001; **24**: 5–10.

99 Sánchez-Barriga JJ, Rangel A, Castaneda R, Flores D, Frati AC, Ramos MA, *et al.* Left ventricular diastolic dysfunction secondary to hyperglycemia in patients with type II diabetes. *Arch Med Res* 2001; **32**:44–47.

100 Di Bonito P, Cuomo S, Moio N, Sibilio G, Sabatini D, Quattrin S, *et al.* Diastolic dysfunction in patients with non-insulin-dependent diabetes mellitus of short duration. *Diabet Med* 1996; **13**:321–324.

101 Annonu AK, Fattah AA, Mokhtar MS, Ghareeb S, Elhendy A. Left ventricular systolic and diastolic functional abnormalities in asymptomatic patients with non-insulin-dependent diabetes mellitus. *J Am Soc Echocardiogr* 2001; **14**:885–891.

102 Henein M, Lindqvist P, Francis D, Mörner S, Waldenström A, Kazzam E. Tissue Doppler analysis of age-dependency in diastolic ventricular behaviour and filling: a cross-sectional study of healthy hearts (the Umea General Population Heart Study). *Eur Heart J* 2002; **23**:162–171.

103 Holzmann M, Olsson A, Johansson J, Jensen-Urstad M. Left ventricular diastolic function is related to glucose in a middle-aged population. *J Intern Med* 2002; **251**:415–420.

104 von Bibra, Thrainsdottir IS, Hansen A, Dounis V, Malmberg K, Rydén L. Tissue Doppler imaging for the detection and quantification of myocardial dysfunction in patients with type 2 diabetes mellitus. *Diabetes Vasc Dis Res* 2005; **2**:24–30.

105 Rydén L, Standl E, Bartnik M, Van den Berghe G, Betteridge J, de Boer MJ, *et al.*; Task Force on Diabetes and Cardiovascular Diseases of the European Society of Cardiology (ESC) and of the European Association for the Study of Diabetes (EASD). Guidelines on diabetes, pre-diabetes, and cardiovascular diseases: executive summary. *Eur Heart J* 2007; **28**:88–136.

106 Acute Infarction Ramipril Efficacy (AIRE) Study Investigators. Effect of ramipril on mortality and morbidity of survivors of acute myocardial infarction with clinical evidence of heart failure. *Lancet* 1993; **342**:821–828.

107 Konstam MA, Rousseau MF, Kronenberg MW, Udelson JE, Melin J, Stewart D, *et al.*; SOLVD Investigators. Effects of the angiotensin converting enzyme inhibitor enalapril on the long-term progression of left ventricular dysfunction in patients with heart failure. *Circulation* 1992; **86**:431–438.

108 Konstam MA, Patten RD, Thomas I, Ramahi T, La Bresh K, Goldman S, *et al.* Effects of losartan and captopril on left ventricular volumes in elderly patients with heart failure: results of the ELITE ventricular function substudy. *Am Heart J* 2000; **139**:1081–1087.

109 CONSENSUS Trial Study Group. Effects of enalapril on mortality in severe congestive heart failure: results of the Cooperative North Scandinavian Enalapril Survival Study (CONSENSUS). *N Engl J Med* 1987; **316**:1429–1435.

110 Pitt B, Poole-Wilson PA, Segal R, Martinez FA, Dickstein K, Camm AJ, *et al.*; ELITE II Investigators. Effect of losartan compared with captopril on mortality in patients with symptomatic heart failure: randomised trial – the Losartan Heart Failure Survival Study ELITE-II. *Lancet* 2000; **355**:1582–1587.

111 SOLVD Investigators. Effect of enalapril on survival in patients with reduced left ventricular ejection fraction and congestive heart failure. *N Engl J Med* 1991; **325**:293–302.

112 Rydén L, Armstrong PW, Cleland JG, Horowitz JD, Massie BM, Packer M, *et al.* Efficacy and safety of high-dose lisinopril in chronic heart failure patients at high cardiovascular risk, including those with diabetes mellitus: results from the ATLAS trial. *Eur Heart J* 2000; **21**:1967–1978.

113 Pfeffer M, Braunwald E, Moyé LA, Basta L, Brown EJ Jr, Cuddy TE, *et al.*; SAVE investigators. Effect of captopril on mortality and morbidity in patients with left ventricular dysfunction after myocardial infarction. *N Engl J Med* 1992; **327**:669–677.

114 Moyé LA, Pfeffer MA, Wun CC, Davis BR, Geltman E, Hayes D, *et al.* Uniformity of captopril benefit in the SAVE study: subgroup analysis. Survival and ventricular enlargement study. *Eur Heart J* 1994; **15**(Suppl B):2–8.

115 Zuanetti G, Latini R, Maggiono AP, Franzosi MG Santoro L, Tognoni G; GISSI 3 Investigators. Effect of the ACE inhibitor lisinopril on mortality in diabetic patients with acute myocardial infarction: data from the GISSI 3 study. *Circulation* 1997; **96**:4239–4245.

116 Herings RMC, deBoer A, Stricker BHC, Leufkens HGM, Porsius A. Hypoglycemia associated with the use of inhibitors of angiotensin-converting enzyme. *Lancet* 1996; **345**:1195–1198.

117 Morris AD, Boyle DIR, McMahon AD, Pearce H, Evans JM, Newton RW, *et al.* ACE inhibitor use is associated with hospitalization for severe hypoglycemia in patients with diabetes. *Diabetes Care* 1997; **20**:1363–1379.

118 Pfeffer MA, Swedberg K, Granger CB, Granger CB, Held P, McMurray JJ, *et al.*; CHARM Investigators and Committees. Effects of candesartan on mortality and morbidity in patients with chronic heart failure: the CHARM-Overall programme. *Lancet* 2003; **362**:759–766.

119 MacDonald MR, Petrie MC, Varyani F, Ostergren J, Michelson EL, Young JB, *et al.*; CHARM Investigators. Impact of diabetes on outcomes in patients with low and preserved ejection fraction heart failure: an analysis of the candesartan in Heart failure: assessment of Reduction in Mortality and morbidity (CHARM) programme. *Eur Heart J* 2008; **29**:1377–1385.

120 Opie LH, Thomas M. Propranolol and experimental myocardial infarction: substrate effects. *Postgrad Med J* 1976; **52**(Suppl 4):124–133.

121 Dávila-Román VG, Vedala G, Herrero P, de las Fuentes L, Rogers JG, Kelly DP, *et al.* Altered myocardial fatty acid and glucose metabolism in idiopathic dilated cardiomyopathy. *J Am Coll Cardiol* 2002; **40**:271–277.

122 CIBIS-II Investigators and Committees. The Cardiac Insufficiency Bisoprolol Study II (CIBIS-II): a randomised trial. *Lancet* 1999; **353**:9–13.

123 Haas SJ, Vos T, Gilberg RE, Krum H. Are β-blockers as efficacious in patients with diabetes mellitus as in patients without diabetes mellitus who have chronic heart failure? A meta-analysis of large-scale clinical trials. *Am Heart J* 2003; **146**:848–853.

124 Hjalmarson A, Goldstein S, Fagerberg B, Wedel H, Waagstein F, Kjekshus J, *et al.*; for the MERIT-HF Study Group. Effects of controlled-release metoprolol on total mortality, hospitalizations, and well-being in patients with heart failure: the Metoprolol CR/XL Randomized Intervention Trial in Congestive Heart Failure (MERIT-HF). *JAMA* 2000; **283**:1295–1302.

125 Deedwania PC, Giles TD, Klibaner M, Ghali JK, Herlitz J, Hildebrandt P, *et al.*; MERIT-HF Study Group. Efficacy, safety and tolerability of metoprolol CR/XL in patients with diabetes and chronic heart failure: experiences from MERIT-HF. *Am Heart J* 2005; **149**: 159–167.

126 Packer M, Coats AJ, Fowler MB, Katus HA, Krum H, Mohacsi P, *et al.*; Carvedilol Prospective Randomized Cumulative Survival Study Group. Effect of carvedilol on survival in severe chronic heart failure. *N Engl J Med* 2001; **344**:1651–1658.

127 Pitt B, Zannad F, Remme WJ, Cody R, Castaigne A, Perez A, *et al.*; Randomized Aldactone Evaluation Study Investigators. The effects of spironolactone on morbidity and mortality in patients with severe heart failure. *N Engl J Med* 1999; **341**:709–717.

128 Kjekshus J, Apetrei E, Barrios V, Böhm M, Cleland JG, Cornel JH, *et al.*; CORONA Group. Rosuvastatin in older patients with systolic heart failure. *N Engl J Med* 2007; **357**:2248–2261.

129 Tavazzi L, Maggioni AP, Marchioli R, Barlera S, Franzosi MG, Latini R, *et al.*; GISSI-HF Investigators. Effect of rosuvastatin in patients with chronic heart failure (the GISSI-HF trial): a randomised, double-blind, placebo-controlled trial. *Lancet* 2008; **372**:1231–1239.

130 Stettler C, Allemann S, Jüni P, Cull CA, Holman RR, Egger M, *et al.* Glycemic control and macrovascular disease in types 1 and 2 diabetes mellitus: meta-analysis of randomized trials. *Am Heart J* 2006; **152**:27–38.

131 Action to Control Cardiovascular Risk in Diabetes Study Group. Effects of intensive glucose lowering in type 2 diabetes. *N Engl J Med* 2008; **358**:2545–2559.

132 Patel A, MacMahon S, Chalmers J, Neal B, Billot L, Woodward M, *et al.*; ADVANCE Collaborative Group. Intensive blood glucose control and vascular outcomes in patients with type 2 diabetes. *N Engl J Med* 2008; **358**:2560–2572.

133 Dormandy JA, Charbonnel B, Eckland DJ, Erdmann E, Massi-Benedetti M, Moules IK, *et al.* Secondary prevention of macrovascular events in patients with type 2 diabetes in the PROactive Study (Prospective Pioglitazone Clinical Trial in Macrovascular Events): a randomised controlled trial. *Lancet* 2005; **366**:1279–1289.

134 Singh S, Loke YK, Furberg CD. Long-term risk of cardiovascular events with rosiglitazone: a meta-analysis. *JAMA* 2007; **298**: 1189–1195.

135 Lincoff AM, Wolski K, Nicholls SJ, Nissen SE. Pioglitazone and risk of cardiovascular events in patients with type 2 diabetes mellitus: a meta-analysis of randomized trials. *JAMA* 2007; **298**:1180–1188.

136 Lipscombe LL, Gomes T, Lévesque LE, Hux JE, Juurlink DN, Alter DA. Thiazolidinediones and cardiovascular outcomes in older patients with diabetes. *JAMA* 2007; **298**:2634–2643.

137 Parsonage WA, Hetmanski D, Cowley AJ. Beneficial haemodynamic effects of insulin in chronic heart failure. *Heart* 2001; **85**:508–513.

138 McNulty PH, Pfau S, Deckelbaum LI. Effect of plasma insulin level on myocardial blood flow and its mechanism of action. *Am J Cardiol* 2000; **85**:161–165.

139 Mellbin L G, Malmberg K, Norhammar A, Wedel H, Rydén L; DIGAMI 2 Investigators. The impact of glucose lowering treatment on long-term prognosis in patients with type 2 diabetes and myocardial infarction: a report from the DIGAMI 2 trial. *Europ Heart J* 2008; **29**:166–176.

140 Smooke S, Horwich TB, Fonarow GC. Insulin-treated diabetes is associated with a marked increase in mortality in patients with advanced heart failure. *Am Heart J* 2005; **149**:168–174.

141 Khoury VK, Haluska B, Prins J, Marwick TH. Effects of glucose–insulin–potassium infusion on chronic ischaemic left ventricular dysfunction. *Heart* 2003; **89**:61–65.

142 Skyler JS, Bergenstal R, Bonow RO, Buse J, Deedwania P, Gale EA, *et al.* Intensive glycemic control and the prevention of cardiovascular events: implications of the ACCORD, ADVANCE, and VA Diabetes Trials: a position statement of the American Diabetes Association and a Scientific Statement of the American College of Cardiology Foundation and the American Heart Association. *Circulation* 2009; **53**:298–304.

143 Rask-Madsen C, Ihlemann N, Krarup T, Christiansen E, Kober L, Nervil Kistorp C, *et al.* Insulin therapy improves insulin-stimulated endothelial function in patients with type 2 diabetes and ischemic heart disease. *Diabetes* 2001; **50**:2611–2618.

144 von Bibra H, Hansen A, Dounis V, Bystedt T, Malmberg K, Ryden L. Augmented metabolic control improves myocardial diastolic function and perfusion in patients with non-insulin dependent diabetes. *Heart* 2004; **90**:1483–1484.

145 Jarnert C, Landstedt-Hallin L, Malmberg K, Melcher A, Ohrvik J, Persson H, *et al.* A randomized trial on the impact of strict glycaemic control on myocardial diastolic function and perfusion reserve: a report from the DADD (Diabetes mellitus And Diastolic Dysfunction) study. *Eur J Heart Fail* 2009; **11**:39–47.

146 Thrainsdottir IS, von Bibra H, Malmberg K, Ryden L. Effects of trimetazidine on left ventricular function in patients with type 2 diabetes and heart failure. *J Cardiovasc Pharmacol* 2004; **44**:101–108.

147 Schmidt-Schweda S, Holubarsch C. First clinical trial with etomoxir in patients with chronic congestive heart failure. *Clin Sci (Lond)* 2000; **99**:27–35.

148 Tuunanen H, Engblom E, Naum A, Någren K, Scheinin M, Hesse B, *et al.* Trimetazidine, a metabolic modulator, has cardiac and extracardiac benefits in idiopathic dilated cardiomyopathy. *Circulation* 2008; **118**:1250–1258.

42 Cerebrovascular Disease

Colum F. Amory & Jesse Weinberger
Mount Sinai School of Medicine, New York, NY, USA

Keypoints

- Diabetes is a strong and independent risk factor for ischemic cerebrovascular disease with a relative risk of around two.
- Ischemic stroke in the patient with diabetes has worse outcomes, including a higher rate of mortality than in patients without diabetes.
- While transient ischemic attacks (TIA) appear to occur less frequently in those with diabetes, people with diabetes who experience a TIA are more likely to go on to have a completed stroke in the immediate period following.
- The patient with diabetes is predisposed to vascular events, including stroke, for a number of reasons including premature atherosclerosis, reduced response to nitric oxide and a general state of hypercoagulability.
- Prevention of stroke in the patient with diabetes is best accomplished through aggressive management of coexisting hypertension and hyperlipidemia, as well as lifestyle modification.
- Reduction of glycated hemoglobin as a proxy for good glycemic control is likely to be associated with a reduction of macrovascular events.
- Aggressive management of hyperglycemia in the acute stroke period may improve outcomes.

Epidemiology of stroke in general

Cerebrovascular disease is a leading cause of morbidity and mortality. It is a highly prevalent disease with approximately 700 000 strokes occurring each year in the USA. Of these, 500 000 are first time events, while 200 000 are recurrent [1].

Stroke is the third leading cause of death in the USA, following heart disease and all forms of cancer. Thus, a woman is more than twice as likely to die from a stroke than she is from breast cancer, and one and a half times as likely as from lung cancer [2]. Furthermore, it is the number one reason listed for discharge diagnosis for patients discharged from hospitals to chronic care facilities. In total, the cost of stroke to the health care system in the USA was $62.7 billion in the year 2007 [1].

Statistics in other countries are similar to those seen in the USA. The Oxford Vascular Study [3], which compiled stroke statistics for every person in the county of Oxfordshire, demonstrated an overall incidence of 1.62 strokes per 1000 patients per year. The WHO MONICA study looked at 21 populations in 11 countries, 10 European countries as well as China, and found an incidence of 125–361/100 000 patients in men, and 61–194/100 000 in women [4].

Textbook of Diabetes, 4th edition. Edited by R. Holt, C. Cockram, A. Flyvbjerg and B. Goldstein. © 2010 Blackwell Publishing.

Diabetes as a risk factor for stroke

There is strong evidence that diabetes mellitus, whether type 1 (T1DM) or type 2 (T2DM), is a strong risk factor for ischemic cerebrovascular disease (Table 42.1). Observational studies have demonstrated associations between the two diseases. A model created from data from the Framingham Heart Study showed that diabetes confers an increased relative risk of 1.4 in men and 1.72 in women [5]. The Honolulu Heart Study showed that diabetes increases the risk of thromboembolic stroke between two- to threefold over those without the disease in Japanese men living in Hawaii [6].

The effect of diabetes is stronger in ethnic minorities in the USA. The Greater Cincinnati and Northern Kentucky Stroke Study found that as a sole risk factor, diabetes increased the odds ratio for having an ischemic stroke by 2.1 in Caucasians; however, in African-Americans that odds ratio was increased by 2.7. These results held true across all age cohorts [7].

Similarly, the Northern Manhattan Study found that diabetes was a stronger risk factor for ischemic stroke among African-Americans and Caribbean Latinos than among Caucasians. In these ethnicities, diabetes increased stroke risk by 1.8 and 2.1, respectively, partly because of increased prevalence of the disease. The fraction of strokes that could be directly attributable to diabetes as a risk factor was 14% among African-Americans and 10% among Caribbean Latinos [8].

The Copenhagen City Heart Study found a difference in the effect of diabetes among men and women. Thus, while diabetes

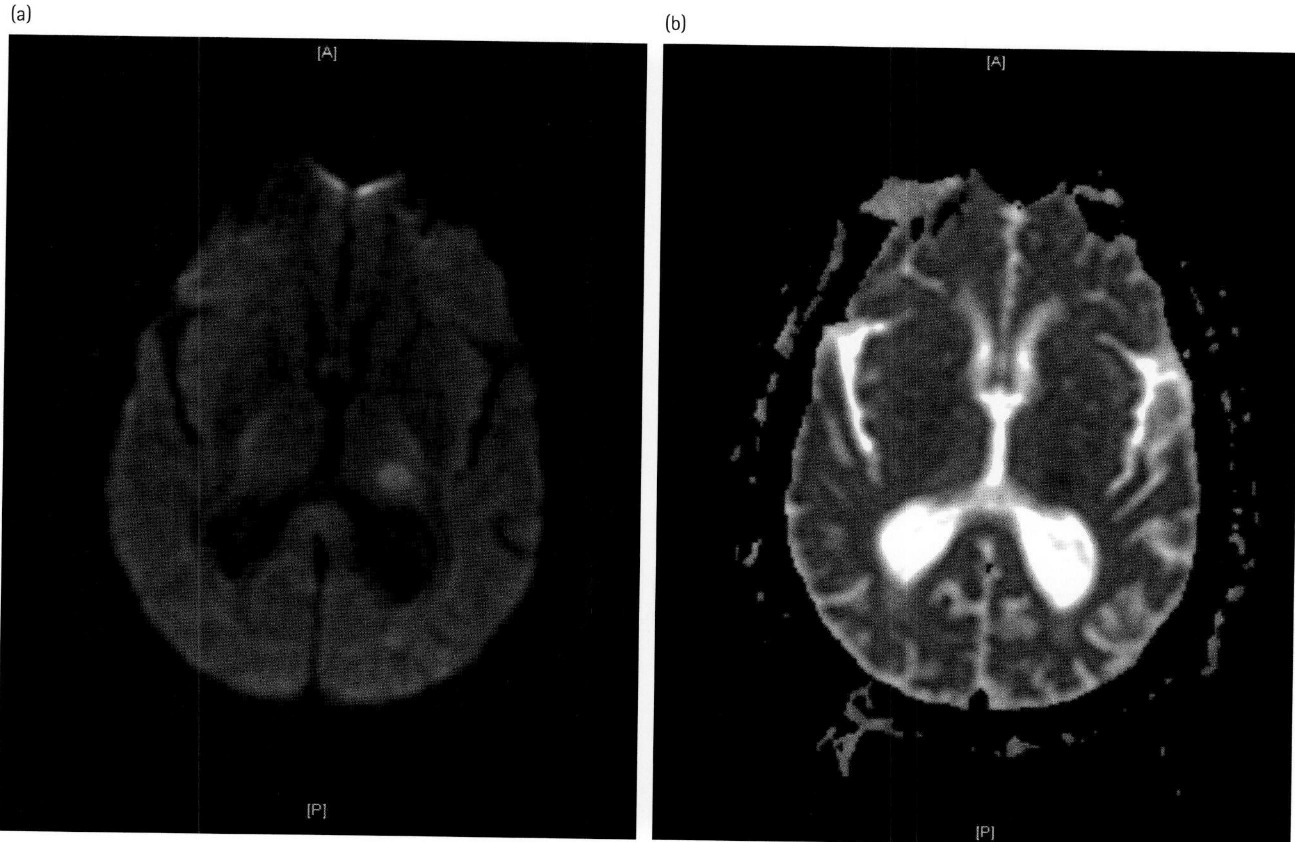

Figure 42.1 Lacunar infarct in the left posterior thalamus. (a) Diffusion weighted imaging, showing hyperintensity in the area of restricted diffusion, corresponding to acute ischemia. (b) Apparent diffusion coefficient image corresponding to the slice seen in (a), demonstrating hypointensity in the same distribution, confirming the presence of acute ischemia.

Table 42.1 Risk factors for stroke.

Hypertension
Diabetes
Tobacco use
Hyperlipidemia
Atrial fibrillation
Carotid artery disease

increased the relative risk of first stroke, incident stroke and hospital admission for stroke among men by 1.5–2, among women the same relative risks were increased by 2–6.5 [9].

In addition to its effects as a sole risk factor, diabetes also exacerbates the effects of other risk factors. Thus, in patients with isolated systolic hypertension, diabetes confers additional risk of ischemic stroke or transient ischemic attack (TIA).

Stroke in patients with diabetes

In epidemiologic studies, ischemic stroke occurs at a younger age in patients who have diabetes. They are also more likely to be African-American. Among other risk factors, those with diabetes who have ischemic stroke are more likely to have hypertension, hyperlipidemia and to have experienced a myocardial infarction (MI) in the past [7].

Furthermore, diabetes increases the risk of death from stroke. In a prospective study in a Finnish cohort, men had an increased relative risk of 6 for mortality from ischemic stroke, while women had a relative risk of 8.2. These relative risks were higher than those for systolic blood pressure (BP), smoking or total serum cholesterol. In this cohort, the fraction of stroke deaths directly attributable to diabetes were 16% in men and 33.3% in women [10].

In terms of stroke subtype, diabetes is most commonly associated with lacunar infarcts. These are small deep infarcts in the territory of a single penetrating arterial branch. Conversely, the highest prevalence of diabetes is found in patients with demonstrable microvascular disease. Similarly, lacunar disease is more likely to be associated with diabetes than hemorrhages in the same location (Figure 42.1) [11–14].

Diabetes is associated with both extracranial and intracranial stenosis. In one study of 510 patients referred for asymptomatic carotid bruits, only 200 had extracranial stenosis by Doppler examination. Sixty-six had asymptomatic intracranial stenosis, of

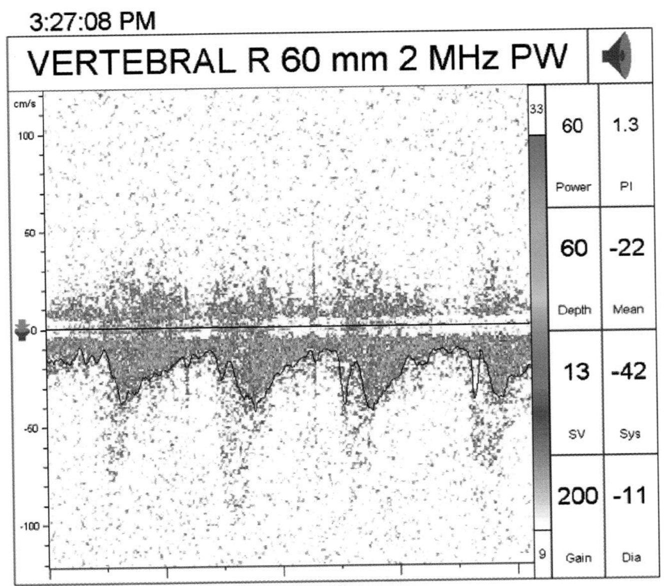

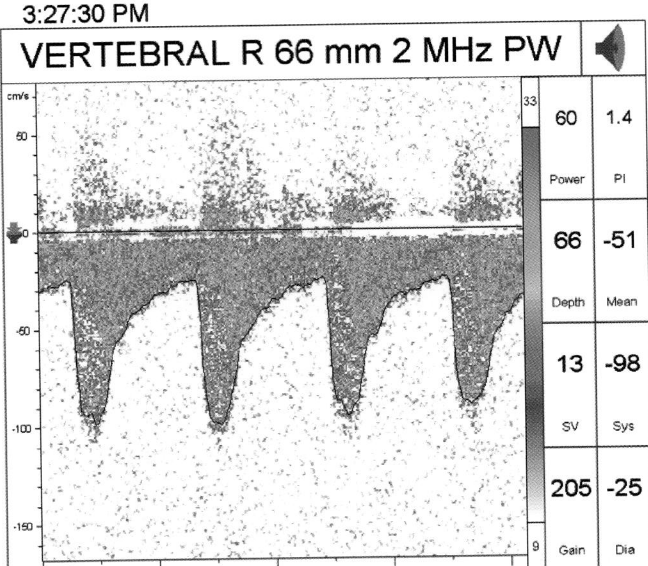

Figure 42.2 Intracranial vertebral artery stenosis as seen by transcranial Dopplers. The first image shows normal flow pre-stenosis, while the second image shows increased velocity of flow post-stenosis.

whom 37 had concurrent extracranial stenosis. Of the patients with intracranial stenosis, 19 had diabetes (Figure 42.2) [15].

TIA is less common in those with diabetes than in those not having the disease. This may indicate that patients with diabetes are more likely to present with completed infarct rather than reversible ischemia [16]; however, patients with diabetes who do present with TIA are more likely to go on to full-blown ischemic stroke in the next 2 days as predicted by the ABCD2 score. This score stratifies patients with TIA by the following factors: age greater than 60 years, BP greater than 140/90 mmHg, clinical features of motor or speech involvement, duration greater than 60 minutes and diabetes [17].

Diabetes is a risk factor for coronary artery disease (CAD), and thus for MI and subsequent development of atrial fibrillation. In one large retrospective study of the relation between diabetes and atrial fibrillation or atrial flutter, diabetes was found after logistic regression to be a strong independent predictor for atrial arrhythmias in a review of over 850 000 charts over a 10-year period. The odds ratio found for diabetes was 2.13, 95% confidence interval (CI) 2.10–2.16 [18]. In turn, atrial fibrillation has been repeatedly demonstrated to be a strong risk factor for cardioembolic stroke, with an estimated 75 000 strokes per year attributable to the arrhythmia [19].

Furthermore, diabetes increases the risk of cardiac embolization. The CHADS2 score is a validated method of stratifying risk of cardioembolic stroke in patients with atrial fibrillation. It assigns one point each for the presence of congestive heart failure (CHF), hypertension, age greater than 75 years, and diabetes, and two points for previous stroke or TIA. Each point increase was associated with a 1.5-fold increased risk of stroke. Diabetes alone, then, would increase the risk of stroke in a patient with atrial fibrillation from 1.9 to 2.8 [20]. While the CHADS2 score is not perfect, and attempts have been made to make it more precise [21], it has the benefit of being very easy to use, thus guiding the non-stroke practitioner towards using anticoagulation in the appropriate section of the population.

In large observational studies, there has not appeared to be an association between diabetes and hemorrhagic strokes. By contrast, in the Hemorrhagic Stroke Project, a case–control study of young patients with intracerebral hemorrhage, diabetes conferred an adjusted odds ration of 2.4. The risk factor with the most impact was, as predicted, hypertension, which outweighed the contribution from diabetes by greater than twofold [22].

Intermediate hyperglycemia and other risk factors

While it is well established that diabetes is a strong risk factor for ischemic stroke, forms of intermediate hyperglycemia are not so clearly indicated as risk factors. Selvin *et al.* [23] looked at people with and without diabetes in the Atherosclerosis Risk In Communities (ARIC) trial and compared hemoglobin A_{1c} (HbA_{1c}) levels drawn at a specified visit, not necessarily related to time of incident stroke. With increasing tertiles of HbA_{1c} across the normal distribution within each group, the risk of stroke increased in both those with diabetes and those without the disease, although it was only in those with diabetes that the difference achieved statistical significance [23].

In contrast, Myint *et al.* [24] abstracted data from the European Prospective Investigation into Cancer (EPIC) on HbA_{1c} levels in patients without known diabetes and correlated these data with stroke risk. In this population, it was only after HbA_{1c} levels were higher than 7.0% (53 mmol/mol) that an increased risk of stroke was demonstrated, compared to those patients with HbA_{1c} less than 5.0% (31 mmol/mol). Given that these patients are most likely to have undiagnosed diabetes, this finding may not implicate chronic hyperglycemia alone as the primary risk factor for stroke [24].

Insulin resistance (IR), another forme fruste of diabetes, likewise has demonstrated conflicting evidence for an association with stroke. The ARIC study investigated hyperinsulinemia in those without diabetes and found a mild increase in risk of stroke of 1.19 with each increase of 50 pmol/L of fasting insulin. After adjustment for other risk factors such as age, systolic BP and smoking, the increase in risk was not as well defined [25].

Obesity, a proxy for insulin resistance and intermediate hyperglycemia, has also been linked to stroke through a number of epidemiologic studies. For example, the Copenhagen City Heart Study found that body mass index (BMI) was independently associated with increased risk of stroke [26]. Similarly, the Nurses' Health Study found, as expected, an increasing risk of stroke with increasing BMI, with a relative risk of stroke of 2.37 (95% CI 1.60–3.50) seen in patients with BMI >32 kg/m^2 [27]; however, ARIC was unable to demonstrate any relationship between BMI and stroke, or between waist : hip ratio, a better measurement of abdominal obesity, and stroke [25]. In addition, when adjustment for cardiovascular risks was performed, the relative risk of BMI for stroke was once again attenuated.

Although these individual forms of intermediate hyperglycemia have not conclusively been shown to predispose people to stroke, the constellation of diseases together called the metabolic syndrome has been. The combination of hypertension, hyperlipidemia, IR and abdominal obesity creates an environment that is highly susceptible to vascular damage and ischemic sequelae.

In a Finnish cohort, the metabolic syndrome in the absence of diabetes or cardiovascular disease (CVD) was associated with stroke with a relative risk of around 2, after adjustment for multiple other risk factors [28]. Similarly, a cohort from the ARIC study who likewise was free of diabetes, coronary heart disease (CHD) or stroke, had an increased risk of 1.5–2.0 for ischemic stroke. In addition, when separating out each risk factor, there appeared to be a synergistic effect from the combination over the relative risks inherent in each component [29].

Pathophysiology of ischemic stroke in diabetes

Diabetes predisposes patients to vascular thrombo-occlusive events in a number of ways. There is accelerated atherosclerosis in both large and medium sized vessels. There is disordered endothelial response and the blood of the patient with diabetes is hypercoagulable [30].

Carotid intima-media thickness (cIMT) is a useful proxy for early atherosclerosis, as it is easily measured by Doppler. Furthermore, cIMT is associated with primary stroke, with an increased relative risk per standard deviation (0.163 mm) of 1.57 in patients who had not had a previous stroke [31]. It also predicts recurrent stroke, with each 0.1 mm of increase in cIMT associated with an increased risk of 18% [32].

Diabetes is associated with increased cIMT. The IR Atherosclerosis Study demonstrated an increase in common cIMT in patients with chronic diabetes, but not in those with newly diagnosed diabetes. Nor was there an association with internal cIMT [33].

Conversely, patients with diabetes and stroke have been found to have greater cIMT. In one study of 438 Japanese patients with T2DM, common cIMT was significantly higher in those who had stroke, even after adjustment for age, BMI and smoking status [34]. Similarly, in a Czech cohort, cIMT was increased in stroke patients with diabetes [35].

Atherosclerosis also affects the ability of endothelium to release nitric oxide (NO), a potent vasodilatator. The diabetic blood vessel has either reduced NO production or altered NO metabolism. In addition to its vasodilatating effects, NO protects against platelet aggregation and enables the blood vessel to withstand ischemic conditions. With decreased NO activity, the vessel will tend more towards vasoconstriction, with predictably poor response to ischemia.

Stroke patients have been demonstrated to have decreased NO in circulating blood, along with increased peroxynitrite ($ONOO^-$), a reactive oxygen species. These results were particularly true in larger strokes. Because the measurements were performed for acute stroke, these levels are likely to represent the outcome of ischemia rather than the cause; however, the correlation supports a role for decreased NO in the effects of stroke [36].

The cerebral vasculature has a diminished response to inhibition of NO synthase (NOS). In a small study of men with diabetes treated with a synthetic NOS inhibitor, NG-monomethyl-L-arginine (L-NMMA), the blood flow through the internal carotid artery was significantly lower than in control subjects treated likewise [37].

As further indirect evidence of the role of NO in stroke, 3-hydroxy-3-methyl-glutaryl coenzyme A (HMG-CoA) reductase inhibitors (statins) have multiple beneficial effects beyond their most common, that of lowering plasma cholesterol. Among these effects is increasing expression of endothelial NOS as well as decreasing the activity of Rho-kinase, a proconstrictor enzyme [38]. Statins have been demonstrated to lower the risk of recurrent stroke in multiple large studies [39–41]. Whether the beneficial effect of statins in stroke is because of their cholesterol lowering effect, their ability to stabilize atherosclerotic plaques, their effects on vascular function or more likely a combination of all of the above, is very difficult to separate.

In addition to the above predisposing factors, the blood of the patient with diabetes is hypercoagulable. Studies have demonstrated increased thrombin generation [42], increased prothrombin fragments and increased thrombin–antithrombin III complexes [43]. Furthermore, the elevated prothrombotic levels were significantly associated with macroangiopathic complications.

Thrombus formation is further promoted by platelet hyper-reactivity in the blood of the patient with diabetes. In patients with metabolic syndrome, platelets have been shown to have increased activity both through closure time as measured by the platelet function analyzer (PFA-100), increased fibrinogen binding after exposure to ADP, implying activation of the GPIIa/IIIb receptors, and by expression of activated ligands on the platelet surface [44]. In full-blown diabetes, platelets were hyperreactive as measured by light transmittance aggregometry and expression of surface ligands [45].

Thus, taken together, the person with diabetes has a vascular environment that is highly susceptible to thrombo-occlusive complications. With early atherosclerosis and disordered endothelial response, the conditions are predisposed to thrombophilia. The blood, in its hypercoagulable state combined with platelets that are highly active in themselves, is far more likely to form clots.

Lacunar strokes are caused by damage to smaller parenchymal vessels. The most common cause is microatheroma, as demonstrated in pathologic case series published by Fisher [46–48], the neurologist responsible for naming the lacunar syndromes. Lipohyalinosis and fibrinoid necrosis also cause microangiopathies, and both are most commonly found in the setting of chronic hypertension of severe acute BP elevations, as seen in hypertensive encephalopathy [49,50].

Primary prevention of stroke in the patient with diabetes

Primary prevention of stroke is of paramount importance as the disability from stroke and health care costs associated with the acute and chronic care of stroke are so extensive. The approach to prevention in the patient with diabetes is of necessity multifactorial.

Medical therapy aimed at achieving normoglycemia is the foundation. The Diabetes Control and Complications Trial (DCCT) investigated intensive insulin regimens including subcutaneous insulin injections and external insulin pumps in those with T1DM. The goal for treatment was HbA_{1c} levels of less than 6.05% (42 mmol/mol). The comparison group had no such goals outside of prevention of hyperglycemia or hypoglycemia [51].

The intensive treatment group achieved a reduction in the combined endpoints of non-fatal MI or stroke, cardiac death or revascularization procedure of 57%. The majority of this improvement was associated with the decrease in HbA_{1c} [51].

Among oral hypoglycemic agents, metformin has been shown to decrease diabetes-related endpoints including stroke by 32% and diabetes-related mortality including stroke by 42% when compared with conventional therapy. Furthermore, it was more effective in reducing these outcomes when compared with other intensive therapies such as sulfonylureas (e.g. chlorpropamide or glibenclamide) or insulin. It should be noted that the HbA_{1c} levels were similar between the treatment groups, and so the benefits obtained were not explicable on the basis of improved glycemic control [52].

Rosiglitazone, a thiazolidinedione, has been linked with increased risk of MI and death from cardiovascular causes. Stroke was not assessed separately in the meta-analysis reporting these findings [53]. In a more recent multicenter, open-label trial directly assessing the effect of rosiglitazone on cardiovascular outcomes, the use of rosiglitazone was associated with a non-significant reduction in stroke (HR 0.72, 95% CI 0.49–1.06) [54]. Pioglitazone, another medication in the same class, was not associated with worse cardiovascular outcomes, including stroke, and, in fact, reduced a secondary outcome of all-cause mortality, non-fatal MI and non-fatal stroke by 16% [55].

The UK Prospective Diabetes Study (UKPDS) failed to show any reduction in macrovascular complications of T2DM despite an 11% reduction in HbA_{1c} in the intensive treatment group. Microvascular complications such as retinopathy and neuropathy were significantly reduced [56]. A 10-year follow-up study of the same cohort after attempts to maintain treatment differences had desisted showed that the original treatment cohort had persistent decreases in microvascular complications as well as in MIs and deaths from any cause but not CVA [57]. Thus, glycemic control, at least in those with T2DM, has not been linked to a reduction in risk for stroke.

Given how susceptible people with diabetes are to the effects of other vascular risk factors such as hypertension and hyperlipidemia, the therapeutic regimen must also address these states. In treating hypertension in people with diabetes, the classes of medications with effects on the renin angiotensin system appear to have the greatest benefit.

The Hypertensive Old People in Edinburgh (HOPE) trial examined patients either with vascular disease (including CAD or stroke) or diabetes plus one other cardiovascular risk factor such as hypertension, tobacco use or elevated low density lipoprotein levels. In this high risk population, ramipril, an angiotensin-converting enzyme inhibitor (ACEi), decreased the risk of death from cardiovascular causes with a relative risk of 0.74 and reduced the risk of stroke with a relative risk of 0.68. As the mean reduction in BP was only 3/2, the benefits were not attributable to the BP lowering effect of the medication. The effect was similar whether or not the patients had had a stroke prior to enrollment [58].

The Losartan Intervention for Endpoint Reduction in Hypertension (LIFE) trial examined patients with diabetes, hypertension and left ventricular hypertrophy. Participants were either treated with losartan, an angiotensin receptor blocker (ARB) or atenolol. Although, once again, both medications achieved the same reduction in BP, the primary endpoint of cardiovascular mortality, MI or non-fatal stroke was reduced with a relative risk of 0.76 in the Losartan group. Notably in this trial, only 40% of participants achieved a systolic BP of less than 140 mmHg, implying that further benefits would likely accrue with more intensive management [59].

A recent trial of intensive multifactorial medical management in patients with diabetes with microalbuminuria showed a reduction in all-cause mortality, cardiovascular mortality and cardiovascular events. The regimen was designed to achieve the following goals: HbA_{1c} levels of less than 6.5% (48 mmol/mol), fasting total serum cholesterol levels of less than 175 mg/dL (4.5 mmol/L), systolic BP less than 130 mmHg and diastolic BP less than 80 mmHg. Stroke was not a pre-specified endpoint in this study; however, there were six strokes in six patients in the intensive medical group, compared with 30 strokes in 18 patients in the control group [60].

While antiplatelet treatment is recommended for the primary prevention of CAD, the Anti-Thrombotic Trialists' Collaboration meta-analysis failed to demonstrate a significant improvement in the primary prevention of ischemic stroke in patients with diabetes. Overall, there were nearly 5000 patients treated with aspirin, with only a 7% reduction in serious vascular events. The confidence interval was wide enough to include a possible 25% risk reduction, a number that is consistent with the prevention of secondary stroke in this population. It may be in this population at high risk, that the potential benefits of prophylactic aspirin outweigh the hemorrhagic complications [61].

Most of the early trials of antithrombotic medications were performed only on men. In the Women's Health Study, a study performed among female health professionals with no history of coronary or cerebrovascular disease, low dose aspirin (100 mg every other day) was associated with a 17% risk reduction in stroke, a result of a 24% risk reduction in ischemic stroke and a non-significant increase in hemorrhagic stroke. These findings were especially pronounced in women older than age 65 at the time of enrollment, as well as in the subgroup with diabetes [62].

Treatment of acute stroke in the patient with diabetes

Treatment of acute stroke is limited by the vulnerability of the neuron to ischemic insult. With decreasing cerebral blood flow (CBF), the parenchyma becomes less likely to recover from even short durations of ischemia. With CBF less than 200 mL/kg of tissue, neurologic dysfunction begins to appear, but it is not until CBF falls below 100 mL/kg of tissue that irreversible ischemia occurs, in a matter of minutes [63].

Thrombolysis has been demonstrated to be effective in the treatment of acute stroke, as long as the medication is given within the first 3 hours after symptom onset, as defined by the last time the patient was seen at their neurologic functional baseline (Table 42.2). The National Institute of Neurologic Disorders (NINDS) trial of intravenous tissue plasminogen activator (t-PA) demonstrated a 30–50% increased likelihood of minimal or no disability 3 months after treatment. The thrombolysis was associated with a 6.4% chance of symptomatic intracranial hemorrhage, but mortality data at 3 months were not statistically different between the treatment and placebo groups [64].

Table 42.2 Management of acute ischemic stroke.

0–3 hours	Intravenous t-PA
0–6 hours	Intra-arterial t-PA
0–8 hours	Mechanical clot retrieval (MERCI device)
Permissive hypertension for the first 3–5 days	
Aspiration precautions	
DVT prophylaxis	
Intravenous t-PA is the only acute intervention approved by the US FDA. Both intra-arterial t-PA and mechanical clot retrieval remain experimental, although widely used. IV t-PA should remain the standard of care when it is not contraindicated, with the other interventions to be used as auxiliary therapy	

DVT, deep venous thrombosis; FDA, Food and Drug Administration; t-PA, tissue plasminogen activator.

Based on this trial, treatment with intravenous t-PA has become standard of care in this early time period. While recent data from the ECASS-III trial suggest that it is not only safe but clinically effective to a lesser degree in a select group of patients to give intravenous t-PA in the window between 3 and 4.5 hours, this has not yet become standard practice. In addition, patients with diabetes who had a previous stroke by history or on imaging were excluded from the trial [65].

Thrombolysis in the patient with diabetes and acute stroke is not as successful as in the general population. In one series of 27 patients treated with intravenous t-PA, none of the patients with diabetes achieved recanalization of the occluded artery as measured by transcranial Doppler [66]. The series was not large enough to demonstrate a significant difference. In another study examining which factors might predict major neurologic improvement in patients treated with intravenous t-PA, there was a trend towards patients with diabetes being less likely to achieve that improvement [67].

Beyond intravenous thrombolysis, intra-arterial thrombolysis has been examined in patients up to 6 hours after the onset of stroke symptoms. The Prolyse in Acute Cerebral Thromboembolism II (PROACT II) trial found that patients treated with intra-arterial urokinase had a 58% relative risk reduction to achieve minimal or no functional disability at 90 days after treatment. Mortality rates were comparable, and recanalization rates were highly improved with the medication [68]. Current guidelines support the use of intra-arterial thrombolysis in the period of time between 3 and 6 hours, but the medication has not been approved by the US Federal Drug Administration (FDA) for this indication [69].

In one case series of 100 patients treated with intra-arterial thrombolysis with urokinase, diabetes was associated with poor functional outcome at 3 months. It was not associated with symptomatic intracranial hemorrhage [70], but because diabetes is independently associated with worse outcomes following acute ischemic stroke, it is not clear whether these data have any meaning for clinical practice.

Hyperglycemia at the time of stroke treatment is associated with worsened outcomes. In a series of 73 patients treated with intravenous t-PA, age, diabetes, admission glucose greater than 140 mg/dL (7.8 mmol/L) and early reocclusion on transcranial Doppler imaging were significantly associated with worsened functional outcome as defined by a score of greater than 3 on the modified Rankin scale, however, after logistic regression, only the hyperglycemia remained as an independent predictor of poor outcome. In particular, it was associated with larger infarct size, lesser degree of neurologic improvement and worse clinical outcome if recanalization was achieved [71].

Similarly, baseline hyperglycemia is associated with a greater likelihood of going on to symptomatic intracranial hemorrhage after intravenous thrombolysis. There appears to be a dose–response relationship between levels of serum glucose and likelihood of hemorrhage. This was especially true when levels were >11.1 mmol/L (200 mg/dL), where 25% of patients had symptomatic intracranial hemorrhage. In a repeat analysis substituting the presence of diabetes for glucose levels, diabetes was associated with an odds ratio of 3.61 for all hemorrhages and 7.46 for symptomatic hemorrhage [72].

Furthermore, both those patients who acutely worsened and those patients who showed lack of improvement at 24 hours were more likely to have elevated blood glucose at baseline. Hyperacute worsening in patients treated with either intravenous or intra-arterial thrombolysis, or both, was not surprisingly associated with intracerebral hemorrhage and lack of recanalization, but it was also associated with higher serum glucose. With every increase of 50 mg/dL glucose, the odds ratio for worsened outcome was 1.50, and the odds ratio for mortality was 1.38. Even in those patients who did achieve recanalization, higher blood glucose predicted worse outcomes [73].

Similarly, serum glucose greater than 144 mg/dL, as well as cortical involvement and time to treatment were independent predictors of lack of improvement at 24 hours after treatment with intravenous thrombolysis. The odds ratio for hyperglycemia was 2.89. Furthermore, lack of improvement at 24 hours predicted poor functional outcome at 3 months [74].

While these data are understandably disheartening, they should by no means be taken to imply that patients with diabetes and acute stroke should not receive thrombolysis, nor that these patients do not benefit from the treatment. Furthermore, it is not clear whether the hyperglycemia that is seen in patients with acute stroke and diabetes is secondary to the ischemic insult as a stress response, or instead part of the chronic diabetic state and thus purely a complicating factor.

Interestingly, one study examined how persistent hyperglycemia differed from transient hyperglycemia in functional outcomes as well as in mortality. When hyperglycemia was present at baseline and when measured 24 hours after admission, it was inversely associated with neurologic improvement in the first 7 days, 30-day functional outcome and 90-day negligible dependence. At the same time, persistent hyperglycemia was positively associated with increased mortality at 90 days, and parenchymal hemorrhage. When hyperglycemia was absent at baseline but present at 24 hours after admission, it was likewise inversely associated with 90-day negligible dependence, and positively associated with death and parenchymal hemorrhage. In this study, baseline hyperglycemia alone (without persistence at 24 hours) was not associated with poor outcomes. These data suggest that it may not be the stress response hyperglycemia that causes damage in the acute stroke setting [75].

Intensive treatment of hyperglycemia may be associated with improved outcomes, as has been demonstrated in the cardiac literature for MIs [76]. A small pilot study found that hyperglycemic patients could be treated with insulin infusions safely, but the numbers were too small to compare functional outcomes at 1 month [77]. The use of insulin drips in another study to maintain glucose levels at 5.0–7.2 mmol/L (90–130 mg/dL) in patients with acute ischemic stroke, started no later than 12 hours after the onset of symptoms, was associated with a trend towards better functional outcomes and minimal or no neurologic symptoms as measured by the Natonal Institutes of Health (NIH) stroke scale. There were hypoglycemic episodes in the group treated with the continuous infusion, but the majority of these were asymptomatic [78]. Clearly, further study is required on this subject.

Hyperglycemia, as defined by serum glucose >400 mg/dL, was a contraindication for inclusion in the NINDS trial for some of the reasons above, as well as that extreme hyperglycemia can cause focal neurologic deficits that mimic stroke [64]. Current guidelines recommend starting aggressive glycemic control if serum glucose is >200 mg/dL, while acknowledging that levels >140–185 mg/dL may still be harmful [69]. While it may be reasonable to attempt to bring down the glucose level and see if any focal symptoms improve or resolve, and then treat with thrombolysis if no improvement is seen, this approach has yet to be tested.

In terms of oral hypoglycemics in the acute stroke setting, one study looked at the role of sulfonylureas taken pre-stroke and during the acute hospitalization. Sulfonylureas have an effect on ATP-sensitive Kir6.2 potassium channels which are regulated by the sulfonylurea receptor 1 (SUR1) receptor, like pancreatic β-cells, and which are open only during ischemic episodes, causing cell death. Theoretically, then, treatment with sulfonylureas should be neuroprotective during ischemia. Although the numbers were small, and patients with more severe strokes (NIH stroke scale greater than 9) were excluded, patients on the medication were more likely to have a decrease of four points on the NIH stroke scale or a score of 0, and were more likely to achieve an excellent functional recovery at discharge. The effect was particularly noticeable in non-lacunar strokes [79].

Further care for the acute stroke patient is best handled in a certified stroke unit, with multidisciplinary care from a team consisting of vascular neurologists, stroke-trained registered nurses, physical therapists, occupational therapists, and speech and swallow specialists. This care results in around a 25% reduction in mortality [80].

BP control in acute ischemic stroke is a subject of ongoing debate. Current thinking still supports the concept of permissive hypertension in the peri-stroke period. Most vascular neurologists would allow the blood pressure to remain untreated until the systolic BP rises >220 mmHg or the diastolic BP >120 mmHg. The period over which permissive hypertension should be allowed is also controversial. Typically, the BP is left untreated for the first 3–5 days after stroke [69].

The majority of medical complications after stroke relate to the disability associated with neurologic deficits. Thus, deep venous thrombosis (DVT) and aspiration pneumonitis are the two complications that stroke units need to prevent. Prevention of DVT is accomplished through subcutaneous anticoagulation with either heparin or low molecular weight heparin with or without external compressive devices [69]. Initiation of treatment is typically immediately on admission, regardless of the size of infarct. One unblinded study looked at heparin versus enoxaparin and found a reduction in thrombosis with the low molecular weight heparin [81].

Prevention of aspiration is more complicated. Protection of the airway is often compromised in the acute period after stroke. Frequent suctioning and positioning helps to prevent aspiration. Swallow evaluations should be undertaken before oral nutrition is started in any patient in whom dysphagia is suspected. Placement of nasogastric tubes (NGT) is often required for nutrition, and frequently patients will require percutaneous endoscopic gastrostomy (PEG) tube for long-term provision of nutrition. Hydration is necessary, either intravenously before enteral access is established, or via NGT or PEG tubes to prevent dehydration and electrolyte abnormalities. Antibiotics should be started in any patient suspected of infection, and fever should prompt aggressive search for a source. Hyperthermia itself causes neurologic deterioration, so antipyrrhetics should be administered [69].

Secondary prevention of stroke in diabetes

The management of the patient with diabetes after stroke is similar to that for primary prevention as outlined above (Table 42.3). The seventh report of the Joint National Committee on prevention and treatment of hypertension recommends that people with diabetes should be maintained at a BP <130/80 mmHg, and that it will likely take multiple antihypertensive medications to achieve this goal [82]. As suggested by the studies described above, ACEi and ARB provide greater protection against cardiovascular events including stroke.

Similarly, the National Cholesterol Education Program [83] and subsequently the Endocrine Society [84] have published guidelines on the management of cholesterol in people with diabetes. Diabetes should be considered a CHD risk equivalent and, as such, cholesterol should be lowered aggressively. This is particularly true in those with diabetes who have had a stroke. These patients are considered high risk for CHD, and their levels should be lowered at least to <100 mg/dL, with <70 mg/dL an ideal. In combination with the data on statins and stroke described above, all those with diabetes and stroke should be started on a statin.

Table 42.3 Prevention of ischemic stroke in the patient with diabetes.

Tight glycemic control
Antihypertensives with ACEi or ARB
Anticholesterol treatment, especially with HMG-CoA-reductase inhibitors (statins)
Lifestyle modifications (e.g. tobacco cessation, weight loss)
Antiplatelet therapy (either aspirin, clopidogrel or dipyridamole) *or*
Anticoagulation in patients with atrial fibrillation

ACEi, angiotensin-converting enzyme inhibitor; ARB, angiotensin receptor blocker; HMG-CoA, 3-hydroxy-3-methyl-glutaryl-Coenzyme A.

Antiplatelet therapy should be started in all patients who have had a non-cardioembolic ischemic stroke (Table 42.3). While the Anti-thrombotic Trialists' Collaboration meta-analysis failed to show benefit in patients with diabetes, post hoc analysis of data from the Clopidogrel versus Aspirin in Patients at Risk of Ischemic Events (CAPRIE) study found that people with diabetes treated with clopidogrel had a decreased rate of stroke, MI or death of 15.6% compared to 17.7% risk in those treated with aspirin [85]. Similarly, in a post hoc subgroup analysis of a study of cilostazol, those with diabetes had a decreased rate of recurrent stroke on the medication when compared with placebo, with a relative risk reduction of 41.7%. This finding was especially true in patients with lacunar stroke [86]. These findings need to be verified by further trials.

In patients who have had ischemic stroke secondary to extracranial carotid stenosis, carotid endarterectomy remains the preferred treatment of choice for carotid artery stenosis greater than 70% (Figure 42.3). For degrees of stenosis of 50–70%, the benefits of surgery are much smaller, and decisions to treat will depend on the complication rate at local institutions [19]. Carotid artery stenting for symptomatic carotid artery stenosis is still being studied. To this point, unless there is significant risk of undergoing the surgery, such as clinically significant cardiac disease or pulmonary disease, contralateral carotid artery occlusion or history of previous radical neck surgery or neck radiation therapy, carotid endarterectomy is still preferable. In these high risk situations, carotid artery stenting is not inferior to the surgery [87]. Diabetes alone is not enough to categorize a patient as high risk.

People with diabetes and atrial fibrillation, paroxysmal or otherwise, should be anticoagulated with warfarin to a goal International Normalized Ratio (INR) of 2.0–3.0. The risk reduction associated with treatment with anticoagulation is 68%, with an absolute risk reduction in the annual stroke rate from 4.5% to 1.4% [88]. This reduction in risk is so strong that one study estimated that a patient would have to fall 295 times in one year for the risk of subdural hematoma secondary to trauma to

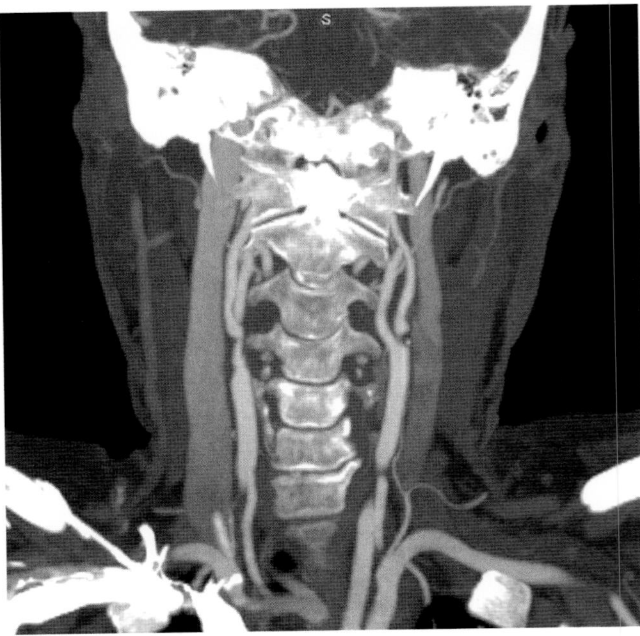

Figure 42.3 Computed tomography angiography with iodinated contrast of the neck. There is mild stenosis seen at the origin of the right internal carotid artery. There is critical stenosis ("string sign") at the origin of the left internal carotid artery, corresponding to severe atherosclerotic plaque.

outweigh the benefits gained from anticoagulation [89]. There is no reason to assume this is any different for patients with diabetes.

Conclusions

Diabetes is a strong risk factor for ischemic stroke, and stroke in patients with diabetes is both more severe in presentation and outcome and more recalcitrant to acute treatment. While many etiologies of stroke are made more common by diabetes, the most common type of stroke found in patients with diabetes is lacunar microvascular infarction. Prevention of stroke in the patient with diabetes is best served through aggressive management of concurrent hypertension and hyperlipidemia. Careful glycemic control likely reduces the risk of stroke as well, but the risk reduction is not nearly as robust. Antiplatelet therapy also has important role; a single antithrombotic agent is sufficient for the prevention of ischemic stroke. Hyperglycemia in the acute phase after ischemic stroke is associated with poor outcomes, and aggressive management likely improves functional recovery.

References

1 Thom T, Haase N, Rosamond W, Howard VJ, Rumsfeld J, Manolio T, *et al.* Heart disease and stroke statistics – 2006 update: a report from the American Heart Association Statistics Committee and the Stroke Statistics Subcommittee. *Circulation* 2006; **113**:e85–e151.

2 Heron MP, Hoyert DL, Xu J, *et al.* Deaths: preliminary data for 2006. *Natl Vital Stat Rep* 2008; **56**:16.

3 Rothwell PM, Coull AJ, Giles MF, Howard SC, Silver LE, Bull LM, *et al.* Change in stroke incidence, mortality, case-fatality, severity, risk factors in Oxfordshire, UK from 1981 to 2004 (Oxford Vascular Study). *Lancet* 2004; **363**:1925–1933.

4 Thorvaldsen P, Asplund K, Kuulaasma K, Rajakangas AM, Schroll M. Stroke incidence, case fatality, and mortality in the WHO MONICA project: World Health Organization Monitoring Trends and Determinants in Cardiovascular Disease. *Stroke* 1995; **26**:361–367.

5 Wolf PA, D'Agostino RB, Belanger AJ, Kannel WB. Probability of stroke: a risk profile from the Framingham Study. *Stroke* 1991; **22**:312–318.

6 Rodriguez BL, D'Agostino R, Abbott RD, Kagan A, Burchfiel CM, Yano K, *et al.* Risk of hospitalized stroke in men enrolled in the Honolulu Heart Program and the Framingham Study. *Stroke* 2002; **33**:230–236.

7 Kissela BM, Khoury J, Kleindorfer D, Woo D, Schneider A, Alwell K, *et al.* Epidemiology of ischemic stroke in patients with diabetes: the Greater Cincinnati and Northern Kentucky Stroke Study. *Diabetes Care* 2005; **28**:355–359.

8 Sacco RL, Boden-Albala B, Abel G, Lin IF, Elkind M, Hauser WA, *et al.* Race ethnic disparities in the impact of stroke risk factors: the northern Manhattan stroke study. *Stroke* 2001; **32**:1725–1731.

9 Almdal T, Scharlik H, Jensen AS, Vestergaard H. The independent effect of type 2 diabetes mellitus on ischemic heart disease, stroke and death. *Arch Intern Med* 2004; **164**:1422–1426.

10 Tuomilehto J, Rastenyte D, Jousilahti P, Sarti C, Vartiainen E. Diabetes mellitus as a risk factor for death from stroke: prospective study of the Finnish middle-aged population. *Stroke* 1996; **27**:210–217.

11 Davis BR, Vogt T, Frost PH, Burlando A, Cohen J, Wilson A, *et al.* Risk factors for stroke and type of stroke in persons with isolated systolic hypertension: Systolic Hypertension in the Elderly Program Cooperative Research Group. *Stroke* 1998; **29**:1333–1340.

12 Grau AJ, Weimar C, Buggle F, Heinrich A, Goertler M, Neumaier S, *et al.* Risk factors, outcome, and treatment in subtypes of ischemic stroke: the German Stroke Data Bank. *Stroke* 2001; **32**:2559–2566.

13 Labovitz DL, Boden-Albala B, Hauser WA, Sacco RL. Lacunar infarct or deep intracerebral hemorrhage: who gets which? The Northern Manhattan Study. *Neurology* 2007; **68**:606–608.

14 Horowitz DR, Tuhrim S, Weinberger JM, Rudolph SH. Mechanisms in lacunar infarction. *Stroke* 1992; **23**:325–327.

15 Elmore EM, Mosquera A, Weinberger J. The prevalence of asymptomatic intracranial large-vessel occlusive disease: the role of diabetes. *J Neuroimaging* 2003; **13**:224–227.

16 Weinberger J, Biscarra V, Weisberg MK, Jacobson JH. Factors contributing to stroke in patients with atherosclerotic disease of the great vessels: the role of diabetes. *Stroke* 1983; **14**:709–712.

17 Johnston SC, Rothwell PM, Nguyen-Huynh MN, Giles MF, Elkins JS, Bernstein AL, *et al.* Validation and refinement of scores to predict very early stroke risk after transient ischemic attack. *Lancet* 2007; **369**:283–292.

18 Movahed M, Hashemzadeh M, Jamal MM. Diabetes mellitus is a strong independent risk for atrial fibrillation and flutter in addition to other cardiovascular disease. *Int J Cardiol* 2005; **105**:315–318.

19 Sacco RL, Adams R, Albers G, Alberts MJ, Benavente O, Furie K, *et al.* Guidelines for prevention of stroke in patients with ischemic stroke or transient ischemic attack: a statement for healthcare profes-

sionals from the American Heart Association/American Stroke Association Council on Stroke. *Stroke* 2006; **37**:577–617.

20 Gage BF, Waterman AD, Shannon W, Boechler M, Rich MW, Radford MJ. Validation of clinical classification schemes for predicting stroke: results from the National Registry of Atrial Fibrillation. *JAMA* 2001; **285**:2864–2870.

21 Rietbrock S, Heeley E, Plumb J, van Staa T. Chronic atrial fibrillation: incidence, prevalence, and prediction of stroke using the congestive heart failure, hypertension, age >75, diabetes mellitus, and prior stroke or transient ischemic attack (CHADS2) risk stratification scheme. *Am Heart J* 2008; **156**:57–64.

22 Feldmann E, Broderick JP, Kernan WN, Viscoli CM, Brass LM, Brott T, *et al.* Major risk factors for intracerebral hemorrhage in the young are modifiable. *Stroke* 2005; **36**:1881–1885.

23 Selvin E, Coresh J, Shahar E, Zhang L, Steffes M, Sharrett AR. Glycemia (haemoglobin A1c) and incident ischaemic stroke: the Atherosclerosis Risk in Communities (ARIC) Study. *Lancet Neurol* 2005; **4**:821–826.

24 Myint PK, Sinha S, Wareham NJ, Bingham SA, Luben RN, Welch AA, *et al.* Glycated hemoglobin and risk of stroke in people without known diabetes in the European Prospective Investigation into Cancer (EPIC)-Norfolk Prospective Population Study: a threshold relationship? *Stroke* 2007; **38**:271–275.

25 Folsom AR, Rasmussen ML, Chambless LE, Howard G, Cooper LS, Schmidt MI, *et al.* Prospective associations of fasting insulin, body fat distribution, and diabetes with risk of ischemic stroke. *Diabetes Care* 1999; **22**:1077–1083.

26 Lindenstrøm E, Boysen G, Nyboe J. Risk factors for stroke in Copenhagen, Denmark. II. Life style factors. *Neuroepidemiology* 1993; **12**:43–50.

27 Rexrode KM, Hennekens CH, Willett WC, Colditz GA, Stampfer MJ, Rich-Edwards JW, *et al.* A prospective study of body mass index, weight change, and risk of stroke in women. *JAMA* 1997; **277**:1539–1545.

28 Kurl S, Laukkanen JA, Niskanen L, Laaksonen D, Sivenius J, Nyyssönen K, *et al.* Metabolic syndrome and the risk of stroke in middle-aged men. *Stroke* 2006; **37**:806–811.

29 McNeill AM, Rosamond WD, Girman CJ, Golden SH, Schmidt MI, East HE, *et al.* The metabolic syndrome and 11-year risk of incident cardiovascular disease in the Atherosclerosis Risk in Communities Study. *Diabetes Care* 2005; **28**:385–390.

30 Air EL, Kissela BM. Diabetes, the metabolic syndrome, and ischemic stroke. *Diabetes Care* 2007; **31**:3131–3140.

31 Bots ML, Hoes AW, Koudstaal PJ, Hofman A, Grobbee DE. Common carotid intima-media thickness and risk of stroke and myocardial infarction: the Rotterdam Study. *Circulation* 1997; **96**:1432–1437.

32 Tsivgoulis G, Vemmos K, Papamichael C, Spengos K, Manios E, Stamatelopoulos K, *et al.* Common carotid intima-media thickness and the risk of stroke recurrence. *Stroke* 2006; **37**:1913–1916.

33 Wagenknecht LE, D'Agostino R Jr, Savage PJ, O'Leary DH, Saad MF, Haffner SM. Duration of diabetes and carotid wall thickness: the Insulin Resistance Atherosclerosis Study. *Stroke* 1997; **28**:999–1005.

34 Matsumoto K, Sera Y, Nakamura H, Miyake S. Correlation between common carotid artery wall thickness and ischemic stroke in patients with type 2 diabetes mellitus. *Metabolism* 2002; **51**:244–247.

35 Chlumsky J, Charvat J. Echocardiography and carotid sonography in diabetic patients after cerebrovascular attacks. *J Int Med Res* 2006; **34**:689–694.

36 Taffi R, Nanetti L, Mazzanti L, Bartolini M, Vignini A, Raffaelli F, *et al.* Plasma levels of nitric oxide and stroke outcome. *J Neurol* 2008; **255**:94–98.

37 Nazir FS, Alem M, Small M, Connell JM, Lees KR, Walters MR, *et al.* Blunted response to systemic nitric oxide synthase inhibition in the cerebral circulation of patients with type 2 diabetes. *Diabet Med* 2006; **23**:398–402.

38 Laufs U, Endres M, Stagliano N, Amin-Hanjani S, Chui DS, Yang SX, *et al.* Neuroprotection mediated by changes in the endothelial actin cytoskeleton. *J Clin Invest* 2000; **106**:15–24.

39 Plehn JF, Davis BR, Sacks FM, Rouleau JL, Pfeffer MA, Bernstein V, *et al.* Reduction of stroke incidence after myocardial infarction with pravastatin: the Cholesterol and Recurrent Events (CARE) study. *Circulation* 1999; **99**:216–223.

40 Sever PS, Dahlöf B, Poulter NR, Wedel H, Beevers G, Caulfield M, *et al.* Prevention of coronary and stroke events with atorvastatin in hypertensive patients who have average or lower-than-average cholesterol concentrations in the Anglo-Scandinavian Cardiac Outcomes Trial – Lipid Lowering Arm (ASCOT-LLA): a multicentre randomised controlled trial. *Lancet* 2003; **361**:1149–1158.

41 Amarenco P, Bogousslavsky J, Callahan A 3rd, Goldstein LB, Hennerici M, Rudolph AE, *et al.* High dose atorvastatin after stroke or transient ischemic attack. *N Engl J Med* 2006; **355**:549–559.

42 Aoki I, Shimoyama K, Aoki N, Homori M, Yanagisawa A, Nakahara K, *et al.* Platelet-dependent thrombin generation in patients with diabetes mellitus: effects of glycemic control on coagulability in diabetes. *J Am Coll Cardiol* 1996; **27**:560–566.

43 Yamada T, Sato A, Nishimori T, Mitsuhashi T, Terao A, Sagai H, *et al.* Importance of hypercoagulability over hyperglycemia for vascular complications in type 2 diabetes. *Diabetes Res Clin Pract* 2000; **49**:23–31.

44 Serebruany VL, Malinin A, Ong S, Atar D. Patients with metabolic syndrome exhibit higher platelet activity than those with conventional risk factors for vascular disease. *J Thromb Thrombolysis* 2008; **25**:207–213.

45 Angiolillo DJ, Fernandez-Ortiz A, Bernardo E, Ramírez C, Sabaté M, Jimenez-Quevedo P, *et al.* Platelet function profiles in patients with type 2 diabetes and coronary artery disease on combined aspirin and clopidogrel treatment. *Diabetes* 2005; **54**:2430–2435.

46 Fisher CM. The arterial lesions underlying lacunes. *Acta Neuropathol* 1969; **12**:1–15.

47 Fisher CM. Thalamic pure sensory stroke: a pathologic study. *Neurology* 1978; **28**:1141–1144.

48 Fisher CM. Capsular infarcts. *Arch Neurol* 1979; **36**:65–73.

49 Chester EM, Agamanolis DP, Banker BQ, Victor M. Hypertensive encephalopathy: a clinicopathologic study of 20 cases. *Neurology* 1978; **28**:928–939.

50 Rosenberg EF. The brain in malignant hypertension: a clinicopathologic study. *Arch Neurol* 1940; **65**:545.

51 Nathan DM, Cleary PA, Backlund JY, Genuth SM, Lachin JM, Orchard TJ, *et al.* Intensive diabetes treatment and cardiovascular disease in patients with type 1 diabetes (DCCT). *N Engl J Med* 2005; **353**:2643–2653.

52 UKPDS Study Group. Effect of intensive blood-glucose control with metformin on complications in overweight patients with type 2 diabetes (UKPDS 34). *Lancet* 1998; **352**:854–865.

53 Nissen SE, Wolski K. Effect of rosiglitazone on the risk of myocardial infarction and death from cardiovascular causes. *N Engl J Med* 2007; **356**:2457–2471.

54 Home PD, Pocock SJ, Beck-Nielsen H, Curtis PS, Gomis R, Hanefeld M, Jones NP, Komajda M, McMurray JJ; RECORD Study Team. Rosiglitazone evaluated for cardiovascular outcomes in oral agent combination therapy for type 2 diabetes (RECORD): a multicentre, randomised, open-label trial. *Lancet* 2009; **373**:2125–2135.

55 Wilcox R, Bousser MJ, Betteridge DJ, Schernthaner G, Pirags V, Kupfer S, *et al.* Effects of pioglitazone in patients with type 2 diabetes with or without previous stroke: results from PROactive (Prospective Pioglitazone Clinical Trial in Macrovascular Events 04). *Stroke* 2007; **38**:865–873.

56 UKPDS. Intensive blood-glucose control with sulphonylureas or insulin compared with conventional treatment and risk of complications in patients with type 2 diabetes (UKPDS 33). *Lancet* 1998; **352**:837–853.

57 Holman RR, Paul SK, Bethel MA, Matthews DR, Neil HA. 10-year follow-up of intensive glucose control in type 2 diabetes. *N Engl J Med* 2008; **359**:1577–1589.

58 Heart Outcomes Prevention Evaluation Study Investigators. Effects of an angiotensin-converting enzyme inhibitor, ramipril, on cardiovascular events in high risk-patients. *N Engl J Med* 2000; **342**:145–153.

59 Dahlöf B, Devereux RB, Kjeldsen SE, Julius S, Beevers G, de Faire U, *et al.* Cardiovascular morbidity and mortality in the Losartan Intervention For Endpoint reduction in hypertension study (LIFE): a randomized trial against atenolol. *Lancet* 2002; **359**:995–1003.

60 Gaede P, Lund-Andersen H, Parving HH, Pedersen O. Effect of a multifactorial intervention on mortality in type 2 diabetes. *N Engl J Med* 2008; **358**:580–591.

61 Antithrombotic Trialists' Collaboration. Collaborative meta-analysis of randomized trials of antiplatelet therapy for prevention of death, myocardial infarction, and stroke in high risk patients. *Br Med J* 2002; **324**:71–86.

62 Ridker PM, Cook NR, Lee IM, Gordon D, Gaziano JM, Manson JE, *et al.* A randomized trial of low-dose aspirin in the primary prevention of cardiovascular disease in women. *N Engl J Med* 2005; **352**:1293–1304.

63 Latchaw RE, Yonas H, Hunter GJ, Yuh WT, Ueda T, Sorensen AG, *et al.* Guidelines and recommendations for perfusion imaging in cerebral ischemia: a scientific statement for healthcare professionals by the writing group on perfusion imaging, from the Council on Cardiovascular Radiology of the American Heart Association. *Stroke* 2003; **34**:1094–1104.

64 National Institute of Neurologic Disorders and Stroke rt-PA Stroke Study Group. Tissue plasminogen activator for acute stroke. *N Engl J Med* 1995; **333**:1581–1587.

65 Hacke W, Kaste M, Bluhmki E, Brozman M, Dávalos A, Guidetti D, *et al.* Thrombolysis with alteplase 3 to 4.5 hours after acute ischemic stroke. *N Engl J Med* 2008; **359**:1317–1329.

66 Tandberg Askevold E, Naess H, Thomassen L. Predictors for recanalization after intravenous thrombolysis in acute stroke. *J Stroke Cerebrovasc Dis* 2007; **16**:21–24.

67 Brown DL, Johnston KC, Wagner DP, Haley EC Jr. Predicting major neurological improvement with intravenous recombinant tissue plasminogen activator treatment of stroke. *Stroke* 2004; **35**:147–150.

68 Furlan A, Higashida R, Wechsler L, Gent M, Rowley H, Kase C, *et al.* Intra-arterial prourokinase for acute ischemic stroke. The PROACT II study: a randomized controlled trial. *JAMA* 1999; **282**:2003–2011.

69 Adams HP, del Zoppo G, Alberts MJ, Bhatt DL, Brass L, Furlan A, *et al.* Guidelines for the early management of adults with ischemic stroke: a guideline from the American Heart Association/American Stroke Association Stroke Council, Clinical Cardiology Council, Cardiovascular Radiology and Intervention Council, and the Atherosclerotic Peripheral Vascular Disease and Quality of Care Outcomes in Research Interdisciplinary Working Groups. *Stroke* 2007; **38**:1655–1711.

70 Arnold M, Schroth G, Nedeltchev K, Loher TJ, Stepper F, Schroth G, *et al.* Intra-arterial thrombolysis in 100 patients with acute stroke due to middle cerebral artery occlusion. *Stroke* 2002; **33**:1828–1833.

71 Alvarez-Sabín J, Molina CA, Montaner J, Arenillas JF, Huertas R, Ribo M, *et al.* Effects of admission hyperglycemia on stroke outcome in reperfused tissue plasminogen activator treated patients. *Stroke* 2003; **34**:1235–1241.

72 Demchuk AM, Morgenstern LB, Krieger DW, Linda Chi T, Hu W, Wein TH, *et al.* Serum glucose level and diabetes predict tissue plasminogen activator-related intracerebral hemorrhage in acute ischemic stroke. *Stroke* 1999; **30**:34–39.

73 Leigh R, Zaidat OO, Suri MF, Lynch G, Sundararajan S, Sunshine JL, *et al.* Predictors of hyperacute clinical worsening in ischemic stroke patients receiving thrombolytic therapy. *Stroke* 2004; **35**:1903–1907.

74 Saposnik G, Young B, Silver B, Legge S, Webster F, Beletsky V, *et al.* Lack of improvement in patients with acute stroke after treatment with thrombolytic therapy. *JAMA* 2004; **292**:1839–1844.

75 Yong M, Kaste M. Dynamic of hyperglycemia as a predictor of stroke outcome in the ECASS II trial. *Stroke* 2008; **39**:2749–2755.

76 Malmberg K, Rydén L, Wedel H, Birkeland K, Bootsma A, Dickstein K, *et al.* Intense metabolic control by means of insulin in patients with diabetes mellitus and acute myocardial infarction. *Eur Heart J* 2005; **26**:650–661.

77 Walters MR, Weir CJ, Lees KR. A randomized, controlled pilot study to investigate the potential benefit of intervention with insulin in hyperglycaemic acute ischaemic stroke patients. *Cerebrovasc Dis* 2006; **22**:116–122.

78 Bruno A, Kent TA, Coull BM, Shankar RR, Saha C, Becker KJ, *et al.* Treatment of hyperglycemia in ischemic stroke (THIS): a randomized pilot trial. *Stroke* 2008; **39**:384–389.

79 Kunte H, Schmidt S, Eliasziw M, del Zoppo GJ, Simard JM, Masuhr F, *et al.* Sulfonylureas improve outcome in patients with type 2 diabetes and acute ischemic stroke. *Stroke* 2007; **38**:2526–2530.

80 Rudd AG, Hoffman A, Irwin P, Lowe D, Pearson MG. Stroke unit care and outcome: results from the 2001 National Sentinel Audit of Stroke (England, Wales, and Northern Ireland). *Stroke* 2005; **36**:103–106.

81 Sherman DG, Albers GW, Bladin C, Fieschi C, Gabbai AA, Kase CS, *et al.* The efficacy and safety of enoxaparin versus unfractionated heparin for the prevention of venous thromboembolism after acute ischemic stroke (PREVAIL Study): an open-label randomized comparison. *Lancet* 2007; **369**:1347–1355.

82 Chobanian AV, Bakris GL, Black HR, Cushman WC, Green LA, Izzo JL Jr, *et al.* The seventh report of the Joint National Committee on prevention, detection, evaluation, and treatment of high blood pressure: the JNC 7 report. *JAMA* 2003; **289**:2560–2572.

83 National Cholesterol Education Program. Third report of the National Cholesterol Education Program (NCEP) Expert Panel on detection, evaluation and treatment of high blood cholesterol in adults (Adult Treatment Panel III) final report. *Circulation* 2002; **106**:3143–3421.

84 Rosenzweig JL, Ferrannini E, Grundy SM, Haffner SM, Heine RJ, Horton ES, *et al.* Primary prevention of cardiac disease and type 2

diabetes in patients at metabolic risk: an Endocrine Society clinical practice guideline. *J Clin Endocrinol* 2008; **93**:3671–3689.

85 Bhatt DL, Marso SP, Hirsch AT, Ringleb PA, Hacke W, Topol EJ. Amplified benefit of clopidogrel versus aspirin in patients with diabetes mellitus. *Am J Cardiol* 2002; **90**:625–628.

86 Shinohara Y, Gotoh F, Tohgi H, Hirai S, Terashi A, Fukuuchi Y, *et al.* Antiplatelet cilostazol is beneficial in diabetic and/or hypertensive ischemic stroke patients. *Cerebrovasc Dis* 2008; **26**: 63–70.

87 Yadav JS, Wholey MH, Kuntz RE, Fayad P, Katzen BT, Mishkel GJ, *et al.* Protected carotid-artery stenting versus endarterectomy in high-risk patients. *N Engl J Med* 2004; **351**:1493–1501.

88 Risk factors for stroke and efficacy of antithrombotic therapy in atrial fibrillation: analysis of pooled data from five randomized controlled trials. *Arch Intern Med* 1994; **154**:1449–1457.

89 Man-Son-Hing M, Nichol G, Lau A, Laupacis A. Choosing antithrombotic therapy for elderly patients with atrial fibrillation who are at risk for falls. *Arch Intern Med* 1999; **159**:677–685.

43 Peripheral Vascular Disease

Henrik H. Sillesen

Department of Vascular Surgery, Rigshospitalet, University of Copenhagen, Copenhagen, Denmark

Keypoints

- Peripheral arterial disease is very common, affecting up to 30% of all people with diabetes.
- Amputations are much more common in patients with diabetes and occur 5–8 times more often than in those without the disease.
- Atherosclerosis is common in people with diabetes, and measurement of ankle blood pressure may identify both people with and without diabetes at an early asymptomatic stage.
- People with diabetes have atherosclerotic lesions located more peripherally than people without diabetes and therefore are more commonly inoperable for technical reasons.
- People with diabetes have more complications to surgery, both locally (infections) and systemically (e.g. cardiac, pulmonary) than people without diabetes.
- Treatment of atherosclerosis in diabetes is basically the same as in patients without diabetes.

Introduction

Peripheral vascular disease includes diseases to arteries and veins outside the thoracic region. Because of the limitations of a chapter in a textbook dealing with diabetes, this chapter mainly covers the three most common arterial diseases: peripheral arterial disease (PAD), carotid artery disease and aortic aneurysmatic disease (AAA). Other, rarer manifestations of atherosclerotic disease (e.g. renovascular hypertension, abdominal angina and ischemia of the upper extremity) are mentioned briefly. Special considerations in patients with diabetes are dealt with in relevant sections; for example, infection in an ischemic foot in a patient with diabetes is described in the section on critical limb ischemia.

Atherosclerosis is the main cause of peripheral arterial vascular disease, and the overall pathogenesis is covered in Chapter 39. It is important to appreciate that the pathogenetic mechanisms of clinical atherosclerosis are dual: chronic obstructive and thrombotic. Whereas the chronic obstructive mechanism is the main cause of lower limb ischemia, also in patients with diabetes, it is often preceeded by a thrombotic event; a patient with mild claudication suddenly experiences significantly shortening of walking distance or sudden onset of rest pain. Or, the seemingly healthy person suddenly develops claudication. Of course, a heart attack or stroke in a patient with claudication is also a thrombotic event in a patient with chronic obstructive disease.

In general, patients with diabetes more often develop symptoms of atherosclerotic complications, they do it at a younger age and they are more difficult to treat and have more complications with treatment (especially with invasive treatment).

Textbook of Diabetes, 4th edition. Edited by R. Holt, C. Cockram, A. Flyvbjerg and B. Goldstein.

Peripheral arterial disease

Peripheral arterial disease is a chronic condition that, like atherosclerosis in other vascular beds, develops over decades. The World Health Organization (WHO) definition includes exercise-related pain and/or ankle brachial index (ABI) <0.9. On average, symptoms from the lower limbs develop 5–10 years later than from the coronary circulation. Acute ischemia may develop because of:

1 Thrombosis in a vessel with pre-existing atherosclerotic plaques and/or stenosis;
2 Embolism (e.g. from mural thrombus in the heart);
3 An arterial lesion upstream; or
4 As a result of trauma.

Diabetes is a major contributor to PAD.

PAD is traditionally divided into four stages (Fontaine):

1 Asymptomatic (ABI <0.9);
2 Functional pain (claudication);
3 Rest pain; and
4 Non-healing ulcers or gangrene.

Incidence

In the most recent population-based studies in Western Europe, the incidence of symptomatic PAD is 3–4% among 60- to 65-year-olds, increasing to 15–20% in persons 85–90 years of age [1–3]. Similar findings have been reported in the USA. Looking at asymptomatic cases where the ABI is <0.9, the incidence is much higher, and approximately 20% of all persons above 65 years of age, ranging from 10% in persons 60–65 years of age to almost 50% of those aged 85–90 years [1–3]. Critical limb ischemia, defined as ABI <0.4 or rest pain and/or non-healing ulcers, occurs in 1% of persons aged 65 years or older.

Incidence of PAD in people with diabetes

The incidence of PAD in people with diabetes depends on the usual atherosclerosis risk factors and duration of diabetes. There are only few demographic studies studying the general population. Using ABI <0.9 as selection criteria, Lange *et al.* [4] found a prevalence of 26.3% in people with diabetes compared to 15.3% in people without diabetes when screening 6880 Germans above 65 years of age, of whom 1743 had diabetes. Similar findings have been reported by others: 20–30% of those with diabetes have PAD [5,6]. Claudication is twice as common in those with diabetes than those who do not have diabetes.

Pathophysiology

It is outside the scope of this chapter to describe the pathophysiology of PAD in detail (see Chapter 39); however, in brief, the pathophysiology of PAD in those with diabetes is similar to that of a non-diabetic population. The abnormal metabolic state that accompanies diabetes directly contributes to the development of atherosclerosis. Pro-atherogenic changes include increases in vascular inflammation and alterations in multiple cell types. Both mechanisms of atherosclerotic complications are of importance in PAD (gradual narrowing resulting in stenosis and acute thrombosis in existing atherosclerotic lesion). Obviously, the long-term accumulation of lipids in the vessel wall is important and sudden local thrombosis can occur at any time, although in most cases this happens after symptoms (claudication) have developed.

To reach the stage of critical limb-threatening ischemia, advanced atherosclerosis has developed. Often, multiple segments of the arterial tree from the aorta to the foot are affected (stenotic and/or occluded). In people with diabetes, the atherosclerotic lesions are more peripherally located than in people without diabetes. Whereas the iliac and femoral arteries are most commonly stenotic and/or occluded in individuals without diabetes, in those with diabetes, it is most often the crural arteries that are severely affected by atherosclerosis. This poses a challenge for revascularization because the results in general are better the more proximal the reconstruction.

In order to develop ischemic non-healing ulcers, perfusion has to be very poor. The most reliable method for assessment of peripheral perfusion in those with diabetes is measurement of toe pressure. A toe pressure below 20–25 mmHg signals a poor chance of healing of a peripherally located ulcer. The special considerations related to the potentially dramatic course of infection in a diabetic foot are dealt with in Chapter 44.

Asymptomatic stage

The asymptomatic stage of PAD is especially interesting because it is associated with an approximately threefold increased mortality compared to matched controls [7,8]. This excess mortality is caused by accompanying cardiovascular disease (CVD). Asymptomatic PAD can be identified by a very simple test: measurement of ankle blood pressure. This test takes only a few minutes and is expressed as the ABI, where the ankle pressure is divided by the highest of the two arm blood pressures (BPs). In this manner, variations in BP between measurements do not influence the test result. Not only is an ABI <0.9 associated with increased mortality from cardiovascular causes, but also the level of ABI reduction is predictive: the lower the ABI the worse prognosis [7].

Identifying an asymptomatic person with an ABI <0.9 is not a case for evaluation with respect to revascularization of the lower limbs, but a case for serious preventive cardiovascular medicine.

Claudication

Claudication is experienced by the patient as pain in lower limb muscles appearing after walking, most often in the calf, the thigh and more rarely in the buttocks. The walking distance eliciting the pain is very variable, beginning after 10–15 meters in severe cases, whereas other patients will report pain only when walking fast uphill for more than 500 meters for example. It is important for both the patient and the treating physician to understand that claudication, although it may be incapacitating for a few, and troublesome for many, signals severe vascular disease systemically, and that cardiovascular morbidity and mortality is high (elevated 3–4 times compared to matched controls).

Rest pain

Rest pain typically begins at night when the patient is in the horizontal position. The positive effect of gravity on lower limb perfusion is then abolished. The patient typically complains about pain in the toes or feet during the night and most have experienced that standing or sitting up relieves the pain. Many patients will sleep sitting in a chair.

In patients with diabetes, symptomatology may differ because of coincidal peripheral neuropathy. Just like myocardial ischemia can be masked, symptoms from the lower extremity may be missing even though peripheral ischemia exists. This is especially important when a patient with diabetes presents with a small ulcer or wound on the lower limb, even if the patient thinks there is a good explanation for developing the ulcer, such as a relevant trauma. The lack of symptoms to signal peripheral ischemia combined with the risk of escalating infection in a diabetic foot has prompted many diabetologists to recommend routine assessment of peripheral circulation at regular intervals in all people with diabetes.

Non-healing ulcers

Non-healing ulcers often begin after minor trauma (e.g. hitting a toe against a chair or by using shoes that are too small). In some cases the ulcers develop without any trauma and those will often progress to gangrene if not treated. Ischemic ulcers develop on

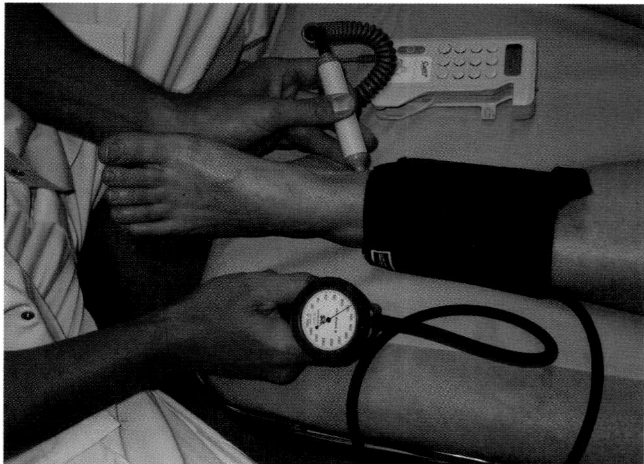

Figure 43.1 Measurement of ankle pressure using Doppler technique.

toes or on the foot, typically at points where shoes are in firm contact. Thus, they are usually easy to discriminate from venous ulcers, which are located at the level of the ankles or lower calf.

Rest pain, non-healing ulcers and/or gangrene are often referred to as critical ischemia. The "diabetic foot" is dealt with in Chapter 44.

Diagnosis

Most often the history and objective findings will ensure the diagnosis, but measurement of ankle blood pressure will quantify the ischemia and can be used to monitor changes in the disease (Figure 43.1). In some patients with diabetes, the media of smaller arteries become calcified making them incompressible. Thus, very high ankle pressures resulting in elevated ABI (>1.3) signals mediasclerosis and should be recognized as a falsely elevated measurement. In fact, ABI >1.3 is associated with a marked increased mortality because media sclerosis is found in patients with diabetes and those with renal failure.

Because small arteries are rarely affected by media sclerosis, measurement of toe pressure is an alternative for assessment of PAD. Use of the strain gauge technique is most commonly used (Figure 43.2). Toe pressure also is useful for prediction of healing of ulcers and amputation wounds.

Prognosis

The risk of amputation is only 1–2% at 5 years. Twenty-five percent of patients with claudication will experience a worsening of their symptoms from the lower legs; however, 75% will be unchanged or improve without revascularization [9]. In contrast the "systemic" risk is huge. Mortality in 5 years will be 15–25% and many more will have non-fatal myocardial infarction (MI) or stroke.

The risk of a patient with diabetes and PAD is much higher than that of the average patient with PAD. The patient with diabetes has an 8 times greater risk of amputation at the level of the transmetatarsal bones or above than the non-diabetic population [10]. In addition to the already severely increased mortality of PAD, patients who additionally have diabetes have a further doubling of their risk of death [10–12].

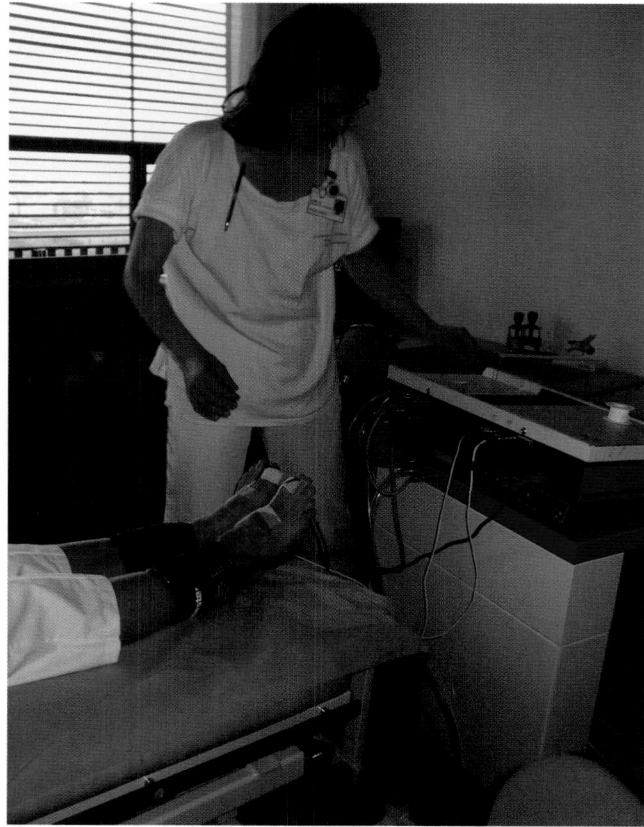

Figure 43.2 Measurement of toe pressure using strain gauge technique.

Treatment

Treatment of patients with symptoms from the lower limb therefore involves two aspects:

- Treatment of symptoms from the lower limb; and
- Prevention of cardiovascular complications

The former includes lifestyle modification, medical therapy and interventional therapy by either percutaneous transluminal angioplasty (PTA) or open surgery, whereas the latter includes lifestyle modification and preventive medical therapy.

It is beyond the scope of this chapter to detail all aspects of lifestyle modification and preventive medical therapy; however, it is extremely important for the reader to understand that patients with PAD derive as much or greater benefit from lifestyle modification and aggressive preventive medical therapy than any other group of patients (see Chapter 40). Most of the lifestyle changes which are beneficial to the patient with diabetes will benefit the PAD aspect as well, especially smoking cessation, regular exercise, weight loss and dietary changes.

Medical prevention follows the same guidelines as that of other clinical atherosclerotic manifestations such as ischemic heart disease and can be summarized as follows: aggressive statin treatment almost irrespective of cholesterol levels (Heart Protection Study and American Heart Association guidelines), antiplatetet therapy and BP control. In this chapter, only details of lifestyle modification and medical therapy relevant to PTA and surgery are discussed.

Treatment of symptoms from the lower limb

The vast majority of patients should be managed without invasive intervention PTA (and/or surgery). Because the risk of cardiovascular complications (cardiac and cerebral) is much higher than the risk of amputation, the main focus should be on preventive measures in order to halt the atherosclerotic process. The conservative approach with respect to revascularization is especially important for patients with diabetes because of the increased risk of surgical complications and poorer results of revascularization. One exception is patients with critical limb ischemia. Early revascularization before widespread infection can be limb-saving.

Exercise therapy has proven effective for improvement of walking distance, and regular exercise for 3 months can be expected to improve walking distance by 200–250% [13]. Because exercise also reduces cardiovascular morbidity and mortality, it cannot be stressed enough (for both the patient and the physician) that this is extremely important. Because the effect on walking distance is so good, and because it is important for survival, exercise therapy should always be tried before considering interventional treatment. There are only few exceptions where interventional treatment may be considered early on:

1 Patients with very short walking distance, not being able to carry out important daily responsibilities such as their work; and
2 Patients at risk of amputation (rest pain and non-healing ulcers).

The dilemma of explaining to patients that the symptoms they are experiencing from the lower limb are signaling high cardiovascular risk rather than lower limb risk is challenging. First of all, there is (or has been) a general perception that atherosclerosis in the limb is less dangerous than in other locations. The author hopes that the introductory remarks in this chapter have changed this potential misperception for the reader. Medical therapy for claudication includes cilostazol and statins. Treatment with both may be expected to improve walking distance by 30–50% and the latter furthermore reduces the cardiovascular risk. Other drugs have not proven useful in improving walking distance significantly [14].

Interventional treatment

Interventional treatment (endovascular or open surgery) for PAD is indicated when:

- Exercise and other lifestyle modification has failed to improve symptoms to an acceptable state;
- Claudication is incapacitating; or
- Critical limb ischemia is present (rest pain, non-healing ulcers and/or gangrene).

Again, for the patient with diabetes, the indication for revascularization should be considered very carefully in patients only with claudication. The choice between PTA and open surgical management depends on the location and extent of disease. In general, endovascular treatment can be expected to perform well in cases of shorter lesions whereas open surgery is preferred in cases of extensive occlusive disease. Obviously, whenever comparable results can be obtained, PTA is preferred for the simple reason that it is less invasive and associated with less complications than open arterial reconstructions. In patients with severe co-morbidity that might complicate the outcome of open surgery, PTA would be preferred even though theoretically surgery would be the treatment of choice if only patency of the revascularization procedure was considered.

The arterial lesions causing obstruction of blood supply to the lower limb are most often located in the distal abdominal aorta just proximally to the aorta–iliac bifurcation, in the iliac arteries, and in the common and superficial femoral arteries. The arteries in the calf, the anterior and posterior tibial and the peroneal artery, are often involved in those with critical ischemia and with diabetes. In general, when patients with diabetes present with symptoms, they have a more distal involvement with open vessels to the level of the popliteal artery and then occlusive disease of the calf vessels and sometimes also the arteries in the foot. The results of revascularization for patients with diabetes with toe or foot ulcers are worse than the general population partly because reconstructions yield better results with respect to patency when the lesions are more centrally located.

Percutaneous transluminal angioplasty

In principle, PTA can be performed anywhere between the heart and the feet. The more centrally located the lesions being treated, the better the results, especially with PTA. Also, the shorter the stenosis or occlusion, the better the results, and stenting improves patency in most cases. Endovascular-treated common iliac arteries, as an example, remain patent in 60–80% of cases after 5 years and thereafter they may be redilatated. Primary stenting has become the preferred treatment in most cases. Obviously, because complications are rare, and this procedure is associated with the best results, the tendency to offer PTA for iliac artery obstruction is greater than for occlusive disease more peripherally located.

PTA of the superficial femoral artery (Figure 43.3) may relieve symptoms, but the results depend on the extent of disease. The longer the lesion, the greater the risk of early reocclusion. Stenting appears to improve patency, at least for longer lesions (Table 43.1) [15]. When the indication for PTA is claudication, patency is better than if the indication is critical ischemia. This difference relates to the more extensive nature of the disease in the case of critical limb ischemia and may also relate to poor run-off vessels. The 3-year patency is 48%, which may be improved to 64% if stenting is added. In case of critical limb ischemia, the results at

(a)

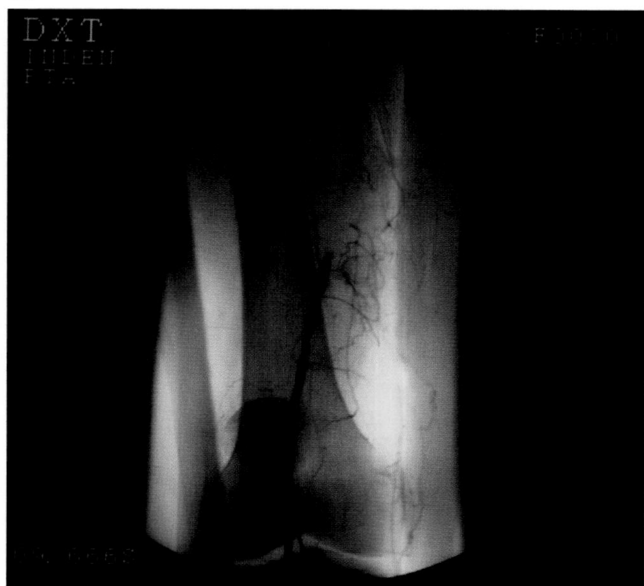

(b)

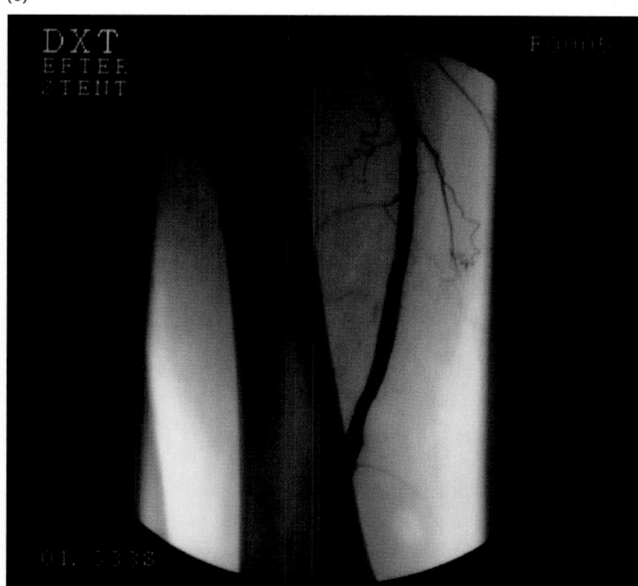

Figure 43.3 Short occlusion of the superficial femoral artery (a) treated with PTA and stenting (b).

Table 43.1 Pooled patency of vascular reconstructions (TASC*II).

	1 year	3 year	5 year	10 year
Endovascular				
Iliac artery	86%	82%	71%	
Fem-pop stenosis PTA	77%	61%	55%	
Fem-pop occl. PTA	65%	48%	42%	
Fem-pop stenosis PTA + stent	75%	66%		
Fem-pop occl. PTA + stent	73%	64%		
Open surgery				
Aorto-bifemoral bypass			90%	80%
Fem-fem cross-over			75%	
Fem-pop vein			80%†	
Fem-pop PTFE†			30–75%†	

fem, femoral; pop, popliteal; PTA, percutaneous transluminal angioplasty; PTFE, polytetrafluoroethylene.

* Inter-Society Consensus for the Management of Peripheral Arterial Disease (TASC).

† Secondary patency.

3 years show a patency of 30% without stenting and 63% with stenting (Table 43.1) [15]. PTA of crural vessels is also feasible; however, the long-term results are not good. Data on limb salvage with PTA of crural vessels alone are scarce. Adjunctive medical therapy to improve patency following PTA and stenting, with anticoagulation and/or antiplatelet therapy, has been tested only in a few trials. Antiplatelet drugs improve patency, and the combination of aspirin and clopidogrel may be beneficial [16].

Open surgical revascularization

Open surgical revascularization still dominates as the treatment of choice in cases of critical limb ischemia, because of the extensive nature of the atherosclerotic lesions in these patients. For claudication, open surgical treatment is rarely performed, while for extensive disease of the distal aorta and iliac arteries, the aorto-bifemoral bypass remains the procedure with the best long-term outcome. In addition, femoral–femoral cross-over bypass may be performed for unilateral iliac artery occlusion. Also, endarterectomy, as described below, may be an option for treatment of claudication. Only one trial has compared open surgery with endovascular treatment of critical limb ischemia, the Bypass versus Angioplasty in Severe Ischaemia of the Leg (BASIL) trial [17]. The primary efficacy outcome measure was amputation-free survival, but because approximately two-thirds of the endpoints were deaths, only one-third of the endpoints really determined which procedure was best. Within 6 months postoperatively, there was no difference in the primary endpoint, but thereafter bypass patients seemed to do better [17].

In general, two surgical techniques are used: endarterectomy and bypass. Endarterectomy is performed by separating the intima from the media, and in this manner the atherosclerotic lesion can be removed. Endarterectomy can be used in cases with severe occlusive lesions of limited anatomic extension, in the external iliac or in the common femoral artery. The advantage of this technique is that it can often be performed without the use of artificial graft material and patency is excellent. Bypass is preferred when the obstructive and/or occlusive lesions are extensive (e.g. total superficial femoral artery occlusion or multiple serial lesions warranting a femoral–crural bypass) (Figure 43.4). Bypass surgery can be performed with artificial materials or with auto-

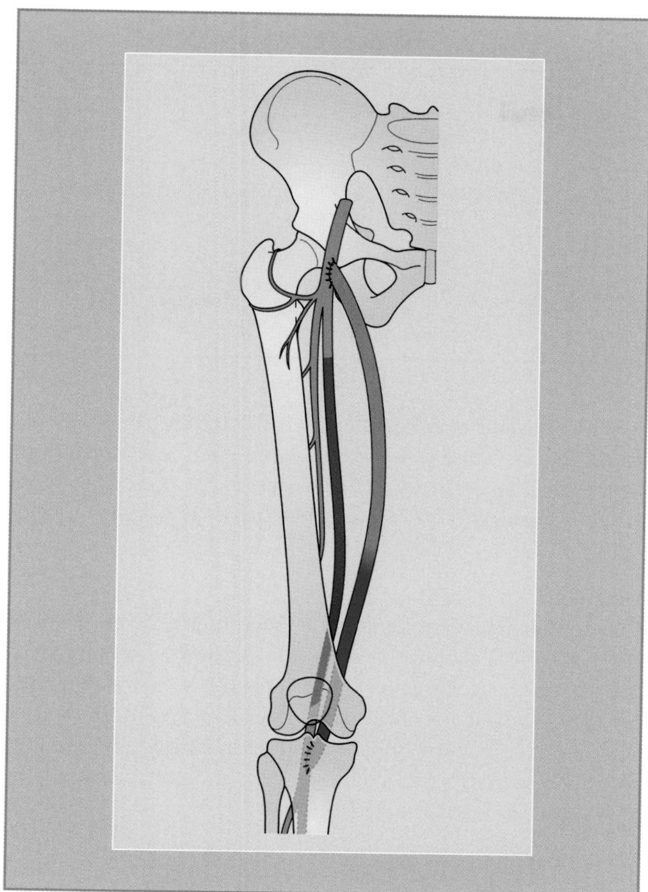

Figure 43.4 Long superficial femoral artery occlusion treated with femoro-popliteal bypass.

logous veins. For bypass of aortic or iliac artery origin, artificial grafts are almost always used. This is because there is no easily removable vein with similar dimensions that can be used in these locations. Also, Dacron or polytetrafluoroethylene (PTFE) grafts perform very well in the aorto-iliac–femoral region. For peripheral bypasses, typically originating from the common femoral artery, autologous vein grafts are preferred for two reasons: they last longer (much better patency) (Table 43.1) and they carry less risk of infection. For longer bypasses, such as from the common femoral to the popliteal artery below the knee, a saphenous bypass is performed leaving the vein *in situ*. This means that the vein is left in its original anatomic location; however, the proximal and distal ends are anatomized to the arterial system. The venous valves are cut with a knife mounted on a catheter and side branches are occluded. In this manner, the vein retains its nervous innervations and native vascularization.

Complications of endovascular treatment

Complications relate mainly to the site of puncture and the risk of peripheral embolization. "Systemic" cardiovascular complications are rare. Hematoma in the groin access point is common; however, it only rarely requires any action to be taken. Development of an iatrogenic pseudo-aneurysm is seen in 0.5–1% of cases and can easily be treated with ultrasound-guided compression or ultrasound-guided thrombin injection.

Complications of open surgical treatment

These can be divided into local and systemic categories. The former relate to the actual incisions and dissections including wound healing and infections. Whereas complications from accidental damage to other organs and/or structures are very rare, wound healing problems and infections are unfortunately quite common. In particular, surgery on the lower limb involving the groin and peripheral incisions have wound complications in 10–20% of cases (e.g. hematoma, lymph oozing or necrosis of the wound) [18]. Infections are seen in 3–5% of cases, approximately one-third involving the vascular reconstruction. Infection of the vascular reconstruction is more frequent when using artificial graft material [18].

Systemic complications to open surgical revascularization relate to the surgical trauma and to the stress response. In vascular reconstructions involving the aorta and other central arteries, the cardiopulmonary complication rate is considerable. Implantation of an aorto-bifemoral bypass graft is associated with a 30-day mortality of 2–5% and a rate of "general" complications of 10–15% (e.g. pulmonary, cardiac, renal, prolonged stay at the intensive care unit, stroke and deep venous thrombosis) [18]. Systemic complications to peripheral revascularizations occur less frequently; however, they are considerable. When the indication is claudication, the morbidity with respect to general complications is low, 2–4%; however, in cases of critical ischemia and peripheral bypass surgery, the morbidity increases to 10% with a 30-day mortality of 3–5%. This difference in morbidity is a reflection of the more advanced level of generalized atherosclerotic disease in patients with critical ischemia. In patients with diabetes, complications are more common especially with open surgery. A doubling of risk should be expected.

Results of endovascular and open surgical reconstructions

These are summarized in Table 43.1. In general, when treating more centrally located arterial obstruction, the long-term results are better. In addition, treating patients with claudication results in better long-term outcome than operating on patients with limb-threatening ischemia. This difference relates to the generally poorer condition of the peripheral circulation in cases of critical ischemia with better run-off vessels in the patient with claudication.

In peripheral reconstructions, vein grafts perform better. It may seem unrewarding to treat patients with critical limb ischemia with a peripheral bypass using an artificial graft when there is only a 50% chance of being patent at 1 year; however, if the alternative is amputation and/or very poor quality of life (i.e. severe rest pain), 1 year with a functioning graft may very well be worthwhile for both the patient and surgeon. Limb salvage as a result is almost always better than patency of the reconstruction

Table 43.2 Separation of threatened from viable extremeties.

Category	Description/prognosis	Findings		Doppler signals	
		Sensory loss	Muscle weakness	Arterial	Venous
Viable	Not immediately threatened	None	None	Audible	Audible
Threatened					
a. Marginal	Salvageable if promptly treated	Minimal (toes) or none	None	(Often) inaudible	Audible
b. Immediate	Salvageable with immediate revascularization	More than toes, associated with rest pain	Mild, moderate	(Usually) inaudible	Audible
Irreversible	Major tissue loss or permanent nerve damage inevitable	Profound, anesthetic	Profound, paralysis (rigor)	Inaudible	Inaudible

because in many cases, once the ischemic limbs with tissue loss have healed, the "need" for amputation becomes less. Patients with diabetes typically have poorer outcome of vascular reconstructions, with patency rates that are inferior to those without diabetes. Patients with diabetes have more complications to treatment, not only infections but also systemic complications are more common.

Acute lower limb ischemia

This condition is most often caused by thrombosis in existing atherosclerosis (i.e. a patient with previous symptoms of chronic PAD). Another common cause is thrombosis of a popliteal aneurysm. Embolism remains a common cause, although not as often as in the past because of better anticoagulant therapy for patients with atrial fibrillation. Eighty percent of emboli are of cardiac origin; however, aneurysms of the aorta or peripheral aneurysms may give rise to peripheral emboli.

Other causes include trauma and iatrogenic lesions (e.g. from arteriography with puncture of the femoral artery). Aortic dissection may cause lower limb ischemia as well as acute deep venous thrombosis (phlegmasia coerulae dolens). Incidence in Western Europe is 300–400 per million per year.

Pathophysiology

Thrombosis is caused by plaque rupture and subsequent thrombosis. Distal to the acute occlusion, arterial flow is slow and when combined with a hypercoagulable condition, it may lead to further thrombosis. The degree of ischemia depends on the location and the degree of collateral development. Therefore, thrombosis is often better tolerated than embolism because patients with existing atherosclerosis most often has developed collaterals.

Emboli will typically occlude an artery at a bifurcation; in the lower limbs, at the aortic bifurcation (saddle embolus), iliac artery and femoral artery bifurcation. Sixty percent of cardiac emboli will end in the lower limbs, 15% in the arms and the rest in the brain and other organs. Microemboli, typically from aneurysms, affect small peripheral arteries, and are thus the cause of "blue toe" syndrome.

Symptoms

Acute ischemia is characterized by pallor, pain, pulselessness, paresthesia and paresis (the 5 P's). Symptoms may begin dramatically and in some cases the late signs of ischemia, paresthesia and paresis occur within a few hours. More often, symptoms begin with pain and paresthesia and later sensory and muscular paresis. Acute ischemia is traditionally divided into three classes (Table 43.2).

Diagnosis

Diagnosis is often easy with typical clinical signs. ABI will be low, if measurable at all. Imaging with either duplex ultrasound, magnetic resonance angiography (MRA) or digital subtraction angiography (DSA) is possible but may delay treatment. In cases of thrombosis, it is most often desirable to perform arteriography with subsequent thrombolysis in order to visualize the underlying pathology causing the thrombosis.

Prognosis

If revascularization is possible before irreversible ischemia has occurred, the limb can be salvaged and normal function regained. Co-morbidity is high in cases of acute ischemia; when acute revascularization is needed the procedure-related mortality is 10–20% because of release of toxic substances from ischemic tissue combined with existing cardiac disease.

Treatment

Thrombosis in existing atherosclerotic lesions may be treated by endovascular or open surgery. The former is preferred if revascularization is not imminent. By catheter-directed intra-arterial thrombolysis, the underlying atherosclerotic lesions will be exposed and may in some cases be treated by PTA and/or stenting. In other cases, bypass surgery may be needed. Inoperable cases may be converted into operable cases by thrombolysis because distal thrombosis most often makes surgery (and PTA) useless when there are no run-off vessels. Another advantage of thrombolysis is that emergency surgery is converted into a less urgent intervention. Emboli can be treated by embolectomy by inserting a balloon catheter, either in the femoral or popliteal artery, and retracting the emboli after inflating the balloon (Figure 43.5). Some cases of embolism may also be treated by thrombolysis.

Prevention

Arterial emboli have a high recurrence rate and the underlying case should be treated, if possible; corrective treatment for atrial

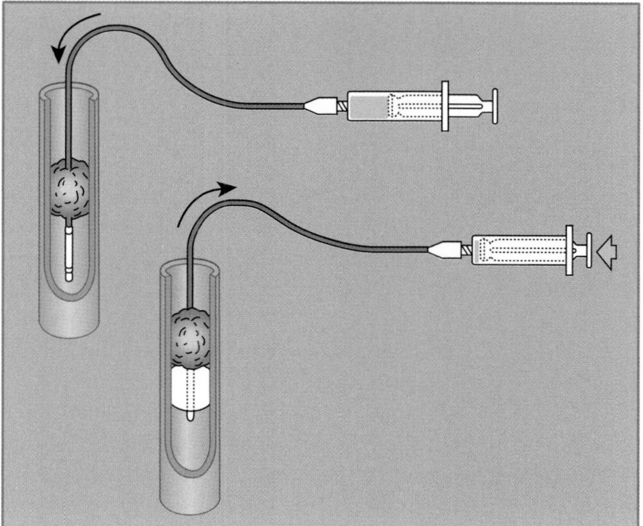

Figure 43.5 Embolectomy performed with a balloon catheter.

fibrillation and resection or exclusion of aneurysms. If the source of embolism cannot be eliminated, anticoagulation must be considered.

Atherosclerosis of renal and mesenteric arteries

Renal artery obstruction

Renal artery obstruction can cause severe hypertension and renal failure but interventional treatment may improve both conditions. Today, open surgical management is only rarely performed because endovascular management is much less invasive and feasible in the majority of cases. Open surgery, thrombo-endarterectomy or bypass, is performed when renal artery disease is combined with other pathology such as aortic occlusion or AAA.

Mesenteric artery occlusive disease

Mesenteric artery occlusive disease may cause abdominal angina. Just like atherosclerotic lesions in other locations, many cases are asymptomatic and probably do not need intervention with regard to the obstructive disease, but lifestyle changes and medical preventive treatment are indicated. Patients with classic symptoms – post-prandial pain occurring 10–20 minutes after a meal and weight loss – often benefit from revascularization; however, many patients have less obvious symptoms, and the mere occurrence of a lesion on one of the three main vessels supplying blood to the gastrointestinal tract (celiac trunk, superior and inferior mesenteric artery) does not warrant interventional treatment. In general, a single lesion in one of the three arteries is seldom thought to cause ischemia. Diagnosis is possible by ultrasound of the suprarenal vessels in most cases, otherwise computed tomography arteriography (CTA), MRA or DSA may be needed. Interventional treatment today is mainly balloon angioplasty and stenting. Long occlusions of the superior mesenteric artery and/or occlusive mesenteric disease combined with other pathology of the aorta may be treated by open surgery (e.g. aorto-mesenteric bypass).

Ischemia of the arms

Atherosclerosis and ischemia of the arm are much less common than in the lower limb. The most common location for development of atherosclerosis in the arteries supplying the upper extremity is in the brachiocephalic trunk and subclavian arteries central for the origin of the vertebral arteries. Rarely, occlusive lesions are located more peripherally in the subclavian or axillary arteries. Takayasu vasculitis may also cause upper extremity ischemia.

Typical symptoms of chronic arm ischemia

Theses include "claudication"; i.e. pain when using the arm. In typical cases pain is encountered when performing tasks with the arms elevated, such as hanging laundry, or other physical use of the arm. Critical ischemia with rest pain or gangrene is rare but may occur. Diagnosis is easy with lack of pulses at palpation. Measurement of bilateral BP and ultrasound may locate and quantitate the stenotic lesion. If BP cannot be measured by auscultation, a Doppler device may be used as for measurement of ankle BP. Additionally, or in case of severe ischemia, finger pressure measurement by strain gauge technique may be used. Upper arm angiography by CT, MRA or DSA may be supplemental.

The prognosis is often good because development of critical ischemia and the necessity for amputation is rare. Patients with finger gangrene should be investigated for vasculitis.

Treatment of upper extremity atherosclerosis is similar to that of atherosclerosis in other vascular distributions: risk factor reduction by lifestyle changes and preventive medications for all, and revascularization in some. In fact, only rarely is interventional treatment indicated, but in cases of incapacitating functional pain and/or critical ischemia, revascularization should be considered. Endovascular treatment dominates because of its less invasive nature for lesions near the origin of the brachiocephalic trunk and subclavian arteries. For lesions that cannot be treated by endovascular techniques, such as long lesions or lesions that cannot be crossed by a guide wire, bypass surgery is indicated (carotid–subclavian bypass). Peripheral bypass of the upper extremity (e.g. at the level of the brachial artery) is rare and patency is poor.

Acute arm ischemia

This is most often caused by embolization, but alternatively can be caused by thrombosis in an existing stenosis such as of the subclavian artery. Whereas the former may be treated easily by embolectomy via a small incision in the cubital fossa, the latter may be more complex to treat, perhaps requiring intra-arterial thrombolysis before vascular reconstruction. Embolism is most often of cardiac origin, either from atrial fibrillation, mural thrombus in the heart or valve disease. Vascular causes include a subclavian aneurysm or stenosis. Microemboli may occur peripherally and present as gangrene of one or more fingers. Extravascular causes include a cervical rib. Obviously, eradication of the embolic source is crucial, if possible. Treatment of the peripheral ischemia may include thrombolysis, but in most cases collaterals develop and amputation does not become necessary.

Aortic aneurysmal disease (abdominal aortic aneurysm)

This section focuses on abdominal aortic aneurysms (AAA) because thoracic aortic aneurysms are not considered part of peripheral vascular disease. The main difference between those with and without diabetes with respect to treatment of aneurysms is that patients with diabetes are more prone to complications after surgery; however, because of the nature of preventive surgery for aneurysms, this only rarely causes changes in management once the risk of surgery has been weighed against non-surgical treatment.

Aneurysm of the aorta is a common condition in the elderly, especially in the infra-renal aorta. An artery by definition becomes aneurysmal when the diameter locally increases more than 50% compared to the "normal" diameter proximal or distal to this site. In case of the infra-renal aorta, an aneurysm is present when the diameter exceeds 30 mm.

The prevalence of AAA is approximately 5% in men over 70 years of age; however, only a minority of them will have a size that mandates surgery (diameter >5–6 cm). In patients with other atherosclerotic manifestations, such as PAD or carotid disease, the incidence of AAA is 2–3 times greater than in persons without. Also, there is a 2 : 1 ratio of AAA occurring in men : women. Finally, the tendency to develop AAA is partly inherited, as the risk for a male with a father or brother with AAA is approximately 20%. People with diabetes seem to have a slightly lower incidence of AAA; approximately 80% of the prevalence of those without diabetes [19].

Pathophysiology

Arteries enlarge with age, and the diameter of the infra-renal aorta is normally below 20 mm in a 70-year-old male. If the wall weakens locally, an aneurysm develops. A true aneurysm develops when all three layers in the arterial wall are involved and dilate as in the case of the typical infra-renal AAA. False aneurysms or pseudo-aneurysms develop after iatrogenic trauma, such as PTA or other transfemoral procedures, and at arterial anastomotic sites. Finally, dissection occurs when a rupture of the intima allows blood to enter between the layers of the artery wall.

Aortic aneurysms may rupture, leading to almost certain death. It is estimated that 80–90% of patients with ruptured AAA die before they get to hospital. Ruptured AAA causes an estimated 2–3% of all deaths among men, whereas the number for women is 1%.

In most AAA there is an atherosclerotic degeneration of the vessel wall that dilates; however, it is unclear why atherosclerosis in some patients results in occlusive disease and in others in aneurysm development. Accelerated breakdown of elastin has a role in AAA development. Simultaneous presence of both occlusive and aneurysmal disease is common in many patients. Inflammatory aneurysms are present in 5–10% of AAA where the aortic wall is thickened as part of perianeurysmal or retroperitoneal fibrosis.

Symptoms from AAA

Symptoms are rare and so most cases are asymptomatic. Diagnosis is often made coincidentally, as when a patient complains of slight upper gastric pain and has an ultrasound of the gallbladder, which discloses the AAA. Also typically, a patient may complain of back pain and have a lumbar X-ray where the AAA is discovered. Whether the patient's pain was really related to the AAA or to gallstones or to the back is often difficult to ascertain.

Some patients will sense a pulsation in the abdomen, while large aneurysms may cause discomfort or compress surrounding organs, mainly the gastrointestinal tract. The main risk is rupture which, when intraperitoneal, most often leads to immediate death. If rupture is into the retroperitoneal space, a hematoma may be contained and the patient may survive for hours. Rupture and development of a hematoma lead to pain in the abdomen and/or back. Chronic rupture is rare because almost all cases will be fatal within hours.

Aneurysms may cause peripheral embolization, causing a cyanotic or gangrenous toe as the first symptom.

Diagnosis

Diagnosis of AAA is easy. Ultrasound is very accurate in making the diagnosis and estimating the diameter of the aneurysm (Figure 43.6). In the few cases where ultrasound is inconclusive, a primary CT scan may be necessary. Otherwise, CT or MR scanning is only performed when the size of the AAA dictates to an extent that intervention should be considered. Arteriography is rarely performed for AAA; however, in cases of both AAA and symptoms of PAD, an arteriogram may be warranted for planning of the revascularization procedure. A patient with acute abdominal pain in pre-shock should always be suspected of ruptured AAA.

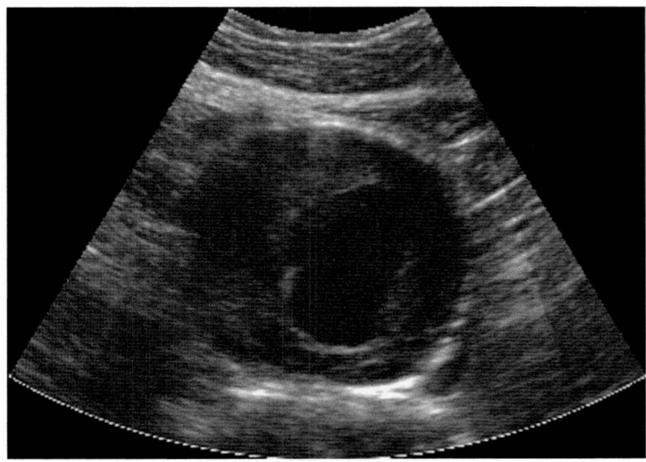

Figure 43.6 Ultrasound image of abdominal aortic aneurysm. Notice the presence of large thrombus inside the aneurysm sac.

Prognosis

The risk of rupture relates to the size of the aneurysm. When the diameter exceeds 6 cm, the annual risk of rupture is 10–20%, whereas the risk of rupture in case of an AAA with a diameter of 3–4 cm is less than 1%. Aneurysms tend to expand; small aneurysms dilate 1–2 mm/year whereas larger aneurysms may expand 2–3 times faster. Smoking and hypertension seem to increase the rate of growth. Rupture is associated with 90% mortality – the survival for those who reach the hospital and have immediate surgery is approximately 50–60%. Concommitent coronary disease is responsible for a 50–100% increased mortality of aneurysm patients even when aneurysm mortality is disregarded.

Treatment

Treatment of AAA involves, in addition to surgery for some, the same preventive treatment that is given to other patients with atherosclerotic manifestations: lifestyle changes and medical therapy with platelet inhibitors, statins and BP control.

Treatment of ruptured AAA is always interventional (open surgical or endovascular) unless the patient's overall condition is considered too poor to attempt rescue. In some cases, a fatal AAA may be a dignified death; for example, in an elderly patient with both end-stage renal failure and heart failure. Symptomatic non-ruptured aneurysms should be treated acutely or subacutely because of the risk of imminent rupture.

Treatment of large asymptomatic AAA reduces AAA mortality [20], and those with asymptomatic AAA should be offered elective interventional treatment if the risk of rupture exceeds the risk of the procedure, and if the patient is fit for the procedure and expected to have some good quality years remaining. Because any procedure for treatment of AAA either carries a considerable perioperative risk or involves a very long postoperative period with potential reinterventions, the decision to offer interventional treatment is not always easy and almost always a decision is made with the patients and their families.

The choice between treatment modalities is made keeping these facts in mind: open surgery is a well-proven procedure with known risks and long-term results, including an overall 3–5% perioperative mortality, but limited AAA morbidity after the procedure. Endovascular aneurysm repair (EVAR) has been shown to have lower perioperative morbidity: 1.5% for EVAR compared to 4.5% for open surgery [21–23]. Because the long-term results of EVAR are unknown (5–10 years), continuous surveillance with annual CT or ultrasound is necessary. Until recently, the number of reinterventions because of either migration or failure of the implanted device, both leading to endo-leak (blood re-entering the excluded aneurysm sac which is thereby again at risk of rupture) were considerable; however, recent data show improvement and is 10–15% at 3 years [23].

As an example of choice of treatment modality, a 65-year-old man with a 6-cm AAA and no other known co-morbidity should be offered treatment, preferentially open surgery, because his perioperative risk will be low (i.e. 2–3%), whereas the annual risk of rupture is approximately 10%. At the other end of the spectrum is the 80-year-old man with previous coronary artery bypass graft surgery and with a similar-sized AAA of 6 cm. His risk with open surgery includes >10% 30-day mortality in addition to a considerable risk of other complications. Endovascular treatment could be a good alternative for this patient if he is expected to live at least 3–5 years.

EVAR has been thought to be a treatment alternative for patients unfit for open surgery. The EVAR-2 trial tested this hypothesis and patients found unfit for open repair were randomized to either conservative management or EVAR. Survival was not improved by EVAR and it was poor in both groups: approximately 50% of patients in both groups were dead at 3 years and only one-quarter of deaths was aneurysm-related [24]. Thus, being found unfit for surgery in this study indicated a poor prognosis in general that EVAR did not affect.

Open surgical treatment with resection of the aneurysm and replacement of the diseased part of aorta with an artificial graft

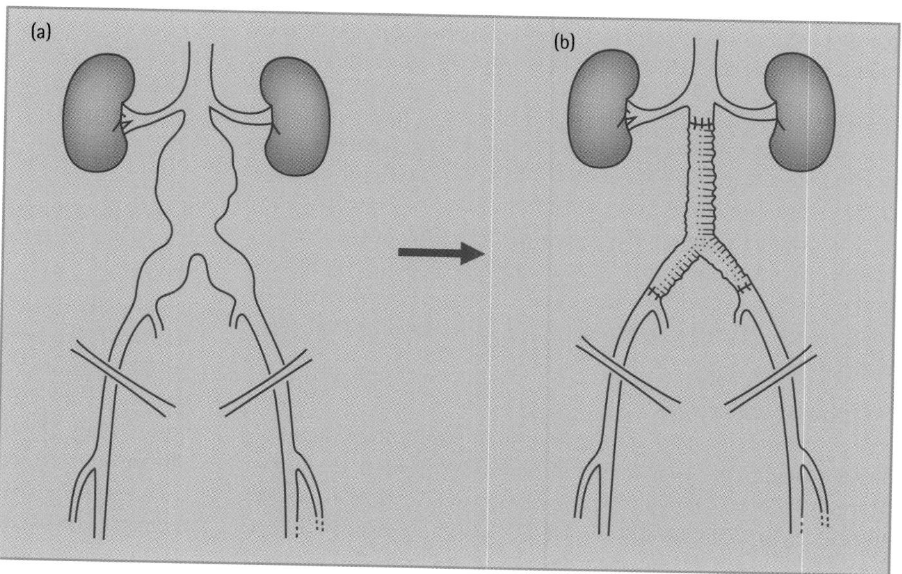

Figure 43.7 Abdominal aortic aneurysm treated by resection and implantation of aorto-bi-iliac bypass graft.

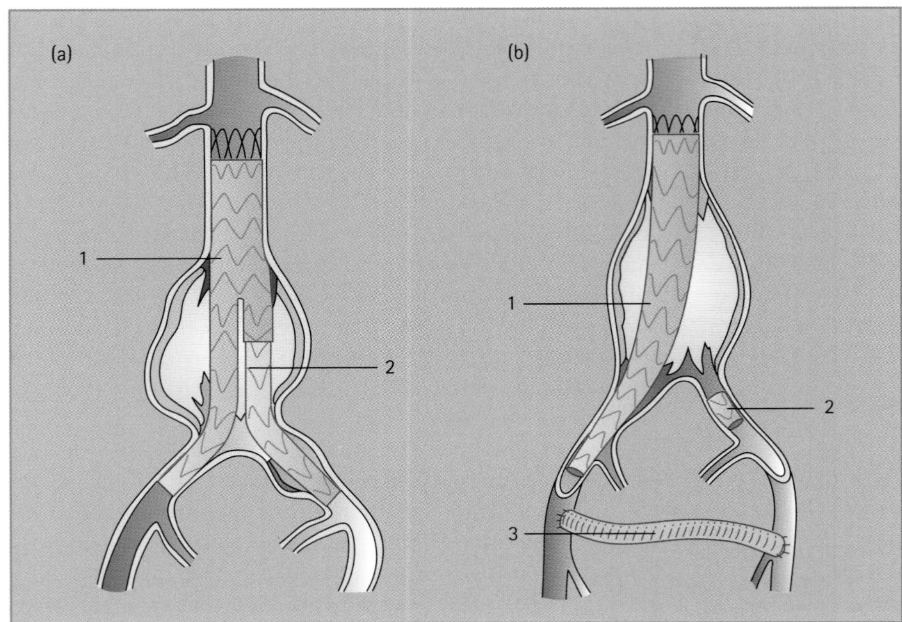

Figure 43.8 Abdominal aortic aneurysm treated by endovascular repair. (A) First the bifurcated graft is inserted via the right femoral artery and fixed by stenting at the proximal and distal end of the graft. The left limb (2) is inserted via the left femoral artery and connected to the main graft. (B) Insertion of an aorto-uni-iliac endograft (1) combined with a femoro-femoral bypass graft (3) is used when one of the iliac arteries (2) cannot be passed.

has been performed for more than 40 years (Figure 43.7). Complications of open surgical repair relate to the considerable surgical trauma of this major procedure. Approximately 10–20% will develop general complications such as cardiac, pulmonary and renal complications in addition to prolonged stay at the intensive care unit and stroke.

Endovascular treatment of AAA involves inserting a collapsed prosthesis via the femoral artery, placing it below the renal arteries, deploying and fixing it (stenting) under X-ray guidance. The technique mostly used today involves inserting a bifurcated graft from one femoral artery and then placing the other limb via the contralateral femoral artery (Figure 43.8). Complications to EVAR are few in the perioperative period, but a considerable number of patients will need reinterventions, which in most cases can be performed by endovascular techniques. These include placement of another proximal stent because of endo-leak and embolization of inferior mesenteric or internal iliac arteries.

Screening

The value of population-based screening for AAA is now well documented. A recent meta-analysis of the four randomized controlled trials found aneurysm-related mortality to be reduced by 43% in people being offered screening [25]. Today, it is recommended in many countries that men older than 65 years and previous smokers undergo ultrasound screening. Family members who are direct descendants of those so affected should also undergo screening.

Peripheral aneurysms

Aneurysms may develop at other locations, popliteal and femoral arteries being the second and third most common locations. More than 50% of patients with peripheral aneurysms also have an AAA. Symptoms are different in the sense that rupture is less common; however, symptoms derived from compression (popliteal vein thrombosis, pain and other symptoms of nerve compression), peripheral embolization or thrombosis of the aneurysm most often bring the patient to medical attention.

Treatment is the same as for AAA: general prevention against atherosclerotic disease and intervention in symptomatic cases. Popliteal aneurysms are generally treated surgically by exclusion and bypass or by resection and replacement by a short graft. Femoral aneurysms are treated by resection and placement of a graft. Endovascular management is possible; however, graft thrombosis and failure of stent graft material have so far made indications unclear. Large asymptomatic peripheral aneurysms should probably be treated by either open or endovascular surgery; however, no documentation is available at this time that such treatment is beneficial.

Aneurysms of visceral or renal arteries may occur but are rare. Treatment is interventional when they are large. Endovascular management is under development, however, its indications are unsettled.

Carotid artery disease

This section focuses on stroke and carotid disease because cerebrovascular disease in general is dealt with in Chapter 42. The relationship to atherosclerosis for many patients with stroke is well documented, although stroke, unlike other ischemic conditions, has other common pathogenetic mechanisms.

It is very important to discriminate between symptomatic disease and asymptomatic cases. Patients with recent cerebrovascular symptoms and an ipsilateral stenosis are comparable with patients with a recent acute coronary event: the risk of a new thromboembolic event is very high and diagnostic workup and treatment should be started immediately. The pathogenetic mechanism is similar to that of an acute coronary event with plaque rupture and subsequent thrombosis; however, in the case of the carotid, embolization into a cerebral artery is much more common than thrombotic occlusion of the carotid artery itself. Perhaps the larger diameter of the carotid artery explains this difference.

The prevalence of carotid stenosis is high. Among patients with acute cerebrovascular symptoms, an ipsilateral stenosis of greater than 50% diameter reduction is found in 15–20% of cases. In patients with other clinical atherosclerotic manifestations, a carotid stenosis is found in 20–30%.

Pathophysiology and symptoms

See Chapter 42, dealing with cerebrovascular disease.

Prognosis

The risk of stroke is increased in the presence of carotid stenosis. For asymptomatic patients with a carotid stenosis exceeding 60% diameter reduction, the annual risk of ipsilateral stroke is approximately 2%. When carotid stenosis is related to recent ipsilateral cerebral ischemic symptoms (symptomatic stenosis), the risk is much higher, especially just after the first event. The 30-day risk of stroke in patients with previous cerebrovascular symptoms is as high as 10% when an ipsilateral carotid stenosis is present. Thereafter, the risk gradually declines and after a year it is approximately 2–3% annually, similar to asymptomatic carotid stenosis. The 3-year risk of ipsilateral stroke is 25–30% in symptomatic patients with a stenosis greater than 70% diameter reduction.

Diagnosis

Diagnosis of carotid disease should be carried out by duplex ultrasound scanning (Figure 43.9). The accuracy of the method is well documented both for identification and quantification of degree of stenosis. Many surgeons will perform endarterectomy based only on ultrasound examination.

Treatment

Treatment of patients with carotid stenosis is like that of any other condition related to atherosclerosis: treatment of the atherosclerotic disease itself and treatment of local manifestations. Risk factor reduction, including changes in lifestyle, is exactly the same as for patients with other clinical manifestations of atherosclerosis, although there may be regional variation in the choice of antiplatelet agents. Aggressive lipid-lowering reduces both the risk of recurrent stroke and the risk of coronary events especially in this patient group [26–28].

It is important to realize that any intervention for carotid stenosis is performed to prevent future "local" events (stroke). Thus, the risk of the intervention itself should be weighed against the absolute risk of an event. Furthermore, the most common complication of surgery and stenting is ipsilateral stroke, the event that the procedure is supposed to prevent. Most important, the overall risk of the patient should be weighed against the absolute risk reduction derived from the procedure.

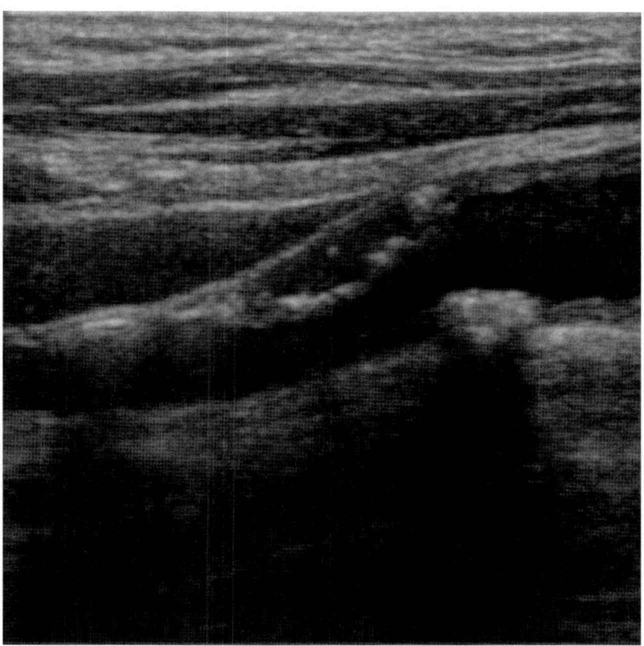

Figure 43.9 B-mode ultrasound image of carotid stenosis. Top part is echolucent indicating high content of lipid/necrotic core; bottom part is echogenic indicating a fibrous plaque.

Symptomatic carotid stenosis

Symptomatic patients with carotid stenosis benefit from endarterectomy when the stenosis is greater than 50–70% diameter reduction and neurologic symptoms are within 6 months of surgery [29,30]. The North American Symptomatic Carotid Endarterectomy Trial (NASCET) and European Carotid Surgery Trialist's Collaborative Group (ECST) trials [29,30] randomized simultaneously, but independently, symptomatic patients with carotid stenosis to best medical treatment or best medical treatment plus endarterectomy. Both trials showed significant benefit (50% relative risk reduction) in patients with greater than 70% stenosis (diameter reduction), whereas the group with 50–69% stenosis had only a marginal effect. Patients with stenoses <50% had no benefit.

Recent reanalysis of the pooled data from these two trials, however, showed that the time interval between onset of neurologic symptoms and surgery was the most important predictive factor of benefit for the patient [31]. The earlier the operation, the greater the benefit. The overall absolute risk reduction of approximately 15% conveyed by endarterectomy could be doubled when patients received surgery within 2 weeks of symptoms. With the knowledge gained during the last 10–15 years concerning the vulnerable plaque and plaque rupture, this finding does not come as a great surprise; however, when these trials were designed, this pathogenetic mechanism of acute ischemia was unknown.

Also, sex, age and degree of stenosis are factors that influence the benefit of surgery [31]. Male sex, older age and severity of stenosis all increase the risk of future stroke in patients with stenosis without any increased risk of the surgical procedure, thus, the overall benefit is greater.

Asymptomatic carotid stenosis

Asymptomatic carotid stenosis is more controversial, although two major trials have shown a small but statistically significant benefit of surgery. First, the Asymptomatic Carotid Atherosclerosis Study (ACAS) trial showed a 50% relative risk reduction of ipsilateral stroke, but the absolute risk reduction was marginal, only 1% per year [32]. Later, the Asymptomatic Carotid Surgery Trial (ACST) reproduced these findings [33]. Taking into consideration that the average annual mortality during the trials were 3–4%, in addition to other ischemic events which were unaffected by the procedure, it may be questioned whether the cost–benefit is reasonable both for the patient and society. The medical treatment offered during these trials was much poorer than that recommended today; thus, the outcomes of these trials may not be reflective of the risk in these patients today. If or when better criteria for selection of patients at higher risk becomes available, selective surgery for high-risk cases of asymptomatic carotid stenosis may yield greater or even much greater benefit.

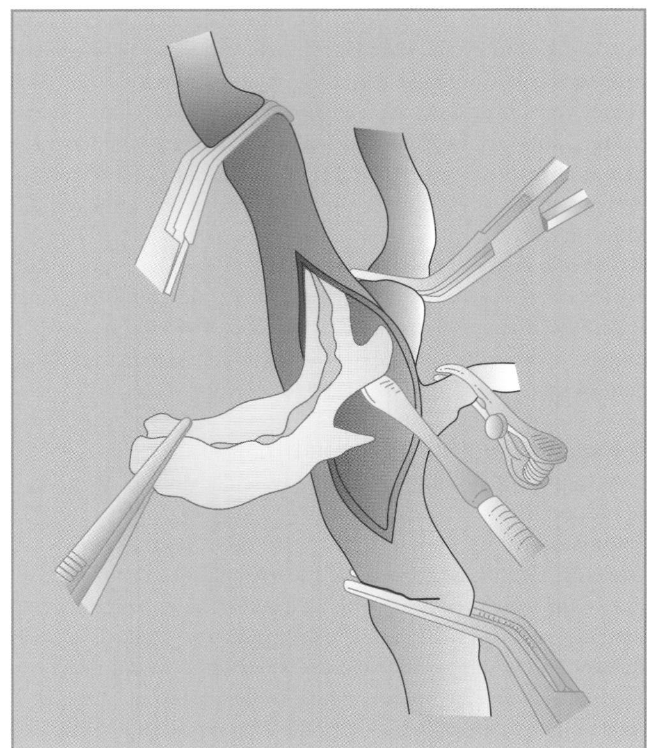

Figure 43.10 Carotid endarterectomy where the intima–media complex is dissected free of the adventitia and removed.

Technical considerations

Technically, carotid endarterectomy may be performed in two ways: classic endarterectomy (Figure 43.10) or eversion endarterectomy. In the latter, the internal carotid artery is divided from the bifurcation, and endarterectomy is performed by everting the vessel wall, thereby removing the carotid lesion. After the stenosis has been removed, the bifurcation is reconstructed by reanastomosing the internal carotid to the bifurcation.

Carotid endarterectomy may be performed under general or local anesthesia. Classically, general anesthesia has been preferred; however, this has carried the challenge of monitoring cerebral circulation during clamping of the carotid artery. A variety of methods have been used ranging from electroencephalography, stump pressure, distal internal carotid artery pressure, evoked potentials, near-infrared spectroscopy, transcranial Doppler and more. None of these methods have proven ideal, so some surgeons use a shunt on a selective basis, whenever their method for monitoring indicates risk of cerebral ischemia during clamping, whereas others use a shunt routinely. By contrast, performing endarterectomy under local anesthesia gives the surgeon the opportunity to communicate with the patient during clamping. Having the patient awake and responsive during surgery may be the best monitoring of cerebral function during clamping. Also, local anesthesia may carry less cardiac and pulmonary risk. Smaller trials and a recent meta-analysis indicate superiority of local anesthesia [34]; however, recently the General Anesthesia versus Local Anesthesia for carotid surgery (GALA) trial reported its results after randomizing 3529 patients to either universal or local anesthesia for carotid endarterectomy – there was no difference in the risk of perioperative stroke or death [35].

Carotid stenting

This has not yet been proven in randomized clinical trials to prevent ipsilateral ischemic events. Seven randomized controlled trials have been published to compare stenting with endarterectomy; however, they have only focused so far on comparison of perioperative complications. The two most recent trials, the EVA-3S and the SPACE trial, failed to show an advantage of the less invasive carotid stenting method with respect to perioperative events [36,37]. In fact, the EVA-3S trial was stopped early because of excess complications in the stenting group [36]. A recent Cochrane meta-analysis, including all seven randomized controlled trials, favors surgery with respect to the primary outcome of perioperative death and ipsilateral stroke [38]. Nevertheless, it is important to acknowledge that technology does develop rapidly and some of the trials may have used devices and/or technologies that are already outdated. Similarly, there may be differences in trial design, and criticism has been raised specifically as to the training of investigators in some studies. Interestingly, stenting appears to be associated with higher complication rates when performed early after neurologic symptoms and in the elderly – the two strongest indications. Finally, it is important to keep in mind that stenting should be evaluated in long-term studies, and not only compared with endarterectomy, but also with medical therapy, which has been improved dramatically the last 10–20 years.

Carotid revascularization prior to coronary artery bypass surgery has been practiced in some institutions whereas others have not found it useful. The potential advantage is avoiding cerebral ischemia during the relative hypotension "on pump"; however, the complications of carotid revascularization have outweighed the gains, as evaluated by recent reviews.

It may be questioned whether the evidence for endarterectomy is outdated. Three of the four major trials proving endarterectomy to be of value for symptomatic and asymptomatic surgery were performed when the only fairly constant preventive medication given was aspirin. The last trial randomized 8–10 years ago and only 30% of patients were taking statins. It is stated in the design of these trials that hypertension and hypercholesterolemia were treated when present; however, in that era, the treatment goals for both hypertension and hypercholesterolemia were much more lax than they are now. Also, new drugs have been introduced and their benefit documented since these trials randomized patients (e.g. statins, newer antiplatelet agents, dual antiplatelet therapy and newer antihypertensive drugs). It may be speculated that if these drugs were used systematically, the risk in patients with carotid stenosis would be much less, not least in those with vulnerable plaques. Therefore, new trials are needed to test how today's medical therapy compares with intervention and if the best medical therapy remains inferior to surgery or stenting. New trials are *not* unethical – it is unethical not to undertake new trials.

References

1 Diehm C, Schuster A, Allenberg J, Darius H, Haberl R, Lange S, *et al.* High prevalence of peripheral arterial disease and co-morbidity in 6880 primary care patients. *Atherosclerosis* 2004; **172**:95–105.

2 Sigvant B, Wiberg-Hedman K, Bergqvist D, Rolandsson O, Andersson B, Persson E, *et al.* A population-based study of peripheral arterial disease prevalence with special focus on critical limb ischemia and sex differences. *J Vasc Surg* 2007; **45**:1185–1191.

3 Eldrup N, Sillesen H, Prescott E, Nordestgaard BG. Ankle brachial index, C-reactive protein, and central augmentation index to identify individuals with severe atherosclerosis. *Eur Heart J* 2006; **27**:316–322.

4 Lange S, Diehm C, Darius H, Haberl R, Allenberg JR, Pittrow D, *et al.* High prevalence of peripheral arterial disease and low treatment rates in elderly primary care patients with diabetes. *Exp Clin Endocrinol Diabetes* 2004; **112**:566–573.

5 Marso SP, Hiatt WR. Peripheral arterial disease in patients with diabetes. *J Am Coll Cardiol* 2006; **47**:921–929.

6 Mostaza JM, Suarez C, Manzano L, Cairols M, López-Fernández F, Aguilar I, *et al.* Sub-clinical vascular disease in type 2 diabetic subjects: relationship with chronic complications of diabetes and presence of cardiovascular disease risk factors. *Eur J Int Med* 2008; **19**:255–260.

7 Lange S, Trampisch HJ, Haberl R, Darius H, Pittrow D, Schuster A, *et al.* Excess 1-year cardiovascular risk in elderly primary care patients with a low ankle–brachial index (ABI) and high homocysteine level. *Atherosclerosis* 2005; **178**:351–357.

8 Criqui MH, Langer RD, Fronek A, Feigelson HS, Klauber MR, McCann TJ, *et al.* Mortality over a period of 10 years in patients with peripheral arterial disease. *N Engl J Med* 1992; **328**:381–386.

9 Dormandy J, Heeck L, Vig S. The natural history of claudication: risk to life and limb. *Semin Vasc Surg* 1999; **12**:123–137.

10 Johannesson A, Larson GU, Ramstrand N, Turkiewicz A, Wiréhn AB, Atroshi I. Incidence of lower limb amputation in the diabetic and nondiabetic general population: a 10-year population-based cohort study of initial unilateral, contralateral and re-amputations. *Diabetes Care* 2009; **32**:275–280.

11 Dormandy JA, Betteridge DJ, Schernthaner G, Pirags V, Norgren L; PROactive Investigators. Impact of peripheral arterial disease in patients with diabetes: results from PROactive. *Atherosclerosis* 2009; **202**:272–281.

12 Norman PE, Davis WA, Bruce DG, Davis TM. Peripheral arterial disease and risk of cardiac death in type 2 diabetes. *Diabetes Care* 2006; **29**:575–580.

13 Leng GC, Fowler B, Ernst E. Exercise for intermittent claudication. *Cochrane Database Syst Rev* 2000; **2**:CD000990.

14 Marso SP, Hiatt WR. Peripheral arterial disease in patients with diabetes. *J Am Coll Cardiol* 2006; **47**:921–929.

15 Norgren L, Hiatt WR, Dormandy JA, Nehler MR, Harris KA, Fowkes FG; TASC II Working Group. Inter-Society Consensus for the Management of Peripheral Arterial Disease (TASC II). *Eur J Vasc Endovasc Surg* 2007; **33**:S1–75.

16 Dörffler-Melly J, Koopman MMW, Prins MH, Büller HR. Antiplatelet and anticoagulant drugs for prevention of restenosis/reocclusion following peripheral endovascular treatment. *Cochrane Database Syst Rev* 2005; **1**:CD002071.

17 Adam DJ, Beard JD, Cleveland T, Bell J, Bradbury AW, Forbes JF, *et al.* Bypass versus angioplasty in severe ischaemia of the leg (BASIL): multicentre, randomised controlled trial. *Lancet* 2005; **366**:1925–1934.

18 www.karbase.dk

19 Le MT, Jamrozik K, Davis TM, Norman PE. Negative association between infrarenal aortic diameter and glycemia: the Health in Men Study. *Eur J Vasc Endovasc Surg* 2007; **33**:599–604.

20 UK Small Aneurysm Trial Participants. Mortality results for randomised controlled trial of early elective surgery or ultrasonographic surveillance for small abdominal aortic aneurysms. *Lancet* 1998; **352**:1649–1655.

21 EVAR Trial Participants. Endovascular aneurysm repair versus open repair in patients with abdominal aortic aneurysm (EVAR trial 1): randomised controlled trial. *Lancet* 2004; **365**:2179–2186.

22 Prinssen M, Verhoeven E, Buth J, Cuypers PW, van Sambeek MR, Balm R, *et al.* A randomized trial comparing conventional and endovascular repair of abdominal aortic aneurysms. *N Engl J Med* 2004; **351**:1607–1618.

23 Schermerhorn ML, O'Malley AJ, Jhaveri A, Cotterill P, Pomposelli F, Landon BE. Endovascular vs. open repair for abdominal aortic aneurysms in the medicare population. *N Engl J Med* 2008; **358**:64–74.

24 EVAR Trial Participants. Endovascular aneurysm repair and outcome in patients unfit for open repair of abdominal aortic aneurysm (EVAR trial 2): randomised controlled trial. *Lancet* 2005; **365**:2187–2192.

25 Fleming C, Whitlock EP, Beil TL, Lederle FA. Screening for abdominal aortic aneurysm: a best-evidence systematic review for the US Preventive Services Task Force. *Ann Intern Med* 2005; **142**:203–211.

26 Amarenco P, Bogousslavsky J, Callahan A 3rd, Goldstein LB, Hennerici M, Rudolph AE, *et al.* High-dose atorvastatin after stroke of transient ischemic attack: the Stroke Prevention with Aggressive Reduction in Cholesterol Levels (SPARCL) study. *N Engl J Med* 2006; **355**:549–559.

27 Sillesen H, Amarenco P, Hennerici MG, Callahan A, Goldstein LB, Zivin J, *et al.* Atorvastatin reduces the risk of cardiovascular events in patients with carotid atherosclerosis: a Secondary Analysis of the Stroke Prevention by Aggressive Reduction in Cholesterol Levels (SPARCL) trial. *Stroke* 2008; **39**:3297–3302.

28 Sillesen H. What does "best medical treatment" really mean? *Eur J Vasc Endovasc Surg* 2008; **35**:139–144.

29 European Carotid Surgery Trialist's Collaborative Group. MRC European carotid surgery trial: interim results for symptomatic patients with severe (70–99%) or with mild (0–29%) carotid stenosis. *Lancet* 1991; **337**:1235–1243.

30 North American Symptomatic Carotid Endarterectomy Trial Collaborators. Beneficial effect of carotid endarterectomy in symptomatic patients with high-grade carotid stenosis. *N Engl J Med* 1991; **325**:445–453.

31 Rothwell PM, Eliasziw M, Gutnikov SA, Warlow CP, Barnett HJ; Carotid Endarterectomy Trialists Collaboration. Endarterectomy for symptomatic carotid stenosis in relation to clinical subgroups and timing of surgery. *Lancet* 2004; **363**:915–924.

32 Executive Committee for the Asymptomatic Carotid Atherosclerosis Study. End-arterectomy for asymptomatic carotid stenosis. *JAMA* 1995; **273**:1421–1428.

33 MRC Asymptomatic Carotid Surgery Trial (ACST) Collaborative Group. Prevention of disabling and fatal strokes by successful carotid endarterectomy in patients without recent neurological symptoms: randomised controlled trial. *Lancet* 2004; **363**:1491–1502.

34 Rerkasem K, Bond R, Rothwell PM. Local versus general anaesthesia for carotid endarterectomy. *Cochrane Database Syst Rev* 2004; **4**:CD000126.

35 Gala Collaborative Group. General anesthesia versus local anesthesia for carotid surgery (GALA): a multicentre, randomized controlled trial. *Lancet* 2008; **372**:2132–2142.

36 Mas JL, Chatellier G, Beyssen B, Branchereau A, Moulin T, Becquemin JP, *et al.* Endarterectomy versus stenting in patients with symptomatic severe carotid stenosis. *N Engl J Med* 2006; **355**:1660–1671.

37 SPACE Collaborative Group. 30 day results from the SPACE trial of stent-protected angioplasty versus carotid endarterectomy in symptomatic patients: a randomized non-inferiority trial. *Lancet* 2006; **368**:1239–1247.

38 Ederle J, Featherstone RL, Brown MM. Percutaneous transluminal angioplasty and stenting for carotid artery stenosis. *Cochrane Database Syst Rev* 2007; **4**:CD000515.

9 Other Complications of Diabetes

44 Foot Problems in Patients With Diabetes

Andrew J.M. Boulton

Department of Medicine, University of Manchester and Manchester Royal Infirmary, Manchester, UK and Miller School of Medicine, University of Miami, Miami, FL, USA

Keypoints

- Diabetic foot problems remain the most common cause of hospital admissions amongst patients with diabetes in Western countries.
- Up to 50% of older patients with type 2 diabetes have risk factors for foot problems.
- Up to 85% of lower limb amputations are preceded by foot ulcers.
- All patients with diabetes should be screened for risk of foot problems on an annual basis: those with risk factors require regular podiatry, patient education and instruction in self-foot care.
- Most foot ulcers should heal if pressure is removed from the ulcer site, the arterial circulation is sufficient and infection is managed and treated aggressively.
- Any patient with a warm unilateral swollen foot without ulceration should be presumed to have an acute Charcot neuroarthropathy until proven otherwise.

Introduction

> *"Superior doctors prevent the disease. Mediocre doctors treat the disease before evident. Inferior doctors treat the full-blown disease."*
> [Huang Dee, China, 2600 BC]

The Chinese proverb suggests that inferior doctors treat the full-blown disease, and until recent years, this was sadly the case with diabetic foot disease. Realizing the global importance of diabetic foot disease, the International Diabetes Federation (IDF) focused on the diabetic foot throughout the year 2005, during which there was a worldwide campaign to "put feet first" and highlight the all too common problem of amputation amongst patients with diabetes throughout the world. To coincide with World Diabetes Day in 2005, *The Lancet* launched an issue almost exclusively dedicated to the diabetic foot: this was the first time that any major non-specialist journal had focused on this worldwide problem; however, major challenges remain in getting across important messages relating to the diabetic foot:

1 Foot ulceration is common, affecting up to 25% of patients with diabetes during their lifetime [1].

2 Over 85% of lower limb amputations are preceded by foot ulcers and diabetes remains the most common cause of non-traumatic amputation in western countries [2].

3 Prevention is the first step towards solving diabetic foot problems. Although it was estimated that a leg is lost to diabetes somewhere in the world every 30 seconds, a more important fact is that up to 85% of all amputations in diabetes should be preventable [2].

4 Reductions in amputations will only be achieved if health care professionals from all specialties realize that, as Brand once stated, "pain is God's greatest gift to mankind": it is the loss of pain that permits patients with neuropathy to develop ulcers and continue walking on them despite the presence of often overwhelming infection [3].

5 Strategies aimed at preventing foot ulcers are cost-effective and can even be cost-saving if increased education and effort are focused on those patients with recognized risk factors for the development of foot problems [4].

6 Diabetes is now the most common cause of Charcot neuroarthropathy in Western countries, another condition that should be generally preventable [3].

Much progress in our understanding of the pathogenesis and management of the diabetic foot has been made over the last quarter century. This has been matched by an increasing number of publications in peer-reviewed journals. Taken as a percentage of all PubMed listed articles on diabetes, those on the diabetic foot have increased from 0.7% in the 1980–1988 period to more than 2.7% in the years 1998–2004 [3]. Prior to 1980, little progress had been made in the previous 100 years despite the fact that the association between gangrene and diabetes was recognized in the mid-19th century [5]. For the first 100 years following these descriptions, diabetic foot problems were considered to be predominantly vascular and complicated by infection. It was not until during the Second World War, for example, that McKeown performed the first ray excision on a patient with diabetes and osteomyelitis but good blood supply: this was performed under

Textbook of Diabetes, 4th edition. Edited by R. Holt, C. Cockram, A. Flyvbjerg and B. Goldstein.

Table 44.1 Epidemiology of foot ulceration and amputation.

Authors [Ref]	Country	Year	N	Prevalence (%)		Incidence (%)		Risk factors for foot ulcers (%)
				Ulcers	Amputation			
Samann *et al.* [9]	Germany	2008	4778	0.8†	1.6	–	–	>40
Al-Mahroos & Al-Roomi [10]	Bahrain	2007	1477	5.9	–	–	–	45
Abbott *et al.* [11]	UK	2002	9710	1.7	1.3	2.2	–	>50
Manes *et al.* [12]	Greece	2002	821	4.8	–	–	–	>50
Muller *et al.* [13]	Netherlands	2002	665	–	–	2.1	0.6	–
Ramsay *et al.* [14]	USA	1999	8965			5.8*	0.9*	–
Vozar *et al.* [15]	Slovakia	1997	1205	2.5	0.9	0.6	0.6	–
Kumar *et al.* [16]	UK	1994	821	1.4†	–	–	–	42
Moss *et al.* [17]	USA	1992	2900	–	–	10.1‡	2.1‡	–

* Incidence figures over 3 years.
† Active ulcers: 5.4% past or current ulcer.
‡ Incidence figures over 4 years.

the encouragement of Lawrence, who had diabetes himself and was co-founder of the British Diabetic Association, now Diabetes UK [6].

In the last two decades many major national and international societies were formed including diabetic foot study groups and the international working group on the diabetic foot was established in 1991. New editions of two leading international textbooks on the diabetic foot have been published in recent years [7,8], and a number of collaborative research groups are now tackling many of the outstanding problems regarding the pathogenesis and management of diabetic foot disease.

In this chapter, the global term "diabetic foot" will be used to refer to a variety of pathologic conditions that might affect the feet of people with diabetes. Initially, the epidemiology and economic impact of diabetic foot disease are discussed, followed by the contributory factors that result in diabetic foot ulceration. The potential for prevention of these late sequelae of neuropathy and vascular disease are discussed, followed by a section on the management of foot ulcers. The chapter closes with a brief description of the pathogenesis and management of Charcot neuroarthropathy, an end-stage complication of diabetic neuropathy. Throughout, cross-referencing will be provided to other chapters that also cover aspects of diabetic foot disease, particularly those on diabetic neuropathy (see Chapter 38), peripheral vascular disease (see Chapter 43), bone and rheumatic disorders in diabetes (see Chapter 48) and infection (see Chapter 50).

Epidemiology and economic aspects of diabetic foot disease

As foot ulceration and amputation are closely inter-related in diabetes [2], they will be considered together in this section. A selection of epidemiologic data for foot ulceration and amputation, originating from studies from a number of different countries [9–17], is provided in Table 44.1. Globally, diabetic foot complications remain major medical, social and economic problems that are seen in all types of diabetes and in every country [18]; however, the reported frequencies of amputation and ulceration vary considerably as a consequence of different diagnostic criteria used as well as regional differences [19]. Diabetes remains a major cause of non-traumatic amputation across the world with rates being as much as 15 times higher than in the non-diabetic population.

Although many of the studies referred to and listed in Table 44.1 were well conducted, methodologic issues remain which make it difficult to perform direct comparisons between studies and/or countries. First, definitions as to what constitutes a foot ulcer vary and, secondly, surveys invariably include only patients with previously diagnosed diabetes, whereas in type 2 diabetes, foot problems may be the presenting feature. In one study from the UK, for example, 15% of patients undergoing amputation were first diagnosed with diabetes on that hospital admission [20]. Third, reported foot ulcers are not always confirmed by direct examination by the investigators involved in the study. Finally, as can be seen from the table, in those studies that assess the percentage of the population that had risk factors for foot ulceration, 40–70% of patients fell into that category. Such observations clearly indicate the need for all diabetes services to have a regular screening program to identify such high risk individuals.

Health economics of diabetic foot disease

In addition to causing substantial morbidity and even mortality, foot lesions in patients with diabetes additionally have substantial economic consequences.

Diabetic foot ulceration and amputations were estimated to cost US health care payers $10.9 billion in 2001 [21,22].

Corresponding estimates from the UK based upon similar methodology suggested that the total annual costs of diabetes-related foot complications was £252 million [23]; however, similar problems to those noted with epidemiology exist when comparing data on the costs of diabetic foot lesions relating to methodology but also as to whether direct and indirect costs were included. Moreover, few studies have estimated costs of the long-term follow-up of patients with foot ulcers or amputations [2].

The most recent data from the USA suggest that in 2007 $18.9 billion was spent on the care of diabetic foot ulcers, and $11.7 billion on lower extremity amputations [24]. Having estimated the total cost of diabetic foot disease to be $30.6 billion in 2007, the authors went on to estimate the potential savings based upon realistic reductions in ulceration and amputation, to be as high as $21.8 billion. Such strong economic arguments may help to drive improvements in preventative foot care which could potentially lead to significant savings for health care systems.

Etiopathogenesis of diabetic foot lesions

"Coming events cast their shadow before." [Thomas Campbell]

If we are to be successful in reducing the high incidence of foot ulcers and ultimately amputation, a thorough understanding of the pathways that result in the development of an ulcer is increasingly important. The words of the Scottish poet, Thomas Campbell, can usefully be applied to the breakdown of the diabetic foot. Ulceration does not occur spontaneously: rather it is the combination of causative factors that result in the development of a lesion. There are many warning signs or "shadows" that can identify those at risk before the occurrence of an ulcer. It is not an inevitable consequence of having diabetes that ulcers occur: ulcers invariably result from an interaction between specific pathologies in the lower limb and environment hazards. The breakdown of the diabetic foot traditionally has been considered to result from an interaction of peripheral vascular disease (PVD), peripheral neuropathy and some form of trauma. Other causes are also briefly described.

Peripheral vascular disease

Although described in detail in Chapter 43, brief mention of the role of PVD in the genesis of foot ulcers must be made here. PVD tends to occur at a younger age in patients with diabetes and is more likely to involve distal vessels. Reports from the USA and Finland have confirmed that PVD is a major contributory factor in the pathogenesis of foot ulceration and subsequent major amputations [25,26]. In the pathogenesis of ulceration, PVD itself in isolation rarely causes ulceration: as will be discussed for neuropathy, it is the combination of risk factors with minor trauma that inevitably leads to ulceration (Figure 44.1). Thus, minor injury and subsequent infection increase the demand for blood supply beyond the circulatory capacity and ischemic ulceration and the risk of amputation ensues. In recent years, neuroischemic ulcers in which the combination of neuropathy and PVD exists in the same patient, together with some form of trauma, are becoming increasingly common in diabetic foot clinics.

Diabetic neuropathy

As discussed in Chapter 38, the diabetic neuropathies represent the most common form of the long-term complications of diabetes, affect different parts of the nervous system and may present with diverse clinical manifestations [27]. Most common amongst the neuropathies are chronic sensorimotor distal symmetrical

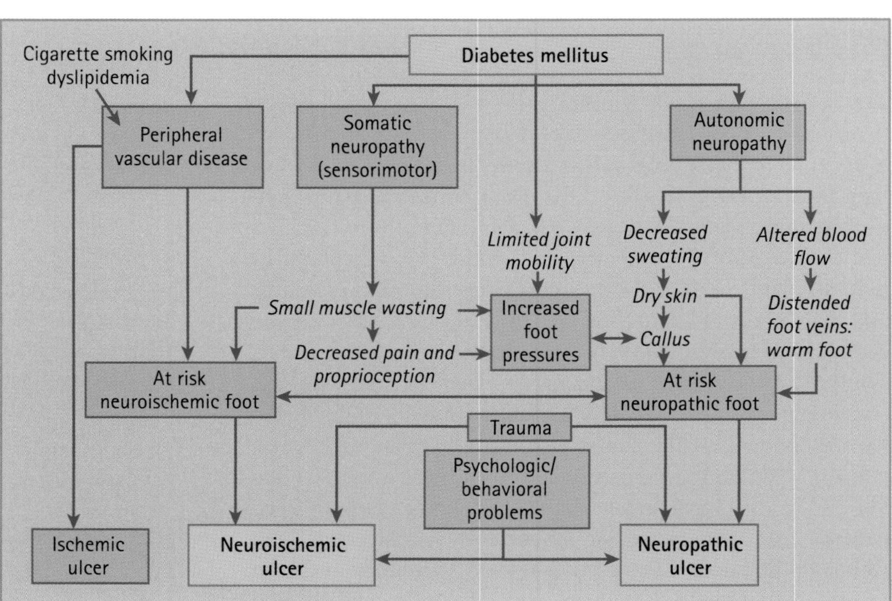

Figure 44.1 Pathways to foot ulceration in diabetes. Reproduced from Boulton *et al.* [7], with permission.

polyneuropathy and the autonomic neuropathies. It is the common sensorimotor neuropathy together with peripheral autonomic sympathetic neuropathy that together have an important role in the pathogenesis of ulceration.

Sensorimotor neuropathy

As noted in Chapter 38, this type of neuropathy is very common and it has been estimated that up to 50% of older patients with type 2 diabetes have evidence of sensory loss on clinical examination and therefore must be considered at risk of insensitive foot injury [27]. This type of neuropathy commonly results in a sensory loss confirmed on examination by a deficit in the stocking distribution to all sensory modalities: evidence of motor dysfunction in the form of small muscle wasting is also often present. While some patients may give a history (past or present) of typical neuropathic symptoms such as burning pain, stabbing pain, paresthesia with nocturnal exacerbation, others may develop sensory loss with no history of any symptoms. Other patients may have the "painful-painless" leg with spontaneous discomfort secondary to neuropathic symptoms but who on examination have both small and large fiber sensory deficits: such patients are at great risk of painless injury to their feet.

From the above it should be clear that a spectrum of symptomatic severity may be present with some patients experiencing severe pain and at the other end of the spectrum, patients who have no spontaneous symptoms but both groups may have significant sensory loss. The most challenging patients are those who develop sensory loss with no symptoms because it is often difficult to convince them that they are at risk of foot ulceration as they feel no discomfort, and motivation to perform regular foot self-care is difficult. The important message is that neuropathic symptoms correlate poorly with sensory loss, and their absence must *never* be equated with lack of foot ulcer risk. Thus, assessment of foot ulcer risk must *always* include a careful foot examination after removal of shoes and socks, whatever the neuropathic history [27].

The patient with sensory loss

A reduction in neuropathic foot problems will only be achieved if we remember that those patients with insensitive feet have lost their warning signal – pain – that ordinarily brings patients to their doctors. Thus, the care of a patient with sensory loss is a new challenge for which we have no training. It is difficult for us to understand, for example, that an intelligent patient would buy and wear a pair of shoes three sizes too small and come to the clinic with extensive shoe-induced ulceration. The explanation is simple: with reduced sensation, a very tight fit stimulates the remaining pressure nerve endings and is thus interpreted as a normal fit – hence the common complaint when we provide patients with custom-designed shoes that "these shoes are too loose". We can learn much about the management of such patients from the treatment of patients with leprosy [28]. Although the cause of sensory loss is very different from that in diabetes, the end result is the same, thus work in leprosy has been very relevant to our understanding of the pathogenesis of diabetic foot lesions. It was Brand (1914–2003) who worked as a surgeon and a missionary in South India, who described pain as "God's greatest gift to mankind" [29]. He emphasized the power of clinical observation to his students and one remark of his that was very relevant to diabetic foot ulceration was that any patient with a plantar ulcer who walks into the clinic without a limp must have neuropathy. Brand also taught us that if we are to succeed, we must realize that with loss of pain there is also diminished motivation in the healing of, and prevention of, injury.

Peripheral sympathetic autonomic neuropathy

Sympathetic autonomic dysfunction of the lower limbs leads to reduced sweating and results in both dry skin that is prone to crack and fissure, and to increased blood flow (in the absence of large vessel obstructive PVD) with arteriovenous shunting leading to the warm foot. The complex interactions of the neuropathies and other contributory factors in the causation of foot ulcers are summarized in Figure 44.1.

Other risk factors

Of all the other risk factors for ulceration (Table 44.2) one of the most important is a past history of similar problems. In many series this has been associated with an annual risk of re-ulceration of up to 50%.

Other long-term complications

Patients with other late complications, particularly nephropathy, have been reported to have an increased foot ulcer risk. Those most at risk are patients who have recently started dialysis as treatment of their end-stage renal disease [30]. It must also be remembered that those patients with renal transplants and more recently combined pancreas–renal transplants are usually at high risk of ulceration even if normoglycemic as a result of the pancreas transplant.

Table 44.2 Factors increasing risk of diabetic foot ulceration. More common contributory factors shown in bold.

Peripheral neuropathy
- **Somatic**
- **Autonomic**

Peripheral vascular disease
Past history of foot ulcers
Other long-term complication
- **End-stage renal disease**
- Visual loss

Plantar callus
Foot deformity
Edema
Ethnic background
Poor social background

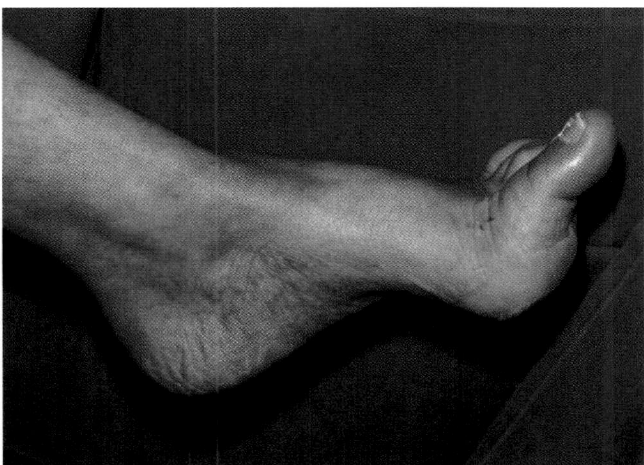

Figure 44.2 The high risk neuropathic diabetic foot demonstrating high arch, prominent metatarsal heads, clawing of toes and callus under first metatarsal head.

Plantar callus

Callus forms under weight-bearing areas as a consequence of dry skin (autonomic dysfunction), insensitivity and repetitive moderate stress from high foot pressure. It acts as a foreign body and causes ulceration [31]. The presence of callus in an insensate foot should alert the physician that this patient is at high risk of ulceration, and callus should be removed by the podiatrist or other trained health care professional.

Elevated foot pressures

Numerous studies have confirmed the contributory role that abnormal plantar pressures play in the pathogenesis of foot ulcers [3,32].

Foot deformity

A combination of motor neuropathy, cheiroarthropathy and altered gait patterns are thought to result in the "high risk" neuropathic foot with clawing of the toes, prominent metatarsal heads, high arch and small muscle wasting (Figure 44.2).

Ethnicity and gender

The male sex has been associated with a 1.6-fold increase of ulcers [11]. With respect to ethnic origin, data from cross-sectional studies in Europe suggests that foot ulceration is more common in Europid subjects than other racial groups: for example, the North-West Diabetes Foot Care Study in the UK showed that the age-adjusted prevalence of diabetic foot ulcers (past or present) for Europeans, South Asians and African-Caribbeans was 5.5%, 1.8% and 2.7%, respectively [33]. Reasons for these ethnic differences certainly warrant further investigation. In contrast, in the southern USA, ulceration was much more common in Latino Americans and Native Americans than in White people of Northern European ancestry [34]; however, more recent data confirmed this increased risk in Latinos, despite the foot pressures being actually lower in this group [35].

Pathway to ulceration

It is the combination of two or more risk factors that ultimately results in diabetic foot ulceration (Figure 44.1). Both Pecoraro *et al.* [25] and later Reiber *et al.* [36] have taken the Rothman model for causation and applied this to amputation and foot ulceration in diabetes. This model is based upon the concept that a component cause (e.g. neuropathy) is not sufficient in itself to lead to ulceration, but when the component causes act together, they result in a sufficient cause which will inevitably result in ulceration. Applying this model to foot ulceration, a small number of causal pathways were identified: the most common triad of component causes, present in nearly two out of three incident foot ulcer cases, was neuropathy, deformity and trauma. Edema and ischemia were also common component causes. Other simple examples of two component causeways to ulceration are loss of sensation and mechanical trauma such as standing on a nail, wearing shoes that are too small; or neuropathy and thermal trauma (e.g. walking on hot surfaces or burning feet in the bath); finally, neuropathy and chemical trauma may result in ulceration from the inappropriate use for example of chemical "corn cures." Similarly, this model can be applied to neuroischemic ulcers where the three component causes comprising ischemia, trauma and neuropathy are often seen.

Prevention of diabetic foot ulcers

Screening

It has been estimated that the vast majority of foot ulcers are potentially preventable, and the first step in prevention is the identification of the "at risk" population. Many countries have now adopted the principle of the "annual review" for patients with diabetes, whereby every patient is screened at least annually for evidence of diabetic complications. Such a review can be carried out either in the primary care center or in a hospital clinic.

A taskforce of the American Diabetes Association recently addressed the question of what should be included for the annual review in the "comprehensive diabetic foot examination (CDFE)" [37]. The taskforce addressed and concisely summarized the recent literature in this area and recommended, where possible using evidence-based medicine, what should be included in the CDFE for adult patients with diabetes. Whereas a brief history was regarded as important, a careful examination of the foot including assessing its neurologic and vascular status was regarded as essential. There is a strong evidence base to support the use of simple clinical tests as predictors of risk of foot ulcers [11,37]. A summary of the key components of the CDFE is provided in Table 44.3. Whereas each potential simple neurologic clinical test has advantages and disadvantages, it was felt that the 10-g monofilament had much evidence to support its use hence the recommendation that assessment of neuropathy should comprise the

Table 44.3 Key components of the diabetic foot examination.

Inspection
Evidence of past/present ulcers?
Foot shape?
- Prominent metatarsal heads/claw toes
- Hallux valgus
- Muscle wasting
- Charcot deformity

Dermatologic?
- Callus
- Erythema
- Sweating

Neurologic
10-g monofilament at four sites on each foot + 1 of the following:
- Vibration using 128 Hz tuning fork
- Pinprick sensation
- Ankle reflexes
- Vibration perception threshold

Vascular
Foot pulses
Ankle brachial index, if indicated

use of a 10 g monofilament plus one other test. In addition to those simple tests listed in Table 44.3, one possible test for neuropathy was assessment of vibration perception threshold. Although this is a semi-quantitative test of sensation, it was included as many centers in both Europe and North America have such equipment. As can be seen from Table 44.3, this is not regarded as essential, but strong evidence does support the use of vibration perception threshold as an excellent predictor of foot ulceration [38,39].

With respect to the vasculature, the ankle brachial index was recommended although it was realized that many centers in primary care may not be able to perform this in day-to-day clinical practice.

Intervention for high-risk patients

Any abnormality of the above screening test would put the patient into a group at higher risk of foot ulceration. Potential interventions are discussed under a number of headings, the most important of which is education.

Education

Previous studies have suggested that patients with foot ulcer risk lack knowledge and skills and consequently are unable to provide appropriate foot self-care [40]. Patients need to be informed of the risk of having insensate feet, the need for regular self-inspection, foot hygiene and chiropody/podiatry treatment as required, and they must be told what action to take in the event of an injury or the discovery of a foot ulcer. Recent studies summarized by Vileikyte *et al.* [41,42] suggests that patients often have distorted beliefs about neuropathy, thinking that this is a circulatory problem and link neuropathy directly to amputation. Thus, an education program that focuses on reducing foot ulcers will be doomed to failure if patients do not believe that foot ulcers precede amputations. It is clear that much work is required in this area if appropriate education is to succeed in reducing foot ulcers and subsequently amputations. The potential for education and self-care at various points on the pathway to neuropathic ulceration is shown in Figure 44.3.

There have been a small number of reports that assess educational interventions, but these have mostly been small single-center studies. In the most recently published study, even though the foot care education program was followed by improved foot care behavior, there is no evidence that such targeted education was associated with a reduced incidence of recurrent foot ulcers [43]. It has been suggested that patients find the concept of neuropathy difficult to understand: they are reassured because they have no discomfort or pain in their feet. It may be that using visual aids (which can also be used for diagnosis of the at risk foot) may help patients to understand that there is something different about their feet compared with their partner's, for example. This might include the use of the administered indicator plaster (Neuropad): when applied to the foot this changes color from blue to pink if there is normal sweating [44]. The absence of sweating such as in a high risk foot, results in no color change enabling patients to see that there is something different about their feet. A similar visual aid is the PressureStat (Podotrack) (Figure 44.4) [45]. This is a simple inexpensive semi-quantitative footprint mat that is able to identify high plantar pressures. The higher the pressure, the darker the color of the footprint. Similarly, this can be used as an educational aid and might help the patient realize that specific areas under their feet are at particular risk of ulceration.

In summary, foot care education is believed to be crucial in the prevention of ulceration, although there is little support for this from randomized controlled trials. Further studies in this area are therefore urgently required.

Podiatry/chiropody

Although not available in every country, regular nail and skin care from a podiatrist/chiropodist is essential in the high-risk neuropathic foot. Attempted self-care has been reported in several cases to cause ulceration and similarly self-care of calluses should be discouraged. Chiropodists and podiatrists should be attached to the foot care team if available and can also educate the patient while treating the feet.

Footwear/othoses/hosiery

Inappropriate footwear is a common cause of foot ulceration in insensitive feet, whereas good footwear can reduce ulcer occurrence [40]. This statement is supported by randomized controlled trials [46]. There is evidence from the literature also to support the use of specialist hosiery which might reduce foot pressures and give all round protection to high risk neuropathic feet [47,48].

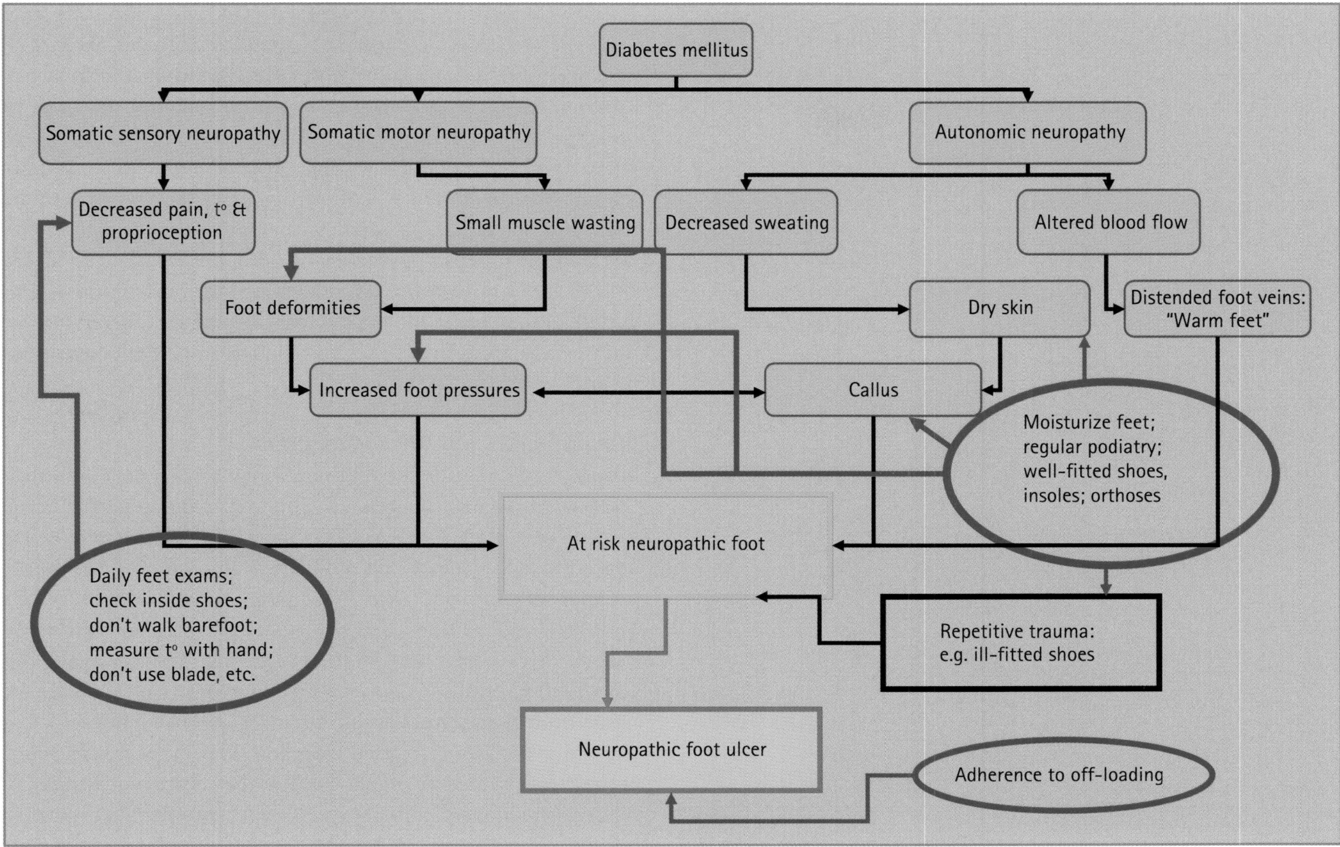

Figure 44.3 The potential for education and self-care in prevention of neuropathic foot ulcers. t°, temperature. Courtesy of L. Vileikyte MD, PhD.

Self-monitoring of skin temperature

It has been known for some time that prior to skin breakdown and ulceration, the involved area of the foot tends to warm up as a consequence of local inflammation. In an appropriately designed, randomized controlled trial, Lavery *et al.* [49] randomized patients with a history of neuropathic foot ulceration to one of three groups, the main intervention being self-monitoring of skin temperature of both feet: those patients who received this skin temperature thermometer were advised to rest or contact their foot clinic should there be a maintained difference in temperature between the two feet. This study clearly showed that those patients who monitored their skin temperatures and followed the advice had a markedly reduced incidence of recurrent ulceration (8% vs 30%). Thus, infrared temperature home monitoring might help to identify the "pre-ulcerative" foot and permit intervention prior to actual skin breakdown. A more recent study has provided further support for this notion [50].

Injected liquid silicone

Injected liquid silicone under high pressure areas of the diabetic foot has been used for some years in the USA and is supported by a randomized controlled trial [51] which confirmed that those patients receiving active agent had reduced foot pressures and increased subcutaneous tissue under the high pressure areas of the forefoot. This therapy is now available in certain European countries, and a follow-up study [52] confirmed that the effect of this "injectable orthosis" lasts for up to 2 years, although booster injections may be required from time to time.

Foot ulcers: diagnosis and management

Foot ulcer classification

Despite increasing efforts in the early identification and preventative foot care education of high risk patients, foot ulcers continue to be a major issue in diabetes management and may indeed be the presenting feature of type 2 diabetes. The principles of management depend up a careful assessment of the causative factors, the presence or absence of infection, the degree of neuropathy and/or ischemia in the foot. Before discussing the management of specific types of ulcers, it is important to consider how to classify foot lesions. Numerous classification systems for diabetic foot ulcers have been proposed [53] but only a few are described here.

The most widely used foot ulcer classification system worldwide at the time of writing is the Meggitt–Wagner grading, as shown in Table 44.4. Despite its wide use, this system does lack specificity and it does not refer to the neuropathic, ischemic or infective status of the ulcers.

The newer University of Texas (UT) wound classification system is currently widely used (Table 44.5) [54]. This is based upon the Meggitt–Wagner system but with the addition of grades of ulcers and stages each grade for the presence or absence of infection and ischemia. In a comparative study of these two systems, the UT system was shown to be a useful predictor of outcome although the Meggitt–Wagner system was still confirmed to be useful [55]. A high risk foot with pre-ulcerative lesions (Wagner 0, UT1A) is shown in Figure 44.5. The two more recently described classification systems, S(AD) SAD system, (size (area, depth), sepsis, arteriopathy and denervation) and the PEDIS (perfusion, extent, depth, infection, sensation) systems appear to have some advantages over the earlier systems, but are not in widespread use [53]. Thus, the UT system will be used to describe ulcer classification here.

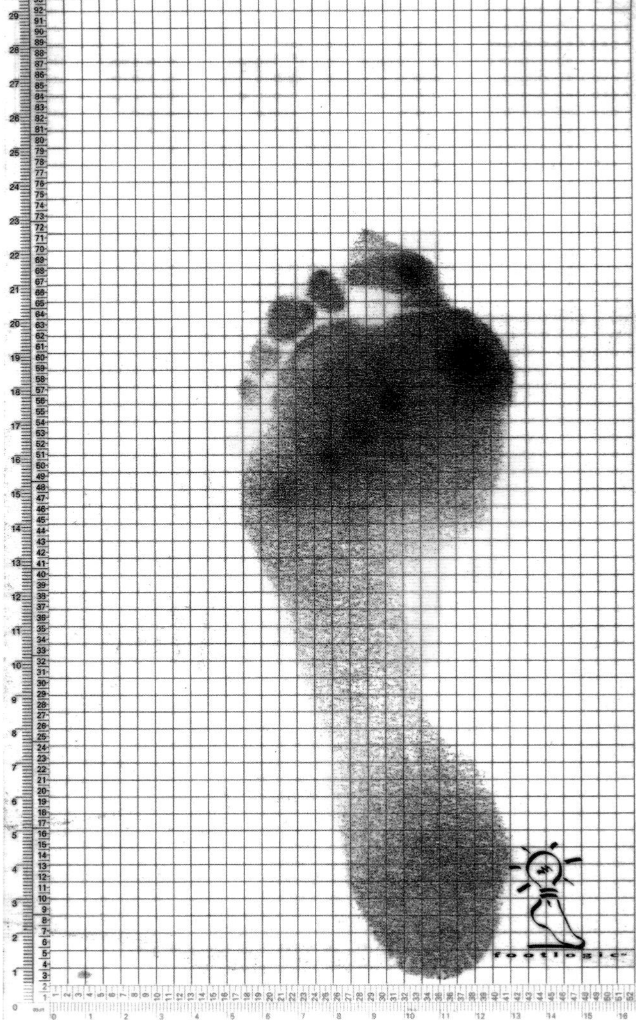

Figure 44.4 A black and white pressure distribution of one footstep using PressureStat: the darkest areas represent highest pressures, in this case under metatarsal heads 1 and 3 and the hallux.

Wound healing in the diabetic foot

Wound healing is a tissue response to injury and passes through the phases of inflammation, chemotaxis, cellular proliferation, extracellular matrix deposition and finally wound remodeling and scarring. Diabetes may influence foot wound healing in a number of different ways including an impairment of the peripheral circulation, altered leukocyte function, disturbed balance of cytokines and proteases and even chronic hyperglycemia itself [3,56]. Thus, foot ulcers in patients with diabetes are recalcitrant to healing because of many cellular and molecular aberrations. When compared with normal acute wound healing, chronic foot ulcers are often stalled in the chronic inflammatory phase with impaired granulation tissue formation. A key question is therefore: is there a fundamental impairment of wound healing in diabetes, and if so, what are the molecular/cellular impairments and are they specific to chronic wounds? A number of studies have reported abnormalities in cytokines and growth factors in tissue from chronic diabetic foot ulcers [57–59]. Most recently, it has been suggested that levels of matrix metallopro-

Table 44.4 Meggitt–Wagner classification. Modified from Oyibo *et al.* [55].

Grade 0	No ulcer, but high risk foot (deformity, callus, etc)
Grade 1	Superficial ulcer
Grade 2	Deep ulcer, may involve tendons but not bone
Grade 3	Deep ulcer with bone involvement, osteomyelitis
Grade 4	Localized gangrene (e.g. toes)
Grade 5	Gangrene of whole foot

Table 44.5 The University of Texas ulcer classification system.

Stage	Grade			
	0	1	2	3
A	High risk foot: no ulcer	Superficial ulcer	Deep ulcer to tendon/capsule	Wound penetrating bone/joint
B	+Infection	+Infection	+Infection	+Infection
C	+Ischemia	+Ischemia	+Ischemia	+Ischemia
D	+Infection and ischemia	+Infection and ischemia	+Infection and ischemia	+Infection and ischemia

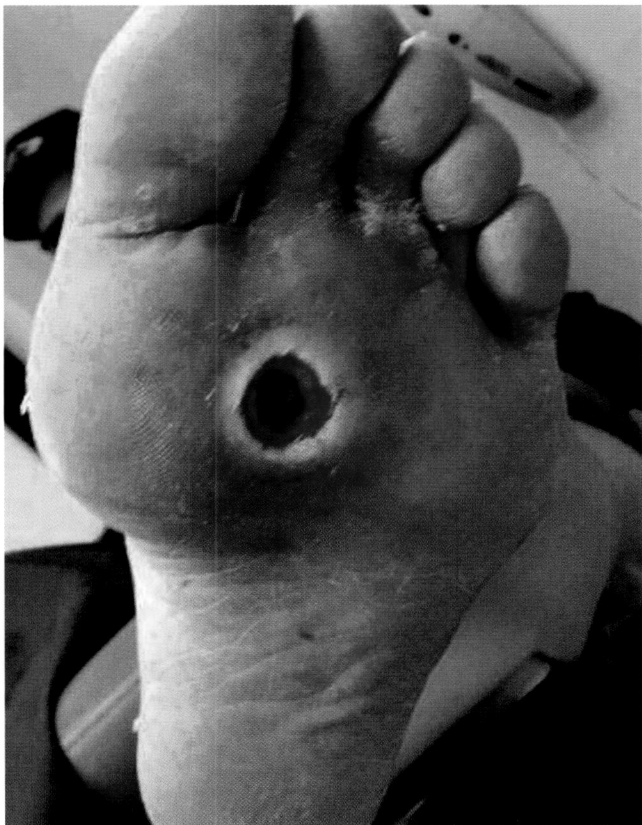

Figure 44.5 Wagner grade I ulcer, UT1A foot ulcer, showing a rim of callus and a punched out neuropathic ulcer in the metatarsal head region with no evidence of infection.

teinases (MMP) are important in predicting the likelihood of wound healing and a high level of MMP-1 seems essential to wound healing [59].

Another contributory factor to impaired wound healing in diabetes appears to be repetitive pressure on the wound. The pivotal role of offloading is therefore considered in the next section.

Offloading

A normal individual with a foot wound will limp: it has been known for some time that neuropathic plantar foot wounds will heal satisfactorily when offloaded in a Total Contact Cast (TCC) [3]. The principle of TCC management is that pressure is mitigated but, in addition, the device is irremovable thus enforcing compliance with therapy. A number of randomized controlled trials have compared the TCC with other removable offloading devices in plantar diabetic foot ulcers and invariably, healing is most rapid in those randomized to TCC treatment [3,60]. As it is known that the Removable Cast Walkers (RCW) redistribute pressure in a similar manner to the TCC, however, the question remained as to why the TCC usually demonstrated superiority in terms of speed of wound closure. The most likely explanation which is that of patient non-compliance, was confirmed in a study of 20 subjects with plantar neuropathic diabetic foot ulcers who were provided with RCWs and their total activity was recorded both from the waist, and from an activity monitor hidden in the RCW. It transpired that patients only wore the RCW for 28% of all footsteps [61]. Subsequent to this observation, it was proposed that an RCW might be rendered irremovable by wrapping it with one or two bands of plaster of Paris, therefore addressing most of the disadvantages of the TCC but preserving irremovability. A subsequent randomized controlled trial of this modified, irremovable RCW versus the TCC showed that healing times were identical [62].

The impact of appropriate offloading on the histopathologic features of neuropathic diabetic foot ulcers was reported by Piaggesi *et al.* [63]. These authors confirm that appropriate offloading resulted in the foot wound appearing more like an acute wound with reparative patterns, angiogenesis and fibroblast proliferation and the presence of granulation tissue. In contrast, biopsies from wounds that had not previously been offloaded confirmed the presence of hyperkeratosis, fibrosis and chronic inflammation. These observations certainly suggest that appropriate offloading is associated with change in the histology of neuropathic foot ulcers including the reduction of inflammatory and reactive components and the acceleration of wound healing.

Another important consideration is the importance of emotional distress (e.g. depression and anxiety) on wound healing in patients with diabetes [64]. Such effects may have direct and indirect effect on wound healing. The direct effects include altered catecholamine and steroid secretion in addition to an imbalance of cytokines which might directly impair wound healing. Indirectly, those patients who are depressed, for example, are less likely to adhere to treatment advice such as wearing an RCW at all times when walking. These important observations have previously been neglected by clinicians and if any patient with a plantar foot ulcer treated by an RCW shows no sign of healing, consideration should be given to compliance and the possibility of rendering the RCW irremovable as noted above.

As might be deduced from the above discussion, offloading is an essential component to the management of predominantly neuropathic plantar foot ulcers. This would include most UT 1A and 2A ulcers. Casts may also be used in the presence of localized infection in neuropathic foot ulcers (Figure 44.6). There is also evidence to support the use of offloading devices in the management of neuroischaemic ulcers but only if they are not clinically infected (UT 1C, 2C) [65].

For those patients treated with irremovable cast walkers, it is recommended that the cast be removed initially on a weekly basis for wound assessment, débridement and cleansing. Healing can generally be a achieved in a period of 6–12 weeks in a cast: it is strongly recommended that after the plantar wound has healed, that the cast be worn for a further 4 weeks to permit the scar tissue to firm up. Thereafter, the patient may be gradually transferred to appropriate footwear which may need extra depth or in the case of severe deformity, custom moulded.

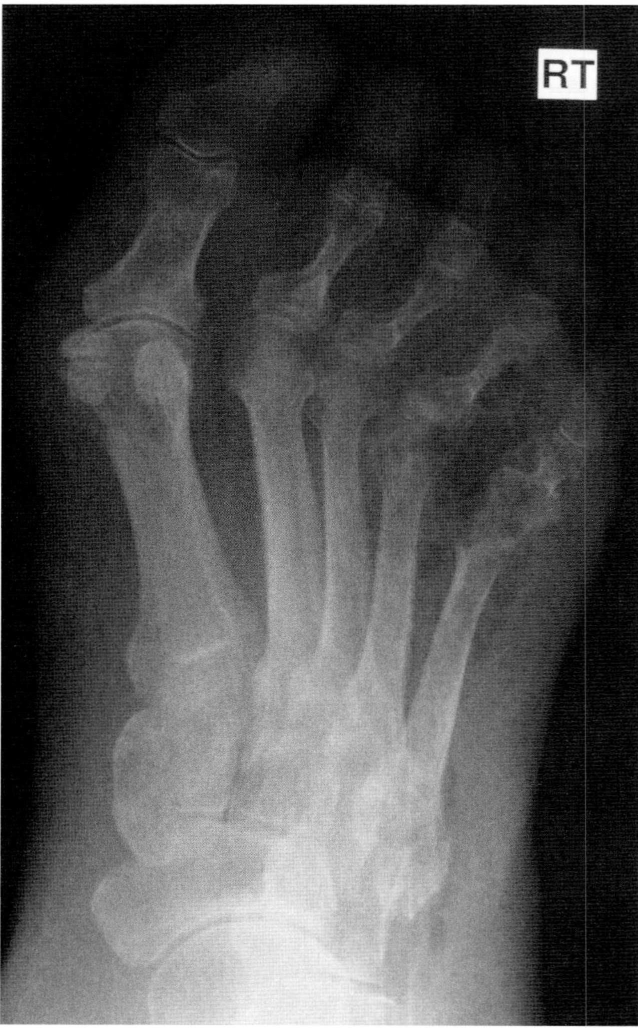

Figure 44.6 Radiograph from a patient with a deep neuropathic ulcer under the right fifth metatarsal head. Gas in the tissues is not uncommon in radiographs of neuropathic foot ulcers as patients lacking pain sensation are able to walk despite the ulcer, "pumping" gas into the tissue. In this example, however, the gas makes it difficult to assess whether osteomyelitis is present.

Dressings

The danger of dressings and bandages is that some health care professionals may draw from them a false sense of security, believing that by dressing an ulcer they are curing it. Nothing could be further from the truth for a neuropathic ulcer. The three most important factors in the healing of a diabetic foot ulcer are: freedom from pressure, freedom from infection and good vascularity. The purpose of dressings is to protect the wound from local trauma, minimize the risk of infection and optimize the wound environment which should be moist in most cases. The evidence base to support the choice of any particular dressing is woefully inadequate with few trials generally hampered by small numbers, inappropriate comparators and poor study design [66,67]. There is little evidence that any specific dressing will have a major impact on the rate of wound healing.

Management of infection

One of the first steps in the management of a foot ulcer is to determine whether infection is present or not: remember that all foot ulcers are colonized with potentially pathogenic organisms and it is generally accepted by the international working group on the diabetic foot that the diagnosis of infection in the diabetic foot ulcer remains a clinical one [68]. Thus, the presence of signs such as purulent discharge, erythema, local warmth and swelling which suggests infection requiring appropriate treatment.

Clinically non-infected ulcers

Where ulcers are not infected and predominantly neuropathic (UT grades 1A, 2A), the use of antibiotics may be withheld as Chantelau *et al.* [69] have shown that with appropriate wound management, patients do equally well with or without systemic antibiotics in a randomized controlled trial. Nevertheless, frequent review, débridement and callus removal together with offloading are essential parts of management of neuropathic foot ulcers and should signs of infection develop, antibiotics may be needed. For those ulcers with an ischemic component which do not have gross signs of infection (UT 1C, 2C) antibiotics should probably be given in most cases as the combination of infection and ischemia in the diabetic foot are a common cause of ultimate lower extremity amputation.

Clinically infected ulcers

Non-limb-threatening infected ulcers (UT 1B, 1D, 2B, 2D) can generally be treated on an outpatient basis, and oral broad-spectrum antibiotics should be used initially until results of sensitivities are obtained. As reviewed by Lipsky, two sets of international guidelines have been published in recent years [68,70,71]. One important aspect of these recent guidelines has been the development of criteria by which to classify the severity of a diabetic foot infection. Generally, mild infections are relatively superficial and limited, moderate infections involve deeper tissues and severe infections are accompanied by systematic signs or symptoms of infection or metabolic disturbances [68]. Any ulcer with clinical evidence of infection should have tissue taken and sent for culture and sensitivity in the microbiology department. Although superficial swabs are commonly taken, deep (preferably tissue) specimens are preferable in terms of accuracy of diagnosis [68]. Most infective ulcers are polymicrobial, often with a mixture of anaerobes and aerobes. Unfortunately, a systematic review of antimicrobial treatments for diabetic foot ulcers revealed that few appropriately designed randomized controlled studies have been conducted and it was difficult to give specific guidelines as to antibiotic regimens for specific infective organisms [72]; however, if there is any suspicion of osteomyelitis (signs such as a sausage-shaped toe or the ability to probe to bone may suggest this diagnosis) should have a radiograph taken of the infected foot and possibly further investigations (see below and Chapter 50). The antibiotic prescription for a clinically infected non-limb-threatening foot ulcer without evidence of osteomyelitis should be guided by sensitivities after these are available from tissue specimens: when sensitivities are known, targeted appropriate narrow-spectrum agents should be prescribed. Suitable broad-spectrum antibiotics to start as soon as the clinical diagnosis of infection is made while waiting for sensitivity from the microbiology department would include drugs such as clindamycin or the amoxicillin–clavulanate combination [68].

Limb-threatening infection

Patients with limb-threatening infection usually have systemic symptoms and signs and require hospitalization with parenteral antibiotics. Deep wound and blood cultures should be taken, the circulation assessed with non-invasive studies initially, and metabolic control is usually achieved by intravenous insulin infusion. Early surgical débridement is often indicated in such cases, and initial antibiotic regimens should be broad-spectrum until sensitivities are determined from cultures. Examples of initial antibiotic regimens include: clindamycin and ciprofloxacin, or flucloxacillin, ampicillin and metronidazole. One problem with interpreting sensitivities is the question as to whether the organism isolated is simply a colonizing bacteria or is it a true infecting organism? One technique, the polymerase chain reaction (PCR) assay has been shown to be effective at identifying many virulent organisms [68]. A recent study from France [73] showed the potential advantages of using this new technique in the rapid distinction between colonizing and virulent infecting organisms.

An increasing problem in diabetic foot clinics is the antibiotic-resistant pathogens such as methacillin-resistant *Staphylococcus aureus* (MRSA). In most cases, MRSA is isolated as an opportunistic colonizing organism following the treatment with often inappropriate long duration broad-spectrum antibiotics. If MRSA is felt to be an infecting organism, there are useful new agents such as linezolid [68], which can be given parenterally or orally and are effective against such organisms. There is a suggestion that larval therapy [74] might be useful in eradicating MRSA that is contaminating diabetic foot wounds.

Osteomyelitis

As discussed in Chapter 50, the diagnosis of osteomyelitis is a controversial topic, and several diagnostic tests have been recommended. Amongst these, "probing to bone" has been shown to have a relatively high predictive value whereas plain radiographs are insensitive early in the natural history of osteomyelitis. In most clinical cases, however, the diagnosis is ultimately made by a plain X-ray of the foot (Figure 44.7). Magnetic resonance imaging (MRI) is having an increasing role in the diagnosis as it has high sensitivity [75]. The combination of an ulcer area $>2 \times 2$ cm, a positive probe to bone test, an elevated sedimentation rate and an abnormal radiograph are most helpful in diagnosing the presence of osteomyelitis in the diabetic foot whereas a negative MRI makes a diagnosis much less likely [76]. The most recent review on this topic suggests that a combination of clinical and laboratory findings together can significantly improve diagnostic accuracy for osteomyelitis in the diabetic foot: the specific combination of ulcer depth with serum inflammatory markers appears to be particularly sensitive [77]. Contrary to traditional teaching, it is increasingly recognized that some cases of localized osteomyelitis can be managed by long-term (10–12 weeks) antibiotic therapy [78]; however, localized bony resection after appropriate antibiotic therapy remains a common approach. Those cases with osteomyelitis confined to one bone without involvement of a joint are most likely to respond to antibiotic therapy particularly in the absence of peripheral vascular disease. It must be pointed out that data to inform treatment choices in osteomyelitis of the diabetic foot for randomized controlled trials are limited and further research is urgently needed [79].

Adjunctive therapies

A number of newer approaches to promote more rapid healing in diabetic foot lesions have been described over the last two decades. Some of those are mentioned below but many were also recently reviewed by the International Working Group on the Diabetic Foot [80].

Growth factors

A number of growth factors and other agents designed to modify abnormalities of the biochemistry of the wound bed or surrounding tissues have been described, but there is still no consensus as their place in day-to-day clinical practice [80]. One example is platelet-derived growth factor (PDGF) which is available for clinical use in a number of countries. Whereas there is some support for their use for randomized clinical studies [81], their expense together with the fact that most neuropathic ulcers can be healed with appropriate offloading, have limited their use. Unfortunately, PDGF together with other topically applied agents such as epidermal growth factor do not have sufficient robust data to support their day-to-day use in routine clinical practice.

Hyperbaric oxygen

Hyperbaric oxygen (HBO) has been widely promoted for the management of non-healing diabetic foot ulcers particularly in the USA, for some years. Many of the reported studies have been poorly designed or anecdotal and have given rise to serious concerns about the widespread use of this treatment [82]; however, there have been several small well-designed randomized controlled trials to assess the efficacy of HBO in ischemic diabetic foot wounds [83]. Whereas the systematic review of the International Working Group that considered HBO accepted that there was some evidence to support its use, it is clear that more data are required from larger controlled trials not only to confirm efficacy but also to clarify which wounds might best benefit from this expensive treatment [80,84].

Negative pressure wound therapy

Over the past several years negative pressure wound therapy (NPWT) using vacuum-assisted closure has emerged as a commonly employed option in the treatment of complex wounds of the diabetic foot [85]. Previous work has suggested that the application of negative pressure optimizes blood flow, decreases local tissue edema and removes excessive fluid and pro-inflammatory exudates from the wound bed. There is now controlled trial evidence for the use of NPWT in both local postoperative wounds in the diabetic foot [86] and, more recently, in the management of complex but non-surgical diabetic foot ulcers [87]. It is clear that this treatment helps promote the formation of granulation tissue, but its cost will limit its use to those complex diabetic foot wounds not responding to standard therapies.

Bioengineered skin substitutes

Similar to other treatments in this group of adjunctive therapies although there is some evidence to support the use of bioengineered skin substitutes in non-infected neuropathic ulcers, its use of somewhat restricted by cost [80]. A systematic review on this topic concluded that the trials assessed were of questionable quality and until high quality studies were performed, recommendations for the use of these skin substitutes could not be made [88].

Charcot neuroarthropathy

Charcot neuroarthropathy (CN) is a non-infective arthropathy that occurs in a well-perfused insensate foot. Although the exact mechanism underlying the development of CN remains unclear, progress has been made in our understanding of the etiopathogenesis of this disorder in the last decade. It is clear that the classic neurotraumatic and neurotrophic theories for the pathogenesis of acute CN in diabetes do not address certain key features of the disease [89]. If the former theory were correct, CN would be much more common and should be symmetrical: in contrast, acute CN is relatively rare amongst patients with neuropathy and is usually asymmetrical, although there is an increased risk of developing CN in the contralateral foot some years later.

CN occurs in a well-perfused insensate foot. Typically, patients present with a warm, swollen foot and contrary to some of the earlier texts, may be accompanied by pain or at least discomfort in the affected limb. The affected patient tends to be slightly younger than is usual for the patient presenting with a diabetic foot ulcer and typically presents with a warm swollen foot which may or may not be painful. Although a history of trauma may be present, the trauma is rarely of sufficient severity to account for the abnormalities observed on clinical examination (Figure 44.7). Although CN is characterized by increased local bone resorption, the exact cellular mechanisms contributing to this condition remain unresolved. Recently, receptor activator of nuclear factor κB ligand (RANKL) has been identified as an essential mediator of osteoclast formation and activation. It has been hypothesized that the RANKL/osteoprotegerin (OPG) pathway may play an important part in the development of acute CN [89]. It has subsequently been confirmed that peripheral blood monocytes isolated from patients with CN and cultured in the presence of macrophage colony-stimulating factor led to an increased osteoclast formation when compared to healthy and diabetic controlled monocytes [90]. These observations suggested that RANKL-mediated osteoclastic resorption occurs in acute CN. Thus, the RANKL-dependent pathway is important in the pathogenesis of acute CN suggesting that in the future, inhibition of RANKL might be useful in management.

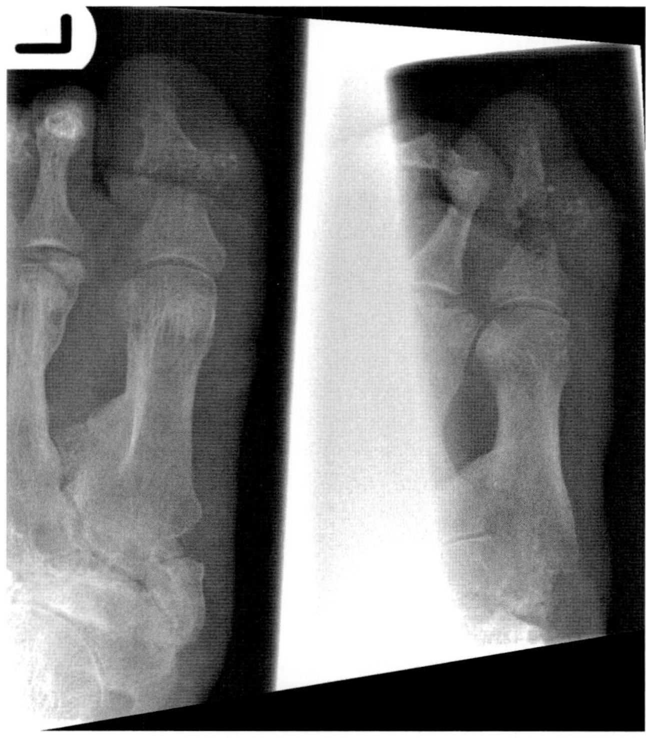

Figure 44.7 This radiograph displays two main abnortmalities: (a) changes of osteomyelitis and septic arthritis involving the first metatarso-phalangeal joint, with destruction of the distal first metatarsal and proximal area of the proximal phalanx of the great toe; and (b) chronic changes of Charcot neuroarthropathy in the first cuneiform/metatarsal area.

As discussed in Chapter 48, the treatment of the foot in CN depends upon the stage in which the disease is diagnosed. In the acute phase, there is evidence that offloading of the affected foot by use of a plaster cast is the most effective method of reducing disease activity and local inflammation. Use of the cast should continue until the swelling and hyperemia have resolved and the skin temperature differential is 1°C or less, at which time custom moulded shoes with appropriate insoles are indicated [91]. Bisphosphonates are potent inhibitors of osteoclast activation and intravenous pamidronate has been shown to be useful in reducing disease activity in acute CN [92]. Larger randomized controlled trials are required to confirm these preliminary observations.

The management of advanced CN with bone deformity requiring reconstructive surgery is beyond the scope of this chapter and the reader is referred to recent reviews [93].

Conclusions

There can be no doubt that despite our efforts in early identification, prevention and aggressive treatment of diabetic foot problems, that the incidence of diabetic foot disease is likely to increase in the next few decades with the global explosion in of the prevalence in type 2 diabetes reviewed elsewhere in this book. It is also clear that diabetic foot disease carries not only a significant morbidity, but even mortality: Armstrong *et al.* [94] pointed out that the outlook for those with diabetic foot disease is worse than many malignant diseases. There is increasing recognition of the multifactorial nature of complications which led Young *et al.* [95] to review the survival of their patients with diabetic foot lesions over the last 13 years. They reported that survival has improved and this has been accompanied by the adoption of an aggressive cardiovascular risk management policy which should be encouraged in all patients with diabetic foot disease. The ultimate prognosis for the limb with a diabetic foot lesion depends upon the presence or absence of an ischemic component: it has been shown that patients with higher Wagner or UT gradings and severity are more likely to end up with minor or even major amputation. Thus, neuropathic foot lesions generally carry a good prognosis, whereas those with a significant ischaemic components are more likely to require the input of the vascular surgeon (see Chapter 43).

The team approach

It should be clear that the spectrum of diabetic foot problems requires the involvement of individuals from many specialties. The diabetic foot cannot be regarded as the sole responsibility of the diabetologist, and a number of reports over the last decade have promoted the benefits of a multidisciplinary approach to diabetic foot care [96]. This started in the early 1990s when the concept of the "annual review" was adopted by most national diabetes societies. This requires that all patients with diabetes be screened on an annual basis for evidence of long-term complications [97]. There is increasing evidence from a number of long-term studies that the adoption of this approach not only in hospital but in community care, has been associated with a reduced incidence of foot problems [98–101]. The improved management of diabetic foot care in the district of Leverkusen, Germany, ultimately resulted in a 37% reduction in non-traumatic amputations in patients with diabetes; however, this took more than 10 years after the establishment of specialist foot care [98]. Two studies from the UK [99,100] have reported reductions of up to 60% in diabetic amputations and both of these followed either the introduction of multidisciplinary team work in the community or the improved organization of general diabetes care. Finally, a sustained reduction in major amputations has been reported from Sweden over the last 20 years suggesting that a substantial decrease in diabetes-related amputations can not only be achieved, but maintained over a long period of time [101].

The team approach, involving diabetologists working together with surgeons (orthopedic and vascular), specialist nurses, podiatrists, orthotists and often many other health care professionals is therefore strongly recommended in the management of complex lesions of the diabetic foot. It should be remenbered, however, it is the patient at risk of, or with foot ulceration, who must be regarded as the most important in this team. Without the patient's willing participation, there is little that other team members can achieve to improve the overall outlook for the diabetic foot in the 21st century.

References

1 Singh N, Armstrong DG, Lipsky BA. Preventing foot ulcers in patients with diabetes. *JAMA* 2005; **293**:217–228.
2 Boulton AJM, Vileikyte L, Ragnarson-Tennvall G, Apelqvist J. The global burden of diabetic foot disease. *Lancet* 2005; **366**:1719–1724.
3 Boulton AJM. The diabetic foot: from art to science: the 18th Camillo Golgi lecture. *Diabetologia* 2004; **47**:1343–1353.
4 Ragnarson-Tennvall G, Apelqvist J. Prevention of diabetes-related foot ulcers and amputations: a cost–utility analysis based on Markov model simulations. *Diabetologia* 2001; **44**:2077–2087.
5 Connor H. Some historical aspects of diabetic foot disease. *Diabet Metab Res Rev* 2008; **24**(Suppl 1):7–13.
6 McKeown KC. The history of the diabetic foot. *Diabet Med* 1995; **12**:19–23.
7 Boulton AJM, Cavanagh PR, Rayman G. *The Foot in DiabetesI*, 4th edn. Chichester: John Wiley & Sons Ltd, 2006.
8 Bowker JH, Pfeifer MA. *Levin & O'Neal's The Diabetic Foot*, 7th edn. Philadelphia: Mosby-Elsevier, 2008.
9 Sämaan A, Tajiyeva O, Müller N, Tschauner T, Hoyer H, Wolf G, *et al.* Prevalence of the diabetic foot syndrome at the primary care level in Germany: a cross-sectional study. *Diabet Med* 2008; **25**:557–563.
10 Al-Mahroos F, Al-Roomi K. Diabetic neuropathy foot ulceration, peripheral vascular disease and potential risk factors among patients with diabetes in Bahrain: a nationwide primary care diabetes clinic-based study. *Ann Saudi Med* 2007; **27**:25–31.
11 Abbott CA, Carrington AL, Ashe H, Bath S, Every LC, Griffiths J, *et al.* The North-West Diabetes Foot Care Study: incidence of, and risk factors for new diabetic foot ulceration in a community-based patient cohort. *Diabet Med* 2002; **19**:377–384.
12 Manes C, Papazoglou N, Sassidou E, Tzounas K. Prevalence of diabetic neuropathy and foot ulceration: a population-based study. *Wounds* 2002; **14**:11–15.
13 Müller IS, de Grauw WJ, van Gerwen WH, Bartelink ML, van Den Hoogen HJ, Rutten GE. Foot ulceration and lower limb amputation in type 2 diabetic patients in Dutch primary health care. *Diabetes Care* 2002; **25**:570–576.
14 Ramsay SD, Newton K, Blough D, McCulloch DK, Sandhu N, Reiber GE, *et al.* Incidence, outcomes and costs of foot ulcers in patients with diabetes. *Diabetes Care* 1999; **22**:382–387.
15 Vozar J, Adamka J, Holeczy P. Diabetics with foot lesions and amputations in the region of Horny Zitmy Ostrov 1993–1995. *Diabetologia* 1997; **40**(Suppl 1):A46.

16 Kumar S, Ashe HA, Parnell LN, Fernando DJ, Young RJ, Tsigos C, *et al.* The prevalence of foot ulceration and its correlates in type 2 diabetic patients: a population-based study. *Diabet Med* 1994; **11**:480–484.

17 Moss S, Klein R, Klein B. The prevalence and incidence of lower extremity amputation in a diabetic population. *Arch Intern Med* 1992; **152**:510–616.

18 Boulton AJM, Vileikyte L. Diabetic foot problems and their management around the world. In: Bowker JH, Pfeifer MA, eds. *Levin & O'Neal's The Diabetic Foot*, 7th edn. Philadelphia: Mosby-Elsevier, 2008: 487–496.

19 Van Houtun WH. Amputations and ulceration: pitfalls in assessing incidence. *Diabet Metab Res Rev* 2008; **24**(Suppl 1):14–18.

20 Deerochanawong C, Home PD, Alberti KG. A survey of lower-limb amputations in diabetic patients. *Diabet Med* 1992; **9**:942–946.

21 Shearer A, Scuffham P, Gordois A, Oglesby A. Predicted costs and outcomes from reduced vibration detection in people with diabetes in the US. *Diabetes Care* 2003; **26**:2305–2310.

22 Gordois A, Scuffham P, Shearer A, Oglesby A, Tobian JA. The health care costs of diabetic peripheral neuropathy in the US. *Diabetes Care* 2003; **26**:1790–1795.

23 Gordois A, Scuffham P, Shearer A, Oglesby A. The healthcare costs of diabetic peripheral neuropathy in the UK. *Diabet Foot* 2003; **6**:62–73.

24 Rogers LC, Lavery LA, Armstrong DG. The right to bear legs. *J Am Podiat Med Assoc* 2008; **98**:166–168.

25 Pecoraro RE, Reiber GE, Burgess EM. Pathways to diabetic limb amputation: basis for prevention. *Diabetes Care* 1990; **13**:510–521.

26 Siitonen OI, Niskanen LK, Laakso M, Siitonen JT, Pyörälä K. Lower extremity amputation in diabetic and non-diabetic patients: a population-based study from Eastern Finland. *Diabetes Care* 1993; **16**:16–20.

27 Boulton AJM, Malik RA, Arezzo JL, Sosenko JM. Diabetic somatic neuropathies: technical review. *Diabetes Care* 2004; **27**:1458–1486.

28 Boulton AJM. Diabetic foot ulceration: the leprosy connection. *Pract Diabet Digest* 1990; **3**:35–37.

29 Boulton AJM. The diabetic foot: grand overview. *Diabet Metab Res Rev* 2008; **24**(Suppl 1):3–6.

30 Game FL, Chipchase SY, Hubbard R, Burden RP, Jeffcoate WJ. Temporal association between the incidence of foot ulceration and the start of dialysis in diabetes mellitus. *Nephrol Dial Transplant* 2006; **21**:3207–3210.

31 Murray HJ, Young MJ, Boulton AJM. The relationship between callus formation, high foot pressures and neuropathy in diabetic foot ulceration. *Diabet Med* 1996; **13**:979–982.

32 Boulton AJM, Kirsner RS, Vileikyte L. Neuropathic diabetic foot ulcers. *N Engl J Med* 2004; **351**:48–55.

33 Abbott CA, Garrow AP, Carrington AL, Morris J, Van Ross ER, Boulton AJM. Foot ulcer risk is lower in South-Asian and African-Caribbean compared with European diabetic patients in the UK: the North-West Diabetes Foot Care Study. *Diabetes Care* 2005; **28**:1869–1875.

34 Lavery LA, Armstrong DG, Wunderlich RP, Tredwell J, Boulton AJM. Diabetic foot syndrome: evaluating the prevalence and incidence of foot pathology in Mexican Americans and non-Hispanic whites from a diabetes disease management cohort. *Diabetes Care* 2003; **26**:1435–1438.

35 Solano MP, Prieto LM, Varon JC, Moreno M, Boulton AJM. Ethnic differences in plantar pressures in diabetic patients with peripheral neuropathy. *Diabet Med* 2008; **25**:505–507.

36 Reiber GE, Vileikyte L, Boyko EJ, del Aguila M, Smith DG, Lavery LA, *et al.* Causal pathways for incident lower-extremity ulcers in patients with diabetes from two settings. *Diabetes Care* 1999; **22**:157–162.

37 Boulton AJM, Armstrong DG, Albert SF, Frykberg RG, Hellman R, Kirkman MS, *et al.* Comprehensive foot examination and risk assessment. *Diabetes Care* 2008; **31**:1679–1685.

38 Abbott CA, Vileikyte L, Williamson S, Carrington AL, Boulton AJ. Multicentre study of the incidence and predictive factors for diabetic foot ulceration. *Diabetes Care* 1998; **21**:1071–1075.

39 Frykberg RG, Lavery LA, Pham H, Harvey C, Harkless L, Veves A. Role of neuropathy and high foot pressures in diabetic foot ulceration. *Diabetes Care* 1998; **21**:1714–1719.

40 Mason J, O'Keeffe C, McIntosh A, Hutchinson A, Booth A, Young RJ. A systematic review of foot ulcer prevention in patients with Type 2 diabetes. 1: Prevention. *Diabet Med* 1999; **16**:801–812.

41 Vileikyte L, Rubin RR, Leventhal H. Psychological aspects of diabetic neuropathic foot complications: an overview. *Diabetes Metab Res Rev* 2004; **20**(Suppl 1):13–18.

42 Vileikyte L. Psychosocial and behavioural aspects of diabetic foot lesions. *Curr Diab Rep* 2008; **8**:119–125.

43 Lincoln NB, Radford KA, Game FL, Jeffcoate WJ. Education for secondary prevention of foot ulcers in people with diabetes: a randomised controlled trial. *Diabetologia* 2008; **51**:1954–1961.

44 Tentolouris N, Achtsidis V, Marinou K, Katsilambros N. Evaluation of the self-administered indicator plaster neuropad for the diagnosis of neuropathy in diabetes. *Diabetes Care* 2008; **31**:236–237.

45 van Schie CH, Abbott CA, Vileikyte L, Shaw JE, Hollis S, Boulton AJM. A comparative study of the Podotrack, a simple semi-quantitative plantar pressure measuring device, and the optical paedobarograph in the assessment of pressures under the diabetic foot. *Diabet Med* 1999; **16**:144–159.

46 Uccioli L, Faglia E, Montocine G, Favales F, Durola L, Aldeghi A, *et al.* Manufactured shoes in the prevention of diabetic foot ulcers. *Diabetes Care* 1995; **18**:1376–1378.

47 Veves A, Masson EA, Fernando DJ, Boulton AJM. Use of experimental padded hosiery to reduce abnormal foot pressures in diabetic neuropathy. *Diabetes Care* 1989; **12**:653–655.

48 Garrow AP, van Schie CH, Boulton AJM. Efficacy of multilayered hosiery in reducing in-shoe plantar foot pressure in high-risk patients with diabetes. *Diabetes Care* 2005; **28**:2001–2006.

49 Lavery LA, Higgins KR, Lanctot DR, Constantinides GP, Zamorano RG, Athanasiou KA, *et al.* Preventing diabetic foot ulcer recurrence in high-risk patients: use of temperature monitoring as a self-assessment tool. *Diabetes Care* 2007; **30**:14–20.

50 Armstrong DG, Holtz-Neiderer K, Wendel C, Mohler MJ, Kimbriel HR, Lavery LA. Skin temperature monitoring reduces the risk for diabetic foot ulceration in high-risk patients. *Am J Med* 2007; **120**:1042–1046.

51 van Schie CHM, Whalley A, Vileikyte L, Wignall T, Hollis S, Boulton AJ. Efficacy of injected liquid silicone in the diabetic foot to reduce risk factors for ulceration: a randomized double-blind placebo-controlled trial. *Diabetes Care* 2000; **23**:634–638.

52 van Schie CH, Whalley A, Armstrong DG, Vileikyte L, Boulton AJM. The effect of silicone injections in the diabetic foot on peak plantar pressure and plantar tissue thickness: a 2-year follow-up. *Arch Phys Med Rehabil* 2002; **83**:919–923.

53 Jeffcoate WJ, Game FL. The description and classification of diabetic foot lesions: systems for clinical care, research and audit. In: Boulton

AJM, Cavanagh PR, Rayman G, eds. *The Foot in Diabetes*, 4th edn. Chichester: John Wiley & Sons Ltd, 2006: 92–107.

54 Armstrong DG, Lavery LA, Harkless LB. Validation of a diabetic wound classification system. *Diabet Med* 1998; **21**:855–859.

55 Oyibo S, Jude EB, Tarawneh I, Nguyen HC, Harkless LB, Boulton AJ. A comparison of two diabetic foot ulcer classification systems. *Diabetes Care* 2001; **24**:84–88.

56 Sibbald RG, Woo KY. The biology of chronic foot ulcers in persons with diabetes. *Diabet Metab Res Rev* 2008; **24**(Suppl 1):25–30.

57 Blakytny R, Jude EB, Gibson M, Boulton AJM, Ferguson MW. Lack of insulin-like growth factor 1 (IGF1) in the basal keratinocyte layer of diabetic skin and diabetic foot ulcers. *J Pathol* 2000; **190**:589–594.

58 Jude EB, Blakytny R, Bulmer J, Boulton AJM, Ferguson MW. Transforming growth factor-beta 1,2,3 and receptor type 1 and 2 in diabetic foot ulcers. *Diabet Med* 2002; **19**:440–447.

59 Müller M, Trocme C, Lardy B, Morel F, Halimi S, Benhamou PY. Matrix metalloproteinases and diabetic foot ulcers: the ratio of MMP-1 to TIMP-1 is a predictor of wound healing. *Diabet Med* 2008; **25**:419–426.

60 Armstrong DG, Nguyen HC, Lavery LA, van Schie CH, Boulton AJM, Harkless LB. Offloading the diabetic foot wound: a randomised clinical trial. *Diabetes Care* 2001; **24**:1019–1022.

61 Armstrong DG, Lavery LA, Kimbriel HR, Nixon BP, Boulton AJM. Activity patterns of patients with diabetic foot ulceration: patients with active ulcers may not adhere to a standard pressure offloading regimen. *Diabetes Care* 2003; **26**:2595–2597.

62 Katz IA, Harlan A, Miranda-Palma B, Preto L, Armstrong DG, Bowker JH, *et al.* A randomised trial of two irremovable offloading devices in the management of plantar neuropathic diabetic foot ulcers. *Diabetes Care* 2005; **28**:555–559.

63 Piaggesi A, Viacava P, Rizzo L, Naccarato G, Baccetti F, Romanelli M, *et al.* Semi-quantitative analysis of the histopathological features of the neuropathic foot ulcers: effects of pressure relief. *Diabetes Care* 2003; **26**:3123–3128.

64 Vileikyte L. Stress and wound healing. *Clin Dermatol* 2007; **25**:49–55.

65 Nabuurs-Franssen MH, Sleegers R, Huijberts MS, Wijnen W, Sanders AP, Walenkamp G, *et al.* Total contact casting of the diabetic foot in daily practice: a prospective follow-up study. *Diabetes Care* 2005; **28**:243–247.

66 Mason J, O'Keeffe CO, Hutchinson A, McIntosh A, Young R, Booth A. A systematic review of foot ulcers in patients with type 2 diabetes. II: Treatment. *Diabet Med* 1999; **16**:889–909.

67 Knowles EA. Dressings: is there an evidence base? In: Boulton AJM, Cavanagh PR, Rayman G, eds. *The Foot in Diabetes*, 4th edn. Chichester: John Wiley & Sons Ltd, 2006: 186–197.

68 Lipsky BA. New developments in diagnosing and treating diabetic foot infections. *Diabet Metab Res Rev* 2008; **24**(Suppl 1):S66–S71.

69 Chantelau EA, Tanudjaja T, Altenhöfer F, Ersanli Z, Lacigova S, Metzger C. Antibiotic treatment for uncomplicated neuropathic forefoot ulcers in diabetes: a controlled trial. *Diabet Med* 1996; **26**:267–276.

70 Lipsky BA. A report from the international consensus on diagnosing and treating the infected diabetic foot. *Diabet Metab Res Rev* 2004; **20**(Suppl 1):68–77.

71 Lipsky BA, Berendt AR, Deery HG, Embil JM, Joseph WS, Karchmer AW, *et al.* Infectious Diseases Society of America guidelines: diagnosis and treatment of diabetic foot infections. *Clin Infect Dis* 2004; **39**:885–910.

72 Nelson EA, O'Meara S, Golder S, Dalton J, Craig D, Iglesias C; DASIDU Steering Group. Systematic review of antimicrobial treatments for diabetic foot ulcers. *Diabet Med* 2006; **23**:348–359.

73 Sotto A, Richard J-L, Jourdan N, Combescure C, Bouziges N, Lavigne J-P. Miniaturised oligonucleotide arrays: a new tool for discriminating colonisation from infection due to *Staphylococcus aureus* in diabetic foot ulcers. *Diabetes Care* 2007; **30**:2819–2828.

74 Bowling FL, Salgami EV, Boulton AJM. Larval therapy: a novel treatment in eliminating methicillin-resistant *Staphylococcus aureus* from diabetic foot ulcers. *Diabetes Care* 2007; **30**:370–371.

75 Rozzanigo U, Tagliani A, Vittorini E, Pacchioni R, Brivio LR, Caudana R. Role of magnetic resonance imaging in the evaluation of diabetic foot with suspected osteomyelitis. *Radiol Med* 2009; **114**:121–132.

76 Butalia S, Palda VA, Sargeant RJ, Detsky AS, Mourad O. Does this patient with diabetes have osteomyelitis of the lower extremity? *JAMA* 2008; **299**:806–813.

77 Fleischer AE, Didyk AA, Woods JB, Burns SE, Wrobel JS, Armstrong DG. Combined clinical and laboratory testing improves diagnostic accuracy for osteomyelitis in the diabetic foot. *J Foot Ankle Surg* 2009; **48**:39–46.

78 Game FL, Jeffcoate WJ. Primarily non-surgical management of osteomyelitis of the foot in diabetes. *Diabetologia* 2008; **51**:962–967.

79 Berendt AR, Peters EJ, Bakker K, Embil JM, Eneroth M, Hinchliffe RJ, *et al.* Diabetic foot osteomyelitis: a progress report on diagnosis and a systematic review of treatment. *Diabet Metab Res Rev* 2008; **24**(Suppl 1):145–161.

80 Jeffcoate WJ, Lipsky BA, Berendt AR, Cavanagh PR, Bus SA, Peters EJ, *et al.* Unresolved issues in the management of ulcers of the foot in diabetes. *Diabet Med* 2008; **25**:1380–1389.

81 Wieman TJ, Smiell JM, Yachin S. Efficacy and safety of a topical gel formulation of recombinant human platelet-derived growth factor-BB (Becaplermin) in patients with chronic neuropathic diabetic foot ulcers. *Diabetes Care* 1998; **21**:822–827.

82 Berendt AR. Counterpoint: hyperbaric oxygen for diabetic foot wounds is not effective. *Clin Infect Dis* 2006; **43**:193–198.

83 Abidia A, Laden G, Kuhan G, Johnson BF, Wilkinson AR, Renwick PM, *et al.* The role of hyperbaric oxygen therapy in ischaemic diabetic lower extremity ulcers: a double-blind randomised-controlled trial. *Eur J Vasc Endovasc Surg* 2003; **25**:513–518.

84 Hinchliffe RJ, Valk GD, Apelqvist J, Armstrong DG, Bakker K, Game FL, *et al.* A systematic review of the effectiveness of interventions to enhance the healing of chronic ulcers of the foot in diabetes. *Diabet Metab Res Rev* 2008; **24**(Suppl 1):119–144.

85 Armstrong DG, Boulton AJM. Negative pressure wound therapy (VAC). In: Boulton AJM, Cavanagh PR, Rayman G, eds. *The Foot in Diabetes*, 4th edn. Chichester: John Wiley & Sons Ltd, 2006: 360–364.

86 Armstrong DG, Lavery LA; Diabetic Foot Study Consortium. Negative pressure wound therapy after partial diabetic foot amputation: a multicentre, randomised controlled trial. *Lancet* 2005; **366**:1704–1710.

87 Blume PA, Walters J, Payne W, Ayala J, Lantis J. Comparison of negative pressure wound therapy using vacuum-assisted closure with advanced moist wound therapy in the treatment of diabetic foot ulcers: a multicentre randomised controlled trial. *Diabetes Care* 2008; **31**:631–636.

88 Blozik E, Scherer M. Skin replacement therapies for diabetic foot ulcers: systematic review and meta-analysis. *Diabetes Care* 2008; **31**:693–694.
89 Jeffcoate WJ. Charcot neuroarthropathy. *Diabet Metab Res Rev* 2008; **24**(Suppl 1):62–65.
90 Mabilleau G, Petrova NL, Edmonds ME, Sabokhar A. Increased osteoclastic activity in acute Charcot osteoarthropathy: the role of receptor activator of nuclear factor-kappa B ligand. *Diabetologia* 2008; **51**:1035–1040.
91 Rathur H, Boulton AJM. The neuropathic diabetic foot. *Natl Clin Pract Endocrinol Metab* 2007; **3**:14–25.
92 Jude EB, Selby PL, Burgess J, Lilleystone P, Mawer EB, Page SR, *et al.* Bisphosphonates in the treatment of Charcot neuroarthropathy: a double-blind randomised controlled trial. *Diabetologia* 2001; **44**:2032–2037.
93 Robinson AH, Pasapula C, Brodsky JW. Surgical aspects of the diabetic foot. *J Bone Joint Surg Br* 2009; **91**:1–7.
94 Armstrong DG, Wrobel J, Robbins JM. Guest editorial: are diabetes-related wounds and amputations worse than cancer? *Int Wound J* 2007; **4**:286–287.
95 Young MJ, McCardle JE, Randall LE, Barclay JI. Improved survival of diabetic foot ulcer patients 1995–2008: possible impact of aggressive cardiovascular risk management. *Diabetes Care* 2008; **31**:2143–2147.
96 Boulton AJM. Why bother educating the multidisciplinary team and the patient: the example of prevention of lower extremity amputation in diabetes. *Patient Educ Coun* 1995; **26**:183–188.
97 Boulton AJM. The annual review: here to stay. *Diabet Med* 1992; **9**:887.
98 Trautner C, Haastert B, Mauckner P, Gatcke LM, Giani G. Reduced incidence of lower-limb amputations in the diabetic population of a German city, 1990–2005: results of the Leverkusen Amputation Reduction Study (LARS). *Diabetes Care* 2007; **30**:2633–2637.
99 Krishnan S, Nash F, Baker N, Fowler D, Rayman. Reduction in diabetic amputations over 11 years in a defined UK population: benefits of multidisciplinary team work and continuous prospective audit. *Diabetes Care* 2008; **31**:99–101.
100 Canavan RJ, Unwin ND, Kelly WF, Connolly VM. Diabetes and non-diabetes-related lower extremity amputation incidence before and after the introduction of better organised diabetes foot care: continuous longitudinal monitoring using a standard method. *Diabetes Care* 2008; 459–463.
101 Larsson J, Eneroth M, Apelqvist J, Stenström A. Sustained reduction in major amputations in diabetic patients: 628 amputations in 461 patients in a defined population over a 20-year period. *Acta Orthop* 2008; **79**:665–673.

45 Sexual Function in Men and Women with Diabetes

David Price
Morriston Hospital, Swansea, UK

Keypoints

- The prevalence of erectile dysfunction (ED) in men with diabetes increases with age and is about 35–50% overall.
- Penile erection occurs as a result of engorgement of the erectile tissue following vascular smooth muscle relaxation in the corpus cavernosum mediated by nitric oxide (NO), which is derived from both parasympathetic nerve terminals and the vascular endothelium.
- ED in diabetes is largely brought about by failure of NO-mediated smooth muscle relaxation secondary to endothelial dysfunction and autonomic neuropathy.
- ED is an early indicator of endothelial dysfunction and a marker of increased cardiovascular risk.
- Phosphodiesterase 5 inhibitors are first-line treatment and act by inhibiting the breakdown of cyclic guanosine monophosphate, the second messenger in the NO pathway, and hence enhance erections under conditions of sexual stimulation.
- Other options are intracavernosal injection of prostaglandin E (alprostadil), transurethral alprostadil, vacuum therapy and surgical insertion of penile prostheses.
- In women with diabetes, sexual dysfunction is less common and usually undeclared, but there is an increased risk of vaginal dryness and arousal disorder.
- Contraception and family planning are especially important in women with diabetes. Although there is little consensus amongst diabetes professionals about the preferred method of contraception for women with diabetes, it appears that most currently available methods of contraception are suitable.
- Hormone replacement therapy (HRT) can be considered for treating menopausal symptoms in women with diabetes on a short-term basis, but HRT is not justified in asymptomatic women.

Male erectile dysfunction

The advent of effective oral treatments has changed the management of erectile dysfunction (ED) in diabetes considerably. Diabetologists and general practitioners can now offer treatments that are easy to use and generally effective. This change, however, has been a long time coming. As recently as 1993, ED was regarded as the most neglected complication of diabetes [1]. Since then, there has been a transformation in attitudes to the subject, in which diabetes professionals have led the way. Previously, ED was generally believed to be psychogenic in origin, even when associated with diabetes, and hence the management was considered to be the preserve of psychosexual counselors. We now accept that ED is a complications of diabetes that can and should be managed by diabetes professionals.

Physiology of erectile function

Tumescence is a vascular process under the control of the autonomic nervous system. The erectile tissue of the corpus cavernosum behaves as a sponge, and erection occurs when it becomes engorged with blood. As shown in Figure 45.1, dilatation of the arterioles and vasculature of the corpus cavernosum leads to compression of the outflow venules against the rigid tunica albuginea [2,3]. Thus, smooth muscle relaxation is the key phenomenon in this process, as it leads to increased arterial inflow and reduced venous outflow [4]. The process is under the control of parasympathetic fibres, which were previously known as non-adrenergic non-cholinergic neurones, as the neurotransmitter was unknown; but it is now clear that nitric oxide (NO) is the agent largely responsible for smooth muscle relaxation in the corpus cavernosum. It is produced both in the parasympathetic nerve terminals and is generated by NO synthase in the vascular endothelium. Within the smooth muscle cell of the corpus cavernosum, NO stimulates guanylate cyclase, leading to increased production of the second messenger, cyclic guanosine monophosphate (cGMP), which induces smooth muscle relaxation, probably by opening up calcium channels (Figure 45.2) [5,6].

There is some evidence that neuronally derived NO is important in initiation, whereas NO from the endothelium is responsible for maintenance of the erection [7].

Pathophysiology of erectile dysfunction in diabetes

In men with diabetes there is evidence that ED is caused by failure of NO-induced smooth muscle relaxation caused by both autonomic neuropathy and endothelial dysfunction [7,8]. Many men with diabetes report that in the early stages they do not have a

Textbook of Diabetes, 4th edition. Edited by R. Holt, C. Cockram, A. Flyvbjerg and B. Goldstein. © 2010 Blackwell Publishing.

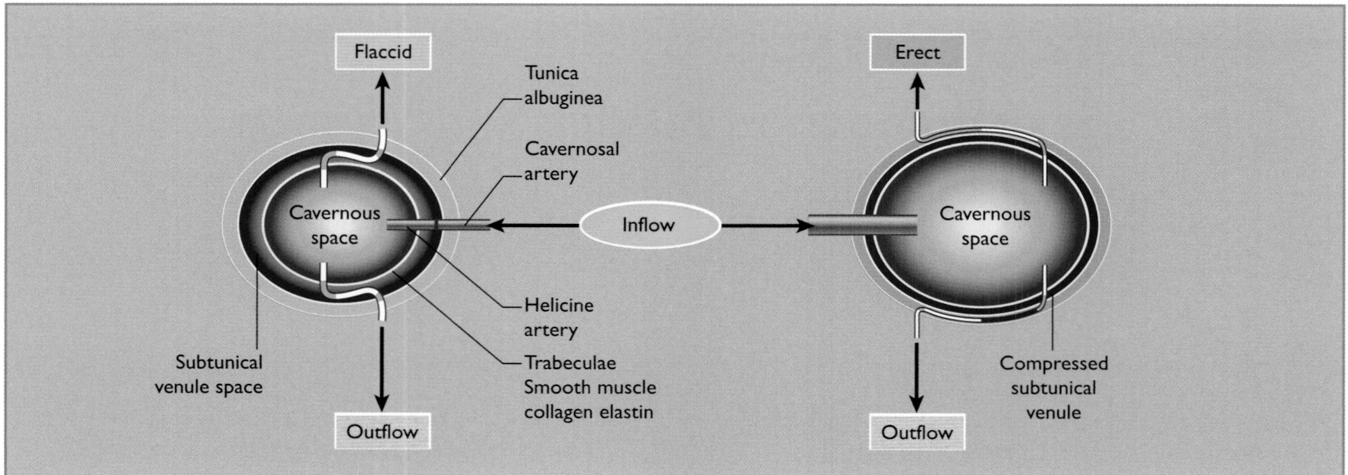

Figure 45.1 Diagrammatic representation of the corpus cavernosum. During tumescence, dilatation of the helicine and cavernosal arteries produces expansion of the cavernosal space and compression of the outflow venules against the rigid tunica albuginea.

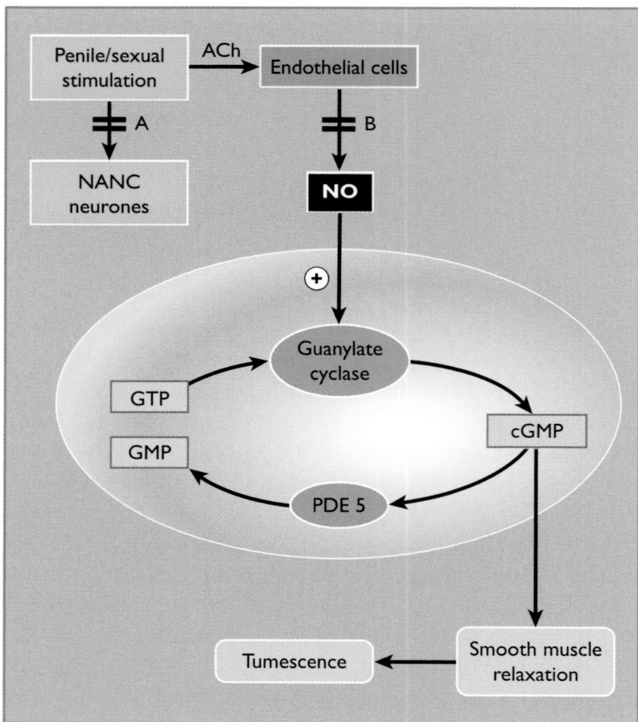

Figure 45.2 Pathophysiology of erectile function in diabetes. Diagrammatic representation of the pathways leading to the relaxation of a corpus cavernosal smooth muscle cell. In diabetes, there are defects in nitric oxide-mediated smooth-muscle relaxation from neuropathy of the non-adrenergic non-cholinergic (NANC) fibers (a) and endothelial dysfunction (b). ACh, acetylcholine; cGMP, cyclic guanosine monophosphate; GTP, guanosine triphosphate; NO, nitric oxide; PDE 5, phosphodiesterase type 5.

problem initially achieving an erection but that they cannot maintain it. This would suggest that in these individuals failure of endothelium-derived NO occurs before significant autonomic neuropathy.

More recently, other potential abnormalities have been described which may contribute to the development of ED in diabetes. Endothelium-derived hyperpolarizing factor (EDHF) has a role in endothelium-dependent relaxation of human penile arteries [9] and this is significantly impaired in penile resistance arteries in men with diabetes [10]. Impaired EDHF responses might therefore contribute to the endothelial dysfunction of diabetic erectile tissue.

A further body of evidence suggests increased oxygen-free radical levels in diabetes may reduce the vasodilator effect of NO. In particular, the formation of products of non-enzymatic glycosylation to produce advanced glycosylation end-products (AGEs) generates reactive oxygen species which impairs NO bioactivity [11]. In animal models, inhibition of AGE formation improves endothelium-dependent relaxation and restores erectile function in diabetic rats [12,13].

Other pathophysiologic changes known to occur in diabetes have been postulated to contribute to ED. Non-enzymatic glycation of proteins has been reported to impair endothelium-dependent relaxation of aorta in rats [13,14].

Other factors, not limited to diabetes, may also contribute to the development of ED in men with diabetes. Structural changes associated with large vessel disease are commonly associated with ED in diabetes; however, this is usually associated with functional changes of widespread endothelial dysfunction in diabetes and it is difficult to separate the relative importance of the two factors.

Other factors contributing to erectile dysfunction in diabetes

In addition to endothelial dysfunction and autonomic neuropathy, ED is associated with other conditions common in diabetes, such as hypertension and large-vessel disease [15]. Furthermore, men with diabetes are more likely to be taking medications that can impair erectile function (Table 45.1). Antihypertensive agents

Table 45.1 Medications associated with erectile dysfunction.

Antihypertensives
Thiazide diuretics
Beta-blockers
Calcium-channel blockers
Angiotensin-converting enzyme (ACE) inhibitors
Central sympatholytics (methyldopa, clonidine)
Antidepressants
Tricyclics
Monoamine oxidase inhibitors
(NB: selective serotonin re-uptake inhibitors can cause ejaculatory problems)
Major tranquillizers
Phenothiazines
Haloperidol
Hormones
Luteinizing hormone-releasing hormone (goserelin, buserelin)
Estrogens (diethylstilbestrol/stilbestrol)
Anti-androgens (cyproterone)
Miscellaneous
5-alpha reductase inhibitors (finasteride)
Statins (simvastatin, atorvastatin, pravastatin)
Cimetidine
Digoxin
Metoclopramide
Allopurinol
Ketoconazole
Non-steroidal anti-inflammatory agents
Fibrates
Drugs of "abuse"/"social" drugs
Alcohol
Tobacco
Marijuana
Amfetamines
Anabolic steroids
Barbiturates
Opiates

are commonly reported to be associated with ED, although much of the evidence is anecdotal; beta-blockers and thiazide diuretics are the most commonly reported culprits [16], alpha-blockers perhaps have the lesser risk [17]. Finally, it should be remembered that there are many other potential causes of ED unrelated to diabetes, from which men with diabetes are not immune (Table 45.2).

Clinical aspects of erectile dysfunction in diabetes

ED becomes more common with age. In a population-based study in Massachusetts, USA, the prevalence of complete erectile failure was reported to be 5% in men in their forties and 15% in those over 70 years [15]. The prevalence in diabetic men is significantly higher and also increases with age. In a survey of men attending a hospital diabetic clinic in the UK, the prevalence of

Table 45.2 Conditions associated with erectile dysfunction.

Psychologic disorders
Anxiety about sexual performance
Psychologic trauma or abuse
Misconceptions
Sexual problems in the partner
Depression
Psychoses
Vascular disorders
Peripheral vascular disease
Hypertension
Venous leak
Pelvic trauma
Neurologic disorders
Stroke
Multiple sclerosis
Spinal and pelvic trauma
Peripheral neuropathies
Endocrine and metabolic disorders
Diabetes
Hypogonadism
Hyperprolactinemia
Hypopituitarism
Thyroid dysfunction
Hyperlipidemia
Renal disease
Liver disease
Miscellaneous
Surgery and trauma
Smoking
Drug and alcohol abuse
Structural abnormalities of the penis

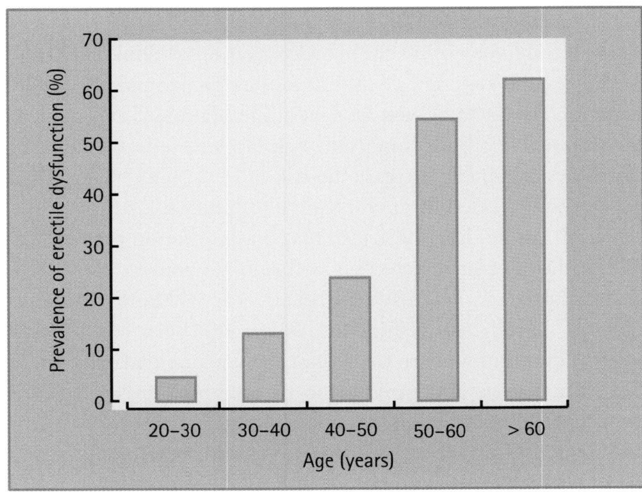

Figure 45.3 The prevalence of erectile dysfunction by age of men attending a hospital diabetic clinic [1].

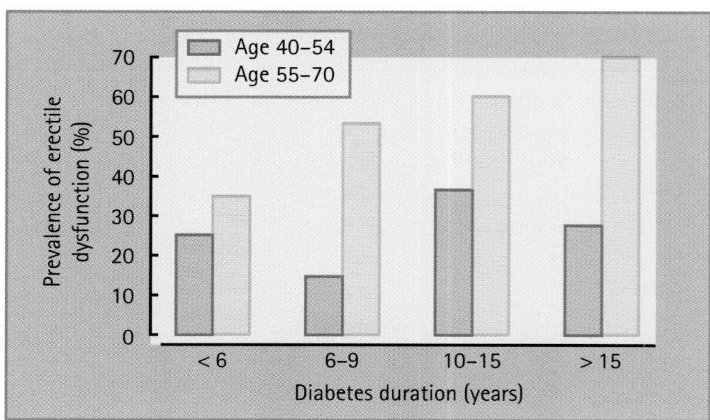

Figure 45.4 The prevalence of erectile dysfunction by duration of diabetes in a population-based study [19].

ED increased from 13% amongst 30-year-olds to 61% amongst men aged over 60 years (Figure 45.3) [1]; overall, the prevalence was 38%. The prevalence of ED in diabetes in a general practice population was reported to be even higher, at 55% [18]. These data would suggest that ED is the most common clinically apparent complication of diabetes in men.

The presence of other medical conditions increases the risk of ED. A population-based survey of 600 men in Brazil, Italy, Japan and Malaysia in 2000 examined the prevalence of ED and its relationship to other diseases and lifestyles. The prevalence of ED among men with diabetes rose from 25% at age 40–44 years to 70% at age 65–70 years [19]. Cardiovascular disease increased the risk of ED. The prevalence was 31.7% in men with diabetes only, 40% in men with diabetes and heart disease and 46.5% in those with diabetes and hypertension. The prevalence also increased with duration of diabetes (Figure 45.4). Men with diabetes who smoked and reported below average levels of physical activity had a fourfold increase in the prevalence of ED.

Erectile dysfunction as a risk factor for cardiovascular disease

There is convincing evidence of an association of between ED and cardiovascular disease [20–22]. This may be because they share common risk factors. Increased waist measurement and reduced physical activity, both important risk factors for ischemic heart disease, considerably increase the risk of ED [23–25]. The risk of ED is also increased in men with hyperlipidemia [26].

Recent studies have suggested that the association between ED and cardiovascular disease may be brought about by more than shared risk factors and may arise because they are both manifestations of endothelial dysfunction. There has been considerable interest in recent years in the role of the vascular endothelium in the pathogenesis and progression of atherosclerosis [27]. It is clear that the endothelium has important and complex endocrine and paracrine functions, and one of its most important products is NO (previously known as endothelium-derived relaxing factor). NO possesses potent antiatherogenic properties, inhibits platelet aggregation and regulates vascular tone [28]. As described above, NO derived from both nerve terminals and the vascular endothelium has a central role in the physiology of erection. Therefore, there are theoretical grounds to believe that the ED might be an early marker of endothelial dysfunction and hence an important risk factor for cardiovascular disease. There is now good evidence that ED is an early marker of endothelial dysfunction [29]. Thus, the association between ED and increased cardiovascular risk may be a case of shared common soil, in particular endothelial dysfunction and microvascular disease. In practical terms this means cardiovascular risk should be assessed in any man with ED whether diabetic or not. A man with type 2 diabetes (T2DM) and ED has approximately double the risk of developing coronary heart disease than a similar man without ED [22].

Smoking and alcohol consumption

Smoking greatly increases the risk of developing ED. A follow-up of the Massachusetts Male Aging Study reported that cigarette smoking almost doubled the risk of developing ED after about 7 years [15]. A similar finding was reported by the large Health Professionals' Follow-up Study [24].

In contrast to tobacco, it is well established that moderate alcohol consumption reduces the risk of a cardiovascular event. It is interesting that drinking alcohol in moderation also appears to reduce the risk of becoming impotent [23].

Quality of life issues

That ED can significantly worsen a man's quality of life is not in doubt. Unfortunately, there are few good data to show objectively the impact ED can have on quality of life measures, and even fewer to show the impact of treating ED. A survey by the Impotence Association found symptoms of lowered self-esteem and depression in 62% of men; 40% expressed concern with either new or established relationships, and 21% blamed it for the break-up of a relationship [30]. In another series in general practice, it was reported that 45% of men with diabetes stated that they thought about their ED all or most of the time, 23% felt that it severely affected their quality of life and 10% felt it severely affected their relationship with their partner [18].

Assessment and investigation of erectile dysfunction in diabetes

Clinical assessment

In most cases, an impotent man will have taken a long time to pluck up the courage to discuss his problem with a doctor and will undoubtedly be anxious. Almost invariably, however, once the subject has been broached, men with ED and their partners do not usually have any difficulty discussing the problem. A description of the nature of the ED should be obtained, not least to ensure that the patient is complaining of ED and not another related problem, such as premature ejaculation. The key features in the history of ED are listed in Table 45.3. Ideally, the man's partner should be present, but most men attend the consultation alone. If the partner is present, talking to her without the patient present can reveal interesting and useful insights into the problem.

Table 45.3 Key features in the clinical history of erectile dysfunction in diabetes.

Onset usually gradual and progressive
Earliest feature often inability to sustain erection long enough for satisfactory intercourse
Erectile failure may be intermittent initially
Sudden onset often thought to indicate a psychogenic cause (but little evidence to support this)
Preservation of spontaneous and early morning erections does not necessarily indicate a psychogenic cause
Loss of libido consistent with hypogonadism, but not a reliable symptom. Impotent men often understate their sex drive for a variety of reasons

Table 45.4 Key physical signs to note on examination of the patient with erectile dysfunction.

Any features of hypogonadism
Manual dexterity – may preclude physical treatment (e.g. intracavernosal injection)
Protuberant abdomen
External genitalia:
Presence of phimosis
Testicular volume

General physical examination may give clues as to the etiology of ED and the choice of treatment. The key features of the physical examination are listed in Table 45.4.

Investigation of erectile dysfunction in diabetes

The suggested investigations of ED in diabetes are listed in Table 45.5. It is now widely accepted that it is not helpful to try to determine whether or not ED is psychogenic in origin, particularly when managing a man with diabetes and ED. Few investigations are needed, but it is worth excluding other treatable causes of ED: in practical terms, hypogonadism is the only treatable one. There is probably no significant relationship between diabetes and hypogonadism, and therefore gonadal function should only be assessed in men with diabetes and ED if it is considered worthwhile looking for a coincidental problem causing hypogonadism. Some men presenting with ED will not have attended any form of clinic for many years, so the consultation provides an opportunity to address other health issues. For the reasons given above, consideration should be given to assessing the patient's cardiovascular status. The consultation also provides an opportunity to address the management of the patient's diabetes.

General advice

Most men with diabetes and their partners seeking treatment for impotence are middle-aged, have been married for many years and require only simple common-sense advice. Specialist psychosexual counseling is not needed for most couples: several series have reported that diabetologists can offer an effective service for the treatment of ED without the support of psychosexual counselors [31–34]. It is important that the cause of the ED is explained, as many patients will blame themselves. They should be advised that if they wish to resume sexual relations they will require long-term treatment, as spontaneous return of erectile function in diabetes occurs only rarely [35].

Table 45.5 Investigation of erectile dysfunction in diabetes.

Serum testosterone if libido reduced or hypogonadism suspected (ideally taken at 9 am)
Serum prolactin and luteinizing hormone if serum testosterone subnormal
Assessment of cardiovascular status if clinically indicated:
Electrocardiography (ECG)
Serum lipids
Glycosylated hemoglobin, serum electrolytes if clinically indicated

Treating ED in an attempt to save a failing relationship is rarely successful and may make the situation worse. The assistance of a suitably qualified psychosexual counselor should be considered in this situation. Referral to a counselor should also be considered if there is any suggestion of severe anxiety, loss of attraction between partners, fear of intimacy or marked performance anxiety. Any other medical problems should be addressed. Improving poor metabolic control may help general well-being, but poor control should not be used as a reason to refuse or delay treatment. Patients who smoke should be advised to stop for reasons of general health, although there is no good evidence that stopping smoking will improve erectile function in a man with diabetes and ED.

Many men with diabetes will be taking medication known to cause ED. Experience has shown that changing the treatment in an attempt to improve sexual function rarely works and may cause delays and frustration for the patient. It is therefore not advisable unless there is a strong temporal relationship between starting treatment and the onset of ED.

Treatment options

The advent of effective oral therapies has transformed the management of ED. These should be offered as first-line therapy to men with diabetes and ED, and the other treatment options should be reserved for those in whom oral therapy is contraindicated or ineffective.

Oral agents

Phosphodiesterase 5 inhibitors

Phosphodiesterase type 5 (PDE 5) is an enzyme found in smooth muscle, platelets and the corpus cavernosum. The mechanism of action of PDE 5 inhibitors is shown in Figure 45.2. During tumescence, there is an increase in the intracellular concentrations of NO, which produces smooth muscle relaxation via the second messenger cGMP. This is broken down in turn by PDE 5. Hence, PDE 5 inhibitors can enhance erections under conditions of sexual stimulation. There are currently three PDE 5 inhibitors licensed for the treatment of ED: sildenafil (Viagra), tadalafil (Cialis) and vardenafil (Levitra).

Clinical trial data. Sildenafil was the first PDE 5 inhibitor. Early small trials showed it was a highly effective treatment for ED in men with and without diabetes [36,37]. The first large study was published in 1998. A total of 532 men with ED of mixed etiology were studied. In the group given sildenafil, 69% of all attempts at intercourse were successful, compared with 22% in those given placebo [38]. Other studies in men with ED of mixed etiology have shown success rates of 65–77% [39,40]. Studies of sildenafil in other patient groups have reported success rates of approximately 70% in hypertension [41], 76% in spinal cord injury [42], 63% in spina bifida [43] and 40% following radical prostatectomy [44].

In men with diabetes, the success rates for sildenafil have been reported to be 56–59% in the treatment of ED [37,45]. A study in elderly men reported success rates of 69% overall and 50% in subjects with diabetes [46]. Most of these studies of sildenafil have been short-term. A trial examining the long-term efficacy of sildenafil in men with ED from a variety of causes reported that only 52% continued to use it after 2 years [47]. This figure may seem surprisingly low, but it is certainly considerably higher than for any other type of ED treatment.

Other PDE 5 inhibitors

Sildenafil was soon followed by tadalafil (Cialis) [48–50] and vardenafil (Levitra) [51,52]. All three appear to be similar in efficacy and safety but there are differences in duration of action and adverse effect profiles as described below.

Adverse effects. The most common adverse effects related to PDE 5 inhibitors are headache, dyspepsia and flushing. Headache and flushing might be expected, as they are vasodilators. The dyspepsia is usually mild and may be caused by relaxation of the cardiac sphincter of the stomach.

Abnormal vision is experienced by about 6% of men taking sildenafil; this may be because the drug has some activity against PDE 6, which is a retinal enzyme. Of more concern are the reports of non-arteritic anterior ischemic optic neuropathy (NAION). This is a rare syndrome characterized by sudden, sometimes unilateral, often reversible, visual loss. Since 2002 there have been case reports of this condition occurring in association with the use of PDE 5 inhibitors, particularly sildenafil [53,54]. NAION is rare but potentially serious as it can, exceptionally, lead to blindness. It would appear it is more common in men with increased cardiovascular risk [55]. The manufacturers of sildenafil estimated the incidence of NAION in 13 000 men receiving sildenafil from pooled safety data from clinical trials and observational studies to be 2.8 cases per 100 000 patient-years of sildenafil exposure [56]. The authors reported this to be similar to estimates reported in general US population samples (2.52 and 11.8 cases per 100 000 men aged over 50 years). It is therefore unknown if PDE 5 inhibitor use increases the risk of NAION but in any case it is a very rare condition and should not discourage the appropriate use of these agents.

The adverse events from the key trials of PDE 5 inhibitors in men with diabetes are given in Table 45.6. In all the studies, the discontinuation rate from adverse effects has been very low.

Table 45.6 Adverse effects of phosphodiesterase 5 (PDE 5) inhibitors (%). The prevalence quoted for each adverse effect is for the top dose used in each study.

	Sildenafil [59,60]	Tadalafil [59,61,62]	Vardenafil [63,64]
Headache	8.1–9.3	8.0–21	5–11
Flushing	7.4–8.1	3.0–9.0	5.4–10
Back pain	2.5	4.6–9.0	0
Dyspepsia	2.7–3.0	4.1–17	2.3
Nasal congestion	2.7–4.1	2.0–5	10
Dizziness	2.5	1.6	
Diarrhea	2.5	0.8	
Abnormal vision	1.4	0	
Muscle cramps	4.1	3–7	

Reasons for PDE 5 inhibitor non-responsiveness. The mechanism of action of sildenafil would suggest that it would be ineffective without the presence of sufficient bioavailable NO in the penile vasculature. Thus, either significant autonomic neuropathy or endothelial dysfunction would be expected to reduce the efficacy of a PDE 5 inhibitor. Slightly surprisingly, two small studies have reported no differences in the presence of autonomic or endothelial function between sildenafil "responders" and "non-responders" [29,57]. It has been reported that failure to respond to sildenafil is more likely in men with long-standing and severe ED [58]; however, no single factor precludes a successful outcome, and in practical terms it is worth trying sildenafil in all men with ED unless there is a contraindication.

Cardiovascular safety of PDE 5 inhibitors. The launch of sildenafil, the first PDE 5 inhibitor, was soon followed by case reports of cardiovascular events and deaths associated with its use. By contrast, there is now good evidence that PDE 5 inhibitors are not associated with increased cardiovascular risk [65,66]. A questionnaire survey of over 5000 sildenafil users reported that adverse cardiovascular events were no more frequent than expected for a comparable population [67]. A retrospective analysis of 36 clinical trials of tadalafil involving over 14 000 men reported no increase in cardiovascular adverse events [68]. Indeed, there is accumulating evidence that PDE 5 inhibitors reduce blood pressure slightly and improve endothelial function [66,69].

Restoring sexual function, however, is not completely without risk. Sexual activity, like any form of physical activity, can precipitate cardiovascular events in those at risk. A large case–control study reported the risk of a cardiovascular event in the 2 hours after intercourse was increased by 2.5 fold in healthy subjects and by 3 fold if there was a history of previous myocardial infarction [70]. Although the absolute risk remains very small, the issue of cardiovascular safety must be addressed in all men before treating ED. Jackson *et al.* [65] have suggested a classification scheme for assessing cardiovascular risk in men undergoing treatment for ED, those with the highest risk should be referred for specialist cardiac evaluation while the lowest risk group could be managed in primary care.

Drug interactions with PDE 5 inhibitors. PDE 5 inhibitors can be used safely in patients taking a wide range of other drugs but there are several potential important interactions. They are contraindicated in the presence of any nitrate therapy (including nicorandil) as the combination can cause profound hypotension. A patient taking nitrates seeking treatment for ED can be offered alternatives to PDE 5 inhibitors or the nitrates can be stopped or changed to an alternative therapy. Nitrates are a symptomatic treatment with no prognostic implications and so this is possible in most cases but should be done in consultation with a cardiologist in all but the most straightforward cases.

Nitrate therapy should not be given within 24 hours of taking sildenafil or vardenafil and at least 48 hours of taking tadalafil. If angina develops during or after sexual activity following the use of a PDE 5 inhibitor, the patient should be advised to discontinue any sexual activity and stand up as this reduces the work of the heart by reducing venous return.

PDE 5 inhibitors should be used with caution in patients who take alpha-blockers because the combination may lead to symptomatic hypotension in some patients. Patients should be stable on alpha-blocker therapy before initiating sildenafil which should be initiated at the lowest dose [66].

Comparison of PDE 5 inhibitors. The three currently available PDE 5 inhibitors, sildenafil, vardenafil and tadalafil, are all similar in efficacy and safety. Their side effect profiles differ slightly but the most notable difference is the longer half-life of tadalafil. Thus, a single dose of tadalafil offers the potential to restore erectile function to normal for 2 days and thereby remove the need for medication to be taken each time prior to sexual activity. The choice between this form of treatment and on-demand dosing is largely a matter of patient choice. Patient preference studies of agents with differing dosing instructions are difficult to perform in a blinded fashion. Several have been reported and have generally shown a preference for tadalafil over sildenafil [59,71–74].

How to use PDE 5 inhibitors. These agents should be taken orally about 1 hour before sexual activity. This period can be shortened if taken on an empty stomach. After the 1-hour period, there is a "window of opportunity" when sexual activity can take place. For sildenafil and vardenafil this is at least 4 hours but may be over 8 hours [75]. For tadalafil the window of opportunity may last 48 hours. Men with diabetes usually require the maximum recommended dose. Patients should be warned that the drug only works in conjunction with sexual stimulation.

Management of PDE 5 inhibitor non-responsiveness. A large proportion of men with diabetes and ED will not respond to PDE 5 inhibitors and there are many potential reasons for this. PDE 5 inhibitors require a degree of NO tone to be effective, therefore severe endothelial dysfunction of autonomic neuropathy might be expected to reduce their efficacy; however, one study reported that neither autonomic neuropathy nor endothelial dysfunction predicted sildenafil responsiveness. The only significant factor that predicted the response to treatment was the initial degree of ED [29]. In practical terms, no single factor should preclude a trial of PDE 5 inhibitor therapy in a man without a contraindication.

Much has been written on the best approach for dealing with men who do not respond to a PDE 5 inhibitor but, unfortunately, mostly based on limited evidence. It has been suggested that if appropriate advice is given and sufficient attempts at intercourse made, many men previously labeled as non-responders can be treated successfully with PDE 5 inhibitors. One study reported that intercourse success rates reached a plateau after eight attempts so men with ED should try at least eight times with a PDE5 inhibitor at the maximum recommended dose before being considered a non-responder [76].

Hypogonadism should always be considered in dealing with men with ED who do not respond. Hypogonadism caused by confirmed pituitary or testicular disease usually responds well to treatment. The management of the borderline hypogonadism of the aging male is more controversial but there is some evidence that testosterone replacement in this situation can improve ED as a sole treatment [77] and enhance the response to PDE 5 inhibitors [78–80].

Other oral therapies

Apomorphine

Apomorphine has been in use for many years. It is a centrally acting D1/D2 dopamine agonist that acts on the paraventricular nucleus of the thalamus early in the cascade that leads to erection. Among its several properties, it is a potent inducer of nausea, and this has previously limited its use as a therapeutic agent. A sublingual formulation is licensed in Europe as a treatment of ED. This preparation has no first-pass metabolism, and it rapidly produces therapeutic blood levels. Studies of the sublingual preparation have suggested that it is effective in inducing erections in about 50% of attempts and has acceptable levels of adverse effects [81]. To date, there have been no published trials of apomorphine in men with diabetes and it is not widely used in diabetic practice.

Various oral agents have been tried as treatments for ED in the past, including trazodone, yohimbine and phentolamine. The data on all of them are limited and none has stood the test of time. Testosterone should only be used to treat ED secondary to confirmed hypogonadism.

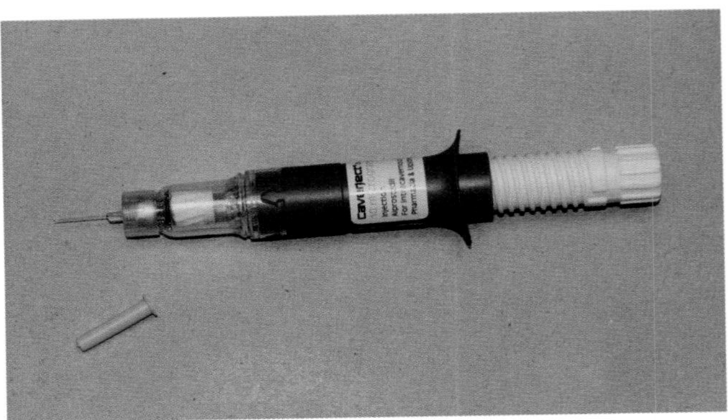

Figure 45.5 Alprostadil self-injection pen device.

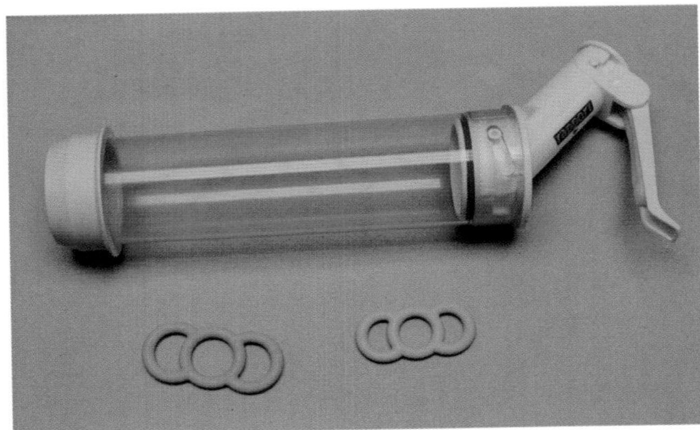

Figure 45.6 A typical vacuum device with constriction rings.

Table 45.7 Instructions to medical staff for treating prolonged erections caused by prostaglandin E1.

- Do not delay treatment beyond 6 hours
- Using aseptic technique, aspirate 20–25 mL blood from the corpus cavernosum (19 or 21 gauge butterfly needle)
- Repeat the above on the opposite side of the penis if detumescence does not occur
- If still unsuccessful, inject 0.5–1.0 mL of a 300-μg/mL solution of phenylephrine every 5–10 minutes (maximum dosage 5 mL) into the corpus cavernosum. If necessary, this may be followed by further aspiration of blood through the same needle. Extreme caution is necessary in those patients taking monoamine oxidase inhibitors, as a hypertensive crisis may result. Use carefully in those with coronary heart disease, uncontrolled hypertension or cerebral ischemia. Monitor pulse rate and blood pressure throughout
- If the above are unsuccessful, refer for urgent surgical treatment, such as a shunt procedure

Intracavernosal injection therapy

The technique of intracavernosal self-injection was first described in 1982 by Brindley [82], using phentolamine, although the French urologist, Virag [83], who used papaverine, was first to publish. Papaverine was more effective than phentolamine, but was an unlicensed treatment; it was superseded by alprostadil (prostaglandin E), which was licensed for the treatment of ED in 1996.

Alprostadil is supplied in a self-injection pen device, which is easy to use, and supplied with excellent instructions (Figure 45.5). In spite of this, most studies show that self-injection therapy has a disappointingly high long-term discontinuation rate [84–86]. Self-injection treatment carries a small risk of priapism (a sustained unwanted erection). Although an infrequent complication, priapism is an important one, as it must be treated within 6 hours by aspirating blood from the corpus cavernosum. Patients undertaking self-injection must be warned of this potential problem and given instructions on what to do should it occur (Table 45.7).

Local adverse reactions, such as penile pain, are relatively common with self-injection therapy. Prolonged papaverine use may lead to fibrosis in the penis, but this has only rarely been reported with alprostadil [87].

More recently the combination of vasoactive intestinal polypeptide and phentolamine has been licensed for use under the name of Invicorp. It appears to be a potentially useful treatment for ED [88,89].

Transurethral alprostadil (MUSE)

Many men find injection therapy unacceptable because it requires injecting the penis. Transurethral administration of the vasoactive agent would appear largely to overcome this problem. The principle is simple. A slender applicator is inserted into the urethra to deposit a pellet containing alprostadil in polyethylene glycol. This gradually dissolves, allowing the prostaglandin to diffuse into the corpus cavernosum. In a placebo-controlled study of 1511 men with ED of mixed etiology, it was reported that 65% were able to have intercourse using this system [90]. The results in the 240 men with diabetes in the study were similar [91]. The most common side effect was penile pain, which occurred in 10.8% of applications. Hypotension was reported by 3.3% of the men receiving alprostadil. Priapism and penile fibrosis were not reported. A more recent study reported that most men found transurethral alprostadil less acceptable and efficacious than intracavernosal injection [92], and the long-term usage has been disappointing [93].

Vacuum therapy

Vacuum devices became widely available in the 1970s. They consist of a translucent tube, which is placed over the penis, and an attached vacuum pump (Figure 45.6). The air is pumped out of the tube, and the negative pressure draws blood into the erectile tissue, producing tumescence. A constriction band (which has previously been placed over the base of the tube) is then slipped off to remain firmly around the base of the penis so as to maintain the erection, and the tube is then removed. The devices require a little practice and some dexterity, but most couples are able to use them satisfactorily. Trials of vacuum therapy have reported success rates of approximately 70% in men with and without diabetes, suggesting it is an effective treatment, provided couples are prepared to use them [94–97].

Vacuum devices are safe and effective treatments, and inexpensive to use after an initial outlay (in the UK) of about £100–250. The side effects are discomfort from the constriction band, failure to ejaculate and a cold penis (reported by the female partner). Many couples find the use of vacuum devices unacceptable, and since the introduction of newer treatments their use has declined; however, they still have a role in men who do not respond or who cannot use other treatments.

Surgery

In spite of recent advances in the management of ED, some men will not be able to use the available treatment options. There will therefore always be a limited role for surgery.

The surgical options available are:

1 The insertion of penile prostheses;

2 Corrective surgery for associated Peyronie disease or post-injection corporal fibrosis;

3 Venous and arterial surgery.

Discussion of vascular and corrective surgery of the penis is best left to a specialist urology textbook, but a general practitioner or diabetes physician needs to know which patients might benefit by referral for insertion of a penile prosthesis. This form of surgery is best reserved for men in whom conventional treatments have failed and who are keen to resume full sexual activity.

Counseling of the patient, and whenever possible his partner, is extremely important, particularly about the choice of prosthesis. The patient's or couple's wishes are very important factors in device selection, as is the cost of the prosthesis. In the UK, many hospital trusts will only pay for the malleable prostheses and not for the insertion of the considerably more expensive inflatable ones.

Patients must be warned regarding postoperative pain or discomfort and the potential for reoperation. Patients will need to restrict physical activity and refrain from intercourse for between 4 and 6 weeks after the operation. They should be warned about the possible complications of infection, erosion and prosthesis failure, and that these problems usually require device removal. It is also very important that the patient and his partner are aware that the erection produced by a prosthesis is different from a normal erection, depending very much on the type of prosthesis chosen. It is useful to show patients examples of the prostheses (Figure 45.7) and to describe how they are inserted and the mechanism of action.

There is uncertainty as to whether men with diabetes are at higher risk of infection than men without diabetes after insertion of a penile prosthesis, but there is a consensus that, should infection occur, it is more serious [98]. Good preoperative control of diabetes is important to minimize the risk. Most published series of well-selected groups of men who have undergone penile prosthesis insertion have reported acceptable results, with good levels of patient satisfaction [99].

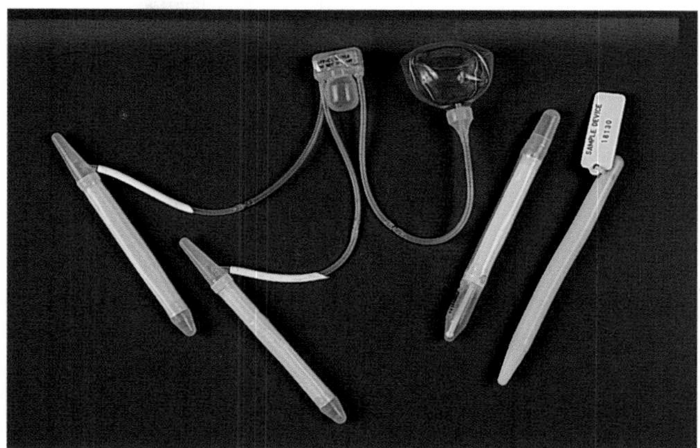

Figure 45.7 Examples of penile prostheses.

Organization of the management of ED

Traditionally, ED has been managed in a dedicated ED clinic, often run by a urologist. The advent of effective oral therapies has made the management much simpler, so that ED in diabetes can usually be managed by any physician or general practitioner. A physician considering treating ED will have to decide whether to run a separate ED clinic or to see the patients in a routine diabetic clinic. Such a decision will depend on local resources and circumstances but it is certainly possible to manage ED in a diabetic clinic. If this is to be done, it is advisable to have patient information literature on ED available. There are several excellent pamphlets produced by pharmaceutical companies and national diabetes organizations such as Diabetes UK. It is often wise to let the patient take away the literature to read and to consider the matter, with treatment being started at a subsequent visit.

Managing ED in primary care

There are considerable advantages for the treatment of ED in general practice. A general practitioner is more likely to know and understand a patient's particular circumstances. Men with ED may be less intimidated in seeking help from their family practitioner than from a hospital specialist or sexual therapist. Little specialized equipment is required, so there is no reason why interested general practitioners should not effectively treat the majority of men presenting with ED.

As with many disorders encountered in primary care, the general practitioner may choose to manage the problem in a standard consultation with the patient. Others may choose to refer their patients to a fellow partner or colleague with a particular interest in ED or to their practice nurse, who may have received appropriate training in the assessment of patients with ED.

When a man presents with ED, his general practitioner has an opportunity to consider other health issues and screen for underlying causes. ED is often associated with conditions that benefit from early detection such as diabetes, hypertension and hyperlipidemia. It is therefore important to consider general health issues and to address lifestyle factors.

The specialist erectile dysfunction service

Although most men with ED will be managed in primary care, there is still a role for a specialist ED service. It is likely that these clinics will mainly treat men who have failed to respond to oral therapies and that they will maintain expertise in the use of other treatments, such as intracavernosal injection therapy and vacuum devices, referring patients when necessary to urologic surgeons for penile prosthesis insertion.

Conclusions on male sexual dysfunction

NO-mediated relaxation of the smooth muscle of the corpus cavernosum is the key phenomenon leading to penile erection. In diabetes, there is impairment of NO production by autonomic nerve terminals (caused by autonomic neuropathy) and by endothelial cells (caused by endothelial cell dysfunction). Sildenafil and other PDE inhibitors work by inhibiting the breakdown of cGMP, the second messenger in the NO pathway, and hence enhance erections under conditions of sexual stimulation. These agents are safe and effective treatments and can be used to treat ED in a diabetic clinic or in general practice.

Female sexual dysfunction

Male sexual dysfunction has been described as the most neglected complication of diabetes. However, there has been considerably more interest in, and research into, the sexual dysfunction of men as compared to women. There may be good reasons for this. In physiologic terms, the female equivalent of male ED is reduced vasocongestion of the vulva and vagina, leading to impaired arousal and reduced vaginal lubrication. Failure to achieve an erection makes sexual intercourse impossible, but reduced vaginal lubrication is easily overcome with simple treatments such as lubricating creams and may not even be considered to be abnormal by a postmenopausal woman.

In a review published in 1998, Enzlin *et al.* [100] undertook an analysis of 15 studies carried out in the area of female sexuality in diabetes since 1971. They reported that the prevalence of impaired sexual arousal and inadequate lubrication was between 14% and 45% in women with diabetes, which was significantly higher than in controls without diabetes [100]. In contrast, there was little evidence of an increased risk of dyspareunia or problems with orgasm in women with diabetes. Thus, it would appear that women with diabetes admit to specific sexual dysfunctions when they are asked, but it is the universal experience of diabetologists that women with diabetes rarely complain of sexual problems. That a problem is not often volunteered by patients does not mean it is not significant or worthy of research.

More recent studies in women with type 1 diabetes (T1DM) have shown similar findings. Enzlin *et al.* [101] reported that 27% of diabetic women had sexual dysfunction compared to 14% in controls but only reduced lubrication was significantly different between the groups. The same group found that in women with T1DM sexual dysfunction was more closely related to psychologic rather than somatic factors [102].

If vaginal lubrication is the female equivalent of tumescence, then vaginal dryness and impaired arousal may be related to failure of NO-mediated smooth muscle relaxation secondary to endothelial dysfunction and autonomic neuropathy. There has been very little research into the pathophysiology of sexual dysfunction in women, but several studies have reported, a little surprisingly, that there does not appear to be a strong relationship between neuropathy and female sexual dysfunction [103–106]. Anecdotally, women with severe autonomic neuropathy can have an excellent sex life, unlike men, so it is likely there are differences between men and women in the way the autonomic nervous system controls genital responses [107]. Little work has been carried out on the effect of other medical conditions or treatments on sexual function in women.

Drug therapy and female sexual dysfunction

The mechanism of action of PDE 5 inhibitors would suggest they might improve arousal and vaginal lubrication; however, trials of sildenafil for this purpose in non-diabetic women have shown conflicting results. In a small cross-over study of 53 premenopausal women, it was reported that sildenafil significantly improved the frequency of intercourse and enjoyment compared with placebo [108]. In contrast, a much larger study of 583 women with female sexual arousal disorder reported no difference between the sildenafil or placebo-treated groups [109]. One of the few studies published to date on the effect of sildenafil on sexual dysfunction in women with diabetes reported that the treated group had improved arousal and sexual enjoyment as well as clitoral blood flow compared with controls [110].

Many women attending a diabetic clinic will be over 50 years of age and some will have problems associated with the menopause, including vaginal dryness and dyspareunia. It can be difficult to distinguish the effects of the menopause from those of diabetes, but in practical terms the treatment is the same. Topical estrogen or simple lubricant gels are usually effective. Managing loss of libido in women with diabetes is more complex and beyond the scope of this chapter. It is much more likely to be caused by psychosocial and relationship issues rather than somatic problems.

Genitourinary infections in women with diabetes

Vaginal candidiasis is a common finding in women with diabetes, particularly if the blood glucose control is poor and probably because yeasts thrive in a glucose-rich environment. Severe infection can be very irritating and painful and can interfere with sexual intercourse. Infections usually respond to conventional antifungal creams and pessaries; resistant cases usually respond to a single oral dose of fluconazole. To reduce the chances of reinfection, attempts should be made to improve diabetic control. The male partner may also need treatment for candidiasis for the same reason.

Other genital infections also occur in women with diabetes, but probably no more frequently than in the general population. These cases should be referred to the appropriate genitourinary service.

Conclusions on female sexual dysfunction

There are differences in the ways in which men and women respond to sexual dysfunction. Traditionally, the view has been expressed that men focus on physiologic function, while the quality of the relationship is more important to women. Such generalizations are now considered a little dangerous, but there is no doubt that in women, psychologic factors are more important than the minor degrees of sexual dysfunction that occur in diabetes. When asked, women with diabetes admit to an increased prevalence of vaginal dryness and impaired arousal, but these are not common problems in the day-to-day management of diabetes. The treatment for these problems is the same for women either with or without diabetes. Other associated problems, such as vaginal candidiasis or estrogen deficiency, should be addressed. If there are relationship problems, referral to a counselor should be considered. The role of PDE 5 inhibitors remains uncertain in female sexual dysfunction, and further research is needed in this area.

Contraception

Contraception and family planning are especially important in women with diabetes. Poor glycemic control during the first trimester of pregnancy is associated with an increased risk of fetal morbidity and mortality [111–113]. It is therefore essential that women with diabetes are advised to plan their pregnancies and achieve strict control of their diabetes prior to conception (see Chapter 53).

Method of contraception

There is little consensus amongst diabetes professionals about the preferred method of contraception for women with diabetes. Neither the American Diabetes Association nor Diabetes UK has published recent guidance on the subject. Surveys of doctors in the UK [114] and Germany [115] have reported considerable variation among physicians for their recommended method of contraception for diabetic women. Most currently available methods of contraception are suitable for women with diabetes; however, certain factors should be taken into consideration before choosing any particular method.

Contraindications to pregnancy

As medical and obstetric care has improved, the list of contraindications to pregnancy in women with diabetes has shrunk (see Chapter 53). If pregnancy is contraindicated, sterilization should be considered.

The oral contraceptive pill

In a survey of 938 women with T1DM undertaken in primary care in the UK, the oral contraceptive pill (OCP) was reported to be the most widely used method of contraception [114]. The combined OCP was used by 17%, and the progesterone-only pill (POP) by 8.6%; however, a more recent survey in general practice in the UK reported women with diabetes were significantly less likely to be prescribed the combined OCP than women without diabetes [116]. In contrast, progesterone-only and depot hormonal contraceptives were relatively more popular in women with diabetes. It seems there is a slight reluctance to prescribe the combined OCP in women with diabetes. The reasons for this are not clear and there are good reasons for using OCP. It is simple to use and, most importantly, very reliable. If properly used, it has the lowest failure rate for any contraceptive method, apart from sterilization [117]. Nevertheless, there have always been concerns about the safety of hormonal contraception in women with diabetes. Both the combined OCP and the POP carry an increased risk of thromboembolic disease and, in theory, can adversely affect glucose metabolism. These concerns are largely unfounded. A systematic review for the Cochrane database reported steroid contraceptive had limited effects of carbohydrate tolerance but strong statements could not be made because of the limited quality of trials [118]. Although a large definitive study examining the effects on cardiovascular morbidity and mortality in women with diabetes has not been performed, several smaller studies have suggested that OCPs with lower doses of estrogen have no greater effect on markers of cardiovascular risk in women with diabetes than women without diabetes [119,120]. Furthermore, there is no evidence that OCPs increase the risk of microvascular complications [121] or worsen metabolic control in women with T1DM [119].

Few studies, if any, have examined the safety of OCPs in T2DM. Two studies have reported that low-dose OCPs have no effect on glucose tolerance or plasma lipids in women with previous gestational diabetes [122,123].

On the available evidence, low-dose (<30 μg estradiol) combined OCPs can be safely used in women with T1DM or T2DM. Any woman taking the OCP should be reviewed regularly for assessment of blood pressure and serum lipids. Women with diabetes can also use the POP. It is not associated with adverse changes in serum lipids or clotting factors and is well tolerated; however, it is associated with menstrual irregularities, particularly intermenstrual bleeding.

Long-acting depot progestin preparations are also effective in women with diabetes. Several small studies have reported that progestins, particularly depot medroxyprogesterone acetate, can worsen carbohydrate tolerance in normal women [124–126], but there is no evidence they have a clinically significant effect on metabolic control in existing diabetes. Depot levonorgestrel (Norplant) appears to have minimal effect on carbohydrate tolerance [125].

Intrauterine contraceptive device

The intrauterine contraceptive device (IUD) is a safe and effective form of contraception in women with diabetes. Early concerns about the risk of pelvic inflammatory disease (PID) in diabetes were largely unfounded; studies have suggested no increased risk of PID in women with T1DM [127] or T2DM [128]. Similarly, early suggestions of an increased failure rate for IUDs in women with diabetes have not been borne out [127].

Barrier methods

Since the advent of AIDS, the condom has been widely advocated to reduce the risk of transmission of sexually transmitted diseases. It has a higher failure rate than OCPs and IUDs and for this reason is not recommended if pregnancy is contraindicated. For high-risk individuals, many genitourinary clinics recommend a combination of the OCP and condom to minimize the risk of pregnancy and sexually transmitted diseases – a technique known as "double-Dutch."

Emergency contraception

Three methods of emergency contraception are licensed in the UK and are available in many other countries: progestogen-only and combined estrogen–progesterone pills, and the copper IUD. The hormonal preparations can be taken up to 72 hours after unprotected intercourse, but are most effective if taken within 24 hours [129]. Nausea was reported in 23% and vomiting in about 6% of the women who used the progesterone-only regimen. Women with T1DM should be warned of these potential side effects. Little work on the use of these agents in women with diabetes has been published, but they may have a role in the prevention of unplanned pregnancies occurring at a time of poor metabolic control.

Conclusions on contraception

All women with diabetes of reproductive age should receive good contraceptive advice, as unplanned pregnancies occurring while glycemic control is poor carry an increased risk of morbidity and fetal abnormalities. Most forms of contraception are safe and effective in women with diabetes, but the OCP remains the most popular as it is very reliable and well tolerated.

Hormone replacement therapy

Attitudes to hormone replacement therapy (HRT) have changed considerably since the start of the new millennium. HRT is well established as an effective treatment for menopausal symptoms and as a treatment for osteoporosis. Until recently there was considerable interest from diabetologists in the potential role of HRT in reducing cardiovascular risk. A survey of general practitioners and hospital doctors in the UK as recently as 2001 suggested the majority would advise HRT for women with diabetes as prophylaxis for cardiovascular disease [130]. This belief was based upon a series of cross-sectional studies and effective marketing by drug companies. Since then the results of a large randomized controlled trials of combined HRT have been published and the results were surprising and interesting. Hulley *et al.* [131] reported that combined HRT did not reduce cardiovascular outcomes in women with established coronary heart disease. The Women's Health Initiative (WHI) study enrolled over 160 000 healthy women and reported in 2002. It was stopped early because of an increase in the risk of breast cancer [132]. Furthermore, there was an significant increase of stroke, coronary heart disease and pulmonary embolus in the group given HRT compared with the control group. There was a reduction in the risk of colorectal cancer and hip fracture. The study also reported an increase in the risk of dementia in the group given HRT [133]. Interestingly, women who took HRT in the WHI had a lower risk of developing diabetes.

Not surprisingly, the WHI study has generated considerable debate and has had a significant impact on practice. Many new guidelines on HRT have been produced, but few in diabetes. A detailed discussion of the benefits of HRT is beyond the scope of this book. The current views of the risks and benefits of HRT are listed in Table 45.8. In brief, in women with diabetes, HRT should be considered for short-term relief of menopausal symptoms, such as hot flushes, but is not indicated for cardiovascular risk reduction.

HRT and glucose tolerance

There is reasonable evidence that HRT does not worsen glucose tolerance in women either with or without diabetes and may produce a slight amelioration. In women without diabetes,

Table 45.8 Risks and benefits of hormone replacement therapy (HRT).

Main benefits of HRT

HRT produces:

- Relief of hot flushes
- Relief of urogenital symptoms
- Reduction of risk of osteoporotic fractures
- Reduction of risk of colorectal cancer

Main risks of HRT

HRT increases the risk of:

- Thromboembolic disease
- Stroke
- Breast cancer (combined HRT)
- Endometrial cancer (estrogen-only HRT)
- Ovarian cancer (estrogen-only HRT)

No change in risk

- Weight gain, headache
- Migraine
- Breast cancer (estrogen-only HRT)
- Colorectal cancer (estrogen-only HRT)

Insufficient evidence

There is incomplete evidence but HRT may worsen:

- Coronary artery disease
- Dementia

estradiol [134] and low-dose conjugated estrogens [135] are associated with an improvement and no effect on insulin sensitivity, while higher doses of conjugated estrogens and alkylated estrogens may cause deterioration of glucose tolerance [134,136–138].

In postmenopausal women with diabetes, estradiol has been reported to improve the fasting blood glucose concentration and glycosylated hemoglobin percentage [139]. A larger prospective study of over 15 000 women with T2DM also reported HRT produced an improvement in HbA_{1c} levels [140]. A recent small randomized trial reported HRT reduced serum fructosamine levels by 5% [141]. Any potential benefit to glucose tolerance is limited to oral HRT preparations: transdermal estradiol does not appear to have any effect on glucose tolerance [142,143].

HRT and lipids

There is now evidence that the effect of HRT on lipid profiles, such as glucose tolerance, is at worst neutral and may be slightly beneficial. In women without diabetes, estrogens reduce total and low density lipoprotein (LDL) cholesterol and increase high density lipoprotein (HDL) cholesterol and triglyceride levels [131,143]. Progestins can reduce triglyceride levels and when given in combination can prevent the estrogen-induced increase. Transdermal estrogen preparations have a beneficial effect on plasma lipids, reducing LDL cholesterol and triglycerides and increasing HDL cholesterol [144].

The effect of HRT on lipid profiles in women with diabetes has been reported to be largely favorable in several studies. In a small randomized cross-over study of overweight women with T2DM, conjugated estrogen therapy reduced central obesity, HbA_{1c} and total cholesterol, and improved physical functioning [145]. In a largert study, 61 postmenopausal women received combined HRT in a randomized cross-over design. HRT reduced total and LDL cholesterol, but there was no change in serum HDL or triglyceride levels [141].

HRT and blood pressure

HRT can be prescribed to hypertensive postmenopausal women under careful supervision. One of the few studies of HRT and blood pressure in diabetes suggested that it can be prescribed without any adverse effect on ambulatory blood pressure measurements in hypertensive and normotensive women [146].

HRT and osteoporosis

There is limited evidence to suggest women with T1DM have reduced bone mineral density at the time of diagnosis [147]. Although women with T2DM might be expected to be protected from osteoporosis because of their increased tendency to obesity, they would appear to be at increased risk of hip fracture (see Chapter 48). A very large prospective cohort study of postmenopausal women in Iowa reported that women with diabetes had a 1.7-fold higher risk of hip fracture than women without diabetes [148]. Thus, the benefits of HRT in reducing the risk of osteoporotic fractures would appear to be at least as great in women with diabetes as women without diabetes. Although HRT can be considered in all postmenopausal women with diabetes and osteoporosis, there are several alternatives including bisphosphonates, raloxifen and strontium which do not have the risks of HRT.

Conclusions on HRT

HRT is an established treatment for the symptoms of the menopause. It is also effective in preventing osteoporosis. It has no adverse effects on glycemic control or lipid profiles. The benefits of HRT do not justify the risks in asymptomatic women and it is not indicated for cardiovascular risk reduction. It can be considered for treating menopausal symptoms in women with diabetes on a short-term basis.

References

1 Price DE, O'Malley BP, Roshan M, James M, Hearnshaw JR. Why are impotent diabetic men not being treated? *Pract Diabetes* 1991; **8**:10–11.

2 Newman HF, Northup JD. Mechanism of human penile erection: an overview. *Urology* 1981; **17**:399–408.

3 Aboseif SR, Lue TF. Hemodynamics of penile erection. *Urol Clin North Am* 1988; **15**:1–7.

4 Krane RJ, Goldstein I, Saenz de Tejada. I. Impotence. *N Engl J Med* 1989; **321**:1648–1659.

5 Bush PA, Aronson WJ, Buga GM, Rajfer J, Ignarro LJ. Nitric oxide is a potent relaxant of human and rabbit corpus cavernosum. *J Urol* 1992; **147**:1650–1655.

6 Rajfer J, Aronson WJ, Bush PA, Dorey FJ, Ignarro LJ. Nitric oxide as a mediator of relaxation of the corpus cavernosum in response to nonadrenergic, noncholinergic neurotransmission. *N Engl J Med* 1992; **326**:90–94.

7 Saenz de Tejada, I, Angulo J, Cellek S, Gonzalez-Cadavid N, Heaton J, Pickard R, *et al.* Physiology of erectile function. *J Sex Med* 2004; **1**:254–265.

8 Saenz de Tejada I, Goldstein I, Azadzoi K, Krane RJ, Cohen RA. Impaired neurogenic and endothelium-mediated relaxation of penile smooth muscle from diabetic men with impotence. *N Engl J Med* 1989; **320**:1025–1030.

9 Angulo J, Cuevas P, Fernandez A, Gabancho S, Videla S, Saenz de Tejada I. Calcium dobesilate potentiates endothelium-derived hyperpolarizing factor-mediated relaxation of human penile resistance arteries. *Br J Pharmacol* 2003; **139**:854–862.

10 Angulo J, Cuevas P, Fernandez A, Gabancho S, Allona A, Martin-Morales A, *et al.* Diabetes impairs endothelium-dependent relaxation of human penile vascular tissues mediated by NO and EDHF. *Biochem Biophys Res Commun* 2003; **312**:1202–1208.

11 Mullarkey CJ, Edelstein D, Brownlee M. Free radical generation by early glycation products: a mechanism for accelerated atherogenesis in diabetes. *Biochem Biophys Res Commun* 1990; **173**:932–939.

12 Seftel AD, Vaziri ND, Ni Z, Razmjouei K, Fogarty J, Hampel N, *et al.* Advanced glycation end products in human penis: elevation in diabetic tissue, site of deposition, and possible effect through iNOS or eNOS. *Urology* 1997; **50**:1016–1026.

13 Cartledge JJ, Eardley I, Morrison JF. Advanced glycation end-products are responsible for the impairment of corpus cavernosal

smooth muscle relaxation seen in diabetes. *BJU Int* 2001; **87**: 402–407.

14 Angulo J, Sanchez-Ferrer CF, Peiro C, Marin J, Rodriguez-Manas L. Impairment of endothelium-dependent relaxation by increasing percentages of glycosylated human hemoglobin: possible mechanisms involved. *Hypertension* 1996; **28**:583–592.

15 Feldman HA, Goldstein I, Hatzichristou DG, Krane RJ, McKinlay JB. Impotence and its medical and psychosocial correlates: results of the Massachusetts Male Aging Study. *J Urol* 1994; **151**:54–61.

16 Hogan MJ, Wallin JD, Baer RM. Antihypertensive therapy and male sexual dysfunction. *Psychosomatics* 1980; **21**:234–237.

17 Kochar MS, Zeller JR, Itskovitz HD. Prazosin in hypertension with and without methyldopa. *Clin Pharmacol Ther* 1979; **25**:143–148.

18 Hackett GI. Impotence: the most neglected complication of diabetes. *Diabetes Res* 1995; **28**:75–83.

19 Nicolosi A, Glasser DB, Moreira ED, Villa M. Prevalence of erectile dysfunction and associated factors among men without concomitant diseases: a population study. *Int J Impot Res* 2003; **15**:253–257.

20 Sullivan ME, Thompson CS, Dashwood MR, Khan MA, Jeremy JY, Morgan RJ, *et al.* Nitric oxide and penile erection: is erectile dysfunction another manifestation of vascular disease? *Cardiovasc Res* 1999; **43**:658–665.

21 Gazzaruso C, Solerte SB, Pujia A, Coppola A, Vezzoli M, Salvucci F, *et al.* Erectile dysfunction as a predictor of cardiovascular events and death in diabetic patients with angiographically proven asymptomatic coronary artery disease: a potential protective role for statins and 5-phosphodiesterase inhibitors. *J Am Coll Cardiol* 2008; **51**:2040–2044.

22 Ma RC, So WY, Yang X, Yu LW, Kong AP, Ko GT, *et al.* Erectile dysfunction predicts coronary heart disease in type 2 diabetes. *J Am Coll Cardiol* 2008; **51**:2045–2050.

23 Bacon CG, Mittleman MA, Kawachi I, Giovannucci E, Glasser DB, Rimm EB. A prospective study of risk factors for erectile dysfunction. *J Urol* 2006; **176**:217–221.

24 Bacon CG, Mittleman MA, Kawachi I, Giovannucci E, Glasser DB, Rimm EB. Sexual function in men older than 50 years of age: results from the health professionals follow-up study. *Ann Intern Med* 2003; **139**:161–168.

25 Bacon CG, Hu FB, Giovannucci E, Glasser DB, Mittleman MA, Rimm EB. Association of type and duration of diabetes with erectile dysfunction in a large cohort of men. *Diabetes Care* 2002; **25**:1458–1463.

26 Schachter M. Erectile dysfunction and lipid disorders. *Curr Med Res Opin* 2000; **16**(Suppl 1):9–12.

27 Ross R. The pathogenesis of atherosclerosis: a perspective for the 1990s. *Nature* 1993; **362**:801–809.

28 Vane JR, Anggard EE, Botting RM. Regulatory functions of the vascular endothelium. *N Engl J Med* 1990; **323**:27–36.

29 Pegge NC, Twomey AM, Vaughton K, Gravenor MB, Ramsey MW, Price DE. The role of endothelial dysfunction in the pathophysiology of erectile dysfunction in diabetes and in determining response to treatment. *Diabet Med* 2006; **23**:873–878.

30 Craig A. *One in Ten*. London: Impotence Association, 1997.

31 Alexander WD. The diabetes physician and an assessment and treatment programme for male erectile impotence. *Diabet Med* 1990; **7**:540–543.

32 Bodansky HJ. Treatment of male erectile dysfunction using the active vacuum assist device. *Diabet Med* 1994; **11**:410–412.

33 Price DE, Cooksey G, Jehu D, Bentley S, Hearnshaw JR, Osborn DE. The management of impotence in diabetic men by vacuum tumescence therapy. *Diabet Med* 1991; **8**:964–967.

34 Ryder RE, Close CF, Moriarty KT, Moore KT, Hardisty CA. Impotence in diabetes: aetiology, implications for treatment and preferred vacuum device. *Diabet Med* 1992; **9**:893–898.

35 McCulloch DK, Young RJ, Prescott RJ, Campbell IW, Clarke BF. The natural history of impotence in diabetic men. *Diabetologia* 1984; **26**:437–440.

36 Boolell M, Gepi-Attee S, Gingell JC, Allen MJ. Sildenafil, a novel effective oral therapy for male erectile dysfunction. *Br J Urol* 1996; **78**:257–261.

37 Price DE, Gingell JC, Gepi-Attee S, Wareham K, Yates P, Boolell M. Sildenafil: study of a novel oral treatment for erectile dysfunction in diabetic men. *Diabet Med* 1998; **15**:821–825.

38 Goldstein I, Lue TF, Padma-Nathan H, Rosen RC, Steers WD, Wicker PA. Oral sildenafil in the treatment of erectile dysfunction. Sildenafil Study Group [see comments]. *N Engl J Med* 1998; **338**:1397–1404.

39 Marks LS, Duda C, Dorey FJ, Macairan ML, Santos PB. Treatment of erectile dysfunction with sildenafil. *Urology* 1999; **53**:19–24.

40 Padma-Nathan H, Steers WD, Wicker PA; Sildenafil Study Group. Efficacy and safety of oral sildenafil in the treatment of erectile dysfunction: a double-blind, placebo-controlled study of 329 patients. *Int J Clin Pract* 1998; **52**:375–379.

41 Price D; Sildenafil Study Group. Sildenafil citrate (Viagra) efficacy in the treatment of erectile dysfunction in patients with common concomitant conditions. *Int J Clin Pract Suppl* 1999; **102**:21–23.

42 Giuliano F, Hultling C, el Masry WS, Luchner E, Stien R, Maytom MC, *et al.* Sildenafil citrate (VIAGRA): a novel oral treatment for erectile dysfunction caused by traumatic spinal cord injury. *Int J Clin Pract Suppl* 1999; **102**:24–26.

43 Palmer JS, Kaplan WE, Firlit CF. Erectile dysfunction in patients with spina bifida is a treatable condition. *J Urol* 2000; **164**: 958–961.

44 Lowentritt BH, Scardino PT, Miles BJ, Orejuela FJ, Schatte EC, Slawin KM, *et al.* Sildenafil citrate after radical retropubic prostatectomy. *J Urol* 1999; **162**:1614–1617.

45 Rendell MS, Rajfer J, Wicker PA, Smith MD; Sildenafil Diabetes Study Group. Sildenafil for treatment of erectile dysfunction in men with diabetes: a randomized controlled trial. *JAMA* 1999; **281**:421–426.

46 Wagner G, Montorsi F, Auerbach S, Collins M. Sildenafil citrate (Viagra) improves erectile function in elderly patients with erectile dysfunction: a subgroup analysis. *J Gerontol A Biol Sci Med Sci* 2001; **56**:M113–M119.

47 El-Galley R, Rutland H, Talic R, Keane T, Clark H. Long-term efficacy of sildenafil and tachyphylaxis effect. *J Urol* 2001; **166**:927–931.

48 Fonseca V, Seftel A, Denne J, Fredlund P. Impact of diabetes mellitus on the severity of erectile dysfunction and response to treatment: analysis of data from tadalafil clinical trials. *Diabetologia* 2004; **47**:1914–1923.

49 Sharlip ID, Shumaker BP, Hakim LS, Goldfischer E, Natanegara F, Wong DG. Tadalafil is efficacious and well tolerated in the treatment of erectile dysfunction (ED) in men over 65 years of age: results from Multiple Observations in Men with ED in National Tadalafil Study in the United States. *J Sex Med* 2008; **5**:716–725.

50 Hatzichristou D, Gambla M, Rubio-Aurioles E, Buvat J, Brock GB, Spera G, *et al.* Efficacy of tadalafil once daily in men with diabetes mellitus and erectile dysfunction. *Diabet Med* 2008; **25**:138–146.

51 Eardley I, Lee JC, Guay AT. Global experiences with vardenafil in men with erectile dysfunction and underlying conditions. *Int J Clin Pract* 2008; **62**:1594–1603.

52 Ziegler D, Merfort F, van AH, Yassin A, Reblin T, Neureither M. Efficacy and safety of flexible-dose vardenafil in men with type 1 diabetes and erectile dysfunction. *J Sex Med* 2006; **3**:883–891.

53 Pomeranz HD, Bhavsar AR. Nonarteritic ischemic optic neuropathy developing soon after use of sildenafil (Viagra): a report of seven new cases. *J Neuroophthalmol* 2005; **25**:9–13.

54 Pomeranz HD, Smith KH, Hart WM Jr, Egan RA. Sildenafil-associated nonarteritic anterior ischemic optic neuropathy. *Ophthalmology* 2002; **109**:584–587.

55 McGwin G Jr, Vaphiades MS, Hall TA, Owsley C. Non-arteritic anterior ischaemic optic neuropathy and the treatment of erectile dysfunction. *Br J Ophthalmol* 2006; **90**:154–157.

56 Gorkin L, Hvidsten K, Sobel RE, Siegel R. Sildenafil citrate use and the incidence of nonarteritic anterior ischemic optic neuropathy. *Int J Clin Pract* 2006; **60**:500–503.

57 Ryder RE, Kitchen MM, Dewsbury JA, Howells MG, Ryan PG, Jones SL, *et al.* Do vascular, neuropathic, hormonal or psychogenic factors identify non-response to Viagra in diabetic impotence? *Diabet Med* 2001; **18**(Suppl 2):108.

58 Jarow JP, Burnett AL, Geringer AM. Clinical efficacy of sildenafil citrate based on etiology and response to prior treatment. *J Urol* 1999; **162**:722–725.

59 Eardley I, Mirone V, Montorsi F, Ralph D, Kell P, Warner MR, *et al.* An open-label, multicentre, randomized, crossover study comparing sildenafil citrate and tadalafil for treating erectile dysfunction in men naive to phosphodiesterase 5 inhibitor therapy. *BJU Int* 2005; **96**:1323–1332.

60 DeBusk RF, Pepine CJ, Glasser DB, Shpilsky A, DeRiesthal H, Sweeney M. Efficacy and safety of sildenafil citrate in men with erectile dysfunction and stable coronary artery disease. *Am J Cardiol* 2004; **93**:147–153.

61 Carson CC, Rajfer J, Eardley I, Carrier S, Denne JS, Walker DJ, *et al.* The efficacy and safety of tadalafil: an update. *BJU Int* 2004; **93**:1276–1281.

62 Brock GB, McMahon CG, Chen KK, Costigan T, Shen W, Watkins V, *et al.* Efficacy and safety of tadalafil for the treatment of erectile dysfunction: results of integrated analyses. *J Urol* 2002; **168**: 1332–1336.

63 Goldstein I, Young JM, Fischer J, Bangerter K, Segerson T, Taylor T. Vardenafil, a new phosphodiesterase type 5 inhibitor, in the treatment of erectile dysfunction in men with diabetes: a multicenter double-blind placebo-controlled fixed-dose study. *Diabetes Care* 2003; **26**:777–783.

64 Valiquette L, Young JM, Moncada I, Porst H, Vezina JG, Stancil BN, *et al.* Sustained efficacy and safety of vardenafil for treatment of erectile dysfunction: a randomized, double-blind, placebo-controlled study. *Mayo Clin Proc* 2005; **80**:1291–1297.

65 Jackson G, Betteridge J, Dean J, Eardley I, Hall R, Holdright D, *et al.* A systematic approach to erectile dysfunction in the cardiovascular patient: a Consensus Statement – update 2002. *Int J Clin Pract* 2002; **56**:663–671.

66 Jackson G, Montorsi P, Cheitlin MD. Cardiovascular safety of sildenafil citrate (Viagra): an updated perspective. *Urology* 2006; **68**(Suppl):47–60.

67 Shakir SA, Wilton LV, Boshier A, Layton D, Heeley E. Cardiovascular events in users of sildenafil: results from first phase of prescription event monitoring in England. *Br Med J* 2001; **322**:651–652.

68 Kloner RA, Jackson G, Hutter AM, Mittleman MA, Chan M, Warner MR, *et al.* Cardiovascular safety update of tadalafil: retrospective analysis of data from placebo-controlled and open-label clinical trials of tadalafil with as needed, three times-per-week or once-a-day dosing. *Am J Cardiol* 2006; **97**:1778–1784.

69 Rosano GM, Aversa A, Vitale C, Fabbri A, Fini M, Spera G. Chronic treatment with tadalafil improves endothelial function in men with increased cardiovascular risk. *Eur Urol* 2005; **47**:214–220.

70 Muller JE, Mittleman A, Maclure M, Sherwood JB, Tofler GH. Triggering myocardial infarction by sexual activity: low absolute risk and prevention by regular physical exertion. Determinants of Myocardial Infarction Onset Study Investigators [see comments]. *JAMA* 1996; **275**:1405–1409.

71 Dean J, Hackett GI, Gentile V, Pirozzi-Farina F, Rosen RC, Zhao Y, *et al.* Psychosocial outcomes and drug attributes affecting treatment choice in men receiving sildenafil citrate and tadalafil for the treatment of erectile dysfunction: results of a multicenter, randomized, open-label, crossover study. *J Sex Med* 2006; **3**: 650–661.

72 Govier F, Potempa AJ, Kaufman J, Denne J, Kovalenko P, Ahuja S. A multicenter, randomized, double-blind, crossover study of patient preference for tadalafil 20 mg or sildenafil citrate 50 mg during initiation of treatment for erectile dysfunction. *Clin Ther* 2003; **25**:2709–2723.

73 Stroberg P, Murphy A, Costigan T. Switching patients with erectile dysfunction from sildenafil citrate to tadalafil: results of a European multicenter, open-label study of patient preference. *Clin Ther* 2003; **25**:2724–2737.

74 von Keitz A, Rajfer J, Segal S, Murphy A, Denne J, Costigan T, *et al.* A multicenter, randomized, double-blind, crossover study to evaluate patient preference between tadalafil and sildenafil. *Eur Urol* 2004; **45**:499–507.

75 McCullough AR, Steidle CP, Klee B, Tseng LJ. Randomized, double-blind, crossover trial of sildenafil in men with mild to moderate erectile dysfunction: efficacy at 8 and 12 hours postdose. *Urology* 2008; **71**:686–692.

76 McCullough AR, Barada JH, Fawzy A, Guay AT, Hatzichristou D. Achieving treatment optimization with sildenafil citrate (Viagra) in patients with erectile dysfunction. *Urology* 2002; **60**(Suppl 2):28–38.

77 Kalinchenko SY, Kozlov GI, Gontcharov NP, Katsiya GV. Oral testosterone undecanoate reverses erectile dysfunction associated with diabetes mellitus in patients failing on sildenafil citrate therapy alone. *Aging Male* 2003; **6**:94–99.

78 Mulhall JP. Treatment of erectile dysfunction in a hypogonadal male. *Rev Urol* 2004; **6**(Suppl 6):S38–S40.

79 Greco EA, Spera G, Aversa A. Combining testosterone and PDE5 inhibitors in erectile dysfunction: basic rationale and clinical evidences. *Eur Urol* 2006; **50**:940–947.

80 Shamloul R, Ghanem H, Fahmy I, El-Meleigy A, Ashoor S, Elnashaar A, *et al.* Testosterone therapy can enhance erectile function response to sildenafil in patients with PADAM: a pilot study. *J Sex Med* 2005; **2**:559–564.

81 Dula E, Bukofzer S, Perdok R, George M. Double-blind, crossover comparison of 3 mg apomorphine SL with placebo and with 4 mg apomorphine SL in male erectile dysfunction. *Eur Urol* 2001; **39**:558–553.

82 Brindley GS. Cavernosal alpha-blockade: a new technique for investigating and treating erectile impotence. *Br J Psychiatry* 1983; **143**:332–337.

83 Virag R. Intracavernous injection of papaverine for erectile failure. *Lancet* 1982; **2**:938.

84 Armstrong DK, Convery AG, Dinsmore WW. Reasons for patient drop-out from an intracavernous auto-injection programme for erectile dysfunction. *Br J Urol* 1994; **74**:99–101.

85 Flynn RJ, Williams G. Long-term follow-up of patients with erectile dysfunction commenced on self injection with intracavernosal papaverine with or without phentolamine. *Br J Urol* 1996; **78**:628–631.

86 Pagliarulo A, Ludovico GM, Cirillo-Marucco E, Corvasce A, Pagliarulo G. Compliance to long-term vasoactive intracavernous therapy. *Int J Impot Res* 1996; **8**:63–64.

87 Padma-Nathan H, Goldstein I, Krane RJ. Treatment of prolonged or priapistic erections following intracavernosal papaverine therapy. *Semin Urol* 1986; **4**:236–238.

88 Kiely EA, Bloom SR, Williams G. Penile response to intracavernosal vasoactive intestinal polypeptide alone and in combination with other vasoactive agents. *Br J Urol* 1989; **64**:191–194.

89 Gerstenberg TC, Metz P, Ottesen B, Fahrenkrug J. Intracavernous self-injection with vasoactive intestinal polypeptide and phentolamine in the management of erectile failure. *J Urol* 1992; **147**:1277–1279.

90 Padma-Nathan H, Hellstrom WJ, Kaiser FE, Labasky RF, Lue TF, Nolten WE, *et al.*; Medicated Urethral System for Erection (MUSE) Study Group. Treatment of men with erectile dysfunction with transurethral alprostadil. *N Engl J Med* 1997; **336**:1–7.

91 Nolten WE, Billington CJ, Chiu KC. Treatment of erectile dysfunction (impotence) with a novel transurethral drug delivery system: results from a multicenter placeb-controlled trial [Abstract]. *10th International Congress of Endocrinology*, 1996.

92 Shabsigh R, Padma-Nathan H, Gittleman M, McMurray J, Kaufman J, Goldstein I. Intracavernous alprostadil alfadex is more efficacious, better tolerated, and preferred over intraurethral alprostadil plus optional actis: a comparative, randomized, crossover, multicenter study. *Urology* 2000; **55**:109–113.

93 Fulgham PF, Cochran JS, Denman JL, Feagins BA, Gross MB, Kadesky KT, *et al.* Disappointing initial results with transurethral alprostadil for erectile dysfunction in a urology practice setting. *J Urol* 1998; **160**:2041–2046.

94 Baltaci S, Aydos K, Kosar A, Anafarta K. Treating erectile dysfunction with a vacuum tumescence device: a retrospective analysis of acceptance and satisfaction. *Br J Urol* 1995; **76**:757–760.

95 Korenman SG, Viosca SP. Use of a vacuum tumescence device in the management of impotence in men with a history of penile implant or severe pelvic disease. *J Am Geriatr Soc* 1992; **40**:61–64.

96 Sidi AA, Becher EF, Zhang G, Lewis JH. Patient acceptance of and satisfaction with an external negative pressure device for impotence. *J Urol* 1990; **144**:1154–1156.

97 Vrijhof HJ, Delaere KP. Vacuum constriction devices in erectile dysfunction: acceptance and effectiveness in patients with impotence of organic or mixed aetiology. *Br J Urol* 1994; **74**:102–105.

98 Kabalin JN, Kessler R. Infectious complications of penile prosthesis surgery. *J Urol* 1988; **139**:953–955.

99 Garber BB. Inflatable penile prosthesis: results of 150 cases. *Br J Urol* 1996; **78**:933–935.

100 Enzlin P, Mathieu C, Vanderschueren D, Demyttenaere K. Diabetes mellitus and female sexuality: a review of 25 years' research. *Diabet Med* 1998; **15**:809–815.

101 Enzlin P, Mathieu C, Van Den BA, Bosteels J, Vanderschueren D, Demyttenaere K. Sexual dysfunction in women with type 1 diabetes: a controlled study. *Diabetes Care* 2002; **25**:672–677.

102 Enzlin P, Mathieu C, Van Den BA, Vanderschueren D, Demyttenaere K. Prevalence and predictors of sexual dysfunction in patients with type 1 diabetes. *Diabetes Care* 2003; **26**:409–414.

103 Ellenberg M. Diabetes and female sexuality. *Women Health* 1984; **9**:75–79.

104 Ellenberg M. Sexual aspects of the female diabetic. *Mt Sinai J Med* 1977; **44**:495–500.

105 Jensen SB. Diabetic sexual dysfunction: a comparative study of 160 insulin treated diabetic men and women and an age-matched control group. *Arch Sex Behav* 1981; **10**:493–504.

106 Tyrer G, Steel JM, Ewing DJ, Bancroft J, Warner P, Clarke BF. Sexual responsiveness in diabetic women. *Diabetologia* 1983; **24**:166–171.

107 Steel JM. Diabetes and female sexuality. *Diabet Med* 1998; **15**:807–808.

108 Caruso S, Intelisano G, Lupo L, Agnello C. Premenopausal women affected by sexual arousal disorder treated with sildenafil: a double-blind, cross-over, placebo-controlled study. *BJOG* 2001; **108**:623–628.

109 Basson R, McInnes R, Smith MD, Hodgson G, Koppiker N. Efficacy and safety of sildenafil citrate in women with sexual dysfunction associated with female sexual arousal disorder. *J Womens Health Gend Based Med* 2002; **11**:367–377.

110 Caruso S, Rugolo S, Agnello C, Intelisano G, Di ML, Cianci A. Sildenafil improves sexual functioning in premenopausal women with type 1 diabetes who are affected by sexual arousal disorder: a double-blind, crossover, placebo-controlled pilot study. *Fertil Steril* 2006; **85**:1496–1501.

111 Peck RW, Price DE, Lang GD, MacVicar J, Hearnshaw JR. Birthweight of babies born to mothers with type 1 diabetes: is it related to blood glucose control in the first trimester? *Diabet Med* 1991; **8**:258–262.

112 Steel JM, Johnstone FD, Smith AF, Duncan LJ. Five years' experience of a "prepregnancy" clinic for insulin-dependent diabetics. *Br Med J (Clin Res Ed)* 1982; **285**:353–356.

113 Steel JM, Parboosingh J, Cole RA, Duncan LJ. Prepregnancy counseling: a logical prelude to the management of the pregnant diabetic woman. *Diabetes Care* 1980; **3**:371–373.

114 Lawrenson RA, Leydon GM, Williams TJ, Newson RB, Feher MD. Patterns of contraception in UK women with type 1 diabetes mellitus: a GP database study. *Diabet Med* 1999; **16**:395–399.

115 Manolopoulos K, Lang U, Schmitt S, Kirschbaum M, Kapellen T, Kiess W. Which contraceptive methods are recommended for young women with type 1 diabetes mellitus? A survey among practitioners in Germany [in German]. *Zentralbl Gynakol* 1998; **120**:540–544.

116 Shawe J, Lawrenson R. Hormonal contraception in women with diabetes mellitus: special considerations. *Treat Endocrinol* 2003; **2**:321–330.

117 Vessey M, Lawless M, Yeates D. Efficacy of different contraceptive methods. *Lancet* 1982; **1**:841–842.

118 Lopez LM, Grimes DA, Schulz KF. Steroidal contraceptives: effect on carbohydrate metabolism in women without diabetes mellitus. *Cochrane Database Syst Rev* 2007; **2**:CD006133.

119 Petersen KR, Skouby SO, Vedel P, Haaber AB. Hormonal contraception in women with IDDM: influence on glycometabolic control and lipoprotein metabolism. *Diabetes Care* 1995; **18**:800–806.

120 Petersen KR, Skouby SO, Sidelmann J, Molsted-Pedersen L, Jespersen J. Effects of contraceptive steroids on cardiovascular risk factors in women with insulin-dependent diabetes mellitus. *Am J Obstet Gynecol* 1994; **171**:400–405.

121 Garg SK, Chase HP, Marshall G, Hoops SL, Holmes DL, Jackson WE. Oral contraceptives and renal and retinal complications in young women with insulin-dependent diabetes mellitus. *JAMA* 1994; **271**:1099–1102.

122 Kjos SL, Shoupe D, Douyan S, Friedman RL, Bernstein GS, Mestman JH, *et al.* Effect of low-dose oral contraceptives on carbohydrate and lipid metabolism in women with recent gestational diabetes: results of a controlled, randomized, prospective study. *Am J Obstet Gynecol* 1990; **163**:1822–1827.

123 Petersen KR, Skouby SO, Jespersen J. Contraception guidance in women with pre-existing disturbances in carbohydrate metabolism. *Eur J Contracept Reprod Health Care* 1996; **1**:53–59.

124 Konje JC, Otolorin EO, Ladipo OA. The effect of continuous subdermal levonorgestrel (Norplant) on carbohydrate metabolism. *Am J Obstet Gynecol* 1992; **166**:15–19.

125 Diab KM, Zaki MM. Contraception in diabetic women: comparative metabolic study of Norplant, depot medroxyprogesterone acetate, low dose oral contraceptive pill and CuT380A. *J Obstet Gynaecol Res* 2000; **26**:17–26.

126 Harvengt C. Effect of oral contraceptive use on the incidence of impaired glucose tolerance and diabetes mellitus. *Diabet Metab* 1992; **18**:71–77.

127 Kimmerle R, Weiss R, Berger M, Kurz KH. Effectiveness, safety, and acceptability of a copper intrauterine device (CU Safe 300) in type I diabetic women. *Diabetes Care* 1993; **16**:1227–1230.

128 Kjos SL, Ballagh SA, La CM, Xiang A, Mishell DR Jr. The copper T380A intrauterine device in women with type II diabetes mellitus. *Obstet Gynecol* 1994; **84**:1006–1009.

129 Task Force on Postovulatory Methods of Fertility Regulation. Randomised controlled trial of levonorgestrel versus the Yuzpe regimen of combined oral contraceptives for emergency contraception. *Lancet* 1998; **352**:428–433.

130 Palin SL, Kumar S, Sturdee DW, Barnett AH. Hormone replacement therapy for postmenopausal women with diabetes. *Diabetes Obes Metab* 2001; **3**:187–193.

131 Hulley S, Grady D, Bush T, Furberg C, Herrington D, Riggs B, *et al.*; Heart and Estrogen/progestin Replacement Study (HERS) Research Group. Randomized trial of estrogen plus progestin for secondary prevention of coronary heart disease in postmenopausal women. *JAMA* 1998; **280**:605–613.

132 Writing Group for the Women's Health Initiative Investigators. Risks and benefits of estrogen plus progestin in healthy postmenopausal women: principal results from the Women's Health Initiative randomized controlled trial. *JAMA* 2002; **288**:321–333.

133 Shumaker SA, Legault C, Rapp SR, Thal L, Wallace RB, Ockene JK, *et al.*; Women's Health Initiative Memory Study. Estrogen plus progestin and the incidence of dementia and mild cognitive impairment in postmenopausal women: a randomized controlled trial. *JAMA* 2003; **289**:2651–2662.

134 Larsson-Cohn U, Wallentin L. Metabolic and hormonal effects of post-menopausal oestrogen replacement treatment. I. Glucose, insulin and human growth hormone levels during oral glucose tolerance tests. *Acta Endocrinol (Copenh)* 1977; **86**:583–596.

135 Lobo RA, Pickar JH, Wild RA, Walsh B, Hirvonen E; Menopause Study Group. Metabolic impact of adding medroxyprogesterone acetate to conjugated estrogen therapy in postmenopausal women. *Obstet Gynecol* 1994; **84**:987–995.

136 Postmenopausal Estrogen/Progestin Interventions (PEPI) Trial. The Writing Group for the PEPI Trial. Effects of estrogen or estrogen/progestin regimens on heart disease risk factors in postmenopausal women. *JAMA* 1995; **273**:199–208.

137 Thom M, Chakravarti S, Oram DH, Studd JW. Effect of hormone replacement therapy on glucose tolerance in postmenopausal women. *Br J Obstet Gynaecol* 1977; **84**:776–783.

138 Ajabor LN, Tsai CC, Vela P, Yen SS. Effect of exogenous estrogen on carbohydrate metabolism in postmenopausal women. *Am J Obstet Gynecol* 1972; **113**:383–387.

139 Andersson B, Mattsson LA, Hahn L, Marin P, Lapidus L, Holm G, *et al.* Estrogen replacement therapy decreases hyperandrogenicity and improves glucose homeostasis and plasma lipids in postmenopausal women with noninsulin-dependent diabetes mellitus. *J Clin Endocrinol Metab* 1997; **82**:638–643.

140 Ferrara A, Karter AJ, Ackerson LM, Liu JY, Selby JV. Hormone replacement therapy is associated with better glycemic control in women with type 2 diabetes: Northern California Kaiser Permanente Diabetes Registry. *Diabetes Care* 2001; **24**:1144–1150.

141 Manning PJ, Allum A, Jones S, Sutherland WH, Williams SM. The effect of hormone replacement therapy on cardiovascular risk factors in type 2 diabetes: a randomized controlled trial. *Arch Intern Med* 2001; **161**:1772–1776.

142 Andersson B, Mattsson LA. The effect of transdermal estrogen replacement therapy on hyperandrogenicity and glucose homeostasis in postmenopausal women with NIDDM. *Acta Obstet Gynecol Scand* 1999; **78**:260–261.

143 Walsh BW, Schiff I, Rosner B, Greenberg L, Ravnikar V, Sacks FM. Effects of postmenopausal estrogen replacement on the concentrations and metabolism of plasma lipoproteins. *N Engl J Med* 1991; **325**:1196–1204.

144 Lobo RA. Clinical review 27: effects of hormonal replacement on lipids and lipoproteins in postmenopausal women. *J Clin Endocrinol Metab* 1991; **73**:925–930.

145 Samaras K, Hayward CS, Sullivan D, Kelly RP, Campbell LV. Effects of postmenopausal hormone replacement therapy on central abdominal fat, glycemic control, lipid metabolism, and vascular factors in type 2 diabetes: a prospective study. *Diabetes Care* 1999; **22**:1401–1407.

146 Hayward CS, Samaras K, Campbell L, Kelly RP. Effect of combination hormone replacement therapy on ambulatory blood pressure and arterial stiffness in diabetic postmenopausal women. *Am J Hypertens* 2001; **14**:699–703.

147 Lopez-Ibarra PJ, Pastor MM, Escobar-Jimenez F, Pardo MD, Gonzalez AG, Luna JD, *et al.* Bone mineral density at time of clinical diagnosis of adult-onset type 1 diabetes mellitus. *Endocr Pract* 2001; **7**:346–351.

148 Nicodemus KK, Folsom AR. Type 1 and type 2 diabetes and incident hip fractures in postmenopausal women. *Diabetes Care* 2001; **24**:1192–1197.

46 Gastrointestinal Manifestations of Diabetes

Adil E. Bharucha & Michael Camilleri

Clinical Enteric Neuroscience Translational and Epidemiological Research Program, Division of Gastroenterology and Hepatology, Mayo Clinic, Rochester, MN, USA

Keypoints

- Gastrointestinal manifestations are frequent in diabetes.
- Diabetes may not be the cause of gastrointestinal symptoms.
- Glycemia influences development of neuropathy and acutely changes gastric emptying.
- Extrinsic and enteric neuropathies are key mechanisms in diabetic gastroenteropathy.
- Motor dysfunctions may affect any region of the gastrointestinal tract in diabetes and cause fast or slow transit.
- Incontinence, a frequently unvoiced symptom, may reflect sphincter or sensation deficits.
- Assessments of hydration, nutrition and metabolic status are essential.
- Measurements of regional transit and anorectal motor and sensory functions are key to management of diabetic gastroenteropathy.
- For management of gastroparesis and dyspepsia, correct hydration, nutrition and metabolic status; exclude any iatrogenic factor, such as GLP-1 analog, and "gastroparesis"; and treat the pathophysiologic process.

Introduction

Although most attention has traditionally focused on the stomach, diabetes can affect the entire gastrointestinal tract. The term diabetic enteropathy refers to all the gastrointestinal complications of diabetes. Gastrointestinal involvement may be asymptomatic or manifest as symptoms (i.e. dysphagia, heartburn, nausea and vomiting, abdominal pain, constipation, diarrhea and fecal incontinence). These manifestations may affect quality of life, impair nutrition, and affect glycemic control.

Epidemiology

Studies in selected patient groups, often from tertiary referral centers, suggest that gastrointestinal symptoms are common in diabetes mellitus [1,2]; however, these studies are prone to selection and other biases, which are avoided by studies conducted among people with diabetes in the community, where the prevalence of gastrointestinal symptoms is either not different, or only slightly higher than people without diabetes. Thus, in the Rochester Diabetic Neuropathy Study, only 1% of patients had symptoms of gastroparesis and only 0.6% had nocturnal diarrhea [3]. In another study from Olmsted County, Minnesota, the prevalence of gastrointestinal symptoms (i.e. nausea and/or vomiting, dyspepsia, heartburn, irritable bowel syndrome, constipation and fecal incontinence) was not significantly different between individuals with either type 1 (T1DM) or type 2 diabetes mellitus (T2DM) and age-matched controls [4]; however, people with T2DM and men with T1DM used laxatives more frequently than in controls. Moreover, that study and a Finnish population-based study reported that people with T1DM had a lower prevalence of heartburn [5].

In contrast to these studies, a study from Australia found that the prevalence of several upper and lower gastrointestinal symptoms was higher in 423 patients with predominantly (95%) T2DM than in controls [6]. Taken together, these data suggest that gastrointestinal manifestations are not uncommon among patients with diabetes presenting for care. In the general population, however, the prevalence of gastrointestinal manifestations is not substantially higher among people with diabetes and matched controls, perhaps partly because the prevalence of gastrointestinal symptoms, mostly attributable to functional gastrointestinal disorders (e.g. irritable bowel syndrome), among people without diabetes in the community is relatively high, and approaches 20%. In Olmsted County, Minnesota, the age-adjusted incidence per 100,000 person-years of definite gastroparesis for the years 1996–2006 was 2.4 (95% confidence interval [CI] 1.2–3.8) for men and 9.8 (95% CI 7.5–12.1) for women. The age-adjusted prevalence of definite gastroparesis per 100 000 persons on January 1, 2007, was 9.6 (95% CI 1.8–17.4) for men and 37.8 (95% CI 23.3–52.4) for women [7].

Textbook of Diabetes, 4th edition. Edited by R. Holt, C. Cockram, A. Flyvbjerg and B. Goldstein.

Diabetic gastroparesis may cause severe symptoms and result in nutritional compromise, impaired glucose control and a poor quality of life, independently of other factors such as age, tobacco use, alcohol use or type of diabetes [8]. Studies of the natural history of gastroparesis have been limited by relatively small numbers of patients, potential referral bias or short follow-up periods. The data suggest that gastric emptying and its symptoms are generally stable during 12 years of follow-up or more [9]. In a study of 86 patients with diabetes who were followed for at least 9 years, gastroparesis was not associated with mortality after adjustment for other disorders [10]. Among patients with gastroparesis, overall survival was significantly lower than the age- and sex-specific expected survival computed from the Minnesota white population [7]; the most common causes of death were cardiovascular disease (24.6%), respiratory failure (23.2%), malignancy (15.9%), chronic renal failure in 11 (15.9%), cerebrovascular accident (10.1%) and other causes (10.1%).

Pathophysiology

Gastrointestinal dysmotility in diabetes is caused by extrinsic (i.e. sympathetic and parasympathetic) neural dysfunction, hyperglycemia and hormonal disturbances. More recently, a role for intrinsic (i.e. enteric) neuronal dysfunctions, resulting from loss of excitatory and inhibitory neurons and interstitial cells of Cajal, has also been implicated [11]. Neural dysfunction has been attributed to several mechanisms (e.g. oxidative stress) described below and detailed elsewhere [12].

Normal gastrointestinal motor functions

Gastrointestinal motor function is primarily controlled by the intrinsic or enteric nervous system (i.e. the "little brain" in the digestive tract) and modulated by the extrinsic (i.e. parasympathetic and sympathetic) nervous system (Figure 46.1) [13]. While intrinsic and extrinsic controls are independent, the prevertebral ganglia integrate afferent impulses between the gut and the central nervous system and provide additional reflex control of the abdominal viscera. The parasympathetic arm is excitatory to non-sphincteric muscle and inhibits sphincters. The sympathetic component has opposite effects. The enteric nervous system consists of 100 million neurons that are organized in distinct ganglionated plexi including the submucous plexus, which is primarily involved in absorption and secretion, and the myenteric plexus, which regulates motility. The interstitial cells of Cajal serve as pacemakers and also convey messages from nerve to smooth muscle. As with the somatic and autonomic nerves elsewhere, the gut's autonomic and enteric nervous system can be affected in diabetes. Derangements of the extrinsic nerves at any level may alter gastrointestinal motility and secretion [14].

Gastrointestinal digestion and absorption require gastrointestinal motility, gastric and pancreatic secretion, and gastrointestinal hormonal release, which in turn, modulate motor, secretory and absorptive functions in the upper gut [15]. Traditionally, these processes are considered in three phases (cephalic, gastric and intestinal), which are integrated and overlap. Normally, liquids, particularly non-caloric liquids, empty rapidly from the stomach in a linear fashion. In contrast, gastric emptying of solids follows an exponential pattern. During the first 45 minute postprandial period (i.e. the lag phase), the gastric antrum grinds

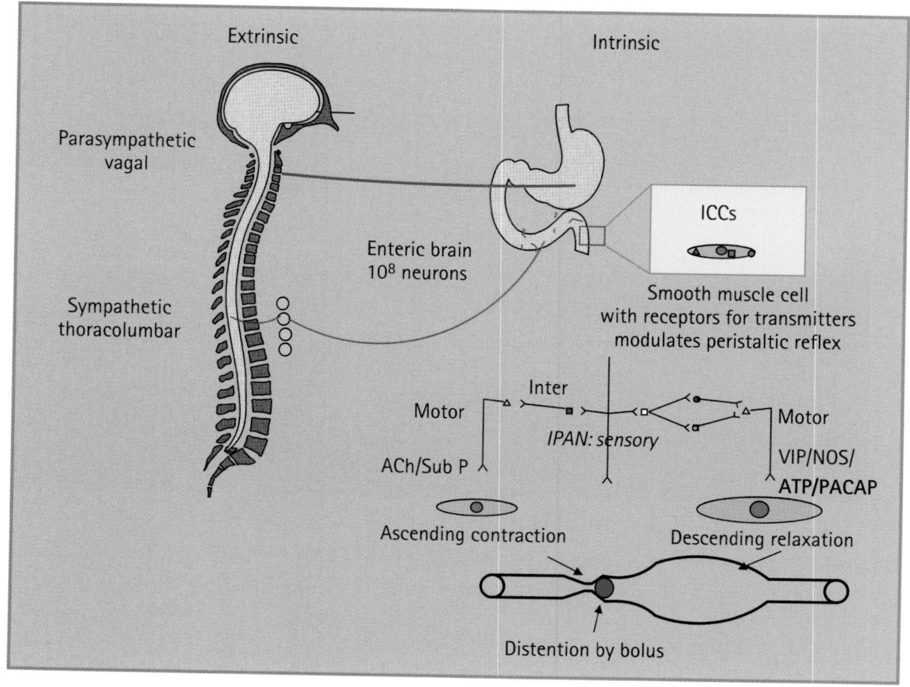

Figure 46.1 Control of gastrointestinal motility. Note the extrinsic or autonomic nervous system modulates the function of the enteric nervous system, which controls smooth muscle cells through excitatory (i.e. acetylcholine [Ach], substance P [Sub P]) or inhibitory (nitric oxide [NO], vasoactive intestinal peptide [VIP], pituitary adenylate cyclase activating peptide [PACAP]) neurotransmitters. ICC, interstitial cells of Cajal; IPAN, intrinsic primary afferent neuron. Adapted from Camilleri M, Phillips SF. Disorders of small intestinal motility. *Gastroenterol Clin North Am* 1989; **18**:405–424.

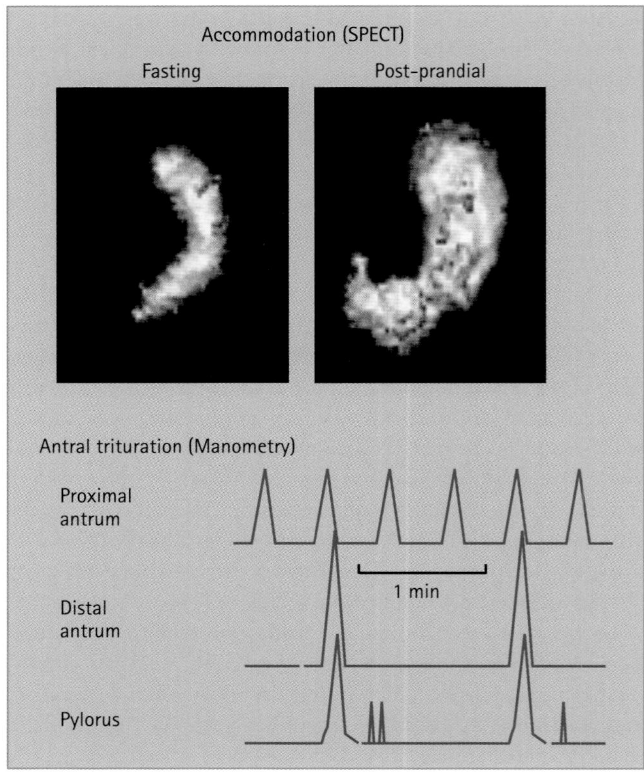

solids into particles smaller than 2 mm in size, so they can be emptied through the pylorus. During the lag phase, the stomach relaxes or accommodates, providing room for digestion to occur (Figures 46.2 & 46.3). Thereafter, solids are emptied in a linear fashion, with approximately 50% emptying in 2 hours and 100% emptying in 4 hours.

Pancreatobiliary secretions and mechanical processes ensure small intestinal digestion, which precedes absorption. The small intestine transports solids and liquids at approximately the same rate; the head of the column of liquid chyme may reach the cecum as early as 30 minutes after ingestion. As a result of the lag phase for the transport of solids from the stomach, liquids typically arrive in the colon before solids. It takes about 150 minutes for half the solid and liquid chyme of similar caloric density (assuming solids are presented in a triturated form to the small bowel) to traverse the small bowel. Complex carbohydrates or fat in the

Figure 46.2 Assessment of gastric motor functions. Gastric accommodation can be assessed by measuring the post-prandial change in gastric volume using single photo emission computed tomography (SPECT). (top panel) The stomach wall is labeled with intravenous ^{99m}Tc pertechnetate. Food is subsequently transferred to the antrum. Manometry (bottom panel) demonstrates that the distal antrum and pylorus contract synchronously to grind food into smaller particles. Only particles 2 mm or smaller can be emptied through the pylorus.

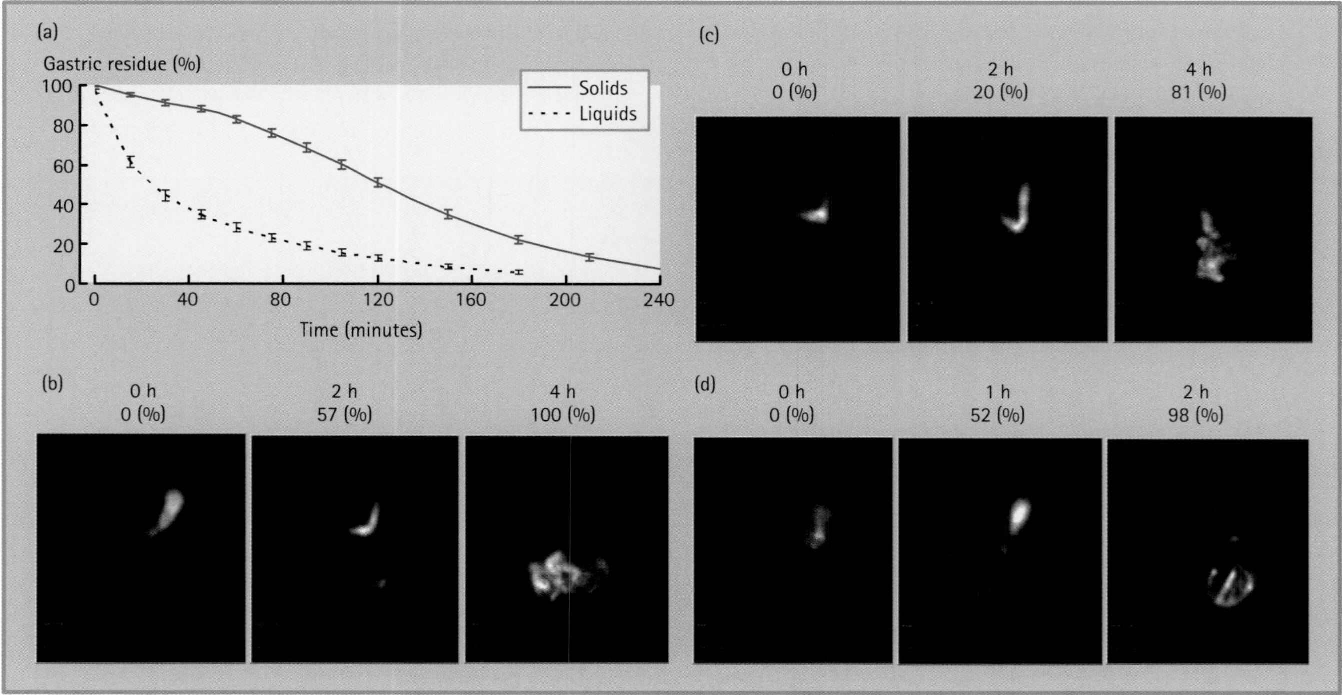

Figure 46.3 Assessment of gastric emptying by scintigraphy. Normally liquids are emptied in a linear manner while solid emptying has an exponential profile, characterized by an initial lag phase, followed by a more rapid, linear emptying (a). The lag phase corresponds to the time required for antral trituration and gastric accommodation, during which approximately 10% of solids are emptied. (b, c, and d) Representative examples of normal, delayed and accelerated gastric emptying respectively of an egg meal, labeled with ^{99m}Tc, in patients with diabetes. At time 0 (i.e. first image in each panel), the entire meal was in the stomach. Thereafter, the normal ranges for gastric emptying are 11–39% at 1 hour, 40–76% at 2 hours and 84–98% at 4 hours.

distal small intestine exert feedback control of proximal small intestinal motility, a process known as the small intestinal brake. Chyme is transferred from the ileum to colon in intermittent boluses. On average, it takes 36 hours, with an upper limit of 65 hours, to transfer contents from the cecum to the rectum. Compared to the stomach and small intestine, colonic transit is relatively prolonged, permitting digestion of fiber and absorption of water and electrolytes to be completed.

Pathophysiology of diabetic enteropathy: insights from animal studies

In animal models, extrinsic neural dysfunction has been primarily implicated to a loss of myelinated and unmyelinated fibers without much neuronal loss [16,17]. The loss of nerve fibers is often multifocal, suggestive of ischemic injury. Within the enteric nervous system, reduced neuronal staining, and to a lesser extent neuronal loss, particularly inhibitory neurons expressing nitric oxide synthase (NOS) have been described in several animal models of diabetes [12]. In theory, this reduction in nitrergic inhibitory functions may contribute to impaired gastric accommodation and accelerated intestinal transit in diabetes. Reduced sympathetic inhibition may also contribute to accelerated intestinal transit. Because nitric oxide (NO) is a mediator of pyloric relaxation, loss of NOS may impair pyloric relaxation and thereby retard gastric emptying. Loss of intestinal cells of Cajal (ICC), documented in several animal models and case reports of diabetes, may also contribute to gut dysmotility [11,18].

Several mechanisms, including apoptosis, oxidative stress, advanced glycation end products and neuroimmune mechanisms may be responsible for neuronal loss and gut dysmotility [12]. The loss of ICC has been attributed to a reduction in heme-oxygenase (HO-1) and other protective mechanisms against hyperglycemia [11]. The effects of diabetes on neuronal morphology and functions are reversible. Insulin or pancreas transplantation improved glycemic control and the axonopathy affecting autonomic nerves in rats with diabetic autonomic neuropathy [19]. Insulin also restored expression of NOS and gastric emptying in animal models of diabetes while insulin and insulin-like growth factors prevented the loss of ICC in cultures [20,21]. Because ICC do not express receptors for either hormone, these effects are perhaps mediated by smooth muscle secretion of stem cell factor, which is the most important growth factor for ICC rather than directly by insulin and insulin-like growth factors [11]. Overexpression of glial cell line-derived neurotrophic factor, a trophic factor for enteric neurons, in transgenic mice reversed hyperglycemia-induced apoptosis of enteric neurons, improved gastric emptying and intestinal transit [22].

Pathophysiology of diabetic enteropathy in humans

Gastric dysfunctions

Neuropathy

Diabetes is associated with accelerated or delayed gastric emptying, increased and reduced gastric sensation, and impaired gastric accommodation (Figure 46.4). A vagal neuropathy can cause antral hypomotility and/or pylorospasm, which may delay gastric emptying [23]. The pathophysiology of rapid gastric emptying in diabetes is less well understood. Conceivably, impaired gastric accommodation resulting from a vagal neuropathy [24] may increase gastric pressure and thereby accelerate gastric emptying of liquids. However, the relationship between rapid gastric emptying and impaired gastric accommodation has not been substan-

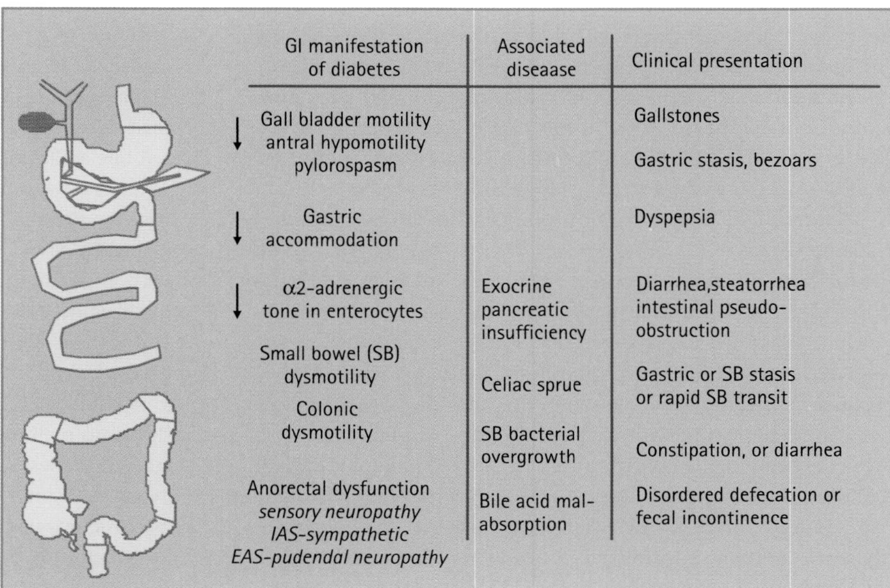

Figure 46.4 Pathophysiology of diabetes enteropathy in humans. Adapted from Camilleri M. Gastrointestinal problems in diabetes. *Endocrinol Metab Clin North Am* 1996; **25**:361–378.

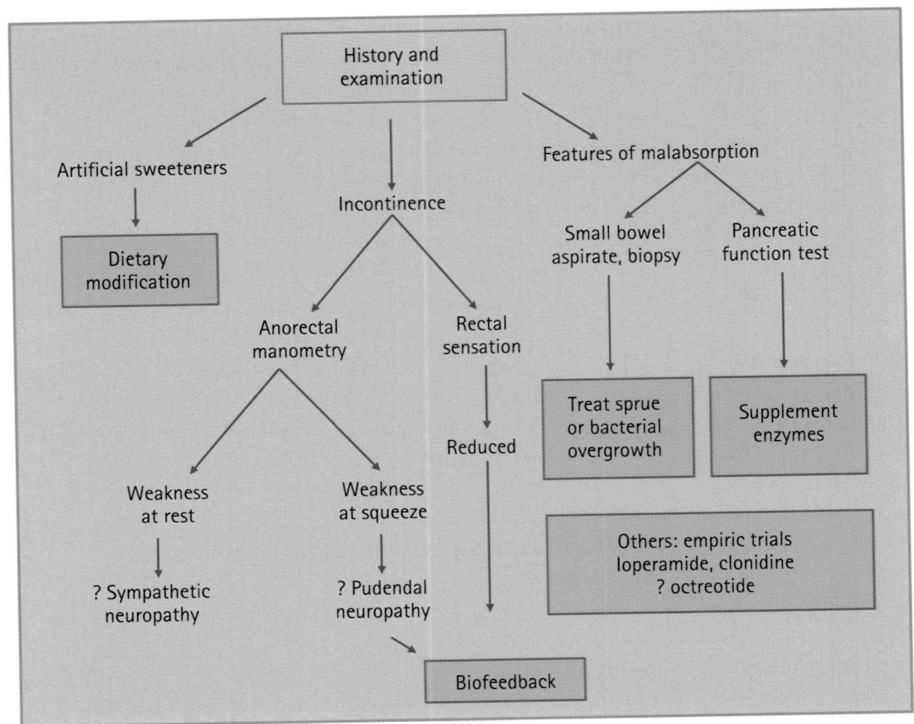

Figure 46.5 Management of diarrhea in diabetes mellitus. Adapted from Camilleri M. Gastrointestinal problems in diabetes. *Endocrinol Metab Clin North Am* 1996; **25**:361–378.

tiated. The relationship between vagal neuropathy and impaired post-prandial accommodation is unclear because accommodation may be preserved even in people with diabetes and vagal neuropathy [25], perhaps reflecting non-vagal adaptive mechanisms involving enteric neurons [26]. Some patients with diabetes and gastroparesis also have small intestinal dysmotility, more frequently characterized by reduced than by increased motility [27]. Small bowel dysmotility may also contribute to gastric stasis.

Hyperglycemia

Acute hyperglycemia delays gastric emptying in healthy subjects and in T1DM [28–31]. These effects may be explained by hyperglycemia-induced suppression of antral motility and migrating motor activity, the so-called intestinal "housekeeper" [32–34]. The effects of acute hyperglycemia on gastric emptying are modest. Indeed, even in T1DM, severe acute hyperglycemia (i.e. 16–20 mmol/L vs 4–8 mmol/L) prolonged the gastric emptying half-time by only 17 minutes from 124 to 141 minutes. Acute modulation of blood glucose within the physiologic postprandial range (4–8 mmol/L) can also delay gastric emptying, to a lesser degree [31]. Cross-sectional studies suggest that higher glycated hemoglobin concentrations are associated with a higher prevalence of gastrointestinal symptoms and slower gastric emptying among people with diabetes in the community [6,35]. While strict glycemic control improves neural, renal and retinal functions in diabetes, the impact on gastric emptying is unclear [36]. Indeed, in the only study that assessed this question, improved glycemic control did not improve gastric emptying 1 week later in 10 patients with T2DM [37]. In addition to hyperglycemia, electrolyte imbalances caused by diabetic ketoacidosis (e.g. hypokalemia) and uremia may also aggravate impaired motor function in patients with diabetes. Iatrogenic gastroparesis may result from treatment with amylin or GLP-1 analogs.

Diabetic diarrhea

It is useful to categorize the pathophysiology of diabetic diarrhea into conditions that are associated with malabsorption and those that are not (Figure 46.5). Involvement of sympathetic fibers, which normally inhibit motility and facilitate absorption via α_2-adrenergic receptors, can result in accelerated small intestinal transit and cause diarrhea [38]. Artificial sweeteners such as sorbitol may also contribute to diarrhea. Patients with rapid ileal transit may have bile acid malabsorption [39,40] and deconjugated bile acids induce colonic secretion.

Features suggestive of malabsorption such as anemia, macrocytosis or steatorrhea should prompt consideration of bacterial overgrowth, small bowel mucosal disease or pancreatic insufficiency. Small intestinal dysmotility predisposes to bacterial overgrowth, which can cause bile salt deconjugation, fat malabsorption and diarrhea. Although T1DM is associated with celiac disease, most patients with celiac disease and T1DM in the community are asymptomatic [41]. Chronic pancreatic insufficiency may result from pancreatic atrophy, disruption of cholinergic enteropancreatic reflexes, or elevated serum hormonal levels of glucagon, somatostatin and pancreatic polypeptide, which reduce pancreatic enzyme secretion [42]. Nevertheless, the association between chronic pancreatic insufficiency and diabetes is uncommon. Moreover, because there is sufficient pancreatic reserve, only 10% of pancreatic function is sufficient for normal digestion.

Fecal incontinence

Loose stools and anorectal dysfunctions contribute to fecal incontinence in diabetic diarrhea. Compared to continent people with diabetes and healthy controls, patients with diabetes and fecal incontinence have a higher threshold for rectal perception of balloon distention, a marker of reduced sensation [43,44]. A sympathetic neuropathy may impair internal anal sphincter function and anal resting pressures while a pudendal neuropathy may result in reduced anal squeeze pressure.

Constipation

The mechanisms of constipation in diabetes have not been carefully studied and are poorly understood. Clinical observations suggest that, similar to idiopathic chronic constipation, both colonic dysmotility and anorectal dysfunctions, such as impaired anal sphincteric relaxation during defecation, may contribute to constipation in diabetes [45]. Patients with colonic dysmotility have an impaired colonic contractile response to a meal and delayed colonic transit [46]. Patients with reduced rectal sensation may not perceive the desire to defecate. Compared to euglycemia, acute hyperglyemia inhibits the colonic contractile response to gastric distention and proximal colonic contraction elicited by colonic distention in healthy subjects [47]. By contrast, acute hyperglycemia did not significantly affect fasting or post-prandial colonic tone, motility, compliance and sensation, or rectal compliance and sensation in healthy people [48].

In addition to these factors, it is also important to consider the role of psychologic factors in the perception of gastrointestinal symptoms. Indeed, psychosomatic symptoms are significantly associated with the reporting of gastrointestinal tract symptoms [4]. Several medications have gastrointestinal side effects; for example, metformin can cause diarrhea while among other medications, verapamil and anticholinergic agents, can cause constipation.

Clinical manifestations

Dysphagia and heartburn

Esophageal dysmotility, typically characterized by impaired peristalsis with simultaneous contractions, is common, may cause dysphagia, and may be related to cardiovascular autonomic neuropathy in diabetic mellitus [49]. The amplitude of peristaltic contractions and basal lower esophageal sphincter pressures are generally normal. Symptoms of gastroesophageal reflux are also common, particularly in patients with impaired gastric emptying who have vomiting. Rarely, recurrent vomiting may lead to Mallory–Weiss tears and bleeding.

Dysphagia and heartburn should prompt upper gastrointestinal endoscopy to exclude reflux and other incidental mucosal diseases, such as candidiasis and neoplasms. While manometry may reveal esophageal peristaltic disturbances in patients with significant dysphagia that is not explained by a structural lesion, it is unlikely to alter management, except for rare patients in whom another disorder, such as achalasia, is responsible for dysphagia. Because of the high prevalence of coronary atherosclerosis in diabetes, testing for coronary artery disease should be considered when necessary in patients with chest pain.

Dyspepsia and gastroparesis

Although gastroparesis refers to a syndrome characterized by symptoms of nausea, vomiting, early satiation after meals and impaired nutrition and objective evidence of markedly delayed gastric emptying, gastric retention may be asymptomatic [50], perhaps because of the afferent dysfunction associated with vagal denervation [51]. Nausea and vomiting often occur in episodes lasting days to months or in cycles. Nausea and vomiting may be associated with impaired glycemic control and often cause hypoglycemia, perhaps because delivery of food into the small bowel for absorption is not sufficient to match the effects of exogenous insulin.

Consistent with the concept of a paralyzed stomach, the term gastroparesis should be restricted to patients with markedly delayed gastric emptying. When the delay in gastric emptying is not severe, the term diabetic dyspepsia is perhaps more appropriate. Dypepsia is characterized by one or more, generally post-prandial, upper gastrointestinal symptoms, including bloating, post-prandial fullness and upper abdominal pain. Typically, vomiting is not severe but significant weight loss secondary to reduced caloric intake is not unusual. In addition to delayed gastric emptying, impaired gastric accommodation and abnormal, either increased or decreased, gastric sensation may also contribute to symptoms in diabetes [52,53]. Nonetheless, the distinction of dyspepsia from gastroparesis is challenging because there is no official distinction between moderately and severely delayed gastric emptying. Perhaps, gastric emptying of less than 65% at 4 hours reflects a significant delay as it is often associated with nutritional consequences, the need for nutritional supplementation, jejunal feeding or gastric decompression [54].

Patients with diabetic gastroparesis frequently have long-standing T1DM with other microvascular complications, including retinopathy, nephropathy, peripheral neuropathy and other forms of autonomic dysfunction. These can present as abnormal pupillary responses, anhidrosis, gustatory sweating, orthostatic hypotension, impotence, retrograde ejaculation and dysfunction of the urinary bladder) (Table 46.1). In contrast, it has been suggested that rapid gastric emptying of liquids is a relatively early manifestation of T2DM [55–59]. Clinicians have relied on these manifestations, and on certain symptoms, such as vomiting of undigested food eaten several hours previously and weight loss, and signs (e.g. a gastric succussion splash or features of an autonomic neuropathy) to predict delayed gastric emptying in patients with diabetes who present with upper and gastrointestinal symptoms. Several studies have shown, however, that symptoms are of limited utility for predicting delayed gastric emptying in diabetes

[60–66]. Similarly, the type and duration of diabetes, glycated hemoglobin levels and extraintestinal complications were, in general, not useful for discriminating normal from delayed or rapid gastric emptying; however, significant weight loss and a neuropathy were risk factors for delayed and rapid gastric emptying, respectively [67].

In patients with upper gastrointestinal symptoms, an upper gastrointestinal endoscopy is necessary to exclude peptic ulcer disease and neoplasms, either of which can cause gastric outlet obstruction. Upper endoscopy may reveal gastric bezoars, which suggest antral hypomotility. Metabolic derangements, such as diabetic ketoacidosis or uremia, and medications, particularly opiates, calcium-channel blockers and anticholinergic agents, may contribute to dysmotility. Rarely, patients with gastroparesis present with retrosternal or epigastric pain and cardiac, biliary or pancreatic disease may be considered.

Table 46.1 Symptoms and signs of autonomic dysfunction. Reproduced from Camilleri M. Disorders of gastrointestinal motility in neurologic disease. *Mayo Clin Proc* 1990; **65**:825–846, with permission.

Sympathetic	Parasympathetic
Failure of pupils to dilate in the dark	Fixed dilated pupils
Fainting, orthostatic dizziness	Lack of pupillary accommodation
Constant heart rate with orthostatic hypotension	Sweating during mastication of certain foods
Absent piloerection	Decreased gut motility
Absent sweating	Dry eyes and mouth
Impaired ejaculation	Dry vagina
Paralysis of dartos muscle	Impaired erection
	Difficulty emptying urinary bladder; recurrent urinary tract infections

Barium X-rays of the small intestine or enterography with computed tomography should be considered only when the clinical features raise the possibility of small intestinal obstruction. Gastric emptying of solids should be quantified by scintigraphy and antroduodenal manometry should be considered in selected circumstances. Measurement of pressure profiles in the stomach and small bowel can confirm the motor disturbance and may facilitate the selection of patients for enteral feeding (Figure 46.6). Patients with selective antral hypomotility may tolerate feeding delivered directly into the small bowel while those with a more generalized motility disorder may not.

Diarrhea and constipation

The term diabetic diarrhea was first coined in 1936 by Bargen at the Mayo Clinic to describe unexplained diarrhea associated with severe diabetes [68]. Diabetic diarrhea is typically chronic, may be episodic and can be severe. Diarrhea can occur at any time but is often nocturnal and may be associated with anal incontinence,

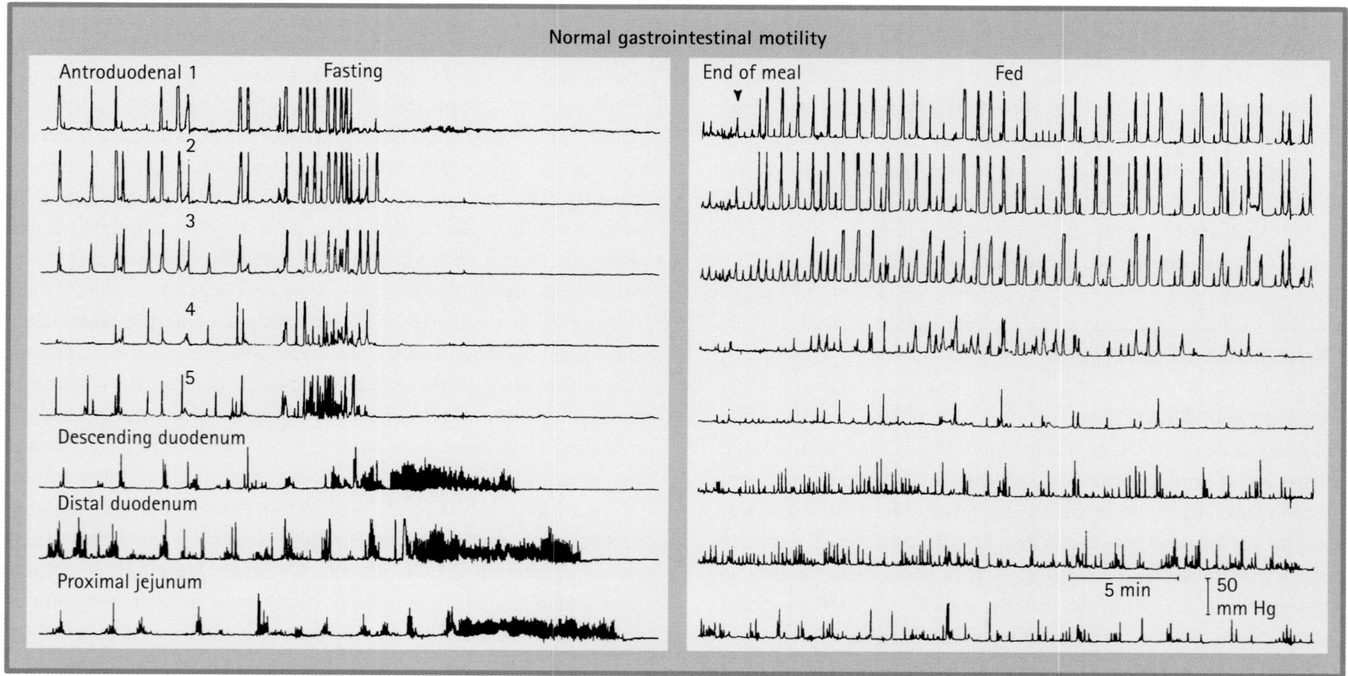

Figure 46.6 Normal manometric profile (fasting and post-prandial). The migrating motor complex characteristic of fasting state is demonstrated by the presence of quiescence (phase I), intermittent activity (phase II) and an activity front (phase III). Post-prandial profile shows high amplitude, irregular but persistent phasic pressure activity at all levels. Reproduced from Malagelada J-R, Camilleri M, Stanghellini V. *Manometric Diagnosis of Gastrointestinal Motility Disorders.* New York: Thieme Publishers, 1986, by permission of Mayo Foundation for Medical Education and Research. All rights reserved.)

which may indicate internal anal sphincter dysfunction. Patients with diarrhea often have symptoms of delayed gastric emptying such as early satiety, nausea and vomiting.

Constipation may occur in isolation or alternate with episodes of diarrhea. Many physicians regard constipation to be synonymous with infrequent bowel movements. It is important to characterize symptoms because many people have misconceptions about normal bowel habits. For example, it is not necessary to have a bowel movement daily – the normal range varies from three bowel movements every week to three every day. Moreover, by constipation, patients refer to one or more of a variety of symptoms including infrequent stools, hard stools, excessive straining during defecation, a sense of anorectal blockage during defecation, the need for anal digitation during defecation and a sense of incomplete evacuation after defecation [69]. Some of these symptoms, such as a sense of anorectal blockage during defecation, may suggest disordered evacuation. A careful rectal examination during relaxation and straining is needed to exclude rectal mucosal lesions and to detect the presence of rectal prolapse, rectocele and disordered defecation. Normally, voluntary contraction is accompanied by upward and anterior motion of the palpating finger toward the umbilicus as the puborectalis contracts. Conversely, the puborectalis should relax and the perineum should descend (by 2–4 cm) during simulated evacuation. The rectal examination may suggest features or defecatory disorders such as reduced or increased perineal descent and paradoxical contraction of puborectalis.

Abdominal pain

Patients with diabetes are obviously susceptible to the usual causes of abdominal pain seen in the general population. There is an increased prevalence of gallstones because of altered gallbladder contractility and of mesenteric ischemia caused by generalized atherosclerosis; however, there is little evidence that altered gallbladder contractility per se (i.e. in the absence of gallstones) causes symptoms. Thoracolumbar radiculopathy may result in pain in a girdle-like distribution which does not cross the midline. Specific tests are indicated in the clinical features of pain suggest these disorders. It is essential to elicit a careful history.

Diagnostic tests

Typically, diagnostic testing is primarily guided by symptom pattern and severity; however, because patients with delayed gastric emptying are often asymptomatic, gastric emptying assessments should also be considered in patients with unexplained hypoglycemia. After initial testing to identify disturbances of transit, more detailed testing with intraluminal techniques, such as manometry and/or a barostat, may be useful for characterizing motor dysfunctions and guiding therapy (Table 46.2). Autonomic function testing is also useful [70]. Delayed gastric emptying can be documented by scintigraphy or the presence of a large amount of retained food in the stomach. Barium studies and scintigraphy using labeled liquid meals are of limited value for identifying dysmotility because the gastric emptying of liquids and semisolids (e.g. mashed potatoes) frequently is normal, even in the presence of moderately severe symptoms. Assessment of solid emptying by means of a radiolabel that tags the solid phase of the meal is a more sensitive test with a well-defined normal range. The proportion of radioisotope retained in the stomach at 2 and 4 hours distinguishes normal function from delayed gastric emptying with a sensitivity of 90% and a specificity of 70% [71]. The importance of obtaining scans for 4 hours after a meal cannot be overemphasized. Because gastric emptying is slow initially, it is not accurate to extrapolate emptying from scans taken for a shorter duration. Another useful test for measuring solid phase gastric emptying utilizes a standardized meal with biscuit enriched with ^{13}C, a substrate containing the stable isotope. When metabolized, the proteins, carbohydrates and lipids of the *S. platensis* or the medium chain triglyceride octanoate give rise to respiratory CO_2 that is enriched in ^{13}C. Measurement of $^{13}CO_2$ breath content (a reflection of the amount of biscuit remaining in the stomach) by isotope ratio mass spectrometry allows an estimation of gastric emptying $t_{1/2}$ [72]. Further validation of this technique is necessary in patients with bacterial overgrowth and small bowel mucosal disease.

For patients with severe upper gastrointestinal symptoms, antropyloroduodenal manometry is a specialized technique that assesses pressure profiles in the stomach and small bowel and also guides management. Manometry may also reveal hypomotility of the gastric antrum and/or an intestinal neuropathy (Figures 46.6 & 46.7). Patients with selective abnormalities of gastric function may be able to tolerate enteral feeding (delivered directly into the small bowel) whereas patients with a more generalized motility disorder may not.

Gastric accommodation in response to meal ingestion may be impaired in diabetes [73]. This may contribute to the gastrointestinal symptoms of nausea, bloating and early satiety. Imaging of the stomach wall using ^{99m}Tc pertechnetate allows measurement of gastric volume after meal ingestion.

For patients with constipation, colonic transit, anorectal manometry and rectal balloon expulsion tests provide a useful start. Anorectal manometry and the rectal balloon expulsion test generally suffice to diagnose or exclude defecation disorders; magnetic resonance imaging (MRI) or barium proctography are only required in selected patients. Colonic transit is often delayed in patients with defecatory disorders. Therefore, in patients with slow colonic transit, slow transit constipation can only be diagnosed after excluding defecatory disorders. Intraluminal assessments of colonic phasic motility (by manometry) and tone (by barostat) often reveal other dysfunctions (e.g. impaired contractile responses to a meal and/or pharmacologic stimuli (e.g. bisacodyl or neostigmine) in patient with slow transit constipation. Colonic transit can be characterized by radiopaque markers, which, depending on the technique, takes 5–7 days, or by scintigraphy, which takes 24–48 hours. Both techniques are equally accurate for identifying slow or rapid colonic transit.

Table 46.2 Commonly performed autonomic tests. Reproduced from Camilleri M, Ford MJ. Functional gastrointestinal disease and the autonomic nervous system: a way ahead? *Gastroenterology* 1994; **106**:1114–1118, with permission.

Test	Physiologic functions tested	Rationale	Comments/pitfalls
Sympathetic Function			
1. Thermoregulatory sweat test (% surface area of anhidrosis)	Preganglionic and postganglionic cholinergic	Stimulation of hypothalamic temp. control centers	Cumbersome, whole body test
2. Quantitative sudomotor axon reflex test (sweat output, latency)	Postganglionic cholinergic	Antidromic stimulation of peripheral fiber by axonal reflex	Needs specialized facilities
3. Heart rate and blood pressure responses			
Orthostatic tilt test	Adrenergic	Baroreceptor reflex	Impaired responses if intra-vascular volume is reduced
Postural adjustment ratio	Adrenergic	Baroreceptor reflex	Impaired responses if intra-vascular volume is reduced
Cold pressor test	Adrenergic	Baroreceptor reflex	Impaired responses if intra-vascular volume is reduced
Sustained hand grip	Adrenergic	Baroreceptor reflex	Impaired responses if intra-vascular volume is reduced
4. Plasma norepinephrine response to:			
Postural changes	Postganglionic adrenergic	Baroreceptor stimulation	Moderate sensitivity, impaired response if intravascular volume is reduced
Intravenous edrophonium	Postganglionic adrenergic	Anticholinesterase "stimulates" postganglionic fiber at prevertebral ganglia	False-negatives caused by contributions to plasma norepinephrine from many organs
Parasympathetic Function			
1. Heart rate (RR) variation with deep breathing	Parasympathetic	Vagal afferents stimulated by lung stretch	Best cardiovagal test available, but not a test of abdominal vagus
2. Supine/erect heart rate	Parasympathetic	Vagal stimulation by change in central blood volume	Cardiovagal test
3. Valsalva ratio (heart rate, max./min.)	Parasympathetic	Vagal stimulation by change in central blood volume	Cardiovagal test
4. Gastric acid secretory or plasma pancreatic polypeptide response to modified sham feeding or hypoglycemia	Parasympathetic	Stimulation of vagal nuclei by sham feeding or hypoglycaemia	Abdominal vagal test, critically dependent on avoidance of swallowing food during test
5. Nocturnal penile tumescence	Pelvic parasympathetic	Integrity of S2-4	Plethysmographic technique requiring special facilities
6. Cystometrographic response to bethanechol	Pelvic parasympathetic	Increase in intra-vesical pressure suggests denervation supersensitivity	Tests parasympathetic supply to bladder, not bowel

Small intestinal dysmotility may manifest as one or more of the following features: abnormal migrating motor complexes; failure to convert from fasting to post-prandial motor pattern and/or features of a vagal neuropathy such as excessive number of fasting migrating motor complexes or persistent post-prandial migrating motor complexes). Assessment of stool fat provides a useful differentiation point for diabetic diarrhea, as it indicates malabsorption as the pathophysiology leading to diarrhea. An upper endoscopy provides an opportunity to obtain duodenal aspirates for bacterial overgrowth and small bowel biopsy to exclude celiac disease. Lactose or glucose hydrogen breath tests rely on substrate metabolism by bacterial overgrowth in the small intestine with hydrogen release and breath excretion; however, studies have shown that the early peak is frequently caused by rapid delivery of the substrate to the colon with bacterial metabolism by normal colonic flora rather than small bowel bacterial overgrowth [74]. To reduce the potential impact of this confounding factor (i.e. rapid intestinal transit), a more restricted definition to diagnose small intestinal overgrowth may be preferable. An early hydrogen peak (20 ppm), caused by small intestinal bacteria, may be seen at least 15 minutes before the later prolonged peak, which corresponds to the passage of the remaining lactulose into the colon. Even with more restricted definitions, the sensitivity and specificity of the lactulose hydrogen breath test in detecting small bowel bacterial overgrowth have been reported to be only 68% and 44% and for the glucose breath test 62% and 83%, respectively [73].

Management

The principles of management are to address fluid and nutritional requirements, improve glycemic control and treat symptoms.

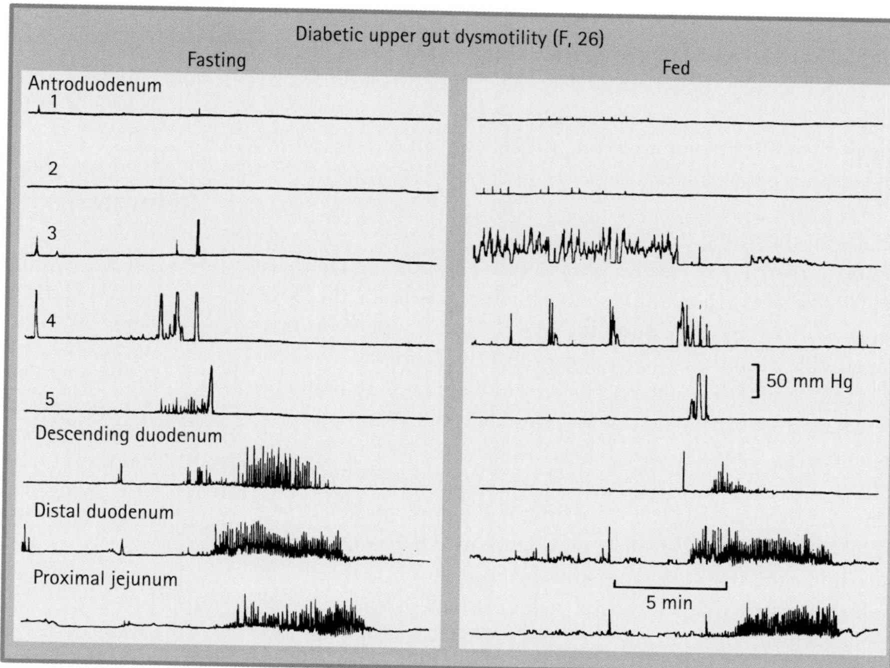

Figure 46.7 Manometric profile in 26-year-old woman with diabetes and autonomic neuropathy, showing abnormal propagation of phase III of interdigestive motor complex and lack of a well-developed antral component in fasting tracing. Post-prandially, note antral hypomotility, pylorospasm, and failure of meal to induce a fed pattern. Reproduced from Colemont LJ, Camilleri M. Chronic intestinal pseudo-obstruction: diagnosis and treatment. *Mayo Clin Proc* 1989; **64**:60–70, with permission.

Gastroparesis and dyspepsia

While nutritional requirements and symptoms can be addressed to a variable extent in patients with mild and compensated gastroparesis, patients with severe gastroparesis often require hospitalization for one or more of the following measures: intravenous hydration and correction of metabolic derangements (ketoacidosis, uremia, hypo-/hyperglycemia), nasoenteric decompression, and/or enteral nutrition to manage vomiting and nutritional requirements [54]. Parenteral nutrition may become necessary in cases of malnutrition. Bezoars may be mechanically disrupted during endoscopy, followed by gastric decompression to drain residual non-digestible particles. Erythromycin at a dose of 3 mg/kg body weight intravenously every 8 hours can accelerate gastric emptying [75,76]. When oral intake is resumed, treatment with oral 250 mg erythromycin t.i.d. for 1–2 weeks is worthwhile. Thereafter, the prokinetic effects of erythromycin are limited by tachyphylaxis. Anecdotal findings suggest that erythromycin may be effective if courses are separated by a drug-free period (e.g. lasting 2 weeks). Hyperglycemia interferes with the prokinetic effect of intravenous erythromycin on gastric emptying in healthy subjects and patients with diabetes [34]. Because both liquids and homogenized solids are more readily emptied from the stomach than solids, liquid or blenderized food will be better tolerated. Frequent monitoring of blood glucose levels is essential during this phase.

For patients with severe gastroparesis who do not respond to the measures outlined above, it may be necessary to bypass the stomach with a jejunal feeding tube. This procedure should be preceded by a trial of nasojejunal feeding for a few days of with infusion rates of at least 60 mL iso-osmolar nutrient per hour. It is preferable to place jejunal feeding tubes directly into the jejunum either by endoscopy, or if necessary by laparoscopy or mini laparotomy, rather than via percutaneous endoscopic gastrostomy tubes. Such tubes allow restoration of normal nutritional status but they are not without adverse effects. There is no evidence to suggest that gastrectomy relieves symptoms or enhances quality of life. Patients with gastroparesis often have concomitant small intestinal denervation which is likely to cause persistent symptoms after gastrectomy [27,77].

If the patient remains symptomatic, other prokinetic agents may be considered as adjuncts. In the USA, the only available medication is metoclopramide, a peripheral cholinergic and antidopaminergic agent. During acute administration, it initially enhances gastric emptying of liquids in patients with diabetic gastroparesis, but its symptomatic efficacy is probably related to its central antiemetic effects. Its long-term use is restricted by a decline in efficacy and by a troubling incidence of central nervous system side effects. Therefore, the authors prefer to prescribe a dose of 10 mg t.i.d., administered 30 minutes before meals, for a short duration; the higher dose is 20 mg t.i.d. A systematic review of trials concluded there was limited evidence to support the use of domperidone, which is another dopaminergic antagonist not approved for use in the USA [78]. Endoscopic injection of botulinum toxin into the pylorus was not effective in controlled studies primarily of patients with idiopathic gastroparesis [79,80].

Although the Food and Drug Administration (FDA) recognizes gastric electrical stimulation as a humanitarian use device for refractory gastroparesis, its use for this indication is controversial. While published data suggest that the device reduces vomiting frequency only when the device is on, data submitted to the FDA concluded that electrical stimulation reduced vomiting frequency to a similar extent with the device turned off or on, suggesting a placebo response [81,82]. Moreover, the device is expensive and does not accelerate gastric emptying. Between 10 and 20% of patients have device-related complications.

Diabetic diarrhea

Diabetic diarrhea is treated symptomatically with loperamide, preferably administered 30 minutes before meals, in the dose range of 2–16 mg/day. Consumption of artificial sweeteners that contain the osmotically active sugar substitute sorbitol should be reduced. Second-line approaches are clonidine, 0.1 mg orally or by patch, in patients who do not experience significant postural hypotension [83]. Amitriptyline, which has anticholinergic effects, may reduce intestinal cramping and transit. Octreotide (25–50 μg subcutaneously 5–10 minutes before meals) delays small intestinal transit [84] and may also reduce secretory diarrhea associated with rapid intestinal transit [85]. While it has been suggested that octreotide reduces small bowel bacterial overgrowth in chronic intestinal pseudo-obstruction [86], this study assessed for bacterial overgrowth by breath testing. Indeed, by delaying small intestinal transit, octreotide may predispose to bacterial overgrowth. Regulating stool consistency may also improve fecal continence. In addition, pelvic floor retraining with biofeedback therapy can improve rectal sensation, and enhance coordination between perception of rectal distention and contraction of the external anal sphincter [44]; however, biofeedback therapy is less effective in patients with markedly reduced rectal sensation. A descending colostomy may be required and may improve the quality of life in patients with severe diarrhea associated with fecal incontinence.

Constipation

For patients without pelvic floor dysfunction, chronic constipation can be generally managed with pharmacologic agents such as osmotic and stimulant laxatives [87]. Pelvic floor retraining by biofeedback therapy is the cornerstone for managing defecatory disorders; laxatives are used as an adjunct to pelvic floor retraining [88]. Fiber supplementation, either with dietary supplementation or with fiber products (e.g. psyllium 15–18 g/day), should be considered in patients with inadequate fiber intake. Of the osmotic laxatives, polyethylene glycol (up to 17 g in 8 ounces of water once or twice per day) is a widely used and safe over-the-counter agent. While lactulose is a poorly absorbed disaccharide, lactulose syrup contains small amounts of absorbable sugars and may increase hyperglycemia. Magnesium compounds are safe but patients with impaired renal function may develop magnesium retention. Bisacodyl or glycerin suppositories are useful rescue agents in patients who do not have a bowel movement for 2 days. If possible, suppositories should be administered 30 minutes after a meal to synergize pharmacologic therapy with the physiologic response to a meal. By activating chloride channels and inducing colonic secretion, lubiprostone accelerates colonic transit in healthy subjects and improves symptoms in functional constipation [89–91]. While there are no studies in patients with diabetes and constipation, lubiprostone should be considered in patients who have not responded to osmotic agents.

References

1 Feldman M, Schiller ER. Disorders of gastrointestinal motility associated with diabetes mellitus. *Ann Intern Med* 1983; 378–384.

2 Clouse RE, Lustman PJ. Gastrointestinal symptoms in diabetic patients: lack of association with neuropathy [see Comment]. *Am J Gastroenterol* 1989; **84**:868–872.

3 Dyck PJ, Karnes JL, O'Brien PC, Litchy WJ, Low PA, Melton LJ 3rd. The Rochester Diabetic Neuropathy Study: reassessment of tests and criteria for diagnosis and staged severity. *Neurology* 1992; **42**: 1164–1170.

4 Maleki D, Locke GR 3rd, Camilleri M, Zinsmeister AR, Yawn BP, Leibson C, *et al.* Gastrointestinal tract symptoms among persons with diabetes mellitus in the community. *Arch Intern Med* 2000; **160**: 2808–2816.

5 Janatuinen E, Pikkarainen P, Laakso M, Pyorala K. Gastrointestinal symptoms in middle-aged diabetic patients. *Scand J Gastroenterol* 1993; **28**:427–432.

6 Bytzer P, Talley NJ, Leemon M, Young LJ, Jones MP, Horowitz M. Prevalence of gastrointestinal symptoms associated with diabetes mellitus: a population-based survey of 15000 adults. *Arch Intern Med* 2001; **161**:1989–1996.

7 Jung HK, Choung RS, Locke GR 3rd, Schleck CD, Zinsmeister AR, Szarka LA, *et al.* The incidence, prevalence, and outcomes of patients with gastroparesis in Olmsted County, Minnesota, from 1996 to 2006. *Gastroenterology* 2009; **136**:1225–1233.

8 Talley NJ, Young L, Bytzer P, Hammer J, Leemon M, Jones M, *et al.* Impact of chronic gastrointestinal symptoms in diabetes mellitus on health-related quality of life. *Am J Gastroenterol* 2001; **96**:71–76.

9 Jones KL, Russo A, Berry MK, Stevens JE, Wishart JM, Horowitz M. A longitudinal study of gastric emptying and upper gastrointestinal symptoms in patients with diabetes mellitus [see Comment]. *Am J Med* 2002; **113**:449–455.

10 Kong MF, Horowitz M, Jones KL, Wishart JM, Harding PE. Natural history of diabetic gastroparesis. *Diabetes Care* 1999; **22**:503–507.

11 Ordog T. Interstitial cells of Cajal in diabetic gastroenteropathy. *Neurogastroenterol Motil* 2008; **20**:8–18.

12 Chandrasekharan B, Srinivasan S. Diabetes and the enteric nervous system. *Neurogastroenterol Motil* 2007; **19**:951–960.

13 Wood JD. Enteric neurophysiology. *Am J Physiol* 1984; **247**: G585–598.

14 Valdovinos MA, Camilleri M, Zimmerman BR. Chronic diarrhea in diabetes mellitus: mechanisms and an approach to diagnosis and treatment. *Mayo Clin Proc* 1993; **68**:691–702.

15 Camilleri M. Integrated upper gastrointestinal response to food intake. *Gastroenterology* 2006; **131**:640–658.

16 Schmidt RE. Neuropathology and pathogenesis of diabetic autonomic neuropathy. *Int Rev Neurobiol* 2002; **50**:257–292.

17 Sinnreich M, Taylor BV, Dyck PJ. Diabetic neuropathies: classification, clinical features, and pathophysiological basis. *Neurologist* 2005; **11**:63–79.

18 Vittal H, Farrugia G, Gomez G, Pasricha PJ. Mechanisms of disease: the pathological basis of gastroparesis – a review of experimental and clinical studies. *Nat Clin Pract Gastroenterol Hepatol* 2007; **4**: 336–346.

19 Schmidt RE, Plurad SB, Olack BJ, Scharp DW. The effect of pancreatic islet transplantation and insulin therapy on experimental diabetic autonomic neuropathy. *Diabetes* 1983; **32**:532–540.

20 Watkins CC, Sawa A, Jaffrey S, Blackshaw S, Barrow RK, Snyder SH, *et al.* Insulin restores neuronal nitric oxide synthase expression and function that is lost in diabetic gastropathy. *J Clin Invest* 2000; **106**:373–384. [Erratum appears in *J Clin Invest* 2000; **106**: 803].

21 Horvath VJ, Vittal H, Lorincz A, Chen H, Almeida-Porada G, Redelman D, *et al.* Reduced stem cell factor links smooth myopathy and loss of interstitial cells of cajal in murine diabetic gastroparesis. *Gastroenterology* 2006; **130**:759–770.

22 Anitha M, Gondha C, Sutliff R, Parsadanian A, Mwangi S, Sitaraman SV, *et al.* GDNF rescues hyperglycemia-induced diabetic enteric neuropathy through activation of the PI3K/Akt pathway [see Comment]. *J Clin Invest* 2006; **116**:344–356.

23 Feldman M, Corbett DB, Ramsey EJ, Walsh JH, Richardson CT. Abnormal gastric function in lonstanding, insulin-dependent diabetic patients. *Gastroenterology* 1979; **77**:12–17.

24 Samsom M, Salet GA, Roelofs JM, Akkermans LM, Vanberge-Henegouwen GP, Smout AJ. Compliance of the proximal stomach and dyspeptic symptoms in patients with type 1 diabetes mellitus. *Dig Dis Sci* 1995; **40**:2037–2042.

25 Delgado-Aros S, Vella A, Camilleri M, Low PA, Burton D, Thomforde G, *et al.* Effects of glucagon-like peptide-1 and feeding on gastric volumes in diabetes mellitus with cardio-vagal dysfunction. *Neurogastroenterol Motil* 2003; **15**:435–443.

26 Takahashi T, Owyang C. Characterization of vagal pathways mediating gastric accommodation reflex in rats. *J Physiol (Lond)* 1997; **504**:479–488.

27 Camilleri M, Malagelada JR. Abnormal intestinal motility in diabetics with gastroparesis. *Eur J Clin Invest* 1984; **14**:420–427.

28 MacGregor IL, Gueller R, Watts HD, Meyer JH. The effect of acute hyperglycemia on gastric emptying in man. *Gastroenterology* 1976; **70**:190–196.

29 Fraser RJ, Horowitz M, Maddox AF, Harding PE, Chatterton BE, Dent J. Hyperglycaemia slows gastric emptying in type 1 (insulin-dependent) diabetes mellitus. *Diabetologia* 1990; **33**:675–680.

30 Oster-Jorgensen E, Pedersen SA, Larsen ML. The influence of induced hyperglycaemia on gastric emptying rate in healthy humans. *Scand J Clin Lab Invest* 1990; **50**:831–836.

31 Schvarcz E, Palmer M, Aman J, Horowitz M, Stridsberg M, Berne C. Physiological hyperglycemia slows gastric emptying in normal subjects and patients with insulin-dependent diabetes mellitus. *Gastroenterology* 1997; **113**:60–66.

32 Barnett JL, Owyang C. Serum glucose concentration as a modulator of interdigestive gastric motility. *Gastroenterology* 1988; **94**:739–744. [Erratum appears in *Gastroenterology* 1988; **95**:262].

33 Hasler WL, Soudah HC, Dulai G, Owyang C. Mediation of hyperglycemia-evoked gastric slow-wave dysrhythmias by endogenous prostaglandins. *Gastroenterology* 1995; **108**:727–736.

34 Samsom M, Akkermans LM, Jebbink RJ, van Isselt H, vanBerge-Henegouwen GP, Smout AJ. Gastrointestinal motor mechanisms in hyperglycaemia induced delayed gastric emptying in type 1 diabetes mellitus. *Gut* 1997; **40**:641–646.

35 Horowitz M, Harding PE, Maddox AF, Wishart JM, Akkermans LM, Chatterton BE, *et al.* Gastric and oesophageal emptying in patients with type 2 (non-insulin-dependent) diabetes mellitus. *Diabetologia* 1989; **32**:151–159.

36 Colwell JA. Intensive insulin therapy in type 2 diabetes: rationale and collaborative clinical trial results. *Diabetes* 1996; **45**(Suppl 3): S87–90.

37 Holzapfel A, Festa A, Stacher-Janotta G, Bergmann H, Shnawa N, Brannath W, *et al.* Gastric emptying in type 2 (non-insulin-dependent) diabetes mellitus before and after therapy readjustment: no influence of actual blood glucose concentration. *Diabetologia* 1999; **42**:1410–1412.

38 Chang EB, Fedorak RN, Field M. Experimental diabetic diarrhea in rats: intestinal mucosal denervation hypersensitivity and treatment with clonidine. *Gastroenterology* 1986; **91**:564–569.

39 Scarpello JH, Hague RV, Cullen DR, Sladen GE. The 14C-glycocholate test in diabetic diarrhoea. *Br Med J* 1976; **2**:673–675.

40 Suhr O, Danielsson A, Steen L. Bile acid malabsorption caused by gastrointestinal motility dysfunction? An investigation of gastrointestinal disturbances in familial amyloidosis with polyneuropathy. *Scand J Gastroenterol* 1992; **27**:201–207.

41 Mahmud FH, Murray JA, Kudva YC, Zinsmeister AR, Dierkhising RA, Lahr BD, *et al.* Celiac disease in type 1 diabetes mellitus in a North American community: prevalence, serologic screening, and clinical features. *Mayo Clin Proc* 2005; **80**:1429–1434.

42 el Newihi H, Dooley CP, Saad C, Staples J, Zeidler A, Valenzuela JE. Impaired exocrine pancreatic function in diabetics with diarrhea and peripheral neuropathy. *Dig Dis Sci* 1988; **33**:705–710.

43 Schiller LR, Schmulen AC. Pathogenesis of fecal incontinence in diabetes mellitus: evidence for internal-anal-sphincter dysfunction. *N Engl J Med* 1982; **307**:1666–1671.

44 Wald A, Tunuguntla AK. Anorectal sensorimotor dysfunction in fecal incontinence and diabetes mellitus: modification with biofeedback therapy. *N Engl J Med* 1984; **310**:1282–1287.

45 Maleki D, Camilleri M, Burton DD, Rath-Harvey DM, Oenning L, Pemberton JH, *et al.* Pilot study of pathophysiology of constipation among community diabetics. *Dig Dis Sci* 1998; **43**:2373–2378.

46 Battle WM, Snape WJ Jr, Alavi A, Cohen S, Braunstein S. Colonic dysfunction in diabetes mellitus. *Gastroenterology* 1980; **79**:1217–1221.

47 Sims MA, Hasler WL, Chey WD, Kim MS, Owyang C. Hyperglycemia inhibits mechanoreceptor-mediated gastrocolonic responses and colonic peristaltic reflexes in healthy humans. *Gastroenterology* 1995; **108**:350–359.

48 Maleki D, Camilleri M, Zinsmeister AR, Rizza RA. Effect of acute hyperglycemia on colorectal motor and sensory function in humans. *Am J Physiol* 1997; **273**:G859–864.

49 Ascaso JF, Herreros B, Sanchiz V, Lluch I, Real JT, Minguez M, *et al.* Oesophageal motility disorders in type 1 diabetes mellitus and their relation to cardiovascular autonomic neuropathy. *Neurogastroenterol Motil* 2006; **18**:813–822.

50 Kassander P. Asymptomatic gastric retention in diabetics: gastroparesis diabeticorum. *Ann Intern Med* 1958; **48**:797–812.

51 Rathmann W, Enck P, Frieling T, Gries FA. Visceral afferent neuropathy in diabetic gastroparesis. *Diabetes Care* 1991; **14**:1086–1089.

52 Mearin F, Malagelada JR. Gastroparesis and dyspepsia in patients with diabetes mellitus. *Eur J Gastroenterol Hepatol* 1995; **7**:717–723.

53 Kumar A, Attaluri A, Hashmi S, Schulze KS, Rao SSC. Visceral hypersensitivity and impaired accommodation in refractory diabetic gastroparesis. *Neurogastroenterol Motil* 2008; **20**:635–642.

54 Camilleri M. Clinical practice: diabetic gastroparesis. *N Engl J Med* 2007; **356**:820–829. [Erratum appears in *N Engl J Med* 2007; **357**:427.]

55 Phillips WT, Schwartz JG, McMahan CA. Rapid gastric emptying of an oral glucose solution in type 2 diabetic patients. *J Nucl Med* 1992; **33**:1496–1500.

56 Frank JW, Saslow SB, Camilleri M, Thomforde GM, Dinneen S, Rizza RA. Mechanism of accelerated gastric emptying of liquids and hyperglycemia in patients with type 2 diabetes mellitus. *Gastroenterology* 1995; **109**:755–765.

57 Schwartz JG, Green GM, Guan D, McMahan CA, Phillips WT. Rapid gastric emptying of a solid pancake meal in type 2 diabetic patients [see Comment]. *Diabetes Care* 1996; **19**:468–471.

58 Weytjens C, Keymeulen B, Van Haleweyn C, Somers G, Bossuyt A. Rapid gastric emptying of a liquid meal in long-term type 2 diabetes mellitus. *Diabet Med* 1998; **15**:1022–1027.

59 Bertin E, Schneider N, Abdelli N, Wampach H, Cadiot G, Loboguerrero A, *et al.* Gastric emptying is accelerated in obese type 2 diabetic patients without autonomic neuropathy. *Diabetes Metab* 2001; **27**:357–364.

60 Keshavarzian A, Iber FL, Vaeth J. Gastric emptying in patients with insulin-requiring diabetes mellitus. *Am J Gastroenterol* 1987; **82**: 29–35.

61 Horowitz M, Maddox AF, Wishart JM, Harding PE, Chatterton BE, Shearman DJ. Relationships between oesophageal transit and solid and liquid gastric emptying in diabetes mellitus. *Eur J Nucl Med* 1991; **18**:229–234.

62 Iber FL, Parveen S, Vandrunen M, Sood KB, Reza F, Serlovsky R, *et al.* Relation of symptoms to impaired stomach, small bowel, and colon motility in long-standing diabetes. *Dig Dis Sci* 1993; **38**:45–50.

63 Jones KL, Horowitz M, Carney BI, Wishart JM, Guha S, Green L. Gastric emptying in early noninsulin-dependent diabetes mellitus. *J Nucl Med* 1996; **37**:1643–1648.

64 Ziegler D, Schadewaldt P, Pour Mirza A, Piolot R, Schommartz B, Reinhardt M, *et al.* [13C] octanoic acid breath test for non-invasive assessment of gastric emptying in diabetic patients: validation and relationship to gastric symptoms and cardiovascular autonomic function. *Diabetologia* 1996; **39**:823–830.

65 Jones KL, Russo A, Stevens JE, Wishart JM, Berry MK, Horowitz M. Predictors of delayed gastric emptying in diabetes. *Diabetes Care* 2001; **24**:1264–1269.

66 Samsom M, Vermeijden JR, Smout AJ, Van Doorn E, Roelofs J, Van Dam PS, *et al.* Prevalence of delayed gastric emptying in diabetic patients and relationship to dyspeptic symptoms: a prospective study in unselected diabetic patients. *Diabetes Care* 2003; **26**: 3116–3122.

67 Bharucha AE, Camilleri M, Forstrom L, Zinsmeister AR. Relationship between clinical features and gastric emptying disturbances in diabetes mellitus. *Clin Endocrinol (Oxf)* 2009; **70**:415–420.

68 Bargen JA, Bollman JL, Kepler EJ. The "diarrhea of diabetes" and steatorrhea of pancreatic insufficiency. *Mayo Clin Proc* 1936; **11**: 737–742.

69 Longstreth GF, Thompson WG, Chey WD, Houghton LA, Mearin F, Spiller RC. Functional bowel disorders. *Gastroenterology* 2006; **130**:1480–1491.

70 Bharucha AE, Camilleri M, Low PA, Zinsmeister AR. Autonomic dysfunction in gastrointestinal motility disorders. *Gut* 1993; **34**(3): 397–401.

71 Camilleri M, Zinsmeister AR, Greydanus MP, Brown ML, Proano M. Towards a less costly but accurate test of gastric emptying and small bowel transit. *Dig Dis Sci* 1991; **36**:609–615.

72 Szarka LA, Camilleri M, Vella A, Burton D, Baxter K, Simonson J, *et al.* A stable isotope breath test with a standard meal for abnormal gastric emptying solids in the clinic and in research. *Clin Gastroenterol Hepatol* 2008; **6**:635–643.

73 Bredenoord AJ, Chial HJ, Camilleri M, Mullan BP, Murray JA. Gastric accommodation and emptying in evaluation of patients with upper gastrointestinal symptoms. *Clin Gastroenterol Hepatol* 2003; **1**:264–272.

74 Simren M, Stotzer PO. Use and abuse of hydrogen breath tests. *Gut* 2006; **55**:297–303.

75 Annese V, Janssens J, Vantrappen G, Tack J, Peeters TL, Willemse P, *et al.* Erythromycin accelerates gastric emptying by inducing antral contractions and improved gastroduodenal coordination. *Gastroenterology* 1992; **102**:823–828.

76 Janssens J, Peeters TL, Vantrappen G, Tack J, Urbain JL, De Roo M, *et al.* Improvement of gastric emptying in diabetic gastroparesis by erythromycin: preliminary studies [see Comment]. *N Engl J Med* 1990; **322**:1028–1031.

77 Jones MP, Maganti K. A systematic review of surgical therapy for gastroparesis. *Am J Gastroenterol* 2003; **98**:2122–2129.

78 Sugumar A, Singh A, Pasricha PJ. A systematic review of the efficacy of domperidone for the treatment of diabetic gastroparesis. *Clin Gastroenterol Hepatol* 2008; **6**:726–733.

79 Friedenberg FK, Palit A, Parkman HP, Hanlon A, Nelson DB. Botulinum toxin A for the treatment of delayed gastric emptying [see Comment]. *Am J Gastroenterol* 2008; **103**:416–423.

80 Arts J, Holvoet L, Caenepeel P, Bisschops R, Sifrim D, Verbeke K, *et al.* Clinical trial: a randomized-controlled crossover study of intrapyloric injection of botulinum toxin in gastroparesis. *Aliment Pharmacol Ther* 2007; **26**:1251–1258.

81 Abell T, McCallum R, Hocking M, Koch K, Abrahamsson H, Leblanc I, *et al.* Gastric electrical stimulation for medically refractory gastroparesis [see Comment]. *Gastroenterology* 2003; **125**:421–428.

82 Jones MP. Is gastric electrical stimulation an effective therapy for patients with drug-refractory gastroparesis? *Nat Clin Pract Gastroenterol Hepatol* 2008; **5**:368–370.

83 Fedorak RN, Field M, Chang EB. Treatment of diabetic diarrhea with clonidine. *Ann Intern Med* 1985; **102**:197–199.

84 von der Ohe MR, Camilleri M, Thomforde GM, Klee GG. Differential regional effects of octreotide on human gastrointestinal motor function. *Gut* 1995; **36**:743–748.

85 Mourad FH, Gorard D, Thillainayagam AV, Colin-Jones D, Farthing MJ. Effective treatment of diabetic diarrhoea with somatostatin analogue, octreotide. *Gut* 1992; **33**:1578–1580.

86 Soudah HC, Hasler WL, Owyang C. Effect of octreotide on intestinal motility and bacterial overgrowth in scleroderma [see Comment]. *N Engl J Med* 1991; **325**:1461–1467.

87 Lembo A, Camilleri M. Chronic constipation [see Comment]. *N Engl J Med* 2003; **349**:1360–1368.

88 Chiarioni G, Whitehead WE, Pezza V, Morelli A, Bassotti G. Biofeedback is superior to laxatives for normal transit constipation due to pelvic floor dyssynergia [see Comment]. *Gastroenterology* 2006; **130**:657–664.

89 Camilleri M, Bharucha AE, Ueno R, Burton D, Thomforde GM, Baxter K, *et al.* Effect of a selective chloride channel activator, lubiprostone, on gastrointestinal transit, gastric sensory, and motor functions in healthy volunteers. *Am J Physiol Gastrointest Liver Physiol* 2006; **290**:G942–947.

90 Johanson JF, Morton D, Geenen J, Ueno R. Multicenter, 4-week, double-blind, randomized, placebo-controlled trial of lubiprostone, a locally-acting type-2 chloride channel activator, in patients with chronic constipation. *Am J Gastroenterol* 2008; **103**:170–177.

91 Johanson JF, Drossman DA, Panas R, Wahle A, Ueno R. Clinical trial: phase 2 study of lubiprostone for irritable bowel syndrome with constipation. *Aliment Pharmacol Ther* 2008; **27**:685–696.

47 The Skin in Diabetes

Graham R. Sharpe & Paul D. Yesudian
Department of Dermatology, Broadgreen Hospital, Liverpool, UK

Keypoints

- Various skin conditions are associated with diabetes, either type 1 or type 2, the specific chronic complications of the disease, the use of antidiabetic drugs and certain endocrine and metabolic disorders that cause diabetes.
- Necrobiosis lipoidica diabeticorum is unrelated to glycemic control. Treatment is difficult, but in the early stages topical steroids may be beneficial.
- Diabetic dermopathy ("shin spots") is the most common skin disorder in patients with diabetes, usually in the pre-tibial region in long-standing diabetes, and tends to resolve within 1–2 years.
- The skin is thickened in diabetes, and irreversible glycation of skin collagen and other proteins may lead ultimately to yellowish skin discoloration especially in the palmar creases.
- Acanthosis nigricans is the presence of hyperpigmented velvety hyperkeratotic plaques in the flexural regions, particularly the axillae or posterior neck. It is associated with various causes of insulin resistance.
- Erythema occurs on the face, around the nail margins and on the lower limbs.
- Calciphylaxis implies advanced vascular damage with a poor prognosis.
- Large vessel injury can lead to recalcitrant leg ulcers.
- Candidal overgrowth is frequently observed in people with poorly controlled diabetes.
- Bacterial infections such as "malignant" otitis externa can be potentially lethal.
- Erythrasma, caused by corynebacteria, is seen more frequently in obese people with diabetes.
- Dermatophytosis is *not* found more frequently in those with diabetes than in those without the disease.
- Vitiligo shares an autoimmune pathogenesis, like type 1 diabetes.
- There is no scientific basis for the assumption that pruritus occurs more commonly in those with diabetes.
- Necrolytic migratory erythema is an unusual rash that is diagnostic of the glucagonoma syndrome.
- Insulin injections can cause both lipoatrophy and lipohypertrophy.
- Allergic insulin reactions, which are now rare because of purer insulin availability, can be subdivided into immediate-local, general, delayed or biphasic responses.
- Sulfonlyureas are well-recognized causes of multiple cutaneous drug reactions.

Introduction

Various skin disorders are associated with diabetes. Some are relatively specific "markers" of the condition, usually caused by the metabolic changes in diabetes or associated with endocrine disorders that cause diabetes. Other skin conditions develop as manifestations of chronic diabetic complications, particularly vascular changes and peripheral neuropathy. Skin infections are more common in people with poorly controlled diabetes, but not specific for the condition. Cutaneous side effects of drug treatments for diabetes may occur, although these are less common with current therapies.

Textbook of Diabetes, 4th edition. Edited by R. Holt, C. Cockram, A. Flyvbjerg and B. Goldstein.

Cutaneous metabolic manifestations

This group includes a number of conditions that appear specific to diabetes (e.g. diabetic thick skin) or are much more common in people with diabetes than the general population (e.g. necrobiosis lipoidica). The cause of many of these conditions remain obscure, although some may be related to the process of non-enzymatic glycation of cutaneous structural proteins, particularly collagens or changes in microvascular structural proteins. A number of cutaneous conditions were previously thought to have an increased incidence in diabetes, but subsequent studies have not substantiated these links (e.g. generalized pruritus) [1]. Likewise, the evidence that granuloma annulare is associated with diabetes is inconclusive [2]. The metabolic manifestations currently regarded as being genuinely associated with diabetes are shown in Table 47.1.

Necrobiosis lipoidica diabeticorum

This is a rare condition with a prevalence of 0.3% in diabetic populations [3]. Although it is much more common in those with diabetes than individuals without diabetes, the relationship to diabetes and the etiology of necrobiosis lipoidica diabeticorum (NLD) remains unclear. An early and much quoted study of 171 patients suggested that about two-thirds of patients with NLD had diabetes, usually type 1 (T1DM) [3], with a further 12–15% having an abnormal glucose tolerance test [4]; however, patient selection may have given an overestimate of the incidence. A more recent retrospective study of 65 patients with NLD in a dermatology clinic found that 11% were known to have diabetes and a further 11% had an abnormal glucose tolerance test [5]. NLD usually develops in young adult or early middle life, but has occasionally been reported in childhood [6]. Women are three times more commonly affected than men.

Table 47.1 Cutaneous metabolic manifestations.

Necrobiosis lipoidica diabeticorum
Diabetic dermopathy ("shin spots")
Diabetic bullae (bullosis diabeticorum)
Diabetic thick skin:
• Diabetic hand syndrome
• Scleredema of diabetes
Acanthosis nigricans (associated with insulin resistance)
Eruptive xanthoma

There is no proven association with glycemic control, but patients with diabetes and NLD do appear to have a higher incidence of chronic diabetic complications such as retinopathy, neuropathy and microalbuminurua [7,8]. This suggests that microangiopathy may have an etiologic role. The presence of immunologic deposits in lesional vessel walls also implicates immune factors in the pathogenesis [9]. Nevertheless, the cause remains unknown.

NLD has a distinctive appearance (Figure 47.1). Early lesions may be rounded, dull red, symptomless papules or plaques which

(a)

(b)

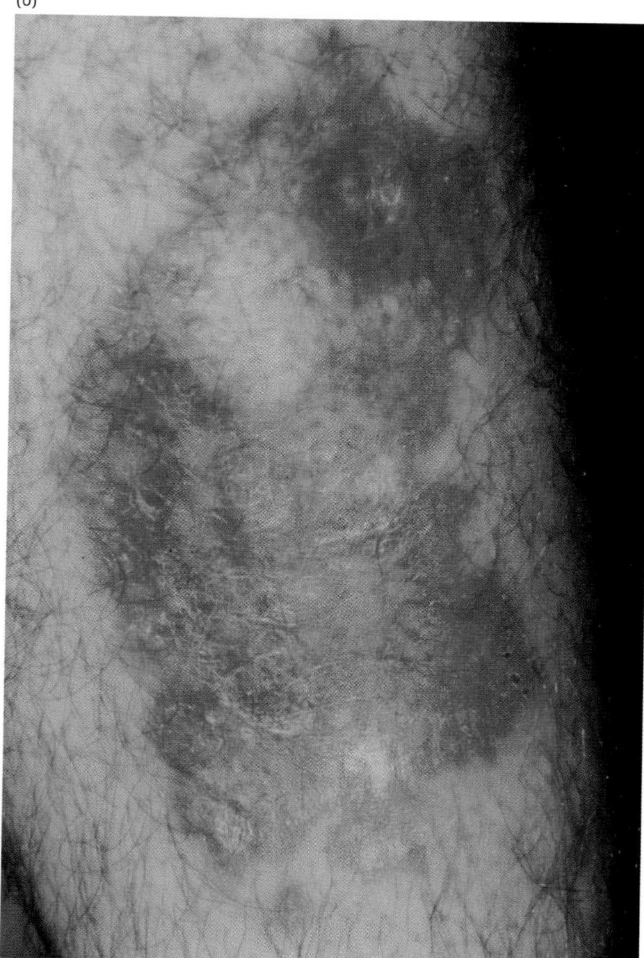

Figure 47.1 Necrobiosis lipoidica diabeticorum (NLD). (a) An early lesion on ankle showing the erythematous stage. (b) A long-standing area of NLD, note the typical yellow atrophic appearance with telangiectasia.

slowly progress to the typical chronic lesion – an oval or irregularly shaped, indurated plaque with central atrophy [3,8]. NLD often has a shiny surface, with prominent telangiectatic vessels crossing over a waxy yellowish central area. The margin of lesions may be brownish or red and sometimes with comedo-like plugs, where necrotic material is extruded through the surface. The shin is the most commonly affected site, but the thighs, ankles and feet may also be affected; lesions rarely occur on the trunk, upper limbs or scalp [10]. Ulceration occurs in 25% of cases and may be very slow to heal. NLD lesions are usually partially or completely anesthetic and alopecia is frequently present [11]. They are variable in number but usually few and most extend slowly over several years, sometimes coalescing with adjacent areas. Long periods of quiescence may occur or occasionally NLD lesions may heal with scarring. The condition can lead to significant morbidity and cosmetic disfigurement. The diagnosis is usually clinical; a diagnostic skin biopsy is not normally required and may heal slowly or risk ulceration in atrophic lesions. The differential diagnosis of early lesions includes granuloma annulare, cutaneous sarcoid, necrobiotic xanthogranuloma and diabetic dermopathy.

Histologically, NLD lesions consist of foci of degenerate collagen bundles with a hyalinized appearance (necrobiosis), surrounded by fibrosis, a diffuse infiltrate of histiocytes and frequently a palisading granulomatous reaction with giant cells similar to those seen in sarcoidosis (Figure 47.2). There is a superficial and deep perivascular infiltrate that is composed of lymphocytes and plasma cells [12,13]. Capillary wall thickening and microvascular occlusion are present, but do not appear central to the pathologic process. These abnormalities occur throughout the dermis. There is considerable overlap between these features and those of granuloma annulare [13], and this similarity undoubtedly contributes to the suggestion that granuloma annulare is associated with diabetes. Despite histologic similarities in the earlier stages of the two conditions they run a very different clinical course and the association has now been discounted [12,14].

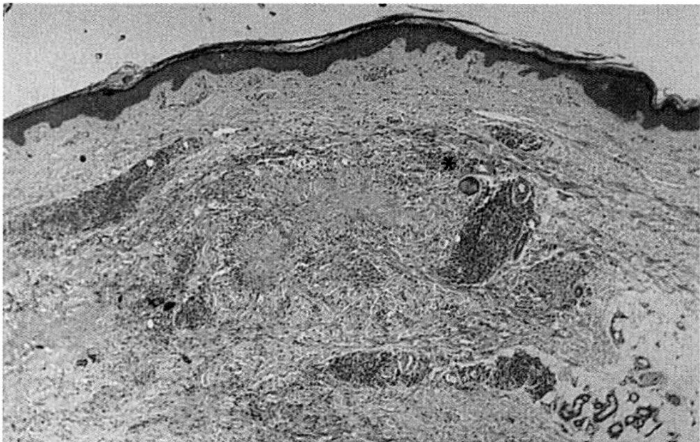

Figure 47.2 Histologic feature of necrobiosis lipoidica diabeticorum showing degeneration of the collagen (necrobiosis), associated with fibrosis and a granulomatous histiocytic infiltrate. A giant cell is indicated by an asterisk. Hematoxylin and eosin stain ×40.

No treatment for NLD has proved effective in double-blind placebo controlled trials and treatment remains unsatisfactory. Spontaneous remission is unusual [3] and good diabetic control does not usually have a significant effect on the course of the condition. Patients should be encouraged not to smoke and to avoid trauma to the area which may result in a painful and recalcitrant ulcer. For early NLD lesions corticosteroids either applied topically (perhaps under occlusion) or by intralesional injection may be beneficial [15,16]. There is evidence that the inflammatory process extends beyond the clinical margins and topical steroids may halt or slow progression if applied to the periphery of lesions [8]. Once atrophy has developed this is irreversible and topical steroids should not be used in chronic lesions because they may worsen skin atrophy. There is a suggestion that topical retinoids may be beneficial in atrophic cases [17]. Oral steroids may be of benefit in a short course of 5 weeks with reduction of disease activity, but not atrophy [18]. Benefit was maintained in a 7-month follow-up but careful monitoring of blood glucose control is essential. The thiazolidinediones or glitazones have been reported to benefit NLD but more experience is required [19]. Various anticoagulants and antiplatelet agents have been tried; including aspirin, dipyridamole, heparin and oxpentifylline, but controlled trials has not shown any of these to be effective [20,21]. Pentoxifylline, ticlopidine, nicotinamide and clofazamine have all been tried [22–24]. There are several reports in small open studies of approximately 50% of the patients responding to topical PUVA (application of 8-methoxypsoralens [methoxsalen] to the skin prior to treatment with ultraviolet A light) [25–27]. Non-steroidal systemic immunosuppression with cyclosporine, mycophenolate mofetil or the tumor necrosis factor α (TNF-α) antagonist infliximab have been reported to be beneficial in a few cases [28–31]. Pulsed dye laser treatment may improve telangiectasia and erythema but there is a risk of skin breakdown [32]. There are reports of good results following excision and grafting [33], although the disease may recur locally. In most cases, cosmetic camouflage is the preferred option.

Diabetic dermopathy (shin spots)

This is the most common dermatologic condition associated with diabetes, occurring in up to 50% of patients with diabetes but also in up to 3% of adults without diabetes; subjects without diabetes usually have only one or two lesions whereas most patients with diabetes have four or more [34,35]. Men are more commonly affected and it is also more prevalent in patients over 50 years of age and in long-standing diabetes. The condition is associated with the three most common microangiopathic complications of diabetes: neuropathy, nephropathy and retinopathy [36]. There is also an association with coronary artery disease and diabetic dermopathy is a subtle sign that suggests more serious complications [37]. The presence of microvascular changes, notably thickening of arterioles and capillaries, led to the term "diabetic dermopathy" [38].

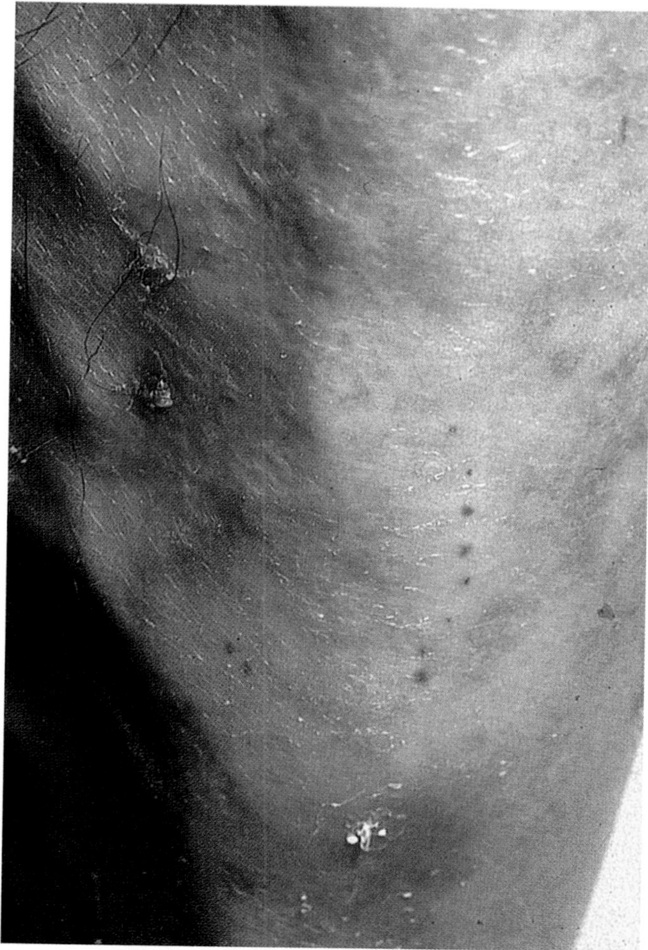

Figure 47.3 Diabetic dermopathy, "shin spots." Courtesy of Professor Julian Verbov, Royal Liverpool University Hospital.

The lesions are well-circumscribed atrophic brownish scars often on the shins, giving the alternative name "diabetic shin spots" (Figure 47.3) [34,35]. The forearms, thighs and bony prominences may also be affected [39]. The lesions are usually bilateral and may appear in crops. Early lesions are oval red papules measuring up to 1 cm in diameter, which slowly develop scaling and a brown color because of the presence of hemosiderin-laden histiocytes and extravasated erythrocytes in the superficial dermis [34]. There is no effective treatment, but the lesions tend to resolve over 1–2 years.

Diabetic bullae (bullosis diabeticorum)

Various forms of bullae have been described in subjects with diabetes, but all are relatively rare [40,41]. Diabetic bullae affect men more than women and are more common in older patients and those with peripheral neuropathy [42]. The conditions usually present as tense blisters, from a few millimeters up to several centimeters in size, on a non-inflammatory base, appearing rapidly and healing over a few weeks without scarring (Figure 47.4). The feet and lower legs are the most common sites, followed by the hands. Electron microscopy studies demonstrate a subepithelial split at the level of the lamina lucida and immunofluorescence studies are negative [43]. Other causes of subepithelial blisters, including the autoimmune blistering diseases porphyria cutanea tarda, pseudoporphyria and infections such as bullous impetigo.

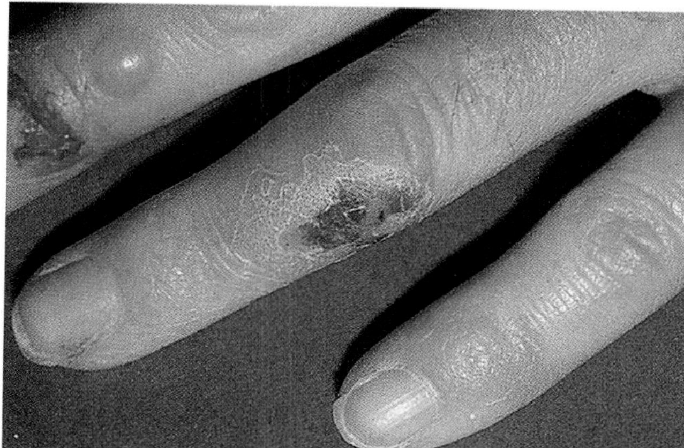

Figure 47.4 Diabetic bullae.

Diabetic thick skin

The thickness of the skin is largely attributable to the filamentous proteins of the dermis, of which collagen is by far the most abundant. Compared with normal subjects, the collagen bundles in the dermis of patients with diabetes are thickened and disorganized, as a result of irreversible non-enzymatic glycation, cross-linking and "browning" of protein. Collagen normally turns over slowly; the formation of advanced glycation end-products (AGEs) damages the protein thereby reducing the ability of enzymes such as collagenase to remodel the collagen fibers [44]. Gradual and irreversible modification of collagen, elastin and other structural dermal proteins is part of the physiologic aging process, but is accelerated in diabetes, especially if poorly controlled.

Browning of collagen results in yellow skin discoloration, best seen on the palms and soles of patients with diabetes. The skin of patients with diabetes is measurably thicker than in subjects without diabetes [45] and shows loss of elasticity [46]. In some studies, skin thickness relates to duration of diabetes [47] and in others to the presence of complications such as neuropathy [48]. Skin thickness is usually clinically insignificant, but may, if advanced, lead to the specific complications of "diabetic hand syndrome" and diabetic scleredema [49]. The combination of thick tight waxy skin and limited joint mobility has been called cheiroarthropathy and is present in 30–40% of patients with T1DM [50].

Diabetic hand syndrome

Up to 75% of subjects with diabetes over 60 years of age are affected, although the incidence is not closely related to the duration of disease or metabolic control [51,52]. Milder skin thickening may develop in up to 20% of individuals without diabetes, but occurs at an older age. The early changes include thickening of the skin over the dorsum of the hands and digits, especially the proximal interphalangeal joints (sclerodactyly). The interphalangeal joints are particularly susceptible and may present as painful stiff fingers. In a minority of patients, the condition progresses to cause a fixed flexion deformity of the fingers and Dupuytren contracture, while soft tissue thickening of the wrist may cause carpal tunnel syndrome by compression of the median nerve. More extreme cases present with a tight waxy appearance together with pebbly pads over the knuckles and distal fingers (Garrod's knuckle pads).

Scleredema of diabetes

This is marked dermal thickening, commonly involving the posterior aspect of the neck and upper parts of the back, and extending to the face, arms and abdomen with more severe involvement. It has a prevalence of 2.5% in type 2 diabetes mellitus (T2DM), and is found particularly in those who are overweight and with poorly controlled diabetes [53]. Histology of the condition shows dermal thickening which contains large collagen bundles and an increased number of mast cells [49]. Scleredema, with similar morphologic changes, may follow chronic streptococcal infection of the skin, often involving the lower legs. Scleredema is reported to respond to ultraviolet light [54].

Acanthosis nigricans

This rare condition is characterized by a velvety papillomatous overgrowth of the epidermis, which is usually hyperpigmented. The flexural areas, particularly the axilla, inguinal region, inframammary region and neck, are most frequently affected (Figure 47.5). Rarely, more generalized changes involve the knuckles and other extensor surfaces, with verrucous patches and hyperkeratosis of the palms and soles. Histologic features include extensive folding and thickening of the epidermis, with increased numbers of melanocytes, which accounts for the dark color.

Severe and widespread acanthosis nigricans is usually a manifestation of internal malignancy, often of the gastrointestinal tract. The more limited presentation is associated with various endocrine disorders, which share the common features of insulin

(a)

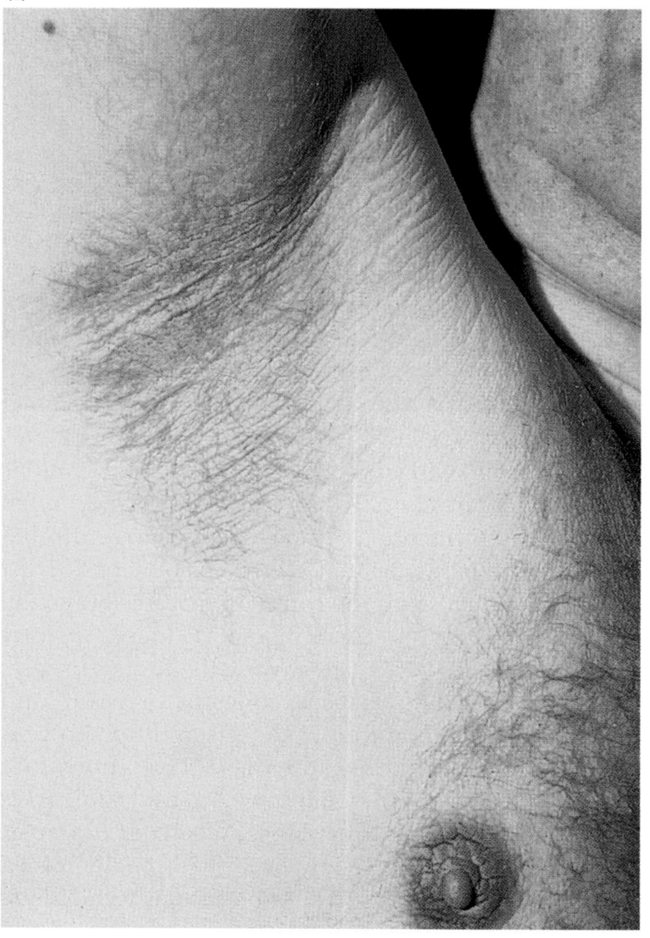

(b)

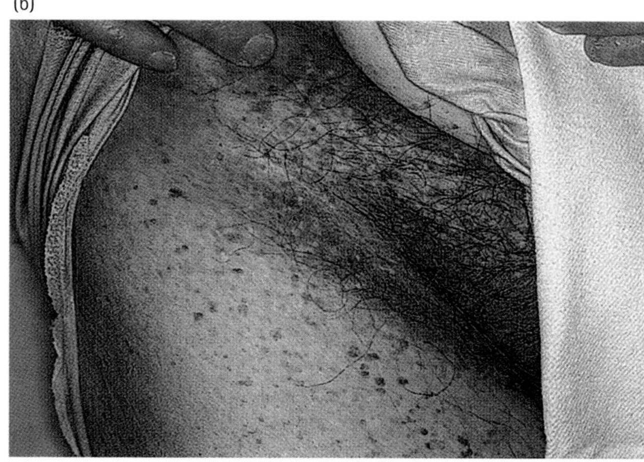

Figure 47.5 Acanthosis nigricans, showing typical dark velvety appearance: (a) in the axilla; (b) in the groin. Figure 47.5(b) courtesy of Dr. S. Mendelsohn, Countess of Chester Hospital, Chester.

resistance and hyperinsulinemia: these include diabetes mellitus, acromegaly, Cushing disease and polycystic ovarian disease, obesity, genetic and autoimmune insulin receptor defects and lipoatrophic diabetes [55–57]. It is presumed that hyperinsulinemia induced by insulin resistance activates insulin-like growth factor I (IGF-I) receptors, which are closely related to insulin receptors, on various tissues [58]. In the skin, stimulation of IGF-I receptors on keratinocytes could lead to excessive epidermal growth (Figure 47.6).

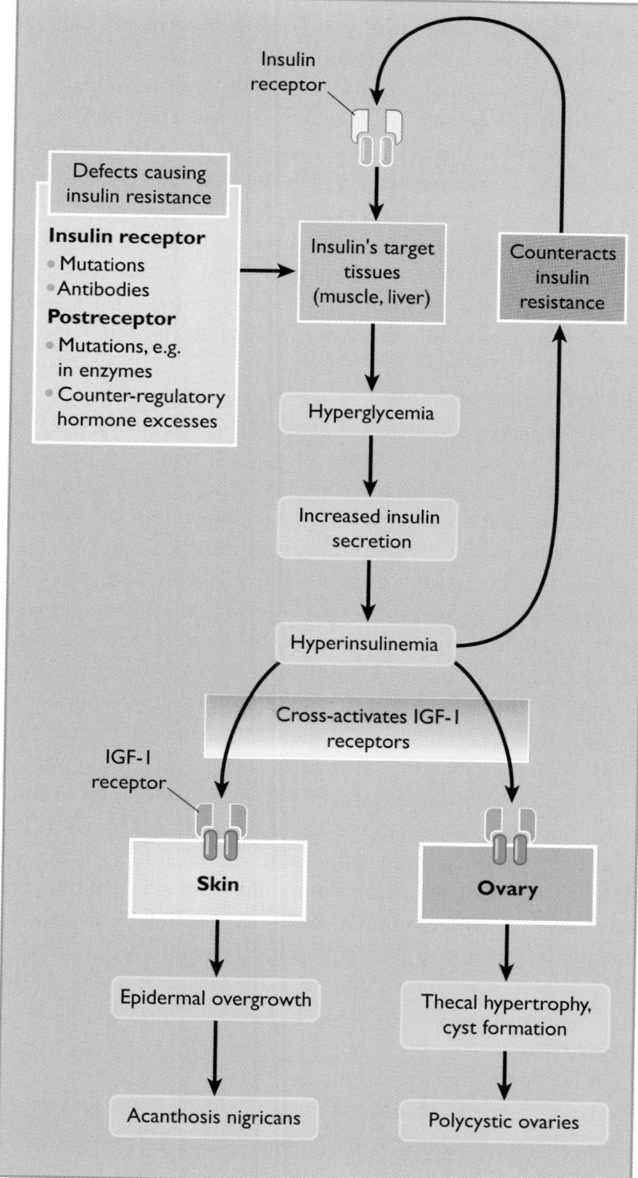

Figure 47.6 Suggested relationship of insulin resistance and hyperinsulinemia to acanthosis nigricans. Raised insulin levels may act on insulin-like growth factor I (IGF-I) receptors in the skin to cause epidermal overgrowth. Similar events in the ovary could lead to polycystic ovary disease which is also associated with insulin-resistant states.

Acanthosis nigricans can be disfiguring and upsetting for the patient. Mild peeling agents such as 5% salicylic acid in a bland cream may be helpful. The condition usually partially regresses if the hyperinsulinemia can be successfully reduced.

Eruptive xanthomas and hypertriglyceridemia

Eruptive xanthomas are caused by hypertriglyceridemia with elevated serum levels of chylomicrons or very low density lipoproteins. This can occur in diabetes, especially if poorly controlled. The lesions are caused by triglyceride deposition in the skin and present as small red or yellow nodules measuring up to 0.5 cm diameter. They occur predominantly on the extensor surfaces of the limbs and buttocks; the onset is usually rapid and lesions frequently occur in groups or crops (Figure 47.7). Men are more commonly affected. Although xanthomas may itch initially, they are usually asymptomatic. Lesions usually regress slowly within months after hypertriglyceridemia has been corrected by lipid lowering drugs or improved glycemic control.

(a)

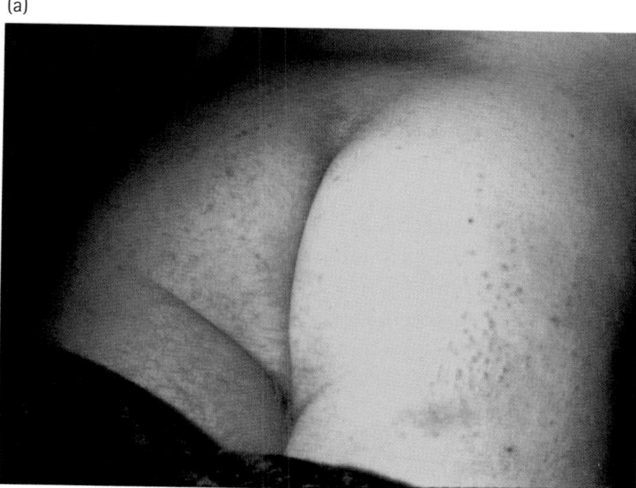

(b)

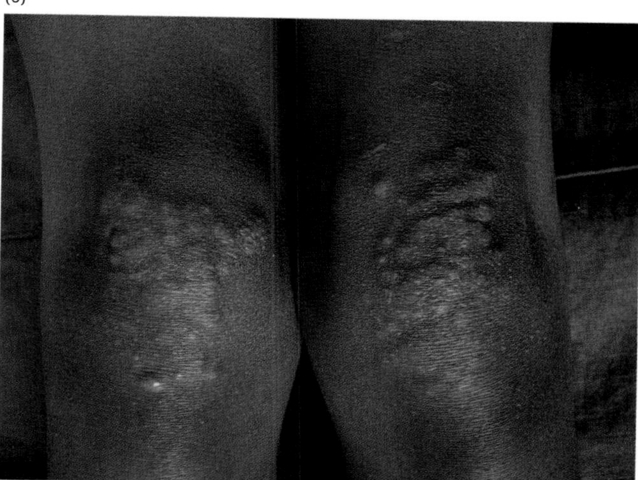

Figure 47.7 Eruptive xanthoma: (a) buttocks; (b) knees.

Table 47.2 Vascular changes.

Diabetic erythema and rubeosis
Periungual telangiectasia
Calciphylaxis
Acral dry gangrene

Vascular changes

Skin conditions develop as manifestations of chronic diabetic complications affecting both small and large vessels. A number of these changes, particularly those causing erythema, are associated with longstanding diabetes (Table 47.2).

Rubeosis faciei

Facial erythema can occur in people with diabetes, with the intensity of coloration dependent on the vascular engorgement in the superficial venous plexus [59]. The changes occur as a result of altered vascular tone or diabetic microangiopathy. Capillary microscopy has demonstrated venular dilatation people with diabetes with this condition. It appears more obvious in fair-skinned individuals and can be difficult to distinguish from normal facial redness in the general population [60]. Hypertension is common in these patients and may exacerbate the capillary damage.

Periungual telangiectasia

Erythema of the skin surrounding the nail bed resulting from the dilatation of proximal nailfold capillaries is an excellent marker of functional microangiopathy [61]. It can occur in up to 49% of those with diabetes. Even though connective tissue diseases can exhibit periungual tengiectases, the lesions are morphologically different. In patients with diabetes, isolated homogenous engorgement of venular limbs is seen; whereas mega-capillaries or irregularly enlarged loops are observed in those with connective tissue disease [62]. Different capillary changes can be observed in those with recently diagnosed diabetes than those with long-standing disease. In patients with advanced microvascular disease or following prolonged periods of poor control, small hemorrhages or vascular occlusion (leading to localized areas of non-perfusion) may occur. Nailfold capillaries are thought to reflect the general status of the microcirculation and have been used in detailed studies of functional changes of diabetic microangiopathy.

Erysipelas-like erythema

This manifests as well-demarcated patches of cutaneous reddening, occurring on the legs and feet of patients with diabetes and microcirculatory compromise. It can be mistaken for erysipelas, but is differentiated by the lack of associated fever, leukocytosis or elevated erythrocyte sedimentation rate. This finding can correlate, in some cases, with destructive lesions of the underlying bone [63]. The pathogenesis of erysipelas-like erythema may be small vessel occlusive disease with compensatory hyperemia.

Table 47.3 Cutaneous infections associated with diabetes.

Yeast infections (candidiasis)
Bacterial infection (boils and sepsis)
Erythrasma
Malignant otitis externa
Necrotizing fasciitis
Phycomyces infections

Calciphylaxis

Calciphylaxis is a small-vessel vasculopathy occurring in patients with renal failure and sometimes in those with diabetes. It is characterized by mural calcification, intimal proliferation, fibrosis and thrombosis [64]. The lesions start as small red tender areas of skin which become ischemic leading to the development of subcutaneous nodules and poorly healing, necrotizing skin ulcers. They can serve as a portal of entry for infectious agents. The prognosis in those with calciphylaxis is poor because of impaired wound healing and infection leading to sepsis. Aggressive analgesic treatment may be required for ischemic pain, along with optimal blood glucose control and weight reduction [65].

Macrovascular changes

Cutaneous signs of ischemia in the lower limbs include cold or cyanosed feet, erythema, hair loss and atrophy. Patients with diabetes and both venous insufficiency of the lower legs and arterial disease are particularly prone to developing non-healing ulcers; these frequently become superinfected and can be very troublesome to manage. Patients with diabetes have a higher incidence of large-vessel disease than the non-diabetic population. A sign of large-vessel disease is dependent rubor with delayed return of color (>15 seconds) after pressure has been applied to the skin. Patients with diabetes are also prone to venous stasis ulcers as many of them are obese and this in turn leads to increased lower extremity venous pressure. Venous hypertension and skin breakdown at sites of increased venous pressure ensues, leading to venous ulcers. Neuropathy, with lack of pain sensation, also contributes to foot ulceration. Repeated trauma and increased shear forces affect the skin without the usual protective mechanisms which are impaired by peripheral neuropathy, leading to further skin breakdown [62].

Infections

Studies have shown that no significant increase in the prevalence of cutaneous infections occurs in most subjects with diabetes and the strength of previously assumed associations have been questioned [66]; however, poor glycemic control can increase the risk of infection by causing abnormal microcirculation, decreased phagocytosis, impaired leukocyte adherence and delayed chemotaxis [67]. Infections occurring at presentation or with poor glycemic control are shown in Table 47.3.

(a)

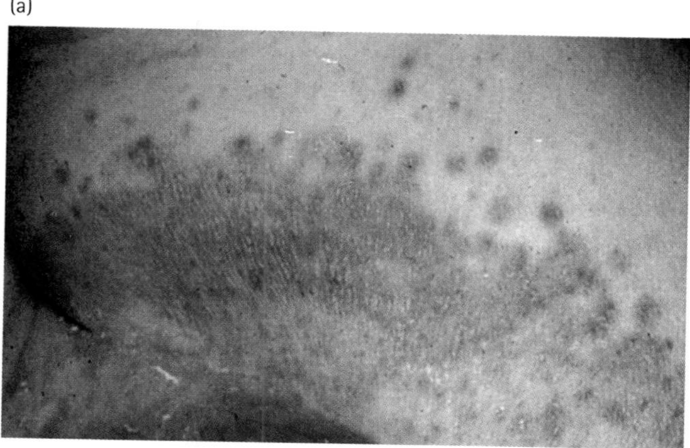

(b)

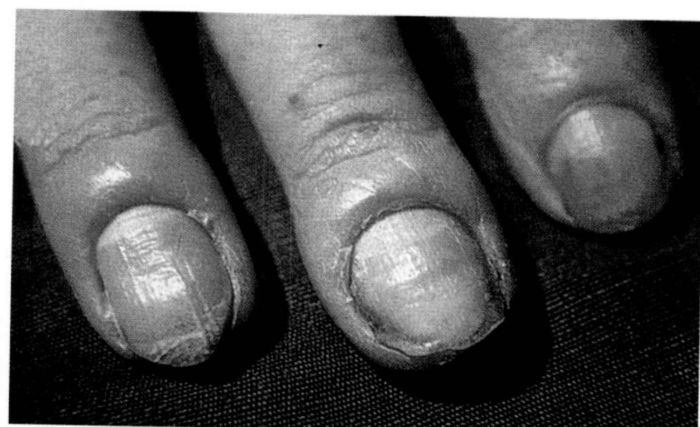

Figure 47.8 *Candida* infections in patients with diabetes. (a) Flexural infection showing satellite lesions. (b) Chronic paronychia caused by *Candida albicans*. Note swollen and erythematous nailfolds.

Candida infection

Infection with *Candida albicans* may be a presenting feature of diabetes or manifest as a complication of poorly controlled diabetes. The infection appears as erythematous papules with satellite pustules and can affect the flexural areas in the body (Figure 47.8a), the vulva and penis, and also the nail margins, causing paronychia (Figure 47.8b). In women, vulvovaginitis is the most common manifestation and presents with pruritus vulvae that can be intense and distressing. The vulva appears erythematous and fissured, with peripheral pustulation in severe cases. It may be particularly troublesome while a patient is hyperglycemic and glycosuric [68]. Candidal balanitis, balanoposthitis and phimosis occur less commonly in men, but could be a presenting feature [69]. Candidal angular stomatitis and an atrophic tongue resembling median rhomboid glossitis are oral manifestations of diabetes. Oral candidiasis occurs more commonly in patients with diabetes who smoke or wear dentures [70]. Candidal intertrigo occurs on opposing surfaces under the breast, in the groins and axillae, or in the folds of the abdominal skin. Scratching of the areas involved with *Candida* infection can result in bacterial superinfection.

Candida infection of the hands and feet are probably equally seen in those with diabetes and the non-diabetic population, but tends to be more severe in the former. Chronic paronychia presents as swelling and erythema around the lateral nailfold, with more severe involvement leading to onycholysis (Figure 47.8b). Microscopic examination and culture of the extruded material will confirm the presence of *Candida*. Less common than paronychia is infection of the web space between the middle and fourth finger (erosion interdigitale blastomycetica) [71]. Exclusion of moisture is an essential aspect to the treatment, and systemic antifungal drugs (e.g. oral fluconazole or itraconazole) rather than topical preparations may be required. Inappropriate treatment with steroids or antibiotics can worsen *Candida* infection at any site.

Bacterial infections

Furuncles, carbuncles, styes and erythrasma were particularly frequent before the introduction of insulin and antibiotics, and skin infections from *Staphylococcus aureus* are still probably more common in the patient with diabetes than in the non-diabetic population. Increased rates of colonization with staphylococci has been reported in those with poorly controlled diabetes [72]. Severe ("malignant") otitis externa is an uncommon but potentially lethal infection caused by invasive *Pseudomonas* spp. The condition occurs in elderly patients with diabetes and manifests as purulent discharge with severe pain in the external ear. It progresses from cellulitis to osteomyelitis, meningitis and cerebritis with a high mortality [73].

Erythrasma, caused by *Corynebacterium minutissimum*, is rare but occurs with increased frequency in obese patients with diabetes. It presents as a red shiny or scaly patch in the intertriginous areas and with ultraviolet light exhibits a characteristic coral-red fluorescence. Topical or systemic erythromycin is curative. Unusual infections with coliforms or anaerobes occur in those with diabetes as can *Pseudomonas* infections of the toe web spaces or nailfold (paronychia) and secondary infection of venous ulcers [74]. Anaerobic cellulitis with *Clostridium* species can occur in patients with diabetic ketoacidosis, requiring treatment with metabolic control, aggressive débridement of devitalized tissue and intravenous antimicrobial therapy [64]. Necrotizing fasciitis is a potentially lethal skin and soft tissue infection that is more common in those with diabetes [68]. *Streptococcus pyogenes*, anaerobic streptococci, *Bacteroides* and *Staphylococcus aureus* are some of the organisms associated with necrotizing fasciitis. This infection can extend from trivial wounds such as furuncles, insect bites and injection sites, or sometimes begin from decubitis ulcers. Rapid progression ensues, with extensive tissue destruction and severe systemic toxicity, leading to death [75]. This condition should be considered in patients with diabetes and cellulitis who have associated systemic features such as tachycardia, leukocytosis, marked hyperglycemia or acidosis. This potentially fatal infection should be treated with urgent surgical débridement of necrotic tissue and intravenous antibiotics, after obtaining blood and tissue culture. The mortality remains high (about 25%) in spite of optimal treatment [76].

Dermatophytosis

Dermatophyte infections are probably not more common in the diabetic population than in their normal counterparts [66]; however, they could serve as a portal of entry for other infectious agents, particularly in those with neurovascular complications. *Trichophyton rubrum* is the most common pathogen, causing erythematous lesions which are often annular with scaly edges. Intertrigo or interdigital infection presents as maceration and superficial scaling. The diagnosis is confirmed by finding fungal hyphae in the superficial scale, ideally taken from the edge of the lesion. Treatment of choice is with the newer topical imidazole antifungal agents, but if extensive, systemic terbinafine, itraconazole or griseofulvin may be required.

Phycomyces infections

Poor metabolic control, resulting in hyperglycemia and ketoacidosis may permit organisms that are normally non-pathogenic to establish infections in traumatized skin. Leg ulcers or non-healing surgical wounds may have super-added phycomycete infections. Deep *Phycomyces* infection such as rhinocerebral mucormycosis is a rare but life-threatening complication of diabetes. It can be a presenting manifestation of diabetes in the elderly and manifests as fever, facial cellulitis, periorbital edema, proptosis and, rarely, blindness [77]. The infection spreads along the turbinates, septum, palate, maxillary and ethmoid sinuses and can extend into the frontal lobe, cavernous sinus or carotid artery. It should be suspected in any patient with diabetes presenting with sinusitis, purulent nasal discharge, altered mental state and infarcted tissue in the nose or palate. Treatment involves correction of acid–base imbalance, aggressive débridement of devitalized tissue and intravenous antifungal therapy.

Associated conditions

These are a group of dermatoses that are reported more commonly in those with diabetes than in the non-diabetic population (Table 47.4). A number of endocrine conditions are associated with diabetes and also cause specific skin changes (Table 47.5).

Table 47.4 Associated conditions.

Vitiligo
Lichen planus
Yellow nails
Clear cell syringoma
Cutaneous neuropathy (pain, neurotrophic ulcers)
Autonomic neuropathy (decreased sweating)
Perforating skin disorders (e.g. folliculitis, Kyrle's disease)

Table 47.5 Associations with other endocrine syndromes.

Hyperlipidemia
Eruptive xanthoma
Hemochromatosis
"Bronzed" pigmentation
Cutaneous signs of liver disease
Glucagonoma syndrome
Necrolytic migratory erythema
Cushing syndrome
Skin atrophy
Striae
Hirsutism
Acromegaly
Thickened skin
Increased sweating
Polycystic ovarian disease
Acanthosis nigricans
Hirsutism
Partial and total lipodystrophy
Absence of subcutaneous fat

Vitiligo

Vitiligo is an autoimmune condition seen more commonly in patients with T1DM, but can also occur in T2DM. Polyglandular autoimmune syndrome type 2 is characterized by adrenal failure, autoimmune thyroid disease and T1DM, and can be associated with vitiligo [78]. There is no evidence that vitiligo occurs specifically in patients with circulating antibodies, and is not associated with any specific human leukocyte antigen type. It manifests as patchy symmetrical depigmented areas of skin and, although asymptomatic, can cause significant emotional distress. Treatment is unsatisfactory but topical steroids and calcineurin inhibitors such as tacrolimus ointment can be used. Patients should be advised on photoprotection and use a high factor sunscreen or cover the area.

Lichen planus

Lichen planus is an inflammatory disorder of the skin recognized by the presence of violaceous flat-topped polygonal papules, distributed in the flexural aspects of the limbs. An increased incidence of diabetes has been reported in patients with lichen planus, particularly the erosive oral lichen planus variant [79,80]; however, most studies have examined the presence of diabetes in patients with lichen planus rather than the reverse. The link between diabetes and lichen planus is therefore still unproven, especially because both are relatively common conditions.

Pruritus

Even though there is a common assumption that itching is a symptom of diabetes, this is highly questionable. Studies have failed to link the presence of generalized pruritus with diabetes [81,82]. Localized itching, particularly in the genital area, can be associated with *Candida* infections which are more common in patients with diabetes. The presence of xerotic skin, a feature present both in those with and without diabetes, can also predispose to pruritus. There is no direct relationship between ichthyosis or xerosis (dry skin) and diabetes [83].

Yellow nails

Yellow nails have frequently been noted in patients with diabetes, particularly the distal hallux [84]. An early sign of diabetes is the presence of a yellowish or brownish discoloration in the distal part of the hallux nail plate. These later change to a canary yellowish color that can affect both the toe and finger nails. Even though yellowish nails are seen in association with onychomycosis, psoriasis and in the elderly, it appears to be a diabetic marker not associated with these causes. A study of finger nails has shown patients with diabetes to have high levels of furosine lysine, another marker of non-enzymatic glycosylation [85].

Clear cell syringomas

Syringomas are adnexal non-neoplastic lesions that are derived from intra-epidermal parts of the sweat duct. Clear cell syringoma is an unusual variant and is clinically undistinguishable from the typical syringomas. They present as yellowish papules distributed around the eyes and are asymptomatic. The clear cell variety has two features of note: the histologic preponderance of clear cell and the frequent coexistence with diabetes [86,87]. It has been postulated that in these patients, there may be a phosphorylase deficiency secondary to elevated glucose levels that in turn results in the formation of clear cells.

Glucagonoma

The glucoganoma syndrome is caused by tumors of the α cells of the pancreas which secrete glucagon (see Chapter 17). Even though the syndrome is extremely rare, it needs to be considered in patients with diabetes who present with diffuse atypical rashes. Most tumors are malignant and have usually metastasized at the time of diagnosis, but tumors grow slowly and patients frequently present with a long history. The syndrome consists of four major components: increased glucagon levels, diabetes (usually mild), weight loss and the pathognomonic rash of necrolytic migratory erythema.

Necrolytic migratory erythema occurs in 70% of patients, manifesting as an annular erythematous and figurate rash. Initial features are a non-specific itchy eczematous rash with a migrating active edge that develops vesicles, superficial blisters, erosions and scaling (Figure 47.9). The eruption waxes and wanes in cycles of up to 2 weeks and occurs particularly on the lower abdomen, buttocks, legs, perineum and intertrigenous areas. The rash can be a presenting sign, occurring 1–6 years before the diagnosis of glucogonoma is made [88]. It can be associated with other physical findings, including glossitis, stomatitis, brittle dystrophic nails and alopecia. A skin biopsy can be contributory, showing suprabasal acantholysis, and psoriasiform hyperplasia with pallor, ballooning and necrosis of the upper spinous layer of the epidermis [89].

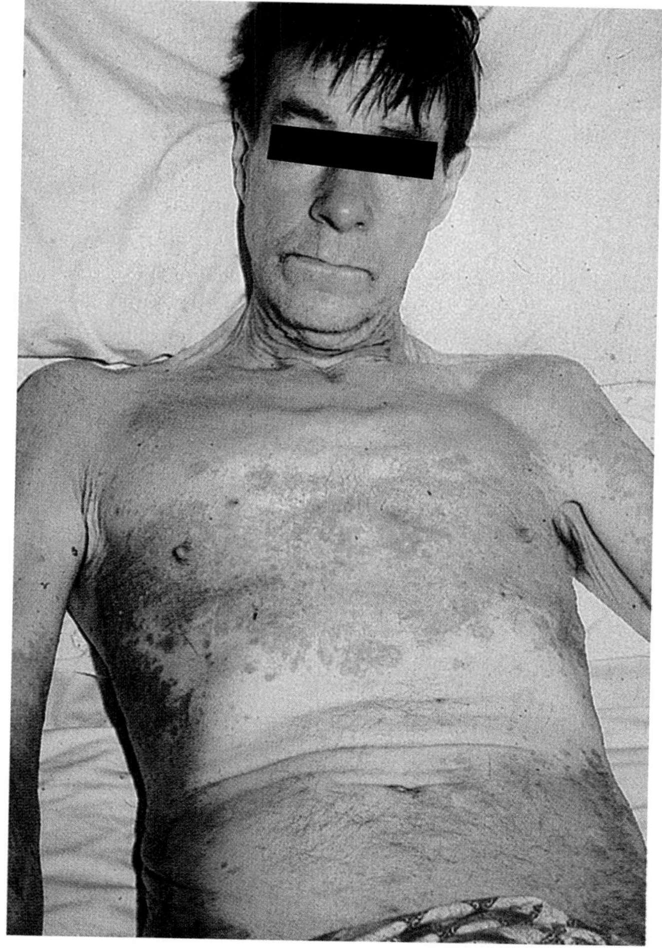

Figure 47.9 Necrolytic migratory erythema in a patient with the glucagonoma syndrome. Courtesy of S. Bloom, Royal Postgraduate Medical School, London, UK.

The role of hyperglucagonemia and the cause of the skin eruption is unclear. Deficiency of essential fatty acids, zinc and amino acids may be important in the pathogenesis. The rash may respond to resection of the pancreatic islet cell tumor, sometimes within 48 hours. Management may also involve chemotherapy, essential amino acid and fatty acid supplementation, and the use of somatostatin or its analog octreotide, which suppresses glucagon levels and may also have an independent action on the skin lesions [90,91].

Perforating dermatoses

Acquired reactive perforating folliculitis, also called Kyrle's disease, is a condition characterized by transepidermal elimina-

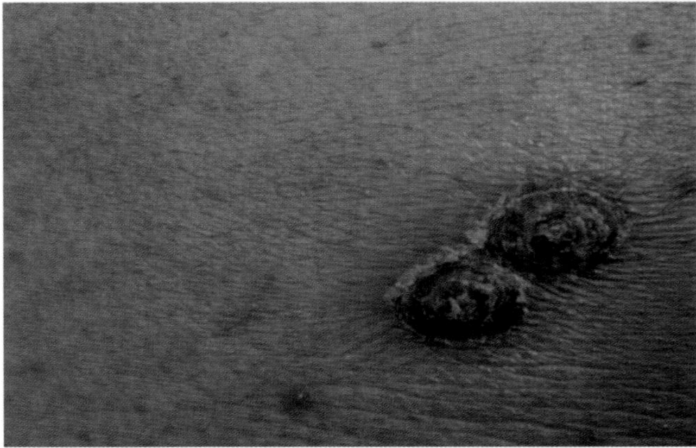

Figure 47.10 Perforating skin disease (Kyrle's disease).

Table 47.6 Cutaneous complications of antidiabetic treatment.

Insulin (especially impure animal preparations)
Localized allergic (urticaria, granuloma)
Systemic allergic (pruritus, urticaria, anaphylactoid)
Lipoatrophy
Lipohypertrophy
Idiosyncratic reactions (pigmentation, keloid formation)
Sulfonylureas
Maculopapular eruptions
Erythema multiforme
Eczematous or lichenoid eruptions
Photosensitivity
Chlorpropamide alcohol-induced flushing

tion of degenerative collagen and is seen in end-stage renal disease caused not only by diabetes but by other conditions as well [92]. Perforating dermatoses have also been associated with T1DM and T2DM, affecting mainly African-American patients on dialysis. It presents with pruritic hyperkeratotic papules on the extensor surfaces of the lower limbs, but can occur on the trunk and face (Figure 47.10). The lesions can occur at sites of trauma (Koebner or isomorphic phenomenon). Histology reveals an atrophic epidermis surrounding a plug of degenerate material consisting of elastin and collagen [62]. It is thought to be a disorder of keratinization which engenders a proliferation of epidermis to eliminate abnormal tissue. Although it appears to be an inflammatory condition, microvasculopathy has been noted in the underlying dermis of biopsy specimens [93]. The lesions can be exacerbated by injury or excoriation. It is notoriously difficult to treat but can be helped by topical steroids or retinoids, failing which phototherapy is a useful option.

Iatrogenic conditions

Both insulin and oral antidiabetic treatments can cause a variety of skin manifestations (Table 47.6).

Reactions to insulin

Lipoatrophy

Lipoatrophy occurs at sites of insulin injections and is particularly prominent with the longer-acting preparations [94]. It is characterized by a loss of subcutaneous fat and can be a cosmetic concern. This complication is less common with the advent of purer insulins. Circumscribed depressed areas of skin are seen at sites of insulin injections 6–24 months after the start of treatment. It is more common in young female subjects with diabetes. The pathogenesis is secondary to an immunologic reaction as biopsies from affected sites show immunoglobulin M and complement. Other theories include mechanical trauma from the angle of injection, surface alcohol contamination or local production of tumor necrosis factor from macrophages induced by injected insulin. Repeated injections to the same site may predispose to this problem [95].

Lipohypertrophy

Lipohypertrophy presents as soft subcutaneous nodules or thickening at sites of repeated injections [96]. It occurs because of the lipogenic action of insulin, with repeated local stimulation of adipocytes being causative. Insulin absorption may be delayed at such sites, potentially resulting in disruption of glycemic control [97]. It resolves spontaneously by changing the site of insulin injections. Hyperkeratotic verrucous variants of lipohypertrophy have also been described [98].

Insulin allergy

Reactions to insulin were previously common because of the presence of impurities such as cow or pig proteins, and preservatives or additives. The use of recombinant human and analog insulin has decreased the incidence of insulin allergy which is now less than 1% of insulin-treated patients [64]. Allergic reactions to insulin can be classified as immediate-local, general, delayed or biphasic. Immediate-local reactions occur within a few minutes of injection and subside within an hour. Erythema with urtication can occur and is possibly immunoglobulin E (IgE) mediated. Treatment of the immediate-local reaction is to change the insulin to a more purified product. Systemic reactions include generalized urticaria and, rarely, anaphylaxis. Generalized urticarial reactions to purified insulins are rare [99], but a few patients sensitized to animal insulins have experienced anaphylaxis with human insulin [100]. Delayed hypersensitivity reactions are the most common, appearing about 2 weeks after the start of insulin therapy. Itchy nodules are evident at the sites of injections, 4–24 hours after injection. Biphasic responses have been reported in some individuals, with immediate urticaria followed by a delayed reaction several hours later. They are considered IgG-mediated immune complex reactions. The hypersensitivity may be to insulin itself, or to preservatives such as aminobenzoic acid or to zinc [101]. Insulin allergic reactions may be managed by antihistamines, addition of glucocorticoids, discontinuation of therapy or a change in the insulin delivery system.

Other cutaneous complications of insulin

Occasionally, lack of simple hygiene leads to infection with abscess formation. Granulomatous lesions that have a furuncular or pustular appearance can occur following insulin injections [102]. Keloids, hyperkeratotic papules, purpura and localized pigmentation can also occur. Patients using insulin pumps for subcutaneous insulin delivery can experience local infections at the site of needle insertion, contact allergy to the associated tape and tubing material and, rarely, subcutaneous nodules [103]. Retention of fluid can occur when insulin therapy is first commenced. This is manifested as edema of the legs and is probably caused by temporary inhibition of sodium excretion.

Reaction to oral hypoglycemic agents

Sulfonyureas

Sulfonylureas are the most common oral hypoglycemic agents that cause skin reactions. About 1–5% of patients taking first-generation sulfonyureas develop cutaneous reactions within 2 months of treatment [64]. Maculopapular, morbilliform, urticarial or generalized erythematous reactions are common and resolve with discontinuation of the medication. Photosensitive reactions, usually of the photoallergic type, as well as lichenoid eruptions have also been reported (Figure 47.11) [104]. Erythema multiforme, characterized by erythematous and hemorrhagic skin lesions associated with "target" lesions, can be a severe manifestation of drug reactions (Figure 47.12). Extensive blistering which includes the mucosal surfaces can occur and if the conjunctiva are involved, urgent ophthalmologic opinion is mandatory. Rarer reactions include erythema nodosum and exacerbation of porphyria cutanea tarda [105].

The chlorpropamide alcohol flush is a disulfiram-like effect occurring in 10–30% of patients taking this drug. Patients experience facial erythema, headache and palpitations about 15 minutes after drinking alcohol and it subsides in about an hour.

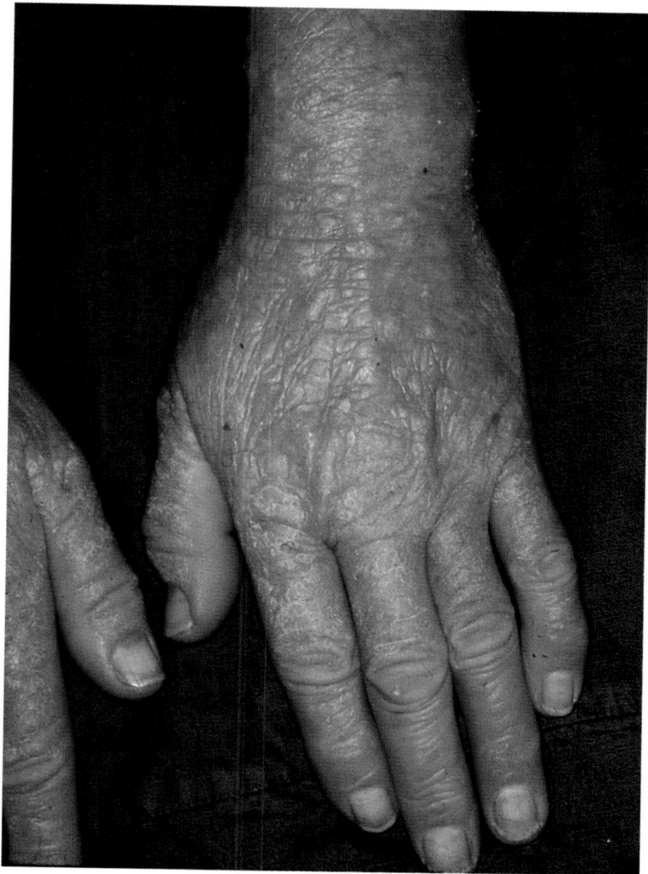

Figure 47.11 Drug rash with chlorpromazine.

(a)

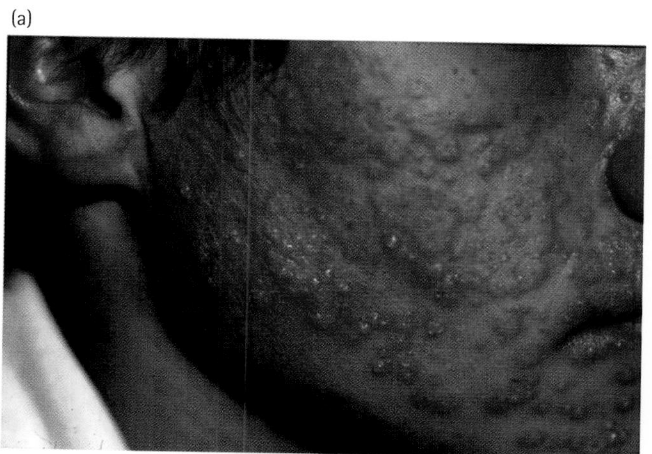

(b)

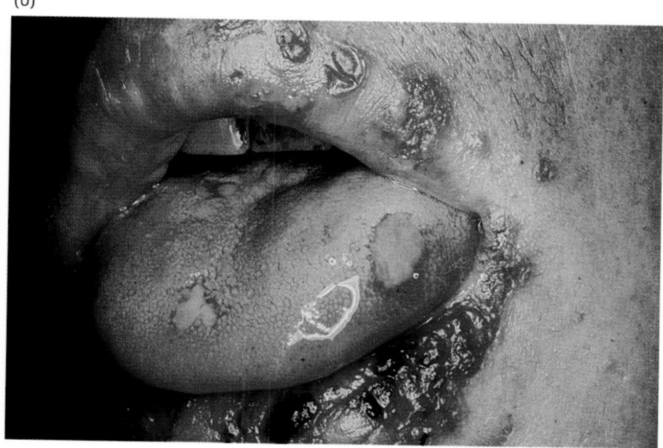

Figure 47.12 Erythema multiforme. (a) Showing the varied appearance of the condition: annular, arcuate and blistering lesions and confluent erythema on the ears. (b) Mouth ulceration in Stevens–Johnson syndrome, the severe form of erythema multiforme.

Endogenous opioids may be important as the flush is blocked by naloxone [106]. Second-generation sulfonylureas such as glipizide and glimepiride are less likely to cause cutaneous side effects. Glipizide has rarely been associated with photosensitivity, rash, urticaria and pruritus. Glimepiride can similarly cause lichenoid skin reactions [107].

Other oral hypoglycemic agents

Rashes with other oral antidiabetic agents are much less common than sulfonylureas. Transient erythema or urticaria may occur with the biguanide metformin. It is also reported to cause a psoriasiform drug eruption, erythema multiforme, photosensitivity and leukocytoclastic vasculitis [108,109]. Acarbose can cause a generalized erythema multiforme, although it is minimally absorbed from the gut. It may be the degradation products of acarbose that causes the allergic reaction [110]. Thiazolidinediones such as rosglitazone and pioglitazone can cause edema, transient erythema and urticaria, as can the glinides such as repaglinide, but such reactions are uncommon.

References

1 Neilly JB, Martin A, Simpson N, MacCuish AG. Pruritus in diabetes mellitus: investigation of prevalence and correlation with diabetes control. *Diabetes Care* 1986; **9**:273–275.

2 Anderson BL, Verdich J. Granuloma annulare and diabetes mellitus. *Clin Exp Dermatol* 1979; **4**:31–37.

3 Muller SA, Winklemann RK. Necrobiosis lipoidica diabeticorum, a clinical and pathological investigation of 171 cases. *Arch Dermatol* 1966; **93**:272–281.

4 Narva WM, Benoit FL, Ringrose EJ. Necrobiosis lipoidica diabeticorum with apparently normal carbohydrate tolerance. *Arch Intern Med* 1965; **115**:718–722.

5 O'Toole EA, Kennedy U, Nolan JJ, Young MM, Rogers S, Barnes L. Necrobiosis lipoidica: only a minority of paients have diabetes mellitus. *Br J Dermatol* 1999; **140**:283–286.

6 Chernosky ME, Guin JD. Necrobiosis lipoidica in a three-year-old girl. *Arch Dermatol* 1961; **84**:135–136.

7 Verrotti AA, Chiarelli F, Amerio P, Morgese G. Necrobiosis lipoidica diabeticorum in children and adolescents: a clue for underlying renal and retinal disease. *Pediatr Dermatol* 1995; **12**:220–223.

8 Boulton AJ, Cutfield RG, Abouganem D, Angus E, Flynn HW Jr, Skyler JS, *et al.* Necrobiosis lipoidica diabeticorum: a clinicopathologic study. *J Am Acad Dermatol* 1988; **18**:530–537.

9 Quimby SR, Muller SA, Schroeter AL. The cutaneous immunopathology of necrobiosis lipoidica diabeticorum. *Arch Dermatol* 1988; **124**:1364–1371.

10 Mackey JP. Necrobiosis lipoidica diabeticorum involving scalp and face. *Br J Dermatol* 1975; **93**:729–730.

11 Mann RJ, Harman RRM. Cutaneous anaesthesia in necrobiosis lipoidica. *Br J Dermatol* 1984; **110**:323–325.

12 Weedon D. *Skin Pathology*. London: Churchill Livingston, 2002: 202–204.

13 Shapiro PE. Non-infectious granulomas. In Elder D, Elenitas R, Jaworsky C, Johnson B Jr, eds. *Lever's Histopathology of the Skin*, 8th edn. Philadephia: Lippincott-Raven, 1999: 330–333.

14 Lowitt MH, Dover JS. Necrobiosis lipoidica. *J Am Acad Dermatol* 1991; **25**:735–748.

15 Volden G. Successful treatment of chronic skin diseases with clobetasol propionate and a hydrocolloid dressing. *Acta Derm Venereol Suppl (Stockh)* 1992; **72**:85–89.

16 Sparrow G, Abel E. Granuloma annulare and necrobiosis lipoidica treated by jet injector. *Br J Dermatol* 1975; **93**:85–89.

17 Heymann WR. Necrobiosis lipoidica treated with topical tretinoin. *Cutis* 1996; **58**:53–54.

18 Petzelbauer P, Wolff K, Tappeiner G. Necrobiosis lipoidica: treatment with systemic corticosteroids. *Br J Dermatol* 1992; **126**:542–545.

19 Boyd AS. Treatment of necrobiosis lipoidica with pioglitazone. *J Am Acad Dermatol* 2007; **57**(Suppl):S120–121.

20 Statham B, Finlay AY, Marks R. A randomized double blind comparison of aspirin dipyridamole combination versus a placebo in the treatment of necrobiosis lipoidica. *Acta Derm Venereol* 1981; **61**:270–271.

21 Beck HI, Bjerring P, Rasmussen I, Zacharie H, Stenberg S. Treatment of necrobiosis lipoidica with low-dose acetylsalicylic acid: a randomized double-blind trial. *Acta Derm Venereol* 1985; **65**:230–234.

22 Noz KC, Korstanje MJ, Vermeer BJ. Ulcerating necrobiosis lipoidica effectively treated with pentoxifylline. *Clin Exp Dermatol* 1993; **18**:78–79.

23 Handfield-Jones S, Jones S, Peachey R. High dose nicotinamide in the treatment of necrobiosis lipoidica. *Br J Dermatol* 1988; **118**: 693–696.

24 Messing H. Clofazamine: therapeutic alternative in necrobiosis lipoidica and granuloma annulare. *Int J Dermatol* 1989; **28**: 195–197.

25 McKenna DB, Cooper EJ, Tidman MJ. Topical PUVA treatment for necrobiosis lipoidica. *Br J Dermatol* 2000; **143**:71.

26 de Rie MA, Sommer A, Hoekzema R, Neumann HAM. Treatment of necrobiosis lipoidica with topical psoralens plus ultraviolet A. *Br J Dermatol* 2002; **147**:743–747.

27 Narbutt J, Torzecka JD, Sysa-Jedrzejowska A, Zalewska A. Long-term results of topical PUVA in necrobiosis lipoidica. *Clin Exp Dermatol* 2006; **31**:65–67.

28 Darvay A, Acland KM, Russell-Jones R. Persistent ulcerated necrobiosis lipoidica responding to treatment with cyclosporine. *Br J Dermatol* 1999; **141**:725–727.

29 Stanway A, Rademaker M, Newman P. Healing of ulcerative necrobiosis lipoidica with cyclosporine. *Australas J Dermatol* 2004; **45**:119–122.

30 Reinhard G, Lohmann F, Uerlich M, Bauer R, Bieber T. Successful treatment of ulcerated necrobiosis lipoidica with mycophenolate mofetil. *Acta Derm Venereol* 2000; **80**:312–313.

31 Kolde G, Muche JM, Schulze P, Fischer P, Lichey J. Infliximab: a promising new treatment option for ulcerated necrobiosis lipoidica. *Dermatology* 2003; **206**:180–181.

32 Moreno-Arias GA, Camps-Fresneda A. Necrobiosis lipoidica diabeticorum treated with pulsed dye laser. *J Cosmet Laser Ther* 2001; **3**:143–146.

33 Dubin BJ, Kaplan EN. The surgical treatment of necrobiosis lipoidica diabeticorum. *Plast Reconstr Surg* 1977; **60**:421–428.

34 Binkley GW. Dermopathy in the diabetic syndrome. *Arch Dermatol* 1965; **92**:625–634.

35 Romano G, Moretti G, Di Benedetto A, Giofrè C, Cesare E, Russo G, *et al.* Skin lesions in diabetes mellitus: prevalence and

clinical correlations. *Diabetes Res Clin Pract* 1998; **39**:101–106.

36 Shemer A, Bergman R, Linn S, Kantor Y, Friedman-Birnbaum R. Diabetic dermopathy and internal complications in diabetes mellitus. *Int J Dermatol* 1998; **37**:113–115.

37 Morgan AJ, Schwartz RA. Diabetic dermopathy: a subtle sign with grave implications. *J Am Acad Dermatol* 2008; **58**:447–451.

38 Bauer M, Levan NE. Diabetic dermangiopathy: a spectrum including pigmented pretibial patches and necrobiosis lipoidica diabeticorum. *Br J Dermatol* 1970; **83**:528–535.

39 Danowski TS, Sabeh G, Sarver ME, Shelkrot J, Fisher ER. Shin spots and diabetes mellitus. *Am J Med Sci* 1966; **251**:570–575.

40 Cantwell AR, Martz W. Idiopathic bullae in diabetics. *Arch Dermatol* 1967; **96**:42–44.

41 Bernstein JE, Medenica M, Soltani K, Griem SF. Bullous eruption of diabetes mellitus. *Arch Dermatol* 1979; **115**:324–325.

42 Lipsky BA, Baker PD, Ahroni JH. Dianetic bullae: 12 cases of a purportedly rare cutaneous disease. *Int J Dermatol* 2000; **39**: 196–200.

43 Basarab T, Munn SE, McGrath J, Russell-Jones R. Bullosis diabeticorum: a case report and review of the literature. *Clin ExpDermatol* 1995; **20**:218–220.

44 Schnider SL, Kohn RR. Effects of age and diabetes mellitus on the solubility and nonenzymatic glucosylation of human skin collagen. *J Clin Invest* 1981; **67**:1630–1635.

45 Huntley AC, Walter RM Jr. Quantitative determination of skin thickness in diabetes mellitus: relationship to disease parameters. *J Med* 1990; **21**:257–264.

46 Nikkels-Tassoudji N, Henry F, Letwe C, Pierard-Franchimont C, Lefebvre P, Pierard GE. Mechanical properties of the diabetic waxy skin. *Dermatology* 1996; **192**:19–22.

47 Collier A, Patrick AW, Bell D, Matthews DM, MacIntyre CC, Ewing DJ, *et al.* Relationship of skin thickness to duration of diabetes, glycemic control, and diabetic complications in male IDDM patients. *Diabetes Care* 1989; **12**:309–312.

48 Forst T, Kann P, Pfützner A, Lobmann R, Schäfer H, Beyer J. Association between "diabetic thick skin syndrome" and neurological disorders in diabetes mellitus. *Acta Diabetol* 1994; **31**:73–77.

49 Huntley AC. Finger pebbles: a common finding in diabetes mellitus. *J Am Acad Dermatol* 1986; **14**:612–617.

50 Collier A, Matthews DM, Kellett HA, Clarke BF, Hunter JA. Change in skin thickness associated with cheiroarthropathy in insulin dependent diabetes mellitus. *Br Med J* 1986; **292**:936.

51 Hanna W, Friesen D, Bombardier C, Gladman D, Hanna A. Pathologic features of diabetic thick skin. *J Am Acad Dermatol* 1987; **16**:546–553.

52 Tüzün B, Tüzün Y, Dinççag N, Minareci O, Oztürk S, Yilmaz MT, *et al.* Diabetic sclerodactyly. *Diabetes Res Clin Pract* 1995; **27**: 153–157.

53 Cole GW, Headley J, Skowsky R. Scleredema diabeticorum: a common and distinct cutaneous manifestation of diabetes mellitus. *Diabetes Care* 1983; **6**:189–192.

54 Kroft EB, de Jong EM. Sclerema diabeticorum case series: successful treatment with UV-A1. *Arch Dermatol* 2008; **144**:947–948.

55 Matsuoka LY, Wortsman J, Gavin JR, Goldman J. Spectrum of endocrine abnormalities associated with acanthosis nigricans. *Am J Med* 1987; **83**:719–725.

56 Barth JH, Ng LL, Wojnarowska F, Dawber RPR. Acanthosis nigricans, insulin resistance and cutaneous virilism. *Br J Dermatol* 1988; **118**:613–619.

57 Kahn CR, Flier JS, Bar RS, Archer JA, Gorden P, Martin MM, *et al.* Syndromes of insulin resistance and acanthosis nigricans. *N Engl J Med* 1976; **294**:739–745.

58 Geffner ME, Golde DW. Selective insulin action on skin, ovary, heart, in insulin-resistant states. *Diabetes Care* 1988; **11**:500–505.

59 Rendell M, Bamisedun O. Diabetic cutaneous microangiopathy. *Am J Med* 1992; **93**:611–618.

60 Gitelson S, Wertheimer-Kapplinski N. Colour of the face in diabetes mellitus; observations on a group of patients in Jerusalem. *Diabetes* 1965; **14**:201–208.

61 Greene RA, Scher RK. Nail changes associated with diabetes mellitus. *J Am Acad Dermatol* 1987; **16**:1015–1021.

62 Ngo BT, Hayes KD, DiMiao DJ, Srinivasan S, Huerter CJ, Rendell MS. Manifestations of cutaneous diabetic microangiopathy. *Am J Clin Dermatol* 2005; **6**:225–237.

63 Lithner F, Heitala SO. Skeletal lesions of the feet in diabetics and their relationship to cutaneous erythema with or without necrosis of the feet. *Acta Med Scand* 1976; **200**:155–161.

64 Van Hattem S, Bootsma AH, Thio HB. Skin manifestations of diabetes. *Cleve Clin J Med* 2008; **75**:772–787.

65 Wilmer WA, Magro CM. Calciphylaxis: emerging concepts in prevention, diagnosis, and treatment. *Dialysis* 2002; **15**:172–186.

66 Lugo-Somolinos A, Sanchez JL. Prevalence of dermatophytosis in patients with diabetes. *J Am Acad Dermatol* 1992; **26**:408–410.

67 Tabor CA, Parlette EC. Cutaneous manifestations of diabetes: signs of poor glycemic control or new-onset disease. *Postgrad Med* 2006; **119**:38–44.

68 Ahmed I, Goldstein B. Diabetes mellitus. *Clin Dermatol* 2006; **24**:237–246.

69 Meurer M, Szeimies RM. Diabetes mellitus and skin diseases. *Curr Probl Dermatol* 1991; **20**:11–23.

70 Tapper-Jones LM, Aldred MJ, Walker DM, Hayes TM. Candidal infections and populations of *Candida albicans* in mouths of diabetics. *J Clin Pathol* 1981; **34**:706–711.

71 Perez MI, Kohn SR. Cutaneous manifestations of diabetes mellitus. *J Am Acad Dermatol* 1994; **30**:519–531.

72 Chandler PT, Chandler SD. Pathogenic carrier rate in diabetes mellitus. *Am J Med Sci* 1977; **273**:259–265.

73 Zaky DA, Bentley DW, Lowy K, Betts RF, Douglas RG Jr. Malignant external otitis: a severe form of otitis in diabetics. *Am J Med* 1976; **61**:298–302.

74 Rajbhandari SM, Wilson RM. Unusual infections in diabetes. *Diabetes Res Clin Pract* 1998; **39**:123–128.

75 Wong CH, Chang HC, Pasupathy S, Khin LW, Tan JL, Low CO. Necrotizing fasciitis: clinical presentation, microbiology, and determinants of mortality. *J Bone Joint Surg Am* 2003; **85-A**:1454–1460.

76 Aye M, Masson EA. Dermatological care of the diabetic foot. *Am J Clin Dermatol* 2002; **3**:463–474.

77 Rajagopalan S. Serious infections in elderly patients with diabetes mellitus. *Clin Infect Dis* 2005; **40**:990–996.

78 Dittmar M, Kahaly GJ. Polyglandular autoimmune syndromes: immunogenetics and long-term follow-up. *J Clin Endocrinol Metab* 2003; **88**:2983–2992.

79 Nigam PK, Singh G, Agarwal JK. Plasma insulin response to oral glycemic stimulus in lichen planus. *Br J Dermatol* 1988; **19**: 128–129.

80 Lundstrom IM. Incidence of diabetes mellitus in patients with oral lichen planus. *Int J Oral Surg* 1983; **12**:147–152.
81 Kantor GR, Lookingbill DP. Generalized pruritus and systemic disease. *J Am Acad Dermatol* 1983; **9**:375–382.
82 Neilly JB, Martin A, Simpson N, MacCuish AC. Pruritus in diabetes mellitus: investigation of prevalence and correlation with diabetes control. *Diabetes Care* 1986; **9**:273–275.
83 DiGiovanna JJ, Robinson-Bostom L. Ichthyosis: etiology, diagnosis and management. *Am J Clin Dermatol* 2003; **4**:81–95.
84 Jelinek JE. Cutaneous manifestations of diabetes mellitus. *Int J Dermatol* 1994; **33**:605–617.
85 Oimomi M, Maeda Y, Hata F, Nishimoto S, Kitamura Y, Matsumoto S, *et al.* Glycosylation levels of nail proteins in diabetic patients with retinopathy and neuropathy. *Kobe J Med Sci* 1985; **31**:183–188.
86 Kudo H, Yonezawa I, Ieki A, Miyachi Y. Generalized eruptive clear-cell syringoma. *Arch Dermatol* 1989; **125**:1716–1717.
87 Furue M, Hori Y, Nakabayashi Y. Clear-cell syringoma: association with diabetes. *Am J Dermatopathol* 1984; **6**:131–138.
88 Edney JA, Hofmann S, Thompson JS, Kessinger A. Glucoganoma syndrome is an underdiagnosed clnical entity. *Am J Surg* 1990; **160**:625–628.
89 Long CC, Laidler P, Holt PJA. Suprabasal acantholysis: an unusual feature of necrolytic migratory erythema. *Clin Exp Dermatol* 1993; **18**:464–467.
90 Bewley AP, Ross JS, Bunker CB, Staughton RCD. Successful treatment of a patient with octreotide-resistant necrolytic migratory erythema. *Br J Dermatol* 1996; **134**:1101–1104.
91 Sohier J, Jeanmougin M, Lombrail P, Passa P. Rapid improvement of skin lesions in glucagonomas with intravenous somatostatin infusion. *Lancet* 1980; **i**:40.
92 Briggs PL, Fraga S. Reactive perforating collagenosis of diabetes mellitus. *J Am Acad Dermatol* 1995; **32**:521–523.
93 Kawakami T, Saito R. Acquired reactive perforating collagenosis associated with diabetes mellitus: eight cases that meet Faver's criteria. *Br J Dermatol* 1999; **140**:521–524.
94 Reeves WG, Allen BR, Tattersall RB. Insulin-induced lipoatrophy: evidence for an immune pathogenesis. *Br Med J* 1980; **280**: 1500–1503.
95 Young RJ, Steel JM, Frier BM, Duncan LPJ. Insulin injection sites in diabetes: a neglected area? *Br Med J* 1981; **283**:349.
96 Johnson DA, Parlette HL. Insulin-induced hypertrophic lipodystrophy. *Cutis* 1983; **32**:273–276.
97 Young RJ, Hannan WJ, Frier BM, Steel JM, Duncan LJ. Diabetic lipohypertrophy delays insulin absorption. *Diabetes Care* 1984; **7**:479.
98 Fleming MJ, Simon SI. Cutaneous insulin reaction resembling acnathosis nigricans. *Arch Dermatol* 1986; **122**:1054–1056.
99 Small P, Lerman S. Human insulin allergy. *Ann Allergy* 1984; **53**:39–41.
100 Fineberg SE, Galloway JE, Fineberg NS, Rathbun MJ, Hufferd S. Immunogenicity of recombinant DNA human insulin. *Diabetologia* 1983; **25**:465–469.
101 Feinglos MN, Jegasothy BV. "Insulin" allergy due to zinc. *Lancet* 1979; **1**:122–124.
102 Jordaan HF, Sandler M. Zinc-induced granuloma: a unique complication of insulin therapy. *Clin Exp Dermatol* 1989; **14**:227–229.
103 Levandoski LA, White NH, Santiago JV. Localized skin reactions to insulin: insulin lipodystrophies and skin reactions to pumped subcuatenous insulin therapy. *Diabetes Care* 1982; **5**:6–10.
104 Dinsdale RC, Ormerod TP, Walker AE. Lichenoid eruption due to chlorpropamide. *Br Med J* 1968; **1**:100.
105 Zarowitz H, Newhouse S. Coproporphyrinuria with cutaneous reaction induced by chlorpropamide. *N Y State J Med* 1965; **65**:2385–2387.
106 Medbak S, Wass JAH, Clement-Jones V, Cooke ED, Bowcock SA, Cudworth AG, *et al.* Chlorpropamide alcohol flush and circulating met-enkephalin: a positive link. *Br Med J* 1981; **283**:937–939.
107 Noakes R. Lichenoid drug eruption as a result of the recently released sulfonylurea glimepiride. *Australas J Dermatol* 2003; **44**:302–303.
108 Burger DE, Goyal S. Erythema multiforme from metformin. *Ann Pharmacother* 2004; **38**:1537.
109 Ben Salem C, Hmouda H, Slim R, Denguezli M, Belajouza C, Bouraoui K. Rare case of metformin-induced leucocytoclastic vasculitis. *Ann Pharmacother* 2006; **40**:1685–1687.
110 Kono T, Hayami M, Kobayashi H, Ishii M, Taniguchi S. Acarbose-induced generalized erythema multiforme. *Lancet* 1999; **354**:396–397.

48 Bone and Rheumatic Disorders in Diabetes

Andrew Grey & Nicola Dalbeth

Department of Medicine, University of Auckland, Auckland, New Zealand

Keypoints

- Musculoskeletal disorders may cause pain and functional impairment, and adversely affect management of diabetes.
- Fibroproliferative disorders of soft tissue such as limited joint mobility, frozen shoulder, Dupuytren contracture, trigger finger and carpal tunnel syndrome occur more commonly in diabetes and can lead to upper limb disability.
- Charcot joint is an infrequent but serious complication of diabetic peripheral neuropathy, and is characterized by disordered osteoclastogenesis. Bisphosphonate therapy may be a useful adjunct to standard treatment.
- Patients with diabetes are at high risk of developing gout, particularly in the presence of renal impairment and diuretic use.
- The prevalence of diffuse idiopathic skeletal hyperostosis is increased in patients with type 2 diabetes (T2DM).
- Fracture risk is increased in both type 1 (T1DM) and T2DM.
- Bone mineral density is decreased in T1DM, and increased in T2DM.
- Disease complications increase fracture risk by increasing risk of falls and causing regional osteopenia.
- Thiazolidinediones decrease bone formation and bone mineral density, and increase fracture risk in T2DM.
- Fracture healing may be impaired in diabetes.

Musculoskeletal disease in diabetes

Background

A variety of musculoskeletal disorders are associated with diabetes. These disorders may cause pain and functional impairment, and influence the ability of patients to adhere to other aspects of diabetes treatment, particularly exercise and weight management. Therapies commonly used in the treatment of rheumatic disease, particularly corticosteroids and non-steroidal anti-inflammatory drugs (NSAIDs), may be particularly problematic in patients with diabetes. The important bone and joint disorders associated with diabetes discussed in this chapter are outlined in Table 48.1.

Fibroproliferative disorders of soft tissue

Limited joint mobility (cheiroarthopathy)

Limited joint mobility refers to a syndrome of joint contractures resulting in decreased passive mobility of the joints in patients with diabetes [1]. Flexion contractures of the proximal interphalangeal (PIP) joints and metacarpophalangeal (MCP) joints of the hands are characteristic, with the fifth PIP joint affected first (Figure 48.1). The skin on the dorsum of the hands typically appears tight and waxy [2]. Large joints such as the wrists, elbows, ankle and cervical spine can also be affected, and reduced lung volumes have been reported in severe cases [3,4]. Pain is usually mild or absent early in disease, and features of synovitis such as joint swelling, effusion, warmth and tenderness are typically absent. The disorder can be readily differentiated from systemic sclerosis by lack of Raynaud phenomenon and other systemic features, normal nailfold capillary examination and negative autoantibodies [5,6].

The presence of limited joint mobility of the hands is detected clinically by assessing for the prayer sign or the table-top sign. The prayer sign is positive if patients are unable to oppose the palmar surfaces at any interphalangeal or MCP joints when the hands are placed in the prayer position. For assessment of the table-top sign, the patient places both hands on a table top with the palms down and the fingers fanned out. The fingers are then viewed at table level. In stage 0, the entire palmer surface of the fingers makes contact with the table. In stage 1, one finger is affected (usually the fifth PIP joint of one or both hands). In stage 2, two or more fingers of both hands are affected (usually the fourth and fifth PIP joints). In stage 3, there is involvement of all the fingers and also restricted movement in a larger joint, usually the wrist or elbow [7]. Passive joint movement should also be assessed to confirm limitation of joint mobility [8].

Prevalence estimates for limited joint mobility in type 1 diabetes mellitus (T1DM) range 9–58%, and 25–75% in type 2 diabetes

Textbook of Diabetes, 4th edition. Edited by R. Holt, C. Cockram, A. Flyvbjerg and B. Goldstein.

Table 48.1 Bone and joint disorders in patients with diabetes.

Fibroproliferative disorders of soft tissue
Cheiroarthropathy
Frozen shoulder
Dupuytren contracture
Stenosing tenosynovitis (trigger finger)
Carpal tunnel syndrome
Disorders of joint tissue
Charcot joint
Gout
Osteoarthritis*
RA genetic risk and type 1 diabetes*
Disorders of bone
Diffuse idiopathic skeletal hyperostosis
Osteoporosis and fractures
Disordered fracture healing

RA, rheumatoid arthritis.
*Direct association not proven.

mellitus (T2DM) [1,9–11]. There is some evidence that prevalence rates have declined in patients with T1DM in the last 20 years because of improvements in glycemic control [12].

Limited joint mobility is an important entity primarily because of its clinical associations. It is one of the earliest complications of diabetes and is strongly associated with the presence of microvascular complications such as retinopathy and nephropathy in T1DM, [1,12–15], and macrovascular complications in T2DM [10]. It is also associated with other fibroproliferative disorders affecting the upper limb such as frozen shoulder, Dupuytren contracture and carpal tunnel syndrome [15–18]. In general, limited joint mobility does not severely impact on hand function, but combinations of these upper limb disorders may cause upper limb disability [19–21]. In addition to microvascular complications, risk factors for the development of limited joint mobility in patients with diabetes include older age, puberty (in T1DM), disease duration and cigarette smoking [10,22–24].

Advanced imaging techniques have demonstrated thickening of skin, tendons and tendon sheaths in patients with limited joint mobility [25,26]. Histologic examination of the skin shows altered mucopolysaccharide distribution, elastin and collagen, and reduced vascular lumen [27]. Non-enzymatic glycosylation and accumulation of collagen have been implicated in the pathogenesis [28]. Disordered glycosaminoglycan (GAG) metabolism is also a feature; skin biopsies from patients with severe limited joint mobility show pronounced hyaluronan expression in the epidermis and diminished expression in the dermis and basement membrane compared with skin from controls without diabetes and controls with diabetes but without limited joint mobility [29]. In addition, increased urinary GAG excretion has been reported in patients with limited joint mobility [30]. Reduced circulating insulin-like growth factor I (IGF-I) is associated with limited joint mobility, implicating the growth hormone–IGF-I axis in the pathogenesis of this complication [31]. Microvascular abnormalities also contribute to disease, with reports of disordered palmar microvascular flow in response to thermal challenge [32].

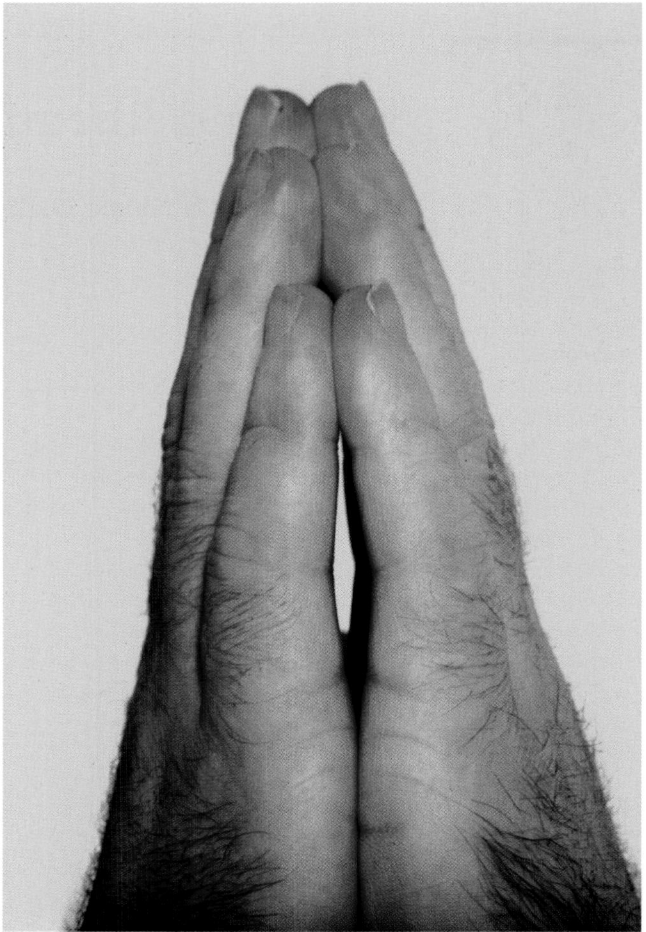

Figure 48.1 Limited joint mobility with flexion contractures affecting the finger proximal interphalangeal joints. Courtesy of Dr. Tim Cundy.

The mainstay of therapy remains obtaining excellent glycemic control, and reduced prevalence of this disorder has been reported with such interventions [12,33]. Physiotherapy, particularly hand therapy, may be of benefit to improve joint contractures and function. Corticosteroid injection of flexor tendon sheaths has been reported to lead to resolution of finger contractures in almost two-thirds of cases related to limited joint mobility, and should also be considered [34].

Frozen shoulder

This disorder is characterized by shoulder pain, stiffness and severely restricted range of motion in all planes [35]. Three phases of the disorder are well-recognized: first, the painful freezing stage with associated nocturnal pain (lasting 4–8 months), followed by the adhesive phase with improvement in pain but severely restricted range of motion (lasting 8–24 months), and finally the resolution phase [36]. The mean time to resolution is 30 months [36]. Plain radiographs of the shoulder are typically normal. Although the condition is usually self-limiting, some patients have persistent shoulder pain and restricted range of motion many years after assessment [37,38].

Imaging and histologic studies have demonstrated that the pathologic features of frozen shoulder are thickening of the capsule and synovium with contracted joint volume. Affected tissue is characterized by dense type I and type III collagen deposition with proliferating fibroblasts and a chronic inflammatory infiltrate comprising T cells, macrophages and mast cells [39,40]. Disordered collagen synthesis and vascular endothelial growth factor 1 (VEGF-1) mediated angiogenesis have also been implicated [41,42].

Treatment is tailored to the stage of the disorder [35]. In the painful freezing stage, analgesics, including NSAIDs if tolerated, are indicated. Early use of intra-articular corticosteroids is associated with improved outcomes, and physiotherapy with exercise within the limits of pain is of greater benefit than more intensive physiotherapy such as stretching and mobilization [43,44]. Although oral corticosteroids provide short-term relief in the painful freezing stage, they are not routinely recommended because of lack of long-term benefit and risk of adverse events [45]. In the adhesive phase, more intensive physiotherapy is indicated. For those who fail to respond to physiotherapy and have persistent shoulder restriction, interventions such as radiographic-guided hydrodilatation, manipulation under anesthesia or arthroscopic release should be considered [46,47].

Diabetes is a major risk factor for frozen shoulder. The prevalence of frozen shoulder is 11–19% of patients with diabetes, compared with 2–3% of age-matched controls [16,19,48,49]. Patients with diabetes are also more likely to have bilateral disease. Key risk factors for frozen shoulder in patients with diabetes are older age, duration of diabetes, previous myocardial infarction, retinopathy and peripheral neuropathy [50]. The presence of other fibroproliferative musculoskeletal disorders such as limited joint mobility and Dupuytren contracture is strongly associated with frozen shoulder in patients with diabetes [50]. Furthermore, frozen shoulder in patients with diabetes is more difficult to treat because of persistent disease and worse outcomes following surgical interventions [47,51,52].

Dupuytren contracture

Dupuytren contracture is a fibroproliferative disorder of the palmar fascia leading to formation of palmar nodules, development of a palmar aponeurosis cord with tethering of the overlying skin and eventually flexion contractures, particularly affecting the ring and little fingers [53]. Elderly men of northern European ancestry are most frequently affected. Disordered fibroblast and myofibroblast function has been described, with deposition of type III collagen, potentially mediated by growth factors such as transforming growth factor β (TGF-β) and basic fibroblast growth factor [54–56].

Surgical treatment is the mainstay of therapy, although non-surgical options, particularly local injection of collagenase, are promising [57]. Splinting and intralesional corticosteroids may be considered, but are frequently ineffective [58]. Surgical referral should be considered in the presence of contracture. Various surgical approaches are available, including fasciotomy (division of the affected palmar fascia) or fasciectomy (excision of the affected palmar fascia). Percutaneous needle fasciotomy is a minimally invasive technique with good short-term outcomes, although recurrence is a frequent problem [59,60].

Risk factors for Dupuytren contracture include advanced age, male sex, cigarette smoking, manual labor and alcohol consumption. Diabetes is also an important risk factor for Dupuytren contracture, which is present in up to 26% of patients with diabetes [19,20,61]. Age and disease duration are the major risk factors for development of Dupuytren contracture in patients with diabetes [62]. Dupuytren contractures are also associated with microvascular complications in T1DM and macroalbuminuria in T2DM [63,64]. Rapidly progressive contractures are less frequently seen in patients with diabetes [62]. Coexistent fibroproliferative disease is frequent in patients with diabetes-associated Dupuytren contracture, with higher rates of limited joint mobility [64].

Stenosing tenosynovitis (trigger finger)

Trigger finger is "a condition in which the flexor tendon is prohibited from gliding through the tendon sheath because of thickening of the synovial sheath over the tendon" [65]. This disorder most frequently affects the ring finger, but can also affect the other fingers and the thumb. The patient may report a clicking sensation when moving the finger, discomfort over the palm or overt triggering when the finger is locked in flexion [66]. Nodular or diffuse flexor tendon sheath swelling may be palpable.

The syndrome occurs as a result of a discrepancy between the flexor tendon and its sheath in the A1 pulley at the level of the metacarpal head [66]. The pulley becomes thickened with increased extracellular matrix and fibrocartilage metaplasia [67]. These pathologic changes may be induced by repetitive trauma.

Corticosteroid injection into the tendon sheath is an effective therapy for the majority of patients, particularly in the presence of nodular disease. For patients with nodular disease of less than 6 months' duration, local injection has a reported success rate of 90% [68]. Splinting and hand therapy are useful adjuncts to local injection. If conservative therapy fails, release using a percutaneous needle approach or open surgery is indicated [69].

Patients with diabetes are at higher risk of trigger finger, with a lifetime risk of 10% compared to 2.6% of the general population [66]. Patient age, diabetes duration and presence of microvascular complications are associated with increased risk of trigger finger in diabetes [62,70]. Outcomes are typically worse when trigger finger is associated with diabetes, with lower responses to corticosteroid injection and greater need for surgery [71–73]. Furthermore, T1DM is associated with higher prevalence of disease, more affected digits, greater need for surgery and higher risk of recurrence [62,71,73].

Carpal tunnel syndrome

Carpal tunnel syndrome is a common compressive neuropathy affecting the median nerve as it traverses with the flexor tendons through the carpal tunnel, an anatomical space comprised of the carpal bones and the transverse carpal ligament [74]. The most common histologic appearance is non-inflammatory tenosynovial fibrosis, with increased fibroblast number and type III collagen deposition, most likely mediated by TGF-β [75]. Compression within the carpal tunnel leads to disordered microvascular supply of the nerve, causing demyelination and axonal degeneration. The typical presentation is hand parasthesia, particularly affecting the thumb, index finger and middle finger. Paresthesia is often more frequent at night, and may wake the patient from sleep. Wrist and hand pain may also occur, and patients frequently report hand clumsiness.

Clinical examination may be normal, but in the presence of severe and prolonged disease there may be features of median nerve denervation, including thenar wasting, weakness of thumb abduction and sensory loss over the median nerve distribution. Provocative tests including Phalen and Tinel tests may be positive, and if present have relatively high specificity for carpal tunnel syndrome. The Phalen test is positive if paresthesia in the median nerve distribution is reported following flexion of the wrist at 90° for 60 seconds. The Tinel test is positive if paresthesia is reported after tapping the volar wrist over the carpal tunnel. The diagnosis is confirmed by nerve conduction testing, with the typical findings of prolonged latencies and delayed conduction velocities affecting the median nerve across the wrist [76].

Treatment consists of maintaining the wrist in a neutral position using a removable wrist splint. Splinting is particularly useful for nocturnal symptoms, and may be sufficient to treat mild disease [77]. Although oral corticosteroids have short-term efficacy, side effects are usually unacceptable [78]. Local corticosteroid injection provides good short-term relief [79]. Surgical release under local anesthesia is a well-tolerated and effective therapy, which should be considered in patients who have failed conservative therapy or have severe symptoms and signs of nerve compression [80]. Open release and endoscopic approaches have similar clinical outcomes [81].

Carpal tunnel syndrome may be caused by a number of factors including non-specific flexor tenosynovitis affecting the wrist, rheumatoid arthritis and other inflammatory synovial arthropathies, obesity, pregnancy and disordered wrist anatomy [74]. Diabetes is one of the most common metabolic disorders associated with carpal tunnel syndrome, being present in 16% of affected patients [82]. Most studies have shown increased risk of carpal tunnel syndrome in patients with both T1DM and T2DM [62,83,84]. A recent survey using clinical and neurophysiologic assessment reported a prevalence of carpal tunnel syndrome of 2% in a reference population without diabetes, 14% in patients with diabetes but no diabetic polyneuropathy, and 30% in patients with diabetic polyneuropathy [85]. Carpal tunnel syndrome is associated with duration of diabetes, and is more frequently present in patients with microvascular complications such as retinopathy, nephropathy and polyneuropathy [62,86]. Carpal tunnel syndrome is also more common in patients with limited joint mobility, and it has been postulated that this disorder occurs at higher frequency in diabetes because of accelerated thickening and fibrosis of the flexor tendon sheaths within the carpal tunnel [18]. Glycosylation of collagen may also reduce compliance of connective tissue within the carpal tunnel [84]. In addition, the presence of existing microvascular disease may further increase the risk of endoneural ischemia as the median nerve travels through the carpal tunnel. Carpal tunnel syndrome may be more difficult to assess in patients with coexistent diabetic neuropathy, because of atypical presentation and neurophysiologic assessment [85,87]. Treatment options for patients with diabetes and carpal tunnel syndrome are similar to those for patients without diabetes, and responses to surgery are usually good [88,89]. One study reported positive results in symptoms scores and neurophysiologic testing using local insulin injections in women with T2DM and carpal tunnel syndrome, in combination with corticosteroid injection [90].

Disorders of joints

Charcot joint

Charcot joint is a destructive arthropathy, most commonly affecting patients with diabetes in the presence of severe peripheral neuropathy. This disorder affects 0.1–0.4% of patients with diabetes and may lead to severe foot deformity and disability, ulceration and limb amputation [91].

Several stages of disease are described [92,93]. The developmental stage presents as acute inflammation with swelling, warmth and erythema of the foot. Pain may be a feature, despite the presence of peripheral sensory neuropathy. Peripheral pulses are usually easily palpable. Gradually worsening deformity occurs, with bone resorption, fracture and dislocation, leading to instability of the foot and the classic rocker-bottom dislocation of the midfoot. Plain radiographs may appear normal early in the acute phase of disease (Stage 0), but magnetic resonance imaging (MRI) scans show florid bone marrow edema, subchondral cysts and microfractures, and bone scintiscan shows increased uptake on the bony phase [93]. As deformity develops, radiographs show severe osteolysis, bone fragmentation and disordered architecture (Stage 1). In the coalescence phase (Stage 2), hyperemia resolves, swelling reduces and skin temperature normalizes. Bone debris is resorbed and bone sclerosis may occur. The reconstructive stage (Stage 3) is characterized by remodeling of bone, ankylosis and proliferation of bone, and formation of a stable foot. The acute phase (Stages 0 and 1) typically lasts 2–6 months, and the reparative phase (Stages 2 and 3) lasts up to 24 months. During both the acute and the reparative phases of disease, bony deformity may lead to abnormal load bearing, with ulceration of overlying skin and secondary osteomyelitis.

Five separate patterns of foot involvement are identified in patients with diabetes [94]: I, affecting the forefoot with osteolysis of the MTP and IP joints of the feet, leading to the "sucked candy" appearance on plain radiography; II, affecting the tarsometatarsal

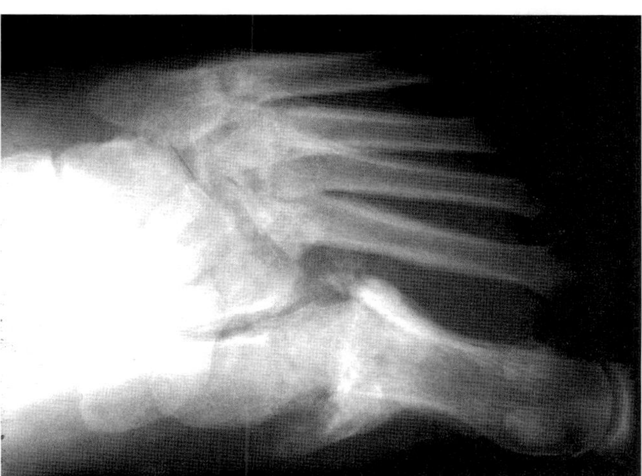

Figure 48.2 Plain radiograph of Charcot foot. Note the osteolysis, bone fragments, subluxation and fracture affecting the tarsometatarsal joints of the foot. Courtesy of Dr. Tim Cundy.

(Lisfranc) joint leading to instability, subluxation and fracture (Figure 48.2); III, dislocation and fracture affecting the midtarsal and naviculocuneiform joints; IV, affecting the ankle and subtalar joints, often with severe osteolysis; V, affecting the calcaneus. The most common patterns are II and III, and combinations of patterns may be present. Bilateral disease is present in one-quarter of patients. Rarely, other joints such as the knees, elbows and shoulders are affected.

The etiology of the disease remains controversial [95]. Minor trauma frequently precipitates onset of disease, and may lead to subclinical bone injury that triggers an aberrant inflammatory response [96]. It is likely that disordered weight-bearing in joints affected by peripheral neuropathy leads to repetitive injury and instability (the neurotraumatic hypothesis). Additionally, autonomic dysfunction causing vasodilatation, arteriovenous shunting and hyperemic bone resorption has been implicated (the neurovascular hypothesis). Development of osteopenia and osteolysis increases risk of fractures in the presence of abnormal load-bearing with a cycle of joint instability and fracture development, causing further abnormal load-bearing [97]. Recent work has focused on the role of local inflammation in disease pathogenesis. Advanced imaging and histologic analysis have demonstrated that inflammation of synovium and bone is evident in Charcot joint, and is characterized by increased expression of the pro-inflammatory cytokines tumor necrosis factor α (TNF-α) and interleukin 1 [98–101]. Large numbers of osteoclasts are present within affected bone, and patients with Charcot joint have increased ability to form peripheral blood derived osteoclasts *in vitro* compared with diabetic and non-diabetic controls [101,102]. Markers of bone resorption are increased in patients with acute Charcot joint [103]. Interestingly, acute phase markers are not significantly elevated, indicating an apparent dissociation between local and systemic inflammatory disease [104]. These data implicate receptor activator of nuclear factor κB ligand (RANKL) mediated osteoclastogenesis, driven locally by pro-inflammatory cytokines, and provide a rationale for the use of agents that target the osteoclast in treatment of the disease.

Management of Charcot joint depends on the stage of disease. Treatment during the acute phase consists of immobilization which reduces inflammation, prevents abnormal load-bearing and stabilizes the foot in a position of least deformity. The standard immobilization method during the acute phase is a non-weightbearing total contact cast. This treatment requires close monitoring and regular adjustment, and should be maintained until swelling and temperature normalize, and radiographs show no further bony destruction [105]. Some recent uncontrolled reports have indicated that use of a weightbearing total contract cast may be an acceptable alternative to the non-weightbearing option, but controlled trials are not yet available [106,107].

The recognition that the acute phase of Charcot joint is associated with excessive osteoclast activity has led to the testing of agents targeting bone turnover for treatment of this condition. Two randomized controlled trials of bisphosphonates have been reported, and both show efficacy. A single intravenous infusion of 90 mg pamidronate in a study of 39 patients with acute Charcot joint led to significant improvements in symptoms and bone turnover markers [108]. In a study of 20 patients with acute Charcot joint, weekly oral administration of 70 mg alendronate for 6 months was associated with significant improvements in pain scores, bone turnover markers and foot bone density [109]. A randomized trial of intranasal calcitonin demonstrated efficacy with respect to bone turnover markers, but no differences in clinical variables were reported [110]. The efficacy of TNF-inhibitors and other antiresorptive agents such as the RANKL inhibitor denosumab has not yet been studied in Charcot joint, although the potential use of these agents has been recently highlighted [96].

Surgery is generally not considered first-line therapy, although one study has reported good surgical outcomes following débridement, open reduction and internal fixation with autologous bone grafting in the acute phase of disease [111]. In general, surgical management is currently recommended for patients in the reparative (rather than the acute) phase of disease, and particularly for patients with deformities associated with chronic foot ulcers and joint instability. Various surgical approaches to arthrodesis may be used, including open reduction with both internal and external fixation, depending on the presence of local infection and other anatomic variables [112]. Other surgery includes exostotomy, osteotomy, intramedullary rodding and amputation. Infection, non-union and triggering of an acute Charcot reaction are important postoperative complications, and careful postoperative management is essential.

Outcomes in patients with Charcot foot are frequently poor. A recent analysis of 115 patients reported that non-operative management was associated with a 2.7% annual rate of amputation, a 23% risk of requiring bracing for more than 18 months and a 49% risk of recurrent ulceration. The presence of open ulcers at

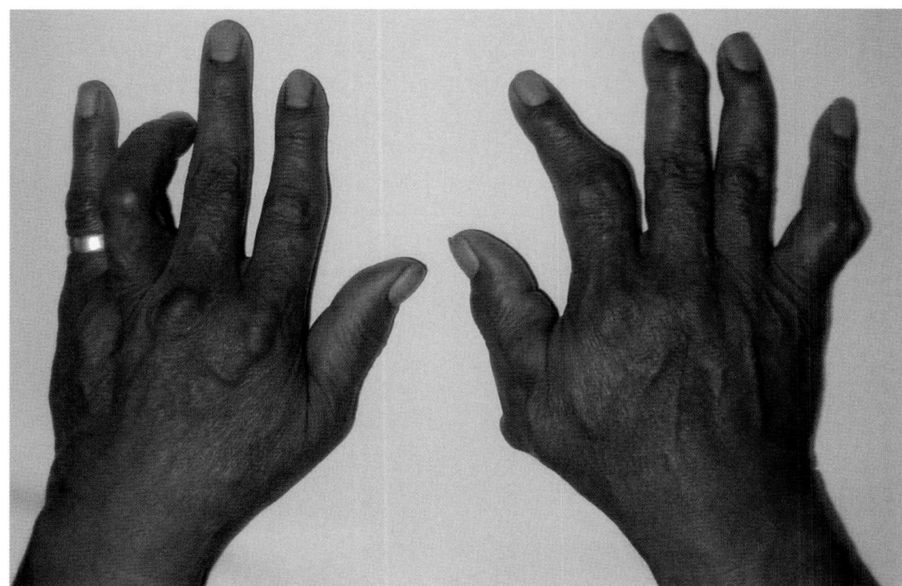

Figure 48.3 Chronic tophaceous gout of the hands in a patient with type 2 diabetes.

initial presentation or chronically recurrent ulcers is associated with increased risk for amputation [113].

Gout

Gout is an inflammatory arthritis caused by intra-articular deposition of monosodium urate (MSU) crystals [114]. This disorder is the most common form of inflammatory arthritis affecting men, and affects 1–2% of the Caucasian adult population [115]. In early disease, gout presents as recurrent episodes of self-limiting acute inflammatory attacks ("flares") of arthritis. These attacks most often affect the first MTP joint, midfoot and ankle. In the presence of prolonged hyperuricemia, some patients develop recurrent polyarticular attacks, chronic tophaceous disease and erosive arthritis (Figure 48.3).

The key risk factors for gout are hyperuricemia, male sex, chronic renal impairment, hypertension, obesity, diuretic use, coronary heart disease, and seafood, meat and alcohol intake [116–118]. The relationship between gout and metabolic syndrome is well-recognized. Serum urate concentrations and gout are strongly associated with abdominal adiposity, and have been shown to predict the development of T2DM [119–121]. Patients with gout have high rates of the metabolic syndrome and T2DM compared to individuals without gout [122]. Promotion of renal tubular reabsorption of uric acid by insulin is thought to mediate this relationship [123]. Recent identification of the glucose and fructose transporter SLC2A9 as a key regulator of serum urate concentrations suggests a further etiologic link between hyperuricemia and hyperglycemia [124]. A recent study reported a prevalence of gout of 22% in patients with T2DM treated in secondary care [125]. Key risk factors for gout in this population were male sex, renal impairment and diuretic use. Fewer than half of the patients with gout and diabetes in this study were prescribed urate-lowering therapy, and only 8% had a serum urate of <0.36 mmol/L. Interestingly, severe hyperglycemia may reduce urate concentrations, as glycosuria has a uricosuric effect. Thus, as glycemic control improves in patients initiating treatment for diabetes, there is a potential risk of worsening gout attacks [126].

Options for treatment of acute gout flares include NSAIDs, corticosteroids and/or colchicine [127]. Long-term urate-lowering therapy is indicated for patients with gout who have recurrent flares, gouty arthropathy, tophi or radiographic damage. Serum urate lowering to a concentration of <0.36 mmol/L (6 mg/dL) is needed to dissolve MSU crystals, prevent flares and achieve tophus regression. Allopurinol is the mainstay of urate-lowering therapy, but may be ineffective at recommended doses. If the serum urate target is not achieved with allopurinol alone, further options include dose escalation of allopurinol, addition of a uricosuric agent such as probenecid or benzbromarone, or consideration of the new xanthine oxidase inhibitor febuxostat [128]. Initiation of urate-lowering therapy is frequently associated with exacerbation of gout flares; this side effect can be avoided by commencement of urate-lowering therapy once the acute flare has resolved, gradual introduction of the urate-lowering drug, and co-prescription of low dose colchicine.

The presence of coexistent gout has several implications for individuals with T2DM. Poorly controlled gout may hinder attempts at exercise and weight loss. In addition to the dietary restrictions required for glycemic control, these patients also need to avoid alcohol and purine-rich foods. Diuretic therapy may exacerbate hyperuricemia and should be avoided in patients with gout unless absolutely required. Drugs such as losartan and fenofibrate have weak urate-lowering effects and may be of particular benefit in patients with diabetes and gout if antihypertensive or lipid-lowering therapy is required [129,130].

Osteoarthritis

Increased load-bearing of articular cartilage is an important risk factor for development of osteoarthritis, and a strong positive relationship has been reported between obesity and the risk of developing osteoarthritis [131–134]. Although some studies have reported an association between T2DM and osteoarthritis, most have not adequately controlled for body mass index (BMI). In most (but not all) studies that have adjusted for BMI, T2DM has not been shown to be an independent risk factor for development of osteoarthritis [131,133,135,136]. Overall, current data indicate that increased BMI, rather than T2DM, is a risk factor for development of osteoarthritis.

Rheumatoid arthritis

Rheumatoid arthritis and T1DM share several genetic associations such as *PTPN22*, *HLA-DR9*, the chromosome 4q27 region, the *IDDM5* region and the *IDDM8* region [137–141]. Furthermore, there is evidence of familial clustering of these disorders; 2.8% of first-degree relatives of probands with rheumatoid arthritis have T1DM, compared with 0.35% of the general population [142]. Despite these observations, there is little evidence that the prevalence of rheumatoid arthritis is increased in patients with T1DM [143].

Skeletal disease in diabetes

Diffuse idiopathic skeletal hyperostosis

Diffuse idiopathic skeletal hyperostosis (DISH) is a disorder characterized by increased bone formation, particularly at the entheses (the insertions of ligaments and tendons into bone) [144]. Ossification of the anterior longitudinal ligament of the spine occurs, most commonly in the thoracic spine (Figure 48.4). Extraspinal ossification may also be identified. The prevalence has been reported to be as high as 15% in women and 25% in men over the age of 50 [145].

Patients may present with back pain and stiffness, although it remains controversial whether DISH is associated with increased back pain, and the disorder is frequently detected as an incidental finding on chest radiographs [146,147]. Rare complications such as dysphagia, vocal cord paralysis, compression of the inferior vena cava and neurologic compression syndromes have been described in patients with florid hyperostosis [148]. Spinal fracture may occur after relatively minor injury and cause significant neurologic compromise [149]. The diagnosis is made radiographically, according to the Resnick criteria, which in brief are:

1 Presence of flowing calcification and ossification along the anterolateral aspects of at least four contiguous vertebral bodies;

2 Relative preservation of intervertebral disc height and the absence of extensive degenerative disc disease;

3 Absence of features of spondyloarthropathy [150].

There have been no controlled trials of therapies in patients with DISH. For symptomatic patients, analgesics and physiotherapy are standard therapy. A small uncontrolled study of patients reported that a physiotherapy program focusing on spinal mobility, stretching and strengthening had some benefits in improving lumbar spinal mobility after 24 weeks, with no significant benefits in pain or functional outcomes [151]. Surgery is rarely required, but may be indicated for compressive syndromes caused by florid hyperostosis.

Most case series have identified both obesity and T2DM as risk factors for DISH [152–154]. The presence of additional metabolic disorders such as dyslipidemia or hyperuricemia further increases the risk of DISH associated with diabetes [155]. Patients with DISH have higher rates of hyperglycemia and higher circulating insulin levels particularly after a glucose load [153,156]. It is likely that obesity has direct biomechanical effects, because of increased load at the entheses. Additionally, systemic factors may contribute to the development of DISH, as patients with this disorder have evidence of increased bone mineral density (BMD) elsewhere in the skeleton [157,158]. Insulin, growth hormone and IGF-I have been implicated in the pathogenesis of DISH, and high circulating concentrations of these hormones may contrib-

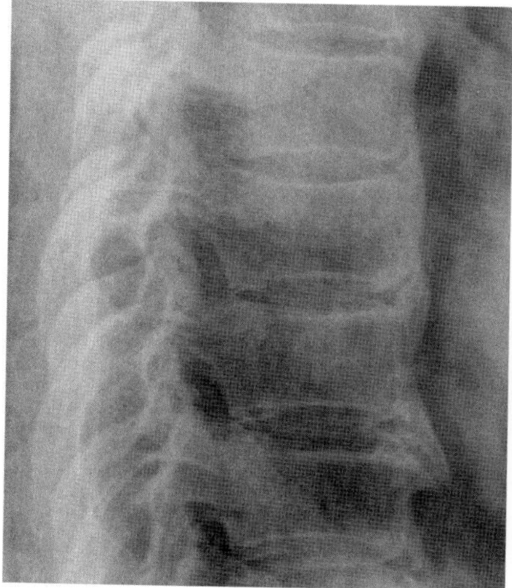

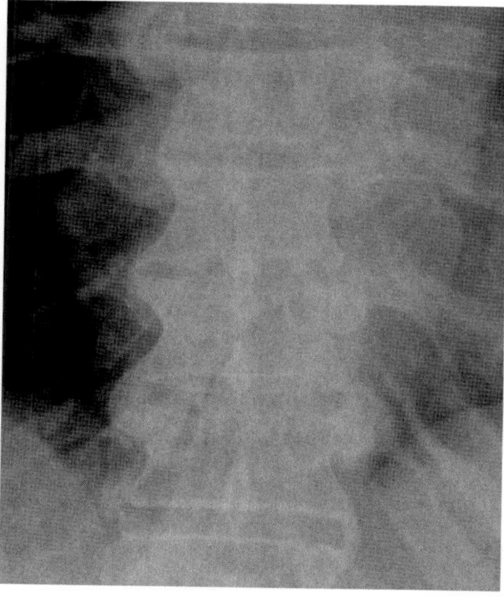

Figure 48.4 Plain radiographs of diffuse idiopathic skeletal hyperostosis (DISH) affecting the thoracic spine. Courtesy of Dr. Anthony Doyle.

ute to the development of hyperostosis [156,159,160]. High expression of nuclear factor κB (NFκB), platelet-derived growth factor BB and TGF-β1 has also been reported in affected tissue in patients with DISH, implicating these factors in osteoblast activation and new bone formation [161].

Osteoporosis and fractures

Background

Fragility fractures are a major cause of morbidity and public health expenditure. The most devastating fracture, that of the proximal femur, is associated with a 20% risk of dying within 6 months of the event, and a substantial risk of loss of independence [162]. Individual fractures are associated with considerable periods of disability and loss of productivity [163]. The number of fractures occurring annually is rising steadily, as a result both of aging of the world population, and of an age-specific increase in some countries [162].

Important risk factors for fragility fracture include low BMD, older age, female gender, light body weight, previous fracture, cigarette smoking and glucocortocoid use [162]. Dual-energy X-ray absorptiometry (DEXA) is currently the preferred modality for measurement of BMD. Recently, absolute fracture risk algorithims have been developed, using these risk factors, to provide 5–10 year estimates of the risk of any osteoporotic fracture, or of hip fracture [164,165].

Insight into the mechanism(s) by which bone loss occurs can be gained by measurement of biochemical markers of bone turnover, which reflect either osteoblast function/bone formation or osteoclast function/bone resorption. At present, bone markers are important tools in evaluating the pathogenesis and treatment of osteoporosis in clinical studies, but their utility in the management of individual patients is limited by assay variability, low predictive value for skeletal events and high cost [166].

In recent years, evidence has accrued that suggests the risk of fragility fractures is increased in both types of diabetes, albeit by different mechanisms. In addition, attention has focused recently on the skeletal effects of treatments for T2DM, in particular the thiazolidinediones.

Fracture epidemiology in diabetes

Type 1 diabetes

Two recent meta-analyses of observational studies have examined the relationship between T1DM and risk of fracture [167,168]. Hip fracture is the only fracture type evaluable in these analyses, because of the paucity of studies of other fracture types. Both meta-analyses demonstrated a substantially increased (six- to ninefold) relative risk of hip fracture in T1DM (Figure 48.5) [167,168]. Studies of other fracture types in T1DM are few in number and many include only a small number of events, but they generally support the notion that non-vertebral fracture risk is increased, with relative risk estimates of 1.3–3 for any fracture [169,170] and of 2.4 for foot fractures [171]. The only study to date to assess vertebral fracture risk in T1DM found no increase [172].

Type 2 diabetes

Until quite recently, little information was available as to the skeletal consequences of T2DM; however, recent epidemiologic studies have suggested that fracture risk is increased in that disease. Meta-analyses of these observational studies report increased risk of all fractures, and also those of the hip, forearm and foot (Figure 48.5) [167,168]. Relative risk estimates for hip fracture are lower in T2DM (1.4–1.7) than in T1DM, and estimates of fracture risk at other sites in T2DM range 1.2–1.4. Since the meta-analyses were published, the Women's Health Initiative (WHI) Observational Study, which included >5000 postmenopausal women with T2DM, reported increased risks of any fracture and of fractures at several specific sites, including the hip, spine, foot and upper arm [173]. Risk estimates ranged 1.2–1.5 across the skeletal sites. The WHI study was one of the few with the capacity to evaluate vertebral fractures. Although there was an increased risk of spine fractures in the WHI study, it remains uncertain whether risk of this fracture type is higher in T2DM, as other studies have not found an association [174].

Mechanisms of skeletal fragility in diabetes

Although fracture risk appears to be increased in both T1DM and T2DM, it is likely that there are important differences in the mechanisms by which skeletal fragility is increased in the two diseases (Table 48.2). At least two mechanisms underlie the increased skeletal fragility in T1DM. The majority of cross-sectional studies of T1DM have reported decreased BMD throughout the skeleton, although there is no consistent association between age of participants or duration of disease and magnitude of BMD deficit [175,176]. Interestingly, studies performed in children and young adults demonstrate lower than normal BMD at hip and spine at the time of diagnosis [177,178]. Taken together with the observations from longitudinal studies that BMD does not progressively decline in T1DM [179–182], and cross-sectional studies of middle-aged subjects with T1DM that report normal levels of markers of bone turnover [183–185], these data suggest that the observed deficit in BMD in T1DM occurs early in the course of the disease, and perhaps prior to its clinical presentation. It is likely that deficiency of insulin and other pancreatic β-cell hormones such as amylin and preptin, each of which has been implicated in skeletal homeostasis [186–189], contributes to the decreased BMD observed in T1DM. Recent data also implicate low levels of IGF-I in the pathogenesis of cortical bone loss in T1DM [190]. Insulin deficiency alone is probably not sufficient to explain the lower BMD, because insulin therapy does not normalize BMD. Lower body weight may also be a factor, as there is a strong positive relationship between weight and BMD [191,192].

The magnitude of the reduction in BMD (3–8%) is probably not sufficient to explain the higher rates of fracture in T1DM [176]. A second mechanism by which skeletal fragility is likely to be increased is via an increased propensity to falls as a result of disease complications. Neuropathy, visual impairment, cerebrovascular disease and hypoglycemia in particular are likely to increase falls risk. In the only study to date that has evaluated this

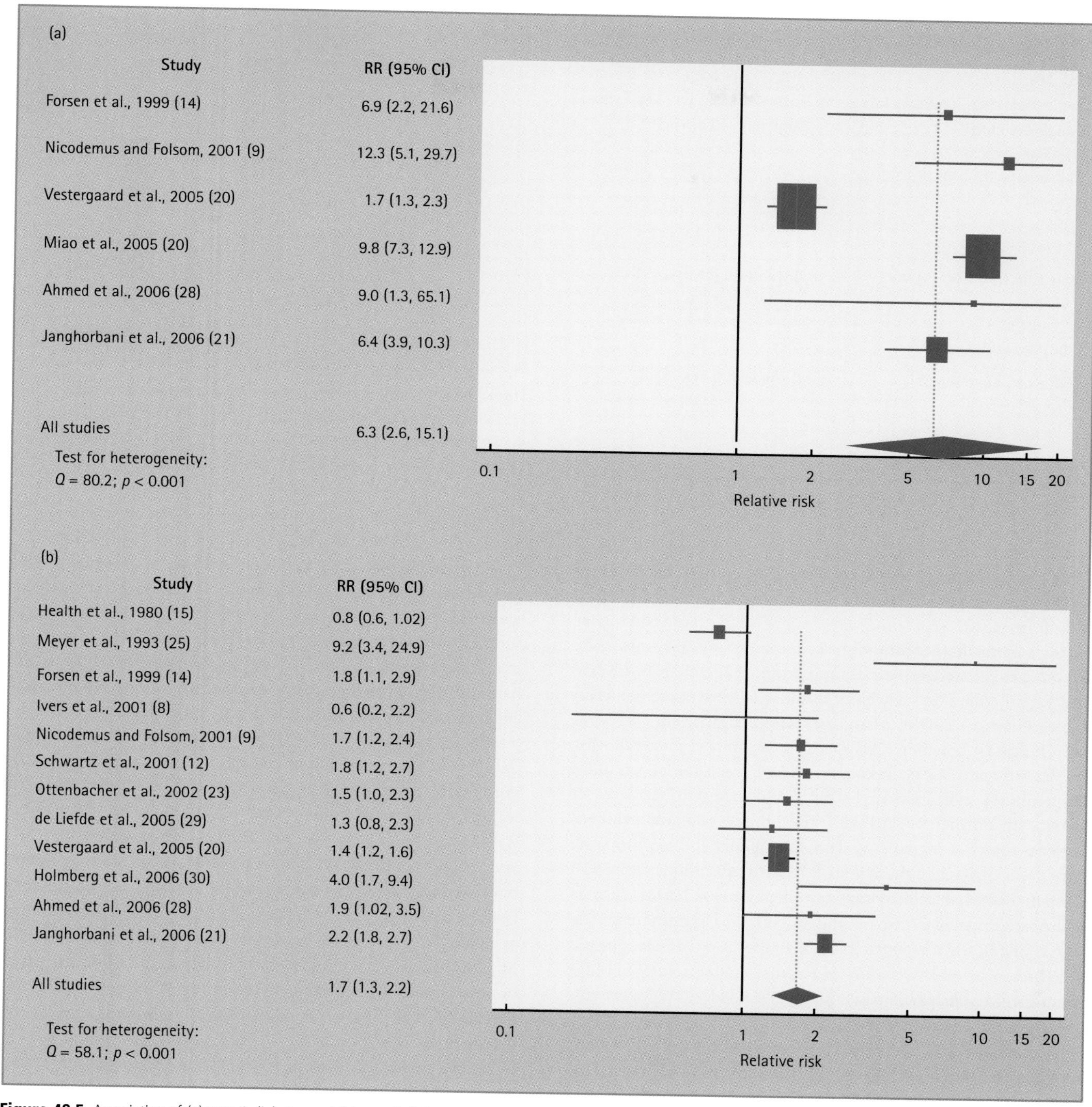

Figure 48.5 Association of (a) type 1 diabetes and (b) type 2 diabetes with hip fracture risk in meta-analyses of case–control and cohort studies. Each square shows the study-specific relative risk (RR) estimate (the size of the square reflects the study-specific statistical weight, i.e. the inverse of the variance), and the horizontal line shows the related 95% confidence interval (CI). The diamond shows the summary RR estimate, and its width represents the corresponding 95% CI. Reproduced from Janghorbani *et al.* [168], with permission from Oxford University Press.

possibility, substantially higher risks of hip fracture were observed in T1DM with a range of disease complications than in those without complications [193]. Neuropathy may also impact adversely on BMD in the distal limbs, as patients with T1DM and neuropathy have lower cortical bone mass in the distal limbs than those without neuropathy [194]. Animal studies suggest that interruption of nerve supply to bone decreases regional bone mass independent of changes in mechanical loading [195]. The presence of regional osteopenia likely contributes to the increased risk of distal limb and foot fractures in T1DM.

Table 48.2 Mechanisms of increased skeletal fragility in diabetes.

Type 1 diabetes	Type 2 diabetes
Decreased BMD	**Regional osteopenia**
Lower body weight	Secondary to neuropathy
Pancreatic β-cell hormone deficiency	
Low levels of IGF-I	
Regional osteopenia secondary to neuropathy	
Increased falls risk	**Increased falls risk**
Disease complications	Disease complications
Hypoglycemia	Hypoglycemia (insulin-treated)
Other medications	Other medications
Decreased bone quality	**Decreased bone quality**
Advanced glycation end-products	Advanced glycation end-products
	Disease treatment
	Thiazolidinediones

BMD, bone mineral density; IGF, insulin-like growth factor.

The mechanism(s) by which skeletal fragility is increased in T2DM is uncertain (Table 48.2). The observation that fracture risk in increased is in some ways surprising, because the higher body weight that commonly accompanies T2DM might be expected to preserve bone mass and protect patients from adverse skeletal outcomes. In fact, BMD in the axial skeleton *is* higher in subjects with T2DM than in subjects without diabetes [167,173,174]; however, BMD remains an important risk factor for fracture in T2DM, because incident fractures occur more frequently in subjects with T2DM and decreased BMD than in those with normal BMD [196]. The limited available evidence suggests that T2DM patients with neuropathy and nephropathy have lower BMD than those free of these complications [167,197].

As in T1DM, it is likely that complications of T2DM, such as neuropathy, vascular disease and impaired vision, increase the risk of falling, and thereby of fracture. In the Study of Osteoporotic Fractures, a prospective study of fracture epidemiology in older American women, participants with T2DM had a 22% higher risk of non-spine fractures than participants without diabetes [174]. Participants with T2DM who were treated with insulin had both a higher prevalence of disease complications and a higher risk of fracture than those with T2DM who were not treated with insulin. In the Health ABC study, a prospective study of older (>70 years) American men and women, there were strikingly higher prevalences of neuropathy, cerebrovascular disease and falls in participants with T2DM who developed a fracture than in those with T2DM who did not fracture [196]. Many risk factors for falls, including use of medications associated with increased falls risk, are more commonly present in those with T2DM than in the population without diabetes [198]. Low-impact falls are more frequent in insulin-treated patients with diabetes than healthy controls [199]. Curiously, adjusting for diabetes complications and/or falls risk did not attenuate the increased fracture risks observed in T2DM [174,196].

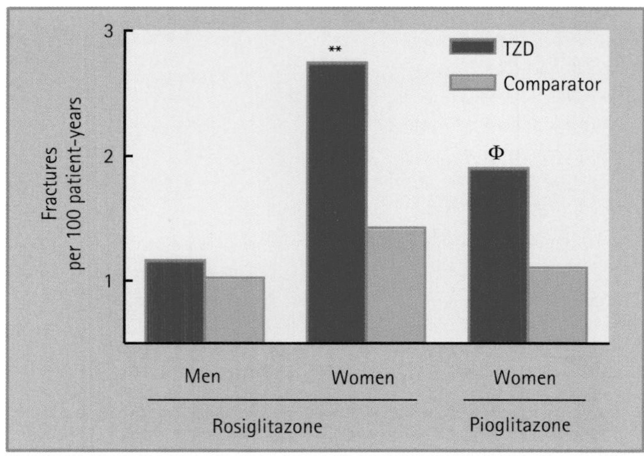

Figure 48.6 Fracture rates, captured as adverse events, in randomized controlled trials of thiazolidinediones (TZDs). **, P <0.01 vs comparator; Φ, significantly higher than comparators. Reproduced from Grey [208], with permission from Wiley-Blackwell Publishing Ltd.

It is possible that aspects of bone strength and/or quality that are not captured by DEXA assessment are abnormal in patients with either type of diabetes, and contribute to increased bone fragility. At present, there is no validated methodology for assessing these aspects of bone quality. Potentially relevant to this hypothesis is a growing body of evidence that advanced glycation end-products (AGE), products of non-enzymatic glycation, are present in greater amounts in the skeletons of diabetic animals than those of non-diabetic animals [200]. The glycation of matrix proteins in bone may alter biomechanical properties in such a way as to decrease bone strength [201,202]. *In vitro* studies suggest that AGEs inhibit differentiation of osteoblasts [200,203] and increase differentiation of osteoclasts [204], thereby potentially altering bone remodeling and/or strength in a detrimental fashion. There may be AGE-specific effects on bone remodeling, as pentosidine decreases osteoclast development *in vitro* [205]; however, mice deficient in the receptor for AGE exhibit increased bone mass and decreased osteoclast function, suggesting that the overall effect of increased AGE signaling in bone is likely to be detrimental [206].

Finally, in T2DM, there is clear evidence that treatment with either of the currently available thiazolidinediones (TZDs), rosiglitazone and pioglitazone, increases fracture risk, at least in women [207,208]. Data collected as adverse events during the conduct of randomized controlled trials of each TZD in middle-aged populations of those with T2DM demonstrated a twofold increase in risk of distal limb fractures in women, although not in men (Figure 48.6) [209–211]. Observational data from an older cohort of patients with T2DM suggest that fracture risk is also increased in men exposed to TZDs, and that the incidence of "classic" osteoporotic fractures (hip, forearm, humerus) is also higher in TZD users [212].

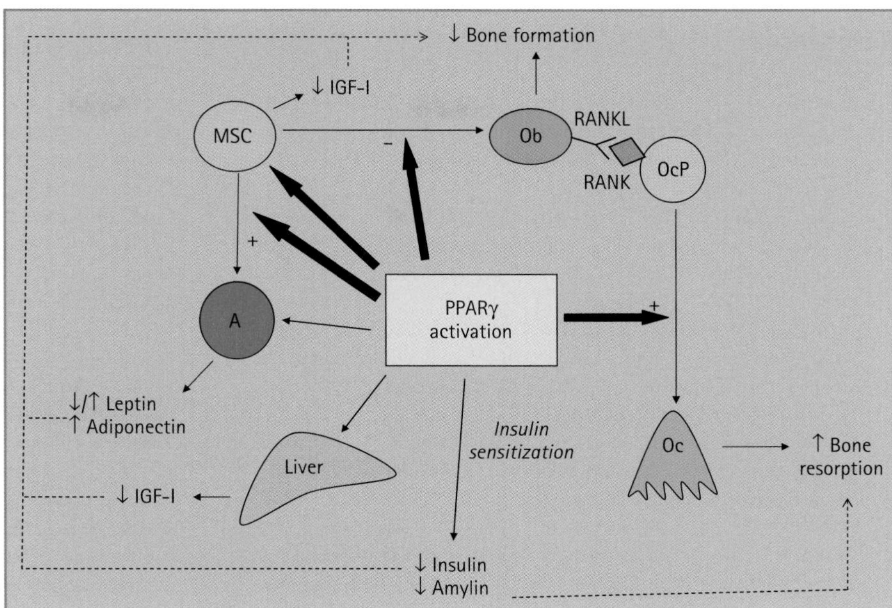

Figure 48.7 Mechanisms by which peroxisome proliferator-activated receptor γ (PPARγ) regulates bone metabolism. Within the bone microenvironment [black arrows], activation of PPARγ signaling promotes differentiation of mesenchymal stem cells (MSC) into adipocytes (A) at the expense of osteoblasts (Ob), decreases stromal cell production of IGF-I, and promotes differentiation of osteoclast precursors (OcP) into mature bone-resorbing osteoclasts (Oc). The net effect is to decrease bone formation and increase bone resorption. Activation of PPARγ signaling at extraskeletal sites such as adipose tissue and the liver, and the ensuing effects of insulin sensitization on the β-cells of the pancreas [regular arrows] may indirectly impact on the skeleton [interrupted arrows] by altering circulating levels of several hormones and cytokines, as indicated. RANK, receptor activator of NFκB; RANKL, receptor activator of NFκB ligand. Reproduced from Grey [208], with permission from Wiley-Blackwell Publishing Ltd.

The mechanisms underlying the adverse skeletal effects of TZDs are complex, and likely to involve both direct and indirect pathways (Figure 48.7). Of primary importance is the effect of the TZDs to inhibit bone formation directly, by diverting mesenchymal stem cell precursors from the osteoblast to the adipocyte lineage [207]. A substantial body of preclinical studies in rodents, and data accruing from studies in humans, demonstrates that TZDs decrease bone formation and BMD *in vivo* [207]. In addition, TZDs increase or maintain bone resorption at inappropriately elevated levels, via direct actions on osteoclast development [207,213]. Indirect actions of TZDs that potentially contribute to their detrimental skeletal effects include decreasing systemic and skeletal production of IGF-I, modulating production of skeletally active adipokines and decreasing levels of pancreatic β-cell hormones with known skeletal activity [208].

The skeletal toxicity of TZDs has prompted interest in the effects of other oral hypoglycemic agents on bone health. At present, the available data suggest that metformin and sulfonylureas are neutral in regard to the skeleton [214].

Investigation and management of osteoporosis in diabetes

Diabetes of either type should be regarded as a risk factor for fragility fracture, and included in clinical fracture risk assessment, along with recognized risk factors such as age, gender, body weight, previous fracture, cigarette smoking, glucocorticoid use and BMD. Recently developed fracture risk algorithms may be helpful in determining an individual patient's short to medium-term absolute fracture risk [164,165]. Although BMD is on average increased in T2DM, measurement of BMD in patients with T2DM is still helpful in defining that person's fracture risk. Prescription of TZDs to patients with T2DM who are found to be at high risk of fracture should be avoided unless there are compelling reasons to do so. Minimizing falls risk is an important component of skeletal management in diabetes – this can be achieved by targeting both macrovascular and microvascular disease complications, minimizing the risk of hypoglycemia, optimizing visual acuity and minimizing use of other medications known to be associated with falls. Although there are no data from interventional studies on the effects of pharmacologic treatments of osteoporosis in diabetes, it is reasonable to assume that agents known to prevent fractures in non-diabetic osteoporotic populations, such as bisphosphonates, will also be effective in those with diabetes [162].

Fracture healing in diabetes

A growing body of evidence suggests that fracture healing is abnormal in those with diabetes. In rat models of T1DM, the mechanical and structural properties of the healing bone are inferior in the diabetic rats when compared with control animals, findings that are accompanied by evidence of both decreased callus size and collagen content [215,216]. Interventional studies demonstrate that therapy with insulin to achieve normoglycemia is associated with fracture healing that is indistinguishable from that observed in non-diabetic animals [217,218]. Subsequently, administration of insulin at the site of skeletal injury was also shown to promote fracture healing, without altering serum glucose, implying a role for insulin in directly mediating bone repair [219]. Few data are available from human studies, but increased rates of fracture non-union in both T1DM and T2DM have been reported [220], as have higher than expected rates of serious complications in patients with diabetes and open ankle fractures [221]. Further investigation of the influence of diabetes and its treatment on fracture repair in humans is needed.

References

1 Rosenbloom AL, Silverstein JH, Lezotte DC, Richardson K, McCallum M. Limited joint mobility in childhood diabetes mellitus indicates increased risk for microvascular disease. *N Engl J Med* 1981; **305**:191–194.

2 Collier A, Matthews DM, Kellett HA, Clarke BF, Hunter JA. Change in skin thickness associated with cheiroarthropathy in insulin dependent diabetes mellitus. *Br Med J (Clin Res Ed)* 1986; **292**: 936.

3 Schulte L, Roberts MS, Zimmerman C, Ketler J, Simon LS. A quantitative assessment of limited joint mobility in patients with diabetes: goniometric analysis of upper extremity passive range of motion. *Arthritis Rheum* 1993; **36**:1429–1443.

4 Schnapf BM, Banks RA, Silverstein JH, Rosenbloom AL, Chesrown SE, Loughlin GM. Pulmonary function in insulin-dependent diabetes mellitus with limited joint mobility. *Am Rev Respir Dis* 1984; **130**:930–932.

5 Trapp RG, Soler NG, Spencer-Green G. Nailfold capillaroscopy in type I diabetics with vasculopathy and limited joint mobility. *J Rheumatol* 1986; **13**:917–920.

6 Gertner E, Sukenik S, Gladman DD, Hanna W, Lee P, Bomardier C, *et al.* HLA antigens and nailfold capillary microscopy studies in patients with insulin dependent and noninsulin dependent diabetes mellitus and limited joint mobility. *J Rheumatol* 1990; **17**: 1375–1379.

7 Grgic A, Rosenbloom AL, Weber FT, Giordano B, Malone JI, Shuster JJ. Joint contracture: common manifestation of childhood diabetes mellitus. *J Pediatr* 1976; **88**:584–588.

8 Rosenbloom AL. Limited joint mobility in insulin dependent childhood diabetes. *Eur J Pediatr* 1990; **149**:380–388.

9 Garza-Elizondo MA, Diaz-Jouanen E, Franco-Casique JJ, Alarcon-Segovia D. Joint contractures and scleroderma-like skin changes in the hands of insulin-dependent juvenile diabetics. *J Rheumatol* 1983; **10**:797–800.

10 Arkkila PE, Kantola IM, Viikari JS. Limited joint mobility in non-insulin-dependent diabetic (NIDDM) patients: correlation to control of diabetes, atherosclerotic vascular disease, and other diabetic complications. *J Diabetes Complications* 1997; **11**:208–217.

11 Larkin JG, Frier BM. Limited joint mobility and Dupuytren's contracture in diabetic, hypertensive, and normal populations. *Br Med J (Clin Res Ed)* 1986; **292**:1494.

12 Lindsay JR, Kennedy L, Atkinson AB, Bell PM, Carson DJ, McCance DR, *et al.* Reduced prevalence of limited joint mobility in type 1 diabetes in a UK clinic population over a 20-year period. *Diabetes Care* 2005; **28**:658–661.

13 Rosenbloom AL, Malone JI, Yucha J, Van Cader TC. Limited joint mobility and diabetic retinopathy demonstrated by fluorescein angiography. *Eur J Pediatr* 1984; **141**:163–164.

14 Arkkila PE, Kantola IM, Viikari JS, Ronnemaa T, Vahatalo MA. Limited joint mobility is associated with the presence but does not predict the development of microvascular complications in type 1 diabetes. *Diabet Med* 1996; **13**:828–833.

15 Eadington DW, Patrick AW, Collier A, Frier BM. Limited joint mobility, Dupuytren's contracture and retinopathy in type 1 diabetes: association with cigarette smoking. *Diabet Med* 1989; **6**:152–157.

16 Pal B, Anderson J, Dick WC, Griffiths ID. Limitation of joint mobility and shoulder capsulitis in insulin- and non-insulin-dependent diabetes mellitus. *Br J Rheumatol* 1986; **25**:147–151.

17 Pal B, Griffiths ID, Anderson J, Dick WC. Association of limited joint mobility with Dupuytren's contracture in diabetes mellitus. *J Rheumatol* 1987; **14**:582–585.

18 Chaudhuri KR, Davidson AR, Morris IM. Limited joint mobility and carpal tunnel syndrome in insulin-dependent diabetes. *Br J Rheumatol* 1989; **28**:191–194.

19 Cagliero E, Apruzzese W, Perlmutter GS, Nathan DM. Musculoskeletal disorders of the hand and shoulder in patients with diabetes mellitus. *Am J Med* 2002; **112**:487–490.

20 Jennings AM, Milner PC, Ward JD. Hand abnormalities are associated with the complications of diabetes in type 2 diabetes. *Diabet Med* 1989; **6**:43–47.

21 Savas S, Koroglu BK, Koyuncuoglu HR, Uzar E, Celik H, Tamer NM. The effects of the diabetes related soft tissue hand lesions and the reduced hand strength on functional disability of hand in type 2 diabetic patients. *Diabetes Res Clin Pract* 2007; **77**:77–83.

22 Silverstein JH, Gordon G, Pollock BH, Rosenbloom AL. Long-term glycemic control influences the onset of limited joint mobility in type 1 diabetes. *J Pediatr* 1998; **132**:944–947.

23 Campbell RR, Hawkins SJ, Maddison PJ, Reckless JP. Limited joint mobility in diabetes mellitus. *Ann Rheum Dis* 1985; **44**:93–97.

24 Rosenbloom AL, Silverstein JH, Lezotte DC, Riley WJ, Maclaren NK. Limited joint mobility in diabetes mellitus of childhood: natural history and relationship to growth impairment. *J Pediatr* 1982; **101**:874–878.

25 Khanna G, Ferguson P. MRI of diabetic cheiroarthropathy. *AJR Am J Roentgenol* 2007; **188**:W94–95.

26 Ismail AA, Dasgupta B, Tanqueray AB, Hamblin JJ. Ultrasonographic features of diabetic cheiroarthropathy. *Br J Rheumatol* 1996; **35**:676–679.

27 Vera M, Shumkov G, Guell R. Histological and histochemical skin changes in insulin-dependent diabetic patients with and without limited joint mobility. *Acta Diabetol Lat* 1987; **24**:101–108.

28 Sell DR, Lapolla A, Odetti P, Fogarty J, Monnier VM. Pentosidine formation in skin correlates with severity of complications in individuals with long-standing IDDM. *Diabetes* 1992; **41**: 1286–1292.

29 Bertheim U, Engstrom-Laurent A, Hofer PA, Hallgren P, Asplund J, Hellstrom S. Loss of hyaluronan in the basement membrane zone of the skin correlates to the degree of stiff hands in diabetic patients. *Acta Derm Venereol* 2002; **82**:329–334.

30 Priestley GC, Collier A, Matthews DM, Clarke BF. Increased urinary excretion of glycosaminoglycans in insulin-dependent diabetic patients with limited joint mobility. *Br J Rheumatol* 1988; **27**:462–464.

31 Amin R, Bahu TK, Widmer B, Dalton RN, Dunger DB. Longitudinal relation between limited joint mobility, height, insulin-like growth factor 1 levels, and risk of developing microalbuminuria: the Oxford Regional Prospective Study. *Arch Dis Child* 2005; **90**:1039–1044.

32 Mitchell WS, Winocour PH, Gush RJ, Taylor LJ, Baker RD, Anderson DC, *et al.* Skin blood flow and limited joint mobility in insulin-dependent diabetes mellitus. *Br J Rheumatol* 1989; **28**:195–200.

33 Infante JR, Rosenbloom AL, Silverstein JH, Garzarella L, Pollock BH. Changes in frequency and severity of limited joint mobility in children with type 1 diabetes mellitus between 1976–78 and 1998. *J Pediatr* 2001; **138**:33–37.

34 Sibbitt WL Jr, Eaton RP. Corticosteroid responsive tenosynovitis is a common pathway for limited joint mobility in the diabetic hand. *J Rheumatol* 1997; **24**:931–936.

35 Dias R, Cutts S, Massoud S. Frozen shoulder. *Br Med J* 2005; **331**:1453–1456.

36 Reeves B. The natural history of the frozen shoulder syndrome. *Scand J Rheumatol* 1975; **4**:193–196.

37 Hand C, Clipsham K, Rees JL, Carr AJ. Long-term outcome of frozen shoulder. *J Shoulder Elbow Surg* 2008; **17**:231–236.

38 Shaffer B, Tibone JE, Kerlan RK. Frozen shoulder: a long-term follow-up. *J Bone Joint Surg Am* 1992; **74**:738–746.

39 Bunker TD, Anthony PP. The pathology of frozen shoulder: a Dupuytren-like disease. *J Bone Joint Surg Br* 1995; **77**:677–683.

40 Hand GC, Athanasou NA, Matthews T, Carr AJ. The pathology of frozen shoulder. *J Bone Joint Surg Br* 2007; **89**:928–932.

41 Kilian O, Pfeil U, Wenisch S, Heiss C, Kraus R, Schnettler R. Enhanced alpha 1(I) mRNA expression in frozen shoulder and Dupuytren tissue. *Eur J Med Res* 2007; **12**:585–590.

42 Ryu JD, Kirpalani PA, Kim JM, Nam KH, Han CW, Han SH. Expression of vascular endothelial growth factor and angiogenesis in the diabetic frozen shoulder. *J Shoulder Elbow Surg* 2006; **15**:679–685.

43 Ryans I, Montgomery A, Galway R, Kernohan WG, McKane R. A randomized controlled trial of intra-articular triamcinolone and/or physiotherapy in shoulder capsulitis. *Rheumatology (Oxford)* 2005; **44**:529–535.

44 Diercks RL, Stevens M. Gentle thawing of the frozen shoulder: a prospective study of supervised neglect versus intensive physical therapy in 77 patients with frozen shoulder syndrome followed up for 2 years. *J Shoulder Elbow Surg* 2004; **13**:499–502.

45 Buchbinder R, Green S, Youd JM, Johnston RV. Oral steroids for adhesive capsulitis. *Cochrane Database Syst Rev* 2006; CD006189.

46 Buchbinder R, Green S, Youd JM, Johnston RV, Cumpston M. Arthrographic distension for adhesive capsulitis (frozen shoulder). *Cochrane Database Syst Rev* 2008; CD007005.

47 Pollock RG, Duralde XA, Flatow EL, Bigliani LU. The use of arthroscopy in the treatment of resistant frozen shoulder. *Clin Orthop Relat Res* 1994; **304**:30–36.

48 Sattar MA, Luqman WA. Periarthritis: another duration-related complication of diabetes mellitus. *Diabetes Care* 1985; **8**:507–510.

49 Aydeniz A, Gursoy S, Guney E. Which musculoskeletal complications are most frequently seen in type 2 diabetes mellitus? *J Int Med Res* 2008; **36**:505–511.

50 Balci N, Balci MK, Tuzuner S. Shoulder adhesive capsulitis and shoulder range of motion in type II diabetes mellitus: association with diabetic complications. *J Diabetes Complications* 1999; **13**:135–140.

51 Moren-Hybbinette I, Moritz U, Schersten B. The clinical picture of the painful diabetic shoulder: natural history, social consequences and analysis of concomitant hand syndrome. *Acta Med Scand* 1987; **221**:73–82.

52 Griggs SM, Ahn A, Green A. Idiopathic adhesive capsulitis: a prospective functional outcome study of nonoperative treatment. *J Bone Joint Surg Am* 2000; **82A**:1398–1407.

53 Townley WA, Baker R, Sheppard N, Grobbelaar AO. Dupuytren's contracture unfolded. *Br Med J* 2006; **332**:397–400.

54 Brickley-Parsons D, Glimcher MJ, Smith RJ, Albin R, Adams JP. Biochemical changes in the collagen of the palmar fascia in patients with Dupuytren's disease. *J Bone Joint Surg Am* 1981; **63**:787–797.

55 Bisson MA, McGrouther DA, Mudera V, Grobbelaar AO. The different characteristics of Dupuytren's disease fibroblasts derived from either nodule or cord: expression of alpha-smooth muscle actin and the response to stimulation by TGF-β1. *J Hand Surg (Br)* 2003; **28**:351–356.

56 Baird KS, Crossan JF, Ralston SH. Abnormal growth factor and cytokine expression in Dupuytren's contracture. *J Clin Pathol* 1993; **46**:425–428.

57 Badalamente MA, Hurst LC. Efficacy and safety of injectable mixed collagenase subtypes in the treatment of Dupuytren's contracture. *J Hand Surg (Am)* 2007; **32**:767–774.

58 Ketchum LD, Donahue TK. The injection of nodules of Dupuytren's disease with triamcinolone acetonide. *J Hand Surg (Am)* 2000; **25**:1157–1162.

59 van Rijssen AL, Gerbrandy FS, Ter Linden H, Klip H, Werker PM. A comparison of the direct outcomes of percutaneous needle fasciotomy and limited fasciectomy for Dupuytren's disease: a 6-week follow-up study. *J Hand Surg (Am)* 2006; **31**:717–725.

60 van Rijssen AL, Werker PM. Percutaneous needle fasciotomy in Dupuytren's disease. *J Hand Surg (Br)* 2006; **31**:498–501.

61 Noble J, Heathcote JG, Cohen H. Diabetes mellitus in the aetiology of Dupuytren's disease. *J Bone Joint Surg Br* 1984; **66**:322–325.

62 Chammas M, Bousquet P, Renard E, Poirier JL, Jaffiol C, Allieu Y. Dupuytren's disease, carpal tunnel syndrome, trigger finger, and diabetes mellitus. *J Hand Surg (Am)* 1995; **20**:109–114.

63 Arkkila PE, Kantola IM, Viikari JS. Dupuytren's disease: association with chronic diabetic complications. *J Rheumatol* 1997; **24**:153–159.

64 Arkkila PE, Kantola IM, Viikari JS, Ronnemaa T, Vahatalo MA. Dupuytren's disease in type 1 diabetic patients: a five-year prospective study. *Clin Exp Rheumatol* 1996; **14**:59–65.

65 Fleisch SB, Spindler KP, Lee DH. Corticosteroid injections in the treatment of trigger finger: a level I and II systematic review. *J Am Acad Orthop Surg* 2007; **15**:166–171.

66 Akhtar S, Bradley MJ, Quinton DN, Burke FD. Management and referral for trigger finger/thumb. *Br Med J* 2005; **331**:30–33.

67 Sampson SP, Badalamente MA, Hurst LC, Seidman J. Pathobiology of the human A1 pulley in trigger finger. *J Hand Surg (Am)* 1991; **16**:714–721.

68 Anderson B, Kaye S. Treatment of flexor tenosynovitis of the hand ('trigger finger') with corticosteroids: a prospective study of the response to local injection. *Arch Intern Med* 1991; **151**:153–156.

69 Gilberts EC, Beekman WH, Stevens HJ, Wereldsma JC. Prospective randomized trial of open versus percutaneous surgery for trigger digits. *J Hand Surg (Am)* 2001; **26**:497–500.

70 Renard E, Jacques D, Chammas M, Poirier JL, Bonifacj C, Jaffiol C, *et al.* Increased prevalence of soft tissue hand lesions in type 1 and type 2 diabetes mellitus: various entities and associated significance. *Diabete Metab* 1994; **20**:513–521.

71 Rozental TD, Zurakowski D, Blazar PE. Trigger finger: prognostic indicators of recurrence following corticosteroid injection. *J Bone Joint Surg Am* 2008; **90**:1665–1672.

72 Baumgarten KM, Gerlach D, Boyer MI. Corticosteroid injection in diabetic patients with trigger finger: a prospective, randomized, controlled double-blinded study. *J Bone Joint Surg Am* 2007; **89**:2604–2611.

73 Stahl S, Kanter Y, Karnielli E. Outcome of trigger finger treatment in diabetes. *J Diabetes Complications* 1997; **11**:287–290.

74 Bland JD. Carpal tunnel syndrome. *Br Med J* 2007; **335**:343–346.

75 Ettema AM, Amadio PC, Zhao C, Wold LE, An KN. A histological and immunohistochemical study of the subsynovial connective tissue in idiopathic carpal tunnel syndrome. *J Bone Joint Surg Am* 2004; **86A**:1458–1466.

76 Jablecki CK, Andary MT, Floeter MK, Miller RG, Quartly CA, Vennix MJ, *et al.* Practice parameter: Electrodiagnostic studies in carpal tunnel syndrome. Report of the American Association of Electrodiagnostic Medicine, American Academy of Neurology, and the American Academy of Physical Medicine and Rehabilitation. *Neurology* 2002; **58**:1589–1592.

77 Piazzini DB, Aprile I, Ferrara PE, Bertolini C, Tonali P, Maggi L, *et al.* A systematic review of conservative treatment of carpal tunnel syndrome. *Clin Rehabil* 2007; **21**:299–314.

78 Wong SM, Hui AC, Tang A, Ho PC, Hung LK, Wong KS, *et al.* Local vs systemic corticosteroids in the treatment of carpal tunnel syndrome. *Neurology* 2001; **56**:1565–1567.

79 Marshall S, Tardif G, Ashworth N. Local corticosteroid injection for carpal tunnel syndrome. *Cochrane Database Syst Rev* 2007; CD001554.

80 Verdugo RJ, Salinas RA, Castillo JL, Cea JG. Surgical versus non-surgical treatment for carpal tunnel syndrome. *Cochrane Database Syst Rev* 2008; CD001552.

81 Scholten RJ, Mink van der Molen A, Uitdehaag BM, Bouter LM, de Vet HC. Surgical treatment options for carpal tunnel syndrome. *Cochrane Database Syst Rev* 2007; CD003905.

82 Phalen GS. Reflections on 21 years' experience with the carpal-tunnel syndrome. *Jama* 1970; **212**:1365–1367.

83 Makepeace A, Davis WA, Bruce DG, Davis TM. Incidence and determinants of carpal tunnel decompression surgery in type 2 diabetes: the Fremantle Diabetes Study. *Diabetes Care* 2008; **31**:498–500.

84 Singh R, Gamble G, Cundy T. Lifetime risk of symptomatic carpal tunnel syndrome in type 1 diabetes. *Diabet Med* 2005; **22**:625–630.

85 Perkins BA, Olaleye D, Bril V. Carpal tunnel syndrome in patients with diabetic polyneuropathy. *Diabetes Care* 2002; **25**:565–569.

86 Comi G, Lozza L, Galardi G, Ghilardi MF, Medaglini S, Canal N. Presence of carpal tunnel syndrome in diabetics: effect of age, sex, diabetes duration and polyneuropathy. *Acta Diabetol Lat* 1985; **22**:259–262.

87 Edwards A. Phalen's test with carpal compression: testing in diabetics for the diagnosis of carpal tunnel syndrome. *Orthopedics* 2002; **25**:519–520.

88 Mondelli M, Padua L, Reale F, Signorini AM, Romano C. Outcome of surgical release among diabetics with carpal tunnel syndrome. *Arch Phys Med Rehabil* 2004; **85**:7–13.

89 Haupt WF, Wintzer G, Schop A, Lottgen J, Pawlik G. Long-term results of carpal tunnel decompression: assessment of 60 cases. *J Hand Surg (Br)* 1993; **18**:471–474.

90 Ozkul Y, Sabuncu T, Yazgan P, Nazligul Y. Local insulin injection improves median nerve regeneration in NIDDM patients with carpal tunnel syndrome. *Eur J Neurol* 2001; **8**:329–334.

91 Hartemann-Heurtier A, Van GH, Grimaldi A. The Charcot foot. *Lancet* 2002; **360**:1776–1779.

92 Eichenholtz SN. *Charcot Joints.* Springfield, IL: Thomas, 1966.

93 Sella EJ, Barrette C. Staging of Charcot neuroarthropathy along the medial column of the foot in the diabetic patient. *J Foot Ankle Surg* 1999; **38**:34–40.

94 Sanders LJ, Frykberg RG. Charcot neuroarthropathy of the foot. In: Bowker JH, Pfeifer MA, eds. *Levin and O'Neal's The Diabetic Foot*, 6th edn. St Louis: Mosby, 2001.

95 Chantelau E, Onvlee GJ. Charcot foot in diabetes: farewell to the neurotrophic theory. *Horm Metab Res* 2006; **38**:361–367.

96 Jeffcoate WJ, Game F, Cavanagh PR. The role of proinflammatory cytokines in the cause of neuropathic osteoarthropathy (acute Charcot foot) in diabetes. *Lancet* 2005; **366**:2058–2061.

97 Chantelau E, Richter A, Ghassem-Zadeh N, Poll LW. "Silent" bone stress injuries in the feet of diabetic patients with polyneuropathy: a report on 12 cases. *Arch Orthop Trauma Surg* 2007; **127**:171–177.

98 Beltran J, Campanini DS, Knight C, McCalla M. The diabetic foot: magnetic resonance imaging evaluation. *Skeletal Radiol* 1990; **19**:37–41.

99 Chantelau E, Poll LW. Evaluation of the diabetic charcot foot by MR imaging or plain radiography: an observational study. *Exp Clin Endocrinol Diabetes* 2006; **114**:428–431.

100 Schlossbauer T, Mioc T, Sommerey S, Kessler SB, Reiser MF, Pfeifer KJ. Magnetic resonance imaging in early stage charcot arthropathy: correlation of imaging findings and clinical symptoms. *Eur J Med Res* 2008; **13**:409–414.

101 Baumhauer JF, O'Keefe RJ, Schon LC, Pinzur MS. Cytokine-induced osteoclastic bone resorption in charcot arthropathy: an immunohistochemical study. *Foot Ankle Int* 2006; **27**:797–800.

102 Mabilleau G, Petrova NL, Edmonds ME, Sabokbar A. Increased osteoclastic activity in acute Charcot's osteoarthropathy: the role of receptor activator of nuclear factor-κB ligand. *Diabetologia* 2008; **51**:1035–1040.

103 Gough A, Abraha H, Li F, Purewal TS, Foster AV, Watkins PJ, *et al.* Measurement of markers of osteoclast and osteoblast activity in patients with acute and chronic diabetic Charcot neuroarthropathy. *Diabet Med* 1997; **14**:527–531.

104 Petrova NL, Moniz C, Elias DA, Buxton-Thomas M, Bates M, Edmonds ME. Is there a systemic inflammatory response in the acute charcot foot? *Diabetes Care* 2007; **30**:997–998.

105 Petrova NL, Edmonds ME. Charcot neuro-osteoarthropathy-current standards. *Diabetes Metab Res Rev* 2008; **24**(Suppl 1): S58–61.

106 Pinzur MS, Lio T, Posner M. Treatment of Eichenholtz stage I Charcot foot arthropathy with a weightbearing total contact cast. *Foot Ankle Int* 2006; **27**:324–329.

107 de Souza LJ. Charcot arthropathy and immobilization in a weight-bearing total contact cast. *J Bone Joint Surg Am* 2008; **90**:754–759.

108 Jude EB, Selby PL, Burgess J, Lilleystone P, Mawer EB, Page SR, *et al.* Bisphosphonates in the treatment of Charcot neuroarthropathy: a double-blind randomised controlled trial. *Diabetologia* 2001; **44**:2032–2037.

109 Pitocco D, Ruotolo V, Caputo S, Mancini L, Collina CM, Manto A, *et al.* Six-month treatment with alendronate in acute Charcot neuroarthropathy: a randomized controlled trial. *Diabetes Care* 2005; **28**:1214–1215.

110 Bem R, Jirkovska A, Fejfarova V, Skibova J, Jude EB. Intranasal calcitonin in the treatment of acute Charcot neuroosteoarthropathy: a randomized controlled trial. *Diabetes Care* 2006; **29**:1392–1394.

111 Simon SR, Tejwani SG, Wilson DL, Santner TJ, Denniston NL. Arthrodesis as an early alternative to nonoperative management of charcot arthropathy of the diabetic foot. *J Bone Joint Surg Am* 2000; **82A**:939–950.

112 Wang JC, Le AW, Tsukuda RK. A new technique for Charcot's foot reconstruction. *J Am Podiatr Med Assoc* 2002; **92**:429–436.

113 Saltzman CL, Hagy ML, Zimmerman B, Estin M, Cooper R. How effective is intensive nonoperative initial treatment of patients with

diabetes and Charcot arthropathy of the feet? *Clin Orthop Relat Res* 2005; **435**:185–190.

114 Choi HK, Mount DB, Reginato AM. Pathogenesis of gout. *Ann Intern Med* 2005; **143**:499–516.

115 Roddy E, Zhang W, Doherty M. The changing epidemiology of gout. *Nat Clin Pract Rheumatol* 2007; **3**:443–449.

116 Klemp P, Stansfield SA, Castle B, Robertson MC. Gout is on the increase in New Zealand. *Ann Rheum Dis* 1997; **56**:22–26.

117 Mikuls TR, Farrar JT, Bilker WB, Fernandes S, Schumacher HR Jr, Saag KG. Gout epidemiology: results from the UK General Practice Research Database, 1990–1999. *Ann Rheum Dis* 2005; **64**:267–272.

118 Choi HK, Atkinson K, Karlson EW, Willett W, Curhan G. Purine-rich foods, dairy and protein intake, and the risk of gout in men. *N Engl J Med* 2004; **350**:1093–1103.

119 Nakanishi N, Okamoto M, Yoshida H, Matsuo Y, Suzuki K, Tatara K. Serum uric acid and risk for development of hypertension and impaired fasting glucose or type II diabetes in Japanese male office workers. *Eur J Epidemiol* 2003; **18**:523–530.

120 Niskanen L, Laaksonen DE, Lindstrom J, Eriksson JG, Keinänen-Kiukaanniemi S, Ilanne-Parikka P, *et al.* Serum uric acid as a harbinger of metabolic outcome in subjects with impaired glucose tolerance: the Finnish Diabetes Prevention Study. *Diabetes Care* 2006; **29**:709–711.

121 Choi HK, De Vera MA, Krishnan E. Gout and the risk of type 2 diabetes among men with a high cardiovascular risk profile. *Rheumatology (Oxford)* 2008; **47**:1567–1570.

122 Choi HK, Ford ES, Li C, Curhan G. Prevalence of the metabolic syndrome in patients with gout: the Third National Health and Nutrition Examination Survey. *Arthritis Rheum* 2007; **57**:109–115.

123 Facchini F, Chen YD, Hollenbeck CB, Reaven GM. Relationship between resistance to insulin-mediated glucose uptake, urinary uric acid clearance, and plasma uric acid concentration. *JAMA* 1991; **266**:3008–3011.

124 Vitart V, Rudan I, Hayward C, Gray NK, Floyd J, Palmer CN, *et al.* SLC2A9 is a newly identified urate transporter influencing serum urate concentration, urate excretion and gout. *Nat Genet* 2008; **40**:437–442.

125 Suppiah R, Dissanayake A, Dalbeth N. High prevalence of gout in patients with type 2 diabetes: male sex, renal impairment, and diuretic use are major risk factors. *N Z Med J* 2008; **121**:43–50.

126 Choi HK, Ford ES. Haemoglobin A1c, fasting glucose, serum C-peptide and insulin resistance in relation to serum uric acid levels: the Third National Health and Nutrition Examination Survey. *Rheumatology (Oxford)* 2008; **47**:713–717.

127 Zhang W, Doherty M, Bardin T, Pascual E, Barskova V, Conaghan P, *et al.* EULAR evidence based recommendations for gout. Part II: Management. Report of a task force of the EULAR Standing Committee for International Clinical Studies Including Therapeutics (ESCISIT). *Ann Rheum Dis* 2006; **65**:1312–1324.

128 Becker MA, Schumacher HR Jr, Wortmann RL, MacDonald PA, Eustace D, Palo WA, *et al.* Febuxostat compared with allopurinol in patients with hyperuricemia and gout. *N Engl J Med* 2005; **353**:2450–2461.

129 Hamada T, Ichida K, Hosoyamada M, Mizuta E, Yanagihara K, Sonoyama K, *et al.* Uricosuric action of losartan via the inhibition of urate transporter 1 (URAT 1) in hypertensive patients. *Am J Hypertens* 2008; **21**:1157–1162.

130 Feher MD, Hepburn AL, Hogarth MB, Ball SG, Kaye SA. Fenofibrate enhances urate reduction in men treated with allopurinol for hyperuricaemia and gout. *Rheumatology (Oxford)* 2003; **42**:321–325.

131 Davis MA, Ettinger WH, Neuhaus JM. Obesity and osteoarthritis of the knee: evidence from the National Health and Nutrition Examination Survey (NHANES I). *Semin Arthritis Rheum* 1990; **20**:34–41.

132 Felson DT, Zhang Y, Hannan MT, Naimark A, Weissman B, Aliabadi P, *et al.* Risk factors for incident radiographic knee osteoarthritis in the elderly: the Framingham Study. *Arthritis Rheum* 1997; **40**:728–733.

133 Bagge E, Bjelle A, Eden S, Svanborg A. Factors associated with radiographic osteoarthritis: results from the population study 70-year-old people in Goteborg. *J Rheumatol* 1991; **18**:1218–1222.

134 Frey C, Zamora J. The effects of obesity on orthopaedic foot and ankle pathology. *Foot Ankle Int* 2007; **28**:996–999.

135 Dahaghin S, Bierma-Zeinstra SM, Koes BW, Hazes JM, Pols HA. Do metabolic factors add to the effect of overweight on hand osteoarthritis? The Rotterdam Study. *Ann Rheum Dis* 2007; **66**:916–920.

136 Frey MI, Barrett-Connor E, Sledge PA, Schneider DL, Weisman MH. The effect of noninsulin dependent diabetes mellitus on the prevalence of clinical osteoarthritis: a population based study. *J Rheumatol* 1996; **23**:716–722.

137 Michou L, Lasbleiz S, Rat AC, Migliorini P, Balsa A, Westhovens R, *et al.* Linkage proof for PTPN22, a rheumatoid arthritis susceptibility gene and a human autoimmunity gene. *Proc Natl Acad Sci U S A* 2007; **104**:1649–1654.

138 Fernando MM, Stevens CR, Walsh EC, De Jager PL, Goyette P, Plenge RM, *et al.* Defining the role of the MHC in autoimmunity: a review and pooled analysis. *PLoS Genet* 2008; **4**:e1000024.

139 Zhernakova A, Alizadeh BZ, Bevova M, van Leeuwen MA, Coenen MJ, Franke B, *et al.* Novel association in chromosome 4q27 region with rheumatoid arthritis and confirmation of type 1 diabetes point to a general risk locus for autoimmune diseases. *Am J Hum Genet* 2007; **81**:1284–1288.

140 Myerscough A, John S, Barrett JH, Ollier WE, Worthington J. Linkage of rheumatoid arthritis to insulin-dependent diabetes mellitus loci: evidence supporting a hypothesis for the existence of common autoimmune susceptibility loci. *Arthritis Rheum* 2000; **43**:2771–2775.

141 Hinks A, Barton A, John S, Shephard N, Worthington J. Fine mapping of genes within the IDDM8 region in rheumatoid arthritis. *Arthritis Res Ther* 2006; **8**:R145.

142 Lin JP, Cash JM, Doyle SZ, Peden S, Kanik K, Amos CI, *et al.* Familial clustering of rheumatoid arthritis with other autoimmune diseases. *Hum Genet* 1998; **103**:475–482.

143 Hakala M, Ilonen J, Reijonen H, Knip M, Koivisto O, Isomaki H. No association between rheumatoid arthritis and insulin dependent diabetes mellitus: an epidemiologic and immunogenetic study. *J Rheumatol* 1992; **19**:856–858.

144 Sarzi-Puttini P, Atzeni F. New developments in our understanding of DISH (diffuse idiopathic skeletal hyperostosis). *Curr Opin Rheumatol* 2004; **16**:287–292.

145 Weinfeld RM, Olson PN, Maki DD, Griffiths HJ. The prevalence of diffuse idiopathic skeletal hyperostosis (DISH) in two large American Midwest metropolitan hospital populations. *Skeletal Radiol* 1997; **26**:222–225.

146 Schlapbach P, Beyeler C, Gerber NJ, Sturzenegger J, Fahrer H, van der Linden S, *et al.* Diffuse idiopathic skeletal hyperostosis (DISH)

of the spine: a cause of back pain? A controlled study. *Br J Rheumatol* 1989; **28**:299–303.

147 Mata S, Fortin PR, Fitzcharles MA, Starr MR, Joseph L, Watts CS, *et al.* A controlled study of diffuse idiopathic skeletal hyperostosis: clinical features and functional status. *Medicine (Baltimore)* 1997; **76**:104–117.

148 Belanger TA, Rowe DE. Diffuse idiopathic skeletal hyperostosis: musculoskeletal manifestations. *J Am Acad Orthop Surg* 2001; **9**:258–267.

149 Hendrix RW, Melany M, Miller F, Rogers LF. Fracture of the spine in patients with ankylosis due to diffuse skeletal hyperostosis: clinical and imaging findings. *AJR Am J Roentgenol* 1994; **162**:899–904.

150 Resnick D, Shaul SR, Robins JM. Diffuse idiopathic skeletal hyperostosis (DISH): Forestier's disease with extraspinal manifestations. *Radiology* 1975; **115**:513–524.

151 Al-Herz A, Snip JP, Clark B, Esdaile JM. Exercise therapy for patients with diffuse idiopathic skeletal hyperostosis. *Clin Rheumatol* 2008; **27**:207–210.

152 Sencan D, Elden H, Nacitarhan V, Sencan M, Kaptanoglu E. The prevalence of diffuse idiopathic skeletal hyperostosis in patients with diabetes mellitus. *Rheumatol Int* 2005; **25**:518–521.

153 Coaccioli S, Fatati G, Di Cato L, Marioli D, Patucchi E, Pizzuti C, *et al.* Diffuse idiopathic skeletal hyperostosis in diabetes mellitus, impaired glucose tolerance and obesity. *Panminerva Med* 2000; **42**:247–251.

154 Julkunen H, Knekt P, Aromaa A. Spondylosis deformans and diffuse idiopathic skeletal hyperostosis (DISH) in Finland. *Scand J Rheumatol* 1981; **10**:193–203.

155 Vezyroglou G, Mitropoulos A, Antoniadis C. A metabolic syndrome in diffuse idiopathic skeletal hyperostosis: a controlled study. *J Rheumatol* 1996; **23**:672–676.

156 Littlejohn GO, Smythe HA. Marked hyperinsulinemia after glucose challenge in patients with diffuse idiopathic skeletal hyperostosis. *J Rheumatol* 1981; **8**:965–968.

157 Di Franco M, Mauceri MT, Sili-Scavalli A, Iagnocco A, Ciocci A. Study of peripheral bone mineral density in patients with diffuse idiopathic skeletal hyperostosis. *Clin Rheumatol* 2000; **19**:188–192.

158 Sahin G, Polat G, Bagis S, Milcan A, Erdogan C. Study of axial bone mineral density in postmenopausal women with diffuse idiopathic skeletal hyperostosis related to type 2 diabetes mellitus. *J Womens Health (Larchmt)* 2002; **11**:801–804.

159 Denko CW, Boja B, Malemud CJ. Growth hormone and insulin-like growth factor-I in symptomatic and asymptomatic patients with diffuse idiopathic skeletal hyperostosis (DISH). *Front Biosci* 2002; **7**:a37–43.

160 Altomonte L, Zoli A, Mirone L, Marchese G, Scolieri P, Barini A, *et al.* Growth hormone secretion in diffuse idiopathic skeletal hyperostosis. *Ann Ital Med Int* 1992; **7**:30–33.

161 Kosaka T, Imakiire A, Mizuno F, Yamamoto K. Activation of nuclear factor κB at the onset of ossification of the spinal ligaments. *J Orthop Sci* 2000; **5**:572–578.

162 Sambrook P, Cooper C. Osteoporosis. *Lancet* 2006; **367**:2010–2018.

163 Fink HA, Ensrud KE, Nelson DB, Kerani RP, Schreiner PJ, Zhao Y, *et al.* Disability after clinical fracture in postmenopausal women with low bone density: the Fracture Intervention Trial (FIT). *Osteoporos Int* 2003; **14**:69–76.

164 FRAX: WHO fracture risk assessment tool. http://www.shef.ac.uk/FRAX/index.htm

165 Dubbo fracture risk calculator. http://www.garvan.org.au/promotions/bone-fracture-risk/

166 Szulc P, Delmas P. Biochemical markers of bone turnover in osteoporosis. In: Favus MJ, ed. *Primer on the Metabolic Bone Diseases and Disorders of Mineral Metabolism*, 7th edn. Washington DC: American Society for Bone and Mineral Research, 2008.

167 Vestergaard P. Discrepancies in bone mineral density and fracture risk in patients with type 1 and type 2 diabetes: a meta-analysis. *Osteoporos Int* 2007; **18**:427–444.

168 Janghorbani M, Van Dam RM, Willett WC, Hu FB. Systematic review of type 1 and type 2 diabetes mellitus and risk of fracture. *Am J Epidemiol* 2007; **166**:495–505.

169 Vestergaard P, Rejnmark L, Mosekilde L. Relative fracture risk in patients with diabetes mellitus, and the impact of insulin and oral antidiabetic medication on relative fracture risk. *Diabetologia* 2005; **48**:1292–1299.

170 Ahmed LA, Joakimsen RM, Berntsen GK, Fonnebo V, Schirmer H. Diabetes mellitus and the risk of non-vertebral fractures: the Tromso study. *Osteoporos Int* 2006; **17**:495–500.

171 Seeley DG, Kelsey J, Jergas M, Nevitt MC. Predictors of ankle and foot fractures in older women: the Study of Osteoporotic Fractures Research Group. *J Bone Miner Res* 1996; **11**:1347–1355.

172 Hanley DA, Brown JP, Tenenhouse A, Olszynski WP, Ioannidis G, Berger C, *et al.* Associations among disease conditions, bone mineral density, and prevalent vertebral deformities in men and women 50 years of age and older: cross-sectional results from the Canadian Multicentre Osteoporosis Study. *J Bone Miner Res* 2003; **18**:784–790.

173 Bonds DE, Larson JC, Schwartz AV, Strotmeyer ES, Robbins J, Rodriguez BL, *et al.* Risk of fracture in women with type 2 diabetes: the Women's Health Initiative Observational Study. *J Clin Endocrinol Metab* 2006; **91**:3404–3410.

174 Schwartz AV, Sellmeyer DE, Ensrud KE, Cauley JA, Tabor HK, Schreiner PJ, *et al.* Older women with diabetes have an increased rsk of facture: a prospective study. *J Clin Endocrinol Metab* 2001; **86**:32–38.

175 Hofbauer LC, Brueck CC, Singh SK, Dobnig H. Osteoporosis in patients with diabetes mellitus. *J Bone Miner Res* 2007; **22**:1317–1328.

176 Strotmeyer ES, Cauley JA. Diabetes mellitus, bone mineral density, and fracture risk. *Curr Opin Endocrinol Diabetes Obes* 2007; **14**:429–435.

177 Lopez-Ibarra PJ, Pastor MM, Escobar-Jimenez F, Pardo MD, González AG, Luna JD, *et al.* Bone mineral density at time of clinical diagnosis of adult-onset type 1 diabetes mellitus. *Endocr Pract* 2001; **7**:346–351.

178 Gunczler P, Lanes R, Paoli M, Martinis R, Villaroel O, Weisinger JR. Decreased bone mineral density and bone formation markers shortly after diagnosis of clinical type 1 diabetes mellitus. *J Pediatr Endocrinol* 2001; **14**:525–528.

179 Campos Pastor MM, Lopez-Ibarra PJ, Escobar-Jimenez F, Serrano Pardo MD, Garcia-Cervigon AG. Intensive insulin therapy and bone mineral density in type 1 diabetes mellitus: a prospective study. *Osteoporos Int* 2000; **11**:455–459.

180 Miazgowski T, Czekalski S. A 2-year follow-up study on bone mineral density and markers of bone turnover in patients with long-standing insulin-dependent diabetes mellitus. *Osteoporos Int* 1998; **8**:399–403.

181 Kayath MJ, Tavares EF, Dib SA, Vieira JG. Prospective bone mineral density evaluation in patients with insulin-dependent diabetes mellitus. *J Diabetes Complications* 1998; **12**:133–139.

182 Gunczler P, Lanes R, Paz-Martinez V, Martins R, Esaa S, Colmenares V, *et al.* Decreased lumbar spine bone mass and low bone turnover in children and adolescents with insulin dependent diabetes mellitus followed longitudinally. *J Pediatr Endocrinol* 1998; **11**:413–419.

183 Strotmeyer ES, Cauley JA, Orchard TJ, Steenkiste AR, Dorman JS. Middle-aged premenopausal women with type 1 diabetes have lower bone mineral density and calcaneal quantitative ultrasound than nondiabetic women. *Diabetes Care* 2006; **29**:306–311.

184 Alexopoulou O, Jamart J, Devogelaer JP, Brichard S, de Nayer P, Buysschaert M. Bone density and markers of bone remodeling in type 1 male diabetic patients. *Diabetes Metab* 2006; **32**:453–458.

185 Mastrandrea LD, Wactawski-Wende J, Donahue RP, Hovey KM, Clark A, Quattrin T. Young women with type 1 diabetes have lower bone mineral density that persists over time. *Diabetes Care* 2008; **31**:1729–1735.

186 Cornish J, Callon KE, Bava U, Watson M, Xu X, Lin JM, *et al.* Preptin, another peptide product of the pancreatic beta-cell, is osteogenic *in vitro* and *in vivo*. *Am J Physiol Endocrinol Metab* 2007; **292**:E117–122.

187 Cornish J, Callon KE, Reid IR. Insulin increases histomorphometric indices of bone formation *in vivo*. *Calcif Tissue Int* 1996; **59**:492–495.

188 Dacquin R, Davey RA, Laplace C, Levasseur R, Morris HA, Goldring SR, *et al.* Amylin inhibits bone resorption while the calcitonin receptor controls bone formation *in vivo*. *J Cell Biol* 2004; **164**:509–514.

189 Thrailkill KM, Lumpkin CK Jr, Bunn RC, Kemp SF, Fowlkes JL. Is insulin an anabolic agent in bone? Dissecting the diabetic bone for clues. *Am J Physiol Endocrinol Metab* 2005; **289**:E735–745.

190 Moyer-Mileur LJ, Slater H, Jordan KC, Murray MA. IGF-1 and IGF-binding proteins and bone mass, geometry, and strength: relation to metabolic control in adolescent girls with type 1 diabetes. *J Bone Miner Res* 2008; **23**:1884–1891.

191 Reid IR, Cornish J, Baldock PA. Nutrition-related peptides and bone homeostasis. *J Bone Miner Res* 2006; **21**:495–500.

192 Reid IR. Relationships between fat and bone. *Osteoporos Int* 2008; **19**:595–606.

193 Miao J, Brismar K, Nyren O, Ugarph-Morawski A, Ye W. Elevated hip fracture risk in type 1 diabetic patients: a population-based cohort study in Sweden. *Diabetes Care* 2005; **28**:2850–2855.

194 Cundy TF, Edmonds ME, Watkins PJ. Osteopenia and metatarsal fractures in diabetic neuropathy. *Diabet Med* 1985; **2**:461–464.

195 Whiteside GT, Boulet JM, Sellers R, Bunton TE, Walker K. Neuropathy-induced osteopenia in rats is not due to a reduction in weight borne on the affected limb. *Bone* 2006; **38**:387–393.

196 Strotmeyer ES, Cauley JA, Schwartz AV, Nevitt MC, Resnick HE, Bauer DC, *et al.* Nontraumatic fracture risk with diabetes mellitus and impaired fasting glucose in older white and black adults: the Health, Aging, and Body Composition study. *Arch Intern Med* 2005; **165**:1612–1617.

197 Strotmeyer ES, Cauley JA, Schwartz AV, de Rekeneire N, Resnick HE, Zmuda JM, *et al.* Reduced peripheral nerve function is related to lower hip BMD and calcaneal QUS in older white and black adults: the Health, Aging, and Body Composition Study. *J Bone Miner Res* 2006; **21**:1803–1810.

198 Lipscombe LL, Jamal SA, Booth GL, Hawker GA. The risk of hip fractures in older individuals with diabetes: a population-based study. *Diabetes Care* 2007; **30**:835–841.

199 Kennedy RL, Henry J, Chapman AJ, Nayar R, Grant P, Morris AD. Accidents in patients with insulin-treated diabetes: increased risk of low-impact falls but not motor vehicle crashes: a prospective register-based study. *J Trauma* 2002; **52**:660–666.

200 Katayama Y, Akatsu T, Yamamoto M, Kugai N, Nagata N. Role of nonenzymatic glycosylation of type I collagen in diabetic osteopenia. *J Bone Miner Res* 1996; **11**:931–937.

201 Hein GE. Glycation endproducts in osteoporosis: is there a pathophysiologic importance? *Clin Chim Acta* 2006; **371**:32–36.

202 Vashishth D, Gibson GJ, Khoury JI, Schaffler MB, Kimura J, Fyhrie DP. Influence of nonenzymatic glycation on biomechanical properties of cortical bone. *Bone* 2001; **28**:195–201.

203 Sanguineti R, Storace D, Monacelli F, Federici A, Odetti P. Pentosidine effects on human osteoblasts *in vitro*. *Ann N Y Acad Sci* 2008; **1126**:166–172.

204 Miyata T, Notoya K, Yoshida K, Horie K, Maeda K, Kurokawa K, *et al.* Advanced glycation end products enhance osteoclast-induced bone resorption in cultured mouse unfractionated bone cells and in rats implanted subcutaneously with devitalized bone particles. *J Am Soc Nephrol* 1997; **8**:260–270.

205 Valcourt U, Merle B, Gineyts E, Viguet-Carrin S, Delmas PD, Garnero P. Non-enzymatic glycation of bone collagen modifies osteoclastic activity and differentiation. *J Biol Chem* 2007; **282**:5691–5703.

206 Zhou Z, Immel D, Xi CX, Bierhaus A, Feng X, Mei L, *et al.* Regulation of osteoclast function and bone mass by RAGE. *J Exp Med* 2006; **203**:1067–1080.

207 Grey A. Skeletal consequences of thiazolidinedione therapy. *Osteoporos Int* 2008; **19**:129–137.

208 Grey A. Thiazolidinedione-induced skeletal fragility: mechanisms and implications. *Diabetes Obes Metab* 2009: **11**:275–84.

209 Kahn SE, Haffner SM, Heise MA, Herman WH, Holman RR, Jones NP, *et al.* Glycemic durability of rosiglitazone, metformin, or glyburide monotherapy. *N Engl J Med* 2006; **355**:2427–2443.

210 Nissen SE, Nicholls SJ, Wolski K, Nesto R, Kupfer S, Perez A, *et al.* Comparison of pioglitazone vs glimepiride on progression of coronary atherosclerosis in patients with type 2 diabetes: the PERISCOPE randomized controlled trial. *JAMA* 2008; **299**:1561–1573.

211 US Food and Drug Administration. http://www.fda.gov/medwatch/safety/2007/Actosmar0807.pdf. Accessed April 15, 2008.

212 Meier C, Kraenzlin ME, Bodmer M, Jick SS, Jick H, Meier CR. Use of thiazolidinediones and fracture risk. *Arch Intern Med* 2008; **168**:820–825.

213 Wan Y, Chong LW, Evans RM. PPARg regulates osteoclastogenesis in mice. *Nat Med* 2007; **13**:1496–1503.

214 Monami M, Cresci B, Colombini A, Pala L, Balzi D, Gori F, *et al.* Bone fractures and hypoglycemic treatment in type 2 diabetic patients: a case–control study. *Diabetes Care* 2008; **31**:199–203.

215 Funk JR, Hale JE, Carmines D, Gooch HL, Hurwitz SR. Biomechanical evaluation of early fracture healing in normal and diabetic rats. *J Orthop Res* 2000; **18**:126.

216 Macey LR, Kana SM, Jingushi S, Terek RM, Borretos J, Bolander ME. Defects of early fracture-healing in experimental diabetes. *J Bone Joint Surg Am* 1989; **71**:722–733.

217 Follak N, Kloting I, Merk H. Influence of diabetic metabolic state on fracture healing in spontaneously diabetic rats. *Diabetes Metab Res Rev* 2005; **21**:288–296.

218 Beam HA, Parsons JR, Lin SS. The effects of blood glucose control upon fracture healing in the BB Wistar rat with diabetes mellitus. *J Orthop Res* 2002; **20**:1210–1216.

219 Gandhi A, Beam HA, O'Connor JP, Parsons JR, Lin SS. The effects of local insulin delivery on diabetic fracture healing. *Bone* 2005; **37**:482–490.

220 Loder RT. The influence of diabetes mellitus on the healing of closed fractures. *Clin Orthop* 1988; **232**:210–216.

221 White CB, Turner NS, Lee GC, Haidukewych GJ. Open ankle fractures in patients with diabetes mellitus. *Clin Orthop* 2003; **414**:37–44.

49 Psychologic Factors and Diabetes

Christopher M. Ryan
University of Pittsburgh School of Medicine, Pittsburgh, PA, USA

Keypoints

- Both type 1 (T1DM) and type 2 diabetes mellitus (T2DM) can affect the psychologic and neuropsychologic status of children and adults. In most instances, these effects are modest in magnitude and are most likely to be associated with certain events that occur during the course of diabetes or its management.
- Children show remarkable psychologic resilience to the diagnosis of diabetes. About one-third report some psychologic distress shortly after diagnosis but this generally subsides within 6 months. This "adjustment disorder" is characterized by increased depressive symptomatology, more anxiety, social withdrawal and sleep disturbances. A similar adjustment reaction is often seen in parents, particularly mothers, of newly diagnosed children. Diagnoses of post-traumatic stress disorder are also more common in parents, occurring at rates comparable with that reported in children diagnosed with cancer. Increased rates of depression are also found in adults newly diagnosed with T1DM, whereas diagnosis of T2DM does not appear to increase the risk of depression unless accompanied by multiple medical co-morbidities.
- During the first 5–10 years of their diabetes, most children and adolescents show adequate psychologic functioning; however, after 10 years of diabetes, their rates of anxiety, depression or eating disorders are markedly increased, with as many as one-third of adolescents with diabetes meeting criteria for one or more psychiatric disorders. Adults with diabetes also show elevated rates of depression which are twice as high as those reported in the general population. At greatest risk are people who have been hospitalized, are older with multiple medical problems, have a history of past psychopathology or are female. Metabolic control is only weakly associated with the occurrence of a mood disorder.
- Macrovascular disease, chronic foot ulceration and proliferative retinopathy increase the risk of psychopathology, an understandable reaction to serious complications; however, lifetime psychiatric disorders such as depression may also increase the risk of later development of complications such as retinopathy. Recurrent diabetic ketoacidosis, particularly in females, is also predicted by poor psychologic functioning, and by high rates of family dysfunction.
- Phobic disorders are more common in adults with diabetes than in the general population. Fear of blood and injury may lead to less blood glucose self-monitoring and poorer control. Fear of hypoglycemia is common and may also lead to premature treatment as blood glucose levels begin to fall, resulting in persisting hyperglycemia.
- Quality of life for those with diabetes does not differ from patients with other chronic conditions, such as arthritis. Poor health-related quality of life is associated with biomedical complications, being female, physical inactivity, low income and recurrently hypoglycemia. Intensive diabetes management is not associated with a deterioration in quality of life.
- Interventions to reduce psychologic distress include individual psychotherapy or counseling, and group therapy; however, the efficacy of either – in terms of affecting mood or metabolic control – has not been studied extensively in clinical trials, but data from smaller studies suggests effects may be weak, at best. A promising technique for depressive symptoms is cognitive–behavior therapy, which teaches patients problem-solving strategies for stressful situations and "thinking away" distorted beliefs. Pharmacotherapy, including selective serotonin reuptake inhibitors and tricyclic antidepressants, has been found to reduce symptom severity but specific drugs may differentially influence glycated hemoglobin values.
- Cognitive dysfunction in diabetes is generally mild, but children diagnosed in the first 5 to 7 years of life have an elevated risk of manifesting clinically significant impairments in all cognitive domains. Those with a later onset of diabetes show modest effects, most evident on measures of intelligence, academic achievement and psychomotor efficiency. Deficits appear early in the course of the disease, and are evident within 2–3 years after diagnosis. Hypoglycemia was long considered to be the cause of this neurocognitive dysfunction but more recent research suggests that adverse effects on cognition may only occur when blood glucose levels are very low for an extended period of time. Although the etiology of neurocognitive changes in children remains poorly understood, a growing body of evidence implicates chronic hyperglycemia and, in particular, the development of microvascular and macrovascular complications.
- In adults with T1DM, neurocognitive deficits are quite modest and are most apparent on measures of intelligence, psychomotor speed and executive function. Older adults with T2DM also manifest marked reductions in memory function and, in both groups, the strongest

Textbook of Diabetes, 4th edition. Edited by R. Holt, C. Cockram, A. Flyvbjerg and B. Goldstein.

predictor of cognitive dysfunction is chronic hyperglycemia and the presence of biomedical complications, particularly retinopathy and peripheral neuropathy.
- Structural damage to the brain is also common in both children and adults with either T1DM or T2DM. Not only is there a reduction in cortical gray matter density, but white matter structures may be disrupted. Cerebral atrophy is often present, neural slowing is evident on electroencephalography and regional cerebral blood flow is altered.
- Diabetes management and health outcomes are influenced by reciprocal relationships between metabolic control and psychologic variables. The latter include enduring psychologic traits such as locus of control, coping style, temperament and transitory psychologic states (stress, anxiety, depression). Diabetes is also strongly related to family functioning, especially in children and adolescents: low family conflict, good communication, cohesion and marital satisfaction relate to better diabetes control.
- Adherence or self-care behaviors (taking medicine, complying with diet, glucose monitoring, exercise regimens) are only weakly related to diabetic control, but this may reflect the inaccuracy of self-reported behavior. For those who are most seriously non-compliant, psychologic interventions include psychotherapy, family therapy and patient empowerment programs to improve goal-setting, problem-solving, coping, managing stress and self-motivation.
- A psychologist or other mental health care professional should be part of the diabetes care team.

Introduction

Diabetes and psychology have long been linked. More than 50 years ago, the psychosomatic model of medical illness postulated that psychosocial factors could trigger or maintain various disorders, including diabetes. This notion was subsequently abandoned by most scientists, yet the person living with diabetes and managing this behaviorally complex condition may nevertheless identify numerous points where diabetes and psychology interact. This chapter examines three major points of intersection: psychologic reactions to the development of diabetes and the appearance of complications, the neuropsychologic or cognitive consequences of diabetes, and psychologic factors that influence, or are influenced by, the everyday management of diabetes.

Psychologic impact of diabetes

Patients with diabetes ought to manifest significant psychologic distress, or so goes conventional clinical wisdom. After all, they have a disorder that shortens their lifespan, leads to debilitating biomedical complications such as blindness or neuropathy, and requires them to take complete daily responsibility for managing their health with drugs or insulin injections and careful monitoring of diet, exercise and blood glucose levels, for the remainder of their lives. Chronic illnesses like diabetes also mark individuals, particularly children, as different from their healthy peers, and burden families with demanding health care responsibilities that they may be unwilling or unable to meet. Given all of these factors, one should not be surprised to find that many people with diabetes, and their families, have elevated rates of emotional disturbances and behavioral problems.

Psychologic distress shortly after diagnosis

Observations in children and their parents

Children and adults show remarkable psychologic resilience in response to a diagnosis of diabetes. In what may be the most comprehensive prospective psychologic study of children with diabetes and their families, Kovacs *et al.* [1] assessed 95 children, 8–13 years of age, shortly after discharge from their initial hospitalization, and followed them for 6–10 years. Within 3 months of diagnosis, 36% of the children experienced sufficient psychologic distress to meet criteria for a diagnosable psychiatric disorder [2]. Most had "adjustment disorder," defined as a transient reaction that exceeds the normal and expectable response to a stressor, develops within 3 months of onset of the stressor and lasts no more than 6 months. The occurrence of such a disorder signals that the child is beginning to come to terms with the diagnosis of diabetes, and can be considered to be a component of the "mourning process" that often accompanies the development of any chronic illness [3]. As one would expect with an adjustment disorder, recovery was rapid, with 93% showing complete remission of these psychiatric symptoms within 9 months. Other investigators, using different outcome measures, have also demonstrated rapid psychologic adaptation to the diagnosis of diabetes [4–6].

Parents of children newly diagnosed with diabetes also manifest psychologic responses that are analogous to an adjustment disorder. For mothers, the strain associated with caring for a school-aged child with diabetes elicited mild levels of depressive symptomatology, anxiety and generalized distress, but this dissipated within 6 months [7]. Less symptomatology was evident in fathers, both shortly after diagnosis and approximately 1 year later; however, if fathers do report experiencing high rates of emotional dysfunction in the first 2 years following their child's diagnosis, their child is more likely to manifest poorer metabolic control and greater blood glucose variability during the first 5 years of diagnosis [8]. Greatly elevated rates of post-traumatic stress disorder (PTSD) have also been reported in a prospective study of parents evaluated at 6 weeks and 6 and 12 months after their child's diagnosis. Depending on time point, 16–22% of mothers met DSM-IV criteria for a PTSD diagnosis, as did 8–14% of fathers [9]. Theses rates were significantly higher than those reported in the general population but are comparable with those seen in mothers of children diagnosed with cancer. The best predictor of PTSD severity at 12 months was PTSD severity at

6 months. Poorer disease outcomes, particularly episodes of hypoglycemia, were associated with an increased level of PTSD severity.

Elevated rates of worry and concern are also present in parents, but these differ by gender: 46% of mothers reported worry all or almost all of the time, whereas only 13% of the fathers reported similarly high levels of concern [10]. Mourning was the primary coping process engaged in by mothers, whose responses most commonly included feeling sad, worried and/or tired, and who manifested bouts of crying and irritability. As duration of illness increased, levels of psychologic distress, particularly depression, showed slight increments, with the greatest increases occurring in those mothers who were most distressed at the time of their child's diagnosis and in those mothers of higher socioeconomic status. The latter finding may reflect the possibility that these women were more knowledgeable about diabetes, and hence may have been more discouraged about its management and long-term outcomes. Despite the stresses and strains that the diagnosis of diabetes exerts on both the child and the family, there is little evidence of major family disruption in the first 2–3 years following diagnosis. Measures of parental perception of overall quality of family life as well as estimates of the quality of parents' marriage show essentially no change during that period [11].

Diagnosis in adulthood

The onset of diabetes during adulthood ought to produce similar adjustment disorders within several months of diagnosis in both the patient as well as the spouse or other family member. A German sample of newly diagnosed, adult patients (aged 17–40 years of age) with type 1 diabetes mellitus (T1DM) had a rate of major depressive episodes that was twice that of a reference group drawn from a representative national population (5.8% vs 2.7%), although more careful analysis shows that these differences were statistically significant only for women with diabetes (9.3% vs 3.2% in reference group) [12]. There were no differences in rates of major depression between men with diabetes and the reference group (3.6% vs 2.2%), nor for other psychiatric disorders. Because this is a cross-sectional study, it is impossible to determine whether this is truly a "classic" depression or whether it is a transient adjustment disorder, as is typically seen in children and adolescents with diabetes. In contrast, several studies of adults with type 2 diabetes mellitus (T2DM) have found little psychologic morbidity in the first year following diagnosis. One smaller clinical study reported that of the 71 subjects studied, more than 50% expressed no emotional reaction to the diagnosis and felt that they could cope with diabetes [13]. Negative emotional reactions, along with feelings of being incapable of coping with this disorder, were expressed by only 26% of the sample, and this may reflect the fact that these individuals had significantly less social support than the others. A larger, more recent study assessing symptoms of depression, similarly found little evidence of a psychologic reaction in 824 patients newly diagnosed with T2DM [14]. Although there were marked gender differences, with women with diabetes reporting higher rates of significant depressive symptomatology than men with diabetes (16.1% and 8.2%, respectively), those values were comparable to UK normative data for women and men (13% and 8%, respectively). Greater depressive symptomatology was associated with more medical co-morbidities: newly diagnosed patients with diabetes taking both lipid-lowering and antihypertensive medications reported more symptoms of depression than those on only one, or on no concurrent medication.

Psychologic reactions emerging in the course of diabetes

Depressive symptomatology in children and adolescents

After resolution of their adjustment disorder, are children able to get on with their lives, or is there an increased likelihood of subsequent psychologic distress in the individual with diabetes? As duration of diabetes continues, it now appears that most children and adolescents with diabetes function well psychologically, although small increases may be evident in depressive symptomatology and internalizing behaviors, such as somatic complaints, social withdrawal, sleep disturbance and symptoms of depression and anxiety). In both school-aged [6,15,16] and pre-school children [17], this was evident after 2–3 years of diabetes, yet the magnitude of these changes was not so large as to be indicative of clinically significant psychopathology. Somewhat higher rates of externalizing, or aggressive, behaviors have also been reported, with this phenomenon especially pronounced in boys with diabetes [15], and strongly associated with consistently elevated blood glucose levels [18]. High levels of family conflict and the occurrence of multiple stressful life events appear to be particularly potent predictors of more aggressive behavior in children and adolescents with diabetes [19].

After 6 years of follow-up, Kovacs *et al.* [16] found trivially small increases in symptoms of depression for all subjects, and increased symptoms of anxiety for girls but not boys. Children who reported more difficulties in managing their diabetes also showed more symptoms of psychologic distress. Level of psychologic distress shortly after diabetes onset was the best predictor of symptomatology 6 years later, whereas the degree of metabolic control, as indexed by glycated hemoglobin (HbA_{1c}) values, was not a viable predictor in this or in most other studies [20,21]. Neither age nor age at onset predicted increased psychologic distress in Kovacs *et al.*'s cohort, although others have found an association between developmental stage and emotional or behavioral problems in so far as adolescents manifested more problems than pre-adolescents [21].

Even after 10 years of diabetes, older adolescents and young adults with childhood onset of diabetes may report little psychologic distress, although they tend to have lower levels of self-esteem and express concerns about their sociability and their physical appearance [22]. What is remarkable, however, is that when patients are formally evaluated with structured psychiatric interviews to assess for clinically significant psychopathology over this extended time period, marked elevations are found in rates of psychiatric disorder. Not only were females more often affected than males [23,24], but their risk of subsequently experiencing a recurrence of depression was nine times greater than males [25]. Kovacs *et al.* [1] reported that 40% of their sample had experienced at least one episode of a psychiatric disorder during the first 10 years of living with diabetes, and 26% had two different psychiatric disorders. Major depression was the most common diagnosis (26% of sample), followed by some form of anxiety disorder (20%). By comparison, similarly aged, subjects without diabetes drawn from the community had rates of depression that ranged from 9–16%, and rates of anxiety that ranged from 11–25% [26].

Remarkably similar rates of clinically significant DSM-IV disorders have been reported more recently by Northam *et al.* [23], who followed a cohort of newly diagnosed Australian children over a 10-year period. By year 10, 37% of those with diabetes received at least one diagnosis; of those, 60% met criteria for two or more disorders and 55% met criteria for three or more disorders [23]. In that study, mood, anxiety and eating disorders were each present in 17% of the sample; nearly 20% of the sample manifested a behavior disorder. Of note is their observation that those adolescents who met criteria for a DSM-IV psychiatric disorder were also more likely to have manifested significant externalizing problems shortly after diagnosis. Although not evaluated by Northam *et al.*, other investigators have identified maternal psychopathology as a potent predictor of subsequent psychiatric disorder [1] and increased depressive symptomatology in children and adults with diabetes [27].

Significantly elevated rates of suicidal ideation have also been reported for adolescents with diabetes, with lifetime prevalence rates noted to be 26%, compared to rates for adolescents without diabetes ranging from 9–12% [28]. Although the rate of actual suicide attempts is low amongst youth with diabetes (4%), suicidal ideation was associated with greatly increased rates of non-compliance with medical treatment.

Clinically significant mood disorders in adults

The process of psychologic adaptation to the diagnosis of diabetes in adulthood remains incompletely understood, largely because few longitudinal studies have been conducted with adults [29]. In what remains the largest follow-up study of adults with T1DM, the Diabetes Control and Complications Trial (DCCT) Research Group [30] found no change in self-reported psychologic symptomatology over a follow-up period of 6–9 years, and found no relationship between type of treatment (conventional or intensive insulin therapy) and levels of psychologic distress [31]. Rates of clinically significant distress were higher in both treatment groups (25%) compared with rates of depression measured by self-report in the general population (14.4%) [32]. A smaller study that followed adults for 2 years from the diagnosis of T1DM also reported either no changes in psychologic state over time, or a significant improvement in functioning (e.g. reduced depressive symptomatology) [33].

Cross-sectional studies of adults with either T1DM or T2DM have demonstrated repeatedly that rates of psychologic distress, particularly depression and anxiety, tend to be higher than the general population, but are usually comparable to those reported in individuals with other chronic diseases [34–38]. Using self-report measures of psychologic symptoms, Peyrot & Rubin [39] found greatly elevated rates of both depressive (41%) and anxiety symptomatology (49%), with 38% of their entire sample showing elevations in both domains; however, repeated reassessment of these patients over a 6-month period indicated that these effects are quite unstable. Across all three assessments, only 13% of the sample was consistently disturbed. The strongest predictors of persisting distress included being female, having less than a high school education, being middle-aged and having more than two diabetes-associated biomedical complications [40]. Prevalence rates for any depressive disturbance were nearly twice as high in this study [39] than DCCT reports (41% vs 25%, respectively), but this is likely to be because of sampling differences. The DCCT study group was comprised of highly motivated patients with minimal diabetes-associated complications who were vigorously followed by a treatment team that included a psychologist or psychiatrist [41], whereas those patients studied by Peyrot & Rubin included a mix of patients with T1DM and T2DM who were recruited during a 1-week diabetes management outpatient program.

Numerous other studies have also demonstrated high rates of anxiety disorder [42] and depressive symptomatology in adults with either T1DM or T2DM [35,43]. An early analysis of 42 studies indicated that the risk of depression was doubled in people with diabetes, as compared to people without diabetes, and this occurred regardless of type of diabetes (Figure 49.1) [32]. Similar results have been reported in a more recent meta-analysis of 10 studies that included 9028 patients with T2DM and 42 272 adults without diabetes; again, rates of self-reported depression were significantly elevated in patients with diabetes (17.6% vs 9.8%) [44].

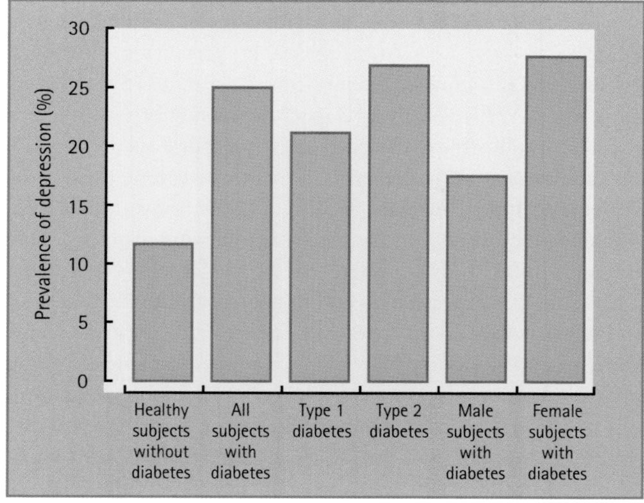

Figure 49.1 The increased prevalence of depression in people with diabetes compared with subjects without diabetes. The data are from a meta-analysis of 42 studies; figures for subjects with diabetes are the aggregate of both controlled and non-controlled studies. Adapted from Anderson *et al.* [32].

Variations in prevalence rates are common across individual studies, and appear to be related to the method used to ascertain depression. Those studies using self-report symptom scales yielded prevalence rates that were nearly three times higher than rates obtained using formal structured interviews with clinically established diagnostic criteria (31% vs 11%) [32]. Discrepancies amongst studies have also been found to be caused by differences in subject characteristics, particularly age and medical history [45,46]. The highest rates of current psychiatric distress tend to be found in hospitalized patients [47] or in older adults with multiple medical co-morbidities [48,49]. Frequently [50,51], but not invariably [45,52], adults with diabetes and more emotional problems also have poorer metabolic control. A review of more than 30 studies indicates that although depression is associated with higher HbA_{1c} values, the magnitude of this effect is extremely small, with the exact value being a function of how depression is ascertained. In studies using symptom self-reports, less than 3% of the variance in HbA_{1c} was explained by depression; when standardized diagnostic interviews are used, approximately 8% of the variance in HbA_{1c} was accounted for by depression [53].

Studies of children with diabetes have indicated that the best predictor of future psychopathology is past psychopathology [16], and the same principle applies to adults. Lustman *et al.* [29] reassessed a group of adults with diabetes 5 years after they had first met criteria for current depression, and found that 67% were depressed at follow-up, whereas only 15% of the initially non-depressed adults met criteria for psychiatric disorder at follow-up. Repeated episodes of depression were common in the initially depressed group, with subjects having an average of 4.2 episodes during the 5-year follow-up period. Recurrence of depression was apparently unrelated to duration of disease, type of diabetes or development of diabetes-associated complications, but it was associated with a family history of psychiatric disorder. A subsequent study found that the severity of recurrent depressive episodes was related to the presence of neuropathy, but no other biomedical complication, at study entry and it has been suggested that the discomfort associated with this complication may serve as a stressor capable of provoking an episode of depression in vulnerable individuals [54]. The generally weak relationship between diabetes-related variables and reoccurrence of a mood disorder suggests that depression is not merely a psychologic reaction to the development of diabetes or its complications, but may be influenced significantly by underlying genetic or constitutional factors [25,55,56].

Depression as a risk factor for subsequent development of type 2 diabetes

Most readers would assume from this literature that the emergence of depression is a direct consequence of coping with its demanding burden of care [48] and/or its associated co-morbid medical conditions [57], but there is growing evidence, at least from studies of older adults with T2DM, that the reverse may be true, and that being depressed greatly increases the risk of subsequently developing diabetes. In a meta-analysis that included 13 comparative prospective studies of depression and T2DM, a robust relationship was noted between depression and the subsequent incidence of T2DM (60% increase in risk), whereas the relationship between having T2DM and subsequently developing depression was modest at best (15% increase in risk) [58]. Although the exact pathologic mechanisms have not yet been established, it is certainly plausible that depression could greatly increase the likelihood of developing diabetes, in so far as depressive symptomatology is associated with a variety of behavioral (e.g. poorer compliance with dietary and weight loss recommendations; less physical activity) [59] and physiologic (e.g. increased activation of the hypothalamic-pituitary-adrenal axis, and increased inflammation) [60] risk factors for T2DM.

The diagnosis and treatment of depression and other psychiatric disorders in patients with diabetes is described in detail in Chapter 55.

Psychologic reactions to biomedical complications

Microvascular and macrovascular complications as triggers for psychologic distress

Diabetic complications may not only disrupt the individual's usual lifestyle and interfere with self-care activities, but may also serve as a reminder that despite their best efforts, patients have failed to manage their disease adequately. In the same way that the child recently diagnosed with diabetes manifests an anxious or depressed mood as part of an adjustment disorder, older patients might be expected to show psychologic distress soon after a complication appears. This conjecture has not been tested empirically: it is not known how adults with diabetes react psychologically shortly after a complication appears, although as a group, adults with complications usually [61], but not invariably [62], have greater levels of psychologic distress.

Three types of diabetic complications are known to increase the risk of psychopathology: macrovascular disorders, chronic foot ulceration and sight-threatening proliferative retinopathy. Adults with diabetes and macrovascular disease often have elevated rates of depression [52] and poorer quality of life [55], although this is not always the case [46,63]. Similarly, patients with chronic unilateral foot ulceration secondary to diabetic neuropathy have higher rates of depression and report greater dissatisfaction with their lives than age-matched adults with diabetes but no history of foot ulceration [64]. Results from a prospective cohort study noted that 24% of adults with diabetes presenting with their first diabetic foot ulcer had clinically significant major depression, and this was associated with a threefold risk of death during an 18-month follow-up period [65]. Other studies have also demonstrated marked increases in depressive symptomatology and peripheral neuropathy, and have attributed this psychologic distress to the physical distress associated with reduced feeling in the feet and unsteadiness, as well as its unpredictability [66,67].

Increased psychiatric symptomatology is also seen in patients with proliferative diabetic retinopathy, compared with those without retinopathy [68]. Both level of visual acuity and duration of visual problems affect mental health. Wulsin *et al.* [69] followed patients with diabetic retinopathy for 8 months, beginning shortly after a vitreous hemorrhage, and found that greater impairment of visual acuity was associated with increased psychologic distress and poorer coping efforts. Unlike a classic adjustment disorder, these relationships grew stronger, rather than weaker, over time. Fluctuations in visual impairment may also increase psychologic distress [70], although that is not inevitable [71], and it is important to keep in mind that the degree of psychologic distress secondary to visual loss is not unique to patients with diabetes; at least one study of older adults has reported no significant difference in psychologic adjustment between those with and without diabetes, either at the onset of visual loss or when re-evaluated 12 months later [72].

Depression exacerbates the development and course of complications

Distress and depression are usually assumed to be a direct response to the occurrence of a complication, but there is growing evidence for the alternative possibility; that depression, at least under certain circumstances, may increase the likelihood that an individual will subsequently develop complications. The most compelling support for this view remains Kovacs' sophisticated statistical analysis of 10-year follow-up data from their childhood-onset cohort study which demonstrated that severity of retinopathy could be predicted from three antecedent variables [73]. These variables had an additive effect in so far as the likelihood of retinopathy increased with increasing duration of diabetes, with length of time spent in poor control and with overall proportion of time depressed. Depression was not a reaction to retinopathy in this cohort but predated the diagnosis of retinopathy by several years.

An analogous pattern of results has been reported more recently in a study of 483 African-Americans with T2DM who were followed over a 6-year period. Patients with high depression scores at both baseline and 6-year follow-up had significantly higher baseline HbA_{1c} values and were more likely to show progression of diabetic retinopathy (odds ratio 2.44) and progression to proliferative diabetic retinopathy (odds ratio 3.19), compared with patients with low depression scores at both visits [74]. Baseline HbA_{1c} values accounted for 21% of the progression to diabetic retinopathy, while being depressed at both visits accounted for an additional 6% in the regression model.

These intriguing findings suggest that depression may be a risk factor, not only for the development of subsequent psychopathology, but also for the development of subsequent diabetes complications, at least in certain individuals. The physiologic basis for this relationship remains unknown but, as discussed below, depression could interfere with patients' ability to manage their diabetes [75], and so contribute to poor metabolic control. It follows that early treatment of depression may not only improve the individual's mental health, but may improve metabolic control and delay the appearance of diabetic complications [76]. Support for that possibility comes from one small placebo-controlled medication trial clinical study that used a selective serotonin reuptake inhibitor (SSRI) in a group of older adults with T2DM [77], but several other studies, taking a "collaborative care" approach have had no impact on metabolic control or other diabetes-related variables despite marked success in reducing depression in people with diabetes [78,79].

Interactions between acute metabolic complications and psychologic distress

Acute complications of diabetes, particularly recurrent diabetic ketoacidosis (DKA), may also be predicted in children from indicators of poor psychologic functioning in the first year following diagnosis [80]. This is particularly true in girls, for whom more behavior problems and lower levels of social competence were associated with higher rates of DKA. Family dysfunction in the first year following diagnosis was also predictive, with higher levels of family conflict and lower levels of family cohesion associated with more recurrent DKA. Again, this relationship is limited to girls and is independent of variations in HbA_{1c} values. Boys showed relatively low rates of recurrent DKA (6% vs 20%) but very high rates of recurrent hypoglycemia (22.6% vs 3%); the latter were unrelated to psychosocial variables shortly after diagnosis. Even after several years of diabetes, family functioning processes can have a major impact on risk for DKA. Adolescents who reported their parents expressed more negativity to their diabetes regimen had a greater risk of experiencing DKA [81]. It is likely that the link between early behavior problems and DKA in girls is mediated by psychosocial factors, such as poor adherence [82], although definitive evidence for that possibility is currently lacking.

Diabetes treatment-induced fears and phobias

Phobic disorders are twice as common in adults with diabetes than the general population [46]. Earlier work failed to explore the possible reasons for that difference, but an increasing body of research has identified injection or blood and injury phobia, and fear of hypoglycemia, as two sequelae of insulin treatment for diabetes [83]. For example, Berlin *et al.* [84] studied more than 100 adults with T1DM and not only found that 94% of their sample reported at least one phobic symptom, but that patients with poorer glycemic control had more symptoms of fear of blood or injury than did those with better control. Those individuals also measured their blood glucose less frequently and endorsed more symptoms of anxiety and depression. Statistical modeling techniques support the possibility that the association between poorer metabolic control and lower rates of daily blood glucose monitoring is mediated by patients' fear of blood and injury. The prevalence of this phobia remains controversial, with estimates ranging from approximately 1.3% [85] to approximately 25% [86], depending on the questionnaire used to ascertain injection phobia and the criterion used operationally to define the severity of the disorder.

Fear of hypoglycemia is also common in children [87] and adults [88,89] with diabetes, as well as in spouses [90] and parents

[91]. The development of hypoglycemic fear, and the corresponding effort to avoid any situation that may lead to a recurrence of a hypoglycemic event, is not at all surprising. Acute hypoglycemic episodes are uncomfortable and unpredictable. They are accompanied by autonomic arousal characterized by aversive symptoms such as trembling, sweating, light-headedness, pounding heart, nervousness [92], feelings of anger and "tense-tiredness" [93,94] and worries that this episode could lead to a seizure, coma or death if not treated promptly.

Individuals who experienced recurrent hypoglycemia [88], or even a single episode of severe hypoglycemia when accompanied by seizure or coma [95], have higher hypoglycemic fear scores, although this is likely to be a consequence of several factors, including pre-existing personality traits, particularly neuroticism [89] or trait anxiety [96], and current level of psychologic distress [88]. In addition to being associated with higher levels of generalized psychologic distress, fear of hypoglycemia may lead patients with diabetes, and the parents of pediatric patients, to avoid hypoglycemia by treating falling blood glucose levels prematurely and hence maintain ambient blood glucose at higher values than desirable [97]. Programs that teach insulin-treated patients to recognize and anticipate blood glucose fluctuations have also been successful in reducing fear of hypoglycemia [98]. One might expect that fear of microvascular and macrovascular complications would also influence the self-management of the diabetes by the patient, but there has been little formal research on this topic. The recent development of a psychometrically sound "fear of complications" scale is an important first step [99].

Quality of life

Psychologic distress has so far been the primary focus of this discussion, but the extent to which diabetes affects the individual's perceived quality of life is also crucially important. Defining and measuring quality of life remains controversial, although it is generally agreed that this concept should include an understanding of how health-related variables affect physical, social and mental functioning as well as the individual's overall feelings of well-being and satisfaction with life [100].

General health-related quality of life

Large-scale studies of groups of individuals with various chronic illnesses have typically found little evidence that quality of life is differentially disrupted in adults with diabetes. Patients with diabetes do not differ from those with arthritis, renal disease, dermatologic disorders or from the general population on measures of anxiety, depression, positive affect, emotional ties, loss of control or overall mental health [101]. When health-related quality of life was assessed in a large cohort of adults with diabetes with the Medical Outcome Study (MOS-36) questionnaire, patients with diabetes reported more problems in physical and social functioning than patients without chronic conditions, but tended to function better than patients with cardiovascular, pulmonary or gastrointestinal disorders [102].

For individuals with T1DM, poorer health-related quality of life is associated with being older, having biomedical complications, being female, being less physically active and having a lower income [103]. Even the presence of a single biomedical complication can have a measurable impact on quality of life, and as the number of complications increase, there is a corresponding decline in quality of life as assessed by virtually all MOS-36 scales [103,104]. Chronic hyperglycemia, as indexed by higher HbA_{1c} levels, is also associated with poorer general health, even after the presence of complications is taken into account statistically [105]. Recurrent hypoglycemia, defined as one or more episodes a month, also predicts poorer health-related quality of life, particularly on measures of mental health and social function [103] and physical health [105,106]. Many of these same variables are associated with poorer health-related quality of life in older adults with T2DM. Among the best predictors are the presence of diabetes-related complications [107], certain demographic characteristics (female, poorly educated, lower income) and lower levels of physical activity [105,108]. The relationship between metabolic control and health-related quality of life remains controversial, with some [105], but not all [109] studies finding statistically reliable correlations.

Diabetes-specific quality of life

The use of diabetes-specific quality of life measures leads to similar conclusions [104]. The Diabetes Quality of Life (DQOL) measure, first developed to assess changes in quality of life during the course of the DCCT, explicitly examines factors such as satisfaction, impact of diabetes, social/vocational worry and diabetes-related worry [110]. When evaluated with either a generic pediatric quality of life measure [111] or with disease-specific questions, adolescents reported a relatively good quality of life which was only moderately affected by their diabetes, yet there was a great deal of inter-individual variation in response [112]. Differences in metabolic control or other biomedical or psychosocial factors may be responsible for this variability, although there is little consistency across studies. For example, improved metabolic control has sometimes [113], but not invariably [112], been found to be associated with better diabetes quality of life in adolescents.

Healthy adults with T1DM also report being satisfied overall with life, and indicate that diabetes has had little impact on their lives [114]. These relationships occur regardless of type of treatment (conventional or intensive insulin therapy) [31], or type of diabetes-associated quality of life measures employed [115]. Despite the demands made on individuals treated with intensive therapy, there is no evidence that treatment over a long period of time (6–9 years) adversely affects quality of life [31]; in fact, over a short-term (4 month) period, it is associated with improvements in diabetes quality of life [116]. The relatively benign experience of intensively treated patients participating in the DCCT may be a consequence of the greater level of psychologic and medical support that is provided to the participants in such clinical trials [41] or, alternately, may reflect the relative insensitivity of a measure like the DQOL to small changes in quality of life over time [100]. More recent studies evaluating changes in quality of life associated with the use of continuous subcutaneous insulin infusion have been mixed, with some indicating no benefit, while others suggesting modest benefit [117], particularly amongst children and their parents [118].

Age at onset of diabetes may also affect certain aspects of life quality. One survey of marital satisfaction found that adults diagnosed with T1DM before 9 years of age were more satisfied with their marriage, and were more likely to have children than those diagnosed later [119]. Those authors suggest that individuals diagnosed earlier in development may be more adept at integrating the disease as part of their lifestyle and thus find less disruption from diabetes later in life. More recent work also suggests that the linkages between marital satisfaction, higher levels of diabetes-related satisfaction and better metabolic control may reflect better psychosocial adaptation to a variety of illness-related and marital role stresses and strains [120].

Diabetes-specific quality of life measures have been used less frequently with older adults with T2DM, but those studies have typically obtained results that do not vary appreciably from those noted in patients with T1DM [104]. When quality of life is operationally defined by measures of mood, cognitive mistakes or work symptoms, most adults with T2DM report little disruption in most areas of life, although an appreciable minority (27%) report loss of enjoyment from previously valued activities, particularly social eating and drinking [121]. Worse quality of life seems to be especially evident in patients with T2DM treated with insulin [122], although several studies, including the UK Prospective Diabetes Study, have found no effect of intensive therapy regimens on quality of life [123].

Interventions to reduce psychologic distress

Traditional psychotherapy

Individual or group psychotherapy or supportive counseling should be as effective in children or adults with diabetes as in individuals without diabetes but with similarly high levels of psychologic distress [124]. Many recommendations have been made for such interventions [16,125], and while there are now a large number of studies that have made use of these, data from several recent meta-analyses have generally found them to have, at best, modest effects in reducing psychologic distress and in improving metabolic control [126–128].

Traditional individualized and group therapy has been used to provide emotional support for both children and adults with diabetes, and may be particularly beneficial for patients who are confronting the development of complications such as blindness [129,130]. Studies of individual psychotherapeutic interventions are rare, but data from a single, very small randomized trial are quite promising. When a time-limited problem-oriented individualized treatment was compared with standard insulin treatment counseling in adults with T1DM, patients receiving the psychotherapeutic treatment showed greater reductions in both problem severity and in HbA_{1c} values than those receiving conventional diabetes care [131].

Group therapy programs, which are far more common, have similarly shown either very small positive effects or no reduction in distress. Such groups are typically led by mental health professionals, have 4–12 participants, meet weekly or fortnightly for 90 minutes; they may run for as long as a year [132], although interventions as brief as 7 weeks have been conducted [129]. A major focus for such groups, at least early on, is to provide participants with more medical information about diabetes [130,132]. Over time, participants become more comfortable in discussing personal concerns, diabetes-related and otherwise. The broad range of topics discussed may include coming to terms with unfinished grieving over diabetes-associated problems, dealing with guilt that they may have caused their own complications and coping with fears about loss of independence [133]. As with individual psychotherapy, the efficacy of formal group therapy, in terms of improved mood or metabolic control, has not been studied extensively in large, carefully designed studies [134] and the quality of the current research is considered "weak" from a methodologic perspective [128]. Anecdotal reports suggest that many participants leave the group happier, or better adjusted, and various "curative factors" have been identified by patients as being a major benefit of group therapy, including interpersonal learning, the experience of catharsis, development of insight into problems and an understanding that the individual is not alone in experiencing disease-related psychologic distress [135,136], but analyses of outcomes from formal clinical trials with children and adults with diabetes have been less sanguine [126,128,137].

Cognitive–behavioral therapy

Of the different psychotherapeutic modalities available, cognitive–behavioral therapy (CBT) appears to be particularly promising in reducing the severity of depressive symptomatology. CBT teaches patients to use problem-solving strategies to reduce stressful situations and trains them to use cognitive techniques to "think away" their distorted beliefs, and replace them with more accurate and adaptive thoughts. Comparing 10 weeks of individualized CBT with non-therapeutic diabetes education (control condition), Lustman *et al.* [138] found that 85% of patients with T2DM receiving CBT achieved remission of depressive symptoms, in contrast to 27% in the control condition; at 6-month follow-up, similar rates of remission were seen (70% vs 33%). Individuals who are most likely to benefit from CBT are those with fewer complications and/or better compliance with blood glucose monitoring [139]. Variations of this approach have been used in studies of adults with T1DM, and while there were marked reductions in diabetes-related distress and in symptoms of depression, they were no differences between those subjects treated with group CBT and those in an active comparator condition who were treated with blood glucose awareness training. In neither group were there meaningful changes in glycemic control at 6 or 12 months after therapy initiation, but both were equally effective in lowering depressive symptoms to a modest degree

[140]. The fact that blood glucose awareness training, which has a minimal psychologic component, is effective in reducing psychologic distress is quite surprising, and emphasizes the potential effects that simple training in diabetes management may have on an individual's level of psychologic distress.

Pharmacotherapy

Diabetes-related depression and anxiety disorders have also been treated successfully with pharmacotherapy [141,142]. Placebo-controlled studies have demonstrated that SSRIs such as fluoxetine [143] and sertraline [77], and tricyclic antidepressants such as nortriptyline [144] effectively reduce severity of depression and its subsequent recurrence in patients with diabetes, whereas the benzodiazepine alprazolam [145] effectively reduces anxiety. These different psychoactive drug classes differentially affect metabolic control. Nortriptyline produces a sustained increase in HbA_{1c} values; in contrast, both fluoxetine and alprazolam reduce HbA_{1c} values significantly. The physiologic basis for these differential effects remains unknown, but most experts believe that pharmcotherapy-induced hyperglycemia can be handled readily with appropriate adjustments to the diabetes management regimen [146].

Pharmacotherapy alone, or paired with a form of psychotherapy such as CBT, may not only improve mental health, but it may also reduce the risk of death, as recently demonstrated in the PROSPECT trial [147]. In that medical practice-based study, older depressed adults with and without diabetes were randomized to usual care or to an intervention in which trained depression-care managers monitored psychopathology, adherence to treatment regimens, patients' responses and side effects, and provided subjects either with a first-line antidepressant medication (an SSRI) or interpersonal psychotherapy. All subjects were followed for a median of 52 months, and only mortality outcomes were reported. There was a significant reduction in all cause mortality, but only for those depressed patients with diabetes who received this simple depression management strategy, demonstrating that even minimal management of depression can have salutary effects in the health of older adults with diabetes. Given the nature of that study's design, however, it is impossible to identify the processes underlying these effects.

Neuropsychologic impact of diabetes

Diabetes has long been thought to affect cognition, as well as emotion, but it was not until the development of clinical neuropsychology (the study of brain–behavior relationships) that researchers were able to demonstrate unequivocally that mental efficiency can be disrupted by diabetes, its complications and its management, and that this neuropsychologic dysfunction reflects changes occurring in the CNS. The magnitude of these effects is relatively modest in most individuals, and few patients with diabetes manifest cognitive changes that would be characterized as being "clinically significant" – unless they developed diabetes early in life. Until very recently, when cognitive dysfunction was found in patients with diabetes it was invariably attributed to the adverse effects of severe and/or recurrent hypoglycemia on the CNS. New research suggests that chronic hyperglycemia, and the metabolic and vascular complications that are associated with it, underlie the development of most structural and functional changes to the CNS, particularly in adults. Although hypoglycemia can never be considered to be entirely benign, it may have a relatively small role in the etiology of neurocognitive changes in patients with diabetes [148,149].

CNS sequelae of diabetes in children and adolescents

Cognitive manifestations

The nature and extent of cognitive dysfunction in children and adolescents differs depending on age of diagnosis. Those diagnosed in the first 5–7 years of life appear to have an elevated risk of manifesting a moderately severe cognitive impairment which is evident across a broad range of cognitive domains, including measures of attention, mental flexibility, psychomotor efficiency, learning, memory, problem-solving and overall intelligence [150–156]. In contrast, those diagnosed after that early "critical period" show very mild cognitive dysfunction which is limited primarily to measures of overall intelligence and to performance on speeded tasks, particularly those having a visuoperceptual component [156]. Learning, memory and problem-solving skills are largely intact in this "later onset" patient population, or are only very minimally [157] and inconsistently affected [158,159]. Regardless of age at diagnosis, children with diabetes also tend to achieve lower scores than their peers without diabetes on measures of academic achievement [157,160], and have somewhat poorer grades in school [161], with these latter effects especially pronounced in children with a very early onset of diabetes [162].

The magnitude of the cognitive dysfunction seen in children with diabetes tends to be quite modest, as demonstrated by a formal meta-analysis of 19 pediatric studies encompassing 1393 children with diabetes and 731 healthy comparison subjects. When effect sizes were calculated (between-group difference divided by pooled standard deviation: "Cohen's **d**" [163]) for studies comparing later-onset children with control subjects, **d** values were approximately 0.20 or less – indicative of "small" to negligible effects. In contrast, effect sizes were more than twice as large when comparing early-onset subjects with diabetes with their peers without diabetes [156]. Using clinical rather than statistical criteria, one similarly finds marked differences between children with an early, as compared with a later, onset of diabetes. One large study found that 24% of children with an early onset of diabetes meet criteria for clinically significant impairment, as compared with only 6% of children with a later onset of diabetes, and 6% of a comparison group without diabetes [153].

This age at onset phenomenon has also been reported in adults diagnosed with diabetes early in life. Young adults who developed diabetes before 7 years of age performed more poorly on measures of information processing speed, and earned lower performance IQ scores than their peers with diabetes diagnosed at or after age 7 [164]. Abnormalities in brain structure are also evident. Magnetic resonance imaging (MRI) scans showed higher rates of mild to moderate ventricular atrophy (61% vs 20%), as well as somewhat higher rates of small punctate white matter lesions within the hippocampus (14% vs 2%). Smaller brain volumes were also correlated with poorer cognitive test performance, supporting the view that cognition dysfunction is necessarily linked to changes in CNS morphology.

Neurocognitive abnormalities appear relatively early in the course of diabetes, having been reported within 2–3 years of diagnosis. In the largest longest prospective pediatric study to date, a representative sample of 90 newly diagnosed youngsters with diabetes and 84 healthy children drawn from the community have been followed over a 12-year period. No between-group differences were evident at study entry [165] but, 2 years later, those children diagnosed before age 4 manifested developmental delays in so far as their scores on both the Wechsler Vocabulary and Block Design subtests improved less over time, relative to either children with a later diabetes onset or to community control subjects [166]. After 6 years of follow-up, children with diabetes – regardless of age at diagnosis – performed worse than their peers without diabetes on measures of intelligence, attention, processing speed, long-term memory and executive skills. Children with an early age at onset were particularly affected, and performed significantly worse on measures of attention and executive function than those with a somewhat later onset of diabetes [151]. After 12 years of follow-up, these children with diabetes – now young adults – continued to earn lower verbal and full-scale IQ scores, demonstrating that these effects are not a "developmental delay," but reflect a true, albeit modest, loss in cognitive efficiency, relative to those without diabetes [167]. Several other reports have also noted gradual decline in IQ scores as diabetes duration increases [161,167,168].

Effects of hypoglycemic episodes on brain function

Hypoglycemia has long been considered to be the cause of these neuropsychologic deficits, particularly in children with an early onset of diabetes [153,155]. Not only are rates of severe hypoglycemia significantly higher in children younger than 5 years of age, compared with children older than 5 (48% vs 13%), but hypoglycemia is also more likely to reccur in this younger group [169]. Behavioral factors could also contribute to the high rates of hypoglycemia early in life. Falling blood glucose levels may go unrecognized and untreated because very young children cannot adequately communicate that they are developing hypoglycemic symptoms. Although that view seems quite plausible, recent large well-designed cross-sectional [164,170] and longitudinal [171,172] studies completely failed to find any relationship between recurrent episodes of hypoglycemia and cognitive impairment, whereas others have reported only very weak and inconsistent findings [159] or have data sets in which severe hypoglycemia and age at onset tend to be confounded [173]. Similarly, both animal neuropathology [174] and human neuroimaging studies [167,175,176] are consistent with that view. For example, no changes in neuronal morphology were found in very young (1 month old) rats despite recurrent bouts of experimentally induced severe hypoglycemia, whereas 2 months of insulin-controlled diabetes caused a reduction in dendritic branching and fewer dendritic spines on neurons, and this was associated with poorer performance on measures of spatial memory [174]. These findings suggest that hypoglycemia is unlikely to be sufficient to induce significant brain dysfunction in most children, at least in those diagnosed with diabetes after the age of 7 years; however, for children with an early onset of diabetes, hypoglycemia may have a contributory role in the development of brain dysfunction [154,159].

Other CNS changes associated with diabetes in childhood

In addition to cognitive dysfunction, children with diabetes manifest multiple other changes in the CNS. Slowed neural activity is a very robust phenomenon. Compared with their peers without diabetes, adolescents with diabetes in good metabolic control showed significant increases in delta and theta (slow wave) activity, significant declines in alpha peak frequency in frontal brain regions, and declines in alpha, beta and gamma fast wave activity in posterior temporal regions [177]. When electroencephalogram (EEG) recordings were evaluated clinically, one large study noted that 26% of their subjects with diabetes had abnormal EEG records, compared to only 7% of healthy controls [178]. Both earlier age of diabetes onset and episodes of severe hypoglycemia were strong predictors of abnormality in that study, as well as in several earlier studies [179]. When auditory or visual evoked potentials were recorded, children and adolescents with a 2 years or more history of diabetes showed significant neural slowing, as evidenced by increased latencies, whereas those with less than 2 years of diabetes had normal latencies [180].

Cerebral blood flow has been measured only infrequently in children with diabetes, but the one study that used single photon emission computed tomography (SPECT) found lower levels of cerebral blood flow in children with diabetes than in healthy comparison subjects [181]. The greatest reductions in brain perfusion were found in the basal ganglia and frontal regions, followed by parietal and temporal areas. This pattern is similar to that reported in adults with T1DM [182], and provides limited support for the view that changes in brain perfusion may occur relatively early in the course of diabetes. The extent to which these cerebrovascular changes contribute to cognitive dysfunction remains to be determined.

Brain structure anomalies, documented with MRI, have only recently been reported in children with diabetes. The one study that focused exclusively on children with an early onset of diabetes noted greatly elevated rates of a very unusual brain anomaly – mesial temporal sclerosis. Within this cohort, 16% manifested this anomaly compared to less than 1% of the general pediatric population [175]. These anomalies apparently developed within a relatively brief period of time (mean duration of diabetes in this sample was approximately 7 years), and were unrelated to a past history of hypoglycemia. By contrast, children who experienced one or more episodes of severe hypoglycemia (seizure or coma) had smaller gray matter volumes than those with no such history (724 vs 764 cm^3), regardless of whether the hypoglycemic event occurred early in life or at a somewhat later age.

A second neuroimaging study used a semi-quantitative voxel-based morphometry technique to ascertain gray and white matter volumes in 108 children with diabetes and 51 age-matched children without diabetes who were 7–17 years of age [176]. Total brain volume was comparable in the two groups, but those children with diabetes who experienced one or more episodes of severe hypoglycemia had a slight reduction in gray matter in the left (but not right) temporal occipital region. This pattern of highly circumscribed effects, localized primarily to the left hemisphere, is consistent with what has been reported in adults with a long history of childhood-onset diabetes [183], as well as in several case reports [184]. Lifetime HbA_{1c} values, used to estimate of chronic hyperglycemia, were associated with less cortical volume in the right posterior brain regions (particularly the right cuneus and precuneus), also replicating findings in adults with diabetes [183]. Chronic hyperglycemia was also associated with less white matter, and these effects were most pronounced in parietal brain regions.

At this point, the underlying pathophysiologic basis for the development of CNS dysfunction in children remains unresolved, because at least some studies have found relationships between neurocognitive outcomes and both hypoglycemia and chronic hyperglycemia; however, there is increasing interest in studying the many metabolic – and potentially neurotoxic – events that occur around the time of diabetes diagnosis such as changes in brain glucose during the peri-onset period, dramatic metabolic perturbations, including the occurrence of DKA, that now seem to have the potential to alter the structure of the developing brain in the child with diabetes [154,185].

Brain structure and function in adults with type 1 diabetes

Neurocognitive manifestations

A highly circumscribed pattern of mild cognitive dysfunction characteristic of adults with T1DM has been identified from a systematic meta-analysis of data from 31 studies published in English between 1980 and 2004 that compared the performance of subjects with and without diabetes on multiple cognitive domains [186]. As illustrated in Table 49.1, subjects with diabetes, who were 18–50 years of age and in relatively good health, performed significantly more poorly on measures of intelligence, attention, psychomotor speed, cognitive flexibility and visual perception, whereas no between-group differences were found on measures of language, learning and memory. Even when differences were detected, they were modest at best, with effect sizes (**d**) ranging from 0.3 to 0.8 standard deviation units. It is important to note that not all cognitive domains were affected. Learning and memory skills, which are generally considered to be sensitive to early brain damage [187], were well preserved in this diverse patient population, despite an average of 20 or more years of T1DM. Moreover, with only one exception ("crystallized intelligence"), virtually all of the cognitive tasks on which patients with diabetes perform more poorly were those that also required rapid responding. That is, mental slowing appears to be the fundamental deficit associated with T1DM in adulthood [188]. A similar pattern of results has been found in adults with T1DM who are over the age of 60 [189]. Remarkably, the magnitude of the cognitive differences found in these older adults was similar (**d** = 0.3–0.5) to that reported in their younger counterparts, despite their longer duration of diabetes.

Table 49.1 Cognitive characteristics of adults with T1DM, based on a meta-analysis of published papers. Standardized effect sizes (Cohen's **d**) for each cognitive domain reflect differences between subjects with and without diabetes. Adapted from Brands *et al.* [186].

Domain	Effect size	Significance	Total number	Studies
Overall cognition	0.40	$P < 0.001$	660	16
Intelligence				
Crystalized	0.80	$P < 0.01$	276	5
Fluid	0.50	$P < 0.01$	168	4
Language	0.05	NS	144	4
Attention				
Visual	0.40	$P < 0.001$	195	5
Sustained	0.30	$P < 0.01$	217	3
Learning and memory				
Working memory	0.10	NS	244	8
Verbal learning	0.20	NS	204	5
Verbal delayed memory	0.30	NS	157	3
Visual learning	0.10	NS	187	5
Visual delayed memory	0.10	NS	157	4
Psychomotor speed	0.60	$P < 0.05$	368	8
Cognitive flexibility	0.50	$P < 0.001$	364	9
Visual perception	0.40	$P < 0.001$	202	5

NS, non-significant.

As noted in studies of children with diabetes, adults with diabetes also manifest slowed neural processing on measures of brainstem auditory evoked potentials [190,191], visual evoked potentials [192] and EEG recordings [193]. The magnitude of these effects is greatest in those individuals who have clinically significant microvascular complications [194–196]. Multiple studies have also demonstrated that cerebral blood flow patterns are abnormal in adults with diabetes, with these effects greatest in frontal and frontotemporal brain regions [197]. Changes in cerebral perfusion, measured by SPECT, are common. In one large study, 85% of middle-aged adults with diabetes showed hypoperfusion in one or more region of interest compared to 10% of controls; similarly, 58% of subjects with diabetes showed hyperperfusion, compared to 20% of controls [182]. Again, these effects were greatest in subjects with microvascular complications.

Changes in gray and white matter

Marked reductions in brain matter density, as demonstrated by voxel-based morphometry, are also associated with T1DM. Compared with a group of healthy individuals without diabetes, young adults with a childhood onset of diabetes manifested significantly less gray matter (approximately 5%) in the right superior temporal gyrus, and in several left hemisphere regions, including the temporal gyrus, angular gyrus, medial frontal gyrus, inferior parietal lobule and thalamus [183]. These structures are especially important for attention, memory and language processing. The strongest predictor of gray matter density reduction was degree of chronic hyperglycemia in so far as higher lifetime HbA_{1c} values were consistently correlated with lower gray matter density.

Similar findings have been reported in a case–control study demonstrating that individuals with diabetic proliferative retinopathy manifest small but statistically reliable reductions in gray matter density in the left middle frontal gyrus, the right inferior frontal gyrus, the right occipital lobe and the left cerebellum, whereas the gray matter values of patients with diabetes without retinopathy were comparable to adults without diabetes [198]. Reductions in white matter volume have also been noted, with effects being greatest amongst adults with a longer history of chronic hyperglycemia and microvascular complications [199].

Retinopathy as a risk factor for CNS abnormalities

In reviewing these structural and functional findings it appears that a long history of chronic hyperglycemia, as indexed by the occurrence of microvascular complications, is a robust risk factor for neurocognitive abnormalities. The most direct support for this possibility comes from a longitudinal study that followed a group of young and middle-aged adults with a childhood onset of T1DM over a 7-year period [200]. Subjects who had clinically significant proliferative diabetic retinopathy at study entry, or who developed retinopathy during the course of the follow-up period, showed a significant decline in psychomotor efficiency, compared to demographically similar subjects without diabetes. In contrast, those without retinopathy at either time showed no evidence of psychomotor slowing. The risk of cognitive change was predicted by four variables: the presence or development of proliferative retinopathy, the presence of autonomic neuropathy, elevated systolic blood pressure and longer duration of diabetes. The resulting statistical model identified, with 83% accuracy, subjects who showed significant cognitive decline and explained 53% of the variance.

Cross-sectional studies of young adults have similarly demonstrated that background retinopathy is associated with white matter abnormalities on MRI and poorer performance on measures of attention, fluid intelligence and information processing speed [201]. Abnormal brain activation patterns during the performance of a working memory task have also been identified in patients with clinically significant retinopathy who were evaluated with functional MRI [202]. Other microvascular complications, particularly peripheral neuropathy, are also associated with changes in brain function and structure [177,193,196,203,204].

Because middle-aged adults without diabetes who have retinal microaneurysms also show a pattern of cognitive decline that is characterized by psychomotor slowing [205], it has been suggested that retinopathy may serve as a general marker of cerebral microangiopathy [148,206]. This is quite plausible, given the well-known homology between the retinal and cerebral microvascular systems [207]. In patients with clinically significant diabetic retinopathy, the resulting microangiopathy could lead to cerebral hypoperfusion and thereby contribute to the development of abnormalities in brain structure and function by interfering with the efficient delivery of glucose and other key substances to neural tissue [148,198]. The relationship often reported between peripheral neuropathy and brain dysfunction in patients with diabetes may simply reflect the fact that microvascular complications tend to appear contemporaneously and have a common origin [208,209]. That is, microvascular disease may be the primary mechanism underlying the development of neurocognitive dysfunction in young and middle-aged adults [150].

Repeated episodes of severe hypoglycemia and cognitive dysfunction

The widespread belief that moderately severe hypoglycemia will induce cognitive impairment in adults with diabetes appears to have little support from a growing body of research on this topic. The most compelling negative data come from the DCCT and its follow-up natural history study, the Epidemiology of Diabetes Interventions and Complications (EDIC). Cognitive functioning was assessed over an 18-year period in 1144 patients with T1DM who were between 29 and 62 years of age (mean 46 years) at the time of their final cognitive evaluation. Lifetime rates of severe hypoglycemia, defined as including a seizure or coma, were high, with a total of 1355 episodes reported in 453 subjects over the course of the study. Despite that, no relationship whatsoever was found between the cumulative number of severe hypoglycemic episodes and performance on a comprehensive battery of cognitive tests [210].

Cross-sectional studies have also failed to find robust relationships between cognition and episodes of severe hypoglycemia [186,201]. Several earlier studies did note a link between hypoglycemia and brain damage [211], but all relied on small samples of highly selected subjects who were assessed with a limited number of cognitive tests which yielded a pattern of results that was not entirely consistent with brain damage. For example, subjects with repeated hypoglycemia performed slower, but no less accurately, on a number of tests, and earned somewhat lower scores on the Performance subtests of the Wechsler Adult Intelligence Scale, yet learning and memory skills were intact. This latter finding is unexpected because of the well-known associations between memory and the hippocampus, a major focus of structural damage following profound hypoglycemia in rodents [212], non-human primates [213] and humans [184,214]. Whether moderately severe bouts of hypoglycemia adversely affect brain structure remains controversial, with some [215] but not all [174] studies finding evidence of neuronal necrosis in rodent models. In human studies it can be quite difficult to make attributions specifically to hypoglycemia, rather than to chronic hyperglycemia, because patients who experience hypoglycemia also have a history of poor metabolic control [177].

As described in Chapter 33, severe and profound hypoglycemia can induce significant structural and function brain damage, but the prevalence of this phenomenon in adults with diabetes seems extremely low.

Hyperglycemia and neurocognitive dysfunction associated with T2DM

Older adults with T2DM also show evidence of psychomotor slowing [216–218] and, in that way, are somewhat similar to young and middle-aged adults with poorly controlled T1DM. In addition, elderly adults with T2DM consistently learn new verbal and non-verbal information more slowly, and remember less of it over a brief delay, compared with subjects without diabetes [219–221]. Interestingly, this phenomenon appears to be limited to individuals over 60 years of age; younger adults with T2DM rarely show memory impairments [222]. Other cognitive skills, particularly problem-solving ability, may also be affected in older adults with T2DM [221], but those skills have been assessed less frequently (for reviews, see [219,223,224]).

The cognitive effects associated with T2DM are similar in magnitude to those reported in younger adults with T1DM. One recent study comparing 119 patients with T2DM (mean age 66 years; mean HbA_{1c} 6.9% [52 mmol/mol]) with 55 age-matched healthy subjects without diabetes found the subjects with diabetes to perform worse only on measures of information processing speed (**d** = 0.50), memory (**d** = 0.43) and attention and executive function (**d** = 0.43) [225]. The strongest predictor of poorer cognitive function was poorer metabolic control; neither duration of diabetes nor severity of peripheral neuropathy were related to any cognitive outcome variable [226]. Other studies have also noted strong negative relationships between HbA_{1c} values and cognition. For example, one very large epidemiologic study has demonstrated that each 1.0% (11 mmol/mol) increase in HbA_{1c} was associated with significantly poorer performance on tests of psychomotor speed, memory and executive function [227].

Despite their often brief duration of diabetes, patients with T2DM also manifest evidence of neural slowing [190,196], overall reductions in cerebral blood flow [228,229] and significant changes in brain structure, including smaller gray matter volumes (apprixmiately 22 mL reduction), greater subcortical atrophy (approximately 7 mL increase in lateral ventricle volume) and larger white matter lesion volume (approximately 57% increase) [230]. Structural changes appeared to be more prominent in women and were associated with higher HbA_{1c} values and older age, but were unrelated to diabetes duration, hypertension or hyperlipidemia. Compared with patients with T1DM, those with T2DM showed significantly greater cortical atrophy and deep white matter lesions, with effect sizes ranging between 0.50 and 0.66 [231], even though the patients with T2DM had diabetes for a shorter period of time (7 vs 34 years) and had lower rates of clinically significant microvascular complications (laser-treated retinopathy: 8% vs 38%). The higher rates of macrovascular disease and atherosclerotic risk factors may underlie the development of the CNS changes seen in the T2DM cohort, although there is evidence to suggest that impairments in glucose and/or insulin regulation may be contributory [232,233]. The hippocampus, which has only infrequently been evaluated in most modern neuroimaging studies, was also found to be reduced in a group of relatively healthy adults with T2DM compared to healthy controls (5.4 vs 6.2 cm^3; **d** = 1.4) [234]. This could explain, at least in part, the poor memory function seen in many older adults with T2DM. The best predictor of hippocampal atrophy was HbA_{1c} values.

Much attention has recently been focused on rates of dementia in older patients with T2DM and it has been argued that diabetes is a significant risk factor for the subsequent development of Alzheimer disease or vascular dementia. Several recent studies and review articles have noted an increased risk of dementia that ranges 1.2–2.3 for Alzheimer disease and 2.2–3.4 for vascular dementia [235–237]. T2DM also has a significant negative impact on activities of daily living, with rates of functional disability doubled (e.g. ability to do housework efficiently and without assistance; walk 2–3 blocks) [238].

The degree of chronic hyperglycemia, as indexed by HbA_{1c} levels, is the best (albeit imperfect) predictor of impairment in the older patient with diabetes, although a growing body of research has identified other diabetes-related conditions, including hyperinsulinemia [239,240], hypertension [220] and hypercholesterolemia [241]. Many patients with T2DM are beset with multiple medical problems or diabetic complications, some of which, such as cerebral atherosclerosis, could contribute to cognitive decline [219,224]. Nevertheless, it is clear that factors other than vascular disease must play a part in the etiology of these cognitive impairments because they can be identified in otherwise healthy adults with T2DM who have no clinically apparent vascular complications [217].

Diabetes management and psychologic processes

The management of diabetes is an extraordinarily complex endeavor. The person with T1DM must take responsibility for injecting insulin two or more times each day, carefully monitor food intake at each meal, periodically measure glucose in blood, and readjust insulin, food and/or exercise during acute illnesses or in response to excessively high or low blood glucose values. Similar demands are placed on those with T2DM. The medication regimen may be less onerous, but dietary and lifestyle changes are often harder to tolerate. In either instance, patients and their families assume primary responsibility for these self-

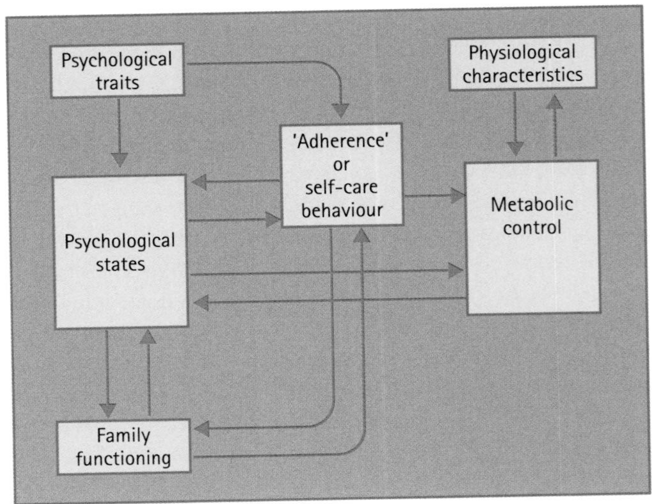

Figure 49.2 A systems model of the relationships between psychological and metabolic variables.

care behaviors, all of which are directed at maintaining optimal metabolic control. Good control signals that the patient's management efforts have been successful, while poor control may be interpreted as evidence that the patient has failed. This latter outcome may adversely affect mood and general psychologic well-being. Conversely, certain personality traits or coping styles that are intrinsic to an individual's psychologic make-up may modulate the patient's ability to manage diabetes self-care activities, as may environmental and psychosocial factors such as peer pressure to engage in certain "forbidden" activities, disruptive interpersonal conflicts and the normal stresses and strains of everyday life. Overall, an individual's "psychology" may influence, and be influenced by, the process of diabetes management.

According to a systems model of health, there is no simple direct relationship between any single psychologic variable and metabolic control [242]. Rather, health outcomes are determined by a system of reciprocal relationships amongst multiple psychologic, behavioral and physiologic variables. Figure 49.2 shows one such model of this process. Psychologic traits are relatively enduring characteristics that include personality, temperament and coping style. These may have a direct impact on self-care behaviors (adherence), and may also have a direct impact on emotional state. Psychologic states are more transitory and reflect emotions or feelings at a given point in time. Both family interactions and self-care behaviors may affect, and be affected by, the individual's mood or level of stress. Theoretically, at least, certain emotional states, especially stress, may also influence metabolic control directly via the autonomic nervous system or, indirectly, by interfering with the patient's ability to manage his/her diabetes. Family functioning, including conflicts and degree of family cohesiveness, can affect psychologic state (and vice versa), but can also influence self-care behaviors. Self-care or adherence behaviors include medication use, diet, exercise and monitoring, and these behaviors serve as the primary final common pathway to metabolic control. The frequently reported absence of a strong relationship between adherence and glycemic levels may reflect the effects of physiologic characteristics, such as intercurrent illness or hormonal fluctuations secondary to puberty.

Psychologic traits and their impact on metabolic control

These encompass a series of overlapping psychologic concepts that include "personality," "temperament" and "coping style." Individuals with personality characteristics indicative of a strong need for achievement and a high level of responsivity to social demands enjoy better metabolic control [243]. By contrast, HbA_{1c} values tend to be higher in adults who are opportunistic and alienated [244] or who have poor impulse control, a propensity for self-destructive behaviors and difficulty maintaining interpersonal relationships [245]. Being a worrier or highly emotional, as reflected by elevated neuroticism scores or higher levels of trait negative affect, may also be associated with poorer metabolic control [246,247], although there is not complete agreement [248,249]. Indeed, in adults with T2DM, higher neuroticism levels were associated with better metabolic control, and it has been suggested that moderate levels of worry may be needed to motivate these older adults to manage their diabetes [250].

Locus of control is another psychologic trait that may affect glycemic state. Individuals who have an "internal" locus of control believe that they are responsible for their health, whereas those who have an "external" locus believe that they are at the mercy of chance, or some other outside force. In general, individuals with an internal locus seem more likely to have better metabolic control [251–253], although that is not invariably the case [33,254,255]. One would expect that individuals with an internal locus of control would do a better job of managing their diabetes, and that this would lead to better metabolic control, yet most studies have failed to demonstrate a strong link between locus of control and adherence [252,256]. Reconciliation of these discrepancies may require a reconceptualization of the locus of control construct. For example, internal locus of control may have multiple dimensions such as autonomy and self-blame that are not typically measured in a systematic fashion yet may lead to somewhat different health outcomes [257]. Multidimensional measures that examine different aspects of sense of control as well as different modes of control and motivation for control may ultimately provide investigators with more accurate insights into the complex inter-relationships between perception of control and optimal diabetes management but, to date, they have been used only infrequently [258].

The complexity of these interactions has recently been underscored in a study that measured locus of control, self-efficacy and outcome expectancy, and used this information to predict patients' HbA_{1c} values. Within a sample of patients with T2DM from a predominantly disadvantaged background, those with an internal locus of control who reported low self-efficacy and low outcome expectancy tended to be in better metabolic control, whereas those with an internal locus of control but also expressed low self-efficacy and high outcome expectancy tended to be in poorer metabolic control [259]. Having an internal locus of control may be particularly beneficial to those patients with little confidence in their ability to follow their physicians' recommendations (i.e. low self-efficacy), as well as little confidence that following those recommendations will actually improve their health (low outcome expectancies).

Coping styles, broadly categorized as emotion-focused and problem-focused [260], serve to modulate the individual's response to stressful situations. Emotion-focused or cognitive coping attempts to reduce threats from the environment by reinterpreting or reappraising the situation ("Stay calm, it really can't hurt you"). Problem-focused coping, in contrast, seeks to change the environment and thereby eliminate the threat (e.g. reduce excessive carbohydrate consumption by removing all high fat snacks). Within each of these categories, specific behavioral strategies may be differentially effective. Some may actually exacerbate stress (e.g. emotion-arousing strategies that include anger, impatience or anxiety), while others (e.g. stoicism) may reduce or "buffer" the effects of stress [261]. In adults with T1DM, higher levels of stress were associated with poorer metabolic control, but only in people who use ineffective coping styles that tend to increase emotional arousal [262]. In adolescents, emotion-focused coping styles (e.g. behavioral and mental disengagement; aggressive coping) was also associated with poorer metabolic control and reduced diabetes-related quality of life, whereas the use of active coping strategies directed at approaching and making a direct effort to change the situation causing psychologic distress was linked to better metabolic control [263]. Data from a meta-analysis of 21 studies have shown that the use of approach coping was associated with both better overall psychologic adjustment and with somewhat better metabolic control [264].

If traits truly reflect enduring behavioral characteristics, they ought to predict long-term adherence. Support for that possibility has been provided by Jacobson *et al.* [256] in their longitudinal study of children and adolescents with diabetes. Coping style assessed soon after diabetes onset predicted adherence behaviors 4 years later. Those children who used more mature defense mechanisms and showed greater adaptive capacity such as higher stress tolerance or greater persistence shortly after diagnosis were most likely to manage their diabetes satisfactorily in the long term.

Psychologic states: stress, depression and anxiety

Many adults with diabetes consider stress to be a powerful determinant of their ability to maintain good metabolic control [265]. Higher levels of stress are associated with poorer glycemic control in adolescents [266,267] and adults [262,268], although there are very high levels of inter-individual variability. Like depression and other negative mood states [269], stress may affect metabolic control indirectly by disrupting the individual's ability to manage diabetes effectively [242,267]. Furthermore, elevated stress levels may affect metabolic control more directly by stimulating the autonomic nervous system to initiate a series of neuroendocrine responses that raise circulating blood glucose and catecholamine levels [270] and alter the activity of the hypothalamic-pituitary-axis, which may, in turn, further disrupt metabolic regulation and brain function [271]. Although this mechanism is theoretically attractive, several physiologic studies using carefully controlled acute stressors failed to find evidence of acute metabolic derangements in children and adults with T1DM [272–274]. No experimental studies have systematically examined the relationship between chronic stress and long-term metabolic changes, and it remains possible that both indirect (behavioral) and direct (neuroendocrine) pathways are involved in mediating the relationship between heightened stress and poor metabolic control [242].

Investigators have also considered the possibility that high levels of stress may trigger the appearance of diabetes in genetically susceptible individuals [275]. Although there is evidence that children with diabetes experienced greater stress (particularly actual or threatened losses within the family) prior to diagnosis than healthy control subjects assessed in the same fashion [276–278], no evidence of a similar relationship has been found in young adults newly diagnosed with T1DM [279]. Nevertheless, the occurrence of major stressful life events [280], or pre-existing depression [281], increases the risk of T2DM by as much as 37% [282]. Although the physiologic basis for this effect remains incompletely understood, it is generally assumed that stress induces a dysregulation of glucose metabolism [283] and/or disrupts insulin signaling processes within the CNS [271] in individuals genetically and constitutionally predisposed to develop diabetes.

Depression and anxiety has been found by some [284–286] but not all studies [45,73,256] to be associated with poorer metabolic control. Some of the strongest evidence for a link between affect and glycemic state comes from an early study in which adults with diabetes were followed during 36 weeks of treatment [287]. As glycemic control improved, symptoms of depression and anxiety declined; as control worsened, depression and anxiety increased, giving the appearance that success (or lack thereof) in managing diabetes led to corresponding changes in mood state. Taking a different approach, more recently researchers focused their attention on the extent to which changes in depressive symptomatology over a 12-month follow-up period influenced HbA_{1c} values [288]. Although there was a marked reduction in depressive symptoms regardless of type of diabetes, there was no corresponding improvement in metabolic control over time, leading to the conclusion that mood state has no meaningful impact on metabolic control.

The absence of an obvious relationship between depression and metabolic control [288] is not only counterintuitive, but it is inconsistent with the growing body of literature that suggests that the presence of depression adversely affects the medication adherence and self-care behaviors of people with diabetes. Particularly in older adults with T2DM, major depression is associated with less physical activity, a more unhealthy diet and poorer adherence to complicated medication regimens that includes taking multiple oral hypoglycemic, antihypertensive and lipid-lowering drugs at various times during the day [75,289–291]. Given those relationships, one would expect that reducing the level of depression would lead to corresponding improvements in their metabolic control as the person with diabetes begins to take better care of themselves but, to the best of our knowledge, no data support that possibility. The only prospective data available demonstrate that the presence of depressive symptoms at baseline predicts poorer adherence 9 months later [292]. Whether adherence would improve as depressive symptoms reduce in severity remains unexamined.

Family characteristics

Diabetes can dramatically disrupt the entire family, particularly when the patient is a child or adolescent [293]. Children, especially younger ones, enjoy better metabolic control when their parents take an active role in managing their diabetes, whereas adolescents are in better control when parents share management responsibilities with them [294–297]. Within the family, low levels of conflict [298], including sibling conflict [299], high levels of cohesion [8,300] and better communication skills [301] are associated with better control, as is a higher level of social support from family and friends [302]. Parental marital satisfaction also predicts control [300], perhaps because it serves as a surrogate for family cohesion and lack of conflict. Maternal trait anxiety [303] and parental intelligence also predict the child's metabolic control [304]; whether this association is mediated by better diabetes management or by less family conflict remains to be determined. Family factors such as lower adherence levels associated and greater levels of family stress, more family conflict and less family cohesion and sociodemographic variables (e.g. single-parent households) are also thought to explain the clinically significant disparity in metabolic control between African-American and Caucasian adolescents in the USA (mean HbA_{1c} 10.1 ± 2.1% [87 ± 2.3 mmol/mol] vs 8.6 ± 1.3% [70 ± 14 mmol/mol], respectively) [305,306]. Consistent with those data is the observation that children raised by single mothers have poorer metabolic control than those from two-parent families [307]. In adults with diabetes, better marital satisfaction is associated with better diabetes-related quality of life and marginally better glycemic control [308] but, not surprisingly, more global variables such as family [309] and work environment [310] do not predict glycemic control, although they do predict degree of psychologic adjustment.

The relationship between family characteristics and glycemic control in children is most likely mediated via a purely behavioral pathway whereby family conflicts disrupt performance of self-care behaviors. Support for this interpretation comes from Jacobson *et al.*'s [311] and Hauser *et al.*'s [312] seminal 4-year follow-up study of recently diagnosed youngsters with diabetes. Degree of family conflict and extent of family organization at diagnosis were the best predictors of both short and long-term adherence to diet, exercise, insulin administration and self-monitoring. Children whose families had less conflict as well as a family structure for planning activities and responses to problems were more likely to manage their diabetes satisfactorily [312] and to have better metabolic control [311]. This pattern of results has subsequently been supported by other large prospective [305] and cross-sectional analyses [313].

Self-care or "adherence" behaviors

The terms "adherence" and "compliance" have been used interchangeably, and refer to the extent to which an individual follows a medical management regimen. Adherence to a diabetes regimen cannot easily be determined, however, because there is no standard against which the person's actual behavior can be compared [314]; for example, few physicians provide a written management plan that specifies all aspects of diabetes care. Because it is the patient, and not the health care professional, who is responsible for nearly all diabetes care [315], an increasing number of writers have suggested that diabetes management efficacy be assessed by determining the extent to which a patient engages in "self-care" behaviors [316,317]. The shift in terminology from "adherence" to "self-care behaviors" acknowledges the behavioral complexity of diabetes management, and takes into account recent data demonstrating that specific self-care behaviors (e.g. taking medication, diet, monitoring and exercise) are not strongly related to one another in either adults [318] or children [319].

Certain self-care behaviors are far more likely to be followed than others. For example, data from a large survey of more than 2000 adults with diabetes indicated that 97% of insulin requiring patients and 93% of oral medication requiring patients always or usually took their medications as recommended, but only 77% reported that they always or usually followed blood glucose self-monitoring recommendations, and even fewer followed diet (63%) and exercise (40%) recommendations [320]. These findings are consistent with earlier studies demonstrating that more behaviorally complex activities such as diet and exercise are performed less consistently than medication-taking and blood glucose monitoring [321]. Not all self-care activities are equally predictive of glycemic control for children or adults [314,322] but, overall, the more self-care behaviors that are performed well, the greater should be the improvement in blood glucose control [257].

Blood glucose self-monitoring frequency ought to be a particularly salient self-care activity. A large medical registry study found that adults with T1DM who self-monitored blood glucose three or more times daily subsequently had HbA_{1c} values that were 1% (11 mmol/mol) lower than those who monitored less frequently; for T2DM adults, the difference was somewhat smaller (0.6%, 7 mmol/mol), albeit statistically significant [323]. Other studies have provided less positive results. For example, studies of patients with T2DM have either failed to find any evidence whatsoever that traditional fingerstick self-monitoring of blood glucose (SMBG) had any impact in reducing HbA_{1c} values over a 1-year period [324] or have noted only weak and inconsistent effects [325]. Similarly pessimistic conclusions have been drawn from several studies of children and adults with T1DM. Data from a recent clinical trial comparing continuous subcutaneous glucose monitoring HbA_{1c} with SMBG technique found the degree of change in HbA_{1c} values to be quite small, ranging from a 0.5% (6 mmol/mol) improvement to essentially no change over a 26-week time period. Moreover, somewhat surprising, the superiority of the CGM technique was limited to those subjects who were 25 years of age or older [326]. These data suggest that simply monitoring blood glucose values, and not using that information to adjust insulin or oral medications frequently and systematically, may have little meaningful impact on patients' long-term metabolic control.

Treatment adherence varies at different ages and changes with time. Younger children with diabetes tend to show better adherence (perhaps because of greater parental involvement) than adolescents [256,322]. Even after controlling for age, however, a longer duration of diabetes tends to be associated with declines in adherence [16,256], at least during adolescence. Other factors associated with better adherence are good family support [296], more shared responsibility between the child with diabetes and parent for self-care behaviors [327], greater cognitive maturity [328], more knowledge of diabetes and its management and better memory skills [319]. The nature of the physician–patient relationship can also influence adherence behaviors [329]. Doctor-centered discussions discourage patients from asking questions and increase their level of uncertainty and discomfort [330], whereas patient-centered communications are predictive of better self-reported adherence [331].

The generally weak relationship between self-care behaviors and metabolic control remains problematic for any model purporting to predict successful diabetes management. To some extent, this could reflect the possibility that the HbA_{1c} concentration is not the most appropriate measure of metabolic control [314], but it is more likely that the unexplained variance in glycemic control reflects unspecified physiologic or situational characteristics, as well as difficulties inherent in measuring self-care behaviors [317]. Because adherence is typically assessed by asking subjects to describe their behavior, rather than by direct observation, it is possible that self-reports may exaggerate or otherwise misrepresent the extent to which patients performed a particular self-care behavior [317].

Psychologic interventions to improve adherence

More traditional psychotherapeutic approaches

Several psychologic interventions have been developed to improve adherence in patients with diabetes. For adults who are most seriously non-compliant and whose consistent refusal to follow medical advice has led to "brittle diabetes," Boehnert & Popkin [332] have recommended a therapeutic approach that begins with crisis management, followed by psychotherapy of the sort typically used with patients diagnosed with "borderline personality." Intensive inpatient psychoanalytic psychotherapy, with 3–5 weekly sessions over a 5–28 week period, has also been found to improve metabolic control over a 1-year period [333], but this may be the least practicable way of treating brittle diabetes, because relatively few hospital settings offer this type of psychotherapy to children.

For less severe adherence problems, a variety of behavioral and psychosocial interventions have been used to improve diabetes management [334,335]. These differ from more traditional group therapy programs in so far as they use several sessions to target one or more self-care behaviors and/or the psychologic factors that may interfere with good adherence. A typical self-management program may meet once or twice monthly for seven or more sessions, discuss specific self-care strategies (e.g. blood glucose monitoring; exercise), role play appropriate behaviors, use homework assignments to practice what has been learned and resolve problems or barriers encountered during diabetes management [336].

Variations on this basic theme include the use of "booster" sessions, scheduled 6 or 12 months following the end of the program and designed to review and reinforce previously learned material. Interventions may include spouses or family members at some or all of the sessions, or incorporate separate but concurrent sessions for parents and adolescents with diabetes [337,338]. The program content also varies. Some focus on basic diabetes management and the acquisition of effective problem-solving skills [336,338] while others emphasize handling stress [339,340] or other psychologic issues that are especially problematic for participants, including fears about hypoglycemia or the development of hyperglycemic complications [130]. Most include homework assignments and extensive self-monitoring [336,340]. Interventions developed initially for patients without diabetes with high levels of psychologic distress are increasingly being applied to patients with diabetes, and both CBT [140] and "motivational interviewing" [341,342] or "motivational enhancement therapy" [127] programs have led to modest improvements in HbA_{1c} levels and in self-reported quality of life.

Family-focused behavioral interventions have been found to be particularly successful in improving diabetes management in children. In one of the largest studies of its kind, Wysocki *et al.* [343] randomized 119 families of adolescents to either 10 sessions of behavioral family systems group therapy, 10 sessions of an education and support group or standard diabetes therapy (with minimal psychologic support). Behavioral family systems therapy included four modules: problem-solving training which focused on conflict resolution; communication skills training; cognitive restructuring to identify and change those attitudes and beliefs that impede effective communication; and specialized family therapy interventions. In the 12 months following treatment, adolescents who participated in behavioral family systems therapy showed long-term improvement in relationships with their parents compared with adolescents in the other two treatment groups, and also manifested improved adherence to their diabetes management regimen, although these behavioral and psychologic changes were not associated with improvements in metabolic control [344]. Similar interventional approaches have also been applied to older adults with T2DM and, as is the case with children and adults with T1DM, there are reductions in psychologic distress and occasionally, but not invariably, small improvements in long-term glycemic control [345].

Cognitive–behavioral approaches

Coping skills training programs have also been found to be effective in improving the diabetes management skills of adolescents treated with intensive insulin therapy [346]. Based on a cognitive–behavioral skills-building model, coping skills training presents participants with a series of social situations that are particularly problematic for adolescents, and asks them to demonstrate how they would resolve that situation (e.g. manage food choices with friends). As implemented by Grey *et al.* [346], groups of 2–3 adolescents role play each scenario with a highly trained group leader who provides correction and models appropriate coping behavior. Sessions last 60–90 minutes and, in the typical training program, subjects participate in six weekly sessions followed by monthly visits. Over a 12-month follow-up period, adolescents randomized to coping skills training plus intensive diabetes management had significantly lower HbA_{1c} values (7.5% vs 8.5%; 58 vs 69 mmol/mol) and reported higher levels of self-efficacy as well as less difficulty in coping with diabetes and less depression when compared with adolescents who received intensive diabetes management alone [297].

Another successful approach is to "empower" patients, and encourage them to take personal responsibility in managing their diabetes [347]. Empowerment programs aim to improve patients' ability to identify and set realistic goals, apply problem-solving strategies to overcome barriers to those goals, develop more effective coping strategies in general, manage stress more effectively, increase levels of social support and improve self-motivation [348,349]. Results from a randomized controlled trial demonstrated that following a 6-week patient empowerment program, adults with diabetes showed a significant decline in HbA_{1c} level as well as increases in ability to set goals, manage stress, obtain external support and make decisions about diabetes management [348].

Individually tailored programs have also been used to help patients manage stress. If elevated levels of stress are a barrier to optimal metabolic control, then the stress-reduction effects of biofeedback-assisted relaxation training ought to reduce blood glucose levels appreciably. Results from various studies are mixed, with some [350], but not all [351,352] reporting significant improvements in glucose control following relaxation training. Results from a recent study suggest that the effectiveness of stress management programs may be determined, at least in part, by the patient's underlying personality. Patients with T2DM who were anxious, angry or hostile showed improved metabolic control following a stress management program that included progressive muscle relaxation training [352].

In their very thoughtful and thorough review of behavioral and psychosocial interventions in diabetes, Peyrot & Rubin [334] discuss the utility of including both problem-focused and emotion-focused interventions as part of an integrated behavior change support program. According to their model, interventions must occur in a particular sequence of five steps:

Table 49.2 Behavioral and/or psychosocial interventions: a step-by-step approach. From Peyrot & Rubin [334].

Intervention	Sample question
Problem-focused interventions	
1 Start with the patient's problem	"What's the hardest thing about managing your diabetes?"
2 Specify the problem	"Can you give me an example?"
3 Negotiate an appropriate goal	"What is your goal for changing your self-care behavior?" "Is that realistic?"
4 Identify barriers to goal attainment	"What could keep you from reaching your goal?" "Why would that keep you from reaching your goal?"
5 Formulate strategies to achieve the goal	"How can you overcome that barrier to reaching your goal?" "How have you successfully dealt with that before; would that work now?"
6 Contract for change	"What are your criteria for defining success?" "How will you reward yourself for success?"
7 Track outcomes	"How will you keep track of your efforts?"
8 Provide on-going support	"What will you do if you slip in your efforts to reach your goal; what can I do to help?"
Emotion-focused interventions	
9 Identify diabetes distress	"Do you feel overwhelmed by diabetes?"
10 Alleviate diabetes distress	"What are you saying to yourself when you deal successfully/unsuccessfully with a diabetes-related challenge?"
11 Identify depression	"In the past 2 weeks have you felt depressed or lost interest or pleasure in things?"
12 Treat disorder or refer for treatment	"Would you like to talk to someone who can help you resolve these problems?"

1 Specify the patient's problem;
2 Translate the patient's intentions to change into concrete, attainable goals;
3 Collaborate with the patient to identify barriers to reach those goals and formulate effective strategies;
4 Establish a "contract" with the patient to meet, or approach, those goals; and
5 Provide continuing support.

The framework provided by these commentators makes much sense from a clinical perspective, and their step-by-step approach is summarized in Table 49.2. The extent to which such an approach will be successful in initiating lasting clinically significant changes in mood, behavior and metabolic control remains unknown at the present time, but it is certainly an approach worth evaluating in formal clinical trials.

Conclusions

This chapter closes with a discussion of psychologic intervention programs because it is here where psychologists and diabetologists can work together effectively to improve their patients' mental as well as their physical health. One of the greatest problems facing mental health professionals is the failure, or inability, of many physicians to identify patients with psychologic distress quickly and provide appropriate treatment. A plethora of complex psychologic tests and questionnaires have been developed for research studies with patients with diabetes [353], yet the easiest way to determine whether a patient is having psychologic problems is to ask them explicitly. When psychologic problems are uncovered, immediate referral should be made to a mental health professional who is familiar with diabetes-related psychologic issues. It has been argued that it is the physicians who should diagnose and treat emotional disorders in their patients with diabetes, but that view is unrealistic. Few physicians have the expertise or the time to provide appropriate psychotherapeutic interventions. A far better solution is to add a psychologist, psychiatrist or social worker to the diabetes treatment team [41]. This approach was taken in the DCCT, and it may be one of the reasons why overall levels of psychopathology were so low, and perceived quality of life was so high, despite the arduous demands made on patients.

From this chapter it is clear that patients with diabetes have a remarkable level of psychologic resilience but, like anyone else, they are likely to experience psychologic distress at some time. Psychologists and diabetologists must continue to develop better ways of delivering psychologic support in order to alleviate their distress.

References

1 Kovacs M, Goldston D, Obrosky DS, Bonar LK. Psychiatric disorders in youths with IDDM: rates and risk factors. *Diabetes Care* 1997; **20**:36–44.

2 Kovacs M, Fineberg TL, Paulauskas S, Finkelstein R, Pollock M, Crouse-Novak M. Initial coping responses and psychosocial characteristics of children with insulin-dependent diabetes mellitus. *J Pediatr* 1985; **106**:827–834.

3 Schiffrin A. Psychosocial issues in pediatric diabetes. *Curr Diab Rep* 2001; **1**:33–40.

4 Northam E, Anderson P, Adler R, Werther G, Warne G. Psychosocial and family functioning in children with insulin-dependent diabetes at diagnosis and one year later. *J Pediatr Psychol* 1996; **21**:699–717.

5 Jacobson AM, Hauser ST, Wertlieb D, Wolfsdorf JI, Orleans J, Vieyra M. Psychological adjustment of children with recently diagnosed diabetes mellitus. *Diabetes Care* 1986; **9**:323–329.

6 Grey M, Cameron ME, Lipman TH, Thurber FW. Psychosocial status of children with diabetes in the first 2 years after diagnosis. *Diabetes Care* 1995; **18**:1330–1336.

7 Kovacs M, Finkelstein R, Feinberg TE, Crouse-Novak M, Paulauskas S, Pollock M. Initial psychologic responses of parents to the diagnosis of insulin-dependent diabetes mellitus in their children. *Diabetes Care* 1985; **8**:568–575.

8 Forsander GA, Persson B, Sundelin J, Berglund E, Snellman K, Hellström R. Metabolic control in children with insulin-dependent diabetes mellitus 5 years after diagnosis: early detection of patients at risk for poor metabolic control. *Acta Paediatr* 1998; **87**:857–864.

9 Landolt MA, Vollrath M, Laimbacher J, Gnehm HE, Sennhauser FH. Prospective study of posttraumatic stress disorder in parents of children with newly diagnosed type 1 diabetes. *J Am Acad Child Adolesc Psychiatry* 2005; **44**:682–689.

10 Kovacs M, Iyengar S, Goldston D, Obrosky DS, Stewart J, Marsh J. Psychological functioning among mothers of children wtih insulin-dependent diabetes mellitus: a longitudinal study. *J Consult Clin Psychol* 1990; **58**:189–195.

11 Kovacs M, Kass RE, Schnell TM, Goldston D, Marsh J. Family functioning and metabolic control of school-aged children with IDDM. *Diabetes Care* 1989; **12**:409–414.

12 Petrak F, Hardt J, Wittchen HU, Kulzer B, Hirsch A, Hentzelt F, *et al.* Prevalence of psychiatric disorders in an onset cohort of adults with type 1 diabetes. *Diabetes Metab Res Rev* 2003; **19**:216–222.

13 Pibernik-Okanovic M, Roglic G, Prasek M, Metelko Z. Emotional adjustment and metabolic control in newly diagnosed diabetic persons. *Diabetes Res Clin Pract* 1996; **34**:99–105.

14 Khunti K, Skinner TC, Heller S, Carey ME, Dallosso HM, Davies MJ, *et al.* Biomedical, lifestyle and psychosocial characteristics of people newly dignosed with type 2 diabetes: baseline data from the DESMOND randomized controlled trial. *Diabet Med* 2008; **25**:1454–1461.

15 Castro D, Tubiana-Rufi N, Fombonne E, Pediab Collaborative Group. Psychological adjustment in a French cohort of type 1 diabetic children. *Diabetes Metab* 2000; **26**:29–34.

16 Kovacs M, Iyengar S, Goldston D, Stewart J, Obrosky DS, Marsh J. Psychological functioning of children with insulin-dependent diabetes mellitus: a longitudinal study. *J Pediatr Psychol* 1990; **15**:619–632.

17 Wysocki T, Huxtable K, Linscheid TR, Wayne W. Adjustment to diabetes mellitus in preschoolers and their mothers. *Diabetes Care* 1989; **12**:524–529.

18 McDonnell CM, Northam EA, Donath SM, Werther GA, Cameron FJ. Hyperglycemia and externalizing behavior in children with type 1 diabetes. *Diabetes Care* 2007; **30**:2211–2215.

19 Holmes CS, Yu Z, Frentz J. Chronic and discrete stress as predictors of children's adjustment. *J Consult Clin Psychol* 1999; **67**:411–419.

20 Blanz BJ, Rensch-Riemann BS, Fritz-Sigmund DI, Schmidt MH. IDDM is a risk factor for adolescent psychiatric disorders. *Diabetes Care* 1993; **16**:1579–1587.

21 Grey M, Cameron ME, Thurber FW. Coping and adaptation in children with diabetes. *Nurs Res* 1991; **40**:144–149.

22 Jacobson AM, Hauser ST, Cole C, Willett JB, Wolfsdorf JI, Dvorak R, *et al.* Social relationships among young adults with insulin-dependent diabetes mellitus: ten-year follow-up of an onset cohort. *Diabet Med* 1997; **14**:73–79.

23 Northam EA, Matthews LK, Anderson PJ, Cameron FJ, Werther GA. Psychiatric morbidity and health outcome in type 1 diabetes: perspectives from a prospective longitudinal study. *Diabet Med* 2004; **22**:152–157.

24 Bryden KS, Peveler RC, Stein A, Neil A, Mayou RA, Dunger DB. Clinical and psychological course of diabetes from adolescence to young adulthood. *Diabetes Care* 2001; **24**:1536–1540.

25 Kovacs M, Obrosky DS, Goldston D, Drash A. Major depressive disorder in youths with IDDM: a controlled prospective study of course and outcome. *Diabetes Care* 1997; **20**:45–51.

26 Giaconia RM, Reinherz HZ, Silverman AB, Pakiz B, Frost AK, Cohen E. Ages of onset of psychiatric disorders in a community population of older adolescents. *J Am Acad Child Adolesc Psychiatry* 1994; **33**:706–717.

27 Jaser SS, Whittemore R, Ambrosino JM, Lindemann E, Grey M. Mediators of depressive symptoms in children with type 1 diabetes and their mothers. *J Pediatr Psychol* 2008; **33**:509–519.

28 Goldston DB, Kelley AE, Reboussin DM, Daniel SS, Smith JA, Schwartz RP, *et al.* Suicidal ideation and behavior and noncompliance with the medical regimen among diabetic adolescents. *J Am Acad Child Adolesc Psychiatry* 1997; **36**:1528–1536.

29 Lustman PJ, Griffith LS, Clouse RE. Depression in adults with diabetes: results of a 5 year follow-up study. *Diabetes Care* 1988; **11**:605–612.

30 Diabetes Control and Complications Trial (DCCT) Research Group. The effect of intensive treatment on the development and progression of long-term complications in insulin-dependent diabetes mellitus. *N Engl J Med* 1993; **329**:977–986.

31 Diabetes Control and Complications Trial (DCCT) Research Group. Influence of intensive diabetes treatment on quality-of-life outcomes in the Diabetes Control and Complications Trial. *Diabetes Care* 1996; **19**:195–203.

32 Anderson RJ, Freedland KE, Clouse RE, Lustman PJ. The prevalence of comorbid depression in adults with diabetes: a meta-analysis. *Diabetes Care* 2001; **24**:1069–1078.

33 Spiess K, Sachs G, Moser G, Pietschmann P, Schernthaner G, Prager R. Psychological moderator variables and metabolic control in recent onset type 1 diabetic patients: a two year longitudinal study. *J Psychosom Res* 1994; **38**:249–258.

34 Engum A, Mykletun A, Midthjell K, Holen A, Dahl AA. Depression and diabetes: a large population-based study of sociodemographic, lifestyle, and clinical factors associated with depression in type 1 and type 2 diabetes. *Diabetes Care* 2005; **28**:1904–1909.

35 Adriaanse MC, Dekker JM, Heine RJ, Snoek FJ, Beekman AJ, Stehouwer CD, *et al.* Symptoms of depression in people with impaired glucose metabolism or type 2 diabetes: the Hoorn Study. *Diabet Med* 2008; **25**:843–849.

36 Hislop AL, Fegan Pg, Schlaeppi MJ, Duck M, Yeap BB. Prevalence and associations of psychological distress in young adults with type 1 diabetes. *Diabet Med* 2008; **25**:91–96.

37 Gavard JA, Lustman PJ, Clouse RE. Prevalence of depression in adults with diabetes: an epidemiological evaluation. *Diabetes Care* 1993; **16**:1167–1178.

38 Lustman PJ, Griffith LS, Clouse RE. Depression in adults with diabetes. *Semin Clin Neuropsychiatry* 1997; **2**:15–23.

39 Peyrot M, Rubin RR. Levels and risks of depression and anxiety symptomatology among diabetic adults. *Diabetes Care* 1997; **20**:585–590.

40 Peyrot M, Rubin RR. Persistence of depressive symptoms in diabetic adults. *Diabetes Care* 1999; **22**:448–452.

41 Lorenz RA, Bubb J, Davis D, Jacobson AM, Jannasch K, Kramer J, *et al.* Changing behavior: practical lessions from the Diabetes Control and Complications Trial. *Diabetes Care* 1996; **19**:648–652.

42 Li C, Barker L, Ford ES, Zhang X, Strine TW, Mokdad AH. Diabetes and anxiety in US adults: findings from the 2006 Behavioral Risk Factor Surveillance System. *Diabet Med* 2008; **25**:878–881.

43 Gendelman N, Snell-Bergeon JK, McFann K, Kinney G, Wadwa RP, Bishop F, *et al.* Prevalence and correlates of depression in individuals with and without type 1 diabetes. *Diabetes Care* 2009; **32**:575–579.

44 Ali S, Stone MA, Peters JL, Davies MJ, Khunti K. The prevalence of co-morbid depression in adults with type 2 diabetes: a systematic review and meta-analysis. *Diabet Med* 2006; **23**:1165–1173.

45 Marcus MD, Wing RR, Guare J, Blair EH, Jawad A. Lifetime prevalence of major depression and its effect on treatment outcome in obese type II diabetic patients. *Diabetes Care* 1992; **15**:253–255.

46 Popkin MK, Callies AL, Lentz RD, Colon EA, Sutherland DE. Prevalence of major depression, simple phobia, and other psychiatric disorders in patients with long-standing type 1 diabetes mellitus. *Am J Psychiatry* 1988; **45**:64–68.

47 Wrigley M, Mayou R. Psychosocial factors and admission for poor glycaemic control: a study of psychological and social factors in poorly controlled insulin dependent diabetic patients. *J Psychosom Res* 1991; **35**:335–343.

48 Knol MJ, Heerdink ER, Egberts CG, Geerlings MI, Gorter KJ, Numans ME, *et al.* Depressive symptoms in subjects with diagnosed and undiagnosed type 2 diabetes. *Psychosom Med* 2007; **69**:300–305.

49 Weyerer S, Hewer W, Pfeifer-Kurda M, Dilling H. Psychiatric disorders and diabetes: results from a community study. *J Psychosom Res* 1989; **33**:633–640.

50 Lustman PJ, Griffith LS, Gavard JA, Clouse RE. Depression in adults with diabetes. *Diabetes Care* 1992; **15**:1631–1639.

51 Lloyd CE, Dyer PH, Barnett AH. Prevalence of symptoms of depression and anxiety in a diabetes clinic population. *Diabet Med* 2000; **17**:198–202.

52 Robinson N, Fuller JH, Edmeades SP. Depression and diabetes. *Diabet Med* 1988; **5**:268–274.

53 Lustman PJ, Anderson RJ, Freedland KE, De Groot M, Carney RM, Clouse RE. Depression and poor metabolic control: a meta-analytic review of the literature. *Diabetes Care* 2000; **23**:934–942.

54 Lustman PJ, Griffith LS, Freedland KE, Clouse RE. The course of major depression in diabetes. *Gen Hosp Psychiatry* 1997; **19**: 138–143.

55 Lloyd CE, Matthews KA, Wing RR, Orchard TJ. Psychosocial factors and complications of IDDM. *Diabetes Care* 1992; **15**:166–172.

56 Talbot F, Nouwen A. A review of the relationship between depression and diabetes in adults: is there a link? *Diabetes Care* 2000; **23**:1556–1562.

57 Egede LE. Effect of comorbid chronic diseases on prevalence and odds of depression in adults with diabetes. *Psychosom Med* 2005; **67**:46–51.

58 Mezuk B, Eaton WW, Albrecht S, Golden SH. Depression and type 2 diabetes over the lifespan: a meta-analysis. *Diabetes Care* 2008; **31**:2383–2390.

59 Golden SH, Lazo M, Carnethon MR, Bertoni AG, Schreiner PJ, Diez Roux AV, *et al.* Examining a bidirectional association between depressive symptoms and diabetes. *JAMA* 2008; **299**: 2751–2759.

60 Musselman DL, Betan E, Larsen H, Phillips LS. Relationship of depression to diabetes types 1 and 2: epidemiology, biology, and treatment. *Biol Psychiatry* 2003.

61 De Groot M, Anderson RA, Freedland KE, Clouse RE, Lustman PJ. Association of depression and diabetes complications: a meta-analysis. *Psychosom Med* 2001; **63**:619–630.

62 Karlson B, Agardh CD. Burden of illness, metabolic control, and complications in relation to depressive symptoms in IDDM patients. *Diabet Med* 1997; **14**:1066–1072.

63 Wilkinson G, Borsey DQ, Leslie P, Newton RW, Lind C, Ballinger CB. Psychiatric morbidity and social problems in patients with insulin-dependent diabetes mellitus. *Br J Psychiatry* 1988; **153**: 38–43.

64 Carrington AL, Mawdsley SKV, Morley M, Kincey J, Boulton AJM. Psychological status of diabetic people with or without lower limb disability. *Diabetes Res Clin Pract* 1996; **32**:19–25.

65 Ismail K, Winkley K, Stahl D, Chalder T, Edmonds M. A cohort study of people with diabetes and their first foot ulcer: the role of depression on mortality. *Diabetes Care* 2007; **30**:1473–1479.

66 Vileikyte L. Psychosocial and behavioral aspects of diabetic foot lesions. *Curr Diabetes Rep* 2008; **8**:119–125.

67 Vileikyte L, Leventhal H, Gonzalez JS, Peyrot M, Rubin RR, Ulbrecht JS, *et al.* Diabetic peripheral neuropathy and depressive symptoms: the association revisited. *Diabetes Care* 2005; **28**:2378–2383.

68 Jacobson AM, Rand LI, Hauser ST. Psychologic stress and glycemic control: a comparison of patients with and without proliferative diabetic retinopathy. *Psychosom Med* 1985; **47**:372–381.

69 Wulsin LR, Jacobson AM, Rand LI. Psychosocial correlates of mild visual loss. *Psychosom Med* 1991; **53**:109–117.

70 Matza LS, Rousculp MD, Malley K, Boye KS, Oglesby A. The longitudinal link between visual acuity and health-related quality of life in patients with diabetic retinopathy. *Health Qual Life Outcomes* 2008; **6**:95.

71 Wulsin LR, Jacobson AM, Rand LI. Psychosocial adjustment to advanced proliferative diabetic retinopathy. *Diabetes Care* 1993; **16**:1061–1066.

72 Robertson N, Burden ML, Burden AC. Psychological morbidity and problems of daily living in people with visual loss and diabetes: do they differ from people without diabetes. *Diabet Med* 2006; **23**:1110–1116.

73 Kovacs M, Mukerji P, Iyengar S, Drash A. Psychiatric disorder and metabolic control among youths with IDDM. *Diabetes Care* 1996; **19**:318–323.

74 Roy MS, Roy A, Affouf M. Depression is a risk factor for poor glycemic control and retinopathy in African-Americans with type 1 diabetes. *Psychosom Med* 2007; **69**:537–542.

75 Gonzalez JS, Peyrot M, McCarl LA, Collins EM, Serpa L, Mimiaga MJ, *et al.* Depression and diabetes treatment nonadherence: a meta-analysis. *Diabetes Care* 2008; **31**:2398–2403.

76 Jackson JL, DeZee K, Berbano E. Can treating depression improve disease outcome? *Ann Intern Med* 2004; **140**:1054–1055.

77 Lustman PJ, Clouse RE, Nix BD, Freedland KE, Rubin EH, McGill JB, *et al.* Sertraline for prevention of depression recurrence in diabetes mellitus: a randomized, double-blind, placebo-controlled trial. *Arch Gen Psychiatry* 2006; **63**:521–529.

78 Williams JW, Katon W, Lin EH, Nöel PH, Worchel J, Connell J, *et al.* The effectiveness of depression care management on diabetes-related outcomes in older patients. *Ann Intern Med* 2004; **140**:1054–1056.

79 Katon WJ, Von Korff M, Lin EHB, Simon G, Ludman E, Russo J, *et al.* The Pathways Study: a randomized trial of collaborative care in patients with diabetes and depression. *Arch Gen Psychiatry* 2004; **61**:1042–1049.

80 Dumont RH, Jacobson AM, Cole C, Hauser ST, Wolfsdorf JI, Willett JB, *et al.* Psychosocial predictors of acute complications of diabets in youth. *Diabet Med* 1995; **12**:612–618.

81 Geffken GR, Lehmkuhl H, Walker KN, Storch EA, Heigderken AD, Lewin A, *et al.* Family functioning processes and diabetic ketoacidosis in youths with type 1 diabetes. *Rehabil Psychol* 2008; **53**:231–237.

82 Liss DS, Waller DA, Kennard BD, McIntire D, Capra P, Stephens J. Psychiatric illness and family suport in children and adolescents with diabetic ketoacidosis: a controlled study. *J Am Acad Child Adolesc Psychiatry* 1998; **37**:536–544.

83 Wild D, von Maltzahn R, Brohan E, Christensen T, Clauson P, Gonder-Frederick L. A critical review of the literature on fear of hypoglycemia in diabetes: implications for diabetes management and patient education. *Patient Educ Couns* 2007; **68**:10–15.

84 Berlin I, Bisserbe JC, Eiber R, Balssa N, Sachon C, Bosquet F, *et al.* Phobic symptoms, particularly the fear of blood and injury, are associated with poor glycemic control in type 1 diabetic adults. *Diabetes Care* 1997; **20**:176–178.

85 Mollema ED, Snoek FJ, Heine RJ, van der Ploeg HM. Phobia of self-injecting and self-testing in insulin-treated diabetes patients: opportunities for screening. *Diabet Med* 2001; **18**:671–674.

86 Zambanini A, Newson RB, Maisey M, Feher M. Injection related anxiety in insulin-treated diabetes. *Diabetes Res Clin Pract* 1999; **46**:239–246.

87 Green LB, Wysocki T, Reineck B. Fear of hypoglycemia in children and adolescents with diabetes. *J Pediatr Psychol* 1990; **15**:633–641.

88 Irvine AA, Cox D, Gonder-Frederick L. Fear of hypoglycemia: relationship to physical and psychological symptoms in patients with insulin-dependent diabetes mellitus. *Health Psychol* 1992; **11**:135–138.

89 Hepburn DA, Deary IJ, MacLeod KM, Frier BM. Structural equation modeling of symptoms, awareness and fear of hypoglycemia, and personality in patients with insulin-treated diabetes. *Diabetes Care* 1994; **17**:1273–1280.

90 Gonder-Frederick L, Cox D, Kovatchev B, Julian D, Clarke W. The psychosocial impact of severe hypoglycemic episodes on spouses of patients with IDDM. *Diabetes Care* 1997; **20**:1543–1546.

91 Clarke WL, Gonder-Frederick LA, Snyder AL, Cox DJ. Maternal fear of hypoglycemia in their children with insulin dependent diabetes mellitus. *J Pediatr Endocrinol Metab* 1998; **11**:189–194.

92 Deary IJ. Symptoms of hypoglycaemia and effects on mental performance and emotions. In: Frier BM, BM Fisher, eds. *Hypoglycaemia in Clinical Diabetes*. London: John Wiley 1999: 29–54.

93 McCrimmon RJ, Frier BM, Deary IJ. Appraisal of mood and personality during hypoglycaemia in human subjects. *Physiol Behav* 1999; **67**:27–33.

94 McCrimmon RJ, Ewing FME, Frier BM, Deary IJ. Anger state during acute insulin-induced hypoglycaemia. *Physiol Behav* 1999; **67**:35–39.

95 Marrero DG, Guare JC, Vandagriff JL, Fineberg NS. Fear of hypoglycemia in the parents of children and adolescents with diabetes: maladaptive or healthy response? *Diabetes Educ* 1997; **23**:281–286.

96 Polonsky WH, Davis CL, Jacobson AM, Anderson BJ. Correlates of hypoglycemic fear in type I and type II diabetes mellitus. *Health Psychol* 1992; **11**:199–202.

97 Gonder-Frederick LA, Clarke WL, Cox DJ. The emotional, social, and behavioral implications of insulin-induced hypoglycemia. *Semin Clin Neuropsychiatry* 1997; **2**:57–65.

98 Cox DJ, Gonder-Frederick L, Polonsky W, Schlundt D, Kovatchev B, Clarke W. Blood glucose awareness training (BGAT-2): long-term benefits. *Diabetes Care* 2001; **24**:637–642.

99 Taylor EP, Crawford JR, Gold AE. Design and development of a scale measuring fear of complications of type 1 diabetes. *Diabetes Metab Res Rev* 2005; **21**:264–270.

100 Speight J, Reaney MD, Barnard KD. Not all roads lead to Rome: a review of quality of life measurement in adults with diabetes. *Diabet Med* 2009; **26**:315–327.

101 Cassileth BR, Lusk EJ, Strouse TB, Miller DS, Brown LL, Cross PA, *et al.* Psychosocial status in chronic illness: a comparative analysis of six diagnostic groups. *N Engl J Med* 1984; **311**:506–511.

102 Stewart AL, Greenfield S, Hays RD, Wells K, Rogers WH, Berry SD, *et al.* Functional status and well-being of patients with chronic conditions: results from the Medical Outcomes Study. *JAMA* 1989; **18**:907–913.

103 Lloyd CE, Orchard TJ. Physical and psychological well-being in adults with type 1 diabetes. *Diabetes Res Clin Pract* 1999; **44**:9–19.

104 Jacobson AM, De Groot M. The evaluation of two measures of quality of life in patients with type 1 and type 2 diabetes. *Diabetes Care* 1994; **17**:267–274.

105 Klein BEK, Klein R, Moss SE. Self-rated health and diabetes of long duration: the Wisconsin Epidemiologic Study of Diabetic Retinopathy. *Diabetes Care* 1998; **21**:236–240.

106 Wikblad K, Leksell J, Wibel L. Health-related quality of life in relation to metabolic control and late complications in patients with insulin dependent diabetes mellitus. *Qual Life Res* 1996; **5**:123–130.

107 Coffey JT, Brandle M, Zhou H, Marriott D, Burke R, Tabaei BP, *et al.* Valuing health-related quality of life in diabetes. *Diabetes Care* 2002; **25**:2238–2243.

108 Glasgow RE, Ruggiero L, Eakin EG, Dryfoos J, Chobanian L. Quality of life and associated characteristics in a large national sample of adults with diabetes. *Diabetes Care* 1997; **20**:562–567.

109 Caldwell EM, Baxter J, Mitchell CM, Shetterly SM, Hamman RF. The association of non-insulin-dependent diabetes mellitus with perceived quality of life in a biethnic population: the San Luis Valley Diabetes Study. *Am J Public Health* 1998; **88**:1225–1229.

110 Jacobson AM, Diabetes Control and Complications Trial (DCCT) Research Group. The Diabetes Quality of Life measure. In: Bradley C, ed. *Handbook of Psychology and Diabetes*. Chur, Switzerland: Harwood Academic, 1994: 65–87.

111 Laffel LMB, Connell A, Vangsness L, Goebel-Fabbri A, Mansfield A, Anderson BJ. General quality of life in youth with type 1 diabetes: relationship to patient management and diabetes-specific family conflict. *Diabetes Care* 2003; **26**:3067–3073.

112 Grey M, Boland EA, Yu C, Sullivan-Bolyai S, Tamborlane WV. Personal and family factors associated with quality of life in adolescents with diabetes. *Diabetes Care* 1998; **21**:909–914.

113 Hoey H, Aanstoot HJ, Chiarelli F, Daneman D, Danne T, Dorchy H, *et al.* Good metabolic control is associated with better quality of life in 2,101 adolescents with type 1 diabetes. *Diabetes Care* 2001; **24**:1923–1928.

114 Jacobson AM. Quality of life in patients with diabetes mellitus. *Semin Clin Neuropsychiatry* 1997; **2**:82–93.

115 Rose M, Burkert U, Scholler G, Schirop T, Danzer G, Klapp BG. Determinants of the quality of life of patients with diabetes under intensified insulin therapy. *Diabetes Care* 1998; **21**:1876–1885.

116 Weinger K, Jacobson AM. Psychosocial and quality of life correlates with glycemic control during intensive treatment of type 1 diabetes. *Patient Educ Couns* 2001; **42**:123–131.

117 Barnard KD, Lloyd CE, Skinner TC. Systematic literature review: quality of life associated with insulin pump use in type 1 diabetes. *Diabet Med* 2007; **24**:607–617.

118 Barnard KD, Speight J, Skinner TC. Quality of life and impact of continuous subcutaneous insulin infusion for children and their parents. *Pract Diabetes Int* 2008; **25**:278–284.

119 Ahlfield JE, Soler NG, Marcus SD. The young adult with diabetes: impact of the disease on marriage and having children. *Diabetes Care* 1985; **8**:52–56.

120 Trief PM, Himes CL, Orendorff R, Weinstock RS. The marital relationship and psychosocial adaptation and glycemic control of individuals with diabetes. *Diabetes Care* 2001; **24**:1384–1389.

121 Mayou R, Peveler R, Davies B, Mann J, Fairburn C. Psychiatric morbidity in young adults with insulin-dependent diabetes mellitus. *Psychol Med* 1991; **21**:639–645.

122 Davis TME, Clifford RM, Davis WA. Effect of insulin therapy on quality of life in type 2 diabetes mellitus: the Fremantle Diabetes Study. *Diabetes Res Clin Pract* 2001; **62**:63–71.

123 UK Prospective Diabetes Study Group. Quality of life in type 2 diabetic patients is affected by complications but not by intensive policies to improve blood glucose or blood pressure control (UKPDS 37). *Diabetes Care* 1999; **22**:1125–1136.

124 Rubin RR, Peyrot M. Psychological issues and treatments for people with diabetes. *J Clin Psychol* 2001; **57**:457–478.

125 Rubin RR, Peyrot M. Psychosocial problems and interventions in diabetes. *Diabetes Care* 1992; **15**:1640–1657.

126 Murphy HR, Rayman G, Skinner TC. Psycho-educational interventions for children and young people with type 1 diabetes. *Diabet Med* 2006; **23**:935–943.

127 Ismail K, Thomas SM, Maissi E, Chalder T, Schmidt U, Bartlett J, *et al.* Motivational enhancement therapy with and without cognitive behavioral therapy to treat type 1 diabetes. *Ann Intern Med* 2008; **149**:708–719.

128 Winkley K, Landau S, Eisler I, Ismail K. Psychological interventions to improve glycaemic control in patients with type 1 diabetes: systematic review and meta-analysis of randomised controlled trials. *Br Med J* 2006; **333**:65.

129 Zettler A, Duran G, Waadt S, Herschbach P, Strian F. Coping with fear of long-term complications in diabetes mellitus: a model clinical program. *Psychother Psychosom* 1995; **64**:178–184.

130 Toth EL, James I. Description of a diabetes support group: lessons for diabetes caregivers. *Diabet Med* 1992; **9**:773–778.

131 Didjurgeit U, Kruse J, Schmitz N, Stückenschneider P, Sawicki PT. A time-limited, problem-orientated psychotherapeutic intervention in type 1 diabetic patients with complications: a randomized controlled trial. *Diabet Med* 2002; **19**:814–821.

132 Pelser HE, Groen JJ, Stuyling de Lange MJ, Dix PC. Experiences in group discussions with diabetic patients. *Psychother Psychosom* 1979; **32**:257–269.

133 Simson U, Nawarotzky U, Friese G, Porck W, Schottenfeld-Naor Y, Hahn S, *et al.* Psychotherapy intervention to reduce depressive symptoms in patients with diabetic foot syndrome. *Diabet Med* 2008; **25**:206–212.

134 Rubin RR. Psychotherapy in diabetes mellitus. *Semin Clin Neuropsychiatry* 1997; **2**:72–81.

135 Tattersall RB, McCulloch DK, Aveline M. Group therapy in the treatment of diabetes. *Diabetes Care* 1985; **8**:180–188.

136 Citrin WS, La Greca AM, Skyler JS. Group interventions in type 1 diabetes mellitus. In: Ahmed PI, N Ahmed, eds. *Coping with Juvenile Diabetes*. Springfield: Charles C. Thomas, 1985: 181–294.

137 Northam EA, Todd S, Cameron FJ. Interventions to promote optimal health outcomes in children with type 1 diabetes: are they effective? *Diabet Med* 2006; **23**:113–121.

138 Lustman PJ, Griffith LS, Freedland KE, Kissel SS, Clouse RE. Cognitive behavior therapy for depression in type 2 diabetes mellitus: a randomized, controlled trial. *Ann Intern Med* 1998; **129**:613–621.

139 Lustman PJ, Freedland KE, Griffith LS, Clouse RE. Predicting response to cognitive behavior therapy of depression in type 2 diabetes. *Gen Hosp Psychiatry* 1998; **20**:302–306.

140 Snoek FJ, Van der Ven NCW, Twisk JWR, Hogenelst MHE, Tromp-Wever AME, Van der Ploeg HM, *et al.* Cognitive behavioural therapy (CBT) compared with blood glucose awareness training (BGAT) in poorly controlled type 1 diabetic patients: long-term effects on HbA1c moderated by depression – a randomized controlled trial. *Diabet Med* 2008; **25**:1337–1342.

141 Lustman PJ, Penckover SM, Clouse RE. Recent advances in understanding depression in adults with diabetes. *Curr Diab Rep* 2007; **7**:114–122.

142 Petrak F, Herpertz S. Treatment of depression in diabetes: An update. *Curr Opin Psychiatry* 2009; **22**:211–217.

143 Lustman PJ, Freedland KE, Griffith LS, Clouse RE. Fluoxetine for depression in diabetes: a randomized double-blind placebo-controlled trial. *Diabetes Care* 2000; **23**:618–623.

144 Lustman PJ, Griffith LS, Clouse RE, Freedland KE, Eisen SA, Rubin EH, *et al.* Effects of nortriptyline on depression and glycemic control in diabetes: results of a double-blind, placebo-controlled trial. *Psychosom Med* 1997; **59**:241–250.

145 Lustman PJ, Griffith LS, Clouse RE, Freedland KE, Eisen SA, Rubin EH, *et al.* Effects of alprazolam on glucose regulation in diabetes: results of a double-blind, placebo-controlled trial. *Diabetes Care* 1995; **18**:1133–1169.

146 Lustman PJ, Clouse RE, Freedland KE. Management of major depression in adults with diabetes: implications of recent clinical trials. *Semin Clin Neuropsychiatry* 1998; **3**:102–114.

147 Bogner HR, Morales KH, Post EP, Bruce ML. Diabetes, depression, and death: a randomized controlled trial of a depression treatment program for older adults based in primary care (PROSPECT). *Diabetes Care* 2007; **30**:3005–3010.

148 Ryan CM. Diabetes and brain damage: more (or less) than meets the eye? *Diabetologia* 2006; **49**:2229–2233.

149 Wessels AM, Scheltens P, Barkhof F, Heine RJ. Hyperglycaemia as a determinant of cognitive decline in patients with type 1 diabetes. *Eur J Pharmacol* 2008; **585**:88–96.

150 Biessels GJ, Deary IJ, Ryan CM. Cognition and diabetes: a lifespan perspective. *Lancet Neurol* 2008; **7**:184–190.

151 Northam EA, Anderson PJ, Jacobs R, Hughes M, Warne GL, Werther GA. Neuropsychological profiles of children with type 1 diabetes 6 years after disease onset. *Diabetes Care* 2001; **24**:1541–1546.

152 Northam EA, Rankins D, Cameron FJ. Therapy insight: the impact of type 1 diabetes on brain development and function. *Nat Clin Pract Neurol* 2006; **2**:78–86.

153 Ryan C, Vega A, Drash A. Cognitive deficits in adolescents who developed diabetes early in life. *Pediatrics* 1985; **75**:921–927.

154 Ryan CM. Why is cognitive dysfunction associated with the development of diabetes early in life? The diathesis hypothesis. *Pediatr Diabetes* 2006; **7**:289–297.

155 Rovet J, Ehrlich R, Hoppe M. Specific intellectual deficits associated with the early onset of insulin-dependent diabetes mellitus in children. *Child Dev* 1988; **59**:226–234.

156 Gaudieri PA, Chen R, Greer TF, Holmes CS. Cognitive function in children with type 1 diabetes: a meta-analysis. *Diabetes Care* 2008; **31**:1892–1897.

157 Kaufman FR, Epport K, Engilman R, Halvorson M. Neurocognitive functioning in children diagnosed with diabetes before age 10 years. *J Diabetes Complications* 1999; **13**:31–38.

158 Hershey T, Lillie R, Sadler M, White NH. Severe hypoglycemia and long-term spatial memory in children with type 1 diabetes mellitus: a retrospective study. *J Intern Neuropsychol Soc* 2003; **9**:740–750.

159 Perantie DC, Lim A, Wu J, Weaver P, Warren SL, Sadler M, *et al.* Effects of prior hypoglycemia and hyperglycemia on cognition in children with type 1 diabetes mellitus. *Pediatr Diabetes* 2008; **9**:87–95.

160 McCarthy AM, Lindgren S, Mengeling MA, Tsalikian E, Engvall JC. Factors associated with academic achievement in children with type 1 diabetes. *Diabetes Care* 2003; **26**:112–117.

161 Kovacs M, Goldston D, Iyengar S. Intellectual development and academic performance of children with insulin-dependent diabetes mellitus: a longitudinal study. *Dev Psychol* 1992; **28**:676–684.

162 Dahlquist G, Källén B; Swedish Childhood Diabetes Study Group. School performance in children with type 1 diabetes: a population-based register study. *Diabetologia* 2007; **50**:957–964.

163 Cohen J. *Statistical Power Analysis for the Behavioral Sciences*, 2nd edn. Hillsdale, NJ: Lawrence Erlbaum, 1988.

164 Ferguson SC, Blane A, Wardlaw JM, Frier BM, Perros P, McCrimmon RJ, *et al.* Influence of an early-onset age of type 1 diabetes on cerebral structure and cognitive function. *Diabetes Care* 2005; **28**:1431–1437.

165 Northam E, Anderson P, Wether G, Adler R, Andrewes D. Neuropsychological complications of insulin dependent diabetes in children. *Child Neuropsychol* 1995; **1**:74–87.

166 Northam EA, Anderson PJ, Werther GA, Warne GL, Adler RG, Andrewes D. Neuropsychological complications of IDDM in children 2 years after disease onset. *Diabetes Care* 1998; **21**:379–384.

167 Northam EA, Rankins D, Lin A, Wellard RM, Pell GS, Finch SJ, *et al.* Central nervous system function in youth with type 1 diabetes 12 years after disease onset. *Diabetes Care* 2009; **32**:445–450.

168 Schoenle EJ, Schoenle D, Molinari L, Largo RH. Impaired intellectual development in children with type 1 diabetes: association with HbA1c, age at diagnosis, and sex. *Diabetologia* 2002; **45**:108–114.

169 Barkai L, Vámosi I, Lukács K. Prospective assessment of severe hypoglycaemia in diabetic children and adolescents with impaired and normal awareness of hypoglycaemia. *Diabetologia* 1998; **41**:898–903.

170 Strudwick SK, Carne C, Gardiner J, Foster JK, Davis EA, Jones TW. Cognitive functioning in children with early onset type 1 diabetes and severe hypoglycemia. *J Pediatr* 2005; **147**:680–685.

171 Musen G, Jacobson AM, Ryan CM, Cleary PA, Waberski BH, Weinger K, *et al.* Impact of diabetes and its treatment on cognitive function among adolescents who participated in the Diabetes Control and Complications Trial. *Diabetes Care* 2008; **31**:1933–1938.

172 Wysocki T, Harris MA, Mauras N, Fox L, Taylor A, Jackso SC, *et al.* Absence of adverse effects of severe hypoglycemia on cognitive function in school-aged children with diabetes over 18 months. *Diabetes Care* 2003; **26**:1100–1105.

173 Rovet J, Alverez M. Attentional functioning in children and adolescents with IDDM. *Diabetes Care* 1997; **20**:803–810.

174 Malone JI, Hanna S, Saporta S, Mervis RF, Park CR, Chong L, *et al.* Hyperglycemia not hypoglycemia alters neuronal dendrites and impairs spatial memory. *Pediatr Diabetes* 2008; **9**:531–539.

175 Ho MS, Weller NJ, Ives FJ, Carne CL, Murray K, vanden Driesen RI, *et al.* High prevalence of structural CNS abnormalities in early onset type 1 diabetes. *J Pediatr* 2008; **153**:385–390.

176 Perantie DC, Wu J, Koller JM, Lim A, Warren SL, Black KJ, *et al.* Regional brain volume differences associated with hyperglycemia and severe hypoglycemia in youth with type 1 diabetes. *Diabetes Care* 2007; **30**:2331–2337.

177 Hyllienmark L, Maltez J, Dandenell A, Ludviggson J, Brismar T. EEG abnormalities with and without relation to severe hypoglycaemia in adolescents with type 1 diabetes. *Diabetologia* 2005; **48**:412–419.

178 Soltész G, Acsádi G. Association between diabetes, severe hypoglycemia, and electroencephalographic abnormalities. *Arch Dis Child* 1989; **64**:992–996.

179 Eeg-Olofsson O. Hypoglycemia and neurological disturbances in children with diabetes mellitus. *Acta Paediatr Scand* 1977:91–95.

180 Seidl R, Birnbacher R, Hauser E, Gernert G, Freilinger M, Schober E. Brainstem auditory evoked potentials and visually evoked potentials in young patients with IDDM. *Diabetes Care* 1996; **19**:1220–1224.

181 Salem MAK, Matta LF, Tantawy AAG, Hussein M, Gad GI. Single photon emission tomography (SPECT) study of regional cerebral blood flow in normoalbuminuric children and adolescents with type 1 diabetes. *Pediatr Diabetes* 2002; **3**:155–162.

182 Quirce R, Carril JM, Jiménez-Bonilla JF, Amado JA, Gutiérrez-Mendiguchía C, Banzo I, *et al.* Semi-quantitative assessment of cerebral blood flow with ^{99m}Tc-HMPAO SPET in type 1 diabetic patients with no clinical history of cerebrovascular disease. *Eur J Nucl Med* 1997; **24**:1507–1513.

183 Musen G, Lyoo IK, Sparks CR, Weinger K, Hwang J, Ryan CM, *et al.* Effects of type 1 diabetes on gray matter density as measured by voxel-based morphometry. *Diabetes* 2006; **55**:326–333.

184 Auer RN, Hugh J, Cosgrove E, Curry B. Neuropathologic findings in three cases of profound hypoglycemia. *Clin Neuropathol* 1989; **8**:63–68.

185 Ryan CM. Searching for the origin of brain dysfunction in diabetic children: going back to the beginning. *Pediatr Diabetes* 2008; **9**:527–530.

186 Brands AMA, Biessels G-J, De Haan EHF, Kappelle LJ, Kessels RPC. The effects of type 1 diabetes on cognitive performance: a meta-analysis. *Diabetes Care* 2005; **28**:726–735.

187 Winblad B, Palmer K, Kivipelto M, Jelic V, Fratiglioni L, Wahlund LO, *et al.* Mild cognitive impairment: beyond controversies, towards a consensus. Report of the International Working Group on Mild Cognitive Impairment. *J Intern Med* 2004; **256**:240–246.

188 Ryan CM. Diabetes, aging, and cognitive decline. *Neurobiol Aging* 2005; **26S**:S21–S25.

189 Brands AMA, Kessels RPC, Biessels GJ, Hoogma RPLM, Henselmans JML, van der Beek Boter JW, *et al.* Cognitive performance, psychological well-being, and brain magnetic resonance imaging in older patients with type 1 diabetes. *Diabetes* 2006; **55**:1800–1806.

190 Durmus C, Yetiser S, Durmus O. Auditory brainstem evoked responses in insulin-dependent (ID) and non-insulin-dependent (NID) diabetic subjects with normal hearing. *Int J Audiol* 2004; **43**:29–33.

191 Virtaniemi J, Laakso M, Kärjä J, Nuutinen J, Karjalainen S. Auditory brainstem latencies in type 1 (insulin-dependent) diabetic patients. *Am J Otolaryngol* 1993; **14**:413–418.

192 Parisi V, Uccioli L. Visual electrophsiological responses in persons with type 1 diabetes. *Diabetes Metab Res Rev* 2001; **17**:12–18.

193 Brismar T, Hyllienmark L, Ekberg K, Johansson BL. Loss of temporal lobe beta power in young adults with type 1 diabetes mellitus. *Neuroreport* 2002; **13**:2469–2473.

194 Bayazit Y, Yilmaz M, Kepekçi Y, Mumbuç S, Kanlikama M. Use of the auditory brainstem response testing in the clinical evaluation of the patients with diabetes mellitus. *J Neurol Sci* 2000; **181**: 29–32.

195 Parisi V, Uccioli L, Monticone G, Parisi L, Manni G, Ippoliti D, *et al.* Electrophysiological assessment of visual function in IDDM patients. *Electroenceph Clin Neurophysiol* 1997; **104**:171–179.

196 Gregori B, Galié E, Pro S, Clementi A, Accornero N. Luminance and chromatic visual evoked potentials in type 1 and type 2 diabetes: relationships with peripheral neuropathy. *Neurol Sci* 2006; **27**:323–327.

197 Jiménez-Bonilla JF, Quirce R, Hernández A, Vallina NK, Guede C, Banzo I, *et al.* Assessment of cerebral perfusion and cerebrovascular reserve in insulin-dependent diabetic patients without central neurological symptoms by means of ^{99m}Tc-HMPAO SPET with acetazolamide. *Eur J Nucl Med* 2001; **28**:1647–1655.

198 Wessels AM, Simsek S, Remijnse PL, Veltman DJ, Biessels GJ, Barkhof F, *et al.* Voxel-based morphometry demonstrates reduced gray matter density on brain MRI in patients with diabetic retinopathy. *Diabetologia* 2006; **49**:2474–2480.

199 Wessels AM, Rombouts SARB, Remijnse PL, Boom Y, Scheltens P, Barkhof F, *et al.* Cognitive performance in type 1 diabetes patients is associated with cerebral white matter volume. *Diabetologia* 2007; **50**:1763–1769.

200 Ryan CM, Geckle MO, Orchard TJ. Cognitive efficiency declines over time in adults with type 1 diabetes: effects of micro- and macrovascular complications. *Diabetologia* 2003; **46**:940–948.

201 Ferguson SC, Blane A, Perros P, McCrimmon RJ, Best JJK, Wardlaw JM, *et al.* Cognitive ability and brain structure in type 1 diabetes: relation to microangiopathy and preceding severe hypoglycemia. *Diabetes* 2003; **52**:149–156.

202 Wessels AM, Rombouts SARB, Simsek S, Kuijer JPA, Kostense PJ, Barkhof F, *et al.* Microvascular disease in type 1 diabetes alters brain activation: a functional magnetic resonance imaging study. *Diabetes* 2006; **55**:334–340.

203 Geissler A, Fründ R, Schölmerich J, Feuerbach S, Zietz B. Alterations of cerebral metabolism in patients with diabetes mellitus studied by proton magnetic resonance spectroscopy. *Exp Clin Endocrinol Diabetes* 2003; **111**:421–427.

204 Ryan CM, Williams TM, Orchard TJ, Finegold DN. Psychomotor slowing is associated with distal symmetrical polyneuropathy in adults with diabetes mellitus. *Diabetes* 1992; **41**:107–113.

205 Wong TY, Klein R, Sharrett AR, Nieto FJ, Boland LL, Couper DJ, *et al.* Retinal microvascular abnormalities and cognitive impairment in middle-aged persons: the Atherosclerosis Risk in Communities Study. *Stroke* 2002; **33**:1487–1492.

206 Wong TY, Klein R, Klein BEK, Tielsch JM, Hubbard L, Nieto FJ. Retinal microvascular abnormalities and their relationship with hypertension, cardiovascular disease, and mortality. *Surv Ophthalmol* 2001; **46**:59–80.

207 Patton N, Aslam T, MacGillivray T, Pattie A, Deary IJ, Dhillon B. Retinal vascular image analysis as a potential screening tool for cerebrovascular disease: a rationale based on homology between cerebral and retinal microvasculatures. *J Anat* 2005; **206**:319–348.

208 Barr ELM, Wong TY, Tapp RJ, Harper CA, Zimmet PZ, Atkins R, *et al.* Is peripheral neuropathy associated with retinopathy and albuminuria in individuals with impaired glucose metabolism? The 1999–2000 AusDiab. *Diabetes Care* 2006; **29**:1114–1116.

209 Orchard TJ, Dorman JS, Maser RE, Becker DJ, Drash AL, Ellis D, *et al.* Prevalence of complications in IDDM by sex and duration: Pittsburgh Epidemiology of Complications Study II. *Diabetes* 1990; **39**:1116–1124.

210 Diabetes Control and Complications Trial/Epidemiology of Diabetes Interventions and Complications (DCCT/EDIC) Study Research Group. Long-term effects of diabetes and its treatment on cognitive function. *N Engl J Med* 2007; **356**:1842–1852.

211 Deary I, Crawford J, Hepburn DA, Langan SJ, Blackmore LM, Frier BM. Severe hypoglycemia and intelligence in adult patients with insulin-treated diabetes. *Diabetes* 1993; **42**:341–344.

212 Auer RN, Wieloch T, Olsson Y, Siesjo BK. The distribution of hypoglycemic brain damage. *Acta Neuropathol (Berl)* 1984; **64**:177–191.

213 Meyers RE, Kahn KJ. Insulin-induced hypoglycemia in the nonhuman primate. II. Long-term neuropathological consequences. In: Brierley JB, Meldrum BS, eds. *Brain Hypoxia*. Philadelphia, PA: JB Lippincott, 1971: 195–206.

214 Fujioka M, Okuchi K, Hiramatsu K, Sakaki T, Sakaguchi S, Ishii Y. Specific changes in human brain after hypoglycemic injury. *Stroke* 1997; **28**:584–587.

215 Ennis K, Tran PV, Seaquist ER, Rao R. Postnatal age influences hypoglycemia-induced neuronal injury in the rat brain. *Brain Res* 2008; **1224**:119–126.

216 Ryan CM, Geckle MO. Circumscribed cognitive dysfunction in middle-aged adults with type 2 diabetes. *Diabetes Care* 2000; **23**:1486–1493.

217 Reaven GM, Thompson LW, Nahum D, Haskins E. Relationship between hyperglycemia and cognitive function in older NIDDM patients. *Diabetes Care* 1990; **13**:16–21.

218 Fontbonne A, Ducimetiere P, Berr C, Alperovitch A. Changes in cognitive abilities over a 4-year period are unfavorably affected in elderly diabetic subjects: results of the Epidemiology of Vascular Aging Study. *Diabetes Care* 2001; **24**:366–370.

219 Strachan MWJ, Deary IJ, Ewing FME, Frier BM. Is type 2 (non-insulin dependent) diabetes mellitus associated with an increased risk of cognitive dysfunction? *Diabetes Care* 1997; **20**:438–445.

220 Elias PK, Elias MF, D'Agostino RB, Cupples LA, Wilson PW, Silbershatz H, *et al.* NIDDM and blood pressure as risk factors for poor cognitive performance. *Diabetes Care* 1997; **20**:1388–1395.

221 Mooradian AD, Perryman K, Fitten J, Kavonian GD, Morley JE. Cortical function in elderly non-insulin dependent diabetic patients: behavioral and electrophysiologic studies. *Arch Intern Med* 1988; **148**:2369–2372.

222 Ryan CM, Geckle M. Why is learning and memory dysfunction in type 2 diabetes limited to older adults? *Diabetes Metab Res Rev* 2000; **16**:308–315.

223 Awad N, Gagnon M, Messier C. The relationship between impaired glucose tolerance, type 2 diabetes, and cognitive function. *J Clin Exp Neuropsychol* 2004; **26**:1044–1080.

224 Stewart RJ, Liolitsa D. Type 2 diabetes mellitus, cognitive impairment and dementia. *Diabet Med* 1999; **16**:93–112.

225 Brands AMA, Van den Berg E, Manschot SM, Biessels GJ, Kappelle LJ, De Haan EHF, *et al.* A detailed profile of cognitive dysfunction and its relation to psychological distress in patients with type 2 diabetes mellitus. *J Intern Neuropsychol Soc* 2007; **13**:288–297.

226 Manschot SM, Biessels GJ, Rutten GEHM, Kessels RPC, Gispen WH, Kappelle LJ, *et al.* Peripheral and central neurologic complications in type 2 diabetes mellitus: no association in individual patients. *J Neurol Sci* 2008; **264**:157–162.

227 Cukierman-Yaffe T, Gerstein HC, Williamson JD, Lazar RM, Lovato L, Miller ME, *et al.* Relationship between baseline glycemic control and cognitive function in individuals with type 2 diabetes and other cardiovascular risk factors: the Action to Control Cardiovascular Risk in Diabetes – Memory in Diabetes (ACCORD-MIND) trial. *Diabetes Care* 2009; **32**:221–226.

228 Last D, Alsop DC, Abduljalil AM, Marquis RP, De Bazelaire C, Hu K, *et al.* Global and regional effects of type 2 diabetes on brain tissue volumes and cerebral vasoreactivity. *Diabetes Care* 2007; **30**: 1193–1199.

229 Novak V, Last D, Alsop DC, Abduljalil AM, Hu K, Lepicovsky L, *et al.* Cerebral blood flow velocity and periventricular white matter hyperintensities in type 2 diabetes. *Diabetes Care* 2006; **29**:1529–1534.

230 Jongen C, Van der Grond J, Kappelle LJ, Biessels GJ, Viergever MA, Pluim JPW, *et al.* Automated measurement of brain and white matter lesion volume in type 2 diabetes mellitus. *Diabetologia* 2007; **50**:1509–1516.

231 Brands AMA, Biessels GJ, Kappelle LJ, De Haan EHF, de Valk HW, Algra A, *et al.* Cognitive functioning and brain MRI in patients with type 1 and type 2 diabetes mellitus: a comparative study. *Dement Geriatr Cogn Disord* 2007; **23**:343–350.

232 Starr VL, Convit A. Diabetes, sugar-coated but harmful to the brain. *Curr Opin Pharmacol* 2007; **7**:638–642.

233 den Heijer T, Vermeer SE, van Dijk EJ, Prins ND, Koudstaal PJ, Hofman A, *et al.* Type 2 diabetes and atrophy of medial temporal lobe structures on brain MRI. *Diabetologia* 2003; **46**:1604–1610.

234 Gold SM, Dziobek I, Sweat V, Tirsi A, Rogers K, Bruehl H, *et al.* Hippocampal damage and memory impairments as possible early brain complications of type 2 diabetes. *Diabetologia* 2007; **50**:711–719.

235 Strachan MWJ, Reynolds RM, Frier BM, Mitchell RJ, Price JF. The relationship between type 2 diabetes and dementia. *Br Med Bull* 2008; **88**:131–146.

236 Kloppenborg PR, Van den Berg E, Kappelle LJ, Biessels GJ. Diabetes and other vascular risk factors for dementia: what factor matters most? A systematic review. *Eur J Pharmacol* 2008; **585**:97–108.

237 Biessels G-J, Staekenborg S, Brunner E, Scheltens P. Risk of dementia in diabetes mellitus: a systematic review. *Lancet Neurol* 2006; **5**:64–74.

238 Gregg EW, Brown A. Cognitive and physical disabilities and aging-related complications of diabetes. *Clin Diabetes* 2003; **21**: 113–118.

239 Stolk RP, Breteler MMB, Ott A, Pols HAP, Lamberts SWJ, Grobbee DE, *et al.* Insulin and cognitive function in an elderly population: the Rotterdam Study. *Diabetes Care* 1997; **20**:792–795.

240 Kalmijn S, Feskens EJM, Launer LJ, Stijnen T, Kromhout D. Glucose intolerance, hyperinsulinaemia, and cognitive function in a general population of elderly men. *Diabetologia* 1995; **38**:1096–1102.

241 Desmond DW, Tatemichi TK, Paik M, Stern Y. Risk factors for cerebrovascular disease as correlates of cognitive function in a stroke-free cohort. *Arch Neurol* 1993; **50**:162–166.

242 Peyrot M, McMurry JF, Kruger DF. A biopsychosocial model of glycemic control in diabetes: stress, coping and regimen adherence. *J Health Soc Behav* 1999; **40**:141–158.

243 Giles DE, Strowig SM, Challis P, Raskin P. Personality traits as predictors of good diabetic control. *J Diabetes Complications* 1992; **6**:101–104.

244 Lustman PJ, Frank BL, McGill JB. Relationship of personality characteristics to glucose regulation in adults with diabetes. *Psychosom Med* 1991; **53**:305–312.

245 Orlandini A, Pastore MR, Fossati A, Clerici S, Sergi A, Balini A, *et al.* Effects of personality on metabolic control in IDDM patients. *Diabetes Care* 1995; **18**:206–209.

246 Gordon D, Fisher SG, Wilson M, Fergus E, Paterson KR, Semple CG. Psychological factors and their relationship to diabetes control. *Diabet Med* 1993; **10**:530–534.

247 Wiebe DJ, Alderfer MA, Palmer SC, Lindsay R, Jarrett L. Behavioral self-regulation in adolescents with type 1 diabetes: negative affectivity and blood glucose symptom perception. *J Consult Clin Psychol* 1994; **62**:1204–1212.

248 Perros P, Deary IJ, Frier BM. Factors influencing preference of insulin regimen in people with type 1 (insulin-dependent) diabetes. *Diabetes Res Clin Pract* 1998; **39**:23–29.

249 Hepburn DA, Langan SJ, Deary IJ, MacLeod KM, Frier BM. Psychological and demographic correlates of glycaemic control in adult patients with type 1 diabetes. *Diabet Med* 1994; **11**: 578–582.

250 Lane JD, McCaskill CC, Williams PG, Parekh PI, Feinglos MN, Surwit RS. Personality correlates of glycemic control in type 2 diabetes. *Diabetes Care* 2000; **23**:1321–1325.

251 Stenström U, Wikby A, Andersson PO, Ryden O. Relationship between locus of control beliefs and metabolic control in insulin-dependent diabetes mellitus. *Br J Health Psychol* 1998; **3**:15–25.

252 Reynaert C, Janne P, Donckier J, Buysschaert M, Zdanowicz N, Lejeune D, *et al.* Locus of control and metabolic control. *Diabete Metab* 1995; **21**:180–187.

253 Peyrot M, McMurry JF. Psychosocial factors in diabetes control: adjustment of insulin-treated adults. *Psychosom Med* 1985; **47**:542–557.

254 Weist MD, Finney JW, Barnard MU, Davis CD, Ollendick TH. Empirical selection of psychosocial treatment targets for children and adolescents with diabetes. *J Pediatr Psychol* 1993; **18**:11–28.

255 Kneckt MC, Syrjälä A-MH, Knuuttila MLE. Locus of control beliefs predicting oral and diabetes health behavior and health status. *Acta Odontol Scand* 1999; **57**:127–131.

256 Jacobson AM, Hauser ST, Lavori P, Wolfsdorf JI, Herskowitz RD, Milley JE, *et al.* Adherence among children and adolescents with insulin-dependent diabetes mellitus over a four-year longitudinal follow-up. I. The influence of patient coping and adjustment. *J Pediatr Psychol* 1990; **15**:511–526.

257 Peyrot M, Rubin RR. Structure and correlates of diabetes-specific locus of control. *Diabetes Care* 1994; **17**:994–1001.

258 Surgenor LJ, Horn JL, Hudson SM, Lunt H, Tennent J. Metabolic control and psychological sense of control in women with diabetes mellitus: alternative considerations of the relationship. *J Psychosom Res* 2000; **49**:267–273.

259 O'Hea EL, Moon S, Grothe KB, Boudreaux E, Bodenlos JS, Wallston K, *et al.* The interaction of locus of control, self-efficacy, and outcome expectancy in relation to HbA1c in medically underserved individuals with type 2 diabetes. *J Behav Med* 2009; **32**:106–117.

260 Lazarus RS. Coping theory and research: past, present, and future. *Psychosom Med* 1993; **55**:234–247.

261 Sultan S, Epel E, Sachon C, Valliant G, Hartemann-Heutier A. A longitudinal study of coping, anxiety and glycemic control in adults with type 1 diabetes. *Psychol Health* 2008; **23**:73–89.

262 Peyrot M, McMurry JF. Stress buffering and glycemic control: the role of coping styles. *Diabetes Care* 1992; **15**:842–846.

263 Graue M, Wentzel-Larsen T, Bru E, Hanestad BR, Sovik O. The coping styles of adolescents with type 1 diabetes are associated with degree of metabolic control. *Diabetes Care* 2004; **27**:1313–1317.

264 Duangdao KM, Roesch SC. Coping with diabetes in adulthood: a meta-analysis. *J Behav Med* 2008; **31**:291–300.

265 Kramer JR, Ledolter J, Manos GN, Bayless ML. Stress and metabolic control in diabetes mellitus: methodological issues and an illustrative analysis. *Ann Behav Med* 2000; **22**:17–28.

266 Farrell SP, Hains AA, Davies WH, Smith P, Parton E. The impact of cognitive distortions, stress, and adherence on metabolic control in youths with type 1 diabetes. *J Adolesc Health* 2004; **34**:461–467.

267 Goldston DB, Kovacs M, Obrosky DS, Iyengar S. A longitudinal study of life events and metabolic control among youths with insulin-dependent diabetes mellitus. *Health Psychol* 1995; **14**: 409–414.

268 Lloyd CE, Dyer PH, Lancashire RJ, Harris T, Daniels JE, Barnett AH. Association between stress and glycemic control in adults with type 1 (insulin-dependent) diabetes. *Diabetes Care* 1999; **22**: 1278–1283.

269 Ciechanowski PS, Katon WJ, Russon JE. Depression and diabetes: impact of depressive symptoms on adherence, function, and costs. *Arch Intern Med* 2000; **160**:3278–3285.

270 Surwit RS, Schneider MS, Feinglos MN. Stress and diabetes mellitus. *Diabetes Care* 1992; **15**:1413–1422.

271 Reagan LP, Grillo CA, Piroli GG. The As and Ds of stress: metabolic, morphological and behavioral consequences. *Eur J Pharmacol* 2008; **585**:64–75.

272 Gilbert BO, Johnson SB, Silverstein J, Malone J. Psychological and physiological rsponses to acute laboratory stressors in insulin-dependent diabetes mellitus adolescents and nondiabetic controls. *J Pediatr Psychol* 1989; **14**:577–591.

273 Delamater AM, Bubb J, Kurtz SM, Kuntze J, Smith JA, White NH, *et al.* Physiologic responses to acute psychological stress in adolescents with type 1 diabetes mellitus. *J Pediatr Psychol* 1988; **13**:69–86.

274 Kemmer FW, Bisping R, Steingrüber H-J, Baar H, Hardtmann F, Schlaghecke R, *et al.* Psychological stress and metabolic control in patients with type 1 diabetes mellitus. *N Engl J Med* 1986; **314**:1078–1084.

275 Wales JK. Does psychological stress cause diabetes? *Diabet Med* 1995; **12**:109–112.

276 Robinson N, Lloyd CE, Fuller JH, Yateman NA. Psychosocial factors and the onset of type 1 diabetes. *Diabet Med* 1989; **6**:53–58.

277 Thernlund GM, Dahlquist G, Hansson K, Ivarsson SA, Ludviggson J, Sjöblad S, *et al.* Psychological stress and the onset of IDDM in children: a case–control study. *Diabetes Care* 1995; **18**:1323–1329.

278 Hägglöf B, Blom L, Dahlquist G, Lönnberg G, Sahlin B. The Swedish childhood diabetes study: indications of severe psychological stress as a risk factor for type 1 (insulin-dependent) diabetes mellitus in childhood. *Diabetologia* 1991; **34**:579–583.

279 Littorin B, Sundkvist G, Nyström L, Carlson A, Landin-Olsson M, Östman J, *et al.* Family characteristics and life events before the onset of autoimmune type 1 diabetes in young adults: a nationwide study. *Diabetes Care* 2001; **24**:1033–1037.

280 Mooy JM, De Vries H, Grootenhuis PA, Bouter LM, Heine RJ. Major stressful life events in relation to prevalence of undetected type 2 diabetes. *Diabetes Care* 2000; **23**:197–201.

281 Eaton WW, Armenian H, Gallo J, Pratt L, Ford DE. Depression and risk for onset of type II diabetes: a prospective population-based study. *Diabetes Care* 1996; **19**:1097–1102.

282 Knol MJ, Twisk JWR, Beekman ATF, Heine RJ, Snoek FJ, Pouwer F. Depression as a risk factor for the onset of type 2 diabetes: a meta-analysis. *Diabetologia* 2006; **49**:837–845.

283 Surwit RS, Schneider MS. Role of stress in the etiology and treatment of diabetes mellitus. *Psychosom Med* 1993; **55**:380–393.

284 Van Tilburg MAL, McCaskill CC, Lane JD, Edwards CL, Bethel A, Feinglos MN, *et al.* Depressed mood is a factor in glycemic control in type 1 diabetes. *Psychosom Med* 2001; **63**:551–555.

285 Nichols GA, Hillier TA, Javor K, Betz Brown J. Predictors of glycemic control in insulin-using adults wtih type 2 diabetes. *Diabetes Care* 2000; **23**:273–277.

286 Lustman PJ, Griffith LS, Clouse RE, Cryer PE. Psychiatric illness in diabetes mellitus: relationship to symptoms and glucose control. *J Nerv Ment Dis* 1986; **174**:736–742.

287 Mazze RS, Lucido D, Shamoon H. Psychological and social correlates of glycemic control. *Diabetes Care* 1984; **7**:360–366.

288 Georgiades A, Zucker N, Friedman KE, Mosunic CJ, Applegate K, Lane JD, *et al.* Changes in depressive symptoms and glycemic control in diabetes mellitus. *Psychosom Med* 2007; **69**:235–241.

289 Lin EHB, Katon W, Von Korff M, Rutter C, Simon GE, Oliver M, *et al.* Relationship of depression and diabetes self-care, medication adherence, and preventive care. *Diabetes Care* 2004; **27**:2154–2160.

290 Gonzalez JS, Safren SA, Cagliero E, Wexler DJ, Delahanty LM, Wittenberg E, *et al.* Depression, self-care, and medication adherence in type 2 diabetes. *Diabetes Care* 2007; **30**:2222–2227.

291 Park HS, Hong YS, Lee HJ, Ha EH, Sung YA. Individuals with type 2 diabetes and depressive symptoms exhibited lower adherence with self-care. *J Clin Epidemiol* 2004; **57**:978–984.

292 Gonzalez JS, Safren SA, Delahanty LM, Cagliero E, Wexler DJ, Meigs JB, *et al.* Symptoms of depression prospectively predict poorer self-care in patients with type 2 diabetes. *Diabetologia* 2008; **25**:1102–1107.

293 Lewin AB, Heidgerken AD, Geffken GR, Williams LB, Storch EA, Gelfand KM, *et al.* The relation between family factors and metabolic control: the role of diabetes adherence. *J Pediatr Psychol* 2006; **31**:174–183.

294 Palmer DL, Berg CA, Butler J, Fortenberry K, Murray M, Lindsay R, *et al.* Mothers', fathers', and children's perceptions of parental diabetes responsibility in adolescence: examining the role of age, pubertal status, and efficacy. *J Pediatr Psychol* 2009; **34**:195–204.

295 Cameron FJ, Skinner TC, de Beaufort CE, Hoey H, Swift PGF, Aanstoot HJ, *et al.* Are family factors universally related to metabolic outcomes in adolescents with type 1 diabetes? *Diabet Med* 2008; **25**:463–468.

296 Anderson BJ, Ho J, Brackett J, Finkelstein D, Laffel L. Parental involvement in diabetes management tasks: relationships to blood glucose monitoring adherencing and metabolic control in young adolescents with insulin-dependent diabetes mellitus. *J Pediatr* 1997; **130**:257–265.

297 Grey M, Davidson M, Boland EA, Tamborlane WV. Clinical and psychosocial factors associated with achievement of treatment goals in adolescents with diabetes mellitus. *J Adolesc Health* 2001; **28**:377–385.

298 Anderson BJ, Brackett J, Ho J, Laffel LMB. An office-based intervention to maintain parent-adolescent teamwork in diabetes management: impact on parent involvement, family conflict, and subsequent glycemic control. *Diabetes Care* 1999; **22**:713–721.

299 Hanson CL, Henggeler SW, Harris MA, Cigrang JA, Schinkel AM, Rodrigue JR, *et al.* Contributions of sibling relations to the adaptation of youths with insulin-dependent diabetes mellitus. *J Consult Clin Psychol* 1992; **61**:104–112.

300 Marteau TM, Bloch S, Baum JD. Family life and diabetic control. *J Child Psychol Psychiatry* 1987; **28**:823–833.

301 Wysocki T. Associations among teen–parent relationships, metabolic control, and adjustment to diabetes in adolescents. *J Pediatr Psychol* 1993; **18**:441–452.

302 Skinner TC, John M, Hampson SE. Social support and personal models of diabetes as predictors of self-care and well-being: a longitudinal study of adolescents with diabetes. *J Pediatr Psychol* 2000; **25**:257–267.

303 Cameron LD, Young MJ, Wiebe DJ. Maternal trait anxiety and diabetes control in adolescents with type 1 diabetes. *J Pediatr Psychol* 2007; **32**:733–744.

304 Ross LA, Frier BM, Kelnar CJH, Deary IJ. Child and parental mental ability and glycaemic control in children with type 1 diabetes. *Diabet Med* 2001; **18**:364–369.

305 Cohen DM, Lumley MA, Naar-King S, Partridge T, Cakan N. Child behavior problems and family functioning as predictors of adherence and glycemic control in economically disadvantaged children with type 1 diabetes: a prospective study. *J Pediatr Psychol* 2004; **29**:171–184.

306 Auslander WF, Thomson S, Dreitzer D, White NH, Santiago JV. Disparity in glycemic control and adherence between African-American and Caucasian youths with diabetes. *Diabetes Care* 1997; **20**:1569–1575.

307 Thompson SJ, Auslander WF, White NH. Comparison of single-mother and two-parent families on metabolic control of children with diabetes. *Diabetes Care* 2001; **24**:234–238.

308 Trief PM, Britton KD, Wade MJ, Weinstock RS. A prospective analysis of marital relationship factors and quality of life in diabetes. *Diabetes Care* 2002; **25**:1154–1158.

309 Trief PM, Grant W, Elbert K, Weinstock RS. Family environment, glycemic control, and the psychosocial adaptation of adults with diabetes. *Diabetes Care* 1998; **21**:241–245.

310 Trief PM, Aquilino C, Paradies K, Weinstock RS. Impact of the work environment on glycemic control and adaptation to diabetes. *Diabetes Care* 1999; **22**:569–574.

311 Jacobson AM, Hauser ST, Lavori P, Willett JB, Cole CF, Wolfsdorf JI, *et al.* Family environment and glycemic control: a four-year prospective study of children and adolescents with insulin-dependent diabetes mellitus. *Psychosom Med* 1994; **56**:401–409.

312 Hauser ST, Jacobson AM, Lavori P, Wolfsdorf JI, Herskowitz RD, Milley JE, *et al.* Adherence among children and adolescents with insulin-dependent diabetes mellitus over a four-year longitudinal follow-up. II. Immediate and long-term linkages with family milieu. *J Pediatr Psychol* 1990; **15**:527–542.

313 Hanson CL, De Guire MJ, Schinkel AM, Kolterman OG. Empirical validation for a family-centered model of care. *Diabetes Care* 1995; **18**:1347–1356.

314 Johnson SB. Methodological issues in diabetes research: measuring adherence. *Diabetes Care* 1992; **15**:1658–1667.

315 Funnell MM, Anderson RM. The problem with compliance in diabetes. *JAMA* 2000; **284**:1709.

316 Lutfey KE, Wishner WJ. Beyond "compliance" is "adherence". *Diabetes Care* 1999; **22**:635–639.

317 McNabb WL. Adherence in diabetes: can we define it and can we measure it? *Diabetes Care* 1997; **20**:215–218.

318 Glasgow RE, Eakin EG. Issues in diabetes self-management. In: Shumaker SA, EB Schron, JK Ockene, WL McBee, eds. *The Handbook of Health Behavior Change*. New York: Springer, 1998: 435–461.

319 Holmes CS, Chen R, Streisand R, Marschall DE, Souter S, Swift EE, *et al.* Predictors of youth diabetes care behaviors and metabolic control: a structural equation modeling approach. *J Pediatr Psychol* 2006; **31**:770–784.

320 Ruggiero L, Glasgow RE, Dryfoos J, Rossi JS, Prochaska JO, Orleans CT, *et al.* Diabetes self-management: self-reported recommendations and patterns in a large population. *Diabetes Care* 1997; **20**:568–576.

321 Glasgow RE, McCaul KD, Schafer LC. Self-care behaviors and glycemic control in type I diabetes. *J Chronic Dis* 1987; **40**:399–412.

322 Johnson SB, Kelly M, Jenretta JC, Cunningham WR, Tomer A, Silverstein J. A longitudinal analysis of adherence and health status in childhood diabetes. *J Pediatr Psychol* 1992; **17**:537–553.

323 Karter AJ, Ackerson LM, Darbinian JA, D'Agostino RB, Ferrara A, Liu J, *et al.* Self-monitoring of blood glucose levels and glycemic control: the Northern California Kaiser Permanent Diabetes Registry. *Am J Med* 2001; **111**:1–9.

324 Farmer A, Wade A, Goyder E, Yudkin P, French D, Craven A, *et al.* Impact of self monitoring of blood glucose in the management of patients with non-insulin treated diabetes: open parallel group randomised trial. *Br Med J* 2007; **335**:132.

325 McAndrews L, Schneider SH, Burns E, Leventhal H. Does patient blood glucose monitoring improve diabetes control? *Diabetes Educ* 2007; **33**:991–1011.

326 Juvenile Diabete Research Foundation Continuous Glucose Monitoring Study Group. Continuous glucose monitoring and intensive treatment of type 1 diabetes. *N Engl J Med* 2008; **359**:1464–1476.

327 Helgeson VS, Reynolds KA, Siminerio L, Escobar O, Becker D. Parent and adolescent distribution of responsibility for diabetes self-care: links to health outcomes. *J Pediatr Psychol* 2008; **33**:497–508.

328 Ingersoll GM, Orr DP, Herrold AJ, Golden MP. Cognitive maturity and self-managment among adolescents with insulin-dependent diabetes mellitus. *J Pediatr* 1986; **108**:620–623.

329 Golin CE, DiMatteo MR, Gelberg L. The role of patient participation in the doctor visit: implications for adherence to diabetes care. *Diabetes Care* 1996; **19**:1153–1164.

330 Mason C. The production and effects of uncertainty with special reference to diabetes mellitus. *Soc Sci Med* 1985; **21**:1329–1334.

331 Rost K, Carter W, Inui T. Introduction of information during the initial medical visit: consequences for patient follow-through with physician recommendations for medication. *Soc Sci Med* 1989; **28**.

332 Boehnert CE, Popkin MK. Psychological issues in treatment of severely noncompliant diabetics. *Psychosomatics* 1986; **27**:11–20.

333 Moran G, Fonagy P, Kurtz A, Bolton A, Brook C. A controlled study of the psychoanalytic treatment of brittle diabetes. *J Am Acad Child Adolesc Psychiatry* 1991; **30**:926–935.

334 Peyrot M, Rubin RR. Behavioral and psychosocial interventions in diabetes: a conceptual review. *Diabetes Care* 2007; **30**:2433–2440.

335 Hampson SE, Skinner TC, Hart J, Storey L, Gage H, Foxcroft D, *et al.* Behavioral interventions for adolescents with type 1 diabetes. *Diabetes Care* 2000; **23**:1416–1422.

336 Delamater AM, Bubb J, Davis SG, Smith JA, Schmidt L, White NH, *et al.* Randomized prospective study of self-management training with newly diagnosed diabetic children. *Diabetes Care* 1990; **13**:492–498.

337 Satin W, La Greca AM, Zigo MA, Skyler JS. Diabetes in adolescence: effects of multifamily group intervention and parent simulation of diabetes. *J Pediatr Psychol* 1989; **14**:259–275.

338 Anderson BJ, Wolf FM, Burkhart MT, Cornell RG, Bacon GE. Effects of peer group intervention on metabolic control of adolescents with IDDM: randomized outpatient study. *Diabetes Care* 1989; **12**:179–183.

339 Boardway RH, Delamater AM, Tomakowsky J, Gutai JP. Stress management training for adolescents with diabetes. *J Pediatr Psychol* 1993; **18**:29–45.

340 Méndez FJ, Beléndez M. Effects of a behavioral intervention on treatment adherence and stress management in adolescents with IDDM. *Diabetes Care* 1997; **20**:1370–1375.

341 Channon S, Smith VJ, Gregory JW. A pilot study of motivational interviewing in adolescents with diabetes. *Arch Dis Child* 2003; **88**:680–683.

342 Channon SJ, Huws-Thomas MV, Rollnick S, Hood K, Cannings-John RL, Rogers C, *et al.* A multicenter randomized controlled trial of motivational interviewing in teenagers with diabetes. *Diabetes Care* 2007; **30**:1390–1395.

343 Wysocki T, Harris MA, Greco P, Bubb J, Danda CE, Harvey LM, *et al.* Randomized, controlled trial of behavior therapy for families of adolescents with insulin-dependent diabetes mellitus. *J Pediatr Psychol* 2000; **25**:23–33.

344 Wysocki T, Greco P, Harris MA, Bubb J, White NH. Behavior therapy for families of adolescents with diabetes: maintenance of treatment effects. *Diabetes Care* 2001; **24**:441–446.

345 Ishmail K, Winkley K, Rabe-Hesketh S. Systematic review and meta-analysis of randomized controlled trials of psychological interventions to improve glycaemic control in patients with type 2 diabetes. *Lancet* 2004; **363**:1589–1597.

346 Grey M, Boland EA, Davidson M, Li JJ, Tamborlane WV. Coping skills training for youth with diabetes mellitus has long-lasting effects on metabolic control and quality of life. *J Pediatr* 2000; **137**:107–113.

347 Feste C. A practical look at patient empowerment. *Diabetes Care* 1992; **15**:922–925.

348 Anderson RM, Funnell MM, Butler PM, Arnold MS, Fitzgerald JT, Feste CC. Patient empowerment: results of a randomized controlled trial. *Diabetes Care* 1995; **18**:943–949.

349 Anderson RM, Funnell MM, Arnold MS. Using the empowerment approach to help patients change behavior. In: Anderson BJ, RR Rubin, eds. *Practical Psychology for Diabetes Clinicians*. Alexandria, VA: American Diabetes Association, 1996: 163–172.

350 McGrady A, Graham G, Bailey B. Biofeedback-assisted relaxation in insulin-dependent diabetes: a replication and extension study. *Ann Behav Med* 1996; **18**:185–189.

351 Feinglos MN, Hastedt P, Surwit RS. Effects of relaxation therapy on patients with type 1 diabetes mellitus. *Diabetes Care* 1987; **10**:72–75.

352 Lane JD, McCaskill CC, Ross SL, Feinglos MN, Surwit RS. Relaxation training for NIDDM: predicting who may benefit. *Diabetes Care* 1993; **16**:1087–1094.

353 Bradley C. *Handbook of Psychology and Diabetes*. Chur, Switzerland: Harwood Academic Publishers, 1994.

50 Diabetes and Infections

Clive S. Cockram[1] & Nelson Lee[2]

[1] Chinese University of Hong Kong, Hong Kong
[2] Department of Medicine and Therapeutics, Prince of Wales Hospital, Chinese University of Hong Kong, Hong Kong

Keypoints

- Diabetes is associated with an increased overall risk of infections.
- The presence of diabetes also modifies the course of many infections and increases morbidity and mortality.
- Multiple disturbances in innate immunity have a role in the pathogenesis of the increased prevalence of infections in people with diabetes.
- Impaired phagocytosis by neutrophils, macrophages and monocytes, impaired neutrophil chemotaxis and bactericidal activity, and impaired innate cell-mediated immunity appear to be the most important disturbances of the immune system.
- Humoral immunity appears relatively unaffected, hence plasma levels of antibodies and responsiveness to vaccination are relatively unaffected.
- In general, better regulation of the diabetes leads to an improvement in cellular immunity and function.
- Increased skin and mucosal carriage of *Staphylcoccus aureus* and *Candida* species may increase risk of infection with these organisms.
- Some microorganisms become more virulent in a high glucose environment; examples include certain *Klebsiella* serotypes and *Burkholderia pseudomallei.*
- Viral infections such as hepatitis C are associated with a higher prevalence of diabetes.
- Highly active antiretroviral therapy therapy for HIV/AIDS may also precipitate diabetes.
- Vascular disease such as microangiopathy can further impair the expression of the immune response as well as affecting the overall function of the microcirculation. It is commonly a factor in severe infections such as malignant otitis externa, emphysematous pyelonephritis and necrotizing fasciitis.
- Urinary tract infections and asymptomatic bacteriuria are more common in people with diabetes. Autonomic neuropathy is a common and important underlying factor.
- Skin and soft tissue infections are more common, with the infected diabetic foot as a prime example. Vascular disease and diabetic neuropathy are important underlying factors in the vulnerability of the foot to infection. Skin infection or infections of the external genitalia are common presenting features of diabetes. Necrotizing fasciitis is also associated with diabetes.
- Some uncommon but life-threatening infections occur almost exclusively in people with diabetes. Examples include the rhinocerebral form of mucormycosis, malignant otitis externa, Fournier gangrene and emphysematous forms of cystitis, pyelonephritis and cholecystitis.
- Diabetes increases the risk of tuberculosis and also increases the risk of treatment failure. Unusual or extrapulmonary sites of infection may be important and cavitatory disease more common.
- Other underlying factors that can predispose to infection include renal failure, obesity, need for hospitalization, indwelling catheters and delayed wound healing.

Introduction

People with diabetes develop infections more often than those without diabetes and the course of the infections is also more complicated. Historically, infections have been well recognized as an important cause of death in diabetes and remain a very important cause of morbidity and mortality in people with diabetes. This is particularly true in less well-developed countries and areas, where infections are commonly the first presenting feature of previously unknown diabetes. The infected diabetic foot remains a prime example of this phenomenon despite its potential preventability.

While the association between diabetes and infections is well recognized, the relationships are complex, not always clear-cut and often controversial. Data on the true incidence of certain infections are lacking and a number of factors complicate efforts to assess risk of infections and outcomes. Studies are often retrospective and uncontrolled in nature.

Some infections, which occur predominantly in people with diabetes, are uncommon and inevitably have limited data. Examples include malignant otitis externa, mucormycosis, emphysematous forms of cholecystitis, cystitis and pyelonephritis, and Fournier gangrene.

Textbook of Diabetes, 4th edition. Edited by R. Holt, C. Cockram, A. Flyvbjerg and B. Goldstein. © 2010 Blackwell Publishing.

In the case of more common infections that, while not limited to people with diabetes, have diabetes as a complicating factor, many potential variables make for considerable heterogeneity in the clinical course. Examples of such factors include duration of disease, presence of diabetic complications, glycemic control (both recent and longer term), access to and provision of medical services, and presence or absence of other concurrent illnesses.

A recent carefully controlled study from Utrecht, the Netherlands, has confirmed that, in general terms, patients with type 1 (T1DM) and type 2 diabetes mellitus (T2DM) are at increased risk of lower (but not upper) respiratory tract infection, urinary tract infection and skin and mucous membrane infections [1]. In this study, the well-documented increased risk of urinary infection was extended to include both risk of recurrence in both sexes and risks in males (perhaps explained by prostatitis).

Another recent study, conducted in Ontario, Canada, compared people with diabetes with matched control subjects without diabetes [2]. The investigators calculated the risk ratios, both for contracting an infection and for death from infection. Forty-six percent of all people with diabetes had at least one hospitalization or outpatient visit for infections compared with 38% of those without diabetes, the relative risk ratio being 1.21. The risk ratios for infectious disease-related hospitalization or death were noticeably higher at 2.17 and 1.92, respectively. This may be attributable to increased severity and presence of complications. In the case of hospitalization, it could also reflect a lower threshold on the part of physicians to admit people with diabetes to hospital when they have intercurrent illnesses. A separate study also from Canada, in this case from the Calgary Health Region, has conducted a population-based assessment of severe bloodstream infections requiring intensive care admission. Demographic and chronic conditions that were significant risk factors for acquiring severe bloodstream infection included diabetes, with a relative risk ratio of 5.9. The most common organisms were *Staphylococcus aureus*, *Escherichia coli* and *Streptococcus pneumoniae* [3].

Data from a study by Bertoni *et al.* [4] suggest that adults with diabetes are at greater risk for infection-related mortality, and that the excess mortality risk may be mediated by cardiovascular disease (CVD). When diabetes was combined with CVD, the relative mortality risk was 3.0 (1.8–5.0), whereas individuals with diabetes without CVD had a risk of 1.0 (0.5–2.2).

Evidence that the presence of diabetes can worsen the outcome or prognosis of infections comes from a number of sources. There is evidence that the presence of T2DM is associated with an increased mortality from community-acquired pneumonia. While much of this may be explained by factors such as age and coexisting comorbid illnesses, admission hyperglycemia has been shown to be a particularly important predictor of death. Also, even in patients without previously diagnosed diabetes, glucose levels in general assume importance [5]. During the outbreaks of severe acute respiratory syndrome (SARS) in 2003 in Toronto, the presence of diabetes was an independent risk factor for poor outcomes (intensive care unit admission, mechanical ventilation and death) with a threefold increase in relative risk [6].

Both host- and organism-specific factors appear to be implicated in the increased susceptibility to particular infections. From the host perspective, defects in innate immunity are important, notably decreased functions (chemotaxis, phagocytosis and killing) of neutrophils, monocytes and macrophages. Other factors include effects of diabetic complications, poor wound healing and the presence of chronic renal failure. Frequent hospitalizations, with the attendant risk of nosocomial infection, can also be contributory.

Infections, as well as leading to considerable morbidity and mortality in people with diabetes, may also precipitate metabolic derangements, producing a bidirectional relationship between hyperglycemic states and infection. Some infections may also be implicated more directly in the etiology of diabetes.

Physicians working in primary care need to have high levels of awareness of the relationships between diabetes and infection, and of the important infections that may be involved. Infections involving the foot, soft tissues, skin and nails, as well as the urinary tract, are of particular importance in the setting of primary care. These infections are commonly encountered in people with diabetes, may be present at diagnosis and may be the presenting feature that leads to the diagnosis of diabetes being suspected. Infections of the foot and skin will receive additional attention elsewhere in this textbook so, in order to avoid duplication, coverage in this chapter is curtailed. This should not be taken as an indication of lack of relative importance, the opposite is the case. The other chapters concerned should be taken as forming part of the overall coverage of the topic of diabetes and infections (see Chapters 44 and 47).

Diabetes, the immune system and host factors

Host immune response

Although the increased susceptibility of people with diabetes to bacterial (and other) infections is well established, the mechanisms remain incompletely understood. Deficiencies in the host innate immune response are apparent and appear more important than changes in adaptive immunity.

The presence of diabetes has multiple effects upon innate immune responses, including effects upon neutrophils, monocytes and other components of innate immunity. These disturbances have important roles in the increased prevalence and enhanced severity of infections in people with diabetes. The effects include reduced chemotaxis, phagocytosis and impaired bactericidal activity.

Some disturbances in the complement system and in cytokine responses have been described in people with diabetes (e.g. low complement factor 4 and decreased cytokine responses after stimulation), but their role in the increased susceptibility to infection is less clear [7]. Consistent defects have not been demonstrated. No clear disturbances in adaptive immunity have been described. Humeral adaptive immunity, in particular, appears relatively unaffected as exemplified by the relatively normal antibody responses to most vaccinations and the fact that serum antibody concentrations and responses in patients with diabetes are generally normal. For example, people with diabetes respond to pneumococcal vaccine equally as well as controls without diabetes [8,9].

The complexity of the component systems involved in the immune system makes comparison between studies difficult and it is obviously simplistic to study individual components of the immune system in isolation given the interdependency of these components. Many studies have relied upon *in vitro* or animal model methodology.

Investigations to identify the mechanisms of immune impairment in animal models of diabetes and *in vitro* experiments have been numerous. A full review of these animal and *in vitro* studies is beyond the scope of this chapter; however, the observations that follow may serve as examples from within the range of abnormalities that have been found, although many questions remain as to the nature of the defects produced by diabetes and their effects upon infection risk.

Neutrophil chemotaxis, neutrophil adherence to vascular endothelium, phagocytosis, intracellular bactericidal activity, opsonization and other aspects of innate immunity are all depressed in hyperglycemic patients with diabetes, although adaptive immunity appears relatively unaffected [10–12]. These changes lead to reduced host defense in response to infection with extracellular bacteria. Both impaired chemotaxis and phagocytosis have been described in monocytes of people with diabetes [13]. Defects in innate immunity have also been shown to predispose *db/db* mice to *S. aureus* infections. Interestingly, these mice show a heightened inflammatory response which occurs in association with an impaired neutrophil respiratory burst, and the recruited neutrophils fail to resolve the infection [14]. A possible role for advanced glycosylation end-products (AGEs) is postulated as a component in the pathogenesis of the impaired neutrophil function.

While release of tumor necrosis factor α and interleukin 1β (IL-1β) from lipopolysaccharide-stimulated macrophages has been shown to be reduced in diabetic mice compared with control mice [15], study of monocytes from patients with diabetes indicates upregulation of the secretion of the same inflammatory mediators [16]. This further illustrates the difficulty in comparing studies conducted in different settings and species. Some innate (e.g. cytokines, complement) immune functions are decreased while others remain the same in patients with diabetes as those without diabetes. For example, while unstimulated cytokine concentrations may be higher, cytokine responses to stimuli are often reduced [17]. Interpretation of the complexity of the underlying mechanisms may also need to take into account potential underlying proinflammatory effects associated with diabetes itself.

The level of macrophage inflammatory protein 2, a mediator of lung neutrophil recruitment, is significantly decreased in diabetic mice compared to control mice [18]. The deficiency causes a delay in neutrophil recruitment in the lungs. This may be an important factor influencing the susceptibility of people with diabetes to infections of the lower respiratory tract.

Hyperglycemia impairs opsonophagocytosis by diverting nicotinic acid adenine dinucleotide phosphate (NADPH) from superoxide production into the aldose reductase-dependent polyol pathway [19], providing one further example of a mechanism by which hyperglycemia directly impairs phagocytosis.

Diabetic mice show greater than twofold induction of genes that directly or indirectly induce apoptosis [20]. By contrast, it is known that blocking of apoptosis allows for a significant improvement in wound healing and bone growth. This may influence many aspects of responses to infection, including impaired wound healing, which are important in the setting of diabetes.

These examples, while somewhat piecemeal, serve to demonstrate the range of abnormalities in the innate immune system that result from hyperglycemia. Of particular importance are those spanning macrophage, monocyte and neutrophil function, and which impair adherence to endothelium, chemotaxis, phagocytosis and bacteriocidal activity. They also point to other abnormalities (e.g. involving apoptosis), wound healing and cytokine responses to infection. The antioxidant systems involved in bacteriocidal activity may be compromised. These impairments, which are exacerbated by hyperglycemia and acidemia, may be reversed substantially, if not entirely, by normalization of pH and blood glucose levels. It needs to be emphasized, however, that the severity of effects correlates somewhat unpredictably with direct contemporaneous measures of glycemic control such as HbA_{1c}, perhaps reflecting longer term or persistent changes such as accumulation of AGEs [21]. In general, a better regulation of the diabetes leads to an improvement of the cellular aspects of immune function.

Other host-related factors

Other host-specific factors, over and above direct diabetes-related impairment of immune defenses, can further the predisposition to infection. These include vascular insufficiency (microangiopathies and macroangiopathies), sensory peripheral neuropathy, autonomic neuropathy, and skin and mucosal colonization with pathogens such as *S. aureus* and *Candida* species. Abnormalities of the structure and function of the microcirculation can also have additional indirect adverse effects on the immune responses themselves. Thus, immunologic responses may be further compromised by microangiopathy, and additional factors related to diabetes complications specifically increase the risks of certain infections, especially those involving the foot and the urinary tract.

While beyond the direct scope of this chapter, obesity, which is commonly associated with diabetes, also increases the risk of certain infections. These include nosocomial infections, wound and surgical site infections, respiratory infections and infections involving the gastrointestinal tract. The presence of obesity also correlates with infected diabetic foot ulcers in people with diabetes [22].

Diabetic complications

Vascular disease is an important component in the etiology of the diabetic foot and the attendant complications of infection, ulceration and gangrene. Vascular disease is very common in diabetes and macrovascular disease may be premature, extensive, severe and present in unusual sites. Vascular insufficiency results in local tissue ischemia that can, in turn, enhance the growth of microaerophilic and anaerobic organisms, while simultaneously depressing the oxygen-dependent bactericidal functions of leukocytes. The antioxidant systems involved in bacteriocidal activity may be compromised by the combination of microvascular disease and the diabetic metabolic derangement itself. Hyperglycemia and acidemia are important predisposing factors to this latter effect and are reversed substantially by normalization of pH and blood glucose levels. Vascular disease related to diabetes may also further impair the local inflammatory response and may also impair the tissue penetration of antibiotics.

Neuropathy, both peripheral and autonomic, also contributes to the risk of foot infections and ulceration, as well as to certain other infections. Sensory peripheral neuropathy masks the recognition of trauma. Minor local trauma in patients with diabetes-associated peripheral neuropathy may result in skin ulcers, which, in turn, lead to diabetic foot infections. Skin lesions are often either unnoticed or ignored until infection occurs. Autonomic neuropathy contributes to the etiology of diabetic foot infections by mechanisms such as decreased sweating, which predisposes to drying and fissuring of the skin, and by further exacerbating abnormalities in the control of the microcirculation. Both sensory and motor neuropathy can lead to deformity and alter the dynamics of the function of the foot. Fuller discussion of the etiologic factors related to sepsis and the diabetic foot is provided in Chapter 44.

Patients with diabetes-associated autonomic neuropathy may develop urinary retention and stasis in association with loss of innervation to the bladder. This predisposes them to urinary tract infections. This risk is particularly high in females. Autonomic neuropathy can also impair the function of the gastrointestinal tract, predispose to certain gastrointestinal tract infections and contribute to risk of aspiration pneumonia in the context of gastroparesis. Renal papillary necrosis can also contribute to the risk of renal failure as well as to infection within the urinary tract.

Thus, a number of factors contribute to the vulnerability of people with diabetes to infections. In addition to the abnormalities of the immune response, vascular disease and neuropathy can greatly enhance susceptibility (e.g. in the lower limb and urinary tract). Hyperglycemia per se may specifically heighten susceptibility to certain fungal and bacterial infections.

Organism-specific factors

Certain organisms may show increased adherence to diabetic cells [12] and others may demonstrate increased virulence in hyperglycemic environments. Specific factors that predispose people with diabetes to infection with specific organisms include the following examples.

Candida albicans and fungi

Glucose-inducible proteins produced by *Candida albicans* are homologous to a complement receptor on phagocytes. These proteins may promote adhesion of *C. albicans* to buccal or vaginal epithelium. This adhesion, in turn, impairs phagocytosis, giving the organism an advantage over the host [12].

Ketone reductases produced by *Rhizopus* species allow these species to thrive in high glucose, acidic conditions typically present in patients with diabetic ketoacidosis [23].

Klebsiella spp.

A bacterial genus of note in the context of diabetes is *Klebsiella*. *Klebsiella* infections are the second most common causes of Gram-negative sepsis (after *E. coli*). In a report from Taiwan, diabetes was the most commonly associated underlying condition in patients presenting with community-acquired *K. pneumoniae* bacteremia (whereas neoplastic diseases were more commonly associated with nosocomial infections) [24]. The percentage of patients with underlying diabetes was 49%, which is even higher than in earlier reports [25,26]. Apart from the high proportion with diabetes, associations were also observed with serotype K1 (associated with impaired phagocytosis), liver abscess and other metastatic complications (endophthalmitis, meningitis, brain abscess) [24]. Primary liver abscess in other parts of Asia is also increasing in incidence, with 40% reportedly associated with diabetes [27]. Bacteremia is present in 50%, and 8–10% have metastatic complications (endophthalmitis, meningitis, brain abscess, pneumonia, skin and soft tissue infections, lung abscess, septic arthritis, renal abscess and prostatic abscess).

Melioidosis

A combination of organism-specific factors together with the changes in innate immunity may explain the increased susceptibility of people with diabetes to melioidosis. About 50% of cases of melioidosis occur in people with diabetes. The responsible organism, *Burkholderia pseudomallei*, has been shown to be selectively resistant to phagocytosis compared to *Salmonella typhimurium* and *E. coli* in subjects with diabetes.

In a study from Thailand, a country where melioidosis is relatively common, neutrophil responses to *B. pseudomallei*, in both healthy subjects and people with diabetes showed that *B. pseudomallei* displayed reduced phagocytosis by neutrophils compared to *S. enterica typhimurium* and *E. coli*. In addition, intracellular survival of *B. pseudomallei* was detected throughout a 24-hour period, indicating intrinsic resistance of *B. pseudomallei* to killing by neutrophils. Furthermore, neutrophils from subjects with diabetes displayed reduced migration in response to IL-8 and an inability to delay apoptosis. Thus, *B. pseudomallei* appears to be intrinsically resistant to phagocytosis and killing by neutrophils. When added to the impaired migration and apoptosis seen in diabetes, the combination seems sufficient to explain the increased susceptibility to melioidosis in people with diabetes [28].

Bidirectionality: the effect of infections on diabetes

Bidirectionality exists in the relationship between diabetes and infections. The effect of infections upon diabetes includes the effects of certain infections on the etiology and pathogenesis of diabetes itself, adverse effects upon hyperglycemia in established diabetes and exacerbation of diabetes complications. The importance of the potential adverse effects upon hyperglycemia in established diabetes needs to be stressed. Infections remain an important predisposing cause of both diabetic ketoacidosis and hyperosmolar hyperglycemia syndrome.

The importance of certain viral infections in the possible etiology of diabetes has received increasing attention in recent years with respect to both T1DM and T2DM.

Viral infections have been implicated in the etiology of T1DM for many years. Although this complicated topic is beyond the general scope of this chapter and is considered in detail in Chapters 3 and 9, it is noteworthy that type 1a (autoimmune) diabetes is increasing in prevalence globally, providing strong evidence that environmental factors are involved in the clinical expression of the disease. Viruses have long been included in the list of putative environmental triggers. Enteroviruses (especially coxsackie B viruses, B4 in particular), rubella, mumps, rotavirus, parvovirus and cytomegalovirus have all been implicated and continue to be reported [29,30]. Although correlations between the presentation of diabetes and the occurrence of a preceding viral infection have been recognized, a direct causal relationship, with fulfillment of Koch postulates, between viral infection and the diabetogenic process, remains difficult to prove, possibly because other inflammatory factors are also required. In this context, it is interesting to note that the process may be associated with a dominant CD4 T-helper type 1 immune response, whereas the dominance of a T-helper type 2 response, as seen in the face of certain infectious and parasitic agents, may protect against T1DM and other autoimmune diseases. Thus, the increasing freedom from such infections, especially in developed areas of the world, may allow the increased expression of an underlying genetic predisposition, and infection by certain viruses, such as the coxsackie B viruses, may then be associated with the appearance of (and persistence of) β-cell antigens, mediated by mechanisms such as molecular mimicry and activation of Toll-like receptors. Lack of exposure to infection and infestation in early childhood appears to dilute the ability of the innate immune system to withstand autoimmune responses and challenges. T1DM is not alone in this respect and the general concept has become known as the "hygiene hypothesis" [31].

The high prevalence of T2DM in association with hepatitis C infection and the progression of certain diabetes complications (e.g. diabetic nephropathy) in association with hepatitis B are other noteworthy examples. The treatment of HIV/AIDS with protease inhibitors predisposes to diabetes, metabolic syndrome and increased cardiovascular risk. The public health implications of these issues are considerable given the concordance of the diabetes epidemic with these other highly prevalent diseases.

All infections, especially if severe, have the potential to exacerbate hyperglycemia by a number of mechanisms (e.g. worsening of insulin resistance by production of "stress" or counter-regulatory hormones and production of cytokines such as IL-1 and tumor necrosis factor) [32]. Infection remains a major factor in the pathogenesis of diabetic ketoacidosis or hyperosmolar hyperglycemia. Infections can also precipitate hypoglycemia if symptoms, such as anorexia, nausea and vomiting, lead to reduced food intake. Malaria and its treatment with quinine can also produce hypoglycemia.

Hepatitis C

A number of reports from North America, Europe and the Middle East consistently demonstrate an increased prevalence of diabetes (ranging from 24% to 62%) among patients with chronic hepatitis C virus (HCV) infection compared both with persons with other forms of liver disease and with other control groups. Among HCV-infected individuals reported prevalence of diabetes (21–50%) is much higher when compared with other forms of chronic liver disease (2–12%) and with control subjects (2–6%) [33–38].

In the USA, T2DM occurs more often in persons with HCV infection who are older than 40 years of age, particularly in the range of 40–49 years where the relative risk ratio is 3.77. Apart from age, the prevalence of diabetes is greatest in subjects who are non-white, have a high body mass index, are below the poverty level and have a family history of diabetes. The prevalence of T1DM appears to be unaffected [39].

The suggestion that HCV infection predisposes to T2DM as a result of the progressive liver damage is supported by the observations that the association is most marked in the older age groups (>40 years), and that there is higher risk among patients with advanced HCV cirrhosis. The presence of diabetes is also associated with worse hepatic fibrosis; however, the higher prevalence of diabetes compared to other forms of liver disease suggests an additional mechanism specific to hepatitis C. Tumor necrosis factor α has been suggested as one possible candidate for this role [40].

HCV infection is also strongly associated with diabetes among intravenous drug users and this is independent of HIV infection or use of highly active antiretroviral therapy (HAART) [41]. Thus, it is important to monitor patients with chronic HCV infection for development of diabetes. Bidirectionality again applies with weight loss and good glycemic control improving hepatitis outcomes.

HIV/AIDS

Although HIV/AIDS has not in itself been reported to increase the risk of diabetes, the treatment of HIV/AIDS with HAART predisposes to T2DM, other metabolic risks and premature cardiovascular disease. This has become a major problem in the management of this already very complicated disease. The effects occur via disturbances in lipid homeostasis and fat partitioning (lipodystrophy), insulin resistance, insulin secretion and mitochondrial function. The underlying cellular mechanisms are complex and incompletely understood. Combination HAART for HIV-1 infection is frequently complicated by lipodystrophy (peripheral fat loss and relative visceral obesity), dyslipidemia and insulin resistance. HIV-infected adults receiving HAART have an increased incidence of elevated blood pressure and cardiovascular morbidity.

Whether antiretroviral therapy-naive patients have altered risk of subsequent CVD or T2DM is unclear, particularly in light of emerging data indicating that rates of CVD may also be higher in people with HIV who are not treated with antiretriviral therapy.

Exposure to antiretroviral therapy for more than 1 year is associated with increasing risk of diabetes. Although the risk is greatest among individuals treated with a protease inhibitors (PI) (attributed to a direct inhibitory effect on cellular glucose transport by PI medications) [41], an increased prevalence of diabetes among those receiving a PI-sparing regimen has also been found and insulin resistance has been reported among PI-naive persons with HIV infection, in association with fat redistribution. Nucleoside analog-induced mitochondrial toxicity is probably of importance. Cessation of PI appears to have little beneficial effect in reversing lipodystrophy, although it may improve the metabolic control in diabetes. Alteration of thymidine analog nucleosidase reverse transcriptase inhibitors may, however, confer benefit on lipodystrophy [42,43].

In a study of almost 900 HIV-infected patients, initiation of antiretroviral therapy was evaluated for prevalence and incidence of metabolic syndrome (using the National Cholesterol Education Program, Adult Treatment Panel III [NCEP ATP-III] and the International Diabetes Federation [IDF] criteria) and subsequent diagnosis of CVD and T2DM over a 3-year period. The prevalence of baseline metabolic syndrome was 8.5% and 7.8% (ATP-III and IDF criteria, respectively). Substantial progression to metabolic syndrome occurred within 3 years following initiation of antiretroviral therapy. The presence of metabolic syndrome at baseline was significantly associated with an increased risk of T2DM while metabolic syndrome occurring during the 3-year period was associated with an increased risk of both CVD and diabetes [44,45].

In another study [46], 123 of 6513 HIV-infected persons developed diabetes during 27 798 person-years of follow-up, resulting in an incidence of 4.4 cases per 1000 person-years of follow-up. An increased incidence rate ratio was found for male subjects, older age, obesity, Afro-American or Asian ethnicity. A weaker, although still significant, association of the incidence rate was also found with Centers for Disease Control and Prevention (CDC) disease stage C. Strong associations were observed with treatment using nucleoside reverse-transcriptase inhibitors (NRTI), NRTI plus PI and NRTI + PI + non-nucleoside reverse-transcriptase inhibitors (NNRTI), but not with an NRTI + NNRTI regimen.

Lipodystrophy is a crucial aspect of the association of HAART with insulin resistance, leading to relative preponderance of visceral fat, hepatic steatosis and fat deposition at other "ectopic" sites. HIV-infected persons with lipodystrophy, compared with those without lipodystrophy, have a reduction in plasma adiponectin and adipose tissue adiponectin mRNA levels of approximately 50%, correlating with insulin resistance and increased cytokine levels [45].

Because baseline and incident metabolic syndrome identifies individuals at risk for both CVD and T2DM, evaluation in all patients commencing HAART is warranted. A fasting plasma glucose concentration should be checked before initiation of therapy and monitored every 3–6 months, especially in patients receiving changes in treatment or who have significant risk factors for insulin resistance. An oral glucose tolerance test may be required, particularly in the presence of risk factors or equivocal glucose concentrations. Dietary guidelines established for the general population remain relevant for the management of glucose disorders in the context of HIV infection. Weight loss through increased activity and caloric restriction should be recommended for overweight HIV-infected patients.

Metformin improves insulin sensitivity in patients with HIV lipodystrophy and is an effective antidiabetic medication; however, it should be used with caution in patients receiving an NRTI, and in persons with impaired renal function because of the possibility of lactic acidosis. Thiazolidinediones also improve insulin sensitivity in patients with HIV lipoatrophy, although rosiglitazone treatment may worsen hyperlipidemia. Insulin therapy should be used according to standard recommendations. Substitution of an NNRTI for a PI has been observed to improve insulin resistance but this needs to be balanced against any risk to virus control. Careful discussion with the HIV physician is therefore essential and it may be deemed safer to increase the antihypoglycemic treatment rather than changing the components of the HAART regime [47–49].

Hepatitis B

Although, in contrast to hepatitis C, hepatitis B virus (HBV) has been less consistently associated with an increased prevalence of diabetes, the presence of hepatitis B markers may nevertheless influence the natural history of diabetes and its complications and the relationship may be bidirectional as the presence of diabetes is associated with more severe fibrosis and cirrhosis. However, there is uncertainty as to cause and effect given the general association of diabetes with liver cirrhosis [50].

Chinese HBV-infected patients with T2DM have been shown to be more likely to develop end-stage renal disease than non-HBV infected patients with T2DM (8.7 vs 6.4%) with a hazard ratio of 4.5. The association of chronic HBV infection with increased risk of end-stage renal disease was independent of other potential confounding factors. HBV-infected patients also reported earlier onset of diabetes and had a higher frequency of diabetic retinopathy than non-HBV-infected patients (28%

compared to 22%). Cardiovascular complications appeared unaffected [51].

Specific infections either strongly associated with diabetes or in which the presence of diabetes is important

Infections involving the head and neck

Two head and neck infections that are associated with high rates of morbidity and mortality, malignant otitis externa and rhinocerebral mucormycosis, are particularly noteworthy in people with diabetes.

Malignant otitis externa

Malignant otitis externa is an invasive infection of the external auditory canal and skull base that typically arises in elderly people with diabetes. An early series of patients was described in 1968 [52]. Most cases (86–90%) have been reported in patients with diabetes. *Pseudomonas aeruginosa* is nearly always the causal organism (>98% of cases) although *Aspergillus* species are occasionally responsible. Microangiopathy in the ear canal has been suggested as a predisposing factor.

Presenting features include severe intractable headache and otalgia, otorrhea and deafness. Patients often report a duration of weeks to months of these symptoms. Intense cellulitis is combined with edema of the ear canal. Focal neurologic signs and cranial nerve palsies may occur. The pain may involve the temporomandibular joint and be aggravated by chewing. Osteomyelitis of the skull base and temporomandibular joint is a potentially life-threatening complication and the mortality in the pre-antibiotic era exceeded 50%. On otoscopy, granulation tissue may be seen in the floor of the ear canal, often in association with edema and intense cellulitis. The tympanic membrane is usually intact. Computed tomography (CT) and magnetic resonance imaging (MRI) studies are essential for defining the extent of bone and soft tissue involvement, together with the bony destruction of the skull base that may be seen in advanced cases.

Systemic antipseudomonal antibiotics are the primary therapy. Early referral to an otorhinolaryngologist is essential and allows diagnostic confirmation by surgical biopsy. Débridement of necrotic tissue can also be carried out if necessary, although the introduction of effective antibiotic therapy has reduced the requirement for surgery. With the introduction of quinolones, the cure rate has increased to 90%, with few adverse effects reported and oral therapy rendered possible. Prolonged treatment for 6–8 weeks is recommended, as for osteomyelitis [53]. Thus, treatment consists of prolonged administration (6–8 weeks) of an antipseudomonal agent (typically, an orally administered quinolone). The emergence of ciprofloxacin resistance is a potential problem. It is recommended that systemic quiniolone use be reserved for treatment of invasive ear infections. An example of invasive aspergillosis involving the skull base is shown in Figure 50.1.

Mucormycosis (zygomycosis)

The term mucormycosis is used to describe a variety of infections caused by fungi of the *Rhizopus* and *Mucor* species which belong to the order Mucorales (class Zygomycetes). These fungi are ubiquitous saprophytes and infections produced by them are essentially confined to immunocompromised individuals. The fungi have a predilection to invade blood vessels. Ketone reductases produced by *Rhizopus* spp. allow them to thrive in high glucose, acidic conditions as are typically present in patients with diabetic ketoacidosis [23]. Rhinocerebral, pulmonary, gastrointestinal, cutaneous and disseminated forms of the infection are described. The rhinocerebral manifestation (and with sinus involvement) has the highest frequency and is potentially the most lethal in the context of people with diabetes (Figure 50.2).

The close connection with diabetes is becoming increasingly diluted as other causes of an immunocompromised state become increasingly common or survivable (notably hematologic cancer and bone marrow transplant recipients). Nevertheless, diabetes remains the most common underlying factor in most reports. In a review of 49 cases of pulmonary mucormycosis, diabetes was the underlying cause of the immunocompromised state in 9 (25%) [54]. In another study, the prevalence and mortality in people with diabetes were 36% and 44%, respectively [55]. It typically, although not exclusively, occurs in association with ketoacidosis, severe hyperglycemia and/or a debilitated state.

Rhinocerebral mucormycosis is a life-threatening fungal infection. Untreated it is universally fatal; if recognized early there is a 20% survival rate. Presenting features include facial or ocular pain and nasal stuffiness. Generalized malaise and fever may also be present. Intranasal black eschars or necrotic turbinates may be found and, if present, provide sites that can be biopsied. Treatment consists of surgical débridement of the involved sinuses and prolonged intravenous therapy with amphotericin B or alternative antifungal agents such as some newer azoles.

Acute invasive fungal sinusitis can also result from aspergillosis, as can malignant otitis externa. Biopsy confirmation of the microbiologic diagnosis is therefore useful [56].

Endophthalmitis

Secondary endophthalmitis may occur as a rare but devastating metastatic complication of septicemia and in this setting is almost entirely confined to people with diabetes. *E. coli* and *Klebsiella* are the more likely pathogens and urinary tract infection is reported as the most common underlying source of infection [57].

People with diabetes are also more prone to postoperative infections following eye surgery or infections secondary to eye trauma. Overall, the most common cause of endophthalmitis is as a postoperative complication of cataract surgery [58], a procedure commonly carried out in patients with diabetes.

Periodontal disease

People with diabetes are very prone to periodontal disease compared to the non-diabetic population, with a two- to fourfold

(a)

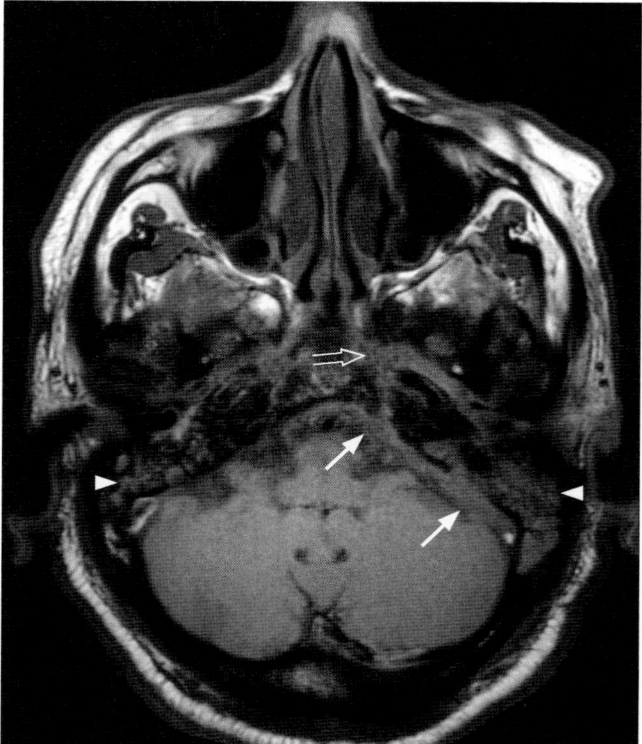

(b)

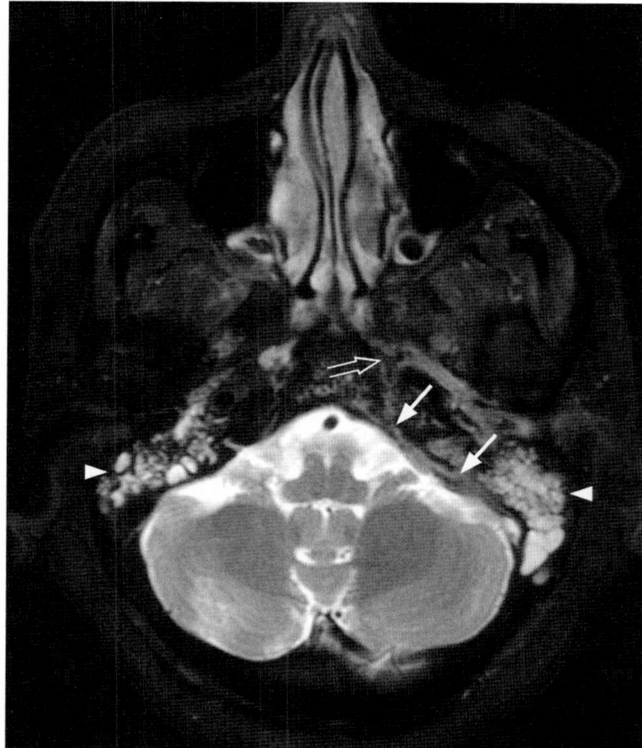

Figure 50.1 Magnetic resonance imaging (MRI) scan of skull base in a 59-year-old male with a 20-year history of diabetes (with nephropathy), treated with insulin who developed severe extensive invasive aspergillosis. He presented with headache and vertigo followed by left sixth and seventh nerve palsies. He subsequently developed bilateral sensorineural hearing impairment and blindness secondary to extensive skull base infiltration by the invasive aspergillosis. MRI demonstrated enhancing soft tissue closely related to the left posterolateral wall of the nasopharynx with parapharyngeal, skull base, perineural and dural infiltration. Biopsy showed inflamed fibrous tissue with degenerated fungal filaments. Culture confirmed *Aspergillus flavus.* He is receiving lifelong therapy with voriconazole. He remains blind. MRI of skull base in the axial plane with: (a) T1-weighted; (b) fat-saturated T2-weighted; and (c) post-gadolinium T1-weighted sequences. These show marked dural thickening (arrows) with enhancement in the left posterior cranial fossa. An abnormal signal with enhancement is also noted in the adjacent left petrous apex (open arrow). Note also the presence of inflammatory fluid within both mastoid air cells (arrowheads). Acknowledgements to Dr. K.T. Wong, Consultant Radiologist, for preparation and reporting of the figures, and to Professor A. Ahuja for permission to use the figures. Both are placed at the Department of Diagnostic Radiology and Organ Imaging, Prince of Wales Hospital, Chinese University of Hong Kong, Hong Kong.

relative increase in prevalence and a particular predilection for those whose diabetes is poorly controlled.

The associated periodontitis, if left untreated, can result in loss of attachment of ligament fibers and supporting alveolar bone, which in turn can increase the mobility of teeth and necessitate extraction. Tooth abscesses and episodes of bacteremia also become more likely. Diabetes may complicate the pathogenesis of periodontitis by causing abnormalities in the vasculature of the gingival tissues, in addition to the effects upon immune responses described earlier. Aggressive and difficult to treat forms of periodontitis are also more common in adults with diabetes. Periodontal health is influenced by glycemic control to the extent that the prevalence of periodontal diseases among people with well-controlled diabetes is not increased [59].

A bidirectional relationship has also been suggested whereby the presence of periodontal disease adds to the overall burden of chronic inflammation, thereby adversely affecting glycemic control as well as overall risk of CVD and diabetic nephropathy.

Respiratory tract infections and tuberculosis

The increased risk of mortality and morbidity from community-acquired pneumonia has been alluded to earlier and includes pneumonia either directly resulting from, or secondary to, common infections such as influenza and *S. pneumoniae* and also includes *Legionella* infections [60]. The risk of bacteremia following pneumococcal infection is increased [61]. Viral shedding may be more prolonged following influenza infections in subjects with co-morbidities including diabetes, which may influence decisions regarding initiation and duration of antiviral therapy [62].

Lower respiratory tract infections, resulting from *S. aureus* and Gram-negative organisms such as *K. pneumoniae*, are more

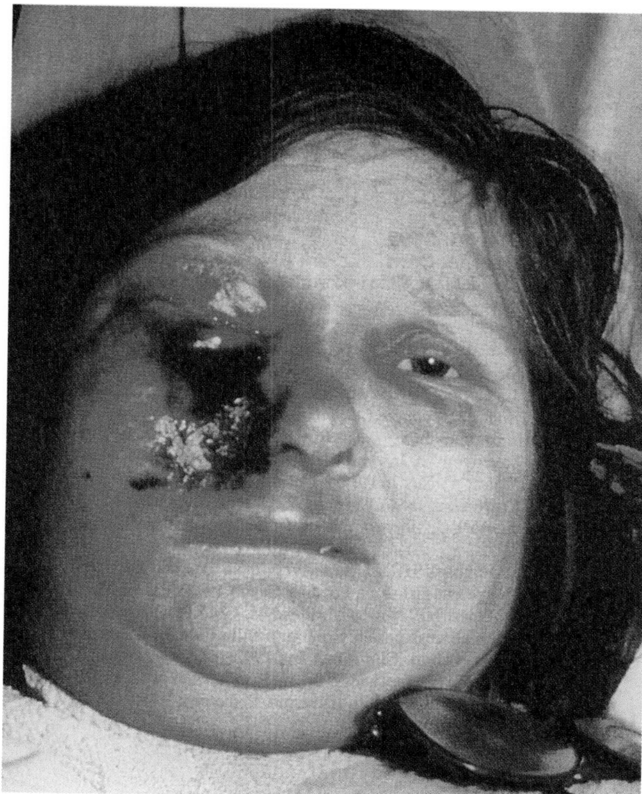

Figure 50.2 Rhinocerebral mucormycosis. Typical appearance in a 45-year-old woman with poorly controlled type 1 diabetes. Periorbital and facial swelling had been present for 3–4 days before admission. Major reconstructive surgery was required. From Rupp ME. Rhinocerebral mucormycosis. *N Engl J Med* 1995; **333**:564.

common in people with diabetes. Melioidosis has also been discussed above as an example of organism-specific factors that interact with diabetes to increase risk of infection. People with diabetes are also thought to be at increased risk for *S. aureus* pneumonia and this may result from the well-documented higher rates of nasal carriage of *S. aureus* in people with diabetes (up to 30%) compared to 11% in healthy individuals [63].

Any respiratory infection in patients with diabetes is associated with increased mortality. In the USA, people with diabetes are reportedly 4 times more likely to die from pneumonia or influenza than are people without diabetes [64].

The importance of diabetes as the most common underlying predisposing factor for thoracic empyema has also long been recognized. A recent report indicates that *Klebsiella* are again notable as the most common pathogens, while other important pathogens include streptococci, *S. aureus* and anaerobes [65].

Diabetes and tuberculosis

An association between diabetes and tuberculosis has been widely accepted in the past, albeit with varying estimates of overall risk (encompassing two- to 11-fold) and variable levels of evidence. The importance of the association is often neglected in the larger arena of public health, for example when compared with the risk of tuberculosis associated with HIV/AIDS.

Diabetes has been confirmed in several recent studies to be associated with increased risk of active tuberculosis. The association of tuberculosis with diabetes presumably reflects impaired innate immunity as well as (in this case at least) a reduced adaptive T-helper type 1 response with reduced secretion of T-helper type 1-related cytokines. A recent review of 13 observational studies published between 1992 and 2007 [66] confirms an increased risk of tuberculosis regardless of study design, population, geographic region and background incidence of tuberculosis, the overall increase in risk being approximately threefold. The risk was greatest among younger people, in areas of high tuberculosis incidence and in non-North American populations. The public health impact may be particularly high in countries such as India and China, which are at the forefront of the diabetes epidemic. The impact of the diabetes epidemic on tuberculosis incidence in India has been modeled by Stevenson *et al.* [67]. They suggest that diabetes accounts for 14.8% (range of uncertainty 7.1–23.8%) of pulmonary tuberculosis and 20.2% (8.3–41.9%) of smear-positive tuberculosis, with an excess risk of the latter in urban areas. This can be compared to an overall estimate of 3.4% for the proportion of adult tuberculosis incidence ascribed to HIV/AIDS in India [68]. Extrapulmonary or unusual manifestations of tuberculosis are also more common in the context of diabetes. In pulmonary tuberculosis, the presence of diabetes, as well as being the most common underlying co-morbidity, has also been reported to increase the risk of cavitatory nodules [69].

In addition to the increased risk, there is also evidence that diabetes leads to worse tuberculosis outcomes and has adverse effects upon responses to treatment. A study from Indonesia indicated a doubling of the risk of remaining smear positive at the end of treatment for pulmonary tuberculosis in people with diabetes compared to those without diabetes [70]. The same group in Indonesia has also shown that the presence of T2DM may adversely affect the bioavailability of rifampicin and lead to an increase in dose requirement [71]. In Hong Kong, an area with much pioneering experience of tuberculosis treatment since the 1950s, the Centre for Health Protection recognizes the risk of a worse outcome, and its guidelines recommend a more prolonged period of treatment for people with diabetes compared to those without. For example, when treating pulmonary tuberculosis using a standard regimen of four drugs for the first 2 months followed by two drugs, a total treatment duration of 9 months, rather than 6 months, is recommended. Bidirectionality again needs to be remembered because the presence of tuberculosis is very likely to have a negative impact upon hyperglycemia. Two examples of individuals with tuberculosis in association with diabetes are shown in Figure 50.3. It is perhaps noteworthy that neither was receiving regular follow-up care for the diabetes.

(a)

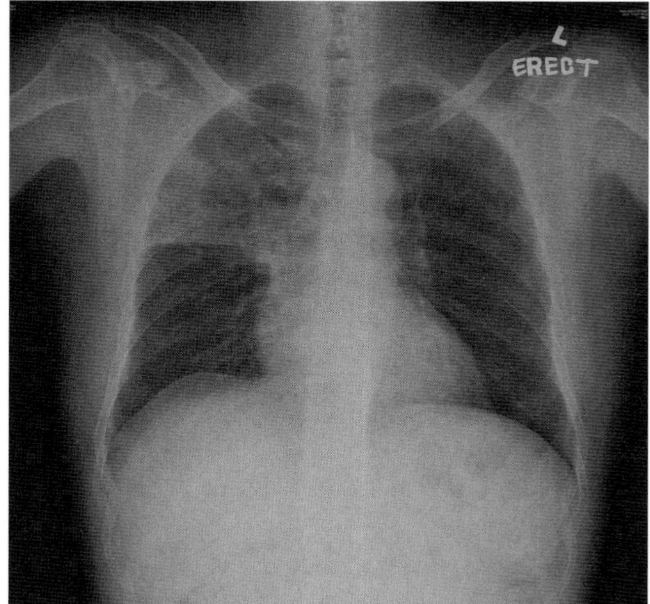

(b)

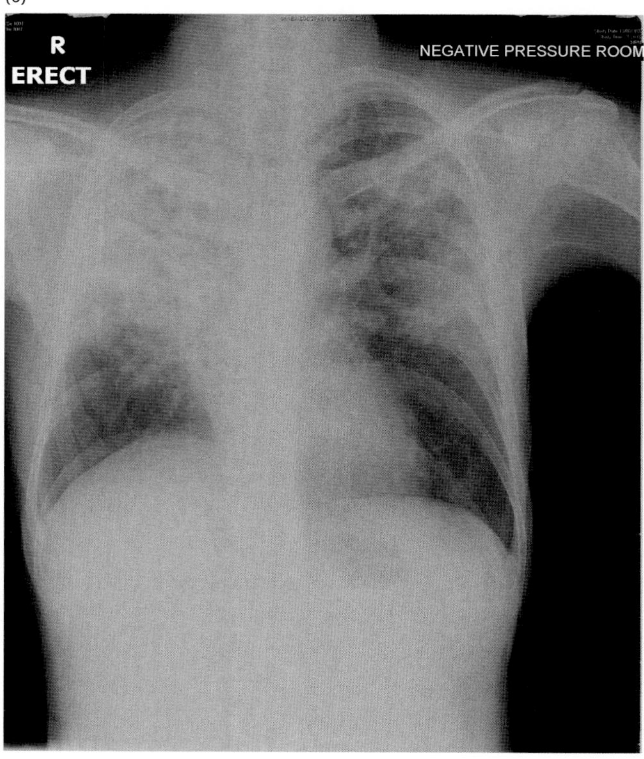

Figure 50.3 (a) A 49-year-old man with diabetes and obesity, not receiving regular follow-up, and presenting with hemoptysis, sputum smear positive for tuberculosis (TB). Chest X-ray shows extensive right upper lobe pneumonic changes. (b) A 30-year-old man with diabetes but no regular follow-up, presents with a cough for 4 months with weight loss, sputum smear positive for TB. Chest X-ray shows extensive bilateral and cavitatory disease.

Infections of the urinary tract

Epidemiology and risk factors

Urinary tract infection (UTI) is frequently encountered in people with diabetes. Asymptomatic bacteriuria also occurs with a higher frequency. One study has demonstrated a prevalence rate for asymptomatic bacteriuria of 26% in women with diabetes, compared to 6% in women without diabetes, a threefold increase [72,73].

A randomized controlled trial of antibiotic treatment for asymptomatic bacteriuria revealed no differences in the development of symptomatic UTI, time to onset of symptoms, risk of pyelonephritis or need for hospitalization [72]. Thus, diabetes does not appear to warrant either screening for, or treating, asymptomatic bacteriuria. This remains a controversial issue and, from the practical standpoint of the physician, ascertaining "asymptomatic status" with confidence, particularly in older women with diabetes, can be difficult or impossible.

A number of studies confirm the increased risk of symptomatic UTI in association with diabetes. In one study of more than 600 women [74], those with T2DM had an overall risk of 20%. A recent study has extended the risk to include recurrence rates as well as risk to males [1].

Diabetes is a risk factor for cystitis in postmenopausal women, leading to a two- to threefold increase in risk [75]. An increased prevalence of asymptomatic vaginal *E. coli* colonization has also been reported in postmenopausal women with diabetes who are receiving insulin treatment. This vaginal colonization may be mediated by greater adherence of type 1 fimbriated *E. coli* to uroepithelial cells in women with diabetes, may be related to impaired cytokine secretion or may reflect a reduced polymorphonuclear inflammatory response [72,76].

Diabetes increases the risk of complications of UTI, serious or unusual forms of infection, and need for prolonged hospitalization [77]. It is a risk factor for acute pyelonephritis in women (odds ratio 4.1), and is the strongest of the various risk factors that have been examined. Among hospitalized patients, 16.7% reported having diabetes compared with 5.8% of non-hospitalized patients [72]. A three- to fivefold increase in risk exists in people with diabetes aged less than 44 years [74].

Diabetic autonomic neuropathy is an important predisposing factor to UTI. This affects the sympathetic and parasympathetic afferent fibers to the bladder and causes decreased reflex detrusor activity. Impaired bladder sensation results in bladder distension, increased residual urine volume, vesicoureteric reflux and recurrent upper UTI [78,79]. Some cases are urinary catheter or instrumentation related [72,78,79]. Additional host factors predisposing to UTI include: glycosuria, sexual intercourse, history of previous UTI, obstruction, longer duration of diabetes, poor glycemic control, decreased urinary cytokine excretion, increased *E. coli* adhesion, macroalbuminuria and neutrophil dysfunction [78,79]. Renal papillary necrosis and chronic renal failure may also contribute to the complex array of risk to the urinary tract.

Microbiology

E. coli is the most commonly reported organism. *Klebsiella* is also a problem, especially among patients with uncommon severe forms of UTI, such as emphysematous pyelonephritis. Other organisms include *Acinetobacter* species, group B streptococci and *P. aeruginosa* [72]. The latter should be suspected particularly if there is a history of recent instrumentation or hospitalization.

C. albicans in the urine can be associated with incomplete bladder emptying and high glucose concentrations in the urine. Diabetes has been shown to be present in 39% of hospitalized patients with funguria [72]. Candiduria may signify contamination of the urine specimen, benign saprophytic colonization (± catheter), or may be indicative of true invasive infection of the upper and/or lower urinary tract [80]. Diabetes is also a risk factor for multidrug-resistant UTI, perhaps related to recurrent or increased exposure to antibiotics [81].

Clinical features of urinary tract infection in diabetes

Uncomplicated UTIs may be asymptomatic. Symptoms, when present, are generally similar to those experienced by the non-diabetic population. Infection of the lower urinary tract usually presents as dysuria, frequency or urgency. Fever, flank pain, chills and rigors, vomiting and costovertebral angle tenderness raise the suspicion of upper tract infection with renal involvement. Bilateral renal involvement is also more frequent and bilateral pyelonephritis is twice as common in people with diabetes. Bacteremia may be present.

A poor response to appropriate antibiotic therapy should raise the suspicion of the presence of complications. These may include renal papillary necrosis and perinephric abscess. The symptoms of renal papillary necrosis include flank and abdominal pain (which mimic both pyelonephritis and ureteric colic), together with fever. Renal functional impairment is commonly found. Features such as a persisting high fever despite antibiotic treatment, hypotension or septicemic shock, and a palpable tender renal mass may point to the presence of a perinephric abscess. In one series of patients with perinephric abscess, 36% had diabetes [82].

Emphysematous cystitis and emphysematous pyelonephritis

Although uncommon, the severity of these infections warrants their special consideration. Emphysematous cystitis is an uncommon complication of lower UTI characterized by the presence of gas in the bladder wall (Figure 50.4). It presents with hematuria, pneumaturia and abdominal pain. Plain abdominal radiography or CT scan are indicated to detect the presence of gas. Surgical intervention may be required in up to 20% of cases and mortality is reportedly up to 10%. Emphysematous cystitis requires aggressive treatment in hospital and intravenous antibiotic therapy [83].

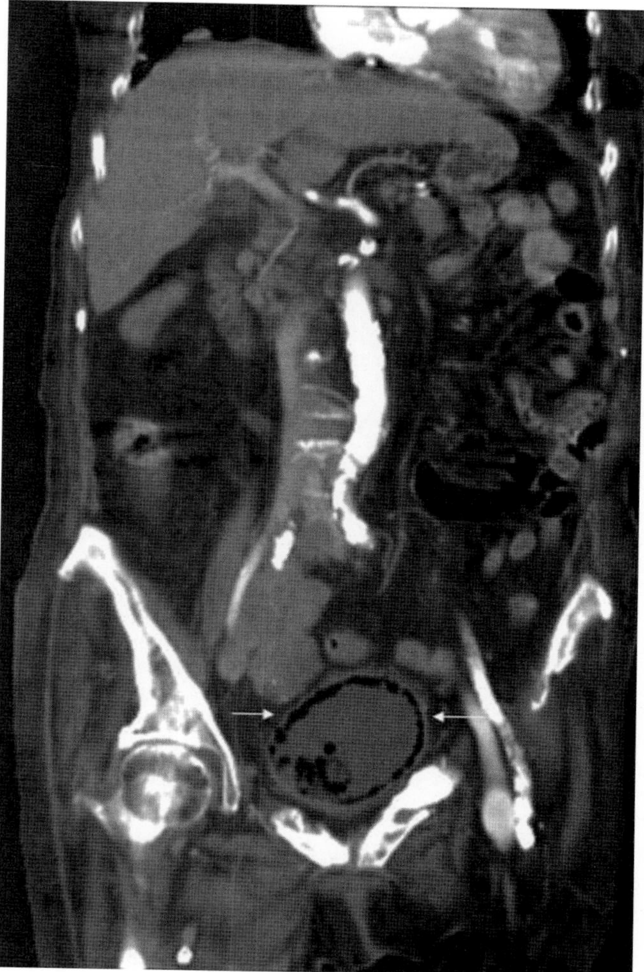

Figure 50.4 Example of emphysematous cystitis in a 67-year-old woman with diabetes and end-stage renal disease (ESRD) requiring hemodialysis. She developed septic shock with lower abdominal tenderness. Blood and urine cultures show *E. coli*. Computed tomography (CT) scan shows air pockets inside the urinary bladder (arrows). From Sun JT, Wang HP, Lien WC. Life-threatening urinary tract infection. *Q J Med* 2009; **102**:223, with permission.

Emphysematous pyelonephritis is an infection that is almost exclusively limited to people with diabetes, who account for 90% of cases (Figure 50.5). It predominantly occurs in females and carries a grave prognosis [84]. It is a necrotizing infection of the renal parenchyma and surrounding areas which can be focal or diffuse and may spread to the collecting system or perinephric tissues. The formation and presence of gas in the renal parenchyma, collecting system or perinephric area may be contributed to by fermentation of glucose when present at high concentra-

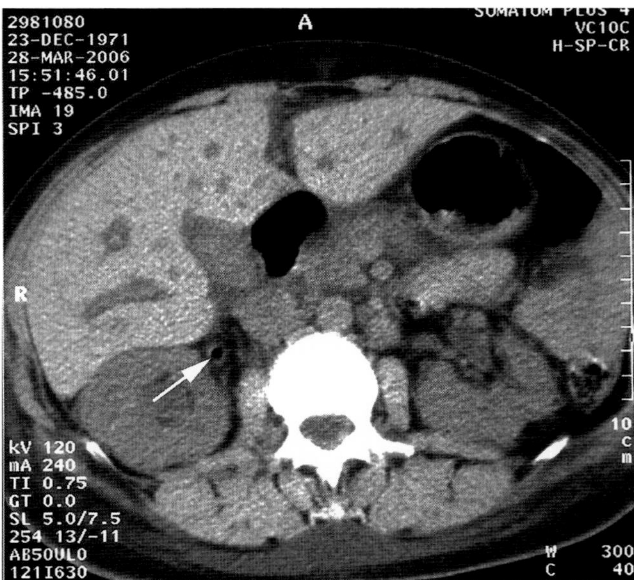

Figure 50.5 Emphysematous pyelonephritis: computed tomography tomography (CT) scan demonstrating gas in the right ureter (indicated by arrow) and a moderate hydronephrosis in a 34-year-old woman with type 1 diabetes. The responsible was organism was *E. coli*. She responded to antibiotics and drainage by nephrostomy, followed by ureteroscopy during which obstructing necrotic slough was removed. From Clark T, Abdalkareem M, Ali K. A case of emphysematous pyelonephritis. *J R Soc Med* 2009; **102**:75–77, with permission.

tions, by the presence of gas-forming organisms and by impaired renal perfusion. Mixed acid fermentation of glucose by Enterobacteriaceae has been suggested as a major pathway of gas formation [85].

A lengthy list of pathogens has been reported; however, as with other UTIs in the context of diabetes, the most common pathogens are *E. coli* (in 70%) and *Klebsiella* (in 30%). Vasculopathy of the renal circulation is believed to be a major factor in the pathogenesis, once again emphasizing the importance of vascular disease in the clinical manifestation of the more severe forms of infection related to diabetes.

Presenting features include fever, abdominal pain, nausea and vomiting and drowsiness or stupor. As a result of these non-specific symptoms the diagnosis is often delayed. The presence of features such as renal angle tenderness, pyuria or pneumaturia should lead to a high index of suspicion. A flank mass may be detected, often accompanied by crepitus. Disseminated intravascular coagulation, septicemic shock and acute renal failure are all associated with a poor prognosis.

The diagnosis is established by radiologic identification of gas in renal tissue. This is best demonstrated by CT. The plain abdominal X-ray sensitivity is lower. Ultrasonography can also be used, but CT should be regarded as the investigation of choice. In a report of 46 cases in Taiwan, 96% had diabetes with HbA_{1c} higher than 8% (>64 mmol/mol), and 22% also had features of obstruction [86]. Mortality can exceed 50% in patients treated with antibiotics alone. Medical therapy alone is therefore not recommended. Patients may require percutaneous drainage (for localized cases with abscess formation or obstruction) or nephrectomy (in extensive cases). The advent of CT has allowed a more rational approach to the use of these surgical interventions, by allowing more accurate delineation of factors such as gas distribution, obstruction and abscess formation [87].

Diagnosis of urinary tract infection

A high index of suspicion is required, with particular attention in the presence of diabetic neuropathy, renal dysfunction or renal papillary necrosis. Microscopic examination of the urine may reveal leukocytosis and pyuria. Urine culture and sensitivity should always be carried out. In febrile patients or in suspected upper tract infection, blood culture is essential to detect bacteremia or Gram-negative septicemia.

Plain abdominal radiography is useful to help rule out obstructive uropathy, stones and emphysematous infection. Ultrasonography is a sensitive, safe and inexpensive technique for initial screening. Ultrasound or CT can confirm the diagnosis of renal abscess, mass, presence of air in the urinary tract and the extent of perinephric spread of infection. The diagnosis of renal papillary necrosis may require ultimate confirmation by retrograde pyelography.

Treatment of urinary tract infection

Treatment should be tailored to take account of local antibiotic resistance patterns (if known), as well as previous history of UTI, previous antibiotic exposure (and possible allergies) together with other risk factors such as recent instrumentation or catheterization. Uncomplicated UTI may be treated with co-trimoxazole (if the local resistance rate is <15–20%), fluoroquinolones, nitrofurantoin, ampicillin, amoxicillin +/– clavulanate, or sulbactam. Increasing resistance to fluoroquinolones has been noted recently. Co-trimoxazole may potentiate the hypoglycemic effect of some oral antihyperglycemic agents and should be used with caution.

Complicated infections require hospitalization and parenteral antibiotics. Intravenous therapy is continued until fever resolves, following which oral antibiotics can be substituted to complete at least 2 weeks of treatment. Second or third-generation cephalosporins, β-lactam/β-lactamase inhibitor combinations, or fluoroquinolones may need to be considered in patients with risk factors, and the possibility of infection with *Pseudomonas* may influence this choice, particularly in the setting of nosocomial exposure or recent instrumentation.

Because upper urinary tract involvement with UTI may be up to 5 times more frequent in patients with diabetes compared with people without diabetes and may be unsuspected or asymptomatic. More prolonged courses of antibiotics (7–14 days) may be considered wise even in the context of apparently uncomplicated UTI [84]. This may also reduce the risk of subsequent relapse. Repeated urine culture to document bacteriologic cure 2–4 weeks post-treatment is advisable given high rates of relapse or treatment failure.

Distinguishing *Candida* infection from colonization is difficult. Removal of an indwelling catheter, if present, is recommended as an initial intervention. Antifungal agents such as fluconazole may be considered in patients with invasive disease.

Intra-abdominal infections other than those within the urinary tract

Emphysematous cholecystitis

Cholecystitis is probably no more common in patients with diabetes than in the general population; however, severe fulminating infection, especially with gas-forming organisms (enteric Gram-negative rods and anaerobes) is more common.

Emphysematous cholecystitis is a rare variant of acute cholecystitis caused by ischemia of the gallbladder wall and infection with gas-producing organisms. It is strongly associated with diabetes (35–55% of cases have underlying diabetes) [88].

Gangrene and perforation of the gallbladder are more frequent, and the overall mortality is substantially higher (at least 15% compared to less than 4%) when compared with acute cholecystitis.

Clostridium perfringens, *E. coli* and *Bacillus fragilis* are the most frequently encountered pathogens. Emphysematous cholecystitis is thought to result from acalculous cystic duct obstruction, associated with inflammatory edema, which can eventually lead to cystic artery occlusion. Colonization by gas-forming organisms contributes to necrosis of the mucosa, venous congestion, gangrene and, eventually, gallbladder perforation. Gallstones are present in only about half of patients.

The early clinical manifestations may be indistinguishable from those of acute cholecystitis. Right hypochondrial pain and fever are present in all cases, and other important features include nausea and vomiting, septic shock, jaundice and peritonitis. Toxicity is marked, and jaundice may develop in the later stages from biliary obstruction. The gallbladder may be palpable in 25–50% of patients. It should be remembered that Murphy sign (pain and inspiratory arrest on palpation of the right upper quadrant) may be absent in patients with underlying diabetic neuropathy. Crepitus on palpation is an ominous sign. Additional complications include pericholecystic abscess, gallbladder necrosis, generalized or biliary peritonitis, and localized perforation sealed by the omentum.

Plain abdominal X-ray or ultrasound can lead to diagnosis in 95% of cases. In a plain radiograph, gas may be visible in the gallbladder lumen or within the gallbladder wall as a gaseous ring. CT is the most sensitive modality for the detection of intraluminal or intramural gallbladder gas and also demonstrate local complications such as pericholecystic inflammatory changes, abscess formation or perforation.

Initiation of appropriate antibiotics and early cholecystectomy is crucial. Emergency surgery is needed because of the high incidence of gangrene and perforation [89,90].

Liver and other intra-abdominal abscesses

Although liver abscesses may occur in many situations not involving diabetes, the issue is of sufficient importance to justify inclusion in this section.

In keeping with the susceptibility to *Klebsiella* infections described earlier, associations between diabetes and *K. pneumoniae* liver abscess have been reported, notably from Taiwan and Korea [91–93]. Examples from Hong Kong are shown in Figure 50.6.

In Korea, invasive liver abscess is particularly associated both with *K. pneumoniae* (78% of the total, 40% of whom have diabetes)) and with the K1 serotype (60%) [27].

Diabetes is the most common underlying risk factor specifically for the virulent K1 serotype, but not for non-*Klebsiella* abscesses [94]. In a population-based series of pyogenic liver abscess reported from Taiwan and including 29 703 subjects [95], diabetes was a risk factor in 33% leading to an odds ratio of 9 and was associated with an increasing incidence. Liver abscess in people with diabetes was not, however, associated with increased mortality, particularly if therapeutic percutaneous drainage procedures are performed. Eighty percent were associated with *K. pneumoniae* and not as a mixed infection with other organisms. Primary liver abscess in other parts of Asia is also increasing in incidence [27], with 40% reportedly associated with diabetes. Bacteremia is present in 50%, and 8–10% of these cases have metastatic complications (e.g. endophthalmitis, meningitis, brain abscess, pneumonia, skin and soft tissue lesions).

In a series from Europe (n = 1448), the presence of diabetes was associated with a 3.6-fold increase in risk for pyogenic liver abscess, and also with a higher 30-day post-discharge mortality rate compared with patients who did not have diabetes [96].

In the context of the K1 serotype of *Klebsiella* species, a pathogenic role for the magA gene in the serotype-specific region of the K1 capsule gene cluster, together with a K1 capsular polysaccharide per se, is considered as one of the virulence determinants essential for the development of invasive liver abscess. MagA, an outer membrane protein contributing to capsular polysaccharide formation, coexists with serotype K1 and has been identified as the major virulence factor of *K. pneumoniae* [95]. Poor glycemic control also has a role by impairing neutrophil phagocytosis of K1/K2 type *K. pneumoniae*, whereas it does not significantly affect the phagocytosis of non-K1/K2 *K. pneumoniae*. An rmpA-associated hypermuco-viscosity phenotype has also been reported in invasive purulent diseases caused by *K. pneumoniae*.

Most isolates are susceptible to cephalosporins (especially third-generation agents) and fluoroquinolones; however, therapeutic drainage is also needed and also assists with obtaining specimens for culture and susceptibility testing.

Metastatic abscesses may occur elsewhere in the abdomen, either singly or in combination with other sites, as well as within the urinary tract. A notorious, although uncommon, example is psoas abscess where responsible organisms are likely to be *S. aureus*, *Mycobacterium tuberculosis*, *E. coli* or *Klebsiella*.

(a)

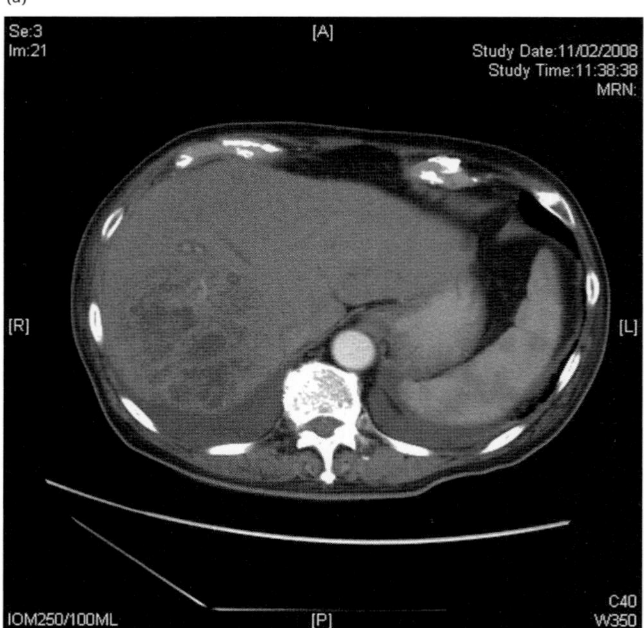

(b)

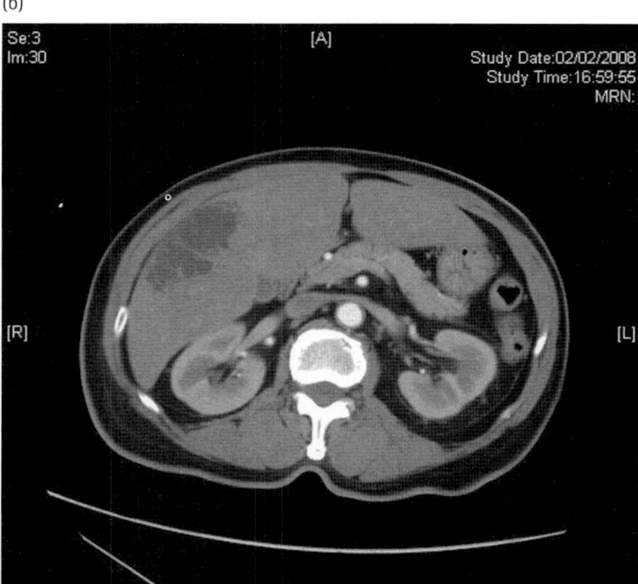

Figure 50.6 (a) CT-scan of an 82-year-old man with fever and newly diagnosed diabetes. Blood culture grew *Klebsiella pneumoniae*. The scan shows an 8 × 8.2 cm heterogeneous lesion in the right lobe of the liver composed of multiple rim enhanced lesions, with septation and hypodense cystic components. A further three smaller similar lesions (1–2.5 cm) were also seen inferiorly. Overall features are suggestive of liver abscesses. The patient recovered with drainage and antibiotics. (b) CT-scan of a 77-year-old woman with underlying diabetes, fever and right upper quadrant pain. Both blood culture and pus (from the liver abscess) grew *K. pneumoniae*. The CT scan shows an irregular ovoid lesion with multiple locules and thin intervening septations in the periphery of liver segment V and measuring 7.3 × 3.2 × 6.1 cm. The features suggest liver abscess with signs of early liquefaction. The patient recovered with drainage and antibiotics. The authors acknowledge the Department of Diagnostic Radiology and Organ Imaging, Prince of Wales Hospital, Chinese University of Hong Kong for kindly supplying the images and permitting their use.

Skin and superficial soft tissue infections

Skin and subcutaneous tissues

Infections involving the skin, nails and subcutaneous tissues are very common, and the skin and subcutaneous tissues are frequent targets of infection in diabetes, particularly in association with poor glycemic control. Candidal infections, bacterial infections such as furunculosis, dermatophycoses and onychophycoses are all commonly seen and may be the reason for diabetes being identified. Cutaneous forms of mucormycosis or other fungal infections may occur and be diagnosed following skin biopsy. More detailed consideration is given to these disorders in Chapter 47 and are not repeated here.

Sensory neuropathy, atherosclerotic vascular disease and hyperglycemia predispose patients with diabetes to skin and soft tissue infections. Additional risk factors for the development of cellulitis include a past history of cellulitis, edema, peripheral vascular disease, tinea infection and dryness of the skin. The predominant organisms involved are group A streptococcus (GAS) and *S. aureus*. Cellulitis can also occur in less usual settings. For example with *S. pneumoniae* (pneumococcal) infections, cellulitis may occur in association with extracutaneous foci of disease, the suggestion being that, in this setting, the cellulitis results from hematogenous spread rather than local infection [97].

People with diabetes, particularly those who inject insulin, often have asymptomatic nasal, mucosal and skin colonization with potential pathogens such as *S. aureus*. Nasal colonization may also contribute to increased risk of staphylococcal pneumonia, for example in association with influenza.

According to data from the National Health and Nutrition Examination Survey (NHANES), people with diabetes who are colonized with *S. aureus* are also more likely to have a methicillin-resistant *S. aureus* isolate than a susceptible one (odds ratio 2.6; 95% CI 1.1–6.1) [98]. A recent increase in community-associated methicillin-resistant *S. aureus* (CA-MRSA) gives additional cause for concern. A recent report evaluating CA-MRSA in three communities found that 77% of skin or soft tissue infections were methicillin-resistant [99]. The underlying conditions identified included smoking (35%), previous skin infection (21%) and diabetes (19%).

Mucosal and skin colonization with *C. albicans* is also common and may involve numerous sites including the genitalia of both sexes as well as the mouth, skin and nails [100]. Balanitis and vulval candidiasis are common presenting features of diabetes.

Colonization may predispose to cutaneous or incisional staphylococcal (or other bacterial) infections as well as transient bacteremia. Entry sites may also include areas of fungal skin infection (e.g. intertrigo). Infection at distant sites with abscess formation or septicemia may then ensue. In two relatively early studies (each from the 1960s) older patients with diabetes were shown both to be at greater risk of staphylococcal septicemia and also to suffer a substantially higher mortality (69% in the diabetic patients compared to 42% overall) [101,102].

Deeper soft tissue infections

Deeper soft tissue infections also occur with increased frequency in people with diabetes. Examples include pyomyositis, necrotizing fasciitis and Fournier gangrene. Pyomyositis, usually associated with infection by *S. aureus*, occurs in muscles that have undergone trauma, especially when associated with hematoma formation.

Necrotizing fasciitis

Necrotizing fasciitis is a deep-seated life-threatening infection of subcutaneous tissue. Progressive destruction of fascia, fat and muscle ensues. Although relatively uncommon, necrotizing fasciitis is a life-threatening condition. Necrotising fasciitis and Fournier gangrene (a form of necrotizing fasciitis involving the perineum), as well as other necrotizing soft tissue infections resulting from a variety of organisms, all have reported associations with diabetes. Diabetes is the most common of a number of conditions predisposing to necrotizing fasciitis, all of which are associated with compromise to the immune system.

As its name indicates, necrotizing fasciitis spreads initially along fascial planes; however, as infection and inflammation progress, necrosis of muscle, subcutaneous tissues and overlying skin occurs. Necrotizing fasciitis usually follows identifiable episodes of trauma such as burns, insect bites or abrasions, or can result from exposure of non-intact skin to a source of infection. The most common sites are the limbs, abdominal wall and perineum. Involvement of the vulva in women with diabetes may begin as a Bartholin gland ductal abscess, usually associated with obesity [103].

Polymicrobial infection is most commonly observed, with streptococci and Enterobacteriaceae being the most common isolates. The great majority of cases result from infection with anaerobes together with one or more facultative aerobes, whereas about 10% are associated with GAS, with or without *S. aureus*. Thus, GAS is the most common cause of infection by a single organism and can also occur in combination with staphylococci, including CA-MRSA. A recent article describing necrotizing fasciitis caused by CA-MRSA showed that although current or past intravenous drug abuse underlay 43% of patients, 21% occurred in people with diabetes [104].

Vibrio, *Aeromonas*, *Haemophilus* and *Salmonella* infections have also been reported. An interesting example is infection by halophilic marine *Vibrios* either following exposure of non-intact skin to seawater [105] or following bites by marine organisms, such as crabs, and this should be considered when a history of appropriate exposure is present.

Necrotizing fasciitis carries a high mortality, particularly when affecting the lower extremities or perineum, and is rapidly fatal unless diagnosed promptly and treated aggressively. It may be initially misdiagnosed as a benign soft tissue infection and a high index of suspicion is therefore required. Skin changes may be minimal in the early phase of infection.

Early disease may be characterized by severe local pain, which is either disproportionate to or precedes other clinical features such as local inflammation and cellulitis, fever and systemic toxicity. Cellulitis may spread rapidly, unseen in deeper fascial planes. Crepitus is present in about half of cases. Violaceous discoloration of the skin may be noticed and may progress into blistering and bullae. Thrombosis and vasculitis each contribute to necrosis of the superficial fascia and suppuration from liquefactive necrosis. Gangrene and ulceration can result. Anesthesia of overlying skin may indicate destruction of subcutaneous nerves.

Plain radiographs, ultrasound, CT and MRI scan can each assist in both diagnosis and management by identifying the presence of gas in the tissues and by delineating the extent of the disease. Aerobic and anaerobic cultures should be taken from within the lesion, as should blood cultures.

Surgical débridement and fasciotomy are the mainstays of therapy. The single most important issue influencing mortality is time to surgical débridement. Thus, timely diagnosis, empirical broad-spectrum antibiotic therapy (including anaerobic cover) and aggressive surgical débridement of affected tissue are crucial components of management. The antibiotic cover can subsequently be tailored according to culture and sensitivity results. Additional supportive therapy in an intensive care environment should be provided where possible and as necessary.

Fournier gangrene

Fournier gangrene is a specific form of necrotizing fasciitis involving the perineum, scrotum and penis. Overall mortality is very high. As with other forms of necrotizing fasciitis, diabetes is the most common of a number of potential predisposing conditions with a reported presence ranging 32–60% of cases [106,107]. Infection is usually polymicrobial with a lengthy list of potential pathogens which is similar to that seen in other forms of necrotizing fasciitis (*E. coli*, *Bacteroides* spp, staphylococci, streptococci, *Proteus* spp, *Pseudomonas* spp, enterococci). *C. perfringens* is present in the great majority (>90%) of cases in which myonecrosis is present.

Initial malaise and scrotal discomfort or pain is followed by systemic toxicity. Blistering ulceration and necrosis of the skin occur and in the later stages progress to scrotal swelling and a foul purulent discharge. Crepitus may be present. Sources of infection include abnormalities of the urogenital system (most notably urethral trauma, instrumentation or a chronic indwelling catheter, scrotal abscess or injury, insect bite) and local gastrointestinal abnormalities (e.g. ischiorectal or perianal abscess, incarcerated inguinal hernia).

Diagnosis is predominantly clinical. Radiologic imaging techniques may reveal subcutaneous gas and delineate the extent of involvement, as with other forms of necrotizing fasciitis.

Fournier gangrene is a surgical emergency, and extensive débridement is required. Urinary or faecal diversion may be required, as may laparotomy. Broad-spectrum antibiotic therapies with anaerobic cover, as well as general supportive measures are indicated as with other forms of necrotizing fasciitis. The results of microbiologic investigation may allow subsequent tailoring of antibiotics.

Infected diabetic foot

Foot infection is the most common soft tissue infection associated with diabetes and therefore is a topic of the utmost importance to all who deal with people with diabetes. Detailed coverage of this topic is provided in Chapter 44. In order to avoid duplication, the topic receives only brief discussion in this chapter.

Disease-related peripheral neuropathy and peripheral vascular disease are both important in the etiology of foot infections, although the clinical presentations of the "predominantly ischemic" and the "predominantly neuropathic" foot differ. Serious complications include osteomyelitis, amputation, or even death. Infection often begins after minor trauma, which may be unnoticed, especially in the presence of sensory neuropathy. Cellulitis, soft tissue necrosis and extension into bone, leading to osteomyelitis, may then follow. Involved organisms most commonly include GAS and *S. aureus*, as well as aerobic Gram-positive cocci, Gram-negative rods and anaerobes.

The mainstays of management include exploration and débridement of the necrotic tissue and administration of appropriate antibiotics. In moderate to severe cellulitis or in the presence of osteomyelitis that places the limb at risk, the patient should be hospitalized for broad-spectrum antibiotic therapy and surgical intervention.

As in most diabetes-related infections, poor glycemic control plays an important part, and foot infections remain a common presenting feature of newly diagnosed diabetes, particularly in less developed parts of the world. Prevention of foot ulcers involves a multidisciplinary team approach. Foot care is an essential component of all diabetes education programs and should include proper foot care habits, protective footwear and pressure reduction.

Bone and joint infections

Bone and joint infections remain a significant problem for people with diabetes and can be very difficult to treat. Diabetes is a risk factor for both osteomyelitis and septic arthritis.

The different types of osteomyelitis require differing medical and surgical therapeutic strategies. The three main types, classified according to etiology, include osteomyelitis secondary to a contiguous focus of infection (e.g. after trauma, surgery or insertion of a joint prosthesis); osteomyelitis secondary to vascular insufficiency (e.g. diabetic foot infections); or osteomyelitis secondary to hematogenous spread of infection. The most common reason for septic arthritis is following insertion of joint prostheses. All are more common in people with diabetes, with osteomyelitis of the foot at the forefront. Taking, as an example, osteomyelitis of the spine, then a recurring theme occurs with a combination of both increased risk of hematogenous vertebral osteomyelitis (two- to sixfold) and predisposition to infection involving unusual organisms [108]. Acute osteomyelitis can respond to antibiotics alone but prolonged courses are required for bone and joint infections given the physiologic and anatomical characteristics of the tissues involved. Early diagnosis, together with bone sampling for microbiologic and pathologic examination to allow targeted and long-lasting antimicrobial therapy, allows the best outcomes. As with the diabetic foot, a multidisciplinary approach is required for success, including expertise in orthopedic surgery and infectious diseases, together with vascular surgery. Surgical intervention should be considered if medical treatment fails, for diagnostic confirmation or in the presence of complications.

Chronic osteomyelitis may be associated with avascular necrosis of bone and formation of sequestrum (dead bone), and surgical débridement is then necessary for cure in addition to antibiotic therapy. It is important to remember the possibility of infection by *M. tuberculosis* [109].

Iatrogenic and surgical site infections

Insulin injections

Infections at the site of insulin injections are very uncommon and remain so even when traditional hygienic practices are not applied. Although not advised, administration of insulin through clothing is also not associated with increased risk of infection. Abscesses at needle sites are occasionally seen in individuals receiving subcutaneous insulin infusions [110]. Likewise, pulp infection over the distal phalanges in association with self blood glucose monitoring is exceedingly unusual.

Surgical site infections

An association between diabetes and an increased risk of surgical site infections has been known to exist for many years. Most of the studies addressing this question have focused on the risk of postoperative infection following coronary artery bypass grafting (CABG). The association has been generally assumed to be causally related to the deleterious effect of hyperglycemia on immune function [111].

Three studies support an increased risk of postoperative infection associated with postoperative hyperglycemia among those with diabetes undergoing CABG [112–114]; however, whether or not hyperglycemia imposes an independent risk for infection remains controversial. In none of the studies was mortality increased and, in one, postoperative hyperglycemia was correlated with a higher risk of infection while an elevated HbA_{1c} was not. The studies do demonstrate, however, that improved glucose control during the operative and perioperative period can reduce the risk of postoperative infections in people with diabetes undergoing cardiac surgery. One retrospective study of 1574 patients undergoing CABG at a single institution found no increase in mortality or rates of infection among those with higher postoperative glucose levels and 34.6% of patients in this series had a diagnosis of diabetes. Nevertheless, increased glucose concentrations were associated with increased hospital charges and a longer postoperative stay.

Both allograft rejection and risk for infection appear to be higher in transplant recipients with diabetes. In one study, the risk of serious infection was higher in diabetic heart transplant recipients in the early postoperative period [115]. In another study, renal transplant recipients had a greater risk of both acute allograft rejection and infection when perioperative glycemic control was poor [116].

Dialysis

Ambulatory peritoneal dialysis is a common form of treatment for end-stage renal disease in people with diabetes. For patients receiving continuous ambulatory peritoneal dialysis (CAPD), episodes of catheter-related peritonitis are common, although variable from patient to patient, with some developing multiple episodes. Overall, however, the rate of infection does not appear to be greater in patients with diabetes than patients without diabetes, perhaps reflecting impairment of immunity associated with end-stage renal disease per se.

The issue of peritonitis in patients receiving CAPD is an important one given the large number of people with diabetes receiving this treatment. It is well recognized that peritonitis, despite significant reductions in the last two decades, remains the most important complication of CAPD with an overall mortality of about 3.5%, irrespective of both the underlying cause of the infection and of the renal failure [117]. The degree to which the presence of diabetes adds to the already considerable infection risk remains uncertain. People with diabetes may, however, be generally more unwell and have additional factors and complications such as macrovascular disease, need for hospitalization and predilection to certain infections, such as candidiasis. All of these may, in principle, contribute to the already very considerable risk.

Principles of treatment, prevention and general care

General principles

A high level of awareness is required in people with diabetes and in all health care providers, both to allow prevention and early, prompt recognition and diagnosis. Education, good glycemic control and general measures to maintain health and nutrition are all important measures aimed at minimizing risk. Careful attention to foot care is particularly emphasized. Vigilant measures should be instituted to prevent infection in patients with diabetes. When infections do occur, evolving antibiotic resistance patterns and other local factors must be considered, with CA-MRSA and tuberculosis both providing obvious examples of the importance of this.

The choice of antibiotic therapy follows the same general principles as for any other individual. Use of empirical broad-spectrum antibiotics is generally recommended until microbiologic results can guide treatment. Due caution should be applied in the presence of diabetic complications. For example, the use of potentially nephrotoxic agents in the context of diabetic nephropathy may aggravate renal dysfunction, and in turn impaired renal function requires caution with doses and monitoring of blood levels. The presence of gastroparesis or autonomic neuropathy may hinder, or render unreliable, the absorption of oral drugs. Patients who are blind or partially sighted as a result of eye complications may also be at increased risk, for example when exposed to drugs that impair hearing or balance. Longer courses of antibiotic therapy may be appropriate, for instance in treating UTI.

Antiviral agents are recommended in the setting of influenza, and a more aggressive treatment approach may be appropriate even when presentation is relatively late [62]. Responses to treatment should also be carefully monitored (e.g. in the case of tuberculosis) [70]. The importance of appropriate referral to surgical or other specialist colleagues has been stressed repeatedly. Examples include surgical débridement in the case of necrotizing fasciitis, and incision and drainage of abscesses.

People with diabetes generally have a normal response to vaccines and should receive immunizations according to established guidelines. None of the vaccines currently available are contraindicated on the basis of diabetes alone. Because of increased susceptibility to complications, routine immunization against pneumococcus and influenza is recommended, particularly for the elderly patient with diabetes or for those with additional co-morbidity such as chronic respiratory disease. Influenza vaccination has been shown to reduce hospital admissions significantly during influenza outbreaks [118]. Hepatitis B vaccination is also important although some populations may require additional or booster doses over and above standard recommended regimens.

Glycemic control

All physicians need to be aware of the importance of careful monitoring of diabetic control in the presence of infection and should be on guard against destabilization of control or development of complications. Interestingly, in people without diabetes following hospitalization, even mild degrees of hyperglycemia are associated with increased mortality in association with severe illness. Although depressed immune function correlates somewhat variably with traditional measures of glycemic control, there is sufficient evidence to indicate an inverse relationship between the two which is potentially reversible. Previously undiagnosed diabetes may also be first detected following hospitalization and then needs to be distinguished from hospital-related hyperglycemia which later reverts to normal.

Patients with T1DM or others receiving insulin need to be aware of the probability of changing insulin requirements in response to infection and to the risk of severe consequences such as diabetic ketoacidosis. Many patients with T2DM, who are not on insulin, need to be transferred temporarily to insulin therapy as the stress of illness frequently adversely affects glycemic control. Hospital admission is mandatory if severe destabilization of glycemic control occurs, or if symptoms such as nausea and vomiting interfere significantly with oral food intake. In this situation, intravenous insulin-glucose regimens are recommended. While good glycemic control is important, it is also important to avoid hypoglycemia. Interaction between the diabetes care team and other involved specialists should be initiated as early as possible.

The importance of perioperative glycemic control in patients with diabetes undergoing surgery also needs to be emphasized in order to minimize negative impacts upon postoperative infection rates and wound healing (see Chapter 32).

Attention to other risk factors (e.g. neurologic and vascular complications) is also important in order to minimize the risk of infections and infection-related complications. The importance of the presence of microangiopathy and neuropathy in the risk of the more severe forms of infection is again emphasized.

For more detailed description of these aspects of care, readers are referred to clinical practice recommendations, for example those of the American Diabetes Association [119] or to other national or international guidelines, as well as to other relevant chapters in this book.

Awareness among physicians needs to be high, especially with regard to the unusual and severe forms of infection that may occur. The general approach to antibiotic treatment is the same as for patients without diabetes, but details may differ (e.g. doses and duration of therapy). Responses to vaccination are generally normal, and influenza and pneumococcal vaccination is recommended. Careful attention to glycemic control and to other underlying factors is essential.

References

1 Muller L, Gorter KJ, Hak E, Goudzwaard WL, Schellevis FG, Hoepelman AI, *et al.* Increased risk of common infections in patients with type 1 and type 2 diabetes mellitus. *Clin Infect Dis* 2005; **41**:281–288.

2 Shah BR, Hux JE. Quantifying the risk of infectious diseases for people with diabetes. *Diabetes Care* 2003; **26**:510–513.

3 Laupland KB, Gregson DB, Zygun DA, Doig CJ, Mortis G, Church DL. Severe bloodstream infections: a population-based assessment. *Crit Care Med* 2004; **32**:992–997.

4 Bertoni AG, Saydah S, Brancati FL. Diabetes and the risk of infection-related mortality in the United States. *Diabetes Care* 2001; **24**:1044–1049.

5 Kornum JB, Thomsen RW, Riis A, Lerving HH, Schonheyder HC, Sorensen HT. Type 2 diabetes and pneumonia outcomes: a population-based cohort study. *Diabetes Care* 2007; **30**:2251–2257.

6 Booth CM, Matukas LM, Tomlinson GA, Rachlis AR, Rose DB, Dwosh HA, *et al.* Clinical features and short-term outcomes of 144 patients with SARS in the Greater Toronto Area. *JAMA* 2003; **289**:2861–2863.

7 Geerlings SE, Hoepelman AIM. Immune dysfunction in patients with diabetes mellitus (DM). *FEMS Immunol Medical Microbiol* 1999; **26**:259–265.

8 Lederman MM, Schifman GA, Rodman, HM. Pneumococcal immunization in adults. *Diabetes* 1981; **30**:119–121.

9 Beam T, Crigler ED, Goldman, JR, Schifmann G. Antibody response to polyvalent pneumococcal polysaccharide vaccine in diabetics. *JAMA* 1980; **244**:2641–2644.

10 Delamaire M, Maugendre D, Moreno M, Le Goff MC, Allannic H, Genetet B. Impaired leucocyte functions in diabetic patients. *Diabet Med* 1997; **14**:29–34.

11 Llorente L, De La Fuente H, Richaud-Patin Y, Alvarado-De La Barrera C, Diaz-Borjón A, López-Ponce A, *et al.* Innate immune response mechanisms in non-insulin dependent diabetes mellitus patients assessed by flow cytoenzymology. *Immunol Lett* 2000; **74**:239–244.

12 Hostetter MK. Handicaps to host defense: effects of hyperglycemia on C3 and *Candida albicans*. *Diabetes* 1990; **39**:271–275.

13 Katz S, Klein B, Elian I, Fishman P, Djaldetti M. Phagocytotic activity of monocytes from diabetic patients. *Diabetes Care* 1983; **6**:479–482.

14 Park S, Rich J, Hanses F, Lee JC. Defects in innate immunity predispose *db/db* mice to infection by *Staphylococcus aureus*. *Infect Immun* 2009; **77**:1008–1014.

15 Zykova SN, Jenssen TG, Berdal M, Olsen R, Myklebust R, Sljelid R. Altered cytokine and nitric oxide secretion *in vitro* by macrophages from diabetic type II-like db/db mice. *Diabetes* 2000; **49**:1451–1458.

16 Offenbacher S, Salvi GE. Induction of prostaglandin release from macrophages by bacterial endotoxin. *Clin Infect Dis* 1999; **28**:505–513.

17 Geerlings SE, Hoepelman AL. Immune dysfunction in patients with diabetes mellitus (DM). *FEMS Immunol Med Microbiol* 1999; **26**:259–265.

18 Amano H, Yamamoto H, Senba M, Oishi K, Suzuki S, Fukushima K, *et al.* Impairment of endotoxin-induced macrophage inflammatory protein 2 gene expression in alveolar macrophages in streptozotocin-induced diabetes in mice. *Infect Immun* 2000; **68**:2925–2929.

19 Mazade MA, Edwards MS. Impairment of type III group B streptococcus-stimulated superoxide production and opsonophagocytosis by neutrophils in diabetes. *Mol Genet Metab* 2001; **73**:259–267.

20 Al-Mashat HA, Kandru S, Liu R, Behl Y, Desta T, Graves DT. Diabetes enhances mRNA levels of proapoptotic genes and caspase activity, which contribute to impaired healing. *Diabetes* 2006; **55**:487–495.

21 Li YM. Glycation ligation binding motif in lactoferrin: implications in diabetic infection. *Adv Exp Med Biol* 1998; **443**:57–63.

22 Falagas ME, Kompoti M. Obesity and infection. *Lancet Infect Dis* 2006; **6**:438–446.

23 Ferguson BJ. Mucormycosis of the nose and paranasal sinuses. *Otolaryngol Clin North Am* 2000; **33**:349–365.

24 Tsay WR, Siu LK, Fung CP, Chang FY. Characteristics of bacteraemia between community-acquired and nosocomial *Klebsiella pneumoniae* infection: risk factor for mortality and the impact of capsular serotypes as a herald for community-acquired infection. *Arch Intern Med* 2002; **162**:1021–1027.

25 Yinnon AM, Butnaru A, Raveh D, Jerassy Z, Rudensky B. *Klebsiella* bacteraemia: community versus nosocomial infection. *Q J Med* 1996; **89**:933–941.

26 Lee KH, Hui KP, Tan WC, Lim TK. *Klebsiella* bacteremia: a report of 101 cases from National University Hospital, Singapore. *J Hosp Infect* 1994; **27**:299–305.

27 Chung DR, Lee SS, Lee HR, Kim HB, Choi HJ, Eom JS, *et al.* Emerging invasive liver abscess caused by K1 serotype *Klebsiella* pneumoniae in Korea. *J Infect* 2007; **54**:578–583.

28 Chanchamroen S, Kewcharoenwong C, Susaengrat W, Ato M, Lertmemongkolchai G. Human polymorphonuclear neutrophil responses to *Burkholderia pseudomallei* in healthy and diabetic subjects. *Infect Immun* 2009; **77**:456–463.

29 Van der Werf N, Kroese FGM, Rozing J, Hillebrands JL. Viral infections as potential triggers of type 1 diabetes. *Diabetes Metab Res Rev* 2007; **23**:169–183.

30 Akatsuka H, Yano EC, Gabazza J, Morser J, Sasaki R, Suzuki T, *et al.* A case of fulminant type 1 diabetes with coxsackie B4 virus infection diagnosed by elevated serum levels of neutralizing antibody. *Diab Res Clin Pract* 2009; **84**:e50–e52.

31 Wills-Karp M, Santeliz J, Karp CL. The germless theory of allergic disease: revisiting the hygiene hypothesis. *Nat Rev Immunol* 2001; **1**:69–74.

32 Ling P, Bistrian B, Mendez B, Istfan NW. Effects of systemic infusion of endotoxin, tumour necrosis factor and interleukin-1 on glucose metabolism in the rat: relationship to endogenous glucose metabolism and peripheral tissue glucose uptake. *Metabolism* 1994; **43**:279–284.

33 Mason AL, Lau JY, Hoang N, Qian K, Alexander GJ, Xu L, *et al.* Association of diabetes mellitus and chronic hepatitis C virus infection. *Hepatology* 1999; **29**:328–333.

34 Grimbert S, Valensi P, Lévy-Marchal C, Perret G, Richardet JP, Raffoux C, *et al.* High prevalence of diabetes mellitus in patients with chronic hepatitis C: a case–control study. *Gastroenterol Clin Biol* 1996; **20**:544–548.

35 Knobler H, Stagnaro-Green A, Wallenstein S, Schwartz M, Roman SH. Higher incidence of diabetes in liver transplant recipients with hepatitis C. *J Clin Gastroenterol* 1998; **26**:30–33.

36 Ozyilkan E, Arslan M. Increased prevalence of diabetes mellitus in patients with chronic hepatitis C virus infection. *Am J Gastroenterol* 1996; **91**:1480–1481.

37 Simo R, Hernandez C, Genesca J, Jardi R, Mesa J. High prevalence of hepatitis C virus infection in diabetic patients. *Diabetes Care* 1996; **19**:998–1000.

38 Caronia S, Taylor K, Pagliaro L, Carr C, Palazzo U, Petrik J, *et al.* Further evidence for an association between non-insulin dependent diabetes mellitus and chronic hepatitis C virus infection. *Hepatology* 1999; **30**:1059–1063.

39 Mehta SH, Brancati FL, Sulkowski MS, Steffanie A, Strathdee MS, Thomas DL. Prevalence of type 2 diabetes mellitus among persons with hepatitis C virus infection in the United States. *Ann Intern Med* 2000; **133**:592–599.

40 Knobler H, Schattner A. TNF-α, chronic hepatitis C and diabetes: a novel triad. *Q J Med* 2005; **98**:1–6.

41 Howard AA, Klein RS, Schoenbaum EE. Association of hepatitis C infection and antiretroviral use with diabetes mellitus in drug users. *Clin Infect Dis* 2003; **36**:1318–1323.

42 Samaras K. Prevalence and pathogenesis of diabetes mellitus in HIV-1 infection treated with combined antiretroviral therapy. *J Acquir Immune Defic Syndr* 2009; **50**:499–505.

43 Tebas P. Insulin resistance and diabetes mellitus associated with antiretroviral use in HIV-infected patients: pathogenesis, prevention, and treatment options. *J Acquir Immune Defic Syndr* 2008; **49**(Suppl 2):S86–S92.

44 Wand H, Calmy A, Carey DL, Samaras K, Carr A, Law MG, *et al.* Metabolic syndrome, cardiovascular disease and type 2 diabetes mellitus after initiation of antiretroviral therapy in HIV infection. *AIDS* 2007; **21**:2445–2453.

45 Samaras K, Wand H, Law M, Emery S, Cooper D, Carr A. Prevalence of metabolic syndrome in HIV-infected patients receiving highly active antiretroviral therapy using International Diabetes Foundation and Adult Treatment Panel III criteria: associations with insulin resistance, disturbed body fat compartmentalization, elevated C-reactive protein, and [corrected] hypoadiponectinemia. *Diabetes Care* 2007; **30**:113–119.

46 Ledergerber B, Furrer H, Rickenbach M, Lehmann R, Elzi L, Hirschel B, *et al.* Factors associated with the incidence of type 2 diabetes mellitus in HIV-infected participants in the Swiss HIV Cohort Study. *Clin Infect Dis* 2007; **45**:111–119.

47 Wohl DA, McComsey G, Tebas P, Brown TT, Glesby MJ, Reeds D, *et al.* Current concepts in the diagnosis and management of metabolic complications of HIV infection and its therapy. *Clin Infect Dis* 2006; **43**:645–653.

48 Lundgren JD, Battegay M, Behrens G, *et al.*; EACS Executive Committee). European AIDS Clinical Society (EACS) guidelines on the prevention and management of metabolic diseases in HIV. *HIV Med* 2008; **9**:72–81.

49 Schambelan M, Benson CA, Carr A, Currier JS, Dubé MP, Gerber JG, *et al.* Management of metabolic complications associated with antiretroviral therapy for HIV-1 infection: recommendations of an International AIDS Society-USA panel. *J Acquir Immune Defic Syndr* 2002; **31**:257–275.

50 Papatheodoridis GV, Chrysanthos N, Savvas S, Sevastianos V, Kafiri G, Petraki K, *et al.* Diabetes mellitus in chronic hepatitis B and C: prevalence and potential association with the extent of liver fibrosis. *J Viral Hepat* 2006; **13**:303–310.

51 Cheng AY, Kong AP, Wong VW, So WY, Chan HL, Ho CS, *et al.* Chronic hepatitis B viral infection independently predicts renal outcome in type 2 diabetic patients. *Diabetologia* 2006; **49**: 1777–1784.

52 Chandler JR. Malignant external otitis. *Laryngoscope* 1968; **78**: 1257–1294.

53 Grandis JR, Branstetter IV BF, Yu VL. The changing face of malignant (necrotising) external otitis: clinical, radiological, and anatomic correlations *Lancet Infect Dis* 2004; **4**:34–39.

54 Lee FYW, Mossad SB, Adal KA. Pulmonary mucormycosis: the last 30 years. *Arch Intern Med* 1999; **59**:1301–1307.

55 Roden MM, Zaoutis TE, Buchana WL, Knudsen TA, Sarkisova TA, Walsh TJ. Epidemiology and outcome of zygomycosis: a review of 929 reported cases. *Clin Infect Dis* 2005; **41**:634–653.

56 Ghadiali MT, Deckard NA, Farooq U, Astor F, Robinson P, Casiano RR. Frozen-section biopsy analysis for acute invasive fungal rhinosinusitis. *Otolarngology* 2007; **136**:714–719.

57 Walmsley RS, David DB, Allan RN, Kirkby GR. Bilateral endogenous *Escherichia coli* endophthalmitis: a devastating complication in an insulin-dependent diabetic. *Postgrad Med J* 1996; **72**: 361–363.

58 Karacal H, Kymes SM, Apte RS. Retrospective analysis of etiopathogenesis of all cases of endophthalmitis at a large tertiary referral center. *Int Ophthalmol* 2007; **27**:251–259.

59 Oliver RC, Tervonen T. Periodontitis and tooth loss: comparing diabetics with the general population. *J Am Dent Assoc* 1993; **124**:71–76.

60 Ljubic S, Balachandran A, Pavlic-Renar I. Pulmonary infections in diabetes mellitus. *Diabetol Croat* 2005; **4**:115–124.

61 Marrie TJ. Bacteraemic pneumococcal pneumonia: a continuously evolving disease. *J Infect* 1992; **24**:247–255.

62 Lee N, Chan PK, Hui DC, Rainer TH, Wong E, Choi KW, *et al.* Viral loads and duration of viral shedding in adult patients hospitalized with influenza. *J Infect Dis* 2009; **200**:492–500.

63 Lipsky BA, Pecoraro RE, Chen MS, Koepsell TD. Factors affecting staphylococcal colonization among NIDDM outpatients. *Diabetes Care* 1987; **10**:483–486.

64 Valdez R, Narayan KM, Geiss LS, Engelgau MM. Impact of diabetes mellitus on mortality associated with pneumonia and influenza among non-Hispanic black and white US adults. *Am J Public Health* 1999; **89**:1715–1721.

65 Cheu KY, Hsueh PR, Liaw YS, Yang PC, Luh K. A 10 year experience with bacteriology of acute thoracic empyema. *Chest* 2000; **117**:1685–1689.

66 Jeon CY, Murray MB. Diabetes mellitus increases the risk of active tuberculosis: a systematic review of 13 observational studies. *PLoS Medicine* 2008;**5**; e152: doi:10.1371/journal.pmed.0050152.

67 Stevenson CR, Forouhi NG, Roglic G, Williams BG, Lauer JA, Dye C, *et al.* Diabetes and tuberculosis: the impact of the diabetes epidemic on tuberculosis incidence. *BMC Public Health* 2007; **7**:234.

68 Corbett EL, Watt CJ, Walker N, Maher D, Williams BG, Raviglione MC, *et al.* The growing burden of tuberculosis: global trends and interactions with the HIV epidemic. *Arch Intern Med* 2003; **163**:1009–1021.

69 Wang JY, Lee LN, Hsueh PR. Factors changing the manifestation of pulmonary tuberculosis. *Int J Tuberc Lung Dis* 2005; **9**:777–783.

70 Alisjahbana B, Sahiratmadja E, Nelwan EJ, Purwa AM, Ahmad Y, Ottenhoff TH, *et al.* The effect of type 2 diabetes on presentation and treatment response of pulmonary tuberculosis. *Clin Infect Dis* 2007; **45**:428–435.

71 Nijland HM, Ruslami R, Stalenhoef JE, Nelwan EJ, Alisjahbana B, Nelwan RH, *et al.* Exposure to rifampicin is strongly reduced in patients with tuberculosis and type 2 diabetes. *Clin Infect Dis* 2006; **43**:848–854.

72 Harding GM, Zhanel GG, Nicolle L, Cheung M. Antimicrobial treatment in diabetic women with asymptomatic bacteriuria. *N Engl J Med* 2002; **347**:1576–1583.

73 Stapleton A. Urinary tract infections in patients with diabetes. *Am J Med* 2002; **113**:80S–84S.

74 Geerlings SE, Stolk RP, Camps MJL, Netten PM, Collet JT, Schneeberger PM, *et al.* Consequences of asymptomatic bacteriuria in women with diabetes mellitus. *Arch Intern Med* 2001; **161**:1421–1427.

75 Hu KK, Boyko EJ, Scholes D, Normand E, Normand E, Chen CL, Grafton J, *et al.* Risk factors for urinary tract infections in postmenopausal women. *Arch Intern Med* 2004; **164**:989–993.

76 Scholes D, Hooton TM, Roberts PL, Gupta K, Stapleton AE, Stamm WE. Risk factors associated with acute pyelonephritis in healthy women. *Ann Intern Med* 2005; **142**:20–27.

77 Efstathiou SP, Pefanis AV, Tsioulos DL, Zacharos ID, Tsiakou AG, Mitromaras AG, *et al.* Acute pelonephritis in aults: prediction of mortality and failure of treatment. *Arch Intern Med* 2003; **163**:1206–1212.

78 Meiland R, Geerlings SE, Hoepelman ALM. Management of bacterial urinary tract infections in adult patients with diabetes mellitus. *Drugs* 2002; **62**:1859–1868.

79 Geerlings SE, Stolk RP, Camps MJL, Netten PM, Collet TJ, Hoepelman AI; Diabetes Women Asymptomatic Bacteriuria Utrecht Study Group. Risk factors for symptomatic urinary tract infection in women with diabetes. *Diabetes Care* 2000; **23**:1737–1741.

80 Vasquez JA, Sobel JD. Fungal infections in diabetes. *Infect Dis Clin North Am* 1995; **9**:97–116.

81 Wright SW, Wrenn KD, Haynes M, Haas DW. Prevalence and risk factors for multidrug resistant uropathogens in ED patients. *Am J Emerg Med* 2000; **18**:143–146.

82 Edelstein H, Mccabe RE. Perinephric abscess: modern diagnosis and treatment in 47 cases. *Medicine (Baltimore)* 1988; **67**:118–131.

83 Grupper M, Kravtsov A, Potasman I. Emphysematous cystitis: illustrative case report and review of the literature. *Medicine* 2007; **86**:47–53.

84 Stamm WE, Hooton TM. Management of urinary tract infections in adults. *N Engl J Med* 1993; **329**:1328–1334.

85 Moutzouris DA, Michalakis K, Manetas S. Severe emphysematous pyelonephritis in a diabetic patient. *Lancet Infect Dis* 2006; **6**: 614.

86 Huang JJ, Tseng CC. Emphysematous pyelonephritis: clinicoradiological classification, management, prognosis, and pathogenesis. *Arch Intern Med* 2000; **160**:797–805.

87 Pontin AR, Barnes RD. Current management of emphysematous pyelonephritis. *Nat Rev Urol* 2009; **6**:272–279.

88 Tellez LG, Rodrigues-Montes JA, de Lis SF, Marten LG. Acute emphysematous cholecystitis: report of twenty cases. *Hepatogastroenterol* 1999; **46**:2144–2148.

89 Elsayes KM, Menias CO, Sierra L, Dillman JR, Platt JF. Gastrointestinal manifestations of diabetes mellitus: spectrum of imaging findings. *J Comput Assist Tomogr* 2009; **33**:86–89.

90 Shrestha Y, Trottier S. Images in clinical medicine: emphysematous cholecystitis. *N Engl J Med* 2007; **357**:1238.

91 Chang FY, Chou MY. Comparison of pyogenic liver abscesses caused by *Klebsiella pneumoniae* and non-*K pneumoniae* pathogens. *J Formos Med Assoc* 1995; **94**:232–237.

92 Chang FY, Chou MY, Fan RL, Shaio MF. A clinical study of *Klebsiella* liver abscess. *J Formos Med Assoc* 1988; **88**:1008–1011.

93 Wang JH, Liu YC, Lee SS, Yen MY, Chen YS, Wang JH, *et al.* Primary liver abscess due to *Klebsiella pneumoniae* in Taiwan. *Clin Infect Dis* 1998; **26**:1434–1438.

94 Kim JK, Chung DR, Wie SH, Yoo JH, Park SW. Risk factor analysis of invasive liver abscess caused by the K1 serotype *Klebsiella pneumoniae. Eur J Clin Microbiol Infect Dis* 2009; **28**:109–111.

95 Tsai FC, Huang YT, Chang LY, Wang JT. Pyogenic liver abscess as endemic disease, Taiwan. *Emerg Infect Dis* 2008; **14**:1592–1600.

96 Thomsen RW, Jepsen P, Sorensen HT. Diabetes mellitus and pyogenic liver abscess: risk and prognosis. *Clin Infect Dis* 2007; **44**:1194–1201.

97 Grau I, Vadillo M, Cisnal M, Pallares R. Bacteremic pneumococcal cellulitis compared with bacteremic cellulitis caused by *Staphylococcus aureus* and *Streptococcus pyogenes. Eur J Clin Microbiol Infect Dis* 2003; **22**:337–341.

98 Graham PL 3rd, Lin SX, Larson EL. A US population-based survey of *Staphylococcus aureus* colonization. *Ann Intern Med* 2006; **144**:318–325.

99 Fridkin SK, Hageman JC, Morrison M, *et al.*; for the Active Bacterial Core Surveillance Program of the Emerging Infections Program Network. Methicillin-resistant *Staphylococcus aureus* disease in three communities. *N Engl J Med* 2005; **352**:1436–1444.

100 Tapper-Jones LM, Aldred MJ, Walker DM, Hayes TM. Candidal infections and populations of *Candida albicans* in mouths of diabetics. *J Clin Pathol* 1981; **34**:706–711.

101 Farrer SM, Macleod CM. Staphylococcal infections in a general hospital. *Am J Hyg* 1960; **72**:38–58.

102 Cluff LE, Reynolds RC, Page DL. Staphylococcal bacteraemia: demographic, clinical and microbiological features of 185 cases. *Trans Am Clin Climatol Assoc* 1968; **79**:905–915.

103 Farley DE, Katz VL, Dotters D. Toxic shock syndrome associated with vulva necrotizing fasciitis. *Obstet Gynaecol* 1993; **82**:660–662.

104 Miller LG, Perdreau-Remington F, Rieg G, Mehdi S, Perlroth J, Bayer AS, *et al.* Necrotizing fasciitis caused by community-associated methicillin-resistant *Staphylococcus aureus* in Los Angeles. *N Engl J Med* 2005; **352**:1445–1453.

105 Howard RJ, Bennett NT. Infections caused by halophilic marine *Vibrio* bacteria. *Ann Surg* 1993; **217**:525–531.

106 Clayton MD, Fowler JE Jr, Sharifi R, Pearl RK. Causes, presentation and survival of 57 patients with necrotizing fasciitis of the male genitalia. *Surg Gynaecol Obstet* 1990:49–55.

107 Smith GL, Bunker CB, Dinneen MD. Fournier's gangrene. *Br J Urol* 1998; **81**:347–355.

108 Cunningham ME, Girardi F, Papadopoulos EC, Cammisa FP. Spinal infections in patients with compromised immune systems. *Clin Orthop Relat Res* 2006; **444**:73–82.

109 Lew DP, Waldvogel FA. Osteomyelitis. *Lancet* 2004; **364**:369–379.

110 Brink SJ, Stewart C. Insulin pump treatment in insulin-dependant diabetic children, adolescents and young adults. *JAMA* 1986; **255**:617–621.

111 Latham R, Lancaster AD, Covington JF, Pirolo JS, Thomas CS. The association of diabetes and glucose control with surgical-site infections among cardiothoracic surgery patients. *Infect Control Hosp Epidemiol* 2001; **22**:607–612.

112 Golden SH, Peart-Vigilance C, Kao WH, Brancati FL. Perioperative glycemic control and the risk of infectious complications in a cohort of adults with diabetes. *Diabetes Care* 1999; **22**:1408–1414.

113 Guvener M, Pasaoglu I, Demircin M, Oc M. Perioperative hyperglycemia is a strong correlate of postoperative infection in type II diabetic patients after coronary artery bypass grafting. *Endocr J* 2002; **49**:531–537.

114 Estrada CA, Young JA, Nifong W, Chitwood WR Jr. Outcomes and perioperative hyperglycemia in patients with or without diabetes mellitus undergoing coronary artery bypass grafting. *Ann Thorac Surg* 2003; **75**:1392–1399.

115 Marelli D, Laks H, Patel B, Kermani R, Marmureanu A, Patel J, *et al.* Heart transplantation in patients with diabetes mellitus in the current era. *J Heart Lung Transplant* 2003; **22**:1091–1097.

116 Thomas MC, Mathew TH, Russ GR, Rao MM, Moran J. Early peri-operative glycaemic control and allograft rejection in patients with diabetes mellitus: a pilot study. *Transplantation* 2001; **72**: 1321–1324.

117 Davenport A. Peritonitis remains the most important complication of peritoneal dialysis: the London, UK, peritonitis audit 2002–2003. *Perit Dial Int* 2009; **29**:297–302.

118 Colquhoun AJ, Nicholson KG, Botha JL, Raymond NT. Effectiveness of influenza vaccine in reducing hospital admissions in people with diabetes. *Epidemiol Infect* 1997; **119**:335–341.

119 American Diabetes Association. Clinical practice recommendations 2009. *Diabetes Care* 2009; **32**(Suppl.1):S13–S61.

10 Diabetes in Special Groups

51 Diabetes in Childhood

Christine Chan & Marian Rewers

Barbara Davis Center for Childhood Diabetes, School of Medicine, University of Colorado Denver, Aurora, CO, USA

Keypoints

- An estimated 700 000 children have diabetes worldwide; 100 000 new cases are diagnosed annually; the incidence has been increasing by up to 5% annually, over decades.
- Type 1a (autoimmune) diabetes mellitus (T1aDM) accounts for almost all cases in children younger than 10 years, for >90% among older children of European ancestry and for 20–70% of diabetes in children older than 10 years from other ethnic groups.
- The presence of two or more of the islet autoantibodies predicts the development of diabetes in those less than 10 years, in most cases; despite enormous research effort, prevention of T1aDM is still elusive.
- Diabetes in children is diagnosed based on polyuria, polydipsia, weight loss, fatigue and random blood glucose >200 mg/dL (11.1 mmol/L). Oral glucose tolerance testing is rarely needed.
- Diabetic ketoacidosis (DKA) in a thin dehydrated child with Kussmaul breathing, abdominal pain, vomiting and impaired neurologic status is present at diagnosis in fewer than 30% of cases in developed countries today.
- There are significant differences in management of DKA in children, compared with adults, with the primary focus on prevention of cerebral edema.
- After diagnosis, childhood diabetes is managed in the outpatient setting by a team including a pediatrician specializing in diabetes, a diabetes nurse educator, a dietitian, a pediatric social worker and/or a pediatric psychologist trained in childhood diabetes.
- In-depth initial and continuing education of parents and patients in the self-management of diabetes is the cornerstone of lowering the risk of acute and long-term complications.
- Insulin pump or basal bolus multiple daily injections are the standard of insulin therapy in children.
- Nutrition planning should be based on carbohydrate counting or exchange system; the macronutrient and micronutrient composition of the diabetic diet is similar to that for healthy children without diabetes.
- While regular exercise is recommended for all children with diabetes, it requires careful planning of insulin and nutritional management to prevent severe hypoglycemia.
- Severe hypoglycemia is largely preventable, but is still the most common serious complication of childhood diabetes.
- Health care providers should equip families with the tools necessary to avoid dehydration, uncontrolled hyperglycemia or DKA, and hypoglycemia during routine infections.
- HbA_{1c} levels below 58 mmol/mol (<7.5%) are the target currently recommended and achievable by most children and adolescents; the gap between recommended and actual HbA_{1c} levels is the widest among adolescents.
- Age-specific psychologic care should include screening for and treatment of family dysfunction, developmental maladjustments, communication problems, disordered eating and sleep patterns, as well as psychiatric disorders both in the patients and their care providers.
- All children with diabetes should be screened at an appropriate age and duration of diabetes for dyslipidemia, microalbuminuria, elevated blood pressure, retinopathy, celiac, thyroid and Addison disease.

Spectrum of diabetes in children

In Europe and North America, 1 in 300 children develops diabetes by the age of 20 years. While the rates are lower elsewhere, there are an estimated 700 000 children with diabetes worldwide and 100 000 new cases are diagnosed annually. Diabetes is a heterogeneous disease at any age. Newborn babies and infants rarely develop the disease (1 in 250 000 in those younger than 6 months) and the etiology is not autoimmune, but usually monogenic (see Chapter 15). From the age of 9 months to 10 years, almost all diabetes is caused by islet autoimmunity (see Chapter 9). Type 1a (autoimmune) diabetes mellitus (T1aDM) accounts also for more than 90% of the cases among older children of European ancestry, but in other ethnic groups 20–70% of older children may have type 2 diabetes mellitus (T2DM; Figure 51.1). With the increasing prevalence of obesity in the general population, a significant proportion of children with T1aDM present with a phenotype that masquerades for T2DM. Measurement of autoantibodies to insulin, GAD_{65}, IA-2 and ZnT8 at diagnosis, C

Textbook of Diabetes, 4th edition. Edited by R. Holt, C. Cockram, A. Flyvbjerg and B. Goldstein.

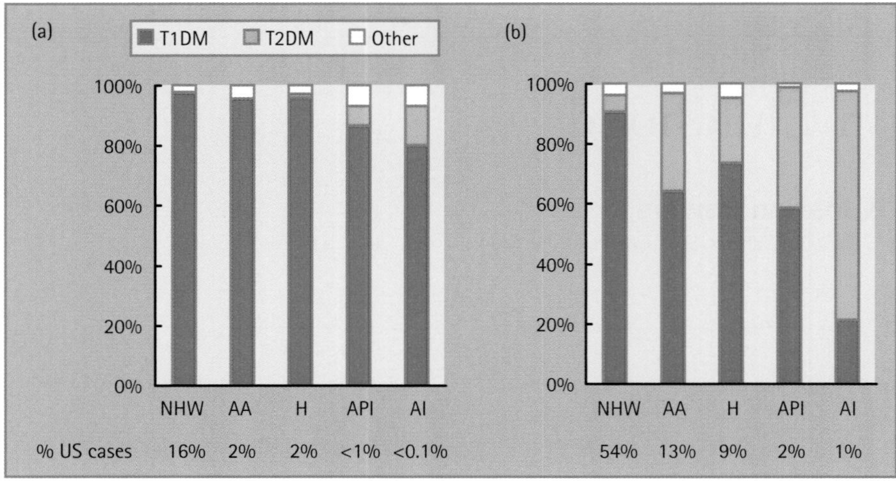

Figure 51.1 Type-specific proportions of prevalent cases of diabetes in the US population, according to age group (a, 0–9 years; b, 10–19 years) and race/ethnicity. AA, African American; AI, American Indian; API, Asian/Pacific Islander; H, Hispanic; NHW, Non-Hispanic White. Adapted from SEARCH for Diabetes in Youth Study, 2001 [30].

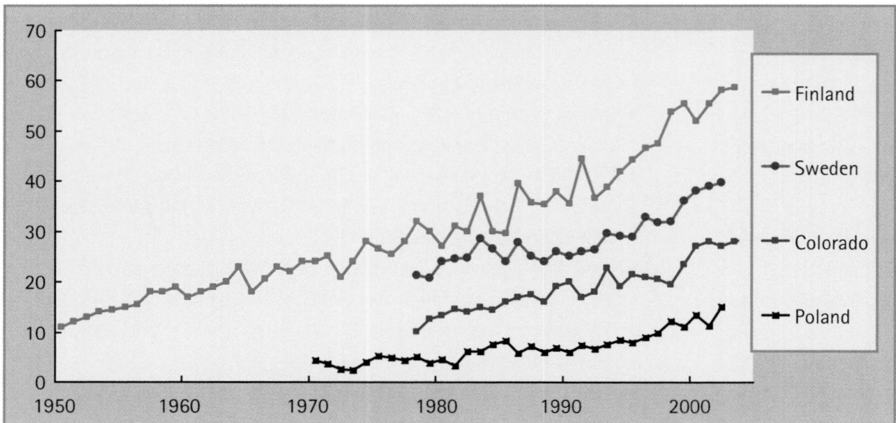

Figure 51.2 Incidence of T1DM has been rising about 3–5% per year.

peptide after the initial metabolic stabilization and HLA-DR,DQ typing may be necessary to assess appropriate long-term treatment.

This chapter focuses on the practical aspects of the management of T1aDM in children, while Chapter 52 addresses management of diabetes in adolescents and transition to adult care. For type 1b diabetes (clinical presentation as in T1aDM, but absent islet autoantibodies) and monogenic diabetes see Chapters 9b and 15, respectively. The epidemiology and etiology of diabetes are addressed in Chapters 3 and 9, respectively. Briefly, T1aDM is caused by the interplay of genetic and environmental factors. The initial step – development of islet autoimmunity marked by the presence of islet autoantibodies – is believed to be driven by one or more environmental triggers [1]. Over the past 40 years, the incidence of childhood T1DM worldwide has increased by 3–5% annually (Figure 51.2). Elimination of the environmental trigger(s) responsible for this epidemic would be the most efficient approach to primary prevention; however, there is lack of consensus about which environmental factors initiate and promote islet autoimmunity. Efforts to prevent T1DM have been recently reviewed elsewhere [2]. After the initiation of islet autoimmunity, most patients have a long preclinical period that offers an opportunity for secondary prevention of the progression to clinical diabetes. The presence of more than one of the autoantibodies combined with susceptibility HLA-DR,DQ genotypes identifies those at high-risk of developing diabetes. There may be a "point of no return" in the autoimmune destruction of the islets, rendering some interventions effective only at the earlier stages of the process. Once tolerance is broken to more than one of islet autoantigens, most individuals progress to diabetes within 10 years. A period of mild asymptomatic hyperglycemia, detectable by oral glucose tolerance testing (OGTT) [3] or HbA_{1c} [4], may precede by months or years overt insulin dependence among persons with islet autoantibodies. Intervention at this "dysglycemic" stage may also theoretically preserve endogenous insulin secretion and prevent the acute and long-term complications of T1DM. Preservation or regaining of residual insulin secretion after diagnosis of diabetes might also help, but the immunomodulatory agents used so far in tertiary prevention may carry unacceptable long-term risks.

Manifestation, diagnosis and initial treatment

Clinical presentation and diagnosis

The cardinal symptoms at the diagnosis of diabetes include polyuria (96% of children, often with nocturia or bed-wetting), polydipsia, weight loss (61%) and fatigue [5]. The classic presentation of diabetic ketoacidosis (DKA) in a thin dehydrated child with Kussmaul breathing, abdominal pain, vomiting and impaired neurologic status affects fewer than 30% of cases presenting in developed countries today [5,6]. With the increasing community recognition of diabetes, most children present with milder hyperglycemia of shorter duration; however, 75% of the children (63% below age 5) have the symptoms for more than 2 weeks, suggesting that the diagnosis could be made earlier in many cases. A young child may have a less specific presentation, for example with vomiting or rapid breathing during the course of an infection. Diabetes should always be considered in ill children; urine or blood testing for glucose and ketones leads to an early diagnosis and may prevent DKA and hospitalization. Nearly all patients admitted with severe DKA have been seen hours or days earlier by health care providers who missed the diagnosis.

While most children do not require intravenous fluids or insulin infusion at the diagnosis of diabetes, many are hospitalized for a few days. These hospitalizations could be avoided if safe outpatient alternatives and adequate reimbursement existed for this initial care. For instance, the availability of an outpatient care center has helped to decrease hospitalization at diagnosis from 88% in 1978–1982 to 46% in 1998–2001, with the proportion of hospitalizations secondary to DKA increasing from 44% to 63% [6].

The diagnostic criteria are the same in children and adults (see Chapter 2); however, most children are quite symptomatic and do not require an extensive work-up. In a symptomatic child, plasma glucose ≥11.1 mmol/L (200 mg/dL) at any time of day, without regard to time since the last meal, or fasting plasma glucose ≥7.0 mmol/L (126 mg/dL) is diagnostic. Blood glucose results obtained using a glucose meter should be immediately confirmed in a laboratory, before the initiation of insulin treatment. By contrast, if marked hyperglycemia and blood or urinary ketones are present, treatment is urgent; waiting another day to confirm the diagnosis may be dangerous if DKA is allowed to develop. In a well child, the diagnosis must not be based on a single plasma glucose test or borderline results obtained using a glucose meter. In such cases, the authors check the HbA_{1c} level; if this is normal, further monitoring of the fasting and/or 2-hour post-prandial blood glucose is recommended for several days. In children progressing to overt diabetes, hyperglycemia after dinner is usually the initial abnormality detectable by self-monitoring of blood glucose at home. OGTT should not be performed if fasting, random or post-prandial criteria are met as it is unnecessary and excessive hyperglycemia can result.

Hyperglycemia detected incidentally or during acute infection, trauma or other illness may be transient, especially if typical symptoms of diabetes are absent or equivocal. Children with transient hyperglycemia may be more likely to develop diabetes, but the reported progression rates vary from 0 to 32%. Testing for islet autoantibodies helps to rule in diabetes in cases with mild presentation; however, it is important to consider that the quality of commercial assays for islet autoantibodies varies widely and testing for at least three autoantibodies (to insulin, GAD_{65} and IA-2) provides 80% predictive value.

Impaired glucose tolerance (IGT) and impaired fasting glucose (IFG) may also be detected in a child with islet autoimmunity progressing to overt diabetes [3]. OGTT is rarely needed in prepubertal children, however, except to reassure the family that a metabolic decompensation is not imminent. In older children, especially obese teenagers with equivocal symptoms, the OGTT may have a role in the earlier diagnosis of T2DM, IGT and IFG.

Diabetic ketoacidosis

The clinical presentation of DKA includes abdominal pain, nausea and vomiting which can mimic an acute abdomen. The patients are mildly to moderately dehydrated (5–10%), may have Kussmaul respiration and become progressively somnolent and obtunded.

DKA results from absolute or relative deficiency of circulating insulin and a corresponding increase in the levels of counter-regulatory hormones, such as catecholamines, cortisol, glucagon and growth hormone (see Chapter 34). This combination leads to a catabolic state with increased glucose production by the liver and kidneys, increased lipolysis, ketogenesis with ketonemia and metabolic acidosis. Absolute insulin deficiency occurs in patients with previously undiagnosed T1DM or in established patients with omission of or inadequate insulin regimens. Relative insulin deficiency occurs during acute illness and stress if the increase in counter-regulatory hormones is not balanced by an appropriate increase in insulin dosage. The severity of DKA is categorized by the degree of acidosis:

- Mild: venous pH 7.2–7.3 or bicarbonate <15 mmol/L
- Moderate: venous pH 7.1–7.2 or bicarbonate <10 mmol/L
- Severe: venous pH <7.1 or bicarbonate <5 mmol/L

Diabetic ketoacidosis at diagnosis of diabetes

In the USA, patients younger than 20 years with a clinical diagnosis of T1DM and T2DM presented in DKA in 29% and 10% of the cases, respectively [6]. In Europe, the rates for T1DM cases ranged 15–67% correlating inversely with the local incidence of T1DM [7]. DKA is more often found among younger children and in children with lower socioeconomic status who encounter barriers in accessing medical care [6]. Intensive community intervention to raise awareness of the signs and symptoms of childhood diabetes among school teachers and primary care providers may help to reduce the prevalence of DKA at diagnosis [8].

Diabetic ketoacidosis in established patients

In a large cohort of children with established T1DM, on average, eight patients per 100 developed DKA every year [9]; however, nearly 60% of the DKA episodes occurred in 5% of children with recurrent events. Recurrent DKA was predicted by poor metabolic control, previous episodes of DKA, psychiatric and eating disorders, difficult family or social circumstances or limited access to medical care.

Treatment of ketoacidosis

Hydration status should be assessed and fluid deficit and osmolality calculated to help guide fluid and electrolyte replacement. Serum electrolytes, glucose, blood urea nitrogen (BUN), creatinine, calcium, magnesium, phosphorous and blood gas testing should be repeated every 2–4 hours or more frequently in severe cases. The calculations are shown below.

$$\text{Anion gap} = \text{Na} - (\text{Cl} + \text{HCO}_3)$$

$$\text{Corrected Na} = \text{measured Na} + [(\text{plasma glucose} - 100\,\text{mg/dL})(1.6)/100]$$

$$\text{Serum osmolality} = 2(\text{Na} + \text{K}) + \text{glucose}/18 + \text{BUN}/2.8\ (\text{mOsm/L})$$

Patients with DKA have a 5–10% deficit in extracellular fluid volume which has developed slowly. Avoid rapid or overzealous fluid replacement. Initial volume expansion should occur over the first 1–2 hours with IV infusion of 10–20 mL/kg normal saline (0.9%) or Ringer solution. The bolus rarely needs to be repeated and should not exceed a total of 40 mL/kg over the first 4 hours of treatment. Subsequent fluid deficit replacement should occur over the next 48 hours using 0.5–0.75 normal saline 0.9%. Once blood glucose concentrations reach 250 mg/dL (14 mmol/L), 5–10% dextrose should be added to the IV solution to maintain the blood glucose concentration between 150 and 250 mg/dL (8–14 mmol/L) and avoid saline overload and hyperchloremic acidosis.

Continuous IV infusion of soluble human insulin at a dose of 0.1 units/kg/hour should commence after the patient has received initial volume expansion. An IV bolus of insulin is unnecessary and may increase the risk of cerebral edema [10]. The insulin infusion should allow for a gradual decrease in blood glucose concentration by 50–100 mg/dL/hour. If the blood glucose levels decrease too quickly or become too low before acidosis has resolved, IV dextrose concentration may be increased to 12.5% to prevent hypoglycemia while continuing to correct the metabolic acidosis with insulin. Unless the patient is truly hypoglycemic, the insulin infusion rate should not be decreased to less than 0.05 U/kg/hour as this is likely to prolong the time needed to suppress ketogenesis. Bedside monitoring of blood ketones (β-hydroxybutyrate) is more helpful than blood gases in adjusting insulin and glucose infusion rates.

Total body potassium is usually depleted, but serum levels at presentation may be normal or high secondary to efflux of intracellular potassium into the extracellular space in the presence of acidosis. Once the serum potassium is found to be normal or low, and urine output is confirmed, IV fluids should include 20–40 mEq/L potassium in the form of K acetate, K_2HPO_4 or a combination of these. No more than half of the potassium replacement should be given as K_2HPO_4 because excessive phosphorous administration may result in hypocalcemia following the suppression of parathyroid hormone.

Similar to serum potassium levels, serum phosphorus levels may be initially elevated only to fall rapidly during treatment of DKA. Clinical problems resulting from low phosphorus levels have not been substantiated; however, severe hypophosphatemia (<1 mg/dL) should be treated. If hypocalcemia develops, administration of phosphate should be decreased or stopped.

Severe acidosis is reversible with fluid and insulin replacement. Bicarbonate therapy may paradoxically cause CNS acidosis and hypokalemia from rapid correction of acidosis and is a risk factor for cerebral edema. Bicarbonate therapy is not recommended unless the acidosis is profound (pH <6.9) and likely to interfere adversely with the action of epinephrine during resuscitation. If bicarbonate is considered necessary, 1–2 mmol/kg can be cautiously administered over 60 minutes.

Cerebral edema

Neurologic status must be monitored at frequent and regular intervals. Subclinical cerebral edema occurs in most children with DKA. Severe clinical edema affects 0.5–1% of the children and is fatal in over 20% [10]. Typically, cerebral edema occurs at 4–12 hours, but has been reported as late as 24–28 hours after the initiation of IV fluid treatment. Potential risk factors for symptomatic cerebral edema in children include:

- More profound dehydration, hyperventilation and acidosis at presentation;
- Bicarbonate therapy;
- Excessive and rapid fluid administration, especially if initial serum osmolality is >320 mOsm/L;
- Failure of serum sodium to rise as hyperglycemia resolves; and
- Initial IV insulin bolus or too early initiation of insulin infusion.

Signs and symptoms of cerebral edema include headache, change in mental status or behavior, incontinence, focal neurologic findings, sudden normalization of heart rate in a previously tachycardic dehydrated patient or a worsening clinical course in a patient with improved laboratory values. Bradycardia, hypertension and irregular respiration (Cushing triad) are signs of greatly increased intracranial pressure. Early intervention is essential. Treatment includes administration of mannitol (1 g/kg over 30 minutes), decreasing fluid rate to 75% or less of maintenance rate, and elevation of head of bed. Mannitol therapy may need to be repeated. Intravenous hypertonic saline has also been used as an alternative to mannitol. Radiographic studies (such as head CT) should be obtained after rather than during treatment of cerebral edema.

Frequent monitoring of blood glucose levels should prevent hypoglycemia. For acute hypoglycemic episodes while on continuous insulin infusion, the insulin infusion may be temporarily discontinued for up to 15 minutes if necessary.

Transition to subcutaneous insulin regimen

Patients may be transitioned to an appropriate subcutaneous insulin regimen once DKA has resolved and they are able to eat. To prevent rebound hyperglycemia, the insulin infusion should not be discontinued until 15–30 minutes after the first subcutaneous injection of rapid-acting insulin has been administered. Long-acting insulin analogs achieve therapeutic levels able to replace insulin infusion 4–6 hours after the subcutaneous injection. Bedside monitoring of blood ketones helps to titrate insulin dose and prevent a relapse.

Pediatric ambulatory diabetes care

Diabetes is primarily managed in the outpatient setting by a team including a pediatrician specializing in diabetes, a diabetes nurse educator, a dietitian, a pediatric social worker trained in childhood diabetes and/or a pediatric psychologist with knowledge of childhood diabetes and chronic illness. In communities with low population density and low prevalence of childhood diabetes, such a care team may not be available and care will primarily be provided by the child's primary care physician. In these instances, these physicians should work closely with and have access to a regional diabetes care team.

Health care providers and the diabetes care team must always be cognizant of and sensitive to the cultural needs and barriers to care that may arise with minority children of recent immigrants. Interpreters should be utilized when needed.

Initial education

Initial education should provide a basic understanding of the pathophysiology of diabetes and its treatment to ensure that families feel confident in providing diabetes care at home (Table 51.1) [11].

At many institutions, initial education at time of diagnosis occurs in an inpatient setting regardless of whether or not the child presents acutely ill in DKA. In some centers with appropriate outpatient resources, initial diabetes education and initiation of insulin therapy can occur in the ambulatory setting which has been shown to be cost effective.

Table 51.1 Initial education curriculum.

An explanation of how the diagnosis was made and reason for symptoms
Discussion regarding normal blood glucose levels and targets, the need for immediate insulin treatment and its mechanism of action
Practical skills including how to draw up and administer insulin, blood glucose testing, blood and urine ketone testing
Basic dietary guidelines
Simple explanation of symptoms and management of hypoglycemia
Diabetes at school
Importance of medical alert identification
Psychologic adjustment to the diagnosis
Emergency telephone contacts

Continuing education

In the first 6 months following diagnosis, close contact in the form of frequent outpatient visits, home visits, telephone communication and other methods of communication is essential for addressing the frequently changing requirements during this time (Table 51.2) [11].

Diabetes education is a continuous process and must be repeated to be effective. It must be adapted and appropriate to the age of the child. Infants and toddlers often have unpredictable eating and activity patterns. There is often more difficulty in distinguishing normal behavior from mood swings related to hypoglycemia or hyperglycemia. Needle phobia can present a significant issue with the perception of pain inflicted by the caregiver. Hypoglycemia is more common in this age group and the prevention, recognition and management of hypoglycemia is a priority. School-aged children will have increased understanding and involvement with their diabetes management. Providers should address school-aged children directly in addition to speaking with their parents or care providers. Education includes monitoring of blood glucose levels and injections at school, particularly during meal times, exercise and extracurricular activities. There should be increased recognition and awareness of hypoglycemic symptoms. Education should also focus on age-appropriate stepwise handover of diabetes responsibilities. This becomes particularly important in adolescence during which there is a critical balance between promoting independent responsible management of diabetes while maintaining parental involvement.

Once established, it is common practice for children to be seen in the ambulatory setting at least every 3 months; visits should be more often if the patient does not meet the treatment goals or intensifies treatment, for example if insulin pump treatment is initiated. During these visits, overall health and well-being is assessed, growth and vital signs are monitored, and a physical

Table 51.2 Continuing education curriculum.

Insulin types, actions and adjustments based on self-monitoring of blood glucose
Monitoring and treatment goals
Mechanisms for coping with and adjusting to the diagnosis of diabetes
Nutrition, including carbohydrate counting
Management of diabetes during illness
Management of hyperglycemia and ketosis and prevention of DKA
Prevention, recognition and management of hypoglycemia
Exercise, travel and holiday planning
Microvascular and macrovascular complications of diabetes and their prevention
Up-to-date information on research in diabetes and new therapies and technologies in diabetes care
When age-appropriate, discuss diabetes and driving, smoking, alcohol, drugs, college and employment

DKA, diabetic ketoacidosis

examination is performed. There should be routine screening for diabetes-associated complications and co-morbidities. Blood glucose records, including a check of HbA_{1c}, medications and school plans are reviewed. This will allow for the insulin doses to be adjusted and provide a template for continued diabetes education.

The dietitian may review dietary habits and provide ongoing nutrition education as needed. The social worker or psychologist assesses and monitors psychosocial problems and family dynamics and the impact of diabetes care. At the conclusion of these visits, an individualized plan should be developed for each child and their family and a written copy of this plan should be provided.

The advent of new technology including downloadable glucometers, insulin pumps and continuous glucose sensors has made it increasingly possible for the diabetes care team to gain insight into home management of diabetes; however, this should not replace self-monitoring and regular review of blood glucose data at home by the patient and their family.

Diabetes management in school

Children with diabetes spend a significant portion of their day in school; therefore, diabetes management in school is a critical portion of their diabetes management plan [12]. The child has the right to receive adult support for diabetes care from school personnel during school hours, outdoor school activities and school-sponsored events away from school. School personnel must be trained to provide or supervise all diabetes care prescribed by the diabetes team and be supportive of providing diabetes care and encourage diabetes management during school hours, including:

- Insulin administration by injection or with an insulin pump;
- Testing blood glucose in young children and older, newly diagnosed children and adolescents until they are capable of performing the task independently; and
- Identification and treatment for hypoglycemia, both mild–moderate and severe.

Children with diabetes should have a school health plan in place. The health plan should include contact information for the child's family as well as their diabetes care providers. It should also contain information regarding routine management of diabetes (blood sugar monitoring, insulin administration and dosing, snack times) and an emergency plan for management of hypoglycemia and hyperglycemia. Issues specific to insulin pumps include remembering to activate insulin bolus with food, disconnecting the pump during vigorous exercise or in the event of severe hypoglycemia, pump failures and pump alarms.

Extracurricular activities are an important component of a child's school experience and children with diabetes should be allowed to participate and their needs accommodated accordingly. Field trips, field days and overnight trips often require advanced planning, but a child's diabetes should never be a cause for exclusion from any school-sanctioned activity.

Insulin treatment

The overarching goal of insulin replacement is to provide just enough insulin at an appropriate time to provide sufficient basal insulin levels as well as higher insulin levels after meals [13]. The choice of insulin regimen depends on the individual's age, duration of diabetes, dietary and activity patterns, ability to cope and metabolic targets. Patient and family preferences should also be respected.

Insulin pump therapy

Insulin pump therapy is the best way to restore the body's physiologic insulin profile. The pump delivers a variable programmed basal rate that corresponds to the diurnal variation in insulin needs. Prepubertal children require a higher basal rate in the early part of night, while post-pubertal patients who experience the "dawn phenomenon" require higher rates in the morning.

The user initiates bolus doses before meals and to correct hyperglycemia. Most pumps can receive wireless transmission of test results from glucose meters, but the patient or caregiver must still manually enter the amount of carbohydrate being consumed. The pump calculates the amount of insulin needed for a meal or correction based on previously entered variables which include: insulin : carbohydrate ratios, insulin sensitivity factor, glycemic target and duration of insulin action (set at 2–8 hours to protect from accumulating too much insulin). The user may override the suggestion or press a button to initiate the bolus.

Rapid-acting insulin analogs perform better in pumps than regular insulin, both in terms of mimicking the first-phase insulin release after meal and avoidance of post-prandial hypoglycemia. Even with the analogs, however, insulin has to be administered at least 10–15 minutes before meal to reach effective levels in time. A longer lead time may be needed if preprandial blood glucose is higher than 150 mg/dL. Young children, picky eaters and disorganized patients may struggle with these requirements. In addition, they are often unable to predict the size of the meal. In these cases, one may administer half of the usual meal bolus in advance, with the other half, if needed, after meal. Compliance problems include infrequent blood glucose testing, not reacting to elevated blood glucose, incorrect carbohydrate counting or missing the boluses altogether.

Patients and their families must be instructed on troubleshooting and treatment of hyperglycemia, particularly if ketones are present, as this may be an indication of a pump malfunction. If the flow of insulin becomes interrupted, ketonemia will develop within 4 hours; this is particularly dangerous at night as there is no long-acting insulin on board. Syringes should always be available so that insulin may be administered via injection in the event of a pump failure.

Most clinical trials have demonstrated better HbA_{1c} and less severe hypoglycemia with pump therapy, compared with multiple daily injections (MDI). Pump therapy can improve the quality of life in children who have trouble with or fear of injections or who desire greater flexibility in their lifestyle (e.g. with sleeping in, sports or irregular eating). Insulin pumps can be particularly helpful in young children or infants who have multiple meals and snacks and require multiple small doses of rapid-acting insulin. The newer generation of insulin pumps can deliver as little as 0.025 U/hour, but higher rates using diluted insulin may be needed for uninterrupted flow.

Disposable pumps are already available and much smaller "patch" pumps are in development. In the near future, one may expect a "closed-loop" system allowing the insulin pump to be directed automatically by a continuous glucose sensor with minimal human input; however, a number of issues remain to be solved, including the biocompatibility of the sensors and infusion sets, limitations of the systemic versus intraportal administration of insulin, lack of counterbalancing delivery of glucagon and optimal delivery algorithms for various meals and activities.

Currently, the most frequent complications of insulin treatment include failures of insulin delivery because of a displaced or obstructed infusion set, local skin infections and DKA. Insulin pump treatment is significantly more expensive than regimens based on injections. For some patients, pumps may be too difficult to operate or comply with the multiple testing and carbohydrate counting requirements, or may be unacceptable because of body image issues or extreme physical activity (e.g. swimming, contact sports).

Subcutaneous insulin injection regimens

Injections regimens, in order of worsening HbA_{1c} outcomes, include:

- Basal bolus regimen: 40–60% of the total daily dose as basal insulin analog (glargine, detemir) in 1–2 doses a day with rapid-acting insulin analog 10–15 minutes before each meal; soluble human insulin is less preferable and requires administration at least 20–30 minutes prior to each meal.
- Intermediate-acting human insulin twice daily and soluble human insulin 20–30 minutes prior to each meal.
- Two injections daily of a mixture of short or rapid and intermediate-acting insulin before breakfast and before the evening meal.
- Three injections using some variation of the following: a mixture of short or rapid and intermediate-acting insulin before breakfast, rapid or soluble human insulin before the afternoon snack or evening meal, and intermediate or basal/long-acting insulin before bed.

Intermediate-acting insulins such as NPH are often mixed with soluble human (regular) or rapid-acting analogs (aspart, lispro or glulisine). Patients and families should be taught how to mix the insulin properly to avoid contamination. It is generally taught to draw up clear (regular or short-acting) insulin prior before drawing up cloudy insulin (NPH). Per the manufacturer's instructions, glargine or detemir insulins should not be mixed with any other insulin.

Premixed insulins contain a mixture of regular (or rapid-acting) insulin and NPH insulin in various fixed ratios. These preparations may be useful for children who do not want to draw insulin from separate vials prior to injecting. They may also be useful in reducing the number of injections when compliance is an issue, especially among teenagers. Premixed insulins are also available for use in pen injector devices. The main disadvantage to using premixed insulin preparations is the lack of flexibility in adjusting the separate insulin doses, which is often necessary with varied food intake or during illness or exercise.

Nutrition

Nutritional management in children with diabetes remains a key component of diabetes care and education; if available, a pediatric dietitian should be a part of the diabetes care team. The management does not require a restrictive diet, just a healthy dietary regimen that the children and their families can benefit from. Current guidelines target optimal glycemic control, reduction of cardiovascular risk, psychosocial well-being and family dynamics [14,15]. A thorough dietary history should be obtained including the family's dietary habits and traditions, the child's typical meal times and patterns of food intake.

Insulin pump and MDI therapy utilize carbohydrate counting in which the grams of carbohydrate to be eaten are counted and a matching dose of insulin is administered. This plan allows for the most freedom and flexibility in food choices, but it requires expert education and commitment and may not be suitable for many families or situations (e.g. school lunches, teenagers). Exchange planning teaches that it is not necessary to count precise grams. Exchanges are taught as either 10 or 15-g servings of carbohydrate. The exchange plan can enable a more consistent daily intake of carbohydrate. The constant carbohydrate meal plan was used often in the past with insulin regimens based on NPH and regular insulin, where carbohydrate intake and the amount of insulin were kept relatively constant from day to day. It has been perceived as too restrictive and a potential source of conflict.

The use of the glycemic index has been shown to provide additional benefit to glycemic control. Low glycemic index carbohydrate foods, such as wholegrain breads, pasta, temperate fruits and dairy products may lower post-prandial hyperglycemia. A glycemic load approach to predicting the post-prandial blood glucose response, based on the glycemic index of the food and the portion size, has not been fully explored in children. Regardless of which meal plan is chosen, helpful principles are shown in Table 51.3.

Age-specific advice

Breastfeeding in infants should be encouraged. Insulin pump therapy should be considered, particularly in patients who require very small doses of insulin. Toddlers are often picky eaters and are more likely to eat frequent smaller meals throughout the day; their insulin regimen should match this eating pattern. Food

Table 51.3 Principles of dietary planning in children with diabetes.

1 Eat a well-balanced diet, with daily energy intake distributed as follows:
- Carbohydrate 50–55% (sucrose intake up to 10% total energy)
- Fat 30–35% (up to 20% monounsaturated fat; <10% polyunsaturated fat; <10% saturated fat and trans fatty acids; n-3 fatty acids 0.15 g/day)
- Protein 10–15%

2 Eat meals and snacks at the same time each day, if possible

3 Use snacks to prevent and treat hypoglycemia, but avoid overtreatment:
- Young children often have a mid or late morning snack
- Most people will have a mid or late afternoon snack
- Many children require a bedtime snack, particularly if the bedtime blood glucose is below 130 mg/dL (7 mmol/L) or if they have been active during the day

4 Gauge energy intake to maintain appropriate weight and body mass index:
- Overinsulinization, "forced" snacking and excess food intake to prevent or treat hypoglycemia promote excessive weight gain and should be avoided
- Eating disorders are common in teenagers with diabetes, particularly girls

5 Recommended fiber intake for children older than 1 year: 2.8–3.4 g/MJ; children older than 2 years should eat = (age in years + 5) g/day fiber

6 Avoid foods high in sodium that may increase the risk of hypertension; target salt intake – to less than 6 g/day (sodium chloride)

7 Avoid excessive protein intake (athletes should not require protein supplements)

8 Children with diabetes have the same vitamin and mineral requirements as other healthy children; however, hypovitaminosis D is common and screening and supplementation are recommended

9 There is no evidence of harm from an intake of artificial sweeteners in doses not exceeding acceptable daily intakes

10 Specially labeled diabetic foods are not recommended because they are not necessary, are expensive, are often high in fat and may contain sweeteners with laxative effects. These include the sugar alcohols such as sorbitol

11 While alcohol intake is generally prohibited in youth, teenagers continue to experiment with and sometimes abuse alcohol. Alcohol may induce prolonged hypoglycemia in young people with diabetes (up to 16 hours after drinking). Carbohydrate should be eaten before, during and/or after alcohol intake. It may be also necessary to lower the insulin dose, particularly if exercise is performed during or after drinking (e.g. dancing)

12 Approximately 10% of patients with type 1 diabetes have serologic evidence of celiac disease. Those with positive intestinal biopsy or symptomatic have to be treated with GFD. Products derived from wheat, rye, barley and triticale are eliminated and replaced with potato, rice, soy, tapioca, buckwheat and perhaps oats. While most of the children are asymptomatic, the long-term consequences of untreated celiac autoimmunity may warrant GFD

GFD, gluten-free diet.

refusal can be a significant source of distress, particularly if an insulin dose has already been administered. In school-aged children, meal plans may need to be adjusted depending on the school schedule. Food intake among teenagers is often chaotic. Breakfasts are skipped and binges may happen at any time of day or night. Weight loss or failure to gain weight may be associated with insulin omission for weight control and may be indicative of a disordered eating behavior. While insulin pump or MDI treatment may help some, simplification of the management plan to avoid extreme mismatches between food intake and insulin are sometimes the only viable option.

Exercise

Children with diabetes derive the same health and leisure benefits from exercise as children without diabetes and should be allowed to participate with equal opportunities and equal safety [16]. Physiologically, during exercise in children without diabetes, there is a decrease in pancreatic insulin secretion and an increase in counter-regulatory hormones resulting in an increase in liver glucose production (see Chapter 23). This matches skeletal muscle uptake of glucose during exercise, maintaining stable blood glucose concentrations under most conditions. In children with T1DM, there is no pancreatic regulation of insulin in response to exercise and there may be impaired counter-regulation. These factors combine to increase the risk of hypoglycemia and hyperglycemia during exercise. It is helpful to keep an exercise record noting the most recent insulin dose, timing and type of exercise, blood glucose levels before and after exercise, snacks eaten and the time of any episode of hypoglycemia.

Factors affecting a child's response to exercise include:
- Duration, type, timing and intensity of activity;
- Overall metabolic control and ambient blood glucose level;
- Type and timing of insulin injections and its absorption;
- Type and timing of food;
- Muscle mass and conditioning; and
- Degree of stress.

Preventing hypoglycemia

Blood glucose levels should be checked before, during and after the exercise. Children should consume carbohydrates prior to exercise, with the amount depending on the blood sugar level prior to exercise and the duration and intensity of exercise. For short duration activity, sports drinks with simple sugars provide optimal absorption and usually prevent hypoglycemia for the next 30–60 minutes. For activity of longer duration, solid foods containing carbohydrates are digested more slowly and should be consumed in addition to a liquid with simple sugars. Extra snacks should always be available to the child during exercise. The child's coaches and teammates or other responsible adult and peers should be aware of the signs and symptoms of hypoglycemia. Often, children will require adjustments to their insulin dosing when exercise is anticipated. The site of insulin injection should also be taken into account. Exercise increases blood flow in the part of the body being used, increasing insulin absorption if that area is where the insulin injection was administered. For example, prior to running the insulin dose should not be administered in the legs.

Insulin adjustments

For exercise anticipated within the first hour after eating, the dose of rapid-acting insulin before the meal may need to be decreased by 25–75% (depending on the intensity of the exercise) in addition to consuming 10–15 g of fast-acting carbohydrate prior to exercise. For day-long activities (such as camps, hiking or skiing), consider a 30–50% reduction in the long-acting insulin dose (or in the basal rate if using an insulin pump) the night before and on the day of the activity. For children using insulin pumps, there are numerous options for insulin adjustments with exercise. If the pump will be worn during exercise, the basal rate can be reduced by 30–50% beginning 30–90 minutes prior to exercise and continuing for up to 30 minutes or longer after the exercise. For some types of activities (e.g. contact sports), children may need to disconnect from the pump and do one of the following:

- Bolus part of the basal insulin to be missed prior to exercise (particularly if the pre-exercise blood sugar level is elevated) and the remainder after exercise;
- Bolus half of the insulin missed while disconnected after exercise;
- Bolus all of the insulin missed while disconnected after exercise.

In general, the pump should not be disconnected for longer than 2 hours. If necessary, the pump should be reconnected briefly and a bolus administered prior to disconnecting again.

Delayed hypoglycemia

Hypoglycemia can occur several hours after exercise secondary to increased glucose transport into the skeletal muscle, the late effect of increased insulin sensitivity, and the delay in replenishing liver and muscle glycogen stores. Blood glucose levels must be monitored for several hours following exercise, at bedtime and sometimes during the night on days with strenuous exercise. Consider a longer lasting snack (containing a solid carbohydrate, protein and fat) at bedtime and reducing the insulin dose as discussed above.

Ketones and exercise

In situations of underinsulinization, whether it be from poor glycemic control or from illness, exercise may be dangerous because of the effect of uninhibited action of the counter-regulatory hormones. Children with diabetes should not participate in strenuous exercise if the pre-exercise blood sugar level is high and urine ketones (small or more) or blood ketones (0.5 mmol/L or more) are present.

Hypoglycemia

Hypoglycemia is the most common acute complication in the treatment of T1DM and responsible for a significant proportion of deaths in people with diabetes aged under 40 years of age (see Chapter 33) [17]. While hypoglycemia in persons with diabetes is defined as plasma glucose below 70 mg/dL (4 mmol/L), severe hypoglycemia (seizure or loss of consciousness) usually does not occur until prolonged exposure to levels of 40–50 mg/dL (2.2–2.7 mmol/L) or lower. Severe hypoglycemia happens to one in five children every year on average, but 80% of the events occur among the 20% of children who have recurrent events [6]. Younger age, longer diabetes duration, barriers in access to care and presence of psychiatric disorders or chaotic family environment increase the risk. While lower HbA_{1c} is generally a risk factor for hypoglycemia, appropriate intensive insulin treatment can lower the risk by improving timing of insulin in relationship to food intake and exercise [18].

Signs and symptoms

- *Autonomic signs and symptoms:* trembling, pounding heart, cold sweatiness, pallor;
- *Neuroglycopenic signs and symptoms:* difficulty concentrating, blurred or double vision, disturbed color vision, difficulty hearing, slurred speech, poor judgment and confusion, problems with short-term memory, dizziness and unsteady gait, loss of consciousness, seizure, death;
- *Behavioral signs and symptoms:* irritability, erratic behavior, nightmares;
- *Non-specific symptoms:* hunger, headache, nausea, tiredness;

Early warning signs and symptoms of hypoglycemia are much more difficult to identify in young children.

Treatment

In mild or moderate symptomatic hypoglycemia, after documenting a blood glucose of ≤70 mg/dL (3.9 mmol/L):

- Provide immediate oral, rapidly absorbed 5–15 g glucose or sucrose: glucose tablets, "Smarties" or 4 oz (100 mL) of sweet drink (juice, soda).
- 1 g glucose should raise the blood glucose by 3 mg/dL (0.17 mmol/L) for the average adult and proportionally more in a child; target the rise of blood glucose level to 100 mg/dL (5.6 mmol/L).
- Retest blood glucose in 10–15 minutes, if no response or inadequate response – repeat as above.
- For initially lower glucose values, as symptoms improve and euglycemia is restored, ingest solid snack or meal (e.g. fruit, bread, cereal) to prevent recurrence.

• Retest blood glucose in 20–30 minutes to confirm that target glucose has been maintained.

In severe hypoglycemia, where the child has an altered mental status and is unable to assist in their care, may be unconscious and/or seizing, urgent treatment with parenteral glucagon or dextrose is required.

Glucagon

Glucagon is given intramuscularly or subcutaneously (10–30 μg/kg body weight):
• 0.3 mg for children younger than 6 years
• 0.5 mg for those 6–12 years
• 1 mg for those older than 12 years or heavier than 100 lb (45 kg)

Glucagon injection may be repeated in 5–10 minutes, if response was inadequate; however, it is likely to be ineffective after prolonged fasting. Side effects include vomiting and tachycardia.

Dextrose

Dextrose can be given intravenously by trained medical staff if glucagon is unavailable or recovery is inadequate in a hospital setting or by paramedics:
• Intravenous dextrose should be administered slowly over several minutes (e.g. dextrose 10–30% at a dose of 200–500 mg/kg; dextrose 10% is 100 mg/mL).
• Rapid administration or higher concentration may result in an excessive rate of osmotic change, phlebitis and extensive tissue damage, if extravasated.

Close observation and monitoring of blood glucose is essential because vomiting is common and hypoglycemia may recur. If recurrent hypoglycemia occurs, the child may ultimately require an IV infusion of dextrose 10% at 2–5 mg/kg/minute until stable.

Severe headache and transient paresis lasting up to 24 hours are not uncommon and generally do not require radiologic work-up.

Hypoglycemia unawareness

Hypoglycemia unawareness occurs when there is reduced awareness of the onset of hypoglycemia. A single hypoglycemic episode can lead to hypoglycemia unawareness secondary to a decrease in counter-regulatory responses, but it is usually seen in patients who have multiple periods of blood glucose <70 mg/dL. Avoiding subsequent hypoglycemia for 2–3 weeks may reverse this loss of awareness.

Prevention

Hypoglycemia occurs more frequently:
• When the treatment regimen or lifestyle is altered (increased insulin, less food, more exercise);
• In younger children;
• With lower HbA_{1c} levels;
• When there are frequent low blood glucose levels;
• When there is hypoglycemia unawareness;
• During sleep; or
• After alcohol ingestion.

Patients and families should be aware of the above risk factors so that glucose monitoring and insulin regimens can be changed accordingly. There is an increased risk for hypoglycemia during, immediately after and up to 2–12 hours after exercise. Untreated celiac disease and Addison disease may also increase the risk of hypoglycemia.

Nocturnal hypoglycemia is often asymptomatic and should be suspected if the morning blood glucose is low and/or there are episodes of confusion, nightmares or seizures during the night, or if there is impaired thinking, altered mood or headaches upon awakening. Nocturnal hypoglycemia can be confirmed with blood glucose monitoring during the night and may be prevented by including more protein and fat in the bedtime snack. Care should be taken that this does not occur at the expense of high overnight blood glucose levels.

Studies have shown an association between hypoglycemia and decrease in cognitive functioning in children with T1DM, particularly in children diagnosed before the age of 5–6 years. More recently, there has been increased interest in the potential role of chronic hyperglycemia on cognitive functioning in young children. Even mild–moderate hypoglycemia may impair school functioning and overall well-being. A reduced awareness of hypoglycemia and the risk of injury or accident often lead to a significant fear of hypoglycemia and decreases in insulin dosing, which in turn results in increased HbA_{1c}. Severe hypoglycemia can increase parental and patient's worry, poor sleep, emergency room visits, hospitalizations, excessive lowering of insulin doses and subsequent worsening of glycemic control. Long-term follow-up of the Diabetes Control and Complications Trial (DCCT) participants has been reassuring that there was no evidence for permanent neurocognitive changes related to hypoglycemia in adolescent and young adult individuals, suggesting that the effect of severe hypoglycemia on long-term neuropsychologic functioning may be age-dependent [19].

Ultimately, hypoglycemia is frequently predictable and should be prevented. Children and their caregivers must be taught to recognize the symptoms of hypoglycemia and treat this immediately and appropriately. Children with diabetes should always carry around a source of rapid-acting glucose and should wear identification noting that they have diabetes. The diabetes care provider should be notified if a child is having recurrent episodes of symptomatic hypoglycemia or if there is hypoglycemia unawareness. This will facilitate discussions to adjust insulin regimens, food intake patterns, blood glucose goals and monitoring. Continuous glucose monitoring helps to detect and to avoid hypoglycemia.

Sick day management

Children with diabetes in good metabolic control should not experience more illness or infections than children without diabetes; however, they will go though their share of routine infections which can be challenging for their caregivers. The influenza vaccine and other routine childhood immunizations are recommended for all children with diabetes.

Health care providers should equip families with the tools necessary to avoid dehydration, uncontrolled hyperglycemia or ketoacidosis, and hypoglycemia. Face to face education and written instructions are important, but most parents require telephone advice when first facing sickness in their child and some may need repeated support. Over time, most parents should be able to manage sick days independently as well as identify appropriate times when to seek help from their diabetes provider or emergency services. Patients should immediately seek medical attention if:

- Blood glucose concentrations continues to rise despite extra insulin;
- Blood glucose concentrations remains persistently below 3.5 mmol/L (70 mg/dL);
- Blood ketones are higher than 1.5 mmol/L or ketonuria is severe and persistent; or
- The child becomes exhausted, confused, dehydrated or develops difficulty in breathing, severe abdominal pain or a severe hypoglycemic reaction.

Missed insulin injection, inactivated insulin or interruption of insulin delivery from pump may lead to "sick days" as well, especially in older children. While treatment is essentially the same as for hyperglycemia in the course of an infection, the differential diagnosis is important for prevention of recurrent events.

Hyperglycemia is seen in many illnesses, particularly those associated with fever, as a result of elevated levels of stress hormones, which promote gluconeogenesis and insulin resistance. Severe illness increases ketone body production secondary to inadequate insulin action or insufficient oral intake of carbohydrates. By contrast, illnesses associated with vomiting and diarrhea can lead to hypoglycemia secondary to decreased food intake, poor absorption and slower gastric emptying.

In general, during illness, blood glucose concentrations must be monitored more frequently – at least every 3–4 hours and more often when blood glucose concentrations are outside the target range (e.g. 80–200 mg/dL). Urinary or blood ketones must be checked at least twice daily and always when blood glucose concentration exceeds 300 mg/dL (17.6 mmol/L). If available, the authors recommend testing blood ketones (β-hydroxybutyrate, using Precision Xtra/Exceed meter) over urine ketone testing as a more specific and timely marker of ketosis:

- The presence of ketones when blood glucose concentrations are persistently elevated above 200 mg/dL (11.1 mmol/L) indicates the need for supplemental insulin and fluids.
- The presence of ketones when blood glucose concentrations are low or normal, especially during gastrointestinal illness, indicate insufficient oral intake of carbohydrates (starvation ketones). In this case, ketones do not reflect insulin deficiency, but rather a physiologic response and may protect the patient from severe hypoglycemia as β-hydroxybutyrate is the only alternative fuel to glucose for the brain. Supplemental insulin is contraindicated as it will likely cause hypoglycemia; the correct treatment includes fluids with glucose.

Insulin therapy must never be stopped during a sick day, although the dose may need to be decreased if the child is vomiting or eating less than usual. A fasting patient still requires approximately 40% of the usual daily insulin dose, as long-acting basal insulin, to cover basic metabolic needs and prevent ketoacidosis; however, infections associated with normal food intake often require an increase of basal insulin by 10–15%. In addition, extra doses of rapid-acting insulin are usually needed to correct hyperglycemia, prevent ketoacidosis and avoid hospital admission. These doses may be repeated every 2–4 hours as needed based on the results of blood glucose and ketone monitoring.

With blood glucose concentrations greater than 200 mg/dL (11.1 mmol/L), the authors recommend:

- Usual high blood glucose correction (e.g. 1 unit of rapid-acting insulin for each 50 mg/dL above 100 mg/dL, if blood ketones <0.6 mmol/L or urine ketones negative/small;
- Injection of rapid-acting insulin in the amount of 10% of the total daily dose, if blood ketones 0.6–1.5 mmol/L or urine ketones are moderate or large;
- Injection of rapid-acting insulin in the amount of 10–20% of the total daily dose if blood ketones >1.5 mmol/L or urine ketones are moderate or large;
- As acidosis is present in most patients with hyperglycemia and blood ketones >3.0 mmol/L, this warrants referral to an emergency department.

Patients using insulin pumps who develop hyperglycemia and moderate or large urine ketones (or greater than 1.0 mmol/L blood ketones) must always take into consideration the possibility of an interruption in insulin delivery. If blood glucose levels do not decrease appropriately after an insulin bolus from the pump, the correction bolus of short-acting insulin should be given as injection by pen or syringe and the pump infusion set should be changed. A temporary increase in the basal rate by 20% or more may be required until blood glucose concentrations begin to normalize and ketones clear.

If hypoglycemia <70 mg/dL (<3.9 mmol/L) persists and the patient is unable to tolerate any oral intake, an injection of low dose glucagon may reverse the hypoglycemia and enable oral fluid intake to resume. Glucagon is mixed as usual but given using an insulin syringe with the dose being one unit per year of age up to 15 years [20]. Upon mixing with water, glucagon remains stable for at least 48 hours at 4°C. The small dose of glucagon can be repeated every 2–4 hours; however, it is likely to be less effective with prolonged fasting. This dose of glucagon is not to be used for the emergency treatment of severe hypoglycemia.

Hydration status must be followed closely. Fever, hyperglycemia with osmotic diuresis, and ketonuria all increase fluid losses. Households should maintain a supply of sugar and electrolyte containing fluids:

• Oral water is sufficient to prevent dehydration in uncomplicated cases of hyperglycemia.
• If there is an ongoing fluid loss from diarrhea or vomiting, hydration liquids should contain salt in addition to water (e.g. Pedialyte, Rehydralate). These preparations contain 25–30 g/L glucose, 45–90 mEq/L sodium, 30 mEq/L bicarbonate and 20–25 mEq/L potassium. Oral rehydration fluid can be made at home by mixing half of a flat teaspoon of salt (~3 g of NaCl = ~50 mEq sodium), 7 teaspoons of sugar (28 g) and (optionally) 100 mL (4 oz) of orange juice into 1 L water.
• If there is difficulty eating or keeping food down and the blood glucose is falling below 200 mg/dL (11.1 mmol/L), sports drinks should be administered. They contain less electrolytes but higher amounts of glucose (e.g. Gatorade contains 255 g/L glucose, 20 mEq/L sodium, 3 mEq/L bicarbonate and 3 mEq/L potassium).
• If the blood glucose is falling below 100 mg/dL (5.6 mmol/L), fluids with higher concentration of sugar are recommended (e.g. juice or non-carbonated regular soda containing approximately 70 g glucose per 100 mL. These fluids contain almost no sodium and are not appropriate in large amounts for children with diarrhea.

The required volume of oral fluid replacement is the sum of maintenance volume, deficit and ongoing losses. In practical terms, infants and toddlers with diabetes who vomited more than twice or have multiple loose stools should be referred to an emergency department for evaluation and intravenous fluids. Those with milder symptoms can be given oral fluid therapy at home; small amounts (5 mL) of cold fluids every 5 minutes. Most children with vomiting can by successfully orally rehydrated with persistent gentle encouragement of parents.

Antiemetic medication at home is generally contraindicated, especially in young children, as it may mask acute abdominal processes such as appendicitis, volvulus or intussusception and may have significant adverse effects. Ondansetron (Zofran) can be used to contain vomiting in patients properly evaluated by a physician and selected older children presenting without abdominal pain.

Estimate of 24-hour maintenance fluid volume

Estimation based on age:

- 0–2 years = 80 mL/kg
- 3–5 years = 70 mL/kg
- 6–9 years = 60 mL/kg
- 10–14 years = 50 mL/kg
- >15 years = 35 mL/kg

Estimation based on body weight:

- 100 mL/kg for the initial 10 kg body weight, plus
- 50 mL/kg for the next 10 kg body weight, plus
- 20 mL/kg for each additional kg body weight

For example, a child weighting 30 kg needs 1000 + 500 + 200 = 1700 mL maintenance water for 24 hours or 70 mL/hour, not counting past or ongoing losses

Monitoring and goals of diabetes management

Hemoglobin A_{1c} (HbA_{1c}) is the only measure of mid to long-term glycemic control for which robust outcome data are available (see Chapter 25). Elevated HbA_{1c} predicts long-term microvascular and macrovascular complications but has its limitations. In the DCCT, an HbA_{1c} of 53 mmol/mol (7.0%) corresponded to a higher average blood glucose concentration (measured seven times a day) of 192 mg/dL in the conventionally treated patients compared with 163 mg/dL in the intensively treated patients. Consequently, the same HbA_{1c} level conferred significantly higher risk of microvascular complications and hypoglycemia in the conventionally treated patients compared with intensively treated patients [21]. HbA_{1c} can only be one of the measures of optimal glycemic control, along with documented hypoglycemia and quality of life. Ideally, there should be four to six measurements per year in younger children and three to four measurements per year in older children.

Self-monitoring of blood glucose (SMBG) provides immediate and daily documentation of hyperglycemia and hypoglycemia, helps to determine immediate and daily insulin requirements and detects hypoglycemia and assists in its management. Blood glucose is best measured during the night, after the overnight fast, at anticipated peaks and troughs of insulin action, 2 hours after a meal and in association with vigorous sport or exercise – typically 4–6 times a day. The frequency of SMBG is associated with improved HbA_{1c} in patients with T1DM [21]. Patient acceptance of SMBG may be enhanced by including the opportunity for testing alternative sites in addition to the fingertips (e.g. the palm of the hand or the forearm); however, alternative sites may be slower to reflect falling blood glucose.

A logbook or some type of electronic memory device has to be used to record patterns of glycemic control and adjustments to treatment. The record book is useful at the time of consultation and should contain time and date of blood glucose reading, insulin dosage, together with a note of special events (e.g. illness, parties, exercise, menses, hypoglycemic episodes and episodes of elevated blood or urinary ketones).

At present, the safest recommendation for glycemic control in children is to achieve the lowest HbA_{1c} that can be sustained without severe hypoglycemia as well as frequent moderate hypoglycemia or prolonged periods of significant hyperglycemia where blood glucose levels exceed 250 mg/dL (14 mmol/L). Each child should have targets individually determined. Targets for HbA_{1c} and SMBG recently proposed by the International Society for Pediatric and Adolescent Diabetes (ISPAD) [21] are summarized in Table 51.4.

Table 51.4 Biochemical targets of glycemic control. These targets are intended as guidelines, each child should have their targets individually determined.

Level of control	Optimal	Suboptimal	High risk
HbA_{1c}			
DCCT standardized (%)	<7.5	7.5–8.9	≥9.0*
IFCC (mmol/mol)	<58	58–74	≥75
SMBG mmol/L (mg/dL)			
Fasting or preprandial BG	5–8.3 (90–150)	>8.3 (>150)	>11.1 (>200)
Post-prandial BG	5–10 (90–180)	10–13.9 (180–250)	>13.9 (>250)
Bedtime BG	6.7–10 (120–180)	<6.7 (<120) or 10–11 (180–200)	<4.4 (<80) or >11.1 (>200)
Nocturnal BG	4.4–9 (80–160)	<4.4 (<80) or >9 >162)	<3.9 (<70) or >11.1 (>200)

BG, blood glucose; DCCT, Diabetes Control and Complications Trial; IFCC, International Federation of Clinical Chemistry; SMBG, self-monitoring of blood glucose.
* DCCT conventional adult cohort had a mean HbA_{1c} value of 8.9% (74 mmol/mol), both DCCT and Epidemiology of Diabetes Interventions and Complications (EDIC) have shown poor outcomes with this level.

Continuous glucose monitoring

Sensors are available and in development that measure interstitial fluid glucose every 1–20 minutes (i.e. "continuously"). Currently, these devices are expensive and insurance coverage is limited. Over time, it is anticipated that these devices will become the standard of care in children with T1DM. The continuous glucose results are available to the user in real-time and are stored in the receiver device or pump for downloading to a computer at a later time. The download allows the patient and health care professional to review the results and make appropriate and educated insulin dosage adjustments. This much more sophisticated approach to SMBG may allow targets to be determined so that an alarm will alert the wearer to a glucose value projected to fall below or above the preset target and inform insulin delivery from a pump. As continuous glucose monitoring becomes more widely available, decreased blood glucose targets may be more safely achieved in children with diabetes.

The average HbA_{1c} is lowest in the youngest age group, perhaps reflecting the more complete caregiver involvement at younger ages. Of all age groups, adolescents are currently the farthest from achieving HbA_{1c} 58 mmol/mol (<7.5%), reflecting the diabetes mismanagement that frequently accompanies the increased independence in diabetes care during the adolescent years, as well as the effect of psychologic and hormonal challenges of adolescence. Too ambitious goals may lead to an unwarranted sense of failure and alienation on part of a teenage person with diabetes. As diabetes technology improves, especially continuous glucose monitoring, recommended target indicators for glycemic control will likely decrease to reflect a new balance of benefits and risks.

Health care providers should be aware that achieving an HbA_{1c} consistently below the target range without extensive personal and national health care resources and outside of a clinical trial structure may be very difficult. As a benchmark, intensively treated adolescents in the DCCT achieved a mean HbA_{1c} of 65 mmol/mol (8.1%), compared to 54 mmol/mol (7.1%) in adults. Older well-educated DCCT participants with excellent access to the newest diabetes technology maintained HbA_{1c} of 62–66 mmol/mol (7.8–8.2%) during 12 years of follow-up in the Epidemiology of Diabetes Interventions and Complications (EDIC) study [22].

Psychologic care

The diagnosis of T1DM brutally changes the lives of affected families and poses relentless challenges. It is impossible to take a "vacation" from diabetes without some unpleasant consequences. It is no wonder that children with T1DM and their parents are at risk for adjustment problems. Persisting adjustment problems may mark underlying dysfunction of the family or psychopathology of the child or caregiver. Young people with T1DM are more frequently diagnosed with and treated for psychiatric disorders, disordered eating, neurocognitive and learning problems, family dysfunction and poor coping skills than the general population. The psychologic care recommendations of the ISPAD [23] are summarized in Table 51.5.

Screening and early treatment of risk factors for complications and associated conditions

Dyslipidemia

Cardiovascular disease (CVD) is a leading cause of morbidity and mortality in adults with T1DM. Preclinical atherosclerosis often starts in childhood. While children with T1DM have generally a favorable lipid profile, this remains a major modifiable CVD risk factor in this population. Screening for dyslipidemia in children with T1DM should commence after the age of 2 years if there is a family history of hypercholesterolemia or CVD or this is unknown, or otherwise at age 12 years, and should be repeated every 5 years thereafter if normal [24]. Glycemic control should be established in newly diagnosed patients prior to screening. Children with low density lipoprotein (LDL) levels 130–159 mg/dL (3.4–4.1 mmol/L) should obtain glucose control, dietary and exer-

Table 51.5 Psychologic care recommendations for families of children with T1DM.

1	Mental health professionals with training in diabetes should be available to interact with patients and families at clinic visits to conduct screening and more complete assessments of psychosocial functioning as well as support the diabetes team in the recognition and management of mental health and behavior problems
2	There should be easy access to consult psychiatrists for cases involving severe psychopathology and the potential need for psychotropic medications
3	Diabetes health care providers should strive to maintain regular, consistent and uninterrupted contact with patients and their families
4	Developmental progress in all domains of quality of life (i.e. physical, intellectual, academic, emotional and social development) should be monitored routinely
5	Routine assessment should be made of developmental adjustment to and understanding of diabetes management, including diabetes-related knowledge, insulin adjustment skills, goal-setting, problem-solving abilities, regimen adherence and self-care autonomy and competence. This is especially important during late childhood and prior to adolescence
6	Psychosocial adjustment problems, depression, eating disorders and other psychiatric disorders should be ruled out or treated, if present, in patients not achieving HbA_{1c} goals or having recurrent severe hypoglycemia or DKA
7	General family functioning needs to be assessed (conflict, cohesion, adaptability and parental psychopathology) and diabetes-related functioning (communication, parental involvement and support, and roles and responsibilities for self-care behaviors) especially when there is evidence of cultural, language or family problems
8	Training parents in effective behavior management skills, especially at diagnosis and prior to adolescence, should emphasize appropriate family involvement and support, effective problem-solving and self-management skills, and realistic expectations
9	Motivational interviewing may be useful in counseling young people and parents regarding intensification of insulin regimens. This may help in clarifying patient and parental goals and resolve ambivalence about regimen intensification. Patients should not be denied access to regimen intensification based on perceptions of limited competence
10	Adolescents should be encouraged to assume increasing responsibility for diabetes management but with continuing, mutually agreed parental involvement and support. The transition to adult diabetes care should be negotiated and carefully planned between adolescents, their parents and the diabetes team well in advance of the actual transfer to adult care

cise counseling for 6 months with consideration of pharmacologic therapy if this fails; pharmacotherapy in addition to diet and lifestyle changes is recommended if LDL is >160 mg/dL (4.1 mmol/L). The treatment goals are LDL <100 mg/dL (2.6 mmol/L), high density lipoprotein (HDL) >35 mg/dL (0.9 mmol/L) and triglycerides <150 mg/dL (1.7 mmol/L).

The use of lipid-lowering drugs in children has been the subject of much discussion. Bile acid sequestrants and statins are currently approved medications [25]. Bile acid sequestrants are not well tolerated and therefore compliance is poor. Several short-term trials of statins have confirmed their safety and efficacy in children and adolescents with familial hypercholesterolemia. The American Heart Association recommends initiating therapy with statins at the lowest dose with emphasis on appropriate patient selection criteria including the presence of other cardiovascular risk factors, age >10 years in boys, Tanner stage II or higher, preferably after menarche in girls. Patient and family preferences should be considered and there should be no contraindication to statin therapy (e.g. hepatic disease) [26]. If therapy with statins is undertaken, regular monitoring of liver function and screening for symptoms of rhabdomyolysis should occur. Appropriate contraceptive advice should be given to girls receiving statins.

Microalbuminuria

Microalbuminuria is the first clinical manifestation of diabetic nephropathy and may be reversible with diligent glycemic and blood pressure control. Microalbuminuria is defined as any of the following [27]:

- Albumin excretion rate 20–200 mg/min, or 30–300 mg/24 hours in 24-hour urine collections.
- Albumin concentration 30–300 mg/L (in early morning urine sample).
- Albumin : creatinine ratio 2.5–25 mg/mmol or 30–300 mg/g (spot urine) in males and 3.5–25 mg/mmol in females (because of lower creatinine excretion).

Screening for microalbuminuria with a random spot urine sample should occur annually in children once they are 10 years of age and have had diabetes for more than 5 years. If values are increasing or borderline, more frequent screening should occur. A timed overnight or 24-hour collection can be obtained for follow-up if needed. Abnormal results should be repeated. The diagnosis of microalbuminuria requires documentation of two abnormal samples out of three samples over a period of 3–6 months. Once persistent microalbuminuria is confirmed, non-diabetes-related causes of renal disease should be excluded. Following this evaluation, treatment with an angiotensin-converting enzyme (ACE) inhibitor should be started, even if the blood pressure is normal. Patients should be counseled about the importance of glycemic control and smoking cessation if applicable.

Elevated blood pressure

Hypertension in adults with diabetes is associated with the development of both microvascular and macrovascular disease. Treatment of blood pressure is critical in reducing these complications in adults and presumably in children and adolescents as well. Blood pressure should be checked and reviewed at each clinic visit. Hypertension is defined as systolic or diastolic blood pressure (measured on at least three separate days) above the 95th percentile for the child's age, sex and height. Care should be taken to ensure use of the appropriate-sized cuff in children to avoid inaccurate readings. If elevated blood pressure is confirmed, non-diabetes causes of hypertension should first be excluded.

Retinopathy

The first dilated ophthalmologic examination should be obtained by an ophthalmologist, optometrist or other health care professional trained in diabetes-specific retinal examination once the child is ≥10 years old and has had diabetes for 3–5 years [24]. The frequency of subsequent examination is generally every 1–2 years, depending on the patient risk profile and advice of an eye care provider.

Celiac disease

The prevalence of biopsy-confirmed celiac disease (CD) in patients with T1DM ranges from 3% to 7%, compared to <1% in the general population [28]. Many children with diabetes are asymptomatic but are positive for specific serologic markers of CD such as autoantibodies to tissue transglutaminase. Most of the children with diabetes and CD still remain undiagnosed, despite intestinal symptoms and/or short stature in about half of the cases.

Clinical manifestations of CD are diverse, vary with age and may overlap with functional disorders. Some of the manifestations, such as delayed growth and puberty, decreased bone mineralization, abdominal pain and abnormal liver function tests, may overlap with those of poorly controlled diabetes. Therefore, physicians and other health care providers need to consider CD in the differential diagnosis and many have argued for a routine transglutaminase screening in children with T1DM.

T1DM and CD share HLA and non-HLA susceptibility genes. The prevalence of transglutaminase autoimmunity is highest in those with the HLA-DR3,DQB1*0201 haplotype. One in four children with diabetes homozygous for this haplotype and 12% of the heterozygotes are positive for transglutaminase autoantibodies.

Most patients with T1DM with CD are transglutaminase-autoantibody-positive at the initial screening, although new cases develop during follow-up. All patients should be screened for immunoglobulin A (IgA) transglutaminase-autoantibodies at onset of diabetes and, if negative and asymptomatic, rescreened every other year. If the transglutaminase-autoantibodies are negative, but the patient has symptoms and/or signs consistent with CD, other causes (e.g. poor glycemic control, or intolerance of milk, soy or salicylates) should be explored. HLA-DQB1 typing and total IgA level measurement may be helpful; if DQB1*0201 is present, IgA <10 mg/dL and, if symptoms persist, biopsy is recommended. Positive transglutaminase autoantibody findings have to be confirmed on another occasion, because transglutaminase autoantibody levels can fluctuate. If transglutaminase autoantibodies are strongly and persistently positive (radioimmunoassay index >0.5 or ELISA >60), biopsy is recommended even in a completely asymptomatic patient. By contrast, patients with low to moderately positive transglutaminase autoantibody levels may have false-negative biopsy and may be falsely reassured that they do not have CD and forego further follow-up. The authors recommend repeating transglutaminase autoantibody testing every 3–6 months as long as the levels are positive.

Untreated CD may pose problems with diabetes management, including increased risk of hypoglycemia and chronic diarrhea which is difficult to differentiate from that caused by autonomic neuropathy in adult patients. It is an open issue whether treating silent CD improves diabetes-related outcomes. To date, results suggest small benefit in growth and bone mineralization, excess weight gain but no diabetes control benefit, or a slight decrease in HbA_{1c}. Gluten-free diets may prevent some of the episodes of hypoglycemia. The benefit of early detection and treatment remains unproven, but is the subject of ongoing investigation.

Thyroid disease

Hypothyroidism is present in 4–18% of children with T1DM. Long-term follow-up suggests that as many as 30% of people with T1DM develop autoimmune thyroiditis [29]. The presence of hypothyroidism has been associated with thyroid autoantibodies, increasing age and diabetes duration and female gender. Hyperthyroidism is not more common in patients with T1DM than in the general population (1%). With follow-up of 20 years, 80% of people with T1DM and thyroid peroxidase (TPO) autoantibodies develop hypothyroidism.

The presence of autoimmune thyroiditis in the population with T1DM has the potential to affect growth, weight gain, diabetes control, menstrual regularity and overall well-being. All children with T1DM should be screened for elevated levels of the thyroid-stimulating hormone after stabilization at onset of diabetes and every 1–2 years thereafter, or sooner if symptoms of hypothyroidism or hyperthyroidism are present. We also recommend measuring TPO and free T4 at the time of thyroid-stimulating hormone screening. Subjects with positive TPO autoantibodies and normal thyroid function should be screened on a more frequent basis (every 6–12 months).

Addison disease

Addison disease affects approximately 1 in 10 000 of the general population and in 1% of subjects with T1DM [29]. The autoimmune process resulting in Addison disease can be identified by the detection of autoantibodies reacting to 21 hydroxylase (21-OH). The presence of this autoantibody in the general population is very rare, in contrast to 1–2% in subjects with T1DM. Of those with positive antibodies but as yet free of Addison disease, 15% develop Addison disease within a few years. Progression to adrenal insufficiency begins with elevated plasma renin activity and then progresses to increased adenocorticotropic hormone, decreased stimulated cortisol, and eventually abnormalities of basal cortisol. The authors' current practice is to screen all children with T1DM for the presence of 21-OH autoantibodies. Those positive are followed for adrenal insufficiency by plasma renin activity and adenocorticotropic hormone stimulation testing. Most subjects who develop disease are mildly symptomatic with decreasing insulin doses and HbA_{1c}.

References

1 Rewers M, Norris J, Kretowski A. Epidemiology of type 1 diabetes mellitus. In: Type 1 Diabetes: Cellular, Molecular & Clinical Immunology. Eisenbarth GS, ed. Online edition version 3.0. http://www.uchsc.edu/misc/diabetes/books/type1/type1_ch9.html. Accessed January 15, 2009.

2 Rewers M, Gottlieb P. Immunotherapy for the prevention and treatment of type 1 diabetes: human trials and a look into the future. *Diabetes Care* 2009; **32**:1769–1782.

3 Sosenko JM, Palmer JP, Rafkin-Mervis L, Krischer JP, Cuthbertson D, Mahon J, *et al.* Incident dysglycemia and the progression to type 1 diabetes among participants in the Diabetes Prevention Trial-Type 1. *Diabetes Care* 2009; **32**:1603–1607.

4 Stene LC, Barriga K, Hoffman M, Kean J, Klingensmith G, Norris JM, *et al.* Normal but increasing hemoglobin A1c levels predict progression from islet autoimmunity to overt type 1 diabetes: Diabetes Autoimmunity Study in the Young (DAISY). *Pediatr Diabetes* 2006; **7**:247–253.

5 Levy-Marchal C, Patterson CC, Green A. Geographical variation of presentation at diagnosis of type 1 diabetes in children: the EURODIAB study. European and Diabetes. *Diabetologia* 2001; **44**(Suppl 3):B75–B80.

6 Rewers A, Klingensmith G, Davis C, Petitti DB, Pihoker C, Rodriguez B, *et al.* Presence of diabetic ketoacidosis at diagnosis of diabetes mellitus in youth: the Search for Diabetes in Youth Study. *Pediatrics* 2008; **121**:e1258–e1266.

7 Dunger DB, Sperling MA, Acerini CL, Bohn DJ, Daneman D, Danne TP, *et al.* European Society for Paediatric Endocrinology/Lawson Wilkins Pediatric Endocrine Society consensus statement on diabetic ketoacidosis in children and adolescents. *Pediatrics* 2004; **113**:e133–e140.

8 Vanelli M, Chiari G, Ghizzoni L, Costi G, Giacalone T, Chiarelli F. Effectiveness of a prevention program for diabetic ketoacidosis in children: an 8-year study in schools and private practices. *Diabetes Care* 1999; **22**:7–9.

9 Rewers A, Chase HP, Mackenzie T, Walravens P, Roback M, Rewers M, *et al.* Predictors of acute complications in children with type 1 diabetes. *JAMA* 2002; **287**:2511–2518.

10 Edge JA, Jakes RW, Roy Y, Hawkins M, Winter D, Ford-Adams ME, *et al.* The UK case–control study of cerebral oedema complicating diabetic ketoacidosis in children. *Diabetologia* 2006; **49**:2002–2009.

11 Swift PG. Diabetes education: ISPAD clinical practice consensus guidelines 2006–2007. *Pediatr Diabetes* 2007; **8**:103–109.

12 Pihoker C, Forsander G, Wolfsdorf J, Klingensmith GJ. The delivery of ambulatory diabetes care: structures, processes, and outcomes of ambulatory diabetes care. *Pediatr Diabetes* 2008; **9**:609–620.

13 Bangstad HJ, Danne T, Deeb LC, Jarosz-Chobot P, Urakami T, Hanas R. Insulin treatment: ISPAD clinical practice consensus guidelines 2006–2007. *Pediatr Diabetes* 2007; **8**:88–102.

14 Aslander-van VE, Smart C, Waldron S. Nutritional management in childhood and adolescent diabetes. *Pediatr Diabetes* 2007; **8**:323–339.

15 Bantle JP, Wylie-Rosett J, Albright AL, Apovian CM, Clark NG, Franz MJ, *et al.* Nutrition recommendations and interventions for diabetes: a position statement of the American Diabetes Association. *Diabetes Care* 2008; **31**(Suppl 1):S61–S78.

16 Robertson K, Adolfsson P, Riddell MC, Scheiner G, Hanas R. Exercise in children and adolescents with diabetes. *Pediatr Diabetes* 2008; **9**:65–77.

17 Clarke W, Jones T, Rewers A, Dunger D, Klingensmith GJ. Assessment and management of hypoglycemia in children and adolescents with diabetes. *Pediatr Diabetes* 2008; **9**:165–174.

18 The effect of intensive treatment of diabetes on the development and progression of long-term complications in insulin-dependent diabetes mellitus: the Diabetes Control and Complications Trial Research Group. *N Engl J Med* 1993; **329**:977–986.

19 Jacobson AM, Musen G, Ryan CM, Silvers N, Cleary P, Waberski B, *et al.* Long-term effect of diabetes and its treatment on cognitive function. *N Engl J Med* 2007; **356**:1842–1852.

20 Chase HP. *Understanding Diabetes: A Handbook for People Who Are Living With Diabetes*, 11th edn. Denver, CO: Children's Diabetes Foundation, 2006.

21 Rewers M, Pihoker C, Donaghue K, Hanas R, Swift P, Klingensmith GJ. Assessment and monitoring of glycemic control in children and adolescents with diabetes. *Pediatr Diabetes* 2007; **8**:408–418.

22 Nathan DM, Cleary PA, Backlund JY, Genuth SM, Lachin JM, Orchard TJ, *et al.* Intensive diabetes treatment and cardiovascular disease in patients with type 1 diabetes. *N Engl J Med* 2005; **353**:2643–2653.

23 Delamater AM. Psychological care of children and adolescents with diabetes. *Pediatr Diabetes* 2007; **8**:340–348.

24 Silverstein J, Klingensmith G, Copeland K, Plotnick L, Kaufman F, Laffel L, *et al.* Care of children and adolescents with type 1 diabetes: a statement of the American Diabetes Association. *Diabetes Care* 2005; **28**:186–212.

25 Maahs DM, Wadwa RP, Bishop F, Daniels SR, Rewers M, Klingensmith GJ. Dyslipidemia in youth with diabetes: to treat or not to treat? *J Pediatr* 2008; **153**:458–465.

26 McCrindle BW, Urbina EM, Dennison BA, Jacobson MS, Steinberger J, Rocchini AP, *et al.* Drug therapy of high-risk lipid abnormalities in children and adolescents: a scientific statement from the American Heart Association Atherosclerosis, Hypertension, and Obesity in Youth Committee, Council of Cardiovascular Disease in the Young, with the Council on Cardiovascular Nursing. *Circulation* 2007; **115**:1948–1967.

27 Donaghue KC, Chiarelli F, Trotta D, Allgrove J, Dahl-Jorgensen K. ISPAD clinical practice consensus guidelines 2006–2007: Microvascular and macrovascular complications. *Pediatr Diabetes* 2007; **8**:163–170.

28 Rewers M, Liu E, Simmons J, Redondo MJ, Hoffenberg EJ. Celiac disease associated with type 1 diabetes mellitus. *Endocrinol Metab Clin North Am* 2004; **33**:197–214, xi.

29 Barker JM. Clinical review. Type 1 diabetes-associated autoimmunity: natural history, genetic associations, and screening. *J Clin Endocrinol Metab* 2006; **91**:1210–1217.

30 Liese AD, D'Agostino RB Jr, Hamman RF, Kilgo PD, Lawrence JM, Liu LL, *et al.* The burden of diabetes mellitus among US youth: prevalence estimates from the SEARCH for Diabetes in Youth Study. *Pediatrics* 2006; **118**:1510–1518.

52 Diabetes in Adolescence and Transitional Care

Debbie Kralik[1] & Maria Kambourakis[2]

[1] Royal District Nursing Service, South Australia and University of South Australia and University of Adelaide
[2] Type 1 Diabetes Program, Diabetes Australia, Victoria, Australia

Keypoints

- Adolescence is characterized by significant and complex biological, social and psychologic changes that occur during the teenage years.
- Adolescents with diabetes establish a long-term positive bond with their pediatric health care team. Consequently, the transition to an adult diabetes service provider is a significant event.
- Adolescents are at risk of dropping away from health care professional contact and follow-up during the time of transition, which may be detrimental to their physical and psychologic well-being.
- Adolescents need support to anticipate the issues they may face when preparing to move from children's services and to identify the solutions that may be available to them.
- The transition must be carefully managed so that the adolescent does not need to make an abrupt adaptation in their move from an environment that is very supportive to one where they are expected to be more independent.

Introduction

Adolescence is a life stage characterized by transition and change regardless of health status. Diabetes in adolescence is a life-changing condition requiring diligent and consistent management by a multidisciplinary team of clinicians in addition to comprehensive care and support provided by the family unit. Many young people with diabetes establish a long-term positive bond with their pediatric health care team. Consequently, the transition to an adult diabetes service provider is a significant event. The seamless transfer of adolescents with diabetes from pediatric to adult services can also be a challenge for health services and clinicians. Young people may mourn the loss of the relationships they had with the pediatric health team and can become distressed about learning to trust new staff [1]. There is evidence to suggest that during the time of transfer, adolescents are at risk of dropping away from health care professional contact and follow-up which may be detrimental to their physical and psychologic well-being [2]. As a result, it has been estimated that 10–60% of adolescents do not make the transition successfully from pediatric to adult health services [3,4]. The purpose of this chapter is to enhance understanding of the key issues presenting for adolescents and clinicians, and to consider effective models of care that will facilitate seamless transition from pediatric to adult diabetes care.

Textbook of Diabetes, 4th edition. Edited by R. Holt, C. Cockram, A. Flyvbjerg and B. Goldstein.

Transition

Transition is the reorientation that people experience to a change event [5]. Events that change our lives occur constantly, but they often go unnoticed, unless we are disrupted by them. These are "change events" that produce an end to one's familiar way of living and require the individual to find new ways of being in the world that incorporate those changes. Change is situational, such as a move to a new job, a new city or a new school. Transition is the way people respond to the changes that are occurring in their lives.

Transition involves moving through the change situation and negotiating one's sense of self in an altered world [6]. Transition is the movement people make through a disruptive life event so that they can continue to live with a coherent and continuing sense of self [7]. Understanding transition involves exploring the person's responses to a passage of change. Health care professionals are frequently in the position of supporting people who are in transition because of the changes associated with the impact of illness.

During the last three decades, the concept of transition has evolved in the social sciences and health disciplines, with nurses contributing to more recent understandings of the transition process as it relates to life and health [8–15]. Transitional definitions alter according to the disciplinary focus, but there is broad agreement that transition involves the way people respond to change. Transition occurs over time and entails change and adaptation, for example developmental, personal, relational, situational, societal or environmental change, but not all change engages transition. Transition is not an event, but rather the inner reorientation and self-redefinition that people go through in order to incorporate changes into their lives [5].

The transition focused on here when discussing adolescent transfer to adult services is when one "chapter" of life is over and the person is unable to go back to the way life was before the change event occurred. The change event under particular focus is the shift to a new and unfamiliar service environment. To enable a "new chapter" to begin these adolescents will need to respond to the changes in their lives, sorting out what can be retained of their former way of living and what has to be released, in order to move forward [15]. This is often the experience of the adolescent moving from child to adult health services. Understanding transition theory will enable health care professionals to assist young people to make this transition during a life stage that is characterized by constant change.

Transition as a process

The terms "transition" and "transfer" have been used interchangeably in the literature when referring to adolescents moving between diabetes services. As a consequence, transition may be interpreted as simply a process of physical transfer to a different service with a failure to acknowledge the psychosocial needs of the adolescent and family members. This oversight may have resulted in a lack of resources to assist the adolescent and parents to make the psychosocial transition between children's and adult services [1]. A clear distinction between the concepts of transition and transfer is needed.

When people experience transition, they look for ways to move through the unfamiliar to create some order in their lives so they can reorient themselves to the new situation [5]. Transition can involve much trial and error, as people work out ways of living and being in their changing world. When young people are learning to live with a chronic illness such as diabetes they are involved in that transitional process. Over time these people redefine their sense of self, redevelop confidence to make decisions about their lives and to respond to the ongoing disruption that so often accompanies chronic illness. When undertaking the work of reclaiming their sense of self and identity, they come to an understanding of what is changing, or has changed in their lives and how this reality is shifting key values and identity markers.

The transitional process takes time, however, as the adolescent will disengage with what was known and familiar and look toward the altered and new situation that lies ahead. At this point it can be helpful for the person to connect with others they can trust. A familiar health professional, support group, a friend or a family member who is a good listener becomes an important asset in the sense-making process. Without such examination of the change event or events, people's understanding of what is changing may be limited. This is particularly the case for adolescents who are engaged in major change in all areas of their lives. For many adolescents, leaving the care of their pediatrician and other familiar health care professionals is a passage from security to uncertainty [16]. These young people need time to examine their perceptions and experiences and to consider the actions that they need or want to take. Adolescents will need support to anticipate the issues they may face when preparing to move from children's services and to identify the solutions that may be available to them. This is a key point in enabling successful transition for adolescents moving to adult diabetes care.

Adolescence as a time of transition

Adolescence is a transitional stage of human development that occurs between childhood and adulthood. This transition is characterized by significant and complex biologic, social and psychologic changes that occur during the teenage years. During this time the adolescent is developing a sense of self and identity, establishing autonomy and understanding sexuality. Adolescence is a stage of life where control–autonomy–dependence are pertinent issues in the lives of young people [16]. There is often anxiety experienced by the adolescent regarding acceptance by peers which may also impact self-care behaviors.

The events and characteristics that mark the end of adolescence and the beginning of adulthood can vary by culture as well as by function. Countries and cultures differ at what age an individual can be considered to be mature enough to undertake particular tasks and responsibilities such as driving a vehicle, having sexual relations, serving in the armed forces, voting or marrying. Adolescence is usually accompanied by an increase in independence allowed by the parents or legal guardians and generally less supervision in daily life. This is true too of adolescents transferring to an adult care service. The intention is to ensure that the adolescent has the practical and cognitive skills required for diabetes self-care and has developed the capability to interact with others such as health care providers; however, age itself may not be a reliable indicator, as adolescents may have different needs and developmental issues at different stages and mature at different rates. The parents of the adolescent must also be prepared to relinquish some of the responsibility for diabetes care which they may have undertaken with a high degree of vigilance for many years. For some parents, this shift in responsibility can be a time of high anxiety. Fundamental to any successful transition program is the work with parents to help them find a balance between shifting the responsibility to the adolescent and continuing to maintain an appropriate level of interest and family cohesion [4].

Adolescence and diabetes

Type 1 diabetes mellitus (T1DM) is the most common metabolic disease that affects children [17]. It occurs when the pancreas is unable to produce insulin. Treatment consists of at least twice daily insulin injections in order to prevent serious short and long-term complications. In addition, children and their families need to ensure that an appropriate diet and lifestyle is followed and blood glucose levels are closely monitored [17].

For an adolescent with diabetes, the rapid changes in physical, sexual, psychologic, social and cognitive function that occur with adolescence can often lead to a decline in self-care behaviors. Glycemic control during adolescence can be suboptimal [18] because of a number of factors such as the physiologic changes associated with puberty [19], a desire to be perceived the same as peers, poor adherence to insulin regimens and decreased attendance at diabetes care clinics [2]. Irregular attendance at clinics has been associated with poor glycemic control and increased rates of diabetes-associated complications [20].

Adolescents who live with T1DM may experience the transition from the children's to the adult health service as an additional burden over and above the everyday challenges of becoming a young adult because achieving glycemic control may have a significant impact on daily life [21–24]. Clinicians working in both children's and adult services have raised concerns that young people transferring between services often fall through service gaps. Scott *et al.* [4] found that 90% of adolescent survey respondents had felt "lost in the shuffle" when making the transition from pediatric to adult diabetes services.

Adolescence is a time when many young people have not received adequate follow-up until a crisis has forced them back into the system [1,3,21]. Transition in this context was defined by Blum *et al.* [25] as "the purposeful, planned movement of adolescents with chronic physical and medical conditions from child-centred to adult-orientated health care systems." This definition has been widely applied within a wide spectrum of clinical practice, guidelines and research studies and focuses on the passage between two points within the health care system. The authors contend, however, that a broadening of this definition is needed because the adolescent's transitional process of inner reorientation also has to be considered in order to provide holistic care.

A systematic review conducted by Fleming *et al.* [21] highlighted the need for collaboration between children and adult services, particularly in light of the well-documented differences between these services [22,26–28]. Some of the differences between services have been identified as decreased parental involvement in adult services and significant differences in clinical practice and culture [29]. While it has been acknowledged that it is necessary for the children's and adult services to have different foci, it is argued that collaboration is needed to help bridge the gap so that transition is experienced by the adolescent as a smoother process [21,22].

Transition in the diabetes care setting

The process of transition in the diabetes care setting involves both the physical transfer of an adolescent from one health care setting to the other (pediatric to adult) as well as the acquisition and practice of self-management skills and the shift of responsibility of care from parent to adolescent. Transition therefore is not only the physical transfer of an individual moving between health services, but also the environmental, emotional and psychologic factors that are encompassed in this process. Transition is a progressive process that involves patient, health care provider and family or carer and effectively commences, in one dimension or another, once a child is diagnosed with diabetes.

Components of transition

It is useful for the purpose of understanding the complexities of transition to investigate the tasks that are accomplished when transition is successfully achieved. Successful transition involves the accomplishment of a number of tasks, as follows.

1 *Acquisition and practice of self-management skills.* The pediatric model of care assumes that young people lack the necessary practical and cognitive skills to undertake some of the tasks imperative to daily diabetes management, such as managing food intake, as well as the broader diabetes management tasks such as interacting with relevant health care professionals and keeping up-to-date with current knowledge. The process of transition involves the acquisition and practice of these skills by the patient, independent of parent or carer.

2 *Acquisition of skills necessary to maximize utility of the adult health care system.* Skills such as self-advocacy, the ability to find and negotiate services and knowledge about general young adult health issues such as substance abuse, mental health, exercise and sexual health prepare the adolescent for self-care [30].

3 *Shift of responsibility of care from parent to individual.* Responsibility of T1DM management must shift from the parent to the adolescent while maintaining an appropriate degree of parental interest and family cohesion [21,31]. Pediatricians who inappropriately foster persistent parental involvement risk promoting dependency in the patient [32]. It is important to note, however, that a shift of responsibility in diabetes management may be perceived as threatening by parent and patient and may result in feelings of neglect and anxiety. Therefore, both too much parental focus and too early a dismissal of parental responsibility can be disadvantageous to the transition process.

4 *Internalization of concept of illness.* Prior to transition, it is likely that responsibility of T1DM management belonged to one or both parents of the young person. Transition involves the shift of responsibility of care from parent to individual, and this shift may trigger or complete the process of internalization (consolidating and accepting illness), offsetting the degree of displacement that is implicit when responsibility of care does not belong to the patient themselves. Consequences of internalization can include loss of identity and subsequent reframing of identity at a time when identity is fluid and in the process of development, and loss of control and personal power, which is important for self-esteem. Again, this occurs during a developmental period when the individual may be struggling with self-esteem issues, because of physical changes and changes in peer significance.

5 *Integration of T1DM management tasks into emerging lifestyle.* In general, the period during which transfer occurs is a time when the adolescent or young adult is adopting a new lifestyle, for

example, leaving secondary school, moving – economically, geographically and emotionally – from the parental home, entering the workforce, attending university or traveling [31]. The adolescent or young adult must learn how to integrate their daily T1DM management tasks into their emerging new lifestyle.

6 *Physical transfer to an adult health care system.* The physical transfer to adult health care services requires the implementation of a specific set of diabetes management skills and knowledge as well as negotiation and self-advocacy skills that are not assumed in the pediatric health care system.

Adolescent needs during transition

Rarely have young people been asked what their needs are during transition. This is surprising given that the transition between diabetes services often occurs concurrently to the time of significant change in the adolescent's life.

A qualitative study undertaken by Visentin *et al.* [33] found that adolescents focused on the medical transfer of care during transition. The focus on medical care may be because many adolescents had not regularly seen any other health care professional. Adolescents stated they were interested in being introduced to the diabetes nurse educator and dietitian at the adult services [33]. Kipps *et al.* [3] reported a higher rate at attendance of adult services when the adolescent had met a member of the adult team before transfer which signifies the importance of prior contact and collaboration.

The precise needs of adolescents will vary according to culture and circumstances [34] and so research at the service level will be required to ensure services are tailored to need. Flexibility seems to be the key, because young people may be ready to transfer to adult services at different times, dependent on their cognitive and physical development, emotional maturity and general health [34]. The role of health professionals in this process is to tailor advice to young people based on their developmental and cognitive level [29].

During this transitional process, adolescents with diabetes need a shared understanding of their needs from their health care provider. This requires consultation with adolescents themselves [33], planning, ongoing contact and feedback between care providers in the two health care systems, and evaluation of services [35].

Promoting self-care

Promoting better management for adolescents with T1DM by developing their capacity to self-care through healthy choices prior to transition to adult services is an optimal goal. Gradual and early promotion of self-care is particularly important during adolescence when young people may try to act out behaviors in order to demonstrate independence. A cross-sectional multisite study of adolescents was conducted with 130 young people, studying factors that affect blood glucose control, such as how they care for themselves, eating problems, relationships, depression and health issues [36]. The research found that poor self-care, disturbed eating behavior, depression and peer relations were all associated with poor blood glucose control. Where there were good family relationships and support from parents, girls achieved better control than boys. The researchers suggest that further research should look at the reasons behind these relationships. The authors propose that monitoring of diabetes knowledge and promotion of self-efficacy from late childhood may optimize the transfer of self-care knowledge and behaviors from parents to adolescents [36].

Adolescence and young adulthood is characterized by a number of cognitive, emotional, behavioral and social changes that can present as barriers to effective self-management, including engagement with health care services. Cognitive changes include a shift in thinking from concrete to abstract and the ability to engage in introspection. These new cognitive skills give the ability to reflect on self-identity (self-concept and self-esteem). Adolescence is also a time of experimenting with new behaviors and, in particular, risk-taking behaviors. Socially, the importance of peers significantly increases at this time and concerns with being accepted by peer group are strong.

Successful transition can only be facilitated by provision of appropriate services, programs and resources. Long-term success is heavily dependent on instilling adequate self-care behaviors and self-advocacy skills so that adolescents can deal appropriately with external factors such as home, school and work life which may present as obstacles to effective diabetes management.

Education programs to promote self-care

A powerful predictor of good self-care is self-efficacy. For the purposes of this chapter, self-efficacy can been seen when adolescents have confidence in their capability to make decisions and take actions that demonstrate diabetes self-care. Education programs that enhance self-efficacy by incorporating personal health care goals and social and peer support have been shown to improve health outcomes and facilitate smooth transition in adolescents and young adults with T1DM [30]. Cook *et al.* [37] describe a pilot study demonstrating how the problem-solving behavior of adolescents with T1DM was improved through participation in a workshop style education program. The Choices Program consisted of six small weekly group workshop style sessions where adolescents came together to discuss major diabetes management problems, including psychosocial issues, and work together to identify solutions. This program demonstrated an increase in the practice of diabetes health care behaviors such as blood glucose monitoring and exercise. Cook *et al.* [37] identified three principles that are key to the success of an education program: parental involvement, integration with clinic (e.g. to allow implementation of regimen changes) and six or more sessions plus multiple follow-up and review sessions.

Education programs should be based on current learning and behavior change theories and should be developed with these key principles in mind. Furthermore, education programs should be part of standard care as well as specific elements in formal transition care programs.

Barriers and facilitators to successful transition

Many authors emphasize the need for collaboration between pediatric and adult diabetes services so as to create a smooth transition for adolescents [1,21,23,28,32]. These authors recommended that transition should be planned and coordinated [21,23,28,32]; however, the reality is that unless there is a transition program in place, adolescents transfer to adult services in an ad hoc manner with little planning, consultation or case management [33]. Hence, the absence of guidelines for the development, implementation and evaluation of transition programs must be viewed as a significant barrier to successful transition. Authors from Australia, the UK and the USA have called for the development of national policies that inform transition for adolescents with chronic conditions [1,21,23,28,32]. More recently, countries such as the UK, Australia and Canada either developed or made progress around developing standards and guidelines for policies in order to improve transition outcomes and experiences. For example, Diabetes Australia – Victoria is undertaking a project to develop a state-wide coordinated transition system for individuals living with T1DM. In addition, some professional organizations have developed best practice guidelines to inform the care of adolescents transferring to adult services. The successful translation of these guidelines into practice, however, remains unclear.

It has been acknowledged that transition to adult services can be difficult for a myriad of reasons. The most reported concern is the notable differences in the approach to care between children's and adult diabetes services. Children's services focus on the whole family and assume the child has little or no knowledge about diabetes and management. The adult sector take a more individual approach and assumes the patient has decision-making capacity and is knowledgable about diabetes and has the necessary skills to navigate the complex health system [26,28]. In addition, adult services expect a much greater degree of independence from young people and encourage communication without parents being present. It may be difficult for adolescents to adapt to this type of relationship, particularly when they have had a long-standing relationship with their pediatrician [22]. The adolescent may experience significant difficulty if the pediatric health care provider has not recognized the need to up-skill the adolescent in self-care behaviors before transfer to an adult service. A helpful approach to assist adolescents to transition is to focus on the location of the actual aspects that are changing, then to explore how the changes are being experienced by the individual, followed by consideration of how the person is responding or may respond [15].

Adult service staff may make the assumption that the adolescent has the necessary skills and maturity to be able to plan their future and have the insight to understand the consequences if they choose not to undertake diabetes self-care [21,22]. Viner [1] argued that adolescents are not served well by either model of diabetes care because the children's clinic may not acknowledge their growing independence while the adult clinic may not acknowledge their growth, development and family concerns. It has been recommended that transition be "a family affair" [27] and that transition in health care is acknowledged as only one aspect of a broader life transition that adolescents move through [1].

If the transition process is not meeting the needs of adolescents then they may choose to drop out of the system. While adolescents may continue to access a primary care physician for the prescription of insulin, it is thought that a multidisciplinary approach to diabetes care provides optimal management [38,39]. If diabetes is poorly managed, young adults are at an increased risk of microvascular and macrovascular complications as well as life-threatening acute complications such as diabetic ketoacidosis (DKA) [40].

The demands of diabetes may be experienced as difficult during the adolescent years and it has been documented that glycemic control at this life stage often deteriorates [21,22,41,42]. The deterioration in glycemic control is thought to be related to an increase in insulin resistance that relates to physiologic changes in puberty coupled with the psychosocial pressures associated with this period [41,42]. Of further concern, glycemic control in young people in the 16–25 year age group was found to be poorer than at other times during the lifespan [43].

The health professionals participating in the study of Visentin *et al.* [33] expressed concern about exposing adolescents to older people with type 2 diabetes, particularly if those older patients had obvious complications of diabetes such as amputations. Interestingly, adolescents claimed that such exposure was not an issue for them.

The experiences of adolescents with diabetes living in rural or remote areas have been rarely reported. There appears to be an assumption that adolescents have easy access to services; however, this may not be the case in many counties. In a study by Cameron *et al.* [44], adolescents in rural areas were found to have poorer outcomes than young adults from metropolitan areas, particularly in the areas of mental health, self-esteem and family cohesion. The authors considered a major factor in the differences in these outcomes was a lack of transition programs and other support services. Another factor was that adolescents with diabetes living in rural and remote areas may have less access to peers who also have diabetes, leading to a lack of peer support.

Models of transition care

While the literature has outlined principles for successful transition and made suggestions for model development, there is limited research that provides outcome data to support one model over another [1,3,30]. A study undertaken in the UK compared different models of transfer within one region using data generated through interviews and retrospective casenote review [3]. The models evaluated were:

1 Direct transfer to an adult clinic;
2 Transfer to a young adult clinic in a different hospital;
3 Transfer to a young adult clinic within the same hospital; and
4 Transfer to an adolescent clinic that was jointly operated by pediatricians and adult physicians.

The most significant declines in clinic attendance were observed when adolescents were either transferred to a young adult clinic in a different hospital or were transferred directly to an adult service. These adolescents were also the most dissatisfied with their care. Consistent with others studied, those adolescents lost to regular follow-up had higher mean HbA_{1c} levels. Variables such as socioeconomic status and geographic location were not included in the analysis. The authors concluded that transfer to a young adult clinic was preferable to direct transfer to an adult-only clinic and providing the opportunity to meet with staff from the adult service prior to transfer may improve outcomes [3].

Another UK-based study [26] surveyed adolescents who were attending an under 25-year-old-clinic. Interestingly, a high number of adolescents in this study did not report difficulties with transition; however, they did feel it would be helpful to have visited the clinic prior to transfer.

A study undertaken in Australia [45] surveyed adolescents aged between 15 and 18 years. The author concluded that a specific transition clinic can provide an important link and that transition needs to be a gradual process. Another study in Australia reported increased effectiveness when a coordinator worked with adolescents during the transition to adult care [46]. Schidlow and Fiel [27] discussed a transition clinic established in the USA where the pediatrician and adult physician conducted joint clinics in pediatrics as a stepping stone to the adult clinic. Unfortunately, there was no reported evaluation of this service.

There has been little qualitative research that has explored how adolescents experience transition. One recent Australian study researched the experiences of six young adults with cystic fibrosis using in-depth interviews [47]. The aim was to reveal the factors that contributed to the experience of transition and potential outcomes. A number of strategies were outlined that may improve the transition process with this patient group. These included a familiar face at adult clinics, orientation tours and the provision of written and verbal information as part of the transition program.

Table 52.1 provides a summary of the recommended stages of transition and includes specific recommendations for improving outcomes at each stage. Seven out of the eight stages of transition identified in Table 52.1 occur prior to transfer to an adult service and constitute the preparation phase (Phase 1). They focus largely on promoting self-care behaviors through education and practice. The stages are sequential, beginning at diagnosis and followed with a detailed introduction of the concepts of transition, assignment of a transition case manager, an assessment of the patient's diabetes and health knowledge, commencement of an education program, demonstration of learned skills and transfer to an adolescent/young adult transition clinic, where the young person is given the opportunity to practice learned skills before transfer to an adult service.

Transition case coordinator

There is sufficient evidence to suggest that successful transition can be facilitated by utilizing a transition case coordinator (TCC) and that the cost benefits from reduced hospital admissions otherwise secondary to preventable complications can cover the cost of establishing and running a TCC program [30,46]. TCCs have also been successfully utilized within juvenile idiopathic arthritis transition programs. An evaluation of a transition program delivered to adolescents and young adults with juvenile arthritis revealed that TCCs are highly valued by both patient and parent [30].

TCCs can be any health care professional with a high level of knowledge of T1DM and its complications as well as knowledge and experience in dealing with adolescents. This includes diabetes nurse educators, diabetes educators, primary care physicians or diabetes specialists such as endocrinologists. One of the most important characteristics of a TCC is the ability to communicate effectively with adolescents and young adults, and one might suggest this as a priority over in-depth knowledge of the condition itself. Research has demonstrated that positive results can be obtained through administrative non-medical case management [48].

The fundamental role of the TCC is to support the adolescent or young adult in becoming their own effective lifelong case manager, by ensuring that an increase in the patient's confidence and skills is a priority of the health care system in which the patient resides. In order to improve health outcomes, TCCs need to be clinically sophisticated advocates of evidence-based care. The tasks of the TCC are to coordinate clinic appointments, follow-ups and appointments with allied health professionals and to ensure accurate adequate information is provided to the patient in a timely manner. TCCs are also responsible for facilitating the patient's engagement with relevant community health organizations. It is the role of the TCC to attempt to re-engage "drop-outs" by identifying barriers to engagement and offering to reactivate and facilitate a referral to an appropriate health care professional or diabetes clinic.

A recent 5-year evaluation of a transition care program in a Sydney-based hospital demonstrated that a TCC program can increase clinic attendance and reduce HbA_{1c} and DKA-related hospital admissions [46]. The transition care program consisted of a TCC (a diabetes educator) who followed up bookings and missed appointments and provided an after-hours sick day phone service. The program also involved a primary care physician and a diabetes specialist. The cost savings from reduced hospital admissions covered the costs of the program. Interestingly, the evaluation revealed that the potential to lose contact with adolescents and young adults is greatest in the first few months after referral; 9 out of 10 young adults (mean age 18) lost to follow-up only attended one appointment.

The effectiveness of an administrative-based non-medical TCC has been demonstrated through evaluation of the Maestro Project, an administrative support and systems navigation service

Table 52.1 Recommended stages of transition.

Action	Description	Stage	Age	Practical and psychosocial achievements	Factors that facilitate success
Diagnosis	Introduction of concepts of illness and care to patient and family/carer Mental health support Introduction of concepts of transition (if age-appropriate) Mental health review	1	NA	Patient and family/carer progress effectively through stages of grief Patient and family/carer understand physical and psychosocial effects of illness Patient and family/carer have a broad notion of the concepts of transition	Information provided at diagnosis should be thorough and of immediate relevance Delivery of information should be by a health professional who is contactable for questions at a later time Incorporate a mental health professional into the diabetes management team who can facilitate understanding of psychosocial impact of illness
Introduction	Introduction of concepts of transition Interactive discussion with input from adolescent and parent, and case manager (see below)	2	12*	Dissemination of patient information First draft transition care plan	Transition care plan should consider and address age, gender and cultural issues
Case coordinator	Appoint a transition case coordinator to coordinate aspects of the process and act as key contact	2	12*	Professional relationship with adolescent and parent	Case coordinator should have significant knowledge of mental health and adolescent-specific issues
Knowledge assessment	Assessment of diabetes knowledge and self-management skills Mental health review	3	12–13*	Second draft care plan, incorporating outcomes of assessment, education goals and mental health review Address any mental health concerns	Transition care plan should consider and address age, gender and cultural issues
Education program	Basic diabetes management Skills development	4a	13–15*	Learning Self-efficacy, problem-solving	Group education including peers and family/carer
	Advanced diabetes management Adolescent-specific and general health issues Dietary review Solo consultations (in part)	4b	13–15*	Gaining independence Active participation in care with parents/carer Solo consultations with parent/carer involvement at end of consultation	Parental/peer involvement Integration with clinic Six or more sessions plus multiple follow-up and review sessions

Continued on p. 882

Table 52.1 *Continued.*

Action	Description	Stage	Age	Practical and psychosocial achievements	Factors that facilitate success
Demonstration	Demonstration of learning outcomes	5a	15–17*	Internalization of concept of illness is complete Adolescent is self-managing Adolescent is self-advocating Solo consultations (with parent/carer involvement at end of consultation if deemed necessary) Responsibility of care has shifted from parent to adolescent/young adult	
	Decide on suitable model of transfer, i.e. private vs. public, transition clinic vs. adult clinic Establish adult diabetes management team	5b	15–17*	Third draft care plan incorporating developed skills and health care goals with patient input Professional relationship with adolescent/young adult transition clinic staff, implying multiple visits to transition clinic	Final diabetes management plan should align health care goals with other life goals
Transfer to adolescent/ young adult clinic	Physical transfer to adolescent/young adult transition clinic to enable patient to practice acquired skills	6	15–25*	Solo consultations Demonstration of acquired skills	Transition clinic staff met prior to transfer First appointment arranged by transition case manager and followed-up Any issues identified addressed immediately
Transfer to adult service	Physical transfer to chosen adult care provider	7	*	Physical transfer to chosen adult care provider	Adult staff met prior to transfer First appointment arranged by transition case manager and followed-up Any issues identified addressed immediately
Support, follow-up and evaluation	Transition case manager provides support and follows up with adolescent/young adult to discuss transition, concerns, etc.	8	*	Minimum 6-monthly follow-ups (2 per year) for 2 years post-transfer	Use multiple vehicles for follow-up, including formal letters via post, telephone calls and SMS reminders

*Age is indicator only. Progression to subsequent stage should occur when it is deemed appropriate by health professional, patient and family/carer.

available to adolescents and young adults aged 18–35 years with T1DM in the province of Manitoba, Canada [49]. The program, Building Connections: The Maestro Project, commenced in 2002 and consists of biannual telephone and email contact by the Maestro, a non-medical TCC who facilitates connections and appointments with relevant health care professionals and follows up bookings and missed appointments. The program also consists of a website through which program participants can locate local services and other relevant educational materials, an e-newsletter, a casual evening drop-in support group and evening group educational dinner events.

The Maestro Project's 2007 Annual Report reveals that the program has significantly increased engagement with health care services. Of the 101 young adults who were referred to the Maestro Project after they had been transferred to an adult service, medical engagement increased from 59.4% having had one or more visits to an endocrinologist to 73.3% after 1 year in the program. Engagement with a diabetes educator also increased, from 25.7% having had one or more visits, to 41.6%. The program has dramatically reduced drop-out rates in the province, from 40.6% to 10.9% [49]. The Maestro Project is one example of how even basic administrative non-medical transition case management can improve outcomes for adolescents and young adults, in terms of increasing their engagement with the adult health care system.

Successful transition: an adolescent perspective

Many studies have identified factors expressed by adolescents and young adults as important for successful transition. A study by the Royal District Nursing Service Research Unit in South Australia [33] revealed that factors most important to adolescents and young adults include feeling secure, safe and trusting (of health care professionals), gaining independence and being able to access accurate and up-to-date information easily. Additionally, earlier discussions on transition and meeting adult staff prior to transfer are two steps that have been consistently reported by adolescents and young adults, not only in the diabetes health care sector but across many chronic illnesses including cystic fibrosis, juvenile rheumatoid arthritis and sickle cell disease [50]. Studies by Court [45] and Scott *et al.* [4] identified several factors as important to adolescents and young adults progressing through transition (Table 52.2). Furthermore, study participants have identified that endocrinologists, dietitians and primary care physician were the top three most important health professionals to have at a transition clinic [4].

Table 52.2 Factors that facilitate transition to adult services.

Preparation process
Earlier discussions surrounding transition
Autonomy and self-direction – 71% of study respondents wanted to set goals with their adult health care team [4]
Important education topics
Research
Stress management
Financial assistance
Cooking
Complications (without direct exposure, as occurs in adult clinics)
Consultation and staff issues
Visits to adult clinic prior to transfer
Longer initial meetings with adult center staff
Ability to talk about personal issues
Continuity of care
Transfer and clinic environment
Clinics not located in a hospital setting
Ideal young adult clinic ages 18–30 years and separate from adult clinic
Evening clinics and opportunities for "drop-in" appointments
Interaction with peers and peer support

Transition in practice

The most effective approach to the transition process is one that is organized and sensitive to the needs of the individual adolescent and family. There is evidence to suggest that a health worker dedicated to facilitate transition between services can have a positive impact on young people [29]. Adolescents in transition from children's to adult diabetes services are involved in a period of critical but forced change. There are variations in the way adolescents engage or fail to engage in transitional processes. For example, adaptation to change often involves undertaking a process of trial and error [10] so that individuals can determine and understand the ways they are responding to change. Sometimes when young people undertake a process of trial and error, health workers may consider that they are engaging in risky behaviors. This may create a problem-orientated approach for adolescents rather than a preventive model of care that may inhibit the promotion of self-care.

Dalton and Gottlieb [51] explored the concept of readiness to embrace change, which they argued was often linked with a person's compliance to a medical regimen. By contrast, previous research revealed that living with long-term illness appears to be about incorporating the consequences of illness into everyday life [10,52]. Dalton and Gottlieb [51] provided an alternative view that conceptualized readiness as a process of *becoming* ready over time. Readiness to change was embedded within a process of learning. Baker and Stern [53] described a process of readiness that involved making the illness a part of life and coming to terms with self-care teaching and having a sense of control. Relationship-building between health care professionals and adolescents, as a means for mapping individual context and identifying shifting values over time, dealing with difference and miscommunication, is perhaps the first step to facilitating this transition.

There have been a number of studies that found that adolescents were keen to receive written and verbal information about transition and that they wanted to be provided with opportunities to meet the new team prior to transition [3,26,45,47]. It is necessary for a transition model to take into account the stakeholders' views (professional, parents and clients). Transition literature from the diabetes and cystic fibrosis fields agree that there is a lack of outcome data that can clearly support one model over another [1,21,32]. Suggestions such as young adult clinics, stepped transition, joint clinics with pediatricians and adult physicians and transition nurses have all been described in the literature.

Health professionals and adolescents in the study by Visentin *et al.* [33] highlighted that transition is frequently focused on the medical transfer of care with the allied health teams having a minor role. Of the four children's services participating in their study, only one had a recall system established to offer adolescents regular education updates at designated intervals. Similarly, only one of the adult services had an established pathway in place to ensure that all of the adolescents were offered dietitian and diabetes nurse educator appointments at the time of the transition. Furthermore, health care professionals reported a poor uptake of these appointments. The ramifications of these findings, which have been replicated in other studies, are that adolescents are not receiving holistic preparation for transition in terms of developing self-management skills required for adaptation to an adult health setting. Adolescents in Visentin *et al.*'s [33] study were keen to be given opportunities to meet staff prior and receive written information. Transition might be easier if adolescents were involved in early planning and informed about what to expect from the adult service and how it may differ to the pediatric service.

Research studies have revealed that transition to adult services is often based on the medical model. Transition needs to be viewed holistically as opposed to focusing solely on the referral from one medical doctor to another. A problem-focused or reactive approach to diabetes care effectively relinquishes the potential for independence and control for the adolescent. If nurses and dietitians are only involved during periods of diabetes instability, then adolescents may not be provided opportunity to learn self-care skills. T1DM is often a family issue with reliance upon parents for information and advice. It is important that diabetes nurses and dietitians become involved in working with adolescents towards self-care as many were diagnosed as children and may never have received first-hand information about diabetes.

The role of diabetes nurse educators in preparation and facilitation of the transition process and follow-up has not been fully realized. Preparation needs to be expanded so that there is a larger focus on developing self-care skills. This approach would assist individuals in taking on the extra responsibilities expected by adult services. Frank [22] stated that a gradual preparation of both youth and parents is an important principle for transition. Blum *et al.* [25] argued that the notion of transition should be discussed as early as diagnosis. One of the transition principles advocated by Rosen *et al.* [32] is to have a designated health professional to coordinate the transition process between children's and adult diabetes services. Diabetes nurse educators are in an excellent position to undertake this role.

Care plans to facilitate a coordinated and planned transition process have been proposed by Weissberg-Benchell *et al.* [31]. The care plans should be developed in consultation with the adolescent and parents, and incorporate all aspects of the transition process such as identifying information regarding specific health services, appointments, and health and education goal planning; however, the effectiveness of the use of care planning as a process to facilitate seamless transition and improve outcomes for adolescents does not appear to have been evaluated.

The optimal goal of transition between services is to provide health care that is uninterrupted, coordinated and developmentally appropriate. The value of early preparation in late childhood from a multidisciplinary team is important for transition. To summarize the evidence, it is proposed that transition programs contain the following elements:

- Early introduction to adolescents of the concept of transition;
- Based on capacity building principles and promotion of confidence and independence and self-advocacy skills;
- Both the pediatric and adult diabetes services have a documented transition program for adolescents;
- Transition care plans incorporating all elements of the transition process;
- Timing of the transition based on maturity and skill rather than age;
- A senior member of the clinical staff from each service is responsible for the successful implementation and maintenance of the transition program;
- A designated professional, who collaborates with the adolescent and family, takes responsibility for the transition of each adolescent;
- The transition program has a multidisciplinary focus with input from consumers, primary care and allied health professionals;
- Adolescents are encouraged to develop a relationship with their primary care physician;
- The transition program should include the details of the process of transition, the expected outcomes and evaluation processes;
- The transition program should promote individualized plans for each adolescent inclusive of expected outcomes and timeframes, opportunity for the adolescent to have a voice in articulating their needs, early involvement with the adult team, opportunity for adolescents and their families to meet with new carers, opportunities to meet with other adolescents who have successfully transitioned to adult services, and access to psychosocial support for adolescents experiencing difficulty in the transition;
- All staff, including clerical and administrative staff as well as clinicians, should be educated in the philosophies and features of the transition program. Parents and children should also have the purpose and principles of structured transition explained and have access to details of the program well before transition commences;
- Include opportunity to address common concerns of adolescents such as growth and development, sexuality, mood and mental health, substance misuse and other high risk behaviors.

Information and communication technology

Modern information and communication technologies such as the Internet and mobile phones have the capacity to provide a unique and effective method of delivering support to adolescents and young adults with chronic illness. Adolescents and young adults are at the developmental age where new technologies are quickly and easily integrated into peer culture and daily life. A study by Rasmussen *et al.* [54] revealed that young women with T1DM use the Internet not only as a means of obtaining information and communicating with others, but also as a means by which to achieve a sense of autonomy and stability.

Text messaging has been recently used in the UK as a way to support young adults with diabetes to achieve goals [55]. The text message provides a weekly reminder of the goal set during clinic, with follow-up messages that reinforce the goal by providing information and reminders. The aim of the program is to optimize self-efficacy and motivate health enhancing behaviors. The program is based on the principles of social cognitive theory and has demonstrated improved metabolic control among participating adolescents [55].

The Internet offers many communication forums that adolescents will be familiar with. Websites, chat forums and various messaging systems are popular and have enormous potential for information sharing and education. For example, Twitter is a free social networking forum that enables users to send and read other users' updates known as "tweets." Tweets are text-based posts and could be used to support self-care and goal achievement for adolescents with diabetes.

There is also major potential for modern technologies such as advanced videoconferencing to provide isolated patients, including those in rural areas, with convenient access to specialist health professionals. The Centre for Online Health commenced a research project in 2000 that aimed to establish and evaluate a telepediatric service in Queensland, Australia [56]. The service operates using a centralized coordination unit, and services regional and remote hospitals. The telepediatric service provides access to specialist pediatric services. A response to the referring clinician is guaranteed within 24 hours. In the first 6 years, more than 4000 consultations were coordinated through the telepediatric service. The consultations have concerned a wide variety of fields including diabetes, endocrinology, burns, cardiology, dermatology, oncology, orthopedics, gastroenterology, neurology and pediatric surgery. A range of communication techniques are used for communicating including email, telephone and videoconferencing. Approximately 90% of referrals result in a consultation via videoconference. The service has demonstrated a significant increase in the number of children accessing specialist services. This type of technology also has significant potential to support adolescents living in rural and remote areas through transition to adult services.

Quality processes

Key performance and clinical indicators developed locally have been identified as being essential for the governance of transition processes [34]. For example, the Australian Clinical Practice Guidelines: Type 1 Diabetes in Children and Adolescents [57] described three phases of transition: preparation, formal transition and evaluation. The guidelines recommend that the preparation phase commences from 12 years of age; however, it is unclear if such early planning actually takes place because evaluation of transition programs has rarely been reported. The findings from studies such as Visentin *et al.* [33] indicated that the three stages of transition programs are often not being fully implemented in health units.

Evaluation of transition programs may include but not be limited to undertaking a satisfaction survey of adolescent clients and their parents, to determine if they are happy with the service, they were able to adopt the treatment regimen, felt involved in and informed about the transition process and attended follow-up appointments [34]. When auditing, it is recommended to consider the availability and effectiveness of policy detailing transition processes and principles, a multidisciplinary education program, processes to enhance coordination between programs and administration and documentation [34]. In summary, some key evaluation measures include:

- Development and documentation of a structured transition program with established review dates;
- Percent of adolescents transitioning with an individualized plan;
- Adolescent and parental satisfaction; and
- Percent of adolescents attending follow-up after 12 months.

Future research

A body of knowledge has developed that has focused on the transition processes, models and adolescent experiences; however, further research is required to enhance our understanding of how best to serve adolescents with diabetes. For example, several studies have explored how developmental stage and lifestyle impact an adolescents' transition and outcomes but research exploring factors such as ethnicity, socioeconomic status, geographic location (e.g. rural and remote) and gendered experiences have not been reported. Rigorous evaluation of variations in transition programs is also needed to inform future program development that promotes long-term engagement with the health system. The promotion of self-care for adolescents with diabetes is an area that would benefit from focused research. There is currently little understanding of care approaches that increase the effectiveness of self-care strategies in adolescents. In addition, research into how to access and re-engage adolescents who drop out of the health care system is urgently needed.

Further research into how modern technologies, resources and networks can be exploited to provide support to adolescents in transition is also necessary. For example, there is potential for developing and implementing an online transition resource that can be integrated into service coordination tools used by health care providers.

Conclusions

Adolescents in transition from pediatric to adult diabetes services are experiencing forced change. Adolescents with diabetes establish a long-term positive bond with their pediatric health care team, so that the transition to an adult diabetes service provider is a significant event in their lives. Evidence has revealed the major elements of successful transition programs; however, there is a need to evaluate the effectiveness of the various transition models. Promoting better management for adolescents with T1DM by developing their capacity to self-care prior to transition to adult services is an optimal goal. There is significant potential to improve practice and outcomes through establishment of transition programs for adolescents with diabetes.

References

1 Viner R. Transition from paediatric to adult care: bridging the gaps or passing the buck? *Arch Dis Child* 1999; **81**:271–275.

2 Nakhla M, Daneman D, Frank M, Guttmann A. Translating transition: a critical review of the diabetes literature. *J Pediatr Endocrinol Metab* 2008; **21**:507–516.

3 Kipps S, Bahu T, Ong K, Ackland FM, Brown RS, Foxt CT, *et al.* Current methods of transfer of young people with type 1 diabetes to adult services. *Diabet Med* 2002; **19**:649–654.

4 Scott L, Vallis M, Charette M, Murray A, Latta R. Transition of care: researching the needs of young adults with type 1 diabetes. *Can J Diabetes* 2005; **29**:203–210.

5 Bridges W. *Transitions: Making Sense of Life's Changes.* Cambridge, MA: Da Capo Press, 2004.

6 Kralik D, Visentin K, van Loon AM. Transition: a literature review. *J Adv Nurs* 2006; **55**:320–329.

7 Kralik D. Transition: qualitative research with people who live with chronic illness and pain. A Satellite Symposium of the 11th World Congress on Pain. Cairns, Australia: 2005.

8 Cantanzaro M. Transitions in midlife adults with long-term illness. *Holistic Nurs Pract* 1990; **4**:65–73.

9 Chick N, Meleis AI. Transitions: a nursing concern. In: Chinn PL, ed. *Nursing Research Methodology: Issues and Implementation.* Aspen: Rockville MD, 1986:237–257.

10 Kralik D. The quest for ordinariness: transition experienced by midlife women living with chronic illness. *J Adv Nurs* 2002; **39**: 146–154.

11 Loveys B. Transitions in chronic illness: the at-risk role. *Holistic Nurs Pract* 1990; **4**:56–64.

12 Meleis AI, Sawyer LM, Im E-O, Hilfinger Messias DK, Schumacher K. Experiencing transitions: an emerging middle-range theory. *Adv Nurs Sci* 2000; **23**:12–28.

13 Meleis AI, Trangenstein PA. Facilitating transitions: redefinition of the nursing mission. *Nurs Outlook* 1994; **42**:255–259.

14 Schumacher KL, Meleis AI. Transitions: a central concept in nursing. *Image J Nurs Sch* 1994; **26**:119–127.

15 van Loon AM, Kralik D. *Facilitating Transition for Survivors of Child Sexual Abuse.* Adelaide, Australia: Royal District Nursing Service Foundation Research Unit, Catherine House Inc, Alcohol Education and Rehabilitation Foundation, 2005.

16 Bartsocas C. From adolescence to adulthood: the transition from child to adult care. *Diabetes Voice* 2007; **52**:15–17.

17 Christian BJ, D'Auria JP, Fox LC. Gaining freedom: self-responsibility in adolescents with diabetes. *Pediatr Nurs* 1999; **25**:255–266.

18 Urbach S, LaFranchi S, Lambert L, Lapidus J, Daneman D, Becker T. Predictors of glucose control in children and adolescents with type 1 diabetes mellitus. *Pediatr Diabetes* 2005; **6**:69–74.

19 Ball G, Huang T, Gower B, Cruz M, Shaibi G, Weigensberg M, *et al.* Longitudinal changes in insulin sensitivity, insulin secretion and beta-cell function during puberty. *J Pediatr* 2006; **148**:16–22.

20 Goyder E, Spiers N, McNally P, Drucquer M, Botha J. Do diabetes clinic attendees stay out of hospital? A matched case–control study. *Diabetes Med* 1999; **16**:687–691.

21 Fleming E, Carter B, Gillibrand W. The transition of adolescents with diabetes from the children's health care service into the adult health care service: a review of the literature. *J Clin Nurs* 2002; **11**:560–567.

22 Frank M. Rights to passage: transition from paediatric to adult diabetes care. *Beta Release* 1992; **16**:85–89.

23 Blum RW. Transition to adult health care: setting the stage. *J Adolesc Health* 1994; **17**:3–5.

24 McGill M. How do we organize smooth, effective transfer from paediatric to adult diabetes care? *Horm Res* 2002; **57**(Suppl 1):66–68.

25 Blum RW, Garell D, Hodgman CH, Jorissen TW, Okinow NA, Orr DP, *et al.* Transition from child-centred to adult health-care systems for adolescents with chronic conditions. *J Adolesc Health* 1993; **14**:570–576.

26 Eiser C, Flynn M, Green E, Havermans T, Kirby R, Sandeman D, *et al.* Coming of age with diabetes: patients' views of a clinic for under-25 year olds. *Diabet Med* 1992; **10**:185–289.

27 Schidlow DV, Fiel SB. Transition of chronically ill adolescents from pediatric to adult health care systems. *Med Clin North Am* 1990; **74**:1113–1120.

28 Sawyer SM, Blair S, Bowes G. Chronic illness in adolescents: transfer or transition to adult services. *J Pediatr Child Health* 1997; **33**:88–90.

29 Jones S, Hamilton S. The missing link: paediatric to adult transition in diabetes services. *Br J Nurs* 2008; **17**:842–847.

30 McDonagh J, Viner R. Lost in transition? Between paediatric and adult services. *Br Med J* 2006; **332**:435–436.

31 Weissberg-Benchell J, Wolpert H, Anderson B. Transitioning from pediatric to adult care: a new approach to the post-adolescent young person with type 1 diabetes. *Diabetes Care* 2007; **30**:2441–2446.

32 Rosen DS, Blum RW, Britto M, Sawyer SM, Siegel DM. Transition to adult health care for adolescents and young adults with chronic illness. *J Adolesc Health* 2003; **33**:309–311.

33 Visentin K, Koch T, Kralik D. Adolescents with type 1 diabetes: transition between diabetes services. *J Clin Nurs* 2006; **15**:761–769.

34 Royal College of Nursing. Adolescent transition care. 2004. http://www.rcn.org.uk/__data/assets/pdf_file/0011/78617/002313.pdf. Accessed April 30, 2009.

35 Lundin C, Danielson E, Ohrn I. Handling the transition of adolexcents with diabetes: participant observations and interviews with care providers in pediatric and adult diabetes outpatient clinics. *Int J Integr Care* 2007; **7**:1–10.

36 Helgeson V, Siminerio L, Escobar O, Becker D. Predictors of metabolic control among adolescents with diabetes: a 4-year longitudinal study. *J Pediatr Psychol* 2009; **34**:254–270.

37 Cook S, Herold K, Edidin D, Briars R. Increasing problem solving in adolescents with type 1 diabetes: the choices diabetes program. *Diabetes Educator* 2002; **28**:115–124.

38 Department of Human Services. *The Strategic Plan for Diabetes in South Australia*. 1999.

39 Parsons J, Wilson D, Scardigno A. *The Impact of Diabetes in South Australia*. South Australian Department of Human Services, 2000.

40 Diabetes Control and Complications Trial (DCCT) Research Group. The effect of intensive treatment of diabetes on the development and progression of long-term complications in insulin-dependent diabetes mellitus. *N Engl J Med* 1993; **329**:977–986.

41 Bryden KS, Peveler RC, Stein A, Neil A, Mayou RA, Dunger DB. Clinical and psychological course of diabetes from adolescence to young adulthood: a Longitudinal Cohort Study. *Diabetes Care* 2001; **24**:1536–1540.

42 Silink M, Clarke C, Couper JJ, Craig M, Crock P, Davies R, *et al.* Adolescent health. In: *Australian Clinical Practice Guidelines: Type 1 Diabetes in Children and Adolescents*. 2003–2004: 176.

43 Wills CJ, Scott A, Swift PGF, Davies MJ, Mackie ADR, Mansell P. Retrospective review of care and outcomes in young adults with type 1 diabetes. *Br Med J* 2003; **327**:260–261.

44 Cameron F, Clarke C, Hesketh K, White E, Boyce D, Dalton V, *et al.* Regional and urban Victorian diabetic youth: clinical and quality of life outcomes. *J Pediatr Health* 2002; **38**:593–596.

45 Court JM. Issues of transition to adult care. *J Pediatr Child Health* 1993; **29**(Suppl 1):53–55.

46 Holmes-Walker D, Llewellyn A, Farrell K. A transition care program which improves diabetes control and reduces hospital admission rates in young adults with type 1 diabetes aged 15–25 years. *Diabetes Med* 2007; **24**:764–769.

47 Brumfield K, Lansbury G. Experiences of adolescents with cystic fibrosis during their transition from paediatric to adult health acre: a qualitative study of young Australian adults. *Disabil Rehabil* 2004; **26**:223–234.

48 Svoren B, Butler D, Levine B, Anderson B, Laffel L. Reducing acute adverse outcomes in youths with type 1 diabetes: a randomised controlled trial. *Pediatrics* 2003; **112**:914–922.

49 Van Walleghem N, MacDonald C, Dean H. Building connections for young adults with type 1 diabetes mellitus in Manitoba: feasibility and acceptability of a transition initiative. *Chron Dis Canada* 2006; **27**:130–134.

50 Tuchman L, Slap G, Britto M. Transition to adult care: experiences and expectations of adolescents with a chronic illness. *Child Care Health Dev* 2008; **34**:557–563.

51 Dalton CC, Gottlieb LN. The concept of readiness to change. *J Adv Nurs* 2003; **42**:108–117.

52 Kralik D, Koch T, Price K, Howard N. Chronic illness self-management: taking action to create order. *J Clin Nurs* 2004; **13**:259–267.

53 Baker C, Stern P. Finding meaning in chronic illness and the key to self care. *Can J Nurs Res* 1993; **25**:23–36.

54 Rasmussen B, Dunning P, O'Connell B. Young women with diabetes: using Internet communication to create stability during life transitions. *J Clin Nurs* 2007; **16**:17–24.

55 Franklin V, Greene A, Waller A, Greene S, Pagliari C. Patients engagement with "sweet Talk": a text messaging support system for young people with diabetes. *J Med Internet Res* 2008; **10**:e20.

56 Smith AC, Scuffham P, Wootton R. The costs and potential savings of a novel telepaediatric service in Queensland. *BMC Health Services Research* 2007; **7**:35.

57 Australasian Paediatric Endocrine Group for the Department of Health and Ageing. *Clinical Practice Guidelines: Type 1 Diabetes in Children and Adolescents*. Australian Government and National Health and Medical Research Council, 2005.

53 Diabetes in Pregnancy

Anne Dornhorst[1] & Anita Banerjee[2]

[1] Department of Medicine, Imperial College Healthcare NHS Trust, Hammersmith Hospital, London, UK
[2] Diabetes and Endocrinology, Princess Royal University Hospital, London, UK

Keypoints

- The number of women with diabetes becoming pregnant is increasing, in line with the increase in type 2 diabetes (T2DM) among women of reproductive age. Rising obesity levels are also contributing to the increasing number of women developing glucose intolerance during pregnancy.
- Perinatal mortality and morbidity is increased in diabetic pregnancies, mainly through increased stillbirths and congenital malformations rates, which are three- to fivefold higher than in non-diabetic pregnancies.
- Metabolic changes occur in pregnancy to facilitate nutrient transfer to the fetus. Maternal insulin resistance helps divert glucose to the fetus. Women with pre-gestational diabetes have insufficient insulin to counter the rise in insulin resistance and require increasing insulin therapy during pregnancy. Women without diabetes before pregnancy become glucose intolerant in pregnancy if they have insufficient insulin reserves.
- Maternal diabetes affects all aspects of pregnancy from conception to the timing and mode of birth. The major early effects are on embryogenesis and the risk of malformations. Glycemic control is critical at this time as glucose is teratogenic to the developing embryo.
- Maternal diabetes affects fetal pancreatic islets and β-cell development which may be a factor in the increased risk of diabetes among children of mothers with diabetes.
- Fetal insulin is an important fetal growth factor and accelerated fetal growth occurs in many diabetic pregnancies as a consequence of maternal hyperglycemia causing fetal hyperinsulinemia. This metabolic environment in later pregnancy may render the fetus susceptible to hypoxia and acidosis and ultimately stillbirth. It also increases the risk of transient neonatal hypoglycemia.
- Good maternal diabetic control lessens the risk to the fetus of malformations, accelerated fetal growth, stillbirth and neonatal hypoglycemia as well as the risk of future obesity and diabetes for the child.
- Pregnancy poses certain risks for the mother with diabetes. Any detrimental effects on retinopathy and nephropathy, however, are limited to those women with significant clinical disease beforehand and are usually self-limiting.
- Proteinuria and microalbuminuria are risk factors for pre-eclampsia and preterm birth.
- Pregnancy in women with underlying cardiovascular disease (CVD) is associated with maternal morbidity and mortality. CVD is likely to increase as more older women with T2DM give birth.
- The increasing prevalence of maternal obesity is having an increasing impact on maternal and fetal pregnancy outcomes.
- The clinical care of women with pre-gestational diabetes and those with previous gestational diabetes mellitus (GDM) should begin before pregnancy. Women who receive pre-pregnancy care have better pregnancy outcomes and it remains a major clinical challenge to ensure that more women with diabetes are properly prepared for pregnancy.
- Preparations include the need to optimize glycemic control, to ensure folic acid supplementation and to stop all unsafe medications for pregnancy. Women should be screened for retinopathy and nephropathy before pregnancy and given relevant information concerning risks to themselves and any unborn child.
- Antenatal management should focus on achieving maternal glucose levels as near to normal as safely possible and close maternal and fetal surveillance for medical and obstetric complications. National evidence-based clinical guidelines for diabetes in pregnancy should be followed to ensure all women have access to the best available care.
- Women at risk of GDM should be screened at 28 weeks' gestation using a 75-g oral glucose tolerance test (OGTT) and the World Health Organization criteria for impaired glucose tolerance.
- Treatment for GDM includes diet and exercise and the use of metformin, glibenclamide or insulin if glucose values cannot be maintained with diet and exercise alone.
- Both women with pre-gestational diabetes and GDM should be offered induction of labor at 38 completed weeks' gestation to reduce the risk of a late stillbirth and the risk of birth injury in a large for gestational age infant. Insulin requirements fall to pre-pregnancy values in the immediate postpartum period and should therefore be reduced.
- The use of insulin pumps, continuous glucose monitors and the basal analog insulin is increasing in clinical practice; however, their use still needs to be fully evaluated in pregnancy.

Textbook of Diabetes, 4th edition. Edited by R. Holt, C. Cockram, A. Flyvbjerg and B. Goldstein.

- Following birth, early breastfeeding reduces the risk of neonatal hypogylcemia and all mothers with diabetes should be encouraged to breastfeed within 30 minutes of birth and then every 3–4 hours until a regular feeding pattern is established.
- Women with GDM should be screened for diabetes before leaving hospital, 6 weeks postpartum and then annually. In low risk populations, a fasting blood glucose value is sufficient and is likely to be associated with greater long-term compliance than an OGTT. All women with a history of GDM should receive lifestyle advice to lessen their long-term risk of future diabetes.

Introduction

Diabetes in pregnancy poses serious problems for both mother and fetus and has long-term health implications for the child. The number of pregnant women with pre-gestational and gestational diabetes mellitus (GDM) is increasing, mainly because of the increasing prevalence of obesity in women of childbearing age.

Despite advances in our scientific knowledge and understanding of the effects of diabetes on fetal growth and development, and improvements in fetal and maternal care, pregnancy outcomes are broadly similar to 1989, when the St. Vincent Declaration pledged to improve pregnancy outcomes to those of women without diabetes [1]. Even in highly developed health care systems, stillbirths and congenital malformations remain three- to fivefold higher than in non-diabetic pregnancies.

Improving pregnancy outcomes depends on improving glycemic control from conception to birth. Newer technologies involving glucose monitoring and insulin pumps may bring promise for the future, but the real challenge today is to ensure all women with diabetes begin their pregnancies well prepared and with optimal glycemic control.

The largest audit of diabetic pregnancies including all 3808 pregnancies of women with type 1 (T1DM) and type 2 diabetes mellitus (T2DM) who delivered or booked in 231 hospitals in England, Wales and Northern Ireland from March 1, 2002 to February 28, 2003 was published in 2005 [2]. These women accounted for 0.38% of all births at this time and provide much of the epidemiologic data in this chapter.

A confidential enquiry reviewing the demographic, social and lifestyle factors and clinical care in 521 pregnancies to women in the original audit was published subsequently [3]. This enquiry included 127 pregnancies with a fetal congenital anomaly, 95 pregnancies with fetal or neonatal death of a normally formed baby, 220 pregnancies with a good outcome and 79 pregnancies in women with T2DM and provides valuable clinical data pertaining to pregnancy outcomes.

The American Diabetic Association (ADA) [4] and the National Institute for Health and Clinical Excellence (NICE) [5] published guidelines on the clinical management of women with pre-existing diabetes in pregnancy in 2008. The clinical guidelines in this chapter are based on these two consensus evidence-based guidelines.

Clinical science and epidemiology of diabetes in pregnancy

Classification of diabetes in pregnancy

The classification of diabetes is discussed in Chapter 2. A uniform classification of diabetic pregnancies is still needed for both epidemiologic and clinical purposes.

Diabetes is recognized as a heterogeneous condition [6] and while most women with pre-gestational diabetes in pregnancy will have T1DM or T2DM, a few will have monogenetic and mitochondrial forms of diabetes, while others will have secondary causes, such as cystic fibrosis. Correctly identifying the type of diabetes during pregnancy can be difficult, especially when the woman is diagnosed with diabetes during pregnancy, as some may be in the early phases of T1DM [7,8], others may have previously undiagnosed T2DM [9], while the most of the remainder have diabetes induced by pregnancy.

Pregnancy may be the first time that asymptomatic forms of monogenetic diabetes are diagnosed, as they are often present in the second and third decade [10,11]. This is true for maturity-onset diabetes of the young (MODY) caused by a mutation in the glucokinase gene (see Chapter 15). While the prevalence of this form of MODY may be less than 2% for the total antenatal population, screening selected women can increase the likelihood of finding a glucokinase gene mutation to approximately 80% in a white population. Clinical features that may suggest MODY includes a combination of:

- Fasting hyperglycemia outside pregnancy (5.5–8 mmol/L);
- A small blood glucose rise (<4.6 mmol/L) during a 2-hour oral glucose tolerance test (OGTT);
- A requirement for insulin treatment during one or more earlier pregnancies but controlled on diet subsequently;
- A first-degree relative with a history of T2DM;
- GDM or fasting hyperglycemia during pregnancy (>5.5 mmol/L) [11].

Many of the fetal complications of a diabetic pregnancy are a direct result of maternal hyperglycemia and therefore are more dependent on glycemic control than the type of maternal diabetes. By contrast, the medical, obstetric and social risk factors differ between women with T1DM and T2DM. Understanding these differences is important for optimizing pregnancy care [3].

The CEMACH audit assessed the outcomes of 3808 pregnancies in 2767 (73%) women with T1DM and 1041 (27%) women with T2DM. Perinatal mortality, stillbirth, neonatal mortality and congenital anomaly rates were similar for both types of diabetes [2]; however, there were significant differences in pre-pregnancy planning, obesity, social deprivation, risks of recurrent and severe hypoglycemia and retinopathy, all of which may affect clinical care before and after pregnancy. Less than 1% (0.73%) of pregnancies were in women identified as either having MODY or another or unknown cause for their diabetes [2].

GDM is defined as glucose intolerance occurring or first recognized during pregnancy [12]. In the general non-diabetic antenatal population, there is no cut off between adverse pregnancy outcomes and either fasting or the 1 or 2-hour OGTT blood glucose values. The Hyperglycemia and Adverse Pregnancy Outcomes study (HAPO) performed 25 505 75-g OGTTs at 24–32 weeks' gestation in women without diabetes and found a continuous relationship between maternal glucose concentrations and increased birth weight and increased cord-blood serum C-peptide levels; both of these measures are surrogate markers for fetal exposure to maternal glucose [13]. These associations occurred at glucose levels below those currently used to diagnose GDM.

Women who develop impaired glucose tolerance (IGT) during pregnancy, share common diabetic risk alleles [14] and have similar insulin secretory defects [15] to women with T2DM. Many of these women develop T2DM in later life [16]. For these reasons, GDM can be considered a forerunner of T2DM, with the caveat that some women diagnosed with GDM are in the preclinical phase of T1DM or have other rarer forms of diabetes.

Historically, the best known classification for diabetes in pregnancy was a Boston classification, named after Priscilla White who published it in 1949 [17]. The White classification was based on maternal and obstetric risk factors, graded from A (best) to F (worst) designed to predict pregnancy outcomes. Subsequent modifications to this classification were introduced in 1965 and 1971 and further updated in 1980 to incorporate ischemic heart disease and renal transplantation [18]. The White classification, like others based on purely pregnancy-related risk factors, "Prognostically Bad Signs in Pregnancy" [19], are no longer used in clinical practice.

Metabolic adaptation to pregnancy

Metabolic changes in normal pregnancy

Metabolic changes occur in pregnancy to ensure sufficient maternal fat deposition in the first half of pregnancy to sustain fetal growth in the second half of pregnancy. By the eighth week of pregnancy, fasting plasma glucose concentrations start to fall and reach a nadir by 12 weeks; by contrast, post-prandial glucose levels rise [20,21]. Fasting and glucose-stimulated insulin concentrations rise throughout pregnancy [22,23]. The fall in fasting glucose precedes changes in insulin secretion or sensitivity, and is partly caused by an increase in renal clearance of glucose early in pregnancy [24].

Maternal insulin sensitivity is reduced in late pregnancy by approximately 50%, becoming comparable with levels seen in T2DM [25–27]. For glucose tolerance to be maintained, maternal β-cells must compensate for this fall in insulin sensitivity by increasing first and second-phase insulin responses approximately threefold by the last trimester [15]. In human pregnancy, increased insulin secretion is associated with morphologic changes in the pancreas, including marked β-cell hypertrophy and hyperplasia [28]. β-Cells are dynamic and increase in both function and mass in rodent pregnancies. Whether this occurs in human pregnancy is unclear [29]. This capability is presumably decreased in women with diabetes [30].

Pregnancy-related maternal insulin resistance benefits fetal growth, because a rise in post-prandial glucose concentration aids glucose transfer to the fetus, a process termed "facilitated anabolism" [31]. Maternal to fetal glucose transfer in the fasting state is enhanced by maternal lipolysis, which occurs in late pregnancy, with free fatty acids becoming the main maternal fuel substrate and diversion of glucose to the fetus. The ability of insulin to suppress lipolysis (via inhibition of hormone-sensitive lipase in adipose tissue) is severely impaired in late pregnancy, when maternal free fatty acid release and fatty acid oxidation are increased in parallel with reduced carbohydrate oxidation [32–34]. This process of enhanced lipolysis has been termed "accelerated starvation" [35] and is attributed to the actions of human placental growth hormone and other placental hormones [36–41]. These metabolic changes facilitate the transfer of glucose and amino acids to the fetus. An increase in hepatic glucose output in late pregnancy, owing to hepatic insulin resistance, ensures that maternal glucose is available to the fetus between meals [26].

Transgenic mice that overexpress human placental growth hormone develop severe peripheral insulin resistance, similar to that found in the third trimester of pregnancy, confirming its importance in the insulin resistance of late pregnancy. This increase in insulin resistance is accompanied by an increase in expression of the p85 regulatory subunit of phosphatidylinositol kinase (PI_3-kinase) and a decrease in insulin receptor substrate 1 (IRS-1) associated PI_3-kinase activity in skeletal muscle [42].

The cytokine tumor necrosis factor α (TNF-α) impairs insulin signaling *in vitro* and is increased in the second and third trimester of human pregnancy. In late pregnancy, circulating TNF-α levels are inversely correlated with insulin sensitivity [43].

The role, if any, of other adipokines including leptin, adiponectin, interleukin-6 (IL-6) and resistin in insulin resistance in pregnancy still needs to be defined. Adiponectin secretion and mRNA levels in white fat decline with advancing gestation in association with decreased insulin-stimulated glucose uptake rather than altered lipid metabolism [44]. Plasma leptin doubles in pregnancy, being produced by both maternal adipose stores and the fetoplacental unit but its role in maternal metabolism is uncertain [45].

Metabolic changes in pregnancy in women with diabetes

Carbohydrate tolerance deteriorates in women with diabetes by the second trimester, in parallel with the physiologic decrease in insulin sensitivity. Women with T1DM therefore need increased insulin to maintain glycemic control from the mid-second trimester [15,46]. By contrast, in the first trimester, insulin sensitivity increases and insulin requirements at 14 weeks' gestation are less than the start of pregnancy for well-controlled women with T1DM [46]. In 237 pregnancies in women with T1DM in Scotland, the rise in insulin requirements was associated with maternal weight at booking and weight gain between 20 and 29 weeks while inversely related to duration of diabetes [47].

The added demand on β-cell secretion may account for the increased presentation of T1DM during pregnancy [7,8]. Women in the prolonged but subclinical phase of T1DM characterized by an active insulitis may have sufficient β-cell function to prevent overt hyperglycemia before pregnancy but insufficient insulin reserve to maintain euglycemia in pregnancy.

Pregnancy-induced lipolysis makes women with T1DM more susceptible to diabetic ketoacidosis (DKA). This can develop rapidly and at relatively low levels of hyperglycemia [48]. If left untreated DKA is associated with high fetal mortality [49].

Women with pre-gestational T2DM are characteristically insulin-resistant before pregnancy with relative insulin deficiency. Further demands on their β-cells often results in a treatment escalation from diet to insulin early in pregnancy to maintain glycemic control. High doses of insulin are frequently needed, and it is not unusual for women to require in excess of 300 U/day by late pregnancy, only to be well controlled with no insulin postpartum [50]. The combination of insulin resistance, decreased insulin secretion and increased lipolysis can precipitate DKA in ketosis-prone obese pregnant women with diabetes, especially among black Afro-Caribbean women, with pre-gestational T2DM or GDM [51,52].

Glucose intolerance in pregnancy

Glucose intolerance in pregnancy as defined by the WHO 1999 criteria [6] develops in a small but increasing percentage of pregnancies. These women have insufficient β-cell capacity to maintain euglycemia and are typically obese and insulin-resistant before pregnancy. They have lower insulin responses to oral glucose at 30 and 60 minutes than glucose-tolerant control subjects [53,54]. Differences in insulin sensitivity between glucose intolerant and glucose-tolerant women are less marked as pregnancy progresses [26].

Glucose intolerance in pregnancy is a continuum [13] and the higher the fasting blood glucose and 2-hour glucose value on an OGTT, the greater the underlying β-cell dysfunction and metabolic derangement. Even lesser degrees of glucose intolerance are accompanied by abnormal glycerol and free fatty acid metabolism [55] and higher circulating pro-insulin concentrations [56].

Women with a history of GDM, who become glucose-tolerant postpartum, continue to have β-cell dysfunction, reduced glucose-stimulated insulin release and impaired suppression of lipolysis [57–61]. As many of these women are obese and insulin-resistant, the persistence of decreased β-cell function postpartum increases their susceptibility to future diabetes [62–64]. Both obesity and increasing weight gain postpartum are major determinants for the development of diabetes [65].

Effect of maternal diabetes on pregnancy

Maternal diabetes influences all aspects of pregnancy, from fertility through to birth, and subsequent health of the child and adult. While hyperglycemia is the most obvious metabolic abnormality of a diabetic pregnancy, other metabolic abnormalities can also influence outcome as implied by the term "fuel-mediated teratogenesis" [31]. In addition, diabetic complications, such as microalbuminuria, can influence the risk of obstetric complications, including hypertension and pre-eclampsia.

Placenta

A healthy pregnancy depends on a healthy placenta but maternal diabetes can cause functional and structural changes in the placenta [66–69]. Insulin receptors are highly expressed in the trophoblast and endothelial cells of the placenta and maternal and fetal insulin regulates nutrient transfer between the maternal and fetal circulation [70]. Placental insulin-binding capacity is increased in macrosomic diabetic pregnancies compared to non-diabetic placentas [71].

Fertility

Before the availability of insulin, most women with diabetes died within 2 years of diagnosis, and pregnancy was rare. In the 1920s, only one diabetic-related pregnancy was recorded in 35 000 deliveries at two London teaching hospitals [72]. Among those women who became pregnant approximately half of mothers and babies died [73].

Nowadays, although most young women with T1DM can be reassured about their fertility, delayed menarche in girls diagnosed before puberty is common, especially if diabetic control is poor [74,75]. More relevant to fertility is the association between T1DM and early menopause [76]. The mean self-reported age at menopause in an USA study of 143 women with T1DM diagnosed before the age of 17 years was 41.6 years, compared to 49.9 years for 186 sisters without diabetes and 48.0 years for 160 unrelated control subjects [76].

Other potential causes of infertility in women with T1DM are weight-related amenorrhea and primary ovarian failure. Eating disorders are more prevalent among young women with T1DM and are commonly associated with anovular cycles and amenorrhea [77]. Premature ovarian failure can have an autoimmune etiology but is seldom associated with T1DM [78].

Obesity and polycystic ovarian syndrome occur more commonly in women with T2DM and both are risk factors for anovulatory cycles and infertility [79–81].

Miscarriage

Obtaining precise data on miscarriage rates is difficult because of selection bias, recall bias and the exact definition of the upper time limit. In the UK, miscarriage is defined as the spontaneous ending of a pregnancy before viability (currently taken as 24 weeks' gestation). Spontaneous miscarriage rates among women with diabetes are broadly similar to the general population, which is 12–15%, although the risk is increased when diabetic control is poor [82–86].

Early fetal loss in non-diabetic pregnancies is often attributable to lethal chromosomal abnormalities and once a viable fetus is confirmed by ultrasound at around 8 weeks, the miscarriage rate falls and continues to fall with increasing gestational age [87,88]. Diabetic pregnancies are not at increased risk of chromosomal abnormalities but non-viable congenital malformations are more common than in non-diabetic pregnancies. These contribute to the early miscarriage rates in women with poorly controlled diabetes.

An observational UK study of 185 pregnancies in women with T1DM found a fourfold increased risk of spontaneous miscarriage when women had a glycated hemoglobin (HbA_{1c}) level >7.5% (58 mmol/mol) compared to those with a HbA_{1c} level <7.5% (58 mmol/mol) (7/48 vs 4/110) [89].

Maternal age and obesity are risk factors for first trimester miscarriage. A threefold increase in recurrent early miscarriage (defined as more than three successive miscarriages before 12 weeks) was found in an UK study of 1644 pregnant obese women (body mass index [BMI] >30 kg/m^2) compared with 3288 age-matched normal weight control subjects (BMI 19–24.9 kg/m^2) [90]. As the number of older obese women with T2DM become pregnant, miscarriage rates are likely to rise.

Embryogenesis and malformations

Maternal hyperglycemia is a major cause of fetal malformation. Clinical and animal studies implicate a combination of metabolic, maternal and fetal factors in the etiologies of diabetic-related malformations [91]. Improved identification and classification of monogenetic and mitochondrial forms of diabetes have shown that some of these rarer forms of diabetes are associated with fetal structural abnormalities, and distinct phenotypes that are independent of maternal glycemic control have been identified (see Chapter 15).

MODY 5 diabetes, which arises from a mutation in the transcription factor hepatocyte nuclear factor-1β, exemplifies this. It is not only associated with early-onset diabetes and renal cysts, but also with a variety of other urogenital and pancreatic anomalies in the offspring [92]. There are well-documented genetic susceptibilities to glucose-mediated malformations in rodents which are likely to occur in human pregnancies [93].

Following improvements in obstetric and neonatal care, congenital malformations now represent the major cause of diabetes-related perinatal morbidity and mortality. Over the last 40 years, diabetes-related congenital malformations rates have been 4–10%. This high rate is especially poignant as good metabolic control around the time of organogenesis lessens this risk [86,94–106].

Multiple anomalies are more common in diabetic pregnancies than in non-diabetic pregnancies. This suggests the teratogenic insult occurs early in embryologic development [107,108]. While heart and CNS congenital abnormalities are the most common diabetes-related abnormalities [106], the caudal regression syndrome (sacral agenesis) is the most pathognonomic of diabetes, being 200 times more common in diabetic pregnancies [109]. A greater than threefold excess of severe cardiac anomalies including transposition of the great arteries, truncus arteriosus and tricuspid atresia occurs in diabetic pregnancies [110].

The prevalence of major congenital anomalies in the CEMACH audit of women with pre-gestational diabetes was 41.8/1000 births [106]. This rate was twofold higher than the rate of major congenital anomalies from non-diabetic pregnancies reported as 21/1000 births in the European Surveillance of Congenital Anomalies (EUROCAT) data for 2002–2003. Anomalies of the circulatory system and neural tube were threefold higher than expected among the diabetic pregnancies.

Congenital malformations – lessons from animal studies

Rodent studies show diabetes-associated fetal malformations that are broadly similar to those of humans, although the susceptibility to particular different diabetes-related malformations depends on the maternal species and strain [93,111].

Apoptosis in the mammalian pre-implantation blastocyst is a natural process that eliminates abnormal cells. Hyperglycemia modifies the expression of key apoptotic regulatory genes and normalizing hyperglycemia in mice during the periconception period normalizes the expression of these genes [112]. In rodents, maternal hyperglycemia reduces the number of blastocysts formed and the total cell mass of those that survive. In a hyperglycemic environment, blastocyst cell mass is reduced predominately from the inner cell layer and insulin treatment of hyperglycemic female dams, starting at the time of conception protects the blastocyst from these changes [113]. Insulin may act as a growth factor during early mammalian embryogenesis, influencing mitosis, apoptosis and differentiation through insulin receptors expressed on blastocysts [114]. Other growth factors and cytokines expressed in early blastocysts that may be involved in embryo development are the insulin-like growth factors (IGFs) and TNF-α [115].

Animal studies, predominantly in the rodent, implicate glucose as the major teratogen in diabetic pregnancies. Many of the cellular processes induce oxygen-derived free radical production and increased oxidative stress which provide a plausible unifying mechanism by which supraphysiologic concentrations of metabolic substrates, including glucose, pyruvate and hydroxybutyrate, could be teratogenic [91,116–118]. Hyperglycemia at the time of embryogenesis exposes the fetal mitochondria to a high influx of glucose-generated pyruvate that, by overwhelming the immature mitochondrial electron transport chain, may result in an excess of reactive oxygen species (mainly superoxide) being generated. The subsequent formation of hydrogen peroxide and hydroxyl radicals in turn leads to increased lipid peroxidation, mitochondrial swelling, DNA damage and altered expression of key genes [91]. Antioxidative agents such as N-acetylcysteine (NAC) and the vitamins E, C and folic acid protect against diabetes-induced malformations in rat embryos [27,119,120].

Myoinositol has an important role as a precursor for a number of secondary messengers and may contribute to diabetic teratogenesis. Cultured rodent embryos in high glucose concentrations have decreased inositol uptake and become inositol deficient [121–125]. Inositol supplementation to embryos cultured in high glucose media or dietary addition to diabetic pregnant rodents protects against glucose-mediated malformation [126,127]. By contrast, the addition of an inositol uptake inhibitor to the culture medium of rodent embryos causes inositol deficiency and embryonic dysmorphogenesis, which is reversible if inositol is added to the culture [128]. Antioxidants diminish both embryonic dysmorphogenesis induced by hyperglycemia and inositol uptake inhibitors, suggesting a possible link between malformations and oxidative stress [129].

Decreased arachidonic acid and several prostaglandins, in particular PGE_2, in diabetic embryogenesis have been implicated as a cause of malformations. Hyperglycemia during the period of neural tube closure reduces embryonic prostaglandin levels secondary to altered arachidonic acid metabolism and phosphatidylinositol turnover, and the downregulation of the embryonic COX-2 gene [130]. Inhibition of rostral neural tube fusion by high glucose concentrations in rat embryos is prevented by the addition of either myoinositol or PGE_2, but not if indometacin, a prostaglandin synthesis inhibitor, is also added to the culture [121]. Intraperitoneal injections of arachidonic acid to diabetic rats reduce the rates of neural tube defects (NTDs) [131]. Reduced yolk sac PGE_2 concentrations have been reported from human pregnancies terminated at 8–10 weeks [132].

There is a possible link between decreased prostaglandin synthesis and oxidative stress in cultured diabetic rat embryos; the reduced PGE_2 concentration seen in day-10 rat embryos and membranes exposed to high glucose concentrations can be restored when the antioxidant NAC amide is added to the culture medium. Superoxide dismutase and NAC can prevent malformations when added to the medium of rat embryos cultured in COX inhibitors, acetylsalicylic acid or high glucose concentrations [118].

NTDs in diabetic pregnancies are 2–5 times higher than in non-diabetic pregnancies [106]. Both genetic and environmental factors are involved in NTD development [133]. Although folic acid supplementation can prevent many cases of NTDs, the cellular mechanism for this protection and the relationship between maternal folate status and genetic susceptibility to NTDs are not known. Low dietary folate is an environmental factor for NTD and the 1996 dietary fortification of enriched grain products with folic acid in the USA coincided with a 20% reduction in NTDs by 1998–1999 [134]. Human studies have not shown any evidence for abnormal folate metabolism in pregnant women with diabetes [135]. In rodent studies, folic acid supplementation protects against diabetes-induced malformations [120].

Diabetic control and malformations

There is a clear association between congenital abnormalities and maternal glucose control in early pregnancy as assessed by HbA_{1c} [2,85,89,95,101,102,136–141]. Despite the evidence that diabetic fetal malformation rates approach those of the general antenatal population when glycemic control from conception through to the end of organogenesis is tightly controlled [142–144], the incidence of serious birth defects has changed little over the last few decades [103,140,145].

In a systematic review of seven cohort studies between 1985 and 2006 that examined 1977 diabetic pregnancies with 117 anomalies, the odds ratio for a congenital malformation increased by 1.2 (95% CI 1.1–1.4) for each one standard deviation (SD) unit rise in HbA_{1c} level at the time of conception [144]. When the pre-conceptional HbA_{1c} concentration was at the mid-normal non-diabetic range, the absolute risk of a congenital anomaly was approximately 2% (95% CI 0.0–4.4) and rose to a risk of 3% (95% CI 0.4–6.1) and 10% (95% CI 2.3–17.8) when the HbA_{1c} levels were 2 and 8 SD above normal range, respectively.

In the CEMACH audit of pre-gestational diabetic pregnancies, 25% of women with a malformation had a first trimester HbA_{1c} level below 53 mmol/mol (7.0%) [2]. This would suggest that at the lower levels of HbA_{1c} this measurement of glycemic control does not assess malformation risk as well as it does at higher HbA_{1c} values, a finding that is supported from continuous glucose monitoring studies [146].

Intensive glycemic management at the time of conception improves malformation rates [142]. In the randomized Diabetes Control and Complication Trial (DCCT), there were 191 live births from 270 pregnancies. HbA_{1c} level at conception was significantly lower in women in the intensive treatment group than in the conventional group (57 ± 9 mmol/mol [7.4% ± 1.3%] and 65 ± 5 mmol/mol [8.1% ± 1.7%], respectively; $P = 0.0001$). There were 92 births (one set of twins) to women in the intensive glycemic management arm and 99 births (two sets of twins) to women in the conventional arm. One (0.7%) congenital malformations occurred in a woman assigned to intensive therapy compared with eight in women in the conventional arm (5.9%; $P = 0.06$).

Fetal pancreatic and β-cell development

Understanding the genetic and intrauterine environmental factors that influence fetal pancreatic and β-cell development and the contribution of maternal diabetes will provide insight into the trans-generational etiology of T2DM.

Immunoreactive insulin is detectable in the human fetal pancreas by 7 weeks after conception and primitive islets by 12–13 weeks, with evidence of functional fetal β-cells by the end of the first trimester [147]. Increased fetal β-cell stimulation and hyperinsulinemia in response to maternal hyperglycemia occurs in early pregnancy and may persist throughout human pregnancy. This early priming of β-cell function may explain why accelerated fetal growth patterns occur even with good metabolic control later in pregnancy [148,149].

β-Cell function and insulin sensitivity in children and young adulthood are influenced by intrauterine growth restriction [150,151]. There are critical spatiotemporal windows in embroyonic and fetal life when maternal diet and placental function affects expression of key developmental pancreatic genes through epigenetic modifications of DNA methylation [152]. While most work has centered on models of growth restriction and subsequent β-cell development, *in utero* exposure to hyperglycemia also affects fetal, neonatal and adult β-cell number and function in rodents [153]; however, these experimental models may be less relevant to human pancreatic β-cell development than those in larger mammals, as the rodent fetal endocrine pancreas is more immature *in utero* and β-cells continue to proliferate postnatally.

The molecular changes linking growth restriction and β-cell mass in the sheep include a normal β-cell mass in fetal and early adult life, corresponding with upregulation of the genes for IGF-II and insulin gene as well as their receptors. By late adult life, however, male sheep have reduced β-cell mass and develop diabetes having lost their ability to upregulate these genes and maintain an adequate β-cell mass [154].

Pancreatic duodenal homeobox-1 (Pdx1) is a pancreatic transcription factor that regulates pancreas development and β-cell differentiation. Decreased Pdx1 expression in humans is associated with T2DM in adulthood. Reduced fetal Pdx1 expression secondary to epigenetic modification occurs in growth-restricted rodents and remains reduced into adulthood, suggesting the window for epigenetic modification of β-cell gene expression extends beyond the embryonic period [152,155].

Abnormal fetal growth

Factors influencing fetal growth include maternal–fetal nutrient transfer, maternal weight and nutritional status [156], placental size, uterine blood flow, and fetal and parental genes [157]. In a healthy non-diabetic pregnancy, parental and fetal genes will be the major contributor to birth weight, while the fetal metabolic intrauterine environment is also a major influence in diabetic pregnancies. The infant of a mother with diabetes is often "growth promoted" [158], a finding confirmed in the CEMACH audit, in which 51% of infants were above the 90th percentile for gestational age [2]. An analysis of 643 singleton babies born after 28 weeks' gestation to mothers with T1DM in Scotland, 1960–1999, found birth weight to be 1.41 SD above the population norm, an increase that remained unchanged over the 40 years of the study [159]. The potential consequences of accelerated growth *in utero* include an increased risk of emergency cesarean section, birth trauma and birth asphyxia [160,161] as well as future childhood and adult obesity.

Glucose is the major fetal and placental fuel substrate and fetal insulin and IGF-I are both fetal anabolic hormones [162], while IGF-II is a placental growth factor. Fetal insulin secretion in humans occurs in response to glucose and the amino acids arginine and leucine by 13 weeks' gestation [147,163]. Maternal hyperglycemia increases placental fetal transfer of glucose and results in fetal hyperinsulineamia [164–166]. The availability of amino acids and lactate is also increased in diabetic pregnancies [167]. The diabetic intrauterine metabolic environment promotes abdominal fat disposition and visceral growth; notably liver, spleen and heart. This type of accelerated growth pattern is visible on routine clinical ultrasound as an increased abdominal circumference from 28 weeks' gestation (Figure 53.1) [168]. Such growth patterns are less common in hypertensive diabetic pregnancies complicated by hypertension or vascular disease which can result in decreased uterine and placental blood flow that compromises nutrient transfer [169].

Maternal glycemic control influences fetal growth as early as the first trimester as shown in a longitudinal study on 136 pregnancies involving 120 women with diabetes in which an elevated first-trimester HbA_{1c} level was the strongest predictor of macrosomia [170].

Accelerated growth patterns occur through maternal hyperglycemia causing fetal hyperinsulinemia, as illustrated by human and animal studies [171]. In human diabetic pregnancies there is a strong association between birth weight and fetal insulin, as assessed by amniotic and umbilical cord insulin, C-peptide and proinsulin [149,172–178].

Inducing hyperinsulinemia in the fetuses of healthy non-diabetic pregnant Rhesus monkeys produces similar accelerated fetal growth to human diabetic pregnancies [163,179]. Conversely, fetal lambs rendered hypoinsulemic *in utero* by streptozocin have decreased somatic and skeletal growth [180].

IGF-I is an important fetal growth factor in humans and a homozygous IGF-I gene deletion results in severe prenatal and postnatal growth restriction and mental retardation [181]. The placental growth factor IGF-II is paternally imprinted, and functions to facilitate maternal–fetal nutrient transfer in late pregnancy, an effect that may depend on fetal insulin [182]. In healthy non-diabetic pregnancies, cord IGF-I and IGF-II are correlated with birth weight [162]. The bioavailability of the IGFs is regulated by the IGF binding proteins (IGFBPs) [183] and proteases that inhibit these binding proteins are increased in human pregnancies [184]. Cord blood IGFBP-1 is lower in T2DM and GDM compared with controls without diabetes, suggesting IGF-I bioavailability is increased in diabetic pregnancies [185].

Stillbirth

Stillbirth in the UK is currently defined as fetal loss occurring after 24 completed weeks' gestation. In both women with and without diabetes, there are identifiable causes for stillbirth that include congenital malformations, chromosomal abnormalities, infection and intrauterine growth restriction. Approximately one-quarter of all cases are unexplained [186]. The risk of stillbirth in diabetic pregnancies is approximately fivefold higher than for non-diabetic pregnancies [101,106,140]. In the CEMACH

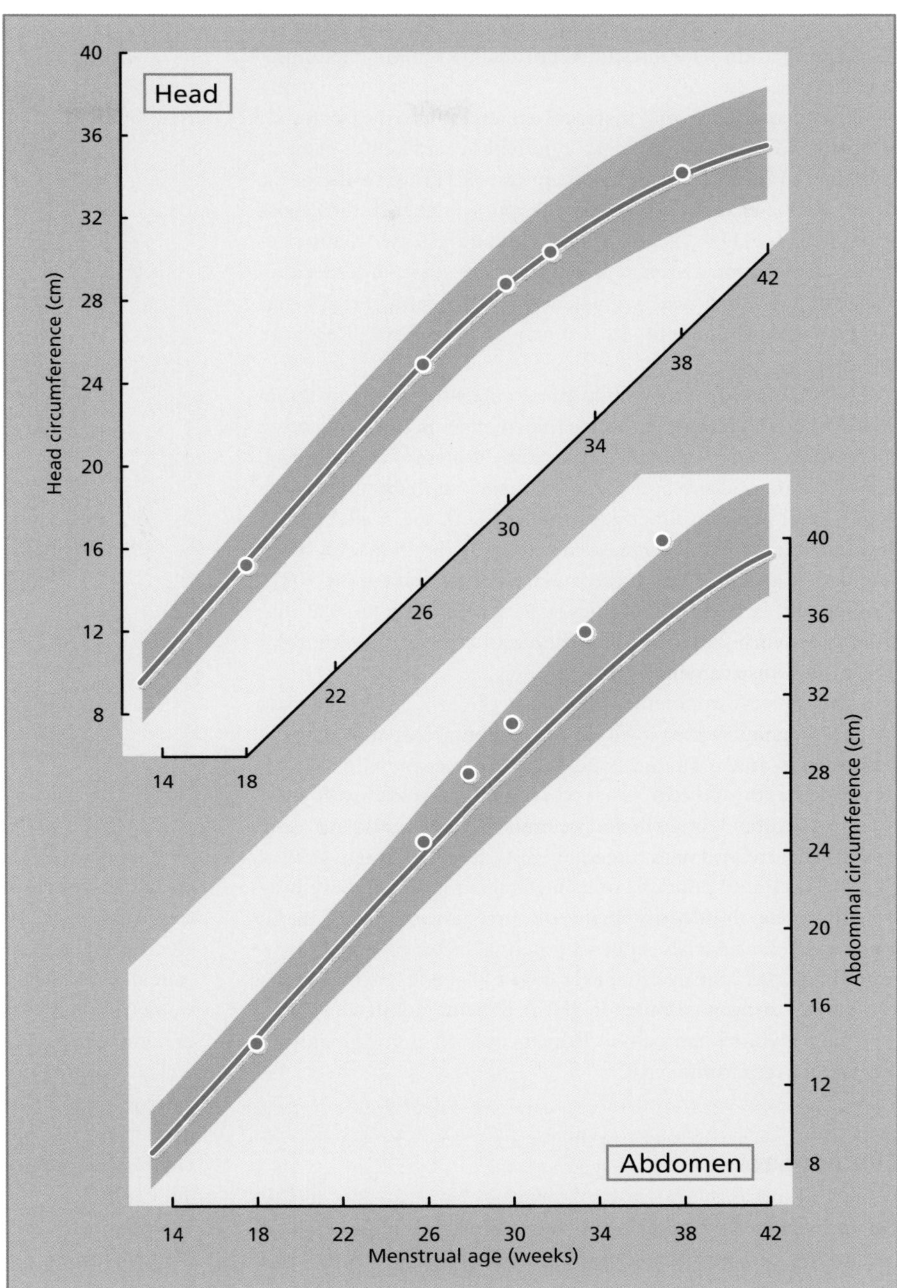

Figure 53.1 Accelerated fetal growth, manifested as a progressive increase in abdominal circumference (lower panel), while head circumference remains on the 50th centile (upper panel). The red line represents the 50th centile and the shaded area represents the 3rd to 97th centile.

audit, there were 63 stillbirths in 2536 births in one calendar year, representing a 4.7 (3.7–6.0) higher risk than for the general UK antenatal population that has a stillbirth rate of 5.7/1000 births. There was no difference in the stillbirth rate between T1DM (25.8/1000) and T2DM (29.2/1000). A similar stillbirth rate of 25/1000 births was seen in an earlier audit of T1DM pregnancies in the north-east of England, 1990–1994, in which there were nine stillbirths among 462 pregnancies in 355 women [102]. In a Danish cohort of 1361 consecutive singleton births to women with T1DM, 1990–1999, 1.8% resulted in stillbirth [187]. Detailed information of these pregnancies including autopsy data was available on all 25 stillbirths (22 women). No anatomical or other identifiable cause was found in 12 cases. Compared with a reference group of 236 consecutive births to women with T1DM, suboptimal glycemic control early and late in pregnancy occurred more frequently; the HbA_{1c} level was above 58 mmol/mol (7.5%) in 64% of the stillbirth group in the first trimester and 67% in the third trimester compared with 33% and 4%, respectively, in the reference group. The CEMACH audit and other earlier studies also identified poor glycemic control throughout pregnancy as a risk factor for stillbirth [2,188]. Other identifiable risk factors in the Danish study were diabetic nephropathy, smoking and lower social status [187].

Obesity and increasing maternal age are other risk factors for stillbirth in the non-diabetic population [189,190]. Among obstetric units that serve extremely obese T2DM women (e.g. South Pacific Islanders), the stillbirth risk is higher in those with T2DM than T1DM [9,191]. As obesity and T2DM trends continue to rise among women of reproductive years, differences in stillbirth rates between women with T2DM and T1DM may become more apparent in women of Northern European ancestry.

The cause for the excess stillbirths in diabetic pregnancies that cannot be attributable to congenital malformations and other identifiable causes remains uncertain, although chronic fetal hypoxia and acidosis appear to be major contributory factors [192]. Fetal hyperinsulinemia combined with the availability of excessive fuel substrate increases oxygen demand in insulin sensitive tissues and this may exceeds placental oxygen supply [193]. Human and large animal studies suggest that the fetuses of diabetic pregnancies are more susceptible to acidosis than those of a non-diabetic pregnancy [194–196].

Amniotic erythropoietin is a marker of chronic fetal hypoxia in late pregnancy and is higher in diabetic than non-diabetic pregnancies [192]. In one study of 156 women with T1DM, amniotic erythropoietin levels correlated inversely with cord blood pH and pO_2 at birth and neonatal hypoglycemia and were positively correlated with maternal HbA_{1c} levels in late pregnancy [178]. The clinical potential of using fetal amniotic fluid erythropoietin levels to identify high-risk pregnancies needs to be assessed in clinical trials. Another potential factor that could have a minimal affect on fetal hypoxia in late diabetic pregnancies is the greater oxygen affinity of glycated hemoglobin compared with non-glycated hemoglobin which could theoretically impair oxygen delivery to the fetus.

The neonate

Neonates born to mothers with diabetes have a higher risk of being born preterm (less than 37 weeks' gestation), being large for gestational age, having a congenital malformation or birth injury and developing hypoglycemia requiring treatment. Neonatal admission to a special care baby unit is common although this often reflects hospital policy rather than clinical need [3].

Approximately half of all neonates born to women with diabetes are large for gestational age (above the 90th percentile) [2]. The increase in subcutaneous fat distribution in these infants combined with their high hematocrit gives them a typical "macrosomic" appearance with plethoric features and an obese body (Figure 53.2).

Hypoglycemia is the most common, albeit usually transient, metabolic condition in infants of women with diabetes and occurs in approximately half of all diabetic pregnancies [197]. Capillary blood glucose readings are often unreliable as many glucose sticks in routine clinical use are not quality assured and validated for neonatal use. It is therefore recommended that ward-based glucose electrode or laboratory analysis is performed to confirm hypoglycemia.

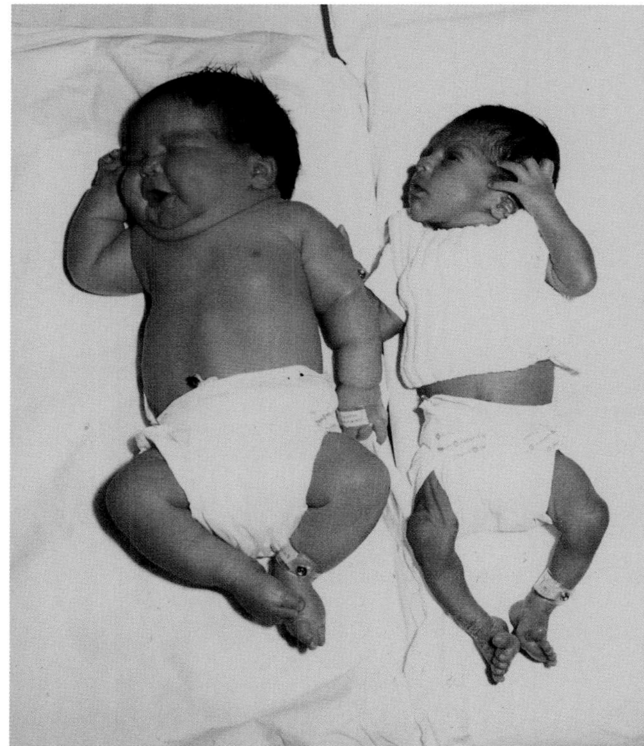

Figure 53.2 Left: A macrosomic baby born to a mother with diabetes. Right: A normal baby born to a mother without diabetes.

The working definition for neonatal hypoglycemia is a blood glucose value <2.6 mmol/L [198,199]. In the majority of healthy neonates, a low blood glucose concentration is merely a normal physiologic response to the metabolic adaptation to extrauterine life [200].

Macrosomic infants are at higher risk of hypoglycemia because of postpartum hyperinsulinemia secondary to *in utero* β-cell hyperplasia. This risk of hypoglycemia is further increased because hyperinsulinemia inhibits hepatic glucose production. Hypoglycemia may also be aggravated by polycythemia (secondary to increased glucose uptake by red blood cells), and possibly by impaired glucagon release.

Preterm infants have more variable swings in blood glucose and are therefore more at risk of hypoglycemia [201] and this may affect subsequent mental and motor development [202]. Early feeding reduces the risk of hypoglycemia [203] and it is therefore recommended that all mothers with diabetes are encouraged to breastfeed within 30 minutes of birth and then every 3–4 hours, until a regular feeding pattern is established.

The current NICE guidelines only recommend the use of intravenous glucose to treat neonatal hypoglycemia when there are clinical signs of hypoglycemia or a persistent blood sugar <2.0 mmol/L that cannot be raised by oral or tube feeding, or when the blood glucose is very low (1.1–1.4 mmol/L). If intravenous glucose is required, this should be continued until the glucose is >2.5 mmol/L [5].

Other transient neonatal complications include polycythemia resulting from enhanced antepartum hemapoiesis [204] in response to fetal hyperinsulinemia [205] and chronic fetal tissue hypoxia [206].

Respiratory distress syndrome was considered to occur more often in diabetic pregnancies but is likely to result from preterm birth and high rate of cesarean section rather than any underlying metabolic effect [207].

Transient hypertrophic cardiomyopathy, characterized by ventricular septal hypertrophy and subaortic stenosis, occurs in up to 30% of all babies of mothers with diabetes [208,209]. Congestive cardiac failure presents in only 5% of babies and this usually has a benign course resolving within a month and without any clinical sequelae.

Both hypocalcemia and hypomagnesemia occur more frequently in the infant of a mother with diabetes, usually as a consequence of prematurity or birth asphyxia. Jaundice is more common in macrosomic babies. The cause of hyperbilirubinemia is probably multifactorial including birth trauma, polycythemia, hemolysis and immature hepatic uptake and conjugation of bilirubin.

Increased risk of diabetes in later life

Both T1DM and T2DM are the result of environmental factors operating in a genetically susceptible individual [210,211]. Diabetes in pregnancy can influence the incidence of obesity and diabetes in the offspring [212,213]. Maternal hyperglycemia during pregnancy predisposes to an earlier presentation of T2DM in the child than when diabetes develops in the mother after the pregnancy [212]. Children and young adults of mothers with T1DM are also more insulin resistant and glucose intolerant than children of mothers without diabetes [214–216]. Similar metabolic abnormalities are not seen in the young adults of fathers with T1DM [215]. An influence of the intrauterine environment on the susceptibility to T2DM is also suggested by the observation that a family history of diabetes is more often reported on the maternal than the paternal side of the family [217–219].

Studies in the Pima population on sibling pairs born before and after the mother had developed diabetes has confirmed the importance of the intrauterine exposure to the risk of future T2DM [213]; over 70% of children with a prenatal exposure to maternal diabetes have themselves developed diabetes by 25–34 years. A prenatal exposure to maternal hyperglycemia is believed to be responsible for 40% of all T2DM in the Pima children (5–19 years) [220,221].

Growth restriction and intrauterine nutritional deprivation predispose to diabetes in later life [222]. Small-for-dates babies are at increased risk of developing T2DM or IGT in middle age [223], suggesting that developing β-cells are programmed by intrauterine events including nutrition and hyperglycemia [224].

Risks of pregnancy for the mother with diabetes

Pregnancy may affect pre-existing microvascular and macrovascular disease but does not usually have any lasting detrimental effect on either retinopathy or nephropathy. In contrast, pregnancy poses a risk for women with established cardiovascular disease, and this risk should be discussed in older women and those with a long duration of disease.

Microvascular complications

Retinopathy

Diabetic retinopathy is more common in women with T1DM of childbearing age than T2DM [3]. It is not a contraindication to pregnancy but retinopathy may progress during pregnancy, especially in women with moderate or severe retinopathy before pregnancy [225,226]. Nevertheless, it rarely has any long-term detrimental effect on the natural history or progression of diabetic retinopathy [227,228]. An analysis of 59 women with T1DM before pregnancy and yearly follow-up for 5 years post pregnancy, with 10-year follow-up data available for 22 women, showed baseline retinopathy status was the only independent risk factor that predicted later progression of retinopathy [228].

Decreased retinal blood flow and retinal arterial constriction occur in the third trimester of a healthy pregnancy, but are more pronounced in diabetic pregnancies [229]. These changes, combined with pregnancy-related hypervolemia and hypercoagulation, could theoretically lower the threshold for retinal ischemia and hypoxia and hence progression of retinopathy. Pregnancy is associated with many circulating growth factors, angiopoietic factors and pro-inflammatory markers, but to date none have been clearly associated with the progression of retinopathy in pregnancy [230–233].

Retinopathy can develop *de novo* in pregnancy [226], although this is unlikely to progress to proliferative retinopathy [225]. Progression to proliferative retinopathy is also uncommon among women with mild or minimal retinopathy at booking. In a prospective study of 169 pregnancies among 139 women with T1DM followed between 1990 and 1998, progression to proliferative retinopathy requiring laser therapy only occurred in 2.2% of pregnancies. Proliferative changes occurred in only two women, one who had occasional microaneurysms at booking and the other who had fewer than four microaneuryms per eye [225]. Progression to proliferative retinopathy requiring laser treatment is more common in women with more advanced retinopathy at booking and longer duration of diabetes [225,226,234]. Laser treatment before pregnancy protects against proliferative changes in pregnancy [226]. Hypertension influence retinopathy progression and optimal blood pressure control is therefore important [235].

Poor glycemic control in early pregnancy and rapid improvement of glycemic control are associated with retinopathy progression [227]. In the DCCT, 180 women with T1DM had 270 pregnancies. All women originally assigned to conventional insulin treatment were switched to intensive therapy in early pregnancy. Compared with non-pregnant control subjects in the intensively treated arm, there was a 1.6-fold increased risk of retinopathy deterioration in pregnancy, while the deterioration in the women originally assigned to conventional treatment was 2.5-fold higher than in the non-pregnant control group. The previously conventionally treated group also had a 2.9-fold increased risk of a three-step progression or more from the baseline retinopathy level than the non-pregnant control group, with the greatest risk occurring in the second trimester (4.3-fold increase) and persisting for 12 months postpartum.

Although individual subjects had transient worsening of retinopathy during pregnancy by the end of the DCCT, levels of retinopathy in subjects who had become pregnant were similar to those who had not, for each treatment group. The worsening of retinopathy in pregnancy in the previously conventionally treated group was attributed to the women entering pregnancy with poor glycemic control experiencing a rapid improvement in their glycemic control [227]. A similar conclusion that rapid intensification of glycemic control was a risk factor for progression of retinopathy was observed in the Diabetes in Early Pregnancy Study [234]. These studies highlight the importance of optimizing glycemic control prior to pregnancy.

Annual retinal screening with digital camera is now part of routine diabetic clinical care, and there is evidence that its introduction into clinical practice is improving the natural history of diabetic retinopathy and reducing blindness [236].

Diabetic nephropathy

Normal pregnancy causes a physiologic increase in glomerular filtration rate (GFR) and creatinine clearance. Estimated GFR formulas based on the Modification of Diet in Renal Disease (MDRD) study equation or the Cockcroft–Gault formulae are consequently unreliable during pregnancy.

Pregnancy is not associated with deteriorating kidney function in most women with diabetes. Among women with established moderate to advanced nephropathy, pregnancy may be associated with a deterioration in kidney function; however, this usually reverts to pre-pregnancy levels in the postpartum period [237].

Women with normal urinary albumin : creatinine ratios (ACR <3.5 mg/mmol) and serum creatinine (<120 μmol/L) seldom experience any adverse effect on renal function during pregnancy. Women with microalbuminuria are not at risk of deteriorating renal function during pregnancy, but are at risk of pregnancy-induced hypertension, pre-eclampsia and preterm birth; early intensive hypertensive management in pregnancy may reduce these risks [238–241], as can good glycemic control [242].

Women with macroalbuminuria or proteinuria (defined as ACR >30 mg/mmol or urinary albumin concentration >200 mg/L) are at increased risk of accelerated deterioration of renal function during pregnancy. The risk of proteinuria on maternal and fetal health increases with increasing proteinuria and declining kidney function. Pre-eclampsia is common within this group. In a prospective study of 203 women with T1DM, pre-eclampsia developed in 6% of women without microalbuminuria, in 42% with microalbuminuria and 64% of women with proteinuria [239].

Women whose protein excretion exceeds 2 g/day or whose serum creatinine concentration exceeds 120 μmol/L before pregnancy require pre-pregnancy advice regarding the risk to themselves and any future unborn child. This should be given by an appropriate specialist who can provide prognostic information on diabetic nephropathy as well as advice on hypertensive management and thromboprophylaxis [5].

Overall survival rates for diabetic nephropathy continue to improve. The Danish National Register on Dialysis and Transplantation reported an increased 5-year overall survival rate of 15% between 1995 and 2005 [243]. These women need to receive realistic and current information on their kidney disease to help them make informed choices to balance a potentially shortened life expectancy and impaired quality of life with the responsibilities of motherhood.

A study of kidney function and end-stage renal replacement requirement in 93 Danish women with T1DM and diabetic nephropathy between 1970 and 1989 followed for 16 years found that the renal outcomes of the 26 women who became pregnant were similar to those who had not become pregnant [244]; however, nine mothers had died during the study period when their children were between 3 and 17 years old (median 9 years), and a further five required renal replacement therapy [244].

Diabetic nephropathy, especially when the serum creatinine is raised, carries a significant risk of preterm birth before 32 weeks' gestation, very low birth weight and neonatal hypoglycemia [245]. Early intensive management of hypertension can lessen this risk [241]. The increased risk of preterm births probably accounts for the mild disturbances in growth and development in early childhood seen in offspring of these pregnancies. A 3-year follow-up study from birth of 10 children of mothers with diabetes and pre-gestational proteinuria and 30 children of mothers without proteinuria found the children of mothers with nephropathy were significantly smaller, had mild linguistic developmental delay and greater susceptibility to infections [246].

The number of women with diabetes undergoing either a renal transplant or a combined renal–pancreatic transplant is increasing. The first report of successful pregnancies following a renal transplant was in 1986 [247]. Successful pregnancies following a transplant are now common [248], with three large registries providing pregnancy outcome data. The National Transplantation Pregnancy Registry in the USA, the European Dialysis and Transplant Association Registry and the UK Transplant Pregnancy Registry all show some increased risk of miscarriages, stillbirths, ectopic pregnancies, preterm births, low birth weight babies and neonatal deaths [248].

Since 1997, the UK has had a dedicated transplant pregnancy registry and live birth rates among renal transplant recipients now approach 80% [249]. Among 176 renal transplant recipients, pregnancy was not associated with any long-term adverse effect on the transplant. When the pre-pregnancy serum creatinine was >150 µmol/L, however, there was a tendency for the serum creatinine to be higher postpartum. The miscarriage rate, intrauterine fetal loss before 24 weeks' gestation and stillbirth rate were 11%, 2% and 2%, respectively. Approximately half of the births occurred before 37 weeks, with a mean gestation of 35.6 weeks. Hypertension occurred in 60–80%, with pre-eclampsia diagnosed in approximately one-third, although this may be over-reported as the diagnosis of pre-clampsia is difficult in women with pre-existing hypertension, renal impairment and proteinuria.

The Toronto Renal Transplant Program is one of the few studies to report follow-up data on 32 children born to renal transplant recipients. Postnatal growth was normal although developmental assessment showed one child had moderate to severe sensorineural hearing loss, another a learning disability and a third a pervasive developmental disorder [250].

It is likely in the future that more women with diabetic nephropathy will have a combined pancreas–kidney transplant before a planned pregnancy. The benefit and risk of a combined pancreas–kidney transplant over a single kidney transplant has not yet been evaluated for pregnancy.

Macrovascular complications

As the general antenatal population becomes more obese and more women give birth in their late reproductive years, ischemic heart disease (IHD) in pregnancy will become more prevalent [251]. Maternal diabetes, obesity and increasing age are all identifiable risk factors for IHD in pregnancy [252,253].

Pregnancy increases the risk of an acute myocardial infarction (MI) three- to fourfold, with the risk being greatest in the peripartum period [252]. The number of pregnant women with IHD and maternal death from IHD has increased in recent years; IHD now represents the most common cause of cardiac death associated with pregnancy in the UK [252–255]. Nevertheless, the mortality rates from acute MI in pregnancy have declined [254,255].

Women with diabetes have a twofold higher risk of dying from IHD than women without diabetes [256,257]. Population studies that capture data on 5–6% of the UK population at any one time have reported that women with T1DM, aged 35–45 years, have a 15-fold higher risk of a major CVD event [258] and women with T2DM, aged 35–54 years, have a fivefold higher risk of an MI than women without diabetes of a similar age [259].

The incidence and maternal mortality rate from acute MI in pregnancy was reported to be 1 in 35 700 deliveries and 7.3% respectively in California between 1991 and 2000 [252]; however, the mortality rate from MI among pregnant women with diabetes is likely to be higher than it is in non-pregnant women [260].

Co-morbidities

Obesity

Obesity is a common co-morbidity in women with diabetes. The antenatal population is becoming more obese, reflecting the secular trend in obesity. It has a major impact on maternal and fetal health as well as on health services and resources [261]. While one expects the majority of women with T2DM and GDM to be obese, an increasing number of women with T1DM are also overweight or obese [262]. In the CEMACH enquiry, 62% of the 137 women with T2DM and 15% of the 181 women with T1DM were obese [3].

Maternal and infant mortality [253] increases with increasing maternal BMI. The risk of congenital malformations and stillbirth are increased [263]. Obesity increases the risk of pre-eclampsia, GDM [264], the need for induction of labor, emergency cesarean section rates, postpartum hemorrhage and infection [265]. Babies of obese mothers are more likely to have birth weight above the 90th percentile [266] and be at risk of birth trauma and adult obesity and diabetes [267].

The first report linking pre-gestational weight and malformations in South Wales between 1964 and 1966 found that mothers of anencephalic infants were significantly heavier than a matched control group [268]. Subsequent epidemiologic and cohort studies have confirmed this finding. A population-based case–control study of mothers of infants born with and without selected birth defects in metropolitan areas of Atlanta, USA, between 1993 and 1997 showed for every incremental unit increase in BMI, the odds ratio for a major malformation increased by 7% [263]. The most common malformations reported occurring as either single or multiple defects, were NTDs, especially spina bifida, omphalocele and heart defects [263].

Although cardiac malformations and NTD are increased in babies of women with diabetes, obtaining euglycemia in obese women with diabetes may not fully protect them against the added risk of a congenital malformation. A cohort study of 2060 infants born to mothers with GDM showed that both diabetes severity and pre-pregnancy BMI were predictors of the 6% minor and 3.8% major malformations, with the BMI being the main contributor [269]. Data from 22 951 pregnant women enrolled in a prospective cohort study reported that major non-chromosomal congenital defects associated with diabetes were more common in obese women [270]. A study of Spanish mothers with GDM also reported that BMI ≥30 kg/m^2 was associated with a two- to threefold greater risk of cardiovascular defects compared with non-obese women [271]. Maternal obesity and GDM may increase the risk of CNS birth defects through shared metabolic mechanisms.

Autoimmune diseases

Women with T1DM are at increased risk of other autoimmune disease, especially thyroid disease and celiac disease. Thyroid function should be monitored in pregnant women with hypothyroidism as small increases in thyroxine replacement are frequently required [272]. This is important as there is some evidence linking mild degrees of hypothyroidism in the first trimester with adverse neurodevelopment [273]. The simultaneous ingestion of iron and thyroxine may inhibit thyroxine absorption, and women should be advised to take any iron supplements at least 2 hours after or before taking thyroxine [274].

Women with a previous history of Graves disease will also need their thyroid function measured before and during pregnancy. Fetal monitoring is also recommended as maternal thyroid-stimulating antibodies can cross the placenta causing transient fetal and neonatal hyperthyroidism [275].

Clinical management

Pre-pregnancy care

Pregnancy care for women with diabetes should begin prior to conception when glycemic control can be optimized, medication reviewed and folic acid started. All health care providers who look after women with diabetes should emphasize the benefits of pre-pregnancy planning and good glycemic control on pregnancy outcomes and encourage women to plan their pregnancies and to engage in pre-pregnancy care.

Discussions about contraception and pregnancy plans should form part of the ongoing care of all pre-menopausal women with diabetes. Once a woman expresses an interest in becoming pregnant she should have access to a pre-pregnancy clinic where specific pre-conceptual advice can be given.

Evidence of effectiveness

There have been no randomized clinical trials of pre-pregnancy counseling nor are there ever likely to be. The evidence of effectiveness is therefore based predominately on observational studies of self-selected women. Furthermore, there is no standardized definition of what constitutes pre-pregnancy care [143]. Nevertheless, pregnancy outcomes are better in women with diabetes who plan their pregnancies [138]. One Scottish study analyzed adverse pregnancy outcomes by markers of pregnancy planning and pre-pregnancy care in 423 singleton T1DM pregnancies. The best pregnancy outcomes were in women who achieved an optimal HbA_{1c} level before conceiving. These women were five times less likely to have an unfavorable outcome than women with suboptimal HbA_{1c} levels prior to conception [276]. Pre-conception care has been shown through economic health care models to be cost effective [5,277].

Clinical studies have shown that planned pregnancies are associated with improved glycemic control in early pregnancy and fewer congenital malformations. A Dutch study of 323 women with T1DM who became pregnant showed a significantly lower incidence of major congenital malformations among the women who had planned their pregnancies (4.2% [11/271] vs 12.2% [6/52]); relative risk 0.34, (95% CI 0.13–0.88) [278].

Accessing pre-pregnancy care

Some 30–80% of women will attend a clinic for pre-pregnancy advice, but this attendance depends on the woman's perception of its benefits [47,279,280]. A study from Michigan, USA, found half of pregnant women with diabetes who had not received pre-pregnancy care claimed they had not been informed of its importance [279]. Women who seek out and engage in pre-pregnancy care tend to have higher educational and economic status and greater family and social support [281,282].

Unplanned pregnancies are common among women with diabetes. In the CEMACH enquiry, only 60% and 62% of women with T1DM and T2DM, respectively, had planned their pregnancy [3]. Overall, 34.5% of the women had received pre-pregnancy care: 38.2% of the women with T1DM and 24.8% of the women with T2DM.

A survey in New Zealand showed 60% of non-pregnant women with diabetes aged 18–40 years would like more information about diabetes and pregnancy [283], suggesting there is an unmet need for good pre-pregnancy advice. It remains a clinical challenge to increase the awareness and uptake of pre-pregnancy care for all women with diabetes planning pregnancy, especially among more hard to reach groups.

Information to cover during pre-pregnancy care

All pre-pregnancy advice should be supported by evidence of its benefit in pregnancy. The advice should be constructive and non-judgmental, and communicated in a way that is appropriate for the individual woman [284].

Women should receive information that covers the following topics:
- The benefits of optimal glycemic control and appropriate and safe glycemic targets;
- Folic acid supplementation;
- General lifestyle advice (e.g. smoking and alcohol);
- Advice on diet and exercise;
- Advice on safe prescription medications;
- General information of pregnancy risk to the woman's health;
- General information of pregnancy risk to the fetus, neonate and their long-term health; and
- General information on diabetic pregnancy management guidelines and the need for extra surveillance.

Benefits of optimal glycemic control prior to conception

The benefits of optimal glycemic control prior to conception on pregnancy outcomes should be explained, stressing the need to continue contraception prior to achieving the agreed glycemic target. While it is important to discuss the strong association between poor pre-conception glycemic control and congenital malformations, this risk should not be exaggerated as malformations only occur in a minority of diabetic pregnancies and may discourage some women in engaging in pre-pregnancy care [280].

There is clinical evidence that pre-pregnancy care is successful in improving glycemic control in the first trimester and reduces

Table 53.1 Recommended pre-pregnancy HbA_{1c} targets in the USA, Australia and the UK.

Country	USA	Australia	UK*
HbA_{1c} upper target			
DCCT	<7.0%	<7.0%	<6.1% if safely possible
IFCC	<53 mmol/mol	<53 mmol/mol	<43 mmol/mol
Reference	[4]	[286]	[5] Available from www.nice.org.uk

* England and Wales.

the risk of malformation, stillbirth and neonatal death; however, it has less effect on the risk of macrosomia in later pregnancy [285]. In a meta-analysis of 14 cohort studies, the major anomaly rate was 2.1% among the 1192 offspring of women who had received preconception care compared with 6.5% in 1459 offspring of non-recipients [143]. In the nine studies that recorded both major and minor congenital anomalies, the relative risk of an anomaly with preconception care was lower (RR 0.32; 95% CI 0.17–0.59). Some of the risk may reflect important demographic differences between women who received preconception care and those who did not.

Appropriate and safe glycemic targets

Pre-conception glycemic control should be assessed by HbA_{1c} and women should be advised to continue using contraception until their HbA_{1c} level reaches the agreed target. An HbA_{1c} test should be performed at 1–3 monthly intervals during this time.

The recommended pre-pregnancy HbA_{1c} targets are lower in the UK NICE guidelines than the national pregnancy guidelines from the USA and Australia (Table 53.1).

A glycemic target of a pre-pregnancy HbA_{1c} <53 mmol/mol (<7%) has been recommended in Denmark after a prospective population-based study of 933 T1DM pregnancies found the risk of a serious adverse outcome, defined as congenital malformations and perinatal mortality, was higher when pre-pregnancy HbA_{1c} values were >52 mmol/mol (>6.9%). In this study, poor pregnancy outcomes correlated with the incremental rise in HbA_{1c}; the risk of a serious adverse outcome was 16% in women whose HbA_{1c} exceeded 90 mmol/mol (10.4%) [141].

The NICE UK guidelines recommend women whose HbA_{1c} exceeds 86 mmol/mol (10%) should be advised against becoming pregnant [5].

The CEMACH study found only 37.1% of the pregnancies had an HbA_{1c} measurement within 6 months of the pregnancy [2]. Evidence of good glycemic control defined as an HbA_{1c} <53 mmol/mol (<7.0%) was found in 24% and 41% of the women with T1DM and T2DM, respectively. Further analysis by the CEMACH enquiry showed pre-pregnancy HbA_{1c} was suboptimal in 88% (165/187) of those women with poor pregnancy outcome, defined as a major congenital anomalies, stillbirths or early neonatal deaths death, compared with 69% (115/167) of those women with a good outcome [2].

When setting glycemic target for the pre-pregnancy period, the risk of hypoglycemia and hypoglycemia unawareness should be discussed. Both are increased during pregnancy, especially in women with T1DM [3]. The risk of hypoglycemia increases with lower HbA_{1c} which may explain why in some studies women who attend pre-pregnancy counseling are at a greater risk of hypoglycemia in the first trimester than women who do not attend [138,287]. The risks and benefits of achieving an HbA_{1c} of <43 mmol/mol (<6.1%) for women with a long history of duration of T1DM [5] need to be discussed and may not be appropriate for all women. Individual HbA_{1c} targets should be set and discussed with the woman concerned, emphasizing that any pre-pregnancy HbA_{1c} reduction reduces the risk of congenital malformations.

Advice to minimize the risk of hypoglycemia should be given to women receiving insulin and ideally women with T1DM should be taught to adjust their insulin dosage according to their dietary carbohydrate intake [288]. Women with T2DM should receive an equivalent form of structured education.

Many women with T2DM attending pre-pregnancy care need to start insulin for the first time, or have their insulin regimen intensified to achieve the recommended HbA_{1c} level. These women need advice on frequency and timing of self-monitoring of blood glucose as well as the need for extra snacks between meals and before bed.

During pre-pregnancy care and insulin intensification, the risk of DKA is low; however, this risk increases during pregnancy and women with T1DM should be taught how to monitor and interpret their blood or urinary ketones.

Folic acid supplementation

Folic acid supplementation in the form of a folate-rich diet plus 400 μg/day folic acid from before conception until 12 weeks is advised for all women planning a pregnancy as this has been shown to reduce the risk of NTD [289]. A dose of 5 mg folic acid is recommended for women with diabetes as the risk of NTD is higher than the background population.

In the CEMACH enquiry, 49% of women with T1DM and 45% of women with T2DM took folic acid in the pre-conception period; however, few women were taking the recommended 5 mg dose [3,5]. A total of 69% (83/120) of women with a poor pregnancy outcome were not taking folic acid in the preconception period compared with 50% (66/131) with a good outcome [3].

It is likely that awareness of the need to take folic acid prior to pregnancy is rising. An earlier study in the UK in the general antenatal population reported less than 10% of women took folic acid supplements in early pregnancy [290].

General advice on lifestyle

Smoking in pregnancy is associated with poor pregnancy outcomes and women seeking pregnancy should be given advice and help to stop smoking. In a study of 211 pregnancies in 132 women with pre-gestational diabetes, women who smoked during the preconception period had an increase risk of a stillbirth, neonatal death or congenital malformation (OR 2.12; 95% CI 1.09–4.10) [291,292].

Advice about alcohol should be similar to the general population, which is to avoid alcohol in the first 3 months of pregnancy [5]. For women with diabetes, this is especially important as alcohol can increase the risk of hypoglycemia and is associated with an increased risk of miscarriage.

Advice on diet and exercise

Pre-pregnancy is a time to provide dietary information that will optimize glycemic control and minimize hypoglycemia during intensive glycemic management. Obese women should be encouraged to achieve a healthy weight prior to pregnancy through diet and exercise if they have BMI >27 kg/m^2 [293,294].

Advice on safe prescription medications

Medication should be reviewed prior to conception. The most common drugs that should be stopped are antihypertensive drugs acting on the renin-angiotensin system, lipid-lowering drugs and certain hypoglycemic oral agents. The continuation of long-acting analog insulin needs to be discussed on an individual basis.

Angiotensin-converting enzyme (ACE) inhibitors cross the placenta [295]. Although the use of ACE inhibitors in the first trimester of pregnancy was initially felt to be safe [296–299], there is sufficient evidence to recommend their discontinuation before conception.

First trimester exposure to ACE inhibitors was linked to malformations in a study of 29 507 infants with no drug exposure and 209 infants exposed to ACE inhibitors but no other drugs in the first trimester from 1985–2000. The risk ratio of major congenital malformations, primarily cardiovascular and CNS anomalies in women who took ACE inhibitors was 2.71 (95% CI 1.72–4.27) compared with infants who had no drug exposure [300].

There is little information on the teratogenic effects of the angiotensin receptor blockers (ARBs). Fetal exposure to losartan at 20–31 weeks' gestation has been linked with oligohydramnios and the intrauterine death of a fetus with hypoplastic lungs and skull bones [301]. A series of five cases exposed to ARBs found one term baby with additional digits, two pregnancies complicated with oligohydramnios and premaurity, another infant with transient abnormal renal function and two babies delivered with no abnormalities [302]. Current recommendations are to avoid ARBs in pregnancy [5,303,304].

The HMGCoA reductase inhibitors, statins, are commonly used in diabetic care. A small number of case reports and surveillance registers have reported congenital malformations following first trimester statin exposure [303,305]. Current guidelines recommend that statins are not to be taken during pregnancy or lactation [5].

Methyldopa remains the first-line antihypertensive agent in pregnancy, but other agents considered to be safe include nifedipine, amlodipine, hydralzine and labetalol. Beta-blockers are usually avoided in the first trimester because of the risk of growth restriction. Other antihypertensive agents should be used on an individual basis and the risks and benefits reviewed. Two small cohort studies suggest calcium-channel blockers are not teratogenic [306,307].

The use of oral hypoglycemic agents other than metformin and glibenclamide are not recommended in pregnancy. Women on oral hypoglycemic therapy during pre-pregnancy care should be switched to insulin if their HbA_{1c} values are above target, although metformin can be continued.

General information on diabetic pregnancy management guidelines and the need for extra surveillance

During pre-pregnancy care, women should be informed of the need to access antenatal care as soon as a pregnancy has been confirmed and the need for additional recommended clinic attendances and fetal monitoring above those for routine antenatal care. The increased fetal monitoring includes ultrasound scanning to assess fetal viability and dating in early pregnancy as well as fetal growth in late pregnancy. General information concerning timing and mode of birth can be given at this time.

Screening for diabetic complications

Women can be reassured that although diabetic retinopathy and nephropathy may progress, it is rare for pregnancy to have long-term detrimental effects. Screening for retinopathy or nephropathy prior to pregnancy is important to assess if any treatment is required before pregnancy and if greater surveillance or treatment will be required during pregnancy. The CEMACH enquiry found that women with T2DM were less likely to have a retinal examination and an assessment of albuminuria in the year prior to pregnancy than women with T1DM [3].

Screening for retinopathy

All women seeking pregnancy should be informed of the importance of retinal screening and the benefits it offers. Any woman with known proliferative retinopathy should be considered for laser treatment prior to pregnancy. Women actively seeking pregnancy should ideally have a dilated digital retinal photograph if one has not been performed in the preceding 12 months.

Women should be informed of the retinal screening guidelines for pregnancy, which include a first trimester screen and a repeat screen at 28 weeks if no retinopathy is present, with an additional screen at 16–20 weeks if retinopathy is present [5]. Women should be reassured that the use of tropicamide to dilate the eye is safe in pregnancy, as is photocoagulation therapy if required. Women who have or develop retinopathy in pregnancy should be aware that retinal follow-up should continue for at least 6 months postpartum [308].

Worsening of retinopathy in pregnancy may be associated with rapid intensification of glycemic control [227,234], emphasizing the importance of optimizing glycemic control prior to pregnancy.

Screening for nephropathy

Women actively seeking pregnancy should be screened for microalbuminuria and have their serum creatinine measured. Women with a normal urinary ACR (<3.5 mg/mmol) and serum creatinine <120 μmol/L can be reassured that their kidney function poses no added risk to the pregnancy. Women with microalbuminuria (ACR 3.5–30 mg/mmol) need to be aware that although pregnancy will not adversely affect their renal function long-term, they are at an increased risk for hypertension and pre-eclampsia in pregnancy [239–241]. For women with macroalbuminuria or proteinuria and established nephropathy, pre-pregnancy advice should cover the evidence that is discussed above.

Screening for autoimmune disorders

Thyroid function should be assessed pre-pregnancy as autoimmune hypothyroidism and hyperthyroidism are more common in women with diabetes and both conditions can affect the fetus and neonate [273,275]. Women with T1DM and celiac disease seeking pregnancy need to be aware that compliance with a gluten-free diet helps fertility rates and during pregnancy lessens the risk of anemia [309].

Ischemic heart disease

Ischemic heart disease in pregnancy is associated with serious mortality and morbidity for the mother and child. Women with a previous or suspected history of IHD should be referred and assessed by a cardiologist prior to pregnancy. Women with T1DM of long duration and older women with T2DM should be informed of their underlying risk for IHD and the added risk this has during pregnancy. A resting and an exercise electrocardiogram (ECG) may be required prior to pregnancy to assess this risk so an informed decision can be made concerning any future pregnancies. For women known to have IHD the potential mortality associated with pregnancy should be discussed.

Antenatal management

Once pregnancy is confirmed women should have easy and immediate access to a combined diabetic and obstetric clinic that can manage and support them throughout the pregnancy. This clinic should comprise a diabetologist with an interest in obstetrics, an obstetrician with an interest in diabetes, a diabetes specialist nurse/educator, a midwife with an interest in diabetes and a dietitian.

The first clinic visit needs to ensure that the woman is taking folic acid and has glycemic management optimized. This will require most women with pre-gestational diabetes not on an insulin pump to be switched to a basal bolus regimen, if not already on one.

Glycemic management

Maternal hyperglycemia from the time of conception to birth affects pregnancy outcome. The aim of glycemic management is to achieve glycemic control as near to that of women without diabetes as possible with due consideration to safety.

In clinical practice the limitations in achieving normoglycemia are the high risk of severe hypoglycemia in women intensively treated with insulin and growth restriction in a fetus of a woman too aggressively treated with hypoglycemic management or dietary restriction.

For women with T1DM, glycemic control is dependent on balancing insulin requirements with the physiologic changes of pregnancy and the risk of hypoglycemia. This can only be achieved through frequent glucose monitoring and flexible insulin dosing, using either a basal bolus regimen or insulin pump.

Women with T2DM will also require intensive insulin management alongside diet and exercise to achieve the required level of glycemic control for pregnancy. For women with GDM, approximately half will be able to achieve the desired glycemic target through diet and exercise, with the remainder requiring the addition of an appropriate oral hypoglycemic agent or insulin.

Risk of hypoglycemia

Insulin sensitivity increases in the first trimester before declining in the second. Insulin requirements for women who become pregnant with good glycemic control will usually fall in the first trimester before rising in the mid-second trimester [46,310–312]. This initial increase in insulin sensitivity occurs at a time when there is a physiologic fall in fasting blood glucose and makes women with T1DM extremely susceptible to hypoglycemia. This may be further exaggerated by a pregnancy-induced decrease in counter-regulatory hormones to hypoglycemia [313,314].

In a prospective observational study of 108 consecutive Danish pregnant women with T1DM, self-reported episodes of hypoglycemia, validated by structured interview within 24 hours, occurred in 49 women (45%) experiencing 178 severe hypoglycemic events requiring third party assistance. Of these severe episodes, 80% occurred in the first 20 weeks of pregnancy and approximately half occurred at night; 11 women had five or more events. Predictors for severe hypoglycemia were a history of similar events in the preceding year, impaired hypoglycemia awareness and long duration of T1DM. There was no evidence that hypoglycemia unawareness changed during the pregnancy or that pregnancy-related nausea was a significant risk factor [46]. In an earlier Danish study in the first trimester, nocturnal hypoglycemia, defined as blood glucose values <3.0 mmol/L, was detected in 16 of 43 women with T1DM who had hourly blood glucose sampling during the night (22.00–07.00). These episodes of hypoglycemia went unrecognized by all but one of the women despite lasting 1–7 hours (mean 2.4 hours) [315].

In the CEMACH enquiry, 61% of women with T1DM had recurrent hypoglycemia during pregnancy, with 33/133 (25%) episodes requiring external help. While women with T2DM are less likely to experience recurrent or severe hypoglycemia, one-fifth of women with T2DM had recurrent hypoglycemia, with 4/102 (4%) requiring external help [3]. Nocturnal hypoglycemia has also been well documented in insulin-treated pregnant women with T2DM undergoing continuous glucose monitoring [316].

The risk of severe hypoglycemia is less after the first 22 weeks of pregnancy when maternal insulin resistance rises and glucose variability and fluctuations become less marked [46].

Maternal mortality from hypoglycemia is extremely rare but well recognized [317] and has been a recurrent cause of death in women with T1DM in the triennial Confidential Enquiry into Maternal Death in the UK over the last 30 years.

All women intensively managed with insulin need to be informed of the added risk of hypoglycemia in pregnancy and given advice to minimize the risk, including advice about whether it is safe to drive. For women with T1DM, their partner or a family member should be given instruction on when and how to give glucagon.

Glucose monitoring

Accurate self-monitoring of blood glucose is required at least five times a day throughout pregnancy. A study comparing blood glucose values obtained using self- monitoring of blood glucose and data from a continuous glucose monitoring (CGM) system found that unless the women were testing 10 or more times a day many episodes where blood glucose values were outside the target range were missed [146]. Monitoring should be increased for women on insulin pumps, those who are dose adjusting their insulin for each meal, experiencing hypoglycemia and when insulin doses are being changed. Glucose monitoring also needs to be carried out before driving and exercising. Monitoring between 02.00 and 04.00 should be performed if nocturnal hypoglycemia is expected.

For women already on insulin, their evening basal insulin is adjusted against their fasting glucose reading, and their bolus insulin against their 1–2 hour post-prandial glucose value. A pre-bed reading may help to calculate the size of the snack required before bed. The use of a 1-hour post-prandial glucose value is more informative for adjusting insulin requirements than a pre-prandial measurement [318]. In an randomized controlled trial of women with GDM, there were fewer large for gestational age babies, fewer cesarean sections for cephalo-pelvic disproportion and less neonatal hypoglycemia in women self-monitoring 1 hour after a meal than immediately before [319].

The use of CGM is currently too expensive for routine use in pregnancy; however, this is likely to change as CGM provides information on the extent of glucose fluctuations and episodes of hyperglycemia and hypoglycemia undetected by self-monitoring of blood glucose [316,320,321].

CGM performed at intervals of 4–6 weeks during pregnancy was associated with a lower HbA_{1c} in the third trimester, lower birth weight and macrosomia compared with standard care in a randomized control trial of 71 pre-gestational pregnant women [322].

The use of CGM in clinical studies in pregnant women with T1DM has also highlighted the extent of glucose fluctuations that are not detected by HbA_{1c} [146]. Intensifying insulin regimens to strict and inflexible glycemic targets based on HbA_{1c} may not be safe using the clinical tools and insulin currently available in routine care.

Glycemic targets in pregnancy

Glycemic targets for pregnancy have been set by national guidelines, and are the same for all women with diabetes regardless of its type; however, there is a need to adjust and discuss these targets individually according to what is safe and achievable for the woman. This is especially true for women with T1DM who experience recurrent hypoglycemia during the first trimester. The current targets for the UK are fasting blood glucose of 3.5–5.9 mmol/L and 1 hour post-prandial blood glucose <7.8 mmol/L, if safely achievable [5].

In women with GDM, active glycemic management with diet, exercise and insulin, if required, using the targets of a fasting blood glucoses <5.5 mmol/L and a 2-hour post-prandial level <7.0 mmol/L was associated with less perinatal morbidity than no active glycemic management (1% vs 4%; RR 0.33; 95% CI 1.03–1.23; $P = 0.01$) in a large randomized trial of 1000 women [323].

Too stringent targets for glycemic control in women with GDM may be potentially detrimental for the infant [324]. In a prospective study of 334 women with GDM who were randomized to maintaining their mean blood glucose levels to <4.8 mmol/L, 4.8–5.8 mmol/L or to >5.8 mmol/L, there was a twofold higher incidence of small for gestational age infants (20%) in the lowest target group compared with a well-matched control group of 334 women without diabetes. In the high glucose group, an approximate twofold increased incidence of large for gestational age infants was seen, while when mean blood glucose values were maintained at 4.8–5.8 mmol/L, the incidence for small and large for gestational age babies was similar to that of the control group.

Insulin management

Women with pre-gestational diabetes who are not using an insulin pump usually require multiple daily injections (MDI) with either short-acting human insulin or quick-acting analog insulin prior to each meal and an intermediate-acting human insulin or long-acting insulin analog before bedtime. In a randomized trial of 60 women with pre-gestational diabetes which compared a MDI regimen with twice daily mixed insulin, the MDI regimen was associated with better glycemic control and less neonatal hypoglycemia [325]. Both US and UK guidelines recommend the use of an MDI regimen for women with pre-gestational diabetes [4,5].

There are theoretical concerns around the use of insulin analogs in pregnancy and no study has yet been sufficiently powered to confirm their complete safety. Quick-acting insulin analogs have been widely used in diabetic pregnancy for over 10 years without any evidence of any harm, and are recommended in both the US and UK guidelines.

Outside pregnancy the use of rapid-acting insulin analogs (Lispro [Eli Lilly], Aspart [Novo Nordisk] and Glulisine Apidra [Sanofi-Aventis]) is beginning to replace short-acting human soluble insulin in MDI regimens, as they potentially offer better post-prandial glycemic control; however, their use puts greater reliance on the basal insulin for glycemic control between meals, for which the pharmacokinetic profiles of the longer-acting insulin analog (Glargine [Sanofi-Aventis] and Determir [Novo Nordisk]) are better suited than the intermediate human insulin (NPH [Neutral Protamine Hagedorn]). In some clinical studies, especially in T1DM, MDI regimens with insulin analogs are associated with less nocturnal hypoglycemia [326]. Rapid-acting insulin analogs are being increasingly used by patients who carbohydrate count and adjust their insulin dose [288].

For these reasons, MDI regimens with insulin analogs are attractive options for diabetic pregnancies. Increasingly, more women with T1DM are treated with insulin analogs prior to pregnancy and switching them to the older human soluble insulin in early pregnancy puts them at potential risk of worsening glycemic control at this critical time. Patient preference may also be important as the women receiving insulin aspart in a randomized controlled trial in pregnancy expressed greater patient satisfaction than women receiving human insulin [327]. Recruiting women with T1DM to participate in future randomized studies will be increasingly difficult as many will be reluctant to be randomized to the older human insulin.

The clinical studies evaluating the efficacy and safety of insulin lispro, the first widely available rapid-acting insulin analog [328–332], all involve small numbers of women, are mostly retrospective and are inadequately designed or powered to evaluate serious adverse pregnancy outcomes. A multinational multicentered retrospective study of 72 women with T1DM treated with insulin lispro for at least 3 months before and 3 months after conception and a control group of 298 women treated with regular human insulin showed a trend towards fewer hypoglycemic episodes and significantly greater reduction in HbA_{1c} during the first trimester in the lispro arm [331]. The early concerns that insulin lispro might be associated with an increased risk of retinopathy progression have not been substantiated by later studies.

An open-labeled randomized control trial compared the safety and efficacy of insulin aspart as part of a MDI regimen with NPH insulin with soluble human insulin in 322 pregnant women with T1DM [327]. Insulin aspart was associated with less nocturnal hypoglycemia and severe hypoglycemia and superior postprandial glycemic control in the third trimester; there were no differences in other pregnancy outcomes between the insulins.

Basal insulin analogs in pregnancy

At present, neither basal analog insulin is recommended in the USA or UK national guidelines for use in pregnancy; instead human intermediate NPH insulin should be used 1–3 times daily to provide adequate basal cover.

Theoretical concerns persist around the long-acting analog insulin glargine because of its higher binding affinity for the IGF-I receptor and potential mitogenic potency compared with human insulin [333,334]. There have been no adequately controlled studies large enough to ascertain its safety in pregnancy. An audit of the use of insulin glargine in 115 women with T1DM and 109 babies was collected over 2 years in 20 diabetic obstetric units in the UK. Insulin glargine was used prior to pregnancy in 69% of women, and stopped at booking in one patient. The bolus insulin used in this audit was insulin aspart (45%), lispro (42%) and human soluble in 8% of women. This audit identified no unexpected or adverse maternal or fetal outcome [335], similar to earlier smaller clinical pregnancy studies [336,337].

The long-acting analog insulin detemir has no increased affinity binding to the IGF-I receptor [334] and may be a more appropriate basal insulin analog than glargine. The outcome of a large randomized control trial is awaited to show if it offers any clinical advantages in diabetic pregnancy.

Continuous subcutaneous insulin pumps in pregnancy

The continuous subcutaneous insulin infusion pumps (CSII) potentially offer the most physiologic form of subcutaneous insulin administration. The technology surrounding the CSII is progressing rapidly, with integrated insulin pumps and continuous glucose monitor systems under development. There are no adequately powered multicentred studies evaluating the use of insulin pumps in pregnancy but clinical experience is increasing.

Outside pregnancy the greatest benefit of insulin pumps over MDI on glycemic control is when control is poor beforehand; this benefit is less apparent when HbA_{1c} approaches the normal range [338].

A systematic review of six randomized trials published between 1974 and 2006 of CSII involving 213 pregnant women (199 T1DM and 14 T2DM) showed no significant differences in pregnancy outcomes or glycemic control including hypoglycemic events between CSII and MDI [339]. A Cochrane review that examined only two studies involving 60 women with 61 pregnancies also concluded that maternal glycemia and pregnancy outcomes were similar between women on CSII and MDI, and concluded more good quality studies were required [340].

In one study that compared the use of CSII in 30 insulin-treated pregnant women with T2DM and GDM with a matched control group on conventional insulin, pump use was associated with larger daily doses of insulin and greater weight gain, without any benefit on pregnancy outcomes. Large multicentered randomized controlled trials are required to identify which women would benefit from CSII in pregnancy. As HbA_{1c} values fall in pregnancy approaching the non-pregnancy range, it is likely that evaluating glycemic control in future trials using CSII will require continuous glucose monitoring systems as these will be more informative than HbA_{1c} values.

CSII may improve overall control and glycemic fluctuations in selected women with poorly controlled T1DM. In an Italian study that compared 25 women with T1DM on CSII with 93 women on MDI, there were no differences in glycemic control and pregnancy outcomes between the groups; however, within the CSII group were women with more retinopathy and nephropathy in whom a poorer pregnancy outcome might have been predicted [341].

Oral hypoglycemic agents

The use of oral agents in the management of diabetic pregnancies remains controversial: the ADA do not currently recommend their use, while the UK NICE guidelines endorse the use of metformin in combination with insulin for the management of women with pre-existing T2DM, as well as metformin and glibenclamide in the management of GDM [4,5].

The number of classes of oral hypoglycemic agents is increasing but the only oral hypoglycemic drugs that have been sufficiently evaluated in pregnancy are sulfonylureas and metformin.

Metformin crosses the placenta, with fetal serum levels being comparable with maternal values [342]; however, there is no evidence of any increased risk for major malformations when metformin is taken during the first trimester of pregnancy [343].

The early introduction of metformin and glibenclamide in the 1970s in South Africa for women with T2DM and GDM was accompanied with a fall in neonatal mortality. Switching women from oral agents to insulin in early pregnancy was associated with better pregnancy outcomes than when women were treated with oral agents alone. In these early observational reports, poor glycemic control rather than oral hypoglycemic agents was thought to be the cause of the high malformation rates and perinatal mortality [344,345]. Many of the later studies in the literature are also observational and involve heterogeneous populations of pregnant women without adequate non-exposed controls, limiting the scope for meta-analysis to be undertaken [346].

More robust clinical randomized trials of the use of metformin and glibenclamide in pregnancy have been conducted in women with GDM than in women with T2DM. A systematic review of four randomized controlled trials (1229 women) and five observational studies (831 women) published prior to January 2007 of maternal and neonatal outcomes when GDM was treated with either glibenclamide or metformin found no differences in outcomes when compared with insulin [347].

A randomized control trial of 751 of women with GDM not controlled with diet alone by 20–33 weeks' gestation compared the efficacy and safety of metformin with insulin [348]. Of the 363 women, 92.6% were assigned to metformin and continued on metformin until the birth. Metformin was increased to a maximum of 2500 mg/day after which insulin was added in 46.3% of women to the metformin if glycemic targets were not met. The mean fasting blood glucose was similar in the metformin and insulin-treated groups but the 2-hour post-prandial blood glucose was lower in the metformin arm. The weight gain in late pregnancy was less in women treated with metformin and was associated with greater weight loss at 6–8 weeks postpartum compared with women treated with insulin alone. Perinatal complications were broadly similar other than a lower incidence of severe hypoglycemia (blood glucose <1.6 mmol/L) in the infants in the metformin group [348]. A total of 76.6% women in the metformin arm compared with 27.2% of the insulin group stated that they would choose to receive their assigned treatment again in a future pregnancy.

A randomized control trial of 404 women with GDM who had failed dietary management alone and were assigned to either glibenclamide or insulin after 15 weeks' gestation reported only 4% of the glibenclamide-treated women required supplemental insulin. The mean blood glucose values were similar in both treatment arms and the incidence of maternal hypoglycemia was lower in the glibenclamide group (2% vs 20%). Perinatal outcome did not differ between the two groups [349].

Oral hypoglycemic agents offer an attractive treatment option for diabetic obstetric clinics serving large numbers of women and their use will grow if future studies of the children of women with GDM treated with these oral agents show the children to be healthy and at no extra risk.

Antenatal care in a diabetic pregnancy

In addition to routine antenatal care, women with diabetes require extra maternal and fetal surveillance in pregnancy. Details in the obstetric and diabetic management of pregnant women with pre-gestational diabetes will vary according to country in which care is being given. The principles of management will be broadly similar and are outlined briefly below, according to trimester.

Antenatal care in the first trimester (1–12 weeks)

All women should be seen at the earliest opportunity once pregnancy is confirmed; this will be earlier than women seen in routine antenatal clinics. At the first clinic visit it is important to review all prescribed and over-the-counter medications for safety and to ensure an appropriate dosage of folic acid has been prescribed.

The importance of optimization of glycemic control during this time requires frequent contact and visits with the members of the multidisciplinary team. This is especially so for women with T2DM who may be starting insulin for the first time. Dietary advice about the avoidance of hypoglycemia should be given, especially to women with T1DM [46].

It is important to confirm viability of the pregnancy at 6–8 weeks; this is before the routine screening for Down syndrome which occurs at 11–13 weeks. The 6–8 week ultrasound provides an accurate gestational age, which is important later in pregnancy when assessing fetal growth and the optimal timing of birth.

The woman's current diet and levels of physical activity should be reviewed and advice given on appropriate food choices taken as snacks for the prevention and management of hypoglycemia. Advice on exercise should be individualized; however, as a general principle, women should be encouraged to take at least 30 min/day of moderate intensity physical activity [4]. This may be modified where there is a risk of exercise-induced hypoglycemia in women with T1DM.

The general advice around diet remains the same as a non-diabetic pregnancy. The ADA guidelines on diet are more prescriptive than those of the UK NICE guidelines, with the former recommending 175 g/day digestible carbohydrate and 28 g/day fiber [4]. Women should be advised to spread their carbohydrate portions throughout the day as this reduces hypoglycemia while avoiding post-prandial hyperglycemia. Low rather than high glycemic index carbohydrates may prevent glycemic excursions. The actual additional calories required to sustain a pregnancy is modest, being approximately 100 kcal in the first trimester rising to 200–300 kcal in the third trimester; this is independent of any reduction in physical activity that might occur [350].

At the start of pregnancy women should be given appropriate weight gain targets. This is especially so for women with T2DM, many of whom will be obese [3]. There is general agreement that for a non-diabetic population a 10–12.5 kg pregnancy weight gain for normal weight women and 12.5–18 kg for underweight women (BMI <19.8 kg/m^2) is associated with fewer pregnancy-related complications. The appropriate weight gain for overweight (25–30 kg/m^2) and obese (>30 kg/m^2) is more controversial and there are no accepted guidelines for morbidly obese women (>40 kg/m^2).

Historically, guidelines around maternal weight gain were focused on preventing low birth weight infants rather than large for gestational age infants. The original and widely accepted recommendations for maternal weight gain were published in 1990 by the US Institute of Medicine. These guidelines were later updated in 2009 when they lowered the recommended upper weight gain limit for overweight and obese women. These guidelines give no specific weight gain targets for morbidly obese women (>40 kg/m^2). This is despite good evidence that little or no weight gain during pregnancy improves many pregnancy outcomes with little increase in the risk of small for gestational age infants [293,351–353]. Gestational weight gain is also directly associated with the risk of obesity in the adolescent offspring [354] and the degree of weight retention postpartum in the mother [355].

Maternal surveillance in the first trimester includes diabetic retinopathy and nephropathy screening. Women with pre-existing hypertension need to be identified and methyldopa initiated if required. Other co-morbidities will need to be screened and treated on an individual basis.

Women with previous GDM should be seen so they can start self-monitoring of blood glucose and be given advice on diet and exercise. The glycemic targets for women with GDM are identical to those with pre-existing diabetes, and pharmacologic treatment should begin if these are not met.

Antenatal care in the second trimester (13–27 weeks)

Glycemic profiles and variability are less labile by the mid-second trimester [46], making insulin intensification easier and safer. Insulin requirements increase and multiple basal insulin doses (2–3 times daily) may be needed to avoid nocturnal hypoglycemia, while ensuring adequate 24-hour cover [4].

It is important to limit excessive weight gain in overweight and obese women in this trimester as appetite and food intake increases. The current UK guidelines recommend women with a pre-pregnancy BMI >27 kg/m^2 to restrict their calorie intake to approximately 25 kcal/kg/day in the second trimester [5].

Fetal surveillance for cardiac anomalies using an appropriate ultrasonography should be performed at 18–22 weeks. It is important to examine the four heart chambers as well as the outflow tract of the aorta and pulmonary artery [5,356]. This scan is in addition to the routine detailed anatomical scan for other congenital anomalies which should be undertaken at around the same time.

For women who had an abnormal retinal screen in the first trimester, repeat digital retinal photographs should be performed at 16 weeks' gestation.

The second trimester is associated with worsening hypertension in women with pre-existing hypertension and the development of pregnancy-induced hypertension in women with microalbuminuria [239]. This trimester is also associated with a number of "minor" complications of pregnancy, many of which can be exacerbated by diabetes, including vaginal candidiasis, heartburn, urinary tract infections and carpal tunnel syndrome, and should be treated on an individual basis.

Antenatal care in the third trimester (28–42 weeks)

Optimizing glycemic control continues to be important as the third trimester continues, because of the risk of stillbirth [2] and accelerated fetal growth at this time [357].

Serial ultrasound scans to assess fetal growth and liquor volume should start at 28 weeks and should be repeated at 32 and 36 weeks' gestation. Accelerated fetal growth patterns in a diabetic pregnancy typically present as serial fetal abdominal circumference measurements that cross percentile lines (Figure 53.1) [168,358]. The 36-week growth scan is one factor the obstetrician takes into consideration when advising on the optimal timing and mode of delivery.

Maternal surveillance in the third trimester includes further digital retinal photographs and regular checks for hypertension and pre-eclampsia.

Gestational diabetes

Screening for gestational diabetes

Glucose intolerance developing *de novo* in pregnancy usually manifests itself by 26–28 weeks' gestation. Both the ADA and NICE guidelines currently recommend selecting women to screen for GDM according to maternal risk factors. The NICE guidelines recommend all women attending the routine antenatal clinic with predefined risk factors (Table 53.2) have a diagnostic 75-g OGTT

Table 53.2 Maternal risk factors for screening women for gestational diabetes.

BMI >30 kg/m^2
Previous macrosomic baby weighing >4.5 kg
Previous GDM
Family history of diabetes – first-degree relative with diabetes
Family origin with high prevalence of diabetes (e.g. South Asian, Afro-Caribbean, Middle Eastern)

BMI, body mass index; GDM, gestational diabetes mellitus.

at around 28 weeks for GDM, with the WHO criteria for IGT being used to establish the diagnosis [5].

The ADA guidelines advocate an initial 50-g glucose challenge test at 24–28 weeks with a glucose measurement 1 hour later. Women with a positive challenge test, defined as an 1-hour plasma glucose >7.8 mmol/L then proceed to a diagnostic OGTT [12]. The ADA guidelines were based on a consensus document last modified in 2005 and are likely to change following the publication of the HAPO trial [13].

Management of gestational diabetes

The glycemic management for women with GDM was discussed previously. All women diagnosed with GDM need to be taught to self-monitor their blood glucose concentrations, and perform daily tests fasting and 1-hour after meals. The glycemic targets for GDM are identical to those for pre-gestational diabetes. Initial management is with diet and exercise, to which many women will respond. If glycemic targets are not met within 2 weeks, or glycemic levels are considered too high to be controlled adequately with diet and exercise alone, hypoglycemic therapy is required.

Increased physical activity combined with dietary modification and intensive glycemic management reduces perinatal complications in women with GDM [323]. Small clinical studies have reported that exercise programs using upper arm exercises and resistance training reduce fasting and post-prandial blood glucose values in obese women with GDM, as well as reducing insulin requirements when compared with women treated with diet alone [359,360].

The use of metformin and glibenclaimide is not recommended by the ADA [12], but has been endorsed in the UK NICE guidelines [5] following the publications of two randomized control trials of their use in the management of GDM [348,349]. Recent case–controlled studies of metformin [361] and glibenclaimide [362] in specialized antenatal clinics where insulin therapy is available if glycemic targets are not met suggest these agents have a role in the pharmacologic management of GDM. Both drugs are well tolerated, and in the case of metformin is associated with less maternal weight gain than insulin [348,361]. Patient preference for oral therapies rather than insulin is likely to increase their future use as first-line pharmacologic therapy after diet and exercise for the management of GDM.

Birth

Timing and mode of delivery

Women with diabetes are at increased risk of a late stillbirth and shoulder dystocia. The observation that the rate of stillbirth rose from 36 weeks' gestation to term prompted Peel and Oakley [363] to advocate delivery at 36 weeks in 1949. By 1980 there was a gradual trend towards later delivery to avoid perinatal morbidity and mortality from prematurity [364]. By 1990, some obstetric units were allowing selected women with T1DM and uncomplicated diabetic pregnancies to go into spontaneous labor irrespective of the gestational age. Experience from Dublin [365], where there was a policy for delivery past 38 weeks in low risk women, suggests that this was associated with increased perinatal deaths. Current UK obstetric guidelines are to offer induction of labor after 38 completed weeks, or an elective cesarean section if indicated to women with both pre-gestational and GDM [5]. The ADA consensus for the obstetric management of GDM puts greater emphasis on the estimated fetal weight when deciding the timing and mode of delivery [12,366].

The only reported randomized controlled trial of induction of labor versus expectant management involved 200 women with insulin-treated diabetes and 187 with GDM, who were all considered to have uncomplicated pregnancies without macrosomia. Of the mothers in the expectant management group, 49% later required induction of labor for obstetric indications, with 31% having a cesarean delivery compared with 25% among the active induction group. More infants in the expectantly managed group were large for gestational age (23% vs 10%). Shoulder dystocia occurred in 3% of births to the women randomized to expectant management compared with none in the women randomized to induction of labor [367].

A prospective case report study that compared an active policy of induction of labor at 38–39 weeks' gestation in 96 women with insulin-treated diabetes with a previous cohort of 164 women who were allowed to progress to spontaneous labor (n = 164), reported an incidence of shoulder dystocia of 1.4% among the women who were induced compared with 10.2% in patients who gave birth beyond 40 weeks' gestation ($P < 0.05$) [368].

In the CEMACH audit, the incidence of shoulder dystocia was two- to threefold higher and for Erb palsy more than 10-fold greater than that reported for the general UK antenatal population. Thirty-nine percent of women had induction of labor compared with 21% in the general maternity population and the cesarean section rate was also higher (67% vs 24%) [2].

The preterm birth rate (birth before 37 completed weeks' gestation) is increased in diabetic pregnancies. In the CEMACH survey, 35.8% of all births were preterm compared with 7.4% in the general maternity population, with 9.4% of all births being spontaneous preterm births [2]. Similarly, 32.2% of births in 323 women with T1DM in the Netherlands between 1999 and 2000 were preterm [278]. Recognized risk factors for spontaneous preterm delivery in women with diabetes are pre-eclampsia [369], nephropathy, poor glycemic control preterm delivery [370] and obesity [352]. It is routine clinical obstetric practice to give steroids (betamethasone or dexamethasone) as two intramuscular injections 24 hours apart to mothers at risk of a preterm birth to accelerate fetal lung maturity. Although not contraindicated in women with diabetes, their use is associated with a worsening of glycemic control, and it is therefore important to increase insulin doses proactively or treat the woman with an insulin infusion to supplement her basal bolus insulin regimen [371,372].

Glycemic management during labor

There is an association between maternal hyperglycemia during labor and neonatal hypoglycemia [373,374], and so it is important to maintain normoglycemia (4–8 mmol/L) during labor [375]. To maintain this, most women with T1DM will require treatment with an insulin infusion with variable dosing from the onset of established labor. The use of insulin pumps in labor has not yet been subjected to critical evaluation, but early observational studies would suggest they may have a place [373].

The need for intravenous insulin for all women with GDM during labor and birth is less certain. A retrospective study of 114 singleton pregnancies of women with GDM (62 insulin-treated) in Australia reported that 37 (93%) of the women who were diet-controlled and 55 (89%) of the women treated with insulin were able to maintain their blood glucose <8 mmol/L throughout the peripartum period without insulin [376].

Immediately following birth, insulin requirement falls precipitously to below the pre-pregnancy levels. Clear instructions need to be given in the clinical notes to reduce the insulin at this time and to monitor blood glucose hourly.

Postnatal management

Breastfeeding

Breastfeeding provides health advantages for both mother and child. In the offspring of mothers without diabetes, breastfeeding protects against early childhood obesity [377,378]. In the Nurses' Health Study, breastfeeding during the first 6 months was inversely associated with overweight in adolescence. This association was also seen among mothers with diabetes during pregnancy (419 with GDM and 56 with pre-gestational diabetes) as well as offspring of normal-weight women (n = 8617) and overweight women (n = 6190) without diabetes during pregnancy [379].

In a case–control study of 80 young people with T2DM and 167 matched control subjects aged 10–21 years, fewer people with T2DM had been breastfed for any duration than control subjects (19.5% vs 27.1% for African-Americans, 50.0% vs 83.8% for Latino and 39.1% vs 77.6% for whites of Northern European ancestry). The overall crude odds ratio for the association of breastfeeding (ever compared with never) and T2DM was 0.26 (95% CI 0.15–0.46) [380].

Earlier concerns that the advantages of breastfeeding on childhood weight might be lost if the mother has diabetes because her milk is more calorie dense have not been substantiated by later studies [381].

All women with diabetes should be encouraged and supported to breastfeed if this is their wish. For women with T1DM, there is an increased risk of hypoglycemia in the postnatal period especially when breastfeeding; they should be advised to have a meal or snack available before or during feeds.

For women with GDM there is no risk of hypoglycemia during breastfeeding, not least because all hypoglycemic treatment should be stopped immediately after birth. If maternal blood glucose remains high and oral agents are needed, metformin and glibenclamide are the only ones currently recommended when breastfeeding [5]. Metformin is excreted into breast milk in clinically insignificant amounts [382] while glibenclamide is undetectable in breast milk and should be used in preference to other sulfonylureas [5,383].

Diabetes following gestational diabetes; screening and prevention

Women with GDM are at increased risk of developing diabetes in the future. Indeed, the original O'Sullivan criteria for diagnosing GDM were based on the risk of future diabetes in the mother [65,384]. While the majority of women who go on to develop diabetes have T2DM, a smaller minority will develop T1DM [62,385].

Progression from IGT to diabetes is more common in women with a history of GDM [386]. In the control arm of the Diabetes Prevention Program (DPP), 122 of the parous women had a prior history of GDM while 487 had no history. Both groups had equivalent degrees of IGT at baseline but within 3 years of randomization, despite the women with a history of GDM being younger, 38% had developed diabetes compared with 25.7% among the women without a history of GDM.

The rate of progression to diabetes following a GDM pregnancy depends on the original criteria for its diagnosis and the length of follow-up [387]. The risk factors for the progression to diabetes are as follow [217,388–394]:

- Family origin with high prevalence of diabetes (e.g. South Asian, Afro-Caribbean, Middle Eastern);
- Treatment with insulin in pregnancy;
- Maternal obesity;
- Weight gain postpartum; and
- Family history of diabetes.

In Latin American women, parity has also been identified as a risk factor for T2DM [395]. The rate of progression is quicker in obese women with high pregnancy fasting blood glucose values and who have an insulinopenic response to oral glucose postpartum [387,392,396].

The time interval between a GDM pregnancy and future T2DM has decreased in recent years because of increasing obesity. The prevalence of diabetes at 10 years among two Danish cohorts diagnosed with GDM between 1978–1985 and 1986–1996 rose from 18.3% to 40.9% [16].

Lifestyle intevention, metformin and thiazolidinediones have all been shown in women with a history of GDM to slow the progression to T2DM [64,386,397]. A subanalysis of the DPP found that the 349 women with prior GDM who received intensive lifestyle (117) or metformin treatment (111) had a 55% and 51% less risk of progression to diabetes within 3 years than the women assigned to the placebo arm. The corresponding risk reductions in the 1416 parous women without a history of GDM were 49% and 14% for intensive lifestyle and metformin, respectively. This suggests that a history of GDM identifies a group of women particularly susceptible to the protective effects of metformin. The DPP investigators estimated that only five to six women with a history of GDM and IGT would need to be treated for 3 years with metformin or lifestyle intervention to prevent one case of diabetes [386].

All women with GDM should be part of a surveillance program to assess glucose tolerance because of the risk of diabetes. Both the ADA [12] and the UK NICE guidelines [5] recommend screening at 6 weeks postpartum and then at regular intervals thereafter. Unfortunately, a high proportion of women fail to attend the postpartum check at 6 weeks and many have no regular checks thereafter [398]. Non-attendance is associated with obesity, higher parity and worse glucose tolerance in pregnancy [399,400].

An OGTT will pick up more women with IGT or diabetes than a fasting glucose test, especially in high risk groups [401]. In low risk groups using a fasting glucose and only performing an OGTT for women with a fasting value equal to or above 6 mmol/L has been shown to have a high sensitivity (100%) and specificity (94%) for detecting postpartum diabetes [402].

In light of the success of lifestyle intervention trials to prevent diabetes, all women with GDM should be offered lifestyle advice on diet and exercise [386,403,404]. Following a GDM pregnancy, women need to be informed of their risk of a recurrence of GDM in any future pregnancy [405], and encouraged to plan any future pregnancy; their glucose status should be checked before conceiving.

References

1 St. Vincent Declaration. Diabetic care and research in Europe. *Diabet Med* 1990; **7**:360.

2 Modder J, ed. *Confidential Enquiry into Maternal and Child Health: Pregnancy in women with type 1 and type 2 diabetes in 2002–03, England, Wales and Northern Ireland*. CEMACH: London, 2005.

3 Modder J, ed. *Confidential Enquiry into Maternal and Child Health, Diabetes in Pregnancy: Are we providing the best care? Findings of a National Enquiry: England, Wales and Northern Ireland*. CEMACH: London, 2007.

4 Kitzmiller JL, Block JM, Brown FM, Catalano PM, Conway DL, Coustan DR, *et al.* Managing preexisting diabetes for pregnancy: summary of evidence and consensus recommendations for care. *Diabetes Care* 2008; **31**:1060–1079.

5 Guideline Development Group. Management of diabetes from preconception to the postnatal period: summary of NICE guidance. *Br Med J* 2008; **336**:714–717.

6 World Health Organization. Definition, diagnosis and classification of diabetes mellitus and its complications. In: *Report of a WHO Consultation. Part 1. Diagnosis and Classification of Diabetes Mellitus*. Geneva: World Health Organization, 1999.

7 Buschard K, Buch I, Mølsted-Pedersen L, Hougaard P, Kühl C. Increased incidence of true type 1 diabetes acquired during pregnancy. *Br Med J* 1987; **294**:275–279.

8 Jarvela IY, Juutinen J, Koskela P, Hartikainen AL, Kulmala P, Knip M, *et al.* Gestational diabetes identifies women at risk for permanent type 1 and type 2 diabetes in fertile age: predictive role of autoantibodies. *Diabetes Care* 2006; **29**:607–612.

9 Cundy T, Gamble G, Neale L, Elder R, McPherson P, Henley P, *et al.* Differing causes of pregnancy loss in type 1 and type 2 diabetes. *Diabetes Care* 2007; **30**:2603–2607.

10 Saker PJ, Hattersley AT, Barrow B, Hammersley MS, McLellan JA, Lo YM, *et al.* High prevalence of a missense mutation of the glucokinase gene in gestational diabetic patients due to a founder-effect in a local population. *Diabetologia* 1996; **39**:1325–1328.

11 Ellard S, Beards F, Allen LI, Shepherd M, Ballantyne E, Harvey R, *et al.* A high prevalence of glucokinase mutations in gestational diabetic subjects selected by clinical criteria. *Diabetologia* 2000; **43**:250–253.

12 Metzger BE, Buchanan TA, Coustan DR, de Leiva A, Dunger DB, Hadden DR, *et al.* Summary and recommendations of the Fifth International Workshop: Conference on Gestational Diabetes Mellitus. *Diabetes Care* 2007; **30**(Suppl 2):251–260.

13 Metzger BE, Lowe LP, Dyer AR, Trimble ER, Chaovarindr U, Coustan DR, *et al.* Hyperglycemia and adverse pregnancy outcomes. *N Engl J Med* 2008; **358**:1991–2002.

14 Lauenborg J, Grarup N, Damm P, Borch-Johnsen K, Jørgensen T, Pedersen O, *et al.* Common type 2 diabetes risk gene variants associate with gestational diabetes. *J Clin Endocrinol Metab* 2009; **94**:145–150.

15 Catalano PM, Huston L, Amini SB, Kalhan SC. Longitudinal changes in glucose metabolism during pregnancy in obese women with normal glucose tolerance and gestational diabetes mellitus. *Am J Obstet Gynecol* 1999; **180**:903–916.

16 Lauenborg J, Hansen T, Jensen DM, Vestergaard H, Mølsted-Pedersen L, Hornnes P, *et al.* Increasing incidence of diabetes after gestational diabetes: a long-term follow-up in a Danish population. *Diabetes Care* 2004; **27**:1194–1199.

17 White P. Infants of mother with diabetes. *Am J Med* 1949; **7**:609–616.

18 Hare JW, White P. Gestational diabetes and the White classification. *Diabetes Care* 1980; **3**:394.

19 Pedersen J, Mølsted-Pedersen LM. Prognosis of the outcome of pregnancies in diabetics: a new classification. *Acta Endocr* 1965; **50**:70–78.

20 Lind T, Billewicz WZ, Brown G. A serial study of changes occurring in the oral glucose tolerance test during pregnancy. *J Obstet Gynaecol Br Commonw* 1973; **80**:1033–1039.

21 Mills JL, Jovanovic L, Knopp R, Aarons J, Conley M, Park E, *et al.* Physiological reduction in fasting plasma glucose concentration in the first trimester of normal pregnancy: the diabetes in early pregnancy study. *Metabolism* 1998; **47**:1140–1144.

22 Spellacy WN, Goetz FC. Plasma insulin in normal late pregnancy. *N Engl J Med* 1963; **268**:988–991.

23 Cousins L. Insulin sensitivity in pregnancy. *Diabetes* 1991; **40**(Suppl 2):39–43.

24 Lind T. Metabolic changes in pregnancy relevant to diabetes mellitus. *Postgrad Med J* 1979; **55**:353–357.

25 Buchanan TA, Metzger BE, Freinkel N, Bergman RN. Insulin sensitivity and β-cell responsiveness to glucose during late pregnancy in lean and moderately obese women with normal glucose tolerance or mild gestational diabetes. *Am J Obstet Gynecol* 1990; **162**: 1008–1114.

26 Catalano PM, Tyzbir ED, Wolfe RR, Calles J, Roman NM, Amini SB, *et al.* Carbohydrate metabolism during pregnancy in control subjects and women with gestational diabetes. *Am J Physiol* 1993; **264**:E60–67.

27 Siman C, Eriksson U. Vitamin E decreases the occurrence of malformations in the offspring of diabetic rats. *Diabetes* 1997; **46**: 1054–1061.

28 Van Assche FA, Aerts L, De Prins F. A morphological study of the endocrine pancreas in human pregnancy. *Br J Obstet Gynaecol* 1978; **85**:818–820.

29 Bonner-Weir S. Perspective: Postnatal pancreatic beta cell growth. *Endocrinology* 2000; **141**:1926–1929.

30 Butler AE, Janson J, Bonner-Weir S, Ritzel R, Rizza RA, Butler PC. Beta-cell deficit and increased beta-cell apoptosis in humans with type 2 diabetes. *Diabetes* 2003; **52**:102–110.

31 Freinkel N. Banting Lecture 1980: Of pregnancy and progeny. *Diabetes* 1980; **29**:1023–1035.

32 Sivan E, Homko CJ, Chen X, Reece EA, Boden G. Effect of insulin on fat metabolism during and after normal pregnancy. *Diabetes* 1999; **48**(4):834–838.

33 Homko CJ, Sivan E, Reece EA, Boden G. Fuel metabolism during pregnancy. *Semin Reprod Endocrinol* 1999; **17**:119–125.

34 Sivan E, Chen X, Homko CJ, Reece EA, Boden G. Longitudinal study of carbohydrate metabolism in healthy obese pregnant women. *Diabetes Care* 1997; **20**:1470–1475.

35 Metzger BE, Freinkel N. Accelerated starvation in pregnancy: implications for dietary treatment of obesity and gestational diabetes mellitus. *Biol Neonate* 1987; **51**:78–85.

36 Martin JW, Friesen HG. Effect of human placental lactogen on the isolated islets of Langerhans. *Endocrinology* 1969; **84**:619–622.

37 Handwerger S, Freemark M. Role of placental lactogen and prolactin in human pregnancy. *Adv Exp Med Biol* 1987; **219**:399–420.

38 Sivan E, Homko CJ, Whittaker PG, Reece EA, Chen X, Boden G. Free fatty acids and insulin resistance during pregnancy. *J Clin Endocrinol Metab* 1998; **83**:2338–2342.

39 Handwerger S, Freemark M. The roles of placental growth hormone and placental lactogen in the regulation of human fetal growth and development. *J Pediatr Endocrinol Metab* 2000; **13**:343–356.

40 Barbour LA, Shao J, Qiao L, Pulawa LK, Jensen DR, Bartke A, *et al.* Human placental growth hormone causes severe insulin resistance in transgenic mice. *Am J Obstet Gynecol* 2002; **186**:512–517.

41 Barbour LA, McCurdy CE, Hernandez TL, Kirwan JP, Catalano PM, Friedman JE. Cellular mechanisms for insulin resistance in normal pregnancy and gestational diabetes. *Diabetes Care* 2007; **30**(Suppl 2):112–119.

42 Barbour LA, Mizanoor Rahman S, Gurevich I, Leitner JW, Fischer SJ, Roper MD, *et al.* Increased P85alpha is a potent negative regulator of skeletal muscle insulin signaling and induces *in vivo* insulin resistance associated with growth hormone excess. *J Biol Chem* 2005; **280**:37489–37494.

43 Kirwan JP, Hauguel-De Mouzon S, Lepercq J, Challier JC, Huston-Presley L, Friedman JE, *et al.* TNF-alpha is a predictor of insulin resistance in human pregnancy. *Diabetes* 2002; **51**:2207–2213.

44 Catalano PM, Hoegh M, Minium J, Huston-Presley L, Bernard S, Kalhan S, *et al.* Adiponectin in human pregnancy: implications for regulation of glucose and lipid metabolism. *Diabetologia* 2006; **49**:1677–1685.

45 Hauguel-de Mouzon S, Lepercq J, Catalano P. The known and unknown of leptin in pregnancy. *Am J Obstet Gynecol* 2006; **194**:1537–1545.

46 Nielsen LR, Pedersen-Bjergaard U, Thorsteinsson B, Johansen M, Damm P, Mathiesen ER. Hypoglycemia in pregnant women with type 1 diabetes: predictors and role of metabolic control. *Diabetes Care* 2008; **31**:9–14.

47 Steel J, Johnstone FD, Hume R, Mao JH. Insulin requirements during pregnancy in women with type 1 diabetes. *Obstet Gynecol* 1994; **83**:253–258.

48 Felig P, Lynch V. Starvation in human pregnancy, hypoglycemia, hypoinsulinaemia and hyperketonaemia. *Science* 1970; **170**:990–992.

49 Kilvert JA, Nicholson HO, Wright AD. Ketoacidosis in diabetic pregnancy. *Diabetes Med* 1993; **10**:278–281.

50 Simmons D, Thompson CF, Conroy C, Scott DJ. Use of insulin pumps in pregnancies complicated by type 2 diabetes and gestational diabetes in a multiethnic community. *Diabetes Care* 2001; **24**:2078–2082.

51 Schneider MB, Umpierrez GE, Ramsey RD, Mabie WC, Bennett KA. Pregnancy complicated by diabetic ketoacidosis: maternal and fetal outcomes. *Diabetes Care* 2003; **26**:958–959.

52 Umpierrez GE, Smiley D, Kitabchi AE. Narrative review: ketosis-prone type 2 diabetes mellitus. *Ann Intern Med* 2006; **144**:350–357.

53 Nicholls JS, Chan SP, Ali K, Beard RW, Dornhorst A. Insulin secretion and sensitivity in women fulfilling WHO criteria for gestational diabetes. *Diabetic Med* 1995; **12**:56–60.

54 Kautzky-Willer A, Prager R, Waldhausl W, Pacini G, Thomaseth K, Wagner OF, *et al.* Pronounced insulin resisitance and inadequate β-cell secretion characterizes lean gestational diabetes diabetes during and after pregnancy. *Diabetes Care* 1997; **20**:1717–1723.

55 Metzger BE, Phelps RL, Freinkel N, Navickas IA. Effects of gestational diabetes on diurnal profiles of plasma glucose, lipids and individual amino acids. *Diabetes Care* 1980; **3**:402–409.

56 Nicholls JS, Ali K, Gray IP, Andres C, Niththyananthan R, Beard RW, *et al.* Increased maternal fasting proinsulin as a predictor of insulin requirement in women with gestational diabetes. *Diabetes Med* 1994; **11**:57–61.

57 Chan SP, Gelding SV, McManus RJ, Nicholls JS, Anyaoku V, Niththyananthan R, *et al.* Abnormalities of intermediate metabolism following a gestational diabetic pregnancy. *Clin Endocrinol* 1992; **36**:417–420.

58 Sakamaki H, Yamasaki H, Matsumoto K, Izumino K, Kondo H, Sera Y, *et al.* No deterioration in insulin sensitivity, but impairment of both pancreatic beta-cell function and glucose sensitivity, in Japanese women with former gestational diabetes mellitus. *Diabet Med* 1998; **15**:1039–1044.

59 Buchanan TA, Xiang AH. Gestational diabetes mellitus. *J Clin Invest* 2005; **115**:485–491.

60 Tura A, Mari A, Winzer C, Kautzky-Willer A, Pacini G. Impaired beta-cell function in lean normotolerant former gestational women with diabetes. *Eur J Clin Invest* 2006; **36**:22–28.

61 Tura A, Mari A, Prikoszovich T, Pacini G, Kautzky-Willer A. Value of the intravenous and oral glucose tolerance tests for detecting subtle impairments in insulin sensitivity and beta-cell function in former gestational diabetes. *Clin Endocrinol* 2008; **69**:237–243.

62 Dornhorst A, Bailey PC, Anyaoku V, Elkeles RS, Johnston DG, Beard RW. Abnormalities of glucose tolerance following gestational diabetes. *Q J Med* 1990; **284**:1219–1228.

63 Buchanan TA, Kjos SL, Schafer U, Peters RK, Xiang A, Byrne J, *et al.* Utility of fetal measurements in the management of gestational diabetes mellitus. *Diabetes Care* 1998; **21**(Suppl 2):B99–106.

64 Buchanan TA, Xiang AH, Peters RK, Kjos SL, Berkowitz K, Marroquin A, *et al.* Response of pancreatic β-cells to improved insulin sensitivity in women at high risk for type 2 diabetes. *Diabetes* 2000; **49**:782–788.

65 O'Sullivan JB. Diabetes mellitus after GDM. *Diabetes* 1991; **40**(Suppl 2):131–135.

66 Desoye G, Hofmann HH, Weiss PA. Insulin binding to trophoblast plasma membranes and placental glycogen content in well-controlled gestational women with diabetes treated with diet or insulin, in well-controlled overt diabetic patients and in healthy control subjects. *Diabetologia* 1992; **35**:45–55.

67 Weiss U, Cervar M, Puerstner P, Schmut O, Haas J, Mauschitz R, *et al.* Hyperglycaemia *in vitro* alters the proliferation and mitochondrial activity of the choriocarcinoma cell lines BeWo, JAR and JEG-3 as models for human first-trimester trophoblast. *Diabetologia* 2001; **44**:209–219.

68 Hiden U, Glitzner E, Ivanisevic M, Djelmis J, Wadsack C, Lang U, *et al.* MT1-MMP expression in first-trimester placental tissue is upregulated in type 1 diabetes as a result of elevated insulin and tumor necrosis factor-alpha levels. *Diabetes* 2008; **57**:150–157.

69 Hiden U, Glitzner E, Hartmann M, Desoye G. Insulin and the IGF system in the human placenta of normal and diabetic pregnancies. *J Anat* 2009; **215**:60–68.

70 Hiden U, Maier A, Bilban M, Ghaffari-Tabrizi N, Wadsack C, Lang I, *et al.* Insulin control of placental gene expression shifts from mother to foetus over the course of pregnancy. *Diabetologia* 2006; **491**:123–131.

71 Takayama-Hasumi S, Yoshino H, Shimisu M, Minei S, Sanaka M, Omori Y. Insulin-receptor kinase is enhanced in placentas from non-insulin-dependent women with diabetes with large-for-gestational-age babies. *Diabetes Res Clin Pract* 1994; **22**:107–116.

72 Walker A. Diabetes mellitus and pregnancy. *Proc R Soc Med* 1928; **21**:337–384.

73 Gabbe SG. A story of two miracles: the impact of the discovery of insulin on pregnancy in women with diabetes mellitus. *Obstet Gynecol* 1992; **79**:295–299.

74 Griffin ML, South SA, Yankov VI, Booth RA Jr, Asplin CM, Veldhuis JD, *et al.* Insulin-dependent diabetes mellitus and menstrual dysfunction. *Ann Med* 1994; **26**:331–340.

75 Danielson KK, Palta M, Allen C, D'Alessio DJ. The association of increased total glycosylated hemoglobin levels with delayed age at menarche in young women with type 1 diabetes. *J Clin Endocrinol Metab* 2005; **90**:6466–6471.

76 Dorman JS, Steenkiste AR, Foley TP, Strotmeyer ES, Burke JP, Kuller LH, *et al.* Menopause in type 1 women with diabetes: is it premature? *Diabetes* 2001; **50**:1857–1862.

77 Engstrom I, Kroon M, Arvidsson CG, Segnestam K, Snellman K, Aman J. Eating disorders in adolescent girls with insulin-dependent diabetes mellitus: a population-based case–control study. *Acta Paediatr* 1999; **88**:175–180.

78 Goswami D, Conway GS. Premature ovarian failure. *Horm Res* 2007; **68**:196–202.

79 Buffington CK, Givens JR, Kitabchi AE. Enhanced adrenocortical activity as a contributing factor to diabetes in hyperandrogenic women. *Metabolism* 1994; **43**:584–590.

80 Morán C, Hernández E, Ruíz JE, Fonseca ME, Bermúdez JA, Zárate A. Upper body obesity and hyperinsulinemia are associated with anovulation. *Gynecol Obstet Invest* 1999; **47**:1–5.

81 Conn JJ, Jacobs HS. The prevalence of polycystic ovaries in women with type 2 diabetes mellitus. *Clin Endocrinol* 2000; **52**:81–86.

82 Wright AD, Nicholson HO, Pollock A, Taylor KG, Betts S. Spontaneous abortion and diabetes mellitus. *Postgrad Med J* 1983; **59**:295–298.

83 Miodovnik M, Skillman C, Holroyde JC, Butler JB, Wendel JS, Siddiqi TA. Elevated maternal glycohemoglobin in early pregnancy and spontaneous abortion among insulin-dependent women with diabetes. *Am J Obstet Gynecol* 1985; **153**:439–442.

84 Mills JL, Simpson JL, Driscoll SG, Jovanovic-Peterson L, Van Allen M, Aarons JH, *et al.* Incidence of spontaneous abortion among normal women and IDDM women whose pregnancies were identified within 21 days of conception. *N Engl J Med* 1988; **319**: 1617–1623.

85 Greene MF, Hare JW, Cloherty JP, Benacerraf BR, Soeldner JS. First trimester hemoglobin A1C and risk for major malformation and spontaneous abortion in diabetic pregnancy. *Teratology* 1989; **39**:225–231.

86 Rosenn B, Miodovnik M, Combs CA, Khoury J, Siddiqi TA. Glycemic thresholds for spontaneous abortion and congenital malformations in insulin-dependent diabetes mellitus. *Obstet Gynecol* 1994; **84**:515–20.

87 Simpson JL, Mills JL, Holmes LB, Ober CL, Aarons J, Jovanovic L, *et al.* Low fetal loss rates after ultrasound-proved viability in early pregnancy. *JAMA* 1987; **258**:2555–2557.

88 Makrydimas G, Sebire NJ, Lolis D, Vlassis N, Nicolaides KH. Fetal loss following ultrasound diagnosis of a live fetus at 6–10 weeks of gestation. *Ultrasound Obstet Gynecol* 2003; **22**:368–372.

89 Temple R, Aldridge V, Greenwood R, Heyburn P, Sampson M, Stanley K. Association between outcome of pregnancy and glycemic control in early pregnancy in type 1 diabetes: population based study. *Br Med J* 2002; **325**:1275–1276.

90 Lashen H, Fear K, Sturdee DW. Obesity is associated with increased risk of first trimester and recurrent miscarriage: matched case–control study. *Hum Reprod* 2004; **19**:1644–1646.

91 Eriksson UJ. Congenital anomalies in diabetic pregnancy. *Semin Fetal Neonatal Med* 2009; **14**:85–93.

92 Bingham C, Hattersley AT. Renal cysts and diabetes syndrome resulting from mutations in hepatocyte nuclear factor-1beta. *Nephrol Dial Transplant* 2004; **19**:2703–2708.

93 Eriksson UJ. Importance of genetic predisposition and maternal environment for the occurrence of congenital malformations in offspring of diabetic rats. *Teratology* 1988; **37**:365–374.

94 Kucera J. Rate and type of congenital anomalies among offspring of women with diabetes. *J Reprod Med* 1971; **7**:61–70.

95 Fuhrmann K, Reiher H, Semmler K, Fischer F, Fischer M, Glöckner E. Prevention of congenital malformations of infants of insulin-dependent mother with diabetes. *Diabetes Care* 1983; **6**: 219–223.

96 Ylinen K. High maternal levels of hemoglobin A1c associated with delayed fetal lung maturation in insulin-dependent diabetic pregnancies. *Acta Obstet Gynecol Scand* 1987; **66**:263–266.

97 Mills JL, Knopp RH, Simpson JL, Jovanovic-Peterson L, Metzger BE, Holmes LB, *et al.* Lack of relation of increased malformation rates in infants of mother with diabetes to glycemic control during organogesis. *N Engl J Med* 1988; **318**:671–676.

98 Lucas JM, Leveno KJ, Williams ML, Raskin P, Whalley PJ. Early pregnancy glycosylated hemoglobin, severity of diabetes, and fetal malformations. *Am J Obstet Gynecol* 1989; **161**:426–431.

99 Hanson U, Persson B, Thunell S. The relationship between HbA1c in early pregnancy and the occurrence of spontaneous abortion and malformation in Sweden. *Diabetologia* 1990; **33**:100–104.

100 Hanson U, Persson B. Outcome of pregnancy complicated by type 1 insulin dependent diabetes in Sweden: acute pregnancy complica-

tions, neonatal mortality, and morbidity. *Am J Perinatol* 1993; **10**:330–333.
101 Hawthorne G, Robson S, Ryall EA, Sen D, Roberts SH, Ward Platt MP. Prospective population based survey of outcome of pregnancy in women with diabetes: results of the Northern Diabetic Pregnancy Audit, 1994. *Br Med J* 1997; **315**:279–281.
102 Casson IF, Clarke CA, Howard CV, McKendrick O, Pennycook S, Pharoah PO, *et al.* Outcomes of pregnancy in insulin dependent women with diabetes: results of a five year population cohort study. *Br Med J* 1997; **315**:275–278.
103 Reece EA, Homko CJ. Why do women with diabetes deliver malformed infants? *Clin Obstet Gynecol* 2000; **43**:32–45.
104 Suhonen L, Hiilesmaa V, Teramo K. Glycemic control during early pregnancy and fetal malformations in women with type I diabetes mellitus. *Diabetologia* 2000; **43**:79–82.
105 Wender-Ozegowska E, Wróblewska K, Zawiejska A, Pietryga M, Szczapa J, Biczysko R. Threshold values of maternal blood glucose in early diabetic pregnancy: prediction of fetal malformations. *Acta Obstet Gynecol Scand* 2005; **84**:17–25.
106 Macintosh MC, Fleming KM, Bailey JA, Doyle P, Modder J, Acolet D, *et al.* Perinatal mortality and congenital anomalies in babies of women with type 1 or type 2 diabetes in England, Wales, and Northern Ireland: population based study. *Br Med J* 2006; **333**:177.
107 Mills JL, Baker L, Goldman AS. Malformations in infants of mother with diabetes occur before the seventh gestational week: implications for treatment. *Diabetes* 1979; **28**:292–293.
108 Martinez-Frias ML. Epidemiological analysis of outcomes of pregnancy in mother with diabetes: identification of the most characteristic and most frequent congenital anomalies. *Am J Med Genet* 1994; **51**:108–113.
109 Mills JL. Malformations in infants of mother with diabetes. *Teratology* 1982; **25**:385–394.
110 Wren C, Birrell G, Hawthorne G. Cardiovascular malformations in infants of mother with diabetes. *Heart* 2003; **89**:1217–1220.
111 Otani H, Tanakao OH, Takewaki R, Naora H, Yoneyama T. Diabetic environment and genetic predisposition as causes of congenital malformations in NOD mouse embryos. *Diabetes* 1991; **40**:1245–1250.
112 Moley KH, Chi MM, Knudson CM, Korsmeyer SJ, Mueckler MM. Hyperglycaemia induces apoptosis in pre-implantation embryos through cell death effector pathways. *Nat Med* 1998; **4**:1421–1424.
113 De Hertogh R, Vanderheyden I, Pampfer S, Robin D, Delcourt J. Maternal insulin treatment improves pre-implantation embryo development in diabetic rats. *Diabetologia* 1992; **35**:406–408.
114 Tonack S, Ramin N, Garimella S, Rao R, Seshagiri PB, Fischer B, *et al.* Expression of glucose transporter isoforms and the insulin receptor during hamster preimplantation embryo development. *Ann Anat* 2009; **191**:485–495.
115 Pampfer S, Vanderheyden I, Wuu YD, Baufays L, Maillet O, De Hertogh R. Possible role of TNF-α in early embryropathy associated with maternal diabetes in the rat. *Diabetes* 1995; **44**:531–536.
116 Eriksson UJ, Borg LA. Protection by free oxygen radical scavenging enzymes against glucose-induced embryonic malformations *in vitro*. *Diabetologia* 1991; **34**:325–331.
117 Eriksson UJ, Borg LA. Diabetes and embryonic malformations: role of substrate-induced free-oxygen radical production for dysmorphogenesis in culture rat embryos. *Diabetes* 1993; **42**:411–419.
118 Wentzel P, Thunberg L, Eriksson UJ. Teratogenic effect of diabetic serum is prevented by supplementation of superoxide dismutase and N-acetylcysteine in rat embryo culture. *Diabetologia* 1997; **40**:7–14.
119 Zaken V, Kohen R, Ornoy A. Vitamins C and E improve rat embryonic antioxidant defense mechanism in diabetic culture medium. *Teratology* 2001; **64**:33–44.
120 Wentzel P, Gareskog M, Eriksson U. Folic acid supplementation diminishes diabetes- and glucose-induced dysmorphogenesis in rat embryos *in vivo* and *in vitro*. *Diabetes* 2005; **54**:546–53.
121 Baker L, Piddington R, Goldman A, Egler J, Moehring J. Myo-inositol and prostaglandins reverse the glucose inhibition of neural tube fusion in cultured mouse embryos. *Diabetologia* 1990; **33**: 593–596.
122 Akashi M, Akazawa S, Akazawa M, Trocino R, Hashimoto M, Maeda Y, *et al.* Effects of insulin and myo-inositol on embryo growth and development during early organogenesis in streptozotocin-induced diabetic rats. *Diabetes* 1991; **40**:1574–1579.
123 Goldman AS, Goto MP. Biochemical basis of the diabetic embryopathy. *Isr J Med Sci* 1991; **27**:469–477.
124 Strieleman PJ, Connors MA, Metzger BE. Phosphoinositide metabolism in the developing conceptus: effects of hyperglycemia and scyllo-inositol in rat embryo culture. *Diabetes* 1992; **41**: 989–997.
125 Reece EA. Maternal fetal fuels, diabetic embryopathy: pathomechanisms and prevention. *Semin Reprod Endocrinol* 1999; **17**: 183–194.
126 Akashi M, Akazawa S, Akazawa M, Trocino R, Hashimoto M, Maeda Y, *et al.* Effects of insulin and myo-inositol on embryo growth and development during early organogenesis in streptozocin-induced diabetic rats. *Diabetes* 1991; **40**:1574–1579.
127 Reece EA, Khandelwal M, Wu YK, Borenstein M. Dietary intake of myo-inositol and neural tube defects in offspring of diabetic rats. *Am J Obstet Gynecol* 1997; **176**:536–539.
128 Hashimoto M, Akazawa S, Akazawa M, Akashi M, Yamamoto H, Maeda Y, *et al.* Effects of hyperglycaemia on sorbitol and myo-inositol contents of cultured embryos: treatment with aldose reductase inhibitor and myo-inositol supplementation. *Diabetologia* 1990; **33**:597–602.
129 Wentzel P, Wentzel CR, Gäreskog MB, Eriksson UJ. Induction of embryonic dysmorphogenesis by high glucose concentration, disturbed inositol metabolism, and inhibited protein kinase C activity. *Teratology* 2001; **63**:193–201.
130 Wentzel P, Welsh N, Eriksson UJ. Developmental damage, increased lipid peroxidation, diminished cyclooxygenase-2 gene expression, and lowered prostaglandin E2 levels in rat embryos exposed to a diabetic environment. *Diabetes* 1999; **48**:813–820.
131 Pinter E, Reece EA, Leranth CZ, Garcia-Segura M, Hobbins JC, Mahoney MJ, *et al.* Arachidonic acid prevents hyperglycemia-associated yolk sac damage and embryopathy. *Am J Obstet Gynecol* 1986; **155**:691–702.
132 Schoenfeld A, Warchaizer S, Erman A, Hod M. Prostaglandin metabolism in the yolk sacs of normal and diabetic pregnancies. *Early Pregnancy* 1996; **2**:129–132.
133 Pani L, Horal M, Loeken MR. Polymorphic susceptibility to the molecular causes of neural tube defects during diabetic embryopathy. *Diabetes* 2002; **51**:2871–2874.
134 Honein MA, Paulozzi LJ, Mathews TJ, Erickson JD, Wong LY. Impact of folic acid fortification of the US food supply on the occurrence of neural tube defects. *JAMA* 2001; **285**:2981–2986.
135 Kaplan JS, Iqbal S, England BG, Zawacki CM, Herman WH. Is pregnancy in women with diabetes associated with folate deficiency? *Diabetes Care* 1999; **22**:1017–1021.

136 Milner E, Hare JW, Clotherty JP. Elevated maternal haemoglobin A1c in early pregnancy and major congenital anomalies in infants of mother with diabetes. *N Engl J Med* 1981; **304**:1331–1334.

137 Goldman JA, Dicker D, Feldberg D, Yeshaya A, Samuel N, Karp M. Pregnancy outcome in patients with insulin-dependent diabetes mellitus with preconceptional diabetic control: a comparative study. *Am J Obstet Gynecol* 1986; **155**:293–297.

138 Steel JM, Johnstone FD, Hepburn DA, Smith AF. Can prepregnancy care of women with diabetes reduce the risk of abnormal babies? *Br Med J* 1990; **301**:1070–1074.

139 Kitzmiller JL, Gavin LA, Gin GD. Preconception management of diabetes continued through early pregnancy prevents the excess frequency of major congenital anomalies in infants of mother with diabetes. *JAMA* 1991; **265**:731–736.

140 Bell R, Bailey K, Cresswell T, Hawthorne G, Critchley J, Lewis-Barned D; Northern Diabetic Pregnancy Survey Steering Group. Trends in prevalence and outcomes of pregnancy in women with pre-existing type I and type II diabetes. *Br J Obstet Gynaecol* 2008; **115**:445–452.

141 Jensen DM, Korsholm L, Ovesen P, Beck-Nielsen H, Moelsted-Pedersen L, Westergaard JG, *et al.* Peri-conceptional A1c and risk of serious adverse pregnancy outcome in 933 women with type 1 diabetes. *Diabetes Care* 2009; **32**:1046–1048.

142 Diabetes Control and Complications Trial Research Group. Pregnancy outcomes in the Diabetes Control and Complications Trial. *Am J Obstet Gynecol* 1996; **174**:1343–1353.

143 Ray JG, O'Brien TE, Chan WS. Preconception care and the risk of congenital anomalies in the offspring of women with diabetes mellitus: a meta-analysis. *Q J Med* 2001; **94**:435–444.

144 Guerin A, Nisenbaum R, Ray JG. Use of maternal GHb concentration to estimate the risk of congenital anomalies in the offspring of women with prepregnancy diabetes. *Diabetes Care* 2007; **30**: 1920–1925.

145 Simmons D, Robertson S. Influence of maternal insulin treatment with insulin on infants of mothers with gestational diabetes. *Diabetes Med* 1997; **14**:762–765.

146 Kerssen A, de Valk HW, Visser GH. Do HbA1c levels and the self-monitoring of blood glucose levels adequately reflect glycemic control during pregnancy in women with type 1 diabetes mellitus? *Diabetologia* 2006; **49**:25–28.

147 Piper K, Brickwood S, Turnpenny LW, Cameron IT, Ball SG, Wilson DI, *et al.* Beta cell differentiation during early human pancreas development. *J Endocrinol* 2004; **181**:11–23.

148 Schwartz R, Gruppuso PA, Petzold K, Brambilla D, Hiilesmaa V, Teramo KA. Hyperinsulinemia and macrosomia in the fetus of the mother with diabetes. *Diabetes Care* 1994; **17**:640–648.

149 Carpenter MW, Canick JA, Hogan JW, Shellum C, Somers M, Star JA. Amniotic fluid insulin at 14–20 weeks' gestation: association with later maternal glucose intolerance and birth macrosomia. *Diabetes Care* 2001; **24**:1259–1263.

150 Veening MA, van Weissenbruch MM, Heine RJ, Delemarre-van de Waal HA. Beta-cell capacity and insulin sensitivity in prepubertal children born small for gestational age: influence of body size during childhood. *Diabetes* 2003; **52**:1756–1760.

151 Mericq V, Ong KK, Bazaes R, Peña V, Avila A, Salazar T, *et al.* Longitudinal changes in insulin sensitivity and secretion from birth to age three years in small- and appropriate-for-gestational-age children. *Diabetologia* 2005; **48**:2609–2614.

152 Simmons RA. Developmental origins of beta-cell failure in type 2 diabetes: the role of epigenetic mechanisms. *Pediatr Res* 2007; **61**:64R–67R.

153 Boloker J, Gertz SJ, Simmons RA. Gestational diabetes leads to the development of diabetes in adulthood in the rat. *Diabetes* 2002; **51**:1499–1506.

154 Gatford KL, Mohammad SN, Harland ML, De Blasio MJ, Fowden AL, Robinson JS, *et al.* Impaired beta-cell function and inadequate compensatory increases in beta-cell mass after intrauterine growth restriction in sheep. *Endocrinology* 2008; **149**:5118–5127.

155 Simmons RA. Developmental origins of adult disease. *Pediatr Clin North Am* 2009; **56**:449–466.

156 Verhaeghe J, van Bree R, Van Herck E. Maternal body size and birth weight: can insulin or adipokines do better? *Metabolism* 2006; **55**:339–344.

157 Hay WW. The role of placental–fetal interaction in fetal nutrition. *Semin Perinatol* 1991; **15**:424–433.

158 Bradley RJ, Nicolaides KH, Brudenell JM. Are all infants of mother with diabetes "macrosomic"? *Br Med J* 1988; **297**:1583–1585.

159 Johnstone FD, Lindsay RS, Steel J. Type 1 diabetes and pregnancy: trends in birth weight over 40 years at a single clinic. *Obstet Gynecol* 2006; **107**:1297–1302.

160 Boyd M, Usher RH, McLean FH. Fetal macrosomia: prediction, risk, proposed management. *Obstet Gynecol* 1983; **61**:715–722.

161 Spellacy WN, Miller S, Winegar A, Peterson PQ. Macrosomia: maternal characteristics and infant complications. *Obstet Gynecol* 1985; **66**:158–161.

162 Verhaeghe J, Van Bree R, Van Herck E, Laureys J, Bouillon R, Van Assche FA. C-peptide, insulin-like growth factors I and II, and insulin-like growth factor binding protein-1 in umbilical cord serum: correlations with birth weight. *Am J Obstet Gynecol* 1993; **169**: 89–97.

163 Schwartz R, Susa J. Fetal macrosomia-animal models. *Diabetes Care* 1980; **3**:430–432.

164 Pedersen B. Hyperglycaemia-hyperinsulinism theory and birth-weight. In: Pedersen J, ed. *The Pregnant Diabetic and her Newborn: Problems and Management*. Baltimore MD: Williams & Wilkins, 1977: 211–220.

165 Cano A, Barcelo F, Fuente T, Martinez P, Parrilla JJ, Abad L. Relationship of maternal glycosylated hemoglobin and fetal beta-cell activity with birth weight. *Gynecol Obstet Invest* 1986; **22**: 91–96.

166 Metzger BE. Biphasic effect of maternal metabolism on fetal growth: quintessential expression of fuel-mediated teratogenesis. *Diabetes* 1991; **40**(Suppl 2):99–105.

167 Challier JC, Schneider H, Dancic J. *In vitro* perfusion of human placenta. V. Oxygen consumption. *Am J Obstet Gynecol* 1976; **126**:261–265.

168 Buchanan TA, Kjos SL, Montoro MN, Wu PY, Madrilejo NG, Gonzalez M, *et al.* Use of fetal ultrasound to select metabolic therapy for pregnancies complicated by mild gestational diabetes. *Diabetes Care* 1994; **17**:275–283.

169 Lauszus FF, Grøn PL, Klebe JG. Pregnancies complicated by diabetic proliferative retinopathy. *Acta Obstet Gynecol Scand* 1998; **77**: 814–818.

170 Rey E, Attie C, Bonin A. The effects of first-trimester diabetes control on the incidence of macrosomia. *Am J Obstet Gynecol* 1999; **181**: 202–206.

171 Katz AI, Lindheimer MD, Mako ME, Rubenstein AH. Peripheral metabolism of insulin, proinsulin, and C-peptide in the pregnant rat. *J Clin Invest* 1975; **56**:1608–1614.

172 Sosenko IR, Kitzmiller JL, Loo SW, Blix P, Rubenstein AH, Gabbay KH. The infant of the mother with diabetes: correlation of increased cord blood C-peptide levels with macrosomia and hypoglycemia. *N Engl J Med* 1979; **301**:859–862.

173 Ogata ES, Freinkel N, Metzger BE, Phelps RL, Depp R, Boehm JJ, *et al.* Perinatal islet function in gestational diabetes: assessment by cord plasma C-peptide and amniotic fluid insulin. *Diabetes Care* 1980; **3**:425–429.

174 Sosenko JM, Kitzmiller JL, Fluckiger R, Loo SW, Younger DM, Gabbay KH. Umbilical cord glycosylated hemoglobin in infants of mother with diabetes: relationships to neonatal hypoglycemia, macrosomia, serum C-peptide. *Diabetes Care* 1982; **5**:566–570.

175 Lin CC, Moawad AH, River P, Blix P, Abraham M, Rubenstein AH. Amniotic fluid C-peptide as an index for intrauterine fetal growth. *Am J Obstet Gynecol* 1981; **139**:390–396.

176 Lin CC, River P, Moawad AH, Lowensohn RI, Blix PM, Abraham M, *et al.* Prenatal assessment of fetal outcome by amniotic fluid C-peptide levels in pregnant women. *Am J Obstet Gynecol* 1981; **141**:671–677.

177 Dornhorst A, Nicholls JSD, Ali K, Andres C, Adamson DL, Kelly LF, *et al.* Fetal proinsulin and birth weight. *Diabet Med* 1994; **11**:171–181.

178 Teramo K, Kari MA, Eronen M, Markkanen H, Hiilesmaa V. High amniotic fluid erythropoietin levels are associated with an increased frequency of fetal and neonatal morbidity in type 1 diabetic pregnancies. *Diabetologia* 2004; **47**:1695–1703.

179 Susa JB, Gruppuso PA, Widness JA, Domenech M, Clemons GK, Sehgal P, *et al.* Chronic hyperinsulinemia in the fetal rhesus monkey: effects of physiologic hyperinsulinemia on fetal substrates, hormones, and hepatic enzymes. *Am J Obstet Gynecol* 1984; **150**:415–420.

180 Philipps AF, Rosenkrantz TS, Clark RM, Knox I, Chaffin DG, Raye JR. Effects of fetal insulin deficiency on growth in fetal lambs. *Diabetes* 1991; **40**:20–27.

181 Woods KA, Camacho-Hübner C, Barter D, Clark AJ, Savage MO. Insulin-like growth factor I gene deletion causing intrauterine growth retardation and severe short stature. *Acta Paediatr Suppl* 1997; **423**:39–45.

182 Gluckman PD. The endocrine role of fetal growth in late gestation: the role of insulin-like growth factors. *J Clin Endocrinol Metab* 1995; **80**:1047–1050.

183 Vatten LJ, Nilsen ST, Odegård RA, Romundstad PR, Austgulen R. Insulin-like growth factor I and leptin in umbilical cord plasma and infant birth size at term. *Pediatrics* 2002; **109**:1131–1135.

184 Byun D, Mohan S, Kim C, Suh K, Yoo M, Lee H, *et al.* Studies on human pregnancy-induced insulin-like growth factor (IGF)-binding protein-4 proteases in serum: determination of IGF-II dependency and localization of cleavage site. *J Clin Endocrinol Metab* 2000; **85**:373–381.

185 Lindsay RS, Westgate JA, Beattie J, Pattison NS, Gamble G, Mildenhall LF, *et al.* Inverse changes in fetal insulin-like growth factor (IGF)-1 and IGF binding protein-1 in association with higher birth weight in maternal diabetes. *Clin Endocrinol* 2007; **66**: 322–328.

186 Silver RM, Varner MW, Reddy U, Goldenberg R, Pinar H, Conway D, *et al.* Work-up of stillbirth: a review of the evidence. *Am J Obstet Gynecol* 2007; **196**:433–444.

187 Lauenborg J, Mathiesen E, Ovesen P, Westergaard JG, Ekbom P, Mølsted-Pedersen L, *et al.* Audit on stillbirths in women with pregestational type 1 diabetes. *Diabetes Care* 2003; **26**:1385–1389.

188 Karlsson K, Kjellmer I. The outcome of diabetic pregnancies in relationship to the mother's blood sugar level. *Am J Obstet Gynecol* 1972; **112**:213–220.

189 Stephansson O, Dickman PW, Johansson A, Cnattingius S. Maternal weight, pregnancy weight gain, and the risk of antepartum stillbirth. *Am J Obstet Gynecol* 2001; **184**:463–469.

190 Cnattingius S, Stephansson O. The epidemiology of stillbirth. *Semin Perinatol* 2002; **26**:25–30.

191 Cundy T, Gamble G, Townend K, Henley PG, MacPherson P, Roberts AB. Perinatal mortality in type 2 diabetes mellitus. *Diabet Med* 2000; **17**:33–39.

192 Teramo KA, Widness JA. Increased fetal plasma and amniotic fluid erythropoietin concentrations: markers of intrauterine hypoxia. *Neonatology* 2009; **95**:105–116.

193 Milley JR, Papacostas JS. Effect of insulin on metabolism of fetal sheep hindquarters. *Diabetes* 1989; **38**:597–603.

194 Myers RE. Brain damage due to asphyxia: mechanism of causation. *J Perinat Med* 1981; **9**:78–86.

195 Philips AF, Dubin JW, Matty PJ, Raye JR. Arterial hypoxemia and hyperinsulinemia in the chronically hyperglycemic fetal lamb. *Pediatr Res* 1982; **16**:653–658.

196 Bradley RJ, Brudenell JM, Nicolaides KH. Fetal acidosis and hyperlacticaemia diagnosed by cordocentesis in pregnancies complicated by maternal diabetes mellitus. *Diabet Med* 1991; **8**:464–468.

197 Fraser RB, Bruce C. Amniotic fluid insulin levels identify the fetus at risk of neonatal hypoglycemia. *Diabet Med* 1999; **16**:568–572.

198 Williams AF. Hyoglycaemia of the newborn: a review. *Bull World Health Organ* 1997; **75**:261–290.

199 Hawdon JM. Hypoglycemia in newborn infants: defining the features associated with adverse outcomes – a challenging remit. *Biol Neonate* 2006; **90**:87–88. [Commentary to Rozance PJ, Hay WW. Hypoglycemia in newborn infants: features associated with adverse outcomes. *Biol Neonate* 2006; **90**:74–86.]

200 Cornblath M, Hawdon JM, Williams AF, Aynsley-Green A, Ward-Platt MP, Schwartz R, *et al.* Controversies regarding definition of neonatal hypoglycemia: suggested operational thresholds. *Pediatrics* 2000; **105**:1141–1145.

201 Hawdon JM, Ward Platt MP, Aynsley-Green A. Patterns of metabolic adaptation for preterm and term infants in the first neonatal week. *Arch Dis Child* 1992; **67**:357–365.

202 Lucas A, Morley R, Cole TJ. Adverse neurodevelopmental outcome of moderate neonatal hypoglycemia. *Br Med J* 1988; **297**:1304–1308.

203 Beard AG, Panos TC, Marasigan BV, Eminians J, Kennedy HF, Lamb J. Perinatal stress and the premature neonate. II. Effect of fluid and calorie deprivation on blood glucose. *J Pediatr* 1966; **68**:329–343.

204 Mimouni F, Tsang RC, Hertzberg VS, Miodovnik M. Polycythemia, hypomagnesemia, and hypocalcemia in infants of mother with diabetes. *Am J Dis Child* 1986; **140**:798–800.

205 Widness JA, Susa JB, Garcia JF, Singer DB, Sehgal P, Oh W, *et al.* Increased erythropoiesis and elevated erythropoietin in infants born to mother with diabetes in hyperinsulinemic rhesus fetuses. *J Clin Invest* 1981; **67**:637–642.

206 Salvesen DR, Brudenell JM, Snijders RJ, Ireland RM, Nicolaides KH. Fetal plasma erythropoietin in pregnancies complicated by maternal diabetes mellitus. *Am J Obstet Gynecol* 1993; **168**:88–94.
207 Mimouni F, Miodovnik M, Whitsett JA, Holroyde JC, Siddiqi TA, Tsang RC. Respiratory distress syndrome in infants of mother with diabetes in the 1980s: no direct adverse effect of maternal diabetes with modern management. *Obstet Gynecol* 1987; **69**:191–195.
208 Gutgesell HP, Speer ME, Rosenberg HS. Characterization of the cardiomyopathy in infants of mother with diabetes. *Circulation* 1980; **61**:441–450.
209 Zielinsky P. Role of prenatal echocardiography in the study of hypertrophic cardiomyopathy in the fetus. *Echocardiography* 1991; **8**:661–668.
210 Hawa MI, Beyan H, Buckley LR, Leslie RD. Impact of genetic and non-genetic factors in type 1 diabetes. *Am J Med Genet* 2002; **115**:8–17.
211 Ridderstrale M, Groop L. Genetic dissection of type 2 diabetes. *Mol Cell Endocrinol* 2009; **297**:10–17.
212 Pettitt D, Aleck KA, Baird HR, Carraher MJ, Bennett PH, Knowler WC. Congenital susceptibility to NIDDM: role of intrauterine environment. *Diabetes* 1988; **37**:622–628.
213 Dabelea D, Hanson RL, Lindsay RS, Pettitt DJ, Imperatore G, Gabir MM, *et al.* Intrauterine exposure to diabetes conveys risks for type 2 diabetes and obesity: a study of discordant sibships. *Diabetes* 2000; **49**:2208–2211.
214 Weiss PA, Scholz HS, Haas J, Tamussino KF. Effect of fetal hyperinsulinism on oral glucose tolerance test results in patients with gestational diabetes mellitus. *Am J Obstet Gynecol* 2001; **184**:470–475.
215 Sobngwi E, Boudou P, Mauvais-Jarvis F, Leblanc H, Velho G, Vexiau P, *et al.* Effect of a diabetic environment *in utero* on predisposition to type 2 diabetes. *Lancet* 2003; **361**:1861–1865.
216 Clausen TD, Mathiesen ER, Hansen T, Pedersen O, Jensen DM, Lauenborg J, *et al.* High prevalence of type 2 diabetes and prediabetes in adult offspring of women with gestational diabetes mellitus or type 1 diabetes: the role of intrauterine hyperglycemia. *Diabetes Care* 2008; **31**:340–346.
217 Martin A, Simpson JL, Ober C, Freinkel N. Frequency of diabetes mellitus in mothers of probands with gestational diabetes: possible maternal influence on the predisposition to gestational diabetes. *Am J Obstet Gynecol* 1985; **151**:471–475.
218 Alcolado JC, Laji K, Gill-Randall R. Maternal transmission of diabetes. *Diabet Med* 2002; **19**:89–98.
219 Ramachandran A, Snehalatha C, Satyavani K, Sivasankari S, Vijay V. Type 2 diabetes in Asian-Indian urban children. *Diabetes Care* 2003; **26**:1022–1025.
220 Dabelea D, Knowler WC, Pettitt DJ. Effect of diabetes in pregnancy on offspring: follow-up research in the Pima Indians. *J Matern Fetal Med* 2000; **9**:83–88.
221 Gautier JF, Wilson C, Weyer C, Mott D, Knowler WC, Cavaghan M, *et al.* Low acute insulin secretory responses in adult offspring of people with early onset type 2 diabetes. *Diabetes* 2001; **50**:1828–1833.
222 Eriksson M, Wallander MA, Krakau I, Wedel H, Svärdsudd K. Birth weight and cardiovascular risk factors in a cohort followed until 80 years of age: the study of men born in 1913. *J Intern Med* 2004; **255**:236–246.
223 Barker DJ, Hales CN, Fall CH, Osmond C, Phipps K, Ckark PM. Type 2 (non-insulin-dependent) diabetes mellitus, hypertension and hyperlipidaemia (syndrome X): relation to reduced fetal growth. *Diabetologia* 1993; **36**:62–67.
224 Gill-Randall R, Adams D, Ollerton RL, Lewis M, Alcolado JC. Type 2 diabetes mellitus: genes or intrauterine environment? An embryo transfer paradigm in rats. *Diabetologia* 2004; **47**:1354–1359.
225 Temple RC, Aldridge VA, Sampson MJ, Greenwood RH, Heyburn PJ, Glenn A. Impact of pregnancy on the progression of diabetic retinopathy in type 1 diabetes. *Diabet Med* 2001; **18**:573–577.
226 Rahman W, Rahman FZ, Yassin S, Al-Suleiman SA, Rahman J. Progression of retinopathy during pregnancy in type 1 diabetes mellitus. *Clin Experiment Ophthalmol* 2007; **35**:231–236.
227 Diabetes Control and Complications Trial Research Group. Effect of pregnancy on microvascular complications in the diabetes control and complications trial. *Diabetes Care* 2000; **23**:1084–1091.
228 Arun CS, Taylor R. Influence of pregnancy on long-term progression of retinopathy in patients with type 1 diabetes. *Diabetologia* 2008; **51**:1041–1045.
229 Larsen M, Colmorn LB, Bønnelycke M, Kaaja R, Immonen I, Sander B, *et al.* Retinal artery and vein diameters during pregnancy in women with diabetes. *Invest Ophthalmol Vis Sci* 2005; **46**:709–713.
230 Loukovaara S, Immonen I, Koistinen R, Rudge J, Teramo KA, Laatikainen L, *et al.* Angiopoietic factors and retinopathy in pregnancies complicated with type 1 diabetes. *Diabet Med* 2004; **21**:697–704.
231 Loukovaara S, Immonen I, Koistinen R, Hiilesmaa V, Kaaja R. Inflammatory markers and retinopathy in pregnancies complicated with type I diabetes. *Eye* 2005; **19**:422–430.
232 Kaaja R, Loukovaara S. Progression of retinopathy in type 1 women with diabetes during pregnancy. *Curr Diabetes Rev* 2007; **3**:85–93.
233 Loukovaara S, Immonen IR, Loukovaara MJ, Koistinen R, Kaaja RJ. Glycodelin: a novel serum anti-inflammatory marker in type 1 diabetic retinopathy during pregnancy. *Acta Ophthalmol Scand* 2007; **85**:46–49.
234 Chew EY, Mills JL, Metzger BE, Remaley NA, Jovanovic-Peterson L, Knopp RH, *et al.* Metabolic control and progression of retinopathy. The Diabetes in Early Pregnancy Study. National Institute of Child Health and Human Development Diabetes in Early Pregnancy Study. *Diabetes Care* 1995; **18**:631–637.
235 Rosenn B, Miodovnik M, Kranias G, Khoury J, Combs CA, Mimouni F, *et al.* Progression of diabetic retinopathy in pregnancy: association with hypertension in pregnancy. *Am J Obstet Gynecol* 1992; **166**:1214–1218.
236 Arun CS, Al-Bermani A, Stannard K, Taylor R. Long-term impact of retinal screening on significant diabetes-related visual impairment in the working age population. *Diabet Med* 2009; **26**:489–492.
237 Kitzmiller JL, Combs CA. Management amd outcome of pregnancy complicated by diabetic nephropathy. In: Dornhorst A, Hadden DR, eds. *Diabetes and Pregnancy: an International Approach to Diagnosis and Management*. Chichester, UK: John Wiley & Sons Ltd, 1996: 167–206.
238 Dunne FP, Chowdhury TA, Hartland A, Smith T, Brydon PA, McConkey C, *et al.* Pregnancy outcome in women with insulin-dependent diabetes mellitus complicated by nephropathy. *Q J Med* 1999; **92**:451–454.
239 Ekbom P, Damm P, Feldt-Rasmussen B, Feldt-Rasmussen U, Mølvig J, Mathiesen ER. Pregnancy outcome in type 1 women with diabetes with microalbuminuria. *Diabetes Care* 2001; **24**:1739–1744.
240 Nielsen LR, Müller C, Damm P, Mathiesen ER. Reduced prevalence of early preterm delivery in women with type 1 diabetes and micro-

albuminuria: possible effect of early antihypertensive treatment during pregnancy. *Diabet Med* 2006; **23**:426–431.

241 Nielsen LR, Damm P, Mathiesen ER. Improved pregnancy outcome in type 1 women with diabetes with microalbuminuria or diabetic nephropathy: effect of intensified antihypertensive therapy? *Diabetes Care* 2009; **32**:38–44.

242 Ekbom P, Damm P, Feldt-Rasmussen B, Feldt-Rasmussen U, Jensen DM, Mathiesen ER. Elevated third-trimester haemoglobin A1c predicts preterm delivery in type 1 diabetes. *J Diabetes Complications* 2008; **22**:297–302.

243 Sorensen VR, Mathiesen ER, Heaf J, Feldt-Rasmussen B. Improved survival rate in patients with diabetes and end-stage renal disease in Denmark. *Diabetologia* 2007; **50**:922–929.

244 Rossing K, Jacobsen P, Hommel E, Mathiesen E, Svenningsen A, Rossing P, *et al.* Pregnancy and progression of diabetic nephropathy. *Diabetologia* 2002; **45**:36–41.

245 Khoury JC, Miodovnik M, LeMasters G, Sibai B. Pregnancy outcome and progression of diabetic nephropathy: what's next? *J Matern Fetal Neonatal Med* 2002; **11**:238–244.

246 Biesenbach G, Grafinger P, Zazgornik J, Helmut, Stöger. Perinatal complications and three-year follow up of infants of mother with diabetes with diabetic nephropathy stage IV. *Ren Fail* 2000; **22**:573–580.

247 Ogburn PL, Kitzmiller JL, Hare JW, Phillippe M, Gabbe SG, Miodovnik M, *et al.* Pregnancy following renal transplantation in class T diabetes mellitus. *JAMA* 1986; **255**:911–915.

248 McKay DB, Josephson MA. Pregnancy in recipients of solid organs: effects on mother and child. *N Engl J Med* 2006; **354**:1281–1293.

249 Sibanda N, Briggs JD, Davison JM, Johnson RJ, Rudge CJ. Pregnancy after organ transplantation: a report from the UK Transplant pregnancy registry. *Transplantation* 2007; **83**:1301–1307.

250 Sgro MD, Barozzino T, Mirghani HM, Sermer M, Moscato L, Akoury H, *et al.* Pregnancy outcome post renal transplantation. *Teratology* 2002; **65**:5–9.

251 Simchen MJ, Yinon Y, Moran O, Schiff E, Sivan E. Pregnancy outcome after age 50. *Obstet Gynecol* 2006; **108**:1084–1088.

252 Ladner HE, Danielsen B, Gilbert WM. Acute myocardial infarction in pregnancy and the puerperium: a population-based study. *Obstet Gynecol* 2005; **105**:480–484.

253 Lewis G, ed. Confidential Enquiry into Maternal and Child Health (CEMACH). *The Confidential Enquiry into Maternal and Child Health (CEMACH). Saving Mothers' Lives: reviewing maternal deaths to make motherhood safer, 2003–2005.* London: CEMACH, 2007.

254 Roth A, Elkayam U. Acute myocardial infarction associated with pregnancy. *J Am Coll Cardiol* 2008; **52**:171–180.

255 Roth A, Elkayam U. Acute myocardial infarction associated with pregnancy. *Ann Intern Med* 1996; **125**:751–762.

256 Gregg EW, Gu Q, Cheng YJ, Narayan KM, Cowie CC. Mortality trends in men and women with diabetes, 1971 to 2000. *Ann Intern Med* 2007; **147**:149–155.

257 Preis SR, Hwang SJ, Coady S, Pencina MJ, D'Agostino RB Sr, Savage PJ, *et al.* Trends in all-cause and cardiovascular disease mortality among women and men with and without diabetes mellitus in the Framingham Heart Study, 1950 to 2005. *Circulation* 2009; **119**:1728–1735.

258 Soedamah-Muthu SS, Fuller JH, Mulnier HE, Raleigh VS, Lawrenson RA, Colhoun HM. High risk of cardiovascular disease in patients with type 1 diabetes in the UK: a cohort study using the general practice research database. *Diabetes Care* 2006; **29**:798–804.

259 Mulnier HE, Seaman HE, Raleigh VS, Soedamah-Muthu SS, Colhoun HM, Lawrenson RA, *et al.* Risk of myocardial infarction in men and women with type 2 diabetes in the UK: a cohort study using the General Practice Research Database. *Diabetologia* 2008; **51**:1639–1645.

260 Dale AC, Nilsen TI, Vatten L, Midthjell K, Wiseth R. Diabetes mellitus and risk of fatal ischaemic heart disease by gender: 18 years follow-up of 74,914 individuals in the HUNT 1 Study. *Eur Heart J* 2007; **28**:2924–2929.

261 Heslehurst N, Lang R, Rankin J, Wilkinson JR, Summerbell CD. Obesity in pregnancy: a study of the impact of maternal obesity on NHS maternity services. *Br J Obstet Gynaecol* 2007; **114**:334–342.

262 Heslehurst N, Ells LJ, Simpson H, Batterham A, Wilkinson J, Summerbell CD. Trends in maternal obesity incidence rates, demographic predictors, and health inequalities in 36,821 women over a 15-year period. *Br J Obstet Gynaecol* 2007; **114**:187–194.

263 Watkins ML, Rasmussen SA, Honein MA, Botto LD, Moore CA. Maternal obesity and risk for birth defects. *Pediatrics* 2003; **111**:1152–1158.

264 Rajasingam D, Seed PT, Briley AL, Shennan AH, Poston L. A prospective study of pregnancy outcome and biomarkers of oxidative stress in nulliparous obese women. *Am J Obstet Gynecol* 2009; **200**:395,e1–9.

265 Sebire NJ, Jolly M, Harris JP, Wadsworth J, Joffe M, Beard RW. Maternal obesity and pregnancy outcome: a study of 287,213 pregnancies in London. *Int J Obes Relat Metab Disord* 2001; **25**:1175–1182.

266 Jolly MC, Sebire NJ, Harris JP, Regan L, Robinson S. Risk factors for macrosomia and its clinical consequences: a study of 350,311 pregnancies. *Eur J Obstet Gynecol Reprod Biol* 2003; **111**:9–14.

267 Catalano PM, Presley L, Minium J, Hauguel-de Mouzon S. Fetuses of obese mothers develop insulin resistance *in utero*. *Diabetes Care* 2009; **32**:1076–1080.

268 Richards ID. Congenital malformations and environmental influences in pregnancy. *Br J Prev Soc Med* 1969; **23**:218–225.

269 García-Patterson A, Erdozain L, Ginovart G, Adelantado JM, Cubero JM, Gallo G, *et al.* In human gestational diabetes mellitus congenital malformations are related to pre-pregnancy body mass index and to severity of diabetes. *Diabetologia* 2004; **47**:509–514.

270 Moore LL, Bradlee ML, Singer MR, Rothman KJ, Milunsky A. Chromosomal anomalies among the offspring of women with gestational diabetes. *Am J Epidemiol* 2002; **155**:719–724.

271 Martinez-Frias ML, Frías JP, Bermejo E, Rodríguez-Pinilla E, Prieto L, Frías JL. Pre-gestational maternal body mass index predicts an increased risk of congenital malformations in infants of mothers with gestational diabetes. *Diabet Med* 2005; **22**:775–781.

272 Lazarus JH, Premawardhana LD. Screening for thyroid disease in pregnancy. *J Clin Pathol* 2005; **58**:449–452.

273 Haddow JE, Palomaki GE, Allan WC, Williams JR, Knight GJ, Gagnon J, *et al.* Maternal thyroid deficiency during pregnancy and subsequent neuropsychological development of the child. *N Engl J Med* 1999; **341**:549–555.

274 Campbell NR, Hasinoff BB, Stalts H, Rao B, Wong NC. Ferrous sulfate reduces thyroxine efficacy in patients with hypothyroidism. *Ann Intern Med* 1992; **117**:1010–1013.

275 Lazarus JH. Thyroid disorders associated with pregnancy: etiology, diagnosis, and management. *Treat Endocrinol* 2005; **4**:31–41.

276 Pearson DW, Kernaghan D, Lee R, Penney GC; Scottish Diabetes in Pregnancy Study Group. The relationship between pre-pregnancy

care and early pregnancy loss, major congenital anomaly or perinatal death in type I diabetes mellitus. *Br J Obstet Gynaecol* 2007; **114**:104–107.

277 Elixhauser A, Kitzmiller JL, Weschler JM. Short-term cost benefit of pre-conception care for diabetes. *Diabetes Care* 1996; **19**:384.

278 Evers IM, de Valk HW, Visser GH. Risk of complications of pregnancy in women with type 1 diabetes: nationwide prospective study in the Netherlands. *Br Med J* 2004; **328**:915.

279 Janz NK, Herman WH, Becker MP, Charron-Prochownik D, Shayna VL, Lesnick TG, *et al.* Diabetes and pregnancy: factors associated with seeking pre-conception care. *Diabetes Care* 1995; **18**:157–165.

280 Holing EV. Preconception care of women with diabetes: the unrevealed obstacles. *J Matern Fetal Med* 2000; **9**:10–13.

281 Steel JM. Personal experience of prepregnancy care in women with insulin dependent diabetes. *Aust N Z J Obstet Gynaecol* 1994; **34**:135–139.

282 Dunne FP, Brydon P, Smith T, Essex M, Nicholson H, Dunn J. Pre-conceptive diabetes care in insulin dependent diabetes mellitus. *Q J Med* 1999; **92**:175–176.

283 Gibb D, Hockey S, Brown LJ, Lunt H. Attitudes and knowledge regarding contraception and prepregnancy counselling in insulin dependent diabetes. *N Z Med J* 1994; **107**:484–486.

284 Holing EV, Beyer CS, Brown ZA, Connell FA. Why don't women with diabetes plan their pregnancies? *Diabetes Care* 1998; **21**:889–893.

285 Temple RC, Aldridge VJ, Murphy HR. Prepregnancy care and pregnancy outcomes in women with type 1 diabetes. *Diabetes Care* 2006; **29**:1744–1749.

286 McElduff A, Cheung NW, McIntyre HD, Lagström JA, Oats JJ, Ross GP, *et al.* The Australasian Diabetes in Pregnancy Society consensus guidelines for the management of type 1 and type 2 diabetes in relation to pregnancy. *Med J Aust* 2005; **183**:373–377.

287 Rosenn BM, Miodovnik M, Holcberg G, Khoury JC, Siddiqi TA. Hypoglycemia: the price of intensive insulin therapy for pregnant women with insulin-dependent diabetes mellitus. *Obstet Gynecol* 1995; **85**:417–422.

288 DAFNE Study Group. Training in flexible, intensive insulin management to enable dietary freedom in people with type 1 diabetes: dose adjustment for normal eating (DAFNE) randomised controlled trial. *Br Med J* 2002; **325**:746–749.

289 MRC Vitamin Research Study Group. Prevention of neural tube defects: the results of the Medical Research Council Vitamin Study. *Lancet* 1991; **388**:131–137.

290 Rogers I, Emmett P. Diet during pregnancy in a population of pregnant women in South West England. ALSPAC Study Team. Avon Longitudinal Study of Pregnancy and Childhood. *Eur J Clin Nutr* 1998; **52**:246–250.

291 Inkster ME, Fahey TP, Donnan PT, Leese GP, Mires GJ, Murphy DJ. The role of modifiable pre-pregnancy risk factors in preventing adverse fetal outcomes among women with type 1 and type 2 diabetes. *Acta Obstet Gynecol Scand* 2009; **88**:1153–1157.

292 McDermott R, Campbell S, Li M, McCulloch B. The health and nutrition of young indigenous women in north Queensland: intergenerational implications of poor food quality, obesity, diabetes, tobacco smoking and alcohol use. *Public Health Nutr* 2009; **12**:2143–2149.

293 Kiel D, Dodson EA, Artal R, Boehmer TK, Leet TL. Gestational weight gain and pregnancy outcomes in obese women: how much is enough? *Obstet Gynecol* 2007; **110**:752–758.

294 Rasmussen K, Yaktine A, eds. *Weight Gain During Pregnancy: Reexamining the Guidelines in Committee to Reexamine Institute of Medicine Pregnancy Weight Guidelines.* Institute of Medicine; National Research Council. Washington, DC: National Academies Press, 2009.

295 Reisenberger K, Egarter C, Sternberger B, Eckenberger P, Eberle E, Weissenbacher ER. Placental passage of angiotensin-converting enzyme inhibitors. *Am J Obstet Gynecol* 1996; **174**:1450–1455.

296 Steffensen FH, Steffensen FH, Olesen C, Nielsen GL, Pedersen L, Olsen J. Pregnancy outcome with ACE-inhibitor use in early pregnancy. *Lancet* 1998; **351**:596.

297 Lip GYH, Churchill D, Beevers M, Auckett A, Beevers DG. Angiotensin-converting-enzyme inhibitors in early pregnancy. *Lancet* 1997; **350**:1446–1447.

298 Bar J, Chen R, Schoenfeld A, Orvieto R, Yahav J, Ben-Rafael Z, *et al.* Pregnancy outcome in patients with insulin dependent diabetes mellitus and diabetic nephropathy treated with ACE inhibitors before pregnancy. *J Pediatr Endocrinol* 1999; **12**:659–665.

299 Burrows RF, Burrows EA. Assessing the teratogenic potential of angiotensin-converting enzyme inhibitors in pregnancy. *Aust N Z J Obstet Gynaecol* 1998; **38**:306–311.

300 Cooper WO, Hernandez-Diaz S, Arbogast PG, Dudley JA, Dyer S, Gideon PS, *et al.* Major congenital malformations after first-trimester exposure to ACE inhibitors. *N Engl J Med* 2006; **354**:2443–2451.

301 Saji H, Yamanaka M, Hagiwara A, Ijiri R. Losartan and fetal toxic effects. *Lancet* 2001; **357**:363.

302 Gersak K, Cvijic M, Cerar L. Angiotensin II receptor blockers in pregnancy: a report of five cases. *Reprod Toxicol* 2009; **28**:109–112.

303 Briggs G, Freeman RA, Yaffe S. *Drugs in Pregnancy and Lactation: A Reference Guide to Fetal and Neonatal Risk*, 7th edn. Philadelphia, PA: Lippincott, Williams and Wilkins, 2007.

304 Joint Formulary Committee. *British National Formulary*, Vol. 53. London: British Medical Association and Royal Pharmaeutical Society of Great Britain, 2007.

305 Edison RJ, Muenke M. Central nervous system and limb anomalies in case reports of first-trimester statin exposure. *N Engl J Med* 2004; **350**:1579–1582.

306 Belfort MA, Anthony J, Buccimazza A, Davey DA. Hemodynamic changes associated with intravenous infusion of the calcium antagonist verapamil in the treatment of severe gestational proteinuric hypertension. *Obstet Gynecol* 1990; **75**:970–974.

307 Magee LA, Schick B, Donnenfeld AE, Sage SR, Conover B, Cook L, *et al.* The safety of calcium channel blockers in human pregnancy: a prospective, multicenter cohort study. *Am J Obstet Gynecol* 1996; **174**:823–828.

308 Chan WC, Lim LT, Quinn MJ, Knox FA, McCance D, Best RM. Management and outcome of sight-threatening diabetic retinopathy in pregnancy. *Eye* 2004; **18**:826–832.

309 Greco L, Veneziano A, Di Donato L, Zampella C, Pecorano M, Paladini D, *et al.* Undiagnosed coeliac disease does not appear to be associated with unfavourable outcome of pregnancy. *Gut* 2004; **53**:149–151.

310 Hare JW. Medical management. In: Hare JW, ed. *Diabetes Complicating Pregnancy: The Joslin Clinic Method.* New York: Alan R. Liss, 1989: 35–51.

311 Langer O, Anyaegbunam A, Brustman L, Guidetti D, Levy J, Mazze R. Pregestational diabetes: insulin requirements throughout pregnancy. *Am J Obstet Gynecol* 1988; **159**:616–621.

312 Jovanovic L, Knopp RH, Brown Z, Conley MR, Park E, Mills JL, *et al.* Declining insulin requirement in the late first trimester of diabetic pregnancy. *Diabetes Care* 2001; **24**:1130–1136.

313 Rosenn B, Miodovnik M, Khoury JC, Siddiqi TA. Counterregulatory hormonal responses to hypoglycemia during pregnancy. *Obstet Gynecol* 1996; **87**:568–574.

314 Cryer PE, Davis SN, Shamoon H. Hypoglycemia in diabetes. *Diabetes Care* 2003; **26**:1902–1912.

315 Hellmuth E, Damm P, Mølsted-Pedersen L, Bendtson I. Prevalence of nocturnal hypoglycemia in first trimester of pregnancy in patients with insulin treated diabetes mellitus. *Acta Obstet Gynecol Scand* 2000; **79**:958–962.

316 Murphy HR, Rayman G, Duffield K, Lewis KS, Kelly S, Johal B, *et al.* Changes in the glycemic profiles of women with type 1 and type 2 diabetes during pregnancy. *Diabetes Care* 2007; **30**:2785–2791.

317 Leinonen PJ, Hiilesmaa VK, Kaaja RJ, Teramo KA. Maternal mortality in type 1 diabetes. *Diabetes Care* 2001; **24**:1501–1502.

318 Manderson JG, Patterson CC, Hadden DR, Traub AI, Ennis C, McCance DR. Preprandial versus postprandial blood glucose monitoring in type 1 diabetic pregnancy: a randomized controlled clinical trial. *Am J Obstet Gynecol* 2003; **189**:507–512.

319 DeVeciana M, Major CA, Morgan MA. Postprandial verses preprandial glucose monitoring in women with gestational diabetes mellitus requiring insulin therapy. *N Engl J Med* 1995; **333**:1237–1241.

320 Yogev Y, Chen R, Ben-Haroush A, Phillip M, Jovanovic L, Hod M. Continuous glucose monitoring for the evaluation of gravid women with type 1 diabetes mellitus. *Obstet Gynecol* 2003; **101**: 633–638.

321 Kerssen A, de Valk HW, Visser GH. Forty-eight-hour first-trimester glucose profiles in women with type 1 diabetes mellitus: a report of three cases of congenital malformation. *Prenat Diagn* 2006; **26**: 123–127.

322 Murphy HR, Rayman G, Lewis K, Kelly S, Johal B, Duffield K, *et al.* Effectiveness of continuous glucose monitoring in pregnant women with diabetes: randomised clinical trial. *Br Med J* 2008; **337**:a1680.

323 Crowther CA, Hiller JE, Moss JR, McPhee AJ, Jeffries WS, Robinson JS; Australian Carbohydrate Intolerance Study in Pregnant Women (ACHOIS) Trial Group. Effect of treatment of gestational diabetes mellitus on pregnancy outcomes. *N Engl J Med* 2005; **352**:2477–2486.

324 Langer O, Levy J, Brustman L, Anyaegbunam A, Merkatz R, Divon M. Glycemic control in gestational diabetes mellitus – how tight is tight enough: small for gestational age versus large for gestational age? *Am J Obstet Gynecol* 1989; **161**:646–653.

325 Nachum Z, Ben-Shlomo I, Weiner E, Shalev E. Twice daily versus four times daily insulin dose regimens for diabetes in pregnancy: randomised controlled trial. *Br Med J* 1999; **319**:1223–1227.

326 Plank J, Siebenhofer A, Berghold A, Jeitler K, Horvath K, Mrak P, *et al.* Systematic review and meta-analysis of short-acting insulin analogues in patients with diabetes mellitus. *Arch Intern Med* 2005; **165**:1337–1344.

327 Mathiesen ER, Kinsley B, Amiel SA, Heller S, McCance D, Duran S, *et al.* Maternal glycemic control and hypoglycemia in type 1 diabetic pregnancy: a randomized trial of insulin aspart versus human insulin in 322 pregnant women. *Diabetes Care* 2007; **30**:771–776.

328 Jovanovic L, Ilic S, Pettitt DJ, Hugo K, Gutierrez M, Bowsher RR, *et al.* Metabolic and immunologic effects of insulin lispro in gestational diabetes. *Diabetes Care* 1999; **22**:1422–1427.

329 Persson B, Swahn ML, Hjertberg R, Hanson U, Nord E, Nordlander E, *et al.* Insulin lispro therapy in pregnancies complicated by type 1 diabetes mellitus. *Diabetes Res Clin Pract* 2002; **58**:115–121.

330 Aydin Y, Berker D, Direktör N, Ustün I, Tütüncü YA, I ik S, *et al.* Is insulin lispro safe in pregnant women: does it cause any adverse outcomes on infants or mothers? *Diabetes Res Clin Pract* 2008; **80**:444–448.

331 Lapolla A, Dalfrà MG, Spezia R, Anichini R, Bonomo M, Bruttomesso D, *et al.* Outcome of pregnancy in type 1 diabetic patients treated with insulin lispro or regular insulin: an Italian experience. *Acta Diabetol* 2008; **45**:61–66.

332 Durnwald CP, Landon MB. A comparison of lispro and regular insulin for the management of type 1 and type 2 diabetes in pregnancy. *J Matern Fetal Neonatal Med* 2008; **21**:309–313.

333 Hirsch IB. Insulin analogues. *N Engl J Med* 2005; **352**:174–183.

334 Kurtzhals P, Schäffer L, Sørensen A, Kristensen C, Jonassen I, Schmid C, *et al.* Correlations of receptor binding and metabolic and mitogenic potencies of insulin analogs designed for clinical use. *Diabetes* 2000; **49**:999–1005.

335 Gallen IW, Jaap A, Roland JM, Chirayath HH. Survey of glargine use in 115 pregnant women with type 1 diabetes. *Diabet Med* 2008; **25**:165–169.

336 Price N, Bartlett C, Gillmer M. Use of insulin glargine during pregnancy: a case–control pilot study. *Br J Obstet Gynaecol* 2007; **114**:453–457.

337 Di Cianni G, Torlone E, Lencioni C, Bonomo M, Di Benedetto A, Napoli A, *et al.* Perinatal outcomes associated with the use of glargine during pregnancy. *Diabet Med* 2008; **25**:993–996.

338 Retnakaran R, Hochman J, DeVries JH, Hanaire-Broutin H, Heine RJ, Melki V, *et al.* Continuous subcutaneous insulin infusion versus multiple daily injections: the impact of baseline A1c. *Diabetes Care* 2004; **27**:2590–2596.

339 Mukhopadhyay A, Farrell T, Fraser RB, Ola B. Continuous subcutaneous insulin infusion vs intensive conventional insulin therapy in pregnant women with diabetes: a systematic review and metaanalysis of randomized, controlled trials. *Am J Obstet Gynecol* 2007; **197**:447–456.

340 Farrar D, Tuffnell DJ, West J. Continuous subcutaneous insulin infusion versus multiple daily injections of insulin for pregnant women with diabetes. *Cochrane Database Syst Rev* 2007; **3**:CD005542.

341 Lapolla A, Dalfrà MG, Masin M, Bruttomesso D, Piva I, Crepaldi C, *et al.* Analysis of outcome of pregnancy in type 1 diabetics treated with insulin pump or conventional insulin therapy. *Acta Diabetol* 2003; **40**:143–149.

342 Vanky E, Zahlsen K, Spigset O, Carlsen SM. Placental passage of metformin in women with polycystic ovary syndrome. *Fertil Steril* 2005; **83**:1575–1578.

343 Hawthorne G. Metformin use and diabetic pregnancy: has its time come? *Diabet Med* 2006; **23**:223–227.

344 Coetzee EJ. Counterpoint: oral hypoglyemic agents should be used to treat diabetic pregnant women. *Diabetes Care* 2007; **30**:2980–2982.

345 Ekpebegh CO, Coetzee EJ, van der Merwe L, Levitt NS. A 10-year retrospective analysis of pregnancy outcome in pregestational type 2 diabetes: comparison of insulin and oral glucose-lowering agents. *Diabet Med* 2007; **24**:253–258.

346 Gilbert C, Valois M, Koren G. Pregnancy outcome after first-trimester exposure to metformin: a meta-analysis. *Fertil Steril* 2006; **86**:658–663.

347 Nicholson W, Bolen S, Witkop CT, Neale D, Wilson L, Bass E. Benefits and risks of oral diabetes agents compared with insulin in women with gestational diabetes: a systematic review. *Obstet Gynecol* 2009; **113**:193–205.

348 Rowan JA, Hague WM, Gao W, Battin MR, Moore MP; MiG Trial Investigators. Metformin versus insulin for the treatment of gestational diabetes. *N Engl J Med* 2008; **358**:2003–2015.

349 Langer O, Conway DL, Berkus MD, Xenakis EM, Gonzales O. A comparison of glyburide and insulin in women with gestational diabetes mellitus. *N Engl J Med* 2000; **343**:1134–1138.

350 Hytten FF. Nutrition. In: Hytten E, Chamberlain G, eds. *Clinical Physiology in Obstetrics*. Oxford, UK: Blackwell Scientific Publications, 1980: 163–192.

351 Bianco A, Smilen SW, Davis Y, Lopez S, Lapinski R, Lockwood CJ. Pregnancy outcome and weight gain recommendations for the morbidly obese woman. *Obstet Gynecol* 1998; **91**:97–102.

352 Nohr EA, Bech BH, Vaeth M, Rasmussen KM, Henriksen TB, Olsen J. Obesity, gestational weight gain and preterm birth: a study within the Danish National Birth Cohort. *Paediatr Perinat Epidemiol* 2007; **21**:5–14.

353 Oken E, Kleinman KP, Belfort MB, Hammitt JK, Gillman MW. Associations of gestational weight gain with short- and longer-term maternal and child health outcomes. *Am J Epidemiol* 2009; **170**:173–180.

354 Oken E, Rifas-Shiman SL, Field AE, Frazier AL, Gillman MW. Maternal gestational weight gain and offspring weight in adolescence. *Obstet Gynecol* 2008; **112**:999–1006.

355 Nohr E, Vaeth M, Baker JL, Sørensen TIa, Olsen J, Rasmussen KM. Combined associations of prepregnancy body mass index and gestational weight gain with the outcome of pregnancy. *Am J Clin Nutr* 2008; **87**:1750–1759.

356 Barboza JM, Dajani NK, Glenn LG, Angtuaco TL. Prenatal diagnosis of congenital cardiac anomalies: a practical approach using two basic views. *Radiographics* 2002; **22**:1125–1137; discussion 1137–1138.

357 Aschwald CL, Catanzaro RB, Weiss EP, Gavard JA, Steitz KA, Mostello DJ. Large-for-gestational-age infants of type 1 mother with diabetes: an effect of preprandial hyperglycemia? *Gynecol Endocrinol* 2009: 1–8.

358 Raychaudhuri K, Maresh M. Glycemic control throughout pregnancy and fetal growth in insulin-dependent diabetes. *Obstet Gynecol* 2000; **95**:190–194.

359 Jovanovic-Peterson L, Durak EP, Peterson CM. Randomized trial of diet versus diet plus cardiovascular conditioning on glucose levels in gestational diabetes. *Am J Obstet Gynecol* 1989; **161**:415–419.

360 Brankston GN, Mitchell BF, Ryan EA, Okun NB. Resistance exercise decreases the need for insulin in overweight women with gestational diabetes mellitus. *Am J Obstet Gynecol* 2004; **190**:188–193.

361 Balani J, Hyer SL, Rodin DA, Shehata H. Pregnancy outcomes in women with gestational diabetes treated with metformin or insulin: a case–control study. *Diabet Med* 2009; **26**:798–802.

362 Holt RI, Clarke P, Parry EC, Coleman MA. The effectiveness of glibenclamide in women with gestational diabetes. *Diabetes Obes Metab* 2008; **10**:906–911.

363 Peel J, Oakley W. The management of pregnancy in diabetics. In: *Transactions of the 12th British Congress of Obstetrics and Gynaecology*. London: Royal College of Obstetricians and Gynaecologists, 1949: 161.

364 Beard RW, Lowy C. The British survey of diabetic pregnancies. *Br J Obstet Gynaecol* 1982: **89**:783–786.

365 McAuliffe FM, Foley M, Firth R, Drury I, Stronge JM. Outcome of diabetic pregnancy with spontaneous labor after 38 weeks. *Ir J Med Sci* 1999; **168**:160–163.

366 Conway DL. Obstetric management in gestational diabetes. *Diabetes Care* 2007; **30**(Suppl 2):175–179.

367 Kjos SL, Henry OA, Montoro M, Buchanan TA, Mestman JH. Insulin-requiring diabetes in pregnancy: a randomized trial of active induction of labor and expectant management. *Am J Obstet Gynecol* 1993; **169**:611–615.

368 Lurie S, Insler V, Hagay ZJ. Induction of labor at 38 to 39 weeks of gestation reduces the incidence of shoulder dystocia in gestational diabetic patients class A2. *Am J Perinatol* 1996; **13**:293–296.

369 Matsushita E, Matsuda Y, Makino Y, Sanaka M, Ohta H. Risk factors associated with preterm delivery in women with pregestational diabetes. *J Obstet Gynaecol Res* 2008; **34**:851–857.

370 Lepercq J, Coste J, Theau A, Dubois-Laforgue D, Timsit J. Factors associated with preterm delivery in women with type 1 diabetes: a cohort study. *Diabetes Care* 2004; **27**:2824–2828.

371 Mathiesen ER, Christensen AB, Hellmuth E, Hornnes P, Stage E, Damm P. Insulin dose during glucocorticoid treatment for fetal lung maturation in diabetic pregnancy: test of an algorithm [correction of analgoritm]. *Acta Obstet Gynecol Scand* 2002; **81**: 835–839.

372 Kaushal K, Gibson JM, Railton A, Hounsome B, New JP, Young RJ. A protocol for improved glycemic control following corticosteroid therapy in diabetic pregnancies. *Diabet Med* 2003; **20**:73–75.

373 Feldberg D, Dicker D, Samuel N, Peleg D, Karp M, Goldman JA. Intrapartum management of insulin-dependent diabetes mellitus (IDDM) gestants: a comparative study of constant intravenous insulin infusion and continuous subcutaneous insulin infusion pump (CSIIP). *Acta Obstet Gynecol Scand* 1988; **67**:333–338.

374 Taylor R, Lee C, Kyne-Grzebalski D, Marchall SM, Davison JM. Clinical outcomes of pregnancy in women with type 1 diabetes. *Obstet Gynecol* 2002; **99**:537–541.

375 Carron Brown S, Kyne-Grzebalski D, Mwnagi B, Taylor R. Effect of management policy upon 120 type 1 diabetic pregnancies: policy decisions in practice. *Diabet Med* 1999; **16**:573–578.

376 Barrett HL, Morris J, McElduff A. Watchful waiting: a management protocol for maternal glycaemia in the peripartum period. *Aust N Z J Obstet Gynecol* 2009; **49**:162–167.

377 Grummer-Strawn LM, Mei Z. Does breastfeeding protect against pediatric overweight? Analysis of longitudinal data from the Centers for Disease Control and Prevention Pediatric Nutrition Surveillance System. *Pediatrics* 2004; **113**:e81–86.

378 Gillman MW, Rifas-Shiman SL, Berkey CS, Frazier AL, Rockett HR, Camargo CA Jr. Breast-feeding and overweight in adolescence: within-family analysis [corrected]. *Epidemiology* 2006; **17**:112–114.

379 Mayer-Davis EJ, Rifas-Shiman SL, Zhou L, Hu FB, Colditz GA, Gillman MW. Breast-feeding and risk for childhood obesity: does maternal diabetes or obesity status matter? *Diabetes Care* 2006; **29**:2231–2237.

380 Mayer-Davis EJ, Dabelea D, Lamichhane AP, D'Agostino RB Jr, Liese AD, Thomas J, *et al.* Breast-feeding and type 2 diabetes in the youth of three ethnic groups: the SEARCh for diabetes in youth case–control study. *Diabetes Care* 2008; **31**:470–475.

381 Plagemann A, Harder T. Breast feeding and the risk of obesity and related metabolic diseases in the child. *Metab Syndr Relat Disord* 2005; **3**:222–232.

382 Briggs GG, Ambrose PJ, Nageotte MP, Padilla G, Wan S. Excretion of metformin into breast milk and the effect on nursing infants. *Obstet Gynecol* 2005; **105**:1437–1441.

383 Feig DS, Briggs GG, Koren G. Oral antidiabetic agents in pregnancy and lactation: a paradigm shift? *Ann Pharmacother* 2007; **41**: 1174–1180.

384 O'Sullivan JB, Mahan CM. Criteria for oral glucose tolerance test in pregnancy. *Diabetes* 1964; **13**:278–285.

385 Damm P, Kühl C, Buschard K, Jakobsen BK, Svejgaard A, Sodoyez-Goffaux F, *et al.* Prevalence and predictive value of islet cell antibodies in women with gestational diabetes. *Diabetic Med* 1994; **1994**:558–563.

386 Ratner RE, Christophi CA, Metzger BE, Dabelea D, Bennett PH, Pi-Sunyer X, *et al.* Prevention of diabetes in women with a history of gestational diabetes: effects of metformin and lifestyle interventions. *J Clin Endocrinol Metab* 2008; **93**:4774–4779.

387 Kim C, Newton KM, Knopp RH. Gestational diabetes and the incidence of type 2 diabetes: a systematic review. *Diabetes Care* 2002; **25**:1862–1868.

388 Beischer NA, Oats JN, Henry OA, Sheedy MT, Walstab JE. Incidence and severity of gestational diabetes mellitus according to country of birth in women living in Australia. *Diabetes* 1991; **40**(Suppl 2):35–38.

389 Henry OA, Beischer NA. Long-term implications of gestational diabetes for the mother. *Baillieres Clin Obstet Gynaecol* 1991; **5**:461–483.

390 Dornhorst A, Paterson CM, Nicholls JS, Wadsworth J, Chiu DC, Elkeles RS, *et al.* High prevalence of gestational diabetes in women from ethnic minority groups. *Diabet Med* 1992; **9**:820–825.

391 Benjamin E, Winters D, Mayfield J, Gohdes D. Diabetes in pregnancy in Zuni Indian women: prevalence and subsequent development of clinical diabetes after gestational diabetes. *Diabetes Care* 1993; **16**:1231–1235.

392 Metzger BE, Cho NH, Roston SM, Radvany R. Prepregnancy weight and antepartum insulin secretion predict glucose tolerance five years after gestational diabetes mellitus. *Diabetes Care* 1993; **16**:1598–1605.

393 Löbner K, Knopff A, Baumgarten A, Mollenhauer U, Marienfeld S, Garrido-Franco M, *et al.* Predictors of postpartum diabetes in women with gestational diabetes mellitus. *Diabetes* 2006; **55**:792–797.

394 Lee AJ, Hiscock RJ, Wein P, Walker SP, Permezel M. Gestational diabetes mellitus: clinical predictors and long-term risk of developing type 2 diabetes: a retrospective cohort study using survival analysis. *Diabetes Care* 2007; **30**:878–883.

395 Peters RK, Kjos SL, Xiang A, Buchanan TA. Long-term diabetogenic effect of single pregnancy in women with previous gestational diabetes mellitus. *Lancet* 1996; **347**:227–230.

396 Buchanan TA, Xiang AH, Kjos SL, Trigo E, Lee WP, Peters RK. Antepartum predictors of the development of type 2 diabetes in Latino women 11–26 months after pregnancies complicated by gestational diabetes. *Diabetes* 1999; **48**:2430–2436.

397 Buchanan TA, Xiang AH, Peters RK, Kjos SL, Marroquin A, Goico J, *et al.* Preservation of pancreatic beta-cell function and prevention of type 2 diabetes by pharmacological treatment of insulin resistance in high-risk hispanic women. *Diabetes* 2002; **51**:2796–2803.

398 Kim C, Tabaei BP, Burke R, McEwen LN, Lash RW, Johnson SL, *et al.* Missed opportunities for type 2 diabetes mellitus screening among women with a history of gestational diabetes mellitus. *Am J Public Health* 2006; **96**:1643–1648.

399 Hunt KJ, Conway DL. Who returns for postpartum glucose screening following gestational diabetes mellitus? *Am J Obstet Gynecol* 2008; **198**:404, e1–6.

400 Ferrara A, Peng T, Kim C. Trends in postpartum diabetes screening and subsequent diabetes and impaired fasting glucose among women with histories of gestational diabetes mellitus: a report from the Translating Research Into Action for Diabetes (TRIAD) Study. *Diabetes Care* 2009; **32**:269–274.

401 Kim C, Herman WH, Vijan S. Efficacy and cost of postpartum screening strategies for diabetes among women with histories of gestational diabetes mellitus. *Diabetes Care* 2007; **30**:1102–1106.

402 Holt RI, Goddard JR, Clarke P, Coleman MA. A postnatal fasting plasma glucose is useful in determining which women with gestational diabetes should undergo a postnatal oral glucose tolerance test. *Diabet Med* 2003; **20**:594–598.

403 Tuomilehto J, Lindström J, Eriksson JG, Valle TT, Hämäläinen H, Ilanne-Parikka P, *et al.* Prevention of type 2 diabetes mellitus by changes in lifestyle among subjects with impaired glucose tolerance. *N Engl J Med* 2001; **344**:1343–1350.

404 Diabetes Prevention Program Research Group. Reduction in the incidence of type 2 diabetes with lifestyle intervention or metformin. *N Engl J Med* 2002; **346**:393–403.

405 Kim C, Berger DK, Chamany S. Recurrence of gestational diabetes mellitus: a systematic review. *Diabetes Care* 2007; **30**:1314–1319.

54 Diabetes in Old Age

Alan J. Sinclair
The Institute of Diabetes for Older People (IDOP), University of Bedfordshire, Luton, UK

Keypoints

- Diabetes affects 10–25% of elderly people (>65 years) worldwide, with particularly high rates in populations such as Pima Indians, Mexican-Americans and South Asians.
- Glucose tolerance worsens with age, the main factor being impairment of insulin-stimulated glucose uptake and glycogen synthesis in skeletal muscle.
- Factors precipitating hyperosmolar hyperglycemic syndrome include infections, myocardial infarction, stroke and drugs such as thiazides or glucocorticoids.
- Episodes of hypoglycemia resulting from insulin or sulfonylureas may be severe and prolonged, particularly because counter-regulatory responses are impaired in the elderly.
- High levels of disability are common in older people with diabetes and lead to heavy usage of health care resources and premature mortality.
- About 16% of elderly people with diabetes in the UK are registered blind or partially sighted (eight times more than the non-diabetic population) which justifies regular screening for undetected eye disease.
- Risk factors for foot ulceration affect 25% of elderly people with type 2 diabetes.
- Management strategies for many elderly people with diabetes are as in the younger population, with similar lipid-lowering and antihypertensive treatment schedules and aspirin or clopidogrel for patients with increased cardiovascular risk.
- Effective delivery of diabetes care depends on close cooperation between hospital and community, the involvement of diabetes specialists and practice nurses, and attention to all causes of disability and ill-health.
- Elderly people with diabetes in care homes are particularly vulnerable and require greater diabetes specialist input.

Introduction

Diabetes, the most common disabling metabolic disorder, imposes considerable economic, social and health burdens [1]. Many of these burdens fall heavily on older patients with diabetes, partly because type 2 diabetes mellitus (T2DM) and its co-morbidities are so much more common in that age group, and partly because of these subjects' special needs. Older people do not accept illness without question, however, and expect equity of access to treatment and services as for younger people. As those who are above pensionable age are, in most Westernized societies, a significant proportion of the voting public, they can be very persuasive in ensuring that there are political commitments to improving the organization and delivery of health care.

Within Europe, T2DM affects 10–30% of subjects above pensionable age and in the USA about 40% of all those with diabetes fall into this category [2]. Older people with diabetes use primary care services two to three times more than their counterparts without diabetes; in one Danish study [3], insulin-treated patients accounted for over half of the services provided, mainly because of macrovascular disease. The burden of hospital care is also increased two to three times in those with diabetes compared with the general aged population [4], with more frequent clinic visits and a fivefold higher admission rate; acute hospital admissions account for 60% of total expenditure in this group [5]. In the UK, some 5–8% of general hospital beds are occupied by patients with diabetes aged 60 years or more [6,7], accounting for 60% of all inpatients with diabetes [7]. Hospital admissions last twice as long for older patients with diabetes compared with age-matched control groups without diabetes, with the totals averaging 7 and 8 days per year for men and women, respectively [4,6,8]. Introducing insulin treatment increases costs fourfold, both in the community and in hospital, where bed occupancy rises to 24 days per year [4].

The management of T2DM and its common co-morbidity of macrovascular disease is complicated in elderly subjects because of the added effects of aging on metabolism and renal function, the use of potentially diabetogenic drugs and low levels of physical activity (Figure 54.1) [9,10]. Cardiovascular risk is particularly high because many risk factors of the metabolic syndrome can be present for up to a decade before T2DM is diagnosed (Figure 54.1) [11].

Textbook of Diabetes, 4th edition. Edited by R. Holt, C. Cockram, A. Flyvbjerg and B. Goldstein.

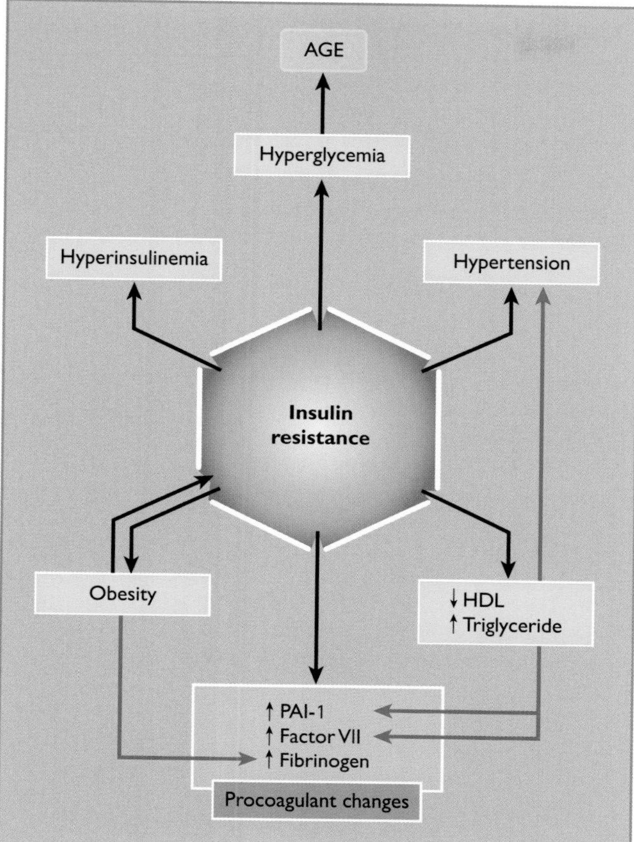

Figure 54.1 Features of the metabolic syndrome. Additional considerations that apply to the elderly population are described in the text. AGE, advanced glycation end-product; HDL, high density lipoprotein; PAI-1, plasminogen activator inhibitor1.

Table 54.1 Special characteristics of older subjects with diabetes.

High level of associated medical co-morbidities
Increased risk of cognitive dysfunction and mood disorder causing more complex decision-making
Varying evidence of impaired activities of daily living and lower limb function
Increased vulnerability to hypoglycemia
Increased risk of inpatient mortality
Unstructured specialist and primary care follow-up
Increased need to involve spouses and informal carers in management

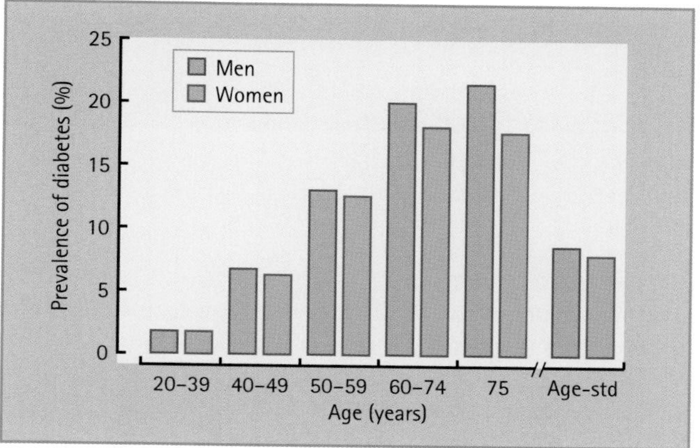

Figure 54.2 Prevalence of diabetes in men and women in the US population aged ≥20 years, based on the NHANES III study [14]. Subjects included those with previously diagnosed and undiagnosed diabetes (defined by fasting plasma glucose ≥7.0 mmol/L). Age-std, age-standardized.

It must be remembered that older people with diabetes, particularly those who are housebound or institutionalized, have special needs (Table 54.1). Overall, the quality of diabetes care for older patients appears to be improving in various countries [12,13], although the UK still seems to be alone in developing geriatric diabetes as a subspecialty.

Epidemiology of diabetes in aging populations

In 1997, there were approximately 124 million people with diabetes worldwide, of whom 97% had T2DM. By the time of publication of this edition, this number is projected to rise to 285 million. Aging is an important factor in the rapid worldwide rise of T2DM. In the USA, the number of new cases of diabetes in people aged 65–79 years was five times higher than in those aged less than 45 years of age [2]. The prevalence of diabetes begins to rise steadily from early adulthood, reaching a plateau in those aged 60 years or older; the data in Figure 54.2, from the Third National Health and Nutrition Examination Survey (NHANES III) in the USA [14], are representative of most developed countries. In some susceptible populations, T2DM may develop earlier; for example, among the Pima Indians prevalence peaks at 40 years of age in men and at 50 years in women, and declines after the ages of 65 and 55 years, respectively.

Overall prevalence rates of diabetes in the elderly are dominated by T2DM, which accounts for 95% of all cases in the UK and European countries, and for virtually all in populations such as the Pima Indians and Mexican-Americans. Some older patients who present clinically with T2DM may have slowly evolving autoimmune β-cell destruction that requires insulin treatment, so-called latent autoimmune diabetes of adults (LADA). This condition appears to be most prevalent in northern Europe and is rare in Asians and Africans.

There are marked ethnic and geographic differences in the prevalence rates of diabetes amongst older people. In the UK and most developed countries, diabetes affects 9–17% of white subjects aged over 65 years and up to 25% of non-white people [15,16]; intriguingly, the prevalence of diabetes in elderly care homes in the UK is also 25% [17]. Among subjects aged over 60 years from NHANES III, Mexican-Americans showed a consist-

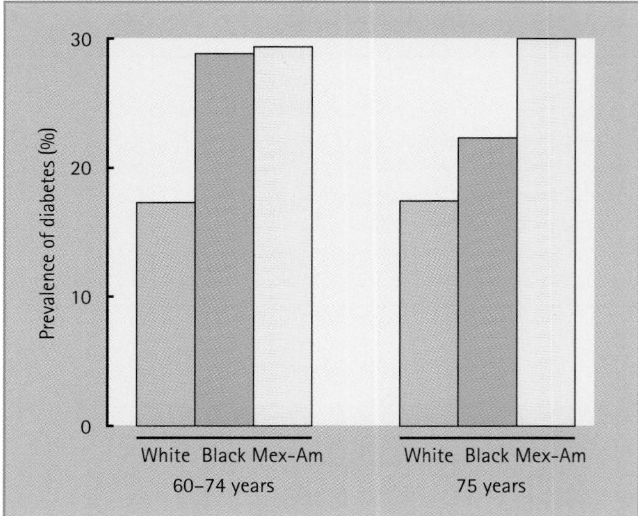

Figure 54.3 Prevalence rates for diabetes among elderly non-Hispanic white, non-Hispanic black and Mexican-American subjects. Data from the NHANES III study [14].

ently higher prevalence of diabetes than non-Latino white and black subjects (Figure 54.3) [14].

Etiology of diabetes in the elderly

T2DM accounts for virtually all of the age-related increase in the prevalence of diabetes. This is attributed to various combinations of insulin resistance and impaired insulin secretion that result in a progressive age-related decline in glucose tolerance, which begins in the third decade and continues throughout adulthood [18,19]. Plasma glucose levels at 1 and 2 hours after the standard 75-g oral glucose challenge rise by 0.3–0.7 mmol/L per decade, the increase being greater in women. Consistent with this, NHANES III found the prevalence of impaired glucose tolerance (IGT) to be 12% in subjects aged 40–49 years, rising to 21% in those aged 60–74 years [14].

Various factors contribute to age-related glucose intolerance (Table 54.2). Perhaps the most important is impairment of insulin-mediated glucose disposal, especially in skeletal muscle [19,20], which is particularly marked in obese subjects (Figure 54.4) [21]. Insulin receptor number and binding are not consistently affected by age, and so post-receptor defects are presumably responsible. Contributory factors in some cases include increased body fat mass, physical inactivity and diabetogenic drugs such as thiazides. In contrast to younger people with T2DM, fasting hepatic glucose production does not appear to be increased in either lean or obese elderly people with T2DM [21]. The ability of insulin to enhance blood flow is also considerably reduced in obese insulin-resistant subjects with diabetes; this may be etiologically important, as insulin-mediated vasodilatation is thought to account for about 30% of normal glucose disposal.

Table 54.2 Factors contributing to glucose intolerance in old age.

Impaired glucose disposal and utilization
• Insulin-mediated uptake into skeletal muscle
• Insulin-mediated vasodilatation in muscle
• NIMGU
Impaired glucose-induced insulin secretion
Other factors
• Obesity
• Physical inactivity
• Reduced dietary carbohydrate
• Diabetogenic drugs (thiazides, glucocorticoids)

NIMGU, non-insulin mediated glucose uptake.

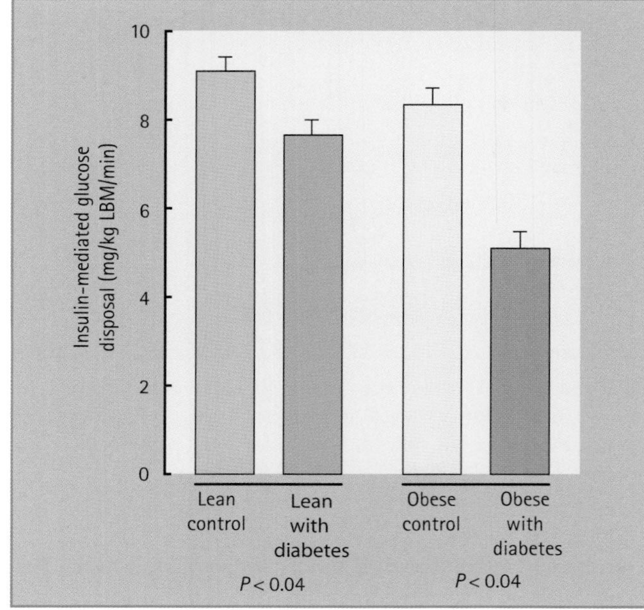

Figure 54.4 Insulin-mediated glucose disposal is decreased in elderly patients with type 2 diabetes. The euglycemic clamp technique was used to measure the glucose disposal rate in healthy lean and obese elderly controls, and in their counterparts with diabetes. LBM, lean body mass. From Meneilly *et al.* [21], with permission.

As well as insulin resistance, many elderly people with glucose intolerance show impairment of glucose-induced insulin secretion, especially in response to oral rather than intravenous glucose. In addition, recent studies have shown that glucose effectiveness (i.e. the ability of glucose to stimulate its own uptake in the absence of insulin) is decreased in healthy elderly subjects [22]. This non-insulin-mediated glucose uptake (NIMGU) accounts for 70% of glucose uptake under fasting conditions (primarily into the CNS) and for 50% of post-prandial glucose uptake (especially into skeletal muscle). This is therefore a potentially important new target for therapeutic intervention, as exercise, anabolic steroids and decreased non-esterified fatty-acid (NEFA) levels can all enhance NIMGU and improve glucose tolerance, at least in younger patients [23].

Acute metabolic complications in elderly people with diabetes

Hyperglycemic states

Older subjects with diabetes can develop diabetic ketoacidosis (DKA) and hyperosmolar hyperglycemic state (formerly known as hyperosmolar non-ketotic coma [HONK]), which occurs predominantly in subjects aged over 50 years. In one study from Birmingham, UK, 22% of admissions with DKA were in subjects aged 60 years or more [24], while 13% of cases of hyperglycemic coma in all ages in Melbourne, Australia, were caused by hyperosmolar hyperglycemic state [25]. Many people with T2DM maintain enough residual insulin secretion to suppress lipolysis and ketogenesis, and so develop hyperosmolar hyperglycemic state instead of DKA; hyperosmolarity can worsen insulin resistance and may also inhibit lipolysis. The tendency to hyperosmolarity may be worsened in elderly people, who may not perceive thirst or drink enough to compensate for the osmotic diuresis, and are often taking diuretics [26].

Causes of hyperglycemia include infection (55% of cases in one series of hyperosmolar hyperglycemic state), myocardial infarction (MI), inadequate hypoglycemic treatment or diabetogenic drug treatment. Thiazide diuretics and glucocorticoids can increase blood glucose levels and may precipitate DKA; thiazide diuretics and furosemide (frusemide) appear particularly likely to cause hyperosmolar hyperglycemic state. A specific cause often cannot be identified – for example, in 38% of DKA cases in Birmingham [24]. Residents of care homes are at increased risk of hyperosmolar hyperglycemic state, which is associated with appreciable mortality [27].

Compared with the young, older patients have higher mortality and longer stays in hospital; they are also less likely to have had diabetes diagnosed previously, and more likely to have renal impairment and to require higher insulin regimens [28]. Death may occur from the metabolic disturbance or concomitant illnesses such as pneumonia and MI.

Investigation and treatment of hyperglycemic comas

The history and examination should pay special attention to previous diabetic symptoms, drug treatment, any precipitating infection (MI), possible MI or medication, evidence of heart failure and the degree of dehydration. Initial investigations are as for younger patients, including arterial blood gases and plasma osmolality (see Chapter 34).

Fluid, insulin and potassium replacement are discussed in general in Chapter 34. In elderly patients, intravenous saline can often be given at a rate of 500 mL/hour for 4 hours, then reducing to 250 mL/hour; faster infusion is needed if the patient is shocked, when a central line is invaluable to monitor filling pressure, particularly in the presence of cardiac failure or recent MI.

Some older subjects with hyperosmolar hyperglycemic state need very small doses of insulin to reduce plasma glucose levels, although hypercatabolic or severely insulin-resistant states will require higher dosages.

Thrombotic complications may occur, especially in subjects with hyperosmolar hyperglycemic state; prophylactic anticoagulation with low dose subcutaneous heparin is therefore recommended.

Hypoglycemia

Older patients are particularly susceptible to hypoglycemia, and this problem is often exacerbated because old people may have been given little knowledge about the symptoms and signs of hypoglycemia [29]. Even health professionals may misdiagnose hypoglycemia as a stroke, transient ischemic attack, unexplained confusion or epileptic fit, as illustrated in the case history below.

Case history

A 76-year-old man was admitted with a left-sided hemiplegia. He was unconscious and the family was told by the emergency room staff that he had had a stroke and his prognosis was very poor. At this point, no-one had thought to assess his glucose concentration. When requested by the medical registrar, it was found to be 1.4 mmol/L. Following treatment with IV glucose, the man regained consciousness and he was able to leave hospital 1 hour later. He had taken his insulin but delayed his meal.

Personal communication from Richard Holt, University of Southampton

Patients with cognitive impairment or loss of the warning symptoms of hypoglycemia are especially vulnerable, as they may not recognize impending hypoglycemia and/or fail to communicate their feelings to their carers. Multiple factors underlie the increased susceptibility to hypoglycemia in the elderly, including recent discharge from hospital with altered sulfonylurea dosages, renal and hepatic impairment, excess alcohol and insulin therapy [30]. In addition, older subjects mount a diminished counter-regulatory response to hypoglycemia [31], and this may delay recovery.

The risk of hypoglycemia is highest with insulin, but prolonged hypoglycemia is an important clinical problem for older subjects taking glibenclamide and chlorpropamide [32]. Glibenclamide-induced hypoglycemia may be more pronounced because the drug accumulates within the β-cell, and its metabolites retain some hypoglycemic activity. The long elimination half-life (approximately 35 hours) of chlorpropamide causes it to accumulate with continued dosing; steady-state is not achieved for 7–10 days. Impaired renal function further prolongs hypoglycemia secondary to sulfonylureas that are cleared through the kidneys. Short-acting sulfonylureas, gliclazide and tolbutamide, are less likely to cause hypoglycemia [33], although glipizide is considered by some to be unsafe in the elderly [34]. Newer oral agents such as the thiazolidinediones and the meglitinides may decrease the risk of hypoglycemia in the elderly, as may both rapid- and prolonged-acting insulin analogs.

In the elderly, serious hypoglycemia appears to carry a worse prognosis and higher mortality; permanent neurologic damage may occur, presumably because of an already compromised cerebral circulation. Most sulfonylureas have caused fatal hypoglycemia, most commonly chlorpropamide or glibenclamide [35]. Other factors predisposing to fatal hypoglycemia include alcohol consumption, poor food intake, renal impairment and potentiation of hypoglycemia by other drugs.

Treatment and prevention of hypoglycemia are as described in Chapter 33. Many old people cannot treat hypoglycemia themselves [28]. The educational program should focus on detecting and treating hypoglycemia, with advice to others about how to manage cases of unresponsive hypoglycemia. In view of the additional vulnerability of older people to hypoglycemia, extra caution is required when there is a history of recurrent symptoms, drowsiness is present, the patient is on relatively large doses of insulin or when their diabetes care is delegated to an informal carer. This increased risk must be balanced by a lower threshold for admission to hospital when hypoglycemia is suspected. In this setting, a glucose level <4 mmol/L may warrant admission.

Chronic diabetic complications in the elderly

Diabetes in older subjects carries considerable morbidity, mainly through its long-term complications. For example, in a 6-year study of 188 patients aged over 60 years in Oxford [36], the reported incidence rates of ischemic heart disease, stroke and peripheral vascular disease (PVD) were 56, 22 and 146 cases per 1000 person-years, respectively. These were slightly higher than the rates in the Framingham study [37], presumably because of the older age of the Oxford patients. Retinopathy occurred at a rate of 60 cases and cataract at 29 cases per 1000 person-years, while the rate of proteinuria (albumin concentration >300 mg/L) was 19 per 1000 person-years. These incidence rates appeared to be unrelated to sex or duration of diabetes, but stroke and PVD rose significantly with age.

The age-dependence of chronic diabetic complications was also investigated in a cross-sectional study of patients with T2DM aged 53–80 years [38]. Logistic regression demonstrated a significant rise in the prevalence of retinopathy with aging, independent of the effects of metabolic control, duration of disease and other risk variables. Age also increased the prevalence of peripheral neuropathy, hypertension and erectile dysfunction. An independent contribution of age per se to retinopathy, however, was not reported by Ballard *et al.* [39] from Minnesota, USA (who found a positive relationship with persistent proteinuria only), or by Knuiman *et al.* [40], who studied patients with both type 1 diabetes (TIDM) and T2DM and found independent associations of age with renal impairment, macrovascular complications and sensory neuropathy only.

Diabetic eye disease and visual loss

Cataract, age-related macular degeneration and diabetic retinopathy remain the major causes of blindness and partial-sight registration in most developed countries (see Chapter 36) [41]. All these conditions are common in elderly patients with diabetes.

Cataract, the most frequent cause of deteriorating vision in the elderly, is more common in subjects with diabetes, even at the time of diagnosis; its presence is associated with premature death [16]. Age-related macular degeneration is also frequent in older patients with diabetes and is an important cause of central visual loss [42]. Risk factors include atherosclerosis, diastolic blood pressure >95 mmHg or antihypertensive medication, and elevated serum cholesterol. Most older patients with diabetes have diabetic retinopathy of some degree, although about 5% show no evidence of retinal damage even after 15 years of the disease [42]. The main sight-threatening consequence of diabetic retinopathy in this population is maculopathy and particularly macular edema (see Chapter 36).

In Nottingham, UK, 16% of elderly people with diabetes are registered blind or partially sighted which is approximately eight times more than among their counterparts without diabetes [43]. The Welsh Community Diabetes Study [44] found that visual acuity was impaired in 40% of elderly subjects with diabetes, compared with only 31% of controls without diabetes (P<0.007). Factors significantly associated with visual loss in people with diabetes included advanced age, duration of diabetes, female sex, a history of foot ulceration and treatment with insulin. Reduced visual acuity was also significantly associated with poorer quality of life, as measured by the SF-36 questionnaire.

Screening for retinopathy

This is particularly important in the elderly, as deteriorating vision may be accepted by the patient as part of aging. Diabetic retinopathy may be the presenting feature of the disease in older people. Elderly people with diabetes need annual measurements of visual acuity and retinal photography; where the latter may not be available or feasible, patients should undergo dilated-pupil fundoscopy by experienced observers. Exudative maculopathy (hard exudates at or within one disc diameter of the macula) is easy to detect, but macular edema is practically impossible to detect by routine ophthalmoscopy; instead, slit-lamp stereoscopic fundoscopy is required to measure retinal thickness. Mydriasis is usually a short-term intervention and, in the great majority of cases, is not associated with any major problems, even in older people. It is always important to know whether patients have a history of glaucoma before mydriasis, as this requires a different approach, often under specialist supervision. This highlights the importance of measuring the corrected visual acuity, which is decreased by maculopathy (see Chapter 36). Indications for referral to an ophthalmologist are generally identical to those in younger patients (see Table 36.3).

Prevention and management of diabetic retinopathy

The benefits of tight glycemic control in slowing the progression of diabetic retinopathy have been convincingly proven in both T1DM and T2DM, by the Diabetes Control and Complications Trial (DCCT) and UK Prospective Diabetes Study (UKPDS) trials, respectively [45,46]. In the UKPDS, the risk of retinopathy progressing was reduced by 25% when HbA_{1c} was maintained at <53 mmol/mol (7.0%) [46], while improved blood pressure control also reduced risk by 37% [47]. Although there have been no specific intervention studies in elderly patients with T2DM, it seems reasonable to extrapolate the general principles to this population. Problems with hypoglycemia and postural hypotension, however, prevent many elderly subjects from achieving tight glycemic and blood pressure control.

Laser photocoagulation should be used as indicated in Chapter 36; it halves the risk of severe visual loss with macular edema and exudative maculopathy (if visual acuity is 6/9 or better), which otherwise reaches 50–70% after 5 years [48–50]. It has been calculated that screening and treating diabetic retinopathy would prevent 56% of blind registrations resulting from this condition.

Diabetic foot disease

Amputation of a limb remains an important and expensive health problem in the diabetic population, with the elderly being particularly affected [51]. A Dutch study [52] identified increasing age and a higher level of amputation as important factors that increased both the duration and costs of hospitalization (estimated at over £10 000 per hospitalization, lasting an average of 42 days). The 3-year survival following lower-extremity amputation is about 50% [53]; in about 70% of cases, amputation is precipitated by foot ulceration [54]. The principal antecedents include peripheral vascular disease, sensorimotor and autonomic neuropathy, limited joint mobility (which especially prevents older people from inspecting their feet) and high foot pressures (Table 54.3) [51]. Most elderly people with diabetes are at increased risk of developing foot ulcers. Peripheral sensorimotor neuropathy, the primary cause or contributory factor in most cases, becomes more common with increasing age and affects 25% of patients with T2DM aged 80 years or more [55]. As well as the common symptoms of numbness, neurogenic pain, "pins and needles" and hyperesthesia (all typically worse at night), peripheral neuropathy often causes gait disturbances, falls and other foot injuries. Concomitant visual loss worsens the situation [56]. A trivial foot injury in a patient with severe neuropathy can eventually lead to Charcot arthropathy; most of these patients have had diabetes for at least 10 years, and many are elderly (see Chapter 44).

Table 54.3 Risk factors for foot ulceration in the elderly.

Peripheral sensorimotor neuropathy
Automatic neuropathy
Peripheral vascular disease
Limited joint mobility
Foot pressure abnormalities, including deformity
Previous foot problems
Visual loss
History of alcohol abuse

Treatment of painful neuropathy in older patients is often difficult. Recent-onset symptoms may remit with improved metabolic control, but pain associated with loss of sensation and of greater than 6 months' duration generally requires specific therapy. Localized pain may respond to topical application of capsaicin cream (0.075%), which depletes pain fibers of the neurotransmitter, substance P. Other drugs include tricyclic antidepressants (e.g. amitriptyline) and antiepileptics, such as carbamazepine and gabapentin (now licensed for this indication). Alternative treatments include transcutaneous nerve stimulation or acupuncture, as described in Chapter 38.

Ischemia, secondary to PVD and perhaps microcirculatory disturbances [57], is the other main contributor to diabetic foot ulceration. Macrovascular disease becomes more common with advancing age. As discussed in Chapter 39, atheromatous lesions in diabetes are more diffuse and involve vessels below the knee more often than in individuals without diabetes. Medial arterial calcification is common, especially in association with somatosensory and autonomic neuropathy; this change can affect Doppler ultrasound measurements of blood pressure in the foot and cause a misleadingly high ankle pressure index.

As in younger patients, many older people with diabetes and critical or worsening limb ischemia, or ischemic ulcers that are slow to heal, will benefit from surgical revascularization (angioplasty or arterial reconstruction). Appropriate cases should be referred early for surgery, ideally through joint protocols developed by the diabetes specialist and the vascular surgeon [58]. A reasonable life expectancy is considered important by surgeons, as concomitant cardiac and cerebrovascular disease kill 50% of patients within 5 years [59]. Following proximal arterial reconstruction, the 5-year patency averages 70% and may exceed life expectancy in patients with major co-morbidities; for distal reconstruction surgery, 5-year limb salvage rates approach 85% [59].

Strategies to prevent diabetic foot ulceration are based on a multidisciplinary approach to identifying, educating and treating high-risk patients; as discussed in Chapter 44, these measures can effectively reduce diabetes-related amputation rates. Many elderly patients have great difficulty in performing the most basic routine foot care [60], often because of poor vision and reduced mobility. In such cases, spouses and other carers must be involved to prevent and treat foot lesions. Education needs to be concise and repeated regularly; video presentations may also be helpful.

Coronary heart disease and arterial disease

Angina, MI, heart failure, stroke and intermittent claudication are substantially more common in elderly subjects with diabetes than in age-matched control groups without diabetes. Mortality is particularly high following MI, especially because of acute pump failure and later onset of left ventricular failure.

Many elderly patients with diabetes may present with atypical symptoms, including "silent ischemia" (which carries a worse prognosis than in the non-diabetic population); even MI may be painless and present non-specifically as a fall, breathlessness, malaise or hypotension.

Investigation and management of cardiovascular disease is covered in detail in Chapter 41.

Erectile dysfunction

Erectile dysfunction becomes more common in older adults and occurs earlier and more commonly in men with diabetes after 60 years of age; 55–95% of men with diabetes are affected, compared with 50% of their counterparts without diabetes [61]. It is often neglected, or attributed to a diminished quality of life or depressive illness. Vasculopathy, autonomic neuropathy, hormonal dysregulation, endothelial dysfunction and psychogenic factors have all been implicated, as have certain drugs (notably cimetidine, beta-blockers and spironolactone) and a high alcohol intake.

Investigation should generally proceed as for younger men, beginning with an interview with the patient and his partner, where appropriate. For many older patients, extensive testing is often avoided. Treatments include oral sildenafil (which achieved erections in 67% of elderly men in one study [61]), a vacuum tumescence device, misoprostol urethral pellets and self-administered intracorporeal injection of vasoactive drugs (e.g. prostaglandin E_1). The latter is relatively successful, but up to 50% of men eventually discontinue because of pain or loss of effect or interest [62].

Mental illness in elderly people with diabetes

Cognitive impairment and dementia

Diabetes and cognitive dysfunction are related and have evoked some interest over the last decade (Table 54.4). Impaired cognitive function has been demonstrated in elderly subjects with diabetes, but these studies were mostly not population-based, excluded subjects with dementia and generally used a large battery of tests to show the deficit [63]. Community-based studies in the UK (Melton Mowbray [64], Nottingham [43] and South Wales [65]) have shown worse cognitive function in elderly subjects with diabetes, using simple instruments such as the Folstein Mini-Mental State Examination (MMSE), Hodkinson's Abbreviated Mental Test (AMT), and the Clock Test. These are easily learned, bedside screening tests of mental status which test several cognitive domains such as memory, orientation, calculation, language and, in the case of the MMSE and Clock Tests, also test planning skills and visuospatial function.

Table 54.4 Background to relationship between diabetes and cognitive disorders. Reproduced from European Diabetes Working Party for Older People [92], with permission.

Professional and public concern about the impact of diabetes on cognition
Long-term influence of hyperglycemia and hypoglycemia on cerebral function unknown
Pathophysiologic mechanisms involved uncertain, but may involve both vascular, inflammatory and neuronal mechanisms
No current agreement on the most optimum method to detect or assess cognitive deficits in diabetes
Clinical relevance of the changes observed uncertain

Impaired glucose tolerance has also been shown to be associated with cognitive dysfunction [66]. It has been suggested that certain components of the metabolic syndrome (hyperglycemia, dyslipidemia, hypertension) may each contribute to memory disturbance in T2DM [67], and that hyperinsulinemia is associated with decreased cognitive function and dementia in women [68]. The Rochester study [69] has demonstrated that the overall risk of dementia is significantly increased for both men and women with T2DM; excess risk for Alzheimer disease achieved significance in men only. Poor glucose control may be associated with cognitive impairment, which recovers following improvement in glycemic control [70]. In other cases, vascular or "mixed" dementias are probably responsible.

Cognitive dysfunction in older subjects with diabetes has wide implications including increased hospitalization, less ability for self-care, reduced likelihood of specialist follow-up and increased risk of institutionalization [71]. Impaired cognitive function should be borne in mind when treating elderly subjects with diabetes, as it has implications for their safe treatment; it may cause difficulty with glycemic control because of erratic taking of diet and medication, including hypoglycemia when the patient forgets earlier administration of hypoglycemic medication and takes more.

Depression

Depression in diabetes is a serious co-morbidity associated with poor outcome and high health care expenditure (see Chapter 55). The presence of a major depressive disorder significantly increases the risk of diabetes [72], this association being apparently independent of age, gender or coexistent chronic disease [73]. Moreover, depression was the single most important indicator of subsequent death in a group of people with diabetes admitted into hospital [74]. Failure to recognize depression can be serious, as this is a long-term life-threatening disabling illness that can significantly damage quality of life. It is also associated with worsening diabetic control [75] and decreased treatment compliance (see Chapter 55) [76].

The relationship between diabetes and depression is complex and may result from the presence of a chronic medical condition in a susceptible individual. There are also complex neuroendocrine and cytokine changes in both conditions that may provide an explanation to link these two conditions (see Chapter 55).

Diabetes and depression share similar symptomatology (e.g. fatigue, irritability and sexual dysfunction). This may delay or confuse the diagnosis, although the commonly used diagnostic assessment scales are unlikely to be invalidated. Enquiries about well-being, sleep, appetite and weight loss should be part of the routine history, with a more comprehensive psychiatric evaluation if appropriate. A Geriatric Depression Scale (GDS) score of >5 can be regarded as indicative of probable depression [77]. While the GDS-15 may be the scale of choice for older people without cognitive impairment, it does not perform as well in those with dementia. Depression in diabetes can be treated successfully with pharmacotherapy, and/or psychologic therapy, but blood glucose levels should be monitored closely especially with pharmacotherapy. Goals for treating patients with depression and diabetes are twofold:

1 Remission or improvement of depressive symptoms; and
2 Improvement of poor glycemic control if present [78].

The preferred first-line treatment is a selective serotonin reuptake inhibitor (SSRI) or a serotonin norepinephrin reuptake inhibitor and psychotherapy. Treatment with SSRIs, such as fluoxetine, may improve symptoms and consequently metabolic control although close observation for side effects and changes to glycemic control are needed [79].

There have been reports of an increase in T2DM following treatment with antipsychotic medication which is often prescribed for older people with mental illness. This use of antipsychotics often goes beyond the license of these drugs but nevertheless has been recommended by groups such as the US Expert Consensus Panel for Using Antipsychotic Drugs in Older Patients to treat psychosis and anxiety [80]. It is estimated that as many as half of all repeat prescriptions for antipsychotics occur in people aged over 65 years [81]. Between 38–43% and 60–80% of all elderly patients living in nursing homes or old age psychiatry units, respectively, receive antipsychotics. Around 20% of people aged over 80 years are affected by dementia and 25–50% of these develop psychotic symptoms that require treatment with antipsychotics.

A systematic review of 17 studies examined the relationship between treatment with several antipsychotic agents and the risk of developing diabetes; olanzapine had an increased odds ratio but the risk for risperidone was small [82]. Data are still relatively limited in the elderly but suggest that the relative risk is less than for younger people with schizophrenia. Nevertheless, it seems prudent to undertake regular monitoring of weight, glucose and lipid profile [83].

Disability

Disability in elderly people with diabetes

Chronic diabetic complications often cause considerable disability in older people. For example, a community-based survey from Nottingham, UK [43], found significant disability in 80% of 98 elderly inner-city patients with diabetes (mean age 73 years); common problems included visual impairment (especially cataract) and previous amputation.

One in four of subjects with diabetes aged over 65 years in the Welsh Community Diabetes Study [65] required assistance with personal care, while older people with diabetes had significantly lower levels of well-being in most of the domains of the SF-36 health status questionnaire. Moreover, one in three subjects with diabetes had been hospitalized in the previous 12 months (twice the rate of those without diabetes), and subjects with diabetes had significantly increased levels of both physical and cognitive disability.

Mortality in elderly subjects with diabetes

People with diabetes die prematurely, mostly from cardiovascular disease. Early reports suggested that excess rates among people with diabetes fell progressively with age, especially in those aged 65 years and over. This has been confirmed largely by the Verona Study, in which the standardized mortality ratio declined from a range of 2–3.5 for middle-aged subjects with diabetes to 1.75 in those aged 65–74 years and 1.3 in patients older than 75 years; at all ages, the impact of diabetes on the standardized mortality ratio was more pronounced in women [84]. A recent systematic review of the relationship between mortality and age has suggested a higher incidence of premature death in older subjects with diabetes [85]. Cardiovascular mortality is primarily responsible, accounting for 42% of the overall mortality in the Verona Study. In the Melton Mowbray, UK, study [86], excess mortality rose substantially in subjects with diabetes aged over 65 years, and impaired glucose tolerance was associated with a relative risk of death of 1.7.

Age remains the strongest predictor of mortality; the contributions of classic cardiovascular risk factors are uncertain in older subjects with diabetes. A Finnish study [87] concluded that smoking, hypertension, low high-density lipoprotein (HDL) cholesterol and high total cholesterol did not affect overall mortality. In the Verona Study, long-term metabolic control was a better predictor of outcome, and subjects with more variable glycemic control (measured by the coefficient of variation of fasting plasma glucose) had lower survival rates, especially in those aged over 75 years [88].

Methodologic variations have prevented a consensus from being reached across different diabetic populations. Unequivocal evidence of increased mortality would argue for a more sustained commitment to diabetic health care provision; otherwise, future care strategies should focus on reducing morbidity and disability.

Clinical features of diabetes in the elderly

The presentation of diabetes in older people is varied and often insidious, which may delay diagnosis (Table 54.5) [1]. Many cases are detected by finding hyperglycemia during investigation for co-morbidities or acute illnesses. Some patients do not have classic features of either DKA or hyperosmolar hyperglycemic state, but present with a "mixed" disturbance of moderate hyperglycemia (blood glucose levels 15–25 mmol/L) and modest acidosis (arterial blood pH ≈7.2), but without marked dehydration or altered consciousness.

Recognition of the diverse, atypical and often cryptic symptom profile of hyperglycemia in older subjects can be helpful in making an early diagnosis (Table 54.5). Worryingly, however, even when hyperglycemia is recognized in hospital, about half of elderly subjects receive no further evaluation or treatment of diabetes [89].

Diagnosis of diabetes in the elderly

Diagnostic criteria are as in younger subjects. Mortality may be higher in those subjects diagnosed with diabetes on the basis of a 2-hour glucose value than with the new fasting criteria alone [90]. Moreover, isolated post-load hyperglycemia with normal fasting glucose (<7.0 mmol/L) is associated with increased fatal cardiovascular disease and heart disease in elderly women [91].

Some elderly patients have hyperglycemia secondary to acute illness, diabetogenic therapy or other stress-inducing disorders. This can be identified because the HbA_{1c} is normal, but the oral glucose tolerance test (OGTT) should be employed where doubt exists. Retesting following an acute illness may sometimes prevent a false diagnosis from being made. Particular difficulties may intrude: a true fasted sample may be difficult to obtain (and may be normal [90]), while an OGTT may be declined because it is time-consuming and inconvenient.

Table 54.5 Presentations of diabetes in older people.

Asymptomatic (coincidental finding)
Classic osmotic symptoms
Metabolic disturbances
- Diabetic ketoacidosis
- Hyperosmolar hyperglycemia syndrome
- "Mixed" metabolic disturbance

Spectrum of vague symptoms
- Depressed mood
- Apathy
- Mental confusion

Development of "geriatric" syndromes
- Falls or poor mobility: muscle weakness, poor vision, cognitive impairment
- Urinary incontinence
- Unexplained weight loss
- Memory disorder or cognitive impairment

Slow recovery from specific illnesses or increased vulnerability
- Impaired recovery from stroke
- Repeated infections
- Poor wound healing

Management of diabetes in the elderly

Prioritizing diabetic care

Ideally, elderly patients with diabetes should be treated as rigorously as younger subjects. Few studies have focused specifically on the elderly but a comprehensive set of evidenced-based clinical guidelines for T2DM in older people has been developed [92], and these provide a logical pathway for clinical decision-making in older people.

In older people, diabetes can cause much physical and mental impairment, and the individual's problems must be targeted effectively. Approaches such as the five-step evaluation shown in Table 54.6 [58] can help to shape the content of the care package.

Despite their numerous problems [65], about two-thirds of older people with diabetes are suitable for strategies to improve or optimize glycemic control (Figure 54.5). It is important to identify "frail" patients (i.e. those who are especially vulnerable to a wide range of diverse outcomes secondary to the effects of aging, chronic diabetic complications, physical and cognitive decline, and the presence of other medical co-morbidities). The Frailty Model of Diabetes [58] can assist clinical decision-making by defining factors (e.g. recurrent hypoglycemia, cardiac disease and reduced recovery from metabolic decompensation), which may herald disability and often directly threaten independence, yet may have preventable or reversible components. In clinical practice, the presence of a mobility disorder or severe restriction of activities of daily living, or the presence of several co-morbid-

Table 54.6 Prioritizing diabetes care in older adults: a five-step approach.

1. Functional assessment, including cognitive testing and screening for depression
2. Vascular risk assessment, especially vascular prophylaxis and lifestyle modification
3. Metabolic targeting ("single disease" or "frailty" models)
4. Devise appropriate interventions for diabetes-related disabilities
5. Assess suitability for self-care or carer assistance

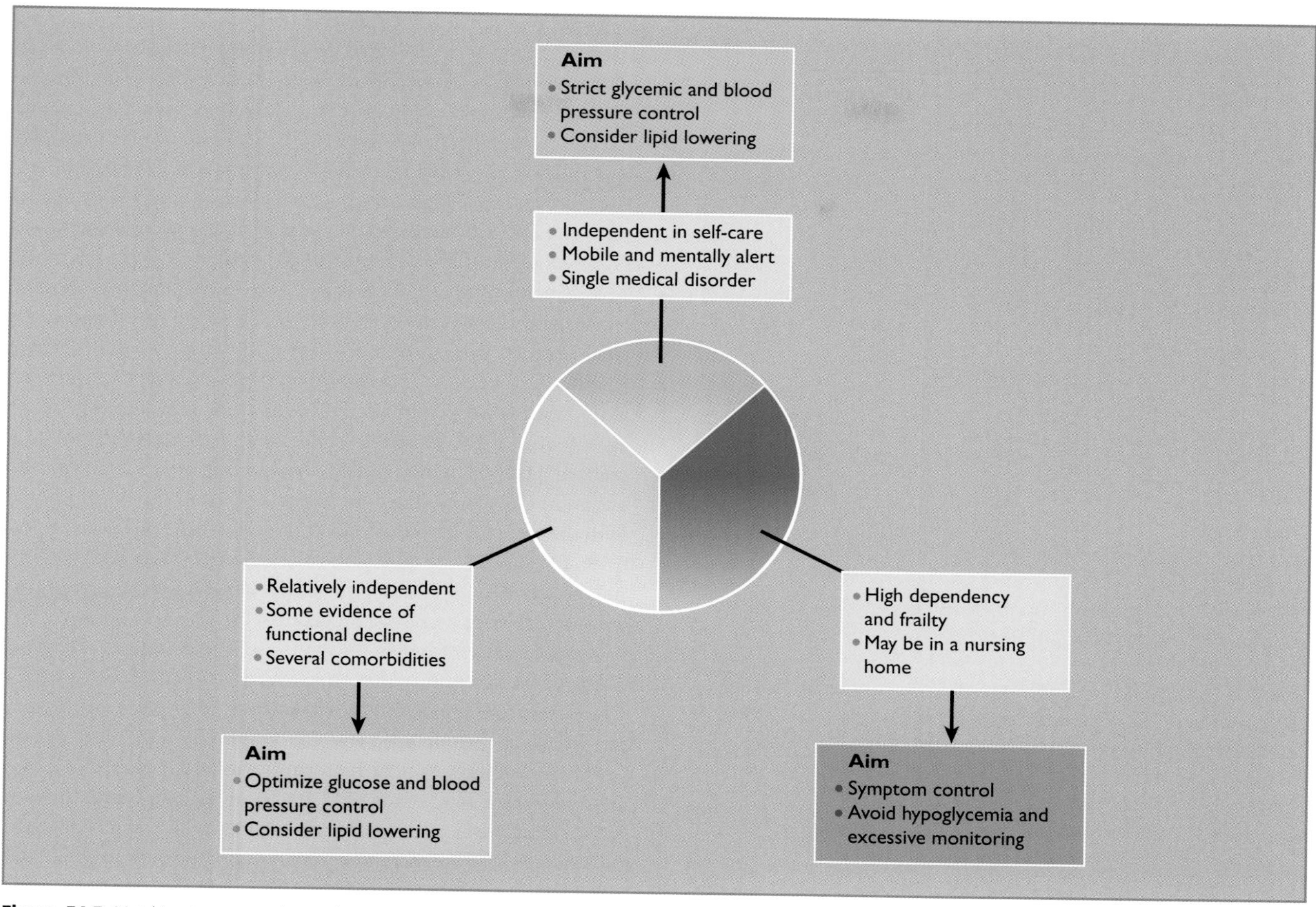

Figure 54.5 Matching treatment aims to functional assessments in elderly people with diabetes.

ities, and/or advanced age (>80 years) will increase the risk of becoming confined to a chair or bed by two- to threefold over 2 years [93].

Treatment targets for older people with diabetes

Table 54.7 lists metabolic and cardiovascular treatment targets appropriate for "strict" and "optimal" therapy, using evidence derived from large-scale clinical trials (referenced in full in Sinclair [58]); caveats about applying these data to the elderly are acknowledged comprehensively in the European Diabetes Working Party for Older People [92]. The European Guidelines have provided a series of glycemic targets to guide treatment (see box).

Because of the increased risk of hypoglycemia, a more realistic target HbA_{1c} in frailer subjects is often <64 mmol/mol (8.0%), which will still reduce hyperglycemic malaise and may decrease the risk of some vascular complications. There are conflicting data about the relationship between advancing age and HbA_{1c}: in a French study of telecom workers aged 18–80 years, HbA_{1c} rose with age but then fell in males [94]. In a smaller study of 93 subjects, however, advancing age was not related to glycated hemoglobin or fasting plasma glucose [95]. This is an area requiring further study.

European guidelines for the management of glycemic control in older people with diabetes

For older patients with T2DM, with single system involvement (free of other major co-morbidities), a target HbA_{1c} (DCCT aligned) range of 7.0–7.5%* should be aimed for. Evidence level 1+; Grade of recommendation A. *The precise target agreed will depend on existing cardiovascular risk, presence of microvascular complications and ability of the individual to self-manage*

For older patients with T2DM, with single system involvement (free of other major co-morbidities), a fasting glucose range of 6.5–7.5 mmol/L can be regarded as indicating good control. Evidence level 2++; Grade of recommendation B

*IFCC HbA_{1c} 53–58 mmol/mol

As well as glycemic and blood pressure control, lipid-lowering therapy should be considered for subjects up to the age of 80 years. Thromboembolic prophylaxis (e.g. with aspirin [75 mg/

Table 54.7 Treatment targets for elderly patients with diabetes.

Blood glucose levels
No specific studies in older people with diabetes
UKPDS: HbA_{1c} <53 mmol/mol (7%); fasting blood glucose <7 mmol/L

Blood pressure
UKPDS: ≤140/80 mmHg (not based on older subjects)
HOT Study: diastolic lowering to ≤83 mmHg
SHEP Study: systolic <150 mmHg
Syst-Eur study: systolic BP <160 mmHg

Blood lipid levels
No specific studies in older people with diabetes
LIPID, CARE, 4S, VA-HIT studies
- Total cholesterol <5 mmol/L
- High density lipoprotein (HDL) cholesterol >1.0 mmol/L
- Triglycerides <2.0 mmol/L

Aspirin use
ATS study: 75–325 mg/day reduced major cardiovascular events in high-risk patients by 25%
HOT study: 75 mg/day reduced major cardiovascular events by 15% and myocardial infarction by 36%

Key to clinical trials: ATS, Antiplatelet Trialists' Study; CARE, Cholesterol and Recurrent Events Study; HOT, Hypertension Optimal Treatment study; LIPID, Long-term Intervention with Pravastatin in Ischemic Disease; 4S, Swedish Simvastatin Survival Study; SHEP, Systolic Hypertension in the Elderly Program (US); Syst-Eur, Systolic Hypertension in Europe Trial; UKPDS, UK Prospective Diabetes Study; VA-HIT, Veterans Affairs High-Density Lipoprotein Cholesterol Intervention Trial.

day] or clopidogrel [75 mg/day] [96] if aspirin is not tolerated) is appropriate in older subjects with diabetes and macrovascular disease or risk factors such as hypertension, obesity, albuminuria or cigarette smoking. Atrial fibrillation is more common in older subjects with diabetes, but there is no specific evidence to support full warfarin anticoagulation in this advanced age group.

Evaluation of cardiovascular risk

Evaluation of cardiovascular risk provides prognostic information and helps to target therapy for the primary and secondary prevention of coronary heart disease (CHD). The available methods estimate risk (e.g. 10–20%) over a 5- or 10-year period, and include the New Zealand tables [97] and data from the Framingham [98] and Seven European Countries studies [99]; all are limited by the lack of data from subjects over 74 years of age.

Reducing triglyceride levels may also help to reduce overall cardiovascular risk in older subjects. In a New Zealand study, subjects with T2DM aged over 70 years had an increased mortality if they were hyperlipidemic [100], while the Veterans Affairs High-Density Lipoprotein Cholesterol Intervention Trial (VA-HIT) study showed that treatment with gemfibrozil lowered cardiovascular mortality by over 20%; three-quarters of the latter subjects were aged 60–74 years, and 25% had diabetes [101].

A more recent study provides convincing evidence of benefit irrespective of age: the Heart Protection Study [102] included adults with diabetes aged 40–80 years treated with 40 mg simvastatin or placebo over a 5-year period. Treatment led to an average fall in low density lipoprotein (LDL) cholesterol of 1.0 mmol/L and resulted in a highly significant reduction of 27% in the incidence of first non-fatal MI or coronary death, and a 25% reduction in first non-fatal or fatal stroke. Evidence of benefit was observed as early as 12 months of treatment.

A relatively recent clinical trial comparing different antihypertensive regimens in the prevention of CHD and other cardiovascular events was terminated early because of the obvious significant benefits on mortality being achieved with an amlodipine-based regimen. This study involved subjects up to age 79 years, and in those with T2DM benefits were similarly realized [103]. These included the incidence of the composite endpoint (total cardiovascular events and procedures) compared with the atenolol-based regimen (hazard ratio 0.86; 95% CI 0.76–0.98; $P = 0.026$). In addition, fatal and non-fatal strokes were reduced by 25% ($P = 0.017$), PVD by 48% ($P = 0.004$) and non-coronary revascularization procedures by 57% ($P < 0.001$).

Angiotensin-converting enzyme (ACE) inhibitors can also improve cardiovascular outcome. The Micro-HOPE study investigated the effects of ramipril on macrovascular and microvascular disease in people aged over 55 years over a 4.5-year period [104]. All subjects were at high cardiovascular risk because of a previous event (e.g. stroke, MI, PVD) or diabetes together with another cardiovascular risk factor such as hypertension or dyslipidemia. Primary endpoints (stroke, or fatal or non-fatal MI) were significantly reduced from 20% to 15%, while all-cause mortality fell by 24%.

Several other recent studies have looked at the benefits of tighter glucose regulation in a wide range of subjects (including older subjects) with T2DM [105–107]. Excess cardiovascular mortality was demonstrated in the Action to Control Cardiovascular Risk in Diabetes (ACCORD) in the intensive group where the average HbA_{1c} was 46 mmol/mol (6.4%) [105], whereas in the Action in Diabetes and Vascular Disease: Preterax and Diamicron MR Controlled Evaluation (ADVANCE) study [106] excess mortality was not demonstrated. Neither study indicated any benefit in reducing cardiovascular outcomes despite similar reductions in HbA_{1c} in the intensive groups. A further study in American veterans [107] with T2DM (average HbA_{1c}: 52 mmol/mol [6.9%] in the intensive group) also failed to show benefit at a level of HbA_{1c} in the range usually aimed for by most clinicians. The rates of hypoglycemia were significantly more common in the intensive groups in all studies.

For older people, these results pose several dilemmas in management: first, they do not answer the important clinical question of how to reduce cardiovascular risk, and, secondly, what is the optimal level to aim for which substantially reduces microvascular risk yet avoids severe hypoglycemia. For now we must continue to aim for realistic targets (similar to younger adults) for all those older patients who do not have marked evi-

Table 54.8 Principal aims in managing older people with diabetes.

Medical
Freedom from hyperglycemic symptoms
Prevent undesirable weight loss
Avoid hypoglycemia and other adverse drug reactions
Screen for and prevent vascular complications
Detect cognitive impairment and depression at an early stage
Achieve a normal life expectancy for patients where possible
Patient-orientated
Maintain general well-being and good quality of life
Acquire skills and knowledge to adapt to lifestyle changes
Encourage diabetes self-care

Table 54.9 Care plan for initial management of diabetes in an elderly person.

1	Establish realistic glycemic and blood pressure targets
2	Provide an estimate of cardiovascular risk over 5 years
3	Ensure consensus with patient, spouse or family, GP, informal carer, community nurse or hospital specialist
4	Define the frequency and nature of diabetes follow-up
5	Organize glycemic monitoring by patient or carer
6	Refer to social or community services as necessary
7	Provide advice on stopping smoking, increasing exercise and alcohol intake

dence of frailty. Intensified treatment in this latter category is not justified at present on the basis of these recent intervention studies.

The principal aims of managing diabetes in older adults are listed in Table 54.8. The priority of each may change with time, the development of complications or the need for external help. An initial diabetes care plan should be drawn up for the individual patient (Table 54.9). The guidelines of the International Diabetes Federation (IDF) for managing T2DM [108] appear equally applicable to older subjects although more detailed specialist guidance is now available [92]. Patients with T1DM are managed as in younger individuals.

Lifestyle modification

Dietary and lifestyle advice are given as for middle-aged subjects, including an exercise program if possible. These measures may be sufficient for subjects with minimal symptoms, whose initial random glucose levels lie between 8 and 17 mmol/L. If metabolic targets are not reached by 6–8 weeks, oral therapy is required [109].

Active management of other cardiovascular risk factors, especially hypertension and dyslipidemia, is necessary from the outset (Table 54.7).

Oral hypoglycemic agents

Sulfonylureas

Sulfonylureas are often used initially in elderly people with diabetes failing on diet, because they are generally well tolerated. Their main hazard is hypoglycemia. This is a particular problem with glibenclamide, the use of which has been associated with more fatalities than other sulfonylureas, including chlorpropamide; it must be strictly avoided in the elderly. Glipizide can cause prolonged hypoglycemia in older people and has been linked to hypoglycemic deaths in elderly Swedish subjects [34]. Gliclazide has a relatively low risk of hypoglycemia; it may be less likely to cause weight gain, the other common problem with sulfonylureas, and it is undoubtedly safer than glibenclamide [33]. A modified-release once-daily preparation of gliclazide is now available. Tolbutamide carries the lowest risk of hypoglycemia and can be used in those with mild renal impairment (serum creatinine <150 µmol/L (estimated glomerular filtration rate [eGFR] <42 mL/min/1.73 m^2 based on a 75-year-old non-black male) [110]. If compliance is uncertain, glimepiride may be useful, because the effective daily dose for all patients is one tablet before breakfast; however, there are no good comparisons between this and gliclazide.

With all sulfonylureas, the maximal glucose-lowering effect is about 4–5 mmol/L. Patients with very high glucose levels will not therefore achieve adequate glycemic control.

Metformin

Metformin is predictable and safe if it is used correctly and its contraindications are respected: these include renal impairment (serum creatinine >120 µmol/L, eGFR <54 mL/min/1.73 m^2 based on a 75-year-old non-black male), hepatic or cardiac failure, critical limb ischemia and severe acute illness. Accordingly, some 40–50% of older subjects are ineligible for the drug.

Particular advantages of metformin are that it does not cause hypoglycemia or weight gain on its own, and is inexpensive. Its glucose-lowering effect is similar to sulfonylureas, including in the elderly. The usual daily dose required is approximately 1.7 g, and it is as effective in the lean as in the overweight. Metformin was the only antidiabetic drug shown to reduce macrovascular events in the UKPDS, and all-cause mortality and combined diabetes-related endpoints were significantly lower with metformin than with insulin or sulfonylurea in obese subjects [111].

Acarbose

Acarbose has a weak hypoglycemic effect, including in elderly subjects. Slow introduction of the drug (e.g. 25 mg with the first mouthful of one meal per day initially) can help to diminish gastrointestinal side effects (bloating and flatulence) which often limit its use. Its main contraindications are inflammatory bowel disease and subacute obstruction. Acarbose can be combined with metformin, sulfonylureas or insulin.

Thiazolidinediones

Thiazolidinediones (TZDs) reduce insulin resistance by activating the peroxisome proliferator activated receptor γ (PPARγ). They lower glucose by 3–4 mmol/L and, as monotherapy, they reduce HbA_{1c} by 5–15 mmol/mol (0.5–1.4%). Although they do not cause hypoglycemia, their main problems are mild edema, dilutional anemia (in <5% of subjects) and weight gain, with a twofold increased risk of heart failure for which they are contraindicated. TZDs can be given in combination with metformin, sulfonylureas and glinides, and pioglitazone can be given with insulin in the UK (see Chapter 29). Several meta-analyses suggest that rosiglitazone treatment may be associated with an increased risk of MI although this has not been demonstrated for pioglitazone. Both TZDs are associated with an increased fracture risk, mainly in women, and this is an additional factor to consider when screening older people with osteoporosis for treatment with a TZD. They are safe in mild to moderate renal impairment; the liver damage associated with troglitazone (now withdrawn) does not appear to extend to rosiglitazone or pioglitazone, but frequent monitoring of liver function is required, especially during the first 12 months of treatment; this is a drawback for many older subjects.

Rosiglitazone and pioglitazone have comparable hypoglycemic effects and the latter shows a modest improvement in lipid profile; up to 6–8 weeks may elapse before the full beneficial actions are seen. These drugs can be given once daily, which is helpful for older patients.

Non-sulfonylurea insulin secretagogues (glinides)

Repaglinide is a benzoic acid derivative of the meglitinide class which predominantly lowers post-prandial hyperglycemia. It has a rapid onset of action and a lower risk of hypoglycemia than the sulfonylureas, and achieves better post-prandial glucose profiles. Repaglinide is predominantly metabolized in the liver to inactive metabolites and is safe in mild to moderate renal impairment. Tablets can be missed if meals are omitted, and it may be effectively combined with metformin and with thiazolidinediones (where license permits). Initially, 0.5 mg can be given with each meal (1 mg for subjects transferring from other oral agents), increasing to 4 mg with each meal.

Nateglinide is a recent meglitinide which has a faster and shorter duration of insulin secretory activity than repaglinide but is less effective as monotherapy or in combination than rapaglinide.

Insulin

Recent improvements in the organization of care between hospital and primary care, and the expanding roles of diabetes specialist nurses and general practice nurses, have made it easier and safer to use insulin in the treatment of older people with diabetes [112]. The main indications in the elderly are T1DM or T2DM where metabolic targets have not been achieved with diet, exercise and oral agents. It should also be used following acute MI (see Chapter 41), acute stroke, hyperglycemic coma and major surgery (see Chapter 32).

The main disadvantage of insulin is hypoglycemia, although the UKPDS found that fewer than 2% of subjects treated with insulin experienced a major hypoglycemic episode. Reported benefits include improvements in well-being and possibly quality of life [113–115] and in cognitive function [70], partly following improved glycemic control; however, others have found lower treatment satisfaction in insulin-treated patients [116].

Some guidelines for insulin treatment in the elderly are suggested in Table 54.10. Rapidly acting insulin analogs such as insulin lispro or insulin aspart may cause less hypoglycemia and weight gain, and can be given after eating where timing may be

Table 54.10 General guidelines for insulin treatment in older people.

	Indications	Advantages	Disadvantages
Once-daily insulin	Frail subjects Very old (>80 years) Symptomatic control	Single injection Can be given by carer or district nurse	Control usually poor Hypoglycemia common
Twice-daily insulin	Preferred if aiming for reasonable glycemic control Suitable for T1DM	Low risk of hypoglycemia Easily managed by most older people with diabetes	Normoglycemia difficult to achieve Fixed meal times reduce flexibility Expensive
Basal/bolus insulin	Well-motivated individuals For acute illness in hospital	Enables tight control Can reduce microvascular complications Flexible meal times	Frequent monitoring required to avoid hypoglycemia
Insulin plus oral agents	If glycemic control is unsatisfactory with oral agents alone To limit weight gain in obese subjects	Limits weight gain by reducing total daily insulin Increased flexibility	May delay conversion to insulin in thin or type 1 patients

unpredictable (e.g. because of memory disorder). In patients with T1DM, premixed insulins given twice daily may achieve reasonable glycemic control, although nocturnal hypoglycemia may be troublesome because of the longer-acting component of the pre-supper dose (see Chapter 27).

In older patients with T2DM, a twice-daily regimen of human isophane insulin can be used, adding short-acting insulin to cover meals if necessary. The newly introduced long-acting insulin analogs (e.g. insulin glargine and insulin detemir) have more reproducible pharmacokinetics and a "peakless" action profile, and may prove safer in older subjects. Once-daily insulin regimens alone are now little used, except where glycemic control is not a priority or injections are impracticable.

Insulin can usefully be combined with an oral agent in patients failing to be controlled by diet and oral agents. A suitable regimen is a night-time dose of intermediate-acting insulin (e.g. isophane) together with metformin, which causes less weight gain and hypoglycemia and better glycemic control than twice-daily insulin or combinations of glibenclamide with insulin or metformin [117]. The use of insulin in the elderly varies enormously even in developed countries. For frail subjects including those within care-home settings, complex regimens should be avoided so the use of longer-acting insulin analogs during the day often combined with oral agents is a feasible alternative.

Low-vision aids are available to help to inject insulin, and some insulin pens have audible clicks for counting doses.

Diabetic patients in care homes

In many developed countries the numbers of care-home residents are increasing and the prevalence of diabetes in this setting will inevitably increase. Recent surveys suggest that 7–27% of care-home residents in the UK and USA have diabetes. The wide range is partly because of differences in the diagnostic criteria used [17,118–120]; the prevalence of IGT may be as high as 30% [17]. People with diabetes in care homes should receive care commensurate with their health and social needs [121]. The best possible quality of life and well-being should be maintained, without unnecessary or inappropriate interventions, while helping residents to manage their own diabetes wherever feasible and worthwhile.

Metabolic control should reduce both hyperglycemic lethargy and hypoglycemia, with a well-balanced dietetic plan that prevents weight loss and maintains nutritional well-being. Foot care and vision require screening and preventive measures to maintain mobility and prevent falls and unnecessary hospital admissions.

At present, residents with diabetes in care homes appear to be generally vulnerable and neglected, with high prevalences of macrovascular complications and infections (especially skin and urinary tract), frequent hospitalization and much physical and cognitive disability. Known deficiencies of diabetes care include lack of individual management care plans and dietary supervision, infrequent review by specialist nurses, doctors and ophthalmologists, and poor knowledge and training for care staff [120,121].

Table 54.11 Some recommendations for improving diabetes management in care homes.

Screen on admission for diabetes and regularly thereafter
Policies must include strategies to minimize hospital admission, metabolic decompensation, pressure-sore development, pain, diabetes-related complications, infections and weight loss
All residents with diabetes must have an annual review and access to specialist services
Care-home diabetes policies must be developed nationally, locally and at the level of the resident with diabetes
Research based on interventional strategies is needed

Various strategies can improve diabetes care in this setting (Table 54.11) [117,122,123]. The impact of these initiatives is being followed on outcomes including well-being, metabolic control, access to regular review, rates of hospitalization and diabetic complications such as amputation and visual loss. A UK Task and Finish Group of Diabetes UK is revising previous guidelines and will be publishing new guidance at the beginning of 2010.

Modern diabetes care for older people

Structured diabetes care is particularly important for older people who are often neglected at present [124]; with the current shift in health care from hospitals to the community, GPs will have an increasingly important role [125,126]. This will require considerable motivation by the GP, effective screening for diabetes program and close liaison with diabetes specialist nurses (see Chapter 56). A shared-care approach, with GPs working in partnership with hospital-based diabetic and surgical specialists and based around agreed clinical protocols, is particularly valuable for older people.

A modern geriatric diabetes service (Figure 54.6) is based on a "multidimensional intervention" model [58]. This emphasizes the importance of early intervention in diabetic complications and of establishing rehabilitation programs for patients disabled by various complications such as amputation, peripheral neuropathy, immobility, falls, stroke and cognitive change. "Critical event monitoring" denotes monitoring periods of ill-health or social care need where patient vulnerability is high and opportunity for intervention is paramount (e.g. admission to hospital, amputation or stroke).

Health care must be cost-effective, which presents a difficult challenge for diabetes, because of its high prevalence, long duration of impact and wide spectrum of complications and emotional and psychologic sequelae; in older subjects, the challenge is even more complex because of the many other confounding factors.

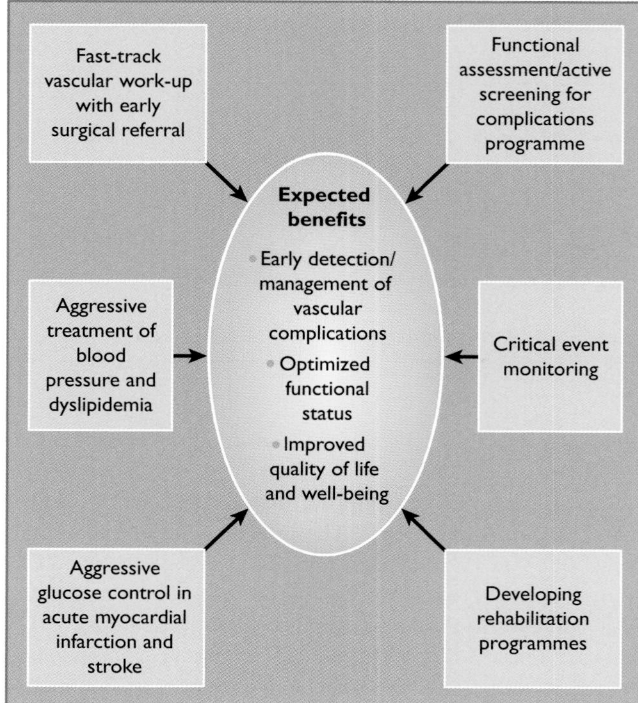

Figure 54.6 Components of a modern strategy for managing diabetes in the elderly.

Recent studies [127–129] have suggested that aggressive treatment of diabetes in older individuals is not warranted because of their reduced life expectancy; however, implementing the strategies outlined above seems likely to reduce acute hospitalization, outpatient costs and long-term disability. Only well-organized prospective clinical trials will be able to determine how best to manage diabetes in older people.

References

1 Sinclair AJ. Issues in the initial management of type 2 diabetes. In: Sinclair AJ, Finucane P, eds. *Diabetes in Old Age*, 2nd edn. Chichester: Wiley, 2001: 155–164.

2 Blaum CS. Descriptive epidemiology of diabetes. In: Munsshi MN, Lipsitz LA, eds. *Geriatric Diabetes*. New York: Informa Healthcare, 2007: 1–10.

3 Damsgaard EM, Froland A, Holm A. Ambulatory medical care for elderly diabetics: the Fredericia survey of diabetic and fasting hyperglycemic subjects aged 60–74 years. *Diabet Med* 1987; **4**:534–538.

4 Damsgaard EM, Froland A, Green A. Use of hospital services by elderly diabetics: the Frederica Study of diabetic and fasting hyperglycemic patients aged 60–74 years. *Diabet Med* 1987; **4**:317–322.

5 Krop JS, Shaffer TJ, Powe NR, Saudek CD, Anderson GF. Patterns of expenditures and use of services among older adults with diabetes. *Diabetes Care* 1998; **21**:747–751.

6 Hudson CN, Lazarus J, Peters J, Beck P, Sinclair AJ. An audit of diabetic care in three district general hospitals in Cardiff. *Pract Diabetes Int* 1995; **13**:29–32.

7 Harrower ADB. Prevalence of elderly patients in a hospital diabetic population. *Br J Clin Pract* 1980; **34**:131–133.

8 Williams DRR. Hospital admissions of diabetic patients: information from hospital activity analysis. *Diabet Med* 1985; **2**:2–32.

9 Beck-Nielsen H; European Group for the study of Insulin Resistance (EGIR). General characteristics of the insulin resistance syndrome. *Drugs* 1999; **1**:7–10.

10 Kamel HK, Morley JE. Metabolic risk factors and their treatment. In: Sinclair AJ, Finucane P, eds. *Diabetes in Old Age*. Chichester: Wiley, 2001: 187–198.

11 Alberti KGMM, Zimmet P, Shaw J. The metabolic syndrome: a new worldwide definition. *Lancet* 2005; **366**:1059–1069.

12 Sinclair AJ. Diabetes in the elderly: a perspective from the United Kingdom. *Clin Geriatr Med* 1999; **15**:225–237.

13 Hendra TJ, Sinclair AJ. Improving the care of elderly diabetic patients: the final report of the St Vincent Joint Task Force for Diabetes. *Age Ageing* 1997; **26**:3–6.

14 Harris MI, Flegal KM, Cowie CC, Eberhardt MS, Goldstein DE, Little RR, *et al.* Prevalence of diabetes, impaired fasting glucose, and impaired glucose tolerance in US adults: the Third National Health and Nutrition Examination Survey, 1988–94. *Diabetes Care* 1998; **21**:518–524.

15 Croxson SCM, Burden AC, Bodington M, Botha JL. The prevalence of diabetes in elderly people. *Diabet Med* 1991; **8**:28–31.

16 Sinclair AJ, Croxson SCM. Diabetes mellitus in the older adult. In: Tallis R, Fillit H, Brocklehurst JC, eds. *Brocklehurst's Textbook of Geriatric Medicine and Gerontology*, 5th edn. Edinburgh: Churchill Livingstone, 1998: 1051–1072.

17 Sinclair AJ, Gadsby R, Penfold S, Croxson SCM, Bayer AJ. Prevalence of diabetes in care home residents. *Diabetes Care* 2001; **24**:1066–1068.

18 Spence JW. Some observations on sugar tolerance with special reference to variations found at different ages. *Q J Med* 1921; **14**:314–326.

19 Jackson RA. Mechanisms of age-related glucose intolerance. *Diabetes Care* 1990; **13**(Suppl. 2):9–19.

20 Muller DC, Elahi D, Tobin JD, Andres R. The effect of age on insulin resistance and secretion: a review. *Semin Nephrol* 1996; **16**:289–298.

21 Meneilly GS, Hards L, Tessier D, Elliott T, Tildesley H. NIDDM in the elderly. *Diabetes Care* 1996; **19**:1320–1375.

22 Meneilly GS, Elahi D, Minaker KL, Sclater AL, Rowe JW. Impairment of noninsulin-mediated glucose disposal in the elderly. *J Clin Endocrinol Metab* 1989; **63**:566–571.

23 Best JD, Kahn SE, Ader M, Watanabe RM, Ni TC, Bergman RN. Role of glucose effectiveness in the determination of glucose tolerance. *Diabetes Care* 1996; **19**:1018–1030.

24 Basu A, Close CF, Jenkins D, Krentz AJ, Nattrass M, Wright AD. Persisting mortality in diabetic ketoacidosis. *Diabet Med* 1993; **10**:282–284.

25 Hamblin PS, Topliss DJ, Chosich N, Lording DW, Stockigt JR. Deaths associated with diabetic ketoacidosis and hyperosmolar coma. *Med J Aust* 1989; **151**:439–444.

26 Small M, Alzaid A, MacCuish AC. Diabetic hyper-osmolar non-ketotic decompensation. *Q J Med* 1988; **66**:251–257.

27 Wachtel TJ, Tetu-Mouradjian LM, Goldman DL, Ellis SE, O'Sullivan PS. Hyper-osmolarity and acidosis in diabetes mellitus: a three-year experience in Rhode Island. *J Gen Intern Med* 1991; **6**:495–502.

28 Croxson SCM. Metabolic decompensation. In: Sinclair AJ, Finucane P, eds. *Diabetes in Old Age*, 2nd edn. Chichester: Wiley, 2001: 53–66.

29 Brierley FJ, Broughton DL, James OFW, *et al.* Awareness of hypoglycemia in the elderly. *Age Ageing* 1993; **22**:9–10.

30 Shorr RI, Ray WA, Daugherty JR, Griffin MR. Incidence and risk factors for serious hypoglycemia in older persons using insulin or sulphonylureas. *Arch Intern Med* 1997; **157**:1681–1686.

31 Meneilly GS, Cheung E, Tuokko H. Counter-regulatory hormone responses to hypoglycemia in the elderly patient with diabetes. *Diabetes* 1994; **43**:403–410.

32 Thomson FJ, Masson EA, Leeming JT, Boulton AJ. Lack of knowledge of symptoms of hypoglycemia by elderly diabetic patients. *Age Ageing* 1991; **20**:404–406.

33 Tessier D, Dawson K, Tetrault JP, Bravo G, Meneilly GS. Glibenclamide vs gliclazide in type 2 diabetes of the elderly. *Diabet Med* 1994; **11**:974–980.

34 Asplund K, Wiholm BE, Lundman B. Severe hypoglycemia during treatment with glipizide. *Diabet Med* 1991; **8**:726–731.

35 Asplund K, Wiholm BE, Lundman B. Glibenclamide-associated hypoglycemia; a report on 57 cases. *Diabetologia* 1983; **24**:412–417.

36 Cohen DL, Neil HAW, Thorogood M, Mann JI. A population-based study of the incidence of complications associated with type 2 diabetes in the elderly. *Diabet Med* 1991; **8**:928–933.

37 Kannel WB, McGee DL. Diabetes and cardiovascular disease: the Framingham Study. *JAMA* 1979; **241**:2035–2038.

38 Naliboff BD, Rosenthal M. Effects of age on complications in adult onset diabetes. *J Am Geriatr Soc* 1989; **37**:838–842.

39 Ballard DJ, Humphrey LL, Melton LJ 3rd, Frohnert PP, Chu PC, O'Fallon WM, *et al.* Epidemiology of persistent proteinuria in type II diabetes mellitus: population based study in Rochester. *Minnesota Diabetes* 1988; **37**:405–412.

40 Knuiman MW, Welborn TA, McCann VJ, Stanton KG, Constable IJ. Prevalence of diabetic complications in relation to risk factors. *Diabetes* 1986; **35**:1332–1339.

41 Grey RHB, Burns-Cox CJ, Hughes A. Blind and partial sight registration in Avon. *Br J Ophthalmol* 1989; **73**:88–94.

42 Butcher A, Dodson P. Visual loss. In: Sinclair AJ, Finucane P, eds. *Diabetes in Old Age*, 2nd edn. Chichester: Wiley, 2001: 119–132.

43 Dornan TL, Peck GM, Dow JDC, Tattersall RB. A community survey of diabetes in the elderly, 1992. *Diabet Med* 1998; **9**:860–865.

44 Sinclair AJ, Bayer AJ, Girling AJ, Woodhouse KW. Older adults, diabetes mellitus and visual acuity: a community-based case–control study. *Age Ageing* 2000; **29**:335–339.

45 Diabetes Control and Complications Trial Research Group. The effect of intensive treatment of diabetes on the development and progression of long-term complications in insulin-dependent diabetes mellitus. *N Engl J Med* 1993; **329**:977–986.

46 UK Prospective Diabetes Study (UKPDS) Group. Intensive blood-glucose control with sulphonylureas or insulin compared with conventional treatment and risk of complications in patients with type II diabetes. *Lancet* 1998; **352**:837–853.

47 UK Prospective Diabetes Study (UKPDS) Group. Tight blood pressure control and risk of macrovascular and microvascular complications in type II diabetes. *Br Med J* 1998; **317**:703–713.

48 Diabetic Retinopathy Research Group. Photocoagulation treatment of proliferative diabetic retinopathy: the second report of Diabetic Retinopathy Study findings. *Ophthalmology* 1978; **85**:82–106.

49 ETDRS (Early Treatment Diabetic Retinopathy Study) Research Group. Treatment techniques and clinical guidelines for photocoagulation of diabetic macular oedema. *Ophthalmology* 1987; **94**:761–764.

50 British Multicentre Study Group. Photocoagulation for diabetic maculopathy. *Diabetes* 1983; **32**:1010–1016.

51 Young MJ, Boulton AJM. The diabetic foot. In: Sinclair AJ, Finucane P, eds. *Diabetes in Old Age*, 2nd edn. Chichester: Wiley, 2001: 67–88.

52 Van Houtum WH, Lavery LA, Harkless LB. The costs of diabetes-related lower extremity amputations in the Netherlands, 1985. *Diabet Med* 1995; **12**:777–781.

53 Palumbo PJ, Melton LJ. Peripheral vascular disease and diabetes. In: National Institutes of Health, eds. *Diabetes in America: Diabetes Data*. 1985; **15**:1–21. Washington, DC: US Government Printing Office, 1985 (NIH publication no. 85–1468).

54 Larsson J, Apelqvist J, Agardh DD, Stenstrom A. Decreasing incidence of major amputation in diabetic patients: a consequence of a multidisciplinary footcare team approach? *Diabet Med* 1995; **12**:770–776.

55 Walters DP, Gatling W, Mullee MA, Hill RD. The prevalence of diabetic distal sensory neuropathy in an English Community. *Diabet Med* 1992; **9**:349–53.

56 Cavanagh PR, Simoneau GG, Ulbrecht JS. Ulceration, unsteadiness and uncertainty: the biomechanical consequences of diabetes mellitus. *J Biomech* 1993; **26**(Suppl. 1):23–40.

57 Flynn FD, Boolell M, Tooke J, Watkins PJ. The effect of insulin infusion on capillary blood flow in the diabetic neuropathic foot. *Diabet Med* 1992; **9**:630–634.

58 Sinclair AJ. Diabetes in old age: changing concepts in the secondary care arena. *J R Coll Physicians Lond* 2000; **34**:240–244.

59 Sigurdsson HH, Macaulay EM, McHardy KC, Cooper GG. Long-term outcome of infra-inguinal bypass for limb salvage: are we giving diabetic patients a fair deal? *Pract Diabetes Int* 1999; **16**:204–206.

60 Thomson FJ, Masson EA. Can elderly diabetic patients cooperate with routine foot care? *Age Ageing* 1992; **21**:333–337.

61 Vinik A, Richardson D. Erectile dysfunction. In: Sinclair AJ, Finucane P, eds. *Diabetes in Old Age*, 2nd edn. Chichester: Wiley, 2001: 89–102.

62 Lakin MM, Montague DK, VanderBrug-Medendorp S, Tesar L, Schover LR. Intravenous injection therapy: analysis of results and complications. *J Urol* 1990; **143**:1138–1141.

63 Strachan MWJ, Deary IJ, Ewing FME, Frier BM. Is type 2 (non-insulin-dependent) diabetes mellitus associated with an increased risk of cognitive dysfunction? *Diabetes Care* 1997; **20**:438–445.

64 Croxson S, Jagger C. Diabetes and cognitive impairment: a community based study of elderly subjects. *Age Ageing* 1995; **24**:421–424.

65 Sinclair AJ, Bayer AJ. *All Wales Research in Elderly (AWARE) Diabetes Study*. Department of Health Report 121/3040. London: UK Government.

66 Vanhanen M, Koivisto K, Kuusisto J, Mykkänen L, Helkala EL, Hänninen T, *et al.* Cognitive function in an elderly population with persistent impaired glucose tolerance. *Diabetes Care* 1998; **21**:398–402.

67 Kumari M, Brunner E, Fuhrer R. Minireview: mechanisms by which the metabolic syndrome and diabetes impair memory. *J Gerontol (Biol Sci)* 2000; **55A**:B228–232.

68 Stolk RP, Breteler MM, Ott A, Pols HA, Lamberts SW, Grobbee DE, *et al.* Insulin and cognitive function in an elderly population: the Rotterdam Study. *Diabetes Care* 1997; **20**:792–795.

69 Leibson CL, Rocca WA, Hanson VA, Cha R, Kokmen E, O'Brien PC, *et al.* Risk of dementia among persons with diabetes mellitus: a population-based cohort study. *Am J Epidemiol* 1997; **145**: 301–308.

70 Gradman TJ, Laws A, Thompson LW, Reaven GM. Verbal learning and/or memory improves with glycemic control in older subjects with non-insulin-dependent diabetes mellitus. *J Am Geriatr Soc* 1993; **41**:1305–1312.

71 Sinclair AJ, Girling AJ, Bayer AJ. Cognitive dysfunction in older subjects with diabetes mellitus: impact on diabetes self-management and use of care services. *Diabetes Res Clin Pract* 2000; **50**:203–212.

72 Eaton WW, Armenian H, Gallo J, Pratt L, Ford DE. Depression and risk for onset of type II diabetes: a prospective population based study. *Diabetes Care* 1996; **19**:1097–1102.

73 Amato L, Padisso G, Cacciatore F; Observatorio Geriatrico of Campania Region Group. Non-insulin dependent diabetes mellitus is associated with a greater prevalence of depression in the elderly. *Diabetes Metab* 1996; **22**:314–318.

74 Rosenthal MJ, Fajarde M, Gilmore S, Morley JE, Naliboff BD. Hospitalisation and mortality of diabetes in older adults. *Diabetes Care* 1998; **21**:231–235.

75 Robinson N, Fuller JH, Edmeades SP. Depression and diabetes. *Diabet Med* 1988; **5**:268–274.

76 Gavard JA, Lustman PJ, Clouse RE. Prevalence of depression in adults with diabetes mellitus. *Diabetes Care* 1993; **16**:1167–1178.

77 Yesavage JA, Brink TA, Rose TL, Lum O, Huang V, Adey M, *et al.* Development and validation of a geriatric depression screening scale; a preliminary report. *J Psychiat Res* 1983; **17**:37–49.

78 Paile-Hyvarinen M, Wahlbeck K, Eriksson JG. Quality of life and metabolic status in mildly depressed women with type 2 diabetes treated with paroxetine: a single-blind randomised placebo controlled trial. *BMC Fam Pract* 2003; **4**:7.

79 Lustman PJ, Freedland KE, Griffith LS. Fluoxetine for depression in diabetes. *Diabetes Care* 2000; **23**:618–623.

80 Alexopoulos GS, Streim J, Carpenter D, Docherty JP. Using antipsychotic agents in older patients. *J Clin Psychiatry* 2004; **65**(Suppl 2):5–99.

81 Feldman PD, Hay LK, Deberdt W, Kennedy JS, Hutchins DS, Hay DP, *et al.* Retrospective cohort study of diabetes mellitus and antipsychotic treatment in a geriatric population in the United States. *J Am Med Dir Assoc* 2004; **5**:38–46.

82 Ramaswamy K, Masand PS, Nasrallah HA. Do certain atypical antipsychotics increase the risk of diabetes? A critical review of 17 pharmacoepidemiologic studies. *Ann Clin Psych* 2006; **18**:183–194.

83 Holt RIG. Antipsychotics, metabolic side effects and the elderly. *Geriatr Med* 2008; **38**:399–402.

84 Muggeo M, Verlato G, Bonora E, Bressan F, Girotto S, Corbellini M, *et al.* The Verona Diabetes Study: a population-based survey on known diabetes mellitus prevalence and 5-year all-cause mortality. *Diabetologia* 1995; **38**:318–325.

85 Sinclair AJ, Robert IE, Croxson SCM. Mortality in older people with diabetes mellitus. *Diabet Med* 1997; **14**:639–647.

86 Croxson SC, Price DE, Burden M, Jagger C, Burden AC. Mortality of elderly people with diabetes. *Diabet Med* 1994; **11**:250–252.

87 Kuusisto J, Mykkanen L, Pyorala K, Laasko M. NIDDM and its metabolic control predict coronary heart disease in elderly subjects. *Diabetes* 1994; **43**:960–967.

88 Muggeo M, Verlato G, Bonora E, Ciani F, Moghetti P, Eastman R, *et al.* Long-term instability of fasting plasma glucose predicts mortality in elderly NIDDM patients: the Verona Diabetes Study. *Diabetologia* 1995; **38**:672–679.

89 Levetan CS, Passaro M, Jablonski K, Kass M, Ratne RE. Unrecognised diabetes among hospital patients. *Diabetes Care* 1998; **21**:246–249.

90 DECODE Study Group/European Diabetes Epidemiology Group. Consequences of the new diagnostic criteria for diabetes in older men and women. *Diabetes Care* 1999; **22**:1667–1671.

91 Barrett-Connor E, Ferrara A. Isolated postchallenge hyperglycemia and the risk of fatal cardiovascular disease in older women and men: the Rancho Bernardo study. *Diabetes Care* 1998; **21**:1236–1239.

92 European Diabetes Working Party for Older People (EDWPOP). Clinical guidelines for type 2 diabetes mellitus, 2004. Available on instituteofdiabetes.org

93 Fried LP, Williamson JD, Kaspar J. The epidemiology of frailty: scope of the problem. In: Perry HM, Morley JE, Coe RM, eds. *Ageing and Musculoskeletal Disorders*. New York: Springer, 1993: 3–15.

94 Simon D, Senan C, Garnier P, Saint-Paul M, Papoz L. Epidemiological features of glycated haemoglobin A1c-distribution in a healthy population: the Telecom Study. *Diabetologia* 1989; **32**:864–869.

95 Kabadi U. Glycosylation of proteins: lack of influence of aging. *Diabetes Care* 1988; **11**:429–432.

96 Jarvis B, Simpson K. Clopidogrel: a review of its use in the prevention of atherothrombosis. *Drugs* 2000; **60**:347–377.

97 Jackson R. Updated New Zealand cardiovascular disease risk–benefit prediction guide. *Br Med J* 2000; **320**:709–710.

98 Wilson PWF, D'Agostino RB, Levy D, Belanger AM, Silbershatz H, Kannel WB. Prediction of coronary heart disease using risk factor categories. *Circulation* 1998; **97**:1837–1847.

99 Menotti A, Lanti M, Puddu PE, Kromhout D. Coronary heart disease incidence in northern and southern European populations: a reanalysis of the Seven Countries Study for a European coronary risk chart. *Heart* 2000; **84**:238–244.

100 Florkowski CM, Scott RS, Moir CL, Graham PJ. Lipid but not glycemic parameters predict total mortality from type 2 diabetes mellitus in Canterbury, New Zealand. *Diabet Med* 1998; **15**:386–392.

101 Rubins HB, Robins SJ, Collins D, Fye CL, Anderson JW, Elam MB, *et al.*; Veterans Affairs High-Density Lipoprotein Cholesterol Intervention Trial Study Group. Gemfibrozil for the secondary prevention of coronary heart disease in men with low levels of high-density lipoprotein cholesterol. *N Engl J Med* 1999; **341**:410–418.

102 Collins R, Armitage J, Parish S, Sleight P, Peto R; Heart Protection Study Collaborative Group. Effects of cholesterol-lowering with simvastatin on stroke and other major vascular events in 20536 people with cerebrovascular disease or other high-risk conditions. *Lancet* 2004; **363**:757–767.

103 Ostergren J, Poulter NR, Sever PS, Dahlöf B, Wedel H, Beevers G, *et al.*; ASCOT Investigators. The Anglo-Scandinavian Cardiac Outcomes Trial: blood pressure-lowering limb – effects in patients with type II diabetes. *J Hypertens* 2008; **26**:2103–2111.

104 Heart Outcomes Prevention Evaluation Study Investigators. Effects of ramipril on cardiovascular and microvascular outcomes in people

with diabetes mellitus: results of the HOPE and MICRO-HOPE substudy. *Lancet* 2000; **355**:253–259.

105 Action to Control Cardiovascular Risk in Diabetes Study Group. Effects of intensive glucose lowering in type 2 diabetes. *N Engl J Med* 2008; **358**:2545–2559.

106 ADVANCE Collaborative Group. Intensive blood glucose and vascular outcomes in patients with type 2 diabetes. *N Engl J Med* 2008; **358**:2560–2572.

107 Duckworth W, Abraira C, Moritz T, Reda D, Emanuele N, Reaven PD, *et al.*; VADT Investigators. Glucose control and vascular complications in veterans with type 2 diabetes. *N Engl J Med* 2009; **360**:129–139.

108 European Diabetes Policy Group. *A Desktop Guide to Type 2 Diabetes Mellitus*. Brussels: International Diabetes Federation (European Region), 1999.

109 Sinclair AJ, Turnbull CJ, Croxson SCM. Document of care for older people with diabetes. *Postgrad Med J* 1996; **72**:334–338.

110 Harrower AD. Pharmacokinetics of oral antihyperglycemic agents in patients with renal insufficiency. *Clin Pharmacokinet* 1996; **31**:111–119.

111 UK Prospective Diabetes Study (UKPDS). Effect of intensive blood-glucose control with metformin on complications in overweight patients with type 2 diabetes. *Lancet* 1998; **352**:854–865.

112 Hendra TJ. Insulin therapy. In: Sinclair AJ, Finucane P, eds. *Diabetes in Old Age*, 2nd edn. Chichester: Wiley, 2001: 165–176.

113 Berger W. Insulin therapy in the elderly type 2 diabetic patient. *Diabetes Res Clin Pract* 1988; **4**(Suppl. 1):24–28.

114 Yki-Jarvinen H, Kauppila M, Kujansuu E, Lahti J, Marjanen T, Niskanen L, *et al.* Comparison of insulin regimens in patients with non-insulin-dependent diabetes mellitus. *N Engl J Med* 1992; **327**:1426–1433.

115 Goddijn PP, Bilo HJ, Feskens EJ, Groeniert KH, van der Zee KI, Meyboom-de Jong B. Longitudinal study on glycaemic control and quality of life in patients with type 2 diabetes mellitus referred for intensified control. *Diabet Med* 1999; **16**:23–30.

116 Petterson T, Lee P, Hollis S, Young B, Newton P, Dorman T. Well-being and treatment satisfaction in older people with diabetes. *Diabetes Care* 1998; **21**:930–935.

117 Yki-Jarvinen H, Ryysy L, Nikkila K, Tulokas T, Vanamo R, Heikkilä M. Comparison of bedtime insulin regimens in patients with type 2 diabetes mellitus. *Ann Intern Med* 1999; **130**:389–396.

118 National Center for Health Statistics. *The National Nursing Home Survey 1977: Summary for the United States*. Hyattsville, MD: US Government Printing Office, 1979.

119 Sinclair AJ, Allard I, Bayer AJ. Observations of diabetes care in long-term institutional settings with measures of cognitive function and dependency. *Diabetes Care* 1997; **20**:778–784.

120 Benbow SJ, Walsh A, Gill GV. Diabetes in institutionalised elderly people: a forgotten population? *Br Med J* 1997; **314**:1868–1869.

121 Sinclair AJ, Gadsby R. Diabetes in care homes. In: Sinclair AJ, Finucane P, eds. *Diabetes in Old Age*, 2nd edn. Chichester: Wiley, 2001: 241–252.

122 Sinclair AJ, Turnbull CJ, Croxson SC. Document of diabetes care for residential and nursing homes. *Postgrad Med J* 1997; **73**:611–612.

123 British Diabetic Association (BDA). *Guidelines of Practice for Residents with Diabetes in Care Homes*. London: British Diabetic Association, 1999.

124 Sinclair AJ, Barnett AH. Special needs of elderly diabetic patients. *Br Med J* 1993; **306**:1142–1143.

125 Goyder EC, McNally PG, Drucquer M, Spiers N, Botha JL. Shifting of care for diabetes from secondary to primary care, 1990–5: a review of general practices. *Br Med J* 1998; **316**:1505–1506.

126 Reenders K. Approaching primary care. In: Sinclair AJ, Finucane P, eds. *Diabetes in Care Homes*, 2nd edn. Chichester: Wiley, 2001: 229–240.

127 Eastman RC, Javitt JC, Herman WH, Dasbach EJ, Zbrozek AS, Dong F, *et al.* Model of complications of NIDDM. 1. Model construction and assumptions. *Diabetes Care* 1997; **20**:725–734.

128 Eastman RC, Javitt JC, Herman WH, Dasbach EJ, Copley-Merriman C, Maier W, *et al.* Model of complications of NIDDM. 2. Analysis of the health benefits and cost-effectiveness of treating NIDDM with the goal of normoglycemia. *Diabetes Care* 1997; **20**:735–744.

129 Vijan S, Hofer TP, Hayward RA. Estimated benefits of glycemic control in microvascular complications in type 2 diabetes. *Ann Intern Med* 1997; **127**:788–795.

55 Psychiatric Disorders and Diabetes

Robert C. Peveler[1] & Richard I.G. Holt[2]

[1] Clinical Neurosciences Division, School of Medicine, University of Southampton and Royal South Hants Hospital, Southampton, UK

[2] Endocrinology and Metabolism Sub-Division, Developmental Origins of Adult Disease Division, School of Medicine, University of Southampton and Southampton General Hospital, Southampton, UK

Keypoints

- The interactions between diabetes and psychiatric disorders are complex: physical illness raises the risk of psychiatric disorder, but mental illness and its treatment also impact on the risks and outcomes of diabetes.
- Because mental health problems are common among people with diabetes, good levels of awareness and knowledge are vital for the health professionals who work with them.
- A strong case has been made for implementation of screening for mental health problems in a range of care settings.
- Increased availability of mental health expertise in the settings where people with diabetes are treated is required.

Introduction

The interaction between mind and body is central to the management and outcome of all chronic diseases, but is perhaps particularly complex and fascinating in the case of diabetes. Diabetes is no longer an invariably fatal condition; however, in order to maintain good health, many patients face high behavioral demands. Psychiatric disorders may significantly compromise the ability of the patient to perform self-care to the required standard for optimum health, leading to increased risks of poor outcomes including complications and premature mortality.

Both diabetes and psychiatric disorders are common conditions, and therefore a degree of co-occurrence would be expected purely by chance; however, there is a considerable body of evidence that diabetes is associated more frequently than expected with a range of psychiatric morbidity. In particular, it appears that patients with mood and psychotic disorders are at increased risk of developing diabetes, and people with diabetes go on to develop a range of psychologic problems at increased rates compared to healthy controls. This was first noted over a century ago; as Henry Maudsley said in his celebrated textbook, *Pathology of Mind*, when discussing the increased rates of diabetes observed among psychiatric patients [1]:

> *"Diabetes is a disease which often shows itself in families in which insanity prevails. Whether one disease predisposes in any way to the other or not, or whether they are independent outcomes of a common neurosis, they are certainly found to run side by side, or alternately with one another more often than can be accounted for by accidental coincidence or sequence".*

Knowledge of the special problems that occur when diabetes and a psychiatric disorder coincide is essential if optimum care is to be provided. Unfortunately, in most countries, services are not well organized to deliver good quality care for both the physical and psychologic needs of patients in the same setting. Clinicians need to be aware of the increased risks of co-morbidity, and the need for screening. Diabetes health care professionals should be able to provide "first response" management, and recognize the needs of those more complex patients for whom specialist management is essential. The topic of co-morbidity is also attracting interest from researchers, and there is the potential for considerable progress in understanding the epidemiology and psychobiologic mechanisms involved. The increased availability of objective measures of glycemic control and diabetes outcomes over the past few decades has opened up the possibility of a wide range of psychobiologic research. This chapter provides an overview of the current state of knowledge of these topics, and highlights needs for further research.

Mood disorders

Until quite recently, any discussion of mood disorders and diabetes would have concentrated solely on the increased rates of depression observed in cohorts of patients with diabetes, and is

Textbook of Diabetes, 4th edition. Edited by R. Holt, C. Cockram, A. Flyvbjerg and B. Goldstein.

likely to have viewed such co-morbidity mainly as an "understandable" reaction to the difficulties resulting from living with a demanding and life-limiting chronic physical illness. We now understand that the interaction between the two conditions is more complex than this:

- Depression may itself be a risk factor for the development of diabetes;
- Biologic aspects of diabetes may contribute to the development of depression;
- Other antecedent factors, such as the early nutritional environment, may have a "common soil effect," thereby contributing to the risks of both conditions.

Depression can also impact on the clinical course of the diabetes, increasing the risk of poor glycemic control and complications. People with both diabetes and depression have been found to have higher symptom burden, poorer functional status, poorer self-care and higher health care costs [2].

Case definition

Depressive symptoms exist on a continuum of severity. Standard definitions of "clinical" depression are based on symptom count and duration; the most widely used diagnostic criteria in current practice are those of the American Psychiatric Association's DSM-IV "major" depression (Table 55.1) [3].

This definition is to some degree arbitrary; however, it approximates to a level of symptomatology that is associated with significant disability and dysfunction, and is very widely accepted as a standard in both clinical practice and research. It is important to note that depressive disorders of lesser severity may still compromise self-care and outcomes in people with diabetes.

The clinical category of mood disorders includes both unipolar depression and bipolar ("manic-depressive") illness. This section focuses on unipolar depression; bipolar illness is included in the section on psychotic disorders.

Table 55.1 DSM-IV "major" depressive episode.

Five or more of the listed symptoms should be present nearly every day, for at least 2 weeks, and should represent a change from normal functioning; at least one of the first two symptoms in the list must be present
Symptoms
1 Depressed mood for most of the day
2 Markedly diminished interest or pleasure in all, or almost all, activities for most of the day
3 Significant weight loss when not dieting, or weight gain (change of 5%), or decrease or increase in appetite
4 Insomnia or hypersomnia
5 Psychomotor agitation or retardation
6 Fatigue or loss of energy
7 Feelings of worthlessness or excessive or inappropriate guilt
8 Diminished ability to think or concentrate
9 Recurrent thoughts of death or suicidal ideation

Epidemiology

Unipolar depression is one of the most common mental health problems in the general population, affecting 3–5% of the population at any time, and its prevalence appears to be increasing, such that the World Health Organization have estimated that it will be the second leading cause of disability (after heart disease) in the world by 2020 [4].

There have been many studies of the prevalence of depressive symptoms and disorders in people with diabetes over the past 40 years. Most of the early studies, however, had significant methodologic shortcomings.

First, they lacked standardized definitions of depressive disorders, mainly using rating scales of unknown reliability and validity in a diabetic population. The "gold standard" for ascertainment of case status is a research diagnostic interview; most rating scales can only give a probabilistic estimate of caseness. In addition, there may be an overlap between symptoms of diabetes and those of depression (e.g. fatigue, weight loss).

Second, studies have tended to ignore the heterogeneity of people with diabetes, studying mixed populations of patients with different forms of diabetes (e.g. type 1 [T1DM] and type 2 [T2DM]). It is important to distinguish between these groups for several reasons:

- Although there is increasing overlap, people with T2DM are older and depression prevalence varies with age;
- There may be differences in pathologic mechanisms;
- The rates of diabetic complications and other co-morbid conditions (e.g. obesity, heart disease) differ; and
- The demands of management are different.

Third, studies have often been based on "convenience" samples of patients, usually drawn from diabetic clinics, where the operation of referral and other biases in sample composition was of unknown effect. Ethnicity is also an important confounder for rates of both depression and diabetes.

Finally, studies have had low or unknown response rates, and because the presence of depressive symptoms may reduce the likelihood of responding in such studies, this biases prevalence estimates further. Not surprisingly, as a result the range of prevalence figures that can be found in the literature is very wide.

More recent studies, using better methods, and meta-analyses, have led to lower estimates of prevalence. For example, one recent review of the prevalence of co-morbid depression in people with T1DM [5] concluded that clinical depression was present in 12%, compared with 3.2% in control subjects without diabetes. Caution is still needed in the interpretation of this finding, because it was based on only 14 studies, of which only four included control groups and only seven were based on interview methods. Excluding studies without control groups and interview ascertainment led to a fall in estimated prevalence to 7.8%, a figure that, although still raised, is no longer statistically significantly different from that found in healthy controls (odds ratio [OR] 2.4; 95% confidence interval [CI] −0.7 to 5.4).

Studies of depression in people with T2DM tend to be based on larger samples, given that around 85% of patients have this disease subtype. A recent study based on clinical diagnoses from a US Health Maintenance Organization [6] concluded that depression was more common in people with T2DM (17.9%) than in matched controls (11.2%), with marked sex differences: depression was nearly twice as common in women, but the effect of the presence of diabetes was greater in men. The effect remained after adjustment for covariates such as cardiovascular disease and obesity.

Depressive disorders as a risk factor for diabetes

The suggestion that emotional factors, such as grief or sadness, could lead to the onset of diabetes was first raised by Thomas Willis in 1684. It is a common clinical observation that the onset of diabetes may follow a depressive episode, although because T2DM often goes undiagnosed for years, the apparent association may be at least partly the result of ascertainment bias – patients with depression are more likely to have a screening test for diabetes than those without.

A recent systematic review has addressed the question of the direction of the association between these conditions, and summarized the evidence that depression may be a risk factor for diabetes [7]. Unfortunately, the vast majority of existing studies are cross-sectional and therefore uninformative about this issue. The reviewers were able to identify nine longitudinal studies, and the analysis suggested that depressed adults have an increased risk of developing T2DM of around 37%; however, this must be regarded as a preliminary finding, and further large well-designed longitudinal studies are needed.

Proposed mechanisms linking depression and diabetes

Psychosocial factors

Most studies confirm that risk factors for depression in otherwise healthy individuals operate equally in people with diabetes. Thus, socioeconomic hardship, poor education, stressful life events and lack of social support are all important [8]. Gender differences are also important. There is relatively little evidence that people with diabetes differ greatly with respect to these types of risk factors, and it can be concluded that much depression in people with diabetes may be "independent" of the presence of the disease, an issue that may be particularly important when it comes to management planning.

Early nutrition

One putative common risk factor that may increase the risks of both of diabetes and depression is that of disrupted nutrition during fetal life. There are now over 38 reports linking poor fetal growth with impaired glucose metabolism in later life [9]. Most of these studies report an inverse relationship or J-shaped relationship between birth weight and plasma glucose and insulin concentrations, the prevalence of T2DM and measures of insulin resistance and secretion. Similarly, the risk of depression has been found to be associated with low birth weight for both young and older adults [10]. Furthermore, data from the Dutch Hunger Winter study showed that exposure to famine during the second or third trimester of fetal life is associated with increased risk of hospital treatment for major affective disorder [11].

The mechanism underlying this association is not clear but one hypothesis proposes that fetal programming of the hypothalamic-pituitary-adrenal (HPA) axis may play a part.

Shared genetic risk

Another suggested mechanism that may link diabetes and psychiatric disorder is that of shared genetic variance. There is some evidence that close relatives of people with some forms of psychiatric disorder have an increased incidence of diabetes [12], and known loci for the disorders occur in overlapping positions within chromosomes [13]. Investigation of this intriguing possibility is in its infancy and further research is needed.

Inflammatory mechanisms

It has been hypothesized that inflammation and increased production of proinflammatory cytokines by activated immune cells may mediate the association between depression and diabetes, with associated perturbation of the HPA axis [14]. Parallels have been noted between depression and so-called "sickness behavior" seen in response to the elevation of cytokines, interleukin 1 (IL-1), IL-6 and tumor necrosis factor α (TNF-α). It is thought that such cytokines may be released in increased amounts from adipose tissue in conditions including diabetes and obesity as people age, and this may interfere with insulin action.

Counter-regulatory hormones

Acute psychologic stress is known to increase circulating concentrations of counter-regulatory hormones including noradrenaline, glucocorticoids and growth hormone (GH), which antagonize the hypoglycemic action of insulin. Although the effects of chronic stress on the HPA axis are somewhat less well understood, the view of depression as a maladaptive prolonged stress reaction has some empirical support.

Loss of normal diurnal variation in cortisol levels together with non-suppression of cortisol release in response to exogenous steroid administration have long been noted as hallmarks of depressive illness, particularly the "melancholic" subtype. It is suggested that this may lead to increased glycogenolysis, gluconeogenesis, lipolysis and inhibition of peripheral glucose transport and utilization [15]. Non-diabetic patients with depression have been shown to have increased insulin resistance, but further investigation of this mechanism is warranted. Glucose transport in the brains of people with depression has also been shown to be abnormal [15].

Depression and glycemic control

Several studies have demonstrated an association between the severity of depressive symptoms and the level of glycemic control as assessed by glycosylated hemoglobin level (HbA_{1c}) [16], although the size of this effect has been generally modest, and may be explained by confounders such as the presence of microvascular complications. Most studies have been cross-sectional in nature, although some treatment studies have suggested that improvements in glycemic control are associated with reduction of depressive symptoms.

Depression and complications

There seems to be little doubt that the risk of depression increases as microvascular and macrovascular complications accrue over the course of the disease [17]. The evidence is less strong that the presence of depression increases the risk of developing complications, although the fact that self-care and resulting glycemic control are impaired would lead to this expectation. One longitudinal cohort study of 66 people with T1DM found that depression was an independent risk factor for retinopathy at 10 years [18], but other studies have had negative results. The meta-analysis of de Groot *et al.* [17] supports a positive association.

One complication that may have a particular association with depression is that of peripheral neuropathic pain. Recent studies suggest that not only is chronic pain a risk factor for depression, but the presence of depression may itself worsen the experience of pain. Common neurotransmitters appear to be involved in both depression and pain [19].

Management of people with diabetes and depression

At present, advice for the management of patients with co-morbid depression and diabetes is based on evidence derived from populations without diabetes because the number of treatment studies in people with diabetes is as yet too small to lead to robust conclusions. Nevertheless, some inroads into this problem are now being made.

The main aims of treatment are to reduce depressive symptoms and to improve self-care, glycemic control and diabetes outcomes. A major difficulty for most clinics is the lack of readily available specialist mental health input, and this has been a disincentive for services to engage actively in tackling this important clinical problem. By contrast, guidelines are now including the issue of psychologic well-being, increasing the need for attention to be paid to it. It should be possible for most clinics to provide "first response" management for simple depressive disorders, although specialist help will still be required for more complex cases, where there is diagnostic uncertainty or lack of response to initial treatment. Assessment and management of suicide risk is a particularly important issue, although fortunately rare in most clinic settings.

Screening for depression

Given the high prevalence of depression in people with diabetes, it is recommended [20] that screening and case finding is worthwhile and this is now recommended by the National Institute for Health and Clinical Excellence (NICE) in the UK [21]. NICE recommends that health care professionals who care for or advise adults with diabetes should be alert to the development or presence of clinical or subclinical depression and anxiety. This is particularly the case where someone reports or appears to be having difficulties with self-management. Health care professionals should ensure they have appropriate diagnostic and management skills for non-severe psychologic disorders in people from different cultural backgrounds. Knowledge of appropriate counseling techniques and appropriate drug therapy is important, as well as an awareness of the need for prompt referral to specialists of those in whom psychologic difficulties continue to interfere significantly with well-being or diabetes self-management.

In the UK, GPs are now reimbursed specifically for carrying out screening in populations with chronic illness, including diabetes. There are several short screening questionnaires that can be used for this purpose including the Patient Health Questionnaire (PHQ-9) [22], Hospital Anxiety and Depression Scale (HADS) [23] and Beck Depression Inventory (BDI) [24], although none of these have been specifically validated for use in diabetic populations, and scores may be inflated by the presence of diabetes-related symptoms. It may be better to use a very brief clinical interview using three questions [25]. Initially, the patient is asked:

- During the past month, have you been bothered by having little interest or pleasure in doing things?
- During the past month, have you been bothered by feeling down, depressed, or hopeless?

If the answer to either of these is "yes," the patient should then be asked if they want help with this problem. If the answer to this is also "yes," then it is reasonable to offer treatment.

Case history 1: A woman with diabetes and depression

Joan is a 62-year-old married woman who has had type 2 diabetes for 15 years, which is treated by diet and oral hypoglycemic medication. She has a body mass index of 32 kg/m^2, and at interview was noticeably low in mood. On direct questioning, she gave a history of significant depressive symptoms lasting for several months, and had a history of previous intermittent depressive episodes dating back to the birth of her first child at the age of 24. She had low self-esteem, and admitted to bouts of "comfort eating" (mainly chocolate) to try to treat her low mood. There was no disturbance of body image. In addition, she was socially isolated, and complained of receiving little support from her husband, who was usually busy at work. Management consisted of antidepressant medication, augmented with advice and support focused on increasing socialization and resumption of pleasurable and rewarding activities, such as spending more time with her grandchildren.

Pharmacotherapy

Many treatment guidelines exist, including those from NICE [26], and similar ones from bodies such as the American Psychiatric Association. Drug treatment is the mainstay of depression management. Effective and well-tolerated antidepressant drugs are widely available and affordable. Choice of agent tends to be based on side effect profile because evidence of differential efficacy is poor. Older families of compounds such as tricyclic antidepressants and monoamine oxidase inhibitors have decreased in popularity because of their toxicity, particularly in patients who might be at increased risk of heart disease.

Selective serotonin reuptake inhibitors are relatively safe and very widely used as first choice agents; however, caution is needed because there are important drug–drug interactions with some members of this class and oral hypoglycemic agents through inhibition of the cytochrome P450 3A4 and 2C9 isoenzymes (see Chapter 26). For example, the use of fluoxetine may lead to hypoglycemia [15]. Weight gain, which occurs with some antidepressants including mirtazepine, is particularly undesirable in overweight people with T2DM.

It is important to have a clear treatment target, and most guidelines now recommend that this should be complete remission of depressive symptoms. To achieve this, treatment must be sustained at an adequate dosage for a sufficient period of time. Once remission has been attained, treatment should be continued for at least 4–6 months to consolidate recovery. There is an increased risk of relapse and recurrence if the course of treatment is given at too low a dosage or for insufficient duration.

In addition to possible direct pharmacologic effects, it should be remembered that treating depression may lead to a change in the patient's behavior and routine that may require adjustment of the diabetic regimen. For example, if the patient's appetite improves, insulin requirements may increase; if the patient becomes more active, they may decrease. It is likely, however, that improvement in depressive symptoms alone will not translate automatically into improved self-care and diabetes outcomes. Additional attention to diabetes management is required as the depression improves.

Clinical management

In most health care systems, depression is managed mostly within primary care by family physicians or GPs. Much emphasis has been placed in recent years on the delivery of evidence-based practice, and this has led to a proliferation of guidelines and educational support designed to improve quality of primary care. In the USA, a case management model known as "collaborative care" has been pursued, whereby family physicians are supported in case management by specialist mental health teams. This approach has been shown to be clinically useful and cost-effective [27,28]. Recently, a large study, the Pathways study [29], has attempted to address the question of whether or not this approach can improve outcomes for patients with both diabetes and depression. In this study over 300 patients were randomly allocated to receive the intensified case management approach or usual care. Contrary to expectations, although depression outcomes were improved, no concomitant improvements in glycemic control were observed over a 12-month period. This finding suggests that when treating depression in people with diabetes, attention also needs to be paid to modifications that are needed in the diabetes regimen such as adjustment of diet, activity and medication if the best possible outcomes are to be attained. Such integrated approaches to management are all too rare at the present time.

Psychologic treatment

The other important aspect of management for depression that has been widely evaluated in diabetic populations is psychologic treatment, which can take a variety of forms. There is some confusion in the literature between approaches that could be broadly described as "educational" – that is, largely based on improving knowledge and understanding of diabetes management – and those with a more psychologic or behavioral basis, such as cognitive–behavior therapy. For most patients with suboptimal self-care, it appears that lack of knowledge of their condition is not the most important cause; rather there are more complex causes, which may have their origins in early life experiences or in current stressful events or circumstances, and it is these that psychologic treatments seek to address.

Educational approaches could be broadly divided into "didactic" and "enhanced"; in the latter form the giving of information and advice is supplemented with behavioral instruction, development of skills such as problem-solving and a range of other techniques such as biofeedback or relaxation. Thus, the boundary between educative approaches and formal psychotherapy has become blurred, and this creates difficulties in evaluating the available literature. The consensus from systematic reviews is that such interventions can improve glycemic control, albeit with a modest effect size of about 0.3 – equivalent to a reduction in HbA_{1c} of around 0.6% (7 mmol/mol) – and can also reduce psychologic distress [30].

There are few trials that have set out to test directly the efficacy of psychologic treatment in treating depression in people with diabetes. Studies of otherwise healthy subjects with depression show that several forms of treatment including cognitive–behavioral therapy, interpersonal psychotherapy and cognitive–analytic therapy can all be of benefit. A recent systematic review evaluated the efficacy of psychologic interventions aimed primarily at improving glycemic control in people with T2DM [30], and found that benefits were seen in terms of reduced psychologic distress and improved long-term glycemic control.

Given that psychologic treatments are potentially very effective, but expensive and limited in availability, there is an urgent need for more evaluation of their benefits and applicability. In the UK, there is currently a large program evaluating the benefits of widening access to psychologic treatment for depression, and a similar initiative in the case of diabetes is warranted. Unfortunately, it appears as if availability of such treatments to people with diabetes is actually decreasing within the UK [31].

Psychotic disorders

Psychotic disorders are the most serious forms of illness within the mental health field, and are often also known as "severe mental illness" (SMI). (Although this term is imprecise because it is perfectly possible for patients to have equally serious forms of other non-psychotic types of illness.) The two main forms of psychotic disorder in working age adults are schizophrenia and

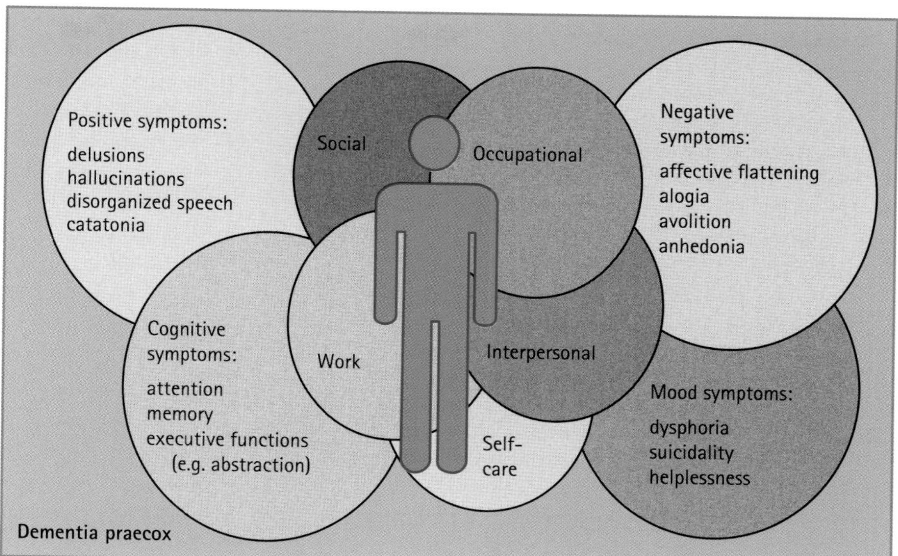

Figure 55.1 Impact of schizophrenia on overall functioning.

bipolar mood disorder or "manic depression." The impact of these disorders on patients' well-being and functioning is particularly severe because of the presence of psychotic symptoms including delusions and hallucinations which have a profound effect on any or all aspects of daily life (Figure 55.1). When they co-occur with a chronic physical illness, they can create significant management challenges, and such patients are amongst the most complex that health care systems encounter.

It has been noted for over a century that abnormalities of glucose metabolism are more common in those with this type of mental illness [32], although only in recent years have efforts been made to establish the precise nature of this association. The situation is complicated by the fact that some forms of treatment for these disorders may also affect metabolic health. It is known that patients with such disorders have reduced life expectancy, and much of the excess early mortality results from physical disease including diabetes and cardiovascular disease. Intensified efforts to improve the physical health of people with long-term mental illness are now underway in most countries, with detection and management of metabolic and cardiovascular risk factors and diabetes at their core [33].

Case definitions

Diagnostic criteria for schizophrenia are shown in Table 55.2. It can be seen that the illness is characterized by psychotic symptoms (delusions, hallucinations), disorganization of speech and other behavior, and so-called "negative" symptoms which include loss of drive and blunting of affect. In the longer term, schizophrenia is also associated with cognitive decline. The illness has marked effects on daily functioning, tends to run a chronic clinical course and most patients with the condition will be under the long-term care of specialist mental health services.

Bipolar disorder is characterized by the occurrence of one or more episodes of mania (elevated mood), with or without a previous history of depressive episodes. Criteria for a manic episode are shown in Table 55.3. The strict diagnostic criteria for bipolar disorders are complex, and there is a degree of overlap with schizophrenia, such that some patients may be characterized as having a "schizo-affective" disorder.

Table 55.2 DSM-IV schizophrenia.

1 Two or more of the following symptoms:
- (i) Delusions
- (ii) Hallucinations
- (iii) Disorganized speech
- (iv) Grossly disorganized or catatonic behavior
- (v) Negative symptoms (affective flattening, alogia or avolition)

2 Social/occupational dysfunction

3 Features continuously present for at least 6 months

Epidemiology

Schizophrenia is estimated to have a point prevalence of 1–7/1000 in the general population, with an annual incidence of 13–70/100 000 and a lifetime risk of 1–2%. Strikingly, this varies very little across the countries of the world. The clinical course of the illness is variable, ranging from a single brief episode (rarely) to a lifelong illness with marked deterioration over time. There are many theories about the causation of schizophrenia. It has a marked genetic risk profile, but is also associated with early cerebral insults (e.g. birth anoxia) and environmental stress.

Bipolar disorder is much less common than unipolar depression, with an estimated lifetime prevalence of 0.5–1.0%. Again, genetic factors are thought to have an important role in the etiology of bipolar disorders, which are among the most heritable of psychiatric disorders.

Table 55.3 DSM-IV manic episode.

1 A distinct period of abnormally and persistently elevated, expansive or irritable mood, lasting at least 1 week
2 During the period of mood disturbance, three or more of the following symptoms have persisted (four if mood only irritable):
  (i) Inflated self-esteem or grandiosity
  (ii) Decreased need for sleep
  (iii) More talkative than usual or pressure to keep talking
  (iv) Flight of ideas or subjective experience that thoughts are racing
  (v) Distractibility
  (vi) Increase in goal-directed activity or psychomotor agitation
  (vii) Excessive involvement in pleasurable activities that have high potential for painful consequences (e.g. spending, sexual activity)
3 Marked impairment in occupational functioning or in usual social activities or relationships with others, or need for hospitalization to prevent harm to self or others, or psychotic symptoms

Mortality of people with psychotic illnesses

The fact that people with psychotic disorders have premature mortality has long been known. A landmark study in this area was that by Brown *et al.* [34], who showed that the standardized mortality ratio of psychiatric patients was increased threefold, and life expectancy reduced by 10–20 years. Although suicide and accidents were important causes of death, "natural causes" accounted for the majority of the excess mortality in this population.

A difficulty in the interpretation of this finding arises from the fact that patients with long-term mental illness are exposed to a wide range of different risk factors from those of the general population. Older studies suggested that hospitalization itself may have been a risk. Most patients are now cared for in community settings, but there are still marked differences in lifestyle, with psychiatric patients being more likely to smoke, being less active and having different diets from the general population, as well as being exposed to a range of pharmacologic agents. Disentangling risks associated with the disease, its treatment and genetic and lifestyle factors has proved to be particularly challenging [35].

As is the case for schizophrenia, there is growing evidence that patients with bipolar illness also have increased all-cause mortality, and evidence of increased cardiovascular disease, when compared with the general population. Again the findings of longitudinal studies in the face of confounders such as lifestyle differences and the effects of treatments can be difficult to interpret. It is likely that those patients with bipolar illness who are exposed to long-term use of antipsychotic drugs (the majority) will have similar outcomes to those of patients with schizophrenia. Other drugs used in bipolar patients such as lithium and sodium valproate are also associated with weight gain, but there has been much less research on their wider metabolic effects to date.

Psychotic disorders and their treatment as a risk factor for diabetes

Papers commenting on the association between schizophrenia and diabetes date back to at least the early part of the 20th century, but the volume of literature exploded in the early years of the 21st century, largely driven by marketing claims related to different antipsychotic drugs. Of course, the early papers demonstrating the association date from the period before the availability of these agents, and provide some of the best evidence we have of an association with the disease alone [32]. This has been supplemented more recently by a small number of studies of drug-naïve patients, but such studies are now very difficult to undertake because of the ethical difficulties of leaving people untreated [36]. Another boost to publication rates occurred when the first antipsychotic agents, the phenothiazines, came into widespread clinical use in the 1950s and 1960s, with many reports of "phenothiazine diabetes" appearing. Unfortunately, interpretation of older studies is hampered by the different diagnostic practices in use for both diabetic and psychotic disorders.

Case history 2: The interaction of schizophrenia and diabetes

Timothy is a 30-year-old man who was admitted to a hospital with an acute psychotic illness. Following a diagnosis of schizophrenia, he was treated with an atypical antipsychotic and after this remained well both physically and mentally. He had a family history of diabetes. He disliked exercise and he tended to eat snacks and smoke 20 cigarettes per day. After 7 years, he developed diabetes. His psychiatrist was concerned that the antipsychotic may have been involved in the development of his diabetes and switched him to an alternative antipsychotic. Unfortunately, the psychosis relapsed and the patient was readmitted to hospital. His diabetes did not resolve and proved more difficult to control until the original medication was restarted and his mental state improved.

A particular difficulty in establishing whether schizophrenia and its treatment increase the risks of diabetes results from the fact that important known risk factors differ between populations, leading to a high degree of confounding in most epidemiologic studies.

The risk factors with large effect sizes include:

- Overweight and obesity;
- Family history;
- Age; and
- Ethnicity.

It is likely that the disease and its treatment have effects that are of smaller size than these, and so failure to match adequately for these confounders can easily yield results that are uninterpretable (Figure 55.2). Added to this is the fact that most studies are retrospective, and that patients tend to be exposed to a wide range of different antipsychotic drugs over the course of their illness. Prospective studies using single agents are much fewer in number, although reviews of such studies are now beginning to appear. Consequently, we are faced with many studies that give inconsistent and often contradictory results.

In order to overcome some of these difficulties, studies in drug naïve, first-episode patients have been instructive in determining the possibility of an underlying abnormality in glucose metabolism associated with schizophrenia. In two small cross-sectional studies of first-episode drug naïve individuals in Ireland, 10–15% of participants had impaired fasting glycemia and were more insulin resistant than healthy control subjects [36,37]. First-episode patients were also found to have significantly higher waist: hip ratios, and over three times as much visceral fat (a predictor of insulin resistance) when assessed by computed tomography scanning [38]. A study from India found that non-fasting blood glucose concentrations were higher in those with first-episode psychosis than healthy controls [39], while other studies have found differences in body composition between first-episode patients and healthy control subjects but without glucose changes [40]. These findings have not been replicated in all studies [41–43].

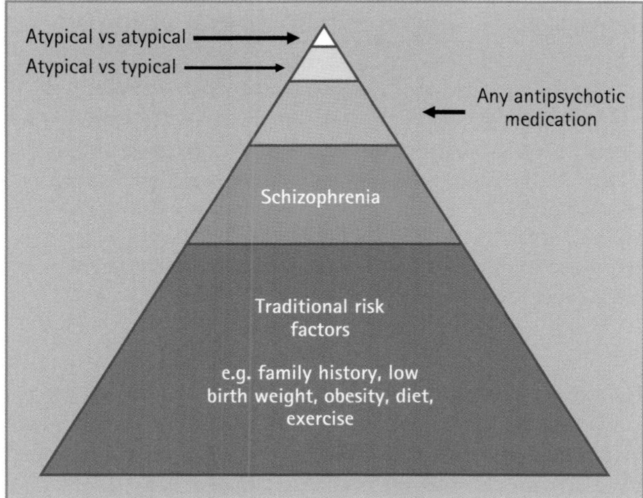

Figure 55.2 The relative contributions of traditional diabetic risk factors, schizophrenia and antipsychotic medication to the development of diabetes in people with serious mental illness. Adapted from Holt RI, Peveler RC. Association between antipsychotic drugs and diabetes. *Diabetes Obes Metab* 2006; **8**:125–135.

The consensus that emerges from the current literature is that having schizophrenia is associated with a two- to fourfold increase in risk of developing diabetes, which leads to an overall prevalence of diabetes of 10–15% in Western populations. Most patients have T2DM and there is some evidence that the rates of T1DM are in fact reduced in people with schizophrenia. Studies conducted in clinical populations suffer from the limitation of screening bias, in that T2DM is often asymptomatic for many years, and ascertainment rates are highly sensitive to such bias. Although subjected to much less systematic study to date, there is a suggestion in the literature that patients with bipolar disorder are also at increased risk of developing diabetes, with a relative risk estimated at two- to threefold. Similar caveats about the effects of treatments and lifestyle differences to those for schizophrenia apply.

By comparing the rates of diabetes at different age groups (Figure 55.3), it is also possible to see that the onset of diabetes appears to occur around 10–20 years earlier in people with SMI than the general population. There are significant numbers of people with diabetes under the age of 40 years and therefore this issue should not be ignored even in those with a recent diagnosis of mental illness.

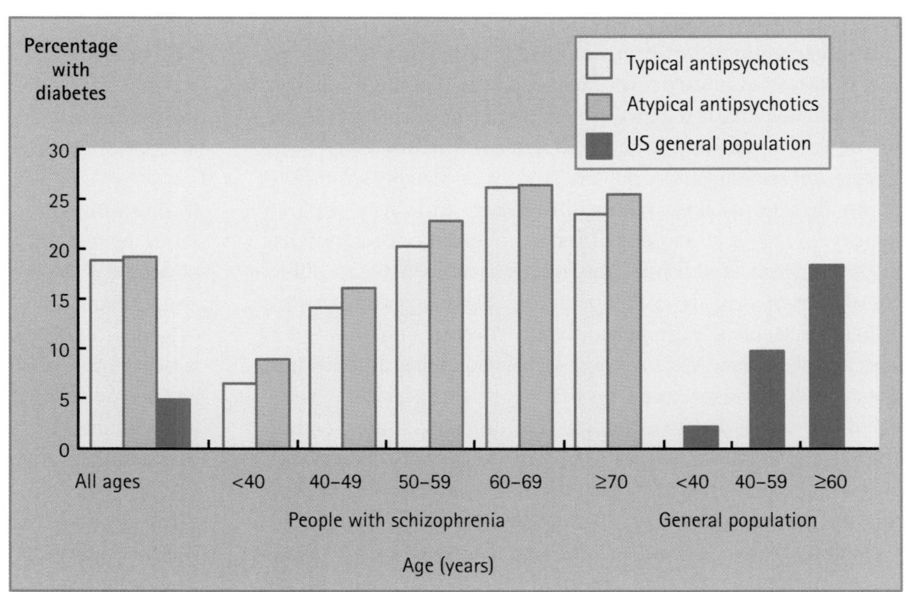

Figure 55.3 Age-specific prevalence rates of diabetes in people with schizophrenia compared with the general US population. Data from Sernyak MJ, Leslie DL, Alarcon RD, Losonczy MF, Rosenheck R. Association of diabetes mellitus with the use of atypical neuroleptics in the treatment of schizophrenia. *Am J Psychiatry* 2002; **159**:561–566 and National Health and Nutritional Examination Survey 2001–2002.

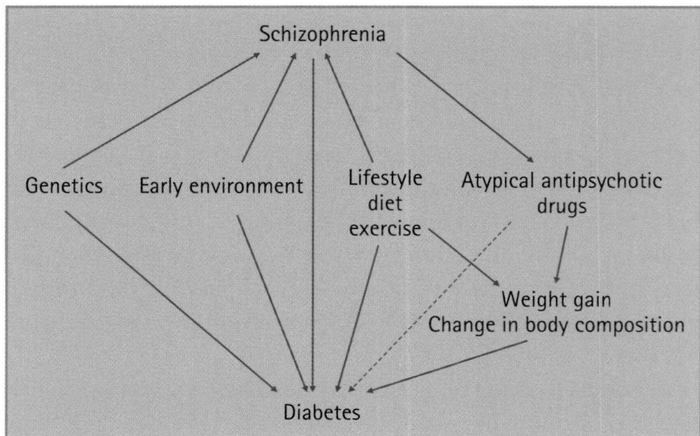

Figure 55.4 The possible mechanisms linking schizophrenia to diabetes. Reproduced from Holt RI, Peveler RC, Byrne CD. Schizophrenia, the metabolic syndrome and diabetes. *Diabet Med* 2004; **21**:515–523.

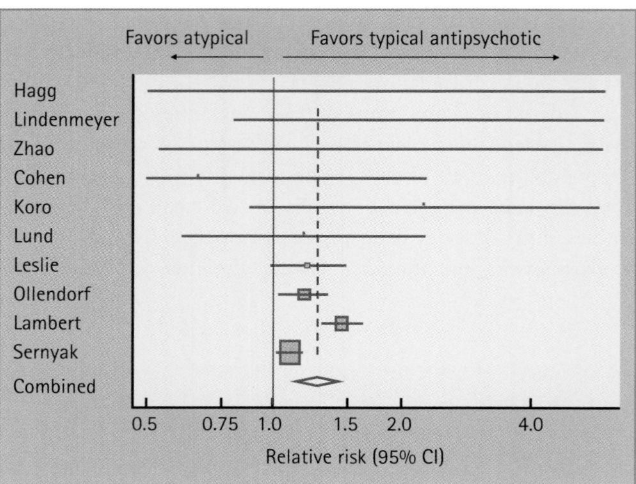

Figure 55.5 Forest plot of relative risks and 95% confidence intervals for diabetes in patients with schizophrenia receiving first-generation antipsychotics compared with second-generation antipsychotics. Adapted from Smith M, Hopkins D, Peveler RC, Holt RI, Woodward M, Ismail K. First- v. second-generation antipsychotics and risk for diabetes in schizophrenia: systematic review and meta-analysis. *Br J Psychiatry* 2008; **192**:406–411.

Mechanisms of the association

There are many difficulties in disentangling the possible mechanisms underlying the apparent associations between psychotic illness and diabetes. Diabetes, schizophrenia and bipolar illness all appear to be strongly heritable, and genetic associations appear to be likely (Figure 55.4). It has been reported that up to 50%, although more commonly 15–30%, of individuals with schizophrenia have a family history of T2DM, compared to 5% of healthy adult controls [12]. Shared susceptibility loci are now being investigated using linkage and candidate gene approaches [13].

Other factors that may underlie the association include a poorer diet, with lower intake of fruit and vegetables and much higher intake of fat, lower levels of physical activity, urbanization and higher rates of smoking among patients [44]. These findings have been documented consistently in several studies; however, it is difficult to assess the size of the effect that they may contribute to the observed association.

Another suggested mechanism involves activation of the HPA axis by stress associated with mental illness, leading to chronic hypercortisolemia and hence an increased risk of diabetes.

The role of antipsychotic medication in contributing to the association remains under debate. There is reasonably strong evidence that most antipsychotic drugs are associated with an increase in risk of developing diabetes, but proof of causation has not been firmly established. Making distinctions between different classes of drug is challenging, and distinguishing between individual agents is extremely difficult. The current consensus is that newer agents (the so-called atypical or second-generation drugs) may have increased propensity to cause diabetes compared to older drugs, although the differences are modest, amounting to perhaps a 10–30% increase in risk (Figure 55.5) [45]. Of the newer agents, clozapine is probably associated with the highest risk but this is not found universally (Figure 55.6). Most antipsychotic drugs induce weight gain, and observational studies suggest that there is a general trend for the drugs with the highest potential for weight gain to also have the highest risk for diabetes, although this is not true in every case. This is in contrast to randomized trials that show no difference in diabetes rates between drugs despite often marked differences in weight gain. Both observational and randomized studies have their pitfalls, which mean that the true risk is difficult to determine [35].

Metabolic syndrome

In recent years investigations in this field have broadened their scope to include assessment of intermediate hyperglycemia and the metabolic syndrome. It appears at this early stage that almost all of the wider range of cardiovascular risk factors, with the possible exception of hypertension, that make up this syndrome are elevated in patients with psychotic disorders, increasing yet further the emphasis on the importance of cardiovascular health promotion in these populations [46].

Management

From the foregoing review it can be seen that the metabolic health of people with psychotic disorders is a wide-ranging public health issue. Historically, it appears that such patients have experienced considerable disadvantage at a time when health promotion as an approach to cardiovascular risk factors in the general population has been developing rapidly. Consideration needs to be given to lifestyle advice, early detection of risk factors, screening for clinical disease and treatment for established disease.

Lifestyle advice and health promotion

National guidelines [33] now stress the importance of physical health promotion for people with long-term mental illness, rec-

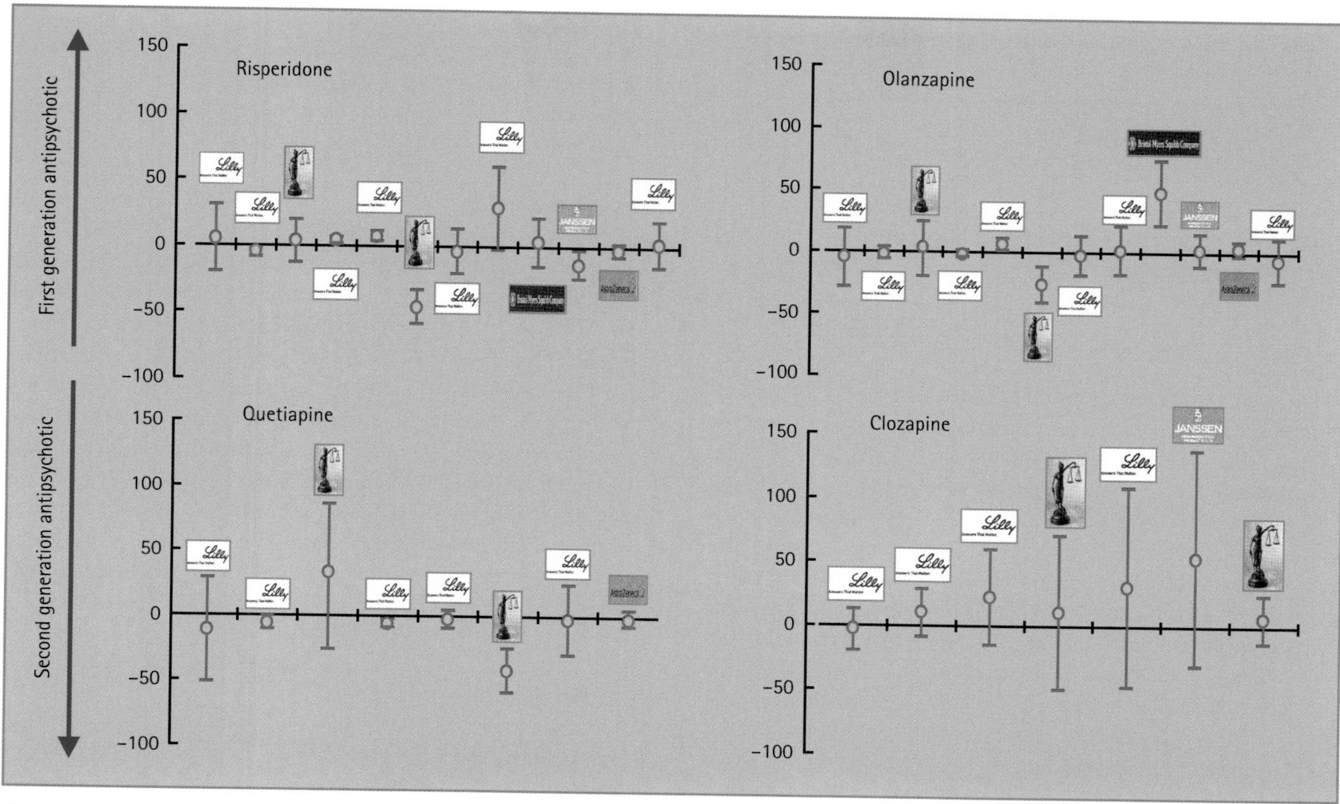

Figure 55.6 Number of cases of diabetes estimated to occur beyond those expected with first-generation antipsychotics per 1000 patients treated with a second-generation antipsychotic, 95% confidence intervals and study sponsorship. Pharmaceutical company sponsorship indicated by figure above or below the upper limit bar in each graph. Independent studies are represented by the scales of justice. Numbers represent additional numbers of cases of diabetes per 1000 treated.

ognizing the health disadvantage that they have experienced in the past. There is still debate about how this is best achieved, with responsibility in many health care systems being split between specialist services and primary care. Primary care is probably the best source of health promotion in most cases, and in many countries this role attracts remuneration, but many patients with long-term mental health problems see their GPs less frequently and depend on the mental health team for most of their health needs. Unfortunately, many such teams have not considered physical health promotion to be part of their remit in the past.

However, there are now signs that this is changing, at least in some countries, and many services are integrating such health promotion into their routine care pathways. Appropriately tailored advice is needed on diet, exercise, weight management, smoking and drug use, supplemented by environmental initiatives such as provision of alternatives to sweetened beverages and "institutional" food in hospital settings, and support for increased activity and body weight monitoring. Contrary to expectation, people with SMI, irrespective of diagnosis or treatment, may well be able to modify their lifestyles with appropriate education and support, and this may result in significant weight loss. Several models to deliver lifestyle education have been proposed but group sessions appear to be both clinically useful and cost-effective. The most important issue is to engage people with mental illness as engagement with the program was the only predictor of long-term weight loss in the longest running program in the UK [47]. A Cochrane review of lifestyle interventions showed modest weight reduction for those currently treated with antipsychotics and a reduction in antipsychotic-induced weight gain in those about to start treatment [48].

Prevention of diabetes

The principles of lifestyle modification have been well established as a means of preventing or at least delaying the onset of diabetes. The lifestyle programs described in the preceding section should provide an effective framework to reduce the incidence of diabetes. These programs are not suitable for all and pharmacologic treatments should be considered for those unable to adapt their lifestyles.

The Diabetes Prevention Program (DPP) has established that the use of metformin is associated with a 31% reduction in the incidence of diabetes. Metformin has been shown to lead to modest reductions in weight in several small studies of people receiving antipsychotics. In one study, metformin treatment

Table 55.4 Drugs that have been tested as potential agents to prevent or reduce weight gain.

Amantadine	Fluoxetine
Nizatidine	Reboxetine
Topiramate	Sibutramine
Metformin	Exenatide
Betahistine	Orlistat

prevented the deterioration in insulin resistance as assessed by homeostasis model assessment in patients treated with antipsychotics [49].

Several other drugs have been tried to prevent or reduce antipsychotic-induced weight gain (Table 55.4). A Cochrane review found that none of the treatments was particularly effective [48] and so none can be recommended without reservation; however, given the long experience with metformin and an understanding of its safety and tolerability, together with its modest cost and proven benefit in reducing incident diabetes, this seems a logical choice for those unable to modify their diet. Further long-term trials are needed, however, to prove that metformin is an effective agent in preventing diabetes in this patient group.

Screening

We now know enough about the scale of risk involved to suggest that patients with psychotic disorders should undergo routine screening for the presence of diabetes. This should be carried out at least annually and possibly more frequently if other risk factors are present. There is debate about the best method of screening – a fasting blood glucose estimation is clearly the ideal, but not easy to obtain in all cases. A random glucose alone, or in combination with an HbA_{1c} test, may be an acceptable substitute, and while its sensitivity and specificity may be lower, it is still preferable to no test at all.

Patients with established diabetes

There are considerable challenges in managing the patient with both a psychotic disorder and established diabetes. The key to success lies in close liaison between the diabetes and mental health services involved with the patient. Management of the mental illness will follow established guidelines, and deploy drug and psychologic treatment, family work, hospital admission and community support as appropriate. It is important to note that most health professionals working in mental health teams are not medically qualified, and will probably have little familiarity with the principles of management of diabetes.

The goals of treating the diabetes should be no different from those in otherwise healthy patients, although achieving these is likely to be much more difficult. Communication with patients with psychotic disorders can be challenging for those with little experience of such work, and patients may find it difficult to report symptoms or extent of self-care to health professionals as clearly as non-psychotic patients might. Extra time and additional training may be needed for health professionals in diabetes teams who are to work with such patients.

Pharmacotherapy

Given what we know about the relative risks of metabolic problems associated with antipsychotic drugs, this aspect of safety must be considered when treatments are being chosen. Unfortunately, there is marked individual variation in clinical response to different antipsychotic agents, and for some patients it will be necessary to continue to use an agent for the sake of obtaining the best result in terms of the patient's mental state, even though metabolic risks may be higher than would be ideal. It is never advisable to discontinue an antipsychotic drug on the grounds that it may be contributing to a metabolic problem without careful consideration of the choices available for treating the psychotic disorder and without discussion with the psychiatric team.

Eating disorders

Case definitions

Three main forms of eating disorder are currently recognized: anorexia nervosa, bulimia nervosa and a residual category of eating disorder not otherwise specified (EDNOS) [3]. The first two conditions have been the subject of much research for many decades; however, the latter category is much less well studied, but is important from a public health perspective as it tends to be more prevalent, and in many cases equally disabling, as the better known forms. As with depressive symptoms, eating disorders exist on a continuum of severity, and there is a lack of good evidence on which to establish a formal boundary or cut-off for "clinical" significance. When an eating disorder co-occurs with a chronic disease such as diabetes, its significance may be increased by the potential for harm resulting from impaired self-care and glycemic control – thus, eating disorders that may be seen as "mild" in an otherwise healthy individual take on increased clinical importance. Because eating disorders are most common in adolescents and young adults, there has been much more research on the co-occurrence of eating disorders and T1DM; far less is known about such problems in the larger population with T2DM [50].

Diagnostic criteria for the common forms of eating disorder are given in Table 55.5 [3].

Clinical features

Anorexia nervosa

The hallmark of anorexia nervosa is weight loss, usually achieved by a combination of extreme dieting, exercise and, less commonly, self-induced vomiting. Misuse of laxatives and other weight-reducing substances (e.g. diuretics, thyroxine) also occurs.

Table 55.5 DSM-IV diagnostic criteria for anorexia nervosa, bulimia nervosa and eating disorder not otherwise specified (EDNOS).

Anorexia nervosa

- A refusal to maintain body weight at or above a minimally normal weight for age and height (e.g. weight loss leading to a maintenance of body weight less than 85% of that expected, or failure to make expected weight gain during period of growth, leading to body weight less than 85% of that expected)
- Intense fear of gaining weight or becoming fat, even though underweight
- Disturbance in the way in which one's body weight or shape is experienced, undue influence of body weight or shape on self-evaluation, or denial of the seriousness of the current low body weight
- In postmenarchal females, amenorrhea (i.e. the absence of at least three consecutive cycles)

Bulimia nervosa

- Recurrent episodes of binge eating. An episode of binge eating is characterized by:
  (i) eating, in a discrete period of time (e.g. within any 2-hour period), an amount of food that is definitely larger than most people would eat during a similar period of time and under similar circumstances; and
  (ii) a sense of lack of control over eating during the episode
- Recurrent inappropriate compensatory behavior in order to prevent weight gain, such as: self-induced vomiting; misuse of laxatives, diuretics, enemas or other medications; fasting or excessive exercise
- The binge eating and inappropriate compensatory behaviors both occur, on average, at least twice a week for 3 months
- Self-evaluation is unduly influenced by body shape and weight
- The disturbance does not occur exclusively during episodes of anorexia nervosa

Eating disorder not otherwise specified

- All the criteria for anorexia nervosa are met except that the individual's current weight is in the normal range or, for females, regular menstruation continues
- All of the criteria for bulimia nervosa are met, except that the binge eating and inappropriate compensatory mechanisms occur at a lower frequency than that required for a full diagnosis
- Use of inappropriate compensatory behaviors by an individual of normal body weight after eating small amounts of food
- Repeatedly chewing and spitting out, but not swallowing, large amounts of food
- Binge eating disorder

Patients have a characteristic set of attitudes and values concerning body shape and weight. They complain of intense feelings of fatness, and extreme fear of loss of control over eating and consequent weight gain. They express a level of dissatisfaction with their shape and weight that is far beyond that seen in the normal population, and tend to judge their self-worth almost solely in terms of weight, shape and ability to control food intake. This is described as the "core psychopathology" of the condition. In some cases there is true body shape misperception, when a thin body shape is actually experienced as fat, although this is not a universal feature.

Anorexia nervosa usually begins in adolescence, although prepubertal and adult onset may occur. For some the natural body changes of adolescence appear to be a risk factor; it has also been reported that weight gain and then loss associated with a diagnosis of T1DM and then commencement of insulin treatment may act as a trigger.

The low weight of patients with anorexia gives rise to the physiologic and psychologic features of starvation, including ritualized eating habits, cognitive rumination about eating, irritability, poor concentration, constant feelings of cold and misery, and decreased activity. Social withdrawal and isolation is common, and anxiety, obsessional features and suicidal thoughts sometimes occur. Foods viewed as fattening are typically avoided and the diet contains an average daily intake of calories in the region of 600–900 kcal/day, with very low fat and mineral intake. In spite of this most patients continue to feel hungry, and as such the term "anorexia" is a misnomer.

Common physical symptoms include gastrointestinal complaints (constipation, fullness after eating, bloating and abdominal pain), lack of energy, reduced libido, early waking and postural dizziness. In postmenarchal females not receiving oral contraceptives, amenorrhoea is often present, with infertility and osteopenia a significant risk. Those with prepubertal onset are often small in stature and show failure of breast development. Bradycardia, hypotension and peripheral neuropathy are also reported, and a range of endocrine abnormalities may be found on investigation, including low sex hormone and tri-iodothyronine levels (with normal thyroxine and thyroid-stimulating hormone), and raised growth hormone and cortisol.

Bulimia nervosa

Bulimia nervosa is characterized by recurrent episodes of binge eating in which large amounts of food are consumed (typically 2000 kcal or more), and the individual has a feeling of being unable to control the eating. This behavior is accompanied by a range of "compensatory" behaviors designed to prevent weight gain, including dietary restriction, vomiting, exercise and misuse of laxatives or diuretics. People with bulimia seem to have broadly the same set of attitudes and beliefs to those seen in anorexia. Although most patients fall within the normal weight range, some will have a past history of underweight and may have met the diagnostic criteria for anorexia in the past, and some are overweight. The vicious cycle of dieting, bingeing, purging and fear of weight gain invariably has a detrimental impact on other aspects of functioning, such as work and social relationships, and can have financial implications resulting from the cost of the food. For some, binge eating seems to serve an important function as a means of regulating unpleasant emotional states. Some individuals also have other impulse control problems and a history of interpersonal difficulties. Depression and self-harming behaviors such as cutting, overdosing or substance misuse may occur.

Physical complications of bulimia include enlargement of the parotid glands, erosion of dental enamel and hypokalemia resulting from vomiting, laxative or diuretic misuse.

Eating disorder not otherwise specified

There is still debate about the best set of criteria to use to define this "residual" category of eating disorder. Patients may either have "partial syndromes" (they may have some but not all the features of anorexia or bulimia) or they may be "subthreshold cases" (they have a full set of clinical features, which fall below the severity threshold currently in use).

The best characterized group of patients are those with recurrent binge eating but no compensatory behavior – usually described as "binge eating disorder." Patients with this syndrome describe:

- Eating rapidly;
- Eating until uncomfortably full;
- Eating when not hungry; and
- Feeling disgusted or guilty after overeating.

Binge eating disorder is associated with obesity, and it appears to affect 5–10% of obese patients in weight loss treatment programs. Physical complications may occur as for anorexia or bulimia, depending on the precise symptom pattern of the presentation and its severity.

Impact on diabetes outcome

In addition to the clinical picture described above, patients who have both an eating disorder and diabetes manifest additional features. Early case reports in the 1970s and 1980s highlighted the fact that people with T1DM have available to them an additional means of weight control in the form of the under-use or omission of insulin. Such "self-induced glycosuria" is common but not universal in patients with eating disorders, and is now known not to be confined to patients with a frank eating disorder, being more widely observed as an occasional phenomenon in a range of weight conscious patients, mostly females. As a means of weight control, the behavior produces rapid but often not sustained weight loss, the main effect being via acute dehydration. Not surprisingly, this behavior is associated with impaired glycemic control, and probably a higher risk of microvascular and macrovascular complications if it persists. Such patients are particularly likely to be admitted to hospital with ketoacidosis [51].

Epidemiology

Estimates of prevalence for eating disorders in the general population remain imprecise because of a lack of systematic study. It is thought that about 1 in 250 females and 1 in 1000 males will experience anorexia, usually during adolescence or early adult life. Bulimia is thought to be much more common: in community studies 0.5–1% of young women have been found to be affected. EDNOS appears to be much more common than anorexia or bulimia, and is the most common presentation seen in routine clinical practice.

Diabetes as a risk factor for the development of an eating disorder

The causes of eating disorders are incompletely understood. Dieting appears to be an important risk factor, although only a small proportion of all those who diet go on to develop a disorder. Other known risk factors include a history of obesity, and premorbid traits including perfectionism and low self-esteem. Family relationships are often disturbed, although this may be either a cause or consequence of the disorder, or both. Genetic risks have also been identified.

Case history 3: Eating disorders and diabetes

Helen is a 20-year-old student with a 3-year history of disturbed eating habits and attitudes. She developed type 1 diabetes at the age of 11. She displayed extreme concerns about her shape and weight, despite have a body mass index well within the normal range. She had experienced weight gain during puberty, which she had found distressing, and had managed by reducing her insulin dosage, diet and exercise. She had continued to reduce or omit her insulin dosage intermittently since, and in the last 3 years had begun to vomit food occasionally, and to have episodes of binge eating. Details of these clinical features remained hidden from the diabetes team until a specialist nurse noticed that she seemed upset at a clinic visit, and arranged a follow-up home visit for a lengthy discussion about her diabetes management. It was subsequently noticed at the next clinic visit that Helen had developed mild retinopathy and proteinuria. Referral to the eating disorder services was made, and a course of cognitive–behavior therapy was offered in an outpatient setting.

There has been a strong clinical impression for many years that eating disorders are over-represented in people with diabetes, and several studies have been conducted to address this. Although both diabetes and eating disorders are common conditions, and so a degree of co-occurrence by chance is expected, there are some theoretical grounds to expect eating disorders to occur more commonly in people with diabetes. The following have been suggested as risk factors:

- The stress of living with a chronic disease;
- The availability of a means of rapid weight control via insulin misuse;
- Prescription of a rigid dietary regimen; and
- The experience of marked weight fluctuation around the time of diagnosis of diabetes.

Insulin treatment itself can lead to weight gain and adjustment of insulin dose through the pubertal period in females is notoriously difficult. In contrast, there may also be protective factors that operate; most notable of these is close medical and family surveillance during the period of highest risk of behaviors such as vomiting and bingeing.

Early studies appeared to support the contention that prevalence was raised in people with diabetes, but these studies had many methodologic shortcomings including use of non-validated assessment measures, recruitment of highly selected populations from specialist diabetes clinics (mainly in the USA) and the absence of well-matched control groups. More recent studies and analyses using better methods of assessing the full range of diagnoses, including EDNOS, have indicated that there may be a slightly raised prevalence in diabetic populations, although the increase in risk appears to be modest if assessed by cross-sectional prevalence comparisons (around a threefold increase for bulimia and a doubling for EDNOS) [50].

Longitudinal studies have now shown that for most patients eating disorder diagnoses are unstable over time, and cross-sectional studies underestimate the proportion of the population that may be affected in the long run. Incidence rates in adolescent and young adult patients are higher than previously estimated, and it is clear that such disorders, especially if persistent, are a major cause of poor outcome in people with diabetes [51]. Rates of serious microvascular and macrovascular complications and mortality are significantly increased in these cohorts, even in those patients whose eating disorder features are relatively short-lived. It appears that adolescence and young adulthood is a particularly vulnerable time for people with T1DM, and even short periods of poor control can have serious consequences in middle and later adult life.

Questions to ask to establish possible eating disorder features

- What is your current weight?
- What would be your ideal weight?
- Are you happy with the shape of your body?
- If not, why not?
- Would you prefer to be a different weight or shape?
- If so, what would you wish to change?
- Do you do anything to control your weight or body shape?
- If so, what do you do?

If appropriate:

- Do you diet?
- Are there any foods that you particularly avoid?
- Do you ever feel that your eating is out of control?
- Have you ever vomited food to avoid weight gain?

Management

Detection

Although some people with diabetes may volunteer information about eating problems, many will be secretive as a result of factors including denial, guilt or shame. Thus, an essential first step in management is successful detection of the problem. It is important to note that, although eating disorders are generally associated with poor self-care and erratic glycemic control, alternating periods of hypoglycemia and hyperglycemia may be undetected by a screening test such as HbA_{1c}. Warning symptoms include the following:

- Marked weight fluctuation or loss;
- Symptoms of hyperglycemia (thirst or tiredness);
- Frequent episodes of ketoacidosis (often requiring hospital admission) or hypoglycemia leading to loss of consciousness;
- Growth retardation and pubertal delay may be seen in younger patients with T1DM.

Unfortunately, most of these features are not specific for eating disorders and are only indicative of poor self-care. The only way to establish a diagnosis of an eating disorder is by means of a clinical interview, although brief self-report scales do exist and may be a useful means of screening. Unfortunately, none have been validated specifically for use with people with diabetes, and many contain items (e.g. "I always avoid foods with sugar in them") that may be contaminated by the presence of diabetes. Sensitive but direct questions related to eating habits and attitudes, concerns about body weight and methods of weight control should be asked.

Principles of treatment

There is a lack of primary research to guide the treatment of patients with an eating disorder and diabetes, and advice is therefore based on existing guidelines for patients without diabetes such as the one by NICE [52]. Dietary counseling by a dietitian or specialist nurse may be a helpful first step, especially for those with milder disorders, but most cases will require specialist help. Guided self-help appears to be a viable option as a first step for patients with bulimia. In all cases, close liaison between the therapist managing the eating disorder and the team managing the diabetes will be required. Eating disorder treatment needs to be enhanced with attention to the following:

- Insulin or medication use;
- Glycemic control;
- Diabetes-related dietary restrictions;
- Relationships with family and medical staff; and
- Feelings about having diabetes.

Although most patients can be managed on an outpatient basis, the risk of impaired physical health necessitating inpatient admission is increased in people with diabetes. Regular physical monitoring is needed to manage the high risk of complications and mortality [53].

Anorexia nervosa

The evidence base for the treatment of anorexia remains surprisingly weak. A necessary first step for all patients is restoration of weight towards normal levels. During this process it is usually necessary to accept that glycemic control may not be perfect, but severe hypoglycemia or hyperglycemia must be avoided. The patient will need to monitor insulin dose and blood glucose levels as eating habits and weight change. It is essential that the eating disorder therapist has a good knowledge of the principles of treatment for diabetes.

Bulimia nervosa

Treatment for bulimia, particularly by means of cognitive–behavioral therapy (CBT) has been widely researched, although the suitability of CBT for people with diabetes has been subjected to much less study. The coexistence of diabetes with bulimia inevitably complicates management. Successfully engaging patients in treatment may itself be more difficult, and approaches such as motivational interviewing may have a role in future [54]. Modification to the standard treatment approach includes the monitoring of self-care behaviors, and it is desirable that the eating disorder therapist has knowledge and experience of the standard management of diabetes. Conflict may arise between the modifications to eating behavior usually advocated for the treatment of bulimia (promoting a more flexible approach to eating) and the dietary advice often given for management of diabetes (regular controlled eating and avoidance of certain food groups). The development of the approach known as DAFNE (diabetes adjusted for normal eating) may offer a solution to this dilemma [55].

Other forms of treatment for bulimia include interpersonal psychotherapy, and the use of antidepressant drugs. Although clinical trials are lacking, there is a clinical impression that medication may be a useful adjunct to psychologic treatment for some patients. A group educational program for patients with bulimia and T1DM was shown to be better than "standard care" in improving eating behavior, but did not lead to improvements in glycemic control [56]. Inpatient treatment has also been evaluated for this group, and appeared to be successful, although the applicability of this approach in most health care systems remains to be tested.

Eating disorder not otherwise specified

Little is known about the optimum management of patients with these more prevalent but less severe forms of eating disturbance. Similar approaches to those used for anorexia and bulimia are usually tried.

Treatment of children and adolescents

Cross-sectional studies investigating the association between family environment, eating problems and diabetes outcomes suggest that family factors have a particularly important role in younger patients. Family-based interventions addressing issues such as limit setting, communication skills and development of self-esteem may be particularly appropriate and helpful for this group. Family interventions in young people without diabetes are known to be more effective in treating eating disorders than individual therapy.

Other disorders

Several other forms of psychiatric or psychological disorder may be important in the management of people with diabetes (see Chapter 49). Needle phobia fortunately appears to be rare among insulin-treated patients, although if it does occur (usually early in treatment) it can create considerable difficulties. It appears to be usually relatively easy to treat using behavioral principles.

Sexual dysfunction is common, and differential diagnosis between organic and psychologic factors can sometimes be difficult, but psychologic factors are usually important and again relatively easy to address using psychologic treatment.

Substance misuse and dependence, and personality disorder, can prove resistant to treatment and create considerable management challenges. Historically, the term "brittle diabetes" has been used to describe patients with unexplained poor metabolic control. It is now recognized that psychologic and behavioral factors are usually the most important causes of this.

Conclusions

This chapter has highlighted the many and various ways in which diabetes and psychiatric disorders can interact. It is clear that such disorders can have a major impact on diabetes outcomes, and health professionals who work with patients with diabetes require good knowledge and awareness of these issues to be able to provide optimal care. There is clearly also a great need for closer working between diabetes services and mental health services. Further research on these topics is clearly required.

References

1 Maudsley H. *The Pathology of Mind.* 1879.

2 Ciechanowski PS, Katon WJ, Russo JE, Hirsch IB. The relationship of depressive symptoms to symptom reporting, self-care and glucose control in diabetes. *Gen Hosp Psychiatry* 2003; **25**:246–52.

3 American Psychiatric Association. *Diagnostic and Statistical Manual of Mental Disorders, 4th edition.* Washington DC: American Psychiatric Association, 2005.

4 Murray CJ, Lopez AD. Alternative projections of mortality and disability by cause 1990–2020: Global Burden of Disease Study. *Lancet* 1997; **349**:1498–1504.

5 Barnard KD, Skinner TC, Peveler R. The prevalence of co-morbid depression in adults with type 1 diabetes: systematic literature review. *Diabet Med* 2006; **23**:445–448.

6 Nichols GA, Brown JB. Unadjusted and adjusted prevalence of diagnosed depression in type 2 diabetes. *Diabetes Care* 2003; **26**:744–749.

7 Knol MJ, Twisk JW, Beekman AT, Heine RJ, Snoek FJ, Pouwer F. Depression as a risk factor for the onset of type 2 diabetes mellitus: a meta-analysis. *Diabetologia* 2006; **49**:837–845.

8 Fisher L, Chesla CA, Mullan JT, Skaff MM, Kanter RA. Contributors to depression in Latino and European-American people with type 2 diabetes. *Diabetes Care* 2001; **24**:1751–1757.

9 Newsome CA, Shiell AW, Fall CH, Phillips DI, Shier R, Law CM. Is birth weight related to later glucose and insulin metabolism? A systematic review. *Diabet Med* 2003; **20**:339–348.

10 Thompson C, Syddall H, Rodin I, Osmond C, Barker DJ. Birth weight and the risk of depressive disorder in late life. *Br J Psychiatry* 2001; **179**:450–455.

11 Brown AS, Susser ES, Lin SP, Neugebauer R, Gorman JM. Increased risk of affective disorders in males after second trimester prenatal exposure to the Dutch hunger winter of 1944–45. *Br J Psychiatry* 1995; **166**:601–606.

12 Mukherjee S, Schnur DB, Reddy R. Family history of type 2 diabetes in schizophrenic patients. *Lancet* 1989; **1**:495.

13 Gough SCL, O'Donovan MC. Clustering of metabolic comorbidity in schizophrenia: a genetic contribution? *J Psychopharmacol Suppl* 2005; **19**:47–55.

14 Ross R. Atherosclerosis: an inflammatory disease. *N Engl J Med* 1999; **340**:115–126.

15 Musselman DL, Betan E, Larsen H, Phillips LS. Relationship of depression to diabetes types 1 and 2: epidemiology, biology, and treatment. *Biol Psychiatry* 2003; **54**:317–329.

16 Lustman PJ, Anderson RJ, Freedland KE, Carney RM, Clouse RE. Depression and poor glycemic control: a meta-analytic review of the literature. *Diabetes Care* 2000; **23**:934–942.

17 de Groot M, Anderson R, Freedland KE, Clouse RE, Lustman PJ. Association of depression and diabetes complications: a meta-analysis. *Psychosom Med* 2001; **63**:619–630.

18 Kovacs M, Mukerji P, Drash A, Iyengar S. Biomedical and psychiatric risk factors for retinopathy among children with IDDM. *Diabetes Care* 1995; **18**:1592–1599.

19 Katona C, Peveler R, Dowrick C, Wessely S, Feinmann C, Gask L, *et al.* Pain symptoms in depression: definition and clinical significance. *Clin Med* 2005; **5**:390–395.

20 Department of Health. *Delivering Investment in General Practice: Implementing the New GMS Contract.* London: Department of Health, 2003.

21 National Collaborating Centre for Chronic Conditions. Royal College of Physicians. *Type 1 Diabetes in Adults: National Clinical Guideline for Diagnosis and Management in Primary and Secondary Care.* London: National Institute for Health and Clinical Excellence, 2004.

22 Kroenke K, Spitzer RL, Williams JB. The PHQ-9: validity of a brief depression severity measure. *J Gen Intern Med* 2001; **16**:606–613.

23 Zigmond AS, Snaith RP. The hospital anxiety and depression scale. *Acta Psychiatr Scand* 1983; **67**:361–370.

24 Beck AT, Ward CH, Mendelson M, Mock J, Erbaugh J. An inventory for measuring depression. *Arch Gen Psychiatry* 1961; **4**:561.

25 Lowe B, Kroenke K, Grafe K. Detecting and monitoring depression with a two-item questionnaire (PHQ-2). *J Psychosom Res* 2005; **58**:163–171.

26 National Collaborating Centre for Mental Health. *Depression: Management of Depression in Primary and Secondary Care.* Clinical Guideline 23. London: National Institue for Health and Clinical Excellence, 2004.

27 Simon GE, Katon WJ, VonKorff M, Unutzer J, Lin EH, Walker EA, *et al.* Cost-effectiveness of a collaborative care program for primary care patients with persistent depression. *Am J Psychiatry* 2001; **158**:1638–1644.

28 Simon GE, Katon WJ, Lin EH, Rutter C, Manning WG, Von KM, *et al.* Cost-effectiveness of systematic depression treatment among people with diabetes mellitus. *Arch Gen Psychiatry* 2007; **64**:65–72.

29 Katon WJ, Von KM, Lin EH, Simon G, Ludman E, Russo J, *et al.* The Pathways Study: a randomized trial of collaborative care in people with diabetesand depression. *Arch Gen Psychiatry* 2004; **61**:1042–1049.

30 Ismail K, Winkley K, Rabe-Hesketh S. Systematic review and meta-analysis of randomised controlled trials of psychological interventions to improve glycaemic control in people with type 2 diabetes. *Lancet* 2004; **363**:1589–1597.

31 Winocour PH, Gosden C, Walton C, Nagi D, Turner B, Williams R, *et al.* Association of British Clinical Diabetologists (ABCD) and Diabetes-UK survey of specialist diabetes services in the UK, 2006. 1. The consultant physician perspective. *Diabet Med* 2008; **25**:643–650.

32 Kohen D. Diabetes mellitus and schizophrenia: historical perspective. *Br J Psychiatry Suppl* 2004; **47**:64–S66.

33 National Institute for Health and Clinical Excellence. *Schizophrenia: Core Interventions in the Treatment and Management of Schizophrenia in Primary and Secondary Care.* London: National Institute for Clinical Excellence, 2002.

34 Brown S, Inskip H, Barraclough B. Causes of the excess mortality of schizophrenia. *Br J Psychiatry* 2000; **177**:212–217.

35 Holt RI, Peveler RC. Antipsychotic drugs and diabetes: an application of the Austin Bradford Hill criteria. *Diabetologia* 2006; **49**:1467–1476.

36 Ryan MC, Collins P, Thakore JH. Impaired fasting glucose tolerance in first-episode, drug-naive patients with schizophrenia. *Am J Psychiatry* 2003; **160**:284–289.

37 Spelman LM, Walsh PI, Sharifi N, Collins P, Thakore JH. Impaired glucose tolerance in first-episode drug-naive patients with schizophrenia. *Diabet Med* 2007; **24**:481–485.

38 Thakore JH, Mann JN, Vlahos I, Martin A, Reznek R. Increased visceral fat distribution in drug-naive and drug-free patients with schizophrenia. *Int J Obes Relat Metab Disord* 2002; **26**:137–141.

39 Saddichha S, Manjunatha N, Ameen S, Akhtar S. Diabetes and schizophrenia: effect of disease or drug? Results from a randomized, double-blind, controlled prospective study in first-episode schizophrenia. *Acta Psychiatr Scand* 2008; **117**:342–347.

40 Sengupta S, Parrilla-Escobar MA, Klink R, Fathalli F, Ying KN, Stip E, *et al.* Are metabolic indices different between drug-naive first-episode psychosis patients and healthy controls? *Schizophr Res* 2008; **102**:329–336.

41 Arranz B, Rosel P, Ramirez N, Duenas R, Fernandez P, Sanchez JM, *et al.* Insulin resistance and increased leptin concentrations in non-compliant schizophrenia patients but not in antipsychotic-naive first-episode schizophrenia patients. *J Clin Psychiatry* 2004; **65**:1335–1342.

42 Zhang ZJ, Yao ZJ, Liu W, Fang Q, Reynolds GP. Effects of antipsychotics on fat deposition and changes in leptin and insulin levels: magnetic resonance imaging study of previously untreated people with schizophrenia. *Br J Psychiatry* 2004; **184**:58–62.

43 Graham KA, Cho H, Brownley KA, Harp JB. Early treatment-related changes in diabetes and cardiovascular disease risk markers in first episode psychosis subjects. *Schizophr Res* 2008; **101**:287–294.

44 McCreadie RG. Diet, smoking and cardiovascular risk in people with schizophrenia: descriptive study. *Br J Psychiatry* 2003; **183**:534–539.

45 Smith M, Hopkins D, Peveler RC, Holt RI, Woodward M, Ismail K. First- v. second-generation antipsychotics and risk for diabetes in schizophrenia: systematic review and meta-analysis. *Br J Psychiatry* 2008; **192**:406–411.

46 Holt RIG, Abdelrahman T, Hirsch M, Dhesi Z, George T, Blincoe T, *et al.* The prevalence of undiagnosed metabolic abnormalities in people with serious mental illness. *J Psychopharmacol* 2009 (March 20, Epub ahead of print).

47 Pendlebury J, Bushe CJ, Wildgust HJ, Holt RI. Long-term maintenance of weight loss in patients with severe mental illness through a

behavioural treatment programme in the UK. *Acta Psychiatr Scand* 2007; **115**:286–294.

48 Faulkner G, Cohn T, Remington G. Interventions to reduce weight gain in schizophrenia. *Cochrane Database Syst Rev* 2007; **1**:CD005148.

49 Knowler WC, Barrett-Connor E, Fowler SE, Hamman RF, Lachin JM, Walker EA, *et al.* Reduction in the incidence of type 2 diabetes with lifestyle intervention or metformin. *N Engl J Med* 2002; **346**:393–403.

50 Peveler R, Turner HM. Eating disorders and type 1 diabetes. In: Norring C, Palmer R, eds. *Eating Disorders Not Otherwise Specified: Scientific and Clinical Perspectives on the Other Eating Disorders*, 1st edn. Hove: Routledge, 2005.

51 Peveler RC, Bryden KS, Neil HA, Fairburn CG, Mayou RA, Dunger DB, *et al.* The relationship of disordered eating habits and attitudes to clinical outcomes in young adult females with type 1 diabetes. *Diabetes Care* 2005; **28**:84–88.

52 National Collaborating Centre for Mental Health. *Eating Disorders: Core Interventions in the Treatment and Management of Anorexia Nervosa, Bulimia Nervosa and Related Eating Disorders.* London: National Institute for Health and Clinical Excellence, 2004.

53 Peveler RC, Fairburn CG. Anorexia nervosa in association with diabetes mellitus: a cognitive–behavioural approach to treatment. *Behav Res Ther* 1989; **27**:95–99.

54 Ismail K, Thomas SM, Maissi E, Chalder T, Schmidt U, Bartlett J, *et al.* Motivational enhancement therapy with and without cognitive behavior therapy to treat type 1 diabetes: a randomized trial. *Ann Intern Med* 2008; **149**:708–719.

55 DAFNE Study Group. Training in flexible, intensive insulin management to enable dietary freedom in people with type 1 diabetes: dose adjustment for normal eating (DAFNE) randomised controlled trial. *Br Med J* 2002; **325**:746.

56 Olmsted MP, Daneman D, Rydall AC, Lawson ML, Rodin G. The effects of psychoeducation on disturbed eating attitudes and behavior in young women with type 1 diabetes mellitus. *Int J Eat Disord* 2002; **32**:230–239.

11 Delivery and Organization of Diabetes Care

56 The Role of Community and Specialist Services

Jane Overland, Margaret McGill & Dennis K. Yue
Diabetes Center, Royal Prince Alfred Hospital, Camperdown, NSW, Australia

Keypoints

- The majority of people with diabetes without complications or co-morbidities can be well managed within the community; however, people with more complicated disease warrant referral to specialists.
- How to design a system to allow most patients to remain in the community, but be referred for specialist treatment at an optimum time, is one of the most important questions in organizing diabetes care. Moreover, to rationalize diabetes care, there are many areas that will need decision-making regarding who is to do what, and at which level. There is no single correct answer as the local situation will influence the decision.
- On a worldwide basis, community care of diabetes by primary care providers is likely to provide the backbone of diabetes treatment. How to improve and support care at this level, and to what extent, is an important strategic question. If it is improved to a specialist level then its cost advantages would be minimized.
- In many areas of the world, specialist care is provided by a hospital, often characterized by a large inpatient unit supported by outpatient clinics. Provision of continuity of care for a chronic disease such as diabetes within hospitals and clinics is a task warranting a great deal of attention.
- Diabetes educators or specialist nurses can complement and enhance what doctors provide. Non-medical staff can be trained to make clinical decisions about the management of diabetes, including the management of glycemic control, hypertension and dyslipidemia, provide self-management education and coordinate team services to meet the patient's health needs, thereby taking the load from the medical staff to allow them to concentrate on more complex cases.
- In some areas of the world, diabetes education centers have been developed to support large diabetes clinics. Staff within these centers have core clinical knowledge of diabetes, as well as understanding teaching and learning principles and behavioral and psychologic strategies to help patients manage their diabetes.
- Some diabetes centers provide integrated specialist diabetes care. Clinical activities undertaken by these centers often include initiation of insulin therapy and stabilization of diabetes without need for hospitalization, screening and management of diabetes complications, management of diabetic foot disease, diabetes in pregnancy, neuropathic pain and insulin pump therapy. This "Rolls Royce" model is expensive and cannot care for every person with diabetes. It must concentrate its role in complementing, not duplicating, what the community doctors can provide. It also has a role in educating community doctors and health care professionals while demonstrating what needs to be done and can be achieved.
- Timely communication is crucial in promoting a seamless interface between community and specialist levels of care. This is most important in improving the skills of primary care health providers, and it involves more than just providing factual information on the level of HbA_{1c} and insulin dosage.

Introduction

The World Health Organization's Declaration of Alma Ata, adopted in 1978, expressed the need to protect and promote the health of all peoples of the world. The Declaration highlighted the inequity between developed and low and middle income countries. Despite the number of decades that has passed since this Declaration, providing appropriate care for all people with diabetes remains problematic. Conclusive evidence now exists that the devastating complications of diabetes can be minimized by timely and effective treatment; however, even in developed countries, with universally funded health services, large proportions of people with diabetes are not routinely monitored either for diabetes or its complications [1]. This is especially so for people living in rural areas [2–5], or for those who are socially disadvantaged [6]. This means that the opportunity to commence early treatment is missed. Today it is estimated that only 5% of people living with diabetes around the world receive optimal care [7]. While clinicians endeavor to provide the best possible treatment, there are often serious limitations stemming from resource availability and/or inadequate models of care.

Textbook of Diabetes, 4th edition. Edited by R. Holt, C. Cockram, A. Flyvbjerg and B. Goldstein.

Globally, the spectrum of diabetes services varies from a single health care provider working in an isolated community setting, to small groups of primary care doctors and nurses working in health centers or district hospitals, through to highly sophisticated tertiary units in major urban areas with access to a range of specialists, nurses and other diabetes team members. In this chapter we explore how diabetes care may be best delivered at these various levels, taking into consideration political, cultural and economic environments. Not every case of diabetes can be looked after at the community level. Likewise, not every case of diabetes can be managed at the specialist level. How to support and to balance these two extremes is one of the most important questions in organizing diabetes care.

Primary care for diabetes

Primary care in the community forms an integral part of health care in most countries and is the first level of contact for most people with diabetes. The sheer number of people with diabetes would dictate this to be a necessity. How we improve diabetes care at this level is therefore a matter of great importance. What is considered primary care may vary a great deal between countries, or within regions of the same country. Likewise, improving primary care for diabetes may take on different meanings in different settings.

On a world basis, primary care is usually provided by a doctor, acting alone and almost invariably also treating many other diseases. In many ways, diabetes is just a condition that the patient "happens to have," and its management can be surreptitiously relegated to a lesser role than the problem of the day. Various attempts have been made to overcome these issues, and it is beyond the scope of this chapter to outline them all, but some examples are mentioned here.

In many countries, primary care is delivered through a system of health centers or clinics which are scattered throughout urban and rural areas. Appropriately supported, these centers can provide routine diabetes management to most people with diabetes within a local area, but require the ability to refer more complicated cases, such as patients with newly diagnosed type 1 diabetes mellitus (T1DM) or those with an active foot problem.

The success of this approach was exemplified by a randomized cluster trial conducted in the Torres Strait, which is located between Australia and Papua New Guinea, and inhabited by indigenous Australians scattered over a wide area in small communities [8]. The study aimed to implement a sustainable system of care by providing basic training in clinical diabetes care to local indigenous health workers employed in randomly selected health centers. The study team also assisted local staff within these centers to establish diabetes registers and recall systems, and to develop diabetes care plans. Diabetes specialist outreach services were established concurrently for all health centers within the Torres Strait, and were designed to facilitate referral and provide care for individuals with more complicated disease. It also provided a secondary benefit for local staff to learn up-to-date diabetes management principles through working alongside the diabetes specialist during visits to the health centers. It was found that diabetes care processes improved in all health centers and the intervention sites showed greatest progress, with significant improvements in weight, blood pressure and glycemic control measures. Moreover, people with diabetes managed by the intervention clinics were 40% less likely to be admitted to hospital for a diabetes-related condition. Over time, local service providers have assumed increasing responsibility for routine diabetes care, thus ensuring sustainability of the service.

The ability of organizational change to improve diabetes care processes and clinical outcomes at the primary care level has been further emphasized by the recently reported TRANSLATE trial [9]. The multicomponent organization intervention adopted within this trial, which included implementation of an electronic diabetes registry, visit reminders and patient-specific physician alerts, resulted in a significant increase in the proportion of patients achieving recommended clinical outcomes.

Tanzania provides a further example of implementing a well-organized system of care at the community level. Prior to 2004, for a general population of 39 million, specialized diabetes care was available in just five referral hospitals nationally, and was provided by a handful of consultant physicians and diabetes educators. Access to diagnosis and treatment, particularly in rural areas, was extremely limited. With support of the Ministry of Health and the Tanzanian Diabetes Association, teams of health care workers from all regional hospitals, comprising a doctor, two nurses and a laboratory technician, were offered comprehensive diabetes training programs. After training, each team was given a starter kit containing diagnostic and educational tools in order to help establish services. By 2006, 29 diabetes clinics had been established, providing accessible and affordable treatment and education services to more than 100 000 people [5]. This model of care is consistent with the World Health Organization's aim of sustainable interventions by helping countries develop their own infrastructure and professional expertise in health care. It will enable Tanzania to continue to progress independently towards providing sustainable and accessible diabetes care in the long term, and can serve as a model for other low and middle income countries.

Since 1993, general practitioners (GPs) in the UK have been encouraged to develop services for diabetes, with a specific payment for doctors offering structured diabetes care. As a result, the proportion of people with diabetes reviewed annually in primary care has increased. Interestingly, Norway also report improvements in processes of diabetes care over a similar time period, without additional incentives for GPs to follow national guidelines. In the case of Norway, the improvement was attributed to ongoing medical education [10]. In Germany, a diabetes management program was introduced in 2003, the core content of which was defined by a national expert panel. Program initiatives included the use evidence-based guidelines and the development of a basic data set, establishment of quality indicators, as well as recall of patients. Fulfilment of program recommendations is compulsory for contracts between health insurers and service providers. By mid-2007, approximately 50% of the estimated population with diabetes, and approximately 65% of family practices, had enrolled in the program. A recently reported survey showed that patients being managed under the program perceived improved care [11].

In Australia, the government funds a chronic disease management program in general practice. Under this program it has been made easier financially for GPs to employ a practice nurse to help with various tasks of managing patients, including but not exclusive to diabetes. Many doctors use these practice nurses to complete the annual cycle of diabetes care, which includes periodic examination of the feet, and ensuring other diabetes complications and metabolic variables are regularly assessed. In recognition of the fact that GPs often encounter difficulties in securing the services of allied health professionals for their patients, the Australian government has also begun a subsidy, through the universal health insurance system, for five allied health visits a year, and made such referrals the prerogative of GPs only. These initiatives are obviously in the right direction from the individual doctor's and patient's point of view. Conceptually, they are elevating primary care for a particular disease to a level close to specialist care. Whether this is true primary care or just specialist care in another guise is debatable. The irony for the health care planner is that if primary care for diabetes becomes progressively better, it may become progressively more like specialist care and thus lose its cost–benefit advantage. Whether this move would translate into better clinical endpoints and provide overall cost–benefits for the treatment of diabetes for the entire community needs to be evaluated.

Traditional specialist care

Hospital clinic

In many areas around the world most diabetes care is provided by a hospital, often characterized by a large inpatient unit supported by outpatient clinics. While some hospitals have diabetes-specific outpatient services, many people with diabetes are seen within the context of a large general medical clinic. Although specialists are often nominally in charge in this setting, and the clinic is considered a specialized diabetes clinic, much of the time the duty of actually seeing people with diabetes is delegated to junior and rotating medical staff. Typically, nursing staff undertake process tasks such as preparing medical records, measuring the patient's height and weight, and testing blood glucose levels. Many of these clinics are not formatted to cope with caring for people with a chronic disease, and entrenched but unsuitable systems, often as a result of hospital regulations, such as only providing patients with a few weeks' supply of medications, mean that clinics are overwhelmed by people attending to have a prescription written. This ultimately leads to shorter consultation times to cope with increased throughput of clinic attendees. As a consequence, care tends not to be patient-focused nor up-to-date, resulting in poor clinical outcomes.

Simple policy changes can improve diabetes care without imposing too much of a cost penalty. For example, if the rationale for writing monthly (or even shorter) prescriptions is because of cost or supply chain issues, doctors can write a prescription valid for several months that can be dispensed monthly by the hospital pharmacist. This will free up the clinic considerably. Another example that can improve continuity of care is to link the rotating junior doctors' clinics with someone more permanent. At least patients will see someone familiar, and if they have a particularly difficult diabetic problem (be it medical, such as insulin allergy, or psychosocial, such as poor family support), at least the junior rotating doctor could be told beforehand about it by the senior consultant who is next door.

A further step that can improve diabetes care within the traditional system is to allocate nurses to the specialized position of diabetes educator or diabetes specialist nurse, so they can complement and enhance what the doctors provide. For this to be successful, it is important their roles are separate to the clinic nurse, and not just be seen as "an additional pair of hands" to help with routine clinic or ward duties. Rather, they should be employed to provide education regarding self-management principles to either inpatients or outpatients, or a combination of both. In some cases their role may be fully dedicated to educating patients; however, with further training, the specialist nurse can well provide many areas of diabetes management [12–16]. These staff can be trained to make clinical decisions about the management of diabetes, including management of glycemic control, hypertension and dyslipidemia, provide self-management education, and coordinate team services to meet the patient's health needs. Utilizing nursing staff to provide many of the routine clinical services is less expensive than using medical staff, and takes the load from the medical staff so they can concentrate on more complex cases. Indeed, studies comparing clinical outcomes from protocol driven, nurse-led clinics with traditional physician-led clinics have shown care is no worse in a nurse or allied health driven system [13–16]; however, the success of this approach may lie in the careful selection of staff. Recognizing the advanced skills of the diabetes specialist nurse, both through a career structure and improved financial incentives, is important to ensure continuity of staff. There is also a need to convince nursing and hospital administrators of the importance of the specialist nurse role so that trained staff are permanently maintained within their specialist area.

Traditional diabetes clinics have often been considered to be antiquated. However, they can be made to work, and realistically they are likely to remain the backbone of specialist diabetes care worldwide. However, for them to be effective, there are organizational and system issues to which the senior doctor in the clinic must pay attention, rather than limiting his/her role to a medical one only.

Private specialist diabetes care

In many areas around the world, a system of private specialist diabetes care exists to offer choice and to reduce some of the burden on public funded services. Subsidy or insurance of private health services is often available, but patients may be faced with a co-payment if their diabetes practitioner charges above the subsidized fee. These costs are a major barrier to many patients receiving the level and type of care they require [17], particularly when multiple specialists are involved. In the majority of cases, private services are run by solo practitioners, and access to support services provided by allied health professionals is also costly. In many ways, similar to their primary care counterparts, the private specialists face the same difficulty of providing multidisciplinary care required by some patients with diabetes.

Integrated specialist care

Specialist diabetes care can also be provided in a more integrated and multidisciplinary manner, addressing not only glucose control, but also complications and co-morbidities of diabetes, involving doctors as well as allied health professionals. The health and cost benefits of such integrated specialist care have been reported by the Steno Hospital [18–26], although it is difficult to evaluate the magnitude of benefits by controlled clinical trials. It is also not clear how much of the reported benefit was brought about by multidisciplinary involvement, and how much by multifaceted treatment.

Such integrated care is often conveniently provided at a diabetes center, an entity that is distinct from the diabetes clinic. To appreciate the full potential of a diabetes center, it is worthwhile noting its heterogeneous nature. Although many facilities may function under the same generic name, they can differ quite considerably. Initially, the role of diabetes centers was to provide diabetes education. For many this remains their primary function, and diabetes education center is perhaps a more appropriate name. These education centers have generally been developed to support large diabetes clinics, and are usually located separately from where medical consultations are made. In this model, clinical care is provided by physicians and patient self-management education is conducted by other diabetes team members. These team members need to have core clinical knowledge of diabetes, understand teaching and learning principles, as well as behavioral and psychologic strategies to help patients to manage their diabetes. It is a system of care repeated in many countries around the world, and can be highly successful in meeting the clinical, educational and psychologic needs of the person with diabetes and their family.

Toward the other end of the spectrum, a diabetes center can incorporate clinical activities. In this manner the duties of doctors and other health professionals become more integrated, co-located and co-dependent. This is the model we have relied on extensively at Royal Prince Alfred Hospital in Sydney for the last two to three decades. Initially, a prime motive of such initiatives was initiation of insulin therapy and stabilization of diabetes without the need for hospitalization, duties largely provided by diabetes nurses, but with the backing of doctors. Over the years more specialized clinical services, such as screening and management of diabetes complications, diabetic foot disease, diabetes in pregnancy, neuropathic pain and use of insulin pump treatment have been progressively added to the services provided by our diabetes center. In many of these activities, nursing and allied health professionals have such a specialized role that the doctor's function can become a supporting as well as a supervisory one. We have found nursing and allied health professionals to be better in these roles than rotating doctors, if for nothing else because patients appreciate more continuity. Conceptually, there is no reason why one good doctor cannot provide all these services to their patients, and we have indeed witnessed some who were able to do so, but in our experience it is logistically difficult. In many ways, in our system there are many specialists that make up the team, but not all of them are doctors. This concept, for example, of a nurse being more "specialized" in a clinical area of diabetes management than a doctor, is sometime difficult for the traditionalist to understand, or with which to feel comfortable.

To provide such specialized services, diabetes center staff members require ongoing training which is at one time more specialized, and yet also broader in scope, philosophically identical to that required by their medical counterparts undergoing specialist training. For example, in addition to understanding general diabetes and dietary principles, dietitians working in a clinical diabetes center need to be expert in insulin adjustment and hypoglycemic unawareness in order to be able to help a patient who is learning carbohydrate counting. Another example is the nurse who is helping the patient to adjust insulin dosage. Such nurses must be familiar with the findings of recent clinical trials such as the ACCORD Study [27] to individualize the level of glycemic control required by that individual.

By its very "Rolls Royce" nature, this type of integrated specialist diabetes care is more resource hungry. By creating such "super centers" there will be constant ambivalence between balancing state of the art services and providing day-to-day diabetes care to a large number of people. Because of resource constraints, this will always be a problem, and it is even worse for a unit that is dependent on throughput for its funding. This dilemma will necessitate a rational debate of who needs specialist care and what this entails.

Sharing the burden of diabetes between community care and specialist care

Many aspects of diabetes management can be very capably provided at the community level [28,29]. It therefore makes sense for the majority of patients without complications or co-morbidities of diabetes to be managed within the community; however, patients with more complicated disease warrant referral to specialists, depending on their individual need. For containment of cost, not surprisingly, virtually all governments embrace this position.

While conceptually sound and obvious, a seamless delivery for such a division of labor is not easy to achieve. It is relatively easy for primary care doctors to notice poor glycemic control. By contrast, patients with complications or risk factors of complications, but who are unaware of their existence, do not readily identify themselves. Various guidelines from learned bodies therefore promote the concept of regular screening for diabetes complications. In Australia, the government rewards primary care doctors with additional remuneration if a patient with diabetes has completed a cycle of care, including assessment for glycemic control and diabetes complications, within a certain timeframe. This push towards primary care, coupled with the natural expectation of a better standard of care, would increase the use of specialized services such as ophthalmology and podiatry, amongst others. Ironically, much of the cost saving of seeing a primary care doctor rather than a specialist may be lost in this manner.

Improving synergism between primary and specialist care

A possible solution is the system we have used at the diabetes center of the Royal Prince Alfred Hospital in Sydney. We rely on a shared care system to partition responsibilities between primary care doctors and specialists, and have established a complication assessment service to underpin such a sharing arrangement [29]. In one visit, patients referred by primary care doctors have examination of the fundi, testing of foot sensation and reflexes, quantitation of albuminuria, assessment of lipid profile and other cardiac risk factors, as well as examination of pedal and carotid pulses. This allows the primary care doctors to provide routine diabetes management for the majority of patients, and to make appropriate referrals to specialists when necessary.

A recent study comparing outcomes of patients managed by our model with those of patients attending traditional specialist services found that the adherence to management guidelines in our shared care model was superior to traditional specialist care. Moreover, a significantly higher proportion of patients managed under the shared care model, achieved an HbA_{1c} within 1% (11 mmol/mol) of normal range, and/or a blood pressure at target [30]. This would suggest that the majority of people with diabetes do not need to see a specialist service in the traditional 3–4 monthly cycle to receive similar quality of care. Apart from achieving good endpoints of glycemic control and complication detection, this system is more cost effective because specialists services such as ophthalmologists and nephrologists are generally only sought when recommended by a diabetes specialist.

It is worthwhile to note particular issues that can make such a system maximally effective. The specialist team that examines the patients and reports to the primary care doctor must have good clinical skills and judgment in managing the various complications of diabetes. This will allow diabetes specialists to provide more precise recommendations about the timing of referrals to other specialists, or indeed to provide appropriate treatment of some complications themselves. For example, the ability of the diabetes specialist to recognize not only retinopathy in a particular patient, but also be confident that it is not vision-threatening for the foreseeable future, may appropriately delay the referral to an ophthalmologist until later. It also offers a cost advantage. During 2008, our center screened over 2400 patients, 237 of whom were found to have retinopathy. The cost to the health system for the screen-negative patients to have been seen by an ophthalmologist would have been close to $AUD150 000. A further example is the ability to identify the occasional patient with non-diabetes-related neuropathic pain; this may save many other patients with typical diabetes neuropathic pain from unnecessary referral to neurologists.

To maximize the effectiveness of this system further, the diabetes center team must also know what a particular primary care doctor is capable of, or willing to do, in the management of diabetes. This will help to decide how much of the care of a patient should be returned to the primary care level. This differential approach to shared care cannot be easily written in a guideline, and can only be established through years of contact with primary care doctors in the community.

There are many other approaches to facilitate complementary primary and specialist diabetes care. For example, telemedicine has been shown to be a useful tool in linking community health services with specialist services. At our center, telemedicine is used in the management of diabetic foot disease, and facilitates routine and urgent consultations between our urban diabetes center and rural sites. Routine consultations are organized by prior arrangement without the patient needing to be present. The process includes the advanced emailing of standardized digital images of the patient's foot for the center's foot team to review before phone linkup. The images are displayed on computer monitors at both sites during the phone linkup and a patient management plan developed, which is then implemented locally. Urgent consultations are booked on demand, and at least one person from the diabetes center foot team is available for immediate advice until further review can be arranged. This system minimizes unnecessary patient travel, facilitates routine clinical care, and allows for urgent consultations, as well as providing ongoing training for community health professionals regarding diabetic foot disease. Such a system has the potential for use in countries where diabetic foot services are limited [31]. Another example is the development of mobile diabetes buses in India [32]. Retinal photographs taken in rural locations are beamed by satellite to specialist diabetes services for their opinion regarding the need for laser therapy. This service is financially supported by local charities and donations from other international organizations, and involves partnerships with government satellite organizations and private medical centers.

Rethinking diabetes care

To rationalize diabetes care, decisions will need to be made in many areas regarding who is to do what, and at which level. There is no single correct answer, since the local situation influences the decision; nevertheless some pertinent examples and relevant points can be raised. For example, emotion would often dictate that the management of gestational diabetes should be at the specialist level; however, the large numbers of women with this diagnosis has the potential to overwhelm diabetes pregnancy clinics. This places increased pressure on staff, and means that women with pre-existing T1DM and type 2 diabetes mellitus (T2DM) may not receive the level of care they need. The morbidity of gestational diabetes is relatively low in comparison with T1DM and T2DM. A better use of resources would be to provide the care for women with gestational diabetes in the community, with appropriate protocols and guidelines to ensure referral to specialist services as required.

Treatment of diabetic foot disease is another example of how care between the community and the specialist services needs to be carefully partitioned, depending on the individual's degree of risk. Guidelines often suggest that all those with diabetes should have their feet assessed and managed by podiatrists. This will place great stress on the availability of podiatrists when their service is better directed to high risk individuals, especially those with active foot lesions. It is better to assign the level of care depending on whether a patient has risk factors for foot ulceration, such as impaired sensation or peripheral circulation, and whether there are active foot lesions. This would allow patients with foot ulceration, severe foot infection and Charcot arthropathy to receive the specialized attention they need.

The care of people with T1DM is challenging. They need more multidisciplinary care, such as dietary counseling of carbohydrate counting or intensive teaching in the use of insulin infusion pumps. These skills are not readily available in the community. The lower prevalence of T1DM also means that most primary care doctors do not have enough exposure to this group of patients to gain experience. Therefore, this group of individuals is probably better managed at the specialist level.

There is also the broader (and economically the most important) question of who should look after the glycemic control for the majority of people with T2DM. There is a great deal of uncertainty about the optimal line of division between primary care and specialist care, both from medical and economic points of view. A reflection of this uncertainty is the ongoing debate on how guidelines on the treatment of T2DM should be framed. There are some who believe that an HbA_{1c} target of <7% (<53 mmol/mol) should be adopted because, amongst other reasons, this is what can reasonably be expected at the primary care level. Others believe that this approach is not individualized enough, and could potentially discourage specialists and patients from aiming for even better glycemic control, even when it is appropriate.

Communication between primary and specialist care

Timely communication is crucial in promoting a seamless interface between primary and specialist care. In our system, we have relied for many years on a report that is a hybrid of a computer report, containing numerical and factual data, supplemented by three free text messages addressing issues related to, respectively:

1 Glycemic control;
2 Complication status and management; and
3 Other important issues.

The messages are intended to provide a management plan and explanation for proposed actions. An example of this report is shown in Figures 56.1 and 56.2. Apart from serving the purpose of documentation and communication, the sending of this report for every patient who attends is, in our opinion, a powerful tool to update our primary care physicians regarding our policy of treatment, and the latest trend in diabetes management. This encourages them to adopt our strategies of diabetes management for other patients; thus, in a de facto way, promoting a more uniform treatment policy for the community. An example of this is our usual practice of maintaining oral antidiabetic agents when we commence someone on insulin treatment. Primary care doctors from out of our area often consider this to be a mistake, and stop the oral agents, while doctors in our area are more than happy to go along with it, having had it explained to them in the past.

In this age of advanced telecommunication, it is possible to communicate through a centralized web-based database, or similar systems to which various health professionals could have access. Technology that enables immediate access to test results means that the clinical consultation is enhanced. For example, a chronic care program conducted in rural Pennsylvania established information systems in the community that allowed for rapid turn around of laboratory results. Local physicians were made responsible for collecting and responding to data, resulting in improved patient outcomes [33]. Patient tracking systems for regular follow-up have also been shown to improve quality of care at the process level and to decrease the number of patients lost to follow-up [13,34–36]; however, while these systems can undoubtedly be helpful in transmitting factual information, they are not as good for individualized advice, which we believe to be the essence of cementing a good community and specialist relationship.

The future challenge

The challenge ahead is to provide accessible and affordable quality care to an increasing number of people with diabetes. If diabetes care is to achieve the health care benefits that the diabetes research described in this textbook has made possible, it must be tackled at both the community and specialist levels. In this regard, the complementarity of primary and specialist care has a pivotal role and is a relationship that must be carefully considered by health care planners.

Diabetes Centre
Royal Prince Alfred Hospital

Prof Dennis K. Yue
Director of Diabetes

Level 6 West Wing, Missenden Road, Camperdown 2050 Australia
Ph:9515 5888 Fax:9515 5820 Email:dice@email.cs.nsw.gov.au

Referring Doctor: REPORT PREPARED BY: Prof Dennis K. Yue

Dr.Harvey NORMAN
22 Weston St
PETERSHAM 2049

DATE OF VISIT: 8/02/2009

Re: Susan Smith
56 Harper Street
CANTERBURY 2193

Date of birth:15/05/1940

COMPLICATIONS THAT WE DRAW YOUR ATTENTION TO ARE:

Diabetic retinopathy
Diabetic nephropathy
Dyslipidaemia
Ischaemic heart disease

Mrs Smith who is 69 years old has had Type 2 diabetes since 1987. Her current weight is 105.1 Kgs and her BMI is 39.6. She is a non smoker.

CURRENT DIABETIC TREATMENT::

Lantus	BB:40 units	BL:	BD:	BBed:49 units
Novorapid	BB:6 units	BL:8 units	BD:12-12 units	BBed:

OTHER RELEVANT MEDICATIONS INCLUDE:
Atacand Plus 16/12.5 mg
Lipitor 40 mg
Actonel 30 mg
Aspirin 100 mg

EYE ASSESSMENT:
**Corrected visual acuity:
Right eye =6/12 Left eye =6/12

**Retina:
**Retinopathy
Right eye: minimal NPDR Left eye: minimal NPDR

**Macular Oedema:
Right eye: Not clinically present
Left eye: Not clinically present

COMMENT: Please see final comments

**No cataracts present

**No evidence of previous laser therapy

Figure 56.1 Example of the computer-generated section of the report to referring primary care physicians. BB, before breakfast; Bbed, before bed; BD, before dinner; BL, before lunch; BMI, body mass index; CAG, coronary artery grafting; CHOL, cholesterol; eGFR, estimated glomerular filtration rate; HDL, high density lipoprotein; LDL, low density lipoprotein; NPDR, non-proliferative diabetic retinopathy; TRIGS, triglycerides.

```
RENAL FUNCTION:
Microalbuminuria: 2.5 mg/L     (Normal: 0-20 mg/L)
Albumin Creatinine Ratio: 0.32 mg/mmol (Normal adjusted for age:<4.0 mg/mmol)
COMMENT: Normal
Haemoglobin: 117 g/L                  (Reference Range:115 - 165 g/L)
eGFR: 34.458 mL/min                   (Normal:>=60 mL/min)
**Blood pressure:
Mean Sitting BP: 120/61 mm/Hg
COMMENT: Her blood pressure is well controlled on treatment

FOOT AND NEUROPATHY ASSESSMENT
**Ankle jerks:
Right foot:  present                 Left foot: present

**Biothesiometer:
This is a measure of large nerve fibre conduction.
Right foot: 24                Left foot : 24 (Normal for age: < 33 volts)

**Monofilament:
Right foot: Can feel          Left foot : Can feel

**Foot pulses:
Right foot:Present                 Left foot:Present

COMMENT: Her vibration perception as measured by biothesiometer is
normal and ankle jerks are present. This makes serious foot problems
unlikely.

MACROVASCULAR STATUS

COMMENT: She has a history of ischaemic heart disease and CAG
surgery.


AUTONOMIC FUNCTION

Symptoms of autonomic neuropathy: Nil

METABOLIC PARAMETERS

HbA1C: 7.2%                          Normal:4.0 - 6.0
Creatinine: 140                      Normal:55 - 120 umol/L
TRIGS: 1.4 mmol/L
CHOL: 4.6 mmol/L
HDL: 0.9 mmol/L
LDL: 2.9 mmol/L
```

Figure 56.1 *Continued*

THE DIABETES COMPLICATION ASSESSMENT SERVICE REPORT

ENQUIRIES: - PH 9515 5888
NAME: Susan Smith DATE OF VISIT: 8/02/2009

COULD YOU PLEASE CONSIDER IMPLEMENTING THE FOLLOWING RECOMENDATIONS:

1. Her glycaemic control has improved relative to last year associated with an ongoing positive approach to lifestyle management and achieved weight loss of 4kg. We have made some slight adjustment to her Novorapid insulin today. If her fasting levels are consistently above 7mmol/l, you might like to gently increase the evening Lantus by a couple of units every few weeks. Overall, I think the current HbA_{1c} of 7.2% is acceptable considering the long history of diabetes and previous ischaemic heart disease. The recently published ACCORD Study suggests that reducing HbA1c to less than 6.5% may paradoxically worsen outcomes.

2. She has minimal diabetic retinopathy which is not surprising in view of the long duration of diabetes. It is stable compared with last year, not vision threatening and no intervention is required. Her eGFR is slightly low even adjusted for her age but stable compared with last year and she is appropriately on an ACE-I. Her cholesterol is also slightly on the high side for someone known to have IHD and you may like to push the Lipitor treatment a bit higher.

3. I note also her problems with osteoarthritis. For someone with marginal renal function, it would be nice to avoid the NSAID as much as possible.

Follow-up: From a diabetes complications perspective, we have not made further plans to review Mrs Pike but recommend she return in approximately twelve months time, or earlier if you require.

REPORT PREPARED BY: Prof Dennis K. Yue
cc: Dice,JO

Note:
To help improve the care we provide your patients, and to shorten the time takes us to forward a detailed report, we would appreciate if you could arrange for the patient to have the following pathology tests when you next refer patients to us. We are happy to accept tests performed within the last 3 months.
1- Cholesterol, triglycerides and HDL cholesterol
2- Serum biochemisty including LFT and creatinine
3- HbA_{1c}
4- Microalbuminuria (spot urine sample)
5- Urine protein
6- Urine creatinine
7- Haemoglobin

Figure 56.2 Example of free text message section of the report to referring primary care physicians. ACEi, angiotensin-converting enzyme inhibitor; eGFR, estimated glomerular filtration rate; HDL, high density lipoprotein; IHD, ischemic heart disease; LFT, liver function test; NSAID, non-steroidal anti-inflammatory drug.

References

1 Overland J, Yue DK, Mira M. The pattern of diabetes care in New South Wales: a five-year analysis using Medicare Occasions of Service Data. *Aust N Z J Public Health* 2000; **24**:389–393.

2 Overland J, Yue DK, Mira M. The use of Medicare services related to diabetes: the impact of rural location. *Aust J Rural Health* 2001; **9**:311–316.

3 Weiner JP, Parente ST, Garnick DW, Fowles J, Lawthers AG, Palmer RH. Variation in office-based quality. *JAMA* 1995; **273**:1503–1508.

4 Mbanya JC. Organization of care: problems in developing countries – sub-Sahara Africa. In: DeFronzo RA, Ferrannini E, Keen H, Zimmet P, eds. *International Textbook of Diabetes Mellitus*, 3rd edn. Chichester: John Wiley & Sons, 2004.

5 Ramaiya K. Setting up diabetes clinics in Tanzania. *Pract Diabetes Int* 2006; **23**:229–240.

6 Overland J, Yue DK, Hayes L. Social disadvantage: its impact on the use of Medicare services related to diabetes in NSW. *Aust N Z J Public Health* 2002; **26**:262–265.

7 *Diabetes Atlas*, 3rd edn. International Diabetes Federation, 2006.

8 McDermott R, Tulip F, Sinha A. Sustaining better diabetes care in remote indigenous Australian communities. *Br Med J* 2003; **327**: 428–430.

9 Peterson KA, Radosevich DM, O'Connor PJ, Nyman JA, Prineas RJ, Smith SA, *et al.* Improving diabetes care in practice: findings of the TRANSLATE trial. *Diabetes Care* 2008; **31**:2238–2243.

10 Cooper JG, Claudi T, Jenum AK, Thue G, Hausken MF, Ingskog W, *et al.* Quality of care for patients with type 2 diabetes in primary care in Norway is improving. *Diabetes Care* 2009; **32**:81–83.

11 Szecsenyi J, Rosemann T, Joos S, Peters-Klimm F, Miksch A. German Diabetes Management Programs are appropriate for restructuring care according to the Chronic Care Model. *Diabetes Care* 2008; **31**:1150–1154.

12 Franz MJ, Splett PL, Monk A, Barry B, McClain K, Weaver T, *et al.* Cost-effectiveness of medical nutrition therapy provided by dietitians for persons with non-insulin dependent diabetes mellitus. *J Am Diet Assoc* 1995; **95**:1018–1024.

13 Aubert RE, Herman WH, Waters J, Moore W, Sutton D, Peterson BL, *et al.* Nurse case management to improve glycaemic control in diabetic patients in a health maintenance organization: a randomized trial. *Ann Intern Med* 1998; **129**:605–612.

14 Peters AL, Davidson MB. Application of a diabetes managed care program: the feasibility of using nurses and a computer system to provide effective care. *Diabetes Care* 1998; **21**:1037–1043.

15 Sikka R, Waters J, More W, Sutton DR, Herman WH, Aubert RE. Renal assessment practices and the effect of nurse case management of health maintenance organization patients with diabetes. *Diabetes Care* 1999; **22**:1–6.

16 Davidson MB, Ansari A, Karlan VJ. Effect of a nurse-directed diabetes disease management program on urgent care/emergency room visits and hospitalisations in a minority population. *Diabetes Care* 2007; **30**:224–227.

17 Simmons D, Peng A, Cecil A, Gatland B. The personal costs of diabetes: a significant barrier to care in South Aukland. *N Z Med J* 2001; **112**:383–385.

18 Gæde P, Vedel P, Parving HH, Pedersen O. Intensified multifactorial intervention in patients with type 2 diabetes and microalbuminuria: the Steno type 2 randomised study. *Lancet* 1999; **353**:617–622.

19 Gæde P, Vedel P, Larsen N, Jensen GVH, Parving HH, Pedersen O. Multifactorial intervention and cardiovascular disease in patients with type 2 diabetes. *N Engl J Med* 2003; **348**:383–393.

20 Pedersen O, Gæde P. Intensified multifactorial intervention and cardiovascular outcome in type 2 diabetes: the Steno-2 study. *Metabolism* 2003; **52**:19–23.

21 Gæde P, Tarnov L, Vedel P, Parving HH, Pedersen O. Remission to normoalbuminuria during multifactorial treatment preserves kidney function in patients with type 2 diabetes and microalbuminuria. *Nephrol Dial Transplant* 2004; **19**:2784–2788.

22 Gæde P, Pedersen O. Intensive integrated therapy of type 2 diabetes: implications for long-term prognosis. *Diabetes* 2004; **53**(Suppl 3): 39–47.

23 Gæde P, Pedersen O. Target intervention against multiple risk markers to reduce cardiovascular disease in patients with type 2 diabetes. *Ann Med* 2004; **36**:355–366.

24 Gæde P, Pedersen O. Multi-targeted and aggressive treatment of patients with type 2 diabetes at high risk: what are we waiting for? *Horm Metab Res* 2005; **37**(Suppl 1):76–82.

25 Gæde P, Lund-Andersen H, Parving HH, Pedersen O. Effect of a multifactorial intervention on mortality in type 2 diabetes. *N Engl J Med* 2008; **358**:580–591.

26 Gæde P, Valentine WJ, Plamer AJ, Tucker DMD, Lammert M, Parving HH, *et al.* Cost-effectivenss of intensified versus conventional multifactorial intervention in type 2 diabetes. *Diabetes Care* 2008; **31**:1510–1515.

27 Action to Control Cardiovascular Risk in Diabetes Study Group. Effects of intensive glucose lowering in type 2 diabetes. *N Engl J Med* 2008; **358**:2545–2559.

28 Whitford DL, Southern AJ, Braid E, Roberts SH. Comprehensive diabetes care in North Tyneside. *Diabet Med* 1995; **12**:691–695.

29 McGill M, Molyneaux LM, Yue DK, Turtle JR. A single visit diabetes complication assessment service: a complement to diabetes management at the primary care level. *Diabet Med* 1993; **10**:366–370.

30 Cheung NW, Yue DK, Kotowicz MA, Jones PA, Flack JR. A comparison of diabetes clinics with different emphasis on routine care, complications assessment and shared care. *Diabet Med* 2008; **25**: 974–978.

31 McGill M, Constantino M, Yue DK. Integrating telemedicine into a National Diabetes Footcare Network. *Pract Diab Int* 2000; **17**: 235–238.

32 Silink M. United Nations Resolution 61/225: what does it mean to the diabetes world? *Int J Clin Pract* 2007; **61**:5–8.

33 Siminerio L, Zgibor J, Solano F. Implementing the chronic care model for improvements in diabetes practices and outcomes in primary care: the University of Pittsburgh Medical Center experience. *Clin Diabetes* 2004; **22**:54–58.

34 Halbert RJ, Leung KM, Nichol JM, Legorreta AP. Effect of multiple patient reminders in improving diabetic retinopathy screening: a randomized trial. *Diabetes Care* 1999; **22**:752–755.

35 Hoskins PL, Fowler PM, Constantino M, Forrest J, Yue DK, Turtle JR. Sharing the care of diabetic patients between hospital and general practitioners: does it work? *Diabet Med* 1993; **10**:81–86.

36 Hurwitz B, Goodman C, Yudkin J. Prompting the clinical care of non-insulin dependent (type II) diabetic patients in an inner city area: one model of community care. *Br Med J* 1993; **306**:624–630.

57 The Role of the Multidisciplinary Team

Wing-Yee So & Juliana C.N. Chan

Department of Medicine and Therapeutics, The Chinese University of Hong Kong, Hong Kong SAR, China

Keypoints

- There is generally low adherence of both people with type 2 diabetes (T2DM) and care providers to recommended treatment guidelines.
- Current opinion advocates a multidisciplinary approach to the treatment of T2DM. This includes system support to encourage use of evidence-based guidelines, reorganization of practice systems and team functions, support for patient self-management, improved access to expertise, and enhanced availability of clinical information to facilitate monitoring and feedback on physicians' performance.
- The key elements of quality diabetes care delivered by a multidisciplinary team include periodic risk stratification, protocol-driven care with regular review, patient empowerment, treatment-to-target, and good record keeping to monitor clinical progress and outcomes.

Introduction

According to the World Health Organization (WHO), four chronic non-communicable diseases – diabetes, cancer, respiratory and cardiovascular diseases (CVD) – account for 60% of global deaths (i.e. 35 million deaths per year) [1]. In Europe and China, 30–40% of patients with acute myocardial infarction have a known history of diabetes. In the remaining subjects, 70% of patients have either diabetes or intermediate hyperglycemia on formal 75-g oral glucose tolerance testing [2,3]. In addition, diabetes and hypertension frequently coexist. Both are important considerations in the majority of cardiovascular deaths worldwide, which are estimated to be 18 million annually. The number of people with diabetes is projected to increase from 285 million in 2010 to 435 million by 2030 [4]. The resulting increase will lead to considerable losses in productivity as well as greatly increasing the burden on health care systems.

Treatment of diabetes and associated complications is costly. In 2006, the WHO estimated that in both developing and developed areas, 2.5–15% of health care budgets were spent on diabetes-related illnesses. The International Diabetes Federation (IDF) also estimated that 7–13% of annual health care expenditure was spent on treatment of diabetic complications [5]. The total direct annual costs of diabetes in eight European countries were estimated at €29 billion, with an estimated yearly cost of €2834 per patient [6]. In the USA, diabetes is associated with an annual direct medical expenditure of $91.8 billion. The per capita cost was estimated to be $13 243 for individuals with diabetes compared to $2560 for those without [7]. In China, one of the countries with the most rapid increase in diabetes prevalence, $558 billion in national income is expected to be lost over the next 10 years as a result of premature deaths caused by non-communicable diseases including heart disease, stroke and diabetes [8].

Early diagnosis and aggressive control of risk factors can prevent complications in both type 1 (T1DM) and type 2 diabetes mellitus (T2DM) [9–11]. International organizations such as the IDF, as well as many national organizations, have published clinical recommendations and set standards to guide clinical practice, in order to optimize metabolic control and prevent complications [12].

Evidence for optimization of diabetes control

To date, most evidence supporting the beneficial effects of optimal diabetes care on clinical outcomes [10,13,14] were collected under closely supervised clinical trial conditions. In the Diabetes and Complications Clinical Trial (DCCT), which lasted for 6.5 years, patients with T1DM treated intensively had an HbA_{1c} level 2% (22 mmol/mol) lower than those who were conventionally treated (7.2% vs 9.1%, 55 vs 76 mmol/mol). After the study was completed, the authors continued to follow these patients in the Epidemiology of Diabetes Interventions and Complications (EDIC) study. There was progressive deterioration in glycemic control once these intensively treated patients returned to their usual care setting; however, patients previously treated conventionally also improved, and both groups converged to achieve HbA_{1c} levels of 8% (64 mmol/mol) [15]. Despite this convergence, patients previously treated intensively maintained over 50% risk reduction in all diabetes-associated complications, including cardiovascular events [16].

Textbook of Diabetes, 4th edition. Edited by R. Holt, C. Cockram, A. Flyvbjerg and B. Goldstein.

Similar findings have also been reported following the post-UK Prospective Diabetes Study (UKPDS). People with T2DM who were previously treated with an intensive regimen continued to have lower rates of complications and all-cause mortality than patients treated conventionally, 10 years after discontinuation of the trial [17]. In the Steno-2 Study, individuals were treated intensively in an attempt to attain control for all major risk factors (HbA_{1c}, blood presssure [BP] and low density lipoprotein [LDL] cholesterol), and had 50–60% risk reduction in microvascular and macrovascular complications compared with those conventionally treated [18]. As in the DCCT and UKPDS, in the post-Steno Study period, people who had been treated intensively in the main trial maintained more than 60% risk reduction in all-cause death compared with those conventionally treated for 13.3 years [19]. Findings from these landmark studies clearly demonstrate the beneficial effects of achieving risk factor control during the early course of disease to achieve long-term benefits.

Diabetes care – the reality

Despite the evidence, national and international surveys have indicated that diabetes management remains suboptimal, regardless of the studied populations and health care settings. It should also be remembered that most of these recommendations, guidelines, surveys and studies emanate from settings, countries and areas that are relatively well-resourced.

According to the National Health and Nutritional Examination Surveys (NHANES), conducted between 1988–1994 and 1999–2002 in the USA, amongst patients with diabetes aged 18–75, although there was a non-significant reduction in the proportion of patients with HbA_{1c} >9% (>75 mmol/mol), since the numbers of patients with HbA_{1c} 6–8% (64–86 mmol/mol) increased, there was no significant change in mean HbA_{1c} between these intervals [20]. In the 1999–2002 survey, there was increased use of multiple antidiabetic agents for control [21], yet nearly half continued to have HbA_{1c} levels greater than the American Diabetes Association (ADA) recommendation, of 7% and 20% had HbA_{1c} >9% (>75 mmol/mol).

There was also no significant change in the distribution of blood pressure, 33% having BP >140/90 mmHg. In the 1999–2002 survey, 60% achieved LDL cholesterol concentrations of <3.4 mmol/L and received annual screening for eye and foot complications. The levels of care were noted to be suboptimal, especially in females and in those under the age of 45 years [22,23]. Thus, between these surveys, some improvements were documented but many problems remained.

Tables 57.1–57.3 summarize the adequacy of glycemic, blood pressure and lipid control in various settings during the last two decades. Despite much data, there has been little change in average values attained or percentage of patients reaching treatment goals.

Table 57.1 summarizes adequacy of glycemic control from the 1988–1994 NHANES, up to the latest International Diabetes Management Practice Study (IDMPS) conducted in 2005 [24]. The latter is a 5-year survey documenting changes in diabetes treatment practice in developing regions including Asia, Eastern Europe and Latin America. It shows that only 37% of people with T2DM achieved HbA_{1c} ≤7% (53 mmol/mol). The results were similar in both developed and low and middle income countries [14,21,24–26], different health care settings, primary care [27–32] and specialist centers [33–36].

Table 57.2 summarizes adequacy of blood pressure control in the same period. The blood pressure target in earlier years was 140/90 mmHg, when approximately 40–60% of people with T2DM achieved target [14,29,37]. There was a tendency to improvement in the study conducted by the Department of Veteran Affairs in the USA. In this study, conducted between 1996 and 2000, the proportion of people with T2DM achieving the target blood pressure increased from 40% to 52% [30]. The DiabCare studies in Asia demonstrated that over 70% and 90% of people with T2DM were able to achieve the target of systolic and diastolic blood pressure of ≤140 and ≤90 mmHg, respectively [34]. Emerging evidence of the importance of blood pressure control led to the target blood pressure being revised to <130/80 mmHg. This is not accompanied by further improvement in terms of rate of achievement of targets. Recent studies in different countries and settings showed that only half of people with T2DM were able to achieve the target of 130/80 mmHg [24,26,31,33].

With regard to lipid control (Table 57.3), there was a slow but gradual improvement, probably because of the availability of effective treatment of LDL cholesterol with 3-hydroxy-3-methyl-glutaryl-coenzyme A (HMG-CoA) reductase inhibitors. In the 1980s and early 1990s, the rate of achievement of target LDL cholesterol <2.6 mmol/L was around 10–15% [14,37]. This had increased to approximately 25–30% subsequently [24,27,29,31,33]. For those on HMG-CoA reductase inhibitors, as illustrated from a study in Sweden, nearly half of patients were able to achieve the target [26].

There are obvious limitations in these studies including heterogeneity of populations in different studies, retrospective reviews, incomplete documentation for medical record review and inaccuracy for claims data. Despite the limitations and lack of comparability of the many studies, the results summarized in Tables 57.1–57.3 indicate the same trend. It should also be noted that, most of these surveys come from well-resourced settings and developed countries, where laboratory assessment for HbA_{1c} is readily available.

The Institute of Medicine has defined quality of care as "the degree to which health services for individuals and populations increase the likelihood of desired health outcomes and are consistent with current professional knowledge" [38,39]. There is ongoing controversy as to the degree to which outcomes can be directly related to processes of care, yet both are considered as important measures of quality. Thus, the degree of adherence to recommended guidelines, based on available clinical evidence, provides guidance to the degree of quality of care. Table 57.4 summarizes attempts to address this issue specifically and includes surveys that assess quality of care as measured by frequency of measurement for HbA_{1c}. In early years, less than one-third of patients received HbA_{1c} monitoring [14,40,41]. Since the early

Table 57.1 Adequacy of glycemic control in various health care settings in patients with type 1 (T1DM) and type 2 diabetes mellitus (T2DM).

Health care setting	Number of patients	Survey year	Method	Findings	Reference
Population-based (US NHANES III and BRFSS)*	4085	1988–1995	Patient survey, clinical examination	42.9% had HbA_{1c} <7% (53 mmol/mol) 18.0% had HbA_{1c} >9.5% (80 mmol/mol)	[14]
Primary care (Netherlands) and managed care organization (USA)	2498 (379 patients from the Netherlands and 2119 patients from USA)	1992–1997	Medical record review and administrative data	In 1996, 43.1% vs. 16.8% of patients had HbA_{1c} <7% (53 mmol/mol); and 85.6% vs 56.7% had HbA_{1c} ≤8.5% (69 mmol/mol) in Netherlands and USA, respectively	[27]
Population survey (USA)	1480	1995	Patient survey, clinical examination	Mean HbA_{1c} 7.6% (60 mmol/mol); 44.6% had HbA_{1c} <7% (53 mmol/mol), 37.1% >8% (64 mmol/mol)	[25]
Community health center (USA)	2865	1995	Medical record review	Mean HbA_{1c} 8.6% (70 mmol/mol) 39% of patients had HbA_{1c} ≤8.0% (64 mmol/mol)	[28]
Primary care (USA)	9557–9985	1995–1997	Medical record review	34–42% with HbA_{1c} >9.5% (80 mmol/mol)	[29]
Veterans' Affairs (USA)	9578 (in 1995) to 25 764 (in 2000)	1995–2000	Medical record review and administrative data	72%, 82% and 87% had HbA_{1c} <10% (86 mmol/mol) from 1995–1998, 59% and 62% had HbA_{1c} <8% (64 mmol/mol) in 1999 and 2000	[30]
Diabetes clinic, general medical (resident) clinic and university (faculty) clinic (USA)	6386	1995–2005	Clinical examination	43.7% of type 2 diabetes had HbA_{1c} <7% (53 mmol/mol)	[33]
Primary care and hospital outpatient clinics (Sweden)	17 547 T2DM in 1996 and 57 119 in 2003	1996 and 2003	Medical record review and administrative data	Mean HbA_{1c} was 7.8% (62 mmol/mol) in 1996 and 7.2% (55 mmol/mol) in 2003. 16% of patients had HbA_{1c} <6.5% (48 mmol/mol) in 2003	[31]
Primary care (UK)	18 642	1997	Questionnaire survey and audit data	42.9% with HbA_{1c} within normal range of local laboratory	[32]
National Diabetes Registry (Sweden)	9424 T1DM in 1997 and 13 612 T2DM in 2004	1997 and 2004	Medical record review	Mean HbA_{1c} was 8 3% (67 mmol/mol) in 1997 and 8% (64 mmol/mol) in 2004 17.4% and 21.1% had HbA_{1c} <7% (53 mmol/mol) respectively in 1997 and 2004	[26]
Primary care and hospital outpatient clinics (Asia)	24 317 T2DM in 230 centers	1998	Medical record review and patient interview	Mean HbA_{1c} was 8.6% (70 mmol/mol) in 18 211 patients, 21% had HbA_{1c} <7% (53 mmol/mol)	[34]
Primary care and hospital outpatient clinic (China)	2246 T2DM in 1998 and 2702 in 2006	1998 and 2006	Medical record review	Mean HbA_{1c} was 8.7% (72 mmol/mol) in 1998 and 7.6% (60 mmol/mol) in 2006	(35)
Population-based survey (US NHANES)	15 332 participants, 16.8% diabetes	1999–2004	Patient interview and administration data	52.2% had HbA_{1c} <7% (53 mmol/mol)	[21]
Specialist pediatric center in Western Pacific Region	2312 T1DM	2001–2002	Medical record review	Mean HbA_{1c} was 8.3% (67 mmol/mol)	[36]
Primary care and specialist center (Asia, Eastern Europe and Latin America)	11 799	2005–2010	Medical record review	Mean HbA_{1c} was 8.3% (67 mmol/mol) in 1898 patients with T1DM, 25.3% had HbA_{1c} ≤7% (53 mmol/mol); Mean HbA_{1c} was 7.8% (62 mmol/mol) in 9901 patients with T2DM, 36.4% had HbA_{1c} ≤7% (53 mmol/mol); % of patients achieved HbA_{1c} ≤7% (53 mmol/mol) by ethnic group (Asia, Eastern Europe, Latin America) was 21.0 vs 31.3 vs 21.1 in T1DM and 37.3 vs 36.0 vs 36.0 in T2DM	[24]

BRFSS, Behavioral Risk Factor Surveillance System; NHANES III, Third National Health and Nutrition Examination Survey.
Interpretation of the adequacy of glycemic control is affected by the laboratory methods used and the corresponding reference range, which might vary across studies. For simplicity, the table only describes the absolute values cited in the original papers, and direct comparisons between studies may not be valid.

Table 57.2 Adequacy of blood pressure control in various health care setting in type 1 (T1DM) and type 2 diabetes (T2DM).

Health care setting	Number of patients	Survey period	Method	Findings	Reference
Population-based (US NHANES III and BRFSS)	4085	1988–1995	Patient survey, clinical examination	65.7% had BP <140/90*	[14]
Population-based (US NHANES III)	733	1991–1994	Patient survey, clinical examination	59% of the hypertensive patients had BP >140/90	[37]
Primary care (USA)	9557–9985	1995–1997	Medical record review	64–66% had BP <140/90	[29]
Veterans Affairs (USA)	9578 (in 1995) to 25 764 (in 2000)	1995–2000	Medical record review and administrative data	40%, 44%, 45% and 52% has BP <140/90 (if hypertensive) from 1996–2000	[30]
Diabetes clinic, general medical (resident) clinic and university (faculty) clinic (USA)	6386	1995–2005	Clinical examination	36.7% of T2DM had BP ≤130/80	[33]
Primary care and hospital outpatient clinics (Swedish)	17 547 T2DM in 1996 and 57 119 in 2003	1996 and 2003	Medical record review and administrative data	Mean BP was 150/82 in 1996 and 143/78 in 2003. 13% of patients had BP <130/80 in 2003	[31]
National Diabetes Registry (Swedish)	9424 T1DM in 1997 and 13 612 T1DM in 2004	1997 and 2004	Medical record review	61.3% had BP ≤130/80 in 2004	[26]
Primary care and hospital outpatient clinics (Asia)	24 317 T2DM in 230 centers in Asia	1998	Medical record review and patient interview	Mean BP was 135/81; with 27% had systolic BP >140 and 10% had diastolic BP >90	[34]
Primary care and specialist center (Asia, Eastern Europe and Latin America)	11 799	2005–2010	Medical record review	44.9% T1DM and 19.2% T2DM patients had BP ≤130/80. By ethnic group (Asia, Eastern Europe and Latin America) was 47.4 vs 43.8 vs 44.1 in T1DM and 21.8 vs 20.1 vs 22.1 in T2DM	[24]

BRFSS, Behavioral Risk Factor Surveillance System; BP, blood pressure; NHANES III, Third National Health and Nutrition Examination Survey.
* BP is expressed in mmHg.

1990s, with the availability of results from the DCCT and UKPDS, the frequency of monitoring has gradually improved [27–29,42–44]. Recently, more than 90% of patients have HbA_{1c} regularly monitored in specialist clinics such as the Steno Diabetes Center [45] and in some primary care settings [30,46]. Elsewhere, monitoring is available in 70–80% of patients [24,32,47].

It is important to note that there is often a discrepancy between doctors' claims of frequency of monitoring and that occurring in practice. Although there appears to have been some improvements in the care processes over time, this has not been matched by improvement in rates of achieving treatment targets (Tables 57.1–57.3).

Discrepancy between evidence-based care and reality

The efficacy of optimization of diabetes control has been confirmed in randomized controlled trials conducted with stringent clinical trial protocols; however, despite improvements in some processes of care such as monitoring of HbA_{1c}, this has not been matched by improvement in rates of achieving treatment targets. In addition, the level of care received by many patients does not meet recommended standards. In a previous survey in USA, only 25% of patients were aware of the term "glycated hemoglobin" or "HbA_{1c}" [43]. Only 72% of the subjects visited a health care provider for diabetes care at least once a year, and approximately 60% received complication screening. Furthermore, despite the proven benefits of many therapeutic agents, many people with diabetes were not prescribed insulin, angiotensin-converting enzyme (ACE) inhibitors or lipid-lowering drugs despite the presence of indications [48–53].

The factors that compromise quality of care have been examined in various studies, but have not been well understood. Nevertheless, some components are obvious.

Patients

Drug compliance by patients receiving chronic medications is consistently reported to be less than 50%, often because of insufficient education and reinforcement [54–56]. Moreover, there is considerable heterogeneity in the patterns and rates of non-adherence to individual components (e.g. diet, exercise, drugs) of a diabetes treatment regimen. Thus, the extent to which people with diabetes adhere to one aspect of the regimen might not cor-

Table 57.3 Adequacy of lipid control in various health care setting in type 1 (T1DM) and type 2 diabetes (T2DM).

Health care setting	Number of patients	Survey period	Method	Findings	Reference
Population-based (US NHANES III and BRFSS)	4085	1988–1995	Patient survey, clinical examination	11.0% had LDL <2.6, 42.0% had LDL <3.4	[14]
Population-based (US NHANES III)	733	1991–1994	Patient survey, clinical examination	15.4% had LDL <2.6, 49.3% had LDL <3.4, 58.4% had TG <2.3. 41% of those known to have dyslipidemia had LDL <3.4	[37]
Primary care (Netherlands) and managed care organization (USA)	2498 (379 patients from Netherlands and 2119 patients from USA)	1992–1997	Medical record review and administrative data	In 1996, 23.1% vs. 40.4% of patients had total cholesterol <5.2 in Netherlands and USA, respectively	[27]
Primary care (USA)	9557–9985	1995–1997	Medical record review	48–52% had TC <5.2, with median TG 2.2	[29]
Veterans Affairs (USA)	9578 (in 1995) to 25 764 (in 2000)	1995–2000	Medical record review and administrative data	62%, 68%, 72% and 76% has LDL <3.4 from 1996–2000	[30]
Diabetes clinic, general medical (resident) clinic and university (faculty) clinic	6386	1995–2005	Clinical examination	28.6% of T2DM had LDL <2.6	[33]
Primary care and hospital outpatient clinics (Swedish)	17 547 T2DM in 1996 and 57 119 in 2003	1996 and 2003	Medical record review and administrative data	28% of patients in 2003 had TC <4.5 mmol/L	[31]
National Diabetes Registry (Swedish)	9424 T1DM in 1997 and 13 612 T1DM in 2004	1997 and 2004	Medical record review	Among those on LLD, 48% had LDL <2.5 mmol/L	[26]
Primary care and specialist center (Asia, Eastern Europe and Latin America)	11 799	2005–2010	Medical record review	39.5% T1DM and 33.2% T2DM had LDL <100 mg/dL; 73.1% T1DM and 49.0% T2DM had TG <150 mg/dL	[24]

BRFSS, Behavioral Risk Factor Surveillance System; LDL, low density lipoprotein cholesterol; LLD, lipid lowering drugs; NHANES III, Third National Health and Nutrition Examination Survey; TC, total cholesterol; TG, triglycerides.
All lipid values in mmol/L unless otherwise stated.
Interpretation of the adequacy of dyslipidemia treatment is affected by the laboratory methods used and thus the corresponding reference range might vary across studies. For simplicity, the table only describes the absolute values cited in the original papers, and direct comparisons between studies may not be valid.

relate with their adherence to other components. Previous studies have shown that only 69% of people with diabetes follow a diet and less than half engage in regular exercise [57]. The reported adherence to self-monitoring of blood glucose ranges from 53% to 70% [58]. Earlier studies have indicated that only 7% of patients with diabetes adhere to all aspects of the treatment regimen [59], while over half made errors with insulin dosage and three-quarters of patients were judged to be in an "unacceptable" category regarding the quality, quantity and timing of meals [60].

In attempts to extrapolate results from clinical trials to daily practice, it is important to individualize interventions taking into account all potential factors. For example, in the elderly, side effects of interventions must be balanced against long-term benefits, limited life expectancy and co-morbidities. Other factors such as education level, access to care, compliance and motivation may also contribute to patient adherence, in addition to treatment-related factors such as adverse effects, polypharmacy and cost [42,43,49]. It is recommended that people with diabetes should be educated about the nature of the disease with particular focus on chronicity and long-term complications, as well as preventability.

Physicians

The key role of health care providers is to equip people with diabetes with knowledge and skills related to self-management, to individualize medical and behavioral regimens, to assist with informed decisions, and provide social and emotional support via a collaborative relationship [61,62]. An important factor is the inertia of physicians in failing to modify the management of patients in response to an abnormal clinical result [63,64]. In a previous study by Kaiser Permanente, one of the major health management organizations in USA, there was on average 15 months and 21 months lapse before escalation of treatment in patients with HbA_{1c} of >8% (64 mmol/mol) on metformin and sulfonlyurea monotherapy, respectively [65]. Despite the complexity and rapid advances in diabetes management, generalists often did not perceive the need for further training in the field of diabetes [66–69]. Involvement of other non-medical health care professionals may also not be welcomed in some traditional settings.

Health care system

Traditional medical practice is organized to respond quickly to acute problems, but does not adequately serve the needs of

Table 57.4 Frequency of HbA_{1c} monitoring in various health care settings in type 1 (T1DM) and type 2 diabetes (T2DM).

Health care setting	Number of patients	Survey period	Method	Performance index (frequency of HbA_{1c} measurements in last year or % of patients with at least 1 HbA_{1c} measured in last year)	Reference
Primary care (USA)	1429 doctors	1989	Mail and telephone questionnaire survey	16–18% of physicians measured every 2–3 months	[40]
Population-based (US NHANES III and BRFSS)	4085	1988–1995	Patient survey, clinical examination	28.8% with monitoring available	[14]
Primary care (USA)	97 388	1990–1991	"Claims-based" profile	16% with monitoring ever	[41]
Primary care (Netherlands) and managed care organization (USA)	2498 (379 patients from Netherlands and 2119 patients from USA)	1992–1997	Medical record review and administrative data	Frequency of measurement improved from 1992 to 1996, with 1.89 in Netherlands and 1.10 tests/year in USA. 80.7% (Netherland) and 57.4% (USA) had more than 1 measurement over last 12 months	[27]
Primary care (USA)	1376	1993	Reimbursement profile	26% had HbA_{1c} in last 1 year; 19% in African Americans and 27% in Caucasians 12% had >1 measurement	[104]
General practitioners or specialist care centers (Hungary)	4824	1993	Administrative database	61.8% had HbA_{1c} in last 1 year	[42]
Population-based (USA)	2118	1994	Patient survey	69.4% had HbA_{1c} in last 1 year	[43]
Community private practices (USA)	30 589	1994	Administrative database	54.6% had HbA_{1c} in last 1 year	[44]
Community health center (USA)	2865	1995	Medical record review	70% had HbA_{1c} in last 1 year	[28]
Primary care (USA)	9557–9985	1995–1997	Medical record review	55, 65 and 80% had HbA_{1c} in last 1 year from 1995–1997	[29]
Steno Diabetes Center (Denmark)	2011 (T1DM)	1995–1997	Patient survey	>99.5%, had HbA_{1c} in last 1 year mean frequency 3 tests/yr	[45]
Veterans Affairs (USA)	9578 (in 1995) to 25 764 (in 2000)	1995–2000	Medical record review and administrative data	59%, 85%, 91%, 93% and 94% had HbA_{1c} in last 1 year from 1995–2000	[30]
Health Management Organization (USA)	3612	1997	Patient survey, administrative database	89.0% had HbA_{1c} in last 1 year	[46]
Primary care (UK)	18 642	1997	Questionnaire survey and audit data	83.0% had HbA_{1c} in last 1 year	[32]
Primary care (Germany)	5057	2001	Medical record review	69.5% of the insulin-treated patients, 64.3% of patients on single oral antidiabetic agent and 41.1% for those on diet had HbA_{1c} in last 1 year	[47]
Primary care and specialist center (Asia, Eastern Europe and Latin America)	11 799	2005–2010	Medical record review	77.6% T1DM and 64.2% T2DM had HbA_{1c} ever monitored. By countries (Asia, Eastern Europe and Latin America) was 81.1 vs 73.1 vs 81.4 for T1DM and 64.0 vs 55.8 vs 75.5 for T2DM	[24]

Data are for patients unless otherwise stated.
BRFSS, Behavioral Risk Factor Surveillance System; NHANES III, Third National Health and Nutrition Examination Survey.

individuals with chronic illnesses, when emphases are to alter behavior and to deal with social and emotional impacts of symptoms as well as disabilities [70]. Health care systems need to ensure that the best possible treatment regimens are administered in order to control disease, alleviate symptoms, inform and support.

Thus, suboptimal quality of care is often caused by combinations of factors relating to the affected individual, to the medical care personnel and to the system of health care delivery. In the IDMPS [24], amongst patients in whom HbA_{1c}, BP and LDL cholesterol measurements were available, only 3.6% of patients attained target values for all three risk factors (BP <130/80 mmHg,

HbA_{1c} <7% (53 mmol/mol) and LDL cholesterol <2.6 mmol/L). In this survey, there was considerable heterogeneity between regions of patient-related factors (e.g. age, disease duration, presence of complications, body weight), health care systems (e.g. health insurance coverage, availability of specialist care, training by diabetes educator) and self-care (e.g. self-adjustment of insulin dosage) all being associated with the likelihood of reaching targets. The problem is particularly marked in low and middle income settings where it is exacerbated by multiple demands upon severely limited resources including those imposed by a continuing burden of infectious diseases and other issues such as accidents and injuries.

The evolving concept of disease management

It will be clear from the previous sections that although optimal care improves clinical outcomes in clinical trial settings, this is often not achieved in real clinical situations for the reasons discussed. This has led to attempts to develop models of care based on multidisciplinary approaches.

In recent years, there has been increasing emphasis on management via coordination and organization of individual components of care into a structured system. The latter is further supported by reinforcement through multiple contacts, including not only physician appointments, but also telephone reminders and visits to other health care professionals such as nurse practitioners, dietitians and pharmacists. According to Wagner *et al.* [70], there are five key elements to improve the outcomes of patients with chronic diseases:

1 A system to support the use of evidence-based guidelines;
2 Reorganization of practice systems and team functions;
3 Patient self-management support;
4 Improved access to expertise; and
5 Improved availability of clinical information to facilitate monitoring and feedback on physician's performance.

The Steno-2 study provides excellent evidence in support of the benefits of protocol-driven multifaceted care using a multidisciplinary approach in T2DM [13,18,19]. Patients randomized to the intensive treatment group were managed by a multidisciplinary team according to a protocol that specified a stepwise implementation of behavior modification, smoking cessation, aggressive control of glycemia, BP, lipids and microalbuminuria, and use of an ACE inhibitor and aspirin. The reductions in HbA_{1c}, BP, serum cholesterol and triglycerides levels and albuminuria were all significantly greater in the intensive care group than in the usual care group. These benefits in metabolic control were translated to risk reductions of cardiovascular morbidity and mortality by 53% (95% confidence interval [CI] 27–76%), nephropathy by 71% (95% CI 13–83%), retinopathy by 58% (95% CI 14–79%) and autonomic neuropathy by 63% (95% CI 21–82%). By the end of 13.3 years, patients previously treated intensively had lower all-cause mortality (hazard ratio [HR] 0.54; 95% CI 0.32–0.89), cardiovascular mortality (HR 0.43; 95% CI 0.19–0.94) and cardiovascular events (HR 0.41; 95% CI 0.25–0.67) than the conventional care group.

In another multicenter randomized study comparing structured care delivered by a diabetologist–nurse team with conventional care, 60% of patients with T2DM with renal impairment receiving structured care attained three or more predefined treatment goals (HbA_{1c} <7% (53 mmol/mol); BP <130/80 mmHg; LDL cholesterol <2.6 mmHg; triglycerides <2 mmol/L and use of ACE inhibitor or angiotensin receptor blocker) compared to 20% in the usual care group. After 2 years, patients who attained three or more treatment goals had 60% risk reduction in all-cause mortality and end-stage renal disease (HR 0.43; 95% CI 0.21–0.86) [71].

Implementation of quality structured care

This concept of disease management emphasizes an organized, proactive multidisciplinary approach to health care in complex and chronic diseases, of which diabetes is a prime example [72,73]. People with chronic diseases should be empowered to improve knowledge and self-management [74,75]. Preferences should be taken into account to individualize treatment plans. Evidence suggests that periodic attendance at a diabetes center [76] and frequent reminders by paramedical staff to reinforce self-management could improve metabolic control, clinical outcomes and survival [13,71,77–84]. Clinical information should be made easily available to provide support. Information technology can be used to monitor adherence to guidelines and provide feedback to the care providers (see Chapter 58) [70,72,85–87].

Provision of structured care to people with T2DM is best implemented through a series of interlinked processes based on these principles. These include risk stratification, protocol-driven care, regular review by a multidisciplinary team, patient empowerment and good record keeping to monitor progress (Figure 57.1).

Risk stratification

Diabetes is characterized by clustering of multiple risk factors that interact in a complex manner to give rise to multiple complica-

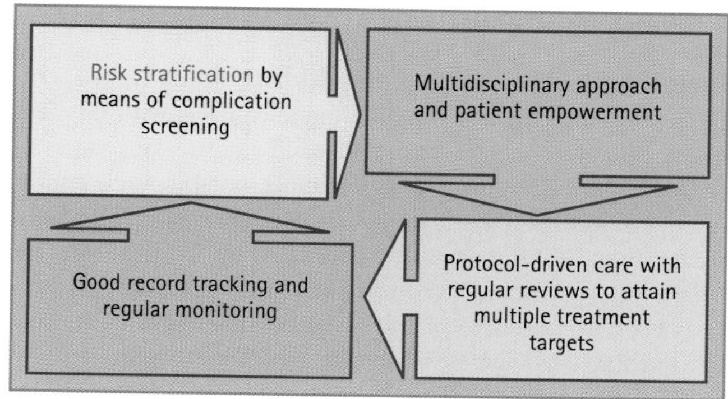

Figure 57.1 Components for quality structured care.

tions [88]. Both the IDF and American Diabetes Association (ADA) recommend that people with diabetes should undergo comprehensive assessment at presentation and annually thereafter to document personal, clinical and laboratory measurements. This enables stratification of risk and placement of patients within different care plans for targeted individualized treatment.

The UKPDS has provided longitudinal data which help to define the natural history of cardiovascular complications in T2DM. Using the UKPDS data, mathematical models have been developed to identify predictors (risk factors) for cardiovascular disease [89]. In addition, the Framingham Heart Study, started in 1948, has prospectively followed a large group of participants in the general population in order to identify factors contributing to development of CVD, and risk engines have also been developed to predict risk of CVD in this population [90]. Both the UKPDS and the Framingham risk equations show moderate effectiveness in risk stratification in UK and USA settings; however, external validation studies show that the performance varies considerably among different countries and ethnic groups [91]. In addition, there were only a few hundred people with diabetes in the original cohort of the Framingham Study, while the UKPDS recruited individuals in the early phase of diabetes. These pose definite limitations in applying the risk engines derived from these two studies to general diabetes populations in Europe, the USA and elsewhere.

Further modification and development of ethnic specific risk equations have now been carried out. For example, equations to predict diabetes complications such as coronary heart disease, stroke, end-stage renal failure, congestive heart failure as well as overall mortality have now been developed for Chinese populations, based on prospective follow-up of approximately 8000 patients, with median follow up of 6 years [89,92–95]. In this particular group of Chinese individuals with diabetes, the Framingham stroke risk engine underestimates, while the UKPDS risk engine overestimates, the risk of stroke. Both of these risk engines for CVD overestimate the risk of CVD in some populations such as Chinese. In addition, it was not possible to develop the UKPDS risk engine to assess risk of end-stage renal disease as an insufficient number of individuals developed this endpoint. Further development in this area is anticipated with expansion of studies into different settings and ethnic-specific areas.

Protocol driven care using a multidisciplinary approach

Diabetes management involves multiple contacts with different health care personnel, each specialized in a particular process or area of expertise. Non-medical personnel, notably nurse educators, nutritionists, pharmacists, physical trainers and podiatrists, are key members of a successful diabetes team. While the doctor adopts the leading and coordinating role in defining problems and needs, the professional knowledge and clinical skills of these non-medical staff are invaluable in providing counseling and holistic care to patients. These health care professionals can also assist physicians to provide follow-up, empower self-management and support carers of patients with cognitive impairment and physical disabilities. This team approach allows physicians to spend more time in discussion of needs, setting of targets and options for management. In high risk individuals, such as those with co-morbidites or those receiving multiple medications, the pharmacist may have a unique role in providing education to patients in collaboration with physicians to improve the safe and effective use of pharmaceutical agents and reduce the risk of drug-related adverse effects and drug–drug interactions.

Given the large number of processes and personnel potentially involved in the delivery of such evidence-based and protocol-driven care, it is important to try to determine which aspects of care can be attributed to which components. In a meta-analysis of 66 publications examining 11 different strategies to improve diabetes care [96], two key strategies were associated with statistically significant incremental reductions in HbA_{1c} value. The first was team changes, which involved either the addition of a team member, shared care between primary care and specialist center, or multidisciplinary team care. This resulted in additional HbA_{1c} reduction by 0.33% (3.6 mmol/mol). The second was case management, which involved coordination in diagnosis, treatment or management by a person or multidisciplinary team in collaboration with or supplementary to the primary care clinician. This was associated with additional HbA_{1c} reduction of 0.22% (2.4 mmol/mol).

This has been replicated in various clinical settings. For example, the Chinese University of Hong Kong Diabetes Group has used different care prototypes since the 1990s to augment delivery of care using nurses and pharmacists. The latter were empowered to run clinics or provide telephone counseling to provide periodic assessments and reinforce treatment compliance. These prototypes consistently showed improved rates of treatment compliance and attainment of multiple treatment targets as well as reduced risk of death and cardiorenal complications by 50–70% in chronic diseases including diabetes with or without complications (Figure 57.2) [82–84]. These two strategies become key components and are applicable globally irrespective of the health care setting. In less resource-rich settings, some of these strategies can be met, at least partially, by appropriate training or relocation of existing staff in response to changing health needs.

Patient empowerment and self-care

In addition to team changes and case management, other processes that have been shown to improve disease control include patient education (effect sizes 0.24 [0.07–0.40]), reminders (0.27 [0.17–0.36]) and financial incentives (0.40 [0.26–0.54]) [86]. While adherence of physicians and care providers to care processes may improve health outcomes, patient adherence is a critical factor in realizing the benefits of these processes. Patients should be encouraged to participate actively in defining and achieving agreed treatment goals rather than conforming to medically defined regimens or instructions. In diabetes, behavioral changes, including adhering to a meal plan, engaging in regular

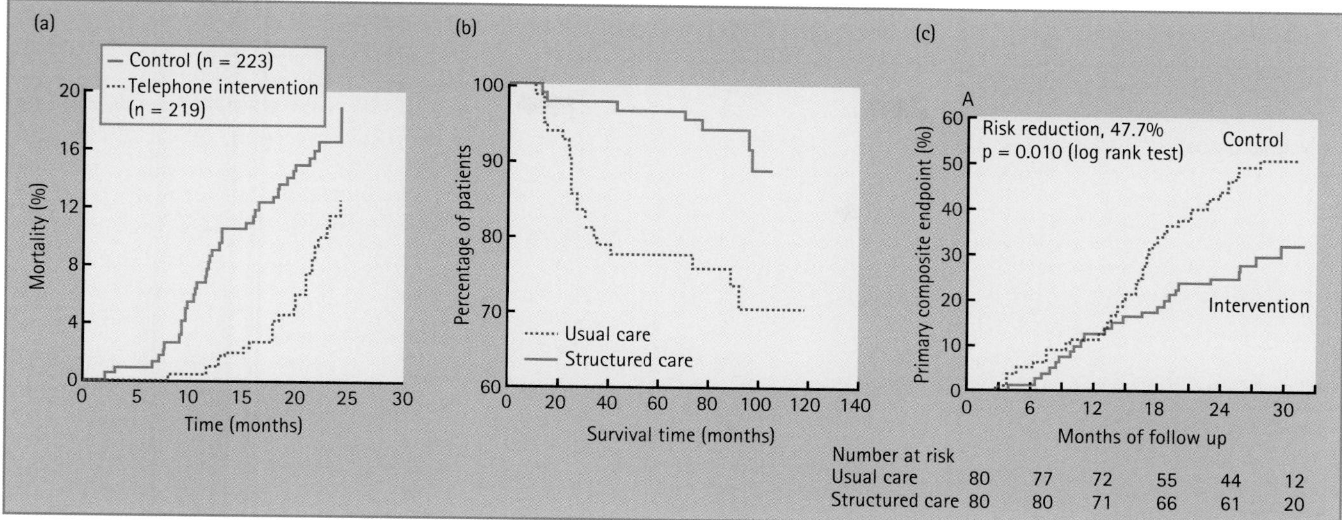

Figure 57.2 Effect of protocol-driven care using a multidisciplinary approach to reduce risk of complications in patients with chronic diseases including type 2 diabetes mellitus (T2DM) [82–84]. (a) Telephone counseling by a pharmacist between clinic visits reduced mortality rate by 50% in patients receiving five or more chronic medications. (b) Patients with T2DM without cardiorenal complications managed in a clinical trial setting was associated with a 70% risk reduction in death rate compared with matched patients followed up in conventional care setting. (c) Patients with T2DM with chronic kidney disease managed by a pharmacist–doctor team had a 50% risk reduction in death and end-stage renal disease compared with patients managed in conventional care setting.

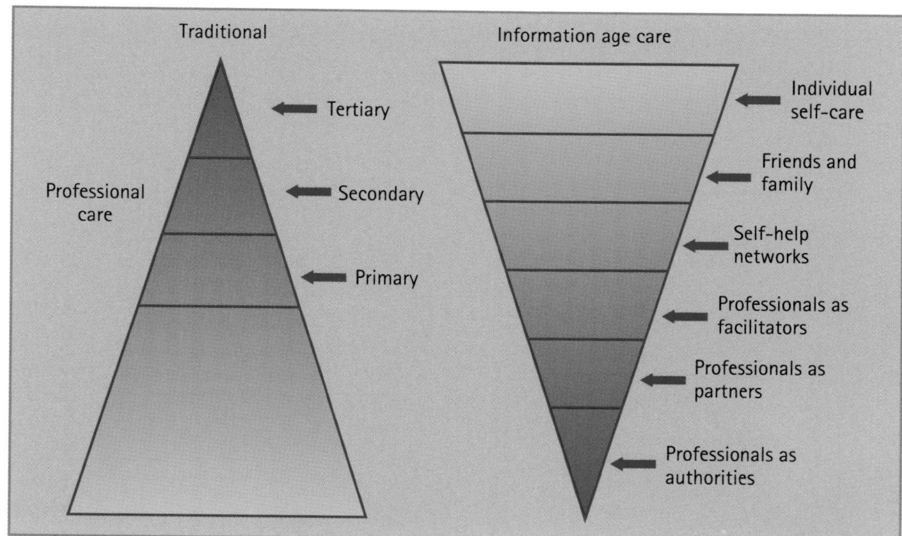

Figure 57.3 Change of paradigm using information technology to improve clinical and self-management. Adapted from Jennings *et al.* [109], with permission from Knowledge Exchange LLC.

physical exercise, taking medications regularly, monitoring blood glucose levels and other complications, and attending to foot care demand high levels of self-discipline and are important components of holistic care models [61].

Given the chronic nature of diabetes and large amount of data collected during contact with care providers, there is a need to develop a system to manage this information effectively and enable health care workers to make decisions, track clinical progress, monitor compliance and benchmark quality of care. The use of information technology can also empower people with diabetes by making information more accessible and understandable. Such technology can also assist individuals with diabetes to keep their own health records, maintain control, and use them to manage their own care in an informed manner (Figure 57.3).

Importance of periodic monitoring and review

Depending on complications and control of risk factors, people with diabetes should be reviewed at intervals ranging from weekly to every few months; however, once stabilized, people with dia-

Table 57.5 Treatment targets, procedures and frequency of monitoring for individual target [12,105–108].

	Frequency	Procedures and targets
Glycemic control		
HbA_{1c}	NGSP of IFCC assay 2–6 monthly	6.5–7% (48–53 mmol/mol) Individualized target based on: • Duration of diabetes • Age/life expectancy • Co-morbid conditions • Known CVD or advanced microvascular complications • Hypoglycemic unawareness
Self-monitoring of blood glucose	≥3 daily for patients on intensive insulin regimen ≥1 daily with weekly profile for those on oral agents ± insulin ≥1 weekly profile for selected patients on diet Additional test with unstable or deteriorating condition	Preprandial BG 5–7 mmol/L Post-prandial <8–10 mmol/L
Blood pressure control		
	At every clinic visit	<130/80 mmHg
Lipid control	Yearly	LDL <2.6 mmol/L; or 30% reduction regardless of baseline LDL Triglycerides <2.3 mmol/L HDL >1.0 mmol/L in men, 1.3 mmol/L in women
Clinic visit	Every 3–6 months	Access progress in achieving treatment goals: • Symptoms • Weight goals • Glycemic, blood pressure and lipid goals • Compliance and side effects of medications • Results of self-monitoring • Adherence to lifestyle including cessation of smoking and avoidance of excessive alcohol use Access complications: • Events including admissions or procedures
Complication screening	Yearly May consider 2–3 yearly for retinopathy in patients with normal examination by experts	Self-care knowledge and beliefs Lifestyle adaptation Psychologic status Self-monitoring skills and equipment Body weight trend Glycemic, blood pressure and lipid control Cardiovascular risk Erectile dysfunction, neuropathy Foot condition Eye condition Kidneys Pre-pregnancy advice Medication review

BG, blood glucose; CVD, cardiovascular disease; HDL, high density lipoprotein; LDL, low density lipoprotein; NGSP, National Glycohemoglobin Standardization Program.

betes should be reviewed by a health care professional at least once a year, no matter how mild the condition may appear. Based on various guidelines, the targets as well as procedures and frequency of monitoring for individual targets are summarized in Table 57.5.

This takes account of the possibility of silent deterioration of metabolic control and development of new risk factors or complications, as proper management cannot be initiated unless indexes of control are measured periodically [97]. In the study shown in Figure 57.2(a), which was conducted in the early 1990s, the omission of the measurement of metabolic indices was associated with a 15-fold increased risk of death. The comparison group in this study had at least one measurement during a 7-year period of observation [82].

These findings are related to adjustment of regimens facilitated by periodic monitoring [97]. Patients receiving structured care have greater utilization of antihypertensive and lipid-lowering agents. Using ACE inhibitors as an example, despite the compelling evidence supporting their protective effects [98], clinicians in conventional care settings often withhold or discontinue these drugs for fear of side effects such as hyperkalemia and deterioration of renal function, especially in high risk patients who are those most likely to benefit [99,100]. This is further supported by the study shown in Figure 57.2(c), in T2DM with nephropathy, in which 60–70% of patients were treated with an ACE inhibitor or ARB at baseline. At the end of a 2-year study period, over 90% of subjects randomized to structured care delivered by a multidisciplinary team persisted with the treatment compared with less than 20% of subjects randomized to conventional care. Together with better risk factor control, increased usage of drugs, more clinical and laboratory assessments, this difference in usage of ACE inhibitor or ARB collectively contributed to the reduction in death and cardiorenal event rates between the structured and conventional care group [71,84].

Importance of attaining multiple targets

As shown in Table 57.5, multiple treatment targets, in addition to glycemic control, need to be taken into consideration when managing people with diabetes. In an observational study of 6386 patients with T2DM in Hong Kong, attainment of ≥2 treatment goals (HbA_{1c}, BP or LDL cholesterol) was associated with 30–50% risk reduction in new onset of CHD, demonstrating the importance of attaining multiple targets [33]. In the Steno-2 study in Denmark, which aimed to achieve multiple risk factor control, the overall relative risk reduction of 59% in composite cardiovascular events accords with the expected cumulative effects of control of individual risk factors in an additive manner [19]. This has been further replicated in another study, in individuals with diabetic nephropathy, in which more people receiving structured care attained ≥3 treatment goals (61%) compared with the conventional care group (28%). This difference translates to a 60–70% reduction in premature death and end-stage renal disease [71].

It has been estimated that use of HMG-CoA reductase inhibitors and blood pressure lowering drugs confers the largest benefit in reducing cardiovascular risk in the initial study period, with optimization of glycemic control and use of aspirin providing additional beneficial effects. The long-term glycemic beneficial effects of glucose lowering on diabetes-related endpoints are expected to occur later. Hence, the attainment of multiple treatment targets might explain the continuing divergence in cardiovascular endpoints, rather than a simple time–effect relationship. The importance of sustained benefits of long-term glycemic control is further supported by the legacy effect associated with intensive blood glucose control, long after the cessation of the UKPDS [101] and the parallel findings of the DCCT/EDIC study [15,16].

Cost-effectiveness of multidisciplinary care

Cost-effectiveness analysis for intensive glycemic and blood pressure control has been performed based on results from the UKPDS [102]. The cost per quality-adjusted life year (QALY) for intensive blood glucose control with insulin or sulfonylureas was £6028 more than conventional treatment, while that with metformin in overweight patients was £1021 less than conventional treatment. These estimates suggest that intensive blood glucose therapy, particularly the use of metformin in obese patients with diabetes, was effective and cost-saving. The cost per QALY gained for tight blood pressure control was £369 based on the UKPDS. Similarly, according to the Centers for Disease Control (CDC) in the USA, the incremental cost : effectiveness ratio for intensive glycemic control was US$41 384 per QALY. The respective costs for intensified blood pressure control and reduction of serum cholesterol were savings of US$1959 and US$51 889 per QALY [103]. Furthermore, these analyses suggested that these interventions were most cost-effective when instituted early during the course of disease.

Similar analysis has also been performed in the Steno-2 Study [19]. The incremental cost : effectiveness ratio for structured care versus conventional treatment was €3927 and €2538 per life year and per QALY gained, respectively. These incremental costs were mainly attributed to increased pharmacy and consultation costs. The author further pointed out that even assuming that patients in the structured care group continued to receive the most expensive treatment in a specialist setting in Denmark and that the treatment effects between the intensive and conventional groups might decline after completion of the 7.8-year intervention period, the incremental costs still represent good value for money. However, because of the multifaceted nature of the intervention, it was difficult to identify the contribution of individual factors to the improved outcome.

Conclusions

In conclusion, T2DM is a massive public health problem and is associated with reduced life expectancy by 10–12 years. It has major implications on quality of life, health care utilization and societal productivity. Diabetes management is complex and effective management requires creation of care models that take account of this complexity and facilitate care providers to attain multiple treatment targets and empower patients to adhere to self-management. Such models should include continuous quality improvement initiatives with measurement of key performance indices, validated outcome measures and risk–benefit analyses of interventions. Landmark trials such as Steno-2 study have demonstrated the cost-effectiveness of the use of protocol-driven multidisciplinary care to manage and prevent diabetes complications. With appropriate organization of care, good clinical governance and patient empowerment, quality diabetes care should eventually become accessible, affordable and sustainable, irrespective of circumstances and resource setting.

References

1 World Health Organization. *2008–2013 Action Plan for the Global Strategy for the Prevention and Control of Noncommunicable Diseases*. World Health Organization, 2008.

2 Hu DY, Pan CY, Yu JM. The relationship between coronary artery disease and abnormal glucose regulation in China: the China Heart Survey. *Eur Heart J* 2006; **19**:19.

3 Bartnik M, Ryden L, Ferrari R, Malmberg K, Pyorala K, Simoons M, *et al.* The prevalence of abnormal glucose regulation in patients with coronary artery disease across Europe: the Euro Heart Survey on diabetes and the heart. *Eur Heart J* 2004; **25**:1880–1990.

4 International Diabetes Federation. Diabetes Facts and Figures http://www.diabetesatlas.org/content/diabetes-and-impaired-glucose-tolerance. Accessed 8 January 2010.

5 International Diabetes Federation (IDF). Diabetes Atlas. http://www.eatlas.idf.org/atlas.html?id=0; 2007.

6 Jonsson B. Revealing the cost of type II diabetes in Europe. *Diabetologia* 2002; **45**:S5–12.

7 American Diabetes Association (ADA). National Diabetes Fact Sheet. http://www.cdc.gov/diabetes/pubs/pdf/ndfs_2005.pdf ed; 2005.

8 He J, Gu D, Wu X, Reynolds K, Duan X, Yao C, *et al.* Major causes of death among men and women in China. *N Engl J Med* 2005; **353**:1124–1134.

9 Implementing the lessons of DCCT. Report of a national workshop under the auspices of the British Diabetic Association. *Diabet Med* 1994; **11**:220–228.

10 UK Prospective Diabetes Study (UKPDS) Group. Intensive blood-glucose control with sulphonylureas or insulin compared with conventional treatment and risk of complications in patients with type 2 diabetes (UKPDS 33). *Lancet* 1998; **352**:837–853.

11 UK Prospective Diabetes Study (UKPDS) Group. Efficacy of atenolol and captopril in reducing risk of macrovascular and microvascular complications in type 2 diabetes: UKPDS 39. *Br Med J* 1998; **317**:713–720.

12 International Diabetes Federation (IDF). Global guideline for type 2 diabetes. 2005 [updated 2005; cited 2009]; Available from: http://www.idf.org/Global_guideline.

13 Gaede P, Vedel P, Parving HH, Pedersen O. Intensified multifactorial intervention in patients with type 2 diabetes mellitus and microalbuminuria: the Steno type 2 randomised study. *Lancet* 1999; **353**:617–622.

14 Saaddine JB, Engelgau MM, Beckles GL, Gregg EW, Thompson TJ, Narayan KM. A diabetes report card for the United States: quality of care in the 1990s. *Ann Intern Med* 2002; **136**:565–574.

15 Diabetes Control and Complications Trial/Epidemiology of Diabetes Interventions and Research Group. Retinopathy and nephropathy in patients with type 1 diabetes four years after a trial of intensive therapy. *N Engl J Med* 2000; **342**:381–389.

16 Nathan D, Cleary P, Backlund J, Genuth S, Lachin J, Orchard T, *et al.* Intensive diabetes treatment and cardiovascular disease in patients with type 1 diabetes. *N Engl J Med* 2005; **353**:2643–2653.

17 Holman RR, Paul SK, Bethel MA, Matthews DR, Neil HA. 10-year follow-up of intensive glucose control in type 2 diabetes. *N Engl J Med* 2008; **359**:1577–1589.

18 Gaede P, Vedel P, Larsen N, Jensen GV, Parving HH, Pedersen O. Multifactorial intervention and cardiovascular disease in patients with type 2 diabetes. *N Engl J Med* 2003; **348**:383–393.

19 Gaede P, Lund-Andersen H, Parving HH, Pedersen O. Effect of a multifactorial intervention on mortality in type 2 diabetes. *N Engl J Med* 2008; **358**:580–591.

20 Saaddine JB, Cadwell B, Gregg EW, Engelgau MM, Vinicor F, Imperatore G, *et al.* Improvements in diabetes processes of care and intermediate outcomes: United States, 1988–2002. *Ann Intern Med* 2006; **144**:465–474.

21 Dodd A, Colby M, Boye K, Fahlman C, Kim S, Briefel R. Treatment approach and HbA1c control among US adults with type 2 diabetes: NHANES 1999–2004. *Curr Med Res Opin* 2009; **25**:1605–1613.

22 Persell SD, Zaslavsky AM, Weissman JS, Ayanian JZ. Age-related differences in preventive care among adults with diabetes. *Am J Med* 2004; **116**:630–634.

23 Wexler DJ, Grant RW, Meigs JB, Nathan DM, Cagliero E. Sex disparities in treatment of cardiac risk factors in patients with type 2 diabetes. *Diabetes Care* 2005; **28**:514–520.

24 Chan JC, Gagliardino JJ, Baik SH, Chantelot JM, Ferreira SR, Hancu N, *et al.* Multifaceted determinants for achieving glycemic control: the International Diabetes Management Practice Study (IDMPS). *Diabetes Care* 2009; **32**:227–233.

25 Harris MI, Eastman RC, Cowie CC, Flegal KM, Eberhardt MS. Racial and ethnic differences in glycemic control of adults with type 2 diabetes. *Diabetes Care* 1999; **22**:403–408.

26 Eeg-Olofsson K, Cederholm J, Nilsson P, Gudbjornsdottir S, Eliasson B. Glycemic and risk factor control in type 1 diabetes: results from 13,612 patients in a national diabetes register. *Diabetes Care* 2007; **30**:496–502.

27 Valk GD, Renders CM, Kriegsman DM, Newton KM, Twisk JW, van Eijk JT, *et al.* Quality of care for patients with type 2 diabetes mellitus in the Netherlands and the United States: a comparison of two quality improvement programs. *Health Serv Res* 2004; **39**:709–725.

28 Chin MH, Auerbach SB, Cook S, Harrison JF, Koppert J, Jin L, *et al.* Quality of diabetes care in community health centers. *Am J Public Health* 2000; **90**:431–434.

29 Acton KJ, Shields R, Rith-Najarian S, Tolbert B, Kelly J, Moore K, *et al.* Applying the diabetes quality improvement project indicators in the Indian Health Service primary care setting. *Diabetes Care* 2001; **24**:22–26.

30 Sawin CT, Walder DJ, Bross DS, Pogach LM. Diabetes process and outcome measures in the Department of Veterans Affairs. *Diabetes Care* 2004; **27**(Suppl 2):B90–94.

31 Eliasson B, Cederholm J, Nilsson P, Gudbjornsdottir S. The gap between guidelines and reality: type 2 diabetes in a National Diabetes Register, 1996–2003. *Diabet Med* 2005; **22**:1420–1426.

32 Khunti K, Ganguli S, Baker R, Lowy A. Features of primary care associated with variations in process and outcome of care of people with diabetes. *Br J Gen Pract* 2001; **51**:356–360.

33 Kong AP, Yang X, Ko GT, So WY, Chan WB, Ma RC, *et al.* Effects of treatment targets on subsequent cardiovascular events in Chinese patients with type 2 diabetes. *Diabetes Care* 2007; **30**:953–959.

34 Chuang LM, Tsai ST, Huang BY, Tai TY. The status of diabetes control in Asia: a cross-sectional survey of 24 317 patients with diabetes mellitus in 1998. *Diabet Med* 2002; **19**:978–985.

35 Pan C, Yang W, Jia W, Weng J, Tian H. Management of Chinese patients with type 2 diabetes, 1998–2006: the Diabcare-China surveys. *Curr Med Res Opin* 2009; **25**:39–45.

36 Craig M, Jones T, Silink M, Ping Y. Diabetes care, glycemic control, and complications in children with type 1 diabetes from Asia and the Western Pacific Region. *J Diabetes Complications* 2007; **21**:280–287.

37 Harris MI. Health care and health status and outcomes for patients with type 2 diabetes. *Diabetes Care* 2000; **23**:754–758.

38 Lohr KN, Schroeder SA. A strategy for quality assurance in Medicare. *N Engl J Med* 1990; **322**:707–712.

39 Lohr KN, Harris-Wehling J. Medicare: a strategy for quality assurance. I. A recapitulation of the study and a definition of quality of care. *QRB Qual Rev Bull* 1991; **17**:6–9.

40 Tuttleman M, Lipsett L, Harris MI. Attitudes and behaviors of primary care physicians regarding tight control of blood glucose in IDDM patients. *Diabetes Care* 1993; **16**:765–772.

41 Weiner JP, Parente ST, Garnick DW, Fowles J, Lawthers AG, Palmer RH. Variation in office-based quality: a claims-based profile of care provided to Medicare patients with diabetes. *JAMA* 1995; **273**: 1503–1508.

42 Tabak AG, Kerenyi Z, Penzes J, Tamas G. Poor level of care among diabetic patients: is that a unique picture? *Diabetes Care* 1999; **22**:533–535.

43 Beckles GL, Engelgau MM, Venkat Narayan KM, Herman WH, Aubert RE, Williamson DF. Population-based assessment of the level of care among adults with diabetes in the US. *Diabetes Care* 1998; **21**:1432–1438.

44 Rosenblatt RA, Baldwin LM, Chan L, Fordyce MA, Hirsch IB, Palmer JP, *et al.* Improving the quality of outpatient care for older patients with diabetes: lessons from a comparison of rural and urban communities. *J Fam Pract* 2001; **50**:676–680.

45 Jensen T, Musaeus L, Molsing B, Lyholm B, Mandrup-Poulsen T. Process measures and outcome research as tools for future improvement of diabetes treatment quality. *Diabetes Res Clin Pract* 2002; **56**:207–211.

46 Simon LP, Albright A, Belman MJ, Tom E, Rideout JA. Risk and protective factors associated with screening for complications of diabetes in a health maintenance organization setting. *Diabetes Care* 1999; **22**:208–212.

47 Hauner H, Koster I, von Ferber L. [Outpatient care of patients with diabetes mellitus in 2001. Analysis of a health insurance sample of the AOK in Hesse/KV in Hesse.] *Dtsch Med Wochenschr* 2003; **128**:2638–2643.

48 Wetzler HP, Snyder JW. Linking pharmacy and laboratory data to assess the appropriateness of care in patients with diabetes. *Diabetes Care* 2000; **23**:1637–1641.

49 Simon LPS, Albright A, Belman MJ, Tom E, Rideout JA. Risk and protective factors associated with screening for complications of diabetes in a health maintenance organisation setting. *Diabetes Care* 1999; **22**:208–221.

50 Ho M, Marger M, Beart J, Yip I, Shekelle P. Is the quality of diabetes care better in a diabetes clinic than in a general medicine clinic? *Diabetes Care* 1997; **20**:472–475.

51 Mayfield JA, Rith-Najarian SJ, Acton KJ, Schraer CD, Stahn RM, Johnson MH, *et al.* Assessment of diabetes care by medical record review. *Diabetes Care* 1994; **17**:918–923.

52 Pommer W, Bressel F, Chen F, Molzahn M. There is room for improvement of preterminal care in diabetic patients with end stage renal failure: the epidemiological evidence in Germany. *Nephrol Dial Transplant* 1997; **12**:1318–1320.

53 el-Kebbi IM, Ziemer DC, Musey VC, Gallina DL, Bernard AM, Phillips LS. Diabetes in urban African-Americans. IX. Provider adherence to management protocols. *Diabetes Care* 1997; **20**: 698–703.

54 Anonymous. Review: medication adherence may reduce mortality and morbidity. *ACP J Club* 1998; **128**:53.

55 Liniger C, Albeanu A, Bloise D, Assal JP. The tuning fork revisited. *Diabet Med* 1990; **7**:859–864.

56 Sackett DL, Snow JC. The magnitude of compliance and non-compliance. In: Haynes RB, Taylor DW, Sackett DL, eds. *Compliance in Health Care*. Baltimore: Johns Hopkins University Press, 1979: 11–22.

57. Kravitz RL, Hays RD, Sherbourne CD, DiMatteo MR, Rogers WH, Ordway L, *et al.* Recall of recommendations and adherence to advice among patients with chronic medical conditions. *Arch Intern Med* 1993; **153**:1869–1878.

58 Hoskins PL, Alford JB, Handelsman DJ, Yue DK, Turtle JR. Comparison of different models of diabetes care on compliance with self-monitoring of blood glucose by memory glucometer. *Diabetes Care* 1988; **11**:719–724.

59 Cerkoney KA, Hart LK. The relationship between the health belief model and compliance of persons with diabetes mellitus. *Diabetes Care* 1980; **3**:594–598.

60 Watkins JD, Williams TF, Martin DA, Hogan MD, Anderson E. A study of diabetic patients at home. *Am J Public Health Nations Health* 1967; **57**:452–459.

61 Glasgow RE, Anderson RM. In diabetes care, moving from compliance to adherence is not enough: something entirely different is needed. *Diabetes Care* 1999; **22**:2090–2092.

62 Fisher E, Brownson C, O'Toole M, Shetty G, Anwuri V, Glasgow R. Ecological approaches to self-management: the case of diabetes. *Am J Public Health* 2005; **95**:1523–1535.

63 Phillips LS, Branch WT, Cook CB, Doyle JP, El-Kebbi IM, Gallina DL, *et al.* Clinical inertia. *Ann Intern Med* 2001; **135**: 825–834.

64 Rodondi N, Peng T, Karter AJ, Bauer DC, Vittinghoff E, Tang S, *et al.* Therapy modifications in response to poorly controlled hypertension, dyslipidemia, and diabetes mellitus. *Ann Intern Med* 2006; **144**:475–484.

65 Brown JB, Nichols GA, Perry A. The burden of treatment failure in type 2 diabetes. *Diabetes Care* 2004; **27**:1535–1540.

66 Larme AC, Pugh JA. Attitudes of primary care providers towards diabetes: barriers to guideline implementation. *Diabetes Care* 1998; **21**:1391–1396.

67 Bernard AM, Anderson L, Cook CB, Phillips L. What do internal medicine residents need to enhance their diabetes care? *Diabetes Care* 1999; **22**:661–666.

68 Lee A, Chan JCN. Shared care in diabetes mellitus: why is it important? *Hong Kong Practitioner* 1997; **19**:315–322.

69 Lee A, Chan JCN. Shared care in diabetes mellutus: what are the obstacles? *Hong Kong Practitioner* 1997; **17**:323–330.

70 Wagner EH, Austin BT, Von Korff M. Organizing care for patients with chronic illness. *Milbank Q* 1996; **74**:511–544.

71 Chan J, So W, Yeung C, Ko G, Lau I, Tsang M, *et al.* Effects of structured versus usual care on renal endpoint in type 2 diabetes.

The SURE study: a randomized multicenter translational study. *Diabetes Care* 2009; **32**:977–982.

72 Ellrodt G, Cook DJ, Lee J, Cho M, Hunt D, Weingarten S. Evidence-based disease management. *JAMA* 1997; **258**:1687–1692.

73 Norris SL, Nichols PJ, Caspersen CJ, Glasgow RE, Engelgau MM, Jack L, *et al.* The effectiveness of disease and case management for people with diabetes: a systematic review. *Am J Prev Med* 2002; **22**(Suppl):15–38.

74 Holman H, Lorig K. Patients as partners in managing chronic disease: partnership is a prerequisite for effective and efficient health care. *Br Med J* 2000; **320**:526–527.

75 Johnson SB. Methodological issues in diabetes research: measuring adherence. *Diabetes Care* 1992; **15**:1658–1667.

76 Verlato G, Muggeo M, Bonora E, Corbellini M, Bressan F, De Marco R. Attending the diabetes center is associated with increased 5-year survival probability of diabetic patients. *Diabetes Care* 1996; **19**:211–213.

77 Haynes RB, McKibbon KA, Kanani R. Systematic review of randomised trials of interventions to assist patients to follow prescriptions for medications. *Lancet* 1996; **348**:383–386.

78 Weinberger M, Kirkman MS, Samsa GP, Shortliffe EA, Landsman PB, Cowper PA, *et al.* A nurse-coordinated intervention for primary care patients with NIDDM: impact on glycemic control and health related quality of life. *J Gen Intern Med* 1995; **10**:59–66.

79 Bero LA, Mays NB, Barjestech K, Bond C. Expanding outpatient pharmacists' roles and health services utilization. *Cochrane Database Syst Rev* 1998; **3**:CD000336.

80 Aubert RE, Herman WH, Waters J, Moore W, Sutton D, Peterson BL, *et al.* Nurse case management to improve glycemic control in diabetic patients in a health maintenance organisation. *Ann Intern Med* 1998; **129**:605–612.

81 Kinmonth AL, Woodcock A, Griffin S, Spiegal N, Campbell J. Randomised controlled trial of patient centred care of diabetes in general practice: impact on current wellbeing and future risk: the Diabetes Care From Diagnosis Research Team. *Br Med J* 1998; **317**:1202–1208.

82 So WY, Tong PC, Ko GT, Leung WY, Chow CC, Yeung VT, *et al.* Effects of protocol-driven care versus usual outpatient clinic care on survival rates in patients with type 2 diabetes. *Am J Manag Care* 2003; **9**:606–615.

83 Wu JY, Leung WY, Chang S, Lee B, Zee B, Tong PC, *et al.* Effectiveness of telephone counselling by a pharmacist in reducing mortality in patients receiving polypharmacy: randomised controlled trial. *Br Med J* 2006; **333**:522.

84 Leung WY, So WY, Tong PC, Chan NN, Chan JC. Effects of structured care by a pharmacist-diabetes specialist team in patients with type 2 diabetic nephropathy. *Am J Med* 2005; **118**:1414.

85 Wagner EH, Groves T. Care for chronic diseases. *Br Med J* 2002; **325**:913–914.

86 Weingarten SR, Henning JM, Badamgarav E, Knight K, Hasselblad V, Gano A Jr, *et al.* Interventions used in disease management programmes for patients with chronic illness-which ones work? Meta-analysis of published reports. *Br Med J* 2002; **325**:925.

87 Bodenheimer T, Wagner E, Grumbach K. Improving primary care for patients with chronic illness. *JAMA* 2002; **288**:1775–1779.

88 Eckel RH, Grundy SM, Zimmet PZ. The metabolic syndrome. *Lancet* 2005; **365**:1415–1428.

89 Adler AI. UKPDS-modelling of cardiovascular risk assessment and lifetime simulation of outcomes. *Diabet Med* 2008; **25**(Suppl 2):41–46.

90 Framingham Heart Study. A Project of the National Heart, Lung and Blood Institute and Boston University. 1948. Available from: http://www.framinghamheartstudy.org/.

91 Simmons R, Coleman R, Price H, Holman R, Khaw K, Wareham N, *et al.* Performance of the UK Prospective Diabetes Study risk engine and the Framingham Risk Equations in estimating cardiovascular disease in the EPIC: Norfolk Cohort. *Diabetes Care* 2009; **32**:708–713.

92 Yang XL, So WY, Kong AP, Clarke P, Ho CS, Lam CW, *et al.* End-stage renal disease risk equations for Hong Kong Chinese patients with type 2 diabetes: Hong Kong Diabetes Registry. *Diabetologia* 2006; **49**:2299–2308.

93 Yang X, Ma RC, So WY, Kong AP, Ko GT, Ho CS, *et al.* Development and validation of a risk score for hospitalization for heart failure in patients with type 2 diabetes mellitus. *Cardiovasc Diabetol* 2008; **7**:9.

94 Yang X, So WY, Tong PC, Ma RC, Kong AP, Lam CW, *et al.* Development and validation of an all-cause mortality risk score in type 2 diabetes. *Arch Intern Med* 2008; **168**:451–457.

95 Yang X, So WY, Kong AP, Ma RC, Ko GT, Ho CS, *et al.* Development and validation of a total coronary heart disease risk score in type 2 diabetes mellitus. *Am J Cardiol* 2008; **101**:596–601.

96 Shojania KG, Ranji SR, McDonald KM, Grimshaw JM, Sundaram V, Rushakoff RJ, *et al.* Effects of quality improvement strategies for type 2 diabetes on glycemic control: a meta-regression analysis. *JAMA* 2006; **296**:427–440.

97 Cagliero E, Levina EV, Nathan DM. Immediate feedback of HbA1c levels improves glycemic control in type 1 and insulin-treated type 2 diabetic patients. *Diabetes Care* 1999; **22**:1785–1789.

98 Investigators HOPES. Effects of ramipril on cardiovascular and microvascular outcomes in people with diabetes mellitus: results of the HOPE study and MICRO-HOPE substudy. *Lancet* 2000; **355**:253–259.

99 Bakris GL, Weir MR. Angiotensin-converting enzyme inhibitor-associated elevations in serum creatinine: is this a cause for concern? *Arch Intern Med* 2000; **160**:685–693.

100 Palmer BF. Managing hyperkalemia caused by inhibitors of the renin-angiotensin-aldosterone system. *N Engl J Med* 2004; **351**:585–592.

101 Holman RR, Paul SK, Bethel MA, Matthews DR, Neil HA. 10-year follow-up of intensive glucose control in type 2 diabetes. *N Engl J Med* 2008; **359**:1577–1589.

102 Gray AM, Clarke P. The economic analyses of the UK prospective diabetes study. *Diabet Med* 2008; **25**(Suppl 2):47–51.

103 CDC Diabetes Cost-effectiveness Group. Cost-effectiveness of intensive glycemic control, intensified hypertension control, and serum cholesterol level reduction for type 2 diabetes. *JAMA* 2002; **287**:2542–2551.

104 Chin MH, Zhang JX, Merrell K. Diabetes in the African-American Medicare population: morbidity, quality of care, and resource utilization. *Diabetes Care* 1998; **21**:1090–1095.

105 American Diabetes Association. Standards of medical care in diabetes, 2009. *Diabetes Care* 2009; **32**(Suppl 1):13–61.

106 Canadian Diabetes Association. Clinical Practice Guidelines, 2008. Available from: http://www.diabetes.ca/for-professionals/resources/2008-cpg/.

107 National Institute for Health and Clinical Excellence (NICE). Type 2 Diabetes: National clinical guideline for management in primary and secondary care (update). 2008. Available from: http://guidance.nice.org.uk/CG66/Guidance/pdf/English.

108 Rodbard HW, Blonde L, Braithwaite SS, Brett EM, Cobin RH, Handelsman Y, *et al.* American Association of Clinical Endocrinologists medical guidelines for clinical practice for the management of diabetes mellitus. *Endocr Pract* 2007; **13**(Suppl 1):1–68.

109 Jennings K, Miller KH, Materna SB. *Changing Health Care: Creating Tomorrow's Winning Health Enterprises Today*. Santa Monica, CA: Knowledge Exchange, 1999.

58 Models of Diabetes Care Across Different Resource Settings

Naomi S. Levitt[1], Bob Mash[2], Nigel Unwin[3], Jean Claude Mbanya[4], Jae-Hyoung Cho[5] & Kun-Ho Yoon[5]

[1] Division of Diabetic Medicine and Endocrinology, University of Cape Town and Groote Schuur Hospital, Cape Town, South Africa
[2] Division of Family Medicine and Primary Care, Stellenbosch University, Tygerberg, South Africa
[3] Faculty of Medicine, University of West Indies, Barbados
[4] Department of Endocrinology, Faculty of Medicine and Biomedical Sciences, University of Yaounde I, Yaounde, Cameroon
[5] Department of Endocrinology, Seoul St. Mary's Hospital, College of Medicine, The Catholic University of Korea, Seoul, Korea

Keypoints

- A comprehensive approach to diabetes prevention and care includes policies and activities outside the formal health sector, particularly for primary prevention.
- Integrated care refers to the need to provide care for conditions coexisting with diabetes within the same primary health care service.
- Continuity of care, a cornerstone of effective health care organization, is associated with improved outcomes.
- Prerequisites for improving outcomes include ensuring that essential medications (including insulin) are either free or highly affordable and that tests for the diagnosis of diabetes, monitoring of control, and equipment to screen for complications are available.
- Living health systems should care for, empower and nurture their staff so that they are enabled to do the same for their patients.
- If no one is responsible for chronic care, the tendency is for it to be overlooked.
- A less qualified professional may offer lower quality care, but there is potential for effective substitution, with the right training and organization.
- A respectful, open and curious stance may help different professionals and people to understand each other better.
- Patient-centeredness improves quality of life, increases patient satisfaction, improves adherence to treatment, enhances the integration of preventive and promotive care, and improves the provider's job satisfaction.
- In low resource settings where large numbers of patients overwhelm facilities, it may make sense to extend care into the community.
- Ideally, a systematic process for reviewing the evidence and updating guidance accordingly should be in place in all countries.
- Advances in the usage of information technology and the internet are likely to provide increasingly important contributions to diabetes care both in well-resourced and less-well resourced settings.

Introduction

Almost no community worldwide remains unaffected by diabetes. Premature mortality and an array of complications, in particular the chronic complications, result in a considerable impact that is experienced by individuals, families and societies. This impact is predicted to increase, primarily in countries such as those in North Africa, sub-Saharan Africa, the Middle East and South Asia. In these countries, lifestyles are transitioning and the populations consume less healthy foods, and have rising levels of physical inactivity and obesity.

Enormous inequalities exist in the provision of health care for people with diabetes, in keeping with the widely disparate socio-economic status that prevails globally. These inequalities are not only found between countries, they occur within countries, for example in rural-versus-urban settings, private-versus-public sectors and hospital-versus-community-based services. Considerable challenges face health planners and providers, especially in less well resourced countries and areas countries, because of the traditional infectious diseases, such as tuberculosis and malaria, coexisting with HIV/AIDS, and the emerging scourge of chronic diseases, including diabetes, producing a multiple disease burden with competition for limited resources. Furthermore, most health care systems have evolved from the basis of dealing with acute medical problems and have been or, in most instances, remain ill-equipped to provide the kind of care that people with chronic diseases require.

That is not to say well-resourced countries do not face challenges with health care delivery. In these countries, there are also problems in ensuring that quality health care is delivered in a

Textbook of Diabetes, 4th edition. Edited by R. Holt, C. Cockram, A. Flyvbjerg and B. Goldstein.

cost-effective manner. Notwithstanding these challenges, each person with diabetes, wherever they live, should have access to the best care that can be provided in their setting and consequently have the opportunity to achieve the outcomes they seek. Unfortunately, this is not the current situation, even in well-resourced countries and settings. The United Nations Resolution on Diabetes "Encourages member states to develop national policies for the prevention, treatment and care of diabetes in line with the sustainable development of the health-care systems, taking into account the internationally agreed upon development goals, including the Millennnium Development Goals" (Resolution 61/225, December 20, 2006). The resolve of the United Nations, together with the policies and influence of the International Diabetes Federation (IDF) and the World Health Organization (WHO), need to be harnessed in order to improve the suboptimal care and outcomes for people with diabetes. After all, it is not that a dearth of evidence exists for the effectiveness of a wide range of interventions to prevent complications associated with diabetes, but rather the reverse. Narayan *et al.* [1] have identified three interventions that are cost-saving and fully feasible in terms of penetration of the target population, technical complexity, amount of capital required and cultural acceptability, even in low and middle income countries and across all regions:

1 Improvement in glycemic control;
2 Blood pressure control; and
3 Foot care.

A fourth intervention, pre-conception care, was found to be cost-saving, but not fully feasible because of concerns of not being able to reach all women with diabetes.

The issue at hand is how to translate the evidence into practice and thus reality, acknowledging that, almost without exception, health services are in need of repair and the specific interventions to be introduced or implemented will undoubtedly vary depending on the health care structure and resources available. There is also the need to recognize that diabetes requires that people not only have access to sufficient resources, such as medication, but also the understanding, motivation and skills to self-manage their condition.

Health care cannot be seen in isolation, occurring as it does within a broad societal framework which places varying degrees of emphasis on ensuring that quality care is prioritized. Thus, in the first instance, for effective health care delivery, a positive policy environment needs to be in place, nationally and locally. The "macro" level of the WHO Innovative Care for Chronic Conditions (ICCC) framework focuses on this very issue (Figure 58.1), highlighting the components that can promote a positive policy environment [2]. Political will, building or strengthening partnerships (e.g. between community-based organizations, patient organizations, health care workers and government), and ensuring consistent funding are key aspects of the process. So too is the need for an inter-sectoral approach or collaboration to building a healthy society, encompassing, for example, urban

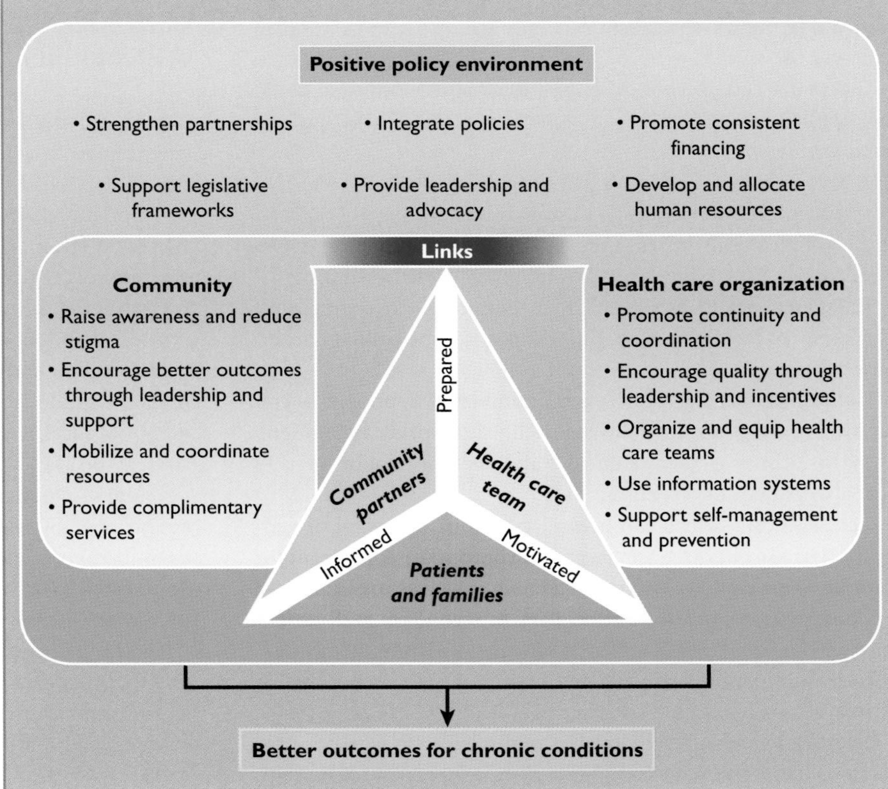

Figure 58.1 Innovotive care for chronic conditions framework. Adapted from WHO [2].

planning (with the provision of green areas, easy public transport, access to sport and recreation facilities), the introduction of health promotion activities within schools and the food industry.

The "meso" level in the ICCC framework relates to health care organization and links to the community. It is at this level that the concept "model of care" comes into play. As coined by Davidson *et al.* [3], a health care model can be regarded as an overarching design for the provision of a service that is ideally underpinned by a theoretical framework, evidence base and clearly defined standards. The model has core principles and elements in addition to an agreed upon agenda for implementation and later evaluation. It is unlikely that a single health care model for diabetes exists that can be used effectively and efficiently in all settings – indeed, the model will take different forms or shapes in different settings. Health planners have to decide whether to pursue a diabetes-specific model of care or to incorporate multiple chronic diseases such as diabetes, hypertension and chronic lung diseases in a common chronic care model. There are salient reasons for pursuing the latter, given the commonality of aspects of care for these conditions, but factors such as the available resources are likely to guide this decision. Regardless of the model selected, changing the value system in which health care is delivered, with the aim of ensuring motivated affirmed health care workers, is perhaps key to equipping or enabling people living with diabetes with the information, motivation and skills to self-manage their diabetes. There is a real need to embrace the lessons that can be learned from the successful highly active antiretroviral therapy (HAART) programs for people with HIV/AIDS, which have yielded levels of adherence to therapy that most clinicians and public health specialists can only dream of in relation to diabetes [4].

There are certain core principles for diabetes care that could be applied across all resource settings [2]. These include establishing:

- A comprehensive approach that provides for health promotion to enable prevention and early diagnosis, management of diabetes and complications when they arise and rehabilitation when needed.
- Integrated health care, such that conditions coexisting with diabetes, can be readily managed within the same primary health care service.
- Continuity of care, which has a number of connotations: in terms of the relationship between health care worker and patient; in terms of management strategies and decision-making; and in terms of patient information.
- Access to care, which can be understood in a physical or geographic sense, but extends to access to appropriate equipment for monitoring, diagnosis and management as well as medication.
- Coordination of care from primary to secondary and tertiary levels, with appropriate referral strategies and role delineation. Where multiple professionals and organizations are involved in primary care, horizontal coordination of care is also important.
- Teamwork: diabetes care involves multiple health workers, professional categories and disciplines, even in low resource settings. Establishment of teams whose focus is on delivering and improving the quality of care permits the development of shared goals, defining and clarifying roles, reflecting on how care can be improved and holding each other accountable for decisions. The identification of a team leader may be a major factor in the success of this element.
- Person-centeredness implies a more collaborative approach and holistic understanding of the patient that elicits, acknowledges and addresses relevant beliefs, concerns and expectations. This is at least partly a paradigm shift in the mind of the health worker from the traditional biomedical, technical and sometimes authoritarian model to a biopsychosocial, holistic and participatory model.
- Family and community orientation are integral to provide support for the individual with diabetes as well as to raise awareness and to extend care from the health centers into the community.
- The use of evidence as far as it is available, accessible and relevant. The evidence base for diabetes is constantly expanding and all resource settings need to look at how they access the latest and ever-changing evidence base.

We now discuss how these principles are being incorporated into care for people with diabetes across different resource settings; low and middle income settings such as encountered in most low and middle income countries as well as in high income countries. Finally, how information technology can be embraced and harnessed appropriately in different settings with the goal of supporting these principles is explored.

A comprehensive approach

Taking a comprehensive approach to diabetes prevention and care implies that polices and activities are put in place to address primary prevention, early diagnosis (including screening if appropriate), management of diabetes and its complications, and rehabilitation for those affected by complications. A comprehensive approach will include policies and activities outside the formal health sector, particularly for the primary prevention of type 2 diabetes mellitus (T2DM). For example, promoting healthier diets and greater physical activity could involve policies on food production, marketing and taxation, and policies on design of local environments and public transport. The WHO's strategy on diet and physical activity provides a framework for developing national and international policy that is relevant to countries at all levels of development [5]. The best indication of a comprehensive approach is a national government-led strategy that covers primary prevention through to rehabilitation, with the caveat that the presence of a strategy does not guarantee that it has been implemented. A recent survey carried out through IDF member organizations [6] found that of the 98 countries from which responses were received, just over 70% claimed that their country had implemented a national diabetes program. The region with the lowest proportion of countries (30%) with a national diabetes program was sub-Saharan Africa, but even in richer regions, such as Europe, over 20% of responding countries did not have a national diabetes program. Examples of national diabetes programs in countries at opposite ends of the economic spectrum include the program in Cameroon [7] and the National Service Framework for Diabetes in England [8].

Integrated health care

Integrated care for people with diabetes refers to the need to provide care for conditions coexisting with diabetes within the same primary health care service. Within most high income countries, primary health care has been developed to provide a range of services covering most of the needs with people with diabetes, and indeed with other chronic conditions. In low and middle income countries, however, integration of care is often a challenge, as donor funding is most often given to specific disease programs such as HIV/AIDS, tuberculosis or malaria, or large-scale government funding is allocated for specific vertical programs, such as HIV/AIDS. For example, in Zambia the donor funding for HIV/AIDS is larger than the total health care budget. While this funding enables higher quality care for a specific disease it can weaken the health care system as a whole. Further, disease-centered programs, through higher salaries and better working conditions, may draw professional staff away from primary care. Therefore, initiatives aimed at strengthening an approach to diabetes should do this with an integrated model of care and with the goal of strengthening the whole approach to chronic care [9,10]. An example of an integrated chronic care clinic for HIV/AIDS, diabetes and hypertension at provincial hospitals in Cambodia has recently been reported (Box 58.1) [11]. There is no reason why such an approach could not be used in primary health care [12].

Box 58.1 Cambodia: integrated chronic disease clinics

Chronic disease clinics for the combined care of HIV/AIDS, diabetes and hypertension were set up in two provincial referral hospitals in Cambodia based on a number of assumptions: a common approach is needed to respond to the needs of chronic disease patients, with the widespread acceptance that HIV/AIDS has become a chronic disease following increasing availability of antiretroviral therapy; attending a combined clinic would minimize the stigma that a specific HIV/AIDS clinic induces; and that the care model should reflect estimates of disease burden. All patients were managed according to standard treatment protocols. A team of counselors promoted adherence and lifestyle changes to complement medical consultations, and peer support groups extended the efforts of the doctors and counselors.

After 2 years

- 70.7% of patients with diabetes (90% of those who attended for >3 months) and 87.7% of patients on highly active retroviral therapy (HAART) remained in active follow-up
- Median HbA_{1c} was 8.6% (70 mmol/mol), but the degree of improvement could not be assessed in the absence of a baseline measurement
- Median CD4 count doubled in patients on HAART

Thus, integrated chronic care is not only feasible, but can produce good patient outcomes

Continuity, access, coordination and teamwork

These four core principles – continuity of care, access to care, coordination between different levels of care and multidisciplinary team work – really belong together, as they concern providing good quality health care for managing diabetes and preventing its complications. A particular challenge in low resource settings is that of moving away from a focus on episodic curative care. High patient numbers, with acute infectious illness and low numbers of trained professionals have nurtured this approach, which will tend to wait for the patient to present with gangrene of the foot rather than invest energy in identifying the patients at risk. Likewise, there is more focus on treating the problem than empowering the person. For example, a patient with elevated blood glucose levels is more likely to receive a change in prescription than a useful exchange of information about diet or exercise and advice about overcoming barriers to adherence.

Continuity of care

Continuity of care in chronic diseases is a cornerstone of effective health care organization and has been associated with lower mortality, better access to care, less hospitalization and referral, fewer emergencies and better detection of adverse medical events [13,14]. Continuity is easier to achieve when services are offered close to communities where access is easier. Care that requires visits to a distant referral hospital is unlikely to support continuity because of the costs and time taken to travel. In many less well resourced countries and areas, diabetes care has not been part of primary health care offered in the community although there is a clear drive by the WHO to change this.

Central to providing continuity of care is continuity of information, such that the status of individuals is known, in terms of when they attended their last appointment, the next appointment due, and what was found, discussed and prescribed at previous appointments. A diabetes register is therefore essential, providing a list of patients with diabetes being treated at that facility, a record of their appointments, linked to a system to follow-up those who fail to attend for an appointment. In higher income situations, electronic diabetes registers are now the norm, and in some situations registers are maintained across more than one level of care, such as primary and secondary care. In low income situations, an adequate register can be kept using "pencil and paper" at the level of the facility at which most diabetes care is delivered. In addition to keeping a register of patients and their appointments, there is the need to provide continuity of relevant information between visits. In high-resource settings, electronic records linked between different levels of care provide a state of the art approach. In low-resource settings, a range of approaches have been tried (e.g. color coding of patient records, the use of annual summary sheets and patient-retained records) [15]. A simple but effective approach in some settings can be a combined "paper and pencil" register and record, recording a small number of core items such as blood pressure, a measure of blood glucose control, whether feet were examined, advice given and current medication.

Continuity of management aims to provide continuity with a specific group of health care providers. The challenge here is to maintain the same team of people for a reasonable period of time. Relational continuity with the same health care provider over time is occasionally possible and would be an ideal [16].

Access to all

Access to care, of any type at all, is still an issue in many low and middle income countries, particularly in more remote areas. A specific example is the lack of availability or access to insulin leading to unnecessary mortality in people with type 1 diabetes (T1DM) [17,18]. Even when available, the cost of purchasing insulin is substantial and can be the equivalent of up to 20 days wages for a 1-month supply of insulin. Thus, addressing the supply chain for medication and ensuring that essential medication is either free or highly affordable is a prerequisite for improving outcomes, but that is not all that is required. Availability of tests for the diagnosis of diabetes, monitoring of control and equipment to screen for complications are also essential.

A shortage of human resources is a serious barrier to providing access to care in many low and middle income countries, the irony being that these countries are often recruiting grounds for high income countries seeking to staff their own health care systems. Given their shortage, health workers in low resource settings often develop a broader scope of practice than their equivalents in high resource settings and as a result need to have a wide range of skills. This is often necessitated by the absence of more highly trained professionals, particularly in rural and remote areas. Although a less qualified professional may offer lower quality care, there is also the potential for effective substitution, with the right training and organization. This has been well demonstrated by Gill *et al.* [19] in rural Africa. Using a wholly primary care level nurse-led program, with key elements of education and drug titration by clinical algorithm and using drugs on the essential drug list, significant improvements in glycemic control were noted and maintained over an 18-month period (HbA_{1c} 11.6 ± 4.5%, 103 ± 49 mmol/mol [SD] at baseline, and 7.7 ± 2.0%, 61 ± 22 mmol/mol at 18 months). The impact of education alone was remarkable, as without any change in drug therapy the HbA_{1c} dropped from 10.6 ± 4.2% (92 ± 46 mmol/mol) baseline to 7.6 ± 2.3% (60 ± 25 mmol/mol) at 18 months.

In primary care, well-trained nurses can offer equivalent care to doctors for routine follow-up of chronic conditions, minor illness and preventative interventions [20]. In diabetes, this may mean the nurse conducting the consultation and reviewing results such as urinalysis, HbA_{1c}, glucose and cholesterol levels. The nurse may also screen the feet, take blood pressure and calculate the body mass index. Nurses will then refer to the generalist doctor for complicated or uncontrolled patients. Patient satisfaction may even be higher as consultations are longer and contain more information. Nurses, however, may not necessarily be cheaper as they are less productive [20]. Similarly, in low resource settings the generalist doctor may need a broader range of procedural and surgical skills at the district hospital and the ability to act as a supportive consultant to nurses. A range of mid-level workers such as health promoters and clinical associates/assistants may also provide effective substitution [21].

Management of diabetes and other chronic diseases involves providing access to screening and early intervention to prevent or at least limit the impact of complications [2]. In low resource settings, some complications are easy to screen for (e.g. using a testing strip dipstick to assess for proteinuria or identifying the at-risk foot with a monofilament) provided the necessary tools are available; however, screening for retinopathy is problematic as health providers seldom succeed in overcoming the many obstacles to effective ophthalmoscopy. Nevertheless, even in low resource settings, appropriate technology using a fundal camera may be possible [22,23].

Further decisions need to be made regarding the relative costs and benefits in different resource settings of macro vs micro albuminuria screening; use (and frequency) of glycated hemoglobin vs random/fasting blood glucose as well as total cholesterol vs high density lipoprotein (HDL) cholesterol and low density lipoprotein (LDL) cholesterol measurements. Effective screening requires a structured and systematic approach by the health care team.

Coordination of care

Coordination of care from primary to secondary and tertiary levels is needed to provide the full range of diabetes care, if resources allow. In well financed and organized systems, this coordination includes well-developed referral pathways within health districts and regions, and well-developed systems of information exchange between the levels, in order to preserve continuity of care. Specialist services likely to be available at a secondary level include the treatment of foot ulcers, retinal laser therapy, and the investigation and medical treatment of renal impairment. Renal dialysis and replacement is an example of services often provided at the tertiary level. In low and middle income settings, and even in some high income countries where universal health insurance does not exist, access to secondary and tertiary care tends to be highly dependent on the ability to pay.

Teamwork

Teamwork is an essential feature of providing diabetes care. Even at primary health care level, particularly in high income situations, several professionals and disciplines can be involved in the routine care people with diabetes – including, for example, doctor, nurse, podiatrist and optometrist. In order to develop chronic care, the people involved in managing chronic conditions need to develop a team that meets regularly to focus on improving the quality of care [2], and one of the team should be appointed as the chronic care coordinator. If no one is responsible for chronic care, the tendency is for it to be overlooked. For example, basic equipment, such as glucometers, monofilaments or obese cuffs for blood pressure measurement, is not provided [15]. In addition, new ideas, initiatives and procedures are not sustained in the absence of a leader who is present over a sufficient time period. Continuously rotating staff, such as nurses, erodes the ability to create effective teams and sustain changes. When teams meet they should develop shared goals, clarify their complementary roles, reflect on how to improve care and hold each other accountable for decisions. Health professionals need to be clearly aligned with the purpose of improving chronic care and not with defending professional identities. A respectful, open and curious stance helps professionals and others to understand each other better [24].

When nurses working in a large informal settlement in Cape Town were asked what would help improve diabetes care they replied "caring for the carers," reminding us that building good teams begins by caring for its members. The nature of the relationship between health workers and managers, and the values embedded in the organizational culture may be reflected in the nature of the relationship between health worker and patient and the culture of caring [25]. Organizations that operate too heavily in a mechanistic and bureaucratic model tend to treat health workers as human resources that can be used and replaced like parts in a machine [26]. Organizations should strive for congruence between individual values and behavior and organizational culture and structures [27]. It is difficult for health workers to empower people for healthy living, motivate change and care for patients when the organization is not congruent with the same values. Wheatley [28] expresses this well when she says, "After years of being bossed around, of being told they're inferior, of power plays that destroy lives, most people are exhausted, cynical and focused only on self-protection … when obedience and compliance are the primary values, then creativity, commitment and generosity are destroyed." Living health systems should care for, empower and nurture their staff so that they are enabled to do the same for their patients.

Patient-centered care

In low resource settings the need to be patient-centered is often dismissed as a luxury in the face of high workloads and sometimes broad differences in education, language and culture between health providers and patients. Nevertheless, patient-centeredness has been found to improve quality of life, increase patient satisfaction, improve adherence to treatment, enhance the integration of preventive and promotive care, and improve the provider's job satisfaction. It does not necessarily imply a longer consultation. Patient-centeredness implies a more collaborative approach and holistic understanding of the patient that elicits, acknowledges and addresses relevant beliefs, concerns, ideas and fears [14].

Patient-centeredness is in part a paradigm shift in the mind of the health worker from a bio-medical, technical and sometimes authoritarian model to a biopsychosocial, holistic and participatory model [14]. It is fundamentally a way of being with the patient. Nevertheless, a range of specific communication skills can be learnt such as the ability to ask open as well as closed questions, to make reflective listening statements, exchange information or invite mutual decision-making [29]. While training of doctors has begun to include these communication skills, even in low resource settings, the training of nurses and mid-level health workers often has not.

Motivational interviewing builds on a patient-centered approach and can best be described as a guiding style. Diabetes, which involves multiple changes in behavior (diet, exercise, smoking, alcohol, medication), particularly lends itself to adaptations of motivational interviewing. A challenge in low resource settings is to see how a range of health workers can incorporate a guiding style into their consultations.

In a model of care that emphasizes patient empowerment and self-care as key components [2], every consultation needs to be seen as an opportunity for this. Health providers need to have the necessary expertise in the relevant topics, useful communication skills and a range of educational materials appropriate to the literacy level of the community. In some settings, group as well as individual approaches may be effective [30].

A family and community orientation

Beyond the individual patient is their family and community context. Clearly, family beliefs and customs and degree of social support will have an impact on the ability of an individual within that family to make lifestyle changes and cope with their diabetes. Involving family members in the consultation or educational program can strengthen the overall response to diabetes [31]. Likewise, an understanding of the patient's environment will inform discussions about appropriate changes and likely constraints.

In low resource settings, where facilities are overwhelmed with large numbers of patients it may make sense to extend care into the community [2]. For example community-based support groups can be run by health promoters or local non-government organizations to offer some aspects of routine chronic care. Patients can then return to the local clinic for periodic or annual review and help with complications. Support groups can also encourage lifestyle change and adherence to medication. Expert patients, an increasingly developed resource in both low and high income situations, may also be useful to enhance self-care, although further evaluation is required [32]. Community health workers have the potential to promote healthy lifestyle, provide home-based care and link selected patients with the local facilities [33].

Communities should not just be seen as additional platforms for care or targets for interventions but representative structures or key leaders should be engaged with in order to understand how local health priorities are perceived and to elicit feedback and involvement in the planning and delivery of services [14].

Primary care workers usually have a responsibility not just for individual patients but for people living within specific communities or health districts [14]. Concern for the growing number of people with diabetes should lead to interventions that address the underlying determinants of obesity and reduced physical activity: for example, school-based healthy lifestyle programs, provision of green spaces in inner cities, marketing of food to children, sale of junk food on public premises and labeling of food. Many of these require health workers to contribute to interventions in other sectors [34].

Making use of evidence

The evidence base for diabetes is constantly expanding and all the above areas need to be informed by the latest evidence base that is relevant to the resource setting in which it is to be applied. Ideally, a systematic process for reviewing the evidence and updating guidance accordingly should be in place in all countries. An example of such a system from a high income setting is the National Institute for Health and Clinical Excellence (NICE) in the UK. This may be beyond the resources of lower income countries but through regional cooperation, such as coordinated by WHO, the IDF and the World Bank, regular reviews of the evidence appropriate to different resource settings do take place. The availability of evidence does not guarantee that it will be used, and there is a strong and growing literature on how to build local ownership and influence local practice, such as through the development of local treatment guidelines.

Information technology – how to embrace it?

Information technology (IT) is a rapidly growing field that has the capacity to strengthen the model of care for diabetes across different resource settings. The potential targets for IT range from people with diabetes to people at risk for diabetes, health workers and managers. Some of the ways in which IT can strengthen the model for diabetes care are improving continuity of information, assisting in running referral systems between different levels of care, and providing tools for education and empowerment.

Numerous IT modalities or systems exist, although these need to be tailored according to the target population and desired outcome. Thus, real-time imaging and audio contact via equipment such as digital cameras, video phones and computers can permit interaction between health workers and individual patients or groups of patients for education sessions. Dietary management and medication adherence support may be provided by mobile phone messaging; self-care may be enabled by technology-mediated feedback on blood glucose levels on a daily basis. Quality of care may be enhanced by access to the latest evidence or decision-support tools; auditing may be supported by software that automates the analysis of raw data and integrates it with district health information systems.

Innovative strategies for clinical management, especially those which address monitoring of patients by technology-mediated communication with the diabetes care team, are being introduced in high resource settings. One of the key issues to be addressed is the cost-effectiveness of such IT-based systems [35] and the amount that an individual is willing to pay may well depend on their perception of risk. Furthermore, even in high resource settings, a patient's age and educational background may place limits on their ability to utilize IT [36]. In contrast, at present IT has limited applicability in low resource settings as these are characterized by no or very limited access to the Internet and a lack of familiarity with computers amongst health care workers. Even when a large health center or hospital has computers and Internet access, these are likely to be available to the managers or possibly large clinical areas, certainly not in individual consulting rooms, while such access in primary care settings is simply not to be had for the most part. Furthermore, patients coming from poor backgrounds are very unlikely to have access to the Internet.

Mobile phone-based telecommunication system to enhance patient self-care

Mobile phones, of all the currently available technologies directed at the patient, are likely to have the greatest potential use in low resource settings. This is because the digital divide along the socioeconomic gradient appears to be less evident with mobile phones than other forms of IT, such as the Internet [37,38]. Mobile phones are even to be found in remote villages, indicating the extent of their penetration in contrast to the lack of access to land lines in many rural areas; however, unlike the situation in well-resourced countries where the majority of mobile phone owners have a contract for a year or so, the usual practice in low income countries is one using prepaid phone cards and sharing of phones. If the IT involvement is simply related to the patient's receipt of messages to support their care, this may not have a negative impact, since even when phone use exceeds the amount paid, the phone may still receive messages, but may not be able to send outgoing comunications.

In countries with better resources, mobile phones have been put to additional uses in diabetes care. A real-time telemedicine transmission system has been developed and tested. One system uses a blood glucose monitor connected to a general packet radio system mobile phone to enable transmission of patients' blood glucose levels [39] with subsequent feedback. Farmer *et al.* [40] demonstrated that real-time telemedicine was feasible and realistic in a randomized controlled trial. Further, the idea of measuring the blood glucose level directly from the mobile phone has also been introduced (Figure 58.2). Cho *et al.* [41] reported that the effect of the mobile communication system using the "diabetes phone" (Figure 58.3b) was not inferior to that of an Internet-

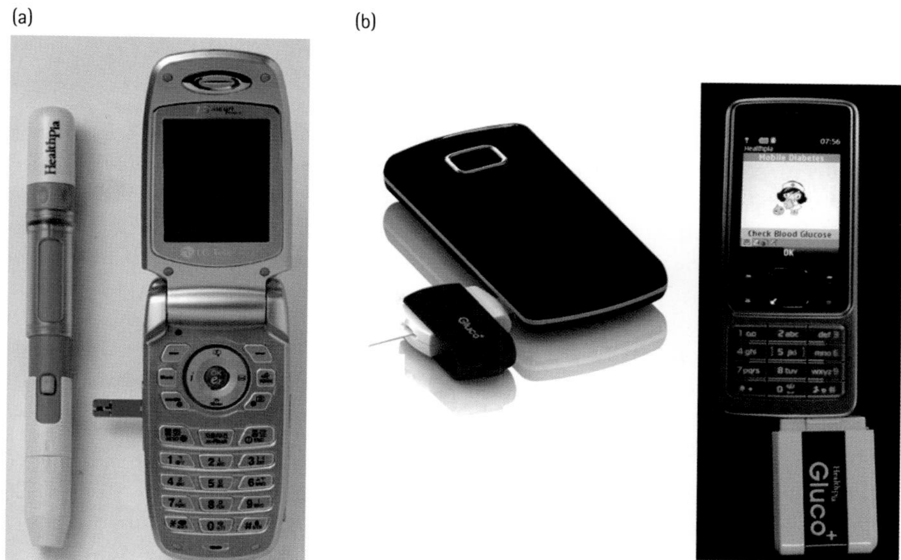

Figure 58.2 Glucometer with telecommunication. Adapted from Cho *et al.* [41]. (a) The Diabetes Phone (Healthpia, Korea) has a glucometer in a battery pack (phone embedded type). (b) The glucometer can be directly connected to a cellular phone (Dongle type). (Gluco plus, Healthpia, Korea.)

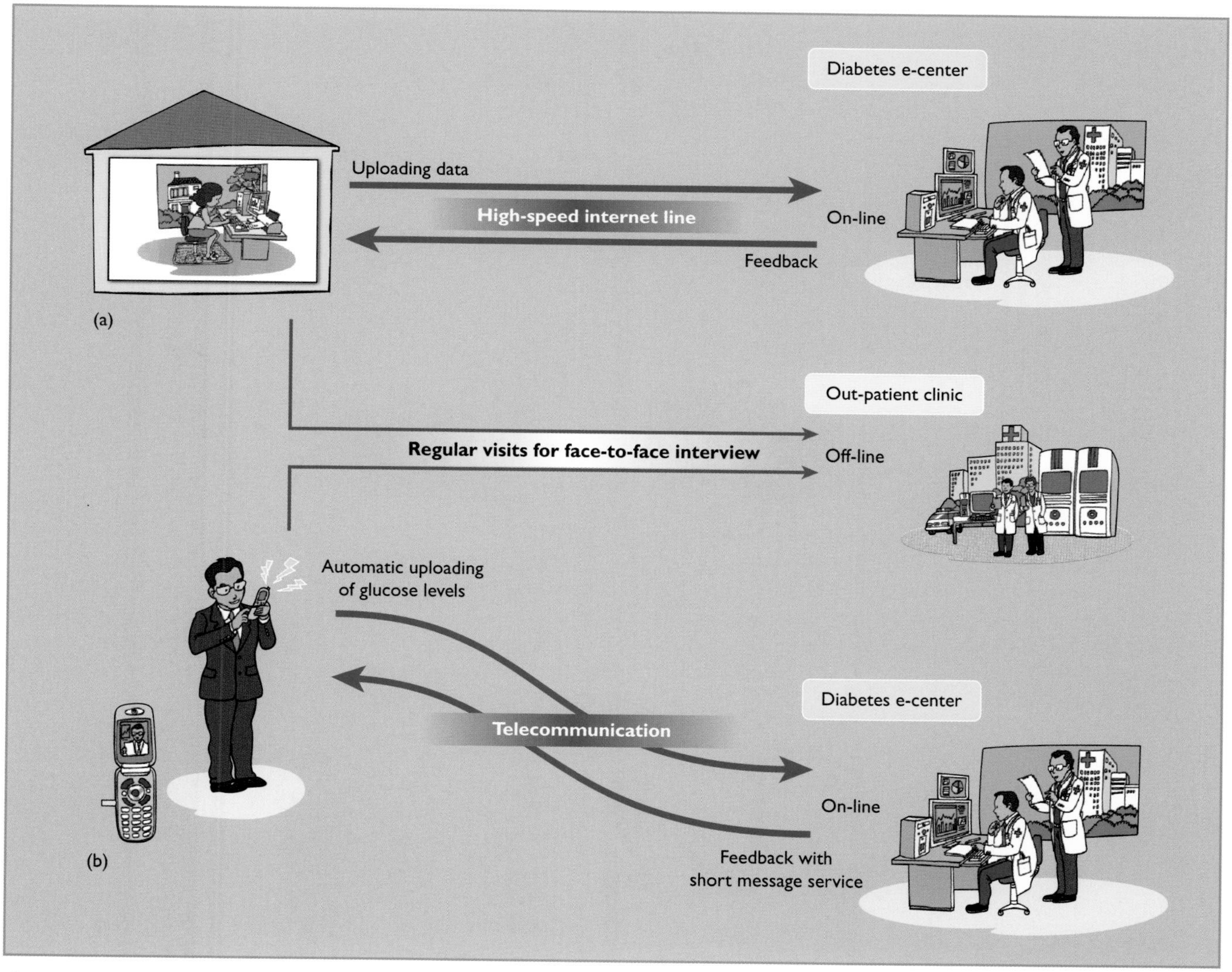

Figure 58.3 (a) The Internet-based glucose monitoring system (IBGMS). Patients logged on to the website from their homes or offices at a time they found convenient and uploaded their glucose data, together with additional information such as current drug information (type and dosage of oral hypoglycemic medications or insulin), lifestyle modifications and hypoglycemic events. In addition, patients recorded any changes in their blood pressure or weight, and any questions or detailed information that they wished to discuss, such as changes in diet, exercise, hypoglycemic events, and other factors that might influence their blood glucose level. (b) The telecommunication-based glucose control system in which mobile devices such as a mobile phone with the capacity to measure blood glucose were adopted. Patients could upload their information through telecommunication automatically and the patient–doctor communication could be achieved practically in real-time by the short message service. Adapted from Yoon *et al.* [42].

based glucose monitoring systems in terms of supervision, care and patient's satisfaction. The fact that text messaging on mobile phones is very limited represents a possible disadvantage for utilizing real-time telemedicine in providing information regarding blood glucose status. It is probable that the integration of medical equipment and mobile phones will be developed within the not-too-distant future.

Technology-based access to the latest evidence and guidelines for health workers

IT can enhance interaction with and use of evidence-based guidelines by health workers even in low resource settings. This can take the form of palm-held stand-alone personal digital assistant (PDA) devices or stand-alone tablets with periodic updating via Internet or CD ROM. The latter has been used sucessfully even in remote areas. Devices can contain reference material, evidence-based guidelines or automated decision trees. If Internet access is available, these devices can be used to access electronic databases from the consulting room. Such technologies need to provide information without interrupting the consultation process for health care workers facing serious time constraints. Additionally, the technology must not have a negative effect on the interaction between the patient and health worker.

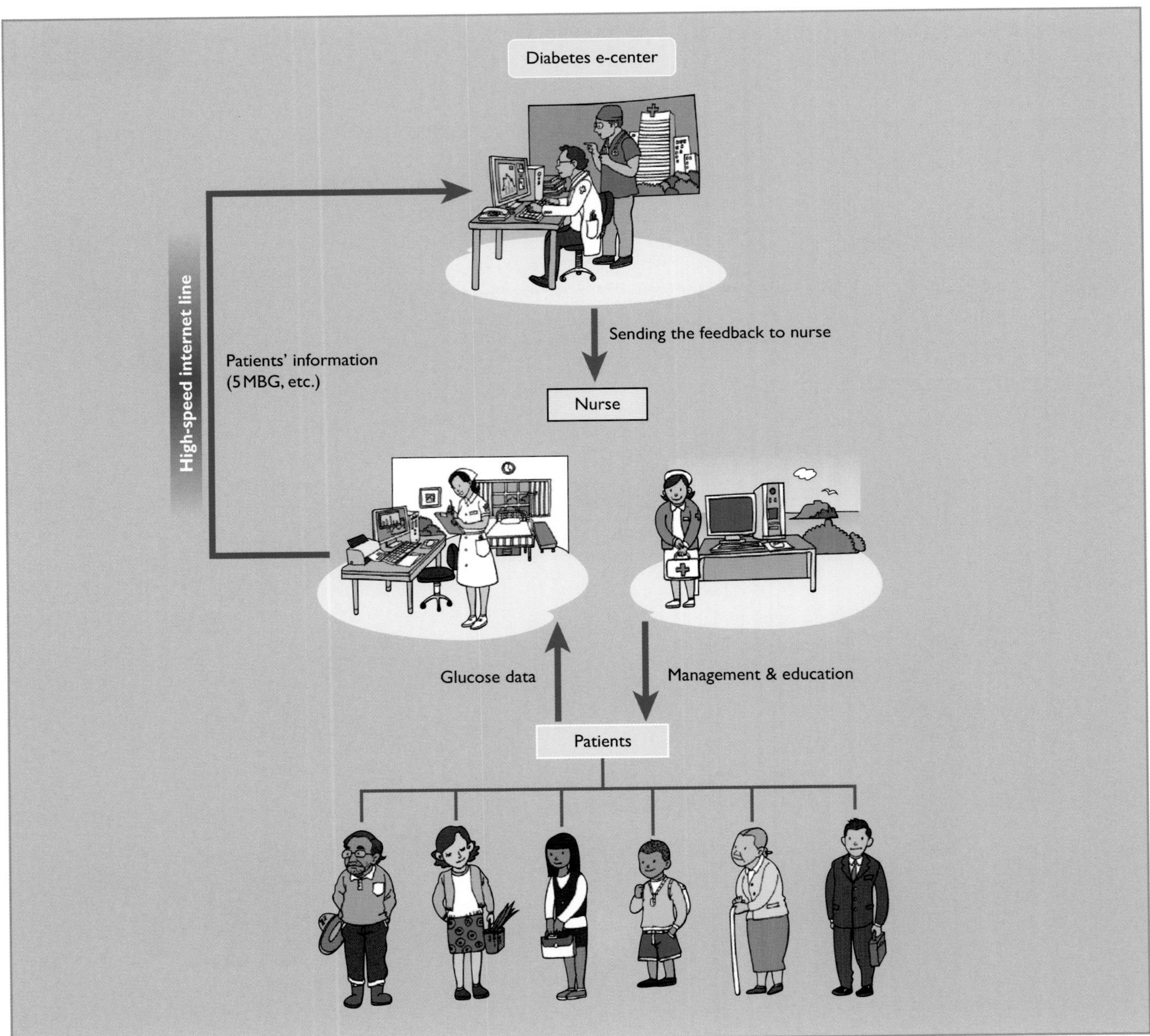

Figure 58.4 Technology-based clinical support. First, a nurse checks the self-monitoring of blood glucose (SMBG) data of patients and sends the patients' data, including SMBG data, to the endocrinologist. The endocrinologist reviews the patients' uploaded information and sends messages to the nurse. The nurse educates and manages the patients according to the endocrinologist's recommendations. Adapted from Yoon *et al.* [42].

Technology-based clinical support

Certain aspects of diabetes care, such as retinal screening, lend themselves to mobile digital photography by fundal camera with transmission of photographs and reports via satellite or Internet between the peripheral and a central reporting site. Examples have been reported from relatively low resource settings in Africa and India [22,23]. Primary care providers can also be supported from referral centers via IT to improve the quality of clinical advice and decision-making. For example, in South Korea a nurse can send information regarding specific patients' glucose readings to an endocrinologist. The specialist can review the data uploaded and send advice on patient management (Figure 58.4) [42]. It is anticipated that the indirect communication system could eventually be applied to health workers living in low resource settings, thereby contributing to the gradual but definite development of universal IT-based diabetes management systems.

Automated feedback systems to enhance patient self-care

People with diabetes can use their own personal computer to receive automated feedback on self-management (Figure 58.5a) [43]. Similar automated feedback on glucose levels can be obtained via the Internet (Figure 58.5b). In this situation, it is imperative to have software or a decision support system that can make an appropriate recommendation on glycemic status. Meigs *et al.* [44] have developed and reported on the clinical applicability of a web-based decision support tool, the diabetes Disease Management Application. Although this system could be highly cost-efficient, long-term compliance and satisfaction could be limited because of lack of flexibility and human contact.

Interactive feedback systems to enhance patient self-care

Internet-based interactive communication systems enable two-way communication between patients and their physicians via the Internet (Figure 58.3a). Systems are still cost-efficient and yet are more personalized [45]. Options range from utilizing e-mail to developing a private homepage to share clinical information [46]. For instance, Kwon *et al.* [47] reported a short-term reduction in HbA_{1c} through the effect of an Internet-based glucose monitoring system (IBGMS), in which patients and doctors shared a web-chart (Figure 58.6). Patients uploaded their glucose data to the remote web server and their doctors provided advice after interpreting the data [47]. The idea of integrating web-based communication with the hospital's own electronic medical record charting system was also introduced [48]. Cho *et al.* [49] reported that the longest prospective study (30 months) of an IBGMS in

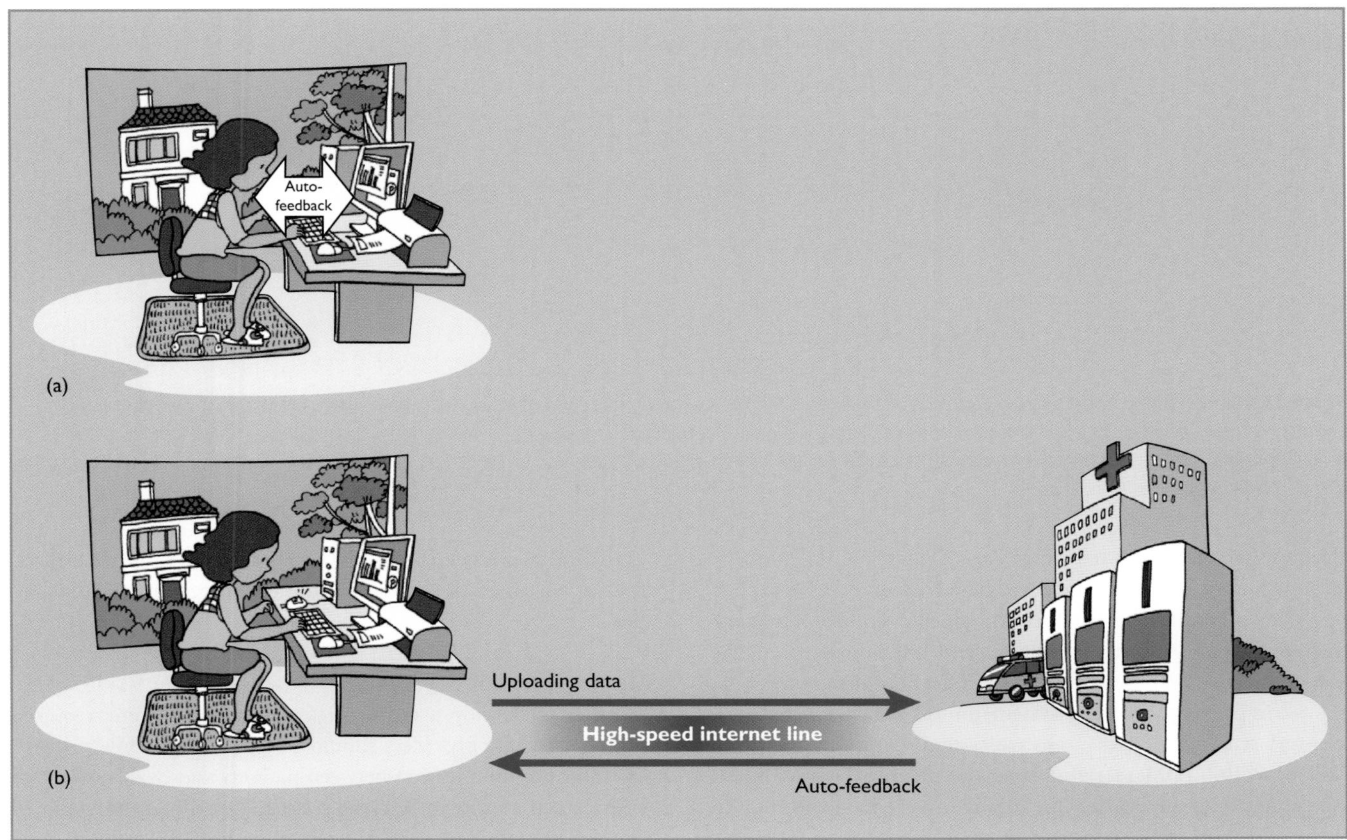

Figure 58.5 (a) Personal computer-based self-management (automated) system. (b) Internet-based auto-feedback system. Adapted from Lehmann [43].

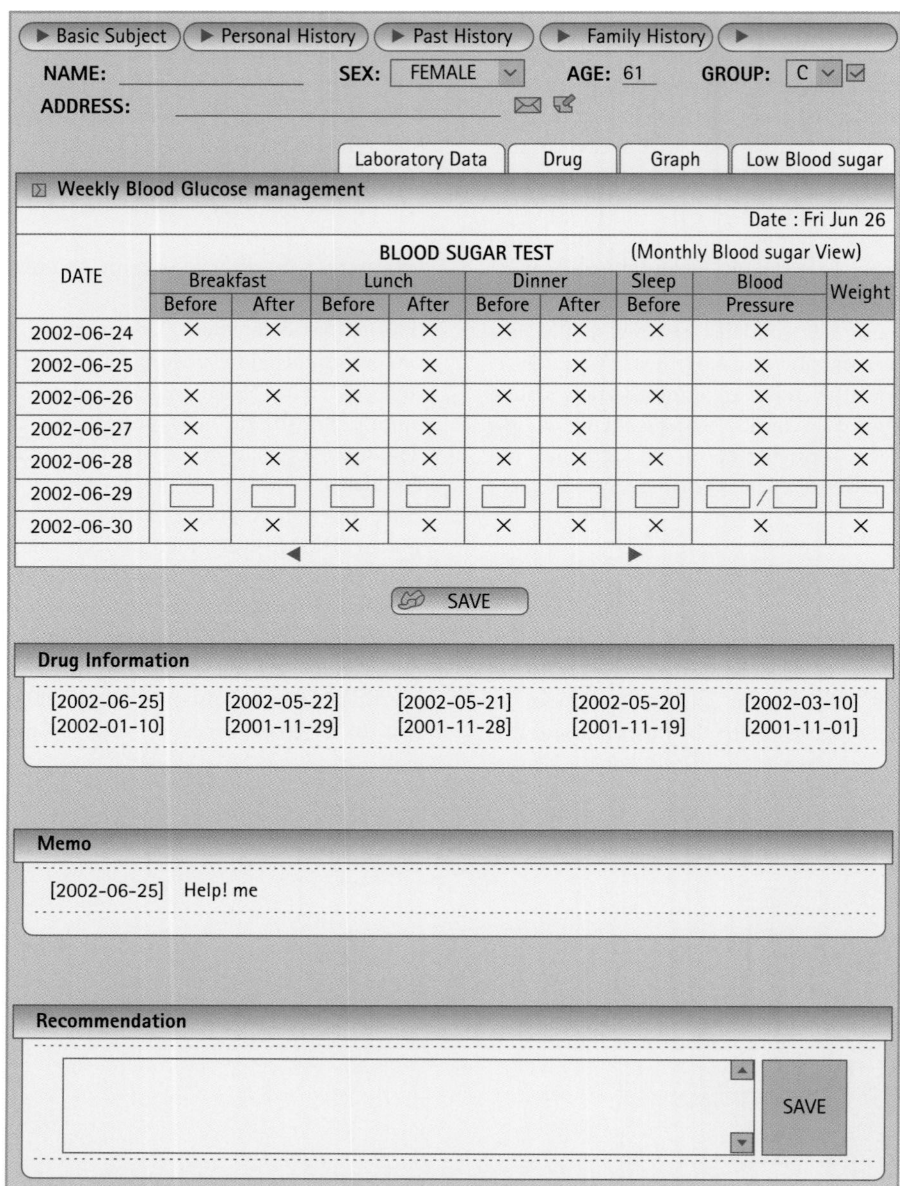

Figure 58.6 Screen viewed by patients and physicians on the website for diabetes management (www.biodang.com). Basic profile, past history, family history and laboratory data are shown on the top. Self-monitored blood glucose levels are shown (middle), which are recorded as fasting or post-prandial (breakfast, lunch and dinner). Drug information, notes from the patients and recommendations from the physicians are shown at the bottom. Reproduced from Kwon *et al.* [47] with permission from the American Diabetes Association.

diabetes was effective in reducing HbA_{1c} (Figure 58.7). Uniquely, this system not only provides periodic advice and feedback, but also allows continuous support for glucose control, frequent encouragement, problem assessment and individualized education about diet, exercise and drug modification, thereby providing a comprehensive caring system for patients with diabetes. Montori *et al.* [50] used a telecare system using a modem for patients with T1DM receiving intensive insulin therapy. When the patient deviated from the desired glycemic control, the glucose analysis software assisted nurses to interpret the patient's status and provide feedback to the patient. Even more specialized systems have been developed for women with gestational diabetes [51].

Merged feedback systems to enhance patient self-care

In order to develop a more efficient system, the time required from health care providers should be minimized, while preserving some communication between patients and health care providers when absolutely necessary. Recently, a system was piloted that will respond automatically when the glucose level is accept-

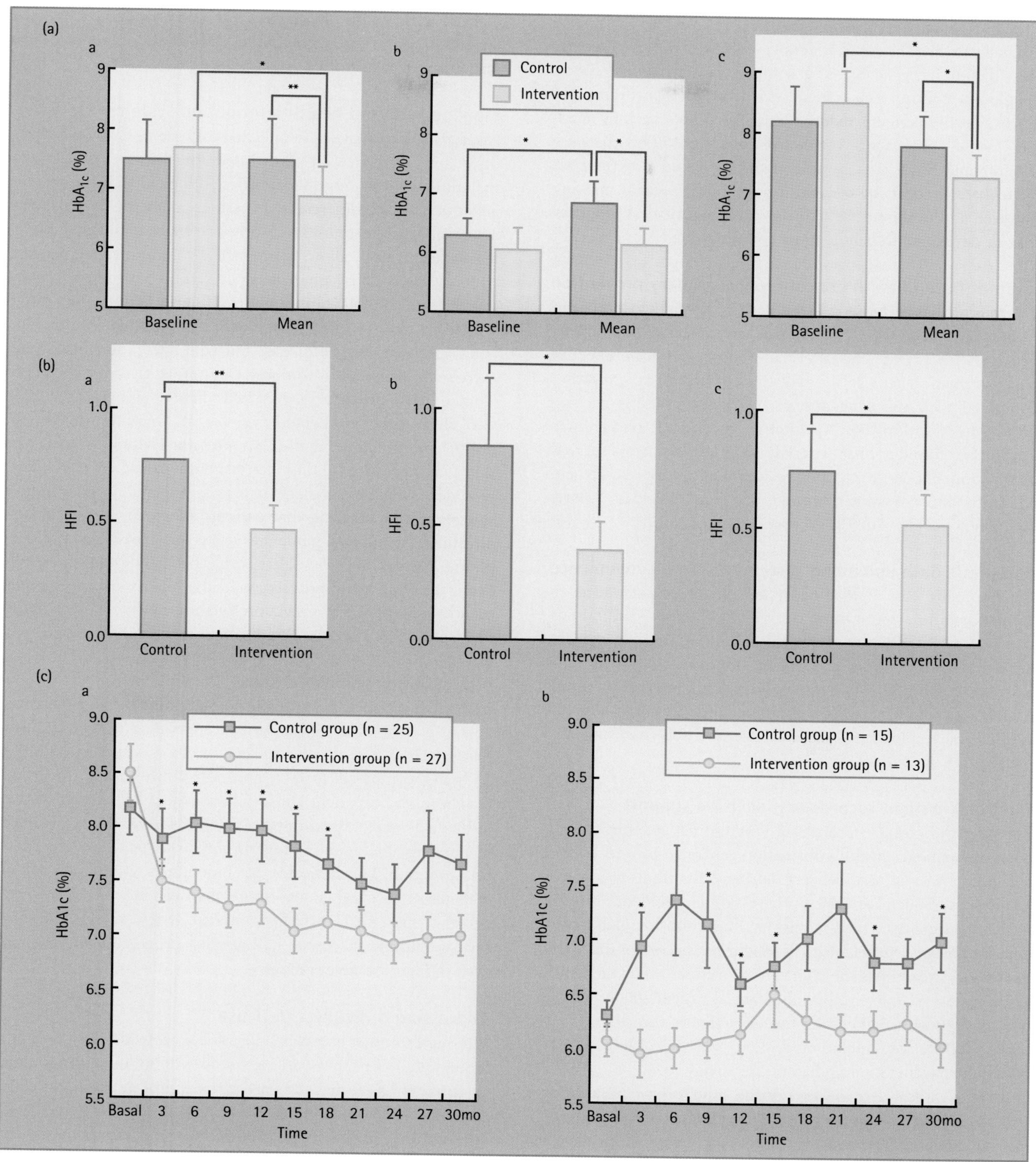

Figure 58.7 The effects of intervention (Internet-based glucose monitoring system [IBGMS]) on changes of HbA_{1c} and glucose stability. A: Baseline HbA_{1c} and mean HbA_{1c} during the study 30-month period. (a) All subjects, control (n = 40) vs intervention (n = 40). (b) Subjects with a basal $HbA_{1c} < 7\%$, control (n = 15) vs intervention (n = 13). (c) Subjects with a basal $HbA_{1c} \geq 7\%$, control (n = 25) vs intervention (n = 27). B: Difference of HbA_{1c} fluctuation index (HFI) between the control and intervention groups. (a) All subjects. (b) Subjects with a basal $HbA_{1c} < 7.\%$. (c) Subjects with a basal $HbA_{1c} \geq 7\%$. C: Fluctuating line of HbA_{1c} for the 30 months. (a) Subjects with a basal $HbA_{1c} \geq 7\%$. (b) Subjects with a basal $HbA_{1c} < 7\%$. At each follow-up point, ≥90% of patients took the test. $*P < 0.05$; $**P < 0.01$. DCCT aligned HbA_{1c} of 7% is equivalent to IFCC HbA_{1c} of 53 mmol/mol. Reproduced from Cho *et al.* [49] with permission from the American Diabetes Association.

able, but which will involve a health care provider for further evaluation when the result is abnormal. Cho *et al.* [52] reported the effect on labor savings of a semi-automatic response system for glucose control. The system, which had an algorithm-based glucose decision engine, reduced physicians' labor time by nearly 50% while preserving interactive communication between patients and physicians. Simple algorithm-based programs are inadequate to meet the complexity of clinical decision-making, however, and in the future artificial intelligence-based programs may be developed to handle more complex data.

Internet-based health education and primary prevention

The Internet has been used as a medium for a weight loss program to prevent diabetes [53] and as part of a walking program for patients with T2DM. The latter had a more significant effect on patients' physical activity and reduction of depressive symptoms, compared with the conventional method of sharing physical activity information [54]. An Internet and mobile phone intervention was found to improve cardiovascular risk factors for both T1DM and T2DM groups [55]. Additionally, a mobile diabetes education and care system brought beneficial effects in children and young people with T1DM in a rural area [56].

Automatic data uploading system for more convenience

An automatic data uploading system has been introduced in South Korea to achieve more convenient IT-based communication system. This system allows for self-monitored glucose data measured with a home glucometer (OneTouchUltra, Lifescan, USA) to be sent to the patient's web chart via Internet by simply connecting it to a personal computer. Physicians can view the automatically uploaded glucose data on the web chart and send messages to the patient.

Electronic patient records and decision support

The electronic health record is a longitudinal electronic document of a patient's health information generated by one or more encounters in any care delivery setting. This information may include patient demographics, progress notes, problems, medications, vital signs, past medical history, immunizations, laboratory data, radiology reports, etc. The electronic health record automates and streamlines the clinician's workflow, it has the ability to generate a complete record of a clinical patient encounter – as well as supporting other care-related activities directly or indirectly via interface – including evidence-based decision support, quality management and outcomes reporting [57].

Various clinical decision supporting systems have been developed, which are able to provide diagnostic and therapeutic services to both clinicians and patients by using electronically recorded health data. Advanced development in IT not only guarantees efficient communication between an individual and a medical institution, but also makes possible for the medical institutions themselves to share information efficiently. Massin *et al.* [58] sent retinal images (non-mydriatic photography) of people with diabetes to a reading center for diagnosis and follow-up of diabetic retinopathy. Recently, efforts to standardize medical terminology and interfaces among devices and communication systems have been made.

Management and health information systems

A variety of personal health information systems have been developed and some are currently used for disease management, including diabetes. Several countries with good IT infrastructure already have commercialized various diabetes management systems. Mycareteam uses web-based software to facilitate diabetes management by allowing interactive communication between patients and their physicians or family members (www.mycareteam.com, Mycareteam Inc, USA). A similar web-based service system in which patients can communicate with the diabetes-specialist care team consisting of a nurse, nutritionist and exercise therapist was introduced to improve glycemic control of women with pregnancy-associated diabetes (www.cared.co.kr, C&I Healthcare Co., Republic of Korea). Growing numbers of health care companies in the USA are using IT tools for their care solutions instead of traditional telephone-based services. Alere provides a diabetes management program mainly focusing on education and ensuring that patients adhere to the physician's directions and clinical guidelines using web-based tool and telephone interactions (www.alere.com, USA). By establishing evidence showing an improvement in the quality of disease care, eventual medical cost reduction and improvement in patients' satisfaction, the IT-based health care market could increase.

Addressing economic hurdles

In the first instance, it is essential to determine the cost-effectiveness of IT. Cho *et al.* [59] reported a simulation study indicating that the IBGMS could save $27 666 of direct cost per person for 35 years compared to a conventional face-to-face interview system in an outpatient clinic. Johnson *et al.* [60] reported that individuals were willing to pay $1500 over 3 years to participate in a lifestyle intervention program similar to the diabetes prevention program. This indicates that individuals with a high risk of diabetes are willing to pay more than individuals with lower perceived risk. An IT-based patient care system sounds tempting but, once again, the key to its feasibility lies in cost-effectiveness even in high resource settings.

Addressing difficulties in IT use

Although Internet access is increasing worldwide, there is still a limited pool of people who can use IT without difficulties. Thus, an Internet-based diabetes care system must address and overcome its limitations before application. Watson *et al.* [61] reported that patients with diabetes with no experience of the Internet or media communication are enthusiastic about adopting future health information technology for their diabetes care. Furthermore, Jackson *et al.* [62] showed that among African-Americans with a lack of computer skills, 66% were willing to learn and 89% were willing to use a computer program to manage their diabetes, if it were offered free of charge. From this evidence, the potential users for IT-based diabetic care should not be underestimated [61].

Advances in the near future

It is believed that the dramatic development of IT and its application to health management systems will have a crucial role. Simple IT management models for controlling blood glucose levels for patients with diabetes will definitely evolve into much more complex models, in which various technologies are integrated in order to provide the complex management required. Technologic gadgets may be directly connected to a communication system to transmit a patient's current status and past data. For example, a physical activity monitor (Lifecoder, Suzuken, Japan; Actical, Philips, USA) could be integrated into the health information system for monitoring real-time physical activity.

These innovative technologies can also be applied to other chronic diseases such as hypertension and rheumatoid arthritis. It is important to develop software that can integrate efficiently and process the constant flow of incoming data. To achieve this, we must keep in mind that simple algorithm-based programs are not enough to meet the challenges of medicine; rather, artificial intelligence-based programs will be necessary to handle the complex data and to provide economic benefits by lowering the human labor and costs. Communication systems that are not hindered by time and space are also needed. Information technology should never be seen as an end in itself, but as a tool to complement other aspects of holistic patient-centered diabetes care.

References

1 Narayan KM, Zhang P, Williams D, Engelgau M, Imperatore G, Kanaya A, *et al.* How should developing countries manage diabetes? *CMAJ* 2006; **175**:733.

2 World Health Organization (WHO). *Innovative Care for Chronic Conditions: Building Blocks for Action: Global Report*. Geneva: WHO, 2002.

3 Davidson P, Halcomb E, Hickman L, Phillips J, Graham B. Beyond the rhetoric: what do we mean by a "model of care"? *Aust J Adv Nurs* 2006; **23**:47–55.

4 Orrell C, Bangsberg DR, Badri M, Wood R. Adherence is not a barrier to successful antiretroviral therapy in South Africa. *AIDS* 2003; **17**:1369–1375.

5 World Health Organization (WHO). *Global Strategy on Diet, Physical Activity and Health*. Geneva: WHO, 2004.

6 International Diabetes Federation (IDF). *Diabetes Atlas*, 4th edn. Brussels: IDF, 2010.

7 Njamnshi A, Bella Hiag A, Mbanya JC. From research to policy: the development of a national diabetes programme. *Diabetes Voice* 2006; **51**:18–21.

8 Department of Health. *Diabetes*. England: Department of Health, 2009.

9 De Maeseneer J, van Weel C, Egilman D, Mfenyana K, Kaufman A, Sewankambo N. Strengthening primary care: addressing the disparity between vertical and horizontal investment. *Br J Gen Pract* 2008; **58**:3–4.

10 Rawaf S, De Maeseneer J, Starfield B. From Alma-Ata to Almaty: a new start for primary health care. *Lancet* 2008; **372**:1365–1367.

11 Janssens B, Van Damme W, Raleigh B, Gupta J, Khem S, Soy Ty K, *et al.* Offering integrated care for HIV/AIDS, diabetes and hypertension within chronic disease clinics in Cambodia. *Bull World Health Organ* 2007; **85**:880–885.

12 Beaglehole R, Epping-Jordan J, Patel V, Chopra M, Ebrahim S, Kidd M, *et al.* Improving the prevention and management of chronic disease in low-income and middle-income countries: a priority for primary health care. *Lancet* 2008; **372**:940–949.

13 Renders CM, Valk GD, Griffin S, Wagner EH, Eijk JT, Assendelft WJ. Interventions to improve the management of diabetes mellitus in primary care, outpatient and community settings. *Cochrane Database Syst Rev* 2001; **1**:CD001481.

14 World Health Organization (WHO). *The World Health Report 2008: Primary Health Care, Now More Than Ever*. Geneva: WHO, 2008.

15 Mash B, Levitt NS, Van Vuuren U, Martell R. Improving the annual review of diabetic patients in primary care: an appreciative inquiry in the Cape Town District Health Services. *S Afri Fam Pract* 2008; **50**:50–50d.

16 Haggerty J, Burge F, Levesque JF, Gass D, Pineault R, Beaulieu MD, *et al.* Operational definitions of attributes of primary health care: consensus among Canadian experts. *Ann Fam Med* 2007; **5**: 336–344.

17 Mendis S, Fukino K, Cameron A, Laing R, Filipe A Jr, Khatib O, *et al.* The availability and affordability of selected essential medicines for chronic diseases in six low- and middle-income countries. *Bull World Health Organ* 2007; **85**:279–288.

18 Beran D, Yudkin JS. Diabetes care in sub-Saharan Africa. *Lancet* 2006; **368**:1689–1695.

19 Gill GV, Price C, Shandu D, Dedicoat M, Wilkinson D. An effective system of nurse-led diabetes care in rural Africa. *Diabet Med* 2008; **25**:606–611.

20 Sibbald B. Should primary care be nurse led? Yes. *Br Med J* 2008; **337**:a1157.

21 Mullan F, Frehywot S. Non-physician clinicians in 47 sub-Saharan African countries. *Lancet* 2007; **370**:2158–2163.

22 Mash B, Powell D, du Plessis F, van Vuuren U, Michalowska M, Levitt N. Screening for diabetic retinopathy in primary care with a mobile fundal camera: evaluation of a South African pilot project. *S Afr Med J* 2007; **97**:1284–1288.

23 Aravind Eye Care System. Activity Report 2007–2008: Diabetic Retinopathy Initiatives. Available from www.aravind.org

24 Mash BJ, Mayers P, Conradie H, Orayn A, Kuiper M, Marais J. How to manage organisational change and create practice teams: experiences of a South African primary care health centre. *Educ Health (Abingdon)* 2008; **21**:132.

25 Couper ID, Hugo JF, Tumbo JM, Harvey BM, Malete NH. Key issues in clinic functioning: a case study of two clinics. *S Afr Med J* 2007; **97**:124–129.

26 Capra F. *The Hidden Connections: A Science for Sustainable Living*. London: Flamingo, 2003.

27 Barrett R. *Building a Values-Driven Organization: A Whole-System Approach to Cultural Transformation*. Butterworth-Heinemann, 2006.

28 Wheatley M. *Turning to One Another: Simple Conversations to Restore Hope to the Future*. Berrett-Koehler, 2002.

29 Rollnick S, Miller WR, Butler CC. *Motivational Interviewing in Health Care: Helping Patients Change Behaviour*. London: Guilford Press, 2008.

30 Deakin T, McShane CE, Cade JE, Williams RD. Group-based training for self-management strategies in people with type 2 diabetes mellitus. *Cochrane Database Syst Rev* 2005: CD003417.

31 McDaniel SH, Campbell TL, Hepworth J, Lorenz A. *Family-Oriented Primary Care*, 2nd edn. Springer, 2004.

32 Foster G, Taylor SJ, Eldridge SE, Ramsay J, Griffiths CJ. Self-management education programmes by lay leaders for people with chronic conditions. *Cochrane Database Syst Rev* 2007: CD005108.

33 Lehmann U, Sanders D. *Community Health Workers: What Do We Know About Them?* WHO, Evidence and Information for Policy. Geneva: World Health Organization, 2007.

34 Unwin N, Alberti KG. Chronic non-communicable diseases. *Ann Trop Med Parasitol* 2006; **100**:455–464.

35 Jackson CL, Bolen S, Brancati FL, Batts-Turner ML, Gary TL. A systematic review of interactive computer-assisted technology in diabetes care: interactive information technology in diabetes care. *J Gen Intern Med* 2006; **21**:105–110.

36 Grant RW, Cagliero E, Chueh HC, Meigs JB. Internet use among primary care patients with type 2 diabetes: the generation and education gap. *J Gen Intern Med* 2005; **20**:470–473.

37 Kaplan WA. Can the ubiquitous power of mobile phones be used to improve health outcomes in developing countries? *Global Health* 2006; **2**:9.

38 Forestier E GJ, Kenny C. Can information and communications policy be pro-poor? *Telecommunications Policy* 2002; **26**:623–646.

39 Farmer A, Gibson O, Hayton P, Bryden K, Dudley C, Neil A, *et al.* A real-time, mobile phone-based telemedicine system to support young adults with type 1 diabetes. *Inform Prim Care* 2005; **13**:171–177.

40 Farmer AJ, Gibson OJ, Dudley C, Bryden K, Hayton PM, Tarassenko L, *et al.* A randomized controlled trial of the effect of real-time telemedicine support on glycemic control in young adults with type 1 diabetes (ISRCTN 46889446). *Diabetes Care* 2005; **28**:2697–2702.

41 Cho JH, Lee HC, Lim DJ, Kwon HS, Yoon KH. Mobile communication using a mobile phone with a glucometer for glucose control in type 2 patients with diabetes: as effective as an Internet-based glucose monitoring system. *J Telemed Telecare* 2009; **15**:77–82.

42 Yoon KH, Kwon HS, Lee JH, Park YM, Lee WC, Cha BY, *et al.* Effect of the Internet-based glucose monitoring system (IBGMS) connected with personal digital assistance (PDA) in rural health subcenter. 6th Diabetes Technology Meeting, USA, 2006.

43 Lehmann ED. Diabetes information technology and WebWatch: general resources. *Diabetes Technol Ther* 1999; **1**:109–112.

44 Meigs JB, Cagliero E, Dubey A, Murphy-Sheehy P, Gildesgame C, Chueh H, *et al.* A controlled trial of web-based diabetes disease management: the MGH diabetes primary care improvement project. *Diabetes Care* 2003; **26**:750–757.

45 Feil EG, Glasgow RE, Boles S, McKay HG. Who participates in Internet-based self-management programs? A study among novice computer users in a primary care setting. *Diabetes Educ* 2000; **26**:806–811.

46 Smith KE, Levine BA, Clement SC, Hu MJ, Alaoui A, Mun SK. Impact of MyCareTeam for poorly controlled diabetes mellitus. *Diabetes Technol Ther* 2004; **6**:828–835.

47 Kwon HS, Cho JH, Kim HS, Song BR, Ko SH, Lee JM, *et al.* Establishment of blood glucose monitoring system using the internet. *Diabetes Care* 2004; **27**:478–483.

48 Ralston JD, Revere D, Robins LS, Goldberg HI. Patients' experience with a diabetes support programme based on an interactive electronic medical record: qualitative study. *Br Med J* 2004; **328**:1159.

49 Cho JH, Chang SA, Kwon HS, Choi YH, Ko SH, Moon SD, *et al.* Long-term effect of the Internet-based glucose monitoring system on HbA1c reduction and glucose stability: a 30-month follow-up study for diabetes management with a ubiquitous medical care system. *Diabetes Care* 2006; **29**:2625–2631.

50 Montori VM, Helgemoe PK, Guyatt GH, Dean DS, Leung TW, Smith SA, *et al.* Telecare for patients with type 1 diabetes and inadequate glycemic control: a randomized controlled trial and meta-analysis. *Diabetes Care* 2004; **27**:1088–1094.

51 Kruger DF, White K, Galpern A, Mann K, Massirio A, McLellan M, *et al.* Effect of modem transmission of blood glucose data on telephone consultation time, clinic work flow, and patient satisfaction for patients with gestational diabetes mellitus. *J Am Acad Nurse Pract* 2003; **15**:371–375.

52 Cho JH, Yoon KH, *et al.* Labor saving effect of the semi-automatic response system for diabetes management (SARS-DM) based on the internet. Poster presentation, American Diabetes Association 68th Scientific Sessions, USA, 2008.

53 McCoy MR, Couch D, Duncan ND, Lynch GS. Evaluating an internet weight loss program for diabetes prevention. *Health Promot Int* 2005; **20**:221–228.

54 McKay HG, King D, Eakin EG, Seeley JR, Glasgow RE. The diabetes network internet-based physical activity intervention: a randomized pilot study. *Diabetes Care* 2001; **24**:1328–1334.

55 Harno K, Kauppinen-Makelin R, Syrjalainen J. Managing diabetes care using an integrated regional e-health approach. *J Telemed Telecare* 2006; **12**(Suppl 1):13–15.

56 von Sengbusch S, Müller-Godeffroy E, Häger S, Reintjes R, Hiort O, Wagner V. Mobile diabetes education and care: intervention for children and young people with type 1 diabetes in rural areas of northern Germany. *Diabet Med* 2006; **23**:122–127.

57 http://www.himss.org/ASP/topics_ehr.asp.

58 Massin P, Aubert JP, Erginay A, Bourovitch JC, Benmehidi A, Audran G, *et al.* Screening for diabetic retinopathy: the first telemedical approach in a primary care setting in France. *Diabetes Metab* 2004; **30**:451–457.

59 Cho JH, Yoon KH, *et al.* Economic impact of the information technology-based diabetes management system on type 2 diabetes: a key for solving world's big problem. American Diabetes Association 67th Scientific Session, 2007.

60 Johnson FR, Manjunath R, Mansfield CA, Clayton LJ, Hoerger TJ, Zhang P. High-risk individuals' willingness to pay for diabetes risk-reduction programs. *Diabetes Care* 2006; **29**:1351–1356.

61 Watson AJ, Bell AG, Kvedar JC, Grant RW. Reevaluating the digital divide: current lack of internet use is not a barrier to adoption of novel health information technology. *Diabetes Care* 2008; **31**:433–435.

62 Jackson CL, Batts-Turner ML, Falb MD, Yeh HC, Brancati FL, Gary TL. Computer and Internet use among urban African Americans with type 2 diabetes. *J Urban Health* 2005; **82**:575–583.

12 Future Directions

59 Future Drug Treatment for Type 1 Diabetes

Helena Elding Larsson, Ahmed J. Delli, Sten-A. Ivarsson & Åke Lernmark
Lund University/Clinical Research Center, Department of Clinical Sciences, University Hospital MAS, Malmö, Sweden

Keypoints

- Insulin replacement therapy is considered the only effective and feasible treatment for type 1 diabetes mellitus (T1DM) as only insulin is capable of reversing the metabolic disturbances and restoring a near-normal quality of life in patients with T1DM.
- Despite rigorous measures and major advances in health care provided for patients with T1DM, increased morbidity and mortality are still common from complications, which commonly develop within 10–12 years after clinical onset.
- Advances in the understanding of the natural history of T1DM and increased abilities to predict the disease have made it possible to design and implement prevention and intervention clinical trials.
- Clinical trials are aimed at: (a) preventing the initiation of islet autoimmunity (primary prevention); (b) reducing autoimmune β-cell killing and progression to clinical diabetes (secondary prevention); or (c) suppressing or modulating the immune response in order to halt β-cell killing and enhance β-cell regeneration (tertiary prevention or intervention).
- Several trials were implemented or are currently ongoing with dietary manipulation, parenteral or oral insulin or immune-suppressing or immune-modulating agents with the aim of preventing the disease or retarding its progression.
- The search for safe, effective and feasible drugs to prevent or cure T1DM is still ongoing. So far, immune modulation with alum-formulated GAD65 has been shown to be the most promising intervention to reduce the loss of β-cells. Anti-CD3 monocloncal autoantibodies also showed some benefits in patients with newly diagnosed T1DM.

Introduction

The pathophysiologic mechanisms in type 1 diabetes mellitus (T1DM) are proposed to progress over several stages, in which autoimmunity is triggered in genetically predisposed individuals and in which β-cell killing by cellular immunity is activated, leading to insulin deficiency [1]. The autoimmune insult, which leads to selective killing of β-cells, may take months to years to develop. Throughout this autoimmune prodrome several genetic, autoimmune and biochemical markers may predict the disease prior to clinical onset. Once the clinical disease is established, the patient will be dependent on exogenous insulin and will require strict control to sustain euglycemia and minimize complications. Shortly after clinical onset of diabetes and initiation of insulin treatment, the remaining β-cells often increase their capacity to produce insulin, thereby decreasing the need for insulin treatment. This period of low insulin requirement, known as "partial remission" or the "honeymoon" period, may last for months or even years and is advantageous for the patient because it simplifies treatment and improves metabolic control, leading to less risk of long-term complications [2]. The "honeymoon" period seems to be longer and appears more frequently in older children and adults than in children diagnosed at a younger age [3].

Several trials seeking to prevent or delay the clinical onset of T1DM in genetically predisposed individuals as well as attempting to spare or even improve residual β-cell function in recently diagnosed patients are planned, implemented or currently ongoing.

Textbook of Diabetes, 4th edition. Edited by R. Holt, C. Cockram, A. Flyvbjerg and B. Goldstein.

Short history of type 1 diabetes prevention trials

Several approaches to modulate the immune system have been tested to prolong the partial remission in newly diagnosed patients. In the 1980s, plasmapheresis was performed in patients newly diagnosed with T1DM. A tendency of improved residual β-cell function and metabolic control was observed [4]. Later, several attempts with immune-modulating drugs were carried out. In order to suppress the immune response against the β-cells, small doses of cyclosporine were administered in a pilot study to autoantibody-positive first-degree relatives (FDR) of patients with T1DM with decreased first-phase insulin release (FPIR). The drug increased the FPIR, suggesting that cyclosporine may delay the onset of T1DM in glucose-intolerant siblings [5]. Cyclosporine was further tested in the Canadian–European Randomized Control Trial [6] as well as in series of controlled or uncontrolled smaller studies [5,7]. It was found that cyclosporine temporarily reduced insulin requirement and enhanced endogenous β-cell function in patients with newly diagnosed T1DM [6]. Although cyclosporine had some effect on preserving β-cell function, further clinical trials were abandoned because of severe kidney lesions [6,8]. Other immunosuppressive drugs such as azathioprine were also tested, either alone [9] or with prednisolone [10]. These immunosuppression trials had verified the immunopathogenic basis of T1DM, indicated by improved indicators of β-cell function in some trials; however, the outcomes were hard to maintain because of concerns about serious side effects [5,7].

Concerns about safety and sustainability of therapeutic effects directed attention towards the search for other preventive agents, with the focus on initiating preventive trials based on the stages of disease progression; however, our understanding of the natural history of T1DM made it possible to identify highly predictive markers (genetic, immunologic and metabolic) and recognize putative etiologic factors and possible intervention methods.

Several studies tested non-antigen-specific agents as possible preventive agents. The Bacille Calmette–Guérin (BCG) vaccine was found to prevent T1DM in experimental animals such as the non-obese diabetic (NOD) mice [11] and the bio-breeding (BB) rat [12]; however, similar results were not achieved in a group of human pilot studies [13,14]. The histamine antagonist, ketotifen [15], used orally in a pilot study in islet cell antibody (ICA) positive children with low FPIR showed no significant effect. Nicotinamide (vitamin B_3) protected β-cells in rodent studies [16] and so the effect of nicotinamide was tested in the European Nicotinamide Diabetes Intervention Trial (ENDIT) [17]. Nicotinamide was administered orally to ICA-positive FDR of patients with T1DM but the drug did not prevent progression to diabetes. High doses of nicotinamide were tested in other efficacy studies such as the DENIS [18] but this study also failed to show beneficial effects among high-risk children. Additionally, a group of pilot studies tested the combination of nicotinamide with cyclosporine [19], vitamin E [20] or intensive insulin regimen [21], none of which showed a preventive effect. These studies showed that nicotinamide could not protect against the loss of β-cells in high-risk subjects and overall no significant beneficial effects were detected.

Insulin, as an antigen-specific agent, has been tested through different routes, parenteral [22], oral [23] or intranasal [24,25] in genetically predisposed individuals, FDR and patients with T1DM in several trials. These trials showed no effect on disease progression or the rate of β-cell loss; however, subanalysis from the oral arm of the Diabetes Prevention Trial-1 (DPT-1) revealed a statistically significant delay in onset of T1DM in subjects with high titer insulin autoantibodies (IAA). A repeat study of the oral insulin trial has therefore been initiated.

Several prevention and intervention trials with long follow-up durations, some even including a combination of therapies, are now ongoing or planned. These trials use different approaches, with goals of preventing the triggering of autoimmunity (primary prevention), halting β-cell destruction (secondary prevention) or preserving remaining β-cells and enhancing their regeneration (tertiary prevention). This chapter presents an evidence-based review of the main ongoing drug clinical trials in subjects at-risk for or in those with newly diagnosed T1DM.

Prediction

Since the late 1970s, several studies have indicated that it is possible to predict T1DM among FDR through testing for human leukocyte antigen (HLA) class II genes and IAA. Several such studies utilized HLA genotyping, islet autoantibody analyses and biochemical indicators, as predictive markers are currently ongoing (Table 59.1). These prospective screening studies, may

Table 59.1 Some of the recent or ongoing screening studies for T1DM in first-degree relatives or high-risk children in the general population.

Study	Screening period	Screening population	Country
German BABYDIAB	1989–2000	Offspring of patients with diabetes	Germany
Australian BABYDIAB	1993	First-degree relatives	Australia
Diabetes Autoimmunity Study in the Young (DAISY)	1993–	First-degree relatives and high-risk children in general population	USA (Colorado)
Diabetes Prediction and Prevention Program (DIPP)	1994–	High-risk children in general population	Finland
Diabetes Evaluation in Washington (DEW-IT)	1995–	High-risk children in general population	USA (Washington)
Prospective Assessment of Newborns for Diabetes Autoimmunity Study (PANDA)	1997–	High-risk children in general population	USA (Florida)
All Babies in south-east Sweden (ABIS)	1997–1999	General population	Sweden
Diabetes Prediction in Skåne (DiPiS)	2000–2004	High-risk children in general population	Sweden
Environmental Triggers of Type 1 Diabetes Study (MIDIA)	2001–	High-risk children in general population	Norway
The Environmental Determinants of Diabetes in the Young (TEDDY)	2004–	Multicenter study of high-risk children in general population	Sweden (Skåne), Finland, Germany, USA (Colorado, Florida, Georgia, Washington)

allow us to define the environmental factors that may trigger islet autoimmunity or accelerate the development of T1DM in subjects with islet autoimmunity. These studies should make it possible to follow the disease process from initiation to the clinical onset of T1DM to help us understand the course of events during β-cell autoimmunity. At the same time, our knowledge about patterns of disease markers during subclinical disease and the predictive value of islet cell autoantibodies should be improved.

Predicting a disease at an early stage of pathologic insult is a prerequisite for attempts to prevent disease progression and initiating interventions to ameliorate symptoms and reduce complications. T1DM fulfils the criteria for predictable disease:

1 Genetic markers, specifically HLA class II genes, assist in recognizing individuals at higher risk who are eligible for autoimmune testing and follow-up [26].

2 T1DM has a prolonged prodrome of islet autoimmunity during which cellular and humoral immune markers may be present as early as the perinatal period [27] and remain detectable for months up to several years before onset.

3 Standardized and validated assays have been developed to detect multiple islet autoantibodies with high degrees of diagnostic sensitivity and specificity [28].

4 The extent of β-cell loss and the remaining function may be indirectly evaluated by assessing FPIR and C-peptide levels, for example [29].

Combining these markers provides highly predictive tools that may help to identify individuals at risk and initiate prevention or intervention at an appropriate point in time.

Currently, exogenous insulin injection is the only therapeutic measure that is able to correct hyperglycemia and enables patients with T1DM to live an almost normal life. Nevertheless, complications are common and may develop within 10–12 years after onset even with adequate metabolic control [30,31]. Prediction of T1DM may provide a window of opportunity to initiate prevention programs to reduce or ideally to prevent β-cell destruction. Identifying susceptible individuals prior to the clinical onset may allow an early and symptom-free diagnosis of diabetes and prevent an otherwise acute T1DM. This is crucially important to prevent the life-threatening condition of diabetic ketoacidosis (DKA) [32], which is commonly seen in children <4 years of age and associated with high morbidity and mortality.

Genetic markers

Much of our knowledge about prediction of T1DM has been generated from studies on FDR of patients with T1DM. These studies have revealed that T1DM can be predicted in siblings of patients with diabetes with analysis of HLA genotypes, number of islet autoantibodies and the titer of IA-2Ab [33]. HLA-identical siblings are at greater risk of developing autoantibodies and T1DM than are non-identical siblings.

Almost 50% of T1DM risk among FDR of Caucasian patients with T1DM is attributed to HLA [34]. One or both of the high-risk class II DQ8 and DQ2 haplotypes were found in more than 90% of patients diagnosed before the age of 30. Additionally, nearly 50% of siblings who carry high-risk HLA genes develop islet autoimmunity by the age of 3 years [35]. By contrast, only 15% of children developing T1DM have FDR with the disease. Therefore, screening of the general population is necessary in order to find a majority of children who are susceptible to T1DM. The diagnostic sensitivity of large-scale genetic screening is low because only 10% of subjects with disease-associated HLA genes develop the disease [36]. Nevertheless, several studies such as the BABYDIAB [37], DAISY [38], DiPiS and TEDDY [39], involving genetically susceptible individuals, continue to improve our understanding of the etiopathologic mechanisms of T1DM. Furthermore, the frequencies of DR-DQ alleles within the high-risk haplotypes DR3-DQ2 (*DRB1*03-DQA1*0501-B1*0201*) and DR4-DQ8 (*DRB1*04-DQA1*0301-B1*0302*) vary among different populations [40]. Indeed, T1DM in Asians is associated with HLA haplotypes other than those in Caucasians, indicating that screening strategies may need to be tailored to the population at hand [41]. Longitudinal studies will identify the relationship between HLA variants and the contribution of environmental factors to risk of T1DM. Other non-HLA genetic markers such as *INS-VNTR, PTPN22, IL2RA* and many others have also been identified [42]. The role of these non-HLA genetic factors in the pathogenesis of islet autoimmunity needs to be clarified, but the relative risk of these genetic factors is shown to be less than that of the HLA genes [42]. HLA and some of the non-HLA genes may be associated with the presence of islet autoantibodies and progression to persistent autoimmunity [43–47]. Combining genetic and autoimmune markers does not improve diagnostic sensitivity of autoantibody testing although the overall positive predictive value may increase.

Autoimmune markers: islet cell autoantibodies

The appearance of diabetes-associated autoantibodies is the first measurable sign of the autoimmune process that eventually leads to T1DM. In 1974, autoantibodies to pancreatic cells were described for the first time [48,49], providing evidence for T1DM being an autoimmune disease. These autoantibodies were named islet cell autoantibodies (ICA) and were detected by immunofluorescence in patients with T1DM. Later, ICA were detected in one patient a year before T1DM onset and in one twin without diabetes who later developed the disease [48], providing the first evidence of an ongoing autoimmune process before the clinical onset of T1DM. ICA are not specific for β-cells and probably represents several different specific autoantigens.

The first autoantigen demonstrated was a Mr64K protein immunoprecipitated by sera from patients with T1DM [50], which was later demonstrated to have glutamic acid decarboxylase (GAD) activity [51], but found not to be a previously recognized isoform of glutamic acid decarboxylase (GAD65) [52]. GAD65 converts glutamic acid to γ-aminobutyric acid (GABA), an inhibitory transmitter in the CNS. GAD65 is primarily present in specific neurons in addition to the pancreatic islet β-cells. Autoantibodies to GAD65 (GAD65Ab) are present in 55–60% of children with T1DM at onset of the disease.

In 1983 autoantibodies to insulin (IAA) were found to be present in patients with diabetes before insulin treatment [53]. This finding suggested that IAA had a role in the autoimmune process of diabetes. IAA are not detected by the immunofluorescence test for ICA. IAA are present in about 35–40% of children with T1DM at onset of the disease.

A third autoantigen, also found to contribute to the ICA reaction, is the insulinoma-associated protein 2 (IA-2), identified in 1996 [54]. IA-2 is a non-functional member of the protein tyrosine phosphatase family. It is localized to the membrane of the secretory vesicles in endocrine and neuronal cells [55]. IA-2 is expressed in both islet α and β-cells, but the function is still unknown because it lacks enzymatic activity. Autoantibodies to IA-2 (IA-2Ab) are directed to the intracellular protein domains [55]. IA-2Ab are present in about 70% of children with T1DM at onset of the disease.

Most recently, autoantibodies to a fourth islet autoantigen, zinc transporter 8 (ZnT8Ab), were reported in patients recently diagnosed with T1DM [56]. This autoantigen is highly β-cell specific. ZnT8 is a protein located in the membrane of the secretory vesicles of the β-cells acting as a zinc ion transporter. Recently, ZnT8Ab have been found in 60–65% of patients with T1DM, compared to <2% in controls [56]. ZnT8Ab are independent markers of islet cell autoimmunity and were detected in otherwise IAA-negative individuals. Furthermore, ZnT8Ab were found to appear and precede disease onset in prospectively studied FDR of patients with T1DM and high-risk individuals from the general population.

Some patients are positive for ICA, but negative for both GAD65Ab and IA-2Ab, suggesting that there are additional, as yet undiscovered, antigens covered by ICA. Some of those patients may have ZnT8Ab. More than 90% of patients with T1DM have previously been reported to have ICA, GAD65Ab, IA-2Ab or IAA at diagnosis. The corresponding number for the general population is about 1% [57]. With the addition of ZnT8Ab to the combined analysis of GAD65Ab, IA-2Ab and IAA, up to 95% of all individuals developing T1DM are positive for at least one autoantibody.

In addition, several other proteins have been proposed as candidate autoantigens (see Chapter 9). Further studies are needed to establish the possible importance of these additional autoantigens for T1DM risk. It is possible that all diabetes-associated autoantibodies have not yet been discovered.

Individuals with clinical T1DM and absence of autoantibodies at diagnosis may still have had an ongoing autoimmune process leading to β-cell destruction. It has been found that 25% of children with T1DM with negative autoantibodies at diagnosis of the disease had autoantibodies present in their cord blood [58].

In genetically predisposed children, detecting islet autoantibodies as early as 3 months of age was associated with high seroconversion rates, where IAA and GAD65Ab often preceded ICA and IA-2Ab appeared last [59,60]. These autoantibodies seem to appear sequentially, with the appearance of additional autoantibodies usually taking place within a year after the detection of the first one [36,61]. While a single autoantibody may be harmless and often represents non-progressive β-cell autoimmunity, the appearance of multiple autoantibodies most often reflects a progressive process [62–66]. The number of detectable autoantibodies is related to the risk of T1DM, both in FDR and in the general population. In studies of family members of patients with T1DM, 60–100% of individuals with three or more autoantibodies develop clinical T1DM over the next 5–6 years and population-based studies indicate that the risk is similar in the general population [67–69]. The autoantibody pattern differs among age groups. It has been suggested that GAD65Ab is a marker of general non-specific autoimmunity, while IA-2Ab and IAA are more specific markers for β-cell death [70]. The recently discovered ZnT8Ab has been reported to appear generally after 3 years of age and thereafter to increase in frequency with age up to adolescence [56].

Titers of the islet autoantibodies need to be taken into consideration for prediction. Higher titers may better predict risk of persistent autoimmunity and T1DM [33,62,64,66], especially in combination with a high-risk HLA genotype [64,71]. Persistent detection of high titer autoantibodies may mirror the intensity of the autoimmune reaction and the rate of progression to clinical diabetes [64].

In studies of the general population, GAD65Ab and IA-2A have been shown to be of equal predictive value as they are in FDR siblings, but for each separate autoantibody a higher cumulative risk was observed among the siblings. Double autoantibody positivity confers a similar cumulative risk among siblings and the general population [69], with additional predictive information provided by the level of the autoantibodies [64]. In one study of school children, the positive predictive value of multiple autoantibodies in the general population was 25–75%, with a sensitivity of 58–100%, not taking HLA genotypes into account [67].

Biochemical (metabolic) markers

Children progressing to T1DM have been shown to have several autoantibodies, high titers of ICA, IA-2Ab and GAD65Ab and decreased FPIR in response to an intravenous glucose tolerance test (IVGTT). A combination of islet autoantibodies and FPIR might therefore potentially predict diabetes [62]. In one study, siblings of children with diabetes were also examined at the time when the index case was diagnosed. Islet autoantibodies alone predicted T1DM in 36%, but when FPIR was taken into account the rate of prediction increased to 56%, with a median observation time of 3.6 years. A young age, a strong humoral response and reduced FPIR seemed to characterize individuals with a progressive process [62]. Additionally, reduced FPIR levels (<50 mU/L) among autoantibody-positive subjects (mainly ICA or IAA) may predict T1DM among FDR by up to 92% over 10 years [29]. C-peptide may predict β-cell functional loss near diagnosis because C-peptide levels may diminish significantly 6 months prior to onset [72]. Therefore, combining these two tests may detect metabolic disturbances and predict the disease prior to clinical onset, especially when monitored in parallel with autoimmune markers. Children developing diabetes in the DPT-1 study had a gradually deteriorating glucose tolerance with declining 2-hour C-peptide levels after an oral glucose tolerance test (OGTT) [73]. These data were seen over a period of at least 2 years before onset of disease, despite the fact that fasting C-peptide levels remained stable [73]. Moreover, among ICA-positive subjects recruited in the DPT-1 trial, an alternative OGTT index (using area-under-the-curve glucose, 60 and 90-minute glucose, instead of 2-hour glucose) was shown to have better predictive criteria than the standard OGTT, especially when combined with C-peptide measurement from the alternative OGTT [74].

Body mass index (BMI) has also been reported to give additional information in T1DM prediction [75]. It has also been reported that a normal but rising HbA_{1c}, a measure that is proportional to the average blood glucose in the previous 120 days, predicts clinical onset of diabetes in autoantibody-positive children [76].

Other markers

The search for additional biomarkers to predict T1DM is ongoing. Cytokines, chemokines and adhesion molecules are proposed as important inflammatory mediators in the pathogenesis of T1DM (for review see Purohit and She [77]). Antigen-specific T-lymphocytes are also proposed markers for T1DM prediction, but standardized tests to detect these markers have yet to be developed.

Prevention and intervention

Several clinical trials aiming to prevent T1DM have been initiated during the past two decades; some have been completed and others are still ongoing. The general aim of prevention is either to prevent islet autoimmunity from happening or retard the autoimmune destruction of β-cells, or alternatively to preserve remaining β-cell secretory capability before clinical diagnosis. The aim of intervention is to interfere with the natural history of T1DM after the clinical diagnosis. The idea of intervention is to stop or halt the killing of β-cells and preserve β-cell secretory function in patients who have already developed clinical diabetes. Therefore, scientists continue to test new drugs with attempts to halt one or both of these stages. The rationale behind reported prevention and intervention has often been obtained from studies on laboratory animals such as the NOD mouse and BB rat [78–80]. Significant differences exist, however, between these animals and humans; therefore a successful intervention in these animals may not have the exact same effects in humans. Moreover, factors such as the duration of the intervention, the stage of enrolment and drug dosage and safety may influence the outcome. These factors, in addition to the complexity of the etiopathogenesis of T1DM, may explain why little success has been achieved so far in prevention or intervention of T1DM.

All three levels of disease prevention (primary, secondary and tertiary) may be applicable to T1DM.

Primary prevention trials

Primary prevention trials aim to prevent the initiation of autoimmune responses among infants with genetic susceptibility (high-risk HLA genes) or history of T1DM among FDR. Several attempts to prevent T1DM in relatives of patients with the disease have been performed over the years. Such trials are often implemented for longer follow-up durations, especially during the main window of autoimmunity triggering (from birth to 6 years) [81]. Primary prevention trials tend to test the effects of safe, mainly non-antigen-specific agents in relation to environmental risk determinants, of which nutritional factors are important. Results from observational studies encouraged trials that use dietary manipulation to prevent T1DM (Table 59.2).

Non-antigen specific primary prevention trials

Gluten-free diet

A gluten-free diet was given to islet autoantibody-positive children without any significant preventive effect neither on the risk of T1DM nor on the titers of T1DM-associated autoantibodies [82].

Cow's milk

There are several suggestions that cow's milk may be associated with higher risk of T1DM [83]. Dietary manipulation using hydrolyzed casein milk formula provided evidence of preventive effect on the risk of T1DM [84,85]. The TRIGR trial is an international effort involving 17 countries to verify if hydrolyzed casein milk formula can reduce T1DM risk among infants at risk (genetically predisposed infants with history of T1DM among FDR), if used instead of cow's milk. Following a period of 6–8 months' breastfeeding, infants are randomized into either receiving hydrolyzed casein-based or conventional cow's milk formulas. This trial is still ongoing and the results of autoantibody analyses are expected in 2012 and the results of T1DM in 2016 [86].

Vitamin D

Supplementary vitamin D has been suggested to protect against T1DM [87], possibly through the effects on the T lymphocytes and through suppression of cytokine production [88]. Lower concentrations of vitamin D have been reported in blood from children with T1DM, and lower vitamin D levels during pregnancy have been suggested to increase the risk for the child to develop T1DM [88,89]. Vitamin D (cholecalciferol) is currently tested in an ongoing randomized feasibility pilot study in Manitoba, Canada, to test if high doses of vitamin D (2000 IU/day) prevent T1DM among genetically susceptible infants ≤4 weeks of age [90].

Nutritional Intervention to Prevent Diabetes study

Supplementation with cod liver oil, an important source of vitamin D and omega-3 fatty acids, during the first year of life led to reduced risk of T1DM in Norwegian children, but no risk

Table 59.2 Primary prevention trials in T1DM. Adapted from Staeva-Vieira *et al.* [94].

Trial name	Agent	Type of trial	Description	Outcome
Non-antigen-specific trials				
PREVFIN	Gluten-free diet	Pilot	Exclusion of dietary gluten	No effects Ended in 2002
TRIGR	Hydrolized casein formulas vs cow's milk	R/PC, DB	To recruited 2800 type infants with FDR and T1DM Implemented in 17 countries	Ongoing NCT00179777
NIP	Oral omega-3 DHA	R/DB Pilot	Infants <5 months and mothers in third trimister (+ve family history) Follow-up until age of 9 years	Primary results awaited NCT00333554
Vitamin D	Cholecalciferol 2000 IU/day	R/OL Pilot	Genetically susceptible infants up to 4 weeks old (Manitoba, Canada)	Phase 1: Results awaited NCT00141986
Antigen-specific trials				
Pre-POINT	Oral/nasal insulin	R, PC	Genetically predisposed FDR infants (18 months to 7 years) No islet autoimmunity	Recruitment started in Germany and USA in 2010 Duration: 3–18 months

DB, double blinded; DHA, docosahexanoic acid; FDR, First-degree relatives; OL, open label; PC, placebo controlled; R, randomized.
For further details, see clinical trial identifier: http://www.clinicaltrials.gov/ct2/search.

reduction was found with other kinds of vitamin D supplementation, suggesting that omega-3 fatty acids were responsible for the effect [91]. In a recent study it was reported that the intake of omega-3 and omega-6 fatty acids were inversely associated with the development of IAA, GAD65Ab and IA-2Ab in children with genetic risk of T1DM [92].

The Nutritional Intervention to Prevent Diabetes (NIP-Diabetes) is a small pilot study to test a proposed preventive effect of oral docosahexanoic acid (DHA) against islet autoimmunity (trial identifier NCT00333554) [93]. Participants included in this trial were infants ≤5 months of age and expected babies of pregnant mothers in their third trimester (>24 weeks) who were genetically predisposed (DR3 or 4) and had family history of T1DM among FDR. DHA is taken in late pregnancy and early infancy and all those infants are followed up for markers of autoimmunity and T1DM (for review see Staeva-Vieira *et al.* [94]).

Antigen-specific primary prevention trials

Pre-POINT Trial

The primary intervention with oral and/or nasal insulin for prevention of T1DM in infants at high genetic risk to develop diabetes (Pre-POINT) is a trial to identify the dose and the type of insulin that can prevent progression to T1DM. Pre-POINT is an ongoing trial, which has two arms: oral and intranasal. This international effort recruits genetically predisposed FDR infants aged 18 months to 7 years with no islet autoimmunity. In this trial, oral insulin dose is almost 10 times higher than that used in the DPT-1 trial (http://www.diabetes-point.org/nav2uk.html).

Secondary prevention trials

Secondary prevention trials are mainly intended for genetically predisposed children in whom autoimmunity has already developed and also for young adults with multiple islet autoantibodies. These trials aim to reduce β-cell killing by autoimmunity and prevent progression to clinical diabetes [95]. Secondary prevention trials may be divided into two groups: non-antigen-specific (Table 59.3) and antigen-specific trials (Table 59.4).

Non-antigen-specific secondary prevention trials

Non-antigen-specific agents were tested in a group of secondary prevention trials including cyclosporine [5,7], BCG vaccine [13], ketotifen [15] and nicotinamide, as in ENDIT [17] and DENIS studies [18]. Although these agents were successful in laboratory animals such as the NOD mice, they failed to show similar benefits in human trials. In regards to immunosuppressive agents, the adverse effects outweighed the temporary benefits observed on indicators of β-cell function [8].

Antigen-specific secondary prevention trials

It is known that an early diabetes diagnosis with mild or no symptoms is associated with good residual capacity of the β-cells to produce insulin and a longer "honeymoon" period [96]. Therefore, it was suggested that insulin therapy in individuals with subclinical diabetes could reduce the β-cell load and be advantageous. Insulin was used in prevention trials as an antigen-specific agent using different routes including parenteral, oral and intranasal insulin. Earlier pilot studies [97,98], which tested parenteral insulin (subcutaneously and intravenously) as prophylaxis among ICA-positive FDR, introduced evidence of delaying disease progression, but the randomized and controlled DPT-1 (parenteral arm) [22] failed to reproduce these results.

It is suggested that insulin given in small doses, either orally or nasally, could induce antigen-specific T-cell tolerance to insulin, which by releasing inhibitory cytokines in the target organ would suppress the autoimmune process against β-cells. This principle

Table 59.3 Non-antigen-specific secondary prevention trials in T1DM. Adapted from Staeva-Vieira *et al.* [94].

Trial name	Agent	Type of trial	Description	Outcome
Cyclosporine	Cyclosporine orally 7.5 mg/kg/day/year	Pilot	FDR with immunologic and metabolic predisposition	Delayed progression, but no prevention
BCG vaccine	BCG vaccine intradermally	Pilot	A group of pilot studies	No effect
Ketotifen	Ketotifen orally	Pilot	ICA +ve subjects with low FPIR	No effect
ENDIT	Nicotinamide Orally 1.2 g/m^2/day	R/PC, DB	ICA +ve FDR of young diabetes onset (<20 years)	No effect
DENIS	Nicotinamide Orally 1.2 g/m^2/day	R, PC	ICA +ve FDR at risk of type 1 diabetes within 3 years	No effect
Nicotinamide combinations	Nicotinamide orally + intensive insulin or cyclosporine or vitamin E	Pilot	Various combinations used with nicotinamide	No effect

BCG, Bacille Calmette–Guérin; DB, double blinded; FDR, first-degree relatives; FPIR, first-phase insulin release; ICA, islet cell autoantibodies; PC, placebo controlled; R, randomized.
For further details, see clinical trial identifier: http://www.clinicaltrials.gov/ct2/search.

Table 59.4 Antigen-specific secondary prevention trials in T1DM. Adapted from Staeva-Vieira *et al.* [94].

Trial name	Agent	Type of trial	Description	Outcome
DPT-1	Parenteral human ultralente insulin s.c. 0.25 U/kg/day + 1 annual infusion	RC/ET	Large multicenter study: FDR with >50% disease risk in 5 years	No effect
DPT-1	Oral insulin 7.5 mg/day	R/PC, DB, ET	Large multicenter study: FDR with 26–50% disease risk in 5 years Follow-up with OGTT for 6 months	No effect (subanalysis showed delay of onset in subjects with IAA >80 U/mL) Phase III is ongoing
DIPP	Intranasal insulin	R/DB/PC PA, ET	Genetically predisposed infants. Tested for ICA, IAA, GAD65Ab and IA-2Ab and IVGTT	No effect after follow-up to 15 years of age
INIT I	Intranasal insulin	OL	Tested effect on autoimmunity among children and young adults	No effect
INIT II	Intranasal insulin 1.6 and 16 mg	R/DB/PC PA, ET	Children and young adults at risk of type 1 diabetes Followed for β-cell function and AAb & OGTT/6 months	Ongoing NCT00336674

AAb, autoantibodies; DB, double blinded; ET, efficacy trial; FDR, first-degree relative; GAD 65Ab, glutamine acid decarboxylase autoantibodies; IAA, insulin autoantibody; IA-2Ab, autoantibody to insulinoma-associated antigen 2; ICA, islet cell autoantibodies; IVGTT, intravenous glucose tolerance test; OGTT, oral glucose tolerance test; OL, open label; PA, parallel assignment; PC, placebo controlled; R, randomized; RC, randomized controlled.
For further details, see clinical trial identifier: http://www.clinicaltrials.gov/ct2/search

has previously been tried in various other autoimmune diseases, with small or inconsistent beneficial effects. The theory is that peptides from orally ingested antigens encounter the lymphoid tissue in the mucosa, which serves to protect the host from reacting against ingested proteins.

Oral insulin

The oral arm of the DPT-1 trial examined a preventive effect of oral insulin (7.5 mg/day) [23]. This placebo-controlled study tested 372 high-risk first and second-degree relatives who were positive for ICA and IAA, but with normal FPIR on IVGTT and glucose tolerance on OGTT. Although the overall results of the DPT-1 showed no significant effect, subanalysis of these data showed a benefit in subjects with IAA >80 U/mL, in whom diabetes was delayed by 4–5 years [23]. This indicates that oral insulin may have a protective effect when given to individuals at risk and having high titers of IAA. No serious study-related adverse events were recorded with oral insulin and the levels of

IAA in the patients did not increase with the administration of oral insulin [99]. Further studies of orally administered insulin in subjects with high titers of IAA are ongoing such as the ongoing repeat of the oral arm of DPT-1 (NCT00419562).

Nasal insulin

Prophylactic administration of insulin nasally has shown to prevent T1DM in NOD mice. In humans, insulin has also been used nasally to induce autoimmune tolerance in prevention trials such as the Intranasal Insulin Trial (INIT) phases I and II and Type 1 Diabetes Prediction and Prevention trial (DIPP). The INIT is a double-blinded cross-over pilot study that recruited T1DM FDR in Australia. INIT-I was completed in 2004 with no significant effect on β-cell function but it showed some indications of mucosal tolerance to insulin [24]. INIT-II (NCT00336674) is an ongoing randomized double-blinded placebo-controlled trial using nasal insulin (1.6 or 16 mg) that aims to assess the effects of nasal insulin on islet autoimmunity. The DIPP study of Finland is a double-blinded prevention trial that used nasal insulin in children with genetic risk and positive ICA and IAA. In 224 children short-acting insulin or placebo was administered intranasally once a day, but no protective effect was seen [25].

In animal studies, oral insulin has shown various results in protecting from T1DM. In BB rats, oral insulin failed to prevent the disease and actually seemed to accelerate the autoimmune process [100,101]. In contrast, studies in the NOD mouse did reveal a protective effect of the drug [102]. Taken together, there is limited evidence that preclinical studies in the NOD mouse and the BB rat can be immediately translated into successful trials in humans.

Intervention (tertiary prevention) trials

Tertiary prevention or intervention trials mainly recruit patients with new-onset T1DM, using interventions intended to preserve β-cells and also to maintain their regeneration [103]. In these studies researchers are trying to suppress or modulate the immune response in order to stop the autoimmune process, which leads to β-cell death and eventually T1DM, or to reduce the β-cell stress, for example by early-introduced insulin therapy. An intensive insulin regimen in patients with new-onset T1DM is proposed to preserve the remaining β-cells and enhance their functionality [104]. Intensive insulin treatment should therefore be used as the basic therapy for all newly diagnosed patients with T1DM who are randomized into intervention trials.

Unlike prevention trials, tertiary interventions mainly test less safe agents over shorter duration of time on subjects who have already developed clinical diabetes. The intervention drug has typically been evaluated in animal studies, and then assessed in small pilot studies to ensure an acceptable route of administration and to verify a safety profile. Intervention trials commonly consider C-peptides as the main outcome for β-cell function, which may reflect the extent of β-cell preservation. Certain trials test combination therapies in which various drug modalities with different modes of action are used in pubertal patients with new-onset T1DM (commonly two drugs in each trial).

Therapeutic agents used in tertiary interventions may also be classified into non-antigen-specific (Table 59.5) or antigen-specific (Table 59.6).

Non-antigen-specific intervention trials

In this set of trials non-antigen-specific drugs are used including immunosuppressive or immunomodulatory agents (Table 59.5). Systemic immunosuppressive drugs such as cyclosporine [7,105] and azathioprine [106] induced remission with signs of improved β-cell function in patients with new-onset T1DM. In spite of that, serious side effects limited prolonged clinical use.

Nicotinamide

Nicotinamide was also used among patients with new-onset T1DM in a group of intervention trials [107–109]. Some of these trials proposed a beneficial effect of nicotinamide reflected in improved C-peptide levels among intervention groups compared with controls [109]. This may indicate that nicotinamide possesses certain therapeutic effects related to β-cell function after onset, but not during the autoimmune prodrome, because prevention trials did not prove a beneficial effect of nicotinamide among high-risk individuals [17,18].

Other agents such as the BCG vaccine [14,110] and diazoxide [111] failed to produce sustained beneficial effect on preserving β-cell function.

Anti-CD3 monoclonal antibodies

Non-specific systemic immunotherapy to modulate T cells has also been attempted with some promising outcomes among this group of drugs. Anti-CD3 monoclonal antibodies (anti-CD3 MoAb), such as teplizumab, have shown some positive effects in postponing the autoimmune destruction of β-cells with preservation of their functionality and enhancement of endogenous insulin [112–114]. Humanized anti-CD3 MoAb were used in order to avoid depleting T-lymphocyte populations. Two variants of these antibodies, mutated Fc region (hOKT3γ1(Ala-Ala) and glycosylated Fc region ChAglyCD3(TRX4)) were used in two already completed trials [112,113]. These trials showed that anti-CD3 MoAb were able to enhance C-peptide levels and improve clinical variables for up to 2 years but they did not induce sustained tolerance of β-cell autoantigens [114]. This effect appears to be transient because the drug only delayed the decline in C-peptide concentration. Despite remission and metabolic enhancement, there were serious adverse effects including bone marrow suppression with cytokine release syndrome or subsequent serious infections or reactivation of Epstein–Barr virus infection with this treatment [113]. Nevertheless, the obtained results encouraged initiating phase II of the anti-CD3 trial (NCT00378508) and planning a third phase.

Antithymocyte globulin

Antithymocyte globulin (ATG) was found to induce short-term benefits in laboratory animals such as the NOD mice, primarily through inducing immunoregulation rather than depleting T-lymphocytes [115]. In humans, ATG is thought to decrease

Table 59.5 Non-antigen-specific intervention trials in T1DM. Adapted from Staeva-Vieira *et al.* [94].

Trial name	Agent	Type of trial	Description	Outcome
Cyclosporine	Cyclosporine-A	R, PC	A group of trials	Remission but with serious side effects
ChAgly CD3	Humanized non-mitogenic CD3 monoclonal Ab 8 mg/day IV/6 days	R, DB, PC, PA, ET	Starts at diagnosis of patients with new onset T1DM 12–45 years	Completed, results awaited NCT00627146
Teplizumab	Anti-CD3 monoclonal Ab hOKT3γ1 (Ala-Ala)	R, DB, PC, PA, ET	Phase II: Single 14 course for 4–12 months after diagnosis of new-onset T1DM, to test effects on insulin secretion	Ongoing NCT00378508
ATG	Antithymocyte globulin	R, SB, PA, ET	Test the effect of ATG plus intensive insulin versus intensive insulin therapy only	Ongoing NCT00190502
STRAT	Anti-thymocyte globulin (ATG) Daily 4-day escalating dose	R, DB, PC, PA, ET	Phase II: Given within 12 weeks of diagnosis to assess effects on insulin secretion (C-peptide) over 12 months	Ongoing ITN028AI
Rituximab	Anti-CD20 monoclonal Ab weekly IV/4 weeks	R, DB, PC, PA, Safety/ET	Phases II & III: 8–45 years patients with T1DM, followed every 3 months/2 years (C-peptide, insulin and HbA_{1c})	Results awaited NCT00279305
Abatacept (CTLA-4)	Cytotoxic T-lymphocyte antigen-4, IV	R, DB, PC, PA, ET	The effect of CTLA-4 on insulin production (C-peptide secretion) over 2 years	Ongoing, not recruiting NCT00505375
HrIFN-α	Oral human recombinant interferon α	R, DB, PC, PA	Phase II: test the effect on counter-regulatory anti-inflammatory cytokines	Ongoing, not recruiting NCT00005665
Anakinra, Kineret®	IL-1 receptor antagonist	E, OL	Whether Anakinra protects β-cells by blocking the IL-1β receptor in children with T1DM	Ongoing NCT00645840
Anakinra, Kineret®	IL-1 receptor antagonist	R, DB, PC, PA, ET	The effect of IL-1β receptor antagonism on insulin secretion in young adults with T1DM	Ongoing NCT00711503

ATG, antithymocyte globulin; DB, double blinded; E, exploratory; ET, efficacy trial; IL, interleukin; OL, open label; PA, parallel assignment; PC, placebo controlled; R, randomized; SB, single blinded.
For further details, see clinical trial identifier: http://www.clinicaltrials.gov/ct2/search.

Table 59.6 Antigen-specific intervention trials in T1DM. Adapted from Staeva-Vieira *et al.* [94].

Trial name	Agent	Type of trial	Description	Outcome
DiaPep77 (HSP60)	Subcutaneous peptide heat shock protein 60	R, PC, DB, PA, ET	An immunomodulatory peptide proposed to protect internal production of insulin through halting β-cell killing	Preserved β-cell over 12–18 months in adults. No similar effect in children Phase III (DIA-AID) is ongoing NCT00615264
Alum-GAD (Diamyd®)	Alhydrogel-formulated GAD65 20 μg s.c.	R, PC, DB, PA, ET	Immuno-modulation effect in LADA (Phase IIa) and 10–18 years old with new-onset T1DM (Phase IIb)	Preserved β-cell and C-peptide levels in patients with <6 months onset Phase III ongoing NCT00723411
NBI-6024	Altered peptide ligand insulin B:9–23 vaccine s.c.	R, DB, PC, PA, ET	Multinational trial used a genetically engineered peptide in adolescents (10–17 years) and adults (18–35 years) with new onset T1DM	Completed NCT00873561
BHT-3021	Pro-insulin-based DNA vaccine weekly i.m. inj./12 weeks	R, DB, PC, OL, CO	Assesses safety in ≥18-year-old patients with T1DM: 12 months blinded treatment, 12 months cross-over and 12 months follow-up	Ongoing NCT00453375

CO, cross-over; DB, double blinded; ET, efficacy trial; i.m. inj., intramuscular injection; LADA, latent autoimmune diabetes of adults; OL, open label; PA, parallel assignment; PC, placebo controlled; R, randomized; RC, randomized controlled; s.c subcutaneous.
For further details, see clinical trial identifier: http://www.clinicaltrials.gov/ct2/search.

insulin requirement in patients with new-onset T1DM; however, serious adverse effects such as transient thrombocytopenia are major drawbacks to be considered. Currently, polyclonal anti-T-lymphocyte globulin is being tested in an ongoing randomized placebo control trial that aims to prevent progression of autoimmune β-cell destruction in patients with new-onset T1DM (NCT00190502).

Anti-CD20 monoclonal antibodies

Anti-CD20 MoAbs are potential non-specific immunoregulatory agents. These monoclonal antibodies induced regulatory B lymphocytes in humanized mice [116]. It is proposed that monoclonal antibodies exert an immunoregulatory effect through reducing B lymphocytes and decreasing their antigen-presentation abilities, cytokine release and antibody production [116]. In humans, anti-CD20 MoAb (rituximab) is currently used in a randomized double-blinded placebo-controlled trial (NCT00279305, phases II and III) to examines whether rituximab can preserve residual insulin and halt β-cell function loss.

Abatacept

The cytotoxic T-lymphocyte antigen 4 (CTLA-4) is thought to be involved in modulating immune responses through inducing co-stimulatory signals, which are important for T-lymphocyte activation [117]. CTLA4 immunoglobulin (CTLA4-Ig) is proposed to regulate, but not delete, T-lymphocytes through inhibiting their stimulatory activation pathway [118], and is therefore considered relatively safer than other immunosuppressive agents. CTLA4-Ig (abatacept) was recently used in a randomized placebo controlled trial to assess the effects of CTLA4-Ig on progression of new-onset T1DM in patients aged 6–45 years (NCT00505375).

Human recombinant interferon α

Several other non-antigen specific interventions are currently ongoing. A randomized double-blinded trial assessing whether orally ingested human recombinant interferon α (hrIFN-α) may prolong the "honeymoon" period in patients with newly diagnosed T1DM aged 3–25 years (NCT00005665) examines whether oral hrIFN-α enhances counter-regulatory anti-inflammatory cytokines such as interleukin-4 (IL-4), IL-10 and peripheral IFN-α, thereby maintaining residual living β-cells.

Interleukin-1 receptor antagonist

Two trials were recently launched to test the anti-inflammatory effect of IL-1 receptor antagonist (Anakinra, Kineret®) on maintaining β-cell function and preserving insulin secretion in children (NCT00645840) and young adults (NCT00711503). Based on results from preclinical T1DM studies and studies in rheumatoid arthritis [119], these trials propose that immune regulation in T1DM may be obtained through blocking the IL-1β receptor, which has an important role in β-cell killing.

Antigen-specific intervention trials

Specific pancreatic antigens have been examined as safe agents to modulate the autoimmune response through inducing immunologic tolerance towards islet antigens. In experimental animals, several antigen-specific molecules are able to induce immunologic tolerance and protection against T1DM [120] using a whole islet protein, peptides taken from islet antigen, or DNA-based vaccines [121]. In humans, only few potential antigen-specific agents may have promising results such as peptide heat shock protein 60 (DiaPep277) and alum-formulated GAD65. The induction of immunologic tolerance using antigen-specific agents is thought to be achieved through the stimulation of antigen-specific regulatory T lymphocyte (T_{reg}); however, standardized specific tools for detecting and measuring these T_{reg} cells are not yet available. A group of intervention trials is currently under way to examine the effect of certain antigen-specific drugs in new-onset T1DM (Table 59.6).

DiaPep277

The humanized DiaPep277 was found to provide protection for β-cells and enhance the levels of C-peptide in a group of trials [122–124]. DiaPep277 was reported to possess a high safety profile; however, the deterioration in β-cell function over an 18-month duration after initiating the intervention was more apparent in children (≤15 years) than in adults [123,124]. A trial with similar design involving newly diagnosed children found no similar beneficial effect on β-cell function and C-peptide levels [125]. DiaPep277 is currently tested in a randomized double-blinded placebo-controlled trial involving patients with new-onset T1DM aged 16–45 years (NCT00615264 phase III).

Alum-GAD65

Another way of trying to induce tolerance to an antigen is to give the antigen subcutaneously in small and repeated doses together with aluminium hydroxide. This adjuvant is commonly used in vaccines. Aluminium salts preferentially induce a humoral (Th2) rather than cellular (Th1) immune response. Because the autoimmune process leading to T1DM is thought to be a mainly cellular (Th1) immune response, aluminium salts could steer the process against a humoral (Th2) response and minimize the likelihood of exacerbating cell-mediated β-cell destruction. This concept is used in the trials of vaccination with Alhydrogel-formulated GAD65 (Diamyd®).

A dose-finding placebo-controlled Phase IIa safety study in 47 patients with latent autoimmune diabetes in adults (LADA) indicated that 20 μg Diamyd reduced β-cell destruction without any serious adverse events. In Phase IIb clinical trial, the efficacy and safety of Diamyd were investigated in children 10–18 years of age, recently diagnosed with T1DM [126]. A total of 70 GAD65 antibody-positive children with a recent diagnosis (<18 months duration) of T1DM were included in the study. All had remaining β-cell capacity measured by C-peptide levels. A total of 35 children received two doses of 20 μg Diamyd and 35 children received placebo. C-peptide levels were measured after mixed meal tolerance tests 3, 9, 15, 21 and 30 months after the first drug injection. Significant differences between groups were found after mixed meal stimulation and fasting C-peptide was different at 30 months only. Furthermore, in a subgroup of children who had been diagnosed with diabetes no longer than 6 months at study-start, the fasting C-peptide levels declined less in children who had received Diamyd compared with the levels in children who received placebo. This indicates that Diamyd may prevent further β-cell destruction in recently diagnosed children, without any serious adverse events. Thus, the study has provided support for the clinical safety of Diamyd and statistically significant and clinically relevant positive effect on the preservation of β-cell function in children diagnosed within 6 months before study start [126]. A Phase III randomized double-blinded placebo-controlled multicenter study is ongoing to evaluate the efficacy and safety of Diamyd further, with a larger number of children diagnosed no longer than 3 months before inclusion in the study.

Studies of the NOD mice indicated that GAD65 prevents the autoimmune destruction of the pancreatic β-cells and T1DM [127–132].

Insulin peptides

It has been observed in animal studies that intermittent immunization with insulin or insulin-β chain coupled with incomplete Freund adjuvant may prevent T1DM progression in NOD mice [133]. Another approach used altered peptide ligand, based on the immunodominant T1DM insulin-β chain:9-23 vaccine (NBI-6024), which was tested in humans based on earlier results from experimental animals [134,135]. This region of insulin-β chain has been shown as a specific T-lymphocyte target antigen in the NOD mouse [134]. A genetically engineered vaccine was prepared based on this peptide region and administered subcutaneously to adolescents and adults with a recent history of T1DM. The Phase I trial showed that NBI-6024 was able to shift the IFN-γ-producing T-helper (Th1) lymphocyte into the Th2 regulatory lymphocyte [135]; however, no preventive effect or metabolic control was observed with this NBI-6024 (NCT00873561).

Pro-insulin-based DNA vaccine (BHT-3021) is an antigen-specific drug which is currently being tested in adults older than 18 years with new-onset T1DM. This randomized blinded placebo-controlled trial is a multicenter study that will test the safety of this drug (NCT00453375).

Combination therapies

The search for a single drug that can modulate the natural history of T1DM continues; however, it is not yet clear to what extent a single agent may be able to modify or retard the progression of T1DM. Therefore, combinations of drugs have also been suggested for patients with new-onset diabetes.

The current direction of research is to combine two immunomodulatory agents: non-specific antibody-based immunotherapy such as anti-CD3 MoAb and specific antigen-based immunoregulatory agent such as proinsulin peptide [136]. This combination may permit reduction of the dose or the duration of one or both drugs to maximize benefits or minimize adverse effects. Bresson and von Herrath suggested two main goals for combination therapy of T1DM [121]. First, ensure rapid interruption of the aggressive autoimmune response with minimum adverse effects. Second, enhance β-cell regeneration to the level of sustaining normal glucose levels independent of exogenous insulin therapy [121].

Among combination therapies aiming at immunoregulation are IL-2 (proleukin) and sirolimus (rapamycin), which are being combined and used in an ongoing open-label uncontrolled safety trial. Participants are adults, 18–45 years old, who were diagnosed with T1DM within 4 years (NCT00525889). This trial was based on results obtained in NOD mice when this therapy combination induced sustained β-cell protection and prevented T1DM progression after omitting the drugs [137]. The synergetic effects of these drugs are thought to be through enhancing shifting Th1 lymphocyte into the protective Th2 regulatory lymphocyte.

A second proposed combination involves anti-CD3 and a proinsulin peptide (B24–C36) nasally. This combination was found to induce proinsulin-specific T_{reg} cells and enhance remission in two experimental animals more than the effect of each single drug alone [136].

Alternatively, an ongoing randomized double-blinded placebo-controlled trial tests two immunosuppressive agents, mycophenolate mofetil (MMF/CellCept) and the anti-IL2 receptor monoclonal antibody, daclizumab (DZB/Zenapax) (NCT00100178). This trial will assess whether this combination preserves the remaining viable β-cells and enhances their regeneration in subjects 8–45 years of age who were diagnosed within a 3-month-period. (For further details on prevention and intervention trials see http://www.ClinicalTrials.gov.)

Future directions

Future drug therapy of T1DM will depend on the success of ongoing and planned intervention trials. Since 1976, patients with newly diagnosed T1DM have been given immunosuppressive agents but none of these have preserved β-cell function. Transient effects have been reported but the benefits have been limited because they had to continue the insulin replacement therapy. Immunomodulation alone, or possibly combined with immunosuppressive therapy, seems to be promising in reducing the loss of C-peptides after diagnosis. It is often questioned whether immunomodulation with a single autoantigen is sufficient. Provided the treatment is safe, it cannot be excluded that the simultaneous administration of GAD65, IA-2 and proinsulin may be more efficacious than GAD65 alone.

The route of administration needs further exploration. Oral insulin has already been tested and it would be interesting to test the efficacy of oral GAD65. Furthermore, it would be interesting to test alum-GAD65 together with alum-formulated proinsulin. Studies of the function of the human immune system lags behind that of the mouse and rat. Safe immune tolerance trials may provide a novel approach to dissect the mechanisms by which the human immune system responds to immune therapy with autoantigens.

Since 2001, TrialNet, an international network of clinical research groups supported by the National Institutes of Health, has established an infrastructure for trials for predicting and preventing T1DM. Within this network, relatives of patients with T1DM will be screened for disease risk and then either followed or randomized into clinical trials. Individuals developing multiple autoantibodies will be eligible for ongoing prevention studies. Networks such as TrialNet will enable different investigators and clinics to cooperate in the attempts to predict and prevent T1DM.

References

1 Gianani R, Eisenbarth GS. The stages of type 1A diabetes: 2005. *Immunol Rev* 2005; **204**:232–249.

2 Steffes MW, Sibley S, Jackson M, Thomas W. Beta-cell function and the development of diabetes-related complications in the Diabetes Control and Complications Trial. *Diabetes Care* 2003; **26**:832–836.

3 Shah SC, Malone JI, Simpson NE. A randomized trial of intensive insulin therapy in newly diagnosed insulin-dependent diabetes mellitus. *N Engl J Med* 1989; **320**:550–554.

4 Ludvigsson J, Heding L, Lieden G, Marner B, Lernmark A. Plasmapheresis in the initial treatment of insulin-dependent diabetes mellitus in children. *Br Med J (Clin Res Ed)* 1983; **286**: 176–178.

5 Carel JC, Boitard C, Eisenbarth G, Bach JF, Bougneres PF. Cyclosporine delays but does not prevent clinical onset in glucose intolerant pre-type 1 diabetic children. *J Autoimmun* 1996; **9**: 739–745.

6 Canadian–European Randomized Control Trial Group. Cyclosporin-induced remission of IDDM after early intervention: association of 1 year of cyclosporin treatment with enhanced insulin secretion. *Diabetes* 1988; **37**:1574–1582.

7 De Filippo G, Carel JC, Boitard C, Bougneres PF. Long-term results of early cyclosporin therapy in juvenile IDDM. *Diabetes* 1996; **45**:101–104.

8 Parving HH, Tarnow L, Nielsen FS, Rossing P, Mandrup-Poulsen T, Osterby R, *et al.* Cyclosporine nephrotoxicity in type 1 diabetic patients: a 7-year follow-up study. *Diabetes Care* 1999; **22**:478–483.

9 Cook JJ, Hudson I, Harrison LC, Dean B, Colman PG, Werther GA, *et al.* Double-blind controlled trial of azathioprine in children with newly diagnosed type I diabetes. *Diabetes* 1989; **38**:779–783.

10 Silverstein J, Maclaren N, Riley W, Spillar R, Radjenovic D, Johnson S. Immunosuppression with azathioprine and prednisone in recent-onset insulin-dependent diabetes mellitus. *N Engl J Med* 1988; **319**:599–604.

11 Shehadeh N, Etzioni A, Cahana A, Teninboum G, Gorodetsky B, Barzilai D, *et al.* Repeated BCG vaccination is more effective than a single dose in preventing diabetes in non-obese diabetic (NOD) mice. *Isr J Med Sci* 1997; **33**:711–715.

12 Sadelain MW, Qin HY, Sumoski W, Parfrey N, Singh B, Rabinovitch A. Prevention of diabetes in the BB rat by early immunotherapy using Freund's adjuvant. *J Autoimmun* 1990; **3**:671–680.

13 Parent ME, Siemiatycki J, Menzies R, Fritschi L, Colle E. Bacille Calmette–Guerin vaccination and incidence of IDDM in Montreal, Canada. *Diabetes Care* 1997; **20**:767–772.

14 Allen HF, Klingensmith GJ, Jensen P, Simoes E, Hayward A, Chase HP. Effect of bacillus Calmette–Guérin vaccination on new-onset type 1 diabetes: a randomized clinical study. *Diabetes Care* 1999; **22**:1703–1707.

15 Bohmer KP, Kolb H, Kuglin B, Zielasek J, Hubinger A, Lampeter EF, *et al.* Linear loss of insulin secretory capacity during the last six months preceding IDDM: no effect of antiedematous therapy with ketotifen. *Diabetes Care* 1994; **17**:138–141.

16 O'Brien BA, Harmon BV, Cameron DP, Allan DJ. Nicotinamide prevents the development of diabetes in the cyclophosphamide-induced NOD mouse model by reducing beta-cell apoptosis. *J Pathol* 2000; **191**:86–92.

17 Gale EA, Bingley PJ, Emmett CL, Collier T. European Nicotinamide Diabetes Intervention Trial (ENDIT): a randomised controlled trial of intervention before the onset of type 1 diabetes. *Lancet* 2004; **363**:925–931.

18 Lampeter EF, Klinghammer A, Scherbaum WA, Heinze E, Haastert B, Giani G, *et al.*; DENIS Group. The Deutsche Nicotinamide Intervention Study: an attempt to prevent type 1 diabetes. *Diabetes* 1998; **47**:980–984.

19 Pozzilli P, Visalli N, Boccuni ML, Baroni MG, Buzzetti R, Fioriti E, *et al.*; IMDIAB Study Group. Randomized trial comparing nicotinamide and nicotinamide plus cyclosporin in recent onset insulin-dependent diabetes (IMDIAB 1). *Diabet Med* 1994; **11**:98–104.

20 Crino A, Schiaffini R, Manfrini S, Mesturino C, Visalli N, Beretta Anguissola G, *et al.* A randomized trial of nicotinamide and vitamin E in children with recent onset type 1 diabetes (IMDIAB IX). *Eur J Endocrinol* 2004; **150**:719–724.

21 Crino A, Schiaffini R, Ciampalini P, Suraci MC, Manfrini S, Visalli N, *et al.* A two year observational study of nicotinamide and intensive insulin therapy in patients with recent onset type 1 diabetes mellitus. *J Pediatr Endocrinol Metab* 2005; **18**:749–754.

22 Diabetes Prevention Trial 1: Type 1 Diabetes Study Group. Effect of insulin in relatives of patients with type 1 diabetes mellitus. *N Engl J Med* 2002; **346**:1685–1691.

23 Skyler JS, Krischer JP, Wolfsdorf J, Cowie C, Palmer JP, Greenbaum C, *et al.* Effects of oral insulin in relatives of patients with type 1 diabetes: the Diabetes Prevention Trial Type 1. *Diabetes Care* 2005; **28**:1068–1076.

24 Harrison LC, Honeyman MC, Steele CE, Stone NL, Sarugeri E, Bonifacio E, *et al.* Pancreatic beta-cell function and immune responses to insulin after administration of intranasal insulin to humans at risk for type 1 diabetes. *Diabetes Care* 2004; **27**: 2348–2355.

25 Nanto-Salonen K, Kupila A, Simell S, Siljander H, Salonsaari T, Hekkala A, *et al.* Nasal insulin to prevent type 1 diabetes in children with HLA genotypes and autoantibodies conferring increased risk of disease: a double-blind, randomised controlled trial. *Lancet* 2008; **372**:1746–1755.

26 Casu A, Trucco M, Pietropaolo M. A look to the future: prediction, prevention, and cure including islet transplantation and stem cell therapy. *Pediatr Clin North Am* 2005; **52**:1779–1804.

27 Nilsson A, Eising S, Hougaard DM, *et al.* Islet antibodies at birth predict development of type 1 diabetes. *Diabetologia* 2006; **49**:1:1–755.

28 Torn C, Mueller PW, Schlosser M, Bonifacio E, Bingley PJ. Diabetes Antibody Standardization Program: evaluation of assays for autoantibodies to glutamic acid decarboxylase and islet antigen-2. *Diabetologia* 2008; **51**:846–852.

29 Vendrame F, Gottlieb PA. Prediabetes: prediction and prevention trials. *Endocrinol Metab Clin North Am* 2004; **33**:75–92, ix.

30 Svensson M, Eriksson JW, Dahlquist G. Early glycemic control, age at onset, and development of microvascular complications in childhood-onset type 1 diabetes: a population-based study in northern Sweden. *Diabetes Care* 2004; **27**:955–962.

31 Henricsson M, Nystrom L, Blohme G, Ostman J, Kullberg C, Svensson M, *et al.* The incidence of retinopathy 10 years after diagnosis in young adult people with diabetes: results from the nationwide population-based Diabetes Incidence Study in Sweden (DISS). *Diabetes Care* 2003; **26**:349–354.

32 Barker JM, Goehrig SH, Barriga K, Hoffman M, Slover R, Eisenbarth GS, *et al.* Clinical characteristics of children diagnosed with type 1 diabetes through intensive screening and follow-up. *Diabetes Care* 2004; **27**:1399–1404.

33 Mrena S, Virtanen SM, Laippala P, Kulmala P, Hannila ML, Akerblom HK, *et al.* Models for predicting type 1 diabetes in siblings of affected children. *Diabetes Care* 2006; **29**:662–667.

34 Noble JA, Valdes AM, Cook M, Klitz W, Thomson G, Erlich HA. The role of HLA class II genes in insulin-dependent diabetes mellitus: molecular analysis of 180 Caucasian, multiplex families. *Am J Hum Genet* 1996; **59**:1134–1148.

35 Redondo MJ, Eisenbarth GS. Genetic control of autoimmunity in type I diabetes and associated disorders. *Diabetologia* 2002; **45**:605–622.

36 Knip M, Veijola R, Virtanen SM, Hyoty H, Vaarala O, Akerblom HK. Environmental triggers and determinants of type 1 diabetes. *Diabetes* 2005; **54**(Suppl 2):125–136.

37 Schenker M, Hummel M, Ferber K, Walter M, Keller E, Albert ED, *et al.* Early expression and high prevalence of islet autoantibodies for DR3/4 heterozygous and DR4/4 homozygous offspring of parents with type I diabetes: the German BABYDIAB study. *Diabetologia* 1999; **42**:671–677.

38 Rewers M, Bugawan TL, Norris JM, Blair A, Beaty B, Hoffman M, *et al.* Newborn screening for HLA markers associated with IDDM: diabetes autoimmunity study in the young (DAISY). *Diabetologia* 1996; **39**:807–812.

39 The Environmental Determinants of Diabetes in the Young (TEDDY) Study. *Ann N Y Acad Sci* 2008; **1150**:1–13.

40 Thomson G, Valdes AM, Noble JA, Kockum I, Grote MN, Najman J, *et al.* Relative predispositional effects of HLA class II DRB1-DQB1 haplotypes and genotypes on type 1 diabetes: a meta-analysis. *Tissue Antigens* 2007; **70**:110–127.

41 Park Y, Eisenbarth GS. Genetic susceptibility factors of type 1 diabetes in Asians. *Diabetes Metab Res Rev* 2001; **17**:2–11.

42 Todd JA, Walker NM, Cooper JD, Smyth DJ, Downes K, Plagnol V, *et al.* Robust associations of four new chromosome regions from genome-wide analyses of type 1 diabetes. *Nat Genet* 2007; **39**:857–864.

43 Serjeantson SW, Kohonen-Corish MR, Rowley MJ, Mackay IR, Knowles W, Zimmet P. Antibodies to glutamic acid decarboxylase are associated with HLA-DR genotypes in both Australians and Asians with type 1 (insulin-dependent) diabetes mellitus. *Diabetologia* 1992; **35**:996–1001.

44 Sanjeevi CB, Hagopian WA, Landin-Olsson M, Kockum I, Woo W, Palmer JP, *et al.* Association between autoantibody markers and subtypes of DR4 and DR4-DQ in Swedish children with insulin-dependent diabetes reveals closer association of tyrosine pyrophosphatase autoimmunity with DR4 than DQ8. *Tissue Antigens* 1998; **51**:281–286.

45 Rajasalu T, Haller K, Salur L, Kisand K, Tillman V, Schlosser M, *et al.* Insulin VNTR I/III genotype is associated with autoantibodies against glutamic acid decarboxylase in newly diagnosed type 1 diabetes. *Diabetes Metab Res Rev* 2007; **23**:567–571.

46 Steck AK, Bugawan TL, Valdes AM, Emery LM, Blair A, Norris JM, *et al.* Association of non-HLA genes with type 1 diabetes autoimmunity. *Diabetes* 2005; **54**:2482–2486.

47 Steck AK, Zhang W, Bugawan TL, Barriga KJ, Blair A, Erlich HA, *et al.* Do non-HLA genes influence development of persistent islet autoimmunity and type 1 diabetes in children with high-risk HLA-DR,DQ genotypes? *Diabetes* 2009; **58**:1028–1033.

48 Bottazzo GF, Florin-Christensen A, Doniach D. Islet-cell antibodies in diabetes mellitus with autoimmune polyendocrine deficiencies. *Lancet* 1974; **2**:1279–1283.

49 MacCuish AC, Irvine WJ, Barnes EW, Duncan LJ. Antibodies to pancreatic islet cells in insulin-dependent diabetics with coexistent autoimmune disease. *Lancet* 1974; **2**:1529–1531.

50 Baekkeskov S, Nielsen JH, Marner B, Bilde T, Ludvigsson J, Lernmark A. Autoantibodies in newly diagnosed diabetic children immunoprecipitate human pancreatic islet cell proteins. *Nature* 1982; **298**:167–169.

51 Baekkeskov S, Aanstoot HJ, Christgau S, Reetz A, Solimena M, Cascalho M, *et al.* Identification of the 64K autoantigen in insulin-dependent diabetes as the GABA-synthesizing enzyme glutamic acid decarboxylase. *Nature* 1990; **347**:151–156.

52 Karlsen AE, Hagopian WA, Grubin CE, Dube S, Disteche CM, Adler DA, *et al.* Cloning and primary structure of a human islet isoform of glutamic acid decarboxylase from chromosome 10. *Proc Natl Acad Sci U S A* 1991; **88**:8337–8341.

53 Palmer JP, Asplin CM, Clemons P, Lyen K, Tatpati O, Raghu PK, *et al.* Insulin antibodies in insulin-dependent diabetics before insulin treatment. *Science* 1983; **222**:1337–1339.

54 Lan MS, Wasserfall C, Maclaren NK, Notkins AL. IA-2, a transmembrane protein of the protein tyrosine phosphatase family, is a major autoantigen in insulin-dependent diabetes mellitus. *Proc Natl Acad Sci U S A* 1996; **93**:6367–6370.

55 Primo ME, Sica MP, Risso VA, Poskus E, Ermacora MR. Expression and physicochemical characterization of an extracellular segment of the receptor protein tyrosine phosphatase IA-2. *Biochim Biophys Acta* 2006; **1764**:174–181.

56 Wenzlau JM, Juhl K, Yu L, Moua O, sarkar SA, Gottlieb P, Rewers M, *et al.* The cation efflux transporter ZnT8 (Slc30A8) is a major autoantigen in human type 1 diabetes. *Proc Natl Acad Sci U S A* 2007; **104**:17040–17045.

57 Notkins AL, Lernmark A. Autoimmune type 1 diabetes: resolved and unresolved issues. *J Clin Invest* 2001; **108**:1247–1252.

58 Elfving M, Lindberg B, Lynch K, Månsson M, Sundkvist G, Lernmark A, *et al.* Number of islet autoantibodies present in newly diagnosed type 1 diabetes children born to non-diabetic mothers is affected by islet autoantibodies present at birth. *Pediatr Diabetes* 2008; **9**:127–134.

59 Kupila A, Keskinen P, Simell T, Erkkilä S, Arvilommi P, Korhonen S, *et al.* Genetic risk determines the emergence of diabetes-associated autoantibodies in young children. *Diabetes* 2002; **51**:646–651.

60 Kimpimaki T, Kupila A, Hamalainen AM, Kukko M, Kulmala P, Savola K, *et al.* The first signs of beta-cell autoimmunity appear in infancy in genetically susceptible children from the general population: the Finnish Type 1 Diabetes Prediction and Prevention Study. *J Clin Endocrinol Metab* 2001; **86**:4782–4788.

61 Yu L, Rewers M, Gianani R, Kawasaki E, Zhang Y, Verge C, *et al.* Antiislet autoantibodies usually develop sequentially rather than simultaneously. *J Clin Endocrinol Metab* 1996; **81**:4264–4267.

62 Mrena S, Savola K, Kulmala P, Akerblom HK, Knip M. Natural course of preclinical type 1 diabetes in siblings of affected children. *Acta Paediatr* 2003; **92**:1403–1410.

63 Kukko M, Kimpimaki T, Korhonen S, Kupila A, Simell S, Veijola R, *et al.* Dynamics of diabetes-associated autoantibodies in young children with human leukocyte antigen-conferred risk of type 1 diabetes recruited from the general population. *J Clin Endocrinol Metab* 2005; **90**:2712–1217.

64 Barker JM, Barriga KJ, Yu L, Miao D, Erlich HA, Norris JM, *et al.* Prediction of autoantibody positivity and progression to type 1 diabetes: Diabetes Autoimmunity Study in the Young (DAISY). *J Clin Endocrinol Metab* 2004; **89**:3896–3902.

65 Redondo MJ, Babu S, Zeidler A, Orban T, Yu L, greenbaum C, *et al.* Specific human leukocyte antigen DQ influence on expression of antiislet autoantibodies and progression to type 1 diabetes. *J Clin Endocrinol Metab* 2006; **91**:1705–1713.

66 Bingley PJ, Christie MR, Bonifacio E, Bonfanti R, Shattock M, Fonte MT, *et al.* Combined analysis of autoantibodies improves prediction of IDDM in islet cell antibody-positive relatives. *Diabetes* 1994; **43**:1304–1310.

67 LaGasse JM, Brantley MS, Leech NJ, Rowe RE, Monks S, Palmer JP, *et al* Successful prospective prediction of type 1 diabetes in schoolchildren through multiple defined autoantibodies: an 8-year follow-up of the Washington State Diabetes Prediction Study. *Diabetes Care* 2002; **25**:505–511.

68 Bingley PJ, Bonifacio E, Williams AJ, Genovese S, Bottazzo GF, Gale EA. Prediction of IDDM in the general population: strategies based on combinations of autoantibody markers. *Diabetes* 1997; **46**:1701–1710.

69 Siljander HT, Veijola R, Reunanen A, Virtanen SM, Akerblom HK, Knip M. Prediction of type 1 diabetes among siblings of affected children and in the general population. *Diabetologia* 2007; **50**:2272–2275.

70 Knip M, Kukko M, Kulmala P, Veijola R, Simell O, Akerblom HK, *et al.* Humoral beta-cell autoimmunity in relation to HLA-defined disease susceptibility in preclinical and clinical type 1 diabetes. *Am J Med Genet* 2002; **115**:48–54.

71 Savola K, Laara E, Vahasalo P, Kulmala P, Akerblom HK, Knip M. Dynamic pattern of disease-associated autoantibodies in siblings of children with type 1 diabetes: a population-based study. *Diabetes* 2001; **50**:2625–2632.

72 Sosenko JM, Palmer JP, Rafkin-Mervis L, Krischer JP, Cuthbertson D, Matheson D, *et al.* Glucose and C-peptide changes in the perionset period of type 1 diabetes in the Diabetes Prevention Trial-Type 1. *Diabetes Care* 2008; **31**:2188–2192.

73 Sosenko JM, Palmer JP, Greenbaum CJ, Mahon J, Cowie C, Krischer JP, *et al.* Patterns of metabolic progression to type 1 diabetes in the Diabetes Prevention Trial-Type 1. *Diabetes Care* 2006; **29**:643–649.

74 Sosenko JM, Palmer JP, Greenbaum CJ, Mahon J, Cowie C, Krischer JP, *et al.* Increasing the accuracy of oral glucose tolerance testing and extending its application to individuals with normal glucose tolerance for the prediction of type 1 diabetes: the Diabetes Prevention Trial-Type 1. *Diabetes Care* 2007; **30**:38–42.

75 Sosenko JM, Krischer JP, Palmer JP, Mahon J, Cowie C, Greenbaum CJ, *et al.* A risk score for type 1 diabetes derived from autoantibody-positive participants in the Diabetes Prevention Trial-Type 1. *Diabetes Care* 2008; **31**:528–533.

76 Stene LC, Barriga K, Hoffman M, Kean J, Klingensmith G, Norris JM, *et al.* Normal but increasing hemoglobin A1c levels predict progression from islet autoimmunity to overt type 1 diabetes: Diabetes Autoimmunity Study in the Young (DAISY). *Pediatr Diabetes* 2006; **7**:247–253.

77 Purohit S, She JX. Biomarkers for type 1 diabetes. *Int J Clin Exp Med* 2008; **1**:98–116.

78 Atkinson MA, Maclaren NK, Luchetta R. Insulitis and diabetes in NOD mice reduced by prophylactic insulin therapy. *Diabetes* 1990; **39**:933–937.

79 Gotfredsen CF, Buschard K, Frandsen EK. Reduction of diabetes incidence of BB Wistar rats by early prophylactic insulin treatment of diabetes-prone animals. *Diabetologia* 1985; **28**: 933–935.

80 Gottlieb PA, Handler ES, Appel MC, Greiner DL, Mordes JP, Rossini AA. Insulin treatment prevents diabetes mellitus but not thyroiditis in RT6-depleted diabetes resistant BB/Wor rats. *Diabetologia* 1991; **34**:296–300.

81 EURODIAB ACE Study Group. Variation and trends in incidence of childhood diabetes in Europe. *Lancet* 2000; **355**:873–876.

82 Hummel M, Bonifacio E, Naserke HE, Ziegler AG. Elimination of dietary gluten does not reduce titers of type 1 diabetes-associated autoantibodies in high-risk subjects. *Diabetes Care* 2002; **25**: 1111–1116.

83 Gerstein HC. Cow's milk exposure and type 1 diabetes mellitus: a critical overview of the clinical literature. *Diabetes Care* 1994; **17**:13–19.

84 Paronen J, Knip M, Savilahti E, Virtanen SM, Ilonen J, Akerblom HK, *et al.*; Finnish Trial to Reduce IDDM in the Genetically at Risk Study Group. Effect of cow's milk exposure and maternal type 1 diabetes on cellular and humoral immunization to dietary insulin in infants at genetic risk for type 1 diabetes. *Diabetes* 2000; **49**:1657–1665.

85 Akerblom HK, Virtanen SM, Ilonen J, Savilahti E, Vaarala O, Reunanen A, *et al.* Dietary manipulation of beta cell autoimmunity in infants at increased risk of type 1 diabetes: a pilot study. *Diabetologia* 2005; **48**:829–837.

86 TRIGR Study Group. Study design of the Trial to Reduce IDDM in the Genetically at Risk (TRIGR). *Pediatric Diabetes* 2007; **8**:117–137.

87 EURODIAB Substudy 2 Study Group. Vitamin D supplement in early childhood and risk for type 1 (insulin-dependent) diabetes mellitus. *Diabetologia* 1999; **42**:51–54.

88 Mathieu C, Badenhoop K. Vitamin D and type 1 diabetes mellitus: state of the art. *Trends Endocrinol Metab* 2005; **16**:261–266.

89 Hypponen E, Laara E, Reunanen A, Jarvelin MR, Virtanen SM. Intake of vitamin D and risk of type 1 diabetes: a birth-cohort study. *Lancet* 2001; **358**:1500–1503.

90 Feasibility study of 2000 IU per day of vitamin D for the primary prevention of type 1 diabetes. Trial NCT00141986. [cited 2009 January 2]; Available from: http://wwwclinicaltrialsgov.

91 Stene LC, Joner G. Use of cod liver oil during the first year of life is associated with lower risk of childhood-onset type 1 diabetes: a large, population-based, case–control study. *Am J Clin Nutr* 2003; **78**:1128–1134.

92 Norris JM, Yin X, Lamb MM, Barriga K, Seifert J, Hoffman M, *et al.* Omega-3 polyunsaturated fatty acid intake and islet autoimmunity

in children at increased risk for type 1 diabetes. *JAMA* 2007; **298**:1420–1428.

93 Nutritional Intervention to Prevent Diabetes (NIP) Study. [cited 2009 February 12]; Available from: http://wwwdiabetestrialnetorg.

94 Staeva-Vieira T, Peakman M, von Herrath M. Translational mini-review series on type 1 diabetes: immune-based therapeutic approaches for type 1 diabetes. *Clin Exp Immunol* 2007; **148**:17–31.

95 Schatz DA, Krischer JP, Skyler JS. Now is the time to prevent type 1 diabetes. *J Clin Endocrinol Metab* 1999; **85**:495–498.

96 Ludvigsson J. Immune intervention at diagnosis: should we treat children to preserve beta-cell function? *Pediatr Diabetes* 2007; **8**(Suppl 6):34–39.

97 Keller RJ, Eisenbarth GS, Jackson RA. Insulin prophylaxis in individuals at high risk of type 1 diabetes. *Lancet* 1993; **341**: 927–928.

98 Fuchtenbusch M, Rabl W, Grassl B, Bachmann W, Standl E, Ziegler AG. Delay of type 1 diabetes in high risk, first degree relatives by parenteral antigen administration: the Schwabing Insulin Prophylaxis Pilot Trial. *Diabetologia* 1998; **41**:536–541.

99 Barker JM, McFann KK, Orban T. Effect of oral insulin on insulin autoantibody levels in the Diabetes Prevention Trial Type 1 oral insulin study. *Diabetologia* 2007; **50**:1603–1606.

100 Mordes JP, Schirf B, Roipko D, Greiner DL, Weiner H, Nelson P, *et al.* Oral insulin does not prevent insulin-dependent diabetes mellitus in BB rats. *Ann N Y Acad Sci* 1996; **778**:418–421.

101 Bellmann K, Kolb H, Rastegar S, Jee P, Scott FW. Potential risk of oral insulin with adjuvant for the prevention of type I diabetes: a protocol effective in NOD mice may exacerbate disease in BB rats. *Diabetologia* 1998; **41**:844–847.

102 Polanski M, Melican NS, Zhang J, Weiner HL. Oral administration of the immunodominant B-chain of insulin reduces diabetes in a co-transfer model of diabetes in the NOD mouse and is associated with a switch from Th1 to Th2 cytokines. *J Autoimmun* 1997; **10**:339–346.

103 Kolb H, Gale EA. Does partial preservation of residual beta-cell function justify immune intervention in recent onset type 1 diabetes? *Diabetologia* 2001; **44**:1349–1353.

104 Diabetes Control and Complications Trial Research Group. Effect of intensive therapy on residual ß-Cell function in patients with type 1 diabetes in the diabetes control and complications trial: a randomized controlled trial. *Ann Intern Med* 1998; **128**:517–523.

105 Feutren G, Papoz L, Assan R, Vialettes B, Karsenty G, Vexiau P, *et al.* Cyclosporin increases the rate and length of remissions in insulin-dependent diabetes of recent onset: results of a multicentre double-blind trial. *Lancet* 1986; **2**:119–124.

106 Harrison LC, Colman PG, Dean B, Baxter R, Martin FI. Increase in remission rate in newly diagnosed type I diabetic subjects treated with azathioprine. *Diabetes* 1985; **34**:1306–1308.

107 Chase HP, Butler-Simon N, Garg S, McDuffie M, Hoops SL, O'Brien D. A trial of nicotinamide in newly diagnosed patients with type 1 (insulin-dependent) diabetes mellitus. *Diabetologia* 1990; **33**: 444–446.

108 Lewis CM, Canafax DM, Sprafka JM, Barbosa JJ. Double-blind randomized trial of nicotinamide on early-onset diabetes. *Diabetes Care* 1992; **15**:121–123.

109 Pozzilli P, Browne PD, Kolb H; The Nicotinamide Trialists. Meta-analysis of nicotinamide treatment in patients with recent-onset IDDM. *Diabetes Care* 1996; **19**:1357–1363.

110 Pozzilli P; IMDIAB Group. BCG vaccine in insulin-dependent diabetes mellitus. *Lancet* 1997; **349**:1520–1521.

111 Ortqvist E, Bjork E, Wallensteen M, Ludvigsson J, Aman J, Johansson C, *et al.* Temporary preservation of beta-cell function by diazoxide treatment in childhood type 1 diabetes. *Diabetes Care* 2004; **27**:2191–2197.

112 Herold KC, Hagopian W, Auger JA, Poumian-Ruiz E, Taylor L, Donaldson D, *et al.* Anti-CD3 monoclonal antibody in new-onset type 1 diabetes mellitus. *N Engl J Med* 2002; **346**:1692–1698.

113 Keymeulen B, Vandemeulebroucke E, Ziegler AG, Mathieu C, Kaufman L, Hale G, *et al.* Insulin needs after CD3-antibody therapy in new-onset type 1 diabetes. *N Engl J Med* 2005; **352**:2598–2608.

114 Herold KC, Gitelman SE, Masharani U, Hagopian W, Bisikirska B, Donaldson D, *et al.* A single course of anti-CD3 monoclonal antibody hOKT3gamma1(Ala-Ala) results in improvement in C-peptide responses and clinical parameters for at least 2 years after onset of type 1 diabetes. *Diabetes* 2005; **54**:1763–1769.

115 Simon G, Parker M, Ramiya V, Wasserfall C, Huang Y, Bresson D, *et al.* Murine antithymocyte globulin therapy alters disease progression in NOD mice by a time-dependent induction of immunoregulation. *Diabetes* 2008; **57**:405–414.

116 Hu CY, Rodriguez-Pinto D, Du W, Ahuja A, henegariu O, Wong FS, *et al.* Treatment with CD20-specific antibody prevents and reverses autoimmune diabetes in mice. *J Clin Invest* 2007; **117**:3857–3867.

117 Alegre ML, Frauwirth KA, Thompson CB. T-cell regulation by CD28 and CTLA-4. *Nat Rev Immunol* 2001; **1**:220–228.

118 Abrams JR, Kelley SL, Hayes E, Kikuchi T, Brown MJ, Kang S, *et al.* Blockade of T lymphocyte costimulation with cytotoxic T lymphocyte-associated antigen 4-immunoglobulin (CTLA4Ig) reverses the cellular pathology of psoriatic plaques, including the activation of keratinocytes, dendritic cells, and endothelial cells. *J Exp Med* 2000; **192**:681–694.

119 Bresnihan B, Alvaro-Gracia JM, Cobby M, Doherty M, Domljan Z, Emery P, *et al.* Treatment of rheumatoid arthritis with recombinant human interleukin-1 receptor antagonist. *Arthritis Rheum* 1998; **41**:2196–2204.

120 Bowman MA, Leiter EH, Atkinson MA. Prevention of diabetes in the NOD mouse: implications for therapeutic intervention in human disease. *Immunol Today* 1994; **15**:115–120.

121 Bresson D, von Herrath M. Moving towards efficient therapies in type 1 diabetes: to combine or not to combine? *Autoimmun Rev* 2007; **6**:315–322.

122 Raz I, Elias D, Avron A, Tamir M, Metzger M, Cohen IR. Beta-cell function in new-onset type 1 diabetes and immunomodulation with a heat-shock protein peptide (DiaPep277): a randomised, double-blind, phase II trial. *Lancet* 2001; **358**:1749–1753.

123 Elias D, Avron A, Tamir M, Raz I. DiaPep277 preserves endogenous insulin production by immunomodulation in type 1 diabetes. *Ann N Y Acad Sci* 2006; **1079**:340–344.

124 Schloot NC, Meierhoff G, Lengyel C, Vándorfi G, Takács J, Pánczel P, *et al.* Effect of heat shock protein peptide DiaPep277 on beta-cell function in paediatric and adult patients with recent-onset diabetes mellitus type 1: two prospective, randomized, double-blind phase II trials. *Diabetes Metab Res Rev* 2007; **23**:276–285.

125 Lazar L, Ofan R, Weintrob N, Avron A, Tamir M, Elias D, *et al.* Heat-shock protein peptide DiaPep277 treatment in children with newly diagnosed type 1 diabetes: a randomised, double-blind phase II study. *Diabetes Metab Res Rev* 2007; **23**:286–291.

126 Ludvigsson J, Faresjo M, Hjorth M, Axelsson S, Chéramy M, Pihi M, *et al.* GAD treatment and insulin secretion in recent-onset type 1 diabetes. *N Engl J Med* 2008; **359**:1909–1920.

127 Agardh CD, Cilio CM, Lethagen A, Lynch K, Leslie RD, Palmér M, *et al.* Clinical evidence for the safety of GAD65 immunomodulation in adult-onset autoimmune diabetes. *J Diabetes Complications* 2005; **19**:238–246.

128 Petersen JS, Karlsen AE, Markholst H, Worsaae A, Dyrberg T, Michelsen B. Neonatal tolerization with glutamic acid decarboxylase but not with bovine serum albumin delays the onset of diabetes in NOD mice. *Diabetes* 1994; **43**:1478–1484.

129 Tian J, Clare-Salzler M, Herschenfeld A, Middleton B, Newman D, Mueller R, *et al.* Modulating autoimmune responses to GAD inhibits disease progression and prolongs islet graft survival in diabetes-prone mice. *Nat Med* 1996; **2**:1348–1353.

130 Tisch R, Liblau RS, Yang XD, Liblau P, McDevitt HO. Induction of GAD65-specific regulatory T-cells inhibits ongoing autoimmune diabetes in nonobese diabetic mice. *Diabetes* 1998; **47**:894–899.

131 Plesner A, Worsaae A, Dyrberg T, Gotfredsen C, Michelsen BK, Petersen JS. Immunization of diabetes-prone or non-diabetes-prone mice with GAD65 does not induce diabetes or islet cell pathology. *J Autoimmun* 1998; **11**:335–341.

132 Jun HS, Chung YH, Han J, Kim A, Yoo SS, Sherwin RS, *et al.* Prevention of autoimmune diabetes by immunogene therapy using recombinant vaccinia virus expressing glutamic acid decarboxylase. *Diabetologia* 2002; **45**:668–676.

133 Muir A, Peck A, Clare-Salzler M, Song YH, Cornelius J, Luchetta R, *et al.* Insulin immunization of nonobese diabetic mice induces a protective insulitis characterized by diminished intraislet interferon-gamma transcription. *J Clin Invest* 1995; **95**:628–634.

134 Alleva DG, Gaur A, Jin L, Kwok WW, Ling N, Gottschalk M, *et al.* Immunological characterization and therapeutic activity of an altered-peptide ligand, NBI-6024, based on the immunodominant type 1 diabetes autoantigen insulin B-chain (9-23) peptide. *Diabetes* 2002; **51**:2126–2134.

135 Alleva DG, Maki RA, Putnam AL, Robinson JM, Kipnes MS, Dandona P, *et al.* Immunomodulation in type 1 diabetes by NBI-6024, an altered peptide ligand of the insulin B epitope. *Scand J Immunol* 2006; **63**:59–69.

136 Bresson D, Togher L, Rodrigo E, Chen Y, Bluestone JA, herold KC, *et al.* Anti-CD3 and nasal proinsulin combination therapy enhances remission from recent-onset autoimmune diabetes by inducing Tregs. *J Clin Invest* 2006; **116**:1371–1381.

137 Rabinovitch A, Suarez-Pinzon WL, Shapiro AM, Rajotte RV, Power R. Combination therapy with sirolimus and interleukin-2 prevents spontaneous and recurrent autoimmune diabetes in NOD mice. *Diabetes* 2002; **51**:638–645.

60 Future Drug Treatment for Type 2 Diabetes

Clifford J. Bailey

Life and Health Sciences, Aston University, Birmingham, UK

Keypoints

- The heterogeneous and progressive nature of type 2 diabetes presents an ongoing requirement for additional and novel blood glucose-lowering agents.
- Longer-acting (once daily and once weekly injected) analogs of the incretin hormone glucagon-like peptide 1 (GLP-1) and new dipeptidyl peptidase 4 inhibitors are being developed.
- Proof of principle studies have shown potential for non-peptide molecules to act as GLP-1 receptor agonists and insulin mimetics.
- Potentiators of insulin action include specific phosphatase inhibitors and other types of compounds that increase insulin receptor and early post-receptor signaling.
- Selective peroxisome proliferator-activated receptor modulators, glucagon receptor antagonists and cellular glucocorticoid inhibitors have shown potential.
- Agents that directly increase glucose disposal (e.g. glucokinase activators) or reduce glucose output (e.g. fructose 1,6-bisphosphatase inhibitors) are receiving attention.
- Sodium-glucose co-transporter 2 inhibitors can facilitate glycemic control through increased renal glucose elimination.

Introduction

Current strategies for managing type 2 diabetes mellitus (T2DM) are described in Part 6. This chapter reviews new therapeutic approaches to address the metabolic disturbances of T2DM. The main focus is on drugs that have recently become available for clinical use or have entered clinical trials, and established agents that have found new applications in patients with diabetes. Some agents in preclinical development that have particular theoretical promise are also considered.

There is a continuing need for new and improved agents to treat diabetes as available therapies do not reinstate normal glucose homeostasis or eliminate the threat of long-term complications. Indeed, patients with T2DM incur chronic tissue damage and suffer premature death, even with assiduous use of the available therapies [1–3]. Lifestyle measures, notably diet and exercise, remain the foundation therapy [4], while pharmacologic interventions are added to provide further recourse against the multiple, heterogeneous and progressive endocrine and metabolic disturbances of the disease [5]. Recent trial outcomes have re-emphasized the importance of comprehensive risk factor management in which early, effective, individualized and sustained glycemic control can defer the onset and reduce the severity of complications [1,2]. In particular, "glycemic memory" requires good glycemic control early after diagnosis to minimize the complications of hyperglycemia much later in the disease process [1,2,6].

Textbook of Diabetes, 4th edition. Edited by R. Holt, C. Cockram, A. Flyvbjerg and B. Goldstein.

Development of new antidiabetic agents

As diabetes must usually be treated for the remainder of the patient's life, any new antidiabetic drug must be safe, well-tolerated, conveniently administered and carry minimal risk of serious hypoglycemia. It should offer durable efficacy and preferably other advantages – for example, a novel mode of action or favorable pharmacokinetics that suit a particular group such as the elderly. Ideally, a new agent will be suited to combination therapy with at least some of the existing agents, and confer benefits against conditions that are commonly associated with diabetes, such as abdominal obesity, dyslipidemia, hypertension and other vascular diseases or risk factors. A new drug might correct at least one of the major underlying endocrine or metabolic disturbances such as counter insulin resistance, improve β-cell function, reduce hyperglucagonemia or act directly to decrease glucotoxicity or lipotoxicity.

The development of a drug from a new chemical entity through to marketing approval involves many stages of rigorous preclinical and clinical evaluation (Table 60.1). The process can take 10–15 years and cost US$ 500–2000 million [7]. If there is evidence of increased adverse cardiovascular outcomes during the

Table 60.1 Stages in the development of a new drug.

Preclinical stages
New chemical entity
- Identification, extraction/synthesis, chemical characterization and patenting of compounds
- Genotoxicity testing: screening for biological activity *in vitro* and *in vivo* in animals
- Preclinical pharmacology, mode of action, pharmacodynamics (activity, safety, tolerance), pharmacokinetics (bioavailability, distribution, metabolism, elimination) and toxicity in ≥ two mammalian species

Clinical stages
Investigational new drug application: permission to begin clinical studies
Phase 1
- First administration to small number of healthy human volunteers
- Dose ranging, vital signs, pharmacodynamics, pharmacokinetics, drug interactions, safety

Phase 2
- First trials in small numbers of patients
- Dose ranging, efficacy, further pharmacodynamics, pharmacokinetics and safety

Phase 3
- Trials in larger numbers of patients
- Multicenter trials, comparative trials with other treatments, efficacy, further pharmacodynamics and safety (including meta-analysis of cardiovascular outcomes)

New drug application: permission to market as a drug
Phase 4
- Use in medical practice
- Additional trials (similar to phase 3), post-marketing surveillance, adverse drug reactions, use in special subgroups (e.g. elderly people)

Table 60.2 Established blood glucose-lowering agents and some other agents with blood glucose-lowering activity.

Agents	Main mode of action
Agents used in the treatment of diabetes	
Metformin (biguanide)	Counters insulin resistance
Sulfonylureas	Stimulate insulin secretion
Prandial insulin releasers (meglitinides)	Stimulate insulin secretion (rapid/short acting)
Thiazolidinediones (glitazones)	Increase insulin sensitivity (PPARγ agonists)
GLP-1 analogs	Potentiate insulin secretion
DPP-4 inhibitors (gliptins)	Potentiate insulin secretion
α-Glucosidase inhibitors	Inhibit carbohydrate digestion
Pramlintide	Satiety, slow gastric emptying, decrease glucagon
Insulin	Decrease glucose production, increase glucose disposal, storage and utilization
Other agents with blood glucose-lowering activity	
Acipimox	Decrease lipolysis, reduce NEFAs
Alcohol	Inhibit gluconeogenesis
Niacin	Decrease lipolysis, reduce NEFAs
Quinine	Stimulate insulin secretion
Salicylates	Stimulate insulin secretion
β-Adrenoceptor blockers*	Inhibit adrenergic counter-regulatory response

DPP-4, dipeptidyl peptidase 4; GLP-1, glucagon-like peptide 1; NEFA, non-esterified fatty acids; PPARγ, peroxisome proliferator-activated receptor γ.
* β-Adrenoceptor blockers usually raise glucose concentrations, but they can contribute to hypoglycemia by inhibiting the acute counter-regulatory response and impairing hypoglycemia awareness.

pre-authorization studies, depending on the circumstances, either additional pre-authorization or post-authorization trials will be required. To extend the period of marketing exclusivity it is not unusual for companies to seek additional indications and develop new formulations post-authorization. Because many patients with T2DM require combination therapy, there is also considerable interest in the production of single-tablet fixed-dose combinations [8].

Classification of new antidiabetic agents

Blood glucose-lowering agents may be either hypoglycemic or antihyperglycemic [9]. Both reduce hyperglycemia, but hypoglycemic agents can lower blood glucose concentrations below the euglycemic range, and therefore carry the risk of clinical hypoglycemia. Such agents include potent inhibitors of hepatic glucose output, insulin secretagogues that act at low glucose concentrations, potent insulin-mimetic drugs and agents that impair counter-regulatory mechanisms. By contrast, antihyperglycemic agents, when used as monotherapy, do not lower blood glucose into the range of overt hypoglycemia. These drugs include the inhibitors of carbohydrate digestion and intestinal glucose absorption, anti-obesity agents, weaker suppressors of hepatic glucose output or counter-regulation, mild or glucose-dependent insulin secretagogues, most insulin-sensitizing agents and modulators of lipid metabolism.

The major glucose-lowering drugs currently used to treat diabetes, and some other agents with glucose-lowering activity, are shown in Table 60.2. Examples of other types of compounds under investigation as potential glucose-lowering drugs are listed in Table 60.3 [10,11] and illustrated in Figure 60.1.

Inhibitors of intestinal carbohydrate digestion and absorption

Delaying the digestion and absorption of dietary carbohydrate in the intestine reduces post-prandial hyperglycemia and may have some "carry-over" benefit to reduce basal glycemia. Efficacy is variable but generally modest, although this approach is usually suitable for combination with most other antidiabetic therapies

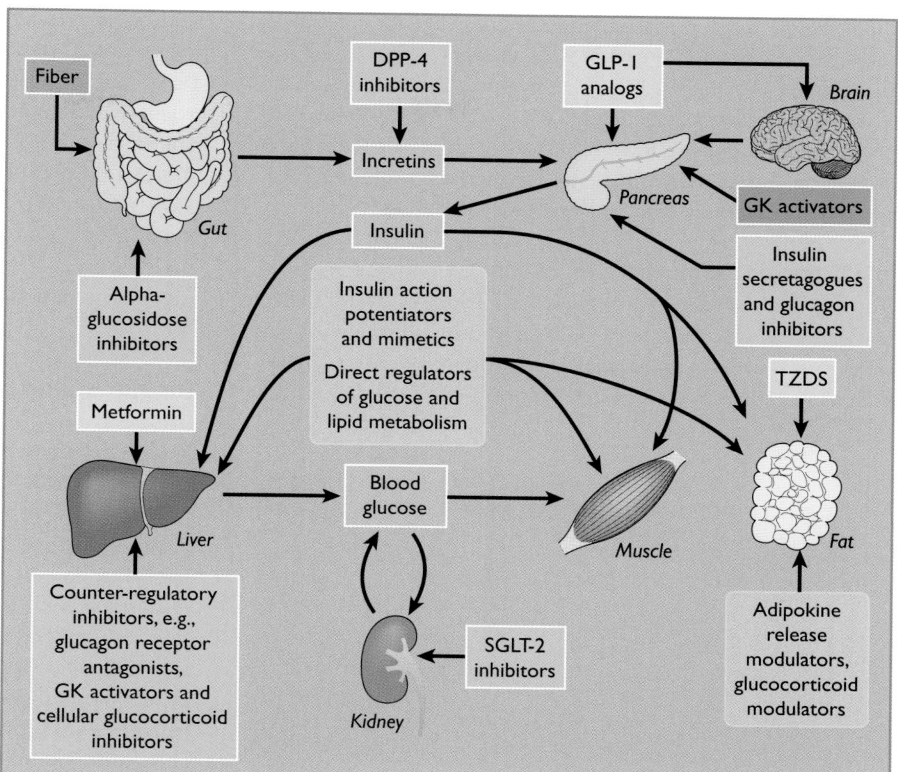

Figure 60.1 Potential sites of action of blood glucose-lowering agents. DPP-4, dipeptidyl peptidase 4; GK, glucokinase; GLP-1, glucagon-like peptide 1; SGLT-2, sodium-glucose co-transporter 2; TZD, thiazolidinedione.

Table 60.3 Examples of some new or investigational blood glucose-lowering agents.

Type of agent	Action	Example
α-glucosidase inhibitors	Inhibit carbohydrate digestion	Voglibose
Insulin secretagogues	Stimulate insulin secretion	Mitiglinide
Insulin secretion potentiators	Enhance nutrient-stimulated insulin secretion	GLP-1 analogs, DPP-4 inhibitors
Insulin mimetics	Insulin-like effects on glucose metabolism	IGF-I
Insulin action potentiators	Enhance actions of insulin	Selective PPAR modulators
Counter-regulatory hormone inhibitors	Suppress secretion/action of counter-regulatory hormones	Glucagon receptor antagonists, cellular glucocorticoid inhibitors
Direct glucose regulators	Increase glucose metabolism	GK activators, F16Pase inhibitors
Lipid regulators	Inhibit oxidation of fatty acids	CPT-1 inhibitors
SGLT2 inhibitors	Increase renal glucose elimination	"Flozins"

CPT-1, carnitine palmitoyl transferase-1; DPP-4, dipeptidyl peptidase 4; F16Pase, fructose 1,6-bisphosphatase; GK, glucokinase; GLP-1, glucagon-like peptide-1; IGF-I, insulin-like growth factor I; PPAR, peroxisome proliferator-activated receptor; SGLT2, secondary active sodium glucose co-transporter 2.

Table 60.4 Soluble and insoluble fiber supplements.

Soluble fiber	Insoluble fiber
Gums	Celluloses
Pectins	Wheat bran
Hemicelluloses	
Mucilages	

including insulin. Extending the period of digestion in this way can also reduce interprandial hypoglycemia in insulin-treated patients. Included here are dietary fiber supplements and inhibitors of digestive enzymes (Table 60.4).

Dietary fiber supplements

Most dietary fiber comprises plant polysaccharides that are not digested or fermented in the large bowel; some are soluble and form bulky viscous gels and gums, while others are coarse and insoluble (Table 60.4). Soluble fiber appears to be more effective than insoluble in reducing post-prandial hyperglycemia and hyperinsulinemia. Fibers can act as a barrier to diffusion within the lumen of the small intestine, where complex starchy carbohydrates are digested. Carbohydrates become entrapped within the matrix, impeding access of digestive enzymes, and restricting the diffusion of liberated saccharides across the unstirred layers of gut contents to the intestinal epithelium [12]. Various fiber supplements have appeared intermittently on the pharmacy shelves. These include common food thickeners such as soluble guar gum (E412), a galactomannan from the Indian cluster bean (*Cyamopsis tetragonoloba*; Figure 60.2) and fruit pectins. The prandial blood glucose-lowering effect of these supplements is usually small, especially if patients are already consuming a balanced diet containing fruit and vegetables [13].

Inhibitors of carbohydrate digestion

Slowing the digestion of complex carbohydrates by inhibiting amylases and glucosidases can reduce post-prandial hyperglycemia, particularly in individuals consuming a high starch diet such as rice (Figure 60.3). Inhibitors of α-amylases impair the hydrolysis of starch, but such agents have been too unpredictable for routine therapeutic use. Reversible competitive inhibitors of brush-border α-glucosidases such as acarbose, miglitol and voglibose are more predictable (Figure 60.4). These still require appropriate titration against the amount of complex carbohydrate in the diet to prevent undigested sugars from entering the large bowel, where bacterial fermentation can produce carbon dioxide and osmotically active glucose, causing flatulence and diarrhea as side effects [14]. There do not appear to be new α-glucosidase inhibitors in clinical development.

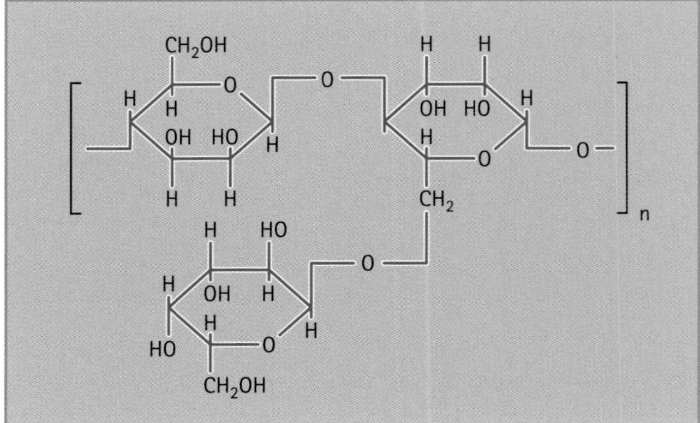

Figure 60.2 Guar, a galactomannan polysaccharide from the Indian cluster bean, *Cyamopsis tetragonoloba*, used as a dietary fiber supplement.

Insulin secretagogues

Several defects in islet β-cell function occur early in the pathogenesis of T2DM: the acute first-phase insulin secretory response to glucose becomes reduced and eventually lost, processing of proinsulin to insulin is impaired, the normal pulsatile rhythm of basal insulin secretion is disturbed, and the second phase of insulin secretion is often extended, albeit diminished in magnitude, as the period of post-prandial hyperglycemia is prolonged (see Chapter 10). In advanced stages of T2DM, β-cell mass and insulin biosynthesis are also compromised. An ideal insulin secretagogue would restore β-cell sensitivity to glucose, and support adequate biosynthesis, processing and secretion of insulin in response to other nutrients, hormones and neural factors. Insulin secretagogues can be categorized into initiators (e.g. sulfonylureas), which stimulate insulin secretion on their own or require only low glucose concentrations, and potentiators (e.g. GLP-1 analogs), which enhance the effect of rising glucose and other secretagogues but do not induce insulin release without glucose.

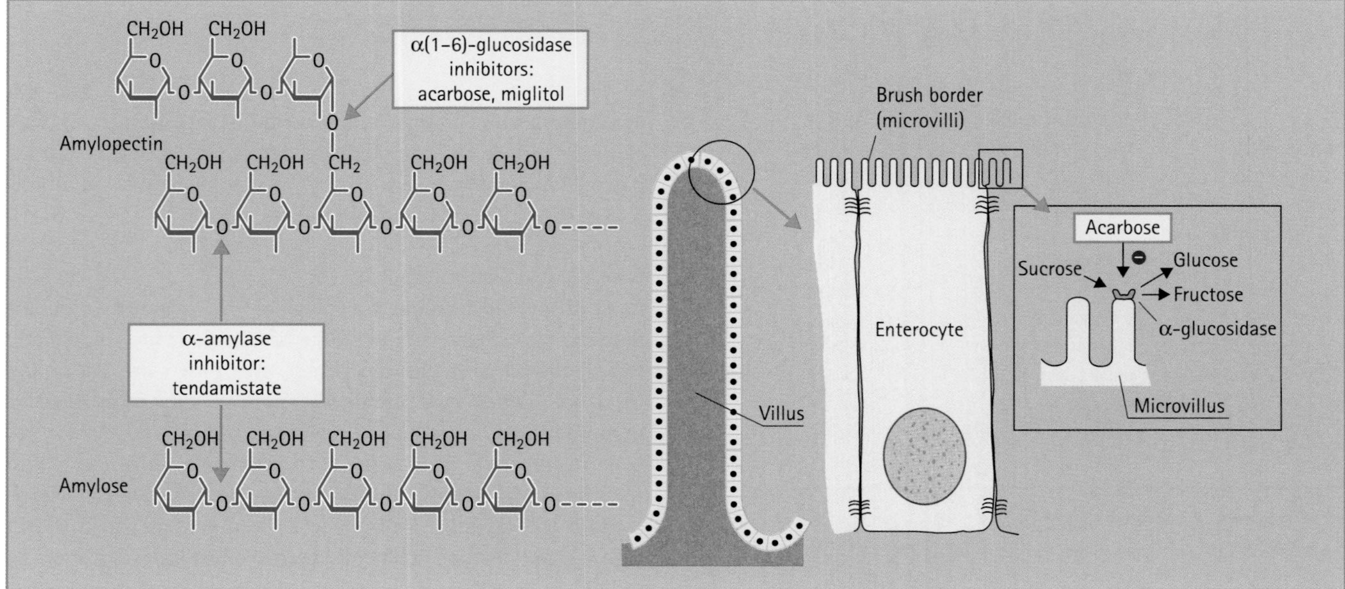

Figure 60.3 Starch digestion and its inhibitors. α(1–6)-glucosidic linkages are cleaved by α(1–6) glucosidases, and α(1–4) linkages by α-amylase. α-Glucosidase inhibitors such as acarbose act by competitive, reversible inhibition of intestinal brush-border α-glucosidase enzymes. This slows the rate of carbohydrate digestion.

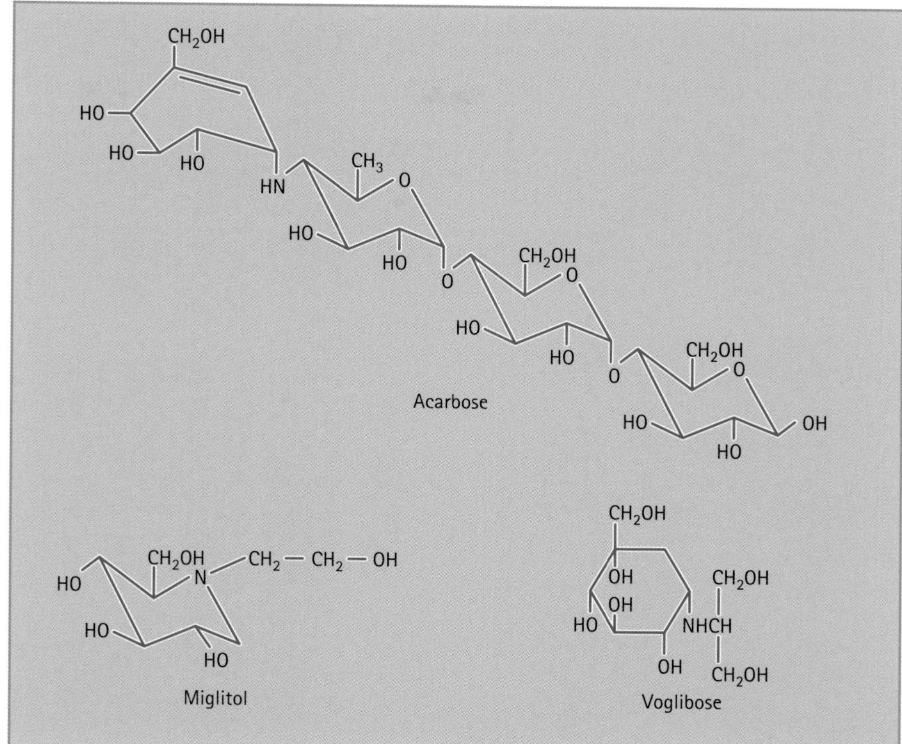

Figure 60.4 α-Glucosidase inhibitors in present use are acarbose and miglitol. Voglibose is available in some countries. These agents have different affinities for specific α-glucosidases: the binding affinity of acarbose is glucoamylase > sucrase > maltase > dextrinase; miglitol and voglibose potently inhibit sucrase, while voglibose shows more potent inhibition of other α-glucosidases than acarbose. Acarbose also weakly inhibits α-amylase.

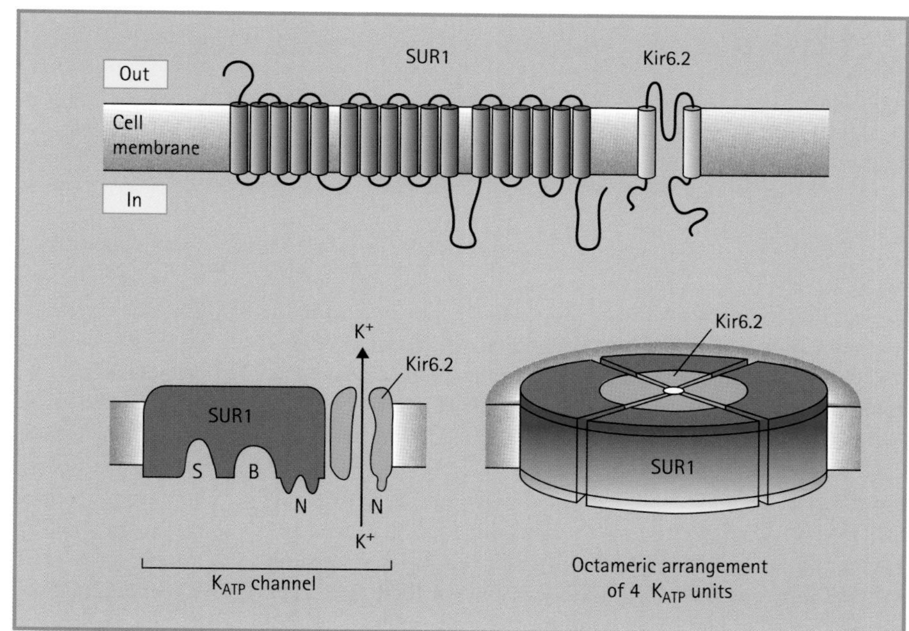

Figure 60.5 The ATP-sensitive (K_{ATP}) channel in the β-cell membrane consists of a large sulfonylurea 1 (SUR1) subunit (17 transmembrane domains) and a smaller pore-forming unit that acts as an inwardly rectifying K channel, Kir6.2. The cytosolic surface of the SUR1 subunit has separate binding sites for sulfonylureas (S), benzamido compounds (B) and the nucleotides, ADP and ATP (N). Four complete channel units self-associate to form an octameric complex in the membrane.

Initiators of insulin secretion

Currently available sulfonylureas and meglitinides are oral insulin secretagogues that initiate insulin secretion (see Chapter 29). They bind to either the sulfonylurea site or the benzamide site (meglitinides) on the sulfonylurea receptor 1 (SUR1) in the plasma membrane of the β-cell. The SUR1 is part of the ATP-sensitive potassium channel (K_{ATP} channel), which consists of an octameric complex of four Kir6.2 pores (inwardly rectifying potassium channels) surrounded by four SUR1 molecules (Figure 60.5). Binding of ligands to the sulfonylurea or benzamide sites

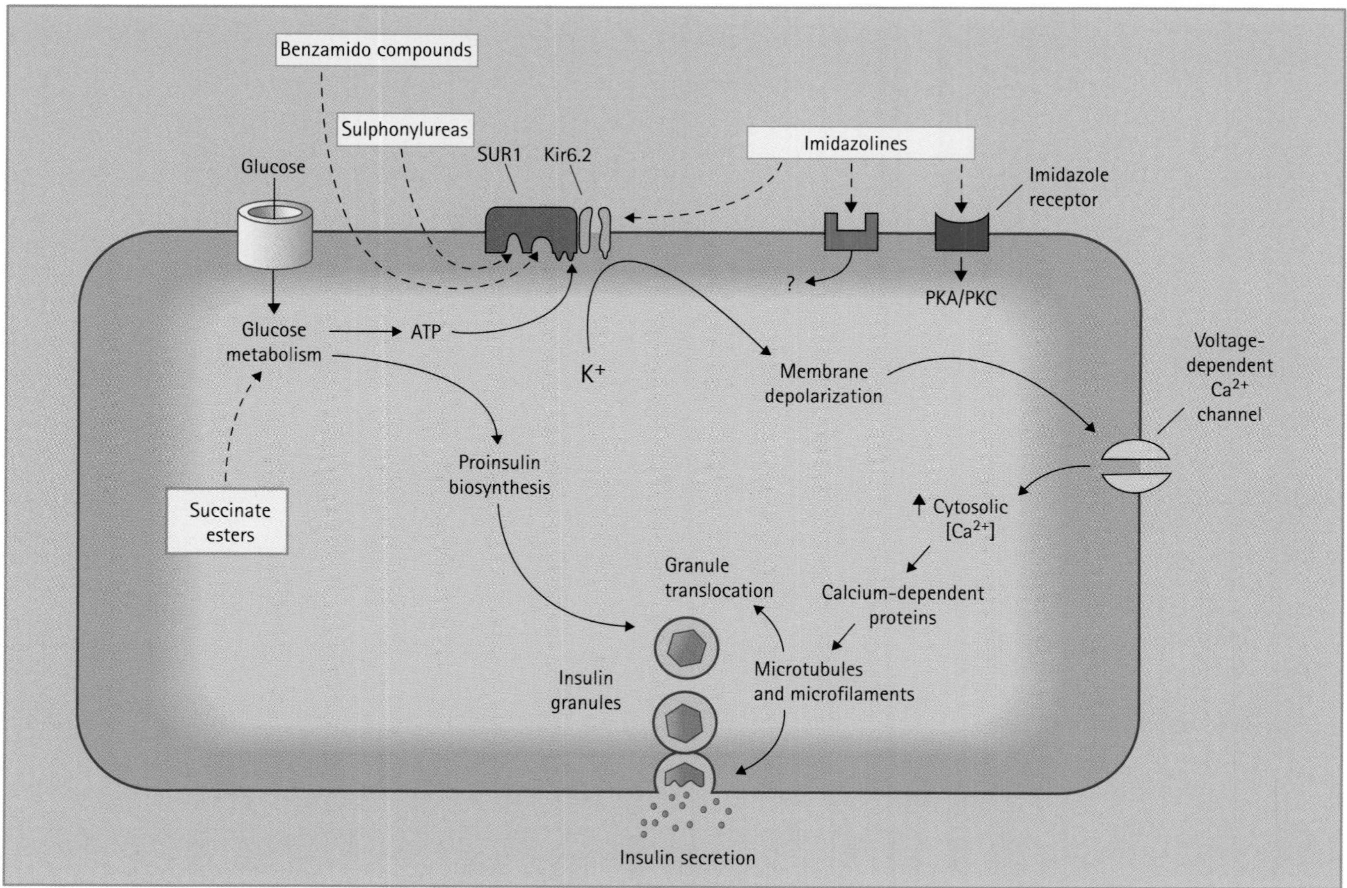

Figure 60.6 Sulfonylureas and benzamido compounds stimulate insulin release mainly by binding to sites on the sulfonylurea receptor 1 (SUR1) of the adenosine triphosphate (ATP)-sensitive potassium channels (K_{ATP} channels). This closes the Kir6.2 pores of the K_{ATP} channels, causing localized depolarization, opening of voltage-dependent calcium channels, increasing Ca^{2+} influx, and activation of calcium-dependent proteins that promote exocytosis of insulin granules. Imidazoline derivatives can act on I_1 and I_2 receptors, as well as other (unclassified) receptors and directly on the Kir6.2 pores to enhance insulin secretion. Succinate esters fuel glucose metabolism.

on SUR1 elicits the same response as binding of ATP to the nucleotide-binding domains of the channel, namely closure of the Kir6.2 pore [15]. This prevents K^+ efflux, which leads to localized depolarization of the plasma membrane. In turn, this opens voltage-gated (L-type) calcium channels, allowing influx of Ca^{2+} ions, which increases the cytosolic calcium ion concentration. Calcium-sensitive proteins are thereby activated, triggering the exocytosis of insulin-containing secretory granules (Figure 60.6). SUR1–Kir6.2 channels have also been identified within the membranes of mitochondria and possibly other organelles, suggesting that sulfonylureas and meglitinides could act at these and other sites in the cell as part of their insulin-releasing action.

Several novel insulin secretagogues have been reported to act by closing the K_{ATP} channels. The meglitinide derivative mitiglinide (KAD-1229) appears to bind at the benzamide site on SUR1 (Figure 60.6), and this agent has proceeded in clinical development [16]. Several other types of compounds have been shown to interact with K_{ATP} channels, but these do not appear to have proceeded beyond early clinical studies (Figure 60.7). These include the morpholinoguanidine BTS67582 [17] and certain imidazolines such as S22068 [18]. Other imidazoline compounds, which bind to I_1, I_2 and probably other receptors, may also close K_{ATP} channels as part of their mechanisms to stimulate insulin secretion [19]; however, there are imidazolines such as BL11282 that stimulate glucose-induced (but not basal) insulin secretion by effects on protein kinases without closing K_{ATP} channels [20]. Various α_2-adrenergic receptor antagonists such as phentolamine, which can reduce the tonic suppression of insulin secretion mediated through α_2-adrenergic activation, may also act to close K_{ATP} channels.

Although closure of K_{ATP} channels initiates insulin secretion, it does not promote insulin biosynthesis. Agents that increase nutrient metabolism, and close K_{ATP} channels through increased ATP production, additionally enhance proinsulin biosynthesis. This capability is illustrated by esters of succinic acid which provide a metabolisable substrate to the mitochondria [21]. These compounds have low enteral bioavailability and a short duration of action, and they also fuel gluconeogenesis in the liver. A related approach could be to stimulate mitochondrial succinyl-

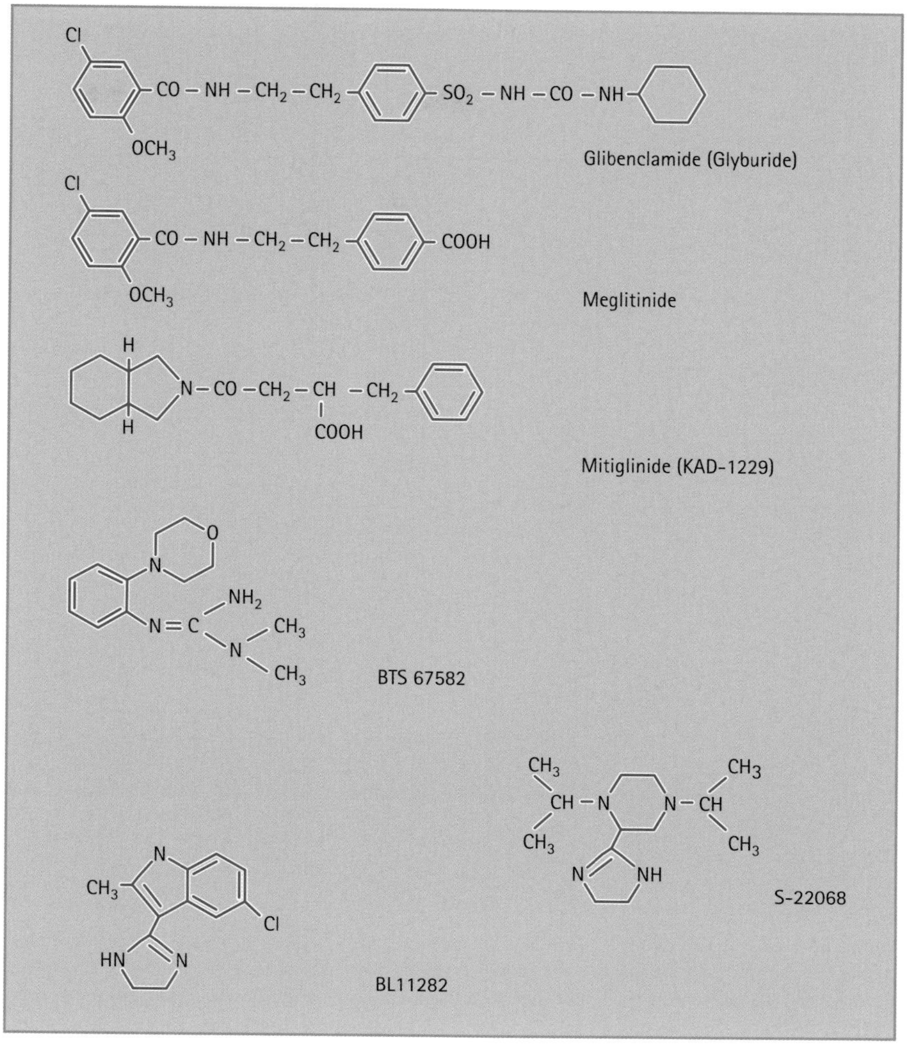

Figure 60.7 Structures of some established and novel insulin secretagogues. Glibenclamide (glyburide) has both a sulfonylurea and a benzamide moiety. Meglitinide derivatives exhibit a benzamide moiety. BTS 67582 is a morpholinoguanidine, while S-22068 and BL11282 are examples of imidazoline compounds.

coenzyme A (CoA) synthetase to generate ATP and guanosine triphosphate (GTP) [22].

Because the islet β-cell takes up glucose approximately in proportion to the circulating glucose concentration and phosphorylates the glucose via glucokinase (GK; EC 2.7.1.1), the β-cell is amenable to stimulation of glycolysis with agents that enhance the activity of GK [23]. Although this effect is actually potentiating the action of glucose (Figure 60.8), it can operate at low glucose concentrations, so it has been categorized here as an initiator. Several specific small molecule activators of GK have been shown to increase insulin secretion and improve glucose homeostasis in models of T2DM. These include allosteric activators and molecules that prevent association of GK with or cause dissociation of GK from inhibitory protein complexes [24–29]. Several of these agents are now in clinical trial, and it will be interesting to see if this approach can benefit other aspects of islet function and be regulated to avoid hypoglycemia. Because liver cells express GK and take up glucose approximately in proportion to the circulating concentration, GK activators will also stimulate hepatic glucose utilization and reduce hepatic glucose production, adding to their blood glucose-lowering potency.

Potentiators of insulin secretion

Potential opportunities to increase nutrient-induced insulin secretion are shown in Figure 60.8. In principle, these agents should predominantly decrease post-prandial hyperglycemia and carry less risk of interprandial hypoglycemia.

Incretins

Insulin secretion is enhanced by several hormones released from the gut during feeding – so-called incretin hormones. The main incretins are glucagon-like peptide 1 (7–36) amide (GLP-1) and gastric inhibitory polypeptide (GIP; also known as glucose-dependent insulinotropic peptide). These hormones activate specific G-protein coupled receptors in the β-cell membrane and potentiate nutrient-induced insulin secretion and insulin biosyn-

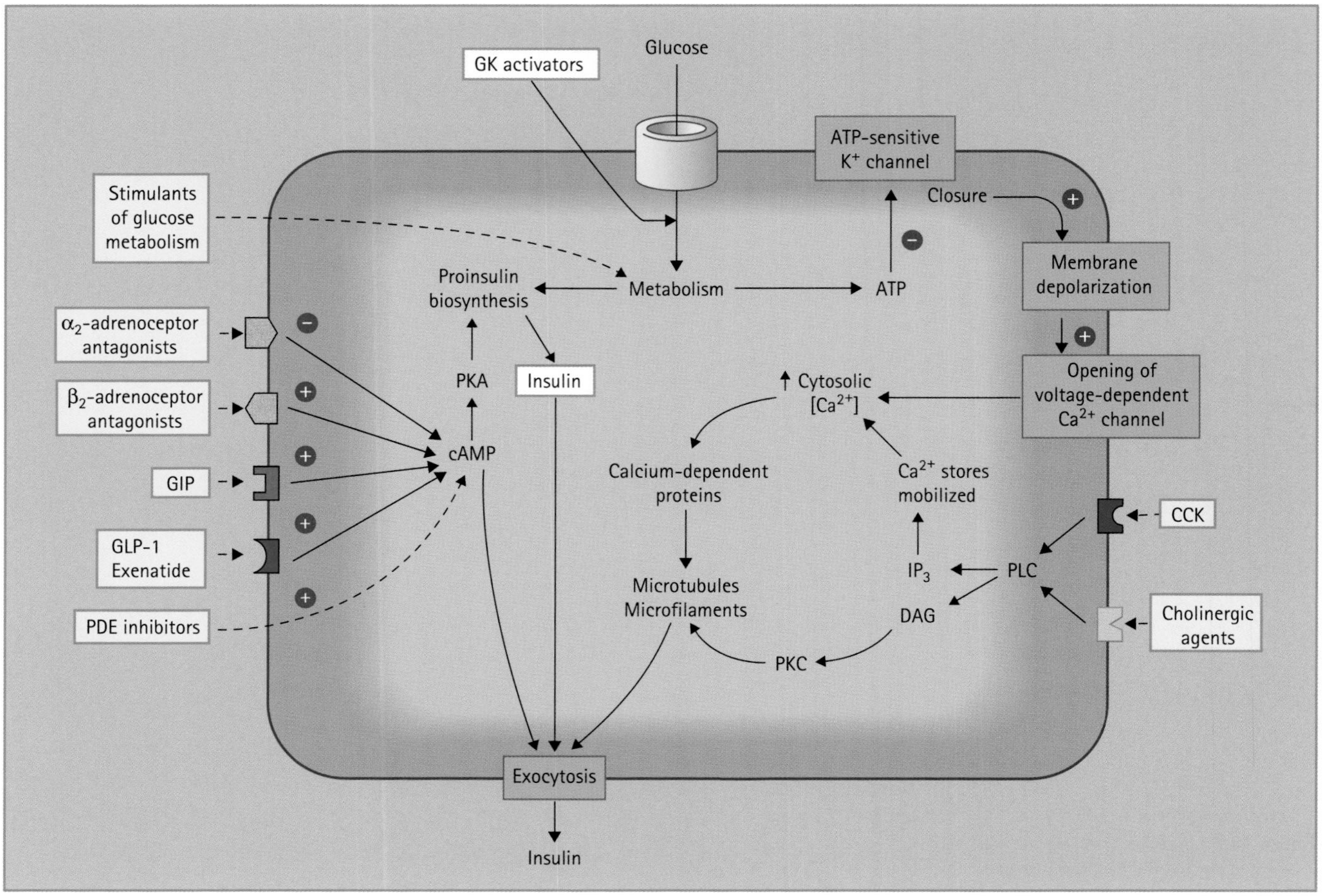

Figure 60.8 Sites on the pancreatic β-cell that offer potential targets to potentiate nutrient-induced insulin secretion. cAMP, cyclic adenosine monophosphate; CCK, cholecystokinin; DAG, diacylglycerol; GIP, gastric inhibitory polypeptide, also known as glucose-dependent insulinotropic peptide; GK, glucokinase; IP_3, inositol-1,4,5-trisphosphate; PDE, phosphodiesterase; PKA, protein kinase A; PKC, protein kinase C; PLC, phospholipase C. Activated β_2-adrenoceptors and GIP and glucagon-like peptide-1 (GLP-1) receptors stimulate insulin secretion, as do antagonists of the inhibitory α_2-adrenoceptors.

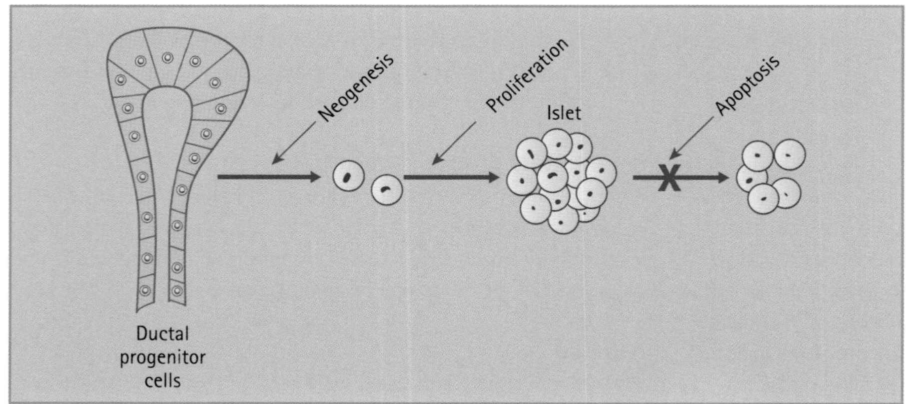

Figure 60.9 Incretin hormones GLP-1 and GIP have been shown to increase β-cell mass in animal models. Possible mechanisms include increased β-cell proliferation and differentiation, slowing of β-cell apoptosis and increased β-cell neogenesis from ductal progenitor cells.

thesis, at least partly through increased cyclic adenosine monophosphate (cAMP) and production of protein kinase A (PKA) [30,31]. Both hormones have also been shown to promote β-cell mass in animal models, possibly slowing β-cell apoptosis and increasing β-cell neogenesis by increased expression of the transcription factor PDX-1 (pancreatic duodenal homeobox 1), which promotes proliferation and differentiation of ductal progenitor cells (Figure 60.9). GLP-1 has been favored as a treatment for T2DM because it also suppresses glucagon secretion in a glucose-dependent manner, slows gastric empting and exerts a satiety effect that can facilitate weight loss [32]. Moreover, GLP-1 concentrations appear to be reduced in T2DM but the ability of the peptide to enhance insulin release is maintained (Table 60.5). Thus, when injected subcutaneously immediately before a meal, GLP-1 can substantially reduce the post-prandial rise in blood glucose concentrations in T2DM (Figure 60.10). However, the rapid degradation of GLP-1, mostly by the enzyme dipeptidyl peptidase 4 (DPP-4) and the renal clearance of GLP-1 (plasma half-life < 2 minutes) makes the peptide itself an inconvenient form of therapy [33].

DPP-4 cleaves off an N-terminal dipeptide where there is an alanine residue (as in GLP-1) or a proline residue at the N2 position. Exenatide (exendin-4) is a GLP-1 analog with a glycine residue at the N2 position (Figure 60.11), making it resistant to degradation by DPP-4, and extending the half-life to several

Table 60.5 Effects of the incretin hormones glucagon-like peptide 1 (7–36) amide (GLP-1) and gastric inhibitory polypeptide (GIP; also known as glucose-dependent insulinotropic peptide).

	GIP	GLP-1
Pancreatic		
Glucose-induced insulin secretion	Increase	Increase
Proinsulin biosynthesis	Increase	Increase
β-Cell mass (rodents)	Increase	Increase
Glucagon secretion	Increase or no effect	Decrease
Other actions		
Gastric emptying	No/slight effect	Decrease
Appetite/feeding	No significant effect	Decrease
Weight gain	No effect or increase	Decrease
Myocardial metabolism	No established effect	Possible benefits
Type 2 diabetes		
Plasma concentrations	Normal or slightly reduced	Reduced late phase
Insulin-releasing effect	Reduced	Mostly retained

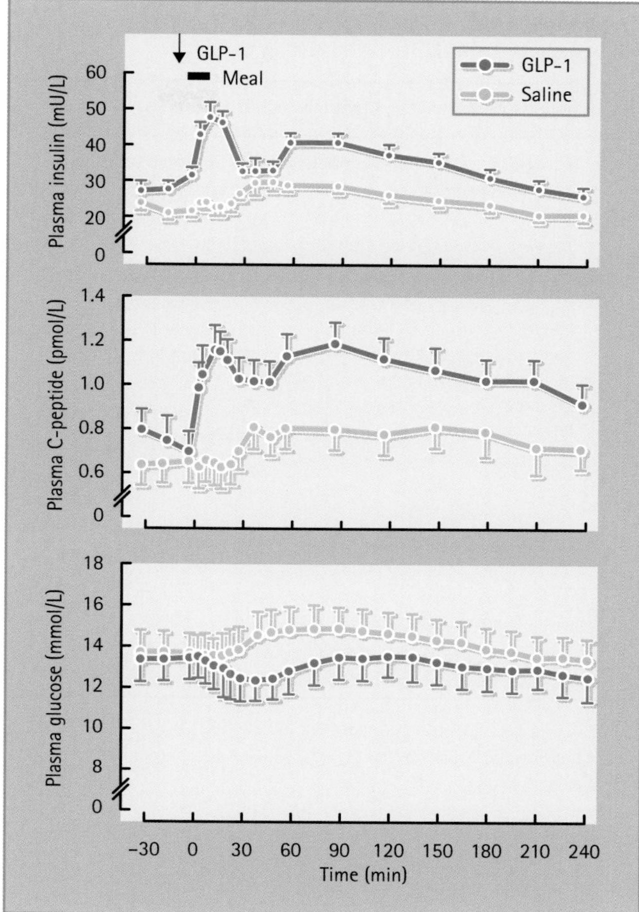

Figure 60.10 Insulin-releasing and glucose-lowering effects of glucagon-like peptide 1 (GLP-1) in eight obese patients with T2DM. A dose of 25 mmol was injected subcutaneously into the gluteal region 5 minutes before a standard meal. The plasma insulin and C-peptide responses were significantly greater, and the plasma glucose response significantly flatter (all $P < 0.001$), compared with a control (saline) injection. Reproduced from Glutniak *et al. Diabetes Care* 1994; 17:1039–1044, with permission from the American Diabetes Association.

```
                   DPP4
Native GLP-1        ↓
 Human GLP-1       HAEGT FTSDV SSYLE GQAAK FFIAW LVKGR G    (7-37)
 Human GLP-1       HAEGT FTSDV SSYLE GQAAK FFIAW LVKGR      (7-36 amide)

GLP-1 Analogs
 Exenatide         HGEGT FTSDL SKQME EEAVR LFIEW LKNGG PSSGA PPPSG
 Liraglutide       HAEGT FTSDV SSYLE GQAAK EFIAW LVRGR G
                                           |
                                       E-palmityl

Related peptides
 Human GIP         YAEGT FISDY SIAMD KIHQQ DFVNW LLAQK GKKND WKHNI TQ
 Human Glucagon    HSQGT FTSDY SKYLD SRRAQ DFVQW LMNT
```

Figure 60.11 The amino acid structure of GLP-1, and the GLP-1 analogs exenatide and liraglutide. GIP and glucagon are shown for comparison. DPP-4 cleaves off an N-terminal dipeptide where there is an alanine residue (as in GLP-1 and GIP) or a proline residue at the N2 position. Liraglutide is protected from degradation by DPP-4 when the palmitoyl fatty acid moiety binds to albumin.

Table 60.6 Peptide glucagon-like peptide 1 (GLP-1) agonists in clinical development.

Compound	Name	Company	Structure
NN2211	Liraglutide* (Victoza)	NovoNordisk	GLP-1 analog linked to palmitoyl fatty acid, t½ 12–13 hours (once daily, s.c.)
Exendin-4	Exenatide-LAR	Amylin/Lilly	Long-acting release exendin (once weekly, s.c.)
?	Albiglutide (Syncria)	GSK	Complex of dimeric GLP-1 bound to albumin (once weekly, s.c.)
LY548806	?	Lilly	DPP-4 resistant GLP-1 analog
LY315902	?	Lilly	GLP-1 analog linked to a fatty acid
BIM-51077, R1583	Taspoglutide	Ipsen/Roche	Long-acting GLP-1 analog (once weekly, s.c.)
CJC-1131	?	ConjuChem	GLP-1 analog linked to a chemical complex
ZP10A, AVE0010	Lixisenatide	Zealand/ Sanofi-Aventis	GLP-1 analog

Other GLP-1 preparations in development include GLP1-INT (GLP-1 analog; Transition Therap/NovoNordisk) and MKC253 (GLP-1-technospheres for inhalation, MannKind Corp).
* Liraglutide was launched in Europe in July 2009.

hours. Because exenatide retains the glucose-lowering efficacy of GLP-1 it has become established as an incretin therapy, injected subcutaneously twice daily before the main meals [34]. The glucose-dependent nature of the insulin-releasing and glucagon-suppressing effects is reflected in the limited risk of hypoglycemia, while the satiety effect has assisted weight loss and favored use in obese patients.

Among other GLP-1 analogs (Table 60.6), liraglutide (NN2211) recognized regulatory approval in Europe in July 2009. Liraglutide is GLP-1 (7-37) with Lys34 replaced by Arg34, and Lys26 attached via a glutamate residue to a C16 hexadecanoyl (palmitoyl) fatty acid chain. The fatty acid chain facilitates association into heptamers and attachment of the molecule to albumin, protecting it from degradation by DPP-4 and enabling once daily injection [35].

A once-weekly depot formulation of exenatide, new long-acting GLP-1 analogs, slow-release formulations and different administration routes (e.g. transdermal, buccal and inhaled) are receiving clinical assessment [32]. Hybrid peptides are also being explored to increase glucose-lowering efficacy, for example DAPD, a peptide that is a GLP-1 receptor agonist and a glucagon receptor antagonist [36]. To circumvent the need for injections, non-peptide GLP-1 receptor agonists (e.g. Boc5) have been identified. These bind to the GLP-1 receptor on islet β-cells and enhance glucose-dependent insulin secretion [37,38].

Although GIP potentiates nutrient-induced insulin secretion it also increases glucagon release and promotes lipid deposition [39]. Moreover, GIP receptor knockout (KO) mice and the administration of GIP receptor antagonists (both peptide and non-peptide) have been shown to prevent the development of obesity, improve glucose homeostasis and reduce insulin resistance in animal models [40–44]. This is consistent with evidence from bariatric surgery: a reduced supply of nutrients through the proximal small intestine (location of GIP-secreting K-cells) rapidly improves glycemic control in obese patients with diabetes [45]. Thus, GIP antagonism by pharmacologic means or "metabolic surgery" may provide a new antidiabetic mechanism [46].

DPP-4 inhibitors

Inhibiting the enzyme DPP-4 (EC 3.4.14.5) prevents the rapid inactivation of the endogenous incretins GLP-1 and GIP, thereby raising their circulating concentrations and increasing nutrient-stimulated insulin release and other effects of these incretins (Table 60.5). DPP-4 is found "loose" in the circulation and tethered to cell membranes, especially endothelia in capillaries of the gastrointestinal tract, a location that facilitates the degradation of incretins. The protease activity of DPP-4 degrades a range of biologically active peptides in addition to incretins, including substance P, bradykinin, peptide YY, neuropeptide Y, pituitary adenylate cyclase-activating peptide, insulin-like growth factor I (IGF-I) and various interleukins and monocyte chemo-attractant proteins [33,47]. Despite affecting this wide range of peptides, to date, specific DPP-4 inhibitors have not shown significant adverse effects during substantial clinical use [32]. Also, DPP-4 is the lymphocyte cell surface protein CD26 required for the co-stimulation response to recall antigens, but its immunologic role does not appear to be interrupted by small molecule inhibitors of its peptidase activity.

Currently available DPP-4 inhibitors (gliptins) include sitagliptin, vildagliptin and saxagliptin (see Chapter 30). These agents improve glycemic control similarly to GLP-1 analogs but there are subtle differences that may partly reflect the concomitantly increased GIP, and the likelihood that raised endogenous incretin concentrations will not achieve the high concentrations of exogenously administered GLP-1 analogs. In consequence, DPP-4 inhibitors are unlikely to cause initial nausea through delayed gastric emptying, and they may exert a lesser satiety effect resulting in little change of body weight. Among the DPP-4 inhibitors in clinical development (Table 60.7), trials with alogliptin are well advanced (Figure 60.12). These agents have shown high specificity for DPP-4 inhibition, and preliminary information indicates that therapeutic concentrations cause almost complete inhibition of DPP-4 activity for about 12 hours, producing similar glucose-lowering efficacy to existing gliptins [32].

Phosphodiesterase inhibitors and other approaches

The β-cell expresses several phosphodiesterases (PDEs) that degrade cAMP and so reduce insulin release. Selective and

Table 60.7 DPP-4 inhibitors recently available and in clinical development.

Compound	Name	Company	Clinical phase	Specificity data (nmol)
MK-0431	Sitagliptin* (Januvia)	MSD	Marketed 2007	$IC_{50} = 18$ $K_i = 9$
LAF237	Vildagliptin (Galvus)	Novartis	Marketed 2008	$IC_{50} = 3.5$ $K_i = 17$
BMS-477118	Saxagliptin (Onglyza)	BMS/AZ	Marketed 2009	$IC_{50} = 26$ $K_i = <1$
SYR-322	Alogliptin	Takeda	3	?
R1438	An aminomethylpyridine	Roche	2	$K_i = 0.1$
P32/98	Isoleucine thiazolidide	Probiodrug	2	$K_i = 80$

AZ, AstraZeneca; BMS, Bristol Myers Squibb; MSD, Merck Sharp Dohme; ?, not reported.
Other compounds under consideration include PSN9301 (Prosidion), GR-8200 (Glenmark), PHX-1149 (Phenomix), SSR-162369 (Sanofi-Aventis), ALS 2-0426 (Alantos/Amgen), and NN-7201 (NovoNordisk).
* Launched in Mexico in 2006, and in USA, UK and several other European countries in 2007.

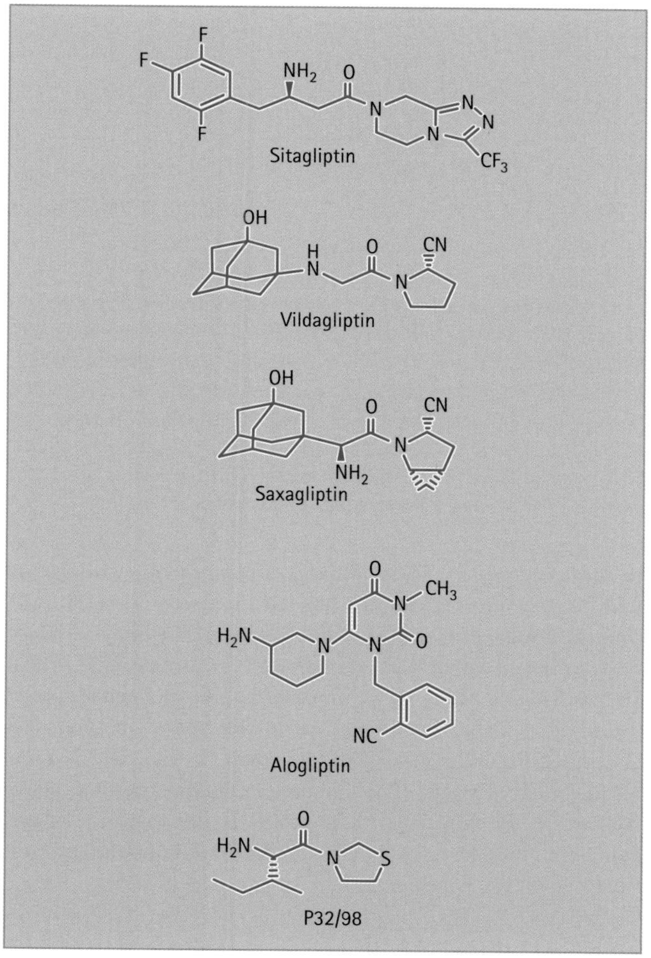

Figure 60.12 Structures of the DPP-4 inhibitors sitagliptin, vildagliptin, saxagliptin, alogliptin and P32/98.

transient inhibition of these enzymes in β-cells, especially isoform PDE-3B, which exerts most influence on glucose-induced insulin secretion, could be a possible intervention [48], but the problem of specifically targeting the β-cells has yet to be overcome. Other theoretical approaches to potentiate insulin secretion (Figure 60.8), such as antagonism of α_2-adrenoceptors and activators of phospholipase C (PLC), have not been possible to target specifically at the β-cell.

Insulin-mimetic drugs

Insulin resistance (impaired insulin action) is a typical feature of T2DM, but it is highly heterogeneous, initially progressive (excepting some monogenic forms), and susceptible to many different genetic and environmental factors [49,50]. Most patients with T2DM probably incur multiple defects that impinge on insulin receptor function and/or various post-receptor signaling pathways, as well as independent disturbances in the activities of substrate transporters and metabolic enzymes consequent to glucotoxicity and lipotoxicity [51]. Indeed, insulin has important genomic effects that determine the expression levels of many cellular components that are directly and indirectly involved in metabolic homeostasis. Defects of insulin receptor structure are uncommon, and reductions in insulin receptor number are not usually rate limiting. Thus, the therapeutic challenge of insulin resistance appears to require interventions at diverse intracellular targets [52].

In theory, agents that address defects of insulin receptor signaling or early post-receptor lesions might be expected to produce a broader spectrum of benefits, but if the rate-limiting defects occur at more distal locations their therapeutic efficacy will be compromised. Potential target sites to obviate cellular defects of insulin action are shown in Figure 60.13.

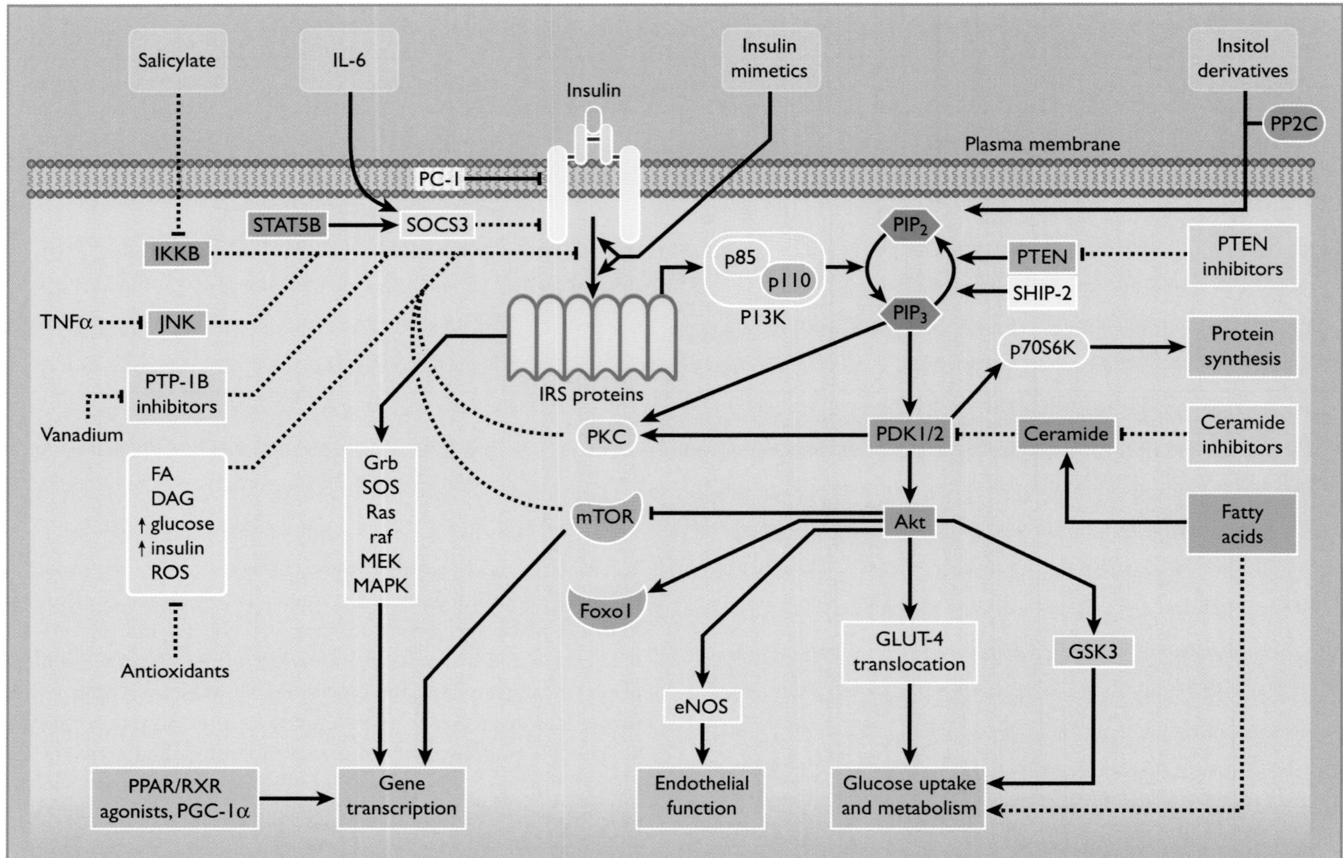

Figure 60.13 Pathways of intracellular insulin signaling showing some of the potential sites for therapeutic intervention. Adapted from Bailey [52]. Akt, protein kinase B (PKB); AMPK, adenosine monophosphate-activated protein kinase; DAG, diacylglycerol; eNOS, endothelial nitric oxide synthase; FA, fatty acid; FOXO1, forkhead box protein O1A; GLUT-4, glucose transporter 4; Grb, growth factor receptor binding protein; GSK3, glycogen synthase kinase 3; IKKB, inhibitor κ-B kinase-β; IL-6, interleukin 6; IRS, insulin receptor substrate; JNK, c-Jun N-terminal kinase; MAPK, mitogen-activated protein kinase; MEK, mitogen-activated protein kinase kinase; mTOR, mammalian target of rapamycin; PC-1/NNP1, glycoprotein-1; PDK, phosphoinositide-dependent protein kinase; PGC-1α, PPAR coactivator 1α; PI3K, phosphatidylinositol 3-kinase; PIP2, phosphatidylinositol-3,4-bisphosphate; PIP3, phosphatidylinositol-3,4,5-trisphosphate; PKC, protein kinase C; PPAR, peroxisome proliferator-activated receptor; PP2C, pyruvate dehydrogenase phosphatase (protein phosphatase 2C); PTEN, protein phosphatase PTEN; PTP-1B, protein tyrosine phosphatase-1B; Raf, a serine-threonine protein kinase; Ras, a guanosine triphosphatase; ROS, reactive oxygen species; RXR, retinoid X receptor; SHIP-2, src homology-2-inositol phosphatase; SOCS-3, suppressor of cytokine signaling-3; SOS, sons of sevenless; STAT, signal transducer and activator of transcription; TNF-α, tumour necrosis factor α; ↑, increase; →, stimulatory effect; ⊣, inhibitory effect.

Insulin receptor activation

Evidence that an orally active, non-peptide molecule can mimic the gluco-regulatory actions of insulin was obtained with L-783,281 (demethylasterriquinone; Figure 60.14), a metabolite from cultures of a *Pseudomassaria* fungus [53]. L-783,281 initiated phosphorylation and tyrosine kinase activity of the β-subunit of the human insulin receptor expressed in Chinese hamster ovary (CHO) cells [54]. This induced tyrosine phosphorylation and activation of insulin receptor substrate 1 (IRS1), increased activity of phosphatidylinositol 3-kinase (PI3K) and increased phosphorylation of Akt (protein kinase B). Studies with mutated subunits of the insulin receptor showed that L-783,281 interacted selectively with the β-subunit (without requiring insulin to bind to the α-subunit), and its activity could not be attributed to inhibition of protein tyrosine phosphatases. Low (3–6) μmol/L concentrations of L-783,281 elicited about 50% of the maximum tyrosine kinase activity (TKA) generated by insulin in CHO cells, and initiated a range of insulin-like effects in normal tissues including increased glucose uptake by isolated rodent adipocytes and skeletal muscle [53]. Oral administration of L-783,281 (5–25 mg/kg/day) lowered blood glucose in insulin-resistant obese-diabetic *db/db* mice providing proof of therapeutic concept, although other features of this particular compound are not suited to clinical development.

Insulin-like growth factor I

IGF-I can weakly mimic the effects of insulin through low affinity binding to the insulin receptor [55]. Cross-talk between the IGF-I

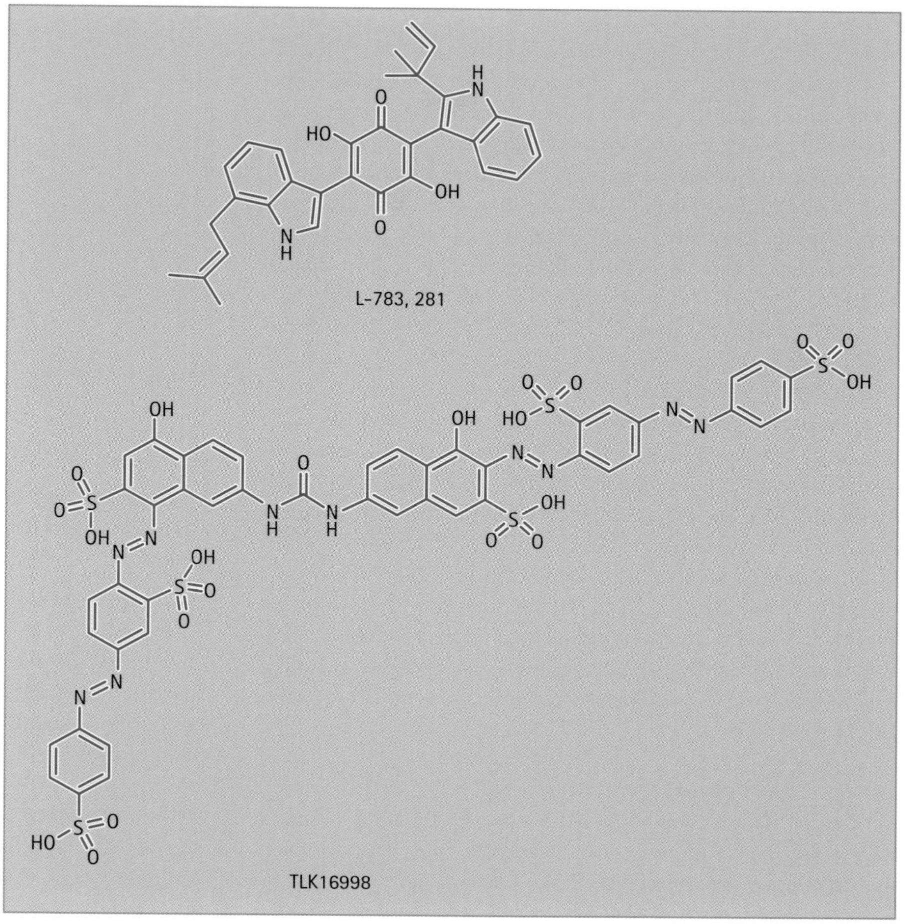

Figure 60.14 Structures of compounds that improve insulin action by direct interaction with insulin receptors: L-783,281 and TLK16998.

receptor and early post-receptor components of the insulin-signaling cascades can ameliorate rare cases of severe insulin resistance caused by genetic defects of the insulin receptor. IGF-I can assist glycemic control in type 1 diabetes mellitus (T1DM) and T2DM, but such therapy is generally discounted by potential proliferative effects and other unwanted side effects of IGF-I. Circulating IGF-I is mostly bound to IGF binding proteins, especially IGFBP-3, and the side effects probably reflect an increase in unbound IGF-I after injection. To address this, mixtures of recombinant human IGF-I and recombinant human IGFBP-3 have been employed [56].

Insulin receptor potentiation

Insulin receptor signaling after initial activation by insulin binding at the α-subunit can be enhanced and/or prolonged by several different mechanisms (Figure 60.13). For example, a non-peptide molecule TLK16998 (Figure 60.14) that does not interact with the insulin receptor α-subunit increased insulin-induced phosphorylation of the insulin receptor β-subunit [54,57]. TLK16998 also potentiated β-subunit phosphorylation initiated by L-783,281. In cultured mouse 3T3-L1 adipocytes, low μmol/L concentrations of TLK16998 increased insulin-induced phosphorylation of IRS-1 and PI3K, increased translocation of GLUT-4 glucose transporters into the plasma membrane and increased glucose uptake during submaximal stimulation by insulin. TLK16998 (30 mg/kg by intraperitoneal injection) also lowered glucose concentrations in insulin resistant obese-diabetic *db/db* mice [57].

C peptide

Insulin C-peptide, which is secreted from pancreatic β-cells along with insulin, appears to bind to G-protein coupled receptors in several insulin-sensitive tissues. In cultured L6 muscle cells, physiologic concentrations of C-peptide (0.3–3.0 nmol/L) increase glycogen synthesis during submaximal (but not maximal) stimulation with insulin, accompanied by increased insulin receptor tyrosine kinase activity and phosphorylation of IRS1 [58]. Activation of PI3K, mitogen activated protein kinase (MAPK) and glycogen synthase kinase 3 (GSK3) was also noted, suggesting that the ability of C-peptide to potentiate insulin receptor signaling might modestly be exploitable as a possible approach to improve insulin action in C-peptide deficient states.

Protein tyrosine phosphatase 1B

Several protein tyrosine phosphatases (PTPs), most notably PTP1B, dephosphorylate the insulin receptor β-subunit, terminating insulin-induced receptor TKA [59]. These phosphatases also dephosphorylate and deactivate IRS1 and IRS2. The therapeutic potential of inhibiting PTP1B has been demonstrated by PTP-1B KO mice which are highly sensitive to insulin [60]. These mice also show an increased metabolic rate and resistance to diet-induced obesity. Antisense oligonucleotides against PTP1B increased insulin sensitivity in *ob/ob* mice, associated with increased phosphorylation of the insulin receptor, IRS1/2 and GSK3, and increased activity of PI3K and Akt [61]. Selective inhibitors of PTP-1B, including certain benzonaphthofurans, thiophenes and acylsulfonamido compounds, improved glycemic control in insulin-resistant diabetic animals and have been considered as templates for potential new therapies [62–64]. PTP-1B inhibitors could also assist weight control by increasing the satiety effect of leptin, because hypothalamic PTP1B normally reduces leptin receptor signaling [65]. Inhibition of PTP1B might also improve endothelial function by improving insulin-induced endothelial nitric oxide synthase (eNOS) production [66]. Vanadium salts inhibit protein tyrosine phosphatases including PTP1B, and have been shown to enhance the actions of insulin and possibly leptin.

Other insulin receptor potentiators

Various substances that increase the number of insulin receptors and/or appear to improve insulin receptor function have been mooted as possible therapeutic leads but have not given rise to new therapeutic entities. These include N-terminal fragments of human growth hormone (GH) and mosapride, a benzamide derivative that activates serotonin 5HT-4 receptors and promotes gastrointestinal motility [52,67].

Insulin receptor and early post-receptor potentiation

The divergent pathways of post-receptor insulin signaling contain many potential rate-limiting steps for insulin action. Most of these pathways are not specific to insulin and impact activities as disparate as cell differentiation and apoptosis. They also include a controlling influence exerted through the feedback of more distal signaling components on more proximal steps [50,51].

Protein kinase C

The IRS–PI3K route of insulin signaling (Figure 60.13) increases the formation of phosphatidylinositol-3,4,5 trisphosphate (PIP3) and phosphoinositide-dependent kinases PDK1/2. These signaling intermediates activate some isoforms of protein kinase C (PKC), which exert a negative feedback on insulin receptor and probably early post-receptor phosphorylation steps [68,69]. Inhibition of specific isoforms of PKC provides a potential means to improve insulin action, although appropriately selective inhibitors have proved difficult. The PKC-β inhibitor LY333531 (ruboxistaurin; Figure 60.15) is in clinical trial as a potential treatment for diabetic retinal and glomerular microvascular disease [70]. Excess fatty acids, diacylglycerol and chronic hyperglycemia also appear to reduce early insulin signaling via activation of PKC isoforms.

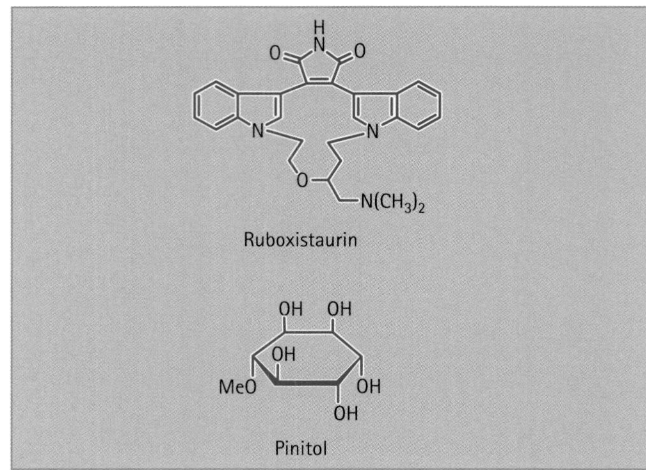

Figure 60.15 Structure of the PKC-β inhibitor LY333531 (ruboxistaurin), the inositol derivative 3-methoxy analog of D-*chiro*-inositol (pinitol).

Other signaling feedbacks

Serine phosphorylation of the insulin receptor β-subunit and IRS proteins, which inhibits their signaling activity, is brought about by several serine kinases such as inhibitor kappa-B kinase-β (IKKβ) and c-Jun N-terminal kinase (JNK; Figure 60.13). These kinases contribute to the insulin resistance produced by the cytokine tumor necrosis factor α (TNF-α) [71,72]. The potential opportunity to prevent these routes of insulin resistance is indicated by the ability of salicylates, which inhibit IKKβ, and a cell-permeable inhibitor of JNK to relieve insulin resistance in part [73,74].

The insulin signaling intermediate Akt appears to participate in a negative feedback effect on the signaling pathway. Akt activates the mammalian target of rapamycin (mTOR) which promotes phosphorylation of serine residues on IRS proteins [75]. The membrane ectoenzyme glycoprotein-1 (PC-1/NNP1) binds to the insulin receptor and prevents the conformational changes required for receptor autophosphorylation [76]. These interactions present potential sites for therapeutic intervention.

Potentiation of phosphatidylinositol-3 kinase

PI3K promotes phosphorylation of phosphatidylinositol 4,5-bisphosphate (PIP2) to the 3,4,5-trisphosphate (PIP3). This step is often reduced in insulin-resistant states [77], but direct targeting of PI3K is difficult because the regulatory (p85) subunit suppresses the catalytic (p110) subunit [78]; however, increasing the availability of precursor inositol substrates and prevention of product breakdown might offer therapeutic mechanisms.

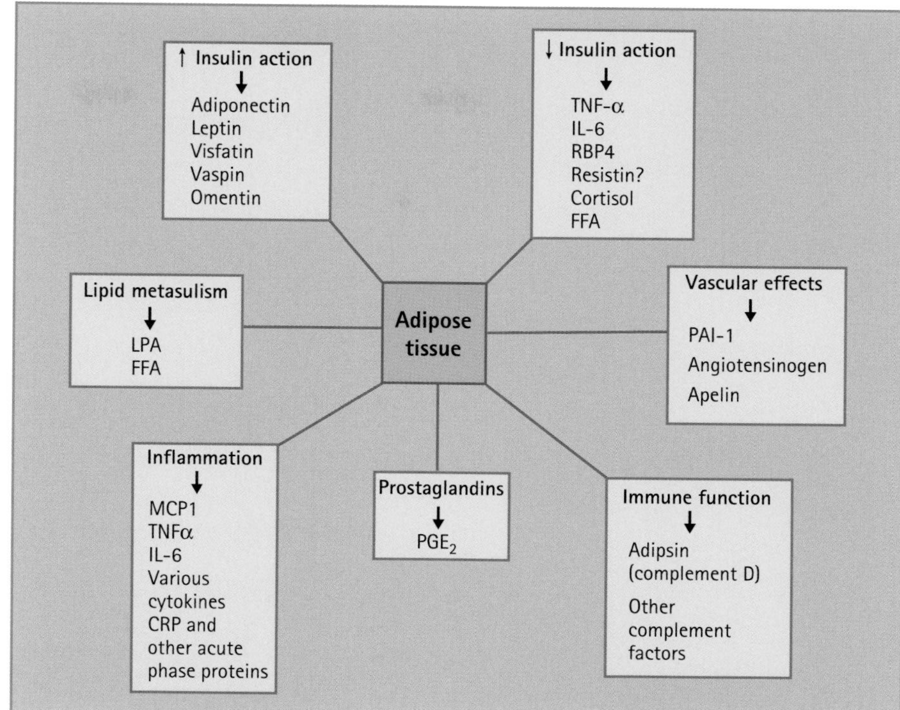

Figure 60.16 Examples of the autocrine, paracrine and endocrine products of adipose tissue that influence insulin action, metabolic control and vascular, inflammatory and immune processes that could impinge on diabetic control. CRP, C-reactive protein; FFA, free fatty acid; IL-6, interleukin 6; LPL, lipoprotein lipase; MCP1, monocyte chemoattractant protein 1; PAI-1, plasminogen activator inhibitor 1; PGE_2, prostaglandin E2; RBP4, retinol-binding protein 4: TNF-α, tumor necrosis factor α.

Inositol derivatives

Inositol derivatives such as D-*chiro*-inositol (INS-1) and the 3-methoxy analog of D-*chiro*-inositol (pinitol; Figure 60.15) improve muscle glucose uptake and reduce hyperglycemia in diabetic animal models and patients with T2DM [79,80]. D-*chiro*-inositol-galactosamine (INS-2) also increased insulin action in diabetic rats, possibly involving direct activation of pyruvate dehydrogenase phosphatase (protein phosphatase 2C [PP2C]) [81].

PTEN and other inositol phosphatases

Preventing the dephosphorylation of PIP3 has been identified as a possible approach to improve insulin action (Figure 60.13). The phosphatase PTEN, which dephosphorylates PIP3, can be inhibited by an antisense oligonucleotide: when administered (ip, once weekly) to *db/db* and *ob/ob* mice, the oligonucleotide increased signaling downstream of PIP3, improved insulin sensitivity and improved glycemic control [82]. Also, an adipose tissue specific PTEN knockout mouse was lean and insulin sensitive with high energy expenditure and increased biogenesis of adipocyte mitochondria [83]; however, substantial disruption of PTEN carries a risk of tumor formation [84]. PIP3 is 5′-dephosphorylated to form phosphatidylinositol 3,4-bisphosphate by the SH2-inositol phosphatases (SHIP-1 and SHIP-2). Partial disruption of the SHIP-2 gene in mice improves insulin sensitivity [85], suggesting another potential target to enhance the effectiveness of PI3K.

Adipokines

Adipose tissue is a source of many autocrine, paracrine and endocrine factors that affect insulin action (Figure 60.16), and obesity is a well-recognized risk factor for insulin resistance and T2DM [86,87]. Thus, some of these factors have been assessed as potential therapeutic targets.

Proinflammatory cytokines

Proinflammatory cytokines produced by adipose tissue, notably TNF-α and interleukin 6 (IL-6), contribute to insulin resistance. They activate or induce JNK, IKKβ and the suppressor of cytokine signaling-3 (SOCS-3), each of which can disrupt TKA of the β-subunit of the insulin receptor (Figure 60.13); however, preliminary evaluation of a TNF-α antibody in patients with T2DM showed little effect on insulin sensitivity, and the risk of susceptibility to infection has called this approach into question [52].

Adipocyte hormones

Leptin

Leptin is an adipocyte hormone that exerts centrally mediated satiety and thermogenic effects, as well as direct effects on cellular nutrient metabolism. Administration of large doses of leptin can produce weight loss and improve insulin action, but the development of leptin resistance and leptin antibodies has compromised long-term efficacy [88]. Leptin analogs and non-peptide receptor agonists remain under consideration.

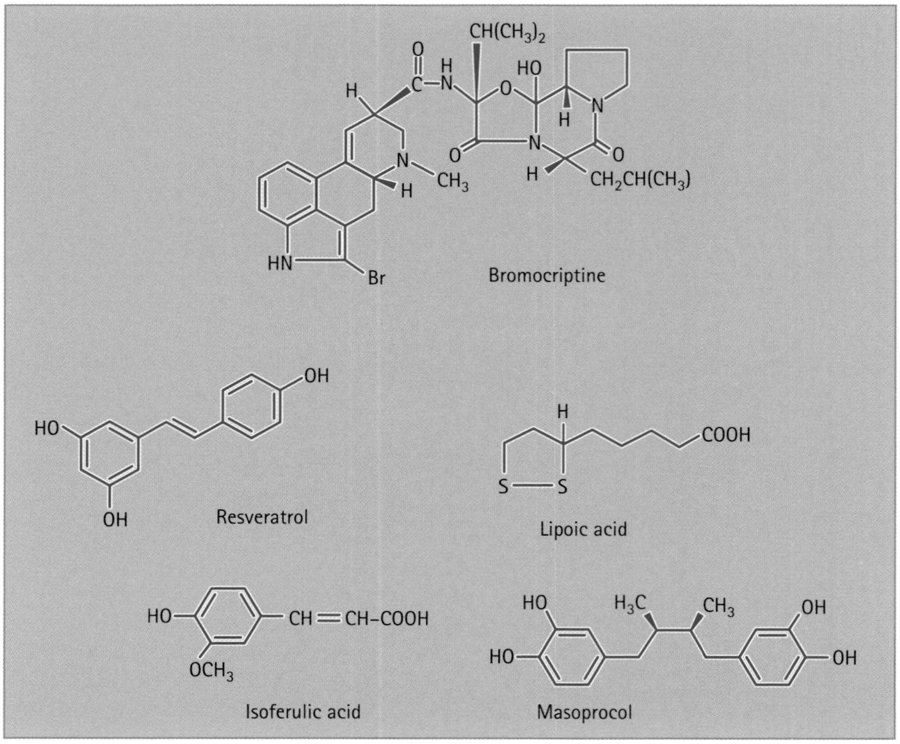

Figure 60.17 Structures of some compounds that potentiate insulin action: bromocriptine, lipoic acid, isoferulic acid, masoprocol and resveratrol.

Resistin

Resistin (FIZZ3), an adipocyte hormone, reduces insulin sensitivity in obese rodents, and immuno-neutralization of resistin improved insulin sensitivity; however, resistin is expressed at low levels by human adipocytes, and may be involved in inflammatory processes, limiting its potential as a therapeutic target [89].

Adiponectin

Adiponectin (Acrp30), produced exclusively and in large amounts by adipocytes, improves insulin sensitivity with increased insulin receptor tyrosine phosphorylation and activation of adenosine monophosphate-activated protein kinase (AMPK) [90]. It also has anti-inflammatory activity and improves vascular reactivity. Adiponectin concentrations become reduced as adipose mass increases, and therapeutic approaches to raise adiponectin levels, develop analogs and non-peptide receptor agonists are under investigation. Part of the insulin-sensitizing effect of thiazolidinediones may reflect increased adiponectin production.

Visfatin

Visfatin (PBEF), mainly from visceral adipocytes, was initially reported to activate insulin receptors. Subsequently, however, no correlation was observed between plasma visfatin concentrations and insulin sensitivity in human subjects [91].

Retinol-binding protein

Retinol-binding protein 4 (RBP4) is one of several retinoid-binding proteins produced by adipocytes and liver that transports retinoids in plasma. Increased RBP4 has been noted in insulin resistant states, while RBP4 gene knockout increases insulin sensitivity [92], suggesting that a reduction of RBP4 might be considered to reduce insulin resistance.

Vaspin

Vaspin (visceral adipose tissue-derived serpin) is an adipocyte serine protease inhibitor which improved insulin sensitivity and glucose homeostasis in obese insulin-resistant rodents, and might therefore offer a therapeutic lead [93].

Omentin

Omentin, a peptide from visceral adipose tissue, increased insulin-stimulated glucose uptake by adipocytes [94], and might indicate a potential therapeutic approach.

Other potentiators of insulin action

Bromocriptine

The dopamine D2 receptor agonist bromocriptine (Figure 60.17), used in the treatment of Parkinson disease, galactorrhea and prolactinomas, has long been known to improve insulin sensitivity and glycemic control in T2DM [95,96]. Bromocriptine as monotherapy or an adjunct to other antidiabetic agents for up to 1 year has reduced HbA_{1c} by 0.5–1.2% (5–13 mmol/mol), lowered triglyceride and non-esterified fatty acid concentrations, reduced some cardiovascular events, not caused serious hypoglycemia, and facilitated weight loss. However, side effects including nausea, hypotension and psychiatric symptoms should be appreciated. Bromocriptine has recently received marketing authorization to treat diabetes in the USA.

Lipoic acid, isoferulic acid and angiotensin-converting enzyme inhibitors

The antioxidant α-lipoic acid (Figure 60.17), used in some countries to treat diabetic neuropathy, increases insulin sensitivity and improves glycemic control, probably brought about in part by its action as a co-factor for dehydrogenases involved in glycolysis and the Krebs cycle. Additionally, α-lipoic acid increases insulin receptor TKA and IRS1 tyrosine phosphorylation, with increased signaling via PI3K and increased GLUT-4 translocation into the plasma membrane [11]. Isoferulic acid increases expression of GLUT-4 and decreases gluconeogenesis by reducing phosphoenolpyruvate carboxykinase (PEPCK) [11].

Modest improvements of insulin sensitivity have been recorded during treatment with angiotensin-converting enzyme (ACE) inhibitors, possibly because of improved hemodynamics resulting from increased bradykinin. ACE is one of the circulating enzymes that normally degrades bradykinin. ACE inhibitors may also help to counter the effects of insulin resistance by reducing inflammation and increasing vascular reactivity [97].

Plant-derived compounds

Plant extracts and herbal preparations remain commonplace as treatments for diabetes, especially in low and middle income countries, and plant-derived compounds have provided templates for the synthesis of potential antidiabetic agents [98]. For example, the herbal use of *Bougainvillaea spectabilis* led to studies on the antidiabetic action of pinitol [79], and the traditional use creosote bush (*Larrea tridentate*) prompted studies on the glucose-lowering effect of masoprocol [99].

Many current pharmaceuticals have their origins in traditional herbal medicines, and phytochemical approaches continue to attract interest. Recent attention has been given to resveratrol (Figure 60.17), a phytophenol (3,4,5 trihydroxystilbene) found in many plants, especially red grape skins [100]. It appears to offer cardioprotective properties, improving the lipid profile, increasing eNOS-dependent vasorelaxation and exerting antioxidant and anti-inflammatory effects. Resveratrol and related phytophenols may improve insulin action and prevent diet-induced obesity by increasing mitochondrial biogenesis through activation of the sirtuin SIRT1 and by increased activity of the PPAR co-activator PGC-1α [101].

Anti-obesity agents

Appetite control, reduced and delayed nutrient absorption and weight loss are well appreciated to reduce insulin resistance and hyperglycemia in the overweight and obese T2DM. Several centrally acting appetite-suppressing and satiety-inducing anti-obesity agents also exert peripheral effects that improve some actions of insulin and assist glycemic control in overweight patients.

Sibutramine

Sibutramine, which is a serotonin-noradrenaline reuptake inhibitor that induces satiety, acts in part through the primary amine metabolite M2. This metabolite increases glucose uptake by muscle tissue independently of weight loss after treatment *in vivo* [102]. Sibutramine was withdrawn in Europe in January 2010.

Rimonabant

Rimonabant (SR141716), an endocannabinoid receptor-1 (CB1) antagonist that suppresses appetite, was recently withdrawn because of neural side effects soon after introduction in some countries as an anti-obesity agent. In overweight and obese diabetic individuals rimonabant induced a greater reduction in HbA_{1c} than expected for the extent of weight loss, possibly explained in part by increased adiponectin production [103].

β_3-Adrenoceptor agonists

β_3-Adrenoceptor agonists act on β_3-adrenoceptors, expressed mainly by brown and white adipose tissue, to assist weight loss by stimulating lipolysis and thermogenesis. Several selective agonists were developed for rodents, but minor differences in the structure of the human form of the receptor rendered these agents relatively ineffective in humans. Various β_3-adrenoceptor agonists have been shown to stimulate insulin release, improve insulin-mediated glucose disposal and improve glycemic control in obese diabetic rodents, but adequate efficacy and a very high level of selectivity have yet to be demonstrated in humans.

Peroxisome proliferator-activated receptor γ agonists

Current thiazolidinediones (pioglitazone and rosiglitazone) exert their "insulin-sensitizing" effects largely by stimulating the peroxisome proliferator-activated receptor γ (PPARγ; Figure 60.18). Stimulation of this nuclear receptor increases transcription of a selection of insulin-sensitive genes and other genes (Table 60.8; see Chapter 29): these collectively increase adipogenesis, enhance insulin sensitivity, improve glycemic control and exert anti-inflammatory and vascular effects [104,105]. Additional thiazolidinediones that stimulate PPARγ continue in development (e.g. rivoglitazone), and non-thazolidinedione PPARγ agonists have been reported (Figure 60.19) [105]. The latter might alter conformation of the PPARγ binding epitope or other regions of the receptor such that different coactivators are recruited, affecting the selection of genes transcribed and the profile of biologic effects. Thus, non-thazolidinedione PPARγ agonists that partially modulate PPARγ, such as halofenate/metaglidasen and FK614, do not activate exactly the same set of genes as a full PPARγ agonist [106]. Through selective modulation of PPARγ binding it should be possible to retain desired therapeutic effects and reduce undesirable side effects [105]. A similar outcome might be achieved by stimulating genes for selected co-activators of PPARγ such as PGC-1α [107].

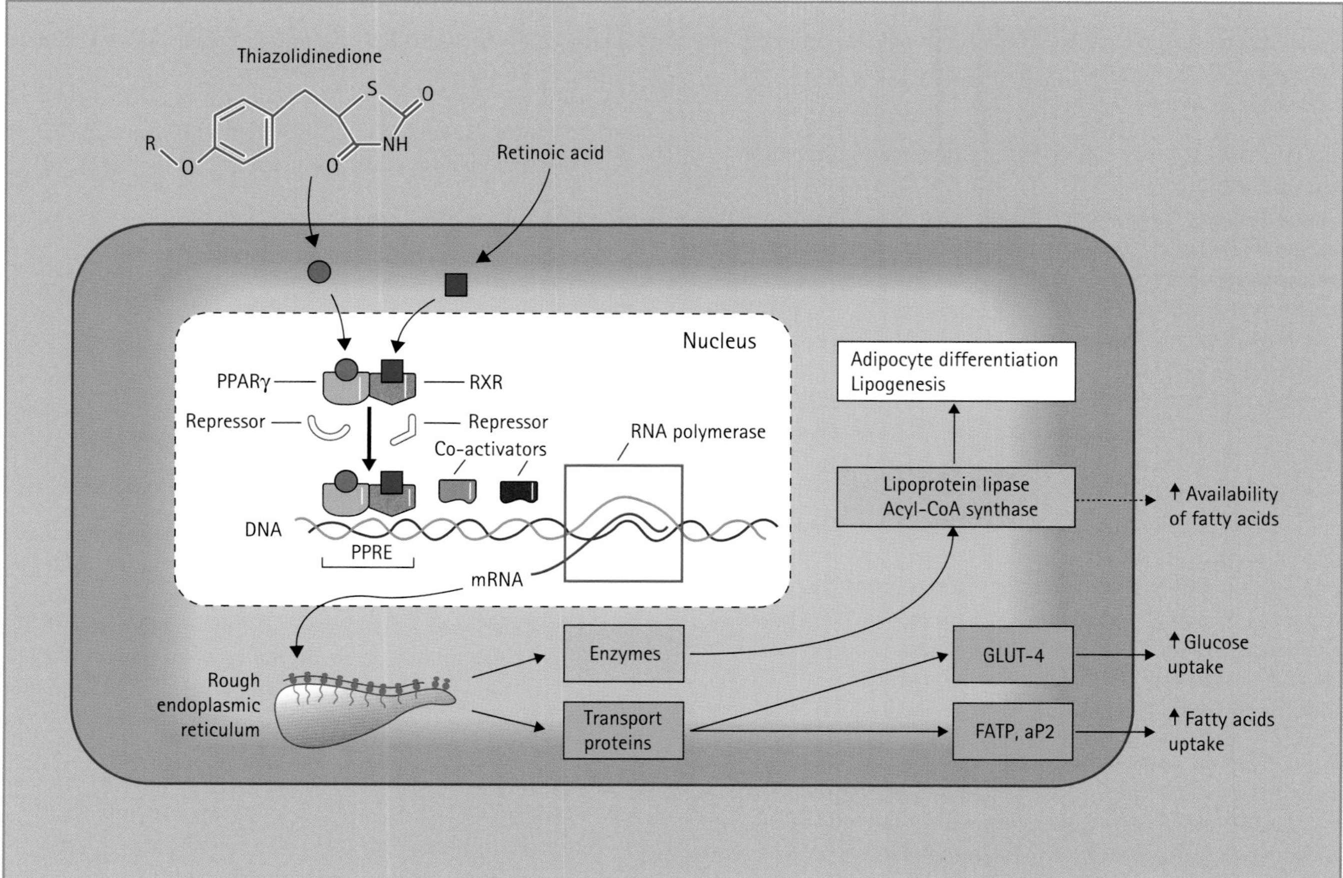

Figure 60.18 Mechanism of action of a thiazolidinedione in an adipocyte. Thiazolidinediones are peroxisome proliferator-activated receptor γ (PPARγ) agonists. They bind to the nuclear PPARγ receptor, which forms a heterodimer with the retinoid X receptor (RXR). Ligand binding releases repressors, attracts co-activators and exposes the active site of the receptors which binds with a specific DNA nucleotide sequence (AGGTCAXAGGTCA) termed the peroxisome proliferator response element (PPRE). RNA polymerase is recruited and transcription of mRNA takes place for genes that carry the PPRE sequence in a promoter region. The mRNA is translated into the enzymes and transporters that bring about the biologic effects of thiazolidinediones in the cell. These include the fatty acid transporter protein (FATP), adipocyte fatty acid binding protein (aP2), acyl-CoA synthase, lipoprotein lipase and glucose transporter 4 (GLUT 4). Stimulation of PPARγ also activates genes encoding proteins with anti-inflammatory and vascular effects.

Other peroxisome proliferator-activated receptor agonists

To take advantage of the blood lipid-lowering and anti-inflammatory effects of low affinity binding to PPARα various thiazolidinediones and non-thiazolidinedione molecules have been described with binding affinities for both PPARγ and PPARα – so-called dual PPARα/γ agonists (glitazars) [105]. The two glitazars most advanced in development (muraglitazar, tesaglitazar) were discontinued because of side effects [108].

Genetic overexpression or selective stimulation of PPARδ (e.g. with GW501516 and L-165041) improves insulin sensitivity, increases fatty acid oxidation, raises thermogenesis and prevents weight gain [109]. Thus, a selective PPARδ agonist or an agent with desired levels of selectivity for PPARα, γ and δ (termed a panPPAR agonist or SPPARM – selective PPAR modulator) could offer therapeutic advantages [105]. Various selective modulators of RXR have been reported to reduce hyperglycemia in animal models, but these tend to have diverse effects including hypertriglyceridemia and interference with thyroid function. Because certain RXR agonists can reduce appetite, increase production of mitochondrial uncoupling proteins and decrease weight gain, combinations of these agents with PPARγ (PPARγ-RXR agonists) have received preclinical consideration [110].

Vitamins and minerals

Vitamins

The pathogenic effect of excess reactive oxygen species has become an accepted part of glucotoxicity, lipotoxicity and insulin resistance, and it is appreciated that anti-oxidant defenses are often depleted in diabetic states [111]. Whether supplementation of the anti-oxidant vitamins C (ascorbic acid), E (α-tocopherol) and β-carotene can measurably benefit insulin sensitivity and reduce cardiovascular risk remains in contention [112]. Adequate concentrations of vitamin D and vitamin D receptor function

Table 60.8 Stimulation of peroxisome proliferator-activated receptor γ increases transcription of a selection of insulin-sensitive and other genes affecting adipogenesis, insulin sensitivity, nutrient metabolism, anti-inflammatory and vascular reactions (so-called "pleitropic" effect).

Lipoprotein lipase (LPL)
Fatty acid transporter protein (FATP/CD36)
Adipocyte fatty acid binding protein (aP2)
Acyl-CoA synthetase (ACS)
Malic enzyme
Glycerol kinase (adipocytes ?)
PEPCK (adipocytes), ↑ perilipin
↑ GLUT-4 (derepression), ↑ GLUT-2
↓ Resistin, ↓ RBP4
↑ Adiponectin (↑ leptin, ↑ IRS2 ?)
↓ TNF-α
↓ CRP and some proinflammatory cytokines, ↓ NFκB, ↓ IFG-γ (T cells)
↓ PAI-1, ↓ MMP-9
↑ UCP1 (?)

↑ increase; ↓ decrease; ? unconfirmed.

CRP, C reactive protein; GLUT-4, glucose transporter 4; IFG-γ, interferon gamma; IRS, insulin receptor substrate; MMP-9, matrix metalloproteinase-9; NKκB, nuclear factor κB; PAI-1, plasminogen activator inhibitor-1; PEPCK, phosphoenolpyruvate carboxy kinase; RBP, retinal binding protein; TNF-α, tumor necrosis factor α; UCP1, uncoupling protein 1.

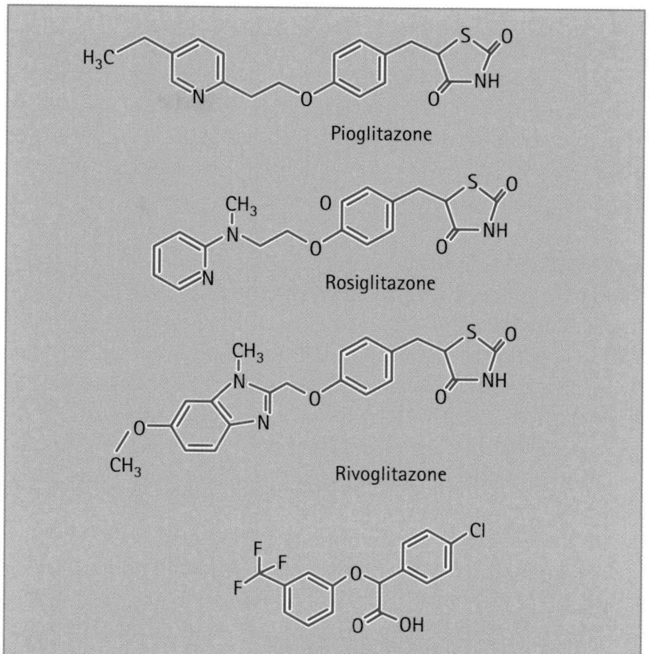

Figure 60.19 Structures of the thiazolidinediones pioglitazone, rosiglitazone, rivoglitazone and the non-thiazolidinedione partial PPARγ agonist metaglidasen.

appear to be necessary for normal insulin production and secretion, and may be required for normal insulin action. Diabetic patients are often deficient in circulating vitamin D_3 (cholecalciferol), and preliminary data suggest that vitamin D supplementation in deficient individuals might benefit glycemic control [113]. Thiamine (vitamin B_1) is a co-factor for pyruvate dehydrogenase and α-ketoglutarate dehydrogenase, and facilitates glucose metabolism, while large amounts of biotin (vitamin H) have been claimed to improve glycemic control and insulin sensitivity in T2DM [52,114]. When interpreting vitamin supplement studies it is pertinent to note that correcting a deficiency is more likely to offer benefit than adding excess in individuals with normal values.

Minerals

Reduced and deficiency levels of several minerals, particularly magnesium, chromium and zinc, are not uncommon amongst older patients with diabetes, and replacement supplements may improve glycemic control in such cases [115]. Supplementation of magnesium (necessary for phosphate transfer and kinase reactions) can enhance insulin action in hypomagnesemic patients [116], and trivalent chromium supplements often improve glycemic control without increasing insulin concentrations in chromium-deficient patients [117]. Insulin-like antidiabetic effects have been reported for zinc, lithium, selenium, molybdenum, tungsten, mercury and cadmium, but the therapeutic index is generally narrow and toxicity risks have limited clinical investigations [115]. Zinc (essential for insulin hexamer formation) appears to assist both the secretion and action of insulin, while molybdenum and tungsten salts act predominantly to decrease hepatic glucose output [13,59,115]. Improved insulin sensitivity with lithium may be offset by decreased insulin secretion resulting in variable effects on glycemic control in T2DM [115].

Vanadium salts have attracted considerable interest because modest vanadium supplements have improved glycemic control and reduced insulin requirements in diabetic animals and in patients with T1DM and T2DM [115,118]. Improved insulin sensitivity has been attributed at least in part to inhibition of protein tyrosine phosphatases, especially PTP-1B, and suppression of glucose 6-phosphatase. Additional effects to reduce appetite and reduce the rate of intestinal glucose absorption may also contribute to the antidiabetic effect of vanadium salts. To address issues of poor absorption and toxicity, low-dose peroxovanadiums, pervanadates and organic vanadium complexes have received attention [119], and an intermittent treatment schedule might be considered because the antidiabetic effects of vanadium salts can persist for weeks after treatment is stopped.

Counter-regulatory hormones

The major counter-regulatory hormones (glucagon, epinephrine, glucocorticoids and GH) raise blood glucose concentrations by increasing hepatic glycogenolysis and gluconeogenesis (see Chapter 13). As hepatic glucose production is inappropriately raised in diabetes, agents that interfere with the secretion or action of counter-regulatory hormones could potentially be therapeutically useful; however, those with highly potent or prolonged actions are undesirable, as they might impair the life-sustaining protection of the liver to produce glucose in response to severe hypoglycemia. Indeed, patients in advanced stages of T2DM often show delayed or deficient counter-regulatory responses to hypoglycemia.

Glucagon antagonists

The concept of reducing hyperglycemia by suppressing glucagon action is illustrated by the use of glucagon antibodies [120], and various peptide antagonists of the glucagon receptor have been described, mostly based on deletion of His1 and replacement of Asp9 with Glu [121]. There are also hybrid peptides that show glucagon receptor antagonism and GLP-1 receptor agonism [36]. Many small molecule glucagon receptor antagonists have been reported. An isopropylfluorobiphenyl (Bay 27–9955) that competitively blocked glucagon binding to its receptor has not proceeded in development [122], but other potent inhibitors such as Cpd1, NNC 25-0926 and MB09975N are being investigated [123,124]. An alternative approach has been to uncouple the glucagon receptor from activation of adenylate cyclase (e.g. with skyrin, a fungal bisanthroquinone) [125]. Inhibitors of glucagon secretion (e.g. MB39890A and somatostatin analogs) have been developed, but have not been sufficiently selective [121]. Thus, the somatostatin analog octreotide (Figure 60.20), suppresses glucagon secretion and delays intestinal glucose absorption as well as preventing GH secretion, but it also inhibits insulin secretion, rendering it unhelpful in T2DM, but potentially useful for glycemic control with insulin in patients with T1DM [121].

Glucocorticoid antagonists

Raised glucocorticoid concentrations can precipitate and aggravate truncal obesity, insulin resistance and hyperglycemia, while maneuvers to reduce glucocorticoid action can prevent and reverse these effects. To avoid lowering overall glucocorticoid production, and to minimize disturbances to the hypothalamic-pituitary-adrenal system, tissue specific inhibition of glucocorticoid action has been investigated. Some inhibitors of glucocorticoid receptor binding show modest degrees of hepatic selectivity [126], but more specific targeting of the liver has been achieved when glucocorticoid receptor inhibitors are conjugated to bile salts. This retains the inhibitor mostly within the entero-hepatic circulation, reducing hyperglycemia and improving hepatic insulin sensitivity in animal models [127].

Another approach to the cellular targeting of glucocorticoid suppression takes advantage of the normal cellular conversion of less active cortisone to more active cortisol (Figure 60.21). This

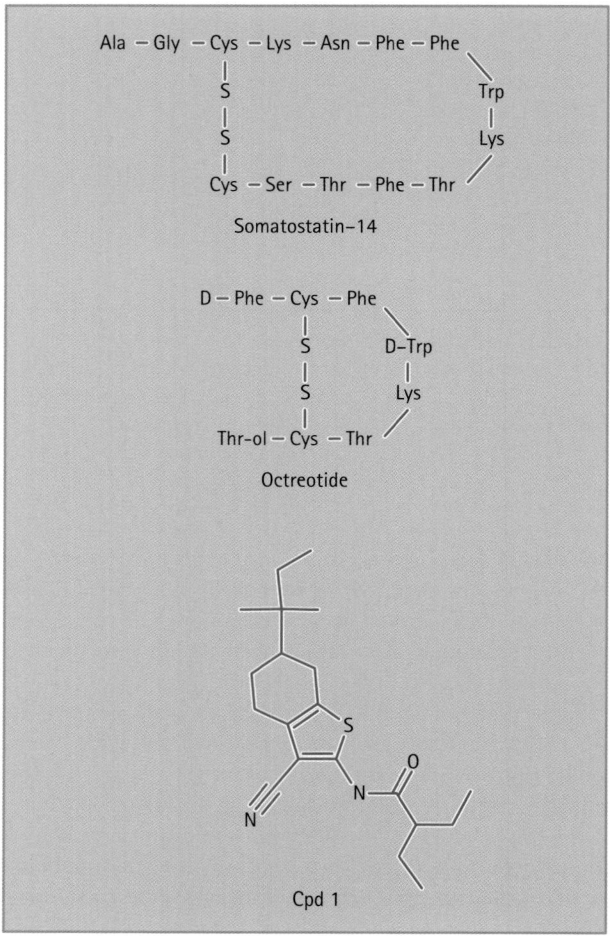

Figure 60.20 Structure of native somatostatin-14, its synthetic octapeptide analog, octreotide, and a non-peptide glucagon receptor antagonist Cpd 1.

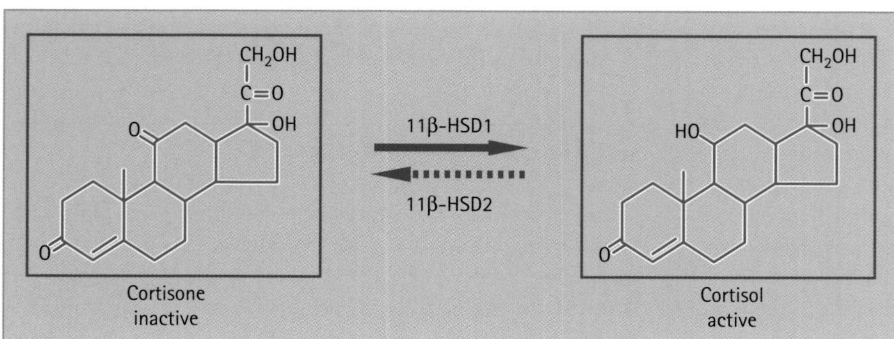

Figure 60.21 Cellular conversion of less active cortisone to more active cortisol through the reductase activity of the enzyme 11β-hydroxysteroid dehydrogenase-1 (11β-HSD1).

reaction is mediated through the predominantly reductase activity of the enzyme 11β-hydroxysteroid dehydrogenase-1 (11β-HSD1) which is strongly expressed in liver and adipose tissue [128]. Selective inhibitors of 11β-HSD1 have been shown to improve insulin sensitivity, glycemic control and plasma lipids in obese-diabetic rodents [129]. Excess glucocorticoids are often associated with some degree of islet hypertrophy, and because 11β-HSD1 is expressed by pancreatic β-cells, possible effects of 11β-HSD1 inhibitors on β-cells require detailed evaluation.

There is a substantial literature documenting that administration of the adrenal androgen dehydroepiandrosterone (DHEA) and an etiocholanolone metabolite (Figure 60.22) can decrease adiposity, improve glycemic control and reduce insulin resistance in obese diabetic animal models [130]. These agents may act in part to elevate tyrosine phosphorylation of IRS proteins and increase translocation of the glucose transporters GLUT-1 and GLUT-4 to the cell membrane [131].

Direct modifiers of glucose metabolism

Many substances directly stimulate glucose uptake and utilization or suppress glucose production. Their metabolic impact is often difficult to control, and their wider effects have precluded therapeutic application for T2DM. Included here are agents that create some insulin-like effects such as deoxyfrenolicin, vitamin K_5, spermine, diamides and peroxides (Figure 60.23) [115]. Okadaic acid and phorbol esters initially imitate certain effects of insulin, but then prevent tissues from responding further to insulin. Dichloroacetate and its esters increase glucose oxidation by stimulating pyruvate dehydrogenase, and suppress hepatic glucose production by inhibiting pyruvate carboxylase, but may adversely affect neural function through the production of glyoxylate and oxylate [115].

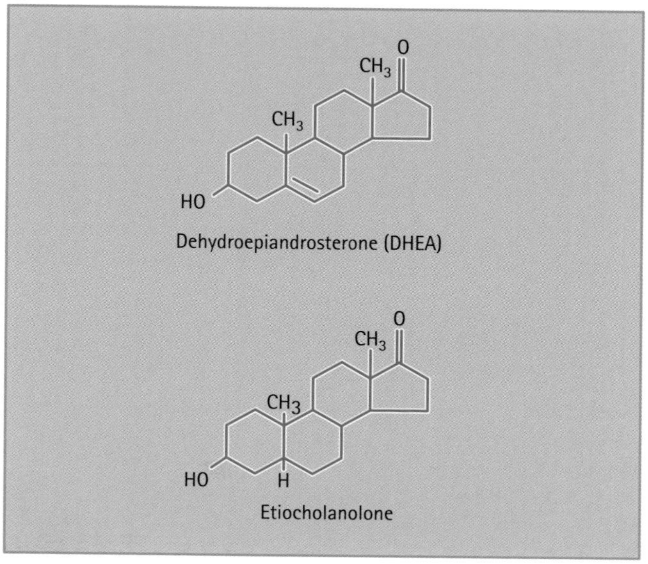

Figure 60.22 Structures of dehydroepiandrosterone (DHEA) and etiocholanolone.

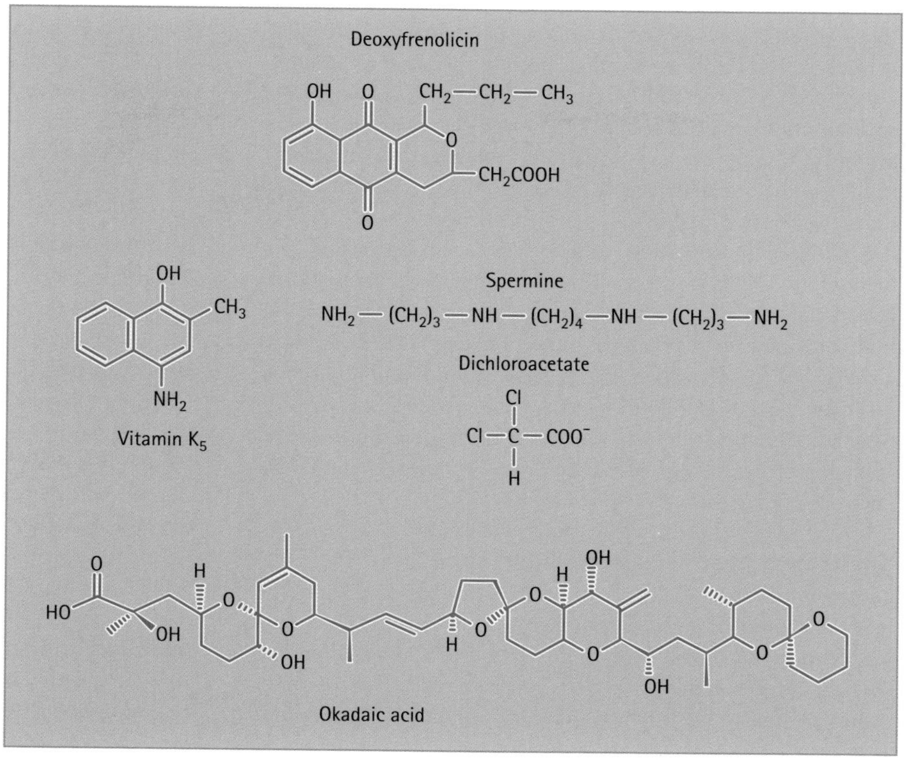

Figure 60.23 Structures of deoxyfrenolicin, vitamin K_5, spermine, okadaic acid and dichloroacetate.

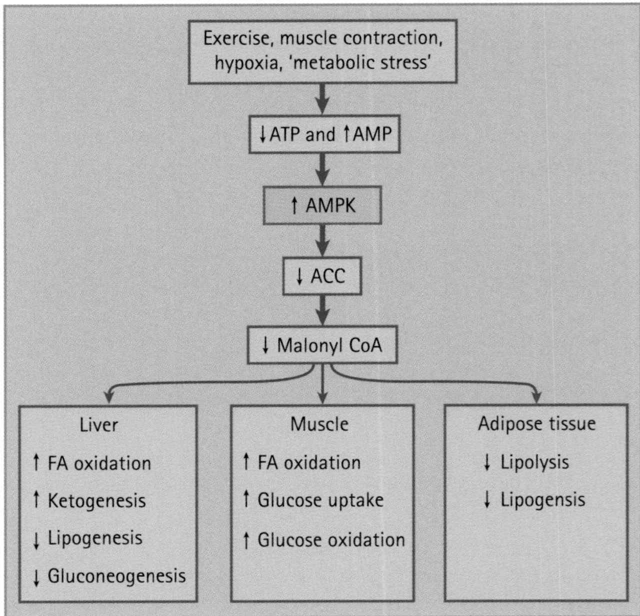

Figure 60.24 Metabolic effects of the energy-regulating enzyme adenosine monophosphate-activated protein kinase (AMPK). ACC, acetyl CoA carboxylase; FA, fatty acid.

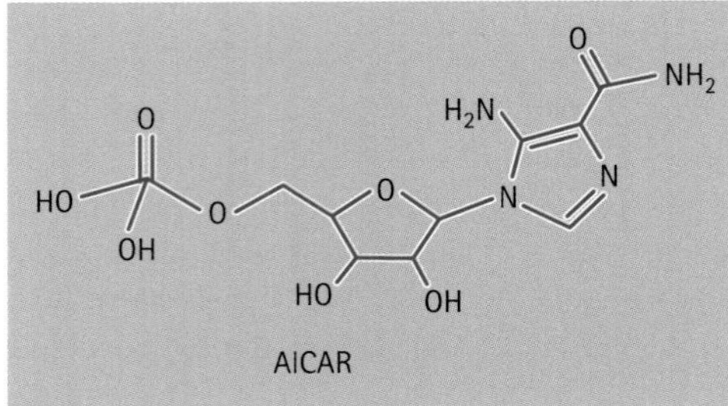

Figure 60.25 Structure of AICAR, 5-aminoimidazole-4-carboxamide-1-B-D-ribofuranoside.

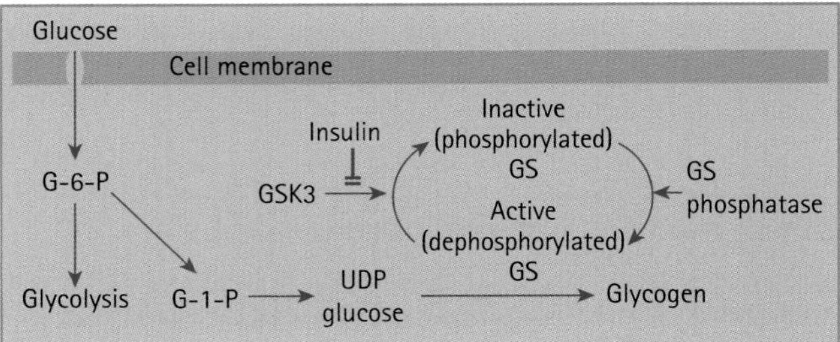

Figure 60.26 Glycogen synthase kinase-3 (GSK3) regulation of glycogen synthase (GS). G-6-P glucose 6-phosphate; G-1-P, glucose 1-phosphate; UDPG, uridine diphosphate glucose.

Adenosine monophosphate-activated protein kinase activators

Adenosine monophosphate-activated protein kinase (AMPK) is a key energy-regulating enzyme that is activated when the energy status of cells declines and/or energy demand escalates [132]. When ATP and creatine phosphate become depleted, for example during exercise, AMP concentrations become raised. Rising AMP concentrations activate AMPK, promoting energy production by increasing the uptake and oxidation of glucose and fatty acids, leading to the restoration of ATP (Figure 60.24). AMPK may also reduce expression of PEPCK (key gluconeogenic enzyme), and depending upon associated regulatory factors, suppress cell proliferation [133]. Metformin, adiponectin and thiaziolidinediones have been shown to activate AMPK amongst other actions that contribute to their glucose-lowering effects [134]. Various analogs of AMP such as AICAR (5-aminoimidazole-4-carboxamide-1-B-D-ribofuranoside) have been shown to activate AMPK and improve glycemic control in insulin-resistant diabetic animals (Figure 60.25) [135, 136], and other activators (e.g. DRL-16536) are being developed.

Glycogen synthase kinase inhibitors

Glycogen synthesis is impaired in T2DM, caused in part by reduced activity of glycogen synthase. Glycogen synthase is normally deactivated through phosphorylation by a serine/threonine kinase – GSK3. Glycogen synthesis proceeds when GSK3 is inactivated by insulin via the PI3K-Akt pathway, but expression and activity of GSK3 are increased in insulin-resistant diabetic states. Small molecule inhibitors of GSK3 have been shown to lower blood glucose and increase insulin-stimulated glucose uptake and glycogenesis by skeletal muscle of insulin-resistant diabetic animals [137,138]. There are two isoforms and several splice variants of GSK3 that have various roles in the signaling of pathways as diverse as cytoskeletal regulation, protein degradation and apoptosis, making it difficult to target glycogen metabolism specifically (Figure 60.26).

Glucokinase activators

Because liver cells, like islet β-cells, can take up glucose approximately in proportion to the circulating glucose concentration, the rate of hepatic glucose disposal is determined mostly through the rate of glucose phosphorylation by GK. Allosteric activators of GK and molecules that prevent GK from binding with its inhibitory regulatory protein have been shown to increase hepatic glucose metabolism and reduce blood glucose concentrations in normal and diabetic rodents [24–29,139]. Clinical studies will establish whether the combined effects of increased hepatic glucose disposal and increased insulin secretion can be titrated to avoid overt hypoglycemia.

Inhibitors of hepatic glucose production

Any therapeutic approach that suppresses gluconeogenesis and/or glycogenolysis should be partial, readily reversible and should not seriously compromise vital actions of counter-regulatory hormones and neural signals in times of rapid and severe hypoglycemia.

Glycogen phosphorylase inhibitors

Glycogen phosphorylase inhibitors have received considerable preclinical attention as possible agents to reduce hyperglycemia by preventing the breakdown of glycogen. The agents studied include inhibitors of the active site, the AMP site and other sites on the enzyme [139–141]. An example is the dihydropyridine derivative BAY R3401, a prodrug that is metabolized to an active agent that binds at the AMP site causing allosteric inhibition and dephosphorylation of active glycogen phosphorylase *a* into the inactive *b* form [141]. While most glycogen phosphorylase inhibitors have been shown to improve glycemic control in animal models of T2DM, there have been few reports of clinical studies, and the limited evidence available suggests only modest or unsustained efficacy.

Glucose 6-phosphatase inhibitors

Glucose 6-phosphatase inhibitors have been considered an attractive approach to address hyperglycemia because they can interrupt the last step in glucose output from both glycogenolysis and gluconeogenesis. Inhibitors of the catalytic subunit and the translocator protein for glucose 6-phosphatase have been shown to reduce hepatic glucose output and lower blood glucose; however, this approach carries a high risk of hypoglycemia. Also, cellular accumulation of glucose 6-phosphate causes excess deposition of glycogen and induction of lipogenic genes which predispose to fatty liver [139].

Fructose 1,6-bisphosphatase (F16BPase) inhibitors

Fructose 1,6-bisphosphatase (F16BPase) inhibitors prevent the dephosphorylation of fructose 1,6-bisphosphate to fructose 6-phosphate as the penultimate step in gluconeogenesis before glucose 6-phosphate. Various F16BPase inhibitors have been described, generally causing only a partial reduction of hepatic glucose output because of increased compensatory glycogenolysis, which helps to guard against hypoglycemia [139]. Although excessive use of a F16BPase inhibitor might cause accumulation of lactate and triglyceride, appropriate titration of such agents in early clinical trials (e.g. MB07803) has given encouraging results.

Modifiers of lipid metabolism

The commonly observed dyslipidemia of T2DM, particularly raised very low density lipoprotein (VLDL), triglyceride and non-esterified fatty acid (NEFA) levels, contribute to insulin resistance and hyperglycemia in several ways [51,142]. These include direct effects of fatty acids and their metabolites to impair cellular insulin signaling pathways, and alterations in fuel selection mediated through the Randle (glucose–fatty acid) cycle. Agents that modify lipid metabolism could therefore benefit glycemic control in T2DM. For example, thiazolidinedione PPARγ agonists act in part through an alteration in fatty acid metabolism, and lipid-lowering fibrates, which act via PPARα agonism, can modestly assist glycemic control in some patients. Other agents that lower plasma triglycerides, such as the fenfluramine analog benfluorex and the long-chain dicarboxylic acid, Medica 16, can lower blood glucose concentrations [121]. Reducing circulating NEFA concentrations with conventional antilipolytic agents such as nicotinic acid (niacin) and its analog acipimox (Figure 60.27) can acutely improve glucose tolerance in T2DM, but the effect is not consistent or sustained [121].

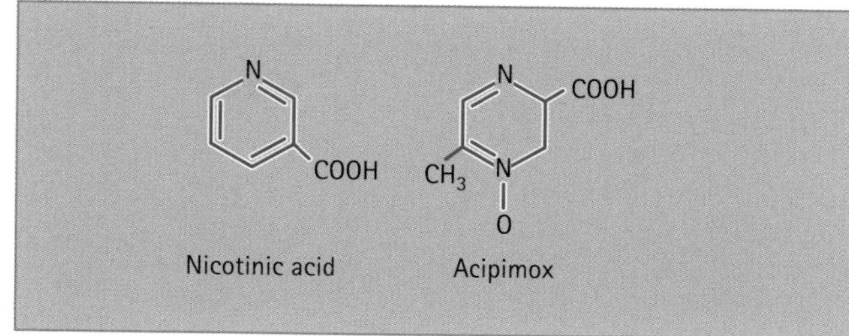

Figure 60.27 Structures of the antilipolytic agents, nicotinic acid and acipimox.

Inhibition of fatty acid oxidation interrupts the supply of energy for hepatic gluconeogenesis and enhances the use of glucose as a source of energy in skeletal muscle. Most inhibitors of fatty acid oxidation act by inhibiting carnitine palmitoyltransferase 1 (CPT-1), the rate-limiting enzyme for transfer of long-chain fatty acyl-CoA into the mitochondria. Irreversible inhibitors of CPT-1 such as the oxirane carboxylates (e.g. etomoxir) and the alkylglycidates (e.g. methyl palmoxirate) have effectively lowered glucose concentrations in diabetic animals, mainly through their antigluconeogenic action, but clinical studies have indicated vulnerability to hypoglycemia. Similar concerns have emerged with agents that inhibit intramitochondrial enzymes of fatty acid oxidation [121].

Sodium-glucose co-transporter 2 inhibitors

Glucose is filtered through the renal glomeruli and (almost) all that has been filtered is reabsorbed in the proximal tubules. Reabsorption is mediated mostly via the sodium-glucose co-transporter 2 (SGLT2) system (Figure 60.28). SGLT2 is expressed only in the first segment of the tubules and enables low affinity secondary active glucose transport into the tubular epithelial cells [143]. Thus, specific and appropriately titrated inhibition of these transporters provides an opportunity to reduce hyperglycemia by elimination of excess glucose in the urine. The potential of this approach has long been appreciated because non-specific inhibitors of sodium-glucose co-transporters such as phlorizin (Figure 60.29) from apple tree bark have been shown to reduce hyperglycemia in animals [144]. Non-specific inhibitors can also inhibit SGLT1 which is responsible for intestinal glucose absorption.

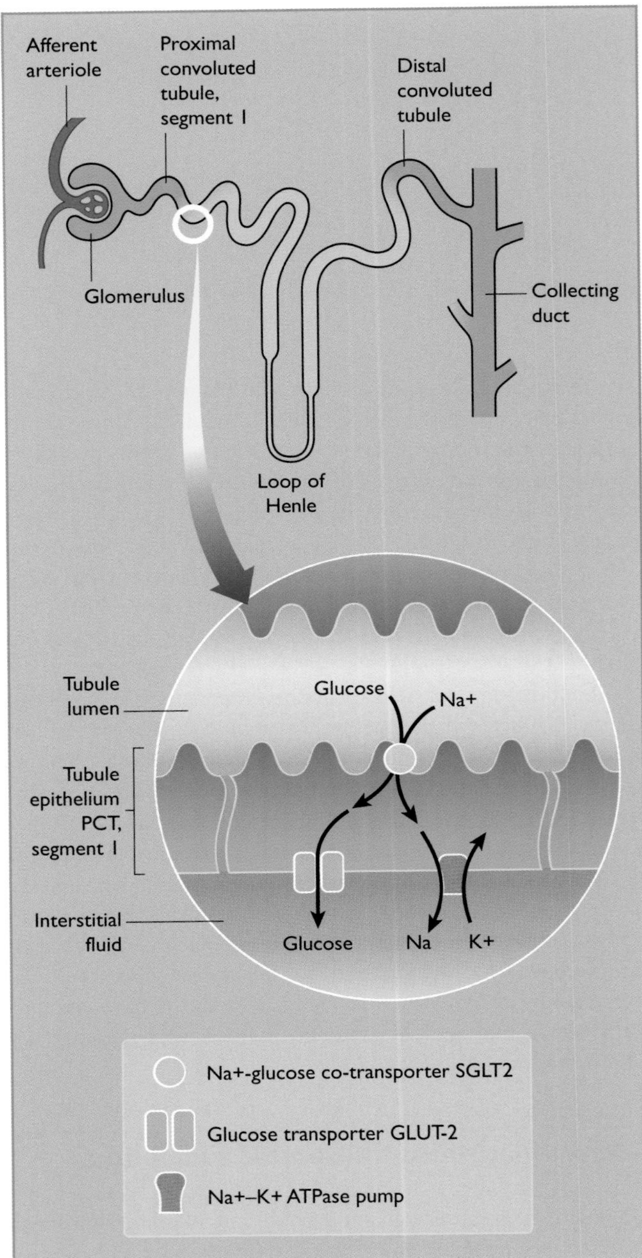

Figure 60.28 After glucose is filtered at the glomerulus into the proximal convoluted tubule (PCT) it is reabsorbed mostly from the first segment of the PCT via the low affinity secondary active sodium glucose co-transporter 2 (SGLT2).

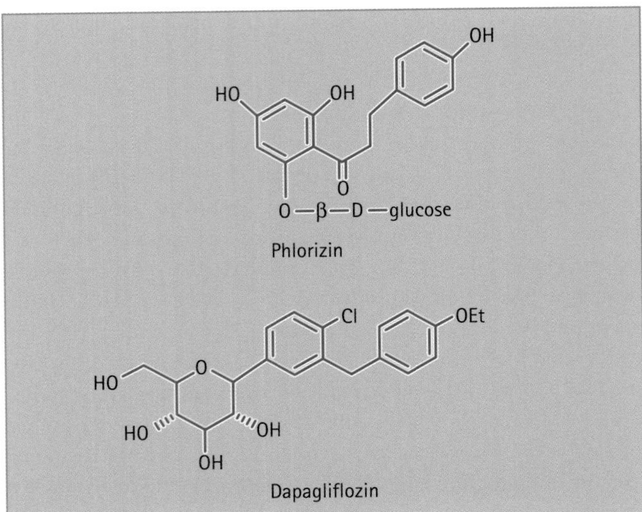

Figure 60.29 Structure of phlorizin (non-specific SGLT1/2 inhibitor) and the selective SGLT2 inhibitor dapagliflozin.

More recently, selective inhibitors of SGLT2 (termed "flozins") have been developed, and these have reduced hyperglycemia in diabetic animals and proceeded into clinical trials [145]. Preliminary evidence suggests that dosages that partially prevent glucose reabsorption to allow elimination of up to about 100 g/day glucose can be used to facilitate glycemic control in patients with T2DM. In principle, reversible SGLT2 inhibitors could be used as adjunctive therapy with any other antidiabetic treatment, and the elimination of glucose should assist weight loss. By lowering glucotoxicity it is anticipated that insulin sensitivity may be improved. Because SGLT2 inhibition does not stimulate insulin secretion or interrupt the counter-regulatory system, serious hypoglycemia should be avoidable if the extent of SGLT2 inhibition is titrated appropriately. Possible adverse effects of osmotic diuresis during SGLT2 inhibition include risk of dehydration and electrolyte imbalance, as well as infection in the urinary tract and urino-genital region.

Sirtuins

Sirtuins comprise a group of seven enzymes that are nicotinamide-adenine-dinucleotide (NAD)-dependent histone deacetylases and/or ADP-ribosyltransferases. They affect gene transcription through chromatin silencing, and mediate metabolic responses that have the potential to extend lifespan similar to chronic caloric restriction [146]. Sirtuin SIRT1 is widely expressed in mammalian tissues including liver, muscle and fat, and appears to promote mitochondrial biogenesis and activity in some tissues, increasing thermogenesis and reducing susceptibility to weight gain, diabetes and cardiovascular disease. AMPK enhances SIRT1 activity, resulting in increased activity of downstream transcription factors such as PGC-1α and the forkhead protein FOXO1 which increase energy production [147]. SIRT1 in pancreatic β-cells may also facilitate insulin secretion. Several small molecule activators of SIRT1 have been described that are structurally unrelated to polyphenols (such as resveratrol). The activators increased mitochondrial capacity, enhanced insulin sensitivity and reduced plasma glucose in animal models [148].

References

1 Holman RR, Paul SK, Bethel MA, Matthews DR, Neil HA. 10-Year follow-up of intensive glucose control in type 2 diabetes. *N Engl J Med* 2008; **359**:1577–1589.

2 Gaede P, Lund-Andersen H, Parving HH, Pedersen O. Effect of a multifactorial intervention on mortality in type 2 diabetes. *N Engl J Med* 2008; **358**:580–591.

3 International Diabetes Federation. *Diabetes Atlas*, 3rd edition. Brussels: International Diabetes Federation, 2006. (www.eatlas.idf.org)

4 American Diabetes Association. Standards of medical care in diabetes – 2009. *Diabetes Care* 2009; **32**(Suppl 1):13–61.

5 Krentz AJ, Bailey CJ. Oral antidiabetic agents: current role in type 2 diabetes mellitus. *Drugs* 2005; **65**:385–411.

6 Bailey CJ, Day C. Glycaemic memory. *Br J Diabetes Vasc Dis* 2008; **8**:242–247.

7 Adams C, Brantner V. Estimating the coast of new drug development. *Health Aff* 2006; **25**:420–428.

8 Bailey CJ, Day C. Fixed-dose single tablet combinations. *Diabetes Obes Metab* 2009; **11**:527–533.

9 Bailey CJ. Hypoglycaemic, antihyperglycaemic and antidiabetic drugs. *Diabet Med* 1992; **9**:492–493.

10 Bailey CJ. Drugs on the horizon for diabesity. *Curr Diabetes Rep* 2005; **5**:353–359.

11 Bailey CJ. Treating insulin resistance: future prospects. *Diabetes Vasc Dis Res* 2007; **4**:20–31.

12 Nuttall FQ. Dietary fiber in the management of diabetes. *Diabetes* 1993; **42**:503–508.

13 Chandalia M, Garg A, Lutjohann D, von Bergmann K, Grundy SM, Brinkley LJ. Beneficial effects of high dietary fibre intake in patients with type 2 diabetes mellitus. *N Engl J Med* 2000; **342**:1392–1398.

14 Lebovitz HE. α-Glucosidase inhibitors as agents in the treatment of diabetes. *Diabetes Rev* 1998; **6**:132–145.

15 Ashcroft FM, Gribble FM. ATP-sensitive K channels and insulin secretion: their role in health and disease. *Diabetologia* 1999; **42**:903–919.

16 Malaisse WJ. Stimulation of insulin release by non-sulphonylurea hypoglycaemic agents: the meglitinide family. *Horm Metab Res* 1995; **27**:263–266.

17 Storey DA, Bailey CJ. Biphasic insulin-releasing effect of BTS67582 in rats. *J Pharm Pharmacol* 1998; **50**:1357–1360.

18 Le Brigand L, Virsolvy A, Manechez D, Godfroid JJ, Guardiola-Lemaître B, Gribble FM, *et al. In vitro* mechanism of action on insulin release of S-22068, a new putative antidiabetic compound. *Br J Pharmacol* 1999; **128**:1021–1026.

19 Morgan NG, Chan SL. Imidazoline binding sites in the endocrine pancreas. *Curr Pharm Des* 2001; **7**:1413–1431.

20 Efanou AM, Zaitsev SV, Mest HJ, Raap A, Appelskog IB, Larsson O, *et al.* The novel imidazoline compound BL11282 potentiates glucose-induced insulin secretion in pancreatic b-cells in the absence of modulation of K_{ATP} channel activity. *Diabetes* 2001; **50**:797–802.

21 Laghmich A, Ladriere L, Malaisse-Lagae F, Dannacher H, Björkling F, Malaisse WJ. Stimulation of biosynthetic activity by novel succinate esters in rat pancreatic islets. *Biochem Pharmacol* 1998; **55**:909–913.

22 Kowluru A. Adenine and guanine nucleotide-specific succinyl-CoA synthetases in the clonal beta-cell mitochondria: implications in the beta-cell high-energy phosphate metabolism in relation to physiological insulin secretion. *Diabetologia* 2000; **44**:89–94.

23 Matschinsky FM, Magnuson MA, Zelent D, Jetton TL, Doliba N, Han Y, *et al.* The network of glucokinase-expressing cells in glucose homeostasis and the potential of glucokinase activators for diabetes therapy. *Diabetes* 2006; **55**:1–12.

24 Grimsby J, Sarabu R, Corbett WL, Haynes NE, Bizzarro FT, Coffey JW, *et al.* Allosteric activators of glucokinase: potential role in diabetes therapy. *Science* 2003; **301**:370–373.

25 Brocklehurst KJ, Payne VA, Davies RA, Carroll D, Vertigan HL, Wightman HJ, *et al.* Stimulation of hepatocyte glucose metabolism by novel small molecule glucokinase activatores. *Diabetes* 2004; **53**:535–541.

26 Efanov AM, Barrett DG, Brenner MB, Briggs SL, Delaunois A, Durbin JD, *et al.* A novel glucokinase activator modulates pancreatic islet and hepatocyte function. *Endocrinology* 2005; **146**:3696–3701.

27 Futamura M, Hosaka H, Kadotani A, Shimazaki H, Sasaki K, Ohyama S, *et al.* An allosteric activator of glucokinase impairs the interation of glucokinase and glucokinase regulatory protein and regulates glucose metabolism. *J Biol Chem* 2006; **281**:37668–37674.

28 Fyfe MC, White JR, Taylor A, Chatfield R, Wargent E, Printz RL, *et al.* Glucokinase activator PSN-GK1 displays enhanced antihyperglycaemic and insulinotropic actions. *Diabetologia* 2007; **50**:1277–1287.

29 Johnson D, Shepherd R, Gill D, Gorman T, Smith DM, Dunne MJ. Glucose-dependent modulation of insulin secretion and intracellular calcium ions by GKA50, a glucokinase activator. *Diabetes* 2007; **56**:1694–1702.

30 Holst JJ. Glucagon-like peptide-1: from extract to agent. *Diabetologia* 2006; **49**:253–260.

31 Drucker DJ. The role of gut hormones in glucose homeostasis. *J Clin Invest* 2007; **117**:24–32.

32 Flatt PR, Bailey CJ, Green BD. Recent advances in antidiabetic drug therapies targeting the enteroinsular axis. *Curr Drug Metab* 2009; **10**:125–137.

33 Holst JJ, Deacon CF. Glucagon-like peptide-1 mediates the therapeutic actions of DPP-IV inhibitors. *Diabetologia* 2005; **48**:612–615.

34 Gentilella R, Bianchi C, Rossi A, Rotella CM. Exenatide: a review from pharmacology to clinical practice. *Diabetes Obes Metab* 2009; **11**:544–556.

35 Garber A, Henry R, Ratner R, Garcia-Hernandez PA, Rodriguez-Pattzi H, Olvera-Alvarez I, *et al.* Liraglutide versus glimepiride monotherapy for type 2 diabetes (LEAD-3 mono): a randomised, 52-week, phase III, double-blind, parallel-treatment trial. *Lancet* 2009; **373**:473–481.

36 Pan CQ, Buxton JM, Yung SL, Tom I, Yang L, Chen H, *et al.* Design of a long acting peptide functioning as both a glucagon-like peptide-1 receptor agonist and a glucagon receptor antagonist. *J Biol Chem* 2006; **281**:12506–12515.

37 Chen D, Liao J, Li N, Zhou C, Liu Q, Wang G, *et al.* A nonpeptidic agonist of glucagon-like peptide-1 receptors with efficacy in diabetic db/db mice. *Proc Natl Acad Sci U S A* 2007; **104**:943–948.

38 Knudsen LB, Kiel D, Teng M, Behrens C, Bhumralkar D, Kodra JT, *et al.* Small-molecule agonists for the glucagon-like peptide 1 receptor. *Proc Natl Acad Sci U S A* 2007; **104**:937–942.

39 Flatt PR. Gastric inhibitory polypeptide (GIP) revisited: a new therapeutic target for obesity-diabetes? *Diabet Med* 2008; **25**:759–764.

40 Miyawaki K, Yamada Y, Ban N, Ihara Y, Tsukiyama K, Zhou H, *et al.* Inhibtion of gastric inhibitory polypeptide signaling prevents obesity. *Nat Med* 2002; **8**:738–742.

41 Hansotia T, Maida A, Flock G, Yamada Y, Tsukiyama K, Seino Y, *et al.* Extrapancreatic incretin receptors modulate glucose homeostasis, body weight and energy expenditure. *J Clin Invest* 2007; **117**:143–152.

42 Gault VA, Irwin N, Green BD, McCluskey JT, Greer B, Bailey CJ, *et al.* Chemical ablation of gastric inhibitory polypeptide receptor action by daily (Pro3)GIP administration improves glucose tolerance and ameliorates insulin resistance and abnormalities of islet structure in obesity-related diabetes. *Diabetes* 2005; **54**: 2436–2446.

43 Irwin N, McClean PL, O'Harte FP, Gault VA, Harriott P, Flatt PR. Early administration of the glucose-dependent insulinotropic polypeptide receptor antagonist (Pro3)GIP prevents the development of diabetes and related metabolic abnormalities associated with genetically inherited obesity in ob/ob mice. *Diabetologia* 2007; **50**:1532–1540.

44 Tsubamoto Y, Nakamura T, Kinoshita H, *et al.* A novel low molecular weight antagonist of glucose-dependent insulinotropic polypeptide receptor, SKL-14959, prevents obesity and insulin resistance. *Diabetologia* 2008; **51**(Suppl 1):S373.

45 Buchwald H, Estok R, Fahrbach K, Banel D, Jensen MD, Pories WJ, *et al.* Weight and type 2 diabetes after bariatric surgery: systematic review and meta-analysis. *Am J Med* 2009; **122**:248–256.

46 Flatt PR. Gastric inhibitory polypeptide (GIP) revisited: a new therapeutic target for obesity-diabetes? *Diabet Med* 2008; **25**:759–764.

47 Flatt PR, Bailey CJ, Green BD. Dipeptidyl peptidase IV (DPP-IV) and related molecules in type 2 diabetes. *Front Biosci* 2008; **13**:3648–3660.

48 Ahmad M, Abdel-Watiab YHA, Tate R, Flatt PR, Pyne NJ, Furman BL. Effect of type sensitive inhibitors on cyclic nucleotide phosphodiesterase activity and insulin secretion in the clonal insulin secreting cell line BRIN-BD11. *Br J Pharmacol* 2000; **129**: 1228–1234.

49 Saltiel AR, Kahn CR. Insulin signalling and the regulation of glucose and lipid metabolism. *Nature* 2001; **414**:799–806.

50 Shulman GI. Cellular mechanisms of insulin resistance. *J Clin Invest* 2000; **106**:171–176.

51 Kahn SE, HullRL, Utzschneider KM. Mechanisms linking obesity to insulin resistance and type 2 diabetes. *Nature* 2006; **444**:840–846.

52 Bailey CJ. Treating insulin resistance: future prospects. *Diabetes Vasc Dis Res* 2007; **4**:20–31.

53 Zhang B, Salituro G, Szalkowski D, Li Z, Zhang Y, Royo I, *et al.* Discovery of a small molecule insulin mimetic with antidiabetic activity in mice. *Science* 1999; **284**:974–977.

54 Li M, Youngren JF, Manchem VP, Kozlowski M, Zhang BB, Maddux BA, *et al.* Small molecule insulin receptor activators potentiate insulin action in insulin resistant cells. *Diabetes* 2001; **50**: 2323–2328.

55 Le-Roith D. Insulin-like growth factors. *N Engl J Med* 1997; **336**:633–640.

56 O'Connell T, Clemmons DR. IGF-1/IGF-binding protein-3 combination improves insulin resistance by GH-dependent and independent mechanisms. *J Clin Endocrinol Metab* 2003; **87**:4356–4360.

57 Manchem VP, Goldfine ID, Kohanski RA, Cristobal CP, Lum RT, Schow SR, *et al.* A novel small molecule that directly sensitizes the insulin receptor *in vitro* and *in vivo*. *Diabetes* 2001; **50**:824–830.

58 Grunberger G, Qiang X, Li Z, Mathews ST, Sbrissa D, Shisheva A, *et al.* Molecular basis for the insulinomimetic effects of C-peptide. *Diabetologia* 2001; **44**:1247–1257.

59 Koren S, Fantus IG. Inhibition of the protein tryosine phosphatase PTP1B: potential therapy for obesity, insulin resistance and type 2 diabetes mellitus. *Clin Endocrinol Metab* 2007; **21**:621–640.

60 Elchebly M, Payette P, Michaliszyn E. Increased insulin sensitivity and obesity resistance in mice lacking the protein tyrosine phosphatase-1B gene. *Science* 1999; **283**:1544–1548.

61 Gum RJ, Gaede LL, Koterski SL, Heindel M, Clampit JE, Zinker BA, *et al.* Reduction of protein tyrosine phosphatase 1B increases insulin-dependent signaling in ob/ob mice. *Diabetes* 2003; **52**:21–28.

62 Zhang ZY, Lee SY. PTP1B inhibitors as potential therapeutics in the treatment of type 2 diabetes and obesity. *Expert Opin Investig Drugs* 2003; **12**:223–233.

63 Lund IK, Andersen HS, Iversen LF, Olsen OH, Moller KB. Structure-based design of selective and potent inhibitors of protein tyrosine phosphatase B. *J Biol Chem* 2004; **279**:24226–24235.

64 Balkan B, Beeler S, Fan C, Orlowski L, Whitehouse D, Dean DJ. Pharmacological inhibition of PTP1B prevents development of diet-induced obesity and insulin resistance. *Diabetes* 2005; **54**(Suppl 1):618-P.

65 Morrison CD, White CL, Wang Z, Lee SY, Lawrence DS, Cefalu WT, *et al.* Increased hypothalamic PTP1B contributes to leptin resistance with age. *Endocrinology* 2007; **148**:435–440.

66 Vercauteren M, Remy E, Devaux C, Dautreaux B, Henry JP, Bauer F, *et al.* Improvement of peripheral endothelial dysfunction by protein tyrosine phosphatase inhibitors in heart failure. *Circulation* 2006; **114**:2498–2507.

67 Ueno N, Inui A, Asakawa A, Takao F, Komatsu Y, Kotani K, *et al.* Mosapride, a 5HT-4 receptor agonist, improves insulin sensitivity and glycaemic control in patients with type II diabetes mellitus. *Diabetologia* 2002; **45**:792–797.

68 Houdali B, Nguyen V, Ammon HP, Haap M, Schechinger W, Machicao F, *et al.* Prolonged glucose infusion into conscious rats inhibits early steps in insulilin signaling and induces translocation of GLUT4 and protein kinase C in skeletal muscle. *Diabetologia* 2002; **45**:356–368.

69 He Z, King GL. Protein kinase C beta isoform inhibitors. *Circulation* 2004; **110**:7–9.

70 Clarke M, Dodson PM. PKC inhibition and diabetic microvascular complications. *Clin Endocrinol Metab* 2007; **21**:573–586.

71 Cai D, Yuan M, Frantz DF, Melendez PA, Hansen L, Lee J, *et al.* Local and systemic insulin resistance resulting from hepatic activation of IKK-beta and NF-KB. *Nat Med* 2005; **11**:183–190.

72 Arkan MC, Hevener AL, Greten FR, Maeda S, Li ZW, Long JM, *et al.* IKK-beta links inflammation to obesity-induced insulin resistance. *Nat Med* 2005; **11**:191–198.

73 Yuan M, Konstantopoulos N, Lee J, Hansen L, Li ZW, Karin M, *et al.* Reversal of obesity- and diet-induced insulin resistance with salicylates or targeted disruption of IkkB. *Science* 2001; **293**:1673–1677.

74 Kaneto H, Nakatani Y, Miyatsuka T, Kawamori D, Matsuoka TA, Matsuhisa M, *et al.* Possible novel therapy for diabetes with cell-permeable JNK-inhibitory peptide. *Nat Med* 2004, **10**:1128–1132.

75 Gual P, Gremeaux T, Gonzalez T, Le Marchand-Brustel Y, Tanti JF. MAP kinases and mTOR mediate insulin-induced phosphorylation of Insulin Receptor Substrate-1 on serine residues 307, 612 and 632. *Diabetologia* 2003; **46**:1532–1542.

76 Dong H, Maddox BA, Altomonte J, Meseck M, Accili D, Terkeltaub R, *et al.* Increased hepatic levels of the insulin receptor inhibitor, PC-1/NNP1, induce insulin resistance and glucose intolerance. *Diabetes* 2005; **54**:367–372.

77 Tanigouchi CM, Emanuelli B, Kahn CR. Critical nodes in signalling pathways: insights into insulin action. *Nat Rev Mol Cell Biol* 2006; **7**:85–96.

78 White MF. IRS proteins and the common path to diabetes. *Am J Physiol* 2002; **283**:E413–422.

79 Bates SH, Jones RB, Bailey CJ. Insulin-like effect of pinitol. *Br J Pharmacol* 2000; **130**:1944–1948.

80 Kim HJ, Ku B, Lee J, Lee SK, Kim Y, Park K. The effects of pinitol on glycaemic control and adipokine levels in type 2 diabetes patients. *Diabetologia* 2006; **49**(Suppl 1):Abs 0857.

81 Brautigan DL, Brown M, Grindrod S, Chinigo G, Kruszewski A, Lukasik SM, *et al.* Allosteric activation of protein phosphatase 2C by D-chiro-inositol-galactosamine, a putative mediator mimetic of insulin action. *Biochemistry* 2005; **44**:11067–11073.

82 Butler M, McKay RA, Popoff IJ, Gaarde WA, Witchell D, Murray SF, *et al.* Specific inhibition of PTEN expression reverses hyperglycaemia in diabetic mice. *Diabetes* 2002; **51**:1028–1034.

83 Komazawa N, Matsuda M, Kondoh G, Mizunoya W, Iwaki M, Takagi T, *et al.* Enhanced insulin sensitivity, energy expenditure and thermogenesis in adipose-specific Pten suppression in mice. *Nat Med* 2004; **10**:1208–1215.

84 Beguinot F. PTEN: targeting the search for novel insulin sensitizers provides new insight into obesity research. *Diabetologia* 2007; **50**:247–249.

85 Clement S, Krause U, Tanti JF, Behrends J, Pesesse X, Sasaki T, *et al.* The lipid phosphatase SHIP2 controls insulin sensitivity. *Nature* 2001; **409**:92–97.

86 Kahn SE, Hull RL, Utzschneider KM. Mechanisms linking obesity to insulin resistance and type 2 diabetes. *Nature* 2006; **444**:840–846.

87 Antuna-Puente B, Feve B, Fellahi S, Bastard P. Adipokines: the missing link between insulin resistance and obesity. *Diabetes Metab* 2008; **34**:2–11.

88 Billyard T, McTernan P, Kumar S. Potential therapies based on antidiabetic peptides. *Clin Endocrinol Metab* 2007; **21**:641–655.

89 Sul HS. Resistin/ADFS/FIZZ3 in obesity and diabetes. *Trends Endocrinol Metab* 2004; **15**:247–249.

90 Kadowski T, Yamauchi T. Adiponectin and adiponectin receptors. *Endocr Rev* 2005; **26**:439–451.

91 Berndt J, Kloting N, Kralisch S, Kovacs P, Fasshauer M, Schön MR, *et al.* Plasma visfatin concentrations and fat-depot specific mRNA expression in humans. *Diabetes* 2005; **54**:2911–2916.

92 Graham TE, Yang Q, Bluher M, Hammarstedt A, Ciaraldi TP, Henry RR, *et al.* Retinal binding protein 4 and insulin resistance in lean, obese and diabetic subjects. *N Engl J Med* 2006; **354**: 2552–2563.

93 Hida K, Wada J, Eguchi J, Zhang H, Baba M, Seida A, *et al.* Visceral adipose tissue-derived serine protease inhibitor: a unique insulin sensitizing adipocytokine in obesity. *Proc Natl Acad Sci U S A* 2005; **102**:10610–10615.

94 Yang RZ, Lee MJ, Hu H, Pray J, Wu HB, Hansen BC, *et al.* Identification of omentin as a novel depot-specific adipokine in human adipose tissue: possible role in modulating insulin action. *Am J Physiol* 2006; **290**:E1253–1261.

95 Pijl H, Ohashi S, Matsuda M, Miyazaki Y, Mahankali A, Kumar V, *et al.* Bromocriptine: a novel approach to the treatment of type 2 diabetes. *Diabetes Care* 2000; **23**:1154–1161.

96 Cincotta AM, Meier AH, Cincotta M. Bromocriptine improves glycaemic control and serum lipid profile in obese type 2 diabetic subjects: a new approach in the treatment of diabetes. *Expert Opin Investig Drugs* 1999; **8**:1683–1707.

97 Das UN. Is angiotensin II an endogenous pro-inflammatory molecule? *Med Sci Monit* 2005; **11**:RA155–162.

98 Day C. Traditional plant treatments for diabetes mellitus. *Acta Chim Ther* 2000; **26**:131–150.

99 Reed MJ, Meszaros K, Entes LJ, Claypool MD, Pinkett JG, Brignetti D, *et al.* Effect of masoprocol on carbohydrate and lipid metabolism in a rat model of type II diabetes. *Diabetologia* 1999; **42**:102–106.

100 Baur JA, Sinclair DA. Therapeutic potential of resveratrol: the *in vivo* evidence. *Nat Rev* 2006; **5**:493–506.

101 Lagouge M, Argmann C, Gerhart-Hines Z, Mexiane H, Lerin C, Daussin F, *et al.* Resveratrol improves mitochondrial function and protects against metabolic diseases by activating SIRT1 and PGC-1 alpha. *Cell* 2006; **127**:1109–1122.

102 Coletta DK, Bates SH, Jones RB, Bailey CJ. The sibutramine metabolite M2 improves muscle glucose uptake and reduces hepatic glucose output: preliminary data. *Diabetes Vasc Dis Res* 2006; **3**:186–188.

103 Scheen AJ, Finer N, Hollander P, Jensen MD, Van Gaal LF. Efficacy and tolerability of rimonabant in overweight or obese patients with type 2 diabetes: a randomized controlled study. *Lancet* 2006; **368**:1660–1672.

104 Desvergne B, Michalik L, Wahli W. Transcriptional regulation of metabolism. *Physiol Rev* 2006; **86**:465–514.

105 Gross B, Staels B. PPAR agonists: multimodal drugs for the treatment of type 2 diabetes. *Clin Endocrinol Metab* 2007; **21**:687–710.

106 Allen T, Zhang F, Moodle SA, Clemens LE, Smith A, Gregoire F, *et al.* Halofenate is a selective peroxisome proliferators-activated receptor g modulator with antidiabetic activity. *Diabetes* 2006; **55**:2523–2533.

107 Puigserver P, Spegelman BM. Peroxisome proliferators-activated receptor-gamma coactivator 1a (PGC-1a): transcriptional coactivator and metabolic regulator. *Endocr Rev* 2003; **24**:78–90.

108 Conlon D. Goodbye glitazars? *Br J Diabetes Vasc Dis* 2006; **6**:135–137.

109 Evans RM, Barish GD, Wang YX. PPARs and the complex journey to obesity. *Nat Med* 2004; **10**:1–7.

110 Cha BS, Ciaraldi TP, Carter L. Peroxisome proliferators-activated receptor (PPAR) γ and retinoid x receptor (RXR) agonists have complimentary effects on glucose and lipid metabolism in human skeletal muscle. *Diabetologia* 2001; **44**:444–452.

111 Houstis N, Rosen ED, Lander ES. Reactive oxygen species have a causal role in multiple forms of insulin resistance. *Nature* 2006; **440**:944–948.

112 Heart Protection Study Collaborative Group. MRC/BHF heart protection study of antioxidant vitamin supplementation in 20,536 high-risk individuals: a randonised placebo-controlled trial. *Lancet* 2002; **360**:23–33.

113 Mathieu C, Gysemans C, Giulletti A, Bouillon R. Vitamin D and diabetes. *Diabetologia* 2005; **48**:1247–1257.

114 Bakker SJL, Hoogeveen EK, Nijpels G, Kostense PJ, Dekker JM, Gans RO, *et al.* The association of dietary fibres with glucose tolerance is partly explained by concomitant intake of thiamine: the Hoorn study. *Diabetologia* 1998; **41**:1168–1175.

115 Bailey CJ. New pharmacological approaches to glycemic control. *Diabetes Revs* 1999; **7**:94–113.

116 American Diabetes Association. Magnesium supplementation in the treatment of diabetes. *Diabetes Care* 1992; **15**:1065–1067.

117 Martin J, Wang ZQ, Zhang XH, Wachtel D, Volaufova J, Matthews DE, *et al.* Chromium picolinate supplementation attenuates body weight gain and increases insulin sensitivity in subjects with type 2 diabetes. *Diabetes Care* 2006; **29**:1826–1832.

118 Tsiani E, Fantus IG. Vanadium compounds: biological actions and potential as pharmacological agents. *Trends Endocrinol Metab* 1997; **8**:51–58.

119 Marti L, Abella A, Carpene C, Palacin M, Testar X, Zorzano A. Combined treatment with benylamine and low dosages of vanadate enhances glucose tolerance and reduces hyperglycemia in streptozotocin-induced diabetic rats. *Diabetes* 2001; **50**:2061–2068.

120 Flatt PR, Swanston-Flatt SK, Bailey CJ. Glucagon antiserum: a tool to investigate the role of circulating glucagon in obese hyperglycaemic (ob/ob) mice. *Biochem Soc Trans* 1979; **7**:911–913.

121 Bailey CJ. New pharmacological approaches to glycaemic control. *Diabetes Rev* 1999; **7**:94–113.

122 Peterson KF, Sullivan JT. Effects of a novel glucagon receptor antagonist (Bay 27–9955) on glucagon-stimulated glucose production in humans. *Diabetologia* 2001; **44**:2018–2024.

123 Rivera N, Everett-Grueter CA, Edgerton DS, Rodewald T, Neal DW, Nishimura E, *et al.* A novel glucagon receptor antagonist, NNC 15-0926, blunts hepatic glucose production in the conscious dog. *J Pharmacol Exp Ther* 2007; **321**:743–752.

124 Van Poelje PD, Potter SC, Liu S, *et al.* Glucagon action is a major determinant of hyperglycemia in animal models of type 2 diabetes. *Diabetes* 2008; **57**(Suppl 1):A406, 1444-P.

125 Parker JC, McPherson RK, Andrews KM, Levy CB, Dubins JS, Chin JE, *et al.* Effects of skyrin, a receptor-selective glucagon antagonist, in rat and human hepatocytes. *Diabetes* 2000; **49**:2079–2086.

126 Link JT, Sorensen B, Patel J, Grynfarb M, Goos-Nilsson A, Wang J, *et al.* Antidiabetic activity of passive nonsteroidal glucocorticoid receptor modulators. *J Med Chem* 2005; **48**:5295–5304.

127 Jacobson PB, von Geldern TW, Ohman L, Osterland M, Wang J, Zinker B, *et al.* Hepatic glucocorticoid antagonism is sufficient to reduce elevated hepatic glucose output and improve glucose control in animal models of type 2 diabetes. *J Pharmacol Exp Ther* 2005; **314**:191–200.

128 Stewart PM, Krozowski ZS. 11B-hydroxysteroid dehydrogenase. *Vitam Horm* 1999; **57**:249–324.

129 Tomlinson JW, Stewart PM. Modulation og glucocoricoid action and the treatment of type 2 diabetes. *Clin Endocrinol Metab* 2007; **21**:607–619.

130 Coleman DL. Hypoglycaemic action of the aetiocholanolones in mice. In: Bailey CJ, Flatt PR, eds. *New Antidiabetic Drugs*. London: Smith-Gordon, 1990: 191–196.

131 Perrini S, Natalicchio A, Laviola L, Belsanti G, Montrone C, Cignarelli A, *et al.* Dehydroepandrosterone stimulates glucose uptake in human and murine adipocytes by inducing GLUT1 and GLUT4 translocation to the plasma membrane. *Diabetes* 2004; **53**:41–52.

132 Hardie DG. The AMP-activated protein kinase cascade: the key sensor of cellular energy status. *Endocrinology* 2003; **144**: 5179–5183.

133 Motoshima H, Goldstein BJ, Igata I, Araki E. AMPK and cell proliferation: AMPK as a therapeutic target for atherosclerosis and cancer. *J Physiol* 2006; **574**:63–71.

134 Schimmack G, DeFronzo RA, Musi N. AMP-activated protein kinase: role in metabolism and therapeutic implications. *Diabetes Obes Metab* 2006; **8**:591–602.

135 Pold R, Jensen LS, Jessen N, Buhl ES, Schmitz O, Flyvbjerg A, *et al.* Long-term AICAR administration and exercise prevents diabetes in ZDF rats. *Diabetes* 2005; **54**:928–934.

136 Iglesias MA, Furler SM, Cooney GJ, Kraegen EW, Ye JM. AMP-activated protein kinase activation by AICAR increases both muscle fatty acid and glucose uptake in white muscle of insulin-resistant rats *in vivo*. *Diabetes* 2004; **53**:1649–1654.

137 Henriksen EJ, Kinnick TR, Teachey MK, O'Keefe MP, Ring D, Johnson KW, *et al.* Modulation of muscle insulin resistance by selective inhibition of GSK3 in Zucker diabetic fatty rats. *Am J Physiol Endocrinol Metab* 2003; **284**:E892–900.

138 Ring DB, Johnson KW, Henrisen EJ, Nuss JM, Goff D, Kinnick TR, *et al.* Selective glycogen synthase kinase inhibitors potentiate insulin activation of glucose transport and utilization *in vitro* and *in vivo*. *Diabetes* 2003; **52**:588–595.

139 Agius L. New hepatic targets for glycaemic control in diabetes. *Clin Endocrinol Metab* 2007; **21**:587–605.

140 Treadway JL, Mendys P, Hoover DJ. Glycogen phosphorylase inhibitors for treatment of type 2 diabetes mellitus. *Expert Opin Investig Drugs* 2001; **10**:439–454.

141 Bergans N, Stalmans W, Goldmann S, Vanstapel F. Molecular mode of inhibition of glycogenolysis in rat liver by the dihydropyridine derivative BAY R3401. *Diabetes* 2000; **49**:1419–1426.

142 McGarry JD. Dysregulation of fatty acid metabolism in the etiology of type 2 diabetes. *Diabetes* 2002; **51**:7–18.

143 Kanai Y, Lee WS, You G, Brown D, Hediger MA. The human kidney low affinity Na^+-glucose transporter SGLT2. *J Clin Invest* 1994; **93**:397–404.

144 Ehrenkranz JRL, Lewis NG, Kahn CR, Roth J. Phlorizin: a review. *Diabetes Metab* 2005; **21**:31–38.

145 Jabbour SA, Goldstein BJ. Sodium glucose co-transporter 2 inhibitors: blocking renal tubular reabsorption of glucose to improve glycaemic control in patients with diabetes. *Int J Clin Pract* 2008; **62**:1279–1284.

146 Lavu S, Boss O, Elliott PJ, Lambert PD. Sirtuins: novel therapeutic targets to treat age-associated diseases. *Nat Rev Drug Discov* 2008; **7**:841–853.

147 Canto C, Gerhart-Hines Z, Feige JN, Lagouge M, Norriega L, Milne JC, *et al.* AMPK regulates energy expenditure by modulating NAD+ metabolism and SIRT1 activity. *Nature* 2009; **458**:1056–1060.

148 Milne JC, Lambert PD, Schenk S, Carney DP, Smith JJ, Gagne DJ, *et al.* Small molecule activators of SIRT1 as therapeutics for the treatment of type 2 diabetes. *Nature* 2007; **450**:712–716.

61 Other Future Directions

Stem Cell Therapy in Diabetes

Shuibing Chen[1], Jayaraj Rajagopal[2,3], Qiao Zhou[3] & Douglas A. Melton[1,3]

[1] Department of Stem Cell and Regenerative Biology, Howard Hughes Medical Institute, Harvard University, Boston, MA, USA
[2] Center for Regenerative Medicine, Massachusetts General Hospital, Boston, MA, USA
[3] Harvard Stem Cell Institute, Harvard University, Cambridge, MA, USA

Islet Transplantation

Angela Koh, Peter Senior & A.M. James Shapiro

Clinical Islet Transplant Program, University of Alberta, Edmonton, USA

Gene Therapy

Andreea R. Barbu & Nils Welsh

Department of Medical Cell Biology, Uppsala University, Uppsala, Sweden

Stem Cell Therapy in Diabetes

Shuibing Chen[1], Jayaraj Rajagopal[2,3], Qiao Zhou[3] & Douglas A. Melton[1,3]

Keypoints

- Stem cells are self-renewing cells that possess the ability to generate daughter cells that produce large numbers of differentiated progeny. They can be divided into two broad categories: embryonic stem cells and adult stem cells.
- Embryonic stem cells are derived from the inner cell mass of mammalian blastocysts and can give rise to all of the differentiated tissues of the embryo proper, including the β-cells of the pancreas.
- Induced pluripotent stem cells are embryonic stem cell-like cells derived from adult cells such as skin fibroblasts in a process called reprogramming.
- Human embryonic stem cells and induced pluripotent stem cells have been shown to produce insulin-producing cells by stepwise approach in culture.
- Adult stem cells have been identified in many organs, where they participate in tissue repair and homeostasis. No definitively identified stem cell population has been described in pancreas.
- Lineage-tracing experiments suggest that β-cell mass is maintained primarily by replication of pre-existing β-cells during normal adult life in mice. After injury, stem/progenitor cells may be recruited to produce additional islet cells, but the identity of these pancreatic stem/progenitor cells remains unclear.
- Pancreatic exocrine cells can be directly converted to become β-cells *in vivo* in a process called lineage reprogramming.

Textbook of Diabetes, 4th edition. Edited by R. Holt, C. Cockram, A. Flyvbjerg and B. Goldstein.

Introduction

The aim of stem cell therapy in the treatment of type 1 diabetes mellitus (T1DM) is to provide a source of cells that are identical or nearly identical to β-cells. Stem cells by definition are self-renewing, and in some cases they can be propagated clonally from a single cell. These properties allow a degree of reproducibility that is unusual for a cell-based therapeutic vehicle. It may be possible to engineer stem cells to evade immune recognition. It is also now possible to derive patient-specific induced pluripotent cells (iPS) that fully match individual patients immunologically. Encouraging progress has been made in recent years to derive insulin-producing cells from either embryonic stem cells or exocrine cells. Future efforts will be focused on continued improvement of the derivation efficiency and fidelity of β-cells, with the ultimate aim of producing sufficient numbers of transplantable mature β-cells that can rescue hyperglycemic conditions.

General definitions: adult and embryonic stem cells

Stem cells are defined functionally. They are capable of self-renewal and possess the ability to generate daughter cells that produce large numbers of differentiated progeny [1]. They can be divided into two broad categories: embryonic stem cells and adult stem cells. Embryonic stem cells are derived from the inner cell mass of the mammalian blastocyst (Figure 61.1) and are said to be pluripotent because they give rise to all of the fully differentiated tissues of the embryo proper, including the products of all three embryonic germ layers and thus the β-cells of the pancreas (Figure 61.2). Fortunately, conditions have been described that permit the long-term culture of these cells *in vitro* without chromosomal aberration or loss of potency to form diverse tissues (Figure 61.3) [2–6]. Indeed, cell lines can be created by the propagation of a single cell, ensuring homogeneous cell populations that can subsequently be used as starting material for β-cell differentiation experiments.

Adult stem cells are thought to be rare cells and are known to participate in the repair or regeneration of certain tissues, most notably in the bone marrow [7,8]. Furthermore, stem cell populations are involved in the tissue homeostasis of the liver, the brain, the skeletal muscle and the skin [9–13]. Adult stem cells, like their embryonic counterparts, are capable of self-renewal and retain the ability to generate large numbers of differentiated progeny, but they are traditionally thought to produce a more limited number of cell types. Although there is some evidence to suggest the existence of a pancreatic stem cell function, no cell type or marker of such a putative cell has been identified. In fact,

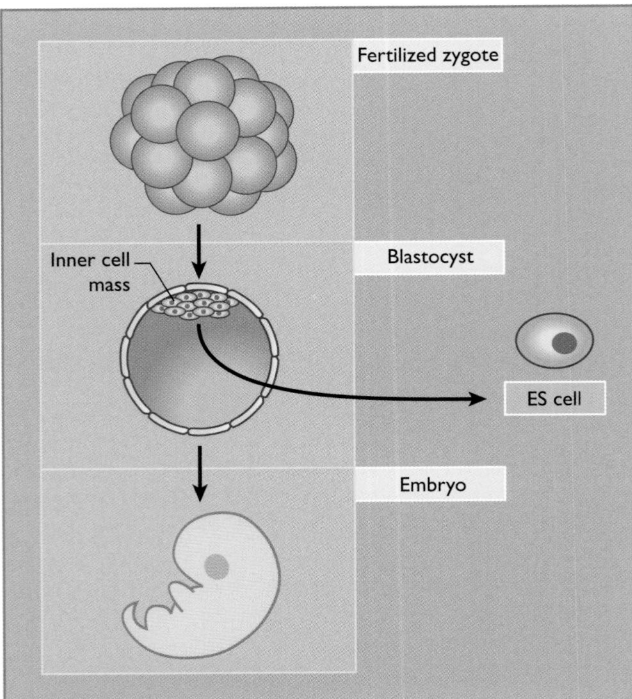

Figure 61.1 Derivation of embryonic stem cells. After fertilization, the single-cell human or mouse zygote undergoes cleavage to produce a multicellular blastocyst. The blastocyst stage of mammalian development occurs well before cytodifferentiation and organogenesis. Cells from the inner cell mass, which normally give rise to the tissues of the embryo proper, can be cultured *in vitro* to produce embryonic stem cells. ES, embryonic stem.

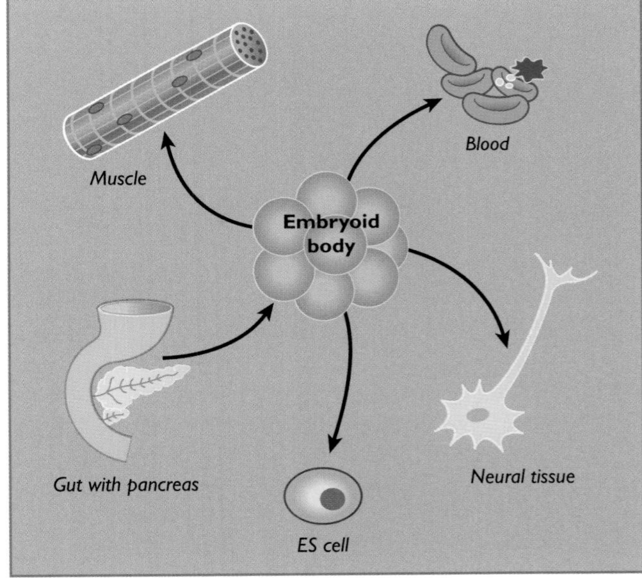

Figure 61.2 The pluripotent nature of embryonic stem (ES) cells. Embryonic stem cells can be cultured *in vitro* indefinitely. When allowed to aggregate in suspension culture, forming embryoid bodies, they differentiate into derivatives of all three embryonic germ layers. This includes ectodermal tissues such as neurons, mesodermal tissues such as muscle cells and blood, and endodermal tissues such as β-cells. Although there are many cell types in embryoid bodies, they are often disorganized and do not adopt the same patterned structure found in mature embryos and adults (e.g. actual muscle, ganglia, gut or islets).

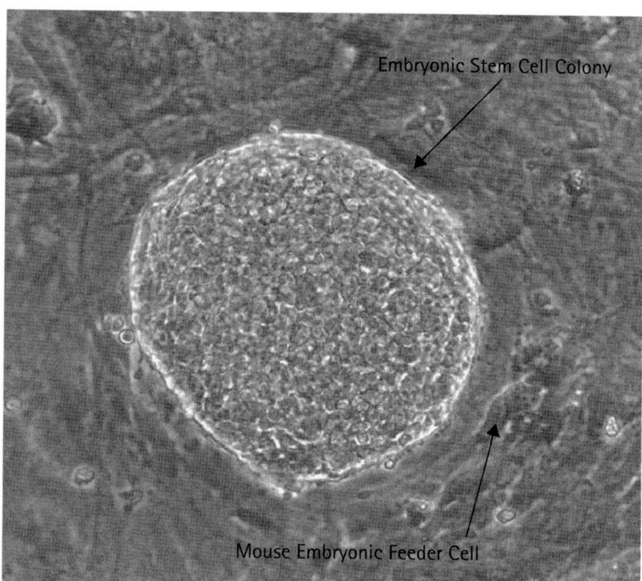

Figure 61.3 A human embryonic stem cell colony is composed of hundreds to thousands of homogeneous cells grown in a Petri dish along with hundreds of other similar stem cell colonies. One colony is shown here. These colonies are grown on mouse embryonic fibroblasts, which provide signals preventing embryonic stem cell differentiation. This allows repeated, near-indefinite subculture of embryonic stem cells. When removed from the murine feeder layer, the stem cells spontaneously differentiate into a wide variety of cell types (not shown).

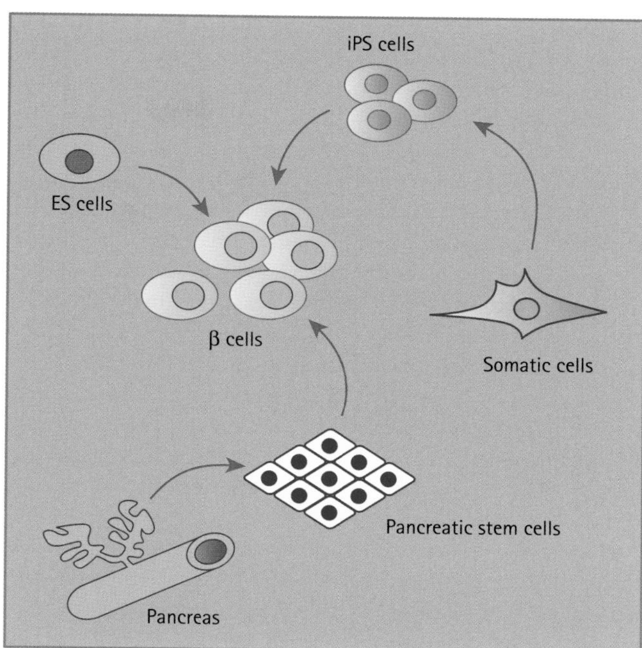

Figure 61.4 Potential stem-cell sources of β-cells. In theory, one can derive pancreatic β-cells from a number of different stem cell sources. Embryonic stem cells from the mammalian blastocyst have the broadest capacity for differentiation. Similarly, induced pluripotent cells (iPS) derived from skin fibroblasts may also give rise to all cell types in the body, including β-cells. Pancreatic stem cells may be the most direct path to β-cells, but their identity is still unclear. ES, embryonic stem.

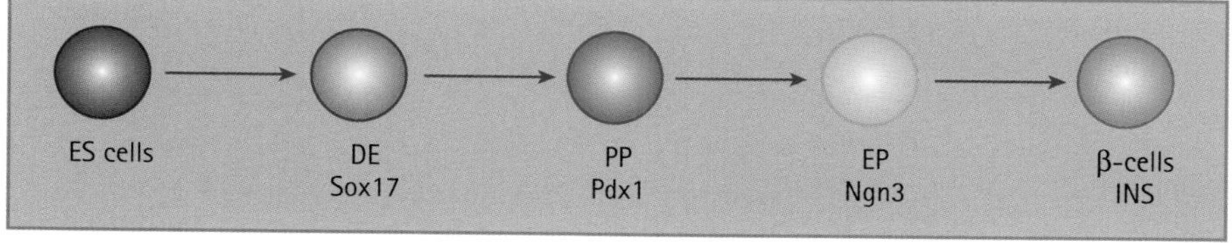

Figure 61.5 Stepwise differentiation from embryonic stem (ES) cells to β-cells. DE, definitive endoderm; PP, pancreatic progenitor; EP, endocrine progenitor; Ngn3, neurogenin 3; INS, insulin.

it is unclear whether the concept of an adult stem cell represents a single well-defined cell type or a common property of a heterogeneous population of different cells [1].

Differentiating β-cells from human embryonic stem cells

Embryonic stem (ES) cells, with a virtually endless replicative capacity and the potential to differentiate into most cell types, provide nearly unlimited starting material to generate differentiated cells for study and clinical therapy [14]. By mimicking signals used during embryonic pancreatic development, to the extent that they are known, a stepwise protocol is being explored to differentiate human ES cells into functional β-cells (Figure 61.4). This involves directing ES cells first to form definitive endoderm, then $Pdx1^+$ pancreatic progenitors, followed by the formation of endocrine progenitors and, finally, $insulin^+$ β-cells (Figure 61.5). Knowledge from pancreatic development provides candidate factors that promote the progression from one step to another, and marker genes that can be used to recognize the cells at each developmental stage.

Using a protocol based on the combination of candidate factors suggested by embryonic pancreatic development, significant advances have been made to produce insulin-producing cells from human ES cells [15–17]. Briefly, human ES cells were first treated with Wnt 3a and Activin A, which can result in approximately 70% of the cells expressing SOX17 [15], a marker of definitive endoderm. In the second step, manipulation of several signaling pathways that include suppression of sonic hedgehog (SHH) and bone morphogenetic protein (BMP), and activation of retinoic acid (RA) [16,17], allow the cells to progress into a pancreatic and endocrine progenitor stage. This heterogeneous progenitor population can be further differentiated and matured into various pancreatic endocrine cell types including insulin-secreting cells either in Petri dish [16] or after being transplanted into mice [17]. The endocrine cells appear to organize into islet-like structures and gain the ability to ameliorate hyperglycemia.

As an alternative to growth factors as inducers, an unbiased chemical screen approach has been used to identify cell-permeable small molecules to direct human ES cells to pancreatic lineage. In the ideal case, as noted by many others, small molecule inducers would be less expensive, more easily controlled, and possibly more efficient than growth factors in directing differentiation. High content chemical screening has led to the identification of a small molecule, (-)-Indolactam V (ILV), that induces human ES cell differentiation to pancreatic progenitors. These pancreatic progenitors can contribute to insulin-secreting cells both *in vitro* and *in vivo* [18].

Despite recent successes with the human ES cell approach, major challenges remain. The efficiency and consistency of β-cell derivation from human ES cells require improvement. The resulting β-like-cells need to be extensively validated to confirm their function [16] and the possibility of tumor formation after transplantation [17] must be fully addressed. New reagents and methodologies of human ES cell differentiation will need to be developed to overcome these challenges.

Human ES cell lines are derived from blastocyst-stage embryos. Recently, significant progress has been made in reprogramming differentiated human skin fibroblasts to a pluripotent state by introducing defined transcription and other reprogramming factors [19–21]. The resulting pluripotent cells are called induced pluripotent stem cells (iPS cells). iPS cells derived from people with diabetes have recently been shown to differentiate into three germ layers [22]. These DiPS cells could provide an important reagent for modeling diabetes pathology and investigating new therapies.

Evidence for the existence of pancreatic stem cells

In principle, tissue turnover in the adult can occur by the differentiation of adult stem cells (e.g. in skin and intestine), or by the replication of existing differentiated cells. In adult pancreas, there is strong evidence suggesting that new β-cells are generated primarily by the replication of pre-existing β-cells during normal adult homeostasis, as well as during β-cell regeneration induced by either partial removal of the pancreas or specific ablation of β-cells [23–27].

The evidence for the existence of adult pancreatic stem cells is indirect and comes from studies of regenerating pancreata. In these models, a chemical or surgical injury is induced in the adult pancreas. After chemical or surgical pancreatectomy in the islet, a burst of replicative activity in the pancreatic duct cells has also been reported. BrdU label disappears from the ducts and then increases in pancreatic exocrine and endocrine tissue, suggesting that cells may be recruited from ducts to form islets and acini [28]. Groups of cells that appear to be budding from the ducts have been suggested to represent cells recruited from a ductal stem cell compartment. The early burst in epithelial duct proliferation following pancreatectomy is reported to be accompanied by an increase in Pdx1 protein in the replicating duct cells [29]. Pdx1 is a protein that is essential for exocrine and endocrine pancreas formation. In the regenerating hamster pancreas, there are nests of cells near ducts that express insulin and glucagon, suggesting that duct cells may differentiate into hormone-producing cells that subsequently migrate into the islets [30]. In addition, after chemical pancreatectomy with streptozocin (streptozotocin), a cell population that coexpress hormones appears in the islets themselves, including Pdx1–somatostatin cells and somatostatin–insulin cells. These double-positive cells have been noted in the developing pancreas, but their exact role in development of the β-cell lineage is unclear. Nonetheless, it has been suggested that the presence of such cells implies neogenesis from a stem cell compartment located within the islets themselves [31].

It has recently been demonstrated that following partial duct ligation, a progenitor population expressing neurogenin 3 (Ngn3), a marker of embryonic endocrine progenitors, appears in adult mice. These Ngn3$^+$ cells can further give rise to new islet cells, including β-cells after transplantation into cultured embryonic pancreata [32]. This study provides an example of the existence of β-cell progenitors in adult pancreas; however, it is not clear whether this event represents the mobilization of existing adult endocrine progenitor cells that already express low levels of Ngn3, activation of dormant stem-like cells, or conversion of other cells into endocrine cells following injury. In addition, the number of Ngn3$^+$ progenitors detected following injury is very low and the molecules triggering the regeneration event remains unknown.

Taken together, the work on regenerating pancreata suggests the possibility of an existing precursor or stem cell; however, no clearly identified subpopulation of cells that has the capacity for self-renewal and β-cell differentiation has yet been identified as the pancreatic stem cell compartment. If such a pancreatic stem cell compartment does exist, its physiologic significance, in terms of the number of new β-cells produced, needs to be compared with the demonstrable capacity of β-cells for self-duplication.

Lineage reprogramming

In rare cases, adult cells of one lineage may be converted directly into cells of another lineage [33]. These phenomena are broadly defined as lineage reprogramming. For the pancreas, there is some experimental evidence suggesting that non-β-cells, such as liver cells, pancreatic duct cells and exocrine cells, may be converted to β-like-cells in culture [34]. In most of these reported cases, however, the extent to which the resulting cells resemble true β-cells is often unclear. The molecular mechanism of these reported conversion events also remain largely unknown.

Recently, it has been shown that mature exocrine cells of the pancreas can be reprogrammed to become β-like-cells *in vivo* with a simple combination of three transcription factors. The induced cells closely resemble endogenous islet β-cells in morphology, ultrastructure, molecular signatures and function [35]. There are several issues that need to be resolved before the *in vivo* lineage reprogramming approach can be applied to clinical therapy. For example, the induced β-cells persist as individual cells or small clusters and do not organize into islets. Moreover, viruses currently used to express the reprogramming factors would need to be replaced by safer reagents such as chemical compounds. Furthermore, given the difficulty of biopsying human pancreas, β-cell reprogramming should be accomplished directly *in vivo*, or alternatively, other more easily accessible starting cell populations, such as adult liver cells and skin fibroblasts, may be used to produce β-cells.

Future issues regarding human transplantation of cell-based therapies

There are several promising strategies for the generation of β-cells, from human embryonic stem cells, putative adult stem cells or lineage reprogramming. Nonetheless, a number of issues must be resolved before cells derived by these methods can be used in human transplantation. Immune rejection is prime amongst these concerns. Although the recent success with non-steroid immunosuppression is encouraging, it may be possible to engineer stem cells to be immunologically silent. The development of iPS technology now allows derivation of patient-specific stem cells and immunologically fully matched β-cells. In addition, considerable work also needs to be done to eliminate the risk of neoplasia. We must demonstrate that cells derived from ES cells are not transformed and that they are free from contaminating undifferentiated cells that could go on to produce teratomas in graft recipients. Cells must also be shown to be free of pathogens. Because human ES cells are currently grown on murine feeder cell lines, pathogens associated with xenotransplantation must be considered. Finally, we must assess the stability of the β-cell phenotype in grafts and the longevity of cells once transplanted. Ideally, these transplants would include not only differentiated β-cells, but also pancreatic stem cells with long-term reconstituting activity.

References

1 Blau HM, Brazelton TR, Weimann JM. The evolving concept of a stem cell: entity or function? *Cell* 2001; **105**:829–841.

2 Evans MJ, Kaufman MH. Establishment in culture of pluripotent cells from mouse embryos. *Nature* 1981; **292**:154–156.

3 Thomson JA, Itskovitz-Eldor J, Shapiro SS, Waknitz MA, Swiergiel JJ, Marshall VS, *et al.* Embryonic stem cell lines derived from human blastocysts. *Science* 1998; **282**:1145–1147.

4 Bongo A, Fong CY, Ng SC, Ratnam S. Isolation and culture of inner cell mass cells from human blastocysts. *Hum Reprod* 1994; **9**:2110–2117.

5 Reubinoff BE, Pera MF, Fong CY, Trounson A, Bongso A. Embryonic stem cell lines from human blastocysts. *Nat Biotechnol* 2000; **18**:399–404.

6 Amit M, Carpenter MK, Inokuma MS, Chui CP, Harris CP, Waknitz MA, *et al.* Clonally derived human embryonic stem cells maintain pluripotency and proliferative potential for prolonged periods in culture. *Dev Biol* 2000; **227**:271–278.

7 Morrison SJ, Weissman IL. The long-term repopulating subset of hematopoietic stem cells is deterministic and isolatable by phenotype. *Immunity* 1994; **1**:661–673.

8 Weissman IL. Stem cells as units of development, units of regeneration, and units of evolution. *Cell* 2000; **100**:157–168.

9 Smythe GM, Hodgetts SI, Grounds MD. Immunobiology and future of myoblast transfer therapy. *Mol Ther* 2000; **1**:304–313.

10 Gage FH. Mammalian neural stem cells. *Science* 2000; **287**:1433–1438.

11 Qian X, Shen Q, Goderie SK, He W, Capela A, Davis AA, *et al.* Timing of CNS cell generation: a programmed sequence of neuron and glial cell production from isolated murine cortical stem cells. *Neuron* 2000; **28**:69–80.

12 Thorgeirsson SS, Evarts RP, Bisgaard HC, Fujio K, Hu Z. Hepatic stem cell compartment: activation and lineage commitment. *Proc Soc Exp Biol Med* 1993; **204**:253–260.

13 Taylor G, Lehrer MS, Jensen PJ, Sun TT, Lavker RM. Involvement of follicular stem cells in forming not only the follicle but also the epidermis. *Cell* 2000; **102**:451–461.

14 *Regenerative Medicine.* Department of Health and Human Services, NIH, Medical and Scientific Illustration Washington, DC Terese Winslow, Washington, DC, 2006.

15 D'Amour KA, Agulnick AD, Eliazer S, Kelly OG, Kroon E, Baetge EE. Efficient differentiation of human embryonic stem cells to definitive endoderm. *Nat Biotechnol* 2005; **23**:1534–1541.

16 D'Amour KA, Bang AG, Eliazer S, Kelly OG, Agulnick AD, Smart NG, *et al.* Production of pancreatic hormone-expressing endocrine cells from human embryonic stem cells. *Nat Biotechnol* 2006; **24**:1392–1401.

17 Kroon E, Martinson LA, Kadoya K, Bang AG, Kelly OG, Eliazer S, *et al.* Pancreatic endoderm derived from human embryonic stem cells generates glucose-responsive insulin-secreting cells *in vivo*. *Nat Biotechnol* 2008; **26**:443–452.

18 Chen S, Borowiak M, Fox JL, Maehr R, Osafune K, Davidow L, *et al.* A small molecule that directs differentiation of human ESCs into the pancreatic lineage. *Nat Chem Biol* 2009; **5**:258–265.

19 Takahashi K, Tanabe K, Ohnuki M, Narita M, Ichisaka T, Tomoda K, *et al.* Induction of pluripotent stem cells from adult human fibroblasts by defined factors. *Cell* 2007; **131**:861–872.

20 Takahashi K, Yamanaka S. Induction of pluripotent stem cells from mouse embryonic and adult fibroblast cultures by defined factors. *Cell* 2006; **126**:663–676.

21 Yu J, Vodyanik MA, Smuga-Otto K, Antosiewicz-Bourget J, Frane JL, Tian S, *et al.* Induced pluripotent stem cell lines derived from human somatic cells. *Science* 2007; **318**:1917–1920.

22 Park IH, Arora N, Huo H, Maherali N, Ahfeldt T, Shimamura A, *et al.* Disease-specific induced pluripotent stem cells. *Cell* 2008; **134**:877–886.
23 Dor Y, Brown J, Martinez OI, Melton DA. Adult pancreatic beta-cells are formed by self-duplication rather than stem cell differentiation. *Nature* 2004; **429**:41–46.
24 Brennand K, Huangfu D, Melton D. All beta cells contribute equally to islet growth and maintanance. *PLoS Biol* 2007; **5**:e163.
25 Lee CS, De Leon DD, Kaestner KH, Stoffers DA. Regeneration of pancreatic islets after partial pancreatectomy in mice does not involve the reactivation of neurogenin-3. *Diabetes* 2006; **55**:269–272.
26 Nir T, Melton DA, Dor Y. Recovery from diabetes in mice by beta cell regeneration. *J Clin Invest* 2007; **117**:2553–2561.
27 Teta M, Rankin MM, Long SY, Stein GM, Kushner JA. Growth and regeneration of adult beta cells does not involve specialized progenitors. *Dev Cell* 2007; **12**:817–826.
28 Bonner-Weir S, Baxter LA, Schuppin GT, Smith FE. A second pathway for regeneration of adult exocrine and endocrine pancreas. *Diabetes* 1993; **42**:1715–1720.
29 Sharma A, Zangen DH, Reitz P, Taneja M, Lissauer ME, Miller CP, *et al.* The homeodomain protein idx1 increases after an early burst of proliferation during pancreatic regeneration. *Diabetes* 1999; **48**:507–513.
30 Rosenberg L, Rafaeloff R, Clas D, Kakugawa Y, Pittenger G, Vinik AI, *et al.* Induction of islet cell differentiation and new islet formation on the hamster: further support for a ductular origin. *Pancreas* 1996; **13**:38–46.
31 Fernandes A, King LC, Guz Y, Stein R, Wright CV, Teitelman G. Differentiation of new insulin-producing cells is induced by injury in adult pancreatic islets. *Endocrinology* 1997; **138**:1750–1762.
32 Xu X, D'Hoker J, Stange G, Bonné S, De Leu N, Xiao X, *et al.* Beta cells can be generated from endogenous progenitors in injured adult mouse pancreas. *Cell* 2008; **132**:197–207.
33 Slack JM. Metaplasia and transdifferentiation: from pure biology to the clinic. *Nat Rev Mol Cell Biol* 2007; **8**:369–378.
34 Minami K, Okuno M, Miyawaki K, Okumachi A, Ishizaki K, Oyama K, *et al.* Lineage tracing and characterization of insulin-secreting cells generated from adult pancreatic acinar cells. *Proc Natl Acad Sci U S A* 2005; **102**:15116–15121.
35 Zhou Q, Brown J, Kanarek A, Rajagopal J, Melton DA. *In vivo* programming of adult pancreatic exocrine cells to beta-cells. *Nature* 2008; **455**:627–632.

Future Directions: Islet Transplantation

Angela Koh, Peter Senior & A.M. James Shapiro

Keypoints

- Islet transplantation is a promising treatment for patients with type 1 diabetes with severe hypoglycemia, hypoglycemia unawareness and/or glycemic lability.
- Successful islet transplantation can lead to insulin independence, but this is usually not maintained in the long term.
- Graft function is preserved for several years beyond the loss of insulin independence, resulting in better glycemic control in spite of a return to insulin use.
- Current immunosuppression protocols include the use of more potent induction agents which may lead to better long-term outcomes.
- The side effects of maintenance immunosuppression are better understood, and appropriate dose titration and/or change to alternative agents have led to fewer and more tolerable side effects.
- The long-term impact of islet transplantation on diabetes-related complications is not fully elucidated, but there appears to be stabilization of microvascular and macrovascular disease.

Introduction

The discovery of insulin dramatically changed the outcome for patients with type 1 diabetes mellitus (T1DM) and the acute lethal complications of diabetes, such as diabetic ketoacidosis, could be effectively treated. The improved survival, however, allowed the development of the secondary complications of diabetes [1]. Typically, the patient with T1DM develops retinopathy, nephropathy, neuropathy or vascular disease over time. It was not until 1993 that definitive proof for the value of good glycemic control was established. The landmark Diabetes Control and Complications Trial (DCCT) study showed that the microvascular complications of diabetes could be delayed or avoided by good glycemic control, which required intensive insulin therapy [2]. Such therapy was associated with a hemoglobin A_{1c} (HbA_{1c}) that was 1% (11 mmol/mol) lower than that of the control group. It should be noted that the HbA_{1c} was not normalized and in the intensively treated group remained at least 1% (11 mmol/mol) above the upper limit of normal. Similar evidence was provided by the UK Prospective Diabetes Study (UKPDS) in T2DM with microvascular disease, showing a significant improvement for a decline of 1% (11 mmol/mol) in the HbA_{1c} [3]. Thus, glycemic control is essential if the microvascular complications of diabetes are to be prevented.

Controlling glycemia with exogenous insulin remains a challenge. Given the non-physiologic subcutaneous route of insulin administration, its inherent delay in absorption, the variability of serum levels obtained and the systemic versus portal venous delivery, it is perhaps remarkable how well the glucose levels are actually controlled. The newer insulin analogs have removed some of the variability and delay in absorption, but even with intensive therapy it is difficult to achieve normoglycemia. Continuous subcutaneous insulin administration helps further, but neither earlier nor more recent studies have managed to normalize glucose values [4,5]. Carbohydrate counting and attention to diet improves the quest for normoglycemia but does not offer a complete solution. The largest study using all available tools to optimize therapy was still associated with an increased risk of hypoglycemia [2]. In the DCCT, the risk for severe hypoglycemia (defined as needing third-party assistance) was increased threefold. Concern about hypoglycemia remains the limiting factor in attempts to achieve optimal glycemic control.

Many efforts have been made to generate a closed-loop system for glucose control. The first successful efforts were with the Biostator®, which involved continuous monitoring of blood glucose and then an insulin infusion using a computer-derived algorithm [6]. Although effective for a short period of time, it was impractical being bulky and plagued with flow problems from the double lumen catheter being used for sensing the glucose level. Insulin infusion pumps especially using insulin analogs (such as lispro or insulin aspart) have helped but are not closed-loop systems and require frequent glucose monitoring and rarely result in normal glycemia without severe hypoglycemia. The goal of any closed-loop system is to have reliable glucose sensing linked to appropriate insulin delivery on a continuous basis. Mechanical closed-loop systems may in the future achieve this but have been fraught with problems despite early promise. Transplantation of islets of Langerhans or of the whole pancreas can achieve a physiologic closed-loop system today.

Background history

Transplantation of pancreatic tissue was first tried in 1890 when a surgeon in England transplanted fragments of a sheep's pancreas into a boy with diabetic ketoacidosis [7]. The immune barriers, unknown at the time, were insurmountable, especially for a xenograft. The modern era of transplantation began in the 1960s when the use of steroids, especially when combined with azathioprine, allowed successful renal transplantation. The steroids block several cytokines and act as inhibitors of antigen presentation, and azathioprine is an inhibitor of purine synthesis and thus impedes the generation of active T cells. Cyclosporine A (CsA), a calcineurin inhibitor, which is associated with an impaired transcription in active T cells and thus blocks interleukin 2 (IL-2) activation, greatly improved transplantation graft survival [8]. In 1972, Ballinger and Lacy [9] demonstrated that chemical diabetes could be "cured" in mice with islet transplantation.

Many groups had been working in rodent and canine models to perfect islet isolation and maintain demonstrable β-cell insulin secretion [10,11]. Experiments in rats and mice showed that success in islet transplantations could be obtained in rodents [8] and the transplanted islets had a biphasic insulin secretory response to glucose [12]. Islet allotransplantation in animals was also successfully performed [13,14] and it has been possible to isolate human islets that would function in diabetic nude mice [15,16].

The results of these studies highlighted the need for purified islets and the importance of the site of transplantation. Multicellular islet tissue comprises 1.5% by weight of the whole pancreas [17]. Careful digestion is necessary to achieve a purified preparation, and collagenase became the mainstay in the digestion [10]. Success with isolation from human pancreases was more problematic than in animal studies [18,19]. Methods used for the dissociation of islets from the exocrine tissue required a combination of mechanical and enzymatic techniques.

The site of transplantation was also an issue. The pancreatic bed, because of the risk of inducing acute pancreatitis, was not a preferred option. Liver, spleen, renal subcapsule and an omental pouch have been the primary locations tried [14,20–22]. Work with immune privileged sites, such as the testes, has been ongoing but has not been routinely adapted [23]. A site with portal drainage has the natural advantage of mimicking the normal route of insulin delivery and is most commonly used for human islet transplantation [24]. The splenic site was associated with infarction [25] and so the liver, renal and omental pouch have been the preferred areas for islet transplantation. Compared to the native islet bed, all sites have the disadvantages that oxygenation is lower [26] and the intra-islet blood pressure is elevated [27]. Vascularization of the liver is advantageous and may help in the angiogenesis of the islets while an advantage of the omental pouch or renal site is the ability to remove the islets for histologic examination. When the liver is used, an unresolved question is whether the venous drainage of the islets appear in the portal sinusoids or the systemic circulation. A possible drawback of the portal site is that it allows more exposure to high levels of immunosuppressive drugs and their potential toxicity as they are absorbed [28].

Early human studies

The first human islet transplants were performed in the 1970s [29], with insulin independence rarely reported [30]. Up to 1998, approximately 260 patients with T1DM had received an islet transplant, with only 12% remaining insulin independent for more than 1 week [24]. The first two patients, transplanted as part of an early cohort transplanted in Edmonton in 1989 [31], received approximately 260 000 islets at the same time as a renal transplantation. Exogenous insulin was used intravenously for 14 days with intensive glucose monitoring in order to maintain euglycemia, which may help preserve β-cell function [32]. The immunosuppression therapy included corticosteroids, azathioprine, CsA, and Minnesota antilymphocyte globulin. Both patients demonstrated positive C-peptide status post-transplant, but both developed cytomegalovirus infection and lost islet mass, never achieving insulin independence. The subsequent five patients had transplants using both fresh and cryopreserved islets so that the total islet mass given exceeded 10 000 islet equivalents per kilogram. One patient obtained insulin independence for 2 years [33]. One patient who was transplanted at this time had a liver transplant with partially purified islets infused. Complete portal vein thrombosis ensued necessitating an urgent repeat liver transplant [34]. Another patient attained insulin independence for a period of time but eventually all patients required insulin again. On long-term follow-up, two of these patients have continued C-peptide production, the longest being more than 9 years since her transplant; however, subsequent technical problems arose in Edmonton, particularly with the collagenase, and so purified islets could not be obtained and thus islet transplantation lapsed as an avenue for treating diabetes. Other major centers, particularly Miami/Pittsburg, St. Louis and Milan, also reported early success [35–38] and demonstrated that the transplanted cells may survive for a prolonged time [39,40].

Pancreas transplantation

With improved immunosuppression the possibility of performing whole pancreas transplants, particularly at the time of renal transplantation for end-stage diabetic nephropathy, became a possibility [41]. Initial efforts were associated with peritonitis from exocrine drainage of the pancreatic duct. These problems were surmounted by using bladder drainage [42] such that success rates reached over 80% for 1-year graft survival accompanied by low mortality rates [43–46]. With newer techniques of anastomosis connecting the transplanted duodenum to an enteric drainage site [47], fewer problems were encountered (especially with the acidosis secondary to bicarbonate loss in the urine associated with the bladder anastomosis [48]). More than 25 000 whole pancreas transplants have been carried out worldwide. The 1-year graft survival rate has improved as a result of reduction in technical and immunologic failure rates [49]; however, the overall 10-year graft survival rate for deceased donor pancreas transplants has not substantially improved over time and was 48% for transplants between 1995 and 1999 [50]. Graft survival is better for simultaneous pancreas–kidney transplantation than either pancreas transplant alone or pancreas transplantation after kidney transplantation. The side effects are diminishing but it remains a technically challenging surgical procedure [51–53] with some morbidity and mortality. The excellent glycemic control [54] can lead to reversal of diabetic renal lesions [55], stabilization or improvement in neuropathy [56,57], vascular status [58,59] and stabilization but not necessarily improvement of retinopathy [60,61].

Islet transplantation in the new millennium

The unimpressive results of islet transplantation in the late 1990s, as illustrated by low rates of insulin independence [39,62,63], were related to the islet preparation (purity of preparations and adequate islet numbers) [64] and immunosuppression (potency and toxicity especially in terms of glucose tolerance), as has been reviewed by Hering and Ricordi [65]. The field of islet transplantation was rejuvenated with our report of seven consecutive cases, achieving insulin independence with islet transplantation using a steroid-free immunosuppression regimen (Edmonton protocol) [66]. Some of the factors associated with this success are discussed below.

Islet isolation

Islet mass availability remained a central issue for success. An adequate islet mass contributed to the success of the Edmonton protocol, with >11 000 islet equivalents per kilogram recipient body weight being transplanted.

The normal pancreas has 1.0–1.7 million islets [67,68], yet early studies showed only 250 000 islets being recovered for allotransplantation. Minimizing warm and cold ischemia time and other donor issues are important [69,70]. Using the University of Wisconsin perfusate solution at the time of organ retrieval enhanced the yield [71]. In addition, the intraductal delivery of collagenase [18,19,72], particularly with improved collagenase preparations [73,74], further enhanced the number of islets obtained. Great strides were made in characterizing the collagenase necessary for purified islet isolation, resulting in much better preparations. The enzyme preparation Liberase was widely used for islet isolation and is a blend of primarily collagenase type 1 and 2, but also has collagenase 3 and 4, clostripain, thermolysin and proteases (trypsin, chymotrypsin and elastase), and is associated with a low endotoxin load [74].

Another major advance was the development of a metal chamber by Ricordi *et al.* [75] allowing disassociation of islets with mechanical digestion and the continuous removal and harvesting of the liberated islets [76]. Purification of islets using a refrigerated COBE centrifuge and Ficoll gradient is also important. While it leads to some loss of cells, it reduces the otherwise substantial risk of intraportal hypertension associated with the infusion of unpurified preparations [34,77]. The increased purification may also have a negative effect because ductal elements, which may be important as a source for islet neogenesis, are removed [78].

Short-term culture of the islets may lead to enhanced purity without excessive loss of islets. In addition, the newer methods of islet isolation have removed all xenoproteins from the process, and this could further reduce the risk of rejection.

Immunosuppression

The importance of the appropriate immunosuppression regimen is demonstrated by the fact that with autotransplantation once 2500 islet equivalents per kilogram are provided then insulin independence can usually be achieved; however, three or four times this number of cells are required for insulin independence in the allotransplant environment [79]. In the Edmonton protocol, daclizumab was used for induction, followed by maintenance immunosuppression therapy with sirolimus (target trough levels of 12–15 μg/L for 3 months, then 10–12 μg/L) and low-dose tacrolimus (target trough levels of 3–6 μg/L) [66]. Such a combination allowed the omission of steroids from the regimen, which was a major advantage in the setting of borderline islet mass by reducing β-cell toxicity. Effective blockade of IL-2 with sirolimus, which inhibits T-cell expression and activation, and daclizumab, an antibody to IL-2 receptors, allows inhibition of T-cell activation and provides potent immunosuppression. Sirolimus can result in lipid abnormalities but was not known to affect glucose tolerance [80,81]. Tacrolimus, a more potent calcineurin inhibitor than CsA, is associated with some diabetogenicity [9,82–84] by inhibiting insulin release [85] in a dose-dependent manner [86], a problem shared by its predecessor CsA [87,88]. Hence, part of the rationale for using sirolimus as the mainstay of immunosuppression with low dose tacrolimus was to reduce diabetogenicity of the maintenance immunosuppression regimen.

Islet transplantation today

Following this initial success, more than 650 islet transplants have been performed worldwide using the Edmonton protocol or variants of it, and incorporating newer advances. Indeed, islet transplantation today is quite different from 10 years ago.

Islet preparation

Pancreas preservation

The University of Wisconsin solution (UW) was effective in pancreas preservation, but prolonged storage before islet isolation led to reduced recovery of viable islets [89]. The two-layer system using perflurodecalin (PFC) and UW for whole pancreas preservation was thus advocated for rescuing ischemically damaged pancreases [90]. This was because of the ability to ensure adequate oxygenation to the pancreas during preservation, and the reduction of cold ischemic injury by promoting adenosine triphosphate production [90]. It was also found that preservation in PFC resulted in the upregulation of anti-apoptotic genes and the downregulation of pro-apoptotic genes [91].

Indeed, islet recovery from pancreases preserved with the two-layer system was double that of UW alone [90,92]. Furthermore, PFC preservation resulted in an islet yield from pancreases procured from marginal donors that was sufficient for clinical transplantation in more cases than with UW alone [92]; however, more recently it was shown that there was no significant difference in islet yield or transplantation outcome regardless of whether the two-layer method or UW alone was used [93]. The authors currently use histidine-tryptophan-ketoglutarate solution alone for pancreas preservation, which appears to be equally effective as UW.

Islet culture

Previously, islets were infused into recipients within 2 hours of isolation to reduce the risk of ischemic injury to the islets [66]; however, this gave little time for appropriate quality control measures to be completed and potential recipients had to live near the transplant center. The authors' current practice is to culture islets for up to 72 hours prior to transplantation. This has numerous advantages because the additional time when the islets are in culture allows for the administration of conditioning or other immunosuppressive therapies, can result in improved safety because transplants can be carried out when the entire transplant team is present and allows for better islet characterization before transplant [94]. In addition, the decrease in total tissue volume with culture may reduce the risk of portal vein thrombosis. Furthermore, the use of regional islet processing centers has been advocated as a means of standardizing the islet product, and hence improving transplant outcomes. Islet culture can result in better islet recovery after shipment [95], and islet culture has now become standard and routine practice at most islet transplant centers worldwide.

Enzyme preparation and digestion protocols

In 2007 it became apparent that the crude collagenase extract in Liberase®, a secretion product of *Clostridium histolyticum* bacteria, could have been contaminated with bovine brain infusion extract, as this extract contains high levels of lipid, carbon and nitrogen which apparently facilitates the proliferation and secretory capacity of the bacteria. The specific risk to an islet patient is the possibility of prion transmission from the cow brain extract through the enzyme and into the pancreas organ during digestion of the gland. The estimated risk is currently unknown, but a working number is currently less than one in ten million – in other words exceedingly remote. Since then, most islet isolation centers have switched to an alternative enzyme manufactured by Serva. This is a GMP (good manufacturing practice) grade enzyme where the potential risk of prion transmission should be dramatically lower as no bovine brain extracts are used in the manufacture process. Using high-pressure liquid chromatography and collagenase activity assay, we found that the Serva collagenase is less pure and less potent than Liberase. With modification of our digestion protocols, we have now managed to achieve a high rate of islet isolation success (defined as >300 000 IEQs, >70% viability and <5 mL packed tissue volume) that is superior to historical outcomes from the Liberase era (unpublished data). Specifically, we use different digestion protocols for younger (≤35 years) versus older donors. For younger donors, we use collagenase and neutral protease simultaneously, while for older donors, a higher amount of collagenase initially, followed by sequential digestion with a lower amount of neutral protease was found to be optimal. Others have found that islet isolation outcomes and islet function are similar with the two enzyme blends [96].

Transplant procedure

Once adequate pure islets are prepared the patient is brought to radiology and percutaneous access is established under midazolam and fentanyl sedation. After infiltration of local anesthetic a 22-gauge Cheba needle is advanced under fluoroscopic guidance into the portal vein. Others have used computer tomography (CT) guidance or it is possible to gain access by the transjugular route or with laparoscopy [97]. A guidewire is then inserted into the main portal vein and a catheter is positioned with confirmation by portal venogram. Purified islets are then infused with frequent monitoring of portal pressure. If the portal pressure doubles or rises above 22 mmHg infusion is halted until it resolves, and if it does not resolve the infusion is discontinued. Initially, we used a 60-mL syringe but quickly adopted the use of an intravenous bag which is prepared in the laboratory [98]. This aids aseptic technique and may also pose less shear pressure on the islets and further provides some constant monitoring of portal pressure during islet infusion.

This percutaneous approach can result in the risk of bleeding from the liver, which was seen in the first report. Subsequently, Gelfoam® pledgets and coils were used to seal the catheter tract, and there was no more bleeding seen in the next 28 cases [99]; however, in 2003, there was a spate of post-procedural bleeding (defined as an acute fall in hemoglobin of 20%, associated with free fluid on ultrasound, the need for blood transfusion or surgical intervention for control of bleeding) [99,100]. Since then, the portal tributary cannulation site was plugged with coils, and the tract ablated using tissue glue (Tisseel®) with no further recurrence of bleeds in the next 35 procedures [100]. More recently, Avitene® paste dissolved in radiologic contrast and saline has been used instead to seal the catheter tract. When adequately deployed, this has eliminated bleeding risks and has the practical advantage of being clearly visible during deployment on fluoroscopy.

Before transplant, intravenous insulin and dextrose infusions are started to maintain euglycemia during transplant. Initially, insulin was discontinued after transplantation and was avoided unless hyperglycemia (serum glucose ≥11.1 mmol/L) occurred [66]. Subsequently, this threshold was lowered and insulin was given if pre-meal glucose was >6.0 mmol/L or 2-hour post-meal glucose was >8.0 mmol/L [99].

Recently, it was shown that maintaining euglycemia in the immediate post-transplant period could contribute to better graft survival [101]. Since mid 2005, it has been our policy to maintain euglycemia (serum glucose 4.0–7.0 mmol/L) following transplant by using intravenous insulin (minimum of 1 unit/hour) with dextrose infusions for the first 48 hours, and subcutaneous insulin thereafter.

Intravenous heparin is also infused to keep the pro-thrombin time 70–90 seconds for 48 hours after transplantation to promote engraftment by reducing the immediate blood mediated inflammatory reaction (IBMIR). Heparin is withheld if there is inadequate tract plugging with Avitene (<3 cm in length) until imaging confirms the absence of bleeding.

After the heparin infusion is discontinued, subcutaneous low molecular weight heparin (30 mg enoxaparin twice daily) is administered for 7 days and 81 mg/day aspirin for 14 days.

In addition, patients receive 400 mg sulfamethozazole–80 mg trimethoprim one tablet daily for 6 months, *Pneumocystis* pneumonia prophylaxis and 900 mg/day valganciclovir for 14 weeks when there is cytomegalovirus status mismatch between donor and recipient, and in patients who have received lymphocyte-depleting induction agents.

Immunosuppression

The immunosuppressive regimen of the original Edmonton protocol is still being used today, but with some modifications. Daclizumab was initially given at a dosage of 1 mg/kg every 2 weeks five times. After 2003, this was changed to 2 mg/kg at transplant and at 5 days post-transplant [99]. This was because the latter regimen was found to be efficacious and was more convenient for patients.

Recently, induction with antithymocyte globulin (6 mg/kg) and etanercept, with maintenance immunosuppression with tacrolimus (target trough level 8–10 μg/L) and mycophenolate mofetil (1 g twice daily), has been used [100]. Also, a lymphocyte depletion protocol consisting of alemtuzumab (Campath-1H), tacrolimus and mycophenolate mofetil is being evaluated. Preliminary data suggest that the use of these potent induction agents have improved short to medium-term graft outcomes [101–103].

Many of the initial patients who were on sirolimus and tacrolimus for maintenance immunosuppression have had intolerable side effects which were attributed to sirolimus, necessitating a switch of immunosuppression to tacrolimus and mycophenolate mofetil. This latter combination appears to be as efficacious and better tolerated [104]. Furthermore, sirolimus impairs β-cell regeneration, and could contribute to the observed gradual loss of graft function seen following islet transplantation [105]. Thus, this combination is increasingly the first-line maintenance immunosuppression choice for islet transplantation.

Islet transplantation outcomes

Glycemic control

Insulin independence was achieved in 11 out of the first 12 patients, after a minimum of 9000 IE/kg were transplanted [66]. HbA_{1c} levels improved in all patients, and this was achieved without hypoglycemia and was accompanied by an improved stability of glucose control [66]. Unfortunately, insulin independence was not sustainable in the long term for the majority of patients. From survival analysis, only approximately 10% of patients remained off insulin at 5 years, although most patients (approximately 80%) still had C-peptide present (Figure 61.6) [99].

In terms of overall blood glucose control, patients who remained off insulin did the best (median HbA_{1c} of 6.2%, 44 mmol/mol), similar to the patients who were back on insulin but still had C peptide (median HbA_{1c} of 6.7%, 50 mmol/mol). Patients who had lost all graft function had relatively poor glucose control (median HbA_{1c} of 9.0%, 75 mmol/mol) and required more insulin than before the transplant (Figure 61.7) [99].

The HYPO score and lability index (LI) were developed to measure the severity of hypoglycemia and glycemic lability. The HYPO score is generated using a combination of 4 weeks of self glucose monitoring results and the patients' self-reported hypoglycemic episodes over the previous year. For every episode of hypoglycemia <3 mmol/L during the 4 weeks, patients were instructed to record all symptoms felt and whether assistance was required for recognition or treatment of the hypoglycemia. Higher scores were given for more severe hypoglycemic episodes (i.e. lower glucose values, absence of symptoms or neuroglycopenic symptoms, needing outside help for recognition/treatment), while from the self-reported episodes during the past year higher points were awarded if an ambulance was called or glucagon given. The LI was also calculated from the 4 weeks of glucose records, using a formula that takes the number of glucose readings, the glucose values and the time interval between testing into account [106]. These scores are now routinely used in the assessment of suitability of a candidate for transplant, as well as for follow-up of patients after transplant. In addition, the Clarke score [107] is also frequently used, with a score of four or more indicating hypoglycemia unawareness.

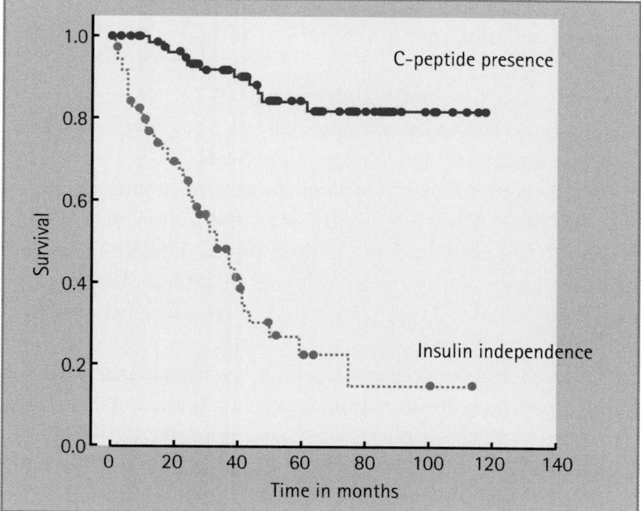

Figure 61.6 Current survival analysis for insulin independence and graft function as indicated by presence of C-peptide.

Both the HYPO score and LI show marked improvement post-transplant. With resumption of insulin use, there was more lability and some episodes of hypoglycemia, but both scores were still better than pre-transplant [99].

A key indication for islet transplantation is hypoglycemia unawareness. Patients who have received a pancreas transplant have restoration of their counter-regulatory response to hypoglycemia [108,109]. The autonomic response and hence hypoglycemia awareness is also improved post-pancreas transplant [110]; however, the same restoration in counter-regulatory responses and symptom recognition was not seen following successful islet transplantation [111]. Conversely, others have found that counter-regulatory hormonal and symptom responses to hypoglycemia do improve after islet transplantation [112–114]. The reasons for these differences are unclear; however, there may be a subset of patients who have return of hypoglycemia awareness, and/or the timing of testing could be critical. Indeed, we have noted that 85% of our cohort of islet transplant recipients reported return of symptoms of hypoglycemia, although 62% of them subsequently lost hypoglycemia awareness.

Diabetes complications

Retinopathy

Retinopathy has been reported to remain stable following islet transplantation [115,116]. The majority of our patients (approxi-

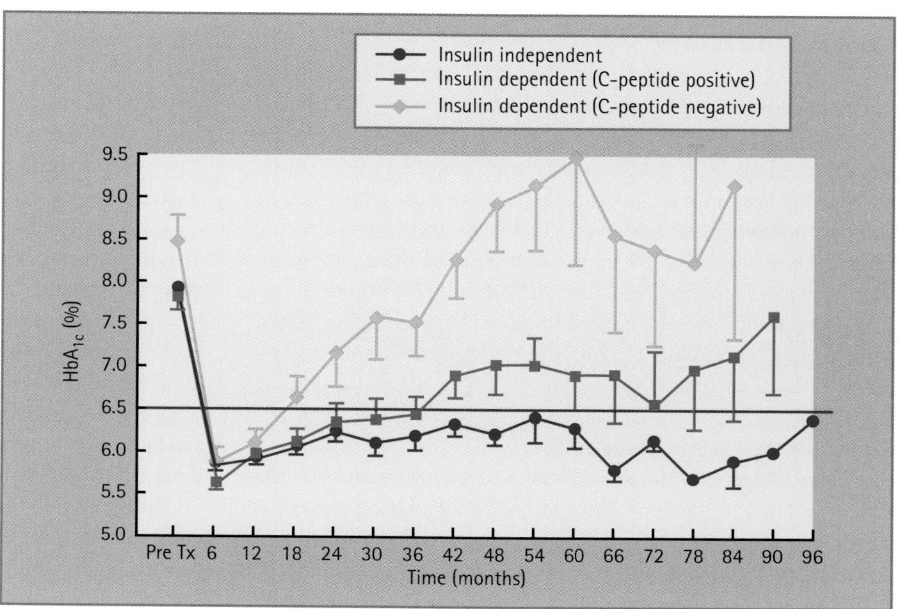

Figure 61.7 Glycemic control is related to islet graft function. DCCT result (%) = (0.0915 × New IFCC result in mmol/mol) + 2.15.

mately 80%) showed either no change or an improvement in retinopathy grade compared with baseline 3 years following islet transplantation; however, in our cohort, 18 of 98 (18.4%) subjects had either vitreous hemorrhage or need for laser photocoagulation after islet transplantation, suggesting that close ophthalmologic follow-up remains necessary.

Nephropathy

We have previously reported that the estimated glomerular filtration rate (eGFR) (by MDRD study equation) declined with time. The median rate of eGFR decline was $-0.39\,mL/min/1.73\,m^2/$month, with wide inter-patient variability [117]. This decline in GFR is comparable to that seen in optimally treated albuminuric patients with T1DM [118]; however, for one-third of the patients, the decline in eGFR exceeded that in untreated diabetic nephropathy [119]. In addition, on follow-up, progression in albuminuria was seen in 24% of the patients, with regression only in 2.4% [117].

When tacrolimus and mycophenolate mofetil were used for maintenance immunosuppression, no difference in the rate of GFR decline was seen compared with either medically treated controls or the general population, nor was there any progression in albuminuria [120].

It is not clear at present whether the decline in renal function in islet alone transplants is brought about by progression of diabetic nephropathy or the effects of immunosuppression, in particular the combination of sirolimus and tacrolimus. Nevertheless, care has to be taken during the patient selection process with regard to the assessment of renal function.

Neuropathy

There was no change in neuropathy status as assessed by vibration perception threshold or neuropathy disability score in our cohort [121], and others have shown stabilization of neuropathy [115].

Cardiovascular disease

A substantial proportion (30%) of islet transplant recipients at our center have pre-existing coronary artery disease (CAD) prior to transplantation. In terms of CAD risk factors, triglyceride levels increased (0.82 ± 0.04 vs $1.09 \pm 0.06\,mmol/L$; $P < 0.001$), while there was a reduction in low density lipoprotein (LDL) cholesterol levels (2.53 ± 0.06 vs $2.14 \pm 0.06\,mmol/L$; $P < 0.001$), likely from an increase in statin use following transplantation. Blood pressure remained unchanged. Following islet transplantation, the rate of incident (new or worse) CAD was similar to the general population with T1DM at 8.9 events/1000 patient years [122].

Procedure-related complications

Complete portal vein thrombosis has not occurred with the use of purified islet allograft preparations, although partial thrombosis (of right or left branch, or peripheral segmental vein) was seen in about 5% of patients, all of whom were treated with anticoagulation without any long-term clinical sequelae [66,99]. The risk of portal vein thrombosis has been minimized by limiting the islet packed cell volume, careful monitoring of portal pressures during islet infusion and intraportal dosing with heparin followed by systemic anticoagulation. Other rare complications include gallbladder puncture and arteriovenous fistulae formation.

Liver enzymes (aspartate transaminase, alanine aminotransferase and alkaline phosphatase) were elevated in more than 50% of transplants and are generally subclinical. These enzymes peak at around 1 week and resolve spontaneously within a month [123].

Changes consistent with fatty liver have also been observed on imaging post-transplantation [124]. These steatotic changes were confirmed with biopsy in some cases, and may be related to the high insulin levels the hepatocytes are exposed to following intrahepatic transplant [124]. It is currently unclear whether these changes may result in any long-term sequelae.

Side effects of immunosuppression

Most patients may have some side effects from immunosuppresion, but it is highly variable among patients.

Mouth ulcers occur in >90% of the patients and is associated with sirolimus. These are usually small and self-limiting, but on occasion may be numerous and/or severe enough to require inpatient care. Most patients respond to topical therapy, dose reduction and switching to the tablet formulation of sirolimus [99].

Gastrointestinal disturbances, either constipation or diarrhea, are also common, occurring in 60% of the patients, while acne was noted in 52%. Peripheral edema was reported by 43% of the patients [100].

Ovarian cysts following transplants have been found to be common [99]. Another study found that among women, ovarian cysts occurred in 62% of the subjects, and menstrual irregularity developed in all six subjects who had regular menstrual cycles before transplant [125]. At our center, new ovarian cysts were found in 33 of 57 (57.9%) women after islet transplantation. Most cysts were asymptomatic but 14 women reported pelvic pain. Sirolimus withdrawal was associated with a reduction in cyst size and resolution of cysts in 80% of the subjects. Also, the use of combined oral contraception appeared to be protective against ovarian cyst development [126].

Other complications related to immunosuppressive therapy include anemia, leukopenia, hypertension, dyslipidemia, weight loss and fatigue [100].

Tacrolimus was associated in a dose-dependent manner with tremor and nephrotoxicity. The combination of sirolimus and tacrolimus could also worsen renal function. Indeed, two patients in whom tacrolimus was switched to mycophenolate mofetil had stabilization of renal impairment [127]. Also, three patients had resolution of proteinuria after sirolimus was withdrawn and replaced by a combination of mycophenolate mofetil and higher dose tacrolimus [128].

Mycophenolate mofetil is generally well tolerated, with the most commonly reported side effect being gastrointestinal in

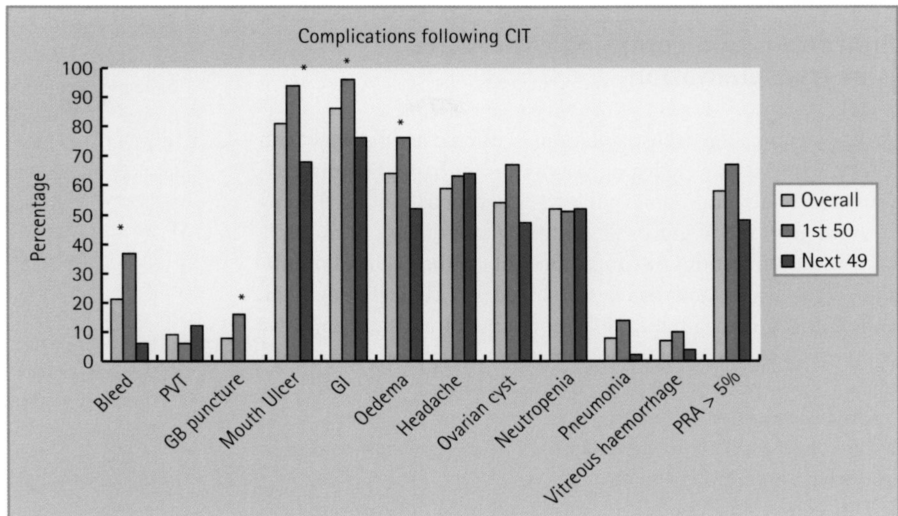

Figure 61.8 Complications following clinical islet transplantation – first 50 vs next 49 patients in Edmonton. * Indicates significant difference ($P < 0.05$) between first 50 and next 49 subjects. GB, gall bladder; GI, gastrointestinal; PRA, panel reactive antibody; PVT, portal vein thrombosis.

nature (bloating, diarrhea, abdominal cramps), which usually subside with dose reduction [129].

Pneumonia occurred in three patients, of whom one was considered fungal in etiology [98].

Cytomegaloviral disease has not occurred, although seroconversion from negative to positive has occurred in 4 of 67 (6%) patients. To date, no lymphoproliferative disease has been observed.

With experience, we have learned to tailor the immunosuppression regimen and target drug levels to minimize side effects without compromising graft function, such that fewer complications are seen in patients transplanted more recently than in earlier patients (Figure 61.8).

A total of 34 patients had undergone immunosuppression change from sirolimus + tacrolimus to tacrolimus + mycophenolate mofetil following islet transplantation. The three most frequent reasons for immunosuppression change were peripheral edema (18/34, 53%), gastrointestinal symptoms (11/34, 32%) and ovarian cysts in women (9/26, 35%). These all improved after the immunosuppression change. Also noteworthy, there were no changes in graft function or immune status following the change (Table 61.1) [104].

Table 61.1 Reasons for and outcomes after immunosuppression (IS) change.

	No. of patients with event before IS change (n = 34)	% with improvement / no change / worsening after IS change	*P* value
Peripheral edema	18	83 / 17 / 0	<0.001
Gastrointestinal symptoms	11	75 / 8 / 17	0.01
Fatigue	9	44 / 55 / 0	0.05
Proteinuria/renal function decline	6	100 / 0 / 0	0.01
Ulcers	4	100 / 0 / 0	0.05
Ovarian cysts/menstrual abnormalities in female patients (n = 26)	9	78 / 22 / 0	0.01

Immune sensitization

The percentage of panel reactive antibodies (PRA) increased in 13% of the patients from levels <15% to ≥15% after transplant [99]. Recently, it has become clear to us that positive PRA does impact islet transplant outcome negatively. Indeed, pre-transplant PRA of >15% in either class I or II is an independent predictor of poor graft survival (in terms of C-peptide) after transplant [130].

For individuals with high PRA, it will be important to determine the specific antibodies causing the positive PRA and a flow cytometry-based cross-match performed against potential donors before transplant. Our current policy is to perform prospective cross-matches for all recipients with PRA above 5% and for those who have received previous transplants.

It has become apparent that high rates of broad PRA sensitization were observed in patients when immunosuppression was slowly and completely withdrawn following complete graft loss [131]. Our current approach is therefore not to withdraw all immunosuppression when a patient loses all islet function, but rather to wean down to single agent therapy with mycophenolate (Myfortic® therapy). We currently plan to continue this for at least 2 years after function is lost in order to reduce the risk of subsequent sensitization. The effectiveness of this strategy is still to be evaluated.

Indications and contraindications for islet transplantation

At our center, islet transplantation is offered to patients with T1DM who have severe hypoglycemia and/or hypoglycemia unawareness, or glycemic lability, in spite of optimal medical therapy with frequent blood glucose monitoring and the use of multiple daily insulin injections or continuous subcutaneous insulin infusion. This is, by and large, still based on clinical judgment, although the use of the HYPO score and LI adds an objective component to the decision. Some patients have progressive complications despite optimization of medical therapy. Although we originally considered this group, they are now the exception, as we are concerned about the potential for immunosuppression to exacerbate renal impairment.

Diabetes-related complications are not absolute contraindications for islet transplantation. For patients with unstable retinopathy, we recommend waiting for 6 months from the last treatment for the disease to stabilize before islet transplantation because there is a risk of worsening following transplantation. The sirolimus and tacrolimus combination is avoided in patients with macroalbuminuria (>300 mg/day). We prefer not to transplant patients with mild to moderate reduction in GFR (<60 mL/min/1.73 m^2). We also recommend waiting for at least 6 months following myocardial infarction, revascularization procedure or evidence of ischemia on functional cardiac testing. A severely reduced left ventricular ejection fraction <30% is a contraindication for islet transplantation.

The current accepted indications and contraindications for islet transplantation in most islet transplantation centers are listed in Table 61.2.

Table 61.2 Indications and contraindications for islet transplantation.

Indications for islet transplantation

Clinical history compatible with type 1 diabetes, with stimulated C-peptide <0.3 μg/L on mixed meal tolerance test

Intensive diabetes management:

- Glucose testing ≥3 times/day
- ≥3 insulin injections/day or insulin pump as directed by endocrinologist, diabetologist or diabetes specialist with ≥3 clinical evaluations during the past year

≥1 severe hypoglycemic event, defined as an event with one of the following symptoms: memory loss; confusion; uncontrollable behavior; irrational behavior; unusual difficulty in awakening; suspected seizure; seizure; loss of consciousness; or visual symptoms, in which the subject was unable to treat him/herself and with blood glucose <54 mg/dL (3 mmol/L) or prompt recovery after oral carbohydrate, intravenous glucose or glucagon in the past 1 year

One of the following:

- Reduced hypoglycemia awareness (Clarke score ≥4 or HYPO score ≥90th percentile or ≥1047) within last 6 months
- Marked glycemic lability with wide swings in glucose levels despite optimal therapy, with glycemic lability index ≥90th percentile or 433 within last 6 months
- Composite Clarke score ≥4 + HYPO score ≥75th percentile (≥423) + lability index ≥75th percentile (≥329)

Contraindications for islet transplantation

Glycated hemoglobin ≥10% (86 mmol/mol)

Untreated proliferative retinopathy

Blood pressure >160/100 mmHg

Glomerular filtration rate <80 mL/min/1.73 m^2

Presence or history of macroalbuminuria >300 mg/day

Presence or history of panel reactive anti-HLA antibodies (by flow cytometry)

Active infections, including:

- Hepatitis B, hepatitis C or HIV
- Tuberculosis requiring treatment within the previous 3 years
- Invasive aspergillus, histoplasmosis or coccidiomycosis within 1 year

Severe cardiac disease:

- Myocardial infarction within 6 months
- Evidence of ischemia on functional cardiac testing within 1 year
- Left ventricular ejection fraction <30%

Any history of malignancy except for completely resected squamous or basal cell carcinoma of the skin

A history of factor V deficiency

Any coagulopathy or medical condition requiring long-term anticoagulant therapy after transplantation

Receiving treatment for a medical condition requiring chronic use of systemic steroids except for the use of ≤5 mg/day prednisolone or equivalent

Any medical condition that could interfere with safe participation in islet transplantation

Desired pregnancy (female recipient)

Patient evaluation

At the assessment visit for islet transplantation the patient should have a realistic expectation of the outcome. If the patient has frequent hypoglycemia and glycemic lability problems, then both of these are readily correctable by islet transplantation. The ability to render the patient free of the progression risk of diabetes complications is unproven at this time, although given good glycemic control this may be expected in the longer term. Patients who have active infection, a history of cancer, severe vascular disease or active foot ulceration, who abuse alcohol or drugs, or who are younger than 18 or older than 65 years are not usually considered. Once the patient meets the entry criteria and is willing to accept the risks of the procedure and immunosuppression, a full evaluation is required. This includes a thorough history and physical examination, the latter concentrating on diabetes complications – retinopathy, neuropathy (autonomic and peripheral) and vascular disease. Our laboratory evaluation includes details of these complications with an ophthalmology report required, 24-hour urine for albuminuria, protein and creatinine clearance; together with a serum creatinine, ECG, stress methoxyisobutylisonitrile (MIBI) scan and a lipid panel. If there is any suggestion of an abnormality either clinically or on vascular testing, coronary angiogram is performed. In addition, the basic transplant screens are required, including blood group, complete blood count, coagulation screen, liver function tests, electrolytes, calcium, magnesium, phosphorus, checks for HIV, hepatitis, Epstein–Barr virus, syphilis, cytomegalovirus and urine culture. An ultrasound of the abdomen and liver is required to ensure that no lesions are present in the liver. A hemangioma on the right side of the liver would place a patient at increased risk of bleeding during the procedure if a percutaneous approach was used. In subjects older than 40 years, mammograms are performed in women and prostate-specific antigen determinations in men. Considerable time is spent reviewing the potential complications with the patients so that each individual can make a personal assessment of the risk : benefit ratio for themselves and decide if they wish to proceed. In most other transplant settings (heart and liver), the issues are life and death but in islet transplantation this is not the case, as continuing to work with other insulin regimens is possible and thus risk : benefit issues are different.

Challenges and future directions

Islet shortage

The shortage of donor pancreases for islet transplantation remains a challenge. Most patients require more than one islet infusion to become insulin independent. Given the limited supply of organs, the ability to achieve insulin independence after infusion of islets from a single donor is an important goal which has been achieved by Hering *et al.* [101] in carefully selected recipients given excellent islet preparations, intensive peri-transplant management and alternative induction immunosuppression. Other alternative sources of islets include xenografts (e.g. porcine islets) or stem cells, but remain in the preclinical experimental phase at present [132–134].

Islet engraftment

Defects in insulin secretion soon after transplantation of what should be an adequate islet mass indicates that many islets were lost at the time of engraftment. This could be because of hypoxia early post-transplant [135], the toxic effects of the immunosuppressive drugs [136] and the IBMIR, which results in immune destruction of islets [137]. It has been estimated that only one-third of islets engraft successfully [138].

Various strategies are being tested in attempts to improve engraftment, including the use of vascular growth factors to promote revascularization [139], inhibitors of IBMIR [140] and anti-apoptotic peptides (e.g. caspase inhibitors) [141]. The use of low molecular weight dextran sulfate was found to block IBMIR to a greater extent than heparin, possibly by its more potent inhibition of the complement system [142]. The use of islet surface heparinization was also shown to attenuate IBMIR significantly *in vitro* and *in vivo*, without systemic side effects [143].

Monitoring the islet graft

A key barrier to understanding what happens to the islet graft after transplantation is the lack of access to the graft. Current methods of monitoring graft function are based on the measurement of markers of glucose homeostasis, which may not be disrupted in early stages of rejection [144]. Immunologic monitoring is limited by the lack of standardized markers for autoimmunity and rejection [145]. Unlike other solid organ transplants, serial protocol liver biopsies may not yield sufficient islet tissue for examination. Several approaches for β-cell imaging have been proposed, but are still in various stages of development [146]. Clearly, it is of vital importance to develop one or more methods to detect graft dysfunction in its early stages or even before it happens, so as to allow intervention in an attempt to rescue the graft.

Promoting graft survival

Islet graft function appears to decline over time, with most patients returning to insulin use. The glucagon-like peptide 1 (GLP-1) agonist, exenatide, when used in islet transplant recipients with failing islet graft function, resulted in reduction in insulin requirements, but this could not be sustained when the drug was discontinued, suggesting that there was no trophic effect on β-cell mass [147]. The lack of detectable changes in markers of allo-immunity or auto-immunity in the majority of islet transplant recipients, together with the absence of significant inflammatory infiltrate in histologic specimens of islet transplants, suggest that non-immunologic mechanisms have an important role in the gradual graft loss [99,148]. Possible culprits include increased metabolic demand and toxicity of immunosuppressants, and certainly warrants further investigation.

Immunosuppression toxicity

While newer immunosuppressant drug combinations are associated with less toxicity, the ideal situation would be the ability to withdraw immunosuppressive drugs after an initial period of use post-transplant. To achieve this, tolerance to the graft must be induced. Co-stimulation blockade has shown promise for tolerance induction. There have been encouraging results with belatacept (LEA29Y), a potent new CTLA4-Ig in primate models of islet transplants [149], and clinical trials in human subjects are being undertaken. Indeed, the use of belatacept for ongoing maintenance immunosuppression, thus allowing the avoidance of calcineurin inhibitors, has been used successfully in the renal transplantation setting and may be the basis for future maintenance therapy [150].

Another strategy would be islet encapsulation, but this has been associated with limited success to date [151].

Conclusions

Islet transplantation can correct problems with glycemic lability and recurrent hypoglycemia. Given its technical ease, it is particularly suitable for those with problems with glycemic control and no other major complications. The more technically difficult whole pancreas transplant provides stable glucose control and is ideal in those undergoing simultaneous renal transplant. The islet transplant procedure has some risks, both acutely (particularly bleeding, and thrombosis in the portal vein circulation) and in the long-term, the unknown but real risk of sepsis and neoplasms. For some patients with major problems, with diabetes control these risks are acceptable. Whether the good glycemic control attained will prevent complications in the long term will take years to resolve. Using the indication of progressive diabetes complications is less suitable at this time, given the problems encountered. Islet transplantation can free a patient with very difficult diabetes from the risks of frequent hypoglycemia or glycemic lability. The decision whether to proceed can only be made by an informed patient who has to cope with difficult diabetes on a daily basis.

Major steps have been taken in islet transplantation but more needs to be done. Significant changes over the past 10 years have resulted in improved outcomes, but many challenges still remain. Islet transplantation has faced hurdles before and overcome them. These new challenges can be met and solved. To quote Sir Winston Churchill, "Now this is not the end. It is not even the beginning of the end. But it is, perhaps, the end of the beginning."

References

1 Banting FG, Best CH, Collip JB, Campbell WR, Fletcher AA. Pancreatic extracts in the treatment of diabetes mellitus: preliminary report. *CMAJ* 1922; **12**:141–146.

2 Diabetes Control and Complications Trial Research Group. The effect of intensive treatment of diabetes on the development and progression of long-term complications in insulin-dependent diabetes mellitus. *N Engl J Med* 1993; **329**:977–986.

3 UK Prospective Diabetes Study (UKPDS) Group. Intensive blood-glucose control with sulphonylureas or insulin compared with conventional treatment and risk of complications in patients with type 2 diabetes (UKPDS 33). *Lancet* 1998; **352**:837–853.

4 Reeves ML, Seigler DE, Ryan EA, Skyler JS. Glycemic control in insulin dependent diabetes mellitus: comparison of outpatient intensified conventional therapy with continuous subcutaneous infusion. *Am J Med* 1982; **72**:673–680.

5 Tsui E, Barnie A, Ross S, Parkes R, Zinman B. Intensive insulin therapy with insulin lispro: a randomized trial of continuous subcutaneous insulin infusion versus multiple daily insulin injection. *Diabetes Care* 2001; **24**:1722–1727.

6 Ratzmann KP, Bruns W, Schulz B, Zander E. Use of the artificial B-cell (Biostator) in improving insulin therapy in unstable insulin-dependent diabetes. *Diabetes Care* 1982; **5**:11–17.

7 Williams P. Notes on diabetes treated with extract and by grafts of sheep's pancreas. *Br Med J* 1894; **2**:1303–1304.

8 Pirsch JD, Miller J, Deierhoi MH, Vincenti F, Filo RS. A comparison of tacrolimus (FK506) and cyclosporine for immunosuppression after cadaveric renal transplantation. *Transplantation* 1997; **7**: 977–983.

9 Ballinger WF, Lacy PE. Transplantation of intact pancreatic islets in rats. *Surgery* 1972; **72**:175–186.

10 Lindall A, Steffes M, Sorensen R. Immunoassayable insulin content of subcellular fractions of rat islets. *Endocrinology* 1969; **85**: 218–223.

11 Lacy PE, Walker MM, Fink CJ. Perifusion of isolated rat islets *in vitro*: participation of the microtubular system in the biphasic release of insulin. *Diabetes* 1972; **21**:987–998.

12 Bromme HJ, Hahn HJ, Blech W. Biphasic release of insulin from islets of Langerhans after their transplantation into the liver of rats. *Horm Metab Res* 1998; **20**:138–140.

13 Bowen KM, Lafferty KJ. Reversal of diabetes by allogenic islet transplantation without immunosuppression. *Aust J Exp Biol Med Sci* 1980; **58**:441–447.

14 Naji A, Silvers WK, Plotkin SA, Dafoe D, Barker CF. Successful islet transplantation in spontaneous diabetes. *Surgery* 1979; **86**:218–226.

15 Ricordi C, Scharp DW, Lacy PE. Reversal of diabetes in nude mice after transplantation of fresh and 7-day culture (24°C) human pancreatic islets. *Transplantation* 1988; **45**:994–996.

16 Gerling IC, Kotb M, Fraga D, Sabek O, Gaber AO. No correlation between *in vitro* and *in vivo* function of human islets. *Transplant Proc* 1998; **30**:587–588.

17 Hellman B. The frequency distribution of the number and volume of the islets of Langerhans in man. *Acta Soc Med Ups* 1959; **64**:432-60.

18 Rajotte RV,Warnock GL, Evans MG, Ellis D, Dawidson I. Isolation of viable islets of Langerhans from collagenase-perfused canine and human pancreata. *Transplant Proc* 1987; **19**:918–922.

19 Gray DWR, McShane P, Grant A, Morris PJ. A method for isolation of islets of Langerhans from the human pancreas. *Diabetes* 1984; **33**:1055–1061.

20 Marchetti P, Scharp DW, Olack BJ, Swanson CJ, Bier D, Cobelli C, *et al.* Glucose metabolism, insulin sensitivity, and glucagon secretion in dogs with intraportal or intrasplenic islet autografts. *Transplant Proc* 1992; **24**:2828–2829.

21 Merani S, Toso C, Emamaullee J, Shapiro AM. Optimal site for pancreatic islet transplantation. *Br J Surg* 2008; **95**:1449–1461.

22 Yasunami Y, Lacy PE, Finek EH. A new site for islet transplantation: a peritoneal–omental pouch. *Transplantation* 1983; **36**:181–182.

23 Selawry HP, Whittington K. Extended allograft survival of islets grafted into intra-abdominally placed testis. *Diabetes* 1984; **33**:405–406.

24 White SA, James RFL, Swift SM, Kimber RM, Nicholson ML. Human islet cell transplantation: future prospects. *Diabet Med* 2001; **18**:78–103.

25 White SA, London NJ, Johnson PR, Davies JE, Pollard C, Contractor HH, *et al.* The risks of total pancreatectomy and splenic islet autotransplantation. *Cell Transplant* 2000; **9**:19–24.

26 Carlsson PO, Palm F, Andersson A, Liss P. Markedly decreased oxygen tension in transplanted rat pancreatic islets irrespective of the implantation site. *Diabetes* 2001; **50**:489–495.

27 Carlsson PO, Jansson L, Andersson A, Källskog O. Capillary blood pressure in syngeneic rat islets transplanted under the renal capsule is similar to that of the implantation organ. *Diabetes* 1998; **47**:1586–1593.

28 Shapiro AM, Gallant H, Hao E, Wong J, Rajotte R, Yatscoff R, *et al.* Portal vein immunosuppressant levels and islet graft toxicity. *Transplant Proc* 1998; **39**:641.

29 Najarian JS, Sutherland DER, Matas AJ, Steffes MW, Simmons RL, Goetz FC. Human islet transplantation: a preliminary report. *Transplant Proc* 1977; **9**:233–236.

30 Largiader F, Kolb E, Binswanger U, Illig R. Successful allotransplantation of an island of Langerhans. *Schweiz Med Wochenschr* 1979; **109**:1733–1736.

31 Warnock GL, Kneteman NM, Ryan EA, Evans MG, Seelis RE, Halloran PF, *et al.* Continued function of pancreatic islets after transplantation in type 1 diabetes. *Lancet* 1989; **2**:570–572.

32 Diabetes Control and Complications Trial Research Group. Effect of intensive therapy on residual β-cell function in patients with type 1 diabetes in the Diabetes Control and Complications Trial. *Ann Intern Med* 1998; **128**:517–523.

33 Warnock GL, Kneteman NM, Ryan EA, Rabinovitch A, Rajotte RV. Long-term follow-up after transplantation of insulin-producing pancreatic islets into patients with type1 (insulin-dependent) diabetes mellitus. *Diabetologia* 1992; **35**:89–95.

34 Shapiro AMJ, Lakey JRT, Rajotte RV, Warnock GL, Friedlich MS, Jewell LD, *et al.* Portal vein thrombosis after transplantation of partially purified pancreatic islets in a combined human liver/islet allograft. *Transplantation* 1995; **59**:1060–1063.

35 Ricordi C, Tzakis A, Alejandro R, Zeng YJ, Demetris AJ, Carroll P, *et al.* Detection of pancreatic islet tissue following islet allotransplantation in man. *Transplantation* 1991; **52**:1079–1080.

36 Tzakis AG, Ricordi C, Alejandro R, Zeng Y, Fung JJ, Todo S, *et al.* Pancreatic islet transplantation after upper abdominal exenteration and liver replacement. *Lancet* 1990; **336**:402–405.

37 Scharp DW, Lacy PE, Santiago JV, McCullough CS, Weide LG, Boyle PJ, *et al.* Results of our first nine intraportal islet allografts in type 1, insulin-dependent diabetic patients. *Transplantation* 1991; **51**:76–85.

38 Socci C, Davalli AM, Vignali A, Bertuzzi F, Maffi P, Zammarchi O, *et al.* Evidence of *in vivo* human islet graft function despite a weak response to *in vitro* perfusion. *Transplant Proc* 1992; **24**: 3056–3057.

39 Alejandro R, Lehmann R, Ricordi C, Kenyon NS, Angelico MC, Burke G, *et al.* Long-term function (6 years) of islet allografts in type 1 diabetes. *Diabetes* 1997; **46**:1983–1989.

40 Robertson RP, Lanz KJ, Sutherland DE, Kendall DM. Prevention of diabetes for up to 13 years by autoislet transplantation after pancreatectomy for chronic pancreatitis. *Diabetes* 2001; **50**:47–50.

41 Kelly WD, Lillehei RC, Merkel FK, Idezuki Y, Goetz FC. Allotransplantation of the pancreas and duodenum along with the kidney in diabetic nephropathy. *Surgery* 1967; **61**:827–837.

42 Cook K, Sollinger HW, Warner T, Kamps D, Belzer FO. Pancreaticocystostomy: an alternative method for exocrine drainage of segmental pancreatic allografts. *Transplantation* 1983; **35**:634–636.

43 Bûsing M, Heimes M, Martin D, Schulz T, Dehof S, Kozuschek W. Simultaneous pancreas-/kidney transplantation: the Bochum experience. *Exp Clin Endocrinol Diabetes* 1997; **105**:92–97.

44 Sutherland DER. Pancreas transplantation as a treatment for diabetes: indications and outcome. In: Bardin CW, ed. *Current Therapy in Endocrinology and Metabolism*, 6th edn. St. Louis: Mosby, 1997: 496–499.

45 Sutherland DE, Gruessner AC, Gruessner RWG. Pancreas transplantation: a review. *Transplant Proc* 1998; **30**:1940–1943.

46 Ryan EA. Pancreas transplants: for whom? *Lancet* 1998; **351**:1072–1073.

47 Kuo PC, Johnson LB, Schweitzer EJ, Bartlett ST. Simultaneous pancreas/kidney transplantation: a comparison of enteric and bladder drainage of exocrine pancreatic secretions. *Transplantation* 1997; **63**:238–243.

48 Nghiem DD, Gonwa TA, Corry RJ. Metabolic effects of urinary diversion of exocrine secretions in pancreatic transplantation. *Transplantation* 1987; **43**:70–73.

49 Gruessner AC, Sutherland DE. Pancreas transplant outcomes for United States (US) and non-US cases as reported to the United Network for Organ Sharing (UNOS) and the International Pancreas Transplant Registry (IPTR) as of June 2004. *Clin Transplant* 2005; **19**:433–455.

50 Waki K, Kadowaki T. An analysis of long-term survival from the OPTN/UNOS Pancreas Transplant Registry. *Clin Transpl* 2007: 9–17.

51 Humar A, Kandaswamy R, Granger D, Gruessner RW, Gruessner AC, Sutherland DER. Decreased surgical risks of pancreas transplantation in the modern era. *Ann Surg* 2000; **231**:269–275.

52 Sutherland DE, Gruessner RW, Gruessner AC. Pancreas transplantation for the treatment of diabetes mellitus. *World J Surg* 2001; **25**:487–496.

53 Sutherland DE, Gruessner RW, Dunn DL, Matas AJ, Humar A, Kandaswamy R, *et al.* Lessons learned from more than 1,000 pancreas transplants at a single institution. *Ann Surg* 2001; **233**:463–501.

54 Robertson RP, Sutherland DE, Lanz KJ. Normoglycaemia and preserved insulin secretory reserve in diabetic patients 10–18 years after pancreas transplantation. *Diabetes* 1999; **48**:1737–1740.

55 Fioretto P, Steffes MW, Sutherland DER, Goetz FC, Mauer M. Reversal of lesions of diabetic nephropathy after pancreas transplantation. *N Engl J Med* 1998; **339**:69–75.

56 Kennedy WR, Navarro X, Goetz FC, Sutherland DER, Najarian JS. Effects of pancreatic transplantation on diabetic neuropathy. *N Engl J Med* 1990; **322**:1031–1037.

57 Martinenghi S, Comi G, Galardi G, Di Carlo V, Pozza G, Secchi A. Amelioration of nerve conduction velocity following simultaneous kidney/pancreas transplantation is due to the glycaemic control provided by the pancreas. *Diabetologia* 1997; **40**:1110–1112.

58 Jukema JW, Smets YFC, van der Pijl JW, Zwinderman AH, Vliegen HW, Ringers J, *et al.* Impact of simultaneous pancreas and kidney transplantation on progression of coronary atherosclerosis in patients with end-stage renal failure due to type 1 diabetes. *Diabetes Care* 2002; **25**:906–911.

59 Fiorina P, La Rocca E, Venturini M, Minicucci F, Fermo I, Paroni R, *et al.* Effects of kidney–pancreas transplantation on atherosclerotic risk factors and endothelial function in patients with uremia and type 1 diabetes. *Diabetes* 2001; **50**:496–501.

60 Wang Q, Klein R, Moss SE, Klein BE, Hoyer C, Burke K, *et al.* The influence of combined kidney–pancreas transplantation on the progression of diabetic retinopathy. *Ophthalmology* 1994; **101**: 1071–1076.

61 Konigsrainer A, Miller K, Steurer W, Kieselbach G, Aichberger C, Ofner D, *et al.* Does pancreas transplantation influence the course of diabetic retinopathy? *Diabetologia* 1991; **34**(Suppl 1):86–88.

62 Brendel MD, Hering BJ, Schulz AO, Bretzel RG. International Islet Transplant Registry Report. *Justus-Liebig-University of Giessen* 1999; 1–20.

63 Benhamou PY, Oberholzer J, Toso C, Kessler L, Penfornis A, Bayle F, *et al.* Human islet transplantation network for the treatment of type 1 diabetes: first data from the Swiss–French GRAGIL consortium (1999–2000). *Diabetologia* 2001; **44**:859–864.

64 Weir GC, Bonner-Weir S, Leahy JL. Islet mass and function in diabetes and transplantation. *Diabetes* 1990; **39**:401–405.

65 Hering B, Ricordi C. Islet transplantation in type 1 diabetes: results, research priorities and reasons for optimism. *Graft* 1999; **2**:12–27.

66 Shapiro AMJ, Lakey JRT, Ryan EA, Korbutt GS, Toth E, Warnock GL, *et al.* Islet transplantation in seven patients with type 1 diabetes mellitus using a glucocorticoid-free immunosuppressive regimen. *N Engl J Med* 2000; **343**:230–238.

67 Korc M. Normal function of the endocrine pancreas. In: Go VLW, Dimagno EP, Gardner JD, Lebenthal E, Reber HA, Scheele GA, eds. *The Pancreas*, 2nd edn. NewYork: Raven Press, 1993: 751–758.

68 Volk BW, Wellmann KF. Quantitative studies of the islets of nondiabetic patients. In: Volk BW, Arquilla ER, eds. *The Diabetic Pancreas*, 2nd edn. New York: Plenum Medical Book Co.; 1985: 117–125.

69 Lakey JRT, Warnock GL, Rajotte RV, Suarez-Alamazor ME, Ao Z, Shapiro AM, *et al.* Variables in organ donors that affect the recovery of human islets of Langerhans. *Transplantation* 1996; **61**:1047–1053.

70 Lakey JRT, Rajotte RV, Warnock GL, Kneteman NM. Human pancreas preservation prior to islet isolation. *Transplantation* 1995; **59**:689–694.

71 Kneteman NM, Warnock GL, Evans MG, Dawidson I, Rajotte RV. Islet isolation from human pancreas stored in UW solution for 6 to 26 hours. *Transplant Proc* 1990; **22**:763–764.

72 Lakey JRT, Warnock GL, Shapiro AMJ, Korbutt GS, Ao Z, Kneteman NM, *et al.* Intraductal collagenase delivery into the human pancreas using syringe loading or controlled perfusion. *Cell Transplant* 1999; **8**:285–292.

73 Johnson PR, White SA, London NJ. Collagenase and human islet isolation. *Cell Transplant* 1996; **5**:437–452.

74 Linetsky E, Bottino R, Lehmann R, Alejandro R, Inverardi L, Ricordi C. Improved human islet isolation using a new enzyme blend, liberase. *Diabetes* 1997; **46**:1120–1123.

75 Ricordi C, Lacy PE, Scharp DW. Automated islet isolation from human pancreas. *Diabetes* 1989; **38**(Suppl 1):140–142.

76 Ao Z, Lakey JRT, Rajotte RV, Warnock GL. Collagenase digestion of canine pancreas by gentle automated dissociation in combination with ductal perfusion optimizes mass recovery of islets. *Transplant Proc* 1992; **6**:2787.

77 Walsh TJ, Eggleston JC, Cameron JL. Portal hypertension, hepatic infarction, and liver failure complication pancreatic islet autotransplantation. *Surgery* 1982; **91**:485–487.

78 Gores PF, Sutherland DER. Pancreatic islet transplantation: is purification necessary? *Am J Surgery* 1993; **166**:538–542.

79 Oberholzer J, Triponez F, Mage R, Andereggen E, Bühler L, Crétin N, *et al.* Human islet transplantation: lesson from 13 autologous and 13 allogenic transplatations. *Transplantation* 2000; **6**:1115–1123.

80 Kahan BD. Efficacy of sirolimus compared with azathioprine for reduction of acute renal allograft rejection: a randomised multicentre study. *Lancet* 2000; **356**:194–202.

81 Kneteman NM, Lakey JRT, Wagner T, Finegood D. The metabolic impact of rapamycin (Sirolimus) in chronic canine islet graft recipients. *Transplantation* 1996; **61**:1206–1210.

82 Panz VR, Bonegio R, Raal FJ, Maher H, Hsu HC, Joffe BI. Diabetogenic effect of tacrolimus in South African patients undergoing kidney transplantation. *Transplantation* 2002; **73**:587–590.

83 Gruessner RW, for the Tacrolimus Pancreas Transplant Study Group. Tacrolimus in pancreas transplantation: a multicenter analysis. *Clin Transplant* 1997; **11**:299–312.

84 Maes BD, Kuypers D, Messiaen T, Evenepoel P, Mathieu C, Coosemans W, *et al.* Posttransplantation diabetes mellitus in FK-506- treated renal transplant recipients: analysis of incidence and risk factors. *Transplantation* 2001; **72**:1655–1661.

85 Tamura K, Fujimura T, Tsutsumi T, Yamamoto T, Nakamura K, Koibuchi Y, *et al.* Transcriptional inhibition of insulin by FK506 and possible involvement of FK506 binding protein-12 in pancreatic β-cell. *Transplantation* 1995; **59**:1606–1613.

86 Ishizuka J, Gugliuzza KK, Wassmuth Z, Hsieh J, Sato K, Tsuchiya T, *et al.* Effects of FK506 and cyclosporine on dynamic insulin secretion from isolated dog pancreatic islets. *Transplantation* 1993; **56**:1486–1490.

87 Cosio FG, Pesavento TE, Osei K, Henry ML, Ferguson RM. Post-transplant diabetes mellitus: increasing incidence in renal allograft recipients transplanted in recent years. *Kidney Int* 2001; **59**: 732–737.

88 Nielsen JH, Mandrup-Poulsen T, Nerup J. Direct effects of cyslosporin A on human pancreatic β-cells. *Diabetes* 1986; **35**:1049–1052.

89 Lakey JR, Rajotte RV, Warnock Gl, Kneteman NM. Pancreas procurement and preservation: impact on islet recovery and viability. *Transplantation* 1995; **59**:689–694.

90 Tsujimura T, Kuroda Y, Kin T, Avila JG, Rajotte RV, Korbutt GS, *et al.* Human islet transplantation from pancreases with prolonged cold ischemia using additional preservation by the two-layer (UW solution/perflurochemical) cold storage method. *Transplantation* 2002; **74**:1687–1691.

91 Ramachandran S, Desai NM, Goers TA, Benshof N, Olack B, Shenoy S, *et al.* Improved islet yields from pancreas preserved in perfluorocarbon is via inhibition of apoptosis mediated by mitochondrial pathway. *Am J Transplant* 2006; **6**:1696–1703.

92 Ricordi C, Fraker C, Szust J, Al-Abdullah I, Poggioli R, Kirlew T, *et al.* Improved human islet isolation outcome from marginal donors following addition of oxygenated perfluorocarbon to the cold-storage solution. *Transplantation* 2003; **75**:1524–1527.

93 Kin T, Mirbolooki M, Salehi P, Tsukada M, O'Gorman D, Imes S, *et al.* Islet isolation and transplantation outcomes of pancreas preserved with University of Wisconsin solution versus two-layer method using preoxygenated perfluorocarbon. *Transplantation* 2006; **82**:1286–1290.

94 Hering BJ, Kandaswamy R, Harmon JV, Ansite JD, Clemmings SM, Sakai T, *et al.* Transplantation of cultured islets from two-layer preserved pancreases in type 1 diabetes with anti-CD3 antibody. *Am J Transplant* 2004; **4**:390–401.

95 Ichii H, Sakuma Y, Pileggi A, Fraker C, Alvarez A, Montelongo J, *et al.* Shipment of human islets for transplantation. *Am J Transplant* 2007; **7**:1010–1020.

96 Sabek OM, Cowan P, Fraga DW, Gaber AO. The effect of isolation methods and the use of different enzymes on islet yield and *in vivo* function. *Cell Transplant* 2008; **17**:785–792.

97 Weimar B, Rauber K, Brendel MD, Bretzel RG, Rau WS. Percutaneous transhepatic catheterization of the portal vein: a combined CT- and fluoroscopy-guide technique. *Cardiovasc Intervent Radiol* 1999; **22**:342–344.

98 Baidal DA, Froud T, Ferreira JV, Khan A, Alejandro R, Ricordi C. The bag method for islet cell infusion. *Cell Transplant* 2003; **12**:809–813.

99 Ryan EA, Paty BW, Senior PA, Bigam D, Alfadhli E, Kneteman NM, *et al.* Five-year follow-up after clinical islet transplantation. *Diabetes* 2005; **54**:2060–2069.

100 Shapiro AMJ, Ryan EA, Lakey JR. Islet transplantation in the treatment of diabetes. In: Barnett AH, ed. *Best Practice and Research Compendium*, Elsevier, 2005.

101 Hering BJ, Kandaswamy R, Ansite JD, Eckman PM, Nakano M, Sawada T, *et al.* Single-donor, marginal-dose islet transplantation in patients with type 1 diabetes. *JAMA* 2005; **293**:830–835.

102 Shapiro AMJ, Koh A, Salam A, *et al.* Impact of different induction therapies on long-term durability of insulin independence after clinical islet transplantation. *Am J Transplant* 2008; Suppl. A212.

103 Shapiro AMJ, Koh A, Kin T, *et al.* Outcomes following alemtuzumab induction in clinical islet transplantation. *Am J Transplant* 2008; Suppl. A213.

104 Koh A, Imes S, Ryan E, Shapiro AMJ, Senior P. Improved tolerability of tacrolimus plus mycophenolate mofetil without graft compromise in islet transplantation. *Diabetes* 2008: **57**(Suppl 1):A541.

105 Berney T, Secchi A. Rapamycin in islet transplantation: friend or foe? *Transpl Int* 2009; **22**:153–161.

106 Ryan EA, Shandro T, Green K, Paty BW, Senior PA, Bigam D, *et al.* Assessment of the severity of hypoglycaemia and glycaemic lability in type 1 diabetic subjects undergoing islet transplantation. *Diabetes* 2004; **53**:955–962.

107 Clarke WL, Cox DJ, Gonder-Frederick LA, Julian D, Schlundt D, Polonsky W. Reduced awareness of hypoglycemia in adults with IDDM: a prospective study of hypoglycemic frequency and associated symptoms. *Diabetes Care* 1995; **18**:517–522.

108 Diem P, Redmon JB, Abid M, Moran A, Sutherland DE, Halter JB, *et al.* Glucagon, cathecholamine and pancreatic polypeptide secretion in type 1 diabetic recipients of pancreas allografts. *J Clin Invest* 1990; **86**:2008–2013.

109 Paty BW, Lanz K, Kendall DM, Sutherland DE, Robertson RP. Restored hypoglycemic counterregulation is stable in successful pancreas transplant recipients for up to 19 years after transplantation. *Transplantation* 2001; **72**:1103–1107.

110 Kendall DM, Rooney DP, Smets YFC, Bolding LS, Robertson RP. Pancreas transplantation restores epinephrine response and symptom recognition during hypoglycaemia in patients with long-standing type 1 diabetes and autonomic neuropathy. *Diabetes* 1997; **46**:249–257.

111 Paty BW, Ryan EA, Shapiro AMJ, Lakey JR, Robertson RP. Intrahepatic islet transplantation in type 1 diabetic patients does not restore hypoglycaemic hormonal counterregulation or symptom recognition after insulin independence. *Diabetes* 2002; **51**: 3428–3434.

112 Meyer C, Hering BJ, Grossmann R, Brandhorst H, Brandhorst D, Gerich J, *et al.* Improved glucose counterregulation and autonomic symptoms after intraportal islet transplants alone in patients with long-standing type 1 diabetes mellitus. *Transplantation* 1998; **66**: 233–240.

113 Rickels MR, Schutta MH, Mueller R, Markmann JF, Barker CF, Naji A, *et al.* Islet cell hormonal responses to hypoglycaemia after human islet transplantation for type 1 diabetes. *Diabetes* 2005; **54**:3205–3211.

114 Rickels MR, Schutta MH, Mueller R, Kapoor S, Markmann JF, Naji A, *et al.* Glycemic thresholds for activation of counterregulatory hormone and symptom responses in islet transplant recipients. *J Clin Endocrinol Metab* 2007; **92**:873–879.

115 Lee TC, Barshes NR, O'Mahony CA, Nguyen L, Brunicardi FC, Ricordi C, *et al.* The effect of pancreatic islet transplantation on progression of diabetic retinopathy and neuropathy. *Transplant Proc* 2005; **37**:2263–2265.

116 Thompson DM, Begg IS, Harris C, Ao Z, Fung MA, Meloche RM, *et al.* Reduced progression of diabetic retinopathy after islet cell transplantation compared with intensive medical therapy. *Transplantation* 2008; **85**:1400–1405.

117 Senior PA, Zeman M, Paty BW, Ryan EA, Shapiro AMJ. Changes in renal function after clinical islet transplantation: four-year observational study. *Am J Transplant* 2007; **7**:91–98.

118 Hoving P, Rossing P, Tarnow L, Parving HH. Smoking and progression of diabetic nephropathy in type 1 diabetes. *Diabetes Care* 2003; **26**:911–916.

119 Bjorck S, Nyberg G, Mulec H, Granerus G, Herlitz H, Aureil M. Beneficial effects of angiotensin converting enzyme inhibition on renal function in patients with diabetic nephropathy. *Br Med J* 1986; **293**:471–474.

120 Fung MA, Warnock GL, Ao Z, Keown P, Meloche M, Shapiro RJ, *et al.* The effect of medical therapy and islet cell transplantation on diabetic nephropathy: an interim report. *Transplantation* 2007; **84**:17–22.

121 Albaker W, Koh A, Ryan EA, Shapiro AM, Senior P. Diabetic peripheral neuropathy is stabilized after clinical islet transplantation: 7 year follow up study. *Endo* 2008; OR26-2.

122 Koh A, Ryan E, Welsh R, Shuaib A, Shapiro AMJ, Senior P. Cardiovascular disease remains stable after islet transplantation. *Diabetes* 2008; **57**(Suppl 1):A108.

123 Rafael E, Ryan EA, Paty BW, Oberholzer J, Imes S, Senior P, *et al.* Changes in liver enzymes after clinical islet transplantation. *Transplantation* 2003; **76**:1280–1284.

124 Bhargava R, Senior PA, Ackerman TE, Ryan EA, Paty BW, Lakey JR, *et al.* Prevalence of hepatic steatosis after islet transplantation and its relation to graft function. *Diabetes* 2004; **53**:1311–1317.

125 Cure P, Pileggi A, Froud T, Norris PM, Baidal DA, Cornejo A, *et al.* Alterations of the female reproductive system in recipients of islet grafts. *Transplantation* 2004; **78**:1576–1581.

126 Alfadhli E, Koh A, Albaker W, Bhargava R, Ackerman T, McDonald C, *et al.* High prevalence of ovarian cysts in pre-menopausal women receiving sirolimus and tacrolimus after clinical islet transplantation. *Transplant Int* 2009; **22**:622–625.

127 Ryan EA, Lakey JR, Paty BW, Imes S, Korbutt GS, Kneteman NM, *et al.* Successful islet transplantation: continued insulin reserve provides long-term glycaemic control. *Diabetes* 2002; **51**:2148–2157.

128 Senior PA, Paty BW, Cockfield SM, Ryan EA, Shapiro AMJ. Proteinuria developing after clinical islet transplant resolves with sirolimus withdrawal and increased tacrolimus dosing. *Am J Transplant* 2005; **5**:2318–2323.

129 van Gelder T, Hilbrands LB, Vanrenterghem Y, Weimar W, de Fijter JW, Squifflet JP, *et al.* A randomized double-blind, multicenter plasma concentration controlled study of the safety and efficacy of oral mycophenolate mofetil for the prevention of acute rejection after kidney transplantation. *Transplantation* 1999; **68**: 261–266.

130 Campbell PM, Salam A, Ryan EA, Senior P, Paty BW, Bigam D, *et al.* Pretransplant HLA antibodies are associated with reduced graft survival after clinical islet transplantation. *Am J Transplant* 2007; **7**:1242–1248.

131 Campbell PM, Senior PA, Salam A, Labranche K, Bigam DL, Kneteman NM, *et al.* High risk of sensitization after failed islet transplantation. *Am J Transplant* 2007; **7**:2311–2317.

132 Rood PPM, Cooper DKC. Islet xenotransplantation: are we really ready for clinical trials? *Am J Transplant* 2006; **6**:1269–1274.

133 Gangaram-Panday ST, Faas MM, de Vos P. Towards stem-cell therapy in the endocrine pancreas. *Trends Mol Med* 2007; **13**:164–173.

134 Bonner-Weir S, Weir GC. New sources of pancreatic β-cells. *Nat Biotech* 2005; **23**:857–861.

135 Davalli AM, Scaglia L, Zangen DH, Hollister J, Bonner-Weir S, Weir GC. Vulnerability of islets in the immediate posttransplantation period: dynamic changes in structure and function. *Diabetes* 1996; **45**:1161–1167.

136 Bell E, Cao X, Moibi H, Greene SR, Young R, Trucco M, *et al.* Rapamycin has a deleterious effect on MIN-6 cells and rat and human islets. *Diabetes* 2003; **52**:2731–2739.

137 Moberg L, Johansson H, Lukinius A, Berne C, Foss A, Källen R, *et al.* Production of tissue factor by pancreatic islet cells as a trigger of detrimental thrombotic reactions in clinical islet transplantation. *Lancet* 2002; **360**:2039–2045.

138 Rickels MR, Schutta MH, Markmann JF, Barker CF, Naji A, Teff KL. β-Cell function following human islet transplantation for type 1 diabetes. *Diabetes* 2005; **54**:100–106.

139 Narang AS, Sabek O, Gaber AO, Mahato RI. Co-expression of vascular endothelial growth factor and interleukin-1 receptor antagonist improves human islet survival and function. *Pharm Res* 2006; **23**:1970–1982.

140 Contreras JL, Eckstein C, Smyth CA, Bilbao G, Vilatoba M, Ringland SE, *et al.* Activated protein C preserves functional islet mass after intraportal transplantation: a novel link between endothelial cell activation, thrombosis, inflammation and islet cell death. *Diabetes* 2004; **53**:2804–2814.

141 Emamaullee JA, Stanton L, Schur C, Shapiro AMJ. Caspase inhibitor therapy enhances marginal mass islet graft survival and preserves long term function is islet transplantation. *Diabetes* 2007; **56**:1289–1298.

142 Johansson H, Goto M, Dufrane D, Siegbahn A, Elgue G, Gianello P, *et al.* Low molecular weight dextran sulfate: a strong candidate drug to block IBMIR in clinical islet transplantation. *Am J Transplant* 2006; **6**:305–312.

143 Cabric S, Sanchez J, Lundgren T, Foss A, Felldin M, Källen R, *et al.* Islet surface heparinization prevents the instant blood-mediated inflammatory reaction in islet transplantation. *Diabetes* 2007; **56**:2008–2015.

144 Faradji RN, Monroy K, Riefkohl A, Lozano L, Gorn L, Froud T, *et al.* Continuous glucose monitoring system for early detection of graft dysfunction in allogenic islet transplant recipients. *Transplant Proc* 2006; **38**:3274–3276.

145 Pileggi A, Ricordi C, Alessiani M, Inverardi L. Factors influencing islets of Langerhans graft function and monitoring. *Clinica Chim Acta* 2001; **310**:3–16.

146 Paty BW, Bonner-Weir S, Laughlin MR, McEwan AH, Shapiro AMJ. Toward development of imaging modalities for islets after transplantation: insights from the National Institutes of Health Workshop on beta cell imaging. *Transplantation* 2004; **77**:1133–1137.

147 Ghofaili KA, Fung M, Ao Z, Meloche M, Shapiro RJ, Warnock GL, *et al.* Effect of exenatide on beta cell function after islet transplantation in type 1 diabetes. *Transplantation* 2007; **83**:24–28.

148 Smith RN, Kent SC, Nagle J, Selig M, Iafrate AJ, Najafian N, *et al.* Pathology of an islet transplant 2 years after transplantation: evidence for a nonimmunological loss. *Transplantation* 2008; **86**:54–62.

149 Adams AB, Shirasugi N, Jones TR, Durham MM, Strobert EA, Cowan S, *et al.* Development of a chimeric anti-CD40 monoclonal antibody that synergizes with LEA29Y to prolong islet allograft survival. *J Immunol* 2005; **174**:542–550.

150 Vincenti F, Larsen C, Durrbach A, Wekerle T, Nashan B, Blancho G, *et al.* Belatacept Study Group. Costimulation blockade with belatacept in renal transplantation. *N Engl J Med* 2005; **353**:770.

151 Beck J, Angus R, Madsen B, Britt D, Vernon B, Nguyen KT. Islet encapsulation: strategies to enhance islet cell functions. *Tissue Eng* 2007; **13**:589–599.

Gene therapy

Andreea R. Barbu & Nils Welsh

Keypoints

- Gene therapy for diabetes can be defined as transfer of DNA to somatic cells in order to understand, treat or prevent the disease or its complications.
- Because the etiology of diabetes is multifactorial in most cases, gene therapy aimed at correcting a single missing or multifunctioning gene will probably not be meaningful. Instead, gene therapy will need to interfere with more distal steps in the pathogenesis of diabetes, correct insulin deficiency or treat secondary complications.
- It is possible to outline several different gene transfer strategies for diabetes; prevention of β-cell destruction could be achieved by manipulating β-cells to produce a protection or survival factor.
- β-Cell destruction might also be prevented by immunomodulation.
- Stimulation of β-cell differentiation and regeneration might involve gene therapy with transcription factors that control β-cell development.
- Ectopic production of insulin by substitute cells has been achieved with fibroblasts, hepatocytes, myocytes, pituitary and exocrine cells.
- Although experimental results are promising, none of the proposed gene therapy models for treatment or prevention of diabetes have reached the stage of clinical testing.
- Clinical trials are in progress with a view to treat diabetic complications such as foot ulcer and limb ischemia.

Gene transfer techniques for genetic modification of pancreatic islets

The ability to engineer pancreatic β-cells is a prerequisite for a successful application of most gene therapy approaches in diabetes. Because pancreatic islets are terminally differentiated cell clusters, gene transfer into islet cells poses significant technical hurdles. To date, several gene therapy vectors have demonstrated their utility in genetic modification of islet cells (Table 61.3). While viral vectors, such as adenovirus [1], lentivirus [2], retrovirus [3] and adeno-associated virus [4], show the most promising gene transfer efficiency into islet cells, it is likely that non-viral vector systems will more easily satisfy biosafety concerns in clinical trials.

Prevention of β-cell destruction in type 1 diabetes

β-Cell survival factors

Prevention of β-cell destruction could be achieved by genetic manipulation of β-cells so that they produce a β-cell protection and/or survival factor. Such an approach would, in general, leave the immune system unaffected as the transgene production is localized to the islets. Targeting of a survival factor to the β-cells could be applied to individuals in whom autoimmune destruction of β-cells has begun, but not reached the end stage. Candidate transgenes currently under investigation include those encoding antioxidant enzymes: glutathione peroxidase, mitochondrial manganese superoxide dismutase (MnSOD), catalase, cytosolic copper-zinc superoxide dismutase, anti-apoptotic proteins (members of the heat shock proteins and Bcl-2 families) and modulators of cytokine signaling pathways (modulation of nuclear factor κB, NFκB), and suppressors of cytokine signaling. Alternative approaches for cytoprotection of β-cells have been envisaged, such as immune modulators; for example, an interleukin-1 (IL-1) receptor antagonist, hepatocyte growth factor, transforming growth factor β (TGF-β), adenoviral E3 and calcitonin gene-related peptide, inhibitors of Fas ligand signaling, and antistress factors such as thioredoxin. These factors have been addressed experimentally and could possibly, when expressed by β-cells in patients with diabetes, promote β-cell survival.

Genetic modulation of the immune system

In individuals with a high risk of developing T1DM, as indicated by genetic and humoral markers, but who have not yet entered the phase of autoimmune β-cell destruction, it might be possible to prevent the progression of the disease by DNA vaccination. In mice, it has already been observed that DNA vaccination with a glutamic acid decarboxylase 65 (GAD65) gene construct generates a protective humoral immune response and significantly delays the onset of diabetes [5]. Other studies of DNA vaccination in non-obese diabetic (NOD) mice were performed with a preproinsulin/glutamic acid decarboxylase 65 (Ins-GAD) fusion construct as the target antigen to introduce a larger number of autoantigenic target epitopes. DNA co-vaccination with Ins-GAD and B7-1wa (a membrane-bound molecule that can engage cytotoxic T-lymphocyte associated antigen 4 [CTLA-4] and promote negative signaling) generated protective regulatory T-cells and ameliorated the disease [6]. Both insulin and GAD65 may be key autoantigens in T1DM, and if the DNA vaccination approach leads to tolerance, β-cell destruction might be avoided.

Furthermore, virus-based IL-10 genetic studies showed beneficial effects on the development of T1DM, both effectively blocking progression of insulitis as well as suppressing autoimmunity in NOD mice transplanted with syngeneic islet grafts [7]. Despite these results, significant immunosuppression, resulting from systemic expression of high levels of IL-10, give rise to serious concerns regarding the applicability of such an approach in clinical settings; however, the development of viral vectors promoting a tightly regulated transgene expression could overcome this obstacle.

Targeted immunomodulation has also been achieved by transducing autoantigen-specific CD4⁺ T-cells *ex vivo* with retrovi-

Table 61.3 Properties of gene therapy vectors with demonstrated utility in islet transduction.

Delivery method		Advantages	Disadvantages
Non-viral vectors	Naked DNA DNA complexes Peptide transduction domains	High clinical safety Easy and inexpensive to produce Non-immunogenic Unlimited capacity	Low transfection efficiency Transient gene expression
Adenovirus		High transduction efficiency High viral titer Infects non-dividing cells	Transient gene expression Immunogenic Clinical safety issues
Adeno-associated virus		Potential site-specific integration Infects non-dividing cells No immune response High clinical safety	Low capacity (5 kb) Very difficult to generate
Lentivirus		High transduction efficiency Long term expression Easy to generate Relatively high titer	Possibility of insertional mutagenesis with clinical effects
Herpes simplex virus		High transduction efficiency Up to 30 kb insertion	Inflammatory and toxic reactions in patients Complicated genome and propagation

ruses that encode immune regulatory proteins [8]. Following intravenous injection of the transduced T-cells, it appears that the cells accumulate at the site of inflammation. Using this site-specific delivery, immune regulatory proteins have been observed to protect against autoimmune reactions, possibly by converting the immune reaction from a Th1 to a Th2 response.

An alternative approach may be targeting expression of disease-specific epitopes to activated B lymphocytes [9]. Antigen presentation by these cells seems to result in immunosupression and therapeutic efficacy. It is not clear why this is the case, but it has been suggested that antigen presentation by B lymphocytes leads to immune downregulation, whereas presentation by macrophages or dendritic cells is immune stimulatory.

Stimulation of β-cell differentiation and regeneration

A better understanding of the cellular sources for the expansion and turnover of β-cells seen in postnatal life could make way for a possible gene therapy approach leading to *in situ* regeneration of β-cells in patients with diabetes. Indirect evidence has suggested that postnatal β-cells derive from adult stem cells, proposed to reside in the pancreatic ducts, bone marrow, spleen or within islets. Lineage tracing experiments, however, demonstrated that the vast majority of adult β-cells derive from preexisting β-cells, suggesting that terminally differentiated β-cells retain a significant proliferative capacity and thus could represent an attractive target for expansion using gene therapy [10]. For example, mice over-expressing gastrin and TGF-α display a significantly increased islet cell mass. In addition, the cyclin-dependent kinase 4 (CDK4) and cyclins D1/D2 emerge as key determinants of β-cell proliferation and β-cell mass. Indeed, mice lacking CDK4 display a selective loss of β-cell function and over-expression of CDK4 results in preferential hyperplasia of the β-cells; however, it is likely that all approaches aiming at regenerating β-cells in patients with T1DM must be combined with a strategy to prevent autoimmune destruction of the newly formed β-cells.

Ectopic production of insulin by substitute cells

With the cloning of the insulin gene in the late 1970s, it was proposed that using a suitable promoter and insulin gene construct, non-insulin-producing cells could be made into insulin-producing substitute cells, and that such cells could restore insulin production in T1DM and some patients with T2DM. The original experiments were carried out on cell lines and fibroblasts, but since then hepatocytes, myocytes, pituitary and exocrine cells have also been made into insulin-producing substitute cells. Proinsulin is only converted into insulin by the prohormone convertases PC2 and PC3, which are not expressed in most substitute cells. This limitation has been overcome by mutating the insulin gene so that a furin cleavable site is generated (INS-FUR). The protease furin, unlike PC2 and PC3, is expressed in most cells. Although processing of proinsulin to insulin can be achieved in substitute cells, none of these cells would be able to respond to insulin secretagogues with a physiologic secretion of insulin. Recent studies showed that both lentivirus [11] and adeno-associated virus vectors [12] were able to deliver INS-FUR cDNA efficiently to hepatocytes *in vitro* and *in vivo*, resulting in long-term correction of diabetes in rats.

Given its role in β-cell maintenance, the transcription factor Pdx-1 was investigated for its ability to induce ectopic insulin production in non β-cells *in vivo*. Ferber and colleagues have used adenoviral-mediated Pdx-1 overexpression for *ex vivo* transduction of adult human hepatocytes for cell-based therapy. In addition to glucagons, insulin and somatostatin, exogenous expression of Pdx-1 induced transcription of several β-cell products, including glucose transporter 2 and glucokinase, endogenous Pdx-1 and multiple downstream pro-endocrine developmental factors [13].

In a recent study Zhou *et al.* describe a way to reprogram pancreatic exocrine cells into insulin producing β-cells [14]. By using adenoviruses, they introduced combinations of nine different genes, previously identified to be essential to the embryonic development of β-cells, into the pancreas of live mice. They found that the transfer of three transcription factors (Ngn3, Pdx1 and Mafa) induces trans-differentiation of up to 20% of the successfully manipulated exocrine cells into β-like cells. By lineage tracing experiments, the authors proved that the trans-differentiated cells were, indeed, exocrine cells. These reprogrammed β-cells had similar morphology, protein expression and the capacity to secrete insulin as their "natural" counterparts. Moreover, they were able to improve hyperglycemia in mice with induced diabetes. This study elegantly shows that adult cells can be directly converted into another type of adult cell, which opens the possibility of directly converting cells *in vivo* for repair and regeneration as a therapeutic tool for diabetes and beyond [14].

Cell therapy using β-cells derived from embryonic stem cells

This topic is discussed in detail in the first part of this chapter.

Ex vivo gene transfer to islets destined for transplantation

Pancreatic islet transplantation has been validated as a realistic alternative to correct the insulin deficiency in T1DM; however, islets are exposed to a plethora of insults before, during, after isolation and at the site of implantation, all of which could result in cellular death and impaired function, therefore reducing the yield of viable islets that engraft after implant. As a result, much effort has been made to understand better the molecular mechanisms involved in all these processes as well as in developing new therapeutic strategies to increase durable functional islet mass. In

Table 61.4 Examples of gene therapy-based strategies leading to improved outcome of islet transplantation in animal models.

Gene product	Delivery method	Animal model	Desired effect
HGF and IL-1Ra	Adenovirus	STZ-induced-diabetic NOD-SCID mice	β-cell survival, β-cell proliferation, increased revascularization
HGF	Adenovirus	Allogeneic transplantation rat model	β-cell survival, β-cell proliferation
IL-10	Adenovirus AAV	STZ-induced diabetic rats (allotransplant) Autoimmune recurrence	Immunotolerance
sCD40-Ig	Adenovirus	Allogeneic transplantation mouse model	Immunotolerance
XIAP	Adenovirus	Chemically diabetic immunodeficient mice STZ-induced diabetic mice (allotransplant)	β-cell survival
Akt	Adenovirus	STZ-induced diabetic SCID mice	β-cell survival
IRAP	Adenovirus	STZ-induced diabetic rats	β-cell survival
TNFR-Ig	Adenovirus	Diabetic mice (allotransplant)	Immunotolerance
VEGF	Non-viral	Diabetic mice	Increased revascularization
MnSOD	Adenovirus	STZ-induced diabetic NODscid mice	β-cell protection against oxidative damage
TGF-β1	Adenovirus	Autoimmune recurrence in NOD mice	β-cell survival
Bcl2	Adenovirus Adenovirus	Xenotransplantation Diabetic SCID mice	β-cell survival

HGF, hepatocyte growth factor; Ig, immunoglobulin; IL, interleukin; IL-1Ra, interleukin-1 receptor antagonist; IRAP, interleukin-1 receptor antagonist protein; MnSOD, manganese superoxide dismutase; NOD, non-obese diabetic; SCID, severe combined immunodeficiency; STZ, streptozotocin; TGF, transforming growth factor; TNFR, tumor necrosis factor receptor; VEGF, vascular endothelial growth factor; XIAP, X-linked inhibitor of apoptosis.

this context, *ex vivo* gene transfer to pancreatic islets represents an attractive approach towards enhancing graft survival after transplantation. Most of the gene therapy strategies described above show promise for the cytoprotection of islets in transplant settings and may ultimately promote significantly enhanced function and survival of transplanted islets leading to an improved outcome of the transplantation procedures (Table 61.4); however, considering the complex pathways involved in β-cell destruction and loss of function following islet transplantation, it is likely that gene therapy strategies targeting multiple genes, using multicistronic vectors, will be more beneficial for the improvement of graft survival. For this purpose, a number of factors still remain to be investigated to find which combination of genes proves optimal, what threshold level of gene expression is required and what delivery strategy is the most efficient for targeting the mechanisms leading to graft failure.

Gene therapy strategies for type 2 diabetes

T2DM is characterized by hyperglycemia combined with variable degrees of insulin resistance. A potential therapeutic approach for the treatment of T2DM is the use of GLP-1, a gut-derived incretin hormone which has important roles in glucose homeostasis. Using an adenoviral vector to express GLP-1 with the insulin leader sequence to ensure secretion, Lee *et al.* [15] have recently demonstrated transient improvement in glucose tolerance using an overt T2DM animal model. Significant therapeutic effects, including improved glucose homeostasis, decreased weight gain, reduced hepatic fat and improved adipokine profile, were also obtained by constitutively expressing exendin-4, a GLP-1 receptor (GLP-1R) agonist in a high fat induced obesity mouse model [16]). These studies suggest that GLP-1/GLP-1R agonist gene therapy may be a promising treatment modality for T2DM.

Another interesting line of research exploits the potential of viral proteins as therapeutic tools for treating glycemic dysregulation in humans. Human adenovirus type 36 (Ad-36) was determined as a novel candidate for improving metabolic profile by expanding adipose tissue while enhancing insulin sensitivity in experimentally infected rats [17]. Recent studies have demonstrated the capacity of Ad-36 to increase glucose uptake by adipose tissue explants obtained from subjects with and without diabetes. Ad-36 upregulated expression of several pro-adipogenic genes, adiponectin and fatty acid synthetase, and reduced the expression of inflammatory cytokine macrophage chemoattractant protein-1 in a phosphotidylinositol 3-kinase dependent manner [18]. Moreover, Ad-36 was also able to enhance glucose uptake in primary skeletal muscle cells from healthy lean subjects and subjects with diabetes [19]. Therefore, the potential of viral proteins to enhance glucose disposal and improve adipose and skeletal muscle tissues metabolic profile could be used as therapeutic targets for humans.

Gene therapy for the treatment of diabetic complications

The gene therapy models for treatment or prevention of T1DM and T2DM outlined above have not yet reached clinical stages. By contrast, the use of gene therapy in the treatment of diabetes complications shows great promise and some projects are in the early stages of clinical testing. Briefly, transduction of nerves by herpes virus expressing nerve growth factor has been investigated for treatment of cystopathy and for peripheral neuropathy. In addition, the effects of gene therapy with vascular endothelial growth factor (VEGF) on coronary artery disease have been studied in a clinical trial. It has been shown that VEGF is required to initiate immature vascular formation, whereas angiopoietin-1 (Ang-1) is essential for the maintenance of endothelial integrity and vascular formation. In this regard, a recent study demonstrated that Ang-1 gene therapy promotes vascular maturation and stabilization and rescues diabetes impaired myocardial angiogenesis and myocardial remodeling in *db/db* mice [20]. Another small clinical trial showed significant improvement in patients with diabetes and diffuse peripheral vascular disease after intramuscular administration of a VEGF gene-carrying plasmid. Furthermore, delivery of insulin-like growth factor I by non-viral gene therapy in combination with autologous cell transplantation improved diabetic wound healing significantly in a preclinical large-animal model [21].

Problems and future directions

Although significant progress is currently being made in the field of gene therapy of diabetes, it should be emphasized that gene therapy is neither a low cost : benefit nor a low risk : benefit approach. For example, there is the obvious risk that the gene therapy could induce severe hypoglycemia if the number of gene modified insulin-producing cells and their insulin release is not under perfect control. In addition, we need to await ongoing developments in gene transfer techniques to achieve therapeutic long-term expression, *in vivo* regulation of transgene expression and lack of immune triggering, in order to conduct gene therapy on β-cells *in vivo*. Because T1DM is usually more severe than T2DM, it is natural to assume that the first gene therapy efforts will be dedicated to the treatment of T1DM, and that the experiences from these trials will be used for later strategies for the treatment of T2DM. Finally, it must be clear that the benefits of gene therapy of diabetes outweigh the risks and offer advantages compared to those of conventional treatment before this approach could become accepted in general practice.

References

1 Gonçalves MA, de Vries AA. Adenovirus: from foe to friend. *Rev Med Virol* 2006; **16**:167–186.

2 Cockrell AS, Kafri T. Gene delivery by lentivirus vectors. *Mol Biotechnol* 2007; **36**:184–204.

3 Dalba C, Bellier B, Kasahara N, Klatzmann D. Replication-competent vectors and empty virus-like particles: new retroviral vector designs for cancer gene therapy or vaccines. *Mol Ther* 2007; **15**:457–466.

4 Wu Z, Asokan A, Samulski RJ. Adeno-associated virus serotypes: vector toolkit for human gene therapy. *Mol Ther* 2006; **14**:316–327.

5 Goudy KS, Wang B, Tisch R. Gene gun-mediated DNA vaccination enhances antigen-specific immunotherapy at a late preclinical stage of type 1 diabetes in nonobese diabetic mice. *Clin Immunol* 2008; **129**:49–57.

6 Prud'homme GJ, Glinka Y, Khan AS, Dragia-Akli R. Electroporation-enhanced nonviral gene transfer for the prevention or treatment of immunological, endocrine and neoplastic diseases. *Current Gene Therapy* 2006; **6**:243–273.

7 Goudy KS, Tish R. Immunotherapy for the prevention and treatment of type 1 diabetes. *Internat Rev Immunol* 2005; **24**:307–326.

8 Fathman CG, Costa GL, Seroogy CM. Gene therapy for autoimmune disease. *Clin Immunol* 2000; **95**:S39–43.

9 Agarwal RK, Kang Y, Zambidis E, Scott DW, Chan CC, Caspi RR. Retroviral gene therapy with an immunoglobulin-antigen fusion construct protects from experimental autoimmune uveitis. *J Clin Invest* 2000; **106**:245–252.

10 Nir T, Dor Y. How to make pancreatic β cells: prospects for cell therapy in diabetes. *Curr Opin Biotechnol* 2005; **16**:524–529.

11 Ren B, O'Brien BA, Swan MA, Koina ME, Nassif N, Wei MQ, *et al.* Long-term correction of diabetes in rats after lentiviral hepatic insulin gene therapy. *Diabetologia* 2007; **50**:1910–1920.

12 Hsu PY, Kotin RM, Yang YW. Glucose- and metabolically regulated hepatic insulin gene therapy for diabetes. *Pharm Res* 2008; **25**:1460–1468.

13 Sapir T, Shternhall K, Meivar-Levy I, Bumenfeld T, Cohen H, Skutelsky E, *et al.* Cell-replacement therapy for diabetes: generating functional insulin-producing tissue from adult human liver cells. *Proc Natl Acad Sci U S A* 2005; **102**:7964–7969.

14 Zhou Q, Brown J, Kanarek A, Rajagopal J, Melton DA. *In vivo* reprogramming of adult pancreatic exocrine cells to β-cells. *Nature* 2008; **455**:627–632.

15 Lee Y, Kwon MK, Kang ES, Park YM, Choi SH, Ahn CW, *et al.* Adenoviral vector-mediated glucagon-like peptide 1 gene therapy improves glucose homeostasis in Zucker diabetic fatty rats. *J Gene Med* 2008; **10**:260–268.

16 Samson SL, Gonzalez EV, Yechoor V, Bajaj M, Oka K, Chan L. Gene therapy for diabetes: metabolic effects of helper-dependent adenoviral exendin 4 expression in a diet-induced obesity mouse model. *Mol Ther* 2008; **16**:1805–1812.

17 Pasarica M, Shin AC, Yu M, Ou Yang HM, Rathod M, Jen KL, *et al.* Human adenovirus 36 induces adiposity, increases insulin sensitivity, and alters hypothalamic monoamines in rats. *Obesity* 2006; **14**:1905–1911.

18 Rogers PM, Mashtalir N, Rathod MA, Dubuisson O, Wang Z, Dasuri K, *et al.* Metabolically favorable remodeling of human adipose tissue by human adenovirus type 36. *Diabetes* 2008; **57**:2321–2331.

19 Wang ZQ, Cefalu WT, Zhang XH, Yu Y, Qin J, Son L, *et al.* Human adenovirus type 36 enhances glucose uptake in diabetic and nondiabetic human skeletal muscle cells independent of insulin signaling. *Diabetes* 2008; **57**:1805–1813.

20 Chen JX, Stinnett A. Ang-1 gene therapy inhibits hypoxia-inducible factor-1α (HIF-1α)-prolyl-4-hydroxylase-2, stabilizes HIF-1α expression, and normalizes immature vasculature in db/db mice. *Diabetes* 2008; **57**:3335–3343.

21 Hirsch T, Spielmann M, Velander P, Zuhaili B, Bleiziffer O, Fossum M, *et al.* Insulin-like growth factor-1 gene therapy and cell transplantation in diabetic wounds. *J Gene Med* 2008; **10**:1247–1252.

62 Future Models of Diabetes Care

Robert A. Gabbay[1] & Alan M. Adelman[2]

[1] Penn State Institute for Diabetes and Department of Medicine and Molecular Medicine, Penn State Milton S. Hershey Medical Center, Hershey, PA, USA

[2] Department of Family & Community Medicine, Penn State Milton S. Hershey Medical Center and Penn State College of Medicine, Hershey, PA, USA

Keypoints

- Future diabetes care will continue to be delivered mainly in the primary care setting.
- Efforts must continue to bridge the gap between evidence-based recommendations and the current outcomes of patients with diabetes.
- The Chronic Care Model (CCM) provides the best evidence-based framework for organizing and improving chronic care delivery to ensure productive interactions between an informed activated patient and a proactive prepared practice team.
- The CCM defines six domains that require attention to optimize outcomes: delivery system design, self-management support, clinical information systems, decision support, community and health system-related issues.
- The most robust results are obtained when multiple elements of the CCM are incorporated together.
- Team-based care is a particularly effective strategy to improve diabetes outcomes.
- Future models for diabetes care need to continue to involve patients in designing the experience of the visit and various aspects of care improvement.

Introduction

The future of diabetes care will be shaped by the projections of increased incidence, producing more devastating complications and higher costs of care. Projections suggest that the worldwide prevalence of 6.6% in 2010 will increase to 7.8% in 2030. This translates into an increase in the number of individuals with diabetes from 285 million in 2010 to 435 million in 2030 [1]. Increased efforts to prevent the development of diabetes will be necessitated by current predictions that one out of three babies born in the USA will develop diabetes in their lifetime [2]. There is expected to be a dramatic increase in incidence of diabetes in low and middle income countries. Current health care costs associated with diabetes and its complications total more than $174 billion in the USA, and worldwide estimates are considerably higher. Despite the necessary efforts towards diabetes prevention, it is clear that with spiraling health care costs the millions of patients with diabetes will require better care models.

Many drivers for new care models are already in place, foremost of which appears to be financial. This is true whether the payer is a government authority, private insurer or purchaser of health care. Nearly a decade after the Institute of Medicine's report describing *Crossing the Quality Chasm* [3], momentum continues to build for an implementation of better models of chronic illness care and diabetes is at the forefront of these efforts. In many ways, diabetes is the hallmark disease for studying quality improvement because of the prevalence, cost and strong evidence-base for specific quality goals. The challenge remains that despite strong agreement about minimum goals for HbA_{1c} < 7% (53 mmol/mol), low density lipoprotein (LDL) cholesterol <100 mg/dL (26 mmol/L) and blood pressure (BP) < 130/80 mmHg, fewer than 7% of Americans with diabetes are currently achieving these goals [4]. Key barriers to achieving these evidence-based patient goals are insufficient patient self-management support to facilitate adherence and clinical inertia. It has become increasingly clear that the systems of care are more responsible for these poorer outcomes than are either providers or patients.

Diabetes is one of the most psychologically and behaviorally challenging chronic illnesses to manage because as much as 95% of the management relies on the patients' self-care efforts [5]. Despite this, the current health care system often does not have in place appropriate resources to foster patient self-management. Limitations in the availability of self-management education and the lack of ongoing self-management support impair patient adherence to self-care. Clinical inertia is defined as the clinician's "recognition of the problem but failure to act" [6]. This refers to the situation where physicians fail to intensify therapy when faced with patients who are not meeting target goals for clinical variables. This inertia certainly has many components including

Textbook of Diabetes, 4th edition. Edited by R. Holt, C. Cockram, A. Flyvbjerg and B. Goldstein. © 2010 Blackwell Publishing.

decreased provider visit time, lack of timely appropriate data, inadequate provider attention to patient adherence and financial barriers. More information is ultimately needed on the basic epidemiology of clinical inertia including a careful analysis of associated patient, physician and clinic characteristics.

Compounding these challenges of self-management and clinical inertia is the plethora of new diabetes management data that is becoming available to the provider. The expanding use of continuous glucose monitoring, personal health records and shared web-based patient portals presents the risk of overwhelming diabetes care providers. Better management systems with appropriate filters and alerts are needed to analyze all these data and to present them in a usable format for providers.

Primary care is an important foundation of care in any health system. Starfield *et al.* [7,8] have shown that residents of countries with strong primary care foundations have improved health outcomes and lower mortality, with lower costs and with fewer health disparities. Despite the highest cost expenditure ($7000 per capita versus less than $3500 for Australia, Canada France, Germany, The Netherlands, New Zealand, and the UK), the USA has a weak primary care base and approximately 50 million uninsured citizens. It comes as no surprise that in a comparison of these eight developed Western nations, the USA had the most negative ratings for access, coordination and safety experiences [9]. What characterized all countries was the need for improved care systems.

For patients with type 2 diabetes mellitus (T2DM) and those at risk for developing the disease, primary care physicians are a critical foundation of the health care delivery system. In the USA, patients with T2DM consulting a primary care physician outnumber those consulting an endocrinologist by almost 10 to 1 [10]. In general, patients at risk for T2DM are seen by primary care physicians and not by endocrinologists. Therefore, any reorganization of care will need to focus on the primary care settings.

Overall, the solutions to these issues will require reorganizing and reinventing diabetes care from a systems approach. In the cross-national Diabetes Attitudes Wishes and Needs (DAWN) study, attitudes towards diabetes care were assessed across 13 countries from Asia, Australia, Europe and North America [11,12]. Although variation existed among countries in terms of both provider and patient perspectives of diabetes care, all respondents (primary care physicians, nurses and specialists) noted lack of care coordination and implementation of chronic disease strategies as an area in need of improvement worldwide. The payment system was also identified as a barrier in most of the countries surveyed, with the USA, Germany and Japan leading the way. Patients reported high ease of access to providers, but patients' ratings of team collaboration among their providers were relatively low. By the same token, primary care physicians noted a lack of multidisciplinary care and a need for more coordination of care. This chapter focuses on the most promising models for diabetes care, provides current examples and attempts to project into the future how these systems will evolve.

The Chronic Care Model

Although several approaches have been utilized to translate evidence-based recommendations into clinical practice, the Chronic Care Model (CCM) has been the most effective model that has been implemented in a variety of clinical settings in the USA and internationally, often with diabetes as the focus disease [13]. The CCM proposes that the productive interactions of a prepared proactive practice team and an informed empowered patient and family will lead to improved outcomes (Figure 62.1). This provides a conceptual framework and roadmap for redesigning care from the typical acute reactive system to one transformed to population-based proactively planned care of individuals with chronic diseases such as diabetes. Mounting evidence from comparison of high and lower performing practices, evaluation of large-scale quality improvement efforts and randomized intervention trials have demonstrated that the implementation of the CCM is feasible by busy practices with resultant improved disease outcomes [14].

The CCM has been employed for diabetes in a number of health care settings and has demonstrated improvement in cardiovascular risk factors [15,16] and reductions in HbA_{1c} [16], along with improvements in complication screening. Although simpler interventions would be attractive, the evidence suggests that high performing practices do best when they incorporate multiple elements of the CCM [17–21].

The CCM focuses on six elements:

1 *Delivery system design.* One of the most critical elements of transforming care relates to the systems for delivery of care. Planned visits are focused to meet the needs of the patient in terms of disease complexity, cognition, social needs, learning style and degree of support needed from providers and staff. Team-based care distributes tasks among the members of the health care

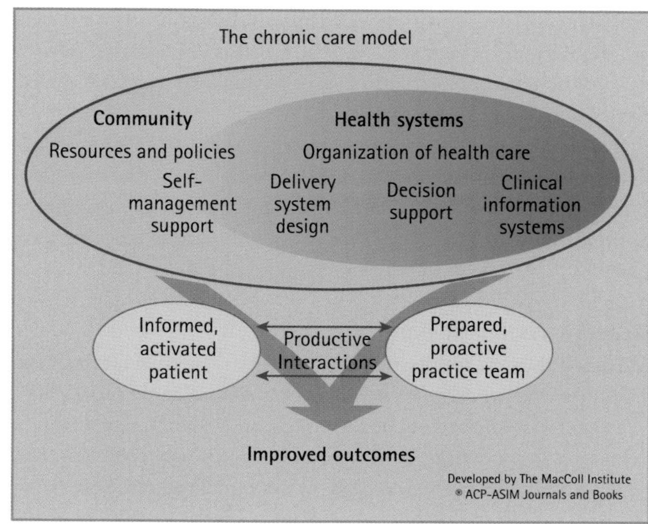

Figure 62.1 The Chronic Care Model. Reproduced from www.improvingchroniccare.org with permission from Group Health Research Institute.

team to optimize care. Reorienting care towards team-based care delivery includes elements such as clinical case management for complex patients, defining and distributing roles amongst team members (nurses, physician assistants, diabetes educators, dietitians, pharmacists and non-medically trained office staff), ensuring follow-up care and identifying patients who "fall between the cracks."

2 *Self-management support.* Self-management support is focused on providing the knowledge needed by the patient to manage their own disease successfully. It also acknowledges patients' central role in their care. This helps to foster the incorporation of effective strategies for living with diabetes and emphasizes the individuals' responsibility for their own health. Although diabetes education has long been recognized as a crucial part of diabetes management, there is increased recognition for the need for ongoing support.

3 *Clinical information systems.* These systems leverage information technology to provide timely reminders to both providers and patients and to identify high-risk subpopulations for proactive care. Diabetes registries that provide searchable information on diabetes populations have proliferated in many health care settings [22].

4 *Decision support.* Embedding evidence-based guidelines into daily clinical practice and sharing those guidelines and information with patients to encourage their participation are the keys to decision support. Guidelines are best integrated through reminder systems that can be embedded into daily care; periodic feedback and standing orders can be used to empower other pratice staff to ensure that evidence-based guidelines are implemented. Although much attention has been given to provider education, better models are needed to integrate specialist expertise and primary care. Innovative approaches that incorporate real-time specialist-based decision support are needed.

5 *Community.* Patients should be encouraged to participate in effective community programs, and this highlights the need of providers to partner with those within the community to fill gaps of care. Partnering becomes even more critical in limited resource environments where extending care beyond the confines of the clinic is essential.

6 *Health systems.* The diabetes care culture must promote effective improvement strategies and support optimal diabetes care. This can include better reimbursement models to encourage optimal care and leadership that stresses the importance of such care.

Delivery system design

Although the best results are obtained when multiple facets of the CCM are implemented together, probably the single most effective quality improvement intervention in diabetes care involves delivery system design to incorporate a team-based approach [23]. Other key elements of delivery system design are case management and shared care.

Realistically, primary care providers have reached their limit in terms of additional tasks that they can undertake, and therefore it is inevitable that the care team needs to be expanded. In many ways, team management has been considered a central feature of superior diabetes care. Diabetes educators and dietitians have long been part of standard diabetes care and the expansion of the roles of these and other individuals within the health care system will likely continue.

Team-based care allows task distribution which includes indentifying team members to:

1 Track longitudinal information through flowsheets or registry data;

2 Perform BP and foot exams; and

3 Ask patients about self-care goals and care barriers prior to the primary health care provider entering the room.

Standing orders can be used to empower office staff to order overdue laboratory screening and eye exam referral, and can even extend to algorithms for medication intensification. Appropriate communication between team members is the key, and the incorporation of clinic "huddles" at the beginning of the day can ensure that appropriately planned care is delivered to all individuals with diabetes.

Diabetes has been a fertile testing ground for case management approaches in which usually either a nurse or pharmacist meets regularly with high-risk patients to provide intensified care [23,24]. Care populations are segmented based on needs to ensure that appropriate care intensity is provided. Key elements of care management include:

1 Defining and identifying high-risk patients;

2 Case assessment;

3 Individualized care plans; and

4 Development, implementation and monitoring of outcomes.

Diabetes registries are an ideal source for identifying high-risk patients either based on clinical measurements (e.g. HbA_{1c} levels), low self-management skills or overdue visits. Intensification of therapy can be facilitated by empowering other health care providers through standing orders to implement changes, and by clearly assessing health management needs and support. Care management is most effective when incorporated within the primary care clinic as opposed to "carve out" models where an outside entity provides telephonic care management for patients and which subsequently leads to ineffective communication with the primary health care provider. Integration of care management with the primary care practice is needed to ensure appropriate information exchange, shared goals and coordination of care.

Diabetes nurses are eager to increase their involvement and take on more responsibility for diabetes care, as recently surveyed internationally through the DAWN study [11]. Pharmacists have also been utilized to work in conjunction with primary care physicians in a case management role. Recent reimbursement changes within the US Medicare system have facilitated billing for these services based on non-randomized trials in which this care has been found to be cost-effective [25].

Care management approaches have been effective at improving glucose control, BP and lipid control in many different settings in the USA and elsewhere [23,24]. One controversy has been the extent to which case management permits medication titration. Two models have been used: one in which the case manager advises the primary care physician who then makes the medication change versus the second in which a standing order algorithm enables a case manager to intensify treatment without routinely checking with the primary care provider. Although studies suggest that standing order algorithms are more effective in lowering HbA_{1c} levels [23,24], some physicians have concerns about nurses or pharmacists making these changes without routine provider input. As more studies and appropriate training programs are developed to allow other health professionals to assist in medication titration, this approach will continue to show promise in improving clinical outcomes while not overburdening the already overtaxed primary care system.

Shared care is defined as "the joint participation of primary care physicians and specialty care physicians in the planned delivery of care, informed by an enhanced information exchange over and above routine discharge and referral notices as the co-management of patients by primary care and subspecialty specialists" [26]. Currently, when most patients are referred to endocrinologists, care is subsumed by the specialists and true co-management is rare. In a recent Cochrane review which examined shared care across multiple chronic illnesses, limited data were available on effective models [27].

Self-management support

A distinction needs to be made between self-management support and self-management education. Self-management education is quite familiar in the diabetes community and encompasses the traditional role of the diabetes educator providing knowledge and skills to patients with diabetes. Self-management support, however, needs not be performed by a diabetes educator and, in fact, peer coaches have been utilized to foster self-management support. Self-management support involves the ongoing collaborative approach between coach and patients to define problems, set priorities, establish goals and create treatment plans. Resources offered to problem solve can include community-based organizations, peer support programs and other groups. Individualized approaches that address the major concerns defined by the patient typically involve a strong element of coaching with the goal of educating and empowering the patient. The challenge for the future is to make self-management support more widely available. Innovative approaches that leverage information technology to provide patient coaching are possible solutions [28].

Self-management has long been recognized as a key determinant of disease outcome. Traditional diabetes education programs have focused on knowledge and specific skills training. It has become increasingly clear, however, that knowledge is necessary but not sufficient to influence behavior. This has led to increased attention to determinants of patient behavior change. In this regard, importance and confidence for a behavior change are key determinants [29].

Importance and confidence

The overall importance of a behavior change is judged by the patients based on their values. Knowledge and education can clearly influence importance by providing the rationale for health improvement. Confidence, also referred to as self-efficacy, is the inherent confidence that a patient can be successful in making the behavior change. This can be augmented through problem-solving and discussion of alternative strategies. Adherence to diet, exercise, monitoring and medication are required for optimal diabetes outcomes. Although many social and societal factors influence patient adherence, clinician counseling style has a profound impact on potential behavior change. Providers can either increase resistance to change or help to facilitate readiness to change on the part of the patient. Patient empowerment and increased self-efficacy are key factors in enabling patients to feel confident in making necessary changes. Recent years have brought to the forefront behavior change approaches from the psychologic literature to be applied to diabetes. One of the most promising approaches is motivational interviewing [29,30].

Motivational interviewing is a directive patient-centered counseling style for eliciting behavior change by helping patients to explore and resolve ambivalence. It is a collaborative patient-provider model that stresses that motivation must come from the patient, not the provider, and honours and respects the patient's autonomy. Initially utilized in the addiction field, it is now being applied to a number of chronic diseases including diabetes [31]. It is a teachable evidence-based approach that holds significant promise to improve patient adherence. Part of the attractiveness of motivational interviewing has been the well-defined set of skills that can be taught to different individuals. Certified trainers are available worldwide [32]. Brief motivational interviewing has adapted many of the skills of traditional motivational interviewing, as used by psychologists, for use in the busy time-pressured health care environment. Meta-analyses have shown this to be a powerful approach which can be learned by people with varying backgrounds and applied to multiple chronic illnesses [31]. Early studies in diabetes are promising [33,34] and larger scale trials are currently underway [35].

Several other behavior change models/theories, which can either explain or help practitioners conceptualize behavior change, have been identified. They include the health belief model, theory of reasoned action or theory of planned behavior, stages of change or transtheoretical model, social cognitive or social learning theory, community organization/building, and social marketing [36].

Clinical information systems

Clinical information systems help to organize patient and population data to facilitate effective and efficient care delivery. Diabetes registries are being adopted in a variety of health care settings involving municipalities, academic health centers, third-party payers, the US Veterans Affairs Health System and international registries in Europe, Canada and elsewhere [37]. A registry is a searchable list of all patients with a particular chronic disease.

The well-designed registry lists all members of the patients' health team and provides key information for patients and providers. The critical impact of the registry is that it can allow timely identification of high-risk subpopulations, permitting the health care team to intensify treatment. A registry can also provide snapshots of care that can collate the many data elements needed for optimal care (e.g. last eye exam, foot exam, nephropathy screen, HbA_{1c}, cholesterol, BP) and can include prompts for care (decision support) as seen in Figure 62.2.

The primary challenges to further adoption of diabetes registries are cost and interoperability issues between different electronic health record systems. Information technology-related issues often receive the most attention by practices in the USA [19]; however, even non-technologic approaches such as incorporation of paper flowsheets can be an effective start. Furthermore, caution is needed to avoid wasting time and resources on implementing information technology solutions to diabetes care without attending to some of the more fundamental practice redesign issues. More robust results are often seen when team-based care and care management are in place.

A new challenge of information overload is entering into diabetes care. The widespread availability of the Internet makes it an attractive communication tool among patients and providers. It has been useful in multiple areas ranging from videoconferencing for diabetes education to tele-ophthalmology to patient support and education websites. Patients desire an effective tool to communicate with their providers in order to receive responsive feedback and advice in a timely manner. Web-based management of diabetes through patient-initiated glucometer uploads can facilitate provider treatment intensification and has demonstrated mixed results in different patient populations [38]. Glucometer uploading is undoubtedly more accurate than patient recorded values. A potential advantage of between visit care offered by this type of telemedicine approach is an improvement in the "velocity to goal" (i.e. how fast the patient reaches good diabetes control). This is particularly important because studies suggest that the average time between treatment intensification in some cases may be as long as 27–35 months [39]. Telemedicine provides a significant opportunity to give providers updated clinical data for more appropriate medication adjustments; however, enthusiasm is tempered by the data burden presented by the frequent communication between patients and providers related to blood glucose values. Reimbursement could facilitate greater adoption of this approach, and future advances could provide clinicians with treatment algorithms that can assist clinical decisions by interpreting data from these glucometer downloads.

The use of computerized glucose predicting engines shows promise in optimizing insulin management [40]. Albisser *et al.* [41] have demonstrated that utilizing a shared central database allowing for patient input of glucose self-monitoring values as well as medication, diet and exercise data, analyzed with a glucose predicting algorithm, enabled providers to reduce iatrogenic hypoglycemic events ninefold compared to that of baseline. The reduction in hypoglycemic events was accomplished without change in HbA_{1c}. Thus, the ability to predict future blood glucose levels improves glycemic stability and may also prove useful in patient self-management. Current research on closed-loop artificial pancreas systems are expected to provide more robust algorithms that will become available to guide patient self-titration of insulin and/or streamline provider titration decisions.

Decision support

The approach frequently used as decision support involves embedding evidence-based guidelines into daily practice to obtain clinical improvement. A number of organizations provide evidence-based clinical guidelines. Although there can be some discrepancies among them, most are generally disagreements on how low goals should be brought down. While these debates are important, overriding evidence suggests that the vast majority of patients are not at minimum clinical care goals. Establishing clinical goals is a first step; however, the best practices to achieve those goals are critically important to ensure positive clinical outcomes. The American Diabetes Association (ADA) and national bodies such as the National Institute for Clinical Excellence (NICE) provide detailed guidelines [42]. This is a necessary first step, but decision support goes beyond the acceptance of consensus guidelines and focuses on the implementation of those guidelines in everyday practice. Although provider education regarding guidelines is important, these interventions typically have had limited impact beyond processes of care (i.e. ensuring that more patients are screened for complications). Effective multifaceted interventions most often include academic detailing, physician reminders, and audit and feedback to improve diabetes outcomes. Patient tracking systems (patient registries) and nurse-led interventions are also effective [43].

Examples of guideline implementation can include incorporating decision support into electronic health records or reviewing the chart prior to a planned visit to identify gaps in care and strategies to intensify treatment plan. Although provider knowledge of guidelines is critical, these guidelines need to be shared with patients to encourage their participation. Empowering patients to "know their numbers" provides the basis for a negotiated treatment plan to achieve those goals.

Given the evidence that BP control can reduce both microvascular and macrovascular complications, future efforts will clearly focus on identifying better approaches for monitoring this outcome. Self or automated BP monitoring offers many of the same advantages as glucose monitoring. An increased number of BP recordings increases the accuracy of the measurement. It may also empower patients to discuss their BP with their physician [44]. Home monitoring, in conjunction with other interventions such as patient education, Internet communication, nurse or pharmacist follow-up, does lead to improved BP control [45,46]. Telemonitoring of BP may lead to reductions in both systolic and diastolic BP [47].

The initial disadvantage of self or automated blood glucose or BP monitorings is that clinicians continue to be bombarded by

PENN STATE INSTITUTE FOR DIABETES & OBESITY

Patient Profile - Confidential

Patient Name: John Doe
Chart Number: 155, 5489
Type of Diabetes: 1
Last Visit: 05/13/2009
Clinic: Palmyra
Provider: Peter Lewis

Printed By: AVIGNATI
Date of Birth: 11/18/1958
Year Diagnosed: 1998
Primary Provider: Dr Unknown
Last Dietitian Visit: *Unknown*
Last Education Visit: 09/17/2008
Flu Status: Refused - 02/22/2008

ACE/ARB Use: *Unknown*
Aspirin Use: Contraindicated
Statin Use: Contraindicated
Weight: 235
BMI: 33 - 05/13/2009
Smoker: No
Pneumovax Status: Vaccinated - 2005

Complications:

___Amputee
___Autonomic Neuropathy
■ Blind
___CAD/MI
___CHF
___CVA/TIAs
___Cataracts
___Charcot Foot
___Depression
___Dialysis
___Erectile Dysfunction
___Gastroparesis
___Hx Foot Ulcer
___Hyperlipidemia
___Hypertension
___Hypoglycemia Unaware
___Hypothyroidism
■ Nephropathy
___PAD (PVD)
___Peripheral Neuropathy
___Retinopathy

HDL: 54 03/16/2006
ALT: 111 03/16/2006
TSH: *Unknown*

Triglycerides: *Unknown*
Microalbumin: 111.00 03/16/2006
Micro/Cr Ratio: 29 05/24/2009

Creatinine: 2.1 06/10/2008
Foot Exam: 05/01/2007 - Sensate
Eye Exam: 11/30/2006 - *Results Unknown*

************ THIS PATIENT IS DUE FOR THE FOLLOWING EXAM(S)/LAB(S): ************
Foot Exam, Creatinine

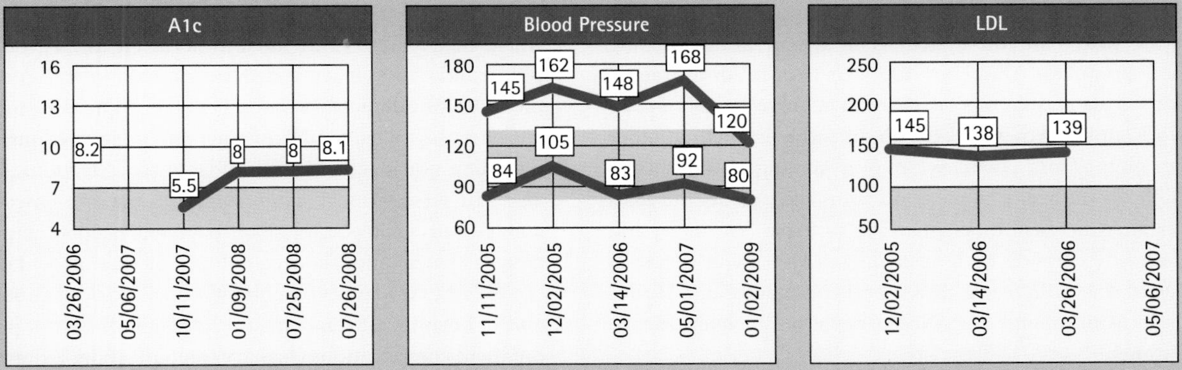

Visit Date: ______________________

Provider: ______________________

Blood Pressure: _______ / _______

Weight: ________

Foot Exam: ____ Sensate ____ Insensate ____ Not Done

Eye Exam: Date ______________________
____ Retinopathy ____ No Retinopathy
____ Results Unknown ____ Refused

Self Care Goals:

___ Diet
■ Exercise
___ Footcare
___ Maintain
___ Medication
___ Monitoring
___ Stress Management
___ Tobacco
___ Other

Figure 62.2 An example of an electronic registry flowsheet. A1c, glycated hemoglobin; LDL, low density lipoprotein cholesterol.

more and more data. The increasing availability of continuous glucose monitoring data, routine self glucose monitoring results that can be shared through web portals, ambulatory BP monitoring and personal health records are all at the expense of potentially overburdening the already busy clinician with too much information. There will clearly be a need to develop more robust data filtering methodologies to analyze and package this information in clear concise summaries that can lead to appropriate clinician and patient action. Some evidence of this is already apparent in software for many of the self glucose monitoring devices that provide ready access to glucose averages, standard deviations and other simple data analytical features. Merging this information with evidence-based decision support tools for providers is likely to increase their overall value to improve quality of care.

Health systems

The overall health care system is an important factor. In suggesting solutions to improving the US health care system, Berwick *et al.* [48] provide insight into important aspects of the health care delivery system that translate into improved outcomes. They propose that an effective health care system that produces outstanding health outcomes pursues three primary goals:

1 Improving the patient's experience of health;
2 Improving the health of a defined population; and
3 Reducing the costs of care for populations.

They refer to this as the Triple Aim. In order to accomplish these goals, Berwick *et al.* define three preconditions. First, the health care system must be focused and responsible for the health of a defined population. Second, monetary and related constraints are placed on the system. The system does not have unlimited resources. The USA has experienced unrestrained health care costs and spends far more than any other developed country's health system, yet its health outcomes lag behind other countries [49]. Third, there is an over-arching entity that is responsible for the health of the population and pursues the goals of the Triple Aim. Health systems such as those in Canada and the UK already embody these principles. There are also several examples in the USA such as Kaiser Permanente and Health Partners in Minneapolis, both closed-panel health maintenance organizations.

Several approaches have been utilized from perspectives to improve clinical outcomes for patients with diabetes. Disease management programs have proliferated in the USA, and worldwide there has been enthusiasm for pay-for-performance (P4P) models that alter reimbursement based on achievement of quality goals.

"Disease management" has been defined by the Disease Management Association of America as "a system of coordinated health care interventions and communications for populations with conditions in which patient self-care efforts are significant" [50]. In the USA, this is a one billion dollar industry that usually is managed by a private company working with a health insurance plan or state health program. Mattke *et al.* [51] question the effectiveness of these programs. They did find that these programs can lower hospitalization rates for patients with congestive heart failure and increase outpatient care and prescriptions for patients with depression and these programs have also lead to improvements in process of care, but it is uncertain if they lead to reduced costs [50]. Linden and Adams [52] found a slight cost savings but cautioned that study design had an influence on the findings. Randomized clinical trials showed a net loss while pre-/post-comparisons and case–control studies demonstrated cost savings. Typically, the severity of illness and intervention intensity varied greatly, and these disease management programs were not fully integrated into the patient's care.

Reimbursement of providers of care may be a mechanism for improving health outcomes of individuals with diabetes. Recently, P4P has been touted as a way of incentivizing clinicians to improve the quality of care that they deliver. Two recent reviews point out that P4P programs may have both benefits and adverse effects [53,54]. Adverse effects include a focusing on only those elements measured and avoiding severely ill patients who may adversely affect performance measures [53]. In a study of the effects of P4P on intermediate outcomes for patients with diabetes in the UK, Millett *et al.* [55] found that while improvements were made, the magnitude of improvements differed according to ethnic group. Comparing P4P between primary care practices in the USA and UK, McDonald and Roland [56] reported that there were unintended consequences resulting from the implementation of P4P. Physicians in the USA were more likely to report that P4P had little impact on their office and voiced feelings of resentment, lack of understanding of the program, loss of autonomy and less satisfaction than their UK counterparts. Design elements such as who is incentivized (individual clinicians, medical groups or hospitals) and what is incentivized (documentation of process of care measures or outcome measures) may be important.

Others suggested models of payment to improve quality of care including non-payment for avoidable complications, case-management fees, primary care capitation, episode-based payment and shared savings [57]. Non-payment models and episode-based payment models usually focus on care provided to inpatients. For example, non-payment models do not pay the provider and/or hospital for removing the wrong body part or preventable inpatient complications (urinary tract infections). Episode-based payment models define a global rate for a specific condition such as diabetes or myocardial infarction and the meeting of predefined process standards such as achieving best practice standards. Case management fees and primary care capitation to primary care physicians have been proposed to coordinate ambulatory care better, particularly in patients with chronic diseases such as diabetes. Lastly, shared savings payment models involve sharing savings from providing improved quality of care with large groups or individual practitioners. Many of these payment models may be specific in the attempt to "fix" the fragmented US health system. Elements of these payment models may already be incorporated into the more integrated single-payor systems of other developed countries.

Another reimbursement model being explored is providing patients with monetary incentives to engage in appropriate self-care and/or removing financial barriers to care. A municipality in the USA (Asheville, North Carolina) eliminated pharmaceutical costs for patients with diabetes in return for mandated regular pharmacist visits and noted significant savings in health care costs [58–60]. Large corporations in the USA have been examining other models whereby patients are incentivized to engage in various programs or activities. To date, there are limited data regarding the efficacy of these initiatives despite their potential promise.

Community

Community resources are often overlooked and not integrated into care for patients with diabetes. Providers can become more familiar with these resources and work collaboratively to make patients aware of opportunities. These can include safe exercise opportunities, healthy food availability, social programs and support services that are available through non-governmental organizations. Communities can partner with health care organizations and governments to improve public awareness about diabetes. For example, recent efforts in the USA between the ADA and the American Heart Association (AHA) publicizing the link between diabetes and heart disease have raised better awareness. Overall, as prevention of diabetes and its complications becomes an increasing public focus, public awareness efforts to empower patients to engage in appropriate diet and exercise will be needed. Social marketing provides a rationale for how this approach can be effective, and an excellent example of success is the change in tobacco use in the USA over the last three decades. Similar public health initiatives are needed to stem the epidemic of obesity that is fueling the rise in diabetes.

Overwhelming evidence now suggests that the simultaneous incorporation of multiple components of the CCM is synergistic and more effective than traditional single intervention approaches [19,23]. Too much past research focused on only a single intervention and therefore missed the potential value of the concurrent implementation of multiple interventions for true "transformation of care."

Transformation of care, according to the CCM, has often been accomplished through "learning collaboratives" either through the Breakthrough Series Collaborative [61,62] or through other similar experiences. Widespread implementation in the USA has generally occurred in large organizations, in part based on supportive reimbursement systems. Nevertheless, external support for practice transformation is being explored in several regional improvement programs [62,63]. Recent position statements from many professional societies have come in strong support for the CCM [64]. Alternatives to the time-consuming learning collaborative model such as practice coaching and web-based learning networks are being developed and tested [65–67].

Another initiative to improve chronic disease management in the USA has focused on the patient-centered medical home. The patient-centered medical home is a concept being developed by the major primary care societies in the USA. It combines the principles of primary care (continuity of care, whole person orientation, quality/safety, prevention, timely access to care) with many of the elements of the CCM (coordinated/integrated care, teams, population health). One of the driving forces behind this concept is to revitalize primary care in the USA.

Although the concept of patient medical home has been attractive and a certification program has been established in the USA, there are concerns that this model may have limited application outside the country. In particular, many of the elements described for the National Center for Quality Assurance certification process require advanced information technology capabilities that generally necessitate an electronic health record. Despite the value of electronic health records, the mere availability of these tools is often insufficient to transform care. Often, practices and health systems can get sidetracked with the formidable information technology and interoperability challenges, losing sight of the overall goal of transforming health care. In comparison, the CCM elements are more easily translatable in low technology environments within the developing world.

In the USA, several states have explored integrated approaches to adopt the CCM. The foremost of these has been initial experience in Pennsylvania where insurers have agreed to provide significant reimbursement and incentives for primary care adoption of the CCM to improve diabetes care. Learning collaboratives are conducted across the state to teach clinicians and office staff the implementation aspects of the CCM. These efforts are supported by practice coaches who meet with practices individually to problem-solve implementation efforts. Clinics are required to report on clinical outcomes and care changes on a monthly basis, and payers have agreed to provide funding for needed practice changes such as case management in the hopes of containing spiraling health care costs [62]. A national initiative is currently underway in Australia to implement the CCM through the Australian National Primary Care Collaboratives [68], and similar initiatives are being explored in Canada, Denmark, Netherlands, New Zealand and elsewhere.

Ideal appointment of the future

One informative exercise is to solicit from patients and providers what the ideal appointment of the future will look like. Certainly, many challenges face health care, but returning the focus to be more patient-centered is a universally adopted goal for patient care. The classic clinical visit can be modified in a variety of ways.

As care moves to be more patient-centered, a key need is to involve patients in designing the type of care and how it could be implemented. This can be rather enlightening to those in the medical community by stretching the medical model in ways not previously considered. The patient's perspective is needed because: "without the inclusion of the affected individual's perspective, it is possible that the information, from the provider's perspective, is incomplete or misleading" [69].

Significant opportunities exist to improve the pre-arrival visit so that patients could spend quality time speaking with their provider, as opposed to providing data. To accomplish this, patients could utilize kiosks in waiting rooms to search for specific disease conditions and receive tailored messages about their health that prompt questions they may want to ask their provider during the visit. Creating such opportunities for "patient activation," which enables patients to become collaborative partners in managing their healths, have had some promising results [40,70,71]. Where kiosks are not feasible, even low-tech (paper) methods to capture current medical histories, patient concerns and symptom screening (e.g. depression) would give patients more time with the provider to focus on the issues they want to address. During the appointment, less time would be spent talking about factual information that could be captured electronically (medications, insurance information, address changes, phone numbers) and more time talking about what matters most to the patient.

A warm inviting environment can have a positive impact on the "ideal" patient appointment [72]. The use of art, particularly art that holds meaning for the patient, is one method to enhance the office environment. Studies have also looked at the creation of art by patients to express their thoughts about having a chronic illness [73,74], which could then be shown to others. The use of art in waiting rooms is an effective way to create an environment that allows for reflection and discussion [75,76]. In fact, the overall patient experience could be improved through providing a service that resembles check-in at a hotel or restaurant. [The word "hospital" comes from Latin *hospes* (host), which is also the root for the English words "hotel," "hostel" and "hospitality".] Imagine being greeted by a concierge, who offers to take the "guest's" coat and find a seat. The guest has the option of reviewing medical information and providing corrected data (phone/address) through either the concierge or a computer station at the concierge's desk. The concierge asks what the main concern of the appointment is today, and makes a note that is forwarded to the provider electronically. Instead of thinking about the patient experience in a clinical way, the model of hospital hospitality opens up the doors for true customer service delivery.

Some may argue that at the core of the issue is how the patient appointment itself should be changed so that patients are treated more like people and less like walking diseases. Contrary to many preconceptions, the clinician may actually gain time by altering current practices, rather than lose time at each appointment [77]. Time is always limited and clinicians can find ways to use interventions or strategies to make most efficient use of the time. Thus, identifying one focused question that connects to the heart of the issue, rather than a dozen that do not, can save time and introduce important matters that otherwise would take years to disclose [78]. The question should be open-ended, not closed, to generate a discussion. If a patient does not have ideal self-management, the clinician could ask a question such as: "Tell me about your struggles (difficulties) with having diabetes?" and then make notes of the patient's response. In turn, the clinician would repeat back the response, and ask, "Did I get it right?" This is a narrative enquiry technique used in medical settings to assist clinicians in understanding the patient's situations, thus being able to offer better suggestions or assist the patient in problem solving on what could be done to overcome those struggles [79]. Other examples of questions used in narrative inquiries include: "How does diabetes impact your life, both negatively and positively?" "What is important to you in your life, besides diabetes?" and "What could I do differently as a provider to help you?" Asking questions such as these often encourages dialogue and deepens the sense of mutual commitment and investment in the learning experience.

In the ideal future appointment, we want to examine critically those things which inhibit our practice from being successful. By asking patients what they want and need from us will improve upon the productive interaction between patients and providers, which is the ultimate goal of the CCM. We want to ask ourselves and our patients "What are the barriers that prevent us from achieving success?" and take action based upon those recommendations. Then we go back to our patients and ask "Did we get it right?" This process will help us redesign our practice to meet needs and provide self-management improvement for patients.

Overall, the future models of diabetes care are in many ways available today. The CCM has been implemented in a number of practice settings with improvements in diabetes quality of care. The model provides a conceptual framework to attend to the many aspects of care required to ensure that productive interactions are achieved between a proactive prepared practice team and an informed activated patient. The assignments of this model to different practice settings and further dissemination of the model are the near-term challenges. Care will inevitably become more patient-centered. Collaboration between patients and practice teams will be required to improve clinical outcomes and subsequently costs. Understanding the needs of patients, creating the ideal environment for their care and using system-based approaches to optimize their care will converge to improve the lives of those with diabetes in the future. Supporting self-management will be critical to achieving these outcomes.

In many ways, the future lies in developing integrated systems of care that are responsible for the outcomes and in getting individuals to take more responsibility to manage their own disease. Diabetes has led the way in many CCM studies and included elements, in part because it represents a costly disease reaching epidemic proportions. Nevertheless, this disease is also blessed with many evidence-based goals of care that can prevent long-term complications, which are the source of most of the overall costs of diabetes.

Acknowledgments

The authors would like to thank Drs. Heather Stuckey and Rena Dearment for their contributions to this chapter and support provided by the National Institute of Diabetes and Digestive and Kidney Diseases (R18-DK067495).

References

1 International Diabetes Federation. Diabetes Facts and Figures http://www.diabetesatlas.org/content/diabetes-and-impaired-glucose-tolerance. Accessed 8 January 2010.

2 Narayan KM, Boyle JP, Thompson TJ, Sorensen SW, Williamson DF. Lifetime risk for diabetes mellitus in the United States. *JAMA* 2003; **290**:1884–1890.

3 Committee on Quality of Health Care in America. *Crossing the Quality Chasm: A New Health System for the 21st Century*. New York, 2001.

4 Saydah SH, Fradkin J, Cowie CC. Poor control of risk factors for vascular disease among adults with previously diagnosed diabetes. *JAMA* 2004; **291**:335–342.

5 Anderson RM. Is the problem of noncompliance all in our heads? *Diabetes Educ* 1985; **11**:31–34.

6 Phillips LS, Branch WT, Cook CB, Doyle JP, El-Kebbi IM, Gallina DL, *et al.* Clinical inertia. *Ann Intern Med* 2001; **135**:825–834.

7 Starfield B, Shi L, Grover A, Macinko J. The effects of specialist supply on populations' health: assessing the evidence. *Health Aff (Millwood)* 2005; Suppl. Web Exclusives:W5-97-W5-107.

8 Starfield B, Shi L, Macinko J. Contribution of primary care to health systems and health. *Milbank Q* 2005; **83**:457–502.

9 Schoen C, Osborn R, How SK, Doty MM, Peugh J. In chronic condition: experiences of patients with complex health care needs, in eight countries. *Health Aff (Millwood)* 2009; **28**:w1–16.

10 Saudek CD. The role of primary care professionals in managing diabetes. *Clin Diabetes* 2002; **20**:65–66.

11 Siminerio LM, Funnell MM, Peyrot M, Rubin RR. US nurses' perceptions of their role in diabetes care: results of the cross-national Diabetes Attitudes Wishes and Needs (DAWN) study. *Diabetes Educ* 2007; **33**:152–162.

12 Peyrot M, Rubin RR, Lauritzen T, Skovlund SE, Snoek FJ, Matthews DR, *et al.* Patient and provider perceptions of care for diabetes: results of the cross-national DAWN Study. *Diabetologia* 2006; **49**:279–288.

13 Wagner EH. Chronic disease management: what will it take to improve care for chronic illness? *Eff Clin Pract* 1998; **1**:2–4.

14 Coleman K, Austin BT, Brach C, Wagner EH. Evidence on the Chronic Care Model in the new millennium. *Health Aff (Millwood)* 2009; **28**:75–85.

15 Wagner EH. A survey of leading chronic disease management programs. *Health Services Research Journal* 2009; In press.

16 UK Prospective Diabetes Study (UKPDS) Group. Intensive blood-glucose control with sulphonylureas or insulin compared with conventional treatment and risk of complications in patients with type 2 diabetes (UKPDS 33). *Lancet* 1998; **352**:837–853.

17 Bodenheimer T, Wagner EH, Grumbach K. Improving primary care for patients with chronic illness. *JAMA* 2002; **288**:1775–1779.

18 Wagner EH, Austin B, Von Korff M. Improving outcomes in chronic illness. *Manag Care Q* 1996; **4**:12–25.

19 Wagner EH, Austin BT, Davis C, Hindmarsh M, Schaefer J, Bonomi A. Improving chronic illness care: translating evidence into action. *Health Aff (Millwood)* 2001; **20**:64–78.

20 Piatt GA, Orchard TJ, Emerson S, Simmons D, Songer TJ, Brooks MM, *et al.* Translating the chronic care model into the community: results from a randomized controlled trial of a multifaceted diabetes care intervention. *Diabetes Care* 2006; **29**:811–817.

21 Siminerio LM, Piatt G, Zgibor JC. Implementing the chronic care model for improvements in diabetes care and education in a rural primary care practice. *Diabetes Educ* 2005; **31**:225–234.

22 Khan L, Mincemoyer S, Gabbay RA. Diabetes registries: where we are and where are we headed? *Diabetes Technol Ther* 2009; **11**:255–262.

23 Shojania KG, Ranji SR, McDonald KM, Grimshaw JM, Sundaram V, Rushakoff RJ, *et al.* Effects of quality improvement strategies for type 2 diabetes on glycemic control: a meta-regression analysis. *JAMA* 2006; **296**:427–440.

24 Norris SL, Engelgau MM, Narayan KM. Effectiveness of self-management training in type 2 diabetes: a systematic review of randomized controlled trials. *Diabetes Care* 2001; **24**:561–587.

25 Young D. Asheville Project improves patient outcomes, cuts medical costs. *Am J Health Syst Pharm* 2003; **60**:868–871.

26 Smith SM, Allwright S, O'Dowd T. Effectiveness of shared care across the interface between primary and specialty care in chronic disease management. *Cochrane Database Syst Rev* 2007; **3**:CD004910.

27 Milnes JP, Cochrane S, Henderson J. Chronic disease in institutionalised patients: using liaison nurses can improve follow-up and care. *Br Med J* 1997; **315**:1540.

28 Welch G, Shayne R. Interactive behavioral technologies and diabetes self-management support: recent research findings from clinical trials. *Curr Diab Rep* 2006; **6**:130–136.

29 Rollnick S, Miller WR, Butler CC. *Motivational Interviewing in Health Care: Helping Patients Change Behavior*. New York: Guilford Press, 2008.

30 Rollnick S, Allison J, Ballasiotes S, *et al.* Variations on a theme: motivational interviewing and its adaptations. In: Miller WR, Rollnick S, eds. *Motivational Interviewing: Preparing People for Change*, 2nd edn. New York: Guilford Press, 2002: 270–283.

31 Hettema J, Steele J, Miller WR. Motivational interviewing. *Ann Rev Clin Psychol* 2005; **1**:91–111.

32 Wagner CC, Conners W. Motivational Interviewing Network of Trainers (MINT). Motivational Interviewing Resources, LLC and the Mid-Atlantic Addiction Technology Transfer Center. Available from: http://www.motivationalinterview.org.

33 Channon S, Smith VJ, Gregory JW. A pilot study of motivational interviewing in adolescents with diabetes. *Arch Dis Child* 2003; **88**:680–683.

34 Doherty Y, Roberts S. Motivational interviewing in diabetes practice. *Diabet Med* 2002; **19**(Suppl 3):1–6.

35 Gabbay RA, Dellasega, C. Patient perceptions of motivational interviewing. *Diabetes Care* 2008; **57**:A522.

36 Whitlock EP, Orleans CT, Pender N, Allan J. Evaluating primary care behavioral counseling interventions: an evidence-based approach. *Am J Prev Med* 2002; **22**:267–284.

37 Gabbay RA, Khan L, Peterson KL. Critical features for a successful implementation of a diabetes registry. *Diabetes Technol Ther* 2005; **7**:958–967.

38 Azar M, Gabbay R. Web-based management of diabetes through glucose uploads: has the time come for telemedicine? *Diabetes Res Clin Pract* 2009; **83**:9–17.

39 Whitlock WL, Brown A, Moore K, Pavliscsak H, Dingbaum A, Lacefield D, *et al.* Telemedicine improved diabetic management. *Mil Med* 2000; **165**:579–584.

40 Williams GC, McGregor H, Zeldman A, Freedman ZR, Deci EL, Elder D. Promoting glycemic control through diabetes self-management: evaluating a patient activation intervention. *Patient Educ Couns* 2005; **56**:28–34.

41 Albisser AM, Wright CE, Sakkal S. Averting iatrogenic hypoglycemia through glucose prediction in clinical practice: progress towards a new procedure in diabetes. *Diabetes Res Clin Pract* 2007; **76**:207–214.

42 Clark MJ, Jr., Sterrett JJ, Carson DS. Diabetes guidelines: a summary and comparison of the recommendations of the American Diabetes Association, Veterans Health Administration, and American Association of Clinical Endocrinologists. *Clin Ther* 2000; **22**:899–910; discussion 898.

43 Renders CM, Valk GD, Griffin S, Wagner EH, Eijk JT, Assendelft WJ. Interventions to improve the management of diabetes mellitus in primary care, outpatient and community settings. *Cochrane Database Syst Rev* 2001; **1**:CD001481.

44 McManus RJ, Glasziou P, Hayen A, Mant J, Padfield P, Potter J, *et al.* Blood pressure self monitoring: questions and answers from a national conference. *Br Med J* 2009; **338**:38–42.

45 Cappuccio FP, Kerry SM, Forbes L, Donald A. Blood pressure control by home monitoring: meta-analysis of randomised trials. *Br Med J* 2004; **329**:145.

46 Green BB, Cook AJ, Ralston JD, Fishman PA, Catz SL, Carlson J, *et al.* Effectiveness of home blood pressure monitoring, web communication, and pharmacist care on hypertension control. a randomized controlled trial. *JAMA* 2008; **299**:2857–2867.

47 Paré G, Jaana M, Sicotte C. Systematic review of home telemonitoring for chronic diseases: the evidence base. *J Am Med Inform Assoc* 2007; **14**:269–277.

48 Berwick DM, Nolan TW, Whittington J. The triple aim: care, health, and cost. *Health Affairs* 2008; **27**:759–769.

49 Commonwealth Fund Commission on a High Performance Health System. *Why not the best? Results from the National Scorecard on US Health System Performance, 2008.* New York: Commonwealth Fund, July 2008.

50 Disease Management Association of America (DMAA). DMAA definition of disease management. Available from: http://www.dmaa.org/dm_definition.asp. Accessed March 1, 2008.

51 Mattke S, Seid M, Ma S. Evidence for the effect of disease management: is $1 billion a year a good investment? *Am J Manag Care* 2007; **13**:670–676.

52 Linden A, Adams JL. Determining if disease management saves money: an introduction to meta-analysis. *J Eval Clin Pract* 2007; **13**:400–407.

53 Mannion R, Davies HTO. Payment for performance in health care. *Br Med J* 2008; **336**:306–308.

54 Petersen LA, Woodard LD, Urech T, Daw C, Sookanan S. Does pay-for-performance improve the quality of health care? *Ann Intern Med* 2006; **145**:265–272.

55 Millett C, Netuveli G, Saxena S, Majeed A. Impact of pay for performance on ethnic disparities in intermediate outcomes for diabetes: a longitudinal study. *Diabetes Care* 2009; **32**:404–409.

56 McDonald R, Roland M. Pay for performance in primary care in England and California: comparison of unintended consequences. *Ann Fam Med* 2009; **7**:121–127.

57 Rosenthal MB. Beyond pay for performance: emerging models of provider-payment reform. *N Engl J Med* 2008; **359**:1197–1200.

58 Cranor CW, Bunting BA, Christensen DB. The Asheville Project: long-term clinical and economic outcomes of a community pharmacy diabetes care program. *J Am Pharm Assoc* 2003; **43**:173–184.

59 Cranor CW, Christensen DB. The Asheville Project: factors associated with outcomes of a community pharmacy diabetes care program. *J Am Pharm Assoc* 2003; **43**:160–172.

60 Cranor CW, Christensen DB. The Asheville Project: short-term outcomes of a community pharmacy diabetes care program. *J Am Pharm Assoc* 2003; **43**:149–159.

61 Kilo CM. A framework for collaborative improvement: lessons from the Institute for Healthcare Improvement's Breakthrough Series. *Qual Manag Health Care* 1998; **6**:1–13.

62 Pennsylvania Chronic Care Management Reimbursement, and Cost Reduction Commission. The Pennsylvania Chronic Care Management, Reimbursement, and Cost Reduction Strategic Plan 2008; p. 9. Available from http://www.rxforpa.com/assets/pdfs/ChronicCareCommissionReport.pdf

63 Newman SP. Chronic disease self-management approaches within the complex organisational structure of a health care system. *Med J Aust* 2008; **189**:S7–8.

64 Siminerio LM, Drab SR, Gabbay RA, Gold K, McLaughlin S, Piatt GA, *et al.* Diabetes educators: implementing the chronic care model. *Diabetes Educ* 2008; **34**:451–456.

65 Dartmouth Institute. Clinical Microsystems. Dartmouth-Hitchcock Medical Center. Available from: dms.dartmouth.edu/cms. Accessed March 27, 2009.

66 American Board of Medical Specialties. Improving Performance in Practice (IPIP), 2008. Available from: www.abms.org/about_abms/ABMS_Research/current.aspx. Accessed March 27, 2009.

67 US Department of Health & Human Services, Agency for Healthcare Research and Quality. Integrating Chronic Care and Business Strategies in the Safety Net, 2008. Available from: www.ahrq.gov/populations/businessstrategies/

68 Eley DS, Del Mar CB, Patterson E, Synnott RL, Baker PG, Hegney D. A nurse led model of chronic disease care: an interim report. *Aust Fam Physician* 2008; **37**:1030–1032.

69 Ravenscroft EF. Diabetes and kidney failure: how individuals with diabetes experience kidney failure. *Nephrol Nurs J* 2005; **32**:502–509.

70 Hibbard JH, Mahoney ER, Stock R, Tusler M. Do increases in patient activation result in improved self-management behaviors? *Health Serv Res* 2007; **42**:1443–1463.

71 Mosen DM, Schmittdiel J, Hibbard J, Sobel D, Remmers C, Bellows J. Is patient activation associated with outcomes of care for adults with chronic conditions? *J Ambul Care Manage* 2007; **30**:21–29.

72 Arneill AB, Devlin AS. Perceived quality of care: the influence of the waiting room environment. *J Environ Psychol* 2002; **22**:345–360.

73 Reynolds F, Prior S. A lifestyle coat-hanger: a phenomenological study of the meanings of artwork for women coping with chronic illness and disability. *Disabil Rehabil* 2003; **25**:785–794.

74 Stuckey H. Healing from dry bones: creative expression and adult learning in diabetes care. Pennsylvania State University, 2007.

75 Homicki B, Joyce EK. Art illuminates patients' experience at the Massachusetts General Hospital Cancer Center. *Oncologist* 2004; **9**:114.

76 Lawson B, Phiri M. Hospital design: room for improvement. *Health Service J* 2000; **24**:20–23.

77 Duffy FD, Gordon GH, Whelan G, Cole-Kelly K, Frankel R, Buffone N, *et al.* Assessing competence in communication and interpersonal skills: the Kalamazoo II report. *Acad Med* 2004; **79**:495–507.

78 Charon R. Narrative and medicine. *N Engl J Med* 2004; **350**:862–865.

79 Charon R. Narrative medicine: a model for empathy, reflection and trust. *JAMA* 2001; **286**:1897–902.

Index

Note: page numbers in *italics* refer to figures; those in **bold** to tables or boxes.

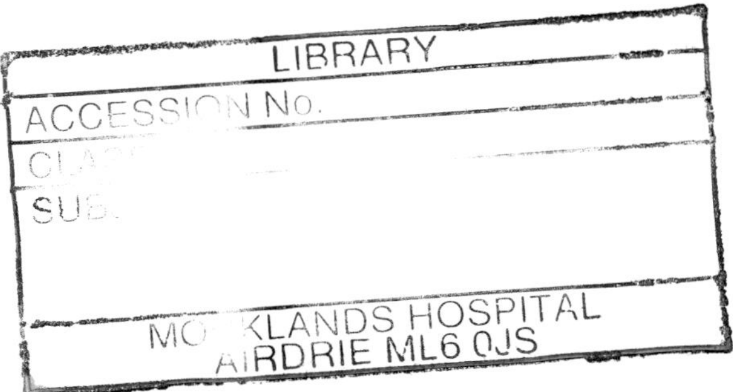